KANSKI'S

A Systematic Approach

John F. Salmon
MD, FRCS, FRCOphth
Consultant Ophthalmic Surgeon
Oxford Eye Hospital
Oxford Radcliffe NHS Trust
Oxford
United Kingdom

KANSKI'S Clinical Ophthalmology

A Systematic Approach

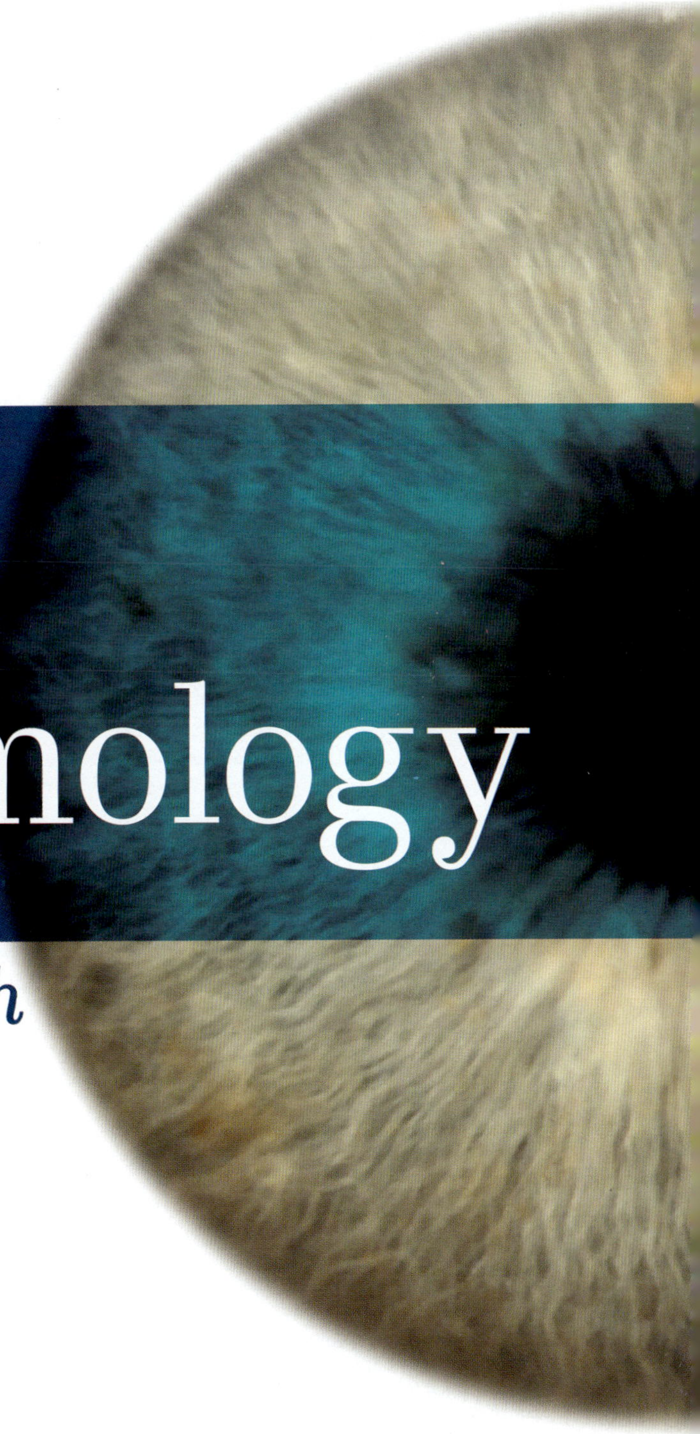

Tenth Edition

ELSEVIER

Notice

Practitioners and researchers must always rely on their own experience and knowledge in evaluating and using any information, methods, compounds or experiments described herein. Because of rapid advances in the medical sciences, in particular, independent verification of diagnoses and drug dosages should be made. To the fullest extent of the law, no responsibility is assumed by Elsevier, authors, editors or contributors for any injury and/or damage to persons or property as a matter of products liability, negligence or otherwise, or from any use or operation of any methods, products, instructions, or ideas contained in the material herein.

ISBN: 978-0-443-11099-3
978-0-443-11109-9

Content Strategist: Kayla Wolfe
Content Development Specialist: Joanie Milnes
Project Manager: Julie Taylor
Design: Amy Buxton
Marketing Manager: Belinda Tudin

Printed in India

Last digit is the print number: 9 8 7 6 5 4 3 2 1

Contents

Dedication

This book is dedicated to my grandsons,
Jack and Sam Spath and Ronan Salmon

Preface to the Tenth Edition

As has been the approach adopted in previous editions of this classic textbook, the tenth edition of *Kanski's Clinical Ophthalmology* is intended to be a useful and comprehensive basis for general ophthalmic and optometric practice. The book is filled with in-depth information on most ophthalmic diseases and includes hundreds of beautiful images and illustrations. I have included sufficient practical information for trainees to manage common ophthalmic conditions in the clinic and enough detail on rare conditions to enable them to prepare for their examinations without resorting to the internet.

The challenge has been to cover the entire field of ophthalmology for a world-wide audience without depending on sub-specialists to prepare each chapter. To do this, I have maintained Jack Kanski's unique approach of presenting core clinical knowledge in a systematic and succinct form. Each chapter has been considerably updated and the latest evidence-based diagnostic and therapeutic approaches have been covered, including genetics and imaging techniques. Many new illustrations have been added and better examples of a range of conditions have been included. An enhanced eBook version is available for rapid access.

I have been extremely fortunate to have received help from colleagues past and present, to whom I wish to express my grateful thanks. Brad Bowling has had a significant influence on previous editions and his accuracy and meticulous attention to detail have been remarkably helpful. Professor Tony Murray provided considerable advice on the text in the strabismus chapter and images of pathology that are not easily found in higher-income countries. Professor Peter Charbel Issa helped to update the text in the inherited eye disease chapter; Dr Christine Kiire the text in the diabetic retinopathy section; Dr Richard Corkin the text in the refractive surgery section; and Professor Gordon Dutton the text in the cerebral visual impairment section. I have received numerous excellent images from Aude Ambresin (medical retina), Trevor Carmichael (cornea), Bertil Damato (ocular oncology), Darius Hildebrand and Manoj Parulekar (paediatrics), Jonathan Norris and Elizabeth Insull (ocular plastics), Geoff Rose and Andy Pearson (orbits/ocular plastics), Martin Leyland (corneal surgery) and Pieter Pretorius (neuroradiology). I have kept many of the outstanding pictures that Chris Barry, Simon Cheng, Mitch Ménage, Stephen Tuft and Pablo Gili have provided for previous editions. Terry Tarrant's beautiful paintings, which have been a characteristic feature of the book in the past, have been maintained in this edition. Images of rare conditions have been generously provided by a number of colleagues throughout the United Kingdom and elsewhere in the world and their contribution has been recognised next to the relevant figures. I wish to thank the team at Elsevier for their meticulous input in the production of the book, especially Kayla Wolfe, Joanie Milnes, Elaine Leek and Julie Taylor.

I have once again had the good fortune to work with Jon Brett, a world-class photographer and artist, whose creativity and genius is present in many of the images included in this edition. I am extremely grateful for his diligence, skill and support.

John F. Salmon
2025

Abbreviations

AAION	arteritic anterior ischaemic optic neuropathy
AAU	acute anterior uveitis
AC	anterior chamber
AC/A ratio	accommodative convergence/accommodation ratio
ACE	angiotensin-converting enzyme
AD	autosomal dominant
AF	autofluorescence
AGIS	Advanced Glaucoma Treatment Study
AHP	abnormal head posture
AI	accommodative insufficiency
AIBSE	acute idiopathic blind spot enlargement syndrome
AIDS	acquired immune deficiency syndrome
AIM	(unilateral) acute idiopathic maculopathy
AION	anterior ischaemic optic neuropathy
AIR	autoimmune retinopathies
AKC	atopic keratoconjunctivitis
ALT	argon laser trabeculoplasty
AMD	age-related macular degeneration
AMN	acute macular neuroretinopathy
ANA	antinuclear antibody
ANCA	antineutrophil cytoplasmic antibodies
APD	afferent pupillary defect
APMPPE	acute posterior multifocal placoid pigment epitheliopathy
AR	autosomal recessive
ARDE	age-related distance esotropia
AREDS	Age-Related Eye Disease Study
ARN	acute retinal necrosis
ARPE	acute retinal pigment epitheliitis
AZOOR	acute zonal occult outer retinopathy
AZOR	acute zonal outer retinopathy
BADI	bilateral acute depigmentation of the iris
BCC	basal cell carcinoma
BCVA	best-corrected visual acuity
BIO	binocular indirect ophthalmoscopy
BP	blood pressure
BRAO	branch retinal artery occlusion
BRVO	branch retinal vein occlusion
BSV	binocular single vision
BUT	breakup time
CAI	carbonic anhydrase inhibitor
CCDD	congenital cranial dysinnervation disorders
CCT	central corneal thickness
C/D	cup/disc
CDCR	canaliculodacryocystorhinostomy
CF	counts (or counting) fingers
CHED	congenital hereditary endothelial dystrophy
CHP	compensatory head posture
CHRPE	congenital hypertrophy of the retinal pigment epithelium
CI	convergence insufficiency
C-MIN	conjunctival melanocytic intraepithelial neoplasia
CMO	cystoid macular oedema (US = CME)
CNS	central nervous system
CNV	choroidal neovascularization
CNVM	choroidal neovascular membrane
COX-2	cyclo-oxygenase-2
CPEO	chronic progressive external ophthalmoplegia
CRAO	central retinal artery occlusion
CRP	C-reactive protein
CRVO	central retinal vein occlusion
CSMO	clinically significant macular oedema (US = CSME)
CSR	central serous chorioretinopathy
CSS	central suppression scotoma
CT	computed tomography
CVI	cerebral visual impairment
CXL	corneal collagen cross-linking
DALK	deep anterior lamellar keratoplasty
DCCT	Diabetes Control and Complication Trial
DCR	dacryocystorhinostomy
DCT	dynamic contour tonometry
DMEK	Descemet membrane endothelial keratoplasty
DMO	diabetic macular oedema (US = DME)
DR	diabetic retinopathy
DRCR.net	Diabetic Retinopathy Clinical Research Network
DRPPT	dark room prone provocative test
DRS	Diabetic Retinopathy Study
DSAEK	Descemet stripping automated endothelial keratoplasty
DVD	dissociated vertical deviation
ECG	electrocardiogram
EDTA	ethylenediaminetetraacetic acid
EGFR	epidermal growth factor inhibitors
EKC	epidemic keratoconjunctivitis
EMGT	Early Manifest Glaucoma Trial
EOG	electro-oculography/gram
ERG	electroretinography/gram
ERM	epiretinal membrane
ESR	erythrocyte sedimentation rate
ETDRS	Early Treatment Diabetic Retinopathy Study
ETROP	Early Treatment of Retinopathy of Prematurity
FA	fluorescein angiography (also FFA)
FAF	fundus autofluorescence
FAP	familial adenomatous polyposis
FAZ	foveal avascular zone
FBA	frosted branch angiitis
FBC	full blood count
FDT	frequency doubling test
FFM	fundus flavimaculatus
FTMH	full-thickness macular hole
5-FU	5-fluorouracil
GA	geographic atrophy

GAT Goldmann applanation tonometry
GCA giant cell arteritis
GDD glaucoma drainage device
GHT glaucoma hemifield test
GPA guided progression analysis
GPC giant papillary conjunctivitis
G-TOP glaucoma tendency orientated perimetry
HAART highly active antiretroviral therapy
HFA Humphrey field analyser
HIV human immunodeficiency virus
HM hand movements
HRT Heidelberg retinal tomography
HSV-1 herpes simplex virus type 1
HSV-2 herpes simplex virus type 2
HZO herpes zoster ophthalmicus
ICE iridocorneal endothelial
ICG indocyanine green
ICGA indocyanine green angiography
ICROP International Classification of Retinopathy of Prematurity
IFIS intraoperative floppy iris syndrome
Ig immunoglobulin
IK interstitial keratitis
ILM internal limiting membrane
IMT idiopathic macular telangiectasia
INO internuclear ophthalmoplegia
INR international normalized ratio
IOFB intraocular foreign body
IOID idiopathic orbital inflammatory disease
IOL intraocular lens
IOP intraocular pressure
IRMA intraretinal microvascular abnormality
IRVAN idiopathic retinal vasculitis, aneurysms and neuroretinitis syndrome
ITC iridotrabecular contact
IU intermediate uveitis
IVTS International Vitreomacular Traction Study
JIA juvenile idiopathic arthritis
KC keratoconus
KCS keratoconjunctivitis sicca
KP keratic precipitate
LA local anaesthetic
LASEK laser (also laser-assisted) epithelial keratomileusis
LASIK Laser (also laser-assisted) *in situ* keratomileusis
LN latent nystagmus
LSCD limbal stem cell deficiency
LV loss variance
MALT mucosa-associated lymphoid tissue
MCP multifocal choroiditis and panuveitis
MEWDS multiple evanescent white dot syndrome
MFC multifocal choroiditis and panuveitis
MIGS minimally invasive glaucoma surgery
MLF medial longitudinal fasciculus
MLT micropulse laser technology
MMC mitomycin C
MNV macular neovascularization
MPS mucopolysaccharidosis
MRI magnetic resonance imaging
MS multiple sclerosis
NF1 neurofibromatosis type 1
NF2 neurofibromatosis type 2
NPDR non-proliferative diabetic retinopathy
NRR neuroretinal rim
NSAID non-steroidal anti-inflammatory drug
NSR neurosensory retina
NTG normal-tension glaucoma
NVD new vessels on the disc
NVE new vessels elsewhere
NVG neovascular glaucoma
NVI new vessels iris
OCT optical coherence tomography/gram
OCTA optical coherence tomography angiography
OHT ocular hypertension
OHTS Ocular Hypertension Treatment Study
OIS ocular ischaemia syndrome
OKN optokinetic nystagmus
OVD ophthalmic viscosurgical devices
PAC primary angle closure
PACG primary angle-closure glaucoma
PACS primary angle-closure suspect
PAM primary acquired melanosis
PAN polyarteritis nodosa
PAS peripheral anterior synechiae
PC posterior chamber
PCO posterior capsular opacification
PCR polymerase chain reaction
PCV polypoidal choroidal vasculopathy
PDR proliferative diabetic retinopathy
PDS pigment dispersion syndrome
PDT photodynamic therapy
PED pigment epithelial detachment
PEE punctate epithelial erosions
PEK punctate epithelial keratitis
PEHCR peripheral exudative haemorrhagic chorioretinopathy
PH pinhole
PHM posterior hyaloid membrane
PIC punctate inner choroidopathy
PIOL primary intraocular lymphoma
PION posterior ischaemic optic neuropathy
PKP penetrating keratoplasty
PMMA polymethyl methacrylate
POAG primary open-angle glaucoma
POHS presumed ocular histoplasmosis syndrome
PP pars planitis
PPCD posterior polymorphous corneal dystrophy
PPDR preproliferative diabetic retinopathy
PPM persistent placoid maculopathy
PPRF paramedian pontine reticular formation
PPV pars plana vitrectomy
PRK photorefractive keratectomy
PRP panretinal photocoagulation
PS posterior synechiae

PSD	pattern standard deviation
PSS	Posner–Schlossman syndrome
PUK	peripheral ulcerative keratitis
PVD	posterior vitreous detachment
PVR	proliferative vitreoretinopathy
PVRL	primary vitreoretinal lymphoma
PXE	pseudoxanthoma elasticum
PXF	pseudoexfoliation
RA	rheumatoid arthritis
RAO	retinal artery occlusion
RAPD	relative afferent pupillary defect
RD	retinal detachment
RNFL	retinal nerve fibre layer
ROCK	Rho-kinase
ROP	retinopathy of prematurity
RP	retinitis pigmentosa
RPC	relentless placoid chorioretinitis
RPE	retinal pigment epithelium
RRD	rhegmatogenous retinal detachment
RS	retinoschisis
RVO	retinal vein occlusion
SACE	serum angiotensin-converting enzyme
SANS	space flight-associated neuro-ocular syndrome
SAP	standard automated perimetry
SCC	squamous cell carcinoma
SCN	suprachiasmic nucleus
SD-OCT	spectral domain optical coherence tomography
SES	sagging eye syndrome
SF	short-term fluctuation
SFU	progressive subretinal fibrosis and uveitis syndrome
SIC	solitary idiopathic choroiditis
SITA	Swedish Interactive Thresholding Algorithm
SJS	Stevens–Johnson syndrome
SLK	superior limbic keratoconjunctivitis
SLT	selective laser trabeculoplasty
SMILE	small incision lenticule extraction
SPARCS	Spaeth Richman contrast sensitivity test
SPK	superficial punctate keratitis
SRF	subretinal fluid
SS	Sjögren syndrome
STIR	short T1 inversion recovery
SWAP	short-wave automated perimetry
TAL	total axial length
TB	tuberculosis
TEN	toxic epidermal necrolysis
TGF	transforming growth factor
TIA	transient ischaemic attack
TM	trabecular meshwork
TRD	tractional retinal detachment
TRP	targeted retinal photocoagulation
TTT	transpupillary thermotherapy
UBM	ultrasonic biomicroscopy
US	ultrasonography
VA	visual acuity
VEGF	vascular endothelial growth factor
VEP	visual(ly) evoked potential(s)
VFI	visual field index
VHL	von Hippel–Lindau syndrome
VKC	vernal keratoconjunctivitis
VKH	Vogt–Koyanagi–Harada syndrome
VMA	vitreomacular adhesion
VMT	vitreomacular traction
VZV	varicella zoster virus
XL	X-linked

Chapter 1

Examination Techniques

OPHTHALMIC HISTORY

Before examining the patient, a thorough ophthalmic history should be taken. A detailed history will depend on the particular visual symptoms and suspected ocular disease. However, a basic history can be divided into the following categories of questioning:

- Main complaint: (a) rapidity of onset, (b) circumstances surrounding the onset, (c) severity, (d) duration of symptoms, (e) frequency of symptoms.
- Past ocular history: e.g. previous surgery, inflammation, trauma.
- Past medical history: e.g. diabetes and hypertension.
- Systemic medication: e.g. corticosteroids, tamsulosin.
- Allergies: e.g. antibiotics, topical glaucoma medications.
- Family history: e.g. glaucoma, macular degeneration, inherited retinal disease.
- Occupation and hobbies

OPHTHALMIC EXAMINATION

Patients with ophthalmic disease must have their vision accurately measured and their eyes need to be examined using specialized techniques. Special investigations should be used to supplement the findings of clinical examination. Electrophysical tests, fluorescein angiography and optical coherence tomography are discussed in later chapters.

PSYCHOPHYSICAL TESTS

Visual acuity

Snellen visual acuity

Distance visual acuity (VA) is directly related to the minimum angle of separation (subtended at the nodal point of the eye) between two objects that allow them to be perceived as distinct. In practice, it is most commonly carried out using a Snellen chart, which utilizes black letters or symbols (optotypes) of a range of sizes set on a white chart (Fig. 1.1), with the subject reading the chart from a standard distance. Distance VA is usually first measured using a patient's refractive correction, generally their own glasses or contact lenses. For completeness, an unaided acuity may also be recorded. The eye reported as having worse vision should be tested first, with the other eye occluded. It is important to push the patient to read every letter possible on the optotypes being tested.

- **Normal monocular VA** equates to 6/6 (metric notation; 20/20 in non-metric 'English' notation) on Snellen testing. Normal corrected VA in young adults is often superior to 6/6.
- **Best-corrected VA** (BCVA) denotes the level achieved with optimal refractive correction.
- **Pinhole VA:** a pinhole (PH) aperture compensates for the effect of refractive error, and consists of an opaque occluder perforated by one or more holes of about 1 mm diameter (Fig. 1.2). However, PH acuity in patients with macular disease and posterior lens opacities may be worse than with spectacle correction. If the VA is less than 6/6 Snellen equivalent, testing is repeated using a pinhole aperture.

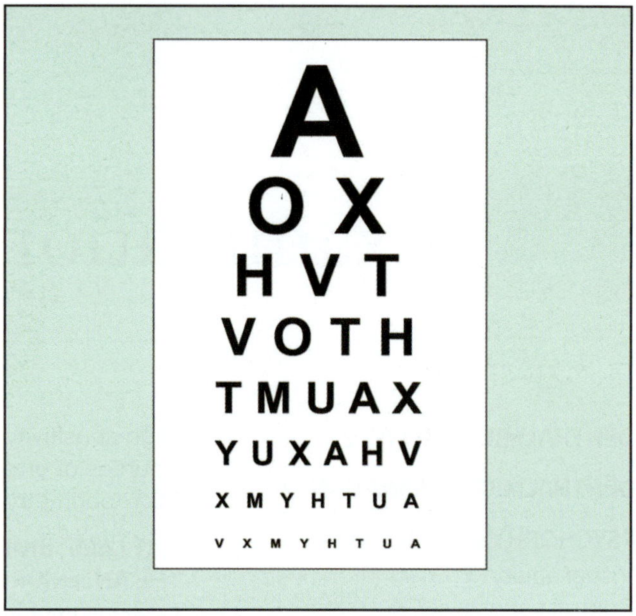

Fig. 1.1 Snellen visual acuity chart.

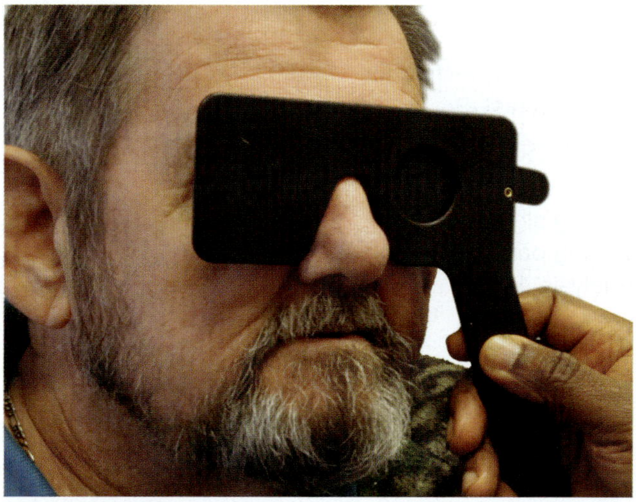

Fig. 1.2 Pinhole.

- **Binocular VA** is usually superior to the better monocular VA of each eye, at least where both eyes have roughly equal vision.

Very poor visual acuity

- **Counting (or counts) fingers (CF)** denotes that the patient is able to tell how many fingers the examiner is holding up at a specified distance (Fig. 1.3), usually 1 metre.
- **Hand movements (HM)** is the ability to distinguish whether the examiner's hand is moving when held just in front of the patient.
- **Perception of light (PL)**: the patient can discern only light (e.g. pen torch), but no shapes or movement. Careful occlusion of the other eye is necessary. If poor vision is due solely to a dense media opacity such as cataract, the patient should readily be able to determine the direction from which the light is being projected (Fig. 1.4).

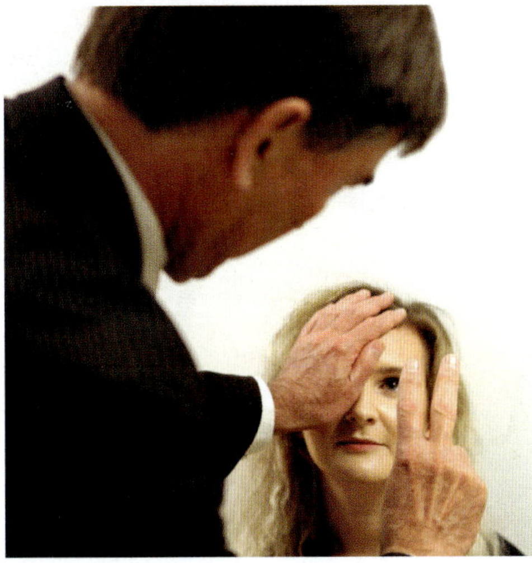

Fig. 1.3 Testing of 'counting fingers' vision.

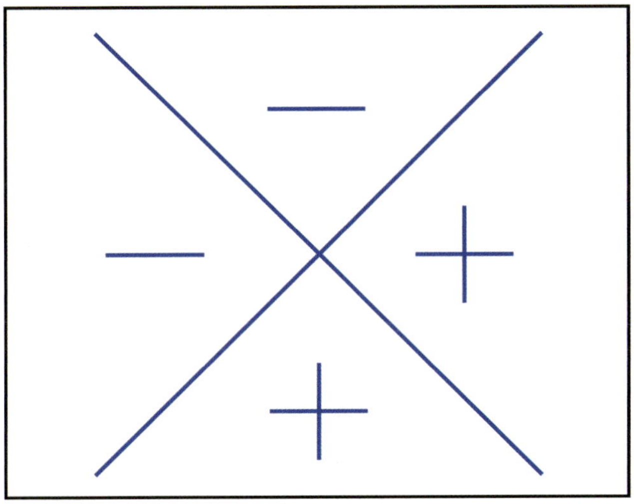

Fig. 1.4 Notation for the projection of light test (right eye); the patient cannot detect light directed from the superior and temporal quadrants.

LogMAR acuity

LogMAR charts address many of the deficiencies of the Snellen chart (Table 1.1), and are the standard means of VA measurement in research and, increasingly, in clinical practice.

- LogMAR is an acronym for the base-10 logarithm of the minimum angle of resolution (MAR) and refers to the ability to resolve the elements of an optotype. Thus, if a letter on the 6/6 (20/20) equivalent line subtends 5′ of arc, and each limb of the letter has an angular width of 1′, a MAR of 1′ is needed for resolution. For the 6/12 (20/40) line, the MAR is 2′, and for the 6/60 (20/200) line it is 10′.
- The logMAR score is simply the base-10 log of the MAR. Because the log of the MAR value of 1′ is zero, 6/6 is equivalent to logMAR 0.00. The log of the 6/60 MAR of 10′ is 1, so 6/60 is equivalent to logMAR 1.00. The log of the 6/12 MAR of 2′ is 0.301, giving a logMAR score of 0.30. Scores better than 6/6 have a negative value.

Table 1.1 Comparison of Snellen and LogMAR Visual Acuity Testing

Snellen	LogMAR
Shorter test time	Longer test time
More letters on the lower lines introduces an unbalanced 'crowding' effect	Equal numbers of letters on different lines controls for 'crowding' effect
Fewer larger letters reduce accuracy at lower levels of VA	Equal numbers of letters on low and higher acuity lines increases accuracy at lower VA
Variable readability between individual letters	Similar readability between letters
Lines not balanced with each other for consistency of readability	Lines balanced for consistency of readability
6m testing distance: longer testing lane (or a mirror) required	4m testing distance on many charts: smaller testing lane (or no mirror) required
Letter and row spacing not systematic	Letter and row spacing set to optimize contour interaction
Lower accuracy and consistency so relatively unsuitable for research	Higher accuracy and consistency so appropriate for research
Straightforward scoring system	More complex scoring
Easy to use	Less user-friendly

- As letter size changes by 0.1 logMAR units per row and there are five letters in each row, each letter can be assigned a score of 0.02. The final score can therefore take account of every letter that has been read correctly and the test should continue until half of the letters on a line are read incorrectly.
- **For conversion of logMAR into metres and feet**: see Table 1.2.

LogMAR charts

- **The Bailey–Lovie** chart (Fig. 1.5)
  - Used at 6 m testing distance.
  - Each line of the chart comprises five letters and the spacing between each letter and each row is related to the width and the height of the letters. The letter signs are rectangular rather than square, as with the EDTRS chart. A 6/6 letter is 5′ in height by 4′ in width.
  - The distance between two adjacent letters on the same row is equal to the width of a letter from the same row, and the distance between two adjacent rows is the same as the height of a letter from the lower of the two rows.
  - Snellen VA values and logMAR VA are listed to the right and left of the rows respectively.
- **The ETDRS (Early Treatment Diabetic Retinopathy Study)** chart is calibrated for 4 m. This chart utilizes balanced rows comprising Sloan optotypes, developed to confer equivalent legibility between individual letters and rows. ETDRS letters

Table 1.2 Conversion of Snellen Visual Acuity from LogMAR

LogMAR	Metre	Foot	Decimal
1.00	6/60	20/200	0.10
0.90	6/48	20/160	0.125
0.80	6/38	20/125	0.16
0.70	6/30	20/100	0.20
0.60	6/24	20/80	0.25
0.50	6/19	20/63	0.32
0.40	6/15	20/50	0.40
0.30	6/12	20/40	0.50
0.20	6/9.5	20/32	0.63
0.10	6/7.5	20/25	0.80
0.00	6/6	20/20	1.00
−0.10	6/4.8	20/16	1.25
−0.20	6/3.8	20/12.5	1.60
−0.30	6/3	20/10	2.00

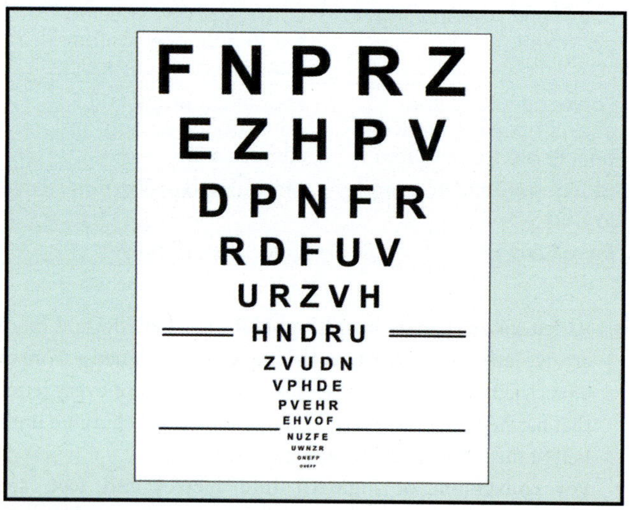

Fig. 1.5 Bailey–Lovie chart.

are square, based on a 5 × 5 grid, i.e. 5′ × 5′ for the 6/6 equivalent letters at 6 m.

- **Computer** charts are available that present the various forms of test chart on display screens, including other means of assessment such as contrast sensitivity (see below).

TIP LogMAR charts are commonly used in clinical trials because they are the most accurate method of measuring visual acuity.

Near visual acuity

Near vision testing can be a sensitive indicator of the presence of macular disease. A range of near vision charts (including logMAR and ETDRS versions) or a test-type book can be used. The book or chart is held at a comfortable reading distance and this is measured and noted. The patient wears any necessary distance correction together with a presbyopia correction if applicable (usually their

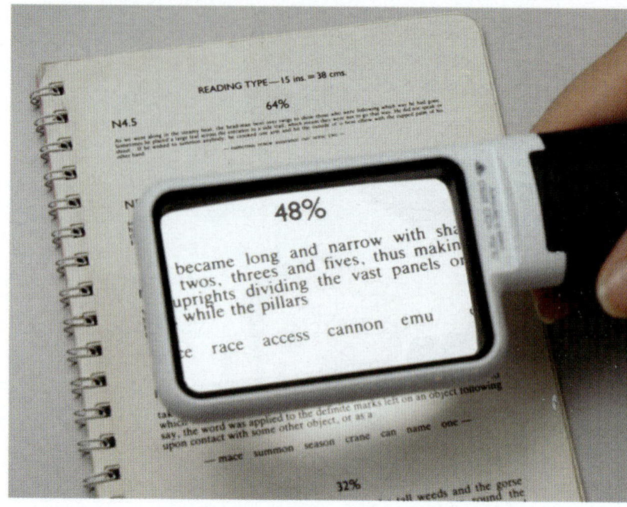

Fig. 1.6 Near visual acuity using a magnifying lens.

own reading spectacles). The smallest type legible is recorded for each eye individually and then using both eyes together (Fig. 1.6).

Contrast sensitivity

- **Principles.** Contrast sensitivity is a measure of the ability of the visual system to distinguish an object against its background. A target must be sufficiently large to be seen, but must also be of high enough contrast with its background. A light grey letter will be less well seen against a white background than a black letter. Contrast sensitivity represents a different aspect of visual function to that tested by the spatial resolution tests described above, which all use high-contrast optotypes.
    - Many conditions reduce both contrast sensitivity and VA, but under some circumstances (e.g. amblyopia, optic neuropathy, some cataracts, and higher-order aberrations), visual function measured by contrast sensitivity can be reduced whilst VA is preserved.
    - Hence, if patients with good VA complain of visual symptoms (typically evident in low illumination), contrast sensitivity testing may be a useful way of objectively demonstrating a functional deficit. Despite its advantages, it has not been widely adopted in clinical practice.
- **The Pelli–Robson** contrast sensitivity letter chart is viewed at 1 metre and consists of rows of letters of equal size (spatial frequency of 1 cycle per degree) but with decreasing contrast of 0.15 log units for groups of three letters (Fig. 1.7). The patient reads down the rows of letters until the lowest-resolvable group of three is reached.
- **Sinusoidal (sine wave) gratings** require the test subject to view a sequence of increasingly lower contrast gratings.
- **Spaeth Richman contrast sensitivity test** (SPARCS) is performed on a personal computer with internet access. It can be accessed online. Each patient is supplied with an identification number and instructions on how to do the test. The test takes 5–10 minutes per eye and measures both central and peripheral contrast sensitivity. Since the test is based on gratings it can be used on illiterate patients.

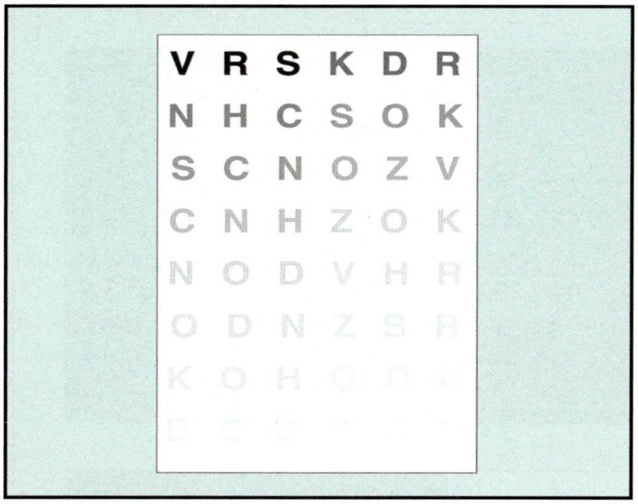

Fig. 1.7 Pelli–Robson contrast sensitivity letter chart.

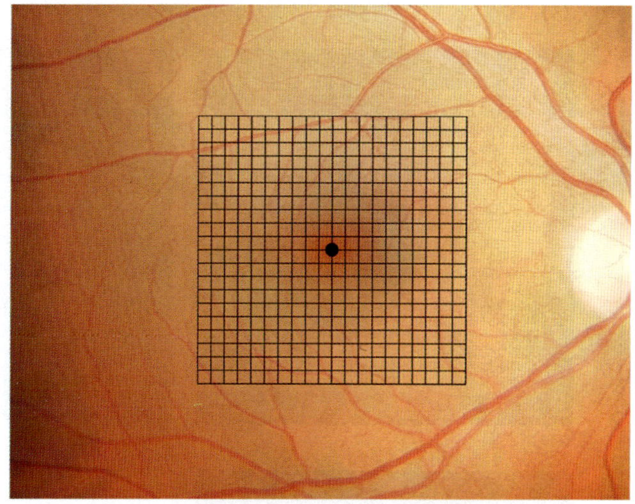

Fig. 1.8 Amsler grid superimposed on the macula.

Amsler grid

The Amsler grid evaluates the 20° of the visual field centred on fixation (Fig. 1.8). It is principally useful in screening for and monitoring macular disease, but will also demonstrate central visual field defects originating elsewhere. Patients with a substantial risk of macular neovascularization (MNV) should be provided with an Amsler grid for regular use at home.

TIP An Amsler grid is a simple and easy method of monitoring central visual field and is commonly abnormal in patients with macular disease.

Charts

There are seven charts, each consisting of a 10-cm outer square (Figs 1.9 and 1.10).

- Chart 1 consists of a white grid on a black background, the outer grid enclosing 400 smaller 5-mm squares. When viewed at about one-third of a metre, each small square subtends an angle of 1°.
- Chart 2 is similar to chart 1 but has diagonal lines that aid fixation for patients with a central scotoma.
- Chart 3 is identical to chart 1 but has red squares. The red-on-black design aims to stimulate long wavelength foveal cones. It is used to detect subtle colour scotomas and desaturation in toxic maculopathy, optic neuropathy and chiasmal lesions.
- Chart 4 consists only of random dots and is used mainly to distinguish scotomas from metamorphopsia, as there is no form to be distorted.
- Chart 5 consists of horizontal lines and is designed to detect metamorphopsia along specific meridians. It is of particular use in the evaluation of patients describing difficulty reading.
- Chart 6 is similar to chart 5 but has a white background and the central lines are closer together, enabling more detailed evaluation.
- Chart 7 includes a fine central grid, each square subtending an angle of a half degree, and is more sensitive.

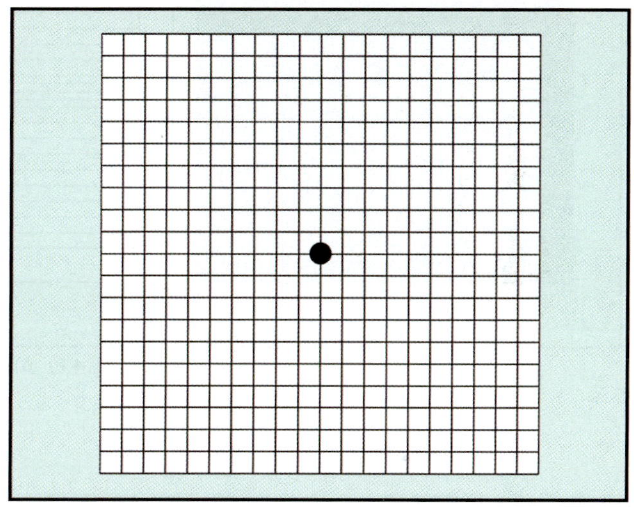

Fig. 1.9 Amsler grid chart.

Technique

The pupils should not be dilated, and in order to avoid a photostress effect, the eyes should not yet have been examined on the slit lamp. A presbyopic refractive correction should be worn if appropriate. The chart should be well illuminated and held at a comfortable reading distance, optimally around 33 cm.

- One eye is covered.
- The patient is asked to look directly at the central dot with the uncovered eye, to keep looking at this, and to report any distortion or waviness of the lines on the grid.
- Reminding the patient to maintain fixation on the central dot, he or she is asked if there are blurred areas or blank spots anywhere on the grid. Patients with macular disease often report that the lines are wavy whereas those with optic neuropathy tend to remark that some of the lines are missing or faint but not distorted.
- The patient is asked if he or she can see all four corners and all four sides of the square – a missing corner or border should raise the possibility of causes other than macular disease, such as glaucomatous field defects or retinitis pigmentosa.
- The patient may be provided with a recording sheet and pen and asked to draw any anomalies (Fig. 1.11).

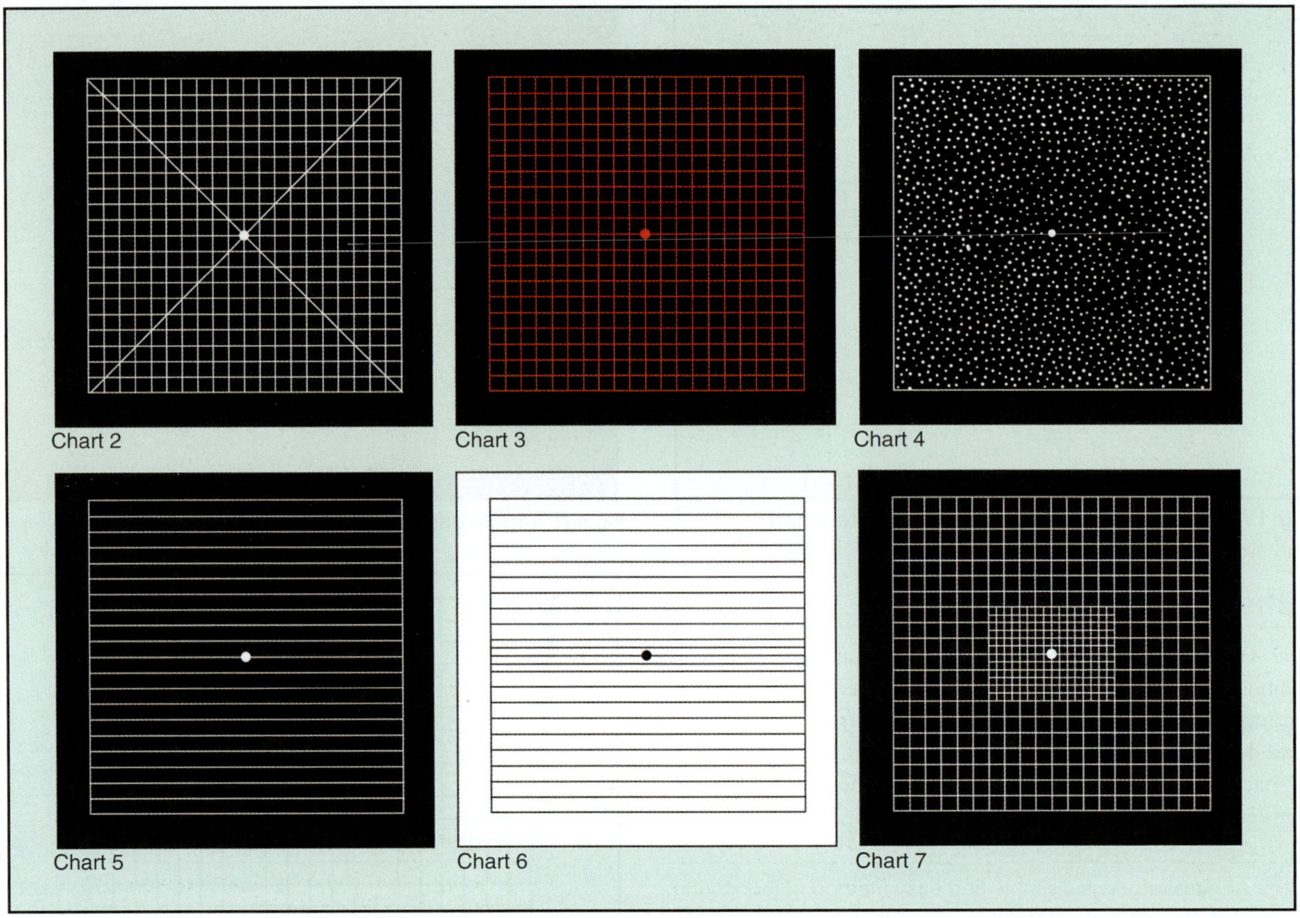

Fig. 1.10 Amsler charts 2–7.

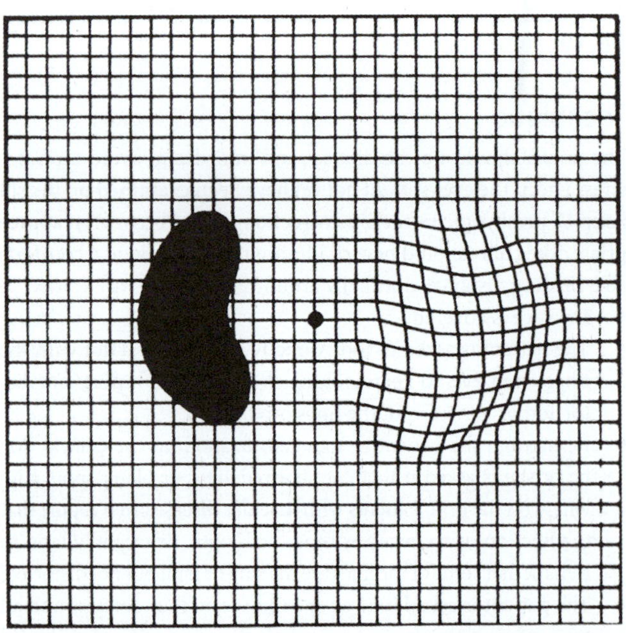

Fig. 1.11 Stylized Amsler recording sheet showing wavy lines indicating metamorphopsia, and a dense scotoma.

Light brightness comparison test

This is a test of optic nerve function, which is usually normal in early and moderate retinal disease. It is performed as follows:

- A light from an indirect ophthalmoscope is shone first into the normal eye and then the eye with suspected disease.
- The patient is asked whether the light is symmetrically bright in both eyes.
- In optic neuropathy the patient will report that the light is less bright in the affected eye.
- The patient is asked to assign a relevant value from 1 to 5 to the brightness of the light in the diseased eye, in comparison to the normal eye.

Photostress test

- **Principles.** Photostress testing is a gross test of dark adaptation in which the visual pigments are bleached by light. This causes a temporary state of retinal insensitivity perceived by the patient as a scotoma. The recovery of vision is dependent on the ability of the photoreceptors to re-synthesize visual pigment. The test may be useful in detecting maculopathy when

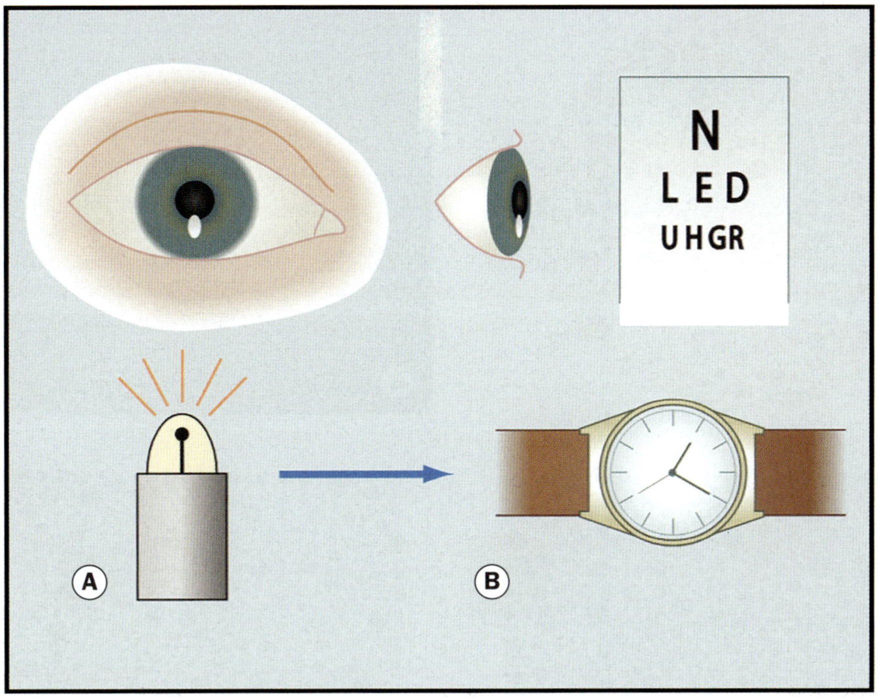

Fig. 1.12 Photostress test. **(A)** The patient looks at a light held about 3 cm away from the eye, for about 10 seconds; **(B)** the photostress recovery time is the time taken to read any three letters of the pre-test acuity line and is normally between 15 and 30 seconds.

ophthalmoscopy is equivocal, as in mild cystoid macular oedema or central serous retinopathy. It may also differentiate visual loss caused by macular disease from that caused by an optic nerve lesion.

- **Techniques**
  - The best-corrected distance VA is determined.
  - The patient fixates on the light of a pen torch or an indirect ophthalmoscope held about 3 cm away for about 10 seconds (Fig. 1.12A).
  - The photostress recovery time (PSRT) is the time taken to read any three letters of the pre-test acuity line and is normally between 15 and 30 seconds (Fig. 1.12B).
  - The test is performed on the other, presumably normal, eye and the results are compared.
  - The PSRT is prolonged relative to the normal eye in macular disease (sometimes 50 seconds or more) but not in an optic neuropathy.

Colour vision testing

Introduction

Assessment of colour vision is useful in the evaluation of optic nerve disease and in determining the presence of a congenitally anomalous colour defect. Congenital colour vision deficiency (CVD) is a common X-linked recessive condition that affects about 8% of Northern European men and 0.5% of women. The prevalence in Black Africans is about 4% for men and 1.5% for women. CVD is the decreased ability to see colour or differences in colour along a red–green axis. It can impair tasks such as choosing clothing and seeing traffic lights. Dyschromatopsia may develop in retinal dystrophies prior to the impairment of other visual parameters. Colour vision depends on three populations of retinal cones, each with a specific peak sensitivity: blue (tritan) at 414–424 nm, green (deuteran) at 522–539 nm and red (protan) at 549–570 nm. Normal colour perception requires all these primary colours to match those within the spectrum. Any given cone pigment may be deficient (e.g. protanomaly – red weakness) or entirely absent (e.g. protanopia – red blindness). Trichromats possess all three types of cones (although not necessarily functioning perfectly), while absence of one or two types of cones renders an individual a dichromat or monochromat, respectively. Most individuals with congenital colour defects are anomalous trichromats and use abnormal proportions of the three primary colours to match those in the light spectrum. Those with red–green deficiency caused by abnormality of red-sensitive cones are protanomalous (2% of men), those with abnormality of green-sensitive cones (6% of men) are deuteranomalous and those with blue–green deficiency caused by abnormality of blue-sensitive cones are tritanomalous. Acquired macular disease tends to produce blue–yellow defects, and optic nerve lesions, red–green defects.

TIP Children who are found to have a congenital colour vision deficiency will find it difficult or impossible to engage in certain occupations and may benefit from early career counselling.

Colour vision tests

- **The Ishihara test** is designed to screen for congenital protan and deuteran defects. It is simple, widely available and frequently used to screen for a red–green colour vision deficit.

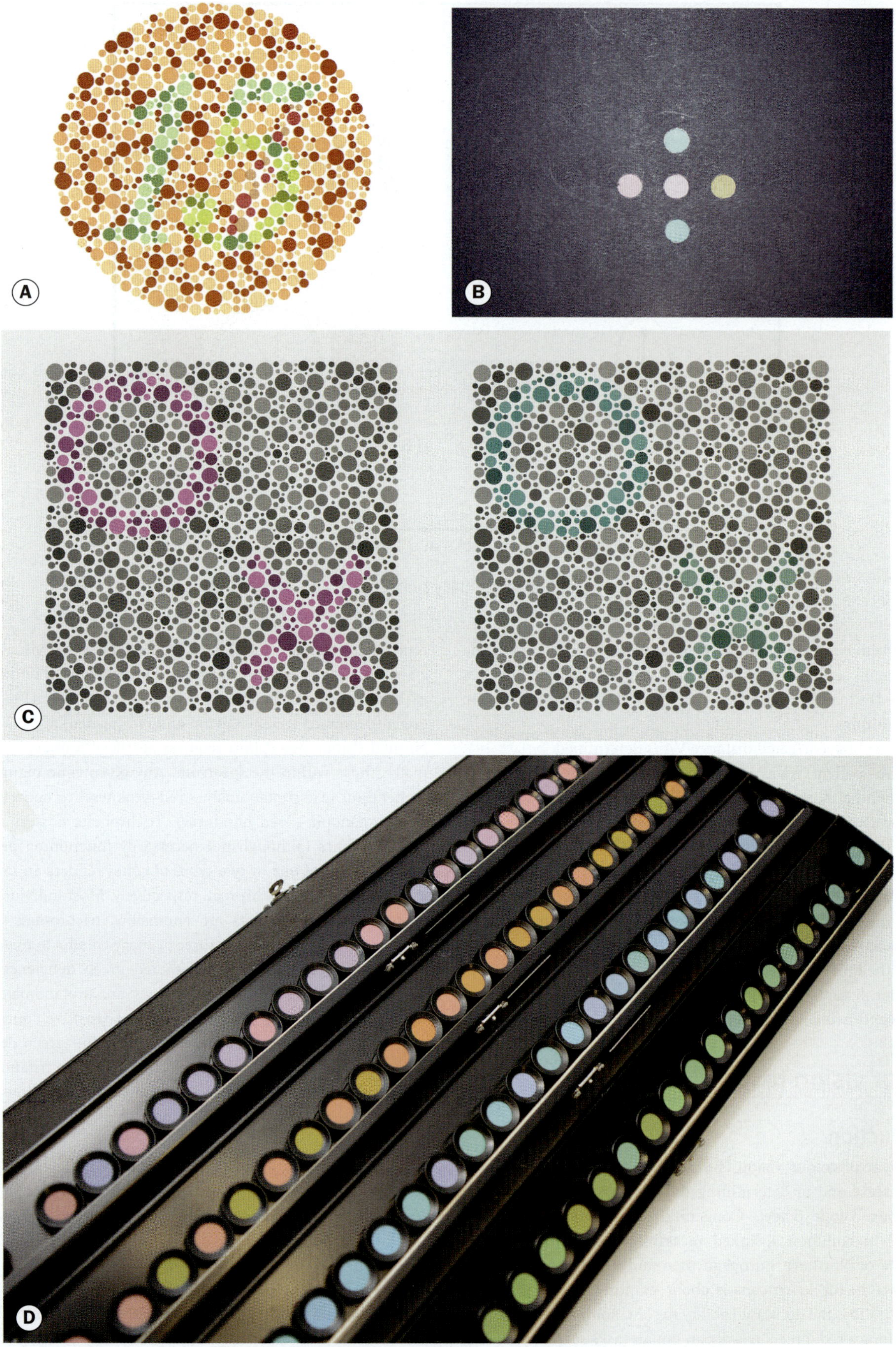

Fig. 1.13 Colour vision tests. **(A)** Ishihara; **(B)** City University; **(C)** Hardy–Rand–Rittler; **(D)** Farnsworth–Munsell 100-hue test.

The test can be used to assess optic nerve function. It consists of a test plate followed by 16 plates, each with a matrix of dots arranged to show a central shape or number that the subject is asked to identify (Fig. 1.13A). A colour-deficient person will be able to identify only some of the figures. Inability to identify the test plate (provided VA is sufficient) indicates non-organic visual loss.

- **The City University test** consists of 10 plates, each containing a central colour and four peripheral colours (Fig. 1.13B) from which the subject is asked to choose the closest match.
- **The Hardy–Rand–Rittler test** is similar to the Ishihara, but can detect all three congenital colour defects (Fig. 1.13C).
- **The Farnsworth–Munsell 100-hue test** is a sensitive but longer test for both congenital and acquired colour defects. Despite the name, it consists of 85 caps of different hues in four racks (Fig. 1.13D). The subject is asked to rearrange randomized caps in order of colour progression, and the findings are recorded on a circular chart. Each of the three forms of dichromatism is characterized by failure in a specific meridian of the chart (Fig. 1.14).

Plus lens test

A temporary hypermetropic shift may occur in some conditions due to an elevation of the sensory retina – the classic example is central serous chorioretinopathy (CSR). A +1.00-dioptre lens will demonstrate the phenomenon.

PERIMETRY

Definitions

- **The visual field** can be represented as a three-dimensional structure akin to a hill of increasing sensitivity (Fig. 1.15A). The outer aspect extends approximately 50° superiorly, 60° nasally, 70° inferiorly and 90° temporally. VA is sharpest at the very top of the hill (i.e. the fovea) and then declines progressively towards the periphery, the nasal slope being steeper than the temporal. The 'bottomless pit' of the blind spot is located temporally between 10° and 20°, slightly below the horizontal.
- **An isopter** is a line connecting points of the same sensitivity, and on a two-dimensional isopter plot encloses an area within which a stimulus of a given strength is visible. When the field is represented as a hill, isopters resemble the contour lines on a map (Fig. 1.15B).
- **A scotoma** is an area of reduced ('relative') or total ('absolute') loss of vision surrounded by a seeing area.
- **Luminance** is the intensity or 'brightness' of a light stimulus, measured in apostilbs (asb). A higher intensity stimulus has a higher asb value; this is related inversely to sensitivity.
- A **logarithmic** rather than a linear scale is used for stimulus intensity and sensitivity, so that for each log unit intensity changes by a factor of 10. With a log scale, greater significance is given to the lower end of the intensity range. The normal eye has a very large sensitivity range, and assessment of the lower end of the scale is of critical significance so that early damage

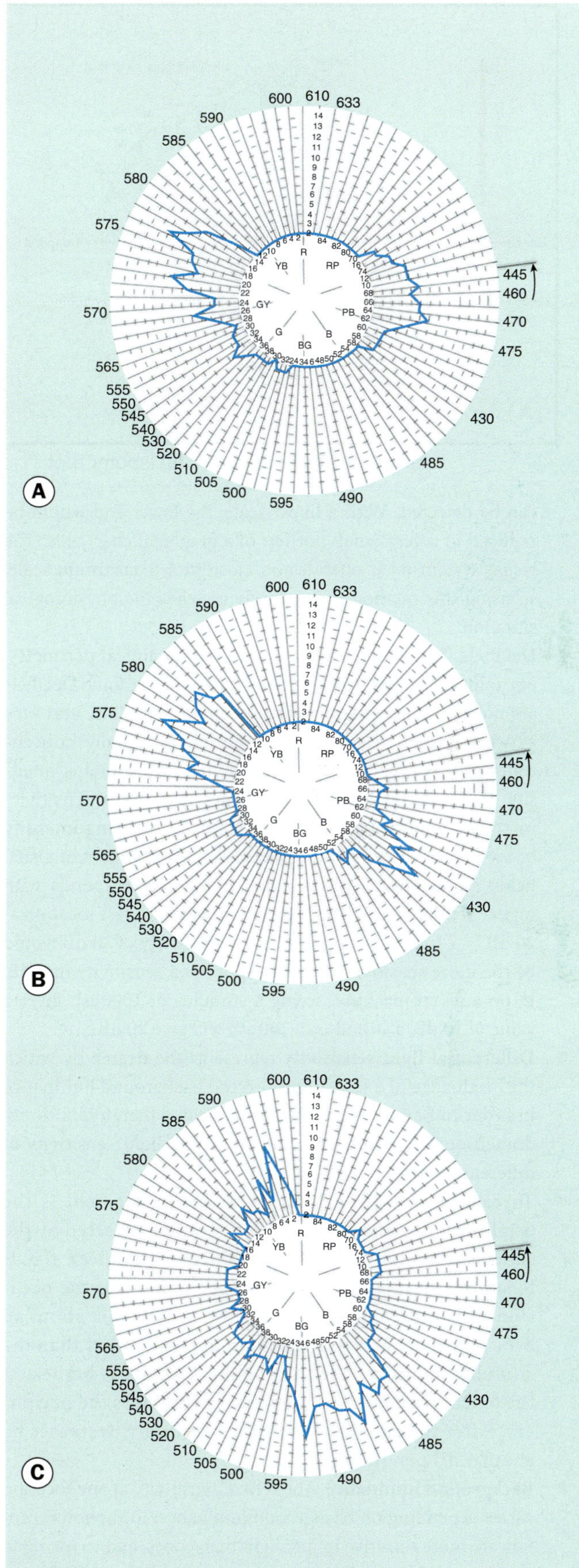

Fig. 1.14 Farnsworth–Munsell test results of colour deficiencies. **(A)** Protanopia; **(B)** deuteranopia; **(C)** tritanopia.

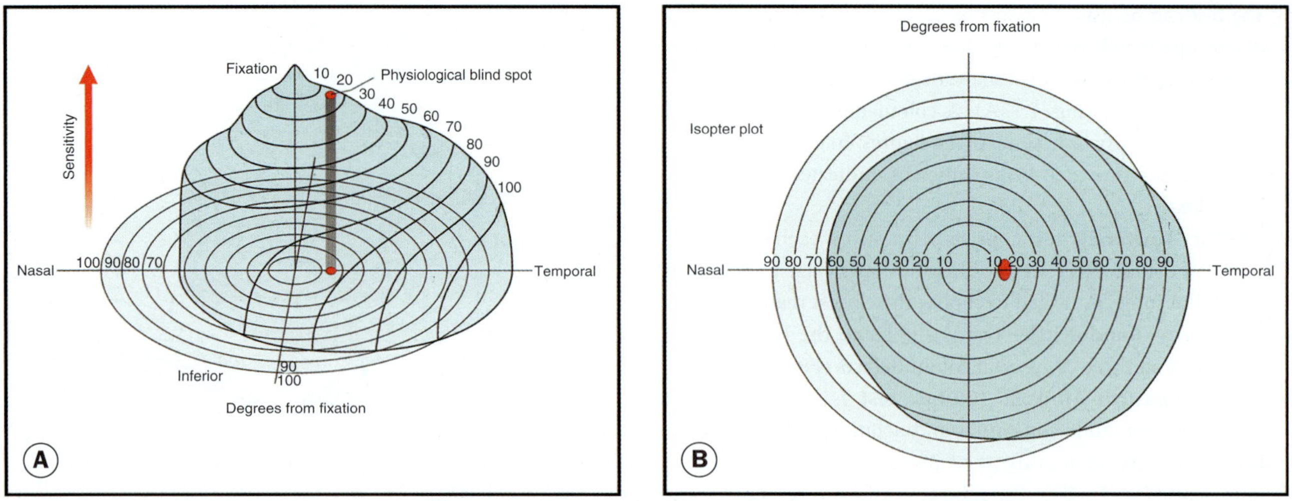

Fig. 1.15 **(A)** Hill of vision; **(B)** isopter plot.

can be detected. With a linear scale, the lower end would be reduced to a very small portion of a graphical chart axis. The visual system itself operates on close to a logarithmic scale, so using this method more closely matches the physiological situation.

- **Decibels.** Simple log units are not used in clinical perimetry, but rather 'decibels' (dB), where 10 dB = 1 log unit. Decibels are not true units of luminance but a representation, and vary between visual field machines. Perimetry usually concentrates on the eye's sensitivity rather than the stimulus intensity. Therefore, the decibel reading goes up as retinal sensitivity increases, which obviously corresponds to reducing intensity of the perceived stimulus. This makes the assessment of visual fields more intuitive, as a higher number corresponds with higher retinal sensitivity. If the sensitivity of a test location is 20 dB (= 2 log units), a point with a sensitivity of 30 dB would be the more sensitive. The blind spot has a sensitivity of 0 dB. If, on a given machine, seeing a stimulus of 1000 asb gives a value of 10 dB, a stimulus of 100 asb will give 20 dB.
- **Differential light sensitivity** represents the degree by which the luminance of a target must exceed background luminance in order to be perceived. The visual field is therefore a three-dimensional representation of differential light sensitivity at different points.
- **Threshold** at a given location in the visual field is the brightness of a stimulus at which it can be detected by the subject. It is defined as 'the luminance of a given fixed-location stimulus at which it is seen on 50% of the occasions it is presented'. In practice we usually talk about an eye's *sensitivity* at a given point in the field rather than the stimulus intensity. The threshold sensitivity is highest at the fovea and decreases progressively towards the periphery. After the age of 20 years the sensitivity decreases by about 1 dB per 10 years.
- **Background luminance.** The retinal sensitivity at any location varies depending on background luminance. Rod photoreceptors are more sensitive in dim light than cones, and so owing to their preponderance in the peripheral retina, at lower (scotopic) light levels the peripheral retina becomes more sensitive in proportion to the central retina. The hill of vision flattens, with a central crater rather than a peak at the fovea due to the high concentration of cones, which have low sensitivity in scotopic conditions. Some diseases give markedly different field results at different background luminance levels, e.g. in retinitis pigmentosa the field is usually much worse with low background luminance. It should be noted that it takes about 5 minutes to adapt from darkness to bright sunlight and 20–30 minutes from bright sunlight to darkness. The HFA (see below) uses a photopic (preferentially cone) level of background luminance at 31.5 asb.
- **Static perimetry.** A method of assessing fields, usually automated, in which the location of a stimulus remains fixed, with intensity increased until it is seen by the subject (threshold is reached – Fig. 1.16A) or decreased until it is no longer detected.
- **Kinetic (dynamic) perimetry** is now much less commonly performed than static perimetry. A stimulus of constant intensity is moved from a non-seeing area to a seeing area (Fig. 1.16B) at a standardized speed until it is perceived, and the point of perception is recorded on a chart. Points from different meridians are joined to plot an isopter for that stimulus intensity. Stimuli of different intensities are used to produce a contour map of the visual field. Kinetic perimetry can be performed by means of a manual (Goldmann) or an automated perimeter if the latter is equipped with an appropriate software program.
- **Manual perimetry** involves presentation of a stimulus by the perimetrist, with manual recording of the response. It was formerly the standard method of field testing but has now largely been superseded by automated methods. It is still used occasionally, particularly in cognitively limited patients unable to interact adequately with an automated system, and for dynamic testing of peripheral fields.
- **Standard automated perimetry (SAP)** is the method used routinely in most clinical situations. Automated perimeters in common use include the Humphrey Field Analyser (HFA),

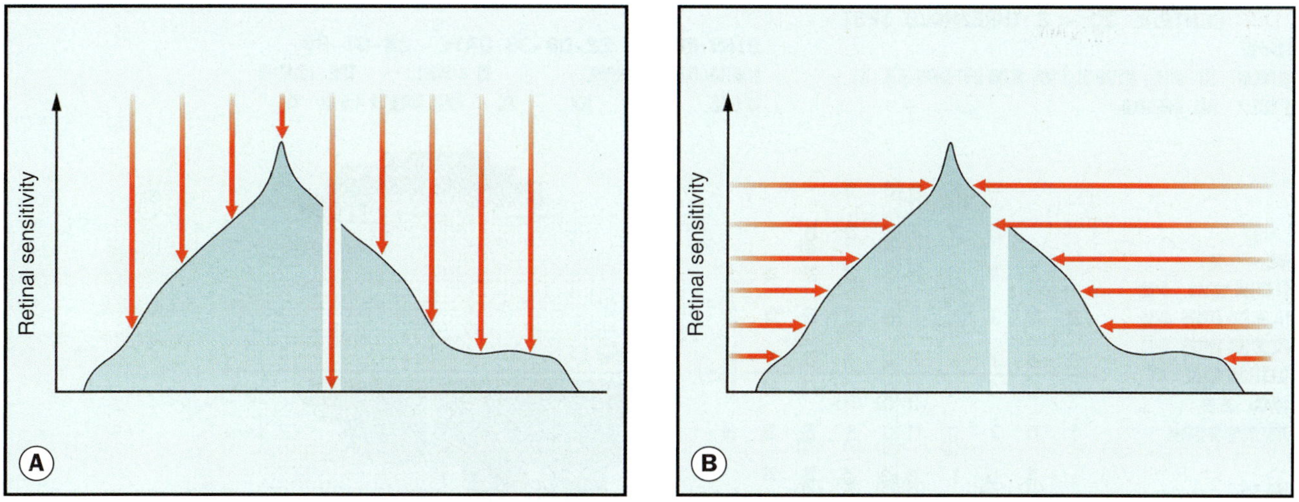

Fig. 1.16 Principles of perimetry. **(A)** Static – stimulus intensity (red arrow) at a single location is increased until perceived – areas of lower sensitivity perceive only stimuli of greater intensity (longer red arrows); **(B)** kinetic – stimulus of constant intensity is moved from a non-seeing area until perceived.

the Octopus, Medmont, Henson and Dicon (Figs 1.17 and 1.18). These predominantly utilize static testing, though software is available on some machines to perform dynamic assessment.

TIP Visual field results should always be used in conjunction with the clinical findings.

Testing algorithms

Threshold

Threshold perimetry is used for detailed assessment of the hill of vision by plotting the threshold luminance value at various locations in the visual field and comparing the results with age-matched 'normal' values. A typical automated strategy is to present a stimulus of higher than expected intensity. If seen, the intensity is decreased in steps (e.g. 4 dB) until it is no longer seen ('staircasing'). The stimulus is then increased again (e.g. 2 dB steps) until seen once more (Fig. 1.19). If the stimulus is not seen initially, its intensity is increased in steps until seen. Essentially, the threshold is crossed in one direction with large increments, then crossed again to 'fine-tune' the result with smaller increments. Threshold testing is commonly used for monitoring glaucoma.

Suprathreshold

Suprathreshold perimetry involves testing with stimuli of luminance above the expected normal threshold levels for an age-matched population to assess whether these are detected. In other words, testing to check that a subject can see stimuli that would be seen by a normal person of the same age. It enables testing to be carried out rapidly to indicate whether function is grossly normal or not and is usually reserved for screening.

Fast algorithms

In recent years, strategies have been introduced with shorter testing times, providing efficiency benefits with little or no detriment to testing accuracy. The HFA offers the SITA (Swedish Interactive Thresholding Algorithm), which uses a database of normal and glaucomatous fields to estimate threshold values and takes responses during the test into account to arrive at adjusted estimates throughout the test. Full-threshold values are obtained at the start of the test for four points. SITA-Standard and SITA-Fast (Fig. 1.20) versions are available. The Octopus Perimeter uses G-TOP (Glaucoma Tendency Oriented Perimetry), which estimates thresholds based on information gathered from more detailed assessment of adjacent points. TOP presents each stimulus once at each location, instead of 4–6 times per location with a standard technique.

Testing patterns

- **Glaucoma**
  - Most important defects in glaucoma occur centrally – within a 30° radius from the fixation point – so this is the area most commonly tested.
  - 24-2 is a routinely used glaucoma-orientated pattern. '24' denotes the extent in degrees to which the field is tested on the temporal side (to 30° on the nasal side). The number after the hyphen (2) describes the pattern of the points tested. 30-2 is an alternative.
  - 10-2 is used to assess a central area of radius 10°. Glaucomatous defects here may threaten central vision. The 10-2 pattern facilitates more detailed monitoring of the extent of damage, especially in advanced glaucoma where there is 'split' fixation.
- **Peripheral field.** Patterns that include central and peripheral points (e.g. FF-120) are typically limited to the assessment of neurological defects.

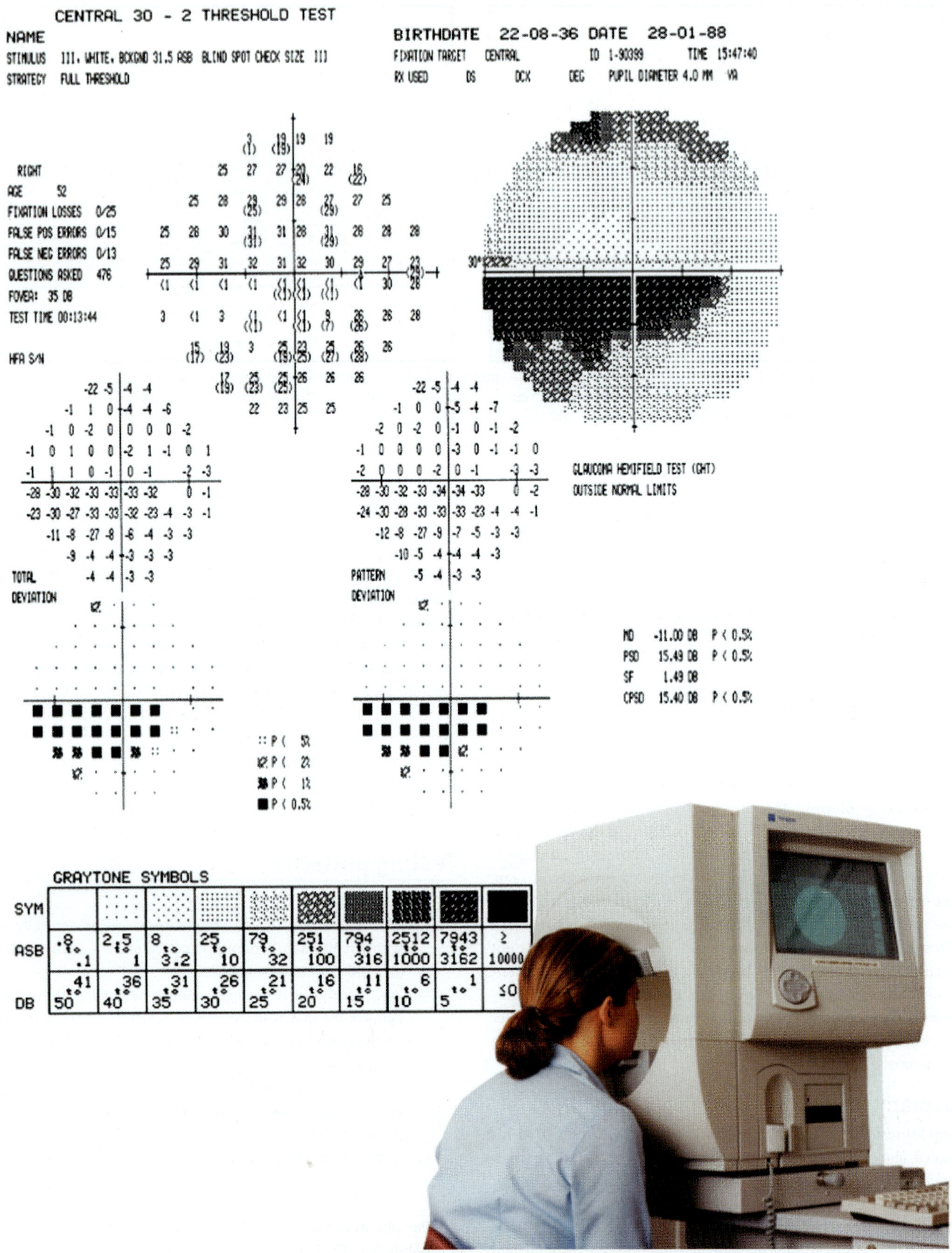

Fig. 1.17 Humphrey perimeter and printout.

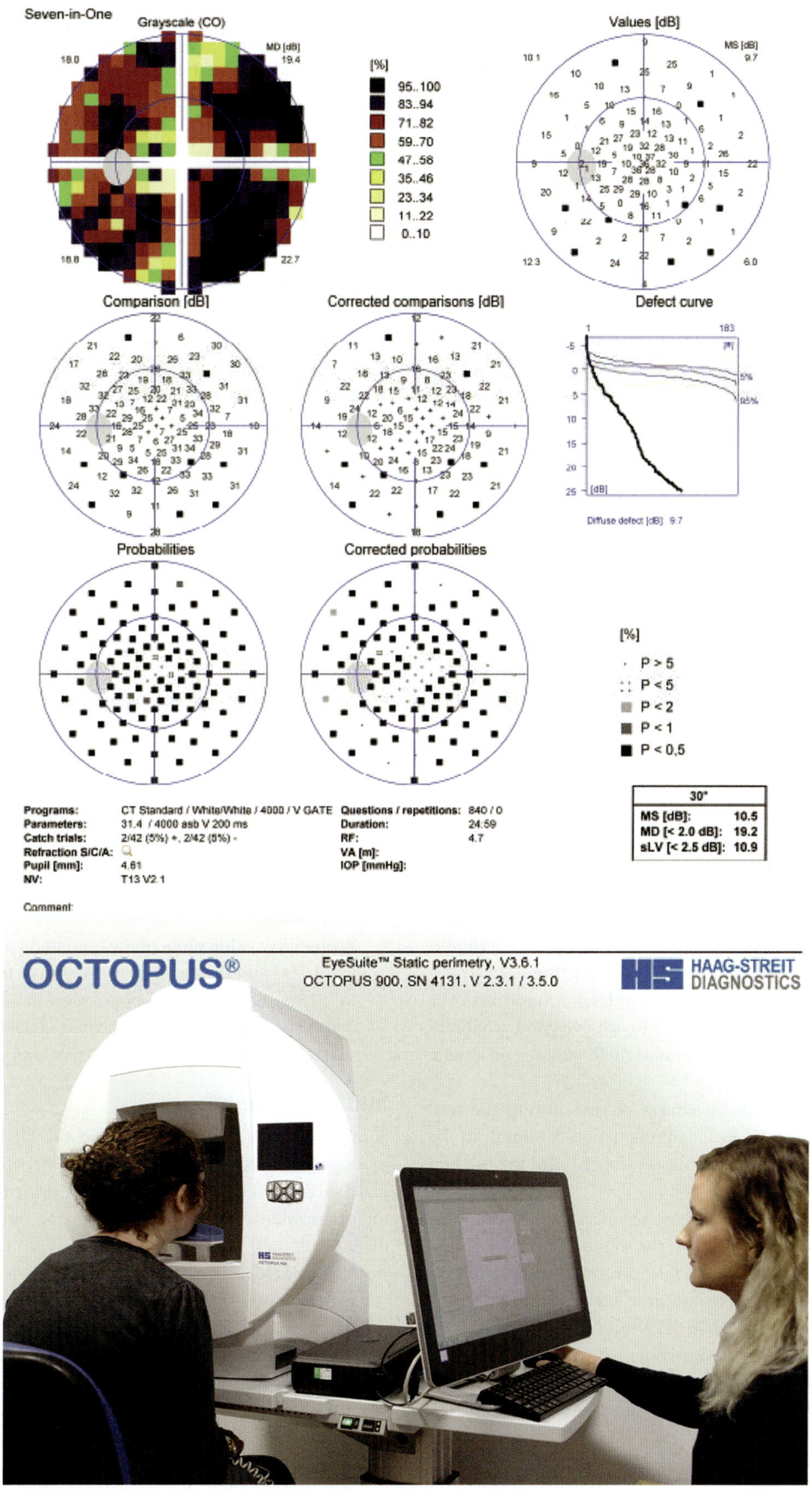

Fig. 1.18 Octopus perimeter and printout.

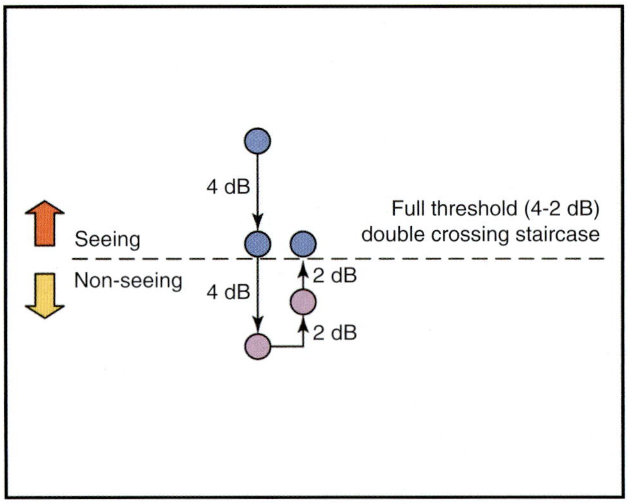

Fig. 1.19 Determination of threshold.

- **Binocular field testing** (e.g. Esterman strategy) is used to assess statutory driving entitlement in many jurisdictions.

Analysis

SAP provides the clinician with an array of clinically relevant information via monitor display or printout. The patient's name and age are confirmed and a check made that any appropriate refractive error compensation was used. General information should be reviewed, such as the type of algorithm performed, the time taken for the test and the order in which the eyes were tested.

Reliability indices

Reliability indices (see Fig. 1.20A) reflect the extent to which the patient's results are reliable. If significantly unreliable, further evaluation of the visual field printout is pointless. With SITA strategies, false negatives or false positives over about 15% should probably be regarded as significant and with full-threshold strategies, fixation losses over 20% and false positives or negatives over 33%. In patients who consistently fail to achieve good reliability it may be useful to switch to a suprathreshold strategy or kinetic perimetry.

- **Fixation losses** indicate steadiness of gaze during the test. Methods of assessment include presentation of stimuli to the blind spot to ensure no response is recorded, and the use of a 'gaze monitor'.
- **False positives** are usually assessed by decoupling a stimulus from its accompanying sound. If the sound alone is presented and the patient still responds, a false positive is recorded. With a high false-positive score the grey scale printout appears abnormally pale (Fig. 1.21). In SITA testing, false positives are estimated based on the response time.
- **False negatives** are registered by presenting a stimulus much brighter than threshold at a location where the threshold has already been determined. If the patient fails to respond, a false negative is recorded. A high false-negative score indicates inattention, tiredness or malingering, but is occasionally an indication of disease severity rather than unreliability. The grey scale printout in individuals with high false-negative responses tends to have a clover leaf shape (Fig. 1.22).

TIP If the reliability indices are poor, be careful when interpreting the results of a visual field test.

Sensitivity values

- **A numerical display** (see Fig. 1.20B) gives the measured or estimated (depending on strategy) threshold in dB at each point. In a full-threshold strategy, where the threshold is rechecked either as routine or because of an unexpected (>5 dB) result, the second result is shown in brackets next to the first.
- **A grey scale** represents the numerical display in graphical form (see Fig. 1.20C) and is the simplest display modality to interpret: decreasing sensitivity is represented by darker tones – the physiological blind spot is a darker area in the temporal field typically just below the horizontal axis. Each change in grey scale tone is equivalent to a 5 dB change in sensitivity at that location.
- **Total deviation** (see Fig. 1.20D) shows the difference between a test-derived threshold at a given point and the normal sensitivity at that point for the general population, correcting for age. Negative values indicate lower than normal sensitivity, positive values higher than normal.
- **Pattern deviation** (see Fig. 1.20E) is derived from total deviation values adjusted for any generalized decrease in sensitivity in the overall field (e.g. lens opacity), and demonstrates localized defects.
- **Probability value plots** of the total and pattern deviation (see Fig. 1.20G and H) are a representation of the percentage (<5% to <0.5%) of the normal population in whom the measured defect at each point would be expected. Darker symbols represent a greater likelihood that a defect is significant.

Summary values

Summary values ('global indices' on the HFA – see Fig. 1.20F) represent distilled statistical information, which considers age-matched normal data. These values are principally used to monitor progression of glaucomatous damage rather than for initial diagnosis.

- **Visual field index (VFI)** in the HFA is a measure of the patient's overall visual field function expressed as a percentage, the normal age-adjusted value being 100%.
- **Mean deviation (MD)** on the HFA (**mean defect** on the Octopus) gives an indication of the overall sensitivity of the field. It is derived from averaging the total deviation values.

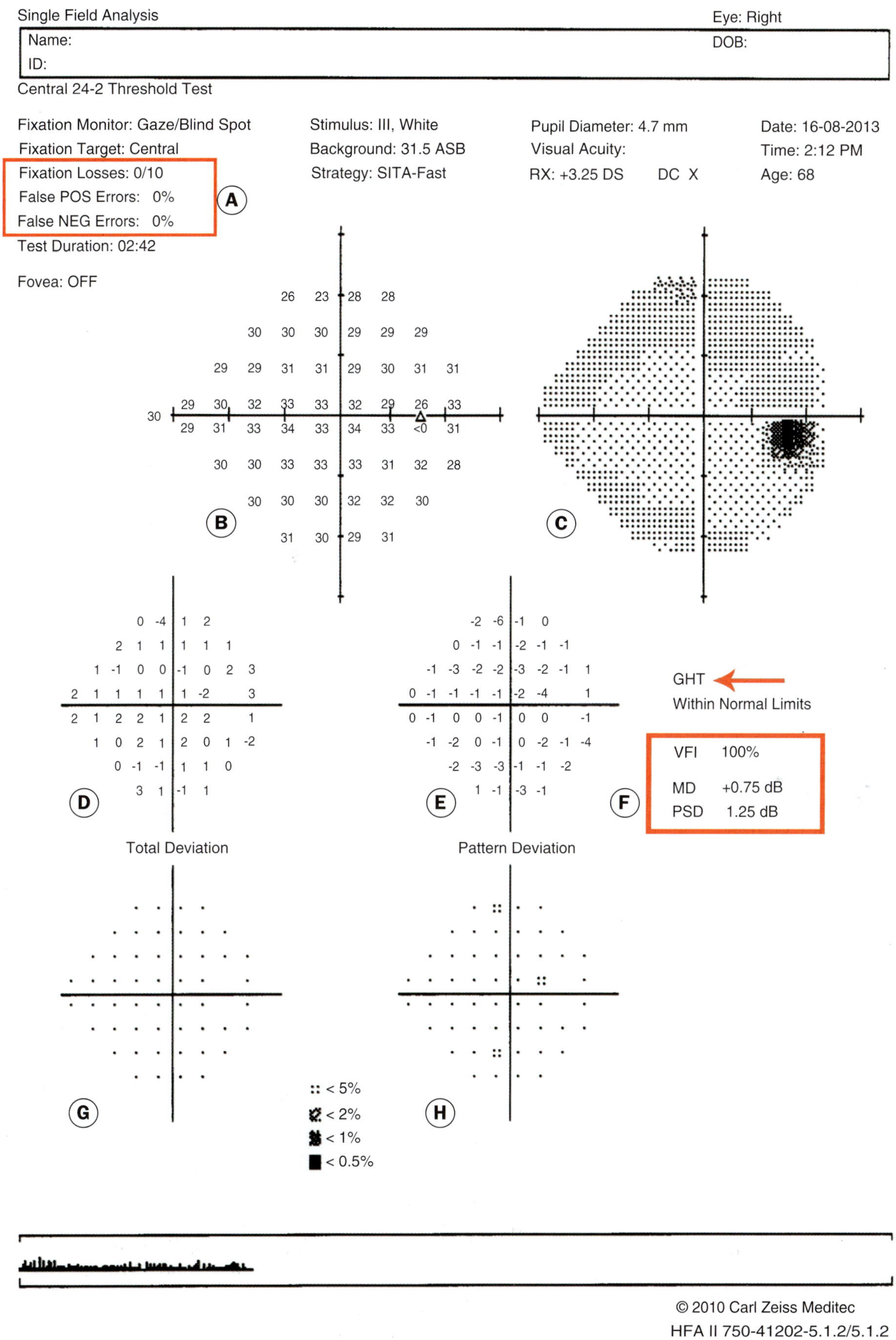

Fig. 1.20 Humphrey perimeter – SITA-Fast printout (see text).

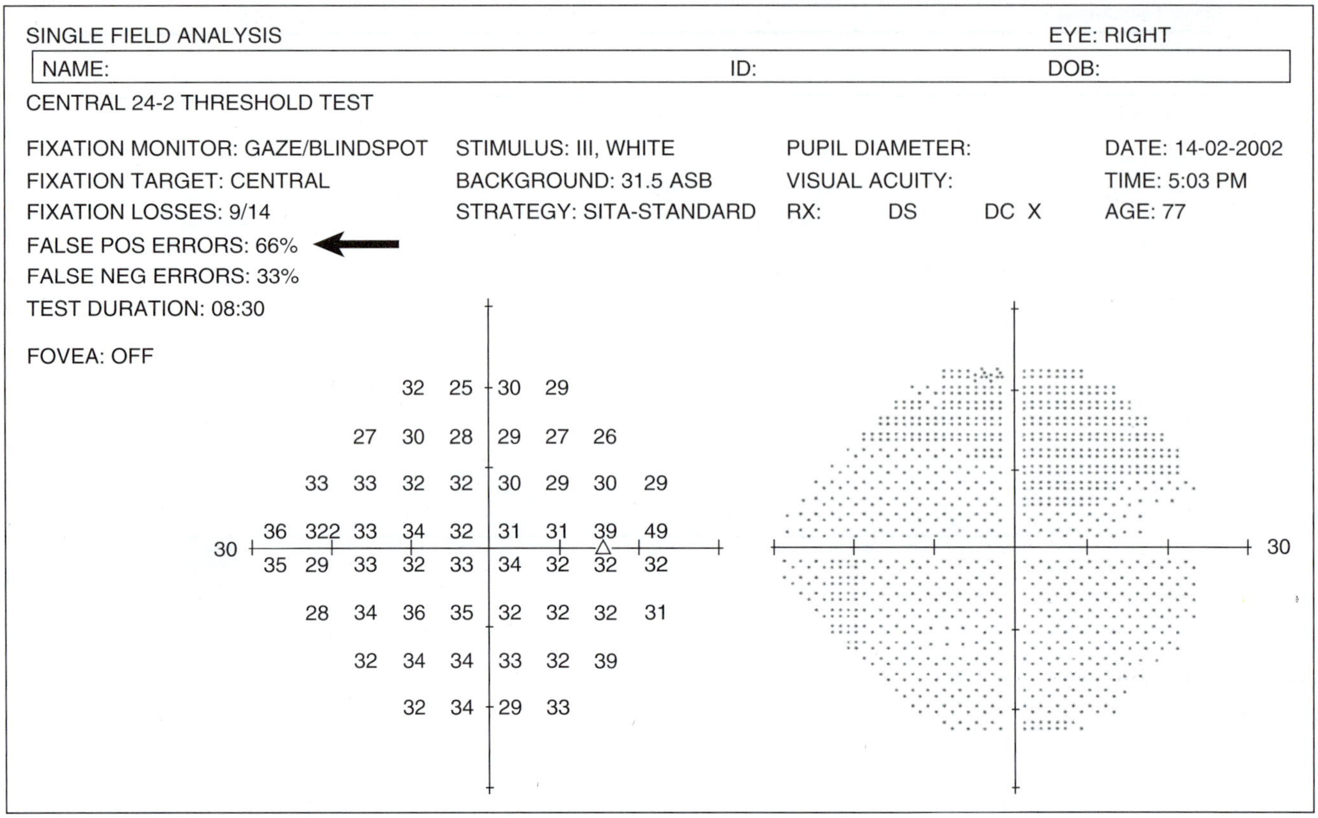

Fig. 1.21 High false-positive score (arrow) with an abnormally pale grey scale display.

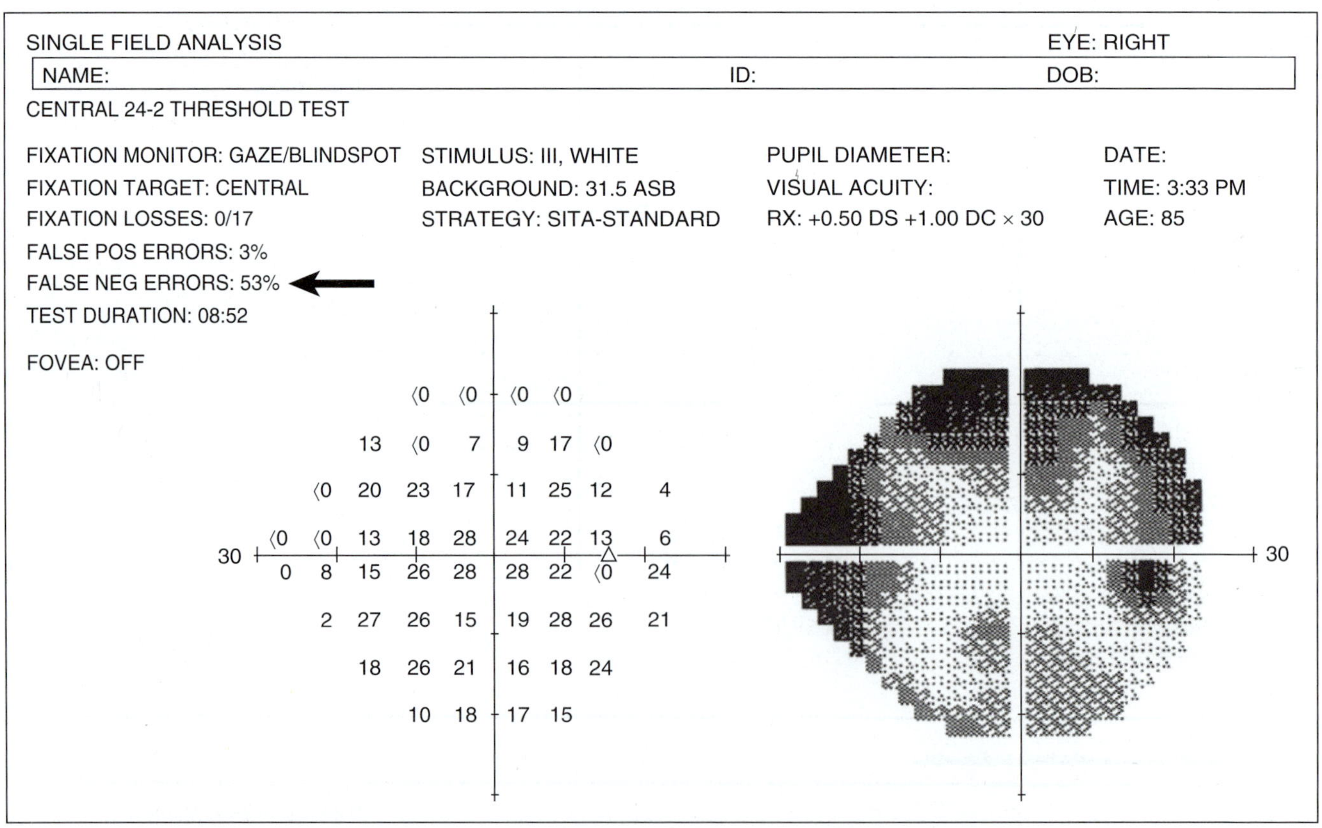

Fig. 1.22 High false-negative score (arrow) with a clover leaf-shaped grey scale display.

- **Pattern standard deviation (PSD)** is a measure of focal loss or variability within the field and considers any generalized depression in the hill of vision. An increased PSD is therefore a more specific indicator of glaucomatous damage than MD.
- **Loss variance (LV)** is a summary measure on the Octopus Perimeter similar to PSD.
- **Probability values.** Abnormal summary values are followed by a probability value, representing the percentage likelihood that an abnormal value of this level will occur in a normal subject. The lower the *P* value, the more likely the result is abnormal.
- The **glaucoma hemifield test (GHT)** compares corresponding areas in the superior and inferior hemifields and relates only to glaucoma.

Computed analysis of serial fields

Computed analysis of serial visual fields for progression is in widespread use. A disadvantage is the requirement for several reliable fields to be carried out before analysis is effective. The quality of available software has been improving steadily, with integrated programs such as GPA (Guided Progression Analysis) on the HFA and several trend analysis options on the Octopus.

High-sensitivity field modalities

SAP tends to detect field damage only after substantial ganglion cell loss is established. Attempts at detecting change at an earlier stage include the adoption of stimuli intended to target specific ganglion cell types.

- **Short-wave automated perimetry (SWAP)** uses a blue stimulus on a yellow background. Sensitivity to blue light (mediated by blue cone photoreceptors) is adversely affected relatively early in glaucoma. SWAP is more sensitive to early glaucomatous defects but has not been widely adopted because cataract decreases sensitivity to blue light (the brunescent lens acts as a yellow filter) and patients frequently dislike the lengthy test. It is available on newer HFA models.
- **Frequency-doubling test (FDT).** Large diameter axon (magnocellular) ganglion cells appear to be preferentially lost in early glaucoma. The frequency-doubling illusion is produced when a low spatial frequency sinusoidal grating undergoes high temporal frequency counter phase flicker (>15 Hz). The rapid alternation in which the light bars become dark and vice versa produces the illusion of the grating having doubled its frequency; magnocellular ganglion cells are believed to mediate the pathways used. Screening (Fig. 1.23) and extended testing (Humphrey Matrix) perimeter versions are available, the latter being suitable for detailed assessment and monitoring of glaucoma.

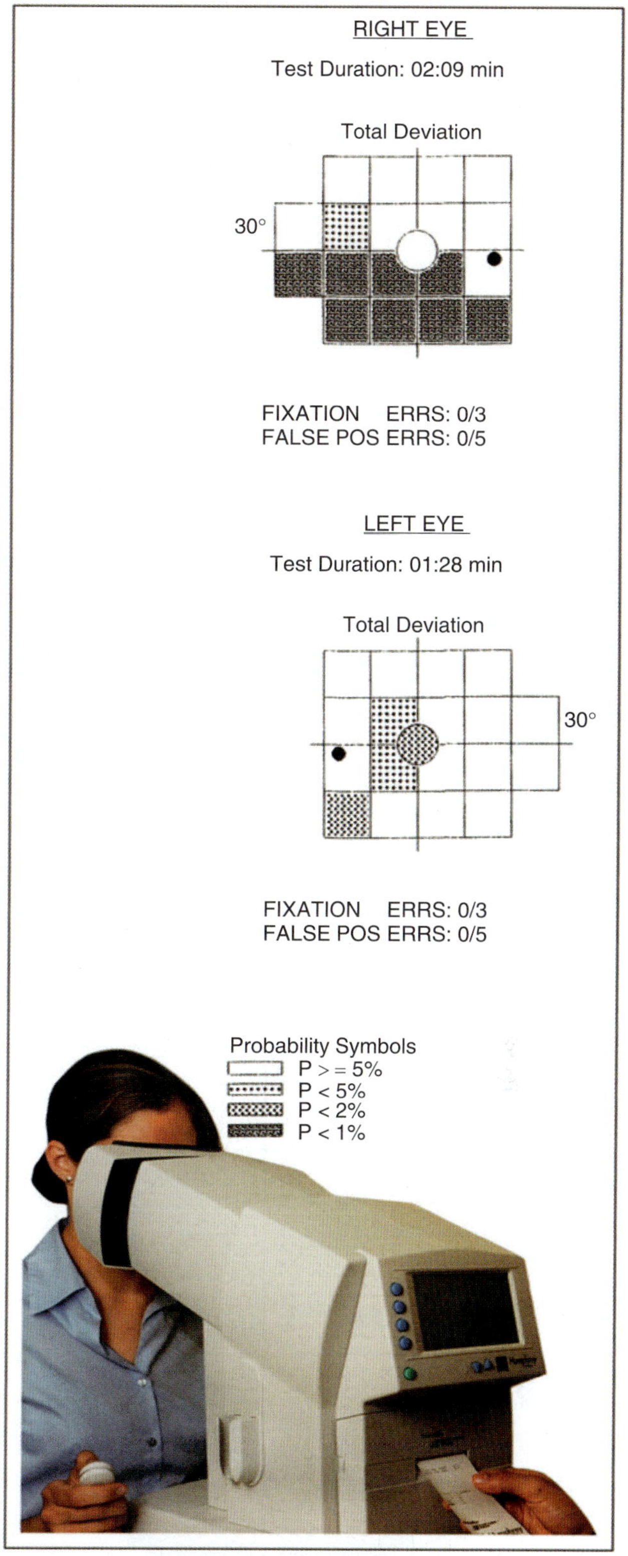

Fig. 1.23 Screening frequency-doubling perimeter with display.

Sources of error

- **Inexperienced or unskilled technician.** Though less important with SAP than manual perimetry, correctly setting up the test, explaining the procedure to and reassuring the patient and monitoring performance are fundamental to obtaining an accurate field.
- **Incorrect patient details.** The patient's date of birth must be entered correctly to facilitate appropriate normative database matching.
- **Poor patient performance.**
- **Uncorrected refractive error** can cause a significant decrease in central sensitivity. If a patient with hypermetropia who usually wears contact lenses is tested wearing spectacles, this will have the effect of magnifying and enlarging any scotomas as compared with contact lenses. Most perimetry is performed with a stimulus at approximately reading distance, so a near correction should be used for individuals who are presbyopic.
- **Spectacle rim artefact.** Spectacles can cause rim scotomas if small aperture lenses are used or if incorrectly dispensed (Fig. 1.24A). Narrow-aperture trial frame lenses are unsuitable for perimetry.
- **Miosis decreases sensitivity** in the peripheral field and increases variability in the central field in both normal and glaucomatous eyes. Pupils less than 3 mm in diameter should therefore be dilated prior to perimetry; a consistent mydriatic should be used for serial tests.
- **Media opacities** (usually cataract) can have a profound effect, exaggerated by miosis.
- **Ptosis**, even if mild, can suppress the superior visual field (Fig. 1.24B). Similar effects result from dermatochalasis, prominent eyelashes and deeply set eyes.
- **Inadequate retinal adaptation** may lead to error if perimetry is performed soon after ophthalmoscopy.

TIP Perimetry is a subjective examination and is not always reliable.

Microperimetry

- Microperimetry is a visual field test that measures retinal sensitivity and fixation behaviour in patients with macular disease and focal glaucoma involving the central visual field. It allows an exact correlation between pathology involving the macula and the corresponding functional abnormality. Microperimetry is more sensitive than SAP in detecting subtle abnormality of visual function.
- The MAIA perimeter is a table-top instrument (Fig. 1.25). The test is usually undertaken after 20 minutes of adaptation in mesopic conditions. Fundus tracking occurs utilizing a line-scanning laser ophthalmoscope (SLO), with super-luminescent diode illumination using a central wavelength of 850 nm.
- Goldmann size 3 stimuli are projected onto the central 9° of the fundus. A 4-2 staircase thresholding technique is used, with each stimulus applied for 200 milliseconds against a white background. Using this instrument normal retinal sensitivity is 18 dB.
- Results are printed, together with reliability indices (fixation loss), probabilities and retinal sensitivity values, which are colour-coded. Microperimetry is particularly useful in assessing the effect of existing and future therapeutic interventions on the macula (Fig. 1.26). It can also be helpful in patients with early glaucoma, particularly when there is subtle change close to fixation.

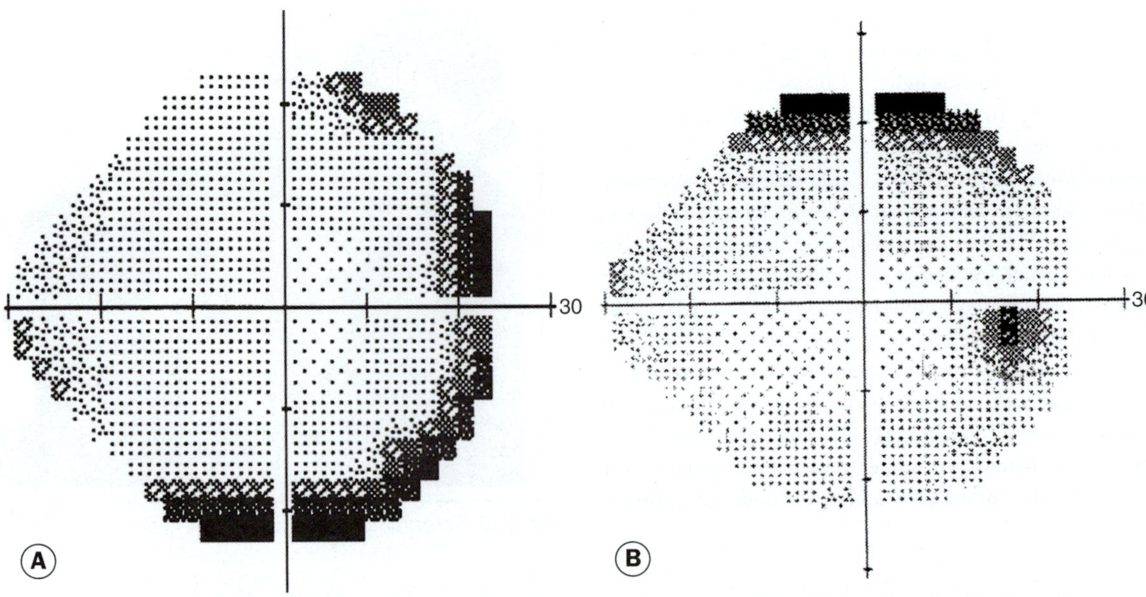

Fig. 1.24 Artefact. **(A)** Grey scale display of spectacle rim artefact; **(B)** grey scale display of upper lid artefact.

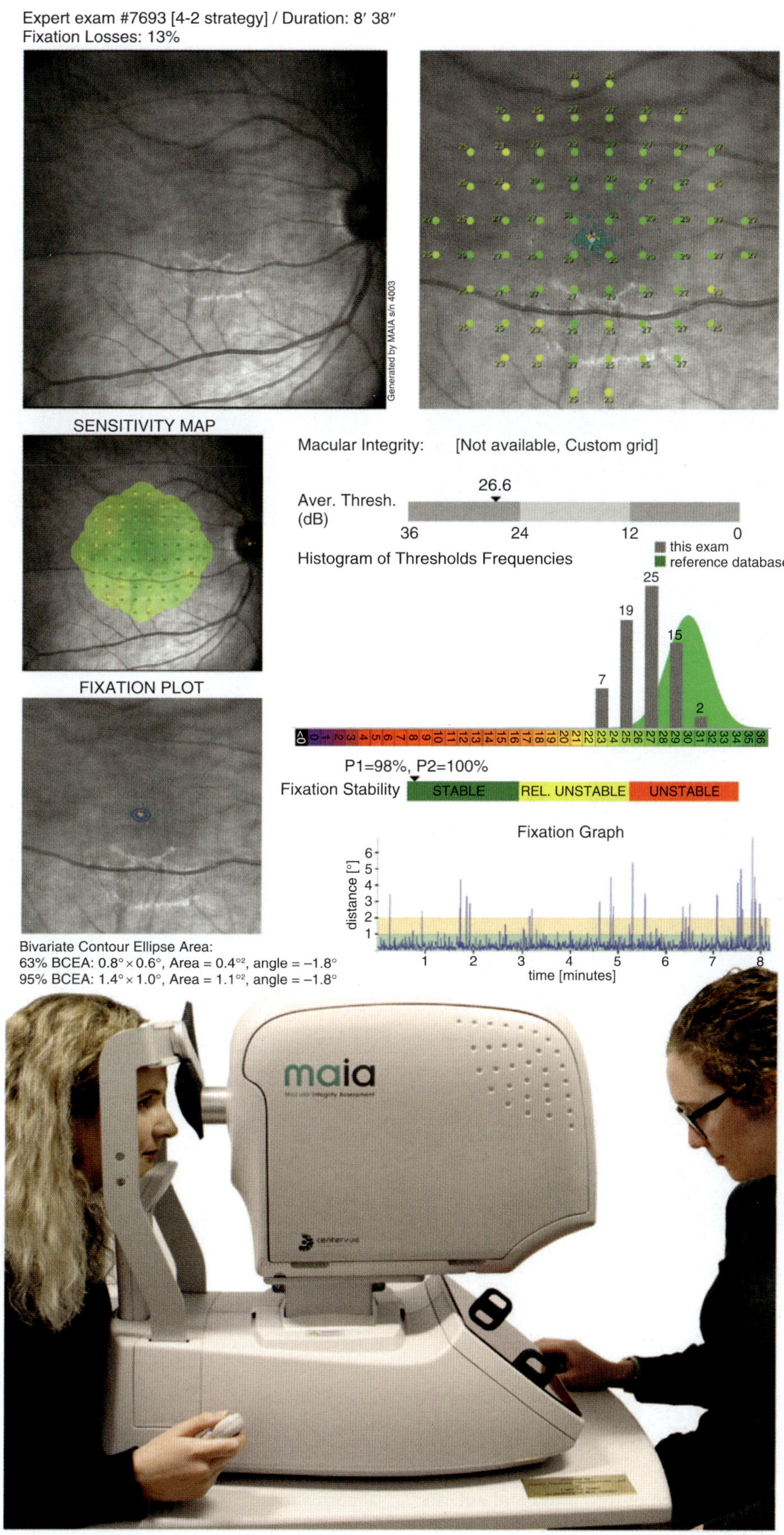

Fig. 1.25 MAIA perimetry and printout.

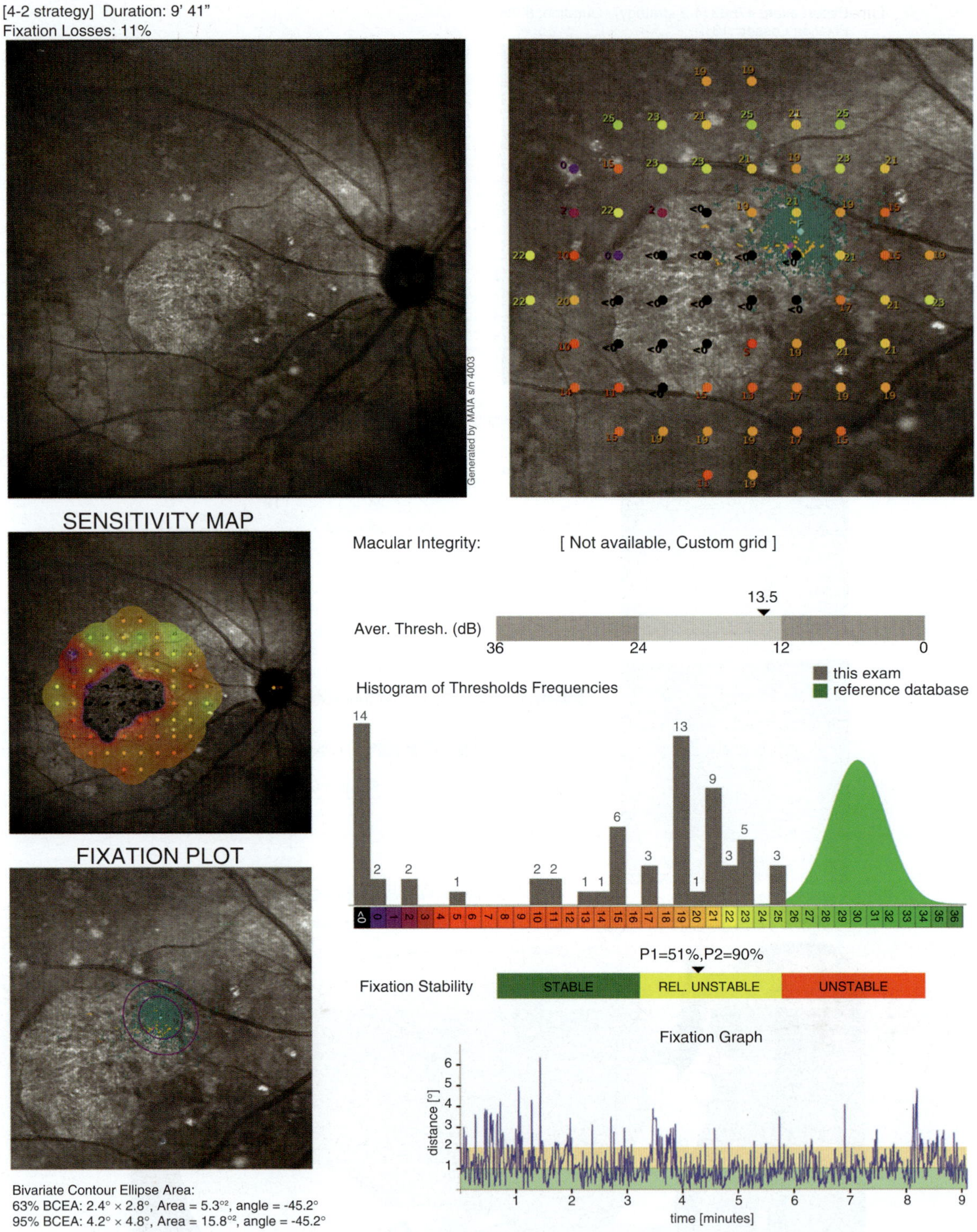

Fig. 1.26 Abnormal microperimetry in a patient with geographic atrophy of the macula.

SLIT LAMP BIOMICROSCOPY OF THE ANTERIOR SEGMENT

The purpose of slit lamp examination of the cornea and anterior segment is to determine the position, depth and size of any abnormality (Fig. 1.27).

Direct illumination

Direct illumination with a diffuse light is used to detect gross abnormalities:

- A narrow obliquely directed slit beam is used to visualize a cross-section of the cornea.

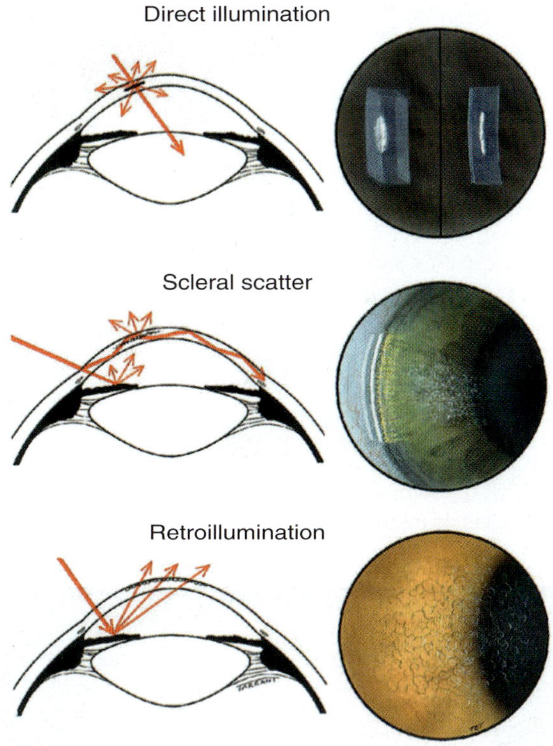

Fig. 1.27 Technique of slit lamp biomicroscopy of the anterior segment.

- Further narrowing of the beam to a very thin optical section moved across the cornea can determine the depth of a lesion.
- The height of the coaxial beam can be adjusted to measure the horizontal and vertical size of a lesion or associated epithelial defect.
- The use of a red-free filter makes red objects appear black, thereby increasing contrast when observing vascular structures. A cobalt blue filter is normally used in conjunction with fluorescein.

Scleral scatter

Scleral scatter involves decentering the slit beam laterally so that the light is incident on the limbus with the microscope focused centrally. Light is transmitted within the cornea by total internal reflection. A corneal stromal lesion will become illuminated because of forward light scatter. This technique is especially useful to detect subtle stromal haze, or cellular or lipid infiltration.

Retroillumination

Retroillumination uses reflected light from the iris or fundus after pupil dilatation to illuminate the cornea. This allows the detection of fine epithelial and endothelial changes, such as epithelial cysts, keratic precipitates and small blood vessels.

Specular reflection

Specular reflection shows abnormalities of the endothelium such as reduced cell density and guttata. Pseudoguttata probably represent reversible endothelial cell oedema and inflammatory cells beneath the endothelial layer.

Portable slit lamp

A hand-held slit lamp allows high-quality examination of the anterior segment in individuals who cannot be examined at a regular slit lamp and is particularly useful when performing eye examinations out of a hospital setting (Fig. 1.28).

FUNDUS EXAMINATION

Direct ophthalmoscopy

- A hand-held slit lamp direct examination of the structures of the fundus using an ophthalmoscope can reveal disease of the eye itself or may reveal an abnormality indicative of disease elsewhere in the body (for example: diabetes, systematic hypertension, raised intracranial pressure). The major advantage of direct ophthalmoscopy is that it can be used at the bedside. The image obtained is significantly magnified (15 times normal) (Fig. 1.29).
- The direct ophthalmoscope can be used to examine the 'red' reflex using retroillumination. By placing a +15 D lens in position and looking at the fundus at a distance of 15–20 cm, lens and vitreous opacities can be detected (Fig. 1.30).
- The light beam can be used to (a) illuminate the cornea, allowing detection of a foreign body, (b) check the pupil for irregularity and (c) determine the light reflexes. Some ophthalmoscopes incorporate a cobalt blue filter, which allows corneal abrasions and ulcers to be seen after the insertion of fluorescein.

TIP A direct ophthalmoscope can be used at the bedside and provides a magnified view of the fundus, but there is no stereopsis and the field of view is small.

Technique

- It is preferable to dilate the pupil if there is no contraindication. However, a good view can be obtained through an undilated pupil by darkening the examination room and by asking the patient to look into the distance.
- When examining the right eye, the clinician should stand at the patient's right side, holding the ophthalmoscope in the right hand. When examining the left eye, the clinician should stand at the left side, holding the ophthalmoscope in the left hand and using the left eye (Fig. 1.31).
- The 'O' on the illuminated lens dial of the ophthalmoscope should be selected.
- To overcome corneal reflection, the small aperture can be used and the light beam directed towards the edge of the pupil, rather than through the centre. The linear polarizing filter may be helpful.
- The examiner's free hand should rest on the patient's forehead.
- The patient is slowly approached at a slight angle, from the temporal side.
- The light beam is directed at the pupil and the optic disc should come into view at a distance of about 3.5 cm from the eye. If the disc is not in sharp focus, the ophthalmoscope lenses should be rotated into the aperture using the index finger until the disc becomes clearly visible.

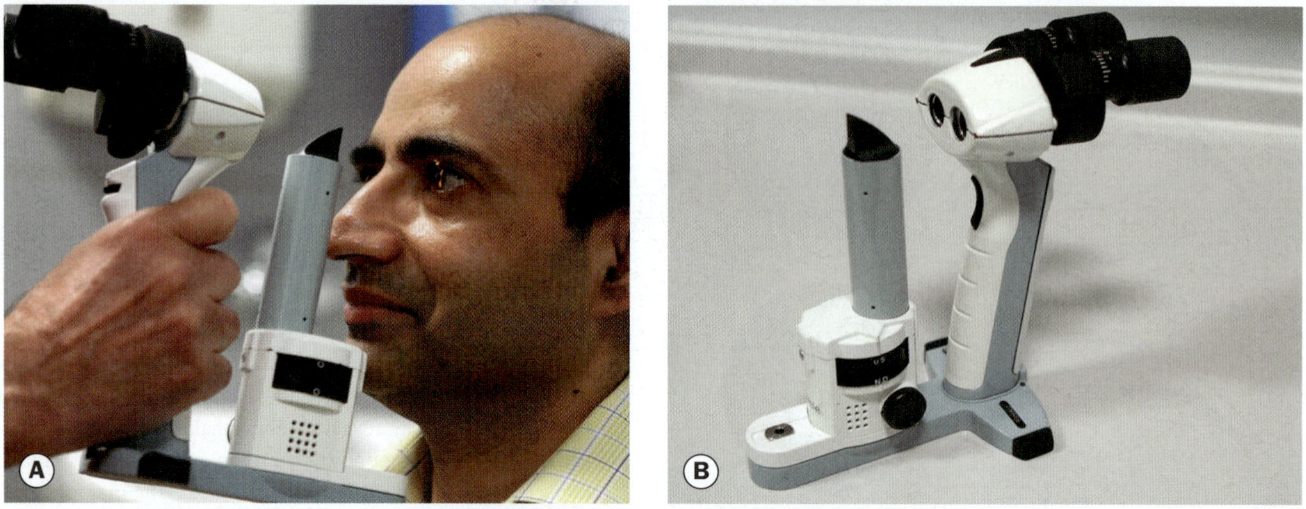

Fig. 1.28 Portable slit lamp. **(A)** Technique; **(B)** Keeler PSL Classic instrument.

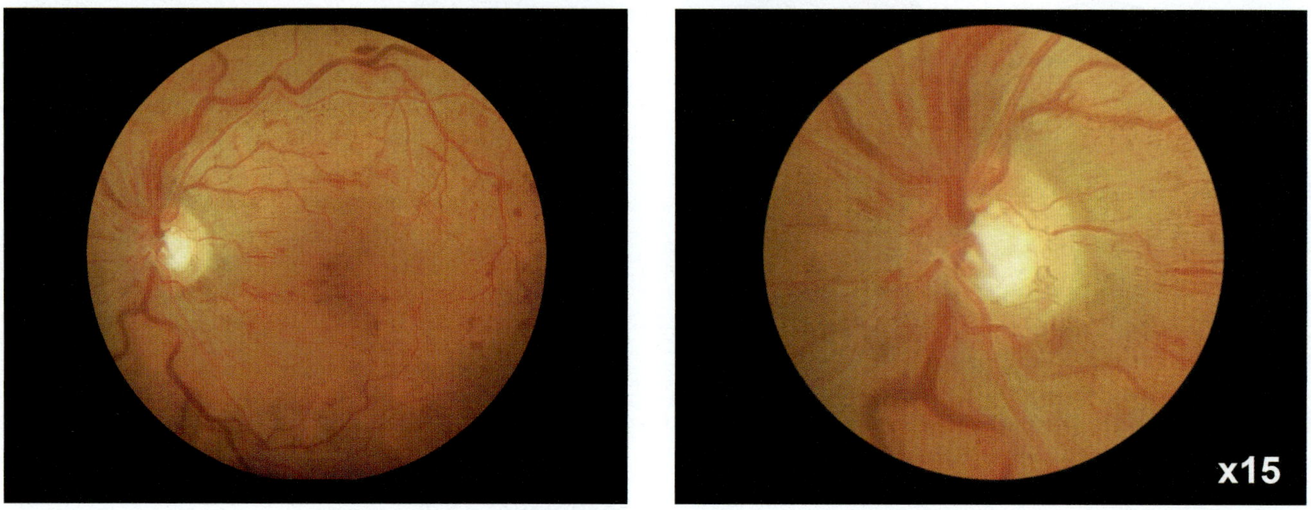

Fig. 1.29 Magnified image obtained from direct ophthalmoscope.

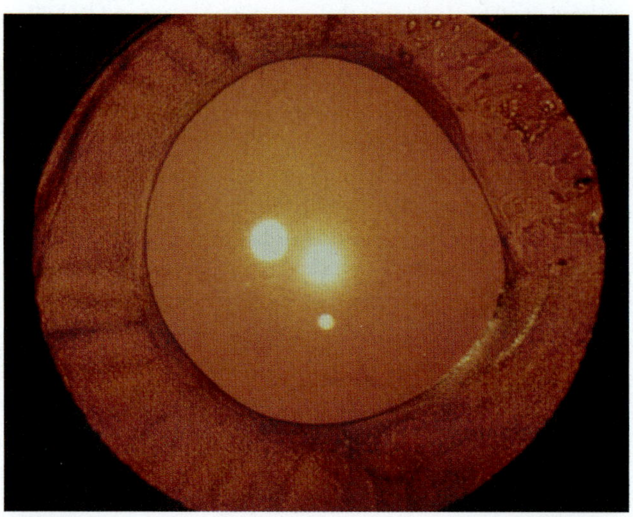

Fig. 1.30 Red reflex showing anterior capsular thickening.

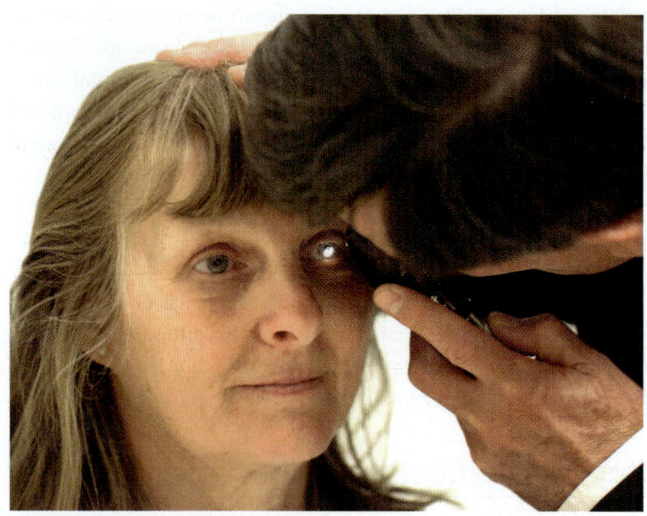

Fig. 1.31 Technique of direct ophthalmoscopy (see text).

- In hyperopic individuals use a plus lens (green) and in myopic individuals a minus lens (red).
- Examine the disc for clarity of outline, colour, elevation and condition of vessels. Check for spontaneous venous pulsation. Follow the vessels as far as possible into the retinal periphery.
- To locate the macula, focus the light on the disc then move the light about 2 disc diameters temporally. Alternatively, ask the patient to look at the light.
- The retinal periphery can be examined by asking the patient to look up/down and to the sides.

Slit lamp biomicroscopy

A range of diagnostic contact and non-contact lenses are available for use with the slit lamp. Contact lenses should not be used if a penetrating injury is suspected or in the presence of corneal trauma, hyphaema or corneal infection.

- **Non-contact lenses**
  - 60 D. High-magnification lens optimized for viewing the posterior pole from a working distance of 13 mm. When estimating optic disc diameter use a correction factor of ×0.88–1.0 for the Volk lens and ×1.0 for the Nikon lens.
  - 90 D. Wide-field lens with lower magnification and shorter (7 mm) working distance. Can be used with smaller pupils. The correction factor is ×1.3 (Fig. 1.32).
  - 78 D. Intermediate properties; ideal for general-purpose examination. The correction factor is ×1.1.
  - Miscellaneous. Numerous other lenses are available, offering qualities such as a very wide field of view and extremely small pupil capability.

Technique

Indirect ophthalmoscopy utilizes a high-power convex lens which is designed to obtain a wide field of view of the fundus. The image is vertically inverted and laterally reversed. The technique is as follows:

- The slit beam is adjusted to a width of about one-quarter of its full round diameter.
- The illumination is set at an angle coaxial with the slit lamp viewing system.
- The magnification and light intensity are adjusted to the lowest settings.
- The light beam should be centred to pass directly through the patient's pupil.
- The lens is held directly in front of the cornea just clearing the lashes so that the light beam passes through its centre.
- The fundus is examined by moving the joystick and vertical adjustment mechanism of the slit lamp whilst keeping the lens still.
- Magnification is increased to show greater detail.
- To view the peripheral retina the patient should be instructed to direct their gaze accordingly.

Using new technology for retinal imaging in rural settings

In areas of the world with few specialist eye-care practitioners, primary health-care workers can take retinal photographs with a smartphone, using a clip-on device (Fig. 1.33). This can then be sent electronically to a specialist centre for an opinion on the further management.

- The Vula Mobile App, which has been fully evaluated in rural settings in Africa, is a successful example of this technology.

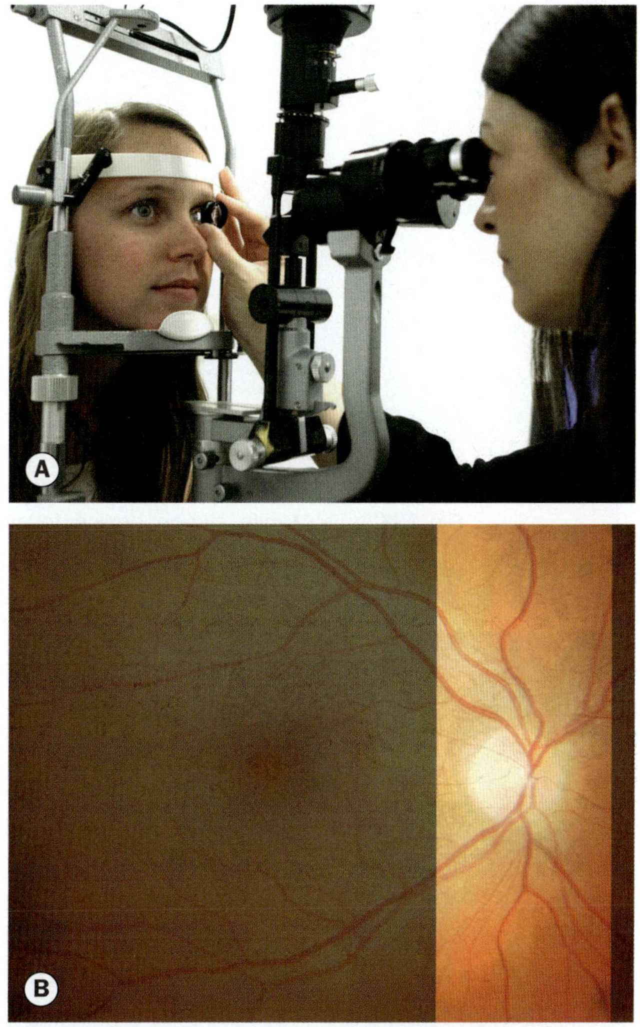

Fig. 1.32 **(A)** Indirect slit lamp biomicroscopy; **(B)** fundus view.

Goldmann three-mirror examination

- **Goldmann three-mirror lens** consists of four parts: the central lens and three mirrors set at different angles. Because the curvature of the contact surface of the lens is steeper than that of the cornea, a viscous coupling substance with the same refractive index as the cornea is required to bridge the gap between the cornea and the goniolens. It is important to be familiar with each part of the lens, as follows (Fig. 1.34A):
  - The central part provides a 30° upright view of the posterior pole.
  - The equatorial mirror (largest and oblong-shaped) enables visualization from 30° to the equator.
  - The peripheral mirror (intermediate in size and square-shaped) enables visualization between the equator and the ora serrata.

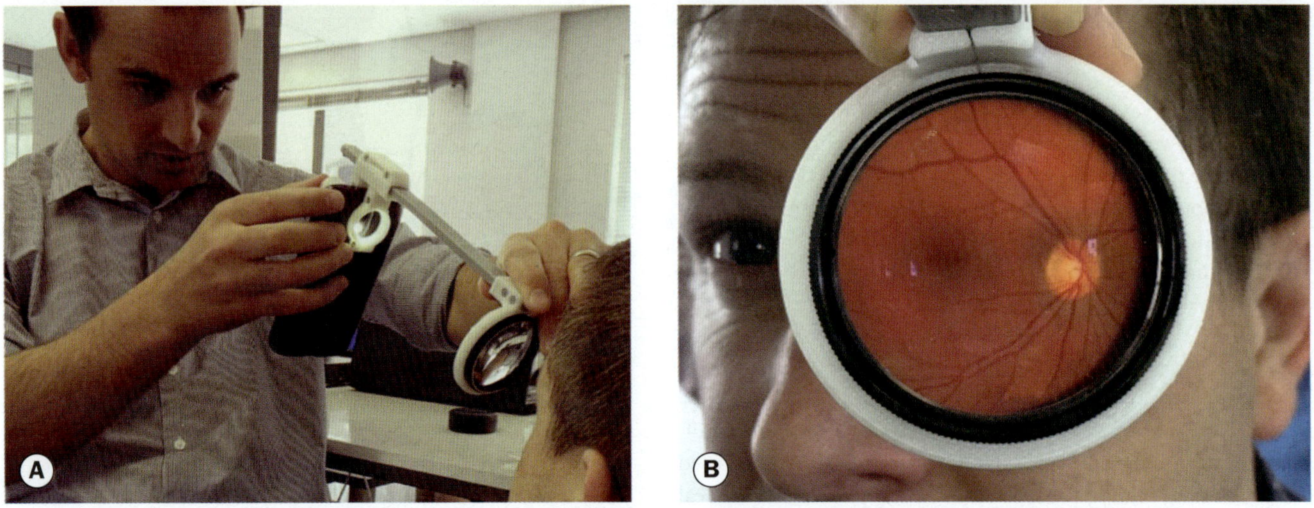

Fig. 1.33 Vula Mobile clip-on device to allow smartphone images of the posterior pole to be taken in a rural setting. **(A)** Technique of use; **(B)** inverted retinal image. *(Courtesy of W Mapham.)*

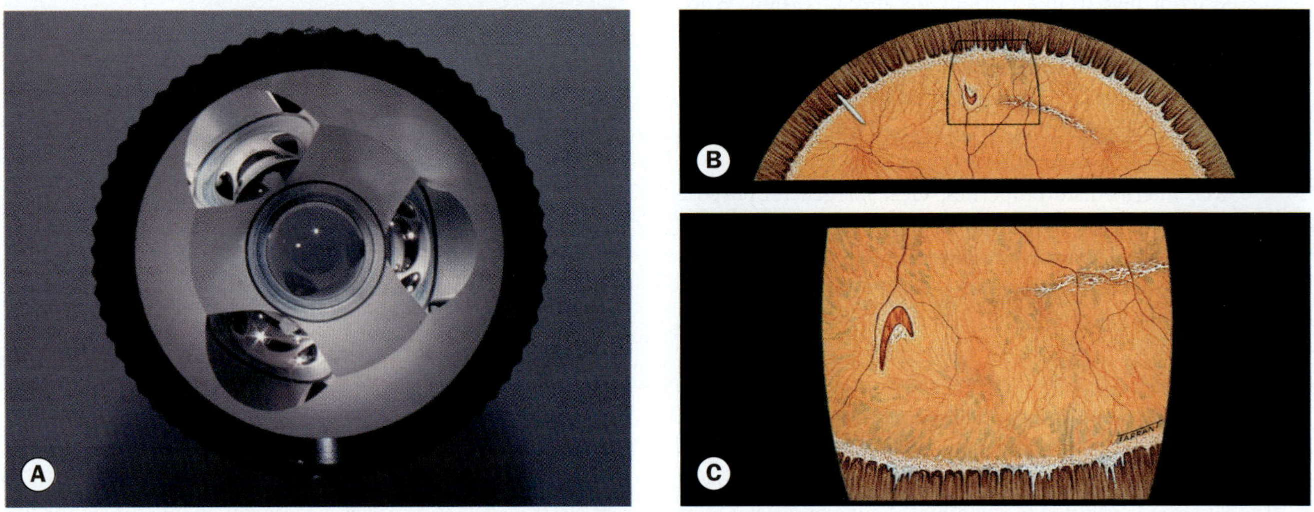

Fig. 1.34 **(A)** Goldmann three-mirror lens; **(B)** U-tear left of 12 o'clock and an area of lattice degeneration right of 12 o'clock; **(C)** the same lesions seen with the three-mirror lens positioned at 6 o'clock.

  - The gonioscopy mirror (smallest and dome-shaped) may be used for visualizing the extreme retinal periphery and pars plana.
  - It is therefore apparent that the smaller the mirror, the more peripheral the view obtained.
- **Mirror positioning**
  - The mirror should be positioned opposite the area of the fundus to be examined. To examine the 12 o'clock position the mirror should be positioned at 6 o'clock.
  - When viewing the vertical meridian, the image is upside down but not laterally reversed, in contrast to indirect ophthalmoscopy. Lesions located to the left of 12 o'clock in the retina will therefore also appear in the mirror on the left-hand side (Fig. 1.34 B and C).
  - When viewing the horizontal meridian, the image is laterally reversed.
- **Technique**
  - The pupils are dilated.
  - The locking screw of the slit lamp is unlocked (Fig. 1.35A) to allow the illumination column to be tilted (Fig. 1.35B).
  - Anaesthetic drops are instilled.
  - Coupling fluid (high viscosity methylcellulose or equivalent) is inserted into the cup of the contact lens; it should be no more than half full.
  - The patient is asked to look up. The inferior rim of the lens is inserted into the lower fornix (Fig. 1.36A) and quickly pressed against the cornea so that the coupling fluid is retained (Fig. 1.36B).
  - The illumination column should always be tilted except when viewing the 12 o'clock position in the fundus (i.e. with the mirror at 6 o'clock).

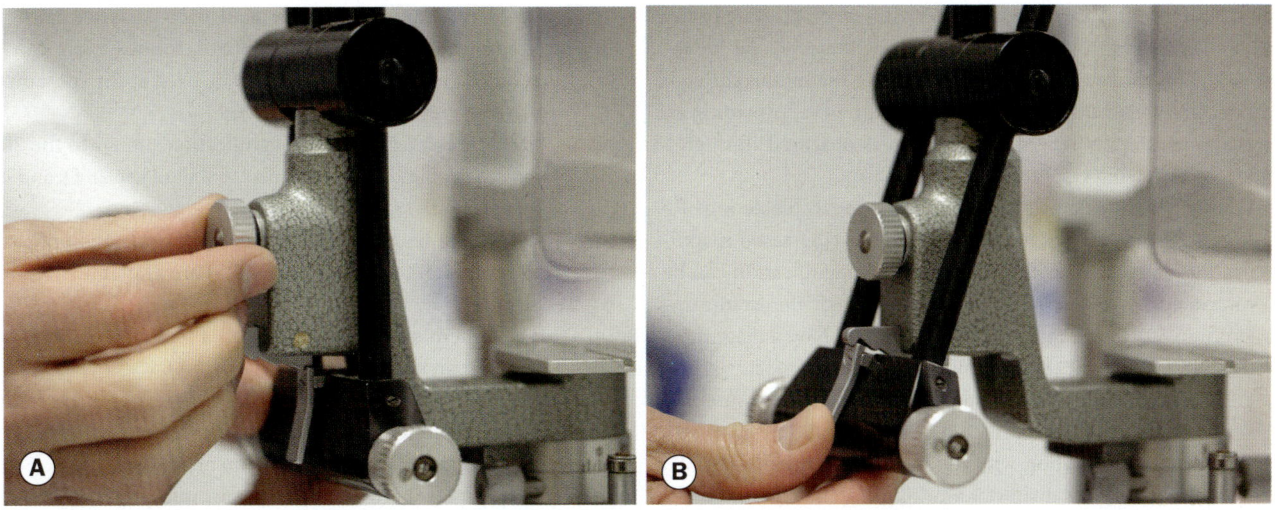

Fig. 1.35 Preparation of the slit lamp for fundus examination. **(A)** Unlocking the screw; **(B)** tilting the illumination column.

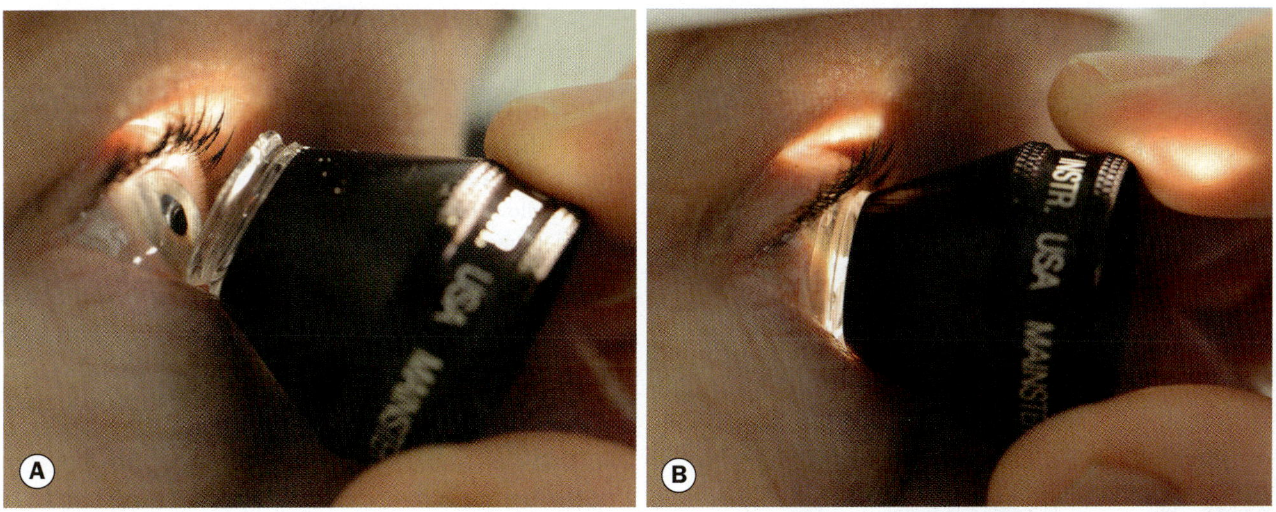

Fig. 1.36 Insertion of contact lens. **(A)** Inserted into the lower fornix with the patient looking up; **(B)** in position for examination of posterior pole.

- When viewing horizontal meridians (i.e. 3 and 9 o'clock positions in the fundus) the column should remain central.
- When viewing the vertical meridians (i.e. 6 and 12 o'clock positions) the column can be positioned left or right of centre.
- When viewing oblique meridians (i.e. 1.30 and 7.30 o'clock) the column is kept right of centre, and vice versa when viewing the 10.30 and 4.30 o'clock positions (Fig. 1.37).
- When viewing different positions of the peripheral retina, the axis of the beam is rotated so that it is always at right-angles to the mirror.
- To visualize the entire fundus the lens is rotated for 360° using first the equatorial mirror and then the peripheral mirrors.
- To obtain a more peripheral view of the retina the lens is tilted to the opposite side asking the patient to move the eyes to the same side. For example, to obtain a more peripheral view of 12 o'clock (with mirrors at 6 o'clock) tilt the lens down and ask the patient to look up.
- The vitreous cavity is examined with the central lens using both a horizontal and a vertical slit beam.
- The posterior pole is examined.

- **Scleral indentation** at the slit lamp can be accomplished using a three-mirror lens with a special attachment (Eisner funnel) or a purpose-made ora serrata contact lens that combines a mirror angled similarly to a gonioscopy lens with an incorporated attachment to facilitate scleral depression (e.g. Goldman One Mirror Glass 904 lens).
- **Miscellaneous** contact lenses are divided principally into those conferring high magnification for an optimal posterior pole view, and those offering a wide field of view, allowing visualization extending to the ora serrata under optimal conditions. Small pupil capability is available, and a flange is offered on many lenses with the aim of improving stability of retention and of lens position on the eye.

Head-mounted binocular indirect ophthalmoscopy

The term binocular indirect ophthalmoscopy (BIO) is by convention used to refer to the head-mounted technique, though strictly it also applies to slit lamp indirect ophthalmoscopy. BIO allows retinal visualization through a greater degree of media opacity than slit lamp biomicroscopy, and readily facilitates scleral indentation. Light is transmitted from the headset to the fundus through a condensing lens held at the focal point of the eye, providing an inverted and laterally reversed image that is observed through a stereoscopic viewing system (Fig. 1.38A).

- **Lenses** of various powers and diameters are available for BIO (Fig. 1.38B). A lens of lower power confers increased magnification, but a smaller field of view. The magnification can be calculated by dividing the dioptric power of the examining lens into 60. (For example, a 20 D lens would have a magnification of 3.) Yellow filters may improve patient comfort.
  - 20 D (magnifies ×3; field about 45°) is the most commonly used for general examination of the fundus.
  - 28 D (magnification with the head-mounted set of ×2.27; field of 53°) has a shorter working distance and is useful when examining patients with small pupils.
  - 40 D (magnification ×1.5; field 65°) is used mainly to examine small children. A broad fundus scan can be acquired rapidly and it can also be used at the slit lamp to provide very high magnification.
  - Panretinal 2.2 combines magnification similar to the 20 D lens with a field of view similar to that of the 28 D, and can be used with small pupils.
  - Ultra-high magnification lenses for macula and optic disc examination (e.g. Macula Plus 5.5) are available.
- **Technique**
  - The patient should be supine on a bed or reclining chair rather than sitting upright (Fig. 1.39A).
  - The pupils should be dilated. Reducing the ambient illumination is often helpful as this improves contrast and allows a lower incident light intensity to be used.
  - The eyepieces are set at the correct interpupillary distance and the beam aligned so that it is located in the centre of the viewing frame.
  - The patient is instructed to keep both eyes open at all times. If necessary, the patient's eyelids are gently separated with the fingers.
  - The lens is taken into one hand with the flat surface facing the patient.
  - The peripheral fundus should be examined first in order to allow the patient to adapt to the light. The patient is asked to move the eyes into optimal positions for examination, e.g. looking away from the examiner to facilitate examination of the retinal periphery.
  - For the examination of small children (e.g. retinopathy of prematurity – see also Ch. 13) a speculum may be utilized to keep the eyelids apart, with an implement such as a squint hook employed to direct the position of the eye.
- **Scleral indentation**
  - The main function of scleral indentation (depression) is to improve visualization of the retina anterior to the equator; it also permits kinetic evaluation (Fig. 1.40).
  - Indentation should be attempted only after the basic technique of BIO has been mastered. It requires practised

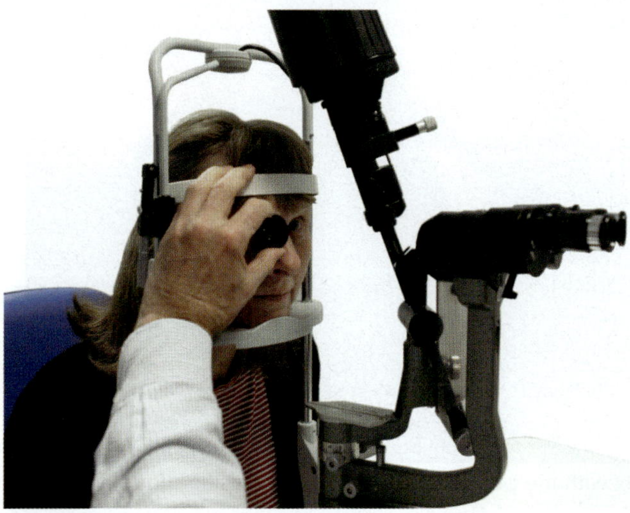

Fig. 1.37 The illumination column is tilted and positioned right of centre to view the oblique meridian at 1.30 and 7.30 o'clock.

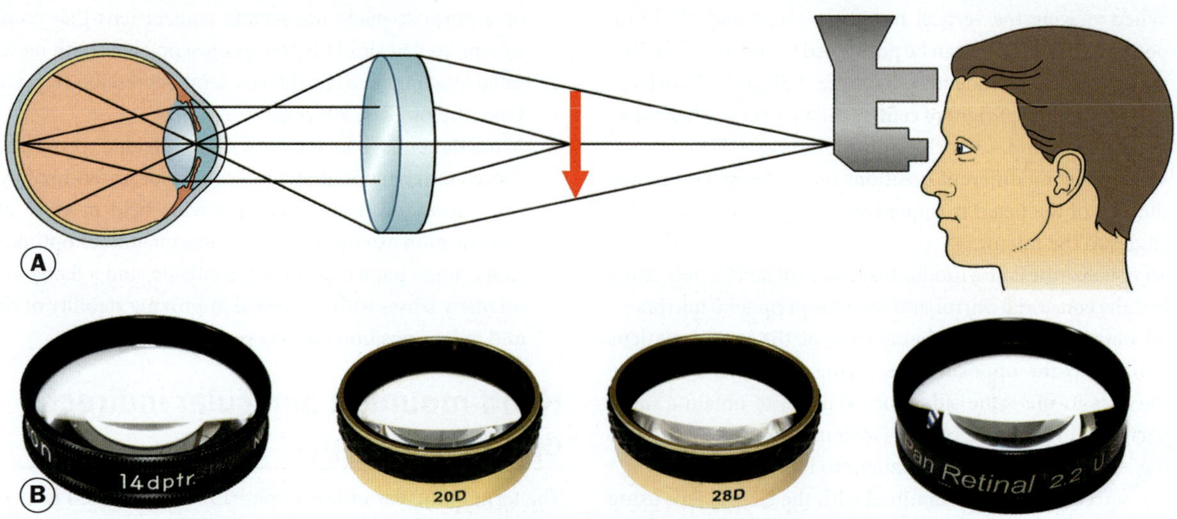

Fig. 1.38 **(A)** Principles of indirect ophthalmoscopy; **(B)** condensing lenses.

coordination between the relative position of the indenter and the viewing apparatus, as well as care to prevent patient discomfort. For example, to view the ora serrata at 12 o'clock, the patient is asked to look down and the scleral indenter (a cotton-tipped applicator is preferred by some practitioners) is applied to the outside of the upper eyelid at the margin of the tarsal plate.

- With the indenter in place, the patient is asked to look up. At the same time the indenter is advanced into the anterior orbit parallel with the globe, and the examiner's eyes are aligned with the condensing lens and indenter (see Fig. 1.39B).
- Gentle pressure is exerted so that a mound is created. After adequate viewing, the indenter is gently moved to an adjacent part of the fundus.
- The indenter should be kept tangential to the globe at all times, as perpendicular indentation will cause pain and even risk perforation if the sclera is very thin.
- For viewing the 3 and 9 o'clock positions, indentation directly on the sclera is sometimes necessary, facilitated by topical anaesthesia. Indentation can also be performed at the slit lamp using some fundus contact lenses.

Fundus drawing

When available, wide-field photographic imaging can be an excellent aid in recording the features of a retinal detachment (Fig. 1.41), but documentation generally takes the form of a manually drawn illustration that optimally is colour-coded (Fig. 1.42). If a retinal detachment is found, the boundaries are drawn by starting at the optic nerve and then extending to the periphery. Detached retina is shaded in blue and flat retina in red. The course of retinal vessels (usually veins) is indicated with blue. Retinal breaks are drawn in red with blue outlines; the flap of a retinal tear is also drawn in blue. Thin retina may be represented by red hatching outlined in blue and lattice degeneration by blue hatching outlined

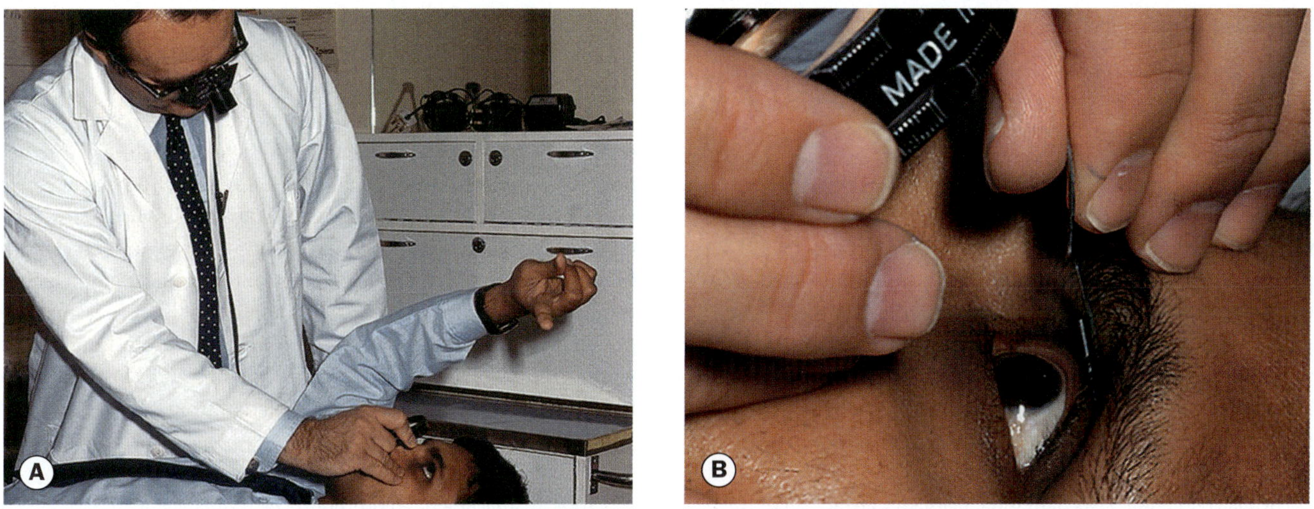

Fig. 1.39 **(A)** Position of patient during indirect ophthalmoscopy; **(B)** scleral indentation.

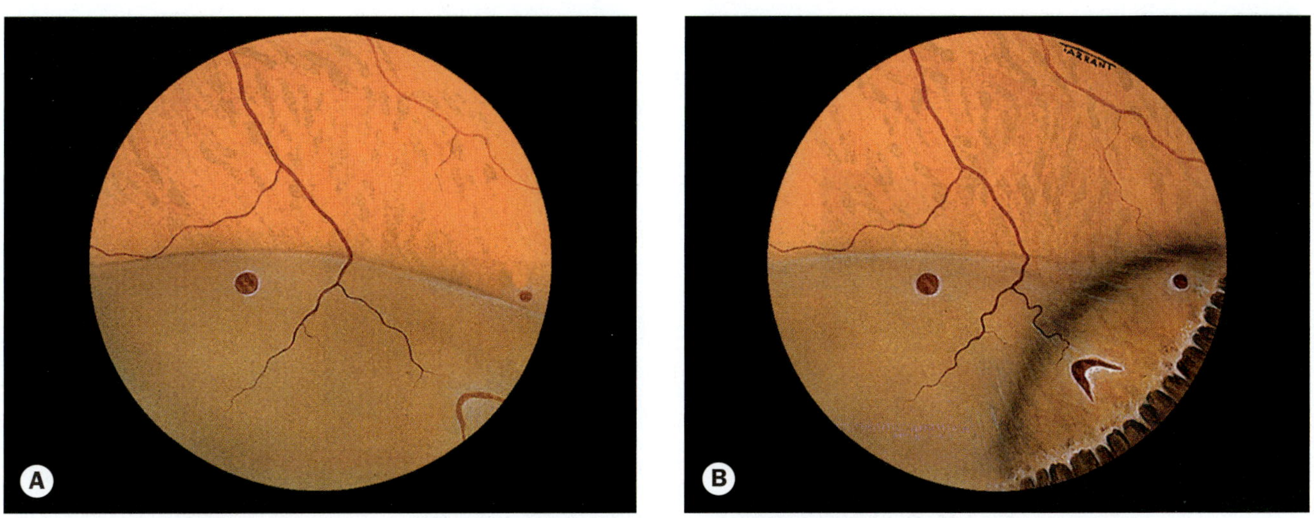

Fig. 1.40 Appearance of retinal breaks in detached retina. **(A)** Without scleral indentation; **(B)** with indentation.

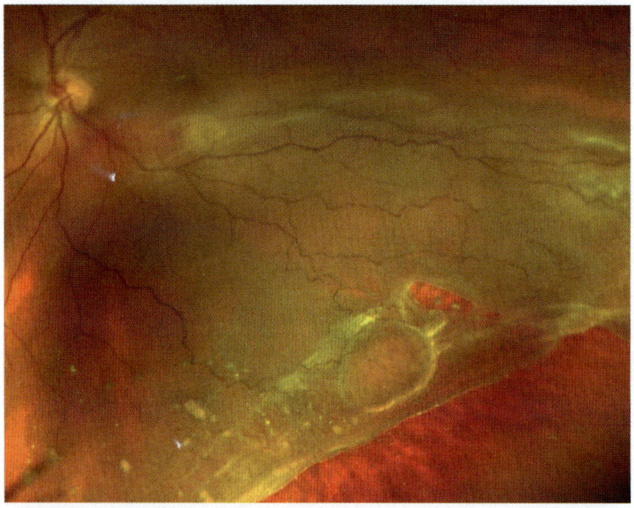

Fig. 1.41 Wide-field fundus photograph showing a peripheral retinal dialysis.

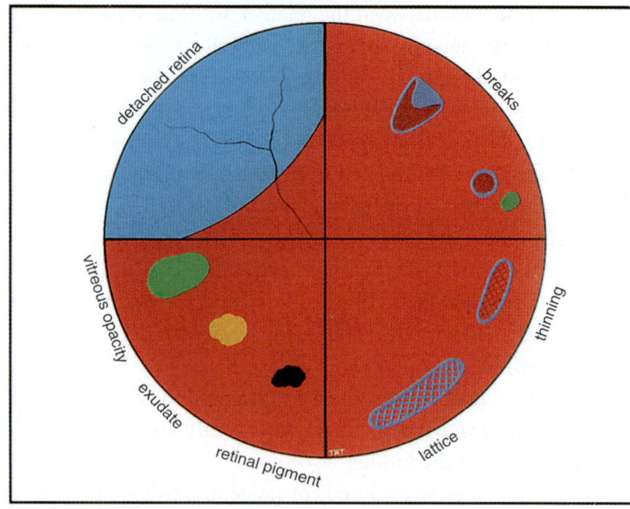

Fig. 1.42 Colour coding for retinal illustration.

in blue. Retinal pigment is indicated in black, retinal exudates in yellow and vitreous opacities in green.

TONOMETRY

Goldmann tonometry

Principles

Goldmann applanation tonometry is based on the Imbert–Fick principle, which states that for an ideal, dry, thin-walled sphere, the pressure inside the sphere (*P*) equals the force necessary to flatten its surface (*F*) divided by the area of flattening (*A*) (i.e. $P = F/A$). The intraocular pressure (IOP) is proportional to the pressure applied to the globe (in practice, the cornea) and the thickness of the wall of the globe (i.e. the thickness of the cornea, which is variable). The human eye, however, is not an ideal sphere – the cornea is rigid and resists flattening. Capillary attraction of the tear meniscus, however, tends to pull the tonometer towards the cornea. Corneal rigidity and capillary attraction cancel each other out when the flattened area has a diameter of 3.06 mm, as in Goldmann tonometry (Fig. 1.43A). The Goldmann tonometer is an accurate variable-force tonometer consisting of a double prism (Fig. 1.43B). The tonometer prism should be disinfected between patients and replaced regularly in accordance with the manufacturer's instructions. Two per cent Na-hypochlorite (dilute bleach) offers effective disinfection against adenovirus and herpes simplex virus. However, disinfectants can cause the tonometer tip to swell and crack with time, which can lead to disinfectant entering the tonometer tip resulting in a corneal abrasion when applied to the cornea. Seventy per cent isopropyl alcohol wipes do not offer protection against viral infections. Disposable tonometer prisms and caps have been introduced to address concerns of infection from reusable prisms.

Technique

- Topical anaesthetic (commonly proxymetacaine 0.5%) and a small amount of fluorescein are instilled into the conjunctival sac.

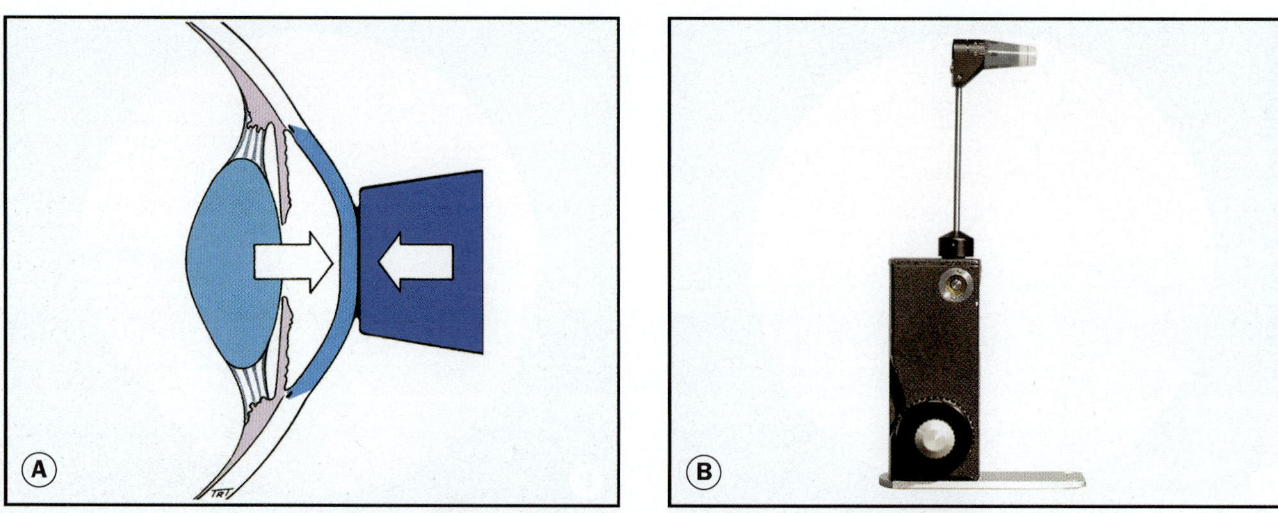

Fig. 1.43 Goldmann tonometry. **(A)** Physical principles; **(B)** tonometer.

- The patient is positioned at the slit lamp with his or her forehead firmly against the headrest and instructed to look straight ahead (often at the examiner's opposite ear) and to breathe normally.
- With the cobalt blue filter in place and illumination of maximal intensity directed obliquely (approximately 60°) at the prism, the prism is centred in front of the apex of the cornea.
- The dial is preset at 1 (i.e. 10 mmHg).
- The prism is advanced until it just touches the apex of the cornea (Fig. 1.44A).
- Viewing is switched to the ocular of the slit lamp.
- A pattern of two green semi-circular mires will be seen, one above and one below the horizontal midline, which represent the fluorescein-stained tear film touching the upper and lower outer halves of the prism. Mire thickness should be around 10% of the diameter of its total arc (Fig. 1.44B). Care should be taken to horizontally and vertically centre the mires so that two centralized semi-circles are observed.
- The dial on the tonometer is rotated to vary the applied force. The inner margins of the semi-circles align when a circular area of diameter precisely 3.06 mm is flattened.
- The reading on the dial, multiplied by 10, gives the IOP in mmHg.

TIP Inadvertent finger pressure applied to the globe when undertaking applanation tonometry or squeezing of the eyelids can cause an anomalously high IOP reading.

Sources of error

- **Inappropriate fluorescein pattern.** Excessive fluorescein will result in the mires being too thick, with consequent overestimation of IOP. Insufficient will make the semi-circles too thin, with consequent underestimation (see Fig. 1.44B, left and centre).
- **Pressure on the globe** from the examiner's fingers, eyelid squeezing or restricted extraocular muscles (e.g. thyroid myopathy) may give an anomalously high reading.
- **Central corneal thickness (CCT).** Calculations of IOP by Goldmann applanation tonometry (GAT) assume that CCT is 520 μm, with minimal normal variation. If the cornea is thinner, an underestimation of IOP is likely to result, and if thicker, an overestimation. Corneas tend to be thicker than average in individuals with ocular hypertension, and thinner in normal-tension glaucoma (NTG). Following refractive surgery procedures, the cornea is both thinner and structurally altered, leading to an underestimation of the IOP. Some methods of IOP measurement (e.g. DCT – see below) may reduce the effect of structural confounding variables. Other corneal mechanical factors may also be important but are less well defined.
- **Corneal oedema** may result in artificial lowering of IOP, hypothesized to be due to a boggy softening; the associated increased CCT seems to be more than offset.
- **Astigmatism**, if significant, may give distorted mires as well as leading to mechanically induced errors. If over 3 dioptres, the average reading of two can be taken with the prism rotated 90° for the second, or optimally the prism is rotated so that the red line on the tonometer housing is aligned with the prescription of the minus axis.
- **Incorrect calibration** of the tonometer can result in a false reading. Calibration should be checked before each clinical session using the manufacturer's calibration arm (Fig. 1.44C).
- **Wide pulse pressure.** It is normal for there to be a small oscillation of IOP in concert with the rhythm of ocular perfusion. If this 'pulse pressure' is substantial, either the midpoint or the highest level observed may be taken.
- **Repeated readings over a short period** will often be associated with a slight fall in IOP due to a massaging effect on the eye.

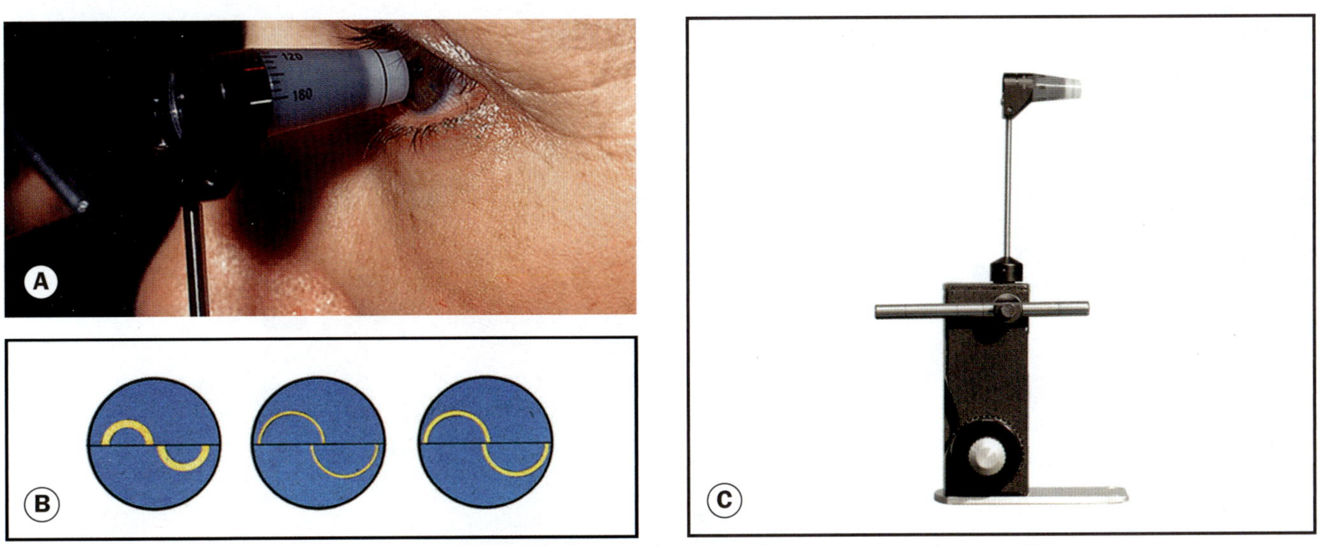

Fig. 1.44 Applanation tonometry. **(A)** Contact between the tonometer prism and the cornea; **(B)** fluorescein-stained semi-circular mires – the diagram at right showing the correct end-point using mires of appropriate thickness; **(C)** tonometer calibration bar in position.

- **Other factors,** including a tight collar and breath-holding, both of which obstruct venous return, can raise IOP.

TIP The Goldmann tonometer loses accuracy with constant use and should be checked for calibration error on a regular basis.

Other forms of tonometry

- **Pneumotonometry** (Fig. 1.45A) is based on the principle of applanation, but the central part of the cornea is flattened by a jet of air rather than a prism. The time required to sufficiently flatten the cornea relates directly to the level of IOP. Contact is not made with the eye and topical anaesthesia is not required, so it is particularly useful for screening in the community. The sudden jet of air can startle the patient. Accuracy is improved if an average of at least three readings is taken.
- **Portable applanation tonometry** (Perkins) uses a Goldmann prism in conjunction with a portable light source (Fig. 1.45B). It is hand-held and can therefore be used in bed-bound or anaesthetized patients.
- **Dynamic contour tonometry (DCT)** (e.g. PASCAL) uses a solid-state sensor and a corneal contour-matching surface, with the aim of measuring IOP relatively independently of corneal mechanical factors such as rigidity. It is mounted on a slit lamp in similar fashion to the Goldmann tonometer and IOP is shown on a digital display. Studies comparing DCT and GAT IOP readings with manometric intracameral IOP seem to confirm DCT as providing a more physiological measurement.
- **Electronic indentation/applanation tonometry** (e.g. Tono-Pen AVIA – Fig. 1.45C) is a hand-held electronic contact tonometer (a modified version of the older Mackay–Marg tonometer). The probe tip contains a transducer that measures applied force. Besides portability, its main advantage is the facility to measure IOP reasonably accurately in eyes with distorted or oedematous corneas and through a soft contact lens.
- **Rebound tonometry** (e.g. iCare – Fig. 1.45D) involves a 1.8 mm plastic ball attached to a wire. Deceleration of the probe upon contact with the cornea is proportional to IOP.

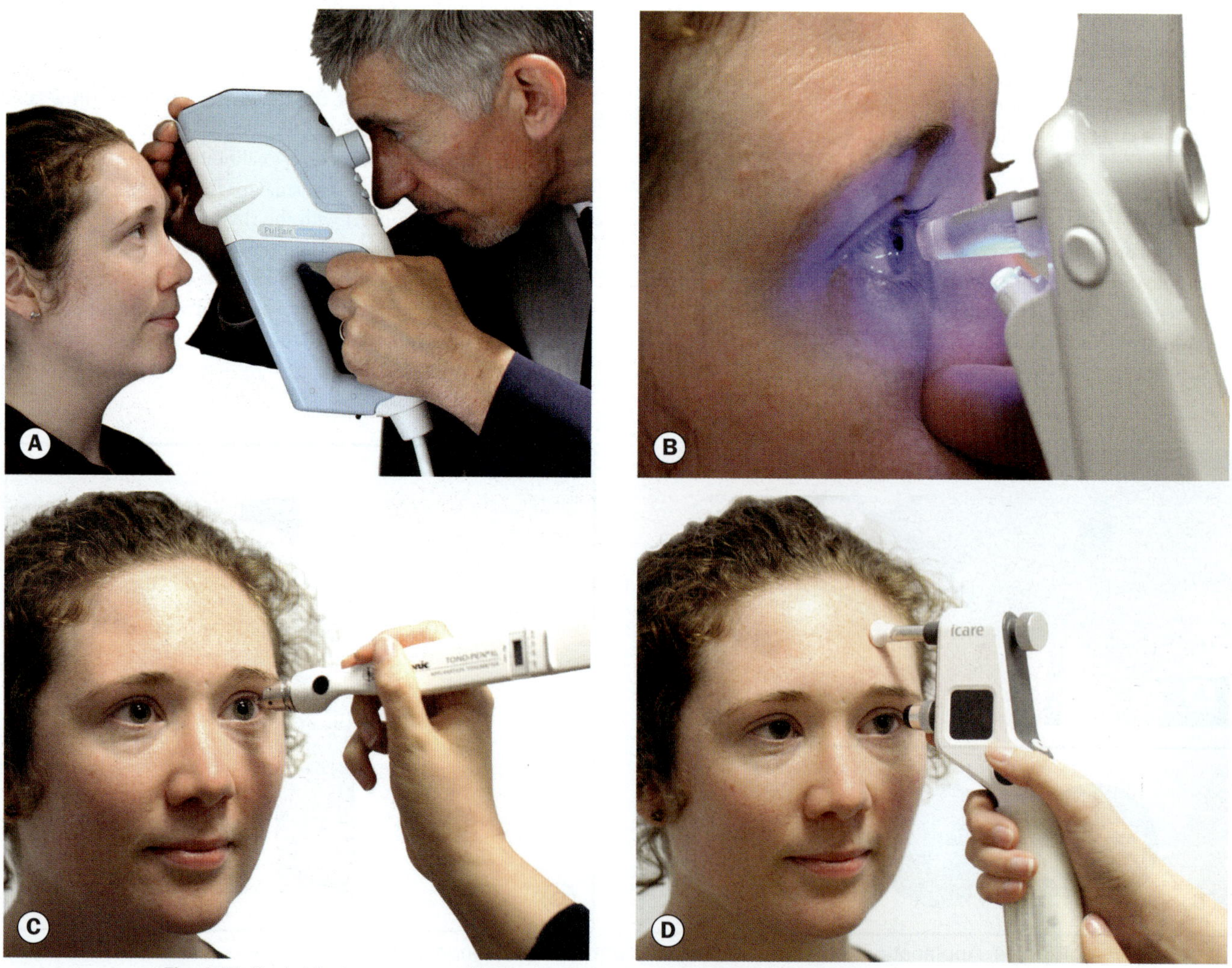

Fig. 1.45 Portable tonometers. **(A)** Keeler Pulsair pneumotonometer; **(B)** Perkins applanation tonometer; **(C)** Medtronic Tono-Pen; (D) iCare IC100.

Anaesthesia is not required. The instrument can be used for self-monitoring and for screening in the community.

- **Home tonometry** (e.g. iCare HOME2) is available for patients who require regular monitoring of their IOP, especially when information is needed on diurnal IOP fluctuation. It is fairly easy to use and provides accurate measurements. It has a positioning system for correct alignment of the instrument and a magnet within the applicator which prevents the probe from falling out.
- **Indentation (impression) tonometry** (e.g. Schiotz) is a seldom-used portable device that measures the extent of corneal indentation by a plunger of known weight.
- **Implantable tonometers** are under development and if a clinically workable device is realized should facilitate accurate lifelong 24-hour IOP measurement.

Ocular response analyser and corneal hysteresis

The ocular response analyser (e.g. Reichert ORA) utilizes air-puff technology to record two applanation measurements: one while the cornea is moving inward and one when the cornea returns to its normal position. The average of these two IOP measurements provides a Goldmann-correlated IOP measurement. The difference between the IOP measurements is called corneal hysteresis (Fig. 1.46). Corneal hysteresis is not a measure of the stiffness of the cornea, but rather a measure of how corneal tissue absorbs and dissipates energy during deformation and return. Corneal hysteresis appears to provide a measurement of IOP that is less affected by factors such as previous laser refractive surgery. It also offers information on which patients with glaucoma are more likely to progress (patients with a low hysteresis value are at a greater risk of glaucoma progression) and it may serve as a biomarker to aid glaucoma case detection. There is also a strong relationship between corneal hysteresis and the magnitude of IOP reduction with topical prostaglandin therapy.

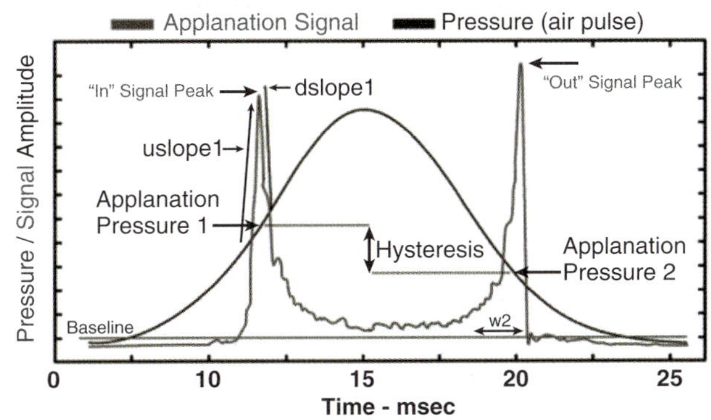

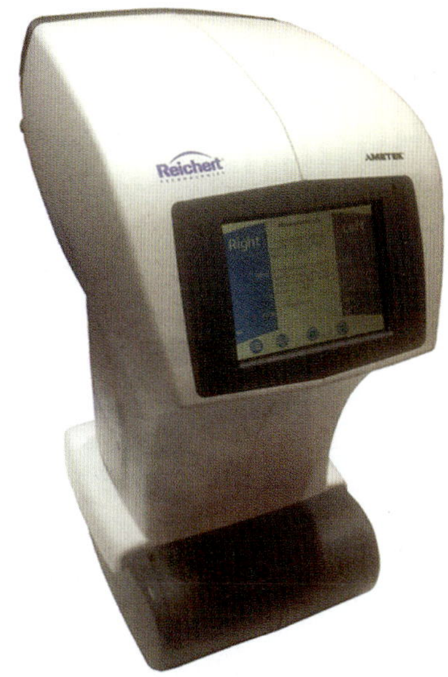

Fig. 1.46 Corneal hysteresis as measured by the Ocular Response Analyzer (Reichert). It is defined as the difference between the pressure at which the cornea bends inward during air-jet applanation and the pressure at which it bends out again.

GONIOSCOPY

Introduction

Overview

- **Gonioscopy** is a method of evaluating the anterior chamber (AC) angle, and can be used therapeutically for procedures such as laser trabeculoplasty and goniotomy.
- **Other means** of angle assessment, such as anterior segment optical coherence tomography (OCT) and high-frequency ultrasound biomicroscopy (UBM), offer advantages in some aspects of angle analysis, but current clinical opinion suggests they should supplement rather than replace gonioscopic evaluation (see Ch. 11).

TIP Gonioscopy is an indispensable technique that allows the filtration angle to be examined in patients with ocular hypertension or glaucoma.

Optical principles

The angle of the AC cannot be visualized directly through the intact cornea because light from angle structures undergoes 'total internal reflection' at the anterior surface of the precorneal tear film (Fig. 1.47, top). When light travels from a medium of higher to one of lower refractive index (such as cornea to air) it will be reflected at the interface between the two unless the angle of incidence is less than a certain 'critical angle' dependent on their refractive index difference (46° for the tear film–air interface). The phenomenon is utilized in optical fibre signal transmission, where it ensures that light is retained within the core of a cable. Because the refractive index of a goniolens is similar to that of the cornea, it eliminates total internal reflection by replacing the tear film–air interface with a tear film–goniolens interface (Fig. 1.47, bottom). Light rays can then be viewed as they exit the contact lens, directly or indirectly (see below).

Disinfection

Lenses must be cleaned between patients to remove any particulate matter and then sterilized. A suggested regimen is to soak the lens

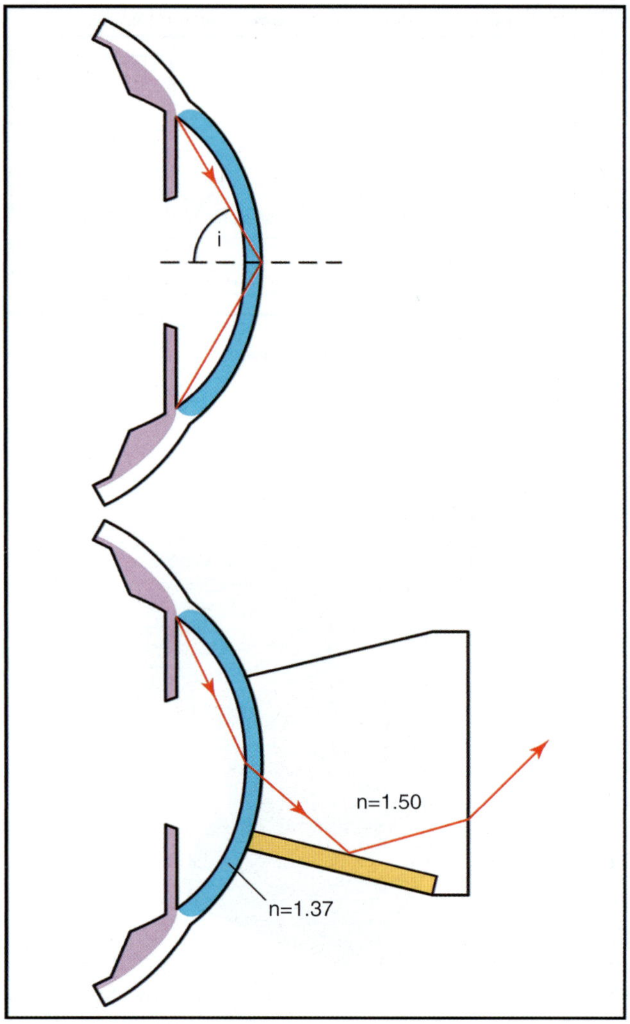

Fig. 1.47 Optical principles of gonioscopy; n = refractive index; i = angle of incidence.

in 2% Na-hypochlorite solution for at least 5 minutes followed by thorough rinsing in sterile saline, then air-drying.

Indirect gonioscopy

Indirect goniolenses use a mirror to reflect rays from the angle such that they exit the goniolens at much less than the critical angle. They provide a mirror image of the opposite angle and can be used only in conjunction with a slit lamp.

Non-indentation gonioscopy

- **Goniolenses**
  - The classic Goldmann lens consists of three mirrors, one of which is specifically for gonioscopy. Some goniolenses have one (Fig. 1.48), two or four mirrors.
  - Lenses of similar basic structure but with modifications include the Magna View, Ritch trabeculoplasty and the Khaw direct view.
  - Because the curvature of the contact surface of the lens is steeper than that of the cornea, a viscous coupling substance of refractive index similar to the cornea is required to bridge the gap between cornea and lens.

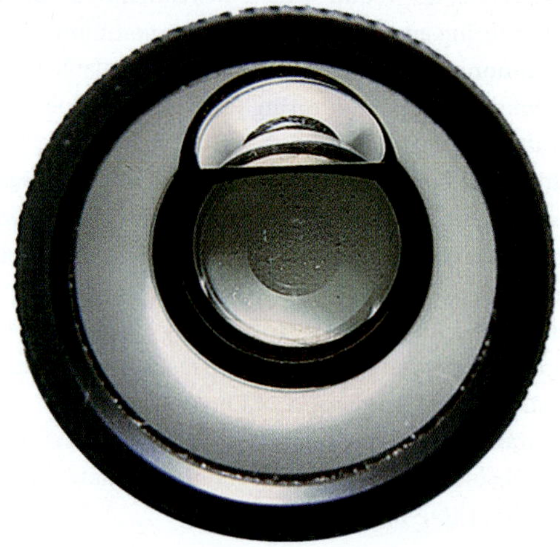

Fig. 1.48 Goldmann single-mirror goniolens.

TIP Gonioscopy should be undertaken in a room where the ambient illumination is low, as pupil size influences the grade of angle closure.

- **Technique**
  - It is essential that the examination takes place in a room in which the ambient illumination is low.
  - The size and intensity of the slit beam should be reduced to the absolute minimum compatible with an adequate view. Do not direct the beam through the pupil.
  - The patient is seated at the slit lamp and advised that the lens will touch the eye but will not usually cause discomfort. The forehead must be kept against the headband and both eyes should remain open.
  - A drop of local anaesthetic is instilled.
  - A drop or two of coupling fluid (e.g. hypromellose 0.3%) is placed on the contact surface of the lens.
  - The patient is asked to look upwards and the lens is inserted rapidly so as to avoid loss of the coupling fluid. The patient then looks straight ahead.
  - Indirect gonioscopy gives an inverted view of the portion of the angle opposite the mirror.
  - Once the initial examination has been performed and the findings noted, increasing the level of illumination may help in defining the angle structures.
  - When the view of the angle is obscured by a convex iris, it is possible to see 'over the hill' by asking the patient to look in the direction of the mirror. Only slight movement is permissible, otherwise the structures will be distorted and a closed angle may appear open.
  - Excessive pressure with a non-indentation lens narrows the angle appearance (in contrast to the effect of pressure during indentation gonioscopy – see below). Excessive

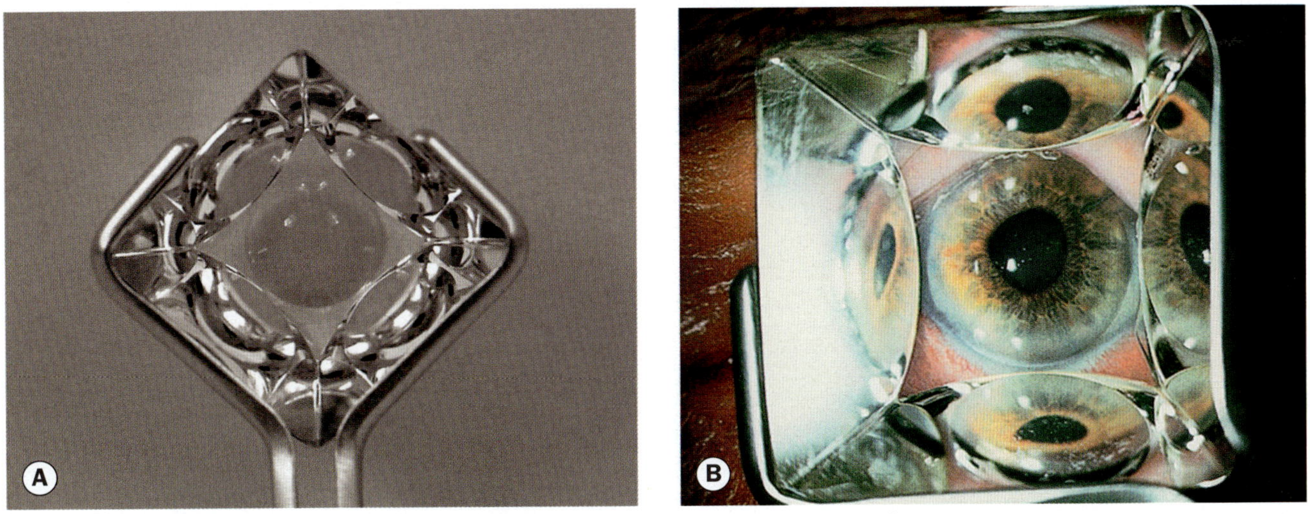

Fig. 1.49 (A) Zeiss goniolens; (B) slit lamp view with lens in place on the cornea.

pressure also causes folds in the cornea that compromise the clarity of the view.

  - In some eyes, suction on the cornea from the lens may artificially open the angle. Awareness of the need to avoid retrograde, as well as anterograde, pressure on the lens will tend to prevent inadvertent distortion.

TIP Indentation gonioscopy is a useful technique to determine the degree of peripheral anterior synechiae in a patient with appositional angle closure.

Indentation (dynamic, compression) gonioscopy

- **Goniolenses** include the Zeiss (Fig. 1.49), Posner and Sussman (no handle), all of which are four-mirror gonioprisms.
  - The contact surface of the lenses has a curvature flatter than that of the cornea, negating the need for a coupling substance.
  - The lenses do not stabilize the globe and are relatively unsuitable for laser trabeculoplasty.
  - The lenses are useful for indentation gonioscopy.
- **Technique**
  - The first stages are as set out above for non-indentation gonioscopy.
  - Indentation is performed by gently pressing the lens posteriorly against the cornea. This forces aqueous into the angle, pushing the peripheral iris posteriorly.
  - If the angle is closed only by apposition between the iris and cornea it will be forced open, allowing visualization of the angle recess (Fig. 1.50).
  - If the angle is closed by adhesions between the peripheral iris and cornea – peripheral anterior synechiae (PAS) – it will remain closed.
  - Dynamic gonioscopy can be invaluable in helping to define the structures in angles that are difficult to assess, such as in distinguishing an extensive or double highly pigmented Schwalbe line from the pigmented meshwork.

Direct gonioscopy

Direct goniolenses work by constructing the viewing surface of the lens in a domed or slanted configuration such that exiting light rays strike the contact lens/air interface at a steeper than critical angle so that they will pass through to the observer. This approach is called 'direct' because light rays from the angle are viewed directly, without reflection inside the lens. They do not require a slit lamp and are used with the patient in the supine position, typically under general anaesthesia in the evaluation and surgical treatment of infantile glaucoma.

- **Direct goniolenses** include the Koeppe (Fig. 1.51A and B), Medical Workshop, Barkan and Swan–Jacob.
- **Technique**
  - Gonioscopy is performed with the patient in the supine position (note that this may deepen the angle) in conjunction with an operating or hand-held microscope or magnifying loupes.
  - The technique cannot be used with a desktop slit lamp so clarity, illumination and variable magnification are not comparable with indirect lenses.

Surgical gonioscopy

- **Technique**
  - The key to successful microinvasive glaucoma surgery is adequate visualization of the filtration angle.
  - This is best achieved by rotating the operating microscope downwards (arrow) (Fig. 1.51C) and by tilting the patient's head away from the surgeon by 30–35° (arrow), until the coaxial light is aligned along the iris plane. Surgical instruments can then approach the angle parallel to the iris plane.
  - A useful surgical landmark is the scleral spur, which separates canal-based surgery (via the trabecular meshwork, anteriorly), from suprachoroidal-based surgery (via the ciliary body band, posteriorly).
  - Pigment within the trabecular meshwork can serve as a visual guide to the Schlemm canal. The canal can also be

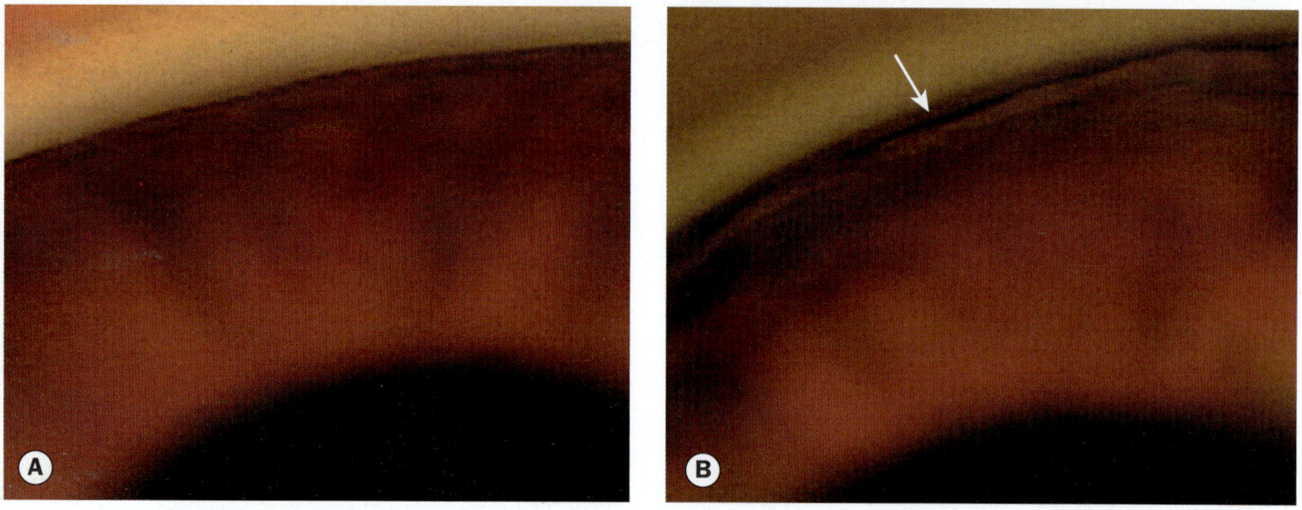

Fig. 1.50 Indentation gonioscopy in appositional angle closure. **(A)** Total angle closure prior to indentation; **(B)** during indentation the structures of the angle become visible (arrow).

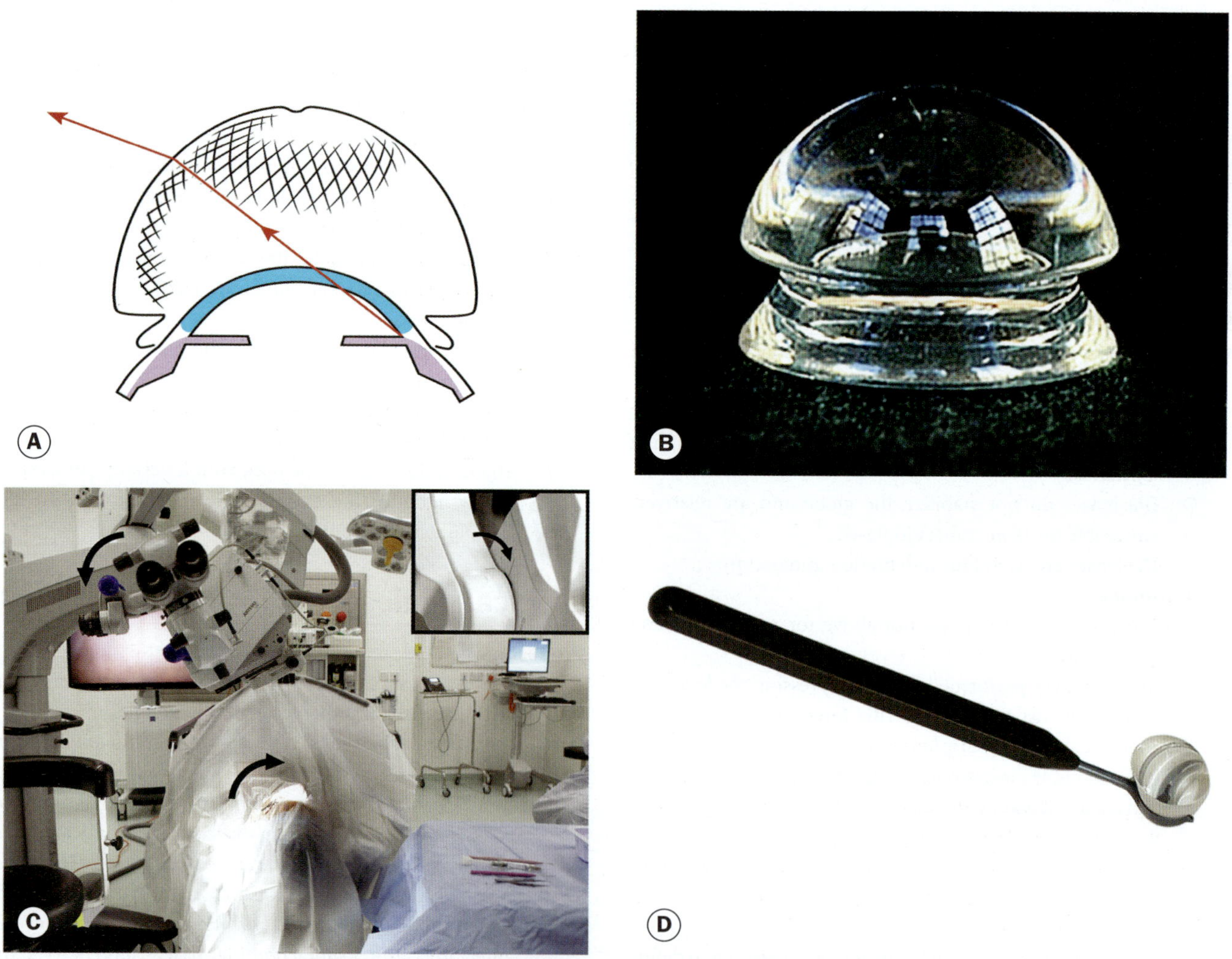

Fig. 1.51 Direct gonioscopy. **(A)** Optical principles of direct gonioscopy; **(B)** Koeppe lens; **(C)** operative gonioscopy: position of microscope (inset) and rotated patient's head when undertaking microinvasive glaucoma surgery (MIGS). Arrows indicate the direction of rotation to obtain an optimum view of the angle; **(D)** Volk Surgical Gonio Lens.

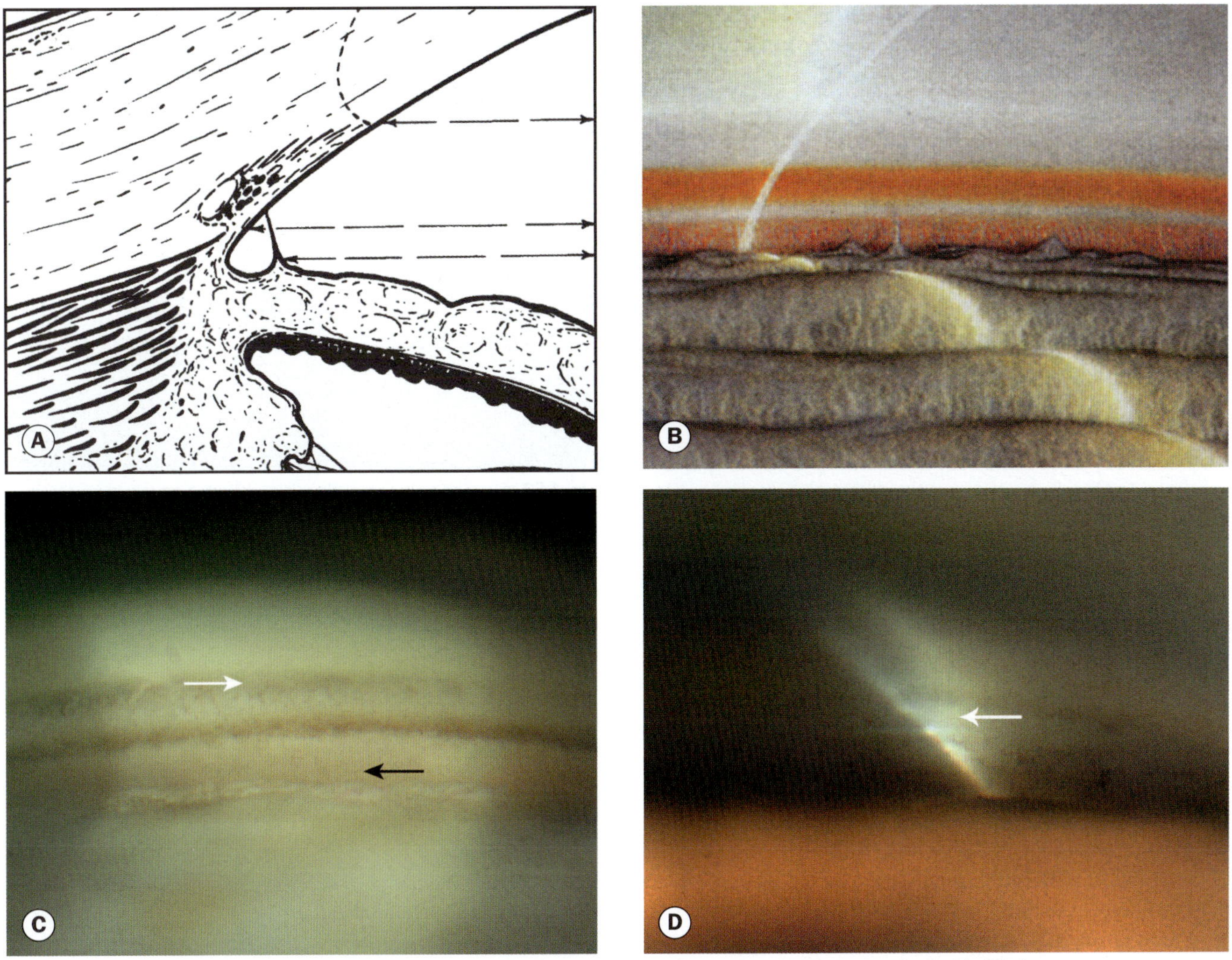

Fig. 1.52 Normal angle structures. **(A)** Schematic cross-sectional representation with **(B)** showing the corneal wedge; **(C)** goniophotograph – a broad Schwalbe line is indicated by the white arrow, below which is the non-pigmented meshwork, the pigmented meshwork, the scleral spur and the ciliary body (black arrow) – the ciliary body is relatively lightly pigmented; **(D)** corneal wedge on gonioscopy (arrow showing Schwalbe line). *(Courtesy of W Alward, from* Color Atlas of Gonioscopy, *Wolfe 1994 – figs A and B; R Tailor – fig. D.)*

located by applying gentle pressure with the edge of the goniolens (Fig. 1.51D) on the perilimbal episcleral vessels nasally, allowing reflux of blood into the canal. Trypan blue can be used to stain the trabecular meshwork when there is limited pigmentation.

Identification of angle structures

Accurate identification of angle structures (Fig. 1.52A–C) is not always straightforward, even for the experienced clinician.

- **Schwalbe line.** This is the most anterior structure, appearing whitish to variably pigmented. Anatomically it demarcates the peripheral termination of Descemet membrane and the anterior limit of the trabeculum. It may be barely discernible in younger patients. In contrast, there may be pigment deposits on or anterior to the Schwalbe line – a Sampaolesi line – especially in heavily pigmented angles (e.g. pseudoexfoliation syndrome). It may have a double-line configuration, when the posterior component may be mistaken for the pigmented meshwork (see Ch. 11).
- **The corneal wedge** is useful in locating an inconspicuous Schwalbe line. Using a narrow slit beam, two distinct linear corneal reflections can be identified, one on the inner and one on the outer corneal surface. The outer reflection will arc round across the corneoscleral interface – due to the sclera being opaque – to meet the inner reflection at the apex of the corneal wedge that coincides with the Schwalbe line (Fig. 1.52D).
- **The trabeculum** extends from the Schwalbe line to the scleral spur, with an average width of 600 μm. In younger people it has a ground-glass translucent appearance. The anterior non-functional part lies adjacent to the Schwalbe line and has a whitish colour. The posterior pigmented functional part lies adjacent to the scleral spur and has a greyish-blue translucent appearance in the young. Trabecular pigmentation is rare prior

to puberty, but in older eyes involves the posterior trabeculum to a variable extent, most marked inferiorly. Patchy trabecular pigmentation in a suspiciously narrow angle raises the possibility of intermittent iris contact.

- **The Schlemm canal** may be identified in the angle, especially if non-pigmented, as a slightly darker line deep to the posterior trabeculum. Blood can sometimes be seen in the canal, either physiologically (sometimes due to excessive pressure on the episcleral veins with a goniolens), or in the presence of low intraocular or raised episcleral venous pressure.
- **The scleral spur** is the most anterior projection of the sclera and the site of attachment of the longitudinal muscle of the ciliary body. Gonioscopically it is situated immediately posterior to the trabeculum and appears as a narrow whitish band that yellows with age.
- **The ciliary body** stands out just behind the scleral spur as a pink, dull brown or slate grey band. Its width depends on the position of iris insertion and it tends to be narrower in hypermetropic eyes and wider in myopic eyes. The angle recess represents the posterior dipping of the iris as it inserts into the ciliary body. It may not be visible in some eyes due to a physiological anterior iris insertion, though fixed pathological angle narrowing due to PAS – adhesions between the iris and angle structures – should be excluded.
- **Iris processes** are small, usually tenuous extensions of the anterior surface of the iris that insert at the level of the scleral spur and cover the ciliary body to a varying extent (Fig. 1.53). They are present in about one-third of normal eyes and are most prominent during childhood and in brown eyes. The processes should not be confused with PAS, which typically extend more anteriorly and are more substantial.
- **Blood vessels.** Radial vessels at the base of the angle recess are often seen in normal eyes. Pathological blood vessels run randomly in various directions. As a general principle, any blood vessel that crosses the scleral spur onto the trabecular meshwork is abnormal. Larger circumferential vessels may also be seen.

Pathological findings

- **Peripheral anterior synechiae**
  - Primary angle-closure glaucoma.
  - Anterior uveitis.
  - Iridocorneal endothelial (ICE) syndrome.
- **Neovascularization**
  - Neovascular glaucoma.
  - Fuchs heterochromic cyclitis.
  - Chronic anterior uveitis.
- **Hyperpigmentation**
  - Physiological variant.
  - Pigment dispersion syndrome.
  - Pseudophakic pigment dispersion.
  - Pseudoexfoliation syndrome.

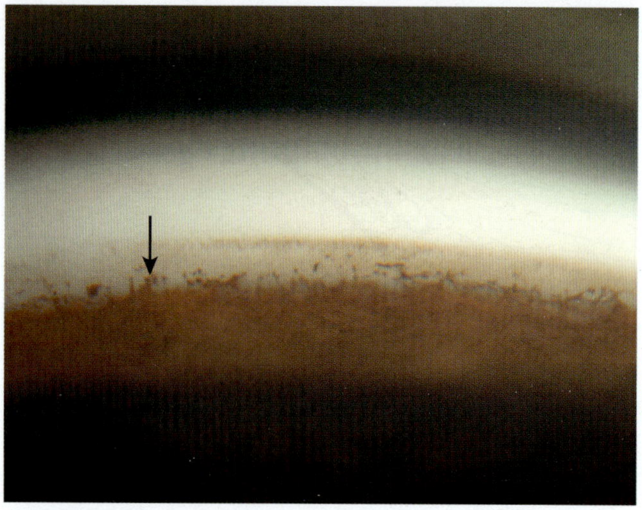

Fig. 1.53 Gonioscopy showing iris processes (arrow).

  - Blunt ocular trauma.
  - Anterior uveitis.
  - Following acute angle-closure glaucoma.
  - Following YAG laser iridotomy.
  - Iris or angle melanoma or naevus.
  - Iris pigment epithelial cysts.
  - Naevus of Ota.
- **Trauma**
  - Angle recession.
  - Trabecular dialysis.
  - Cyclodialysis.
  - Foreign bodies.
- **Blood in the Schlemm canal**
  - Physiological variant.
  - Carotid–cavernous fistula and dural shunt.
  - Sturge–Weber syndrome.
  - Obstruction of the superior vena cava.

CENTRAL CORNEAL THICKNESS

Central corneal thickness (CCT) can be measured using pachymetry or by Orbscan (see Fig. 11.5). The normal distribution is 540±30 µm (mean ±1 standard deviation). CCT influences GAT readings. Eyes with a thin cornea have a true IOP that is greater than the measured IOP. Conversely, eyes with a thick cornea have a true IOP that is lower than the measured IOP. There is no validated and useful correction algorithm for these two measurements. Patients with NTG tend to have thin CCT measurements. It is an important value when determining risk of conversion to glaucoma in individuals with raised IOP (see Ch. 11). It is also an easy and practical indicator of corneal endothelial function.

TIP CCT should be measured in individuals with ocular hypertension, as it helps to determine the risk of conversion to glaucoma.

Chapter

Eyelids 2

INTRODUCTION

Anatomy

The skin (Fig. 2.1A) consists of the epidermis, dermis and related structures (adnexa).

Epidermis

The epidermis comprises four layers of keratin-producing cells (keratinocytes). It also contains melanocytes, Langerhans cells and Merkel cells. The layers of the epidermis around the eye are described below. Cells migrate superficially, undergoing maturation and differentiation through successive layers.

- **Keratin layer** (stratum corneum or horny layer) consists of flat cells devoid of nuclei.
- **Granular cell layer** (stratum granulosum) typically consists of one or two layers of flattened cells containing keratohyaline granules.
- **Prickle cell layer** (stratum spinosum) is approximately five cells deep. The cells are polygonal in cross-section and have abundant eosinophilic cytoplasm. Their free borders are united by spiny-appearing desmosomes (cellular junctions).
- **Basal cell layer** (stratum basale) comprises a single row of columnar-shaped proliferating cells containing melanin derived from adjacent melanocytes.

Dermis

The dermis is much thicker than the epidermis. It is composed of connective tissue and contains blood vessels, lymphatics and nerve fibres in addition to fibroblasts, macrophages and mast cells. Upward dermal extensions (papillae) interdigitate with downward epidermal projections (rete ridges). In the eyelid the dermis lies on the orbicularis muscle. Adnexa lie deep in the dermis or within the tarsal plates.

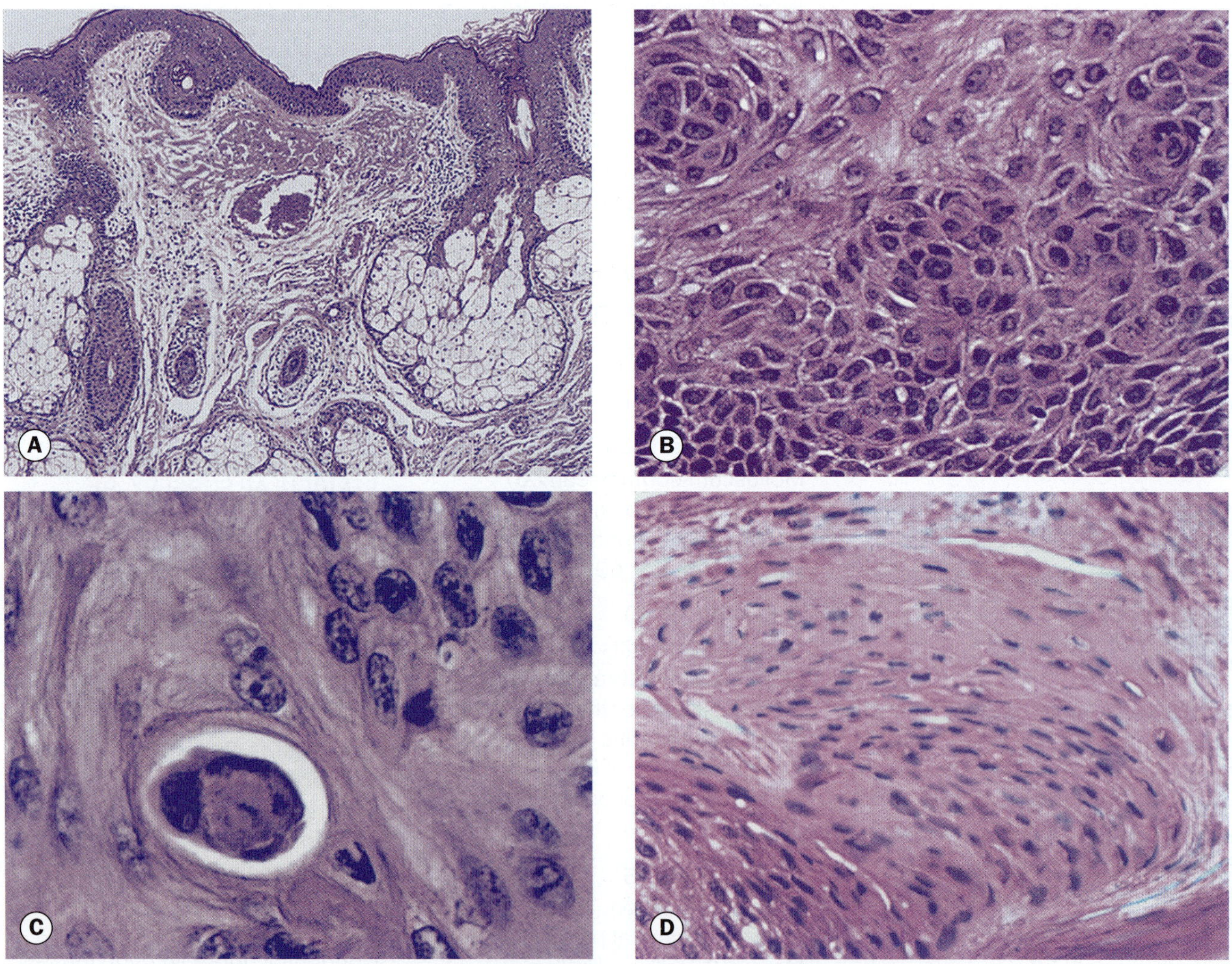

Fig. 2.1 Eyelid skin. **(A)** Normal skin is composed of keratinized stratified epithelium that covers the surface; pilosebaceous elements are conspicuous in the dermis and a few blood vessels and sweat glands are also seen; **(B)** dysplasia with loss of cell polarity; **(C)** dyskeratosis – a non-surface epithelial cell producing keratin; **(D)** parakeratosis – retention of cell nuclei into the surface keratin layer. *(Courtesy of J Harry and G Misson, from* Clinical Ophthalmic Pathology, *Butterworth-Heinemann, 2001.)*

- **Sebaceous glands** are located in the caruncle and within eyebrow hairs. Tiny sebaceous glands are associated with the thin (vellus) hairs covering periocular skin.
- **Meibomian glands** are modified sebaceous glands found in the tarsal plates. They empty through a single row of 20–30 orifices on each lid. A gland consists of a central duct with multiple acini, the cells of which synthesize lipids (meibum) that form the outer layer of the tear film.
- **Glands of Zeis** are modified sebaceous glands associated with lash follicles.
- **Glands of Moll** are modified apocrine sweat glands opening either into a lash follicle or directly onto the anterior lid margin between lashes. They are more numerous in the lower lid.
- **Eccrine sweat glands** are distributed throughout eyelid skin and are not confined to the lid margin, in contrast to glands of Moll.
- **Pilosebaceous units** comprise hair follicles and their sebaceous glands (see Fig. 2.1A).

Terminology

Clinical

- **Macule.** Localized area of colour change without infiltration, depression or elevation, less than 1 cm in diameter.
- **Papule.** A solid elevation less than 1 cm in diameter.
- **Vesicle.** Circumscribed lesion containing serous fluid (less than 0.5 cm across).
- **Bulla.** A large (more than 0.5 cm) serous fluid-filled lesion (plural – bullae).
- **Pustule.** A pus-filled elevation less than 1 cm in diameter.
- **Crust.** Solidified serous or purulent exudate.
- **Nodule.** A palpable solid area measuring more than 1 cm.
- **Cyst.** A nodule consisting of an epithelial-lined cavity filled with fluid or semi-solid material.
- **Plaque.** A solid elevation of the skin, greater than 1 cm in diameter.
- **Scale.** Readily detached fragments of shed keratin layer.
- **Papilloma.** A benign neoplastic warty or tag-like projection of the skin or mucous membrane.
- **Ulcer.** A circumscribed area of epithelial loss. In skin an ulcer extends through the epidermis into the dermis.

Histological

- **Tumour** strictly refers only to a swelling, though is commonly used to denote a neoplasm.
- **Neoplasia.** Abnormal tissue growth, either benign (localized, non-invasive and non-spreading) or malignant (progressive growth with the potential for distant spread).
- **Atypia** refers to an abnormal appearance of individual cells, e.g. abnormal mitotic figures.
- **Dysplasia** is an alteration of the size, morphology and organization of cellular components of a tissue. There is disturbance of normally structured and recognized layers of tissue (e.g. loss of cell polarity – Fig. 2.1B).
- **Carcinoma *in situ*** (intraepidermal carcinoma, Bowen disease) exhibits dysplastic changes throughout the thickness of the epidermis.
- **Hyperkeratosis.** An increase in thickness of the keratin layer that appears clinically as scaling. Hyperkeratosis can be a feature of benign or malignant epithelial tumours.
- **Acanthosis.** Thickening of the prickle cell layer.
- **Dyskeratosis** is keratinization other than on the epithelial surface (Fig. 2.1C).
- **Parakeratosis** is the retention of nuclei into the keratin layer (Fig. 2.1D).

General considerations

- **Classification.** Epidermal, adnexal or dermal.
- **Diagnosis.** The clinical characteristics of benign lesions are a tendency to a lack of induration and ulceration, uniform colour, limited growth, regular outline and preservation of normal lid margin structures. Biopsy may be required if the appearance is suspicious.
  - Incisional biopsy involves removal of a portion of a lesion for histopathology.
  - Excision biopsy is performed on small tumours and fulfils both diagnostic and treatment objectives.
- **Treatment** options include:
  - Excision of the entire lesion and a small surrounding portion of normal tissue.
  - Marsupialization involves the removal of the top of a cyst allowing drainage of its contents and subsequent epithelialization.
  - Ablation with laser or cryotherapy.

NON-NEOPLASTIC LESIONS

Chalazion (meibomian cyst)

Pathogenesis

A chalazion is a sterile chronic granulomatous inflammatory lesion (lipogranuloma) of the meibomian, or sometimes Zeis, glands caused by retained sebaceous secretions. Histopathology shows a lipogranulomatous chronic inflammatory picture with extracellular fat deposits surrounded by lipid-laden epithelioid cells, multinucleated giant cells and lymphocytes (Fig. 2.2A). Blepharitis is commonly present; rosacea can be associated with multiple and recurrent chalazia. Bortezomib, a proteasome inhibitor used in the treatment of multiple myeloma, predisposes to the formation of chalazia within 3 months of initiation of treatment. A recurrent chalazion should be biopsied to exclude masquerading malignancy.

TIP If a chalazion recurs in the same lid position in an older patient, consider undertaking a biopsy to exclude malignancy.

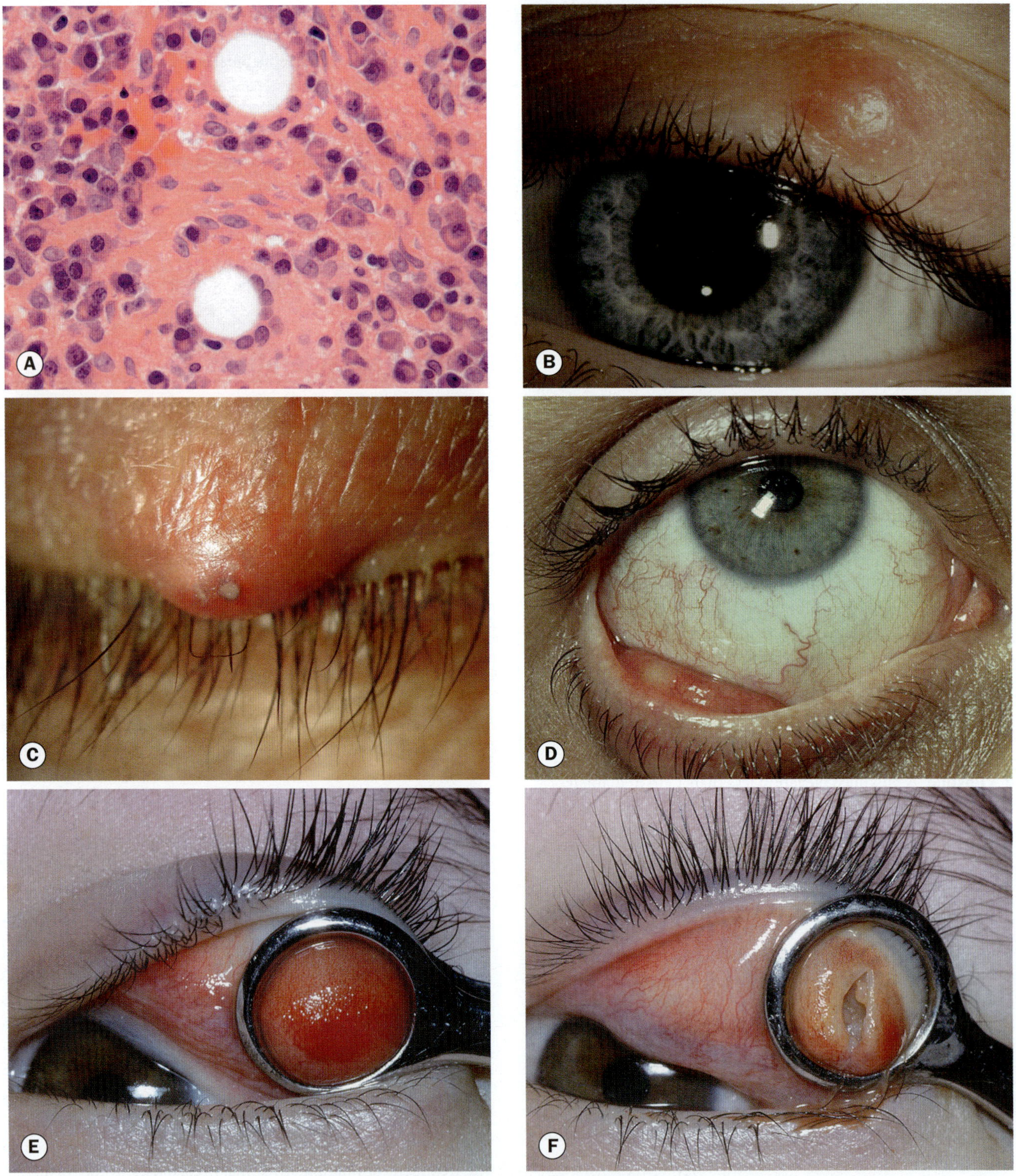

Fig. 2.2 Chalazion. **(A)** Histopathology showing a lipogranuloma; the large pale cells are epithelioid cells and the well-demarcated empty space contained fat dissolved out during processing; **(B)** uninflamed chalazion; **(C)** marginal chalazion with superimposed bacterial infection; **(D)** conjunctival chalazion; **(E)** conjunctival view of chalazion clamp in place; **(F)** after curettage. *(Courtesy of J Harry and G Misson, from* Clinical Ophthalmic Pathology, *Butterworth-Heinemann 2001 – fig. A.)*

Diagnosis

- **Symptoms**
  - Subacute/chronic: gradually enlarging painless rounded nodule (Fig. 2.2B).
  - Acute: sterile inflammation or bacterial infection with localized cellulitis. A secondarily infected meibomian gland is referred to as an internal hordeolum (Fig. 2.2C).
- **Signs**
  - A nodule within the tarsal plate, sometimes with associated inflammation (Fig. 2.2D).
  - Bulging inspissated secretions may be visible at the orifice of the involved gland.
  - There may be an associated conjunctival granuloma.
  - A lesion at the anterior lid margin may be connected to a typical chalazion deeper in the lid or be due to isolated involvement of a gland of Zeis.

Treatment

- **Oral antibiotics** are required for significant bacterial infection, but not for sterile inflammation.
- **Conservative.** At least a third resolve spontaneously so observation may be appropriate, especially if the lesion is showing signs of improvement.
- **Hot compress** application several times daily may aid resolution, particularly in early lesions.
- **Expression.** Compression between two cotton-tipped applicators is sometimes effective in expressing the contents of a fresh lesion near the lid margin.
- **Steroid injection** into or around the lesion has been reported to give similar resolution rates to incision and curettage (see below). It may be preferred for marginal lesions or lesions close to structures such as the lacrimal punctum because of the risk of surgical damage.
  - Reported regimens include 0.2–2 ml of triamcinolone acetonide aqueous suspension diluted with lidocaine to a concentration of 5 mg/ml and 0.1–0.2 ml of 40 mg/ml, injected with a 27- or 30-gauge needle.
  - The success rate following one injection is about 80%. A second can be given 1–2 weeks later.
  - Local skin depigmentation and fat atrophy are uncommon complications, which are less likely to occur by utilizing a conjunctival approach.
  - Retinal vascular occlusion is a rare complication.
- **Surgery**
  - Following local anaesthesia infiltration, the eyelid is everted with a specialized clamp (Fig. 2.2E), the cyst is incised vertically through the tarsal plate and its contents curetted (Fig. 2.2F).
  - Limited excision of solid inflammatory material (sent for histopathology) with fine scissors may be helpful in some cases, especially if there is no focus of secretions.
  - A suture should not be used.
  - Topical antibiotic is used three times daily for 5 days following curettage.
- **Marginal lesions** can be managed by steroid injection, by curettage of an associated deeper chalazion, by shave curettage or by incision and curettage via a horizontal incision on the conjunctival surface or vertically through the grey line.
- **Prophylaxis**
  - Treatment of blepharitis, e.g. daily lid hygiene regimen.
  - Systemic tetracycline may be required as prophylaxis in patients with recurrent chalazia, particularly if associated with acne rosacea.

Other eyelid cysts

- **Cyst of Zeis** is a small, non-translucent cyst on the anterior lid margin arising from obstructed sebaceous glands associated with the eyelash follicle (Fig. 2.3A).
- **Cyst of Moll** (apocrine hidrocystoma) is a small retention cyst of the lid margin apocrine glands. It appears as a round, non-tender, translucent fluid-filled lesion on the anterior lid margin (Fig. 2.3B).
- **Sebaceous (pilar)** cyst is caused by a blocked pilosebaceous follicle and contains sebaceous secretions; the gland orifice will often be visible (Fig. 2.3C). It is only rarely found on the eyelid although it may occasionally occur at the inner canthus.
- **Comedones** are plugs of keratin and sebum within the dilated orifice of hair follicles that often occur in patients with acne vulgaris. They may be either open (blackheads), containing a darkened plug of oxidized material (Fig. 2.3D), or closed (whiteheads).
- **Milia** are caused by occlusion of pilosebaceous units resulting in retention of keratin. They are tiny, white, round, superficial papules that tend to occur in crops (Fig. 2.3E).
- **Epidermal inclusion** cyst is usually caused by implantation of epidermis into the dermis following trauma or surgery. It is a slow-growing, round, firm, superficial or subcutaneous lesion containing keratin (Fig. 2.3F).
- **Epidermoid** cyst is uncommon and usually developmental, occurring along embryonic lines of closure. It is similar in appearance to an epidermal inclusion cyst.
- **Dermoid** cyst is usually subcutaneous or deeper and is typically attached to the periosteum at the lateral end of the brow (Fig. 2.3G). It is caused by skin sequestered during embryonic development.
- **Eccrine hidrocystoma** is less common but similar in appearance to a cyst of Moll except that it is usually located along the medial or lateral aspects of the lid and is close to, but does not involve, the lid margin itself (Fig. 2.3H).

Xanthelasma

Introduction

Xanthelasma (plural – xanthelasmata) is a common, frequently bilateral condition typically affecting middle-aged and elderly individuals. It is a subtype of xanthoma. Hyperlipidaemia is found in about one-third of patients, in whom corneal arcus may also be present. In contrast to chalazion, fat in xanthelasmata is mainly intracellular, with lipid-laden histiocytes (foam cells) in the dermis.

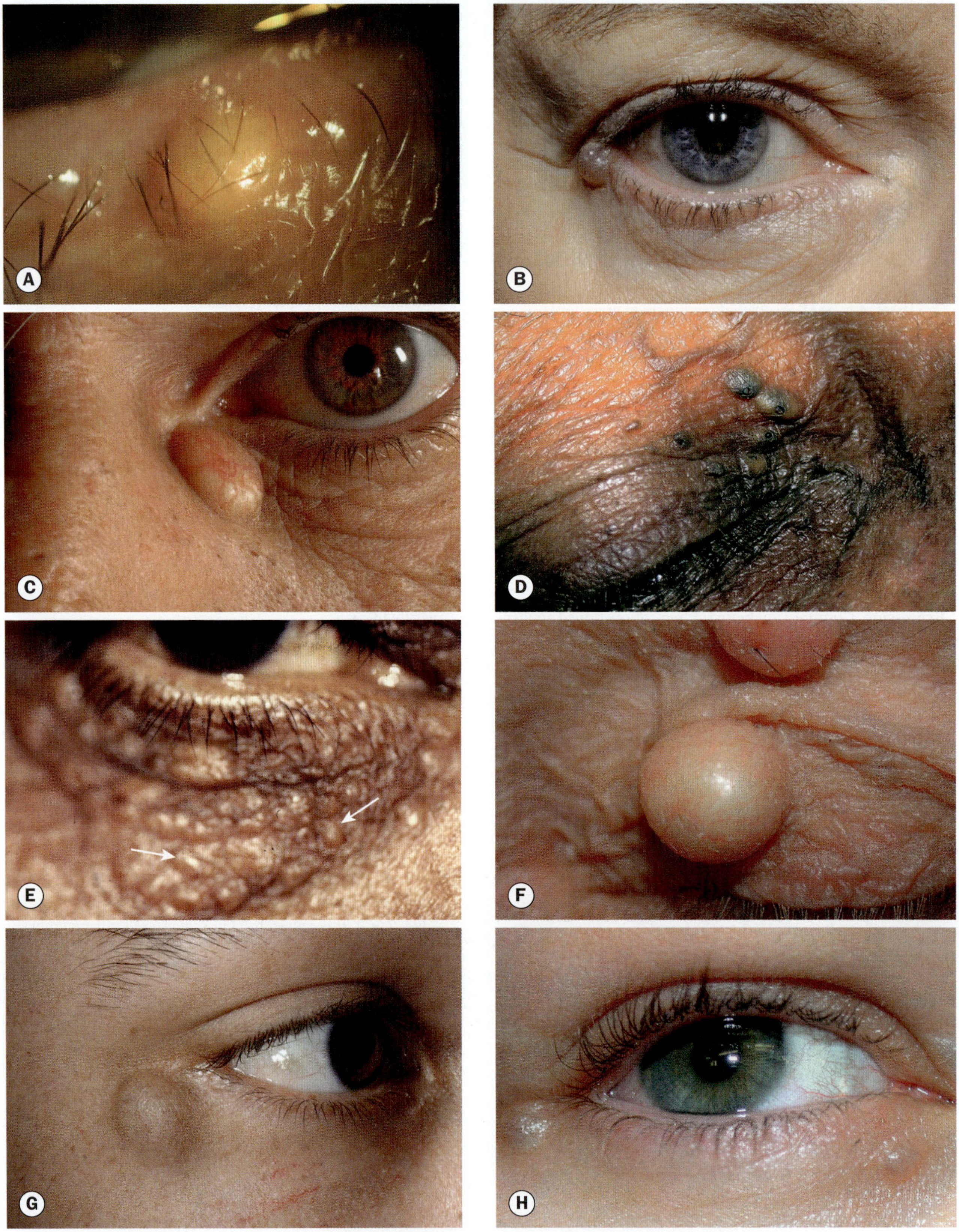

Fig. 2.3 Eyelid cysts. **(A)** Cyst of Zeis; **(B)** cyst of Moll; **(C)** sebaceous cyst; **(D)** comedones – blackheads; **(E)** milia (arrows); **(F)** epidermal inclusion cyst; **(G)** dermoid cyst; **(H)** eccrine hidrocystomas. *(Courtesy of A Pearson – figs D and H.)*

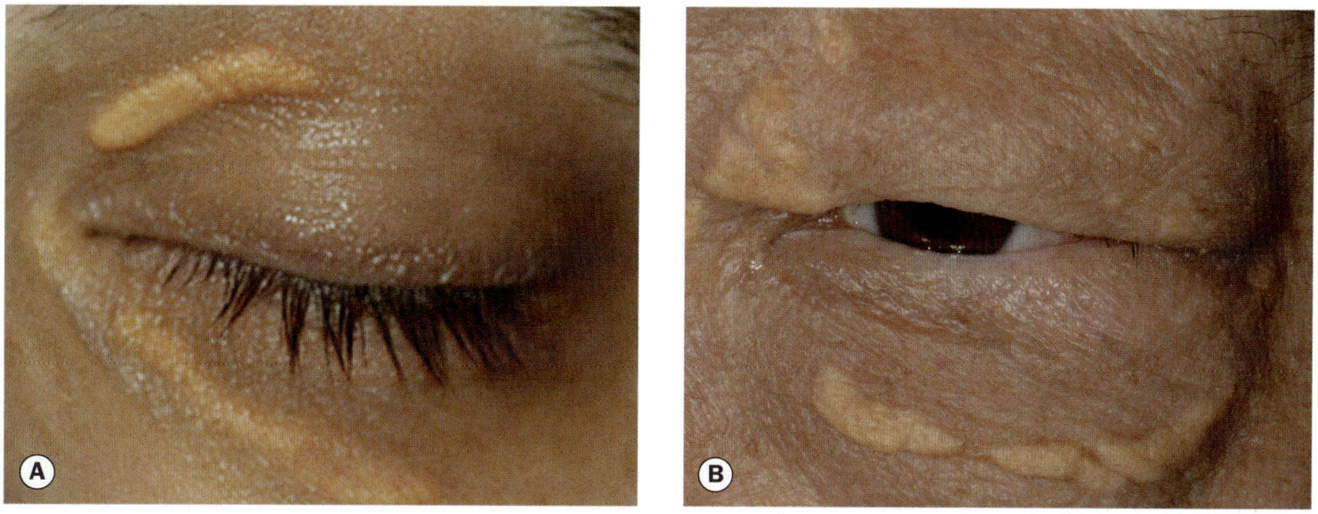

Fig. 2.4 Xanthelasma. **(A)** Large isolated lesions; **(B)** multiple smaller lesions.

Diagnosis

Xanthelasmata are yellowish subcutaneous plaques, usually in the medial aspects of the eyelids (Fig. 2.4A), commonly bilateral and are multiple (Fig. 2.4B).

Treatment

This is principally for cosmesis. Recurrence occurs in up to 50% and is most common in patients with hypercholesterolaemia.

- **Simple excision** is commonly performed where adequate excess skin is present.
- **Microdissection.** Larger lesions can be raised in a flap, the fatty deposits dissected from overlying skin under a surgical microscope using micro scissors and the skin replaced.
- **Other methods.** Good results can be obtained using chemical peeling with bi- or trichloroacetic acid. Laser ablation and cryotherapy have advantages but may be more prone to scarring, including pigmentary changes.

BENIGN EPIDERMAL TUMOURS

Squamous cell papilloma

Histopathology in all clinical types is similar, showing finger-like projections of fibrovascular connective tissue covered by irregular acanthotic and hyperkeratotic squamous epithelium (Fig. 2.5A). Squamous cell papilloma is a very common benign epithelial tumour with a range of clinical appearances, including narrow-based (pedunculated or 'skin tag' – Fig. 2.5B), pink broad-based (sessile – Fig. 2.5C) and whitish thread-like (filiform) hyperkeratotic lesions (Fig. 2.5D). The incidence increases with age. Some cases result from human papilloma virus infection. Treatment usually involves simple excision, but other options include cryotherapy and laser or chemical ablation.

Seborrhoeic keratosis

Histopathology shows expansion of the squamous epithelium of the epidermis by proliferating basal cells, sometimes with keratin-filled horns or cystic inclusions (Fig. 2.6A). Seborrhoeic keratosis (basal cell papilloma) is an extremely common slowly growing lesion found on the face, trunk and extremities of elderly individuals as a discrete light- to dark-brown plaque with a friable, greasy, verrucous surface and a 'stuck-on' appearance (Fig. 2.6B). They are frequently numerous. The differential diagnosis includes pigmented basal cell carcinoma, naevus and melanoma. Treatment involves shave biopsy (occasionally simple excision), electrodesiccation with curettage, laser ablation, cryotherapy with liquid nitrogen and chemical peeling.

Actinic keratosis

Histopathology (Fig. 2.7A) shows irregular dysplastic epidermis with hyperkeratosis, parakeratosis and occasionally cutaneous horn formation. Actinic (solar, senile) keratosis is a common slowly growing lesion that rarely develops on the eyelids. It typically affects elderly, fair-skinned individuals on areas of sun-damaged skin, such as the forehead and backs of the hands, and appears as a hyperkeratotic plaque with distinct borders and a scaly surface that may become fissured (Fig. 2.7B). Occasionally the lesion is nodular or wart-like and may give rise to a cutaneous horn. It has potential, though low, for transformation into squamous cell carcinoma. Treatment involves biopsy followed by excision or cryotherapy.

BENIGN PIGMENTED LESIONS

Freckle

A freckle (ephelis, plural ephelides) is a small (generally 1–5 mm) brown macule due to increased melanin in keratinocytes, typically in sun-exposed skin. This is particularly common in fair-skinned individuals and children with red hair, where the *MC1R* gene is involved (Fig. 2.8A). The number of freckles varies with the level of sun exposure and can sometimes regress completely. Histopathology shows hyperpigmentation of the basal layer of the epidermis, with a normal melanocyte population.

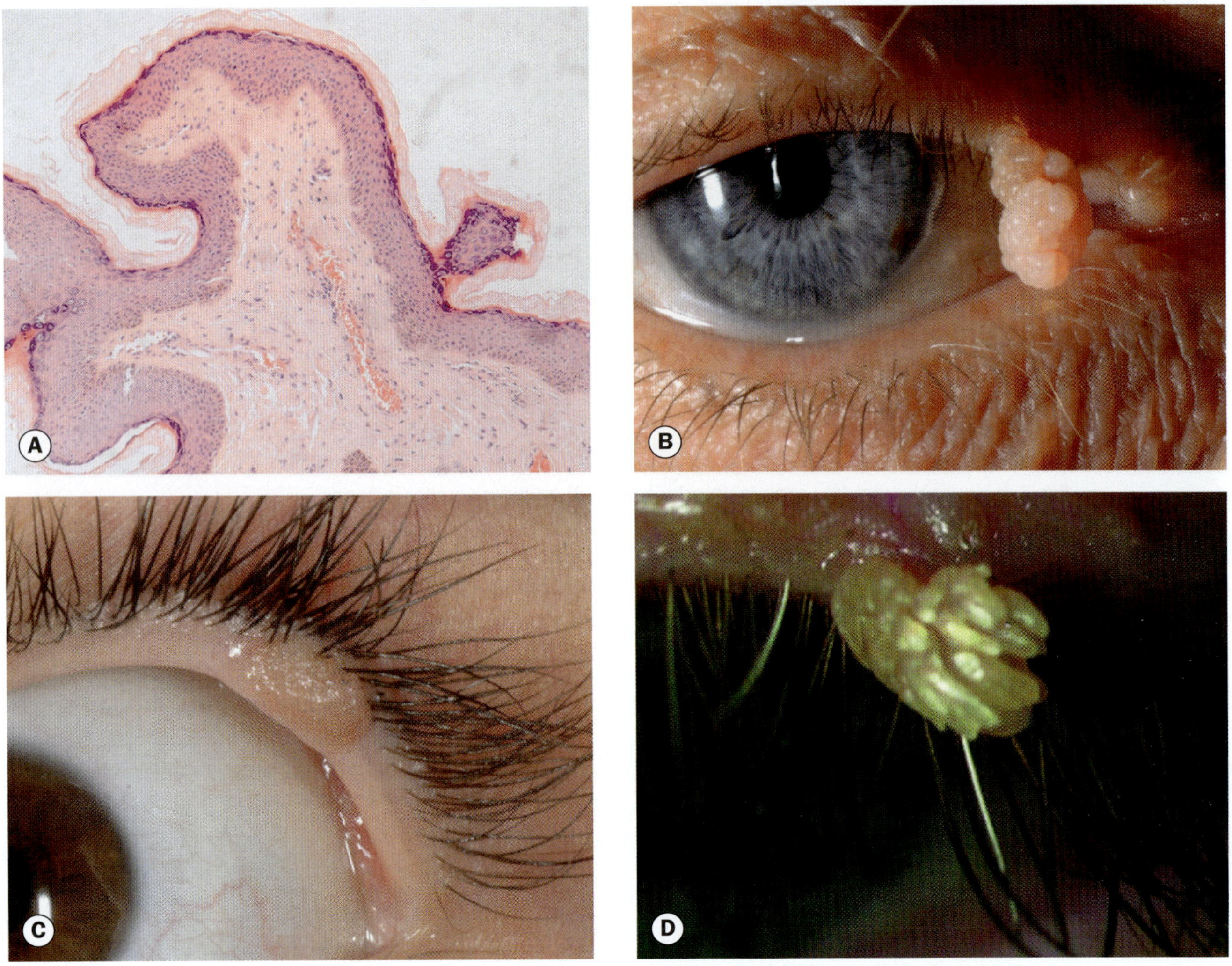

Fig. 2.5 Squamous cell papilloma. **(A)** Histopathology showing finger-like projections of fibrovascular connective tissue covered by irregular acanthotic and hyperkeratotic squamous epithelium; **(B)** pedunculated 'skin tag'; **(C)** sessile lesion; **(D)** hyperkeratotic filiform lesion.

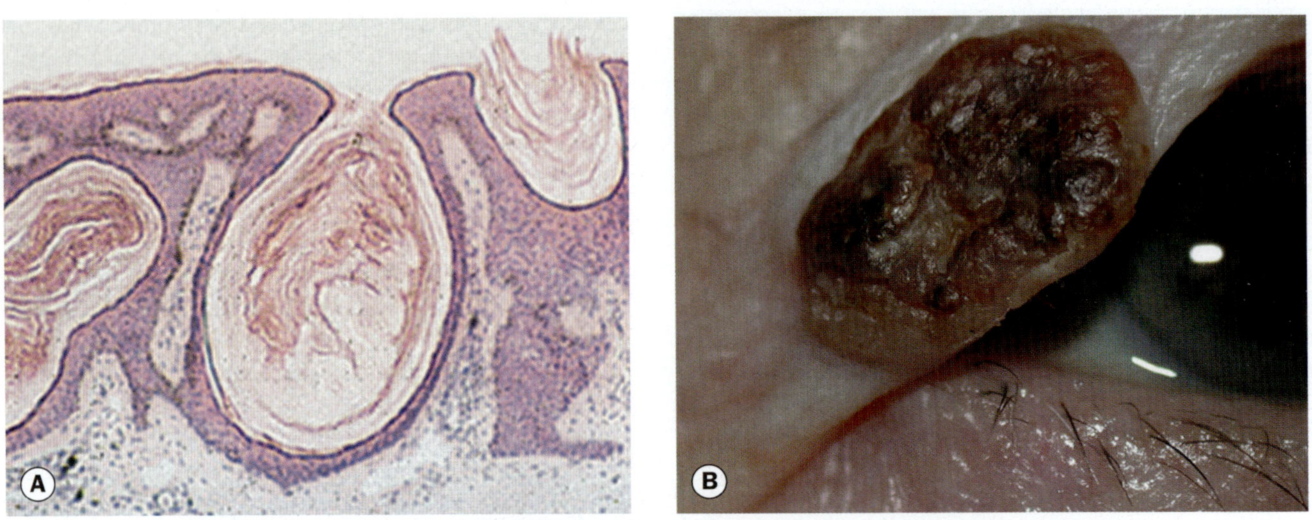

Fig. 2.6 Basal cell papilloma. **(A)** Histopathology showing an elevated expansion of the epidermis with proliferation from basal cells – horn cysts and pseudo-horn cysts are present; **(B)** typical 'stuck-on' appearance. *(Courtesy of A Pearson – fig. B.)*

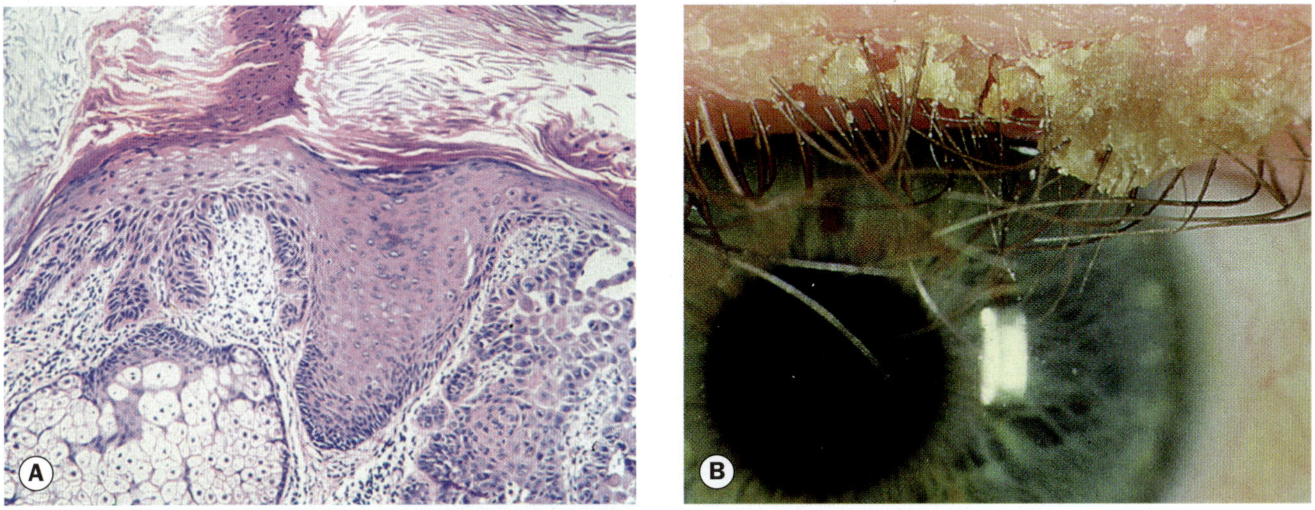

Fig. 2.7 Actinic keratosis. **(A)** Histopathology showing irregular dysplastic epidermis with hyperkeratosis and parakeratosis; **(B)** clinical appearance. *(Courtesy of J Harry and G Misson, from* Clinical Ophthalmic Pathology, *Butterworth-Heinemann 2001 – fig. A.)*

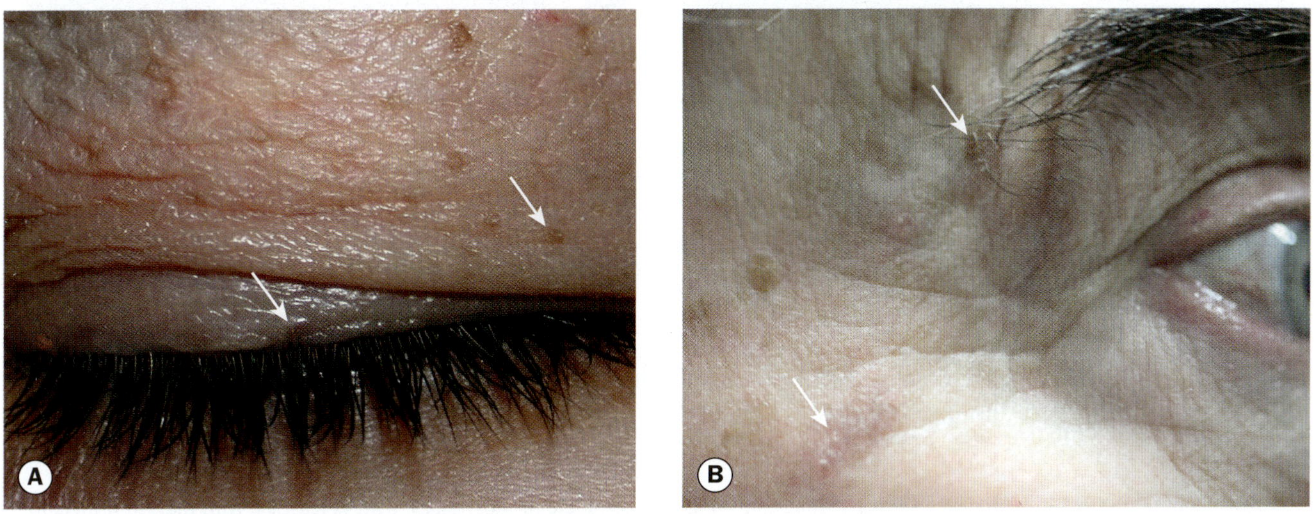

Fig. 2.8 Benign pigmented lesions. **(A)** Freckle (ephelis) (arrows); **(B)** lentigo (arrows).

Lentigo

Lentigo (plural: lentigines) are harmless flat, brownish lesions with a clearly defined scalloped edge that are larger than freckles. They may have a dry or slightly scaly surface. Solar lentigines occur in middle-aged individuals and result from sun damage. They are persistent and do not disappear in the winter (Fig. 2.8B). Histopathology shows a proliferation of keratinocytes and an increase in the number of melanocytes.

Congenital melanocytic naevus

Congenital naevi are uncommon and histologically resemble their acquired counterparts (see below). They are usually small and of uniform colour. Rare variants include a 'kissing' or split naevus that involves the upper and lower eyelid (Fig. 2.9A) and may occasionally contain numerous hairs (Fig. 2.9B), and a large lesion covering the face (Fig. 2.9C) or an extensive area of the body ('giant hairy naevus'). Large lesions have the potential for malignant transformation (up to 15%). Treatment, if necessary, involves complete surgical excision.

Acquired melanocytic naevus

Diagnosis

The clinical appearance and potential for malignant transformation of a naevus is determined by the histological location within the skin.

- **Junctional** naevus occurs in young individuals as a uniformly brown macule or plaque (Fig. 2.10A). The naevus cells are located at the junction of the epidermis and dermis and have a low potential for malignant transformation (Fig. 2.10B).
- **Compound** naevus occurs in middle age as a raised papular lesion. The shade of pigment varies from light tan to dark

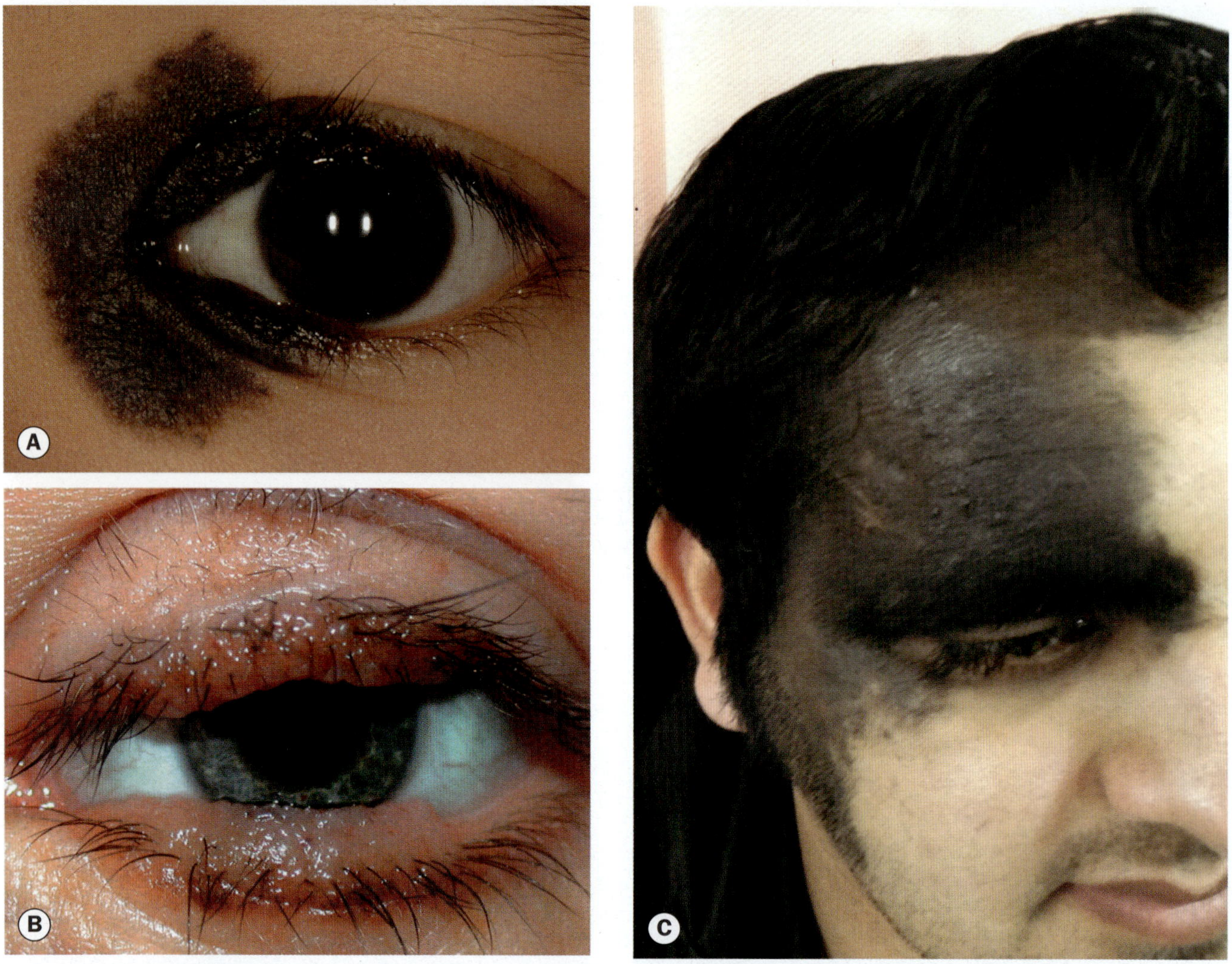

Fig. 2.9 Congenital melanocytic naevus. **(A)** Split naevus; **(B)** split naevus containing hair; **(C)** large facial naevus. *(Courtesy of A Pearson – fig. B; RSR Naik – fig. C.)*

brown but tends to be relatively uniform throughout (Fig. 2.10C). The naevus cells extend from the epidermis into the dermis (Fig. 2.10D). It has a low malignant potential related to the junctional component.

- **Intradermal** naevus, the most common, typically occurs in older patients. It is a papillomatous lesion, with little or no pigmentation (Fig. 2.10E). Histologically, naevus cells are confined to the dermis and have no malignant potential (Fig. 2.10F).
- **Variants** of naevus include balloon cell naevus, halo naevus, Spitz naevus (juvenile melanomas) and dysplastic naevus (atypical moles). Multiple dysplastic naevi constitute the dysplastic naevus syndrome (atypical mole syndrome – AMS). Individuals with AMS are at increased risk of developing conjunctival and uveal naevi and cutaneous, conjunctival and uveal melanomas.

Treatment

Treatment is indicated for cosmesis or if the naevus has unusual features that raise concern about malignancy. Excision should be complete in most cases, with at least a 3 mm margin if melanoma is suspected.

BENIGN ADNEXAL TUMOURS

Syringoma

Syringomas are benign proliferations arising from eccrine sweat glands. They are characterized by small papules that are often multiple and bilateral (Fig. 2.11A).

Pilomatricoma

Pilomatricoma (pilomatrixoma, calcifying epithelioma of Malherbe) is derived from the germinal matrix cells of the hair bulb and is the commonest hair follicle proliferation seen by ophthalmologists. It affects children and young adults and is more common in females. Histopathology shows irregular epithelial islands exhibiting viable basophilic cells at the periphery and degenerate 'shadow' cells centrally. Clinically it appears as a mobile purplish

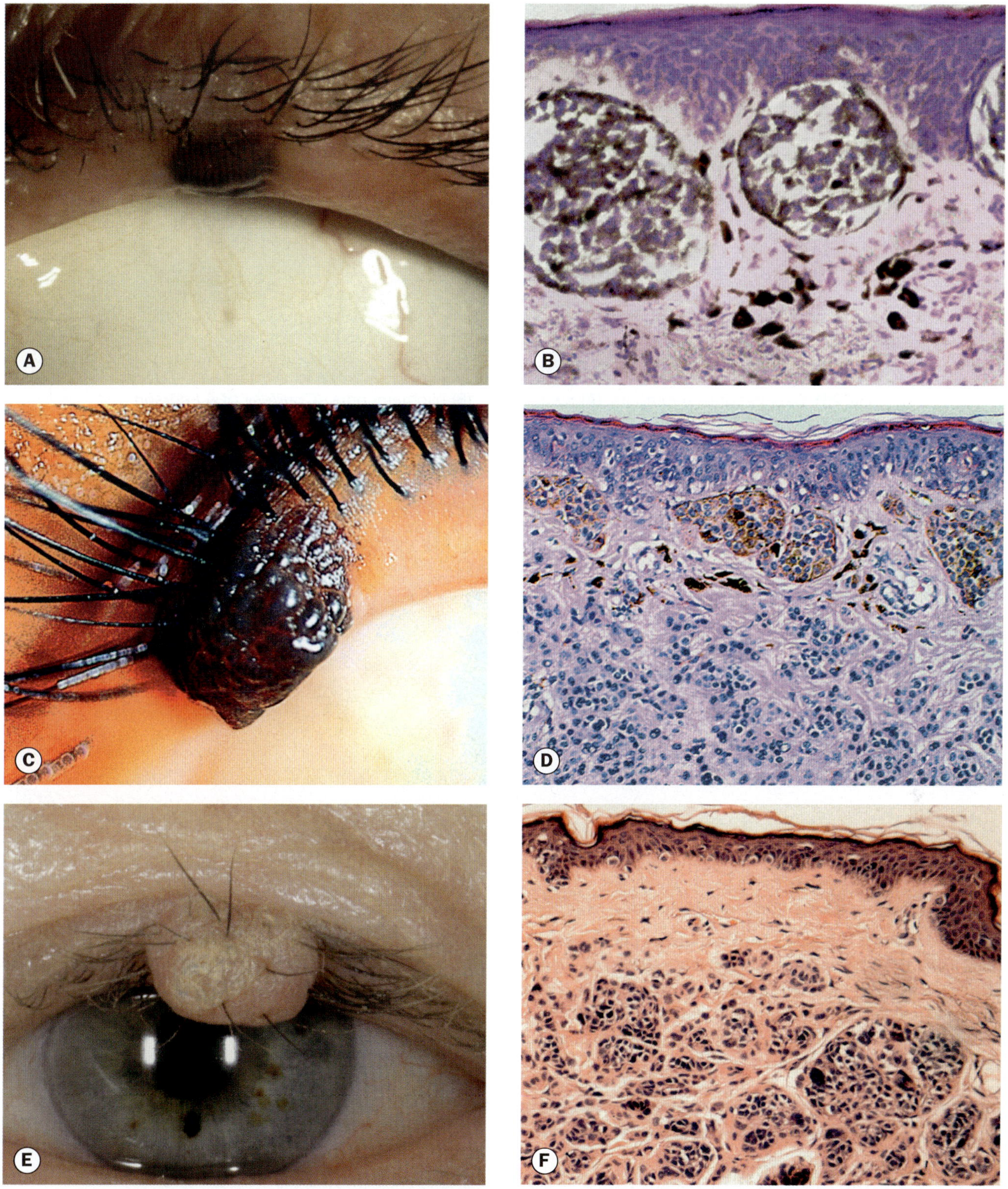

Fig. 2.10 Acquired melanocytic naevus. **(A)** Junctional naevus; **(B)** histopathology showing heavily pigmented naevus cells at the epidermal/dermal junction; **(C)** compound naevus; **(D)** histopathology showing naevus cells both at the epidermal/dermal junction and within the dermis; **(E)** intradermal naevus showing little pigmentation and eccentric lashes; **(F)** histopathology showing naevus cells within the dermis separated from the epidermis by a clear zone.

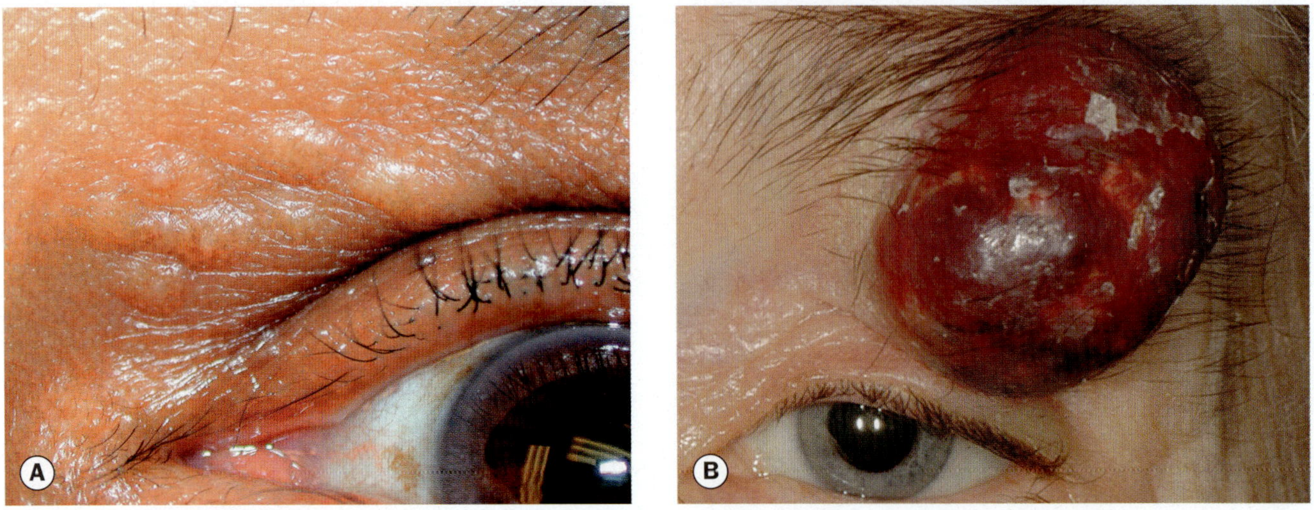

Fig. 2.11 Benign adnexal tumours. **(A)** Syringomas; **(B)** pilomatricoma. *(Courtesy of A Pearson – fig. A.)*

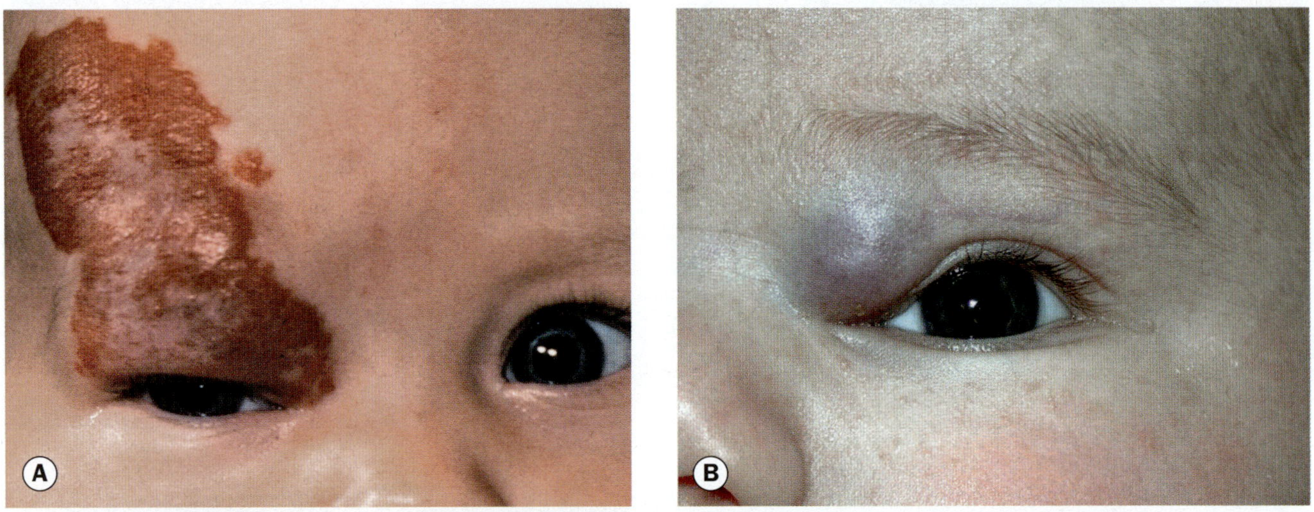

Fig. 2.12 Capillary haemangioma. **(A)** Unilateral, raised and bright red lesion; **(B)** mechanical ptosis.

dermal nodule that may have a hard consistency due to calcification (Fig. 2.11B). Calcification is frequently present and there is often a foreign body giant cell reaction. Malignant change is rare. The lesion is usually removed surgically. Other less common disorders of hair follicle proliferation include trichofolliculoma, trichoepithelioma and trichilemmoma.

MISCELLANEOUS BENIGN TUMOURS

Capillary haemangioma

Capillary haemangioma (strawberry naevus) is one of the most common tumours of infancy. It is three times as common in girls as boys. Histopathology shows proliferation of varying-sized vascular channels in the dermis and subcutaneous tissue. It presents shortly after birth as a unilateral, raised bright red lesion (Fig. 2.12A), usually in the upper lid. A deeper lesion appears purplish (Fig. 2.12B). The lesion blanches on pressure and may swell on crying. Ptosis is frequent and there may be orbital extension (see Ch. 4). Occasionally the lesion may involve the skin of the face and some patients have strawberry naevi on other parts of the body. It is important to be aware of an association between multiple cutaneous lesions and visceral haemangiomas and to consider systemic assessment in appropriate cases. Treatment is described in Chapter 4.

TIP A capillary haemangioma can be easily and successfully treated by regular application of a topical beta-blocker to the affected lesion.

Port-wine stain

Introduction

Port-wine stain (naevus flammeus) is a congenital malformation of vessels within the superficial dermis, consisting histopathologically

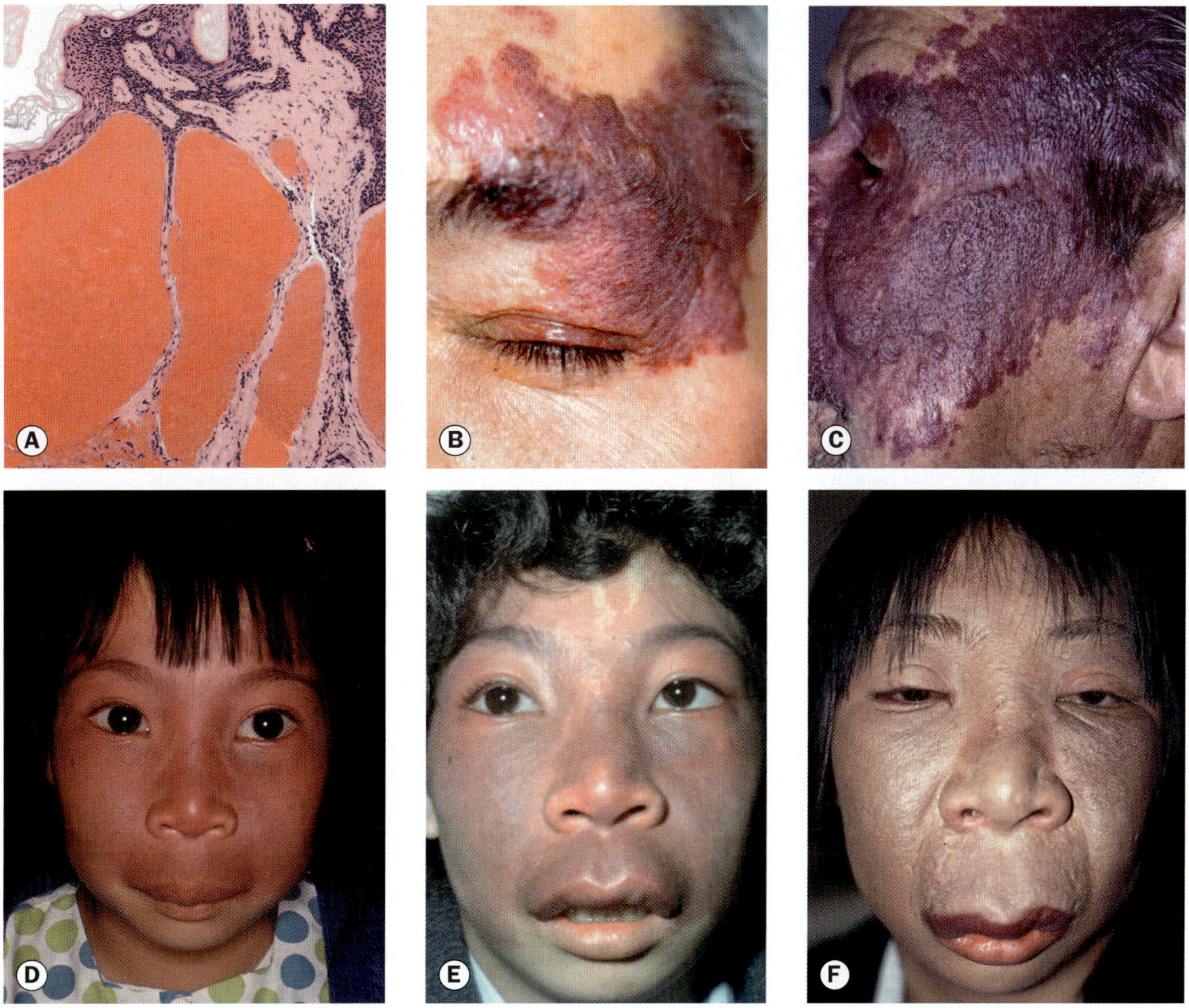

Fig. 2.13 Port-wine stain. **(A)** Histopathology showing widely dilated blood-filled spaces separated by fibrous septa; **(B)** and **(C)** clinical appearance; **(D–F)** progression of port-wine stain over time, with associated underlying soft tissue hypertrophy.

of vascular spaces of varying calibre separated by thin fibrous septa (Fig. 2.13A). About 10% have associated ocular or CNS involvement, including Sturge–Weber (see below) and other defined syndromes.

Diagnosis

Port-wine stain manifests clinically as a sharply demarcated soft pink patch that does not blanch with pressure, most frequently located on the face. It is usually unilateral and tends to be aligned with the skin area supplied by one or more divisions of the trigeminal nerve (Fig. 2.13B and C). Darkening to red or purple takes place with age and there is commonly associated soft tissue hypertrophy (Fig. 2.13D–F). Bleeding may occur from focal overlying lobulations (pyogenic granulomas – see below).

Treatment

Treatment with laser (e.g. pulsed-dye) is effective in decreasing skin discoloration, particularly if undertaken early. Topical preparations such as imiquimod and rapamycin, alone or with adjuvant laser, show promise. Soft tissue debulking is used in a small number of cases. Screening for glaucoma should begin in infancy. Systemic investigation is considered in some patients, particularly those with a lesion of the lumbar area.

Sturge–Weber syndrome

Sturge–Weber syndrome (encephalotrigeminal angiomatosis) is a congenital, sporadic phacomatosis.

- **Port-wine stain**, extending over the area corresponding to the distribution of one or more branches of the trigeminal nerve.
- **Leptomeningeal haemangioma** involving the ipsilateral parietal or occipital region may cause contralateral focal or generalized seizures, hemiparesis or hemianopia.
- **Ocular** features may include ipsilateral glaucoma, episcleral haemangioma, iris heterochromia and diffuse choroidal haemangioma (see Ch. 20).

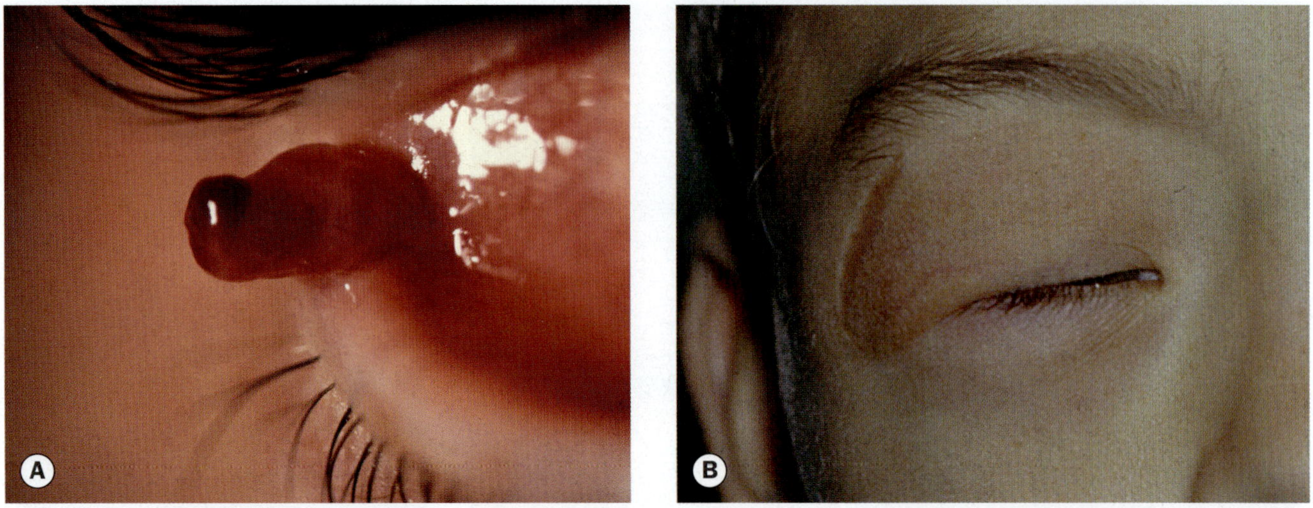

Fig. 2.14 Other benign tumours. **(A)** Pyogenic granuloma of the tarsal surface of the lower lid; **(B)** plexiform neurofibroma – characteristic S-shaped upper lid.

Pyogenic granuloma

Pyogenic granuloma is a rapidly growing vascularized proliferation of granulation tissue that is usually antedated by surgery, trauma or infection, although some cases are idiopathic. Clinically there is a painful, rapidly growing, vascular granulating polypoidal lesion (Fig. 2.14A) that may bleed following relatively trivial trauma. Cutaneous lesions should be excised. Conjunctival pyogenic granuloma is discussed in Chapter 6.

Neurofibroma

Cutaneous neurofibromas are benign nerve tumours, usually nodular or pedunculated, that can be found anywhere on the skin. An isolated neurofibroma is common in normal individuals, but if multiple lesions are present, neurofibromatosis (see Ch. 19) should be excluded. Plexiform neurofibromas typically present in childhood as a manifestation of neurofibromatosis type 1 with a characteristic S-shaped deformity of the upper eyelid (Fig. 2.14B). Treatment of solitary lesions involves simple excision, but removal of the more diffuse plexiform lesions may be difficult.

MALIGNANT TUMOURS

The treatment of malignant eyelid tumours in general is discussed at the end of this section.

Rare predisposing conditions

Young patients who suffer from one of the following conditions may develop eyelid malignancies.

- **Xeroderma pigmentosum** is characterized by skin damage on exposure to sunlight, leading to progressive cutaneous abnormalities (Fig. 2.15A). More than 90% have ocular or periocular involvement and 65% experience photophobia. It is inherited in an autosomal recessive (AR) fashion. Affected patients have a bird-like facial appearance and a significant propensity to the development of basal cell carcinoma (BCC), squamous cell carcinoma (SCC) and melanoma, which are commonly multiple. Conjunctival malignancies have also been reported.
- **Gorlin–Goltz syndrome** (naevoid BCC syndrome) is a rare autosomal dominant (AD) disorder characterized by extensive congenital deformities of the eye, face, bone and central nervous system. Many patients develop multiple small BCC during the second decade of life (Fig. 2.15B) and are also predisposed to medulloblastoma, breast carcinoma and Hodgkin lymphoma.
- **Muir–Torre syndrome** is a rare AD condition that predisposes to cutaneous and internal malignancies. Cutaneous tumours include BCC, sebaceous gland carcinoma and keratoacanthoma. Colorectal and genitourinary carcinomas are the most common systemic tumours.
- **Bazex syndrome** can be used to describe two distinct conditions: Bazex–Dupré–Christol syndrome, an X-linked dominant condition characterized by multiple BCCs, commonly facial including the eyelids, associated with skin changes including follicular indentations without hairs on extensor surfaces (follicular atrophoderma), hypohidrosis and hypotrichosis and acrokeratosis paraneoplastica of Bazex, in which eczema-like and psoriasiform lesions are associated with an underlying malignancy of the upper respiratory or digestive tract.
- **Other predispositions** include immunosuppression, prior retinoblastoma and albinism.

Basal cell carcinoma

Introduction

BCC is the most common human malignancy and typically affects older people. The most important risk factors are fair

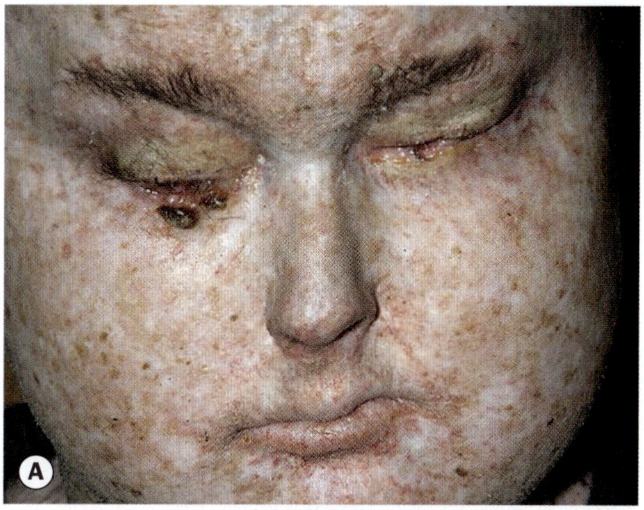
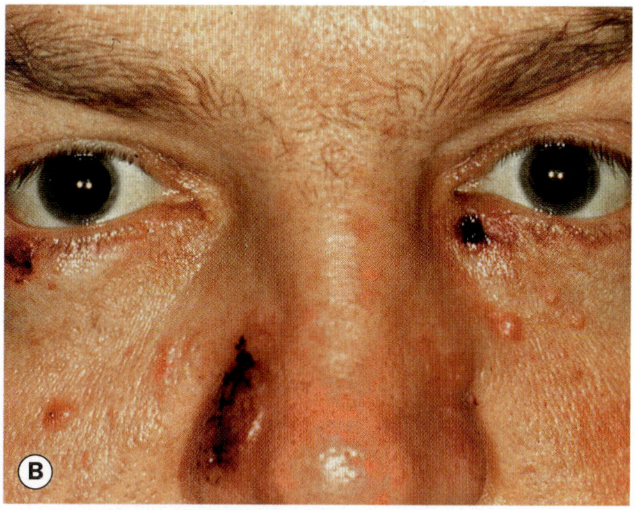

Fig. 2.15 Predispositions to eyelid malignancies. **(A)** Xeroderma pigmentosum; **(B)** Gorlin–Goltz syndrome. *(Courtesy of J Krachmer, M Mannis and E Holland, from* Cornea*, Mosby 2005 – fig. B.)*

skin, inability to tan and chronic exposure to sunlight. Ninety per cent of cases occur in the head and neck and about 10% of these involve the eyelid. BCC is by far the most common malignant eyelid tumour, accounting for 90% of all cases. It most frequently arises from the lower eyelid, followed in relative frequency by the medial canthus, upper eyelid and lateral canthus. Madarosis is commonly seen in association with the tumour, which is slow-growing and locally invasive, but non-metastasizing. Tumours located near the medial canthus are more prone to invade the orbit and sinuses, are more difficult to manage than those arising elsewhere and carry the greatest risk of recurrence. Tumours that recur following incomplete treatment tend to be more aggressive.

Histopathology

The tumour arises from the cells that form the basal layer of the epidermis. The cells proliferate downwards (Fig. 2.16A) and characteristically exhibit palisading at the periphery of a tumour lobule of cells (Fig. 2.16B). Squamous differentiation with the production of keratin results in a hyperkeratotic type of BCC. There can also be sebaceous and adenoid differentiation while the growth of elongated strands and islands of cells embedded in a dense fibrous stroma result in a sclerosing (morphoeic) type of tumour.

Clinical features

Eyelid BCC conforms to one of the morphological patterns below.

- **Nodular BCC** is a shiny, firm, pearly nodule with small overlying dilated blood vessels. Initially, growth is slow and it may take the tumour 1–2 years to reach a diameter of 0.5 cm (Fig. 2.16C and D).
- **Nodulo-ulcerative BCC (rodent ulcer)** is centrally ulcerated with pearly raised rolled edges and dilated and irregular blood vessels (telangiectasis) over its lateral margins (Fig. 2.16E). With time it may erode a large portion of the eyelid (Fig. 2.16F).
- **Sclerosing (morphoeic) BCC** is less common and may be difficult to diagnose because it infiltrates laterally beneath the epidermis as an indurated plaque (Fig. 2.16G and H). The margins of the tumour may be impossible to delineate clinically and the lesion tends to be much more extensive on palpation than inspection. On cursory examination a sclerosing BCC may simulate a localized area of chronic blepharitis.
- **Other types** not usually found on the lid are cystic, adenoid, pigmented and multiple superficial.

TIP Sclerosing BCC can mimic a localized area of unilateral chronic blepharitis.

Squamous cell carcinoma

Introduction

SCC is a much less common, but typically more aggressive tumour than BCC, with metastasis to regional lymph nodes in about 20% of cases. Histopathology shows dysplastic changes throughout the thickness of the epidermis (Fig. 2.17A). Careful surveillance of regional lymph nodes is therefore an important aspect of initial management. The tumour may also exhibit perineural spread to the intracranial cavity via the orbit. SCC accounts for 5–10% of eyelid malignancies and may arise *de novo* or from pre-existing actinic keratosis or carcinoma *in situ* (Bowen disease, intraepidermal carcinoma – Fig. 2.17B). Immunocompromised individuals, such as those with acquired immunodeficiency syndrome (AIDS) or following renal transplantation are at increased risk, as are those with a predisposing syndrome such as xeroderma pigmentosum. The tumour has a predilection for the lower eyelid and the lid margin. It occurs most commonly in older individuals with a fair complexion and a history of chronic sun exposure. The diagnosis of SCC may sometimes be difficult because

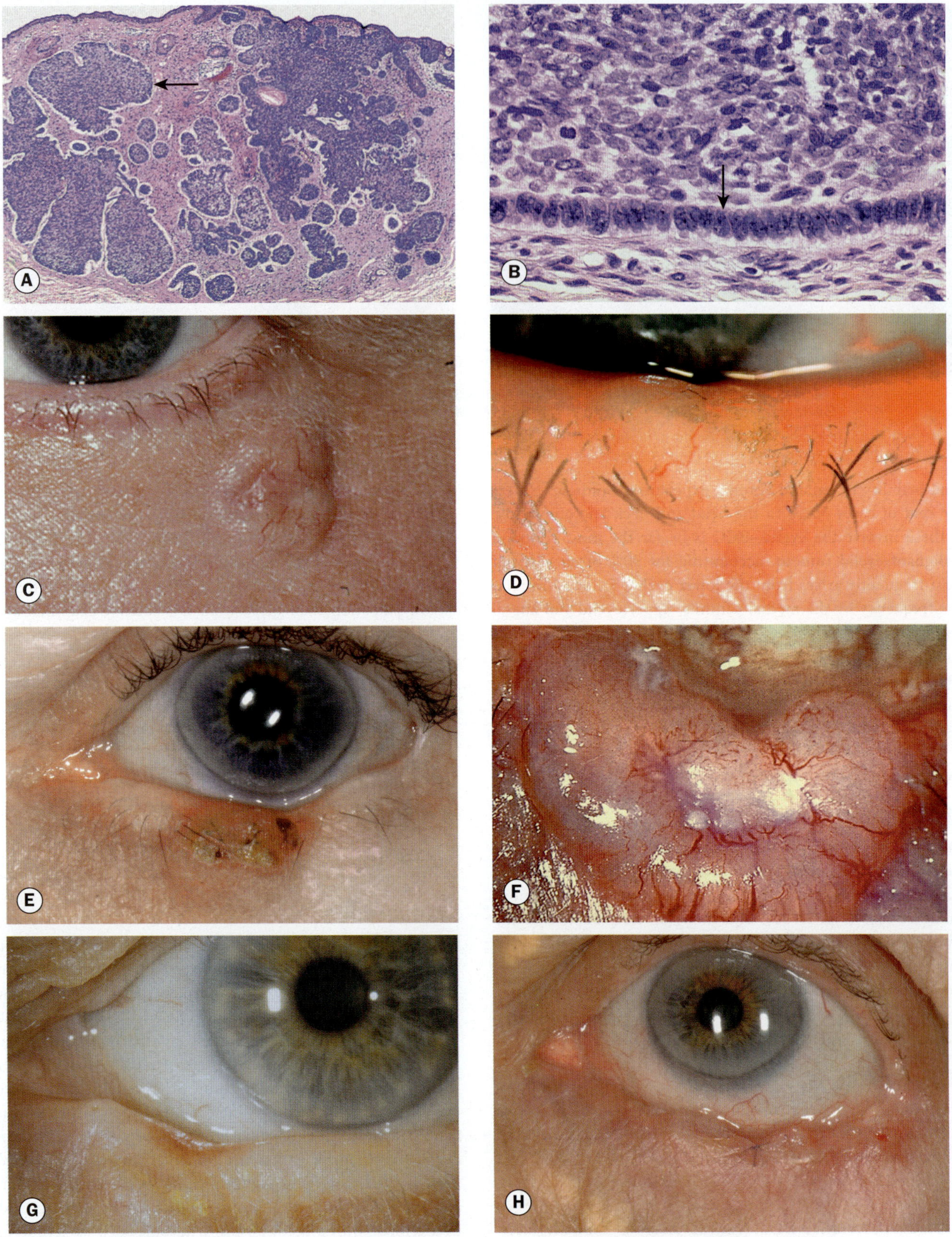

Fig. 2.16 Basal cell carcinoma. **(A)** Histopathology showing downward proliferation of lobules of basophilic (blue) cells (arrow); **(B)** palisading of cells at the periphery of a tumour lobule (arrow); **(C)** small lid margin tumour; **(D)** larger nodular tumour; **(E)** rodent ulcer; **(F)** large rodent ulcer; **(G)** sclerosing tumour; **(H)** extensive sclerosing tumour.

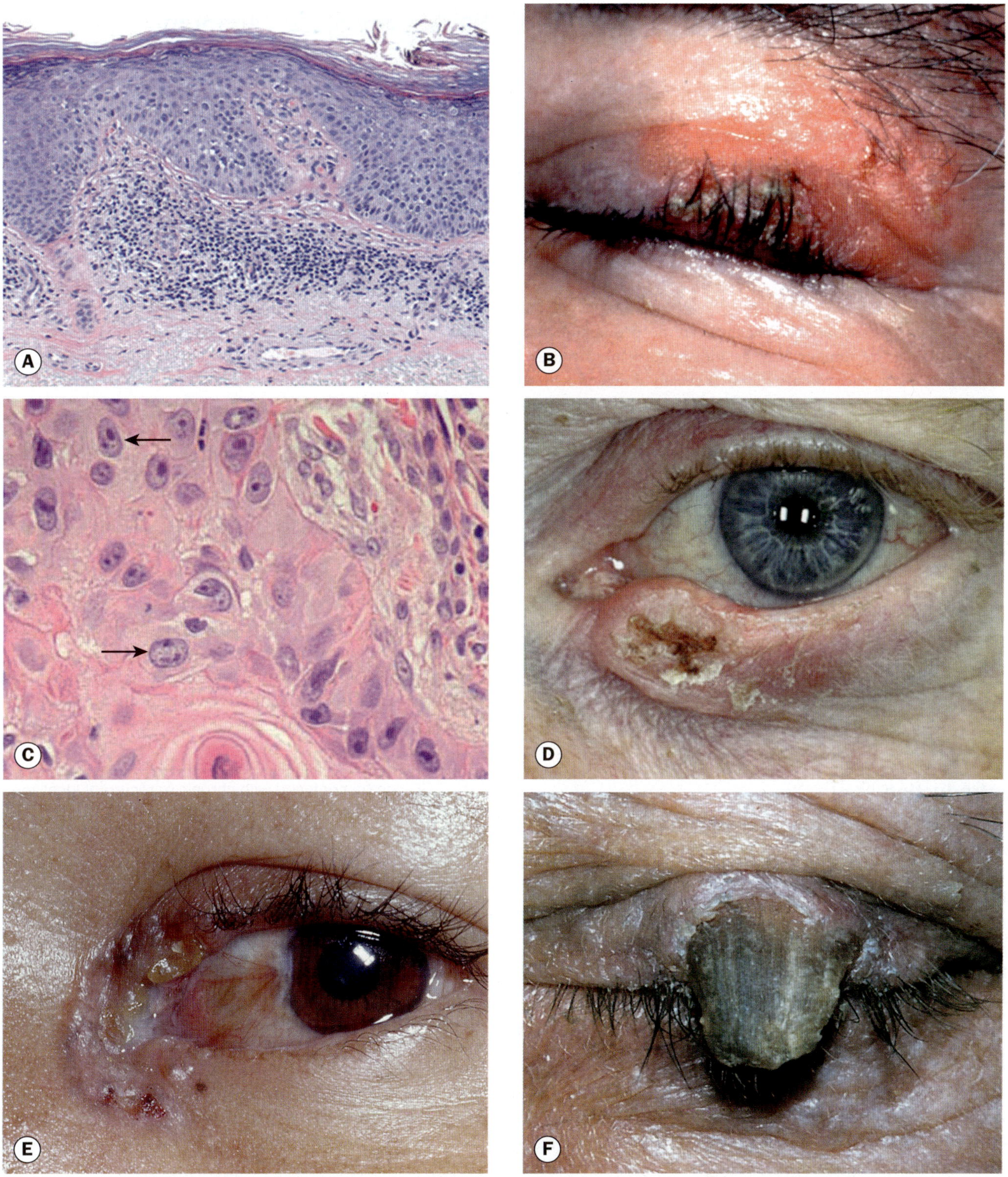

Fig. 2.17 Squamous cell carcinoma. **(A)** Histopathology of carcinoma *in situ* showing dysplastic changes throughout the thickness of the epidermis; **(B)** Bowen disease; **(C)** histopathology of squamous cell carcinoma showing acanthotic squamous epithelium and eosinophilic (pink) islands of dysplastic squamous epithelium within the dermis. Note the large nucleus with more than one large purple nucleoli (arrows); **(D)** nodular tumour with surface keratosis; **(E)** ulcerating tumour; **(F)** cutaneous horn. *(Courtesy of ADN Murray – fig. E.)*

certain ostensibly benign lesions such as keratoacanthoma and cutaneous horn may reveal histological evidence of invasive SCC at deeper levels of sectioning.

Histopathology

The tumour arises from the squamous cell layer of the epidermis. It is composed of variably sized groups of atypical epithelial cells with prominent nuclei and abundant eosinophilic cytoplasm within the dermis (Fig. 2.17C). Well-differentiated tumours may show characteristic keratin 'pearls' and intercellular bridges (desmosomes).

Clinical features

The clinical types are variable and there are no pathognomonic characteristics. The tumour may be indistinguishable clinically from a BCC but surface vascularization is usually absent, growth is more rapid and hyperkeratosis is more common.

- **Nodular SCC** is characterized by a hyperkeratotic nodule that may develop crusting, erosions and fissures (Fig. 2.17D).
- **Ulcerating SCC** has a red base and sharply defined, indurated and everted borders, but pearly margins and telangiectasia are not usually present (Fig. 2.17E).
- **Cutaneous horn** with underlying invasive SCC (Fig. 2.17F).

TIP Ostensibly benign lesions such as keratoacanthoma and cutaneous horn may reveal histological evidence of SCC in deeper levels of sectioning.

Keratoacanthoma

Introduction

Keratoacanthoma is a rare, rapidly growing but subsequently regressing tumour that usually occurs in fair-skinned individuals with a history of chronic sun exposure. Immunosuppressive therapy is also a predisposing factor. Invasion and metastasis are rare. Histopathological examination reveals irregular thickened epidermis surrounded by acanthotic squamous epithelium. A sharp transition from the thickened involved area to normal adjacent epidermis is referred to as shoulder formation (Fig. 2.18A) and a keratin-filled crater may be seen.

Diagnosis

A pink dome-shaped hyperkeratotic lesion develops, often on the lower lid (Fig. 2.18B) and may double or treble in size within weeks (Fig. 2.18C). Growth then ceases for 2–3 months, after which spontaneous involution occurs, when a keratin-filled crater may develop (Fig. 2.18D). Complete involution may take up to a year and usually leaves an unsightly scar.

Treatment

Treatment involves complete surgical excision with a margin of at least 3 mm or utilizing Mohs surgery. Radiotherapy, cryotherapy or local chemotherapy are sometimes used.

Sebaceous gland carcinoma

Introduction

Sebaceous gland carcinoma (SGC) is a very rare, slowly growing tumour that most frequently affects the elderly, with a predisposition for females. It usually arises from the meibomian glands, although on occasion it may arise from the glands of Zeis or elsewhere. Histopathology demonstrates lobules of cells with pale foamy vacuolated lipid-containing cytoplasm and large hyperchromatic nuclei. Pagetoid spread refers to extension of a tumour within the epithelium and is not uncommon. Overall mortality is 5–10%. Adverse prognostic features include upper lid involvement, tumour size of 10 mm or more and duration of symptoms of more than 6 months.

Clinical features

In contrast to BCC and SCC, SGC occurs more commonly on the upper eyelid where meibomian glands are more numerous. There may be simultaneous involvement of the lower and upper lid on one side (5%).

- **Yellowish material** within the tumour is highly suggestive of SGC.
- **Nodular SGC** presents as a discrete, hard nodule, most commonly within the upper tarsal plate (Fig. 2.19A) and may exhibit yellow discoloration due to the presence of lipid; it can be mistaken for a chalazion.
- **Spreading SGC** infiltrates into the dermis and causes a diffuse thickening of the lid margin (Fig. 2.19B) often with eyelash distortion and loss and can be mistaken for blepharitis.

TIP SGC can be confused with chronic or recurrent localized meibomian gland inflammation.

Lentigo maligna and melanoma

Introduction

Melanoma rarely develops on the eyelids but is potentially lethal. Although pigmentation is a hallmark of skin melanomas, half of lid melanomas are non-pigmented and this may give rise to diagnostic difficulty. Features suggestive of melanoma include recent onset of a pigmented lesion, change in an existing pigmented lesion, irregular margins, asymmetrical shape, colour change or presence of multiple colours and diameter greater than 6 mm.

Lentigo maligna

Lentigo maligna (melanoma *in situ*, intraepidermal melanoma, Hutchinson freckle) is an uncommon condition that develops in sun-damaged skin in elderly individuals (Fig. 2.20A). Malignant melanoma arises within lentigo maligna in 3–10% of cases. Histopathology shows intraepidermal proliferation of spindle-shaped atypical melanocytes replacing the basal layer of the epidermis. Clinically lentigo maligna presents as a slowly expanding

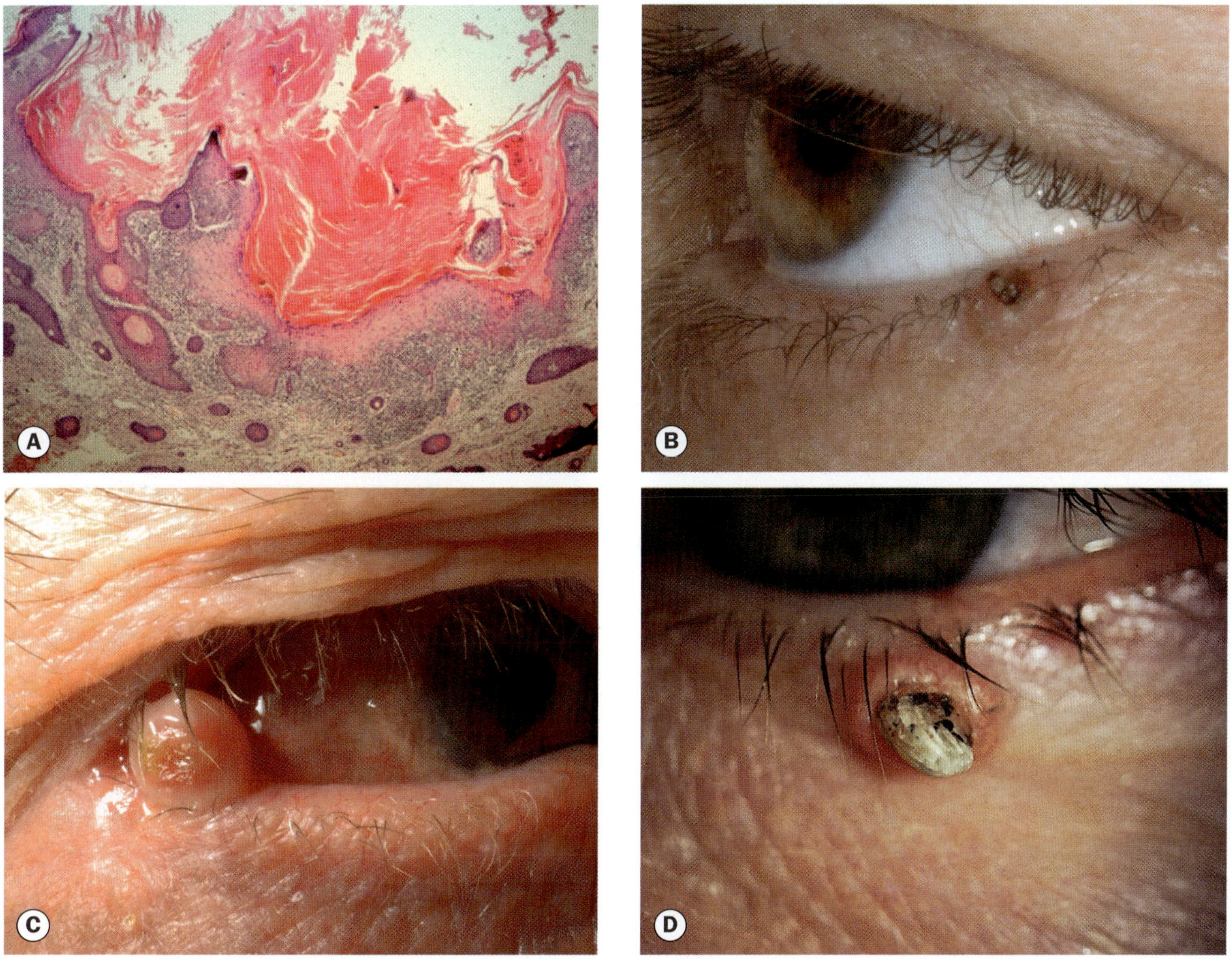

Fig. 2.18 Keratoacanthoma. **(A)** Histopathology showing irregularly thickened eosinophilic epidermis with a keratin-containing cup; **(B)** small nodule on lid margin; **(C)** hyperkeratotic nodule; **(D)** keratin-filled crater during involution.

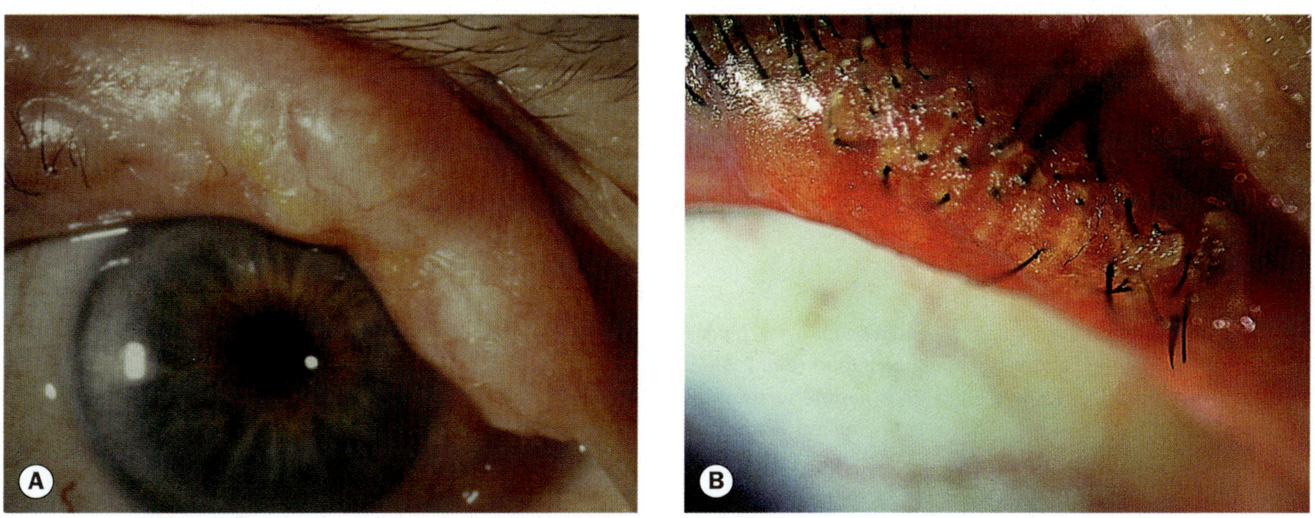

Fig. 2.19 Sebaceous gland carcinoma. **(A)** Nodular tumour; **(B)** spreading tumour.

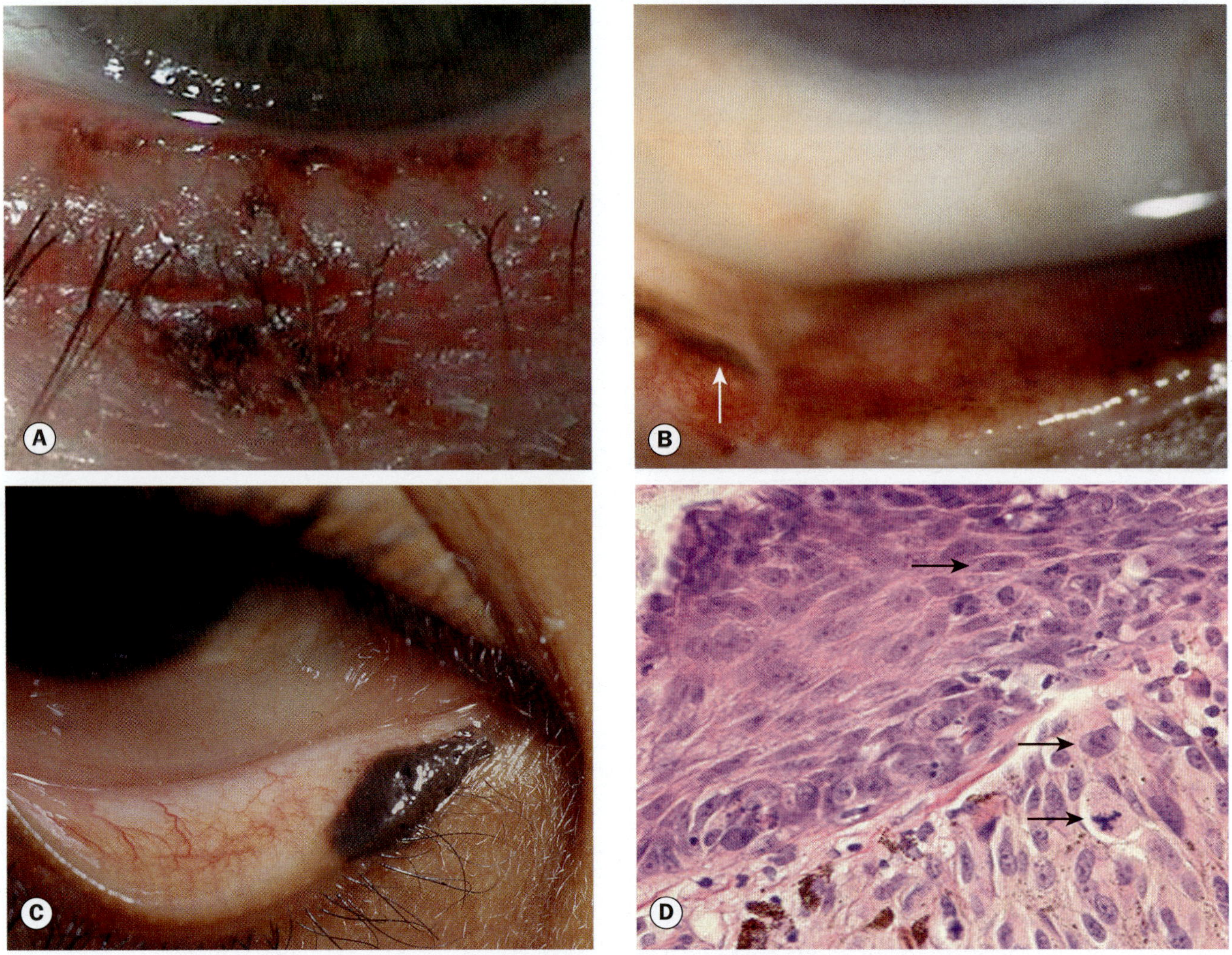

Fig. 2.20 Melanoma. **(A)** Clinical appearance of early lentigo maligna; **(B)** melanoma (arrow) arising from lentigo maligna; **(C)** spreading melanoma onto tarsal conjunctiva; **(D)** histopathology showing melanoma cells (arrows) within the dermis. Note the large nucleus with irregular nuclear border and large, purple nucleoli. *(Courtesy of ADN Murray – fig. C.)*

pigmented macule with an irregular border and variable pigmentation. Nodular thickening and areas of irregular pigmentation are highly suggestive of malignant transformation (Fig. 2.20B).Treatment is usually by complete excision with large margins. Imiquimod 5% topical cream is a reasonable alternative in those with extensive involvement or in those who decline surgery.

Melanoma

Superficial spreading melanoma is characterized by a plaque with an irregular outline and variable pigmentation (Fig. 2.20C). Nodular melanoma is typically a blue–black nodule surrounded by normal skin. Histopathology shows large atypical epithelioid melanocytes scattered throughout the epidermis and invading the dermis (Fig. 2.20D). Treatment is usually by wide excision and may include local lymph node removal. Early detection carries a good prognosis and surgical excision is often curative, but long-term survival for patients with metastatic disease is poor. Radiotherapy and chemotherapy are of limited efficacy. However, new approaches using immunotherapy (ipilimumab, nivolumab, pembrolizumab, talimogene laherparepvec) are showing considerable promise. Targeted treatment for advanced melanoma exhibiting the *BRAF* gene is also available (verumurafenib, dadrafenib, trametinib). Research is under way to produce a vaccine for cutaneous melanoma.

Merkel cell carcinoma

Merkel cells are a form of sensory receptor concerned with light touch. Merkel cell carcinoma is a rapidly growing, highly malignant tumour that typically affects older adults. Its rarity may lead to difficulty in diagnosis and delay in treatment and 50% of patients have metastatic spread by presentation. Factors involved in the development include exposure to the Merkel cell polyomavirus, a weakened immune system and sun exposure. Histopathology shows a sheet of Merkel cells. A violaceous, well-demarcated nodule with intact overlying skin is seen, most frequently involving

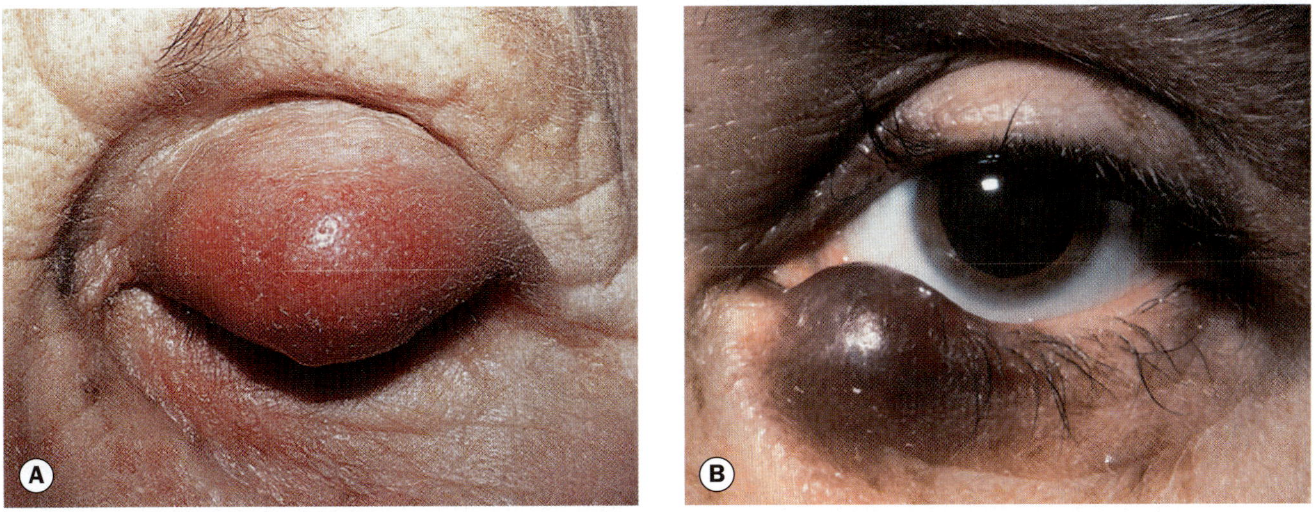

Fig. 2.21 Rare malignant tumours. **(A)** Merkel cell carcinoma; **(B)** Kaposi sarcoma.

the upper eyelid (Fig. 2.21A). Treatment is by excision, often with adjuvant therapy.

Kaposi sarcoma

Kaposi sarcoma is a vascular tumour that typically affects individuals with AIDS. Many patients have advanced systemic disease although in some instances the tumour may be the only clinical manifestation of human immunodeficiency virus (HIV) infection. Histopathology shows proliferating spindle cells, vascular channels and inflammatory cells within the dermis. Clinically a pink, red-violet to brown lesion (Fig. 2.21B) develops, which may be mistaken for a haematoma or naevus. Treatment is by radiotherapy or excision and by optimal control of AIDS.

Treatment of malignant tumours

Biopsy

Biopsy can be either *incisional*, using a blade or a biopsy punch, in which only part of the lesion is removed for histological diagnosis, or *excisional*, in which the entire lesion is removed. The latter may consist of shave excision using a blade to remove shallow epithelial tumours, such as a papilloma and seborrhoeic keratosis, or full-thickness skin excision for tumours that are not confined to the epidermis.

Surgical excision

Surgical excision aims to remove the entire tumour with preservation of as much normal tissue as possible. Smaller tumours can be removed via an excision biopsy and the defect closed directly, whilst awaiting histological confirmation of complete clearance. Most small BCCs can be cured by excision of the tumour together with a 2–4 mm margin of clinically normal tissue. More radical surgical excision is required for a large BCC and aggressive tumours such as SCC, SGC and melanoma. It may not be possible to close all defects at the time of initial removal, but it is necessary to ensure complete clearance of tumour prior to undertaking any reconstruction. There are several options for the coordination of histopathological diagnosis and tumour clearance with excision.

- **Conventional paraffin-embedded specimen.** Rapid processing can reduce the interval to confirmation of histological clearance but still requires that reconstruction be performed as a separate procedure. Faster confirmation can be achieved using either frozen-section control or micrographic surgery (see next) and reconstruction can then take place on the same day.
- **Standard frozen section** involves histological examination of the margins of the excised specimen at the time of surgery to ensure that they are tumour-free. If no tumour cells are detected, the eyelid is reconstructed on the same day. However, if residual tumour is present, further excision is performed at the appropriate edge of the surgical site until no tumour is detected.
- **Mohs micrographic surgery** involves layered excision of the tumour; specimens are usually examined frozen. Processing of each layer enables a map of the edges of the tumour to be developed. Further tissue is taken in any area where tumour is still present until clearance is achieved. Although time-consuming, this technique maximizes the chances of total tumour excision whilst minimizing sacrifice of normal tissue. This is a particularly useful technique for tumours that grow diffusely and have indefinite margins with finger-like extensions, such as sclerosing BCC, SCC, recurrent tumours and those involving the medial or lateral canthi. The irregular contours around the eyelids and extension of tumours into orbital fat can make interpretation difficult.

Reconstruction

The technique of reconstruction depends on the extent of tissue removed. It is important to reconstruct both anterior and posterior lamellae, each of which must be reconstructed with similar tissue. Anterior lamellar defects may be closed directly or with a local flap or skin graft. Options for the repair of full-thickness defects are set out below.

- **Small defects** involving less than one-third of the eyelid can usually be closed directly, provided the surrounding tissue is sufficiently elastic to allow approximation of the cut edges (Fig. 2.22A–D). If necessary, a lateral cantholysis can be performed for increased mobilization.
- **Moderate size defects** involving up to half of the eyelid may require a flap (e.g. Tenzel semi-circular) for closure (Fig. 2.23A–D).
- **Large defects** involving over half of the eyelid may be closed by one of the following techniques:
  - Posterior lamellar reconstruction may involve an upper lid free tarsal graft, buccal mucous membrane or hard palate graft, or a Hughes tarsoconjunctival flap from the upper lid, which is left attached for 4–6 weeks before transection (Fig. 2.24A–F).
  - Anterior lamellar reconstruction may involve skin advancement, a local skin flap or a free skin graft (Fig. 2.24D). The patient must be made aware that grafted skin is unlikely to be a perfect match. At least one reconstructed lamella requires its own blood supply to maximize the viability of a free graft component.

Laissez-faire

Full reconstruction of the defect created by tumour removal may not always be required. In the *laissez-faire* approach the wound edges are approximated as far as possible and the defect is allowed to granulate and heal by secondary intention. Even large defects can often achieve a satisfactory outcome with time.

Radiotherapy

The recurrence rate following irradiation alone is higher than after surgery, and radiotherapy does not allow histological confirmation of tumour eradication. Recurrences following radiotherapy are difficult to treat surgically because of the poor healing properties of irradiated tissue.

- **Indications**
  - Patients who are either unsuitable for, or refuse, surgery.
  - Highly radiosensitive tumours, such as Kaposi sarcoma.

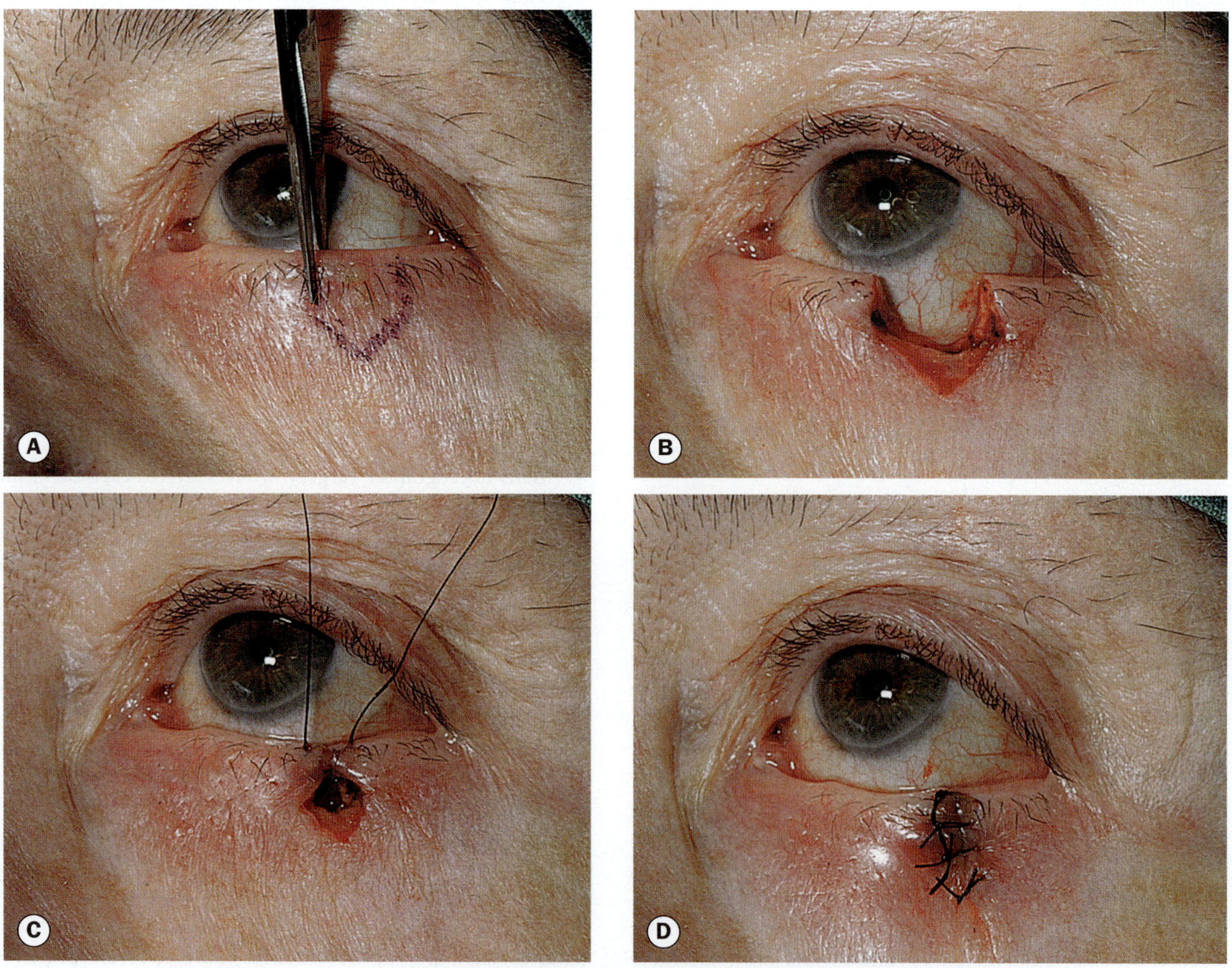

Fig. 2.22 Direct closure. **(A)** Preoperative appearance of a basal cell carcinoma, showing lid marking; **(B)** first cut at right-angles to lid margin; **(C)** excision of pentagon and first suture at posterior lid margin; **(D)** tarsal plate closure with lid margin suture *in situ. (Courtesy of AG Tyers and JRO Collin, from* Colour Atlas of Ophthalmic Plastic Surgery, *Butterworth-Heinemann 2001.)*

- Adjunctive therapy in some cases.
- Palliative treatment.

- **Relative contraindications**
  - Medial canthal lesions due to the high probability of lacrimal canalicular damage.
  - Upper eyelid tumours – conjunctival keratinization is common and difficult to manage.
  - Aggressive tumours such as SGC are relatively radioresistant, but higher-dose treatment may be effective.
- **Complications.** Many of these can be minimized by appropriate shielding.
  - Skin damage and madarosis (eyelash loss).
  - Nasolacrimal duct stenosis following irradiation to the medial canthal area.
  - Conjunctival keratinization, dry eye, keratopathy and cataract.
  - Retinopathy and optic neuropathy.

Cryotherapy

Cryotherapy may be considered for a small superficial BCC and can be a useful adjunct to surgery in some patients. Complications include skin depigmentation, madarosis and conjunctival overgrowth.

Immunotherapy

Vismodegib (administered orally) has been approved for use in patients with extensively advanced BCC. Overall response rates in up to two-thirds of patients have been reported. The initial response to treatment can predict a complete response outcome. However, systemic side effects are common and are the main reason for treatment failure.

Oral nicotinamide for non-melanoma skin cancers

Nicotinamide in a dose of 500 mg once daily appears to reduce the incidence of skin malignancies. Because of its favourable safety

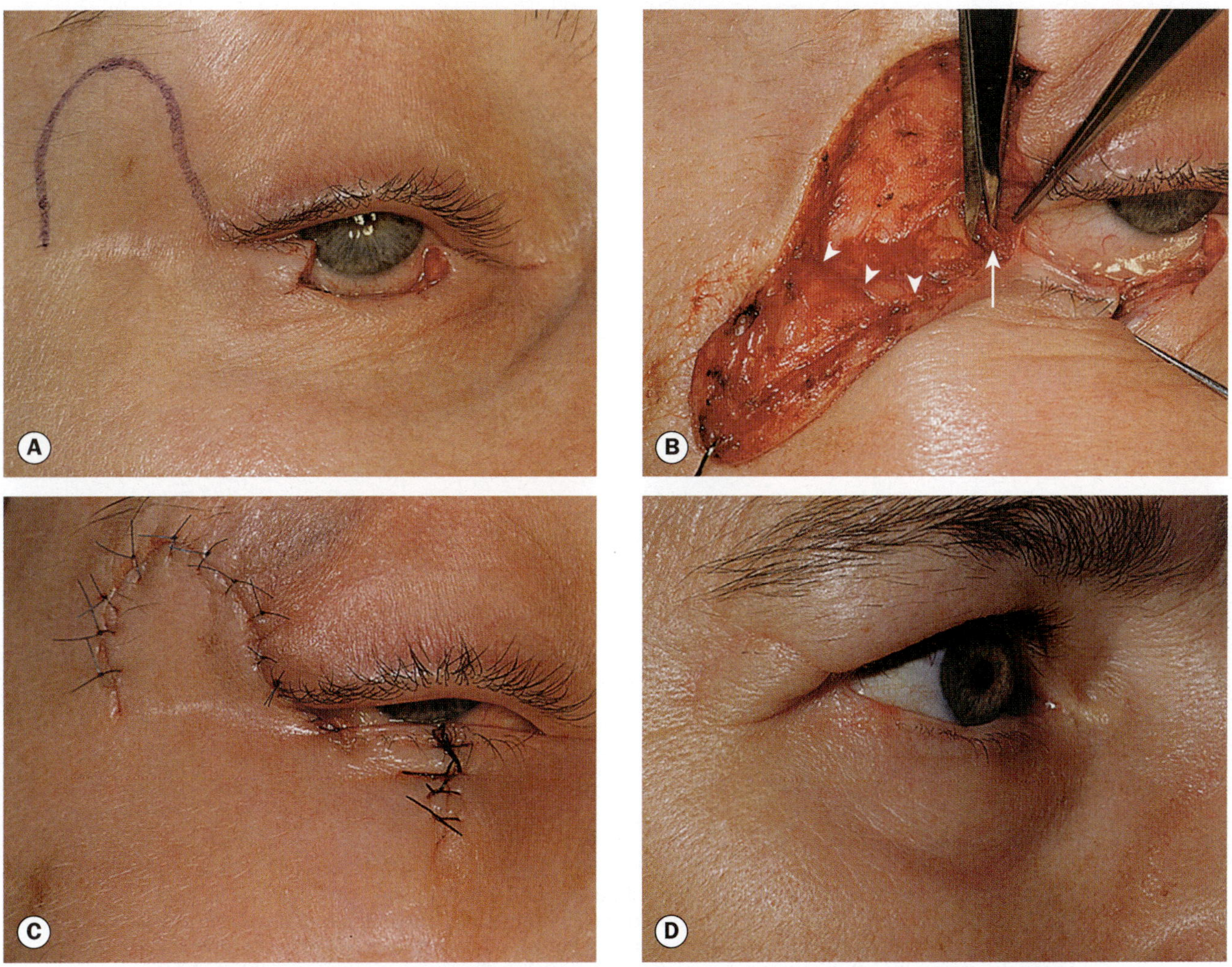

Fig. 2.23 Tenzel flap. **(A)** Incision marks and excision of tumour; **(B)** flap reflected deep to orbicularis muscle (arrowheads) and cut lower limb of lateral canthal tendon (arrow); **(C)** flap edge fixed to the opposite limb of the lateral canthal tendon; eyelid defect and flap closed; **(D)** 6 months after surgery. *(Courtesy of AG Tyers and JRO Collin, from* Colour Atlas of Ophthalmic Plastic Surgery, *Butterworth-Heinemann 2001.)*

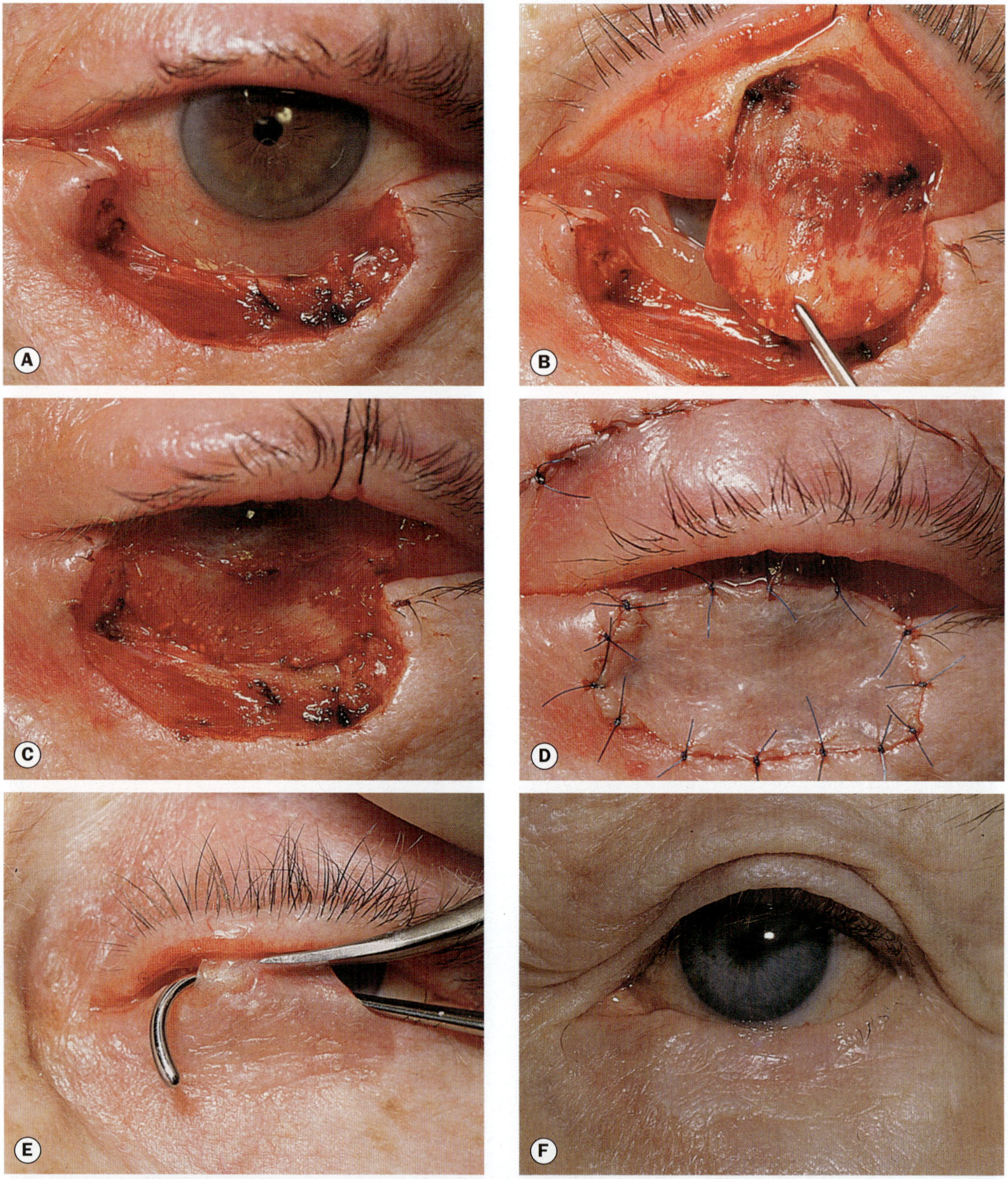

Fig. 2.24 Posterior lamellar reconstruction with a Hughes upper lid flap. **(A)** Lower lid defect; **(B)** tarsoconjunctival flap cut and turned into the defect; Müller muscle separated from the superior tarsal border; **(C)** tarsoconjunctival flap sutured into the defect; **(D)** anterior lamellar reconstruction with full-thickness skin graft from upper lid; **(E)** division of conjunctival pedicle; **(F)** 3 months after surgery. *(Courtesy of AG Tyers and JRO Collin, from* Colour Atlas of Ophthalmic Plastic Surgery, *Butterworth-Heinemann 2001.)*

profile regular supplementary nicotinamide should be considered in individuals who are at high risk of further skin tumours.

DISORDERS OF THE EYELASHES

Misdirected lashes

Introduction

The roots of the eyelashes (cilia) lie against the anterior surface of the tarsal plate. The cilia pass between the main part of the orbicularis oculi and its more superficial part (Riolan muscle), exiting the skin at the anterior lid margin and curving away from the globe. It is particularly important to be familiar with the normal anatomical appearance of the lid margin in order to be able to identify the cause of eyelash misdirection. From anterior to posterior:

- **Eyelashes** (cilia).
- **The grey line**, by definition the border between the anterior (lashes, skin and orbicularis) and posterior (tarsal plate and conjunctiva) lamellae.
- **The meibomian gland orifices** are located just anterior to the mucocutaneous junction. The edge of the tarsal plate is deep to the gland orifices; the glands themselves run vertically within the plate.
- **The mucocutaneous junction** is where keratinized epithelium of the skin merges with conjunctival mucous membrane.
- **Conjunctiva** lines the posterior margin of the lid.

Clinical features

Trauma to the corneal epithelium may cause punctate epithelial erosions, with ocular irritation often worsened by blinking. Corneal ulceration and pannus formation may occur in severe cases. The clinical appearance varies with the cause.

- **Trichiasis** refers to misdirection of growth from individual follicles (Fig. 2.25A and B), rather than a more extensive inversion of the lid or lid margin. The follicles are at anatomically normal sites. It is commonly due to inflammation such as chronic blepharitis or herpes zoster ophthalmicus, but can also be caused by an injury or by surgery, such as incision and curettage of a chalazion (Fig. 2.25C).

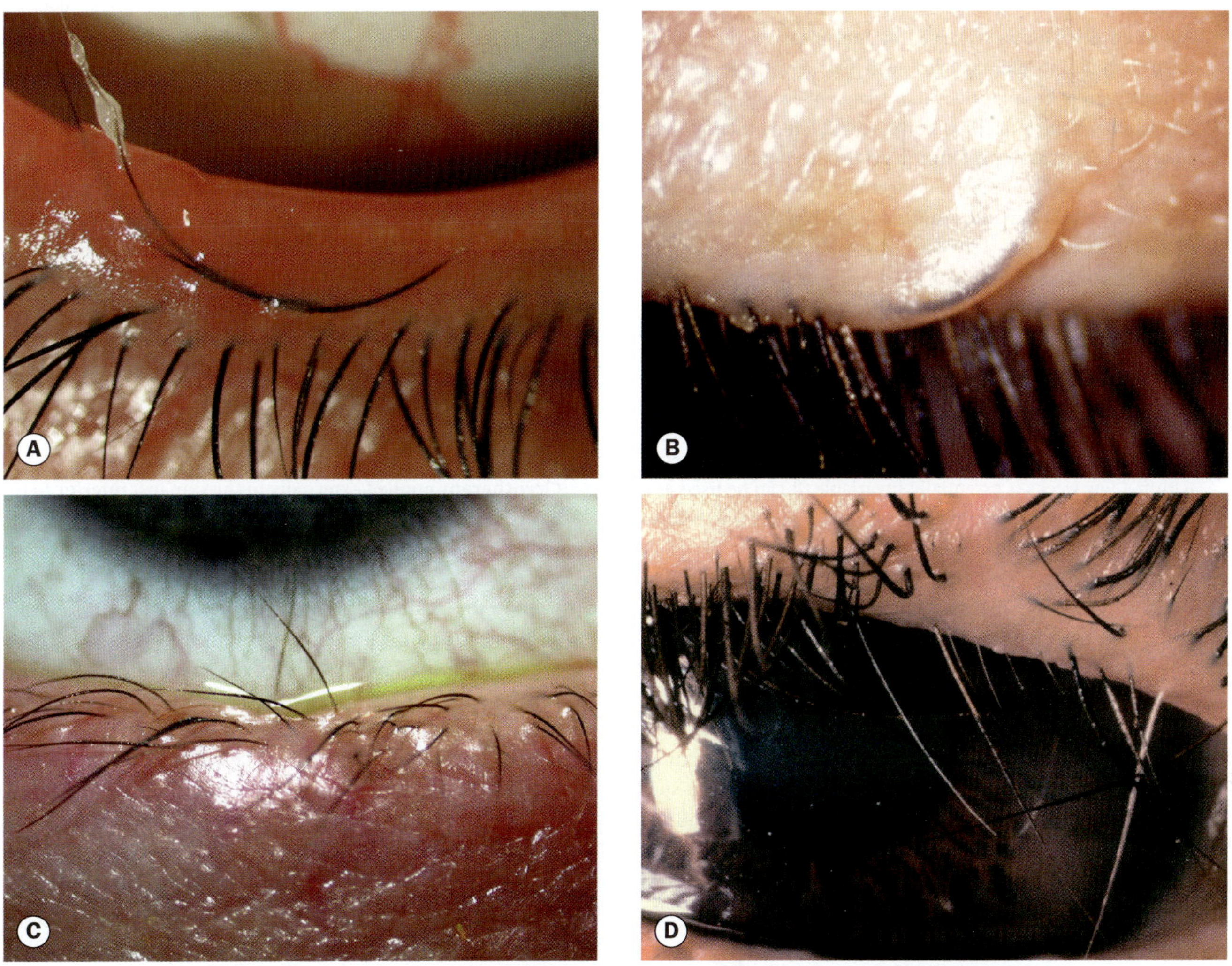

Fig. 2.25 Misdirected lashes. **(A)** Single trichiatic lash; **(B)** ingrown lash; **(C)** group of misdirected lashes secondary to chronic lid inflammation; **(D)** acquired distichiasis. *(Courtesy of R Bates – fig. D.)*

- **Marginal entropion** has increasingly been recognized as a very common cause of eyelash misdirection, secondary to subtle cicatricial posterior lamellar shortening that rotates a segment of the lid margin towards the eye. The mucocutaneous junction migrates anteriorly and the posterior lid margin becomes rounded rather than physiologically square. Typically, numerous aligned lashes are involved.
- **Congenital distichiasis** is a rare condition that occurs when a primary epithelial germ cell destined to differentiate into a meibomian gland develops instead into a complete pilosebaceous unit. The condition is frequently inherited in an AD manner with high penetrance but variable expressivity. The majority of patients also manifest primary lymphoedema of the legs (lymphoedema–distichiasis syndrome). A partial or complete second row of lashes is seen to emerge at or slightly behind the meibomian gland orifices. The aberrant lashes tend to be thinner and shorter than normal cilia and are often directed posteriorly. They are usually well tolerated during infancy and may not become symptomatic until the age of about 5 years.
- **Acquired distichiasis** is caused by metaplasia of the meibomian glands into hair follicles such that a variable number of lashes grow from meibomian gland openings. The most important cause is intense conjunctival inflammation (e.g. chemical injury, Stevens–Johnson syndrome, ocular cicatricial pemphigoid). In contrast to congenital distichiasis, the cilia tend to be non-pigmented and stunted (Fig. 2.25D) and are usually symptomatic.
- **Epiblepharon** – see later.
- **Entropion.** In contrast to marginal entropion, profound inversion of a substantial width of the lid is readily identified – see later.

Treatment

- **Epilation** with forceps is simple and effective but recurrence within a few weeks is essentially invariable. It can be used as a temporizing measure or in the occasional patient who refuses or cannot tolerate surgery.
- **Electrolysis** or electrocautery (hyfrecation) are broadly similar electrosurgical techniques in which, under local anaesthesia, a fine wire is passed down the hair follicle to ablate the lash. It is generally useful for a limited number of lashes, but scarring can follow. Frequently multiple treatments are required to obtain a satisfactory result.
- **Laser ablation** is also useful for the treatment of a limited number of aberrant eyelashes and is performed using a spot size of 50 μm, duration of 0.1–0.2 s and power of 800–1000 mW. The base of the lash is targeted and shots are applied to create a crater that follows the axis of the follicle (Fig. 2.26). Success is broadly comparable to that achieved with electrosurgery.

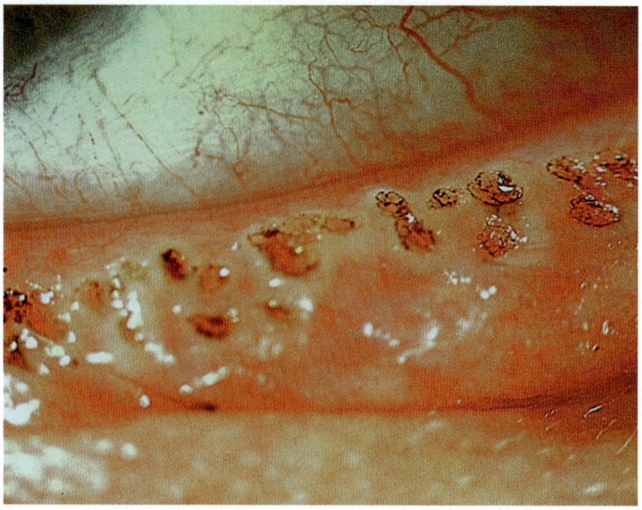

Fig. 2.26 Appearance following laser ablation of multiple lashes.

- **Surgery**
  - Tarsal fracture (transverse tarsotomy) is performed for marginal entropion. After placing a 4-0 traction suture, a horizontal incision is made through the tarsal plate via the conjunctiva, at least halfway down the plate, along the affected length of the lid and extended to 2–3 mm either side of the involved region. Depending on the extent of lid involvement, either two or three double-armed absorbable sutures are passed through the upper edge of the lower section of the tarsal plate to emerge just anterior to the lashes, leaving the lid margin very slightly everted (Fig. 2.27A–D). The sutures are left in place following the surgery. Occasionally short-term use of a bandage contact lens is required to prevent corneal abrading.
  - A full-thickness eyelid pentagon resection can be used for a focal group of aberrant lashes, typically after trauma, or for localized marginal entropion.
  - Other options include lid splitting (see next) with follicle excision and anterior lamellar rotation surgery.
- **Cryotherapy** applied externally to the skin just inferior to the base of the abnormal lashes, or – especially in distichiasis – to the internal aspect of the anterior lamella of the lid following splitting of the margin at the grey line (Fig. 2.28A), can be used for numerous lashes. After separation of the anterior and posterior lamellae under local anaesthesia (Fig. 2.28B), the cryoprobe is applied to the posterior lamella (Fig. 2.28C), using a double freeze–thaw cycle at −20 °C with a plastic eye protector in place. Full-thickness sutures hold the anterior lamella recessed on the posterior lamella (Fig. 2.28D). Suturing of the lid margin is not usually necessary following limited splitting. The method is effective, but **carries a high rate of local adverse effects**, especially loss of lashes and entropion of the upper lid if there is inadequate recession of the anterior lamella. It is less commonly performed now than in previous years.

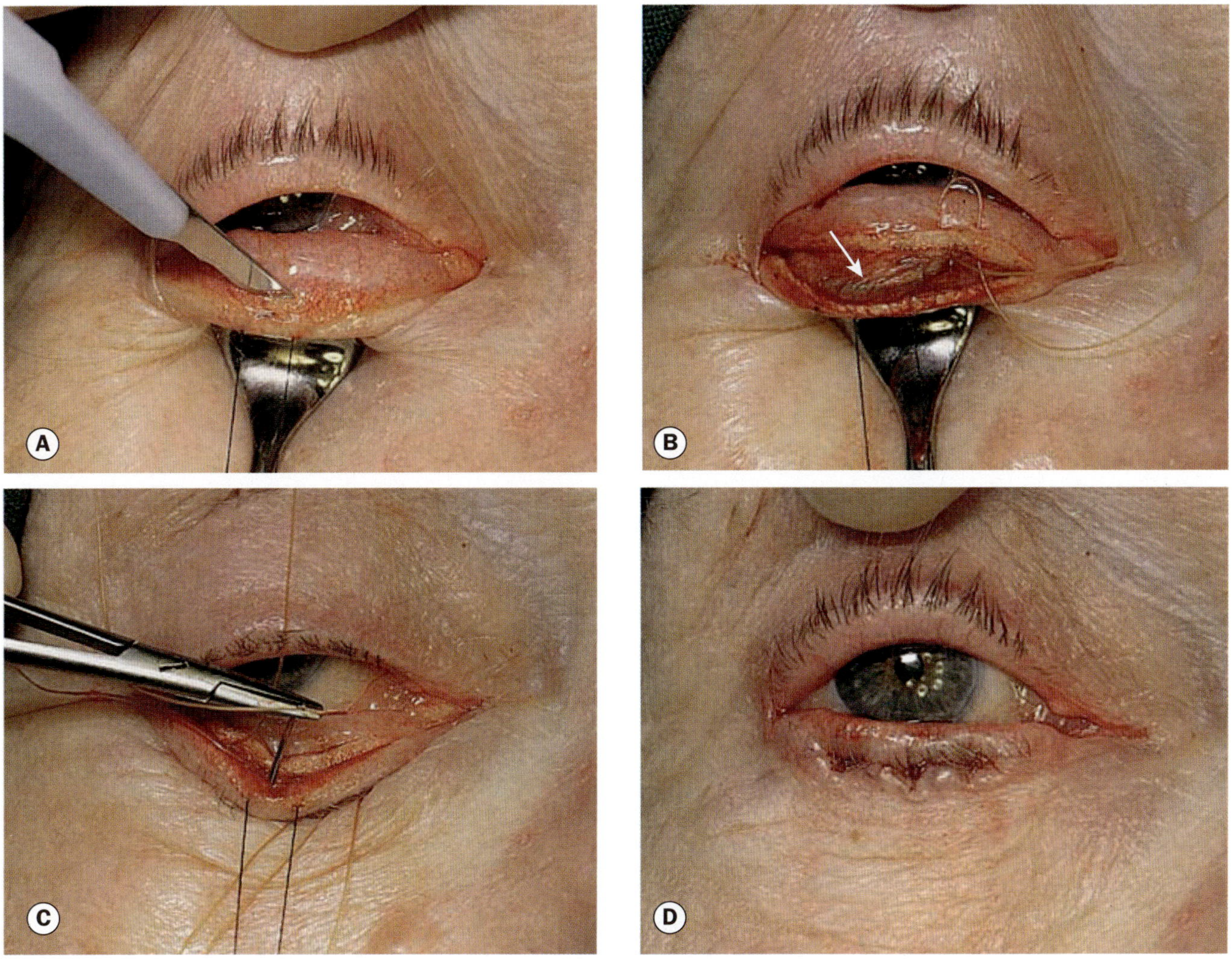

Fig. 2.27 Tarsal fracture for repair of mild entropion of lower lid. **(A)** Transverse, full-thickness incision along the middle of the tarsal plate; **(B)** double-armed 4-0 sutures passed through conjunctiva and lower lid retractors. Note the posterior surface of the pretarsal muscle (arrow); **(C)** sutures are passed anterior to the marginal strip of tarsus, emerging just below the lashes; **(D)** everting sutures tied with slight over-correction. *(Courtesy of AG Tyers and JRO Collin, from* Colour Atlas of Ophthalmic Plastic Surgery, *Butterworth-Heinemann 2001.)*

Eyelash ptosis

Eyelash ptosis refers to a downward sagging of the upper lid lashes (Fig. 2.29A). The condition may be idiopathic or associated with floppy eyelid syndrome, dermatochalasis with anterior lamellar slip or long-standing facial palsy.

Trichomegaly

Trichomegaly is excessive eyelash growth (Fig. 2.29B). The main causes are listed in Table 2.1.

Madarosis

Madarosis is the term used for the loss of lashes (Fig. 2.29C). The main causes are shown in Table 2.2.

Table 2.1 Causes of Trichomegaly
Drug-induced – topical prostaglandin analogues, phenytoin and ciclosporin
Malnutrition
AIDS
Porphyria
Hypothyroidism
Familial
Congenital: Oliver–McFarlane, Cornelia de Lange, Goldstein–Hutt, Hermansky–Pudlak syndromes

Poliosis

Poliosis is a premature localized whitening of hair, which may involve the lashes and eyebrows (Fig. 2.29D). The main causes are shown in Table 2.3.

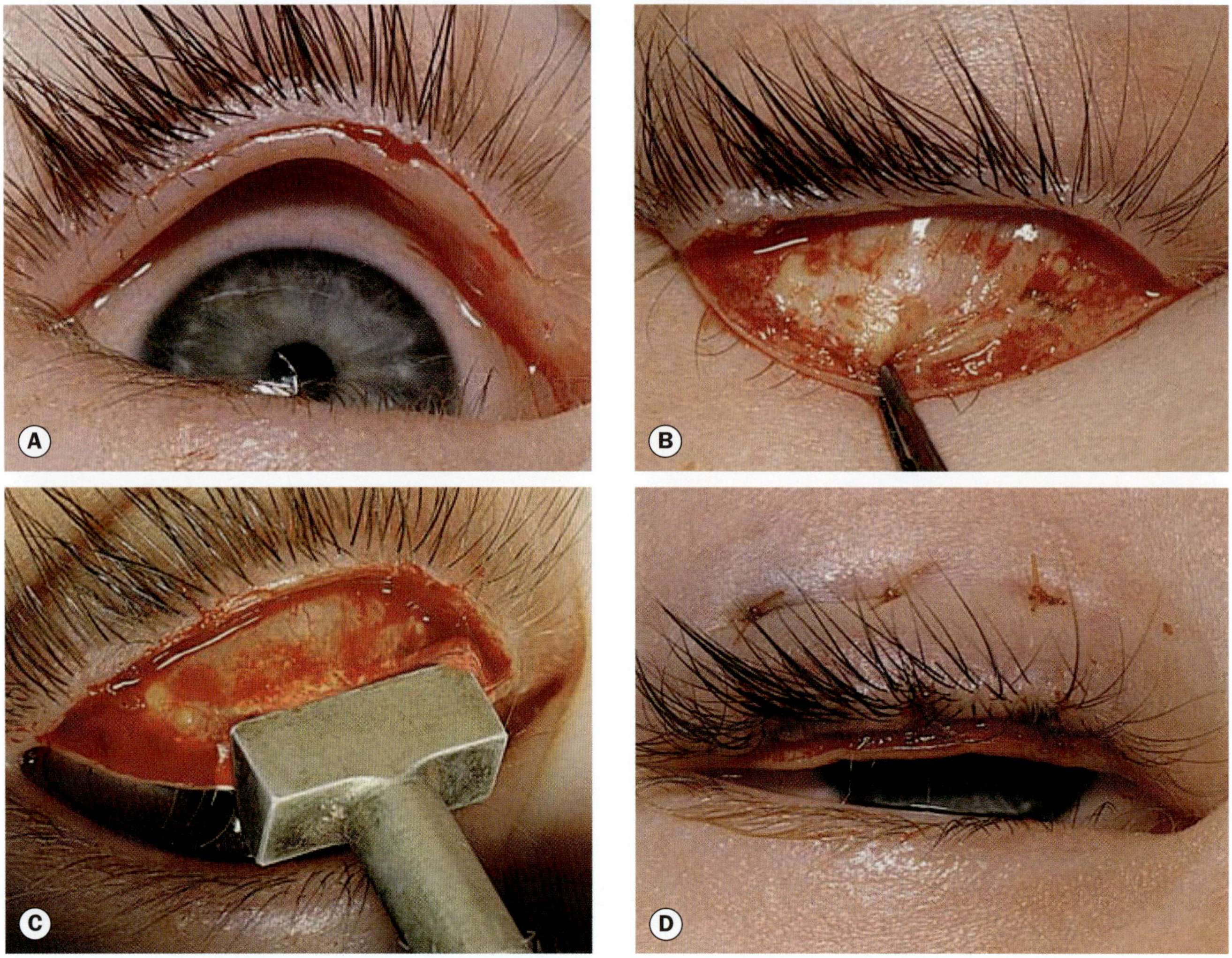

Fig. 2.28 Cryotherapy to the eyelid in distichiasis. **(A)** Incision in the grey line; **(B)** separation of the anterior and posterior lamellae; **(C)** application of cryoprobe to the posterior lamella; **(D)** full-thickness sutures hold the anterior lamella recessed on the posterior lamella. *(Courtesy of AG Tyers and JRO Collin, from* Colour Atlas of Ophthalmic Plastic Surgery, *Butterworth-Heinemann 2001.)*

ALLERGIC DISORDERS

Acute allergic oedema

Acute allergic oedema may occur rapidly in a child exposed to cat or dog hairs (Fig. 2.30A). When it is caused by exposure to pollen or by insect bites it manifests with the sudden onset of bilateral boggy periocular oedema (Fig. 2.30B), often accompanied by conjunctival swelling (chemosis – see Ch. 6). Treatment is often unnecessary, but systemic antihistamines are sometimes given.

Contact dermatitis

Contact dermatitis is an inflammatory response that usually follows exposure to a medication such as eye drops, cosmetics or metals. An irritant can also cause a non-allergic toxic dermatitis. The individual is sensitized on first exposure and develops an immune reaction on further exposure; the mediating reaction is type IV (delayed type) hypersensitivity. Signs consist of lid skin scaling, angular fissuring, oedema and tightness (Fig. 2.30C). There may be chemosis, redness and papillary conjunctivitis. Corneal involvement is usually limited to punctate epithelial erosions. Treatment consists primarily of avoidance of allergen exposure, provided it can be identified. Cold compresses provide symptomatic relief. Topical steroids and oral antihistamines can be used but are rarely required.

IDIOPATHIC DERMATITIS

Atopic dermatitis

Atopic dermatitis (eczema) is a very common idiopathic condition, typically occurring in patients who also suffer from asthma and hay fever. Eyelid involvement is relatively infrequent but when present is invariably associated with generalized dermatitis. Thickening, crusting and fissuring of the lids (Fig. 2.30D) is typical and staphylococcal blepharitis, vernal or atopic keratoconjunctivitis are also commonly present. Herpetic blepharitis and keratoconjunctivitis

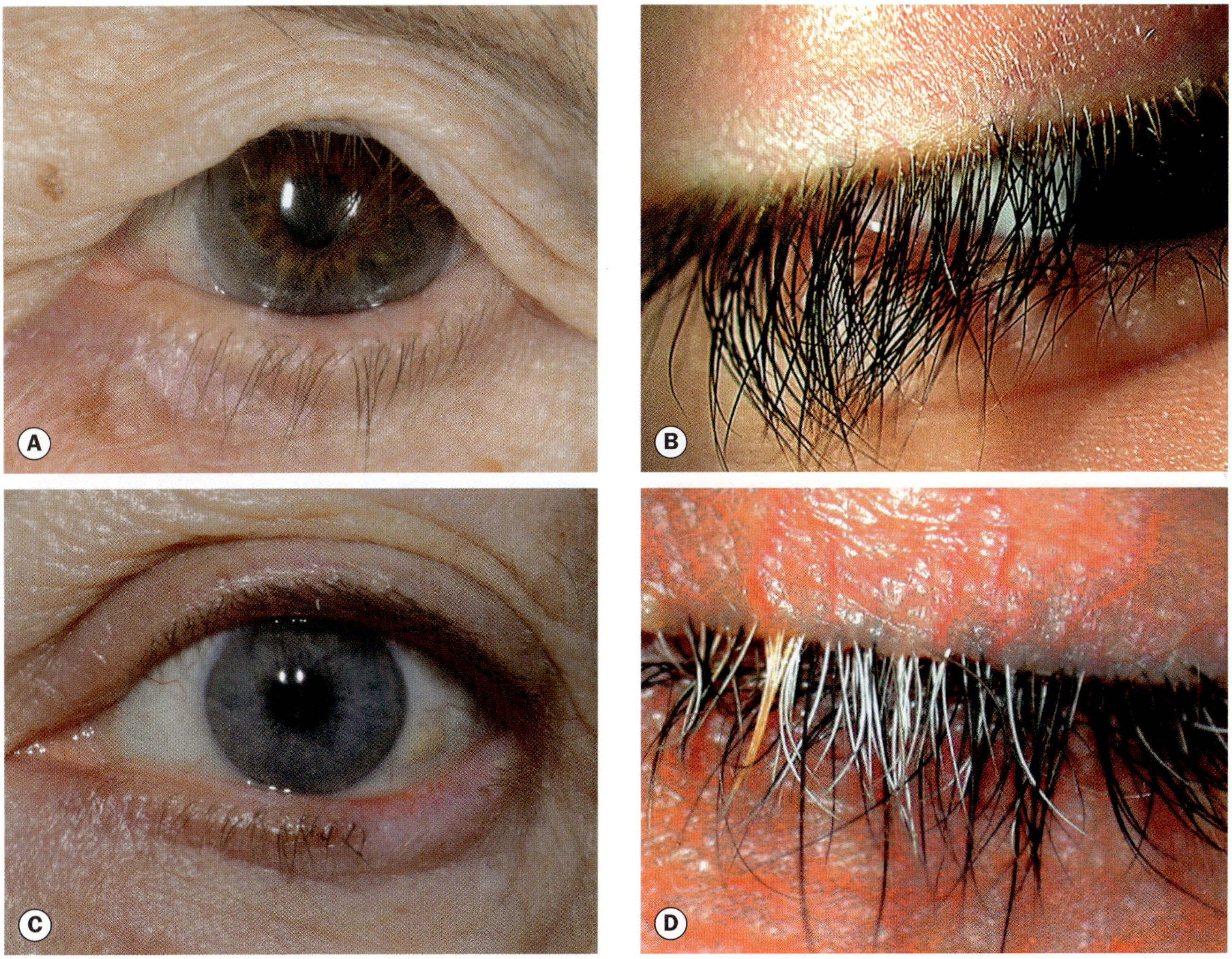

Fig. 2.29 Miscellaneous eyelash disorders. **(A)** Eyelash ptosis; **(B)** trichomegaly; **(C)** madarosis; **(D)** poliosis.

Table 2.2 Causes of Madarosis

1. Local
Chronic anterior lid margin disease
Infiltrating lid tumours
Burns
Radiotherapy or cryotherapy of lid tumours
2. Skin disorders
Generalized alopecia
Psoriasis
3. Systemic diseases
Myxoedema
Systemic lupus erythematosus
Acquired syphilis
Lepromatous leprosy
4. Following removal
Procedures for trichiasis
Trichotillomania – psychiatric disorder of hair removal

are more common and more severe in patients with atopy (eczema herpeticum). Treatment of the lid features is with emollients to hydrate the skin and the judicious use of mild topical steroid such as hydrocortisone 1%. Uncommon ocular associations include keratoconus, cataract and retinal detachment (see also Ch. 6).

Table 2.3 Causes of Poliosis

1. Ocular
Chronic anterior blepharitis
Sympathetic ophthalmitis
Idiopathic uveitis
2. Systemic
Vogt–Koyanagi–Harada syndrome
Waardenburg syndrome
Vitiligo
Marfan syndrome
Tuberous sclerosis
Systemic monoclonal antibody treatment

Periorificial dermatitis

This is a common chronic inflammatory skin eruption of unknown cause that can affect the periocular region. It resembles rosacea and allergic dermatitis, but is considered a disease of the hair follicle, with biopsy samples showing a lymphohistiocytic infiltrate. Clusters of red papules, vesicles and pustules with an erythematous base and a sharp border are seen, with dry surrounding skin. It usually affects young

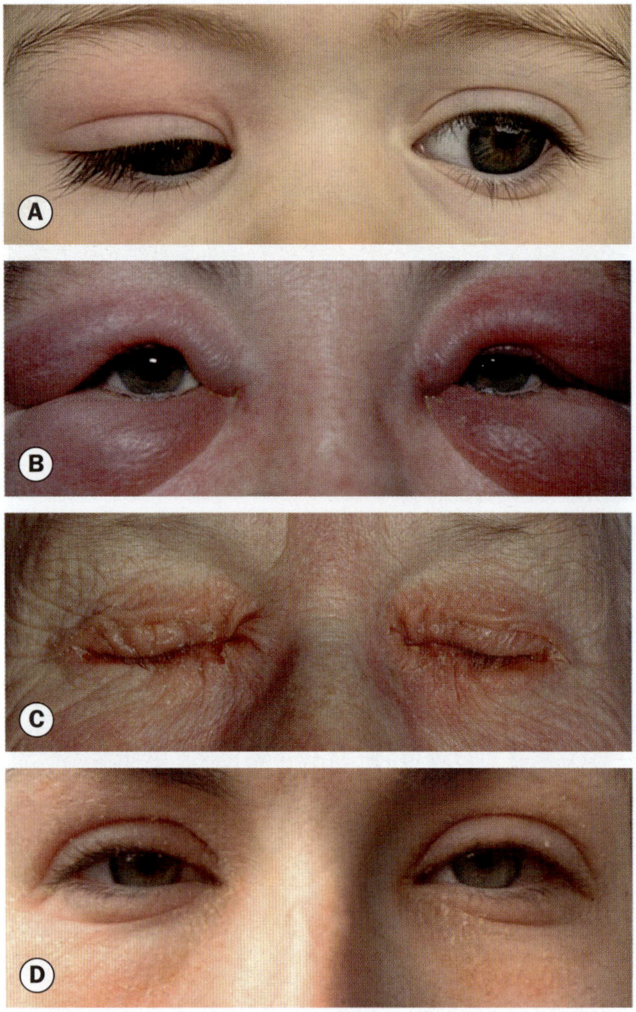

Fig. 2.30 Allergic disorders. **(A)** Unilateral acute allergic oedema in a child; **(B)** bilateral acute allergic oedema; **(C)** contact dermatitis; **(D)** atopic dermatitis in a young adult.

to middle-aged women. Exposure to sunlight, heat and wind can exacerbate the inflammation. The condition is benign and self-limiting. If topical steroids have been used, they should be slowly discontinued and replaced with a bland emollient without preservatives. Specific treatment includes topical metronidazole 0.75%, topical erythromycin 1% and oral tetracycline for 4–8 weeks.

IMMUNE-RELATED INFLAMMATION

Dermatomyositis

Dermatomyositis is a chronic inflammatory disorder of muscles which can present in an acute or chronic fashion with muscle weakness and a skin rash. In children, about half develop eyelid swelling and a heliotrope rash (Fig. 2.31). In adults it may be associated with ovarian, breast or lung cancer, as an autoimmune response. The condition is treated with systemic steroids or immunosuppressive medication (methotrexate, azathioprine).

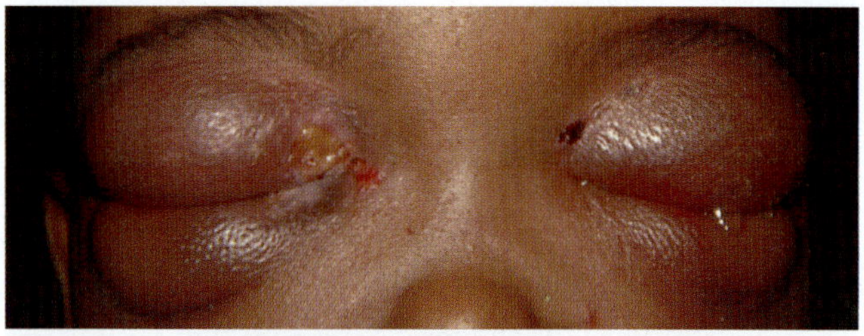

Fig. 2.31 Acute lid swelling secondary to dermatomyositis in a child.

Systemic monoclonal antibody therapy

See Chapter 21.

BACTERIAL INFECTIONS

External hordeolum

An external hordeolum (stye) is an acute staphylococcal abscess of a lash follicle and its associated gland of Zeis that is common in children and young adults. A stye presents as a tender swelling in the lid margin pointing anteriorly through the skin, usually with a lash at its apex (Fig. 2.32A). Multiple lesions may be present and occasionally an abscess may involve the entire lid margin. Treatment involves topical (occasionally oral) antibiotics, hot compresses and epilation of the associated lash.

Impetigo

Impetigo is a superficial skin infection caused by *Staphylococcus aureus* or *Streptococcus pyogenes*, typically affecting children. Involvement of the eyelids is usually associated with infection of the face. Painful erythematous macules rapidly develop into thin-walled blisters, which develop golden-yellow crusts on rupturing (Fig. 2.32B). There may be fever, malaise and local lymphadenopathy. Treatment is with topical and sometimes oral antibiotics (beta-lactamase resistant) and preventative measures to reduce transmission as the condition is highly contagious. It is particularly dangerous to neonates, contact with whom should be avoided.

Erysipelas

Erysipelas (St Anthony's fire) is an uncommon acute, potentially severe, dermal and superficial lymphatic infection usually caused by *S. pyogenes*. Diabetes, obesity and alcohol abuse are predisposing factors. An inflamed erythematous plaque develops (Fig. 2.32C). A well-defined raised border distinguishes erysipelas from other forms of cellulitis. Complications such as metastatic infection are rare. Treatment is with oral antibiotics, but recurrence is common.

Necrotizing fasciitis

Necrotizing fasciitis is a rare but commonly very severe infection involving subcutaneous soft tissue and the skin, with associated

TIP In a patient with chronic follicular conjunctivitis that does not respond to topical antibiotics, look for molluscum contagiosum involving the lid margin.

Mpox (Monkey pox)

Mpox is caused by a zoonotic virus in the genus *Orthopoxvirus.* It was once considered rare in humans, but the quantity and severity of outbreaks is increasing, possibly as a consequence of waning immunity since the stopping of routine smallpox vaccination. In July 2022 the World Health Organization declared the outbreak a Public Health Emergency of International Concern.

- It is spread from animals by handling infected meat and from human-to-human through exposure to contaminated body fluids and intimate contact with the pox lesions. Sexual transmission occurs predominantly in a man who has sex with a man who carries the virus. The virus is spread from the onset of symptoms until all the lesions have scabbed and fallen off.
- Early symptoms include headache, fever and fatigue. This is followed a few days later by the development of vesicles on the face and then elsewhere on the body, particularly on the palms of the hand and soles of the feet.
- Approximately one in five cases have ocular lesions. Pustules on the lid margin can result in follicular conjunctivitis, secondary lid swelling (Fig. 2.33E) and preauricular lymph gland enlargement. In those with conjunctivitis there is a higher frequency of other systemic symptoms, compared to those without conjunctivitis. Corneal involvement in the form of keratitis may range from mild to severe. Loss of vision has been reported in about 5%.
- The lesions on the body resemble chickenpox (Fig. 2.33F), except that swollen glands are found. They start as small spots which become bumps that fill with clear fluid; then umbilicated pustules which subsequently burst and scab.
- The illness is usually mild and most will recover within a few weeks without treatment. There is no cure, but the antiviral drugs cidofovir and tecovirimat and vaccinia immune globulin may be used in severe cases. The smallpox vaccine is 85% protective in preventing infection in close contacts.

Herpes zoster ophthalmicus

Herpes zoster ophthalmicus (HZO – Fig. 2.34A and B) is a common, generally unilateral infection caused by varicella-zoster virus. It is discussed in detail in Chapter 7.

Herpes simplex

Introduction

Herpes simplex skin rash results from either primary infection or reactivation of herpes simplex virus previously dormant in the trigeminal ganglion. Prodromal facial and lid tingling lasting about 24 hours is followed by the development of eyelid and periocular skin vesicles (Fig. 2.35A) that break down over 48 hours. Although typically confined to a single dermatome and with individual lesions that are often similar in appearance, the distribution of the herpes simplex skin rash contrasts with the sharply delineated unilateral involvement in HZO (see Fig. 2.34). There is commonly an associated papillary conjunctivitis, discharge and lid swelling. Dendritic corneal ulcers can develop, especially in atopic patients, in whom skin involvement can be extensive and very severe (eczema herpeticum – Fig. 2.35B).

Treatment

In many patients the inflammation will gradually settle without treatment over about a week. If treatment is necessary, a topical (aciclovir cream five times daily for 5 days) or oral (oral aciclovir, famciclovir or valaciclovir) antiviral agent can be used. Antibiotics

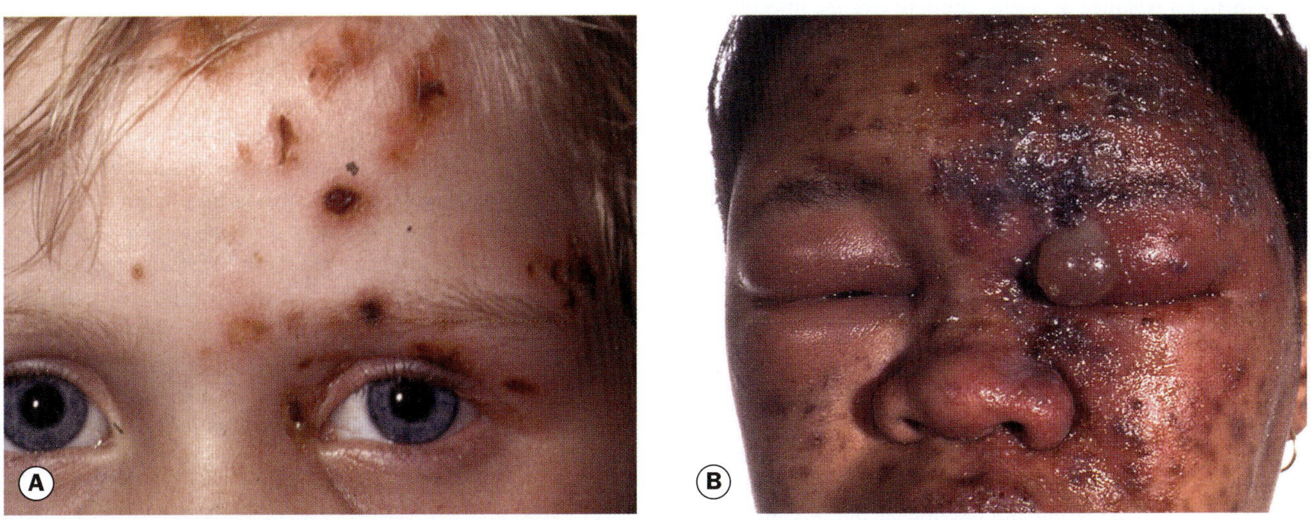

Fig. 2.34 Herpes zoster ophthalmicus. **(A)** Healing rash in a child; **(B)** left maculopapular crusting rash with periocular oedema; the right side shows passive swelling. *(Courtesy T Carmichael – fig. B.)*

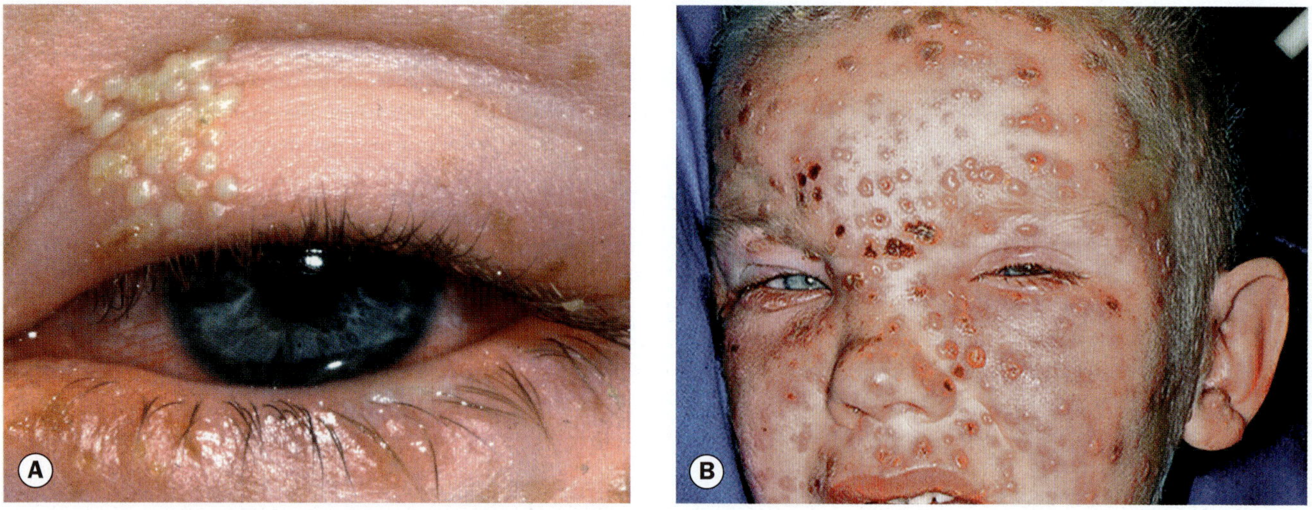

Fig. 2.35 Herpes simplex. (A) Vesicles; (B) eczema herpeticum.

(e.g. co-amoxiclav, erythromycin) may also be required in patients with secondary bacterial infection. This is particularly common in eczema herpeticum.

BLEPHARITIS

Chronic blepharitis

Introduction

Chronic blepharitis (chronic marginal blepharitis) is a common cause of ocular discomfort and irritation. The poor correlation between symptoms and signs, the uncertain aetiology and mechanisms of the disease process all combine to make management difficult. Blepharitis may be subdivided into anterior and posterior forms, although there is considerable overlap and both types are often present (mixed blepharitis).

- **Anterior blepharitis** affects the area surrounding the bases of the eyelashes and may be staphylococcal or seborrhoeic. It is sometimes regarded as related more to chronic infective elements and hence more amenable to treatment and remission than the posterior form. An aetiological factor in staphylococcal blepharitis may be an abnormal cell-mediated response to components of the cell wall of *S. aureus,* which may also be responsible for the red eyes and peripheral corneal infiltrates seen in some patients. It is more common and more marked in patients with atopic dermatitis. Seborrhoeic blepharitis is strongly associated with generalized seborrhoeic dermatitis that characteristically involves the scalp, nasolabial folds, skin behind the ears and the sternum.
- **Posterior blepharitis** is caused by meibomian gland dysfunction and alterations in meibomian gland secretions. Bacterial lipases may result in the formation of free fatty acids. This increases the melting point of the meibum, preventing its expression from the glands, contributing to ocular surface irritation and possibly enabling growth of *S. aureus*. Loss of the tear film phospholipids that act as surfactants results in increased tear evaporation and osmolarity and an unstable tear film. Posterior blepharitis is commonly thought of as a more persistent and chronic inflammatory condition than anterior blepharitis; there is an association with acne rosacea.
- **Demodex.** A reaction to the extremely common hair follicle and sebaceous gland-dwelling mite *Demodex* and other microorganisms may play a causative role in some patients – *Demodex folliculorum longus* in anterior blepharitis and *Demodex folliculorum brevis* in posterior blepharitis – though the mite can be found normally in a majority of older patients, most of whom do not develop symptomatic blepharitis. Collarettes, a combination of partially digested epithelial cells, keratin, waste and mite eggs, are considered a pathognomonic sign of *Demodex* infection. It has been proposed that circumstances such as overpopulation or hypersensitivity (perhaps to a bacillus carried symbiotically by *Demodex*) may lead to symptoms. *Demodex* mites are a major cause of the animal disease mange.

The characteristics of the different forms of blepharitis are set out in Table 2.4.

Diagnosis

Involvement is usually bilateral and symmetrical, with no visual disturbance.

- **Symptoms** are caused by disruption of normal ocular surface function and reduction in tear stability and are similar in all forms of blepharitis, though stinging may be more common in posterior disease. Because of poor correlation between the severity of symptoms and signs it can be difficult to objectively assess the benefit of treatment. Burning, grittiness, mild photophobia and crusting and redness of the lid margins with remissions and exacerbations are characteristic. Symptoms are usually worse in the mornings although in patients with associated dry eye they may increase during the day. Contact lenses may be poorly tolerated.
- **Signs – staphylococcal blepharitis**
  - Hard scales and crusting are found, mainly located around the bases of the lashes and are associated with collarettes, which are cylindrical collections around lash bases (Fig. 2.36A).

Table 2.4 Summary of Characteristics of Chronic Blepharitis

	Feature	Anterior blepharitis		Posterior blepharitis
		Staphylococcal	Seborrhoeic	
Lashes	Deposit	Hard	Soft	
	Loss	++	+	
	Distorted or trichiasis	++	+	
Lid margin	Ulceration	+		
	Notching	+		++
Cyst	Hordeolum	++		
	Meibomian			++
Conjunctiva	Phlyctenule	+		
Tear film	Foaming			++
	Dry eye	+	+	++
Cornea	Punctate erosions	+	+	++
	Vascularization	+	+	++
	Infiltrates	+	+	++
Commonly associated skin disease		Atopic dermatitis	Seborrhoeic dermatitis	Acne rosacea

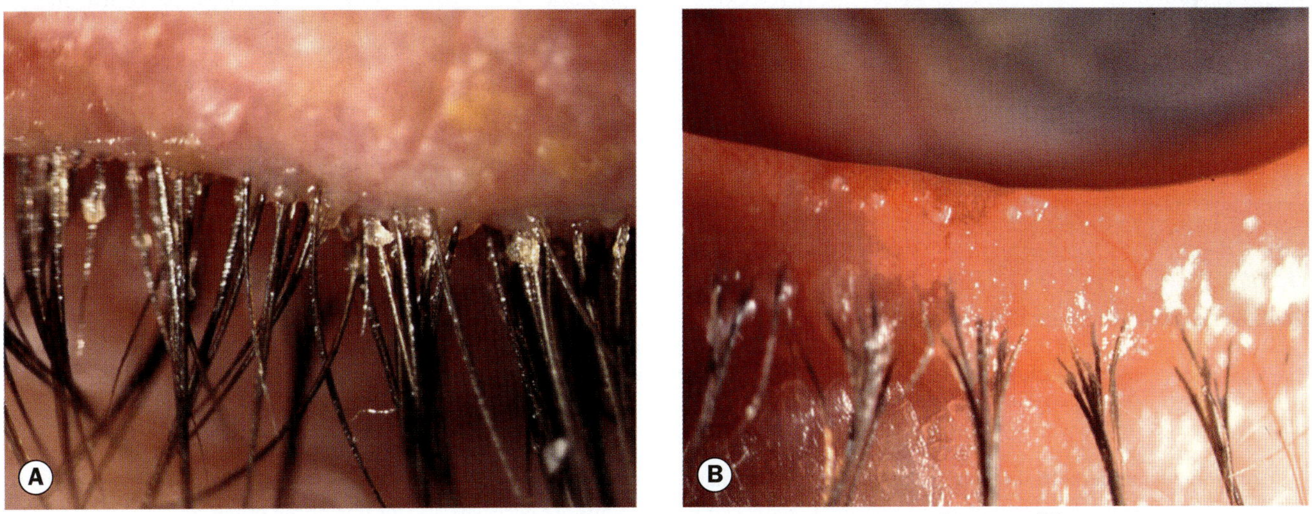

Fig. 2.36 Chronic anterior blepharitis. **(A)** Scales and crusting including collarettes; **(B)** greasy lid margin with sticky lashes in seborrhoeic blepharitis.

  - Mild papillary conjunctivitis and chronic conjunctival hyperaemia are common.
  - Long-standing cases may develop scarring and notching of the lid margin, madarosis, trichiasis and poliosis.
  - Associated tear film instability and dry eye syndrome are common.
  - Atopic keratoconjunctivitis may be present in patients with atopic dermatitis.
- **Signs – seborrhoeic blepharitis**
  - Hyperaemic and greasy anterior lid margins with soft scales and adherence of lashes to each other (Fig. 2.36B).
- **Signs – posterior blepharitis** (meibomian gland disease)
  - Excessive and abnormal meibomian gland secretion, manifesting as capping of meibomian gland orifices with oil globules (Fig. 2.37A).
  - Pouting, recession, or plugging of meibomian gland orifices (Fig. 2.37B).
  - Hyperaemia and telangiectasis of the posterior lid margin.
  - Pressure on the lid margin results in expression of meibomian fluid that may be turbid or toothpaste-like (Fig. 2.37C). In severe cases the secretions become so inspissated that expression is impossible.
  - Lid transillumination may show gland loss and cystic dilatation of meibomian ducts.
  - The tear film is oily and foamy and often unstable, and froth may accumulate on the lid margins (Fig. 2.37D) or inner canthi.
- ***Demodex* infestation** may lead to cylindrical dandruff-like scaling (collarettes) around the base of eyelashes, though this is not always present (see Fig. 2.36A). The mites can be

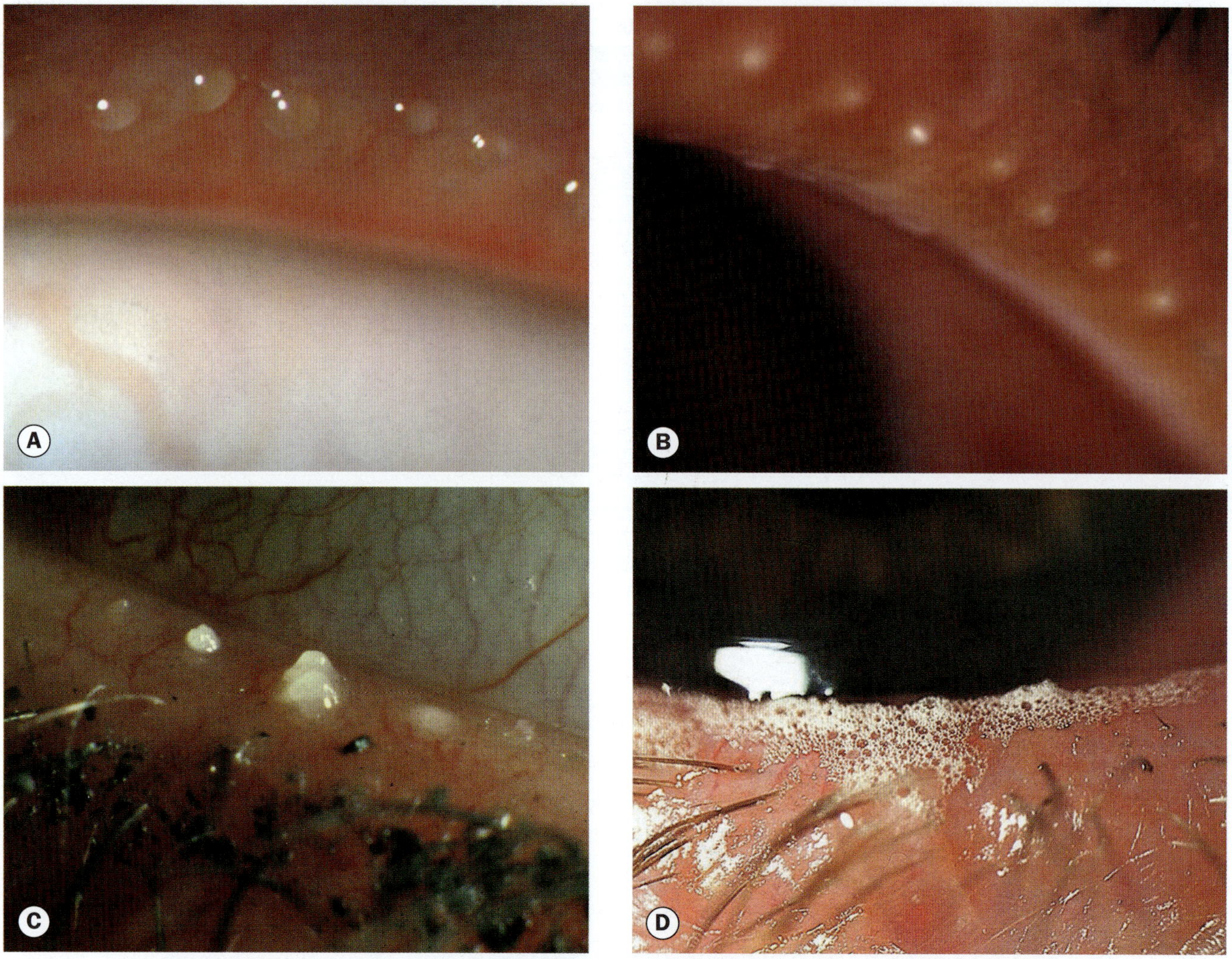

Fig. 2.37 Chronic posterior blepharitis. **(A)** Capping of meibomian gland orifices by oil globules; **(B)** plugged meibomian gland orifices; **(C)** expressed toothpaste-like material; **(D)** froth on the eyelid margin.

demonstrated under ×16 slit lamp magnification by first manually clearing around the base of an eyelash and then by gently rotating the lash or moving it from side to side for 5–10 seconds with fine forceps. If one or more mites (0.2–0.4 mm long) do not emerge, the lash should be gently epilated. Slide microscopy can be performed on the mites or lashes if necessary.

- **Secondary changes** include papillary conjunctivitis, inferior corneal punctate epithelial erosions, corneal scarring and vascularization including Salzmann nodular degeneration and advancing wave-like epitheliopathy-type changes, stye formation, marginal keratitis and occasionally bacterial keratitis (especially in contact lens wearers) and phlyctenular eye disease.

Treatment

There is limited evidence to support any particular treatment protocol for blepharitis. Patients should be advised that a permanent cure is unlikely, but control of symptoms is usually possible. The treatment of anterior and posterior disease is similar for both types, particularly as they commonly co-exist, but some treatments are fairly specific for one or the other.

- **Lid hygiene** can be carried out once or twice daily initially, although compliance and technique are highly variable.
  - A warm compress should first be applied for several minutes to soften crusts at the bases of the lashes.
  - Lid cleaning is subsequently performed to mechanically remove crusts and other debris, scrubbing the lid margins with a wet cotton bud or clean, wet face-cloth. Contrary to popular belief, baby shampoo should not be recommended, as it destabilizes the tear film and is a common cause of contact dermatitis.
  - Commercially produced soap/alcohol impregnated pads for lid scrubbing are available and are often highly effective, but care should be taken not to induce mechanical irritation.
  - When substantial meibomian gland disease is present, the regimen may include expression of accumulated meibum by rolling the finger anteriorly over the margin.

- The putative action of lid hygiene against *Demodex* is via prevention of reproduction.
- Lid hygiene can be performed less frequently as the condition is brought under control.

- **Antibiotics**
  - Topical sodium fusidic acid, erythromycin, bacitracin, azithromycin or chloramphenicol is used to treat active folliculitis in anterior disease and is occasionally used for an extended period. Following lid hygiene, the ointment should be rubbed onto the anterior lid margin with a cotton bud or clean finger.
  - Oral antibiotic regimens include doxycycline (50–100 mg twice daily for 1 week and then daily for 6–24 weeks), lymecycline (one 408 mg capsule daily for up to 3 months), other tetracyclines, or azithromycin (500 mg daily for 3 days for three cycles at 1-week intervals). Antibiotics are thought to reduce bacterial colonization and may also exert other effects such as a reduction in staphylococcal lipase production with tetracyclines. Tetracyclines may be more effective in the treatment of posterior disease and azithromycin in anterior. Tetracyclines should not be used in children under the age of 12 years or in pregnant or breastfeeding women because they are deposited in growing bone and teeth. Patients should also be made aware of the possibility of increased sun sensitivity. Erythromycin 250 mg once or twice daily is an alternative.
- **Plant and fish oil supplements** have been shown to be of substantial benefit in some cases.
- **Topical steroid.** A low potency preparation such as fluorometholone 0.1% or loteprednol four times daily for 1 week is useful in patients with substantial active inflammation, especially papillary conjunctivitis; occasionally a higher strength preparation is used.
- **Tear substitutes** and other dry eye treatments are typically helpful for associated tear insufficiency and instability.
- **Tea tree oil** has been suggested as a treatment based primarily on its activity against *Demodex* infestation *in vitro*, although there remains some uncertainty to the effectiveness *in vivo*. The optimal vehicle and regimen have not been established, but lid, eyebrow and periocular skin cleansing once daily with a 50% scrub and application of 5% ointment has been described. Preservative-free, sterile, ready-to-use wipes containing 2.5% terpinen-4-ol are available and can be applied once or twice daily to the lid margins (depending on severity) for 4 weeks. People should be educated on how to accurately apply tea tree oil products, because adherence and method of application are likely to affect efficacy. Topical permethrin and topical (1% cream) or oral (two doses of 200 μg/kg 1 week apart) ivermectin have also been used by some practitioners. Early pre-clinical results using lotilaner 0.25% ophthalmic solution (TP-03) are encouraging, as it is well tolerated and effective in reducing collarettes and *Demodex* density within 4 weeks of commencing treatment. High temperature cleaning of bedding, the use of tea tree shampoo and facial soap, and treating the patient's partner may all help to reduce recurrences.
- **Novel therapies** include topical ciclosporin, pulsed light application and purpose-designed devices to probe, heat and/or express the meibomian glands (e.g. LipiFlow) in posterior disease.
- **Complications** are treated specifically.

TIP *Demodex* infection is characterized by itching and the presence of collarettes, a combination of partially digested epithelial cells, keratin, waste and mite eggs. The infestation can be treated with accurately applied tea tree oil products.

Phthiriasis palpebrarum

The crab louse *Phthirus pubis* is adapted to living in pubic hair, but is also commonly found in other hair-covered body areas such as the chest, axillae and eyelids (phthiriasis palpebrarum). Symptoms consist of chronic irritation and itching of the lids, but the lice are often an incidental discovery. Conjunctivitis is uncommon. The lice are readily visible anchored to lashes (Fig. 2.38A); lice have six legs rather than the eight possessed by ticks (see next). Ova and their empty shells appear as oval, brownish, opalescent pearls adherent to the base of the cilia (Fig. 2.38B). Treatment consists of mechanical removal of the lice and their attached lashes with fine forceps. If necessary, topical yellow mercuric oxide 1% or petroleum jelly can be applied to the lashes and lids twice a day for 10 days. Delousing of the patient, family members, clothing and bedding is important to prevent recurrence.

Tick infestation of the eyelid

Ticks can attach themselves to the eyelid and should be removed at the earliest opportunity in order to minimize the risk of contracting a tick-borne zoonosis such as Lyme disease, Rocky Mountain fever, African tick bite fever (Fig. 2.39) or tularaemia. If the tick is attached some distance from the eye such that spray can safely be applied, an insect repellent containing pyrethrin or a pyrethroid should be sprayed on the tick twice at intervals of a minute. Alternatively, a scabies cream containing permethrin can be applied. These have a toxic effect that prevents the tick from injecting saliva and after 24 hours it should drop off or can be removed with fine-tipped forceps at the slit lamp (blunt-tipped needle-holders are an alternative in restrained small children). It is critical that the tick is detached as close to its skin attachment as possible in order to remove its head and mouthparts, following which it might be retained in sealed packaging to permit identification if necessary. In areas endemic for Lyme disease, some authorities suggest routine antibiotic prophylaxis with doxycycline following a confirmed deer tick bite. Patients should be told to seek medical advice urgently at the onset of suspicious symptoms, particularly erythema migrans, over the subsequent few weeks. Lyme disease transmission is thought to require attachment of the tick for at least 36 hours. African tick bite fever is a rickettsial infection, which is fairly common in sub-Saharan Africa. The onset of symptoms occurs 4–10 days after the bite.

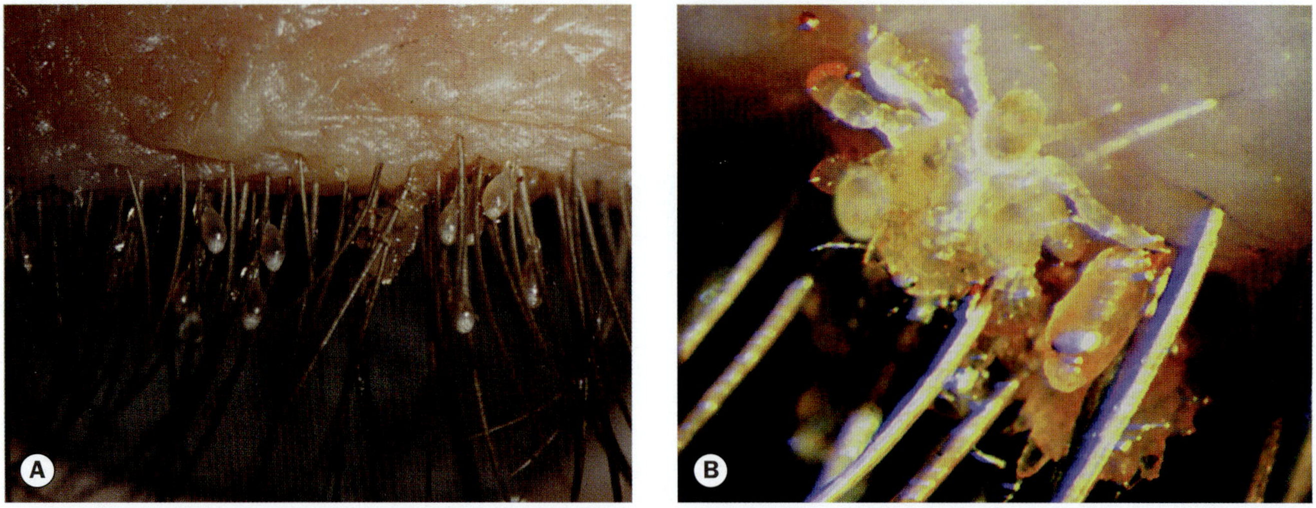

Fig. 2.38 Phthiriasis palpebrarum. **(A)** Louse anchored to lashes with ova; **(B)** close-up appearance of a louse.

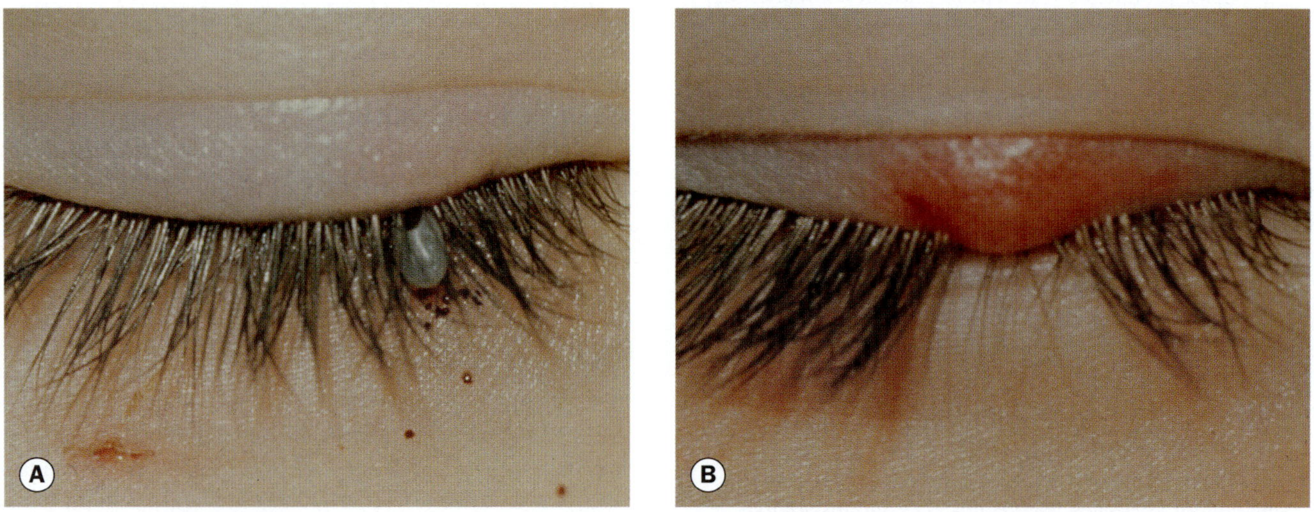

Fig. 2.39 **(A)** African tick on lid margin; **(B)** 2 weeks after removal. *(Courtesy of ADN Murray.)*

Angular blepharitis

The infection is usually caused by *Moraxella lacunata* or *S. aureus* although other bacteria and, rarely, herpes simplex have also been implicated. Red, scaly, macerated and fissured skin is seen at the lateral and/or medial canthi of one or both eyes (Fig. 2.40). Skin chafing secondary to tear overflow, especially at the lateral canthus, can cause a similar clinical picture and may also predispose to infection. Associated papillary and follicular conjunctivitis may occur. Treatment involves topical chloramphenicol, bacitracin or erythromycin.

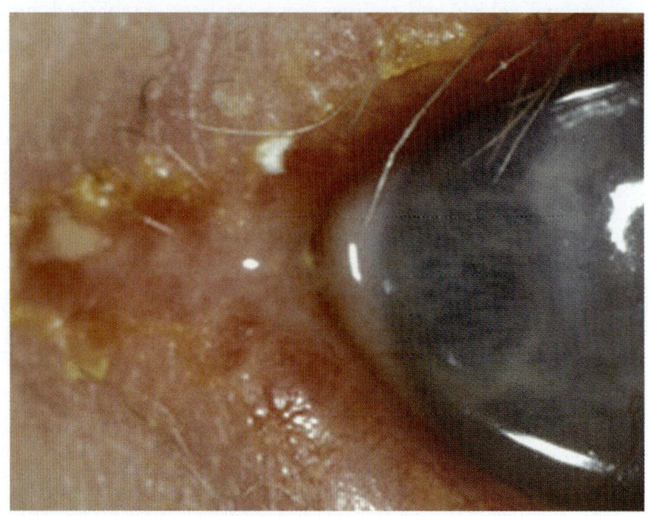

Fig. 2.40 Angular blepharitis. *(Courtesy of S Tuft.)*

Childhood blepharokeratoconjunctivitis

Childhood blepharokeratoconjunctivitis is a poorly defined condition that tends to be more severe in Asian and Middle Eastern populations. Presentation is usually at about 6 years of age with recurrent episodes of anterior or posterior blepharitis, sometimes associated with recurrent styes or chalazia. Constant eye rubbing and photophobia may lead to misdiagnosis as allergic eye disease. Conjunctival changes include diffuse hyperaemia, bulbar phlyctens and follicular or papillary hyperplasia.

Corneal changes include superficial punctate keratopathy, marginal keratitis, peripheral vascularization and axial subepithelial haze. Treatment is with lid hygiene and topical antibiotic ointment at bedtime. Topical low-dose steroids (prednisolone 0.1% or fluorometholone 0.1%) and erythromycin syrup 125 mg daily for 4–6 weeks may also be used.

PTOSIS

Classification

Ptosis is an abnormally low position of the upper lid, which may be congenital or acquired.

- **Neurogenic** ptosis is caused by an innervational defect such as third nerve paresis and Horner syndrome (see Ch. 19) (Fig. 2.41A).
- **Myogenic** ptosis is caused by a myopathy of the levator muscle itself, or by impairment of transmission of impulses at the neuromuscular junction (neuromyopathic). Acquired myogenic ptosis occurs in myasthenia gravis, myotonic dystrophy and progressive external ophthalmoplegia (see Ch. 19) (Fig. 2.41B).
- **Aponeurotic** or involutional ptosis is caused by a defect in the levator aponeurosis (Fig. 2.41C).
- **Mechanical** ptosis is caused by the gravitational effect of a mass or by scarring (Fig. 2.41D).

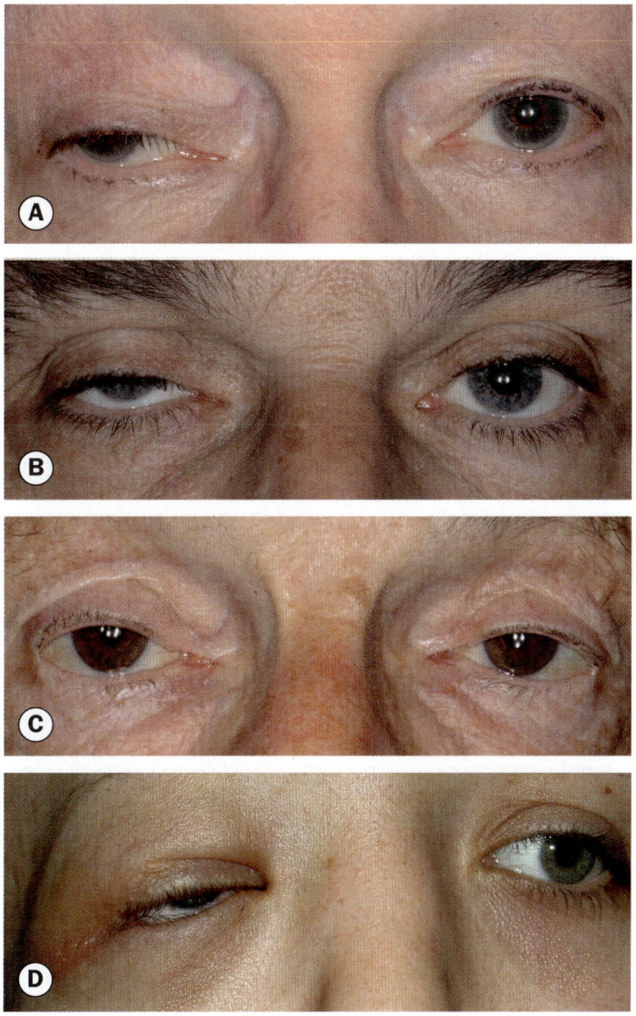

Fig. 2.41 Causes of ptosis. **(A)** Neurogenic (third nerve palsy); **(B)** myogenic (myasthenia gravis); **(C)** aponeurotic (age-related); **(D)** mechanical (neurofibroma).

Clinical evaluation

General

The age at onset of ptosis and the duration will usually distinguish congenital from acquired cases. If the history is ambiguous, old photographs may be helpful. It is also important to enquire about symptoms of possible underlying systemic disease, such as associated diplopia, variability of ptosis during the day and excessive fatigue.

Pseudoptosis

A false impression of ptosis may be caused by the following:

- **Lack of support** of the lids by the globe may be due to an orbital volume deficit associated with an artificial eye (Fig. 2.42A), microphthalmos, phthisis bulbi, or enophthalmos.
- **Contralateral lid retraction**, which is detected by comparing the levels of the upper lids, remembering that the margin of the upper lid normally covers the superior 2 mm of the cornea (Fig. 2.42B).
- **Ipsilateral hypotropia** causes pseudoptosis because the upper lid follows the globe downwards (Fig. 2.42C). It disappears when the hypotropic eye assumes fixation on covering the normal eye.
- **Brow ptosis** due to excessive skin on the brow, or seventh nerve palsy, which is diagnosed by manually elevating the eyebrow.
- **Dermatochalasis.** Overhanging skin on the upper lids (Fig. 2.42D) may be mistaken for ptosis, but may also cause mechanical ptosis.

Measurements

- **Margin–reflex distance** is the distance between the upper lid margin and the corneal reflection of a pen torch held by the examiner on which the patient fixates (Fig. 2.43). The normal measurement is 4–5 mm.
- **Palpebral fissure height** is the distance between the upper and lower lid margins, measured in the pupillary plane (Fig. 2.44). The upper lid margin normally rests about 2 mm below the upper limbus and the lower 1 mm above the lower limbus. This measurement is shorter in males (7–10 mm) than in females (8–12 mm). Unilateral ptosis can be quantified by comparison with the contralateral side. Ptosis may be graded as mild (up to 2 mm), moderate (3 mm) and severe (4 mm or more).
- **Levator function** (upper lid excursion) is measured by placing a thumb firmly against the patient's brow to negate

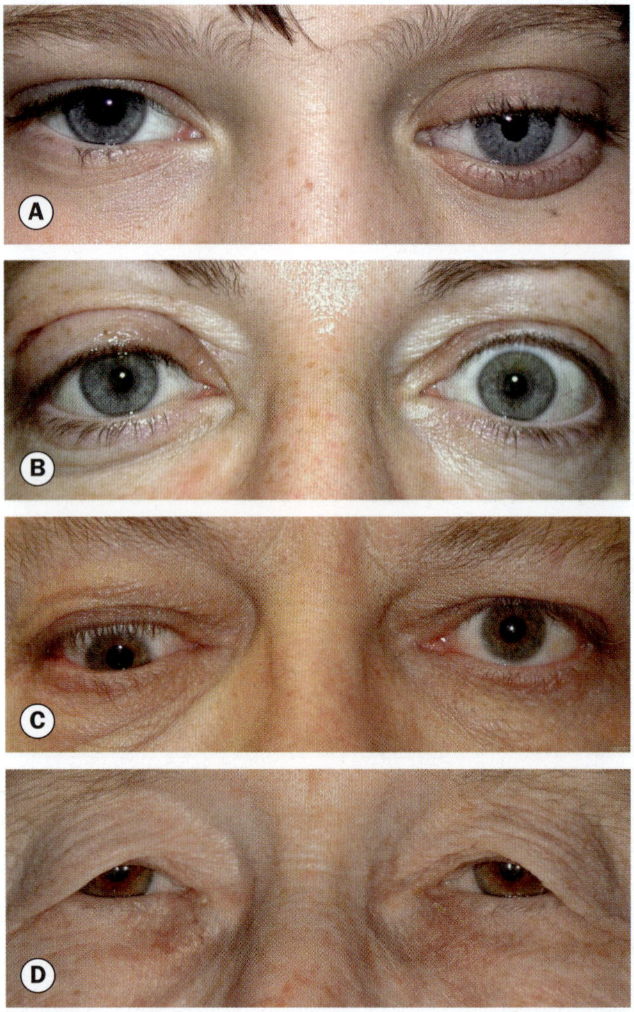

Fig. 2.42 Causes of pseudoptosis. **(A)** Left ill-fitting artificial eye; **(B)** asymmetrical lid position with contralateral lid retraction; **(C)** ipsilateral hypotropia which disappears on covering the normal left eye; **(D)** bilateral brow ptosis with marked dermatochalasis.

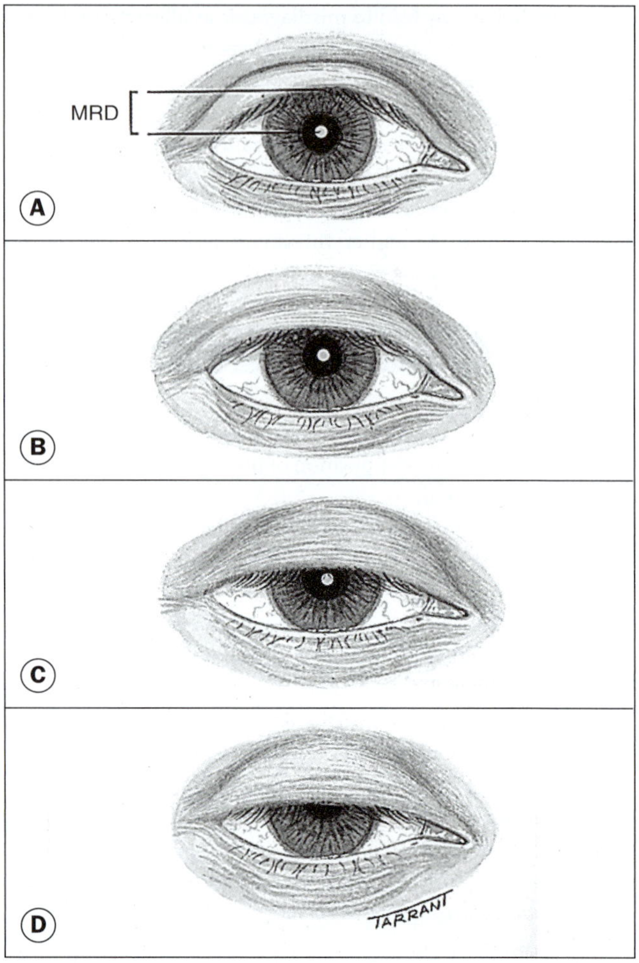

Fig. 2.43 Margin–reflex distance (MRD). **(A)** Normal; **(B)** mild ptosis; **(C)** moderate ptosis; **(D)** severe ptosis.

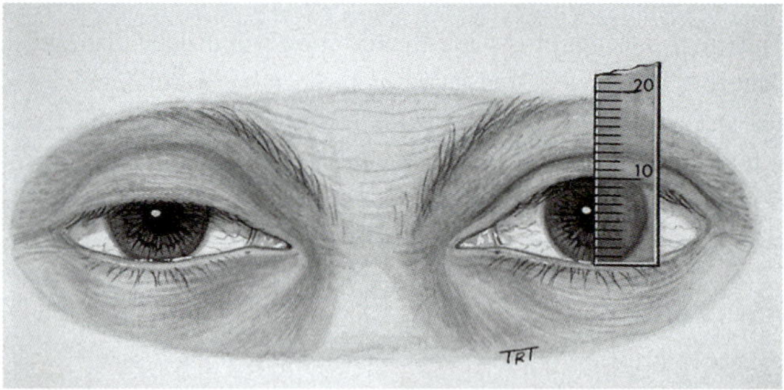

Fig. 2.44 Measurement of palpebral fissure height.

the action of the frontalis muscle, with the eyes in downgaze (Fig. 2.45A). Alternatively, the brow can be lifted above the orbit and held firmly against the forehead to reduce frontalis function. The patient then looks up as far as possible and the amount of excursion is measured with a rule (Fig. 2.45B). Levator function is graded as normal (15 mm or more), good (12–14 mm), fair (5–11 mm) and poor (4 mm or less).

- **Upper lid crease** is taken as the vertical distance between the lid margin and the lid crease in downgaze. In females it measures about 10 mm and in males 8 mm. Absence of the crease in a patient with congenital ptosis is evidence of poor levator function, whereas a high crease suggests an aponeurotic defect (usually involutional). The skin crease is also used as a guide to the initial incision in some surgical procedures.
- **Pretarsal show** is the distance between the lid margin and the skin fold with the eyes in the primary position.

Associated signs

- **The pupils** should be examined to exclude Horner syndrome and a subtle pupil-involving third nerve palsy – the latter is an unlikely acute clinical presentation (see Ch. 19).
- **Increased innervation** may flow to the levator muscle of a unilateral ptosis, particularly in upgaze. Associated increased innervation to the contralateral normal levator will result in lid retraction. The examiner should therefore manually elevate the lid and look for drooping of the opposite lid. If this occurs, the

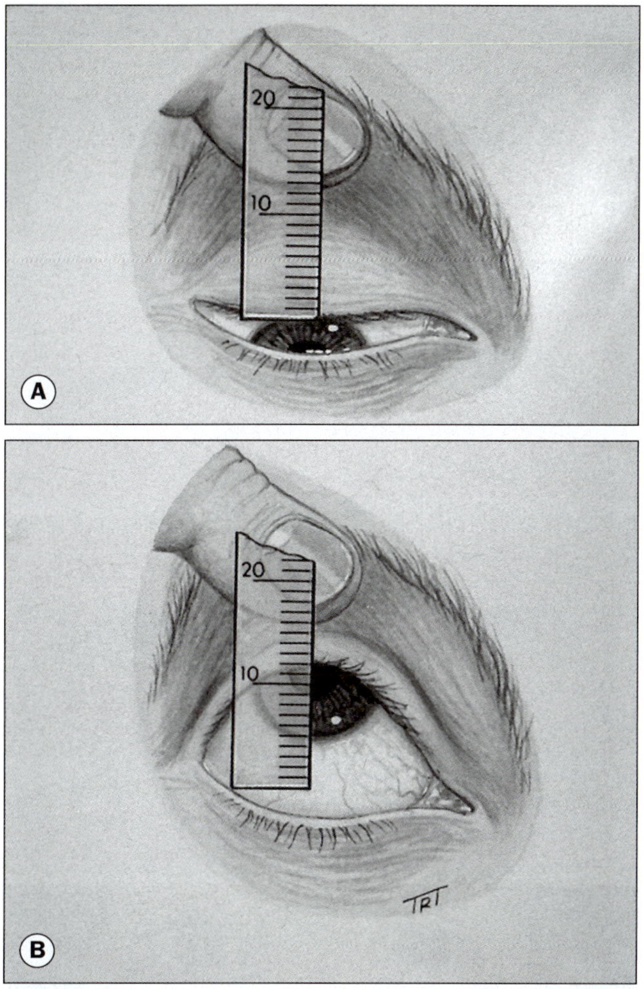

Fig. 2.45 Measurement of levator function. **(A)** Place a thumb firmly against the brow to reduce the effect of the frontalis muscle and ask the patient to look down; **(B)** the patient then looks up as far as possible and the amount of excursion is measured with a ruler.

patient should be warned that surgical correction may induce a lower position in the opposite lid.

- **Fatigability** is tested by asking the patient to look up without blinking for 30–60 seconds. Progressive drooping of one or both lids, or an inability to maintain upgaze, is suggestive of myasthenia gravis (see Ch. 19). Myasthenic ptosis may show an overshoot of the upper lid on saccade from downgaze to the primary position (Cogan twitch sign) and a 'hop' on side-gaze.
- **Ocular motility defects**, particularly of the superior rectus, must be evaluated in patients with congenital ptosis. Correction of an ipsilateral hypotropia may improve the degree of ptosis. Deficits consistent with a subtle or partial third nerve paresis should be identified.
- **Jaw-winking** can be identified by asking the patient to chew and move the jaws from side to side (see below).
- **Bell phenomenon** is tested by manually holding the lids open, asking the patient to try to shut the eyes and observing upward and outward rotation of the globe. A weak Bell phenomenon carries a variable risk of postoperative exposure keratopathy, particularly following large levator resections or suspension procedures.
- **The tear film** should be inspected – a poor volume or unstable film may be worsened by ptosis surgery and should be addressed preoperatively as far as possible.

Simple congenital ptosis

Diagnosis

Congenital ptosis probably results from a failure of neuronal migration or development with muscular sequelae secondary to this. A minority of patients have a family history.

- **Signs**
  - Unilateral or bilateral ptosis of variable severity (Fig. 2.46A and B).
  - Absent upper lid crease and poor levator function (Fig. 2.46C–F).
  - In downgaze the ptotic lid is higher than the normal because of poor relaxation of the levator muscle. This is in contrast to acquired ptosis, in which the affected lid is either level with or lower than the normal lid on downgaze.
  - Following surgical correction, the lid lag in downgaze may worsen.
- **Associations**
  - Superior rectus weakness may be present because of its close embryological association with the levator.
  - Compensatory chin elevation in severe bilateral cases.
  - Refractive errors are common and more frequently responsible for amblyopia than the ptosis itself.

Treatment

Treatment should be carried out during the preschool years once accurate measurements can be obtained, but may be considered earlier in severe cases to prevent amblyopia. Levator resection (see below) is usually required.

TIP A weak Bell phenomenon can result in exposure keratopathy after ptosis surgery.

Marcus Gunn jaw-winking syndrome

Introduction

About 5% of all cases of congenital ptosis are associated with the Marcus Gunn jaw-winking phenomenon. Most are unilateral. Although the exact aetiology is unclear, it has been postulated that a branch of the mandibular division of the fifth cranial nerve is misdirected to the levator muscle.

Diagnosis

- **Signs**
  - Retraction of the ptotic lid in conjunction with stimulation of the ipsilateral pterygoid muscles by chewing,

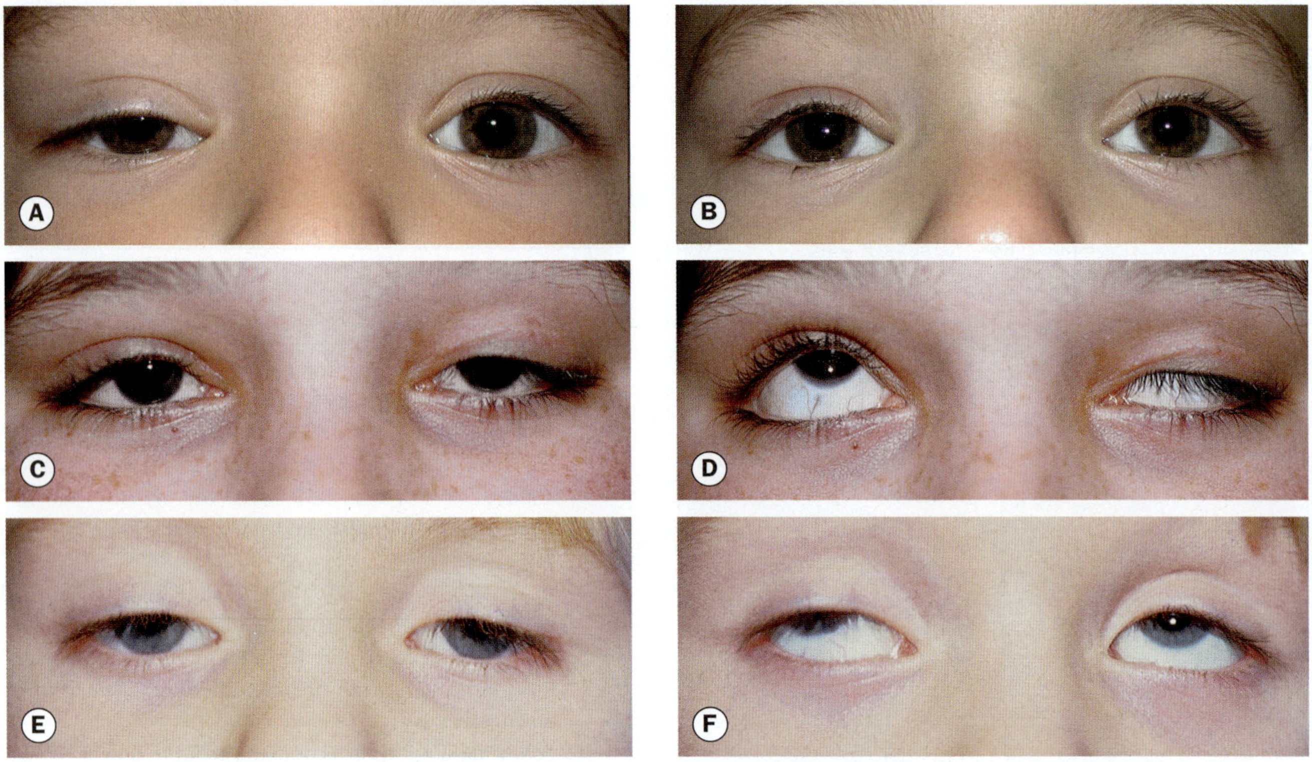

Fig. 2.46 Congenital ptosis. **(A)** Mild right ptosis; **(B)** good levator function; **(C)** severe left ptosis with absent skin crease; **(D)** poor levator function; **(E)** severe bilateral ptosis; **(F)** poor levator function.

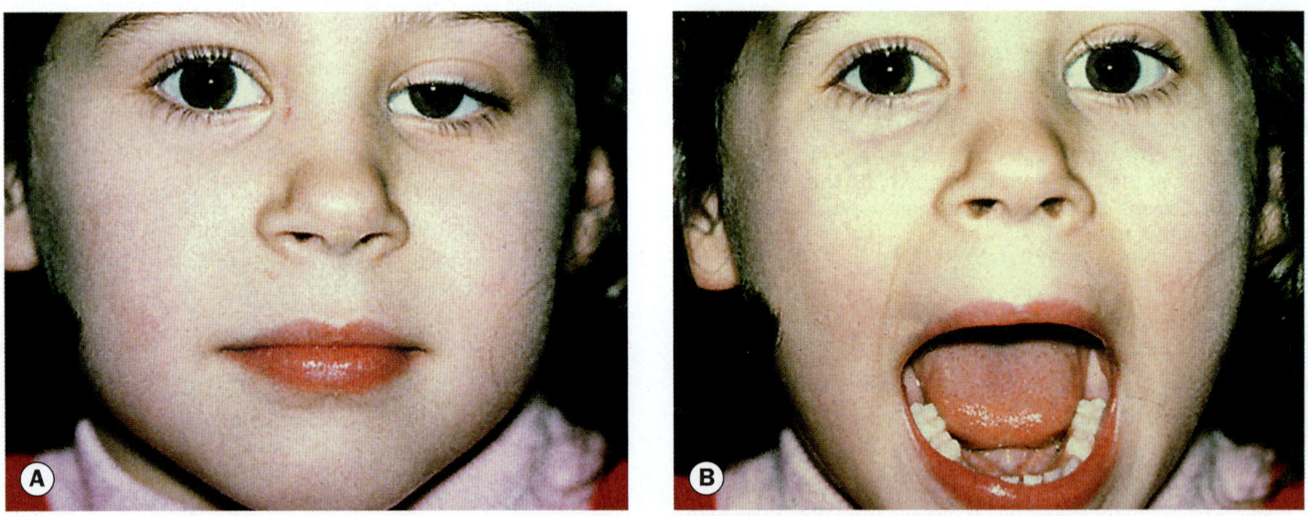

Fig. 2.47 Marcus Gunn jaw-winking syndrome. **(A)** Moderate left ptosis; **(B)** retraction of the lid on opening the mouth.

sucking, opening the mouth (Fig. 2.47) or contralateral jaw movement.

- ○ Less common stimuli to winking include jaw protrusion, smiling, swallowing and clenching of teeth.
- ○ Jaw-winking does not improve with age, although patients may learn to mask it.

Treatment

Surgery should be considered if jaw-winking or ptosis represents a significant functional or cosmetic problem.

- **Mild cases** with reasonable levator function of 5 mm or better and little synkinetic movement may be treated with unilateral levator advancement.
- **Moderate cases.** Unilateral levator disinsertion can be performed to address the synkinetic winking component, with ipsilateral brow (frontalis) suspension so that lid elevation is due solely to frontalis muscle elevation.
- **Bilateral surgery.** Bilateral levator disinsertion with bilateral brow suspension may be carried out to produce a symmetrical result.

Third nerve misdirection syndromes

Third nerve misdirection syndromes may be congenital, but more frequently follow acquired third nerve palsy. Bizarre movements of the upper lid accompany various eye movements (Fig. 2.48). Ptosis may also occur following aberrant facial nerve regeneration. Treatment is by levator disinsertion and brow suspension.

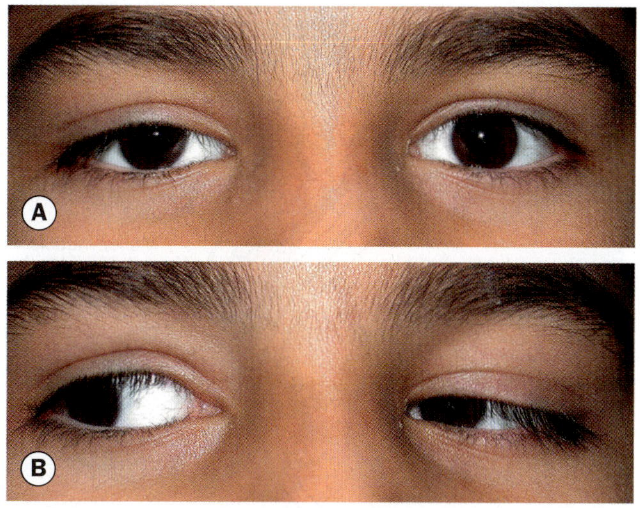

Fig. 2.48 Third nerve redirection. **(A)** Moderate right ptosis; **(B)** retraction of the right lid on right gaze. *(Courtesy of A Pearson.)*

Involutional ptosis

Involutional (aponeurotic) ptosis is an age-related condition caused by dehiscence, disinsertion or stretching of the levator aponeurosis, limiting the transmission of force from a normal levator muscle to the upper lid. Due to fatigue of the Müller muscle, it frequently worsens towards the end of the day, so that it can sometimes be confused with ptosis secondary to myasthenia. There is a variable, usually bilateral, ptosis with a high upper lid crease and good levator function. In severe cases the upper lid crease may be absent, the eyelid above the tarsal plate is very thin and the upper sulcus deep (Fig. 2.49). Treatment options include levator resection, advancement with reinsertion or anterior levator repair.

TIP Involutional ptosis may be confused with ocular myasthenia gravis because it frequently gets worse towards the end of the day.

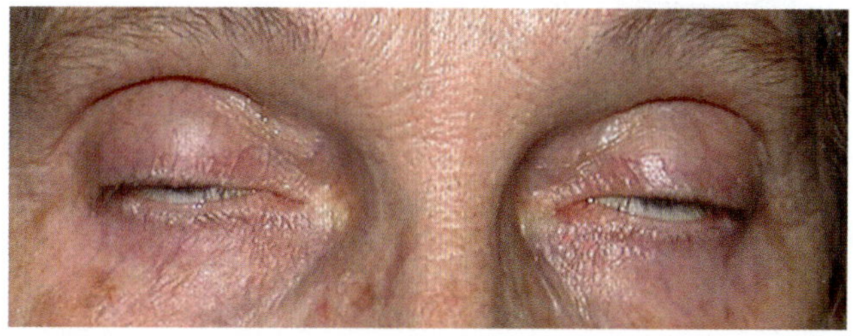

Fig. 2.49 Severe bilateral involutional ptosis with absent skin creases and deep sulci.

Mechanical ptosis

Mechanical ptosis is the result of impaired mobility of the upper lid. It may be caused by dermatochalasis, large tumours such as a neurofibroma, heavy scar tissue, severe oedema and anterior orbital lesions.

Surgery

Anatomy

- **The levator aponeurosis** fuses with the orbital septum about 4 mm above the superior border of the tarsal plate (Fig. 2.50A). Its posterior fibres insert into the lower third of the anterior surface of the tarsal plate. The medial and lateral horns are expansions that act as check ligaments (Fig. 2.50B). Surgically, the aponeurosis can be approached through the skin or conjunctiva.
- **Eyelids of Asians.** The main difference in the upper lid appearance is a low or absent skin crease in about 50% of Asians due to the low insertion of the levator aponeurosis, close to the lashes. The septum also inserts lower on the aponeurosis. The presence of a medial canthal fold can cause lash ptosis (Fig. 2.51).
- **Müller muscle** is inserted into the upper border of the tarsal plate and can be approached transconjunctivally.
- **The inferior tarsal aponeurosis** consists of the capsulopalpebral expansion of the inferior rectus muscle and is analogous to the levator aponeurosis.
- **The inferior tarsal muscle** is analogous to Müller muscle.

Conjunctiva–Müller resection

This involves excision of Müller muscle and overlying conjunctiva with reattachment of the resected edges (Fig. 2.52A–C). The maximal elevation achievable is 2–3 mm, so it is used in cases of mild ptosis with good (at least 10 mm) levator function, which includes most cases of Horner syndrome and mild congenital ptosis.

Levator advancement (resection)

In this technique the levator complex is shortened through either an anterior – skin (Fig. 2.53A–C) – or posterior – conjunctival – approach. Indications include ptosis of any cause, provided residual levator function is at least 5 mm. The extent of resection is determined by the severity of the ptosis and the amount of levator function. The predictability of correcting height is the same whether an anterior or posterior approach is used. However, the advantage of a posterior approach is the predictability of the lid contour.

Brow (frontalis) suspension

Brow (frontalis) suspension is used for severe ptosis (>4 mm) with very poor levator function (<4 mm) from a variety of causes. Typical indications include ptosis associated with third nerve palsy,

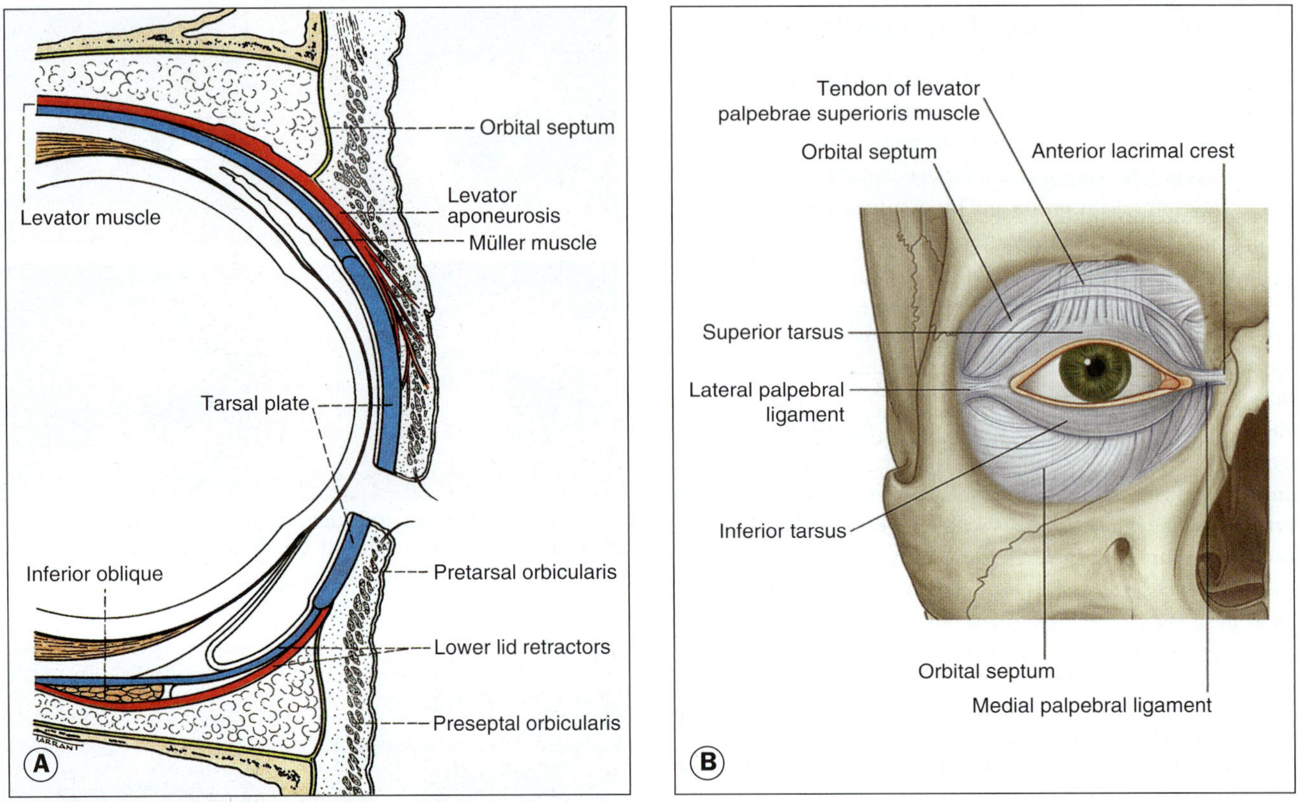

Fig. 2.50 Anatomy of the eyelid. **(A)** Cross-sectional diagram; **(B)** anterior view.

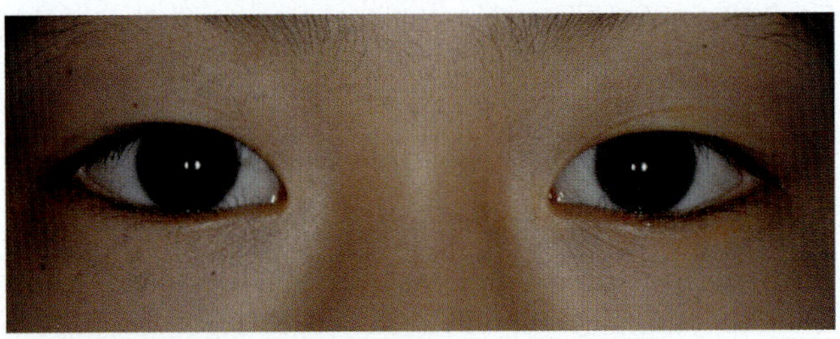

Fig. 2.51 Appearance of eyelids in an Asian child.

blepharophimosis syndrome and following an unsatisfactory result from previous levator resection. The tarsal plate is suspended from the frontalis muscle with a sling consisting of non-absorbable material such as silicone or less commonly in recent years, autologous fascia lata (Fig. 2.54A–C).

ECTROPION

Involutional ectropion

Introduction

Involutional (age-related) ectropion affects the lower lid of elderly individuals. It causes epiphora (tear overflow) and may exacerbate ocular surface disease. The red appearance of the exposed conjunctiva is cosmetically poor. In long-standing cases the tarsal conjunctiva may become chronically inflamed, thickened and keratinized (Fig. 2.55A). Aetiological factors include:

- **Horizontal lid laxity,** demonstrated by pulling the central part of the lid 8 mm or more from the globe, with a failure to snap back to its normal position on release without the patient first blinking.
- **Lateral canthal tendon laxity**, characterized by a rounded appearance of the lateral canthus and the ability to pull the lower lid medially more than 2 mm.
- **Medial canthal tendon laxity**, demonstrated by pulling the lower lid laterally and observing the position of the inferior punctum. If the lid is normal the punctum should not be displaced more than 1–2 mm. If laxity is mild the punctum reaches the limbus and if severe it may reach the pupil.

Treatment

The approach to repair depends on apparent causation and the predominant location of the ectropion.

- **Generalized ectropion is treated with repair of horizontal lid laxity.** This is achieved with a lateral tarsal strip procedure, in which the lower canthal tendon is tightened by shortening and reattachment to the lateral orbital rim (Fig. 2.56). This is particularly helpful if the lateral canthus is rounded and lax, with associated tear overflow. Excision of a tarsoconjunctival pentagon is an alternative that can be placed to excise an area of misdirected lashes or keratinized conjunctiva (Fig. 2.57).
- **Medial** ectropion, if mild, may be treated with a medial conjunctival diamond excision (medial spindle procedure). It is often combined with a tarsal strip or lateral canthal sling (see 'Treatment'), or pentagon excision as significant horizontal laxity frequently co-exists.

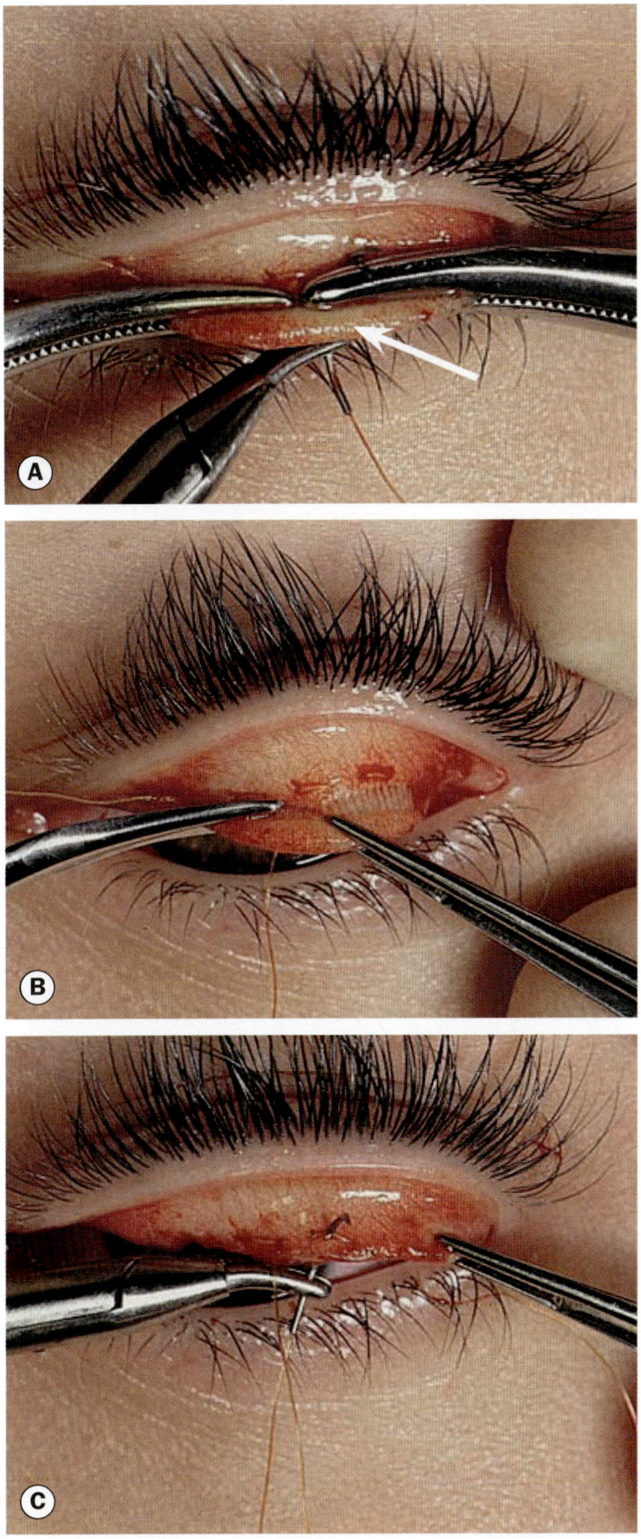

Fig. 2.52 Conjunctiva–Müller resection (Fasanella-Servat). **(A)** Forceps applied parallel to the superior border (arrow) of the tarsal plate. A 6-0 absorbable suture is inserted medially and passed continuously through the full thickness of the lid behind the forceps; **(B)** superior tarsal plate and smooth muscle are excised; **(C)** the second arm of the suture runs continuously over the cut edge. The two sutures are brought out through a lateral skin incision and tied. *(Courtesy of AG Tyers and JRO Collin, from* Colour Atlas of Ophthalmic Plastic Surgery, *Butterworth-Heinemann 2001.)*

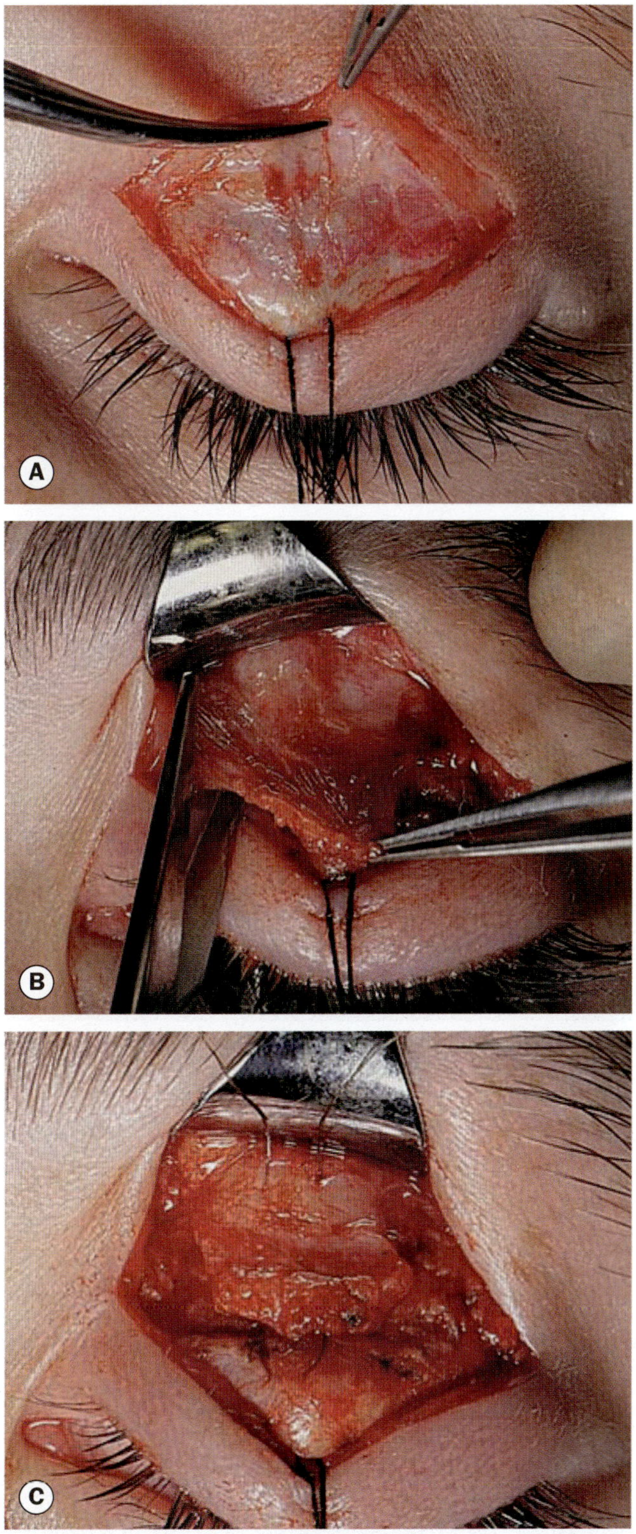

Fig. 2.53 Anterior levator resection. **(A)** Skin incision; **(B)** dissection and resection of levator aponeurosis; **(C)** levator reattachment to the tarsal plate. *(Courtesy of AG Tyers and JRO Collin, from* Colour Atlas of Ophthalmic Plastic Surgery, *Butterworth-Heinemann 2001.)*

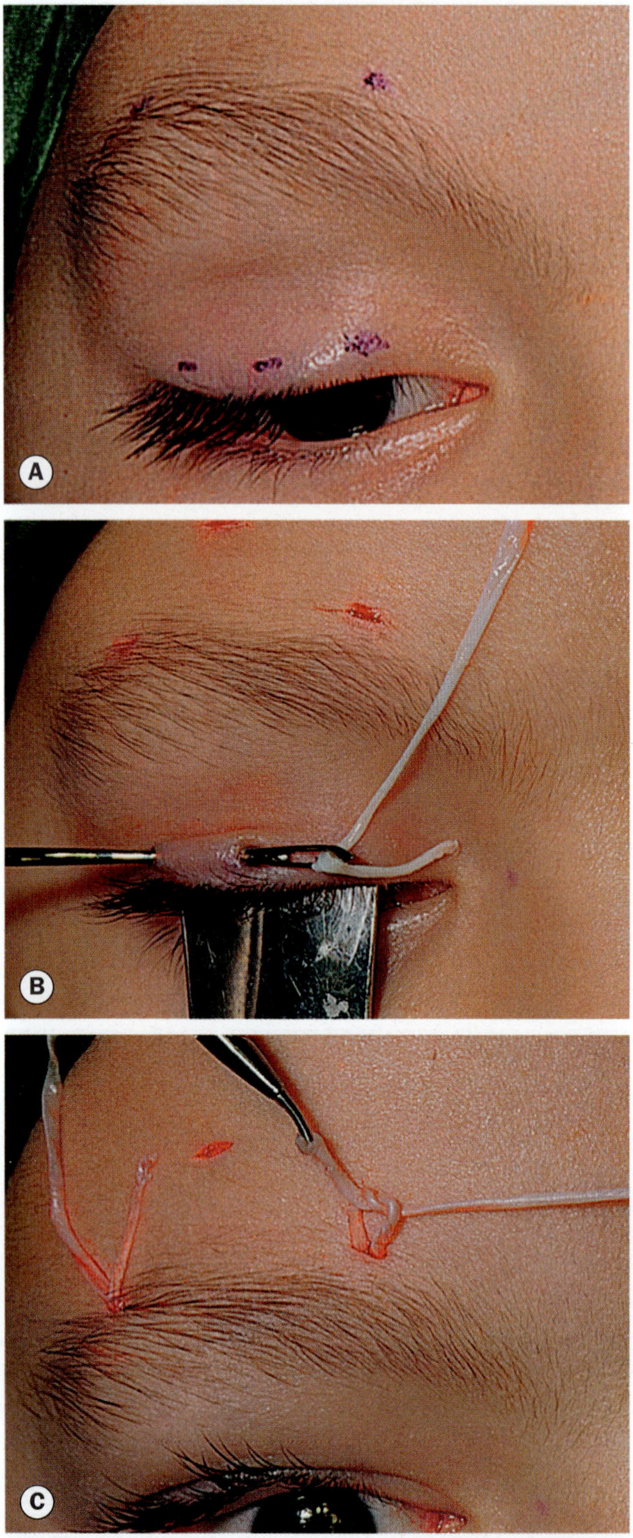

Fig. 2.54 Brow suspension. **(A)** Site of incisions marked; **(B)** threading of fascia lata strips; **(C)** tightening and tying of strips. *(Courtesy of AG Tyers and JRO Collin, from* Colour Atlas of Ophthalmic Plastic Surgery*, Butterworth-Heinemann 2001.)*

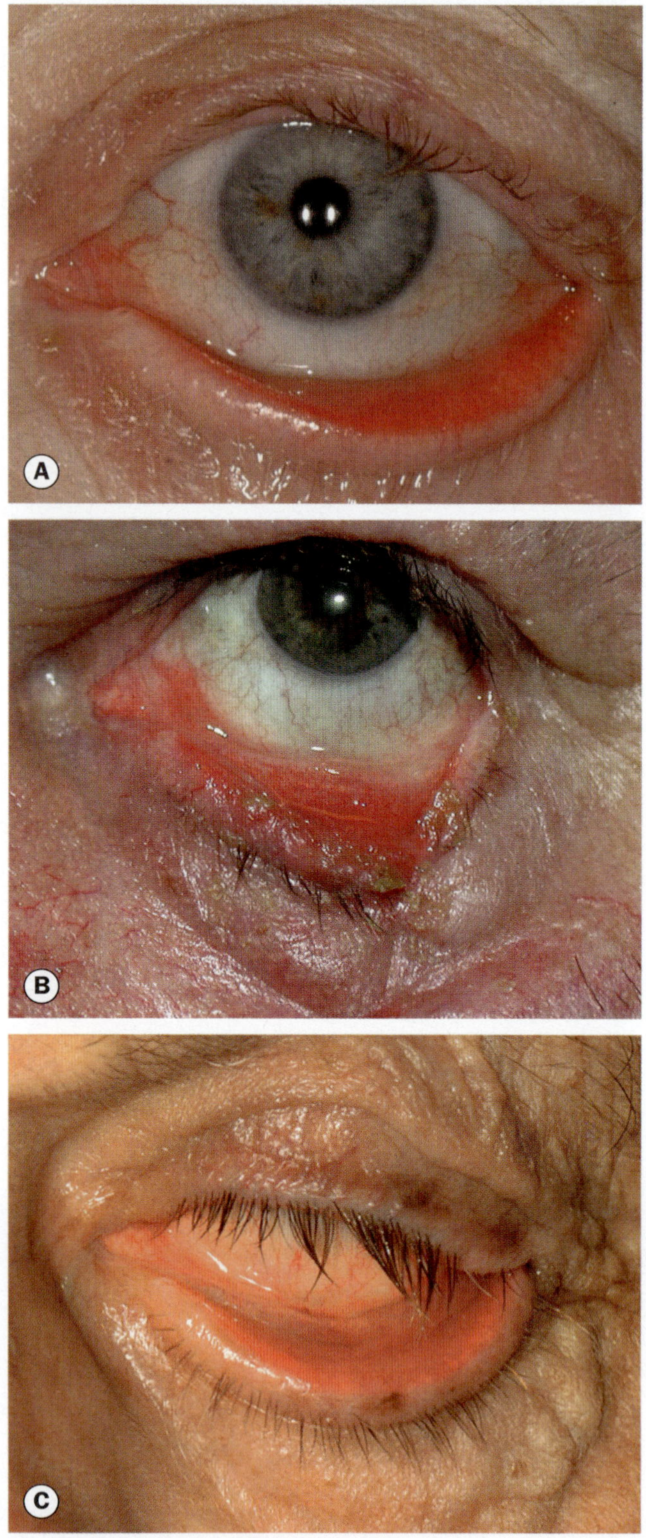

Fig. 2.55 Ectropion. **(A)** Severe long-standing involutional ectropion with keratinization of the marginal conjunctiva; **(B)** cicatricial; **(C)** paralytic secondary to a facial nerve palsy. *(Courtesy of C Barry – fig. A; A Pearson – fig. B; JH Norris – fig. C.)*

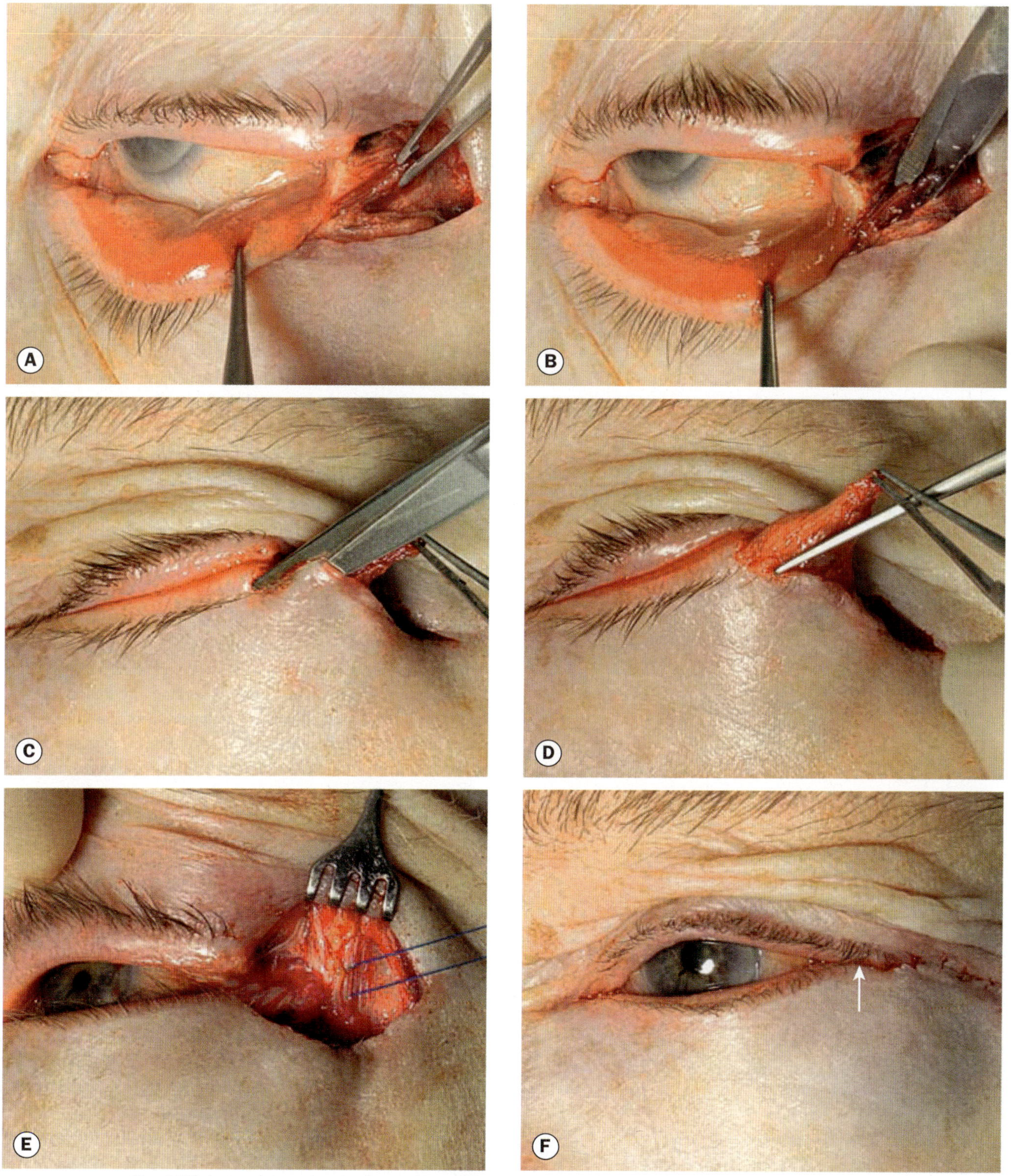

Fig. 2.56 Lateral tarsal strip procedure. **(A)** Lower limb of the lateral canthal tendon is isolated; **(B)** the tendon is cut close to the orbital rim; **(C)** lid margin skin is excised, then skin and orbicularis tissue are separated from the tarsal plate; **(D)** a lateral tarsal strip is created; **(E)** this is sutured to periosteum anterior to the orbital rim; **(F)** a new canthus is formed (arrow). *(Courtesy of AG Tyers and RJO Collin, from* Colour Atlas of Ophthalmic Plastic Surgery, *Butterworth-Heinemann 2001.)*

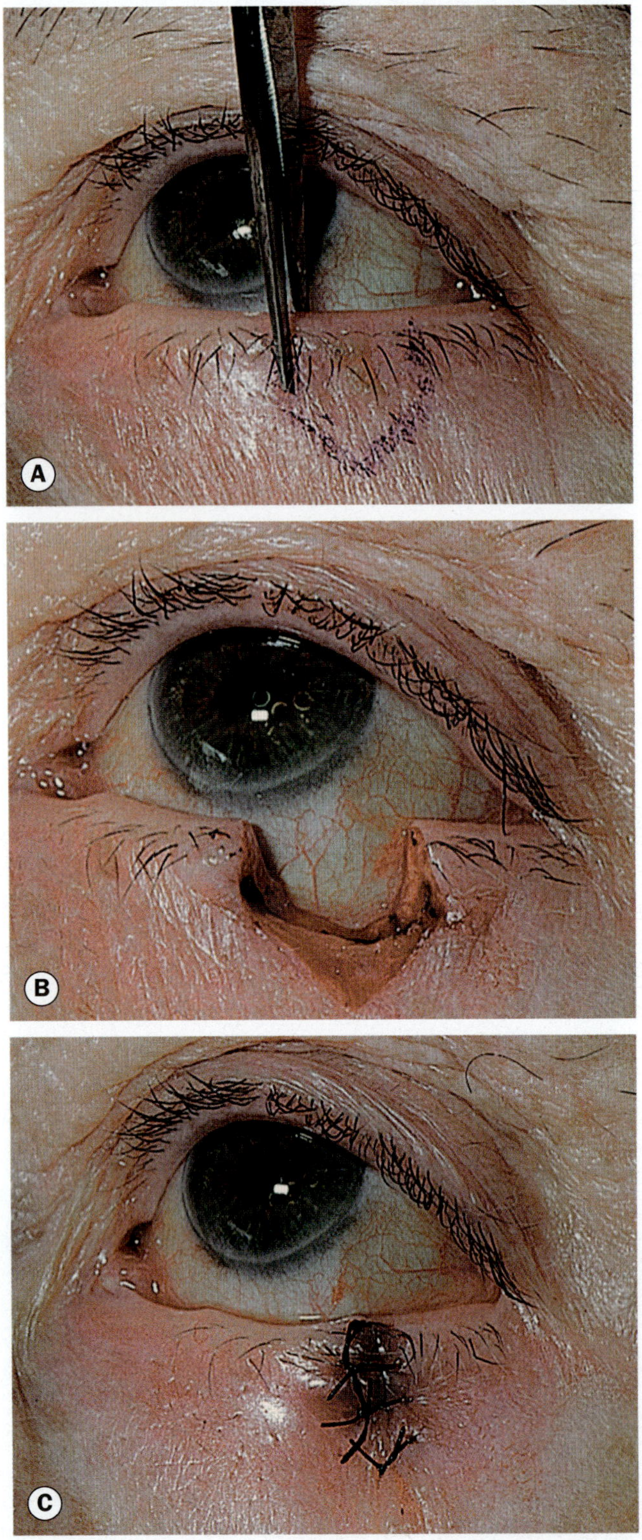

Fig. 2.57 Horizontal lid shortening to correct ectropion. **(A)** Marking; **(B)** excision of a pentagon; **(C)** closure. *(Courtesy of AG Tyers and JRO Collin, from* Colour Atlas of Ophthalmic Plastic Surgery, *Butterworth-Heinemann 2001.)*

- **Medial canthal tendon laxity**, if marked, requires stabilization prior to horizontal shortening to avoid excessive dragging of the punctum laterally.
- **Punctal ectropion** without more extensive lid involvement is considered in Chapter 3.

Cicatricial ectropion

Cicatricial ectropion is caused by scarring or contracture of the skin and underlying tissues, which pulls the eyelid away from the globe (see Fig. 2.55B). If the skin is pushed up over the orbital margin with a finger the ectropion will be relieved. Opening the mouth tends to accentuate the eversion. Depending on the cause, both lids may be involved, and the defect may be local (e.g. trauma) or general (e.g. burns, dermatitis, ichthyosis). Mild localized cases are treated by excision of the offending scar tissue combined with a procedure that lengthens vertical skin deficiency, such as Z-plasty. Severe generalized cases require transposition flaps or free skin grafts. Sources of skin include the upper lids, posterior auricular, preauricular and supraclavicular areas.

Paralytic ectropion/facial nerve palsy

Introduction

Paralytic ectropion is caused by ipsilateral facial nerve palsy (see Fig. 2.55C) and is associated with retraction of the upper and lower lids and brow ptosis. The latter may mimic narrowing of the palpebral aperture.

Complications include exposure keratopathy due to lagophthalmos and watering caused by malposition of the inferior lacrimal punctum, failure of the lacrimal pump mechanism and an increase in tear production resulting from corneal exposure.

Treatment

- **Temporary** measures may be instituted to protect the cornea in anticipation of spontaneous recovery of facial nerve function.
  - Lubrication with high viscosity tear substitutes during the day, with instillation of ointment and taping shut of the lids during sleep, are usually adequate in mild cases.
  - Botulinum toxin injection into the levator to induce temporary ptosis.
  - Temporary tarsorrhaphy may be necessary, particularly in patients with a poor Bell phenomenon where the cornea remains exposed when the patient attempts to blink. The lateral aspects of the upper and lower lids are sutured together.
- **Permanent** treatment should be considered when there is irreversible damage to the facial nerve which may occur following removal of a vestibular schwannoma, or when no further improvement has occurred for 6–12 months in a Bell palsy.
  - Medial canthoplasty may be performed if the medial canthal tendon is intact. The eyelids are sutured together medial to the lacrimal puncta (Fig. 2.58A) so that the

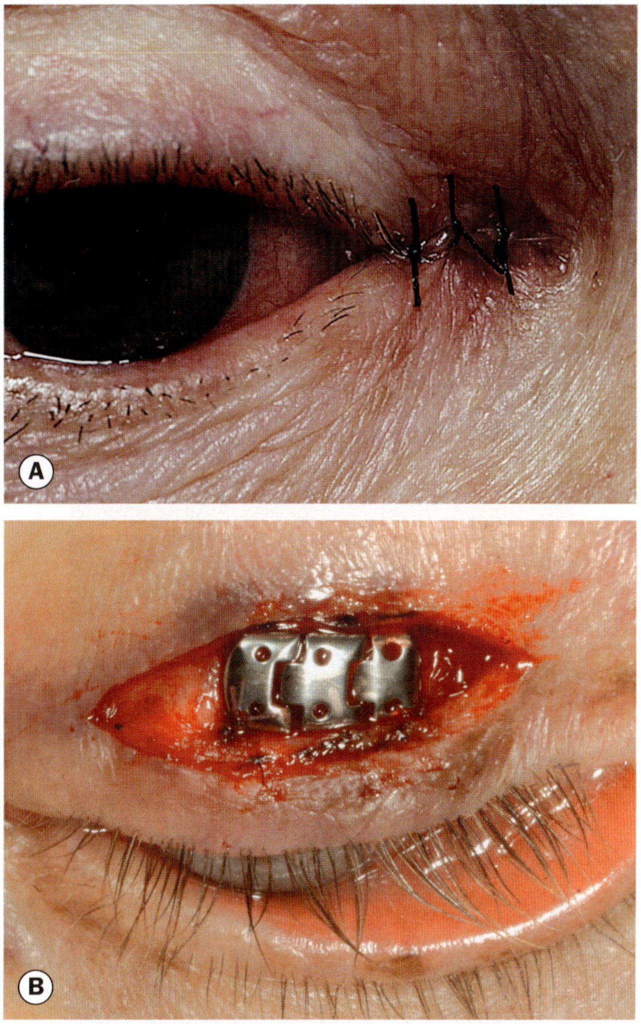

Fig. 2.58 (A) Medial canthoplasty as permanent treatment of paralytic ectropion; **(B)** platinum weight used to correct lagophthalmos. *(Courtesy JH Norris – fig. B.)*

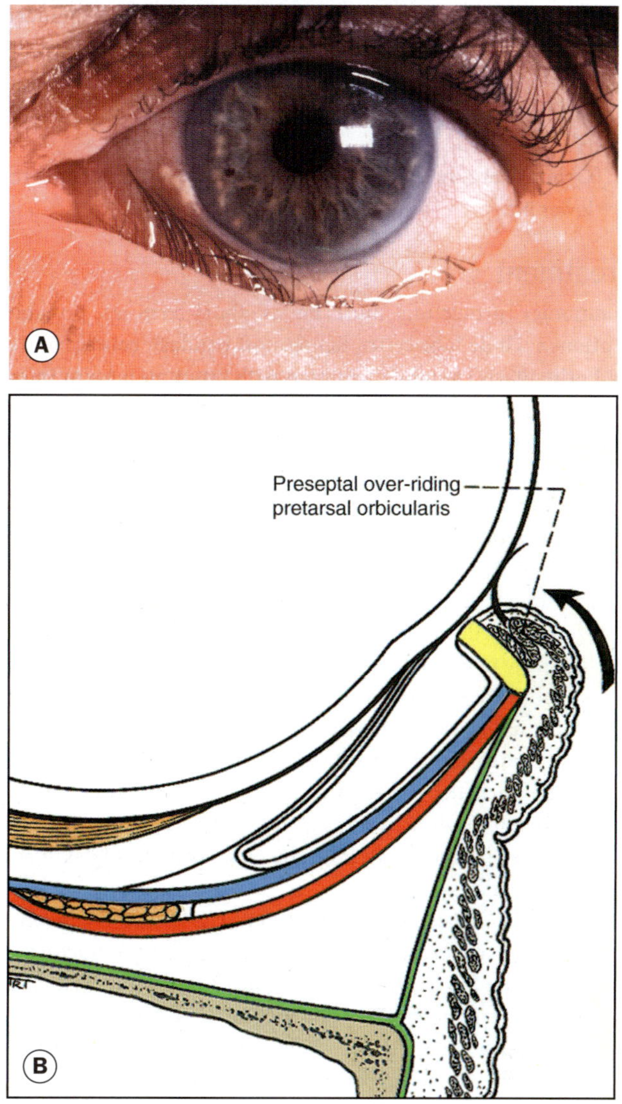

Fig. 2.59 (A) Involutional entropion and pseudotrichiasis; **(B)** preseptal orbicularis over-riding the pretarsal orbicularis.

puncta become inverted and the fissure between the inner canthus and puncta is shortened.

- A lateral canthal sling or tarsal strip may be used to correct residual ectropion and raise the lateral canthus.
- Upper eyelid lowering by levator disinsertion.
- In patients with lagophthalmos either gold or platinum weights can be implanted into the upper lid. Platinum weights are preferred because they are less bulky than gold weights, provide a better eyelid contour and are less likely to need long-term revisional surgery (Fig. 2.58B).
- A small lateral tarsorrhaphy is usually cosmetically acceptable.

Mechanical ectropion

Mechanical ectropion is caused by tumours on or near the lid margin that mechanically evert the lid. Treatment involves removal of the cause if possible and correction of significant horizontal lid laxity.

ENTROPION

Involutional entropion

Introduction

Involutional (age-related) entropion affects mainly the lower lid. The constant rubbing of the lashes on the cornea in long-standing entropion (pseudotrichiasis – Fig. 2.59A) may cause irritation, corneal punctate epithelial erosions and, in severe cases, pannus formation and ulceration. Aetiological factors include:

- **Horizontal lid laxity** caused by stretching of the canthal tendons and tarsal plate.
- **Vertical lid instability** caused by attenuation, dehiscence or disinsertion of the lower lid retractors. Weakness of the latter is recognized by decreased excursion of the lower lid in downgaze.

- **Over-riding of the pretarsal** by the preseptal orbicularis during lid closure tends to move the lower border of the tarsal plate anteriorly, away from the globe and the upper border towards the globe, thus tipping the lid inwards (Fig. 2.59B).
- **Orbital septum laxity** with prolapse of orbital fat into the lower lid.

Treatment

Temporary protection must be as short-term as possible. Options include lubricants, taping, soft bandage contact lenses and orbicularis chemodenervation with botulinum toxin injection. Surgical treatment aims to correct the underlying problems as follows:

- **Over-riding** and disinsertion
  - Transverse everting sutures prevent over-riding of the preseptal orbicularis. They are quick and easy to insert (Fig. 2.60A–C), providing a correction that typically lasts several months and may be used in circumstances (e.g. a confused patient) where a more intricate procedure is not likely to be tolerated.
  - The Wies procedure gives a durable correction. It consists of full-thickness horizontal lid splitting and insertion of everting sutures (Fig. 2.61A–D). The scar creates a barrier between the preseptal and pretarsal orbicularis and the everting suture fairly effectively transfers the pull of the lower lid retractors from the tarsal plate to the skin and orbicularis.
  - Lower lid retractor reinsertion (Fig. 2.62A–D) involves direct exposure and advancement of the retractors as opposed to the less precise approach used in the Wies procedure. The subciliary skin incision used and its repair also create a barrier to over-riding of the preseptal orbicularis muscle. It can be performed as a primary treatment but may be reserved for recurrence.
- **Horizontal lid laxity** is usually present and can be corrected with a lateral canthal sling (tarsal strip –see Fig. 2.56) or, less commonly, a full-thickness lateral pentagon excision (see Fig. 2.57). Tightening serves also to retain the lid in apposition against the globe, preventing over-correction.

Cicatricial entropion

Scarring of the palpebral conjunctiva can rotate the upper or lower lid margin towards the globe. Causes include cicatrizing conjunctivitis, trachoma, trauma and chemical injuries (see Figs 6.7F, 6.18C, 6.20D). Treatment of mild cases is by tarsal fracture (transverse tarsotomy) with anterior rotation of the lid margin, as for marginal entropion of the lower lid. Treatment of severe cases is difficult and is directed at replacing deficient or keratinized conjunctiva and replacing the scarred and contracted tarsal plate with composite grafts.

TIP Horizontal lid laxity should be corrected with a lateral tarsal sling procedure.

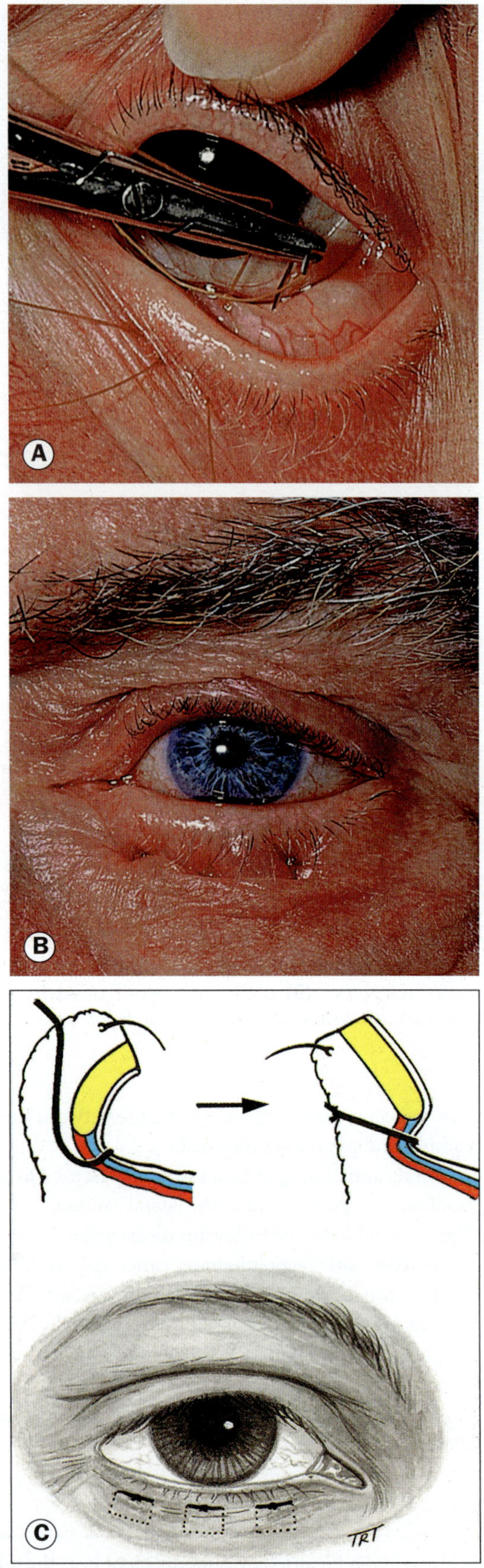

Fig. 2.60 Lid-everting sutures for entropion. **(A)** Three double-armed sutures are passed as shown; **(B)** sutures are tied; **(C)** schematic. *(Courtesy of AG Tyers and JRO Collin, from* Colour Atlas of Ophthalmic Plastic Surgery, *Butterworth-Heinemann 2001 – figs A and B.)*

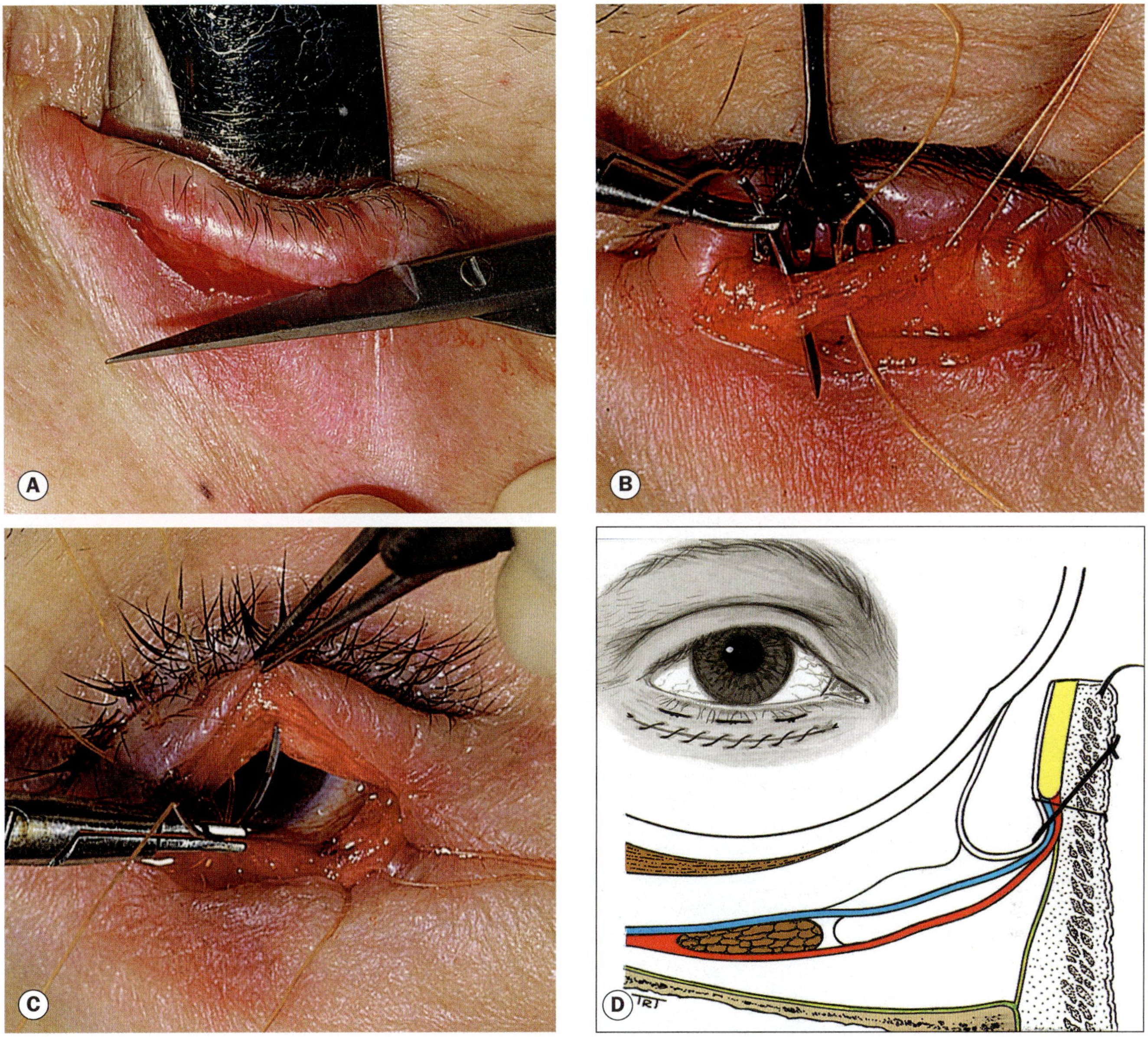

Fig. 2.61 Wies procedure for entropion. **(A)** Full-thickness incision; **(B)** sutures are passed through the conjunctiva and lower lid retractors; **(C)** sutures are passed anterior to the tarsal plate to exit inferior to the lashes; **(D)** schematic. *(Courtesy of AG Tyers and JRO Collin, from* Colour Atlas of Ophthalmic Plastic Surgery, *Butterworth-Heinemann 2001 – figs A–C.)*

MISCELLANEOUS ACQUIRED DISORDERS

Varix

An eyelid varix (plural – varices) is a common lesion that may be mistaken for a naevus or haemangioma. A varix is commonly an isolated lesion, but may be associated with orbital involvement (see Ch. 4). It appears as a dark red or purple subcutaneous compressible (unless thrombosed) lesion (Fig. 2.63A), which in some cases becomes apparent only with a Valsalva manoeuvre (Fig. 2.63B and C). It is clinically and histologically similar to a lymphangioma. Simple excision may be performed for diagnostic or cosmetic reasons. The possibility of orbital communication should be borne in mind during surgery.

Dermatochalasis

This is described in the discussion of pseudoptosis (above) and upper lid blepharoplasty (below).

Floppy eyelid syndrome

Introduction

Floppy eyelid syndrome (FES) is an uncommon unilateral or bilateral condition that is often overlooked as a cause of persistent ocular surface symptoms. It typically affects obese middle-aged and older men who sleep with one or both eyelids against the pillow, which results in the lid pulling away from the globe. Consequent nocturnal exposure

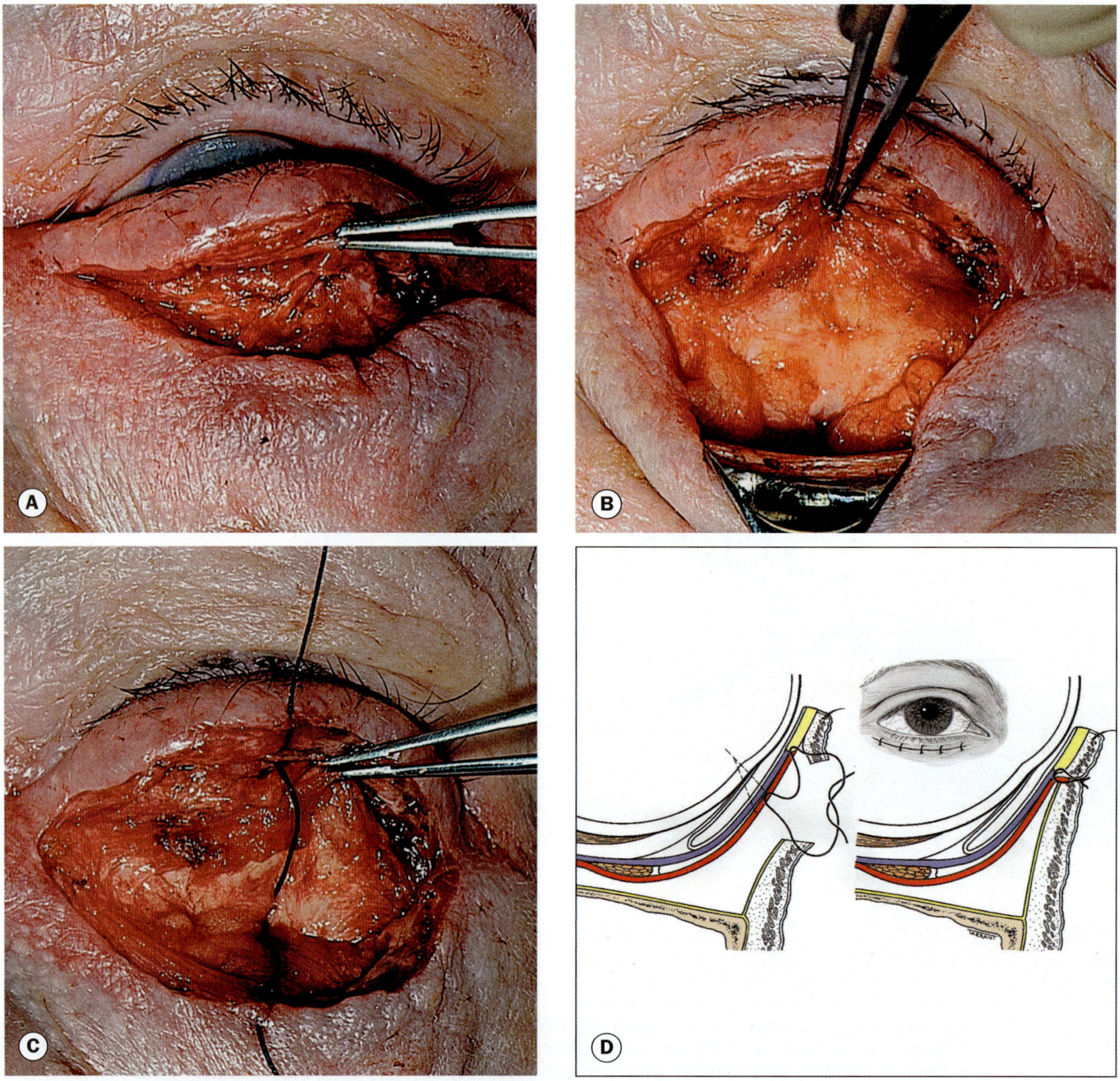

Fig. 2.62 Lower retractor reinsertion. **(A)** Incision to expose the lower border of the tarsal plate; **(B)** reflection of the orbital septum and fat pad to expose the lower lid retractors; **(C)** tightening of retractors by plication; **(D)** schematic. *(Courtesy of AG Tyers and JRO Collin, from* Colour Atlas of Ophthalmic Plastic Surgery, *Butterworth-Heinemann 2001 – figs A–C.)*

and poor contact with the globe, often exacerbated by other ocular surface disease such as dry eye and blepharitis, result in chronic keratoconjunctivitis. Obstructive sleep apnoea (OSA) is strongly associated and is linked to significant morbidity, including cardiopulmonary disease and subtle but irreversible mental dysfunction.

Diagnosis

- **The upper eyelid** is typically extremely lax, often with substantial excess loose upper lid skin (Fig. 2.64A). The tarsal plate has a rubbery consistency (Fig. 2.64B). The lid is very easy to evert (Fig. 2.64C), to fold and to pull away from the eye.
- **Papillary conjunctivitis** of the superior tarsal conjunctiva may be intense (Fig. 2.64D).
- **Keratopathy.** Punctate keratopathy, filamentary keratitis and superior superficial vascularization may be present.
- **Other findings** may include eyelash ptosis, lacrimal gland prolapse, ectropion and aponeurotic ptosis. Patients with both FES and OSA are at greater risk of developing glaucoma.
- **Investigation for OSA** should be considered in most cases of FES, particularly if the patient reports substantial snoring and/or excessive daytime sleepiness.

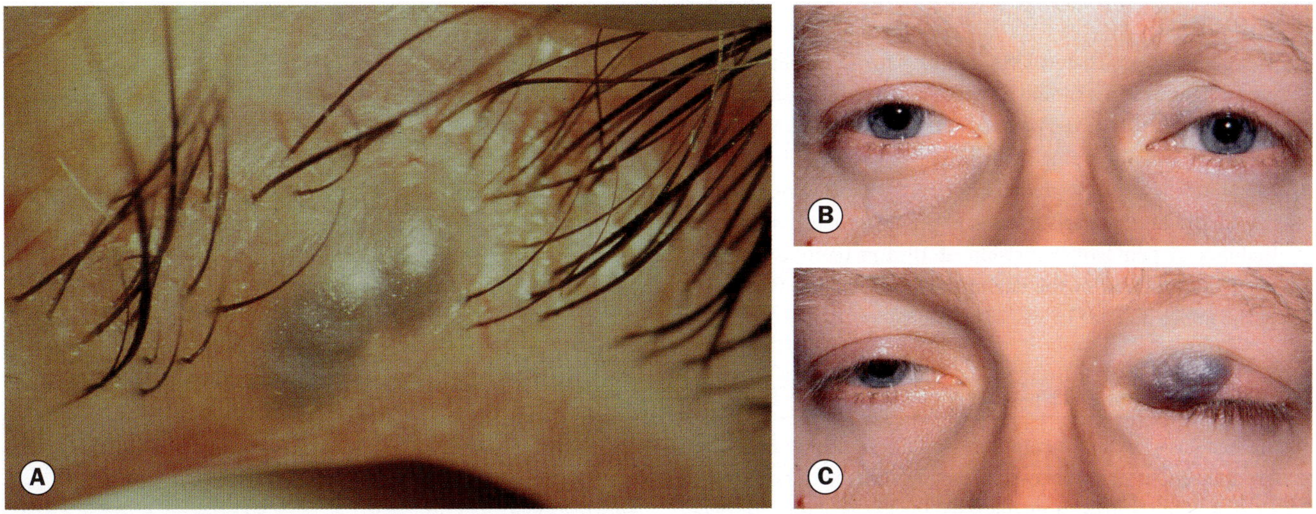

Fig. 2.63 Eyelid varices. **(A)** Typical appearance of a commonly seen small varix; **(B)** larger lesion, probably with orbital involvement, before Valsalva manoeuvre; **(C)** during Valsalva. *(Courtesy of G Rose – figs B and C.)*

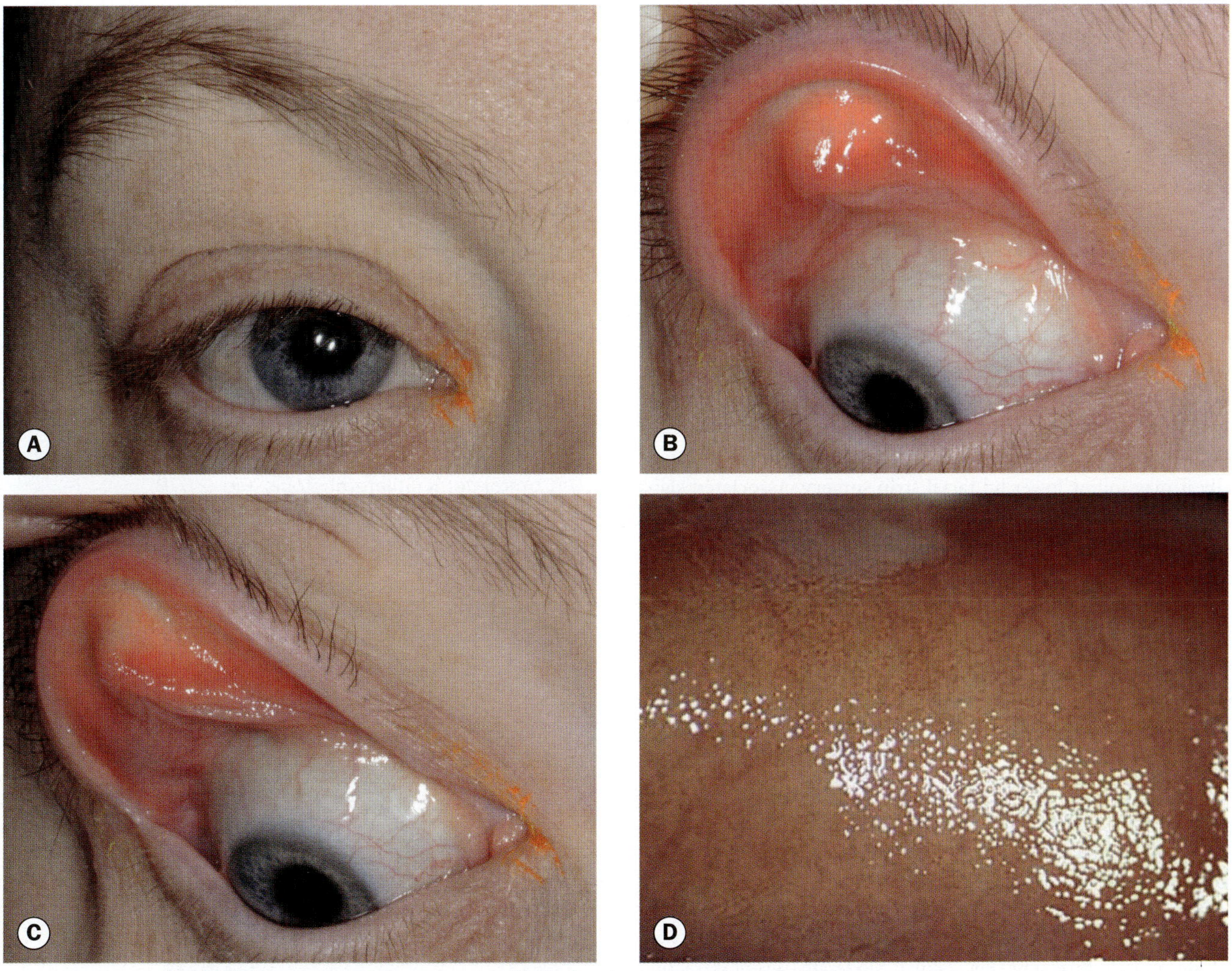

Fig. 2.64 Floppy eyelid syndrome. **(A)** Redundant upper lid skin; **(B)** loose and rubbery tarsal plates; **(C)** very easily everted eyelid; **(D)** superior tarsal papillary conjunctivitis.

Treatment

- Treatment of associated OSA is likely to be of benefit, and overweight patients should be encouraged to lose weight.
- Mild cases may respond to lubrication together with nocturnal eye shield wear or taping of the lids.
- Moderate–severe cases require horizontal shortening to stabilize the lid and ocular surface and prevent nocturnal lagophthalmos. A pentagonal excision of 10 mm or more is taken from the junction of the lateral third and medial two-thirds of the upper lid.

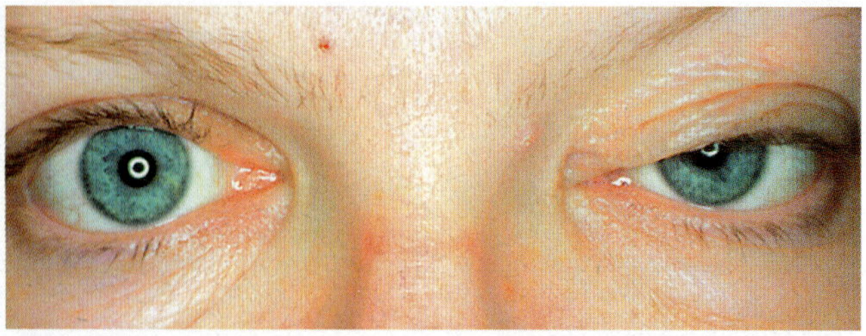

Fig. 2.65 Blepharochalasis – left aponeurotic ptosis and thinned upper lid skin.

Blepharochalasis

Blepharochalasis is an uncommon condition characterized by recurrent episodes of painless, non-pitting oedema of both upper lids that usually resolves spontaneously after a few days. Presentation is usually around puberty, episodes becoming less frequent with time. Eyelid skin becomes stretched and atrophic, characteristically said to resemble wrinkled cigarette paper. Severe cases may give rise to stretching of the canthal tendons and levator aponeurosis resulting in ptosis (Fig. 2.65) and lacrimal gland prolapse may occur. A hypertrophic form with orbital fat herniation and an atrophic form with absorption of orbital fat have been described. The differential diagnosis includes similarly episodic conditions, particularly drug-induced urticaria and angioedema. Treatment involves blepharoplasty for redundant upper lid skin and correction of ptosis.

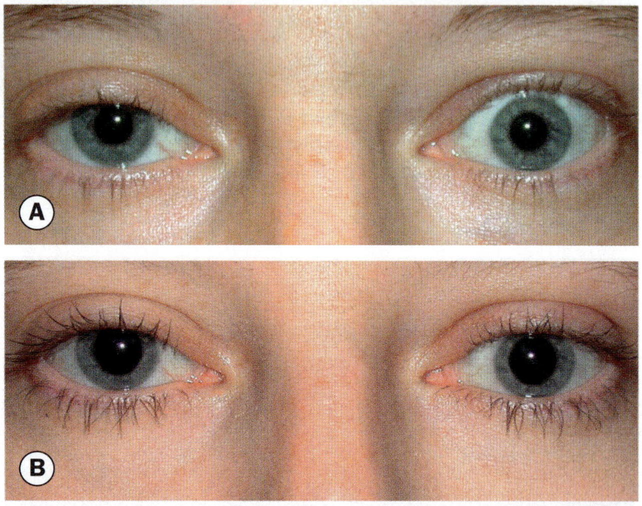

Fig. 2.66 **(A)** Left lid retraction in thyroid eye disease; **(B)** following Müller muscle recession. *(Courtesy of A Pearson.)*

Eyelid imbrication syndrome

Eyelid imbrication syndrome is an uncommon and frequently unrecognized disorder in which the upper lid overlaps the lower on closure so that the lower lashes irritate the superior marginal tarsal conjunctiva. It may be unilateral or bilateral and the major symptom is ocular irritation. It can be acquired, commonly associated with FES, or – very rarely – can be congenital. Occasionally it may follow lower lid tarsal strip surgery. Associated signs include superior tarsal papillary conjunctivitis and rose Bengal staining of the superior marginal conjunctiva. Definitive treatment consists of upper lid pentagon resection and/or lateral canthal tightening.

Upper lid retraction

Upper lid retraction is suspected when the upper lid margin is either level with or above the superior limbus (Fig. 2.66A). Intermittent upper lid retraction may occur in healthy infants and disappears by 6 months. Other causes are listed in Table 2.5 and selected examples are illustrated in Fig. 2.67. Where there is no loss or tightness of the upper eyelid skin, retraction is corrected by surgical release of the eyelid retractors, usually via a transconjunctival posterior approach. Mild retraction may be treated with Müller muscle recession (Fig. 2.66B). Moderate–severe retraction may require levator aponeurosis recession.

Table 2.5 Causes of Lid Retraction

1. Thyroid eye disease (Fig. 2.67A)
2. Neurogenic
Contralateral unilateral ptosis (Fig. 2.67B)
Unopposed levator action due to facial palsy
Third nerve misdirection
Marcus Gunn jaw-winking syndrome
Collier sign of the dorsal midbrain (Parinaud syndrome – see Fig. 19.85D)
Infantile hydrocephalus (setting sun sign – Fig. 2.67C)
Parkinsonism (Fig. 2.67D)
Sympathomimetic drops
3. Mechanical
Surgical over-correction of ptosis
Scarring of upper lid skin
4. Congenital
Isolated
Duane retraction syndrome
Down syndrome
Transient 'eye popping' reflex in normal infants
5. Miscellaneous
Prominent globe (pseudo-lid retraction)
Severe liver disease (Summerskill sign)
Idiopathic

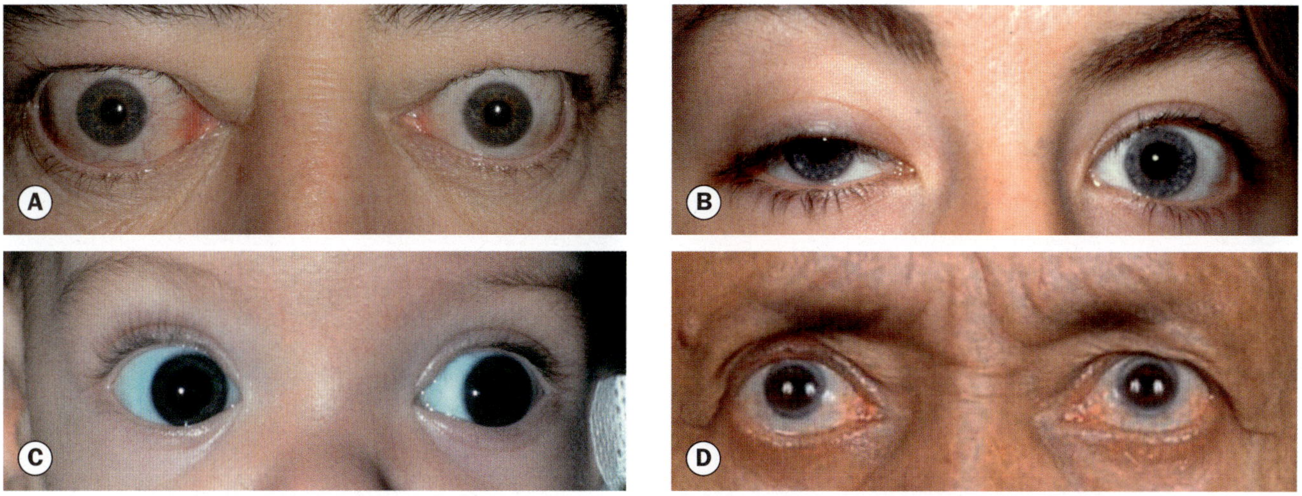

Fig. 2.67 Causes of lid retraction. **(A)** Thyroid eye disease; **(B)** unilateral myasthenic ptosis with contralateral lid retraction; **(C)** 'setting sun' sign in infantile hydrocephalus; **(D)** Parkinson disease. *(Courtesy of R Bates – fig. C.)*

Lower lid retraction

Inferior scleral show may be physiological in patients with large eyes or shallow orbits, but is commonly involutional or secondary to some of the conditions in Table 2.5. It may follow lower lid blepharoplasty, when aggressive upward massage of the lid for 2 or 3 months may be curative for minor degrees. In other cases, a tarsal strip operation may raise the lid slightly but when moderate elevation is required, inferior retractor recession with a posterior lamellar spacer is likely to be necessary. More aggressive procedures have been described for severe cases.

COSMETIC EYELID AND PERIOCULAR SURGERY

Involutional changes

Involutional (age-related) changes around the eyes can lead to functional and cosmetic concerns that may require treatment.

- **Reduction in cutaneous elasticity** and thickness results in loose, wrinkled skin.
- **Weakening of the orbital septum** may lead to orbital fat prolapse.
- **Thinning and stretching** of the canthal tendons, levator aponeurosis and lower lid retractors may cause eyelid laxity and ptosis.
- **Atrophy of orbital and eyebrow fat pads** can give enophthalmos and eyebrow sagging.
- **Weakening of the frontalis muscle** and epicranial aponeurosis may cause descent of the eyebrows and increasing looseness of upper eyelid skin.
- **Thinning and stretching of midfacial support** leads to descent with formation of a tear trough depression and exacerbation of lower eyelid changes.
- **Thinning and resorption of periorbital bone** exacerbates the appearance of surplus overlying tissues.

Non-surgical techniques

Botulinum toxin injection to periocular muscles

Botulinum toxin injection can be used to reduce wrinkling, particularly for 'crows' feet' at the lateral canthus and for glabellar frown lines and 'brow lift' by a reduction in the action of brow depressors. Complications include temporary ptosis, lagophthalmos, ectropion and diplopia.

Tissue fillers

These are used to address age-related wrinkles and, less commonly, defects from other causes such as trauma. Complications include hypersensitivity reactions.

- **Hyaluronic acid** is the most commonly used tissue filler and can be used to temporarily fill in hollows and replace lost volume. This is injected deep to orbicularis and the effects generally last 3–12 months depending on the agent used.
- **Autologous fat** gives a more permanent replacement.
- **Others** include collagen, microspheres of calcium hydroxyapatite and synthetic fillers.

Skin resurfacing

Removal of the superficial layers of the skin, by chemical peels or laser, can lead to a reduction in wrinkling, increased evenness of pigmentation, removal of blemishes and improved texture by generating new epidermis and increasing collagen production in the dermis.

Surgical techniques

Upper eyelid blepharoplasty

Upper eyelid involutional changes are characterized by surplus upper eyelid skin (dermatochalasis) that leads to baggy lids with indistinct creases and pseudo- or mechanical ptosis. It may cause a heavy sensation around the eyes, brow-ache and, in more advanced cases, obstruction of the superior visual field (Fig. 2.68A). Upper lid blepharoplasty (Fig. 2.68B) is effective for the removal of

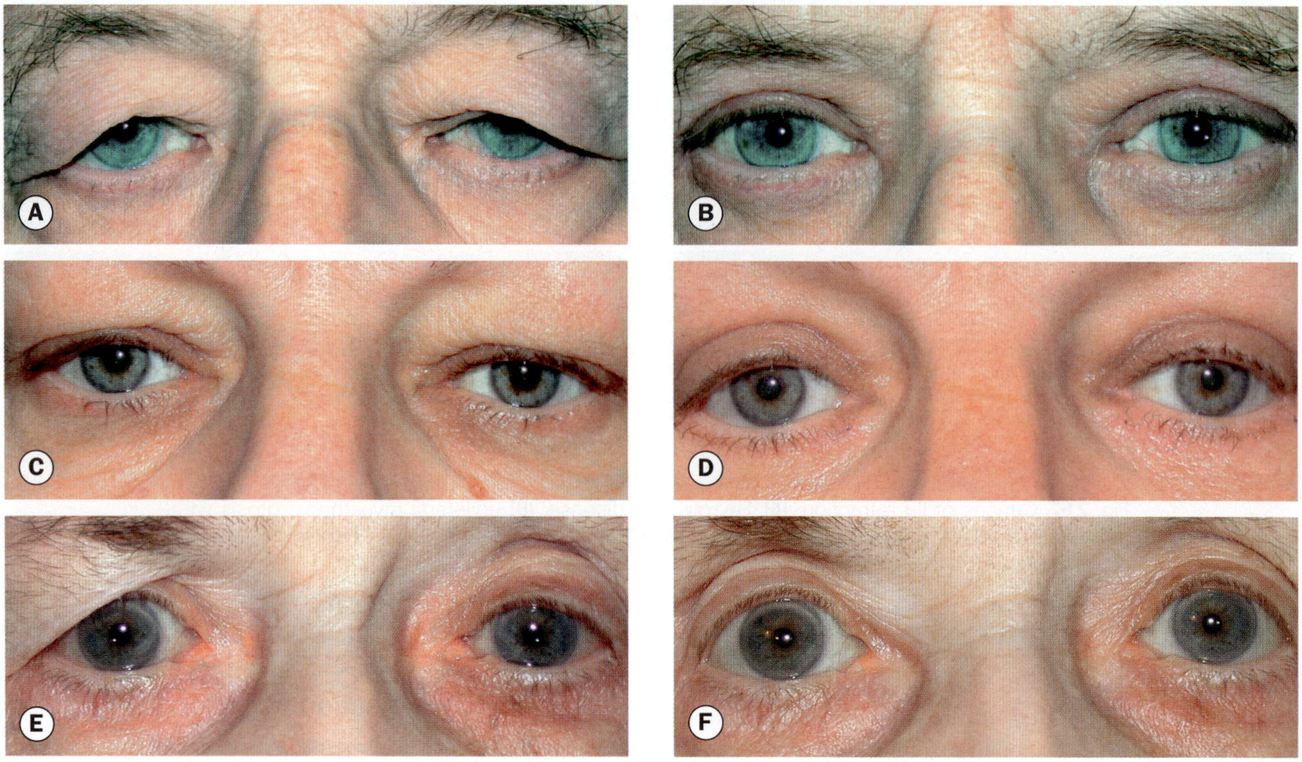

Fig. 2.68 **(A)** Severe dermatochalasis causing reduction of upper visual field; **(B)** appearance following surgery; **(C)** mild dermatochalasis and excess lower lid skin; **(D)** appearance following upper and lower lid blepharoplasty; **(E)** right brow ptosis and dermatochalasis; **(F)** following direct brow lift. *(Courtesy of A Pearson.)*

surplus skin and can be combined with reduction of the superior orbital fat pads. Care must be taken prior to surgery to look for ptosis of the eyelid or eyebrow and ocular surface dryness. Complications include removal of excess skin leading to lagophthalmos and corneal drying and removal of excess orbital fat leading to an unattractive hollowed out upper eyelid sulcus.

Lower eyelid blepharoplasty

Lower lid involutional changes are characterized by excess skin and/or prolapsed orbital fat (Fig. 2.68C) which can be addressed with blepharoplasty (Fig. 2.68D).

- **Anterior approach.** Where there is excess skin, an anterior approach is used to raise a skin/muscle flap that can be lifted and re-draped on the lid with the surplus removed. At the same time the inferior orbital fat pads can be reduced by a small incision through the septum.
- **Posterior approach.** Bulging of the lower eyelid fat pads without eyelid laxity or surplus skin is best reduced by a posterior, transconjunctival approach. Complications include lower eyelid retraction, contour abnormalities (particularly lateral drooping) and ectropion.

Brow ptosis correction

Brow ptosis frequently accompanies dermatochalasis (Fig. 2.68E) and may also follow facial nerve palsy or localized trauma. Lifting of the brow needs to precede or occasionally be combined with upper lid blepharoplasty.

- **Direct brow lift.** An incision is made above the eyebrow hairs and an ellipse of skin is removed (Fig. 2.68F).
- **Endoscopic brow lift.** Small incisions within the hair-line enable endoscopic elevation of the whole forehead tissues and release at the eyebrow periosteum to allow lifting of the eyebrows through sutures supported on frontal bone anchors within the hair-line.

CONGENITAL MALFORMATIONS

Epicanthic folds

Epicanthic folds are bilateral vertical folds of skin that extend from the upper or lower lids towards the medial canthi (Fig. 2.69A). They may give rise to pseudoesotropia. The folds may involve the upper or lower lids or both. Lower lid folds extending upwards to the medial canthal area (epicanthus inversus – Fig. 2.69B) are associated with the blepharophimosis syndrome. Treatment is by V–Y or Z-plasty.

Blepharophimosis, ptosis and epicanthus inversus syndrome

Blepharophimosis, ptosis and epicanthus inversus syndrome (BPES) is a complex of eyelid malformations consisting of moderate–severe symmetrical ptosis with poor levator function, telecanthus, epicanthus inversus, manifesting with small palpebral

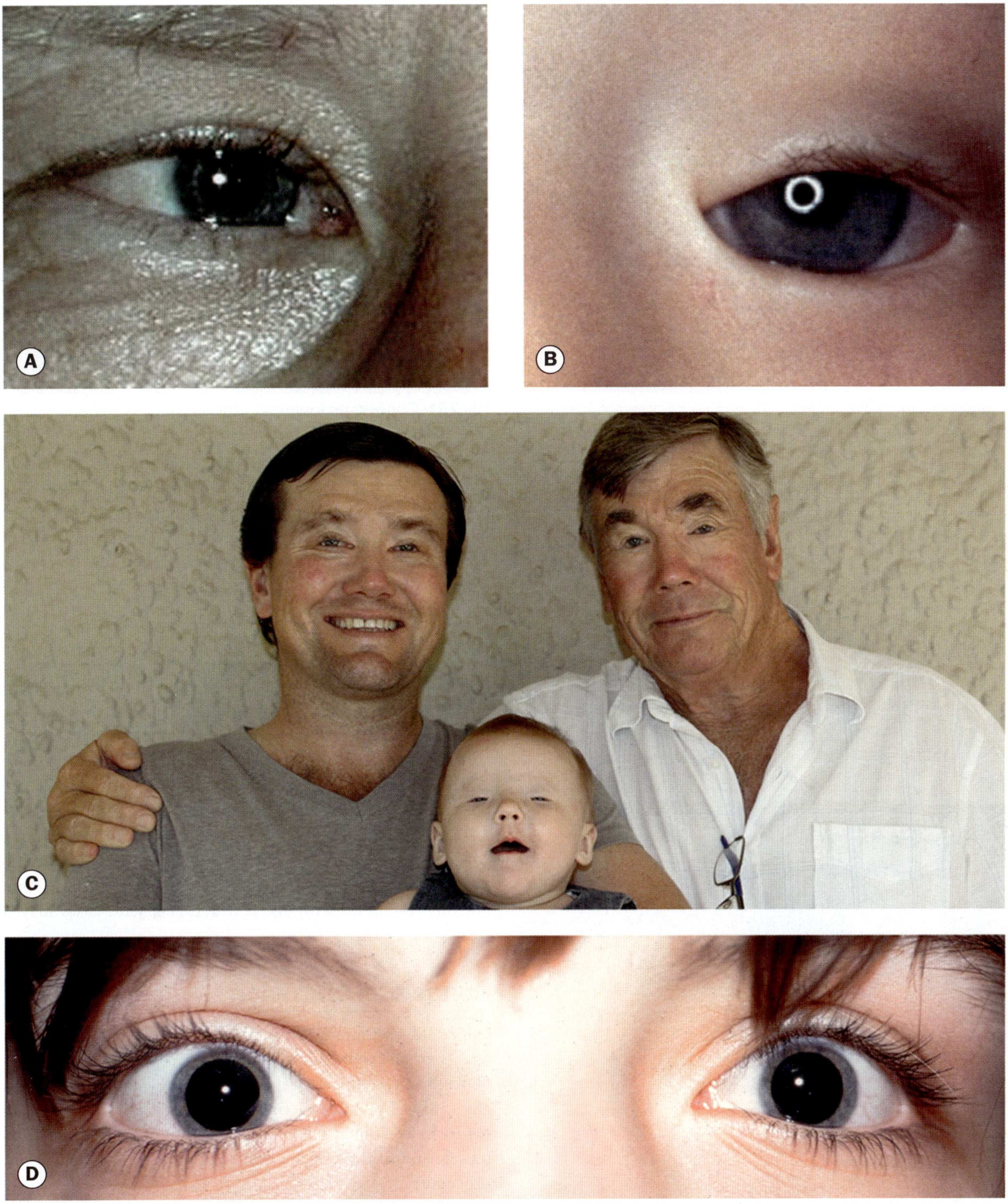

Fig. 2.69 Congenital malformations. **(A)** Epicanthic fold; **(B)** epicanthus inversus; **(C)** dominantly inherited blepharophimosis – the child's grandfather and father have undergone surgery to correct the defect; **(D)** telecanthus.

fissures (Fig. 2.69C). Other minor facial anomalies are commonly present. Inheritance is usually AD. Both BPES type I (with premature ovarian failure) and BPES type II (without premature ovarian failure) are caused by mutations in the *FOXL2* gene on chromosome 3. Treatment initially involves correction of epicanthus and telecanthus, followed later by bilateral frontalis suspension. It is also important to treat amblyopia, which is present in about 50%.

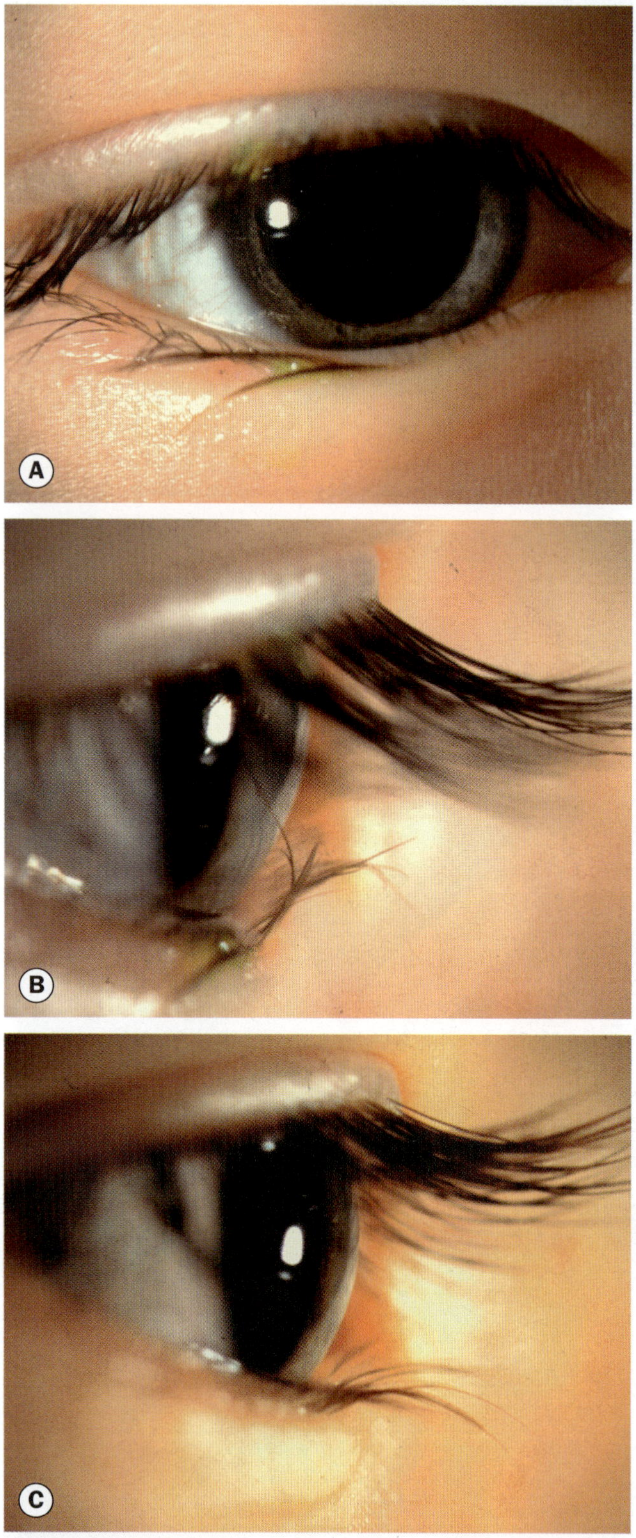

Fig. 2.70 **(A)** Epiblepharon; **(B)** lashes pointing upwards; **(C)** normal position of lashes following manual correction.

Telecanthus

Telecanthus is an uncommon condition that may occur in isolation or in association with blepharophimosis and some systemic syndromes. It manifests with increased distance between the medial canthi due to abnormally long medial canthal tendons (Fig. 2.69D). It should not be confused with hypertelorism in which there is wide bony separation of the orbits. Treatment involves shortening and refixation of the medial canthal tendons to the anterior lacrimal crest, or insertion of a trans-nasal suture.

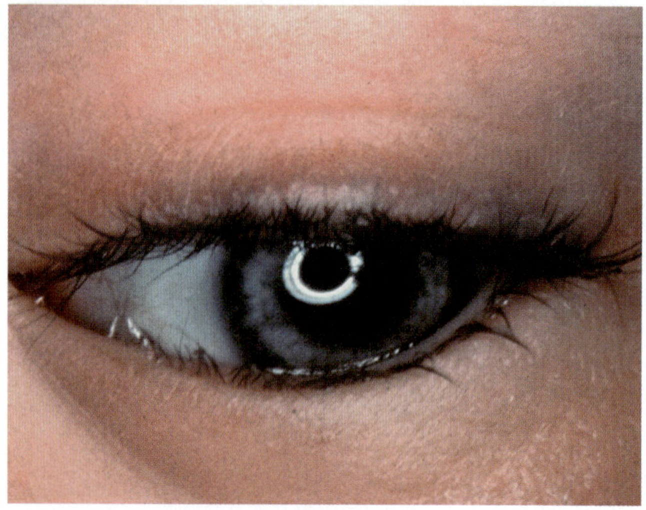

Fig. 2.71 Congenital lower lid entropion.

Epiblepharon

Epiblepharon comprises an extra horizontal fold of skin stretching across the anterior lid margin and is commonly found in individuals of Eastern Asian ethnicity. The lashes are directed vertically, especially in the medial part of the lid (Fig. 2.70A and B). When the fold of skin is pulled down the lashes turn out and the normal location of the lid becomes apparent (Fig. 2.70C). It should not be confused with the much less common congenital entropion (see next). Treatment is not required in the majority of individuals of European origin because spontaneous resolution with age is usual. Persistent cases may be treated surgically.

Congenital entropion

Upper lid entropion is usually secondary to the mechanical effects of microphthalmos, which cause variable degrees of upper lid inversion. Lower lid entropion (Fig. 2.71) is generally caused by maldevelopment of the inferior retractor aponeurosis. Treatment involves the excision of a strip of skin and muscle and fixation of the skin crease to the tarsal plate (Hotz procedure).

Coloboma

A congenital coloboma is an uncommon, unilateral or bilateral, partial- or full-thickness eyelid defect. It occurs when eyelid development is incomplete, due to either failure of migration of lid ectoderm to fuse the lid folds or to mechanical forces such as amniotic bands. Coloboma elsewhere in the eye (see Figs 19. 26 and 19.27),

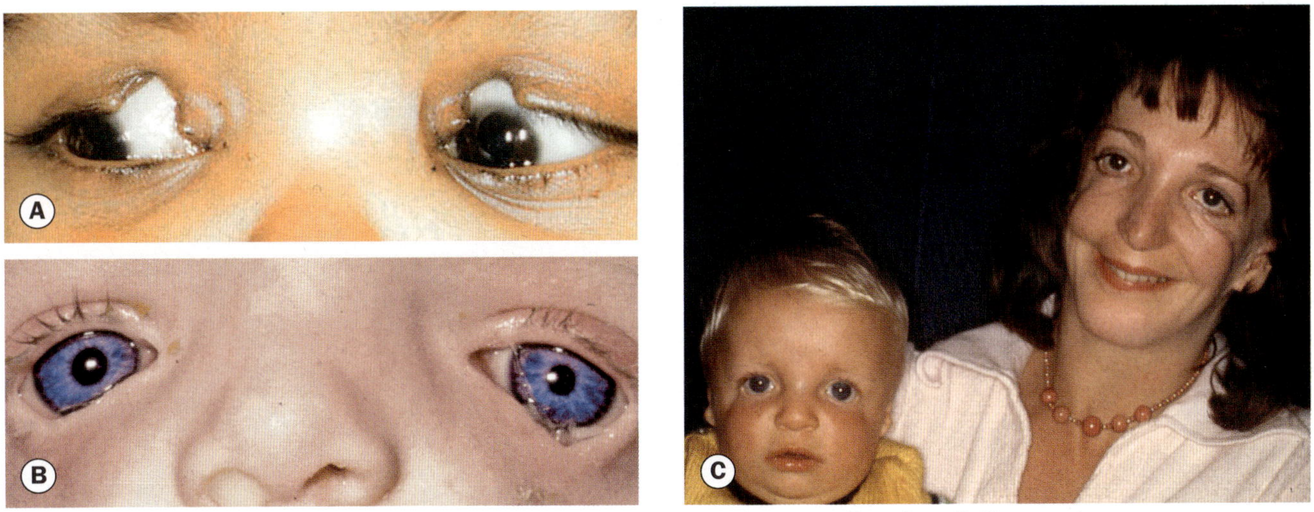

Fig. 2.72 (A) Upper lid coloboma; **(B)** lower lid coloboma in Treacher Collins syndrome; **(C)** Treacher Collins syndrome.

as well as a range of other associations, may be present. The treatment of small defects involves primary closure, while large defects require skin grafts and rotation flaps.

- **Upper lid coloboma** occurs at the junction of the middle and inner thirds (Fig. 2.72A). Relatively strong associations include cryptophthalmos (see below), facial abnormalities and Goldenhar syndrome.
- **Lower lid coloboma** occurs at the junction of the middle and outer thirds (Fig. 2.72B) and is frequently associated with systemic conditions.
- **Treacher Collins syndrome** (mandibulofacial dysostosis) is a genetically heterogeneous condition characterized by malformation of derivatives of the first and second branchial arches, principally mandibular and ear anomalies. Lower eyelid coloboma is a feature. Ocular anomalies also described include slanted palpebral apertures, cataract, microphthalmos and lacrimal atresia (Fig. 2.72C).

Cryptophthalmos

Cryptophthalmos is a rare congenital anomaly in which the eyelids are absent, replaced by a continuous layer of skin.

- **Complete cryptophthalmos.** A microphthalmic eye (Fig. 2.73A) is covered by a fused layer of skin with no separation between the lids.
- **Incomplete cryptophthalmos** is characterized by rudimentary lids and microphthalmos (Fig. 2.73B).
- **Fraser syndrome** is a recessively inherited condition in which cryptophthalmos is a common finding. Other features can include syndactyly, urogenital and craniofacial anomalies.

Euryblepharon

Euryblepharon refers to horizontal enlargement of the palpebral fissure with associated lateral canthal malposition and lateral ectropion (Fig. 2.73C), which may result in lagophthalmos and exposure keratopathy. Euryblepharon is present at birth and there are no other associated ocular abnormalities. It is usually dominantly inherited, but may occur sporadically. Systemic conditions associated with euryblepharon include: Kabuki syndrome, Down syndrome and blepharocheilodontic syndrome. Most cases do not require treatment, as the condition becomes less pronounced with facial growth. Surgical treatment may be needed to protect the cornea.

Microblepharon

Microblepharon is characterized by small eyelids, often associated with anophthalmos.

Congenital upper lid eversion

Congenital upper lid eversion is a rare condition more frequently seen in infants of Afro-Caribbean origin, in Down syndrome and in congenital ichthyosis (collodion skin disease – Fig. 2.73D). It is typically bilateral and symmetrical. It may resolve spontaneously with conservative treatment or require surgery.

Ablepharon

Ablepharon consists of deficiency of the anterior lamellae of the eyelids (Fig. 2.73E). Treatment involves reconstructive skin grafting. Ablepharon-macrostomia syndrome is characterized by an enlarged fish-like mouth, ear, skin and genital anomalies.

Ankyloblepharon filiforme adnatum

In ankyloblepharon filiforme adnatum the upper and lower eyelids are joined by thin tags (Fig. 2.73F). Most cases are sporadic. Treatment involves transection with scissors, usually without anaesthesia.

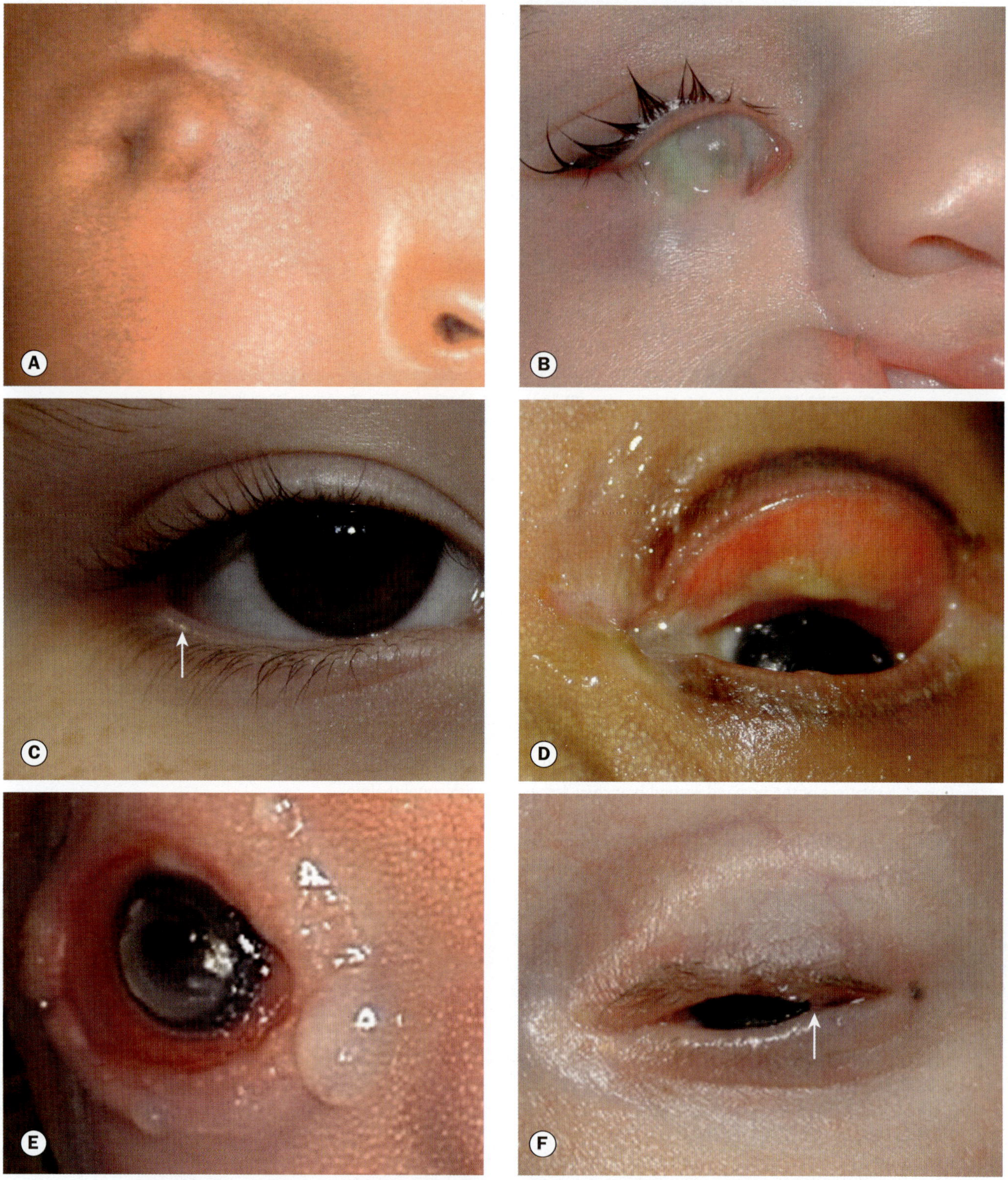

Fig. 2.73 **(A)** Complete cryptophthalmos; **(B)** incomplete cryptophthalmos; **(C)** euryblepharon (arrow shows slightly everted lateral lower lid); **(D)** congenital upper lid eversion in a patient with ichthyosis; **(E)** ablepharon; **(F)** ankyloblepharon filiforme adnatum (arrow shows adhesion). *(Courtesy of D Meyer – figs A and D; M Parulekar – figs C, E and F.)*

Chapter 3

Lacrimal Drainage System

INTRODUCTION

Anatomy

The lacrimal drainage system consists of the following structures (Fig. 3.1):

- **The puncta** are located at the posterior edge of the lid margin, at the junction of the lash-bearing lateral five-sixths (pars ciliaris) and the medial non-ciliated one-sixth (pars lacrimalis). The punctum and vertical canaliculus are part of the tarsal plate. Normally the puncta face slightly posteriorly and can be inspected by everting the medial aspect of the lids. Treatment of watering caused by punctal stenosis or malposition is relatively straightforward.
- **The canaliculi** pass vertically from the lid margin for about 2 mm (ampullae). They then turn medially and run horizontally for about 8 mm to reach the lacrimal sac. The horizontal canaliculus is surrounded by the palpebral part of the orbicularis oculi muscle (Horner muscle). The superior and inferior canaliculi usually (>90%) unite to form the common canaliculus, which opens into the lateral wall of the lacrimal sac. Uncommonly, each canaliculus opens separately into the sac. A small flap of mucosa (Rosenmüller valve) overhangs the junction of the common canaliculus and the lacrimal sac (the internal punctum) and prevents reflux of tears into the canaliculi. Treatment of canalicular obstruction may be complex.
- **The lacrimal sac** is 10–12 mm long and lies in the lacrimal fossa between the anterior and posterior lacrimal crests. The lacrimal bone and the frontal process of the maxilla separate the lacrimal sac from the middle meatus of the nasal cavity. In a dacryocystorhinostomy (DCR) an anastomosis is created between the sac and the nasal mucosa to bypass an obstruction in the nasolacrimal duct.
- **The nasolacrimal duct** is 12–18 mm long and is the inferior continuation of the lacrimal sac. It descends and angles slightly laterally and posteriorly to open into the inferior nasal meatus, lateral to and below the inferior turbinate. The opening of the duct is partially covered by a mucosal fold (valve of Hasner).

Physiology

Tears secreted by the main and accessory lacrimal glands pass across the ocular surface. A variable amount of the aqueous component of the tear film is lost by evaporation, with the remainder of the tears hypothesized to drain substantially as follows (Fig. 3.2):

- Tears flow along the upper and lower marginal strips (Fig. 3.2A), pooling in the lacus lacrimalis medial to the lower puncta, then entering the upper and lower canaliculi by a combination of capillarity and suction.
- With each blink, the pretarsal orbicularis oculi muscle compresses the ampullae, shortens and compresses the horizontal canaliculi and closes and moves the puncta medially, resisting reflux. Simultaneously, contraction of the lacrimal part of the orbicularis oculi creates a positive pressure that forces tears down the nasolacrimal duct and into the nose, mediated by helically arranged connective tissue fibres around the lacrimal sac (Fig. 3.2B).
- When the eyes open, the canaliculi and sac expand, creating negative pressure that draws tears from the canaliculi into the sac (Fig. 3.2C).

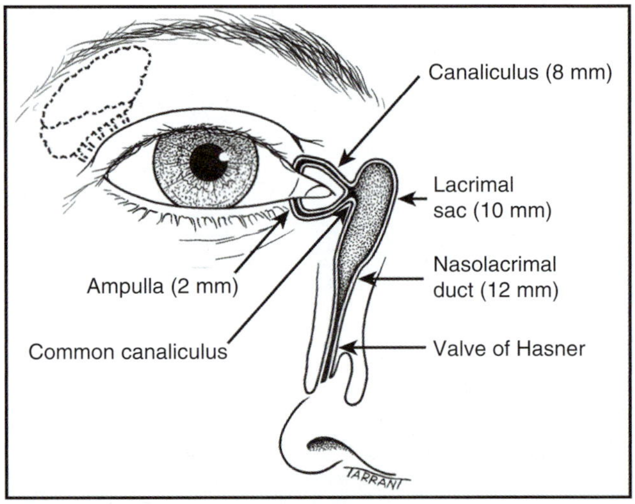

Fig. 3.1 Anatomy of the lacrimal drainage system.

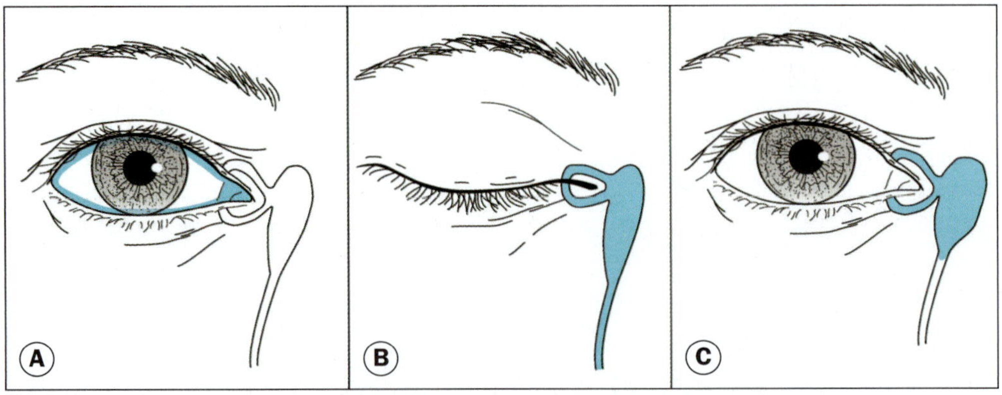

Fig. 3.2 Physiology of the lacrimal drainage system. **(A)** Tears flow along the marginal strips, pooling in the lacus lacrimalis; **(B)** contraction of the orbicularis oculi muscle with each blink forces tears down the nasolacrimal duct; **(C)** when the eyes open, the canaliculus and sac expand creating a negative pressure that draws tears from the canaliculus into the sac.

Causes of a watering eye

Epiphora is the overflow of tears at the eyelid margin. There are two mechanisms:

- **Hypersecretion** secondary to anterior segment disease such as dry eye ('paradoxical watering') or inflammation. In these cases, watering is associated with symptoms of the underlying cause and treatment is usually medical.

TIP It is common for a watering eye to be caused by reflex hypersecretion of tears secondary to a dry ocular surface.

- **Defective drainage** due to a compromised lacrimal drainage system. This may be caused by:
    - Malposition (e.g. ectropion) of the lacrimal puncta.
    - Obstruction at any point along the drainage system, from the punctal region to the valve of Hasner.
    - Lacrimal pump failure, which may occur secondarily to lower lid laxity or weakness of the orbicularis muscle (e.g. facial nerve palsy).

Evaluation

History

Enquiry should be made about ocular discomfort and redness to aid in excluding hypersecretion. Drainage failure tends to be exacerbated by a cold and windy environment and to be least evident in a warm, dry room. A complaint of the tears overflowing onto the cheek is likely to indicate drainage failure rather than hypersecretion.

External examination

Punctal abnormality is the most common cause of lacrimal drainage failure.

- **The puncta and eyelids** should be examined using a slit lamp. It is critical that examination of the puncta is performed prior to cannulation for diagnostic irrigation, which temporarily dilates the punctal opening and masks stenosis.
    - There will often be obvious tear overflow from the medial, or less commonly the lateral, canthal region.
    - Visible mucopurulent discharge is more likely to occur with nasolacrimal duct obstruction than a blockage more proximally.
    - Punctal stenosis (Fig. 3.3A). This is extremely common and has been reported as present in up to about half of the general population. Over half of patients with evident stenosis are asymptomatic, in many cases due to insufficiency of tear production or increased evaporation.
    - Ectropion, either localized to the punctal region or involving the wider lid, is often associated with secondary stenosis (Fig. 3.3B).
    - Punctal obstruction, usually partial, by a fold of redundant conjunctiva (conjunctivochalasis – Fig. 3.3C) is common but underdiagnosed.
    - Occasionally an eyelash may lodge in the ampulla (Fig. 3.3D).
    - A large caruncle may displace the punctum away from the globe (Fig. 3.3E).
    - In the presence of substantial lid laxity, the puncta may rarely over-ride each other.
    - A pouting punctum (Fig. 3.3F) is typical of canaliculitis.
    - The eyelid skin will often be moderately scaly and erythematous in chronic epiphora.
    - Centurion syndrome is characterized by anterior malposition of the medial part of the lid, with displacement of puncta out of the lacus lacrimalis due to a prominent nasal bridge.
    - Occasionally a child with congenital glaucoma can present with a watery eye.
- **The lacrimal sac** should be palpated. Punctal reflux of mucopurulent material on compression is indicative of a mucocoele (a dilated mucus-filled sac; US spelling – mucocele) with a patent canalicular system, but with an obstruction either at or distal to the lower end of the lacrimal sac. In acute dacryocystitis, palpation is painful and should be avoided. Rarely, palpation of the sac will reveal a stone or tumour.

Fluorescein disappearance test

The marginal tear strip of both eyes should be examined on the slit lamp prior to any manipulation of the eyelids or instillation of topical medication. Many patients with watering do not have obvious overflow of tears but merely show a high meniscus (marginal tear strip) of 0.6 mm or more (Fig. 3.4) versus 0.2–0.4 mm normally. The fluorescein disappearance test is performed by instilling fluorescein 1% or 2% drops into both conjunctival fornices. Normally, little or no dye remains after 5–10 minutes. Prolonged retention is indicative of inadequate lacrimal drainage. This should be distinguished from the 'fluorescein clearance test' used to assess tear turnover in dry eye, in which retained stain is measured in the meniscus 15 minutes after instillation of 5 μl of fluorescein.

Lacrimal irrigation

Lacrimal irrigation should be performed only after ascertaining punctal patency. If absent or severely stenosed, surgical enlargement of the punctum may be needed before canalicular and nasolacrimal duct patency can be confirmed. It is contraindicated in acute infection.

- Local anaesthetic is instilled into the conjunctival sac.
- A punctum dilator is used to enlarge the punctal orifice (Fig. 3.5A), entering vertically and then tilting the instrument horizontally whilst exerting lateral tension on the lid (Fig. 3.5B and C).
- A gently curved, blunt-tipped 26- or 27-gauge lacrimal cannula on a 3 ml saline-filled syringe is inserted into the lower punctum and, whilst keeping a gentle stretch laterally on the eyelid, advanced a few millimetres, following the contour of the canaliculus (Fig. 3.5D).
- **A hard stop** occurs if the cannula enters the lacrimal sac, coming to a stop at the medial wall of the sac, through which can be felt the rigid lacrimal bone (Fig. 3.6A). This excludes complete obstruction of the canalicular system. Gentle saline irrigation

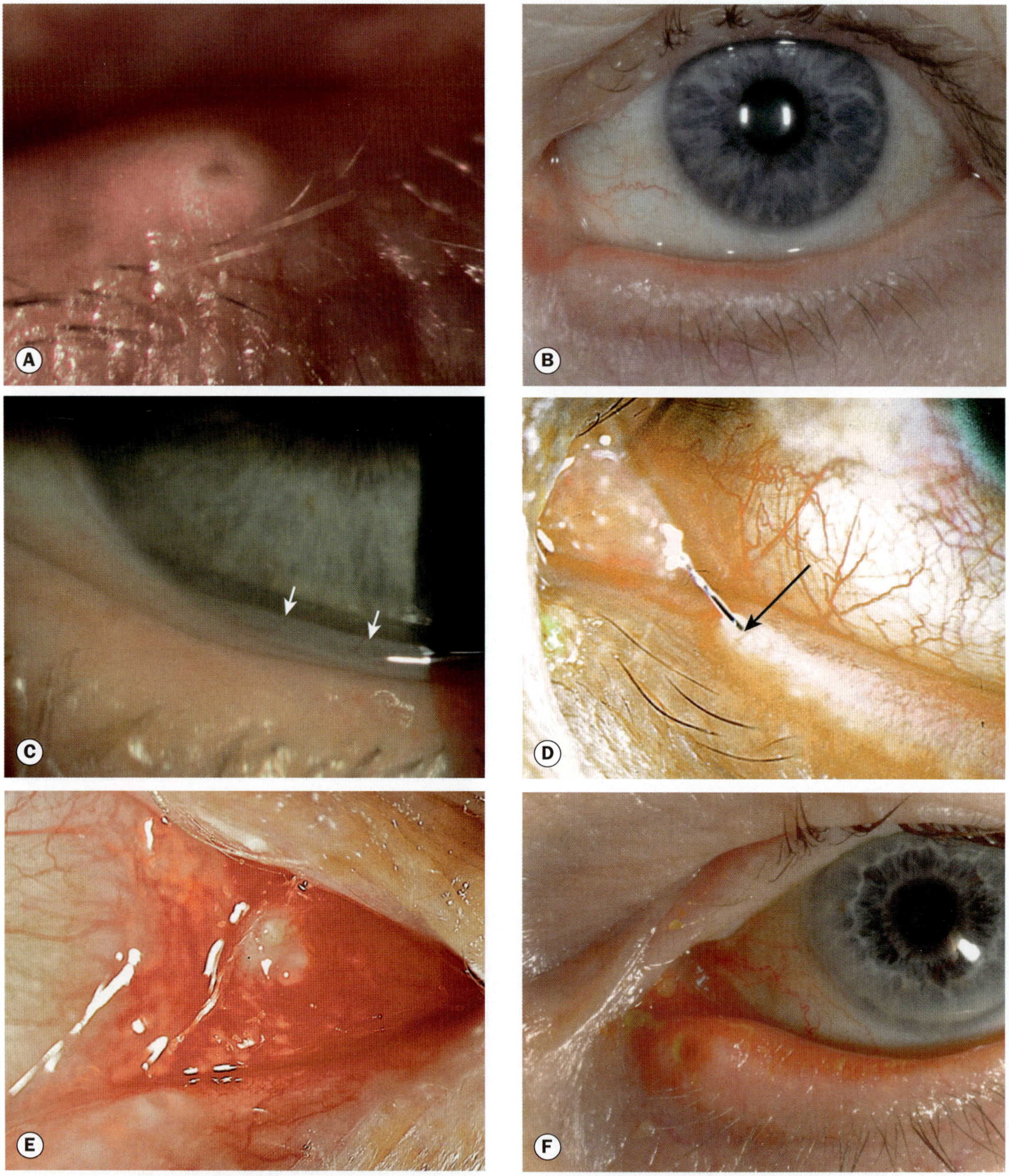

Fig. 3.3 (A) Marked punctal stenosis; **(B)** mild medial ectropion; **(C)** conjunctivochalasis (arrows); **(D)** punctal obstruction by an eyelash (arrow); **(E)** large caruncle; **(F)** pouting punctum.

is then attempted. If saline passes into the nose and throat, when it will be tasted by the patient, a patent lacrimal system is present, although there may still be stenosis; alternatively, symptoms may be due to subtle lacrimal pump failure. Failure of saline to reach the throat is indicative of total obstruction of the nasolacrimal duct. In this situation, the lacrimal sac will distend slightly during irrigation and there will be reflux, usually through both the upper and lower puncta. The regurgitated material may be clear, mucoid or mucopurulent, depending on the contents of the lacrimal sac.

- **A soft stop** is experienced if the cannula stops at or proximal to the junction of the common canaliculus and the lacrimal sac. The sac is thus not entered – a spongy feeling is experienced as the cannula presses the soft tissue of the common canaliculus and the lateral wall against the medial wall of the sac and the lacrimal bone behind it (Fig. 3.6B). As a crimped canaliculus with occlusion of the cannula tip against the canalicular wall can also give this impression, it is worthwhile slightly retracting the tip, increasing the lateral tension on the lid and gently repeating the attempt to advance the probe. In the case of lower canalicular obstruction, a soft stop will be associated with reflux of saline through the lower punctum. Reflux through the upper punctum indicates patency of both upper and lower canaliculi, but obstruction of the common canaliculus.

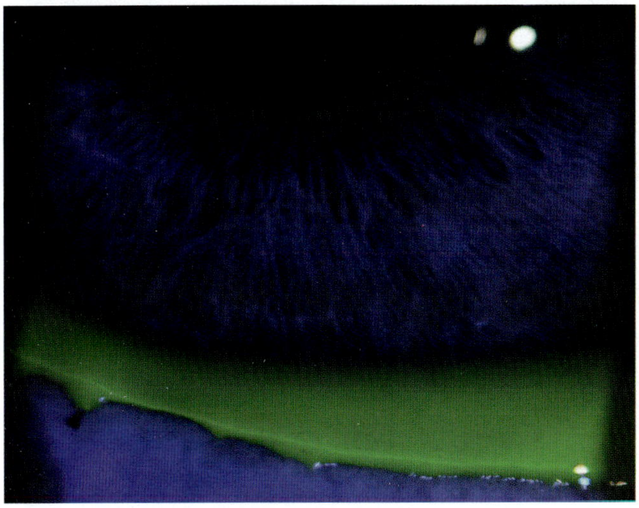

Fig. 3.4 High marginal tear strip stained with fluorescein.

Jones dye testing

Dye testing is indicated only in patients with suspected partial obstruction of the drainage system. Epiphora is present, but there is no punctal abnormality and the patient tastes saline in his or her throat on irrigation.

- **The primary test** (Fig. 3.7A) differentiates partial obstruction of the lacrimal passages and lacrimal pump failure from primary hypersecretion of tears. A drop of 2% fluorescein is instilled into the conjunctival sac of one eye only. After about 5

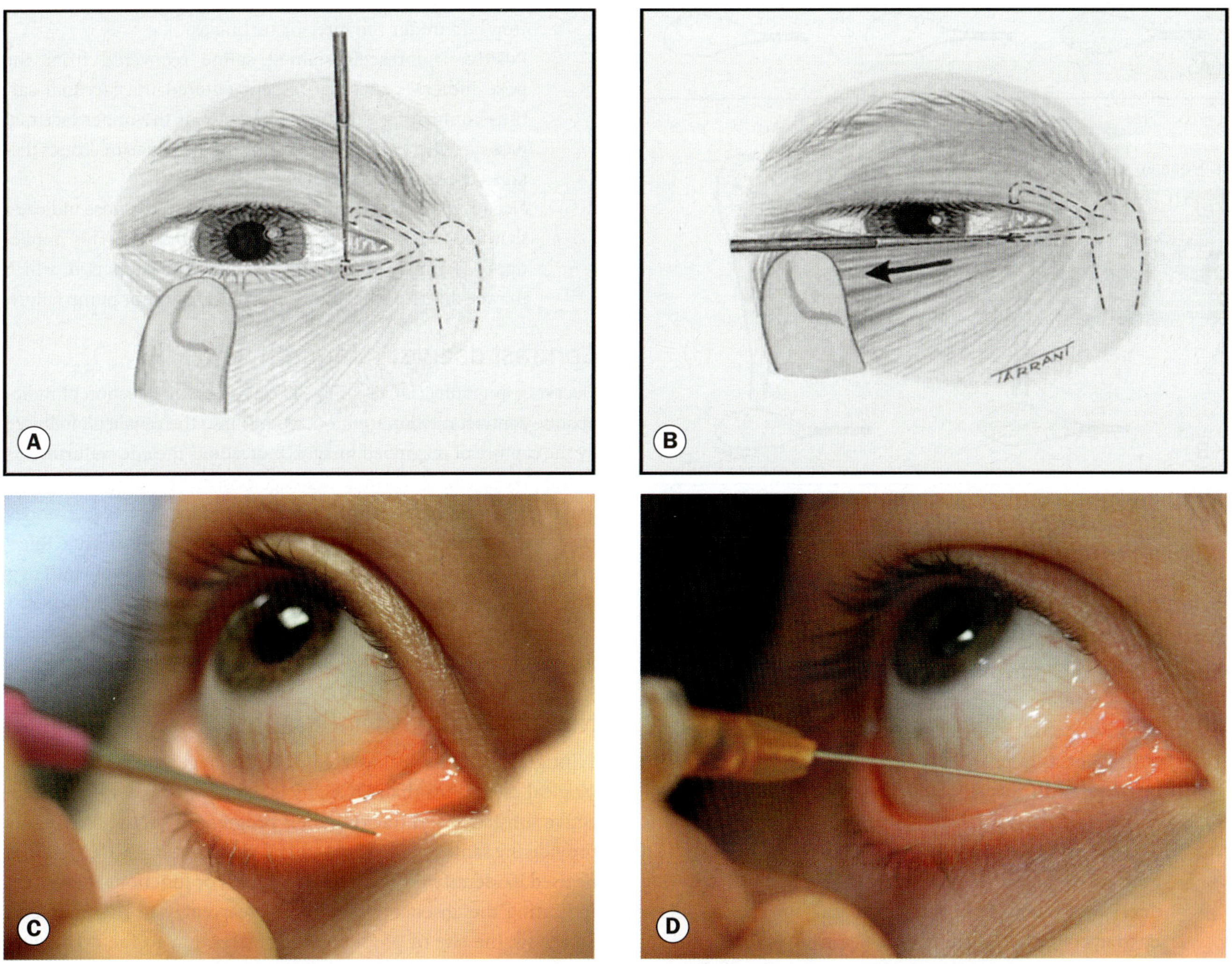

Fig. 3.5 **(A)** Dilatation of the inferior punctum; **(B)** and **(C)** dilatation technique; **(D)** irrigation.

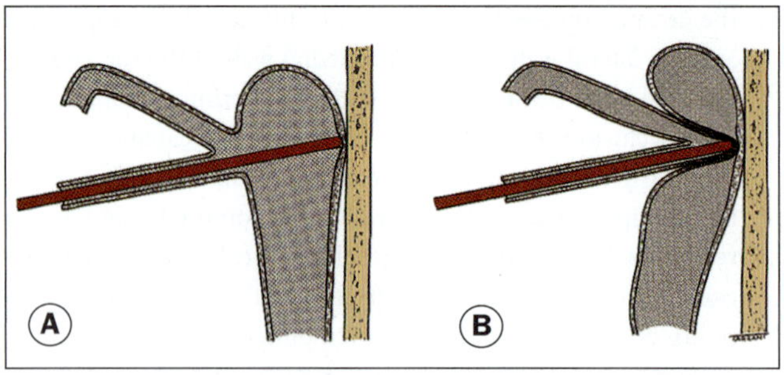

Fig. 3.6 Possible results of probing. **(A)** Hard stop; **(B)** soft stop.

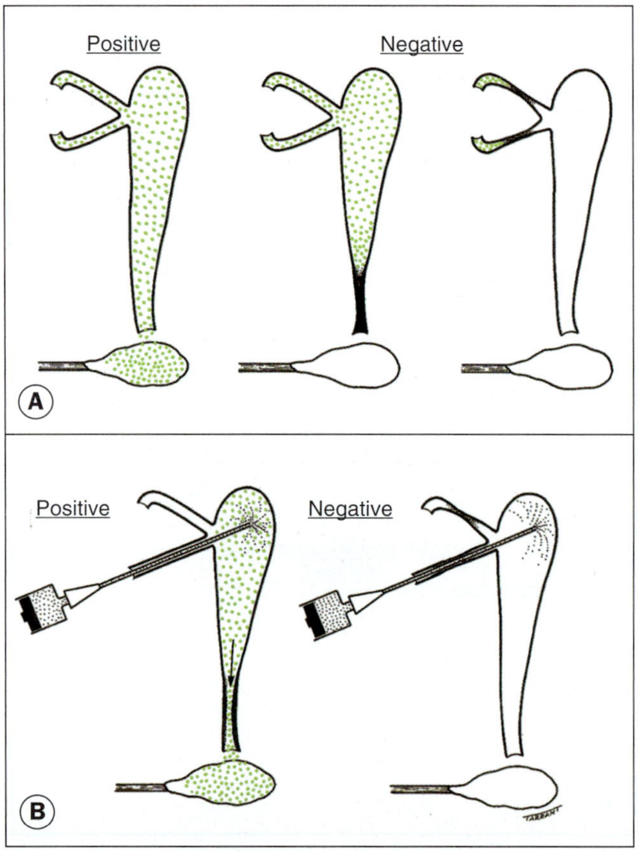

Fig. 3.7 Jones dye testing. **(A)** Primary; **(B)** secondary.

minutes, a cotton-tipped bud moistened in local anaesthetic is inserted under the inferior turbinate at the nasolacrimal duct opening. The results are interpreted as follows:

- Positive: fluorescein recovered from the nose indicates patency of the drainage system. Watering is due to primary hypersecretion and no further tests are necessary.
- Negative: no dye recovered from the nose indicates a partial obstruction (site unknown) or failure of the lacrimal pump mechanism. In this situation the secondary dye test is performed immediately. There is a high false-negative rate – that is, dye is commonly not recovered even in the presence of a functionally patent drainage system. Modifications involving direct observation of the oropharynx using cobalt blue light for up to an hour may reduce the false-negative rate almost to zero.

- **The secondary (irrigation) test** (Fig. 3.7B) identifies lacrimal pump failure or the probable site of partial obstruction,

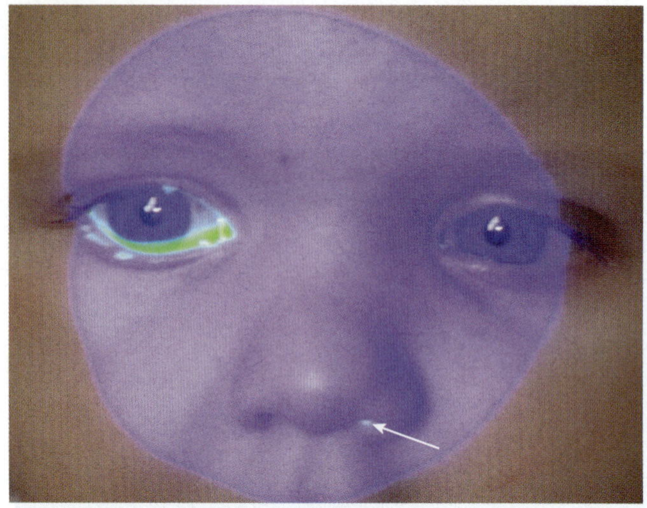

Fig. 3.8 Drainage test showing 2% fluorescein in the left nostril only (arrow), confirming a patent nasolacrimal duct on that side. *(Courtesy of D Hildebrand.)*

on the basis of whether the topical fluorescein instilled for the primary test entered the lacrimal sac. Topical anaesthetic is instilled and any residual fluorescein washed out from the conjunctival fornix. The drainage system is then irrigated with a cotton bud under the inferior turbinate.

- Positive: fluorescein-stained saline recovered from the nose indicates that fluorescein entered the lacrimal sac, thus confirming functional patency of the upper lacrimal passages. Partial obstruction of the nasolacrimal duct distal to the sac is inferred (Fig. 3.8).
- Negative: unstained saline recovered from the nose indicates that fluorescein did not enter the lacrimal sac. This implies upper lacrimal (punctal or canalicular) dysfunction, which may be due to partial physical occlusion and/or pump failure.

Contrast dacryocystography

Dacryocystography (DCG – Fig. 3.9) involves the injection of radio-opaque contrast medium (ethiodized oil) into the canaliculi followed by the capture of magnified images. Indications include confirmation of the precise site of lacrimal drainage obstruction to guide surgery and the diagnosis of diverticuli, fistulae and filling defects (e.g. stones, tumours). It should not be performed in the presence of acute infection. A DCG is unnecessary if the site of obstruction is obvious (e.g. regurgitating mucocoele). A normal dacryocystogram in the presence of subjective and objective epiphora suggests failure of the lacrimal pump, though this is more readily demonstrated by simple irrigation.

Nuclear lacrimal scintigraphy

Scintigraphy (Fig. 3.10) assesses tear drainage under more physiological conditions than DCG, by labelling the tears with a radioactive substance and tracking their progress. Although it does not provide the same detailed anatomical visualization as DCG, it may be used to identify the location of a partial or functional block (e.g. indicating the absence of significant tear entry to the canaliculi, localizing the site of physiological obstruction to the eyelids), to confirm functional obstruction, or sometimes to confirm the presence of normal drainage such that surgery is not indicated.

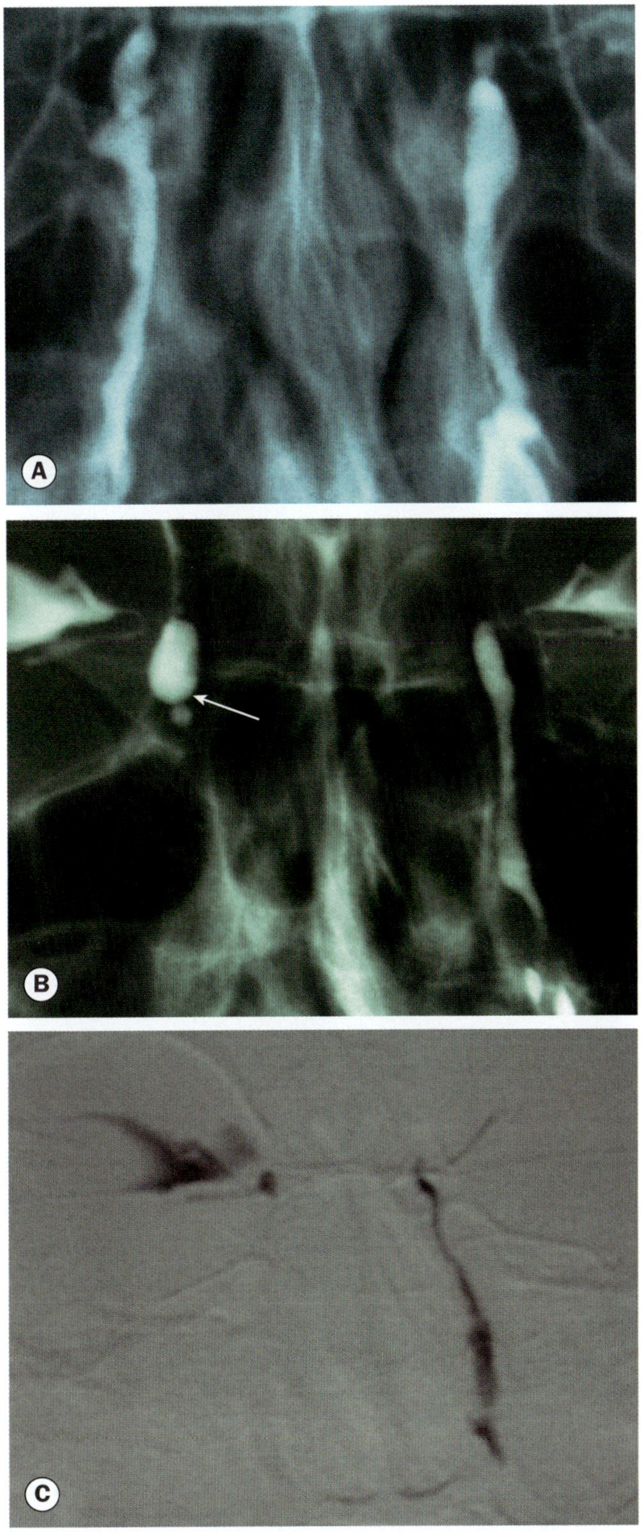

Fig. 3.9 Dacryocystography (DCG). **(A)** Conventional DCG without subtraction showing normal filling on both sides; **(B)** normal left filling and obstruction at the junction of the right sac and nasolacrimal duct (arrow); **(C)** digital subtraction DCG showing similar findings to (B). *(Courtesy of A Pearson.)*

TIP Scintigraphy allows tear drainage to be assessed under physiological conditions and may be helpful to identify the location of a partial or functional block.

CT and MRI

Computed tomography (CT) and magnetic resonance imaging (MRI) are occasionally employed in the assessment of lacrimal obstruction, for instance in the investigation of paranasal sinus or suspected lacrimal sac pathology.

Internal nasal examination

Assessment of the nasal cavity, especially with endoscopy, can be invaluable in the detection of obstructions such as nasal polyps or a deviated septum.

ACQUIRED OBSTRUCTION

Conjunctivochalasis

Conjunctivochalasis is characterized by one or more folds of redundant conjunctiva prolapsing over the lower eyelid margin (see Fig. 3.3C). It can exacerbate the symptoms of dry eye and commonly contributes to epiphora, of which it can be an under-recognized cause. It is thought to be predominantly an involutional process involving the loss of conjunctival adhesion to underlying Tenon capsule and episclera and may be analogous to the conjunctival abnormalities leading to superior limbic keratoconjunctivitis (see Ch. 6). Chronic low-grade ocular surface inflammation (e.g. dry eye, blepharitis) is likely to play a role. If severe, exposure of a redundant fold can occur (Fig. 3.11).

- **Observation or lubricants** alone may be appropriate in mild cases.
- **Topical steroids** or other anti-inflammatories.
- **Surgical options** include securing the bulbar conjunctiva to the sclera with three absorbable sutures (e.g. 6-0 polyglactin) placed 6–8 mm from the limbus, or excision of a crescent-shaped area of excess bulbar conjunctiva, with an anterior limit of around 6 mm from the limbus. Suturing the edges of the excised patch together, or replacement with amniotic membrane have been described.

Primary punctal stenosis

Primary stenosis (see Fig. 3.3A) occurs in the absence of punctal eversion. The most common causes are chronic blepharitis and idiopathic stenosis. Other causes include herpes simplex and herpes zoster lid infection, local radiotherapy, cicatrizing conjunctivitis, chronic topical glaucoma treatment, systemic cytotoxic drugs such as 5-fluorouracil and rare systemic conditions such as porphyria cutanea tarda.

- **Dilatation** of the punctum alone can be tried, but rarely gives sustained benefit. The results are significantly improved by inserting a mini-Monoka stent (FCI Ophthalmics) after simple dilatation. The stent is removed after one month (see Fig. 22.3B).
- **Punctoplasty** may be needed, but it is important to remember that surgical intervention has the potential to disrupt the normal anatomical and physiological punctal tear drainage function. A number of techniques have been described, including one-, two- (Fig. 3.12) or three-snip enlargement with removal

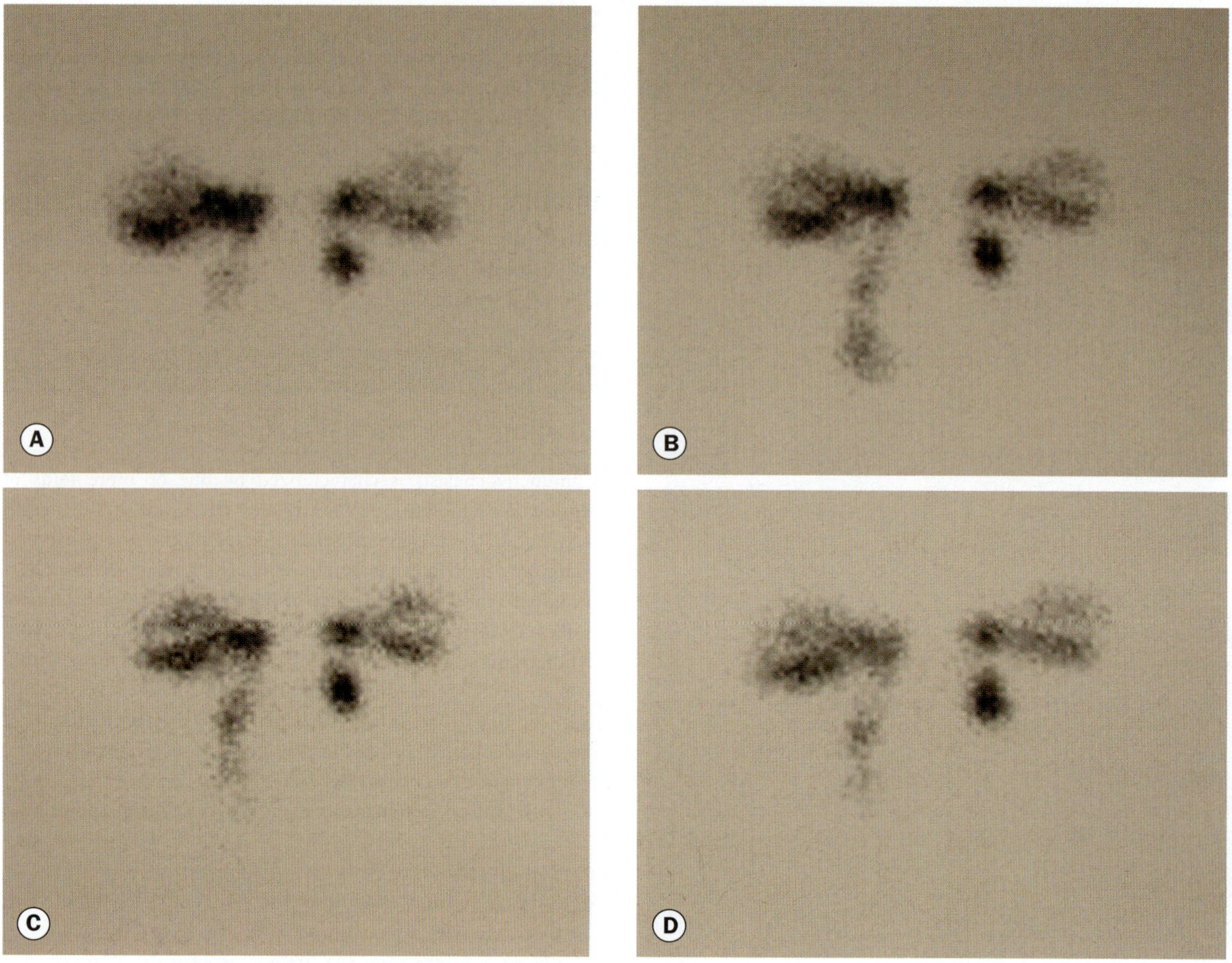

Fig. 3.10 (A–D) Nuclear lacrimal scintigraphy showing passage of tracer via the right lacrimal system but obstructed drainage in the left nasolacrimal duct. *(Courtesy of A Pearson.)*

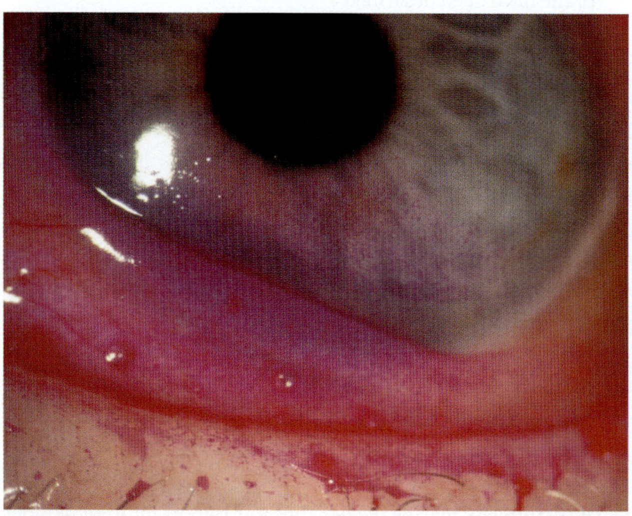

Fig. 3.11 Conjunctivochalasis. Substantial exposed fold with conjunctival and corneal rose Bengal staining. *(Courtesy of S Tuft.)*

of the posterior ampulla wall and procedures using a mechanical punch (e.g. Kelly punch), laser or microsurgery; a temporary stent can be used.

Secondary punctal stenosis

Secondary stenosis occurs after punctal eversion leads to chronic failure of tear entry and punctoplasty is usually performed in conjunction with correction of the eversion.

- **Retropunctal (Ziegler) cautery** can be used for pure punctal eversion. Burns are applied to the palpebral conjunctiva at approximately 5 mm below the punctum. Subsequent tissue shrinkage should invert the punctum.
- **Medial conjunctivoplasty** can be used in medial ectropion of a larger area of lid if there is no substantial horizontal laxity. A diamond-shaped piece of tarsoconjunctiva is excised, about 4 mm high and 8 mm wide, parallel with and inferolateral to the canaliculus and punctum, followed by approximation of the superior and inferior wound margins with sutures (Fig. 3.13).

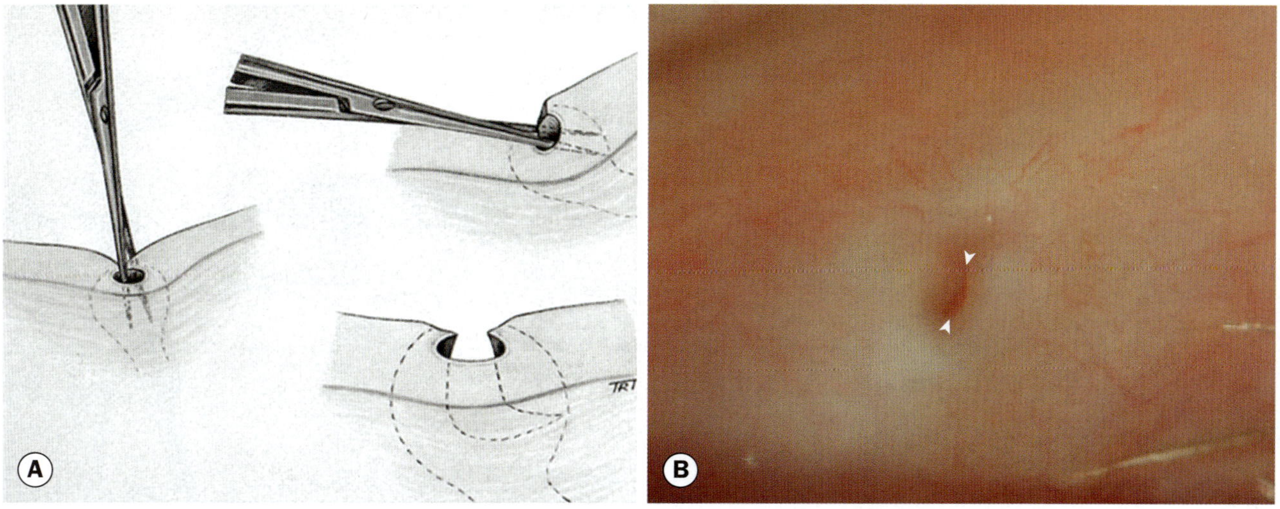

Fig. 3.12 Two-snip punctoplasty. **(A)** Technique; **(B)** postoperative appearance (arrowheads).

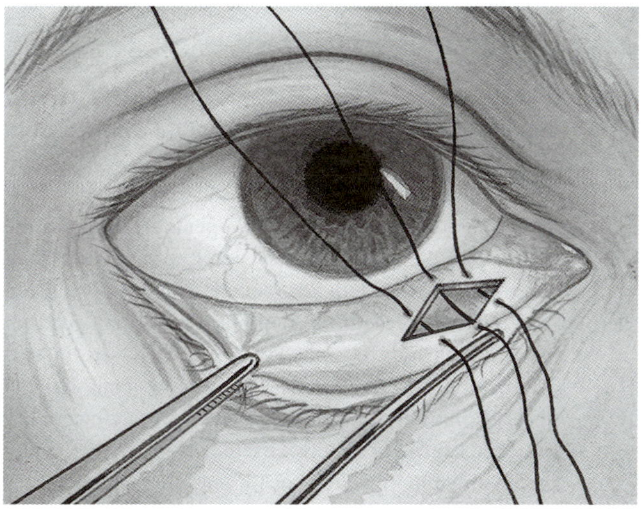

Fig. 3.13 Medial conjunctivoplasty.

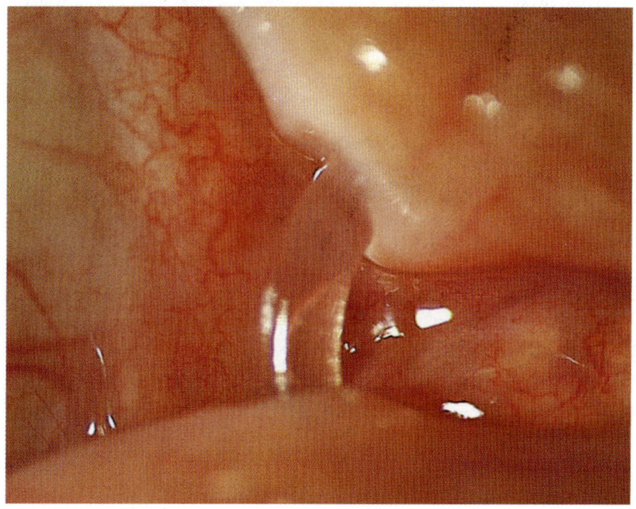

Fig. 3.14 Silicone lacrimal stent *in situ*.

Incorporation of the lower lid retractors in the sutures further aids repositioning.

- **Lower lid tightening,** usually with a tarsal strip, is used to correct lower lid laxity and may be combined with medial conjunctivoplasty where there is a significant medial ectropion component.

Canalicular obstruction

Causes include congenital, trauma, herpes simplex infection, drugs and irradiation. Chronic dacryocystitis can cause a membrane to form in the common canaliculus. The initial surgical approach has tended over recent years to attempt to preserve the physiological anatomy.

- **Partial obstruction** of the common or individual canaliculi, or anywhere in the lacrimal drainage system, may be treated by simple intubation of one or both canaliculi with silicone stents. These are left *in situ* for 6 weeks to 6 months (Fig. 3.14).
- **Total individual canalicular obstruction**
  - Canalicular trephination using a purpose-made minitrephine (Sisler), followed by intubation. Trephination has also been described using an intravenous catheter with a retracted introducer needle used as a stent and then advanced to overcome the obstruction. Balloon canaliculoplasty and endoscopic laser techniques are available. These less invasive options may have lower success rates than more aggressive surgery.
  - With 6–8 mm of patent normal canaliculus between the punctum and the obstruction, anastomosis of the patent part of the canaliculus into the lacrimal sac, with intubation, can be performed.
  - Where obstruction is severe or it is not possible to anastomose functioning canaliculi to the lacrimal sac, conventional surgery consists of

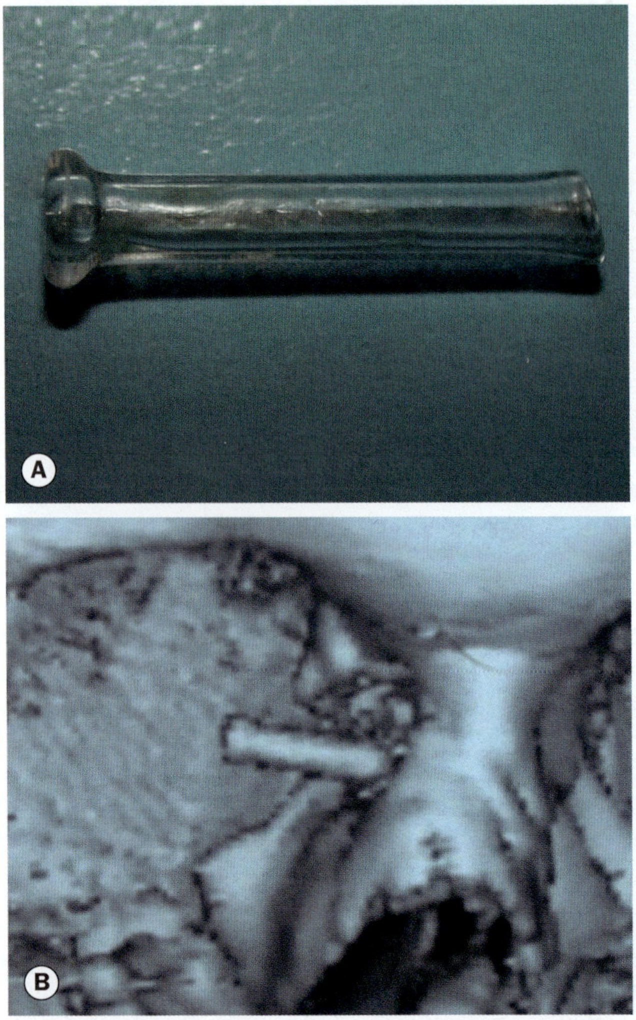

Fig. 3.15 **(A)** Lester Jones tube; **(B)** CT scan 3D reconstruction of tube *in situ*.

conjunctivodacryocystorhinostomy and the insertion of a toughened glass (Lester Jones) tube (Fig. 3.15). This may also be used when the lacrimal system is intact but non-functioning due to failure of the physiological pump (e.g. facial nerve palsy). The surgery is performed as for an external approach dacryocystorhinostomy (DCR – see below) but the caruncle is excised and a track for the tube created between the lacus lacrimalis and the lacrimal sac. Patient satisfaction is variable.

Nasolacrimal duct obstruction

- **Causes**
  - Idiopathic stenosis – by far the most common.
  - Naso-orbital trauma, including nasal and sinus surgery.
  - Granulomatous disease such as granulomatosis with polyangiitis and sarcoidosis.
  - Infiltration by nasopharyngeal tumours.
- **Treatment**
  - Conventional (external approach) dacryocystorhinostomy (DCR) is indicated for obstruction distal to the medial

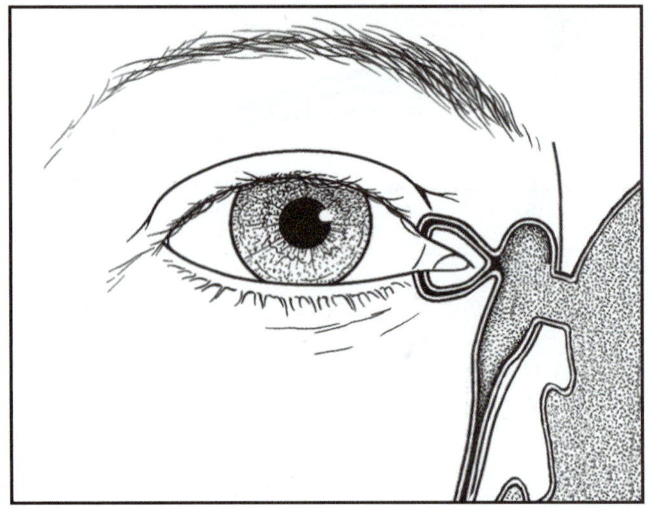

Fig. 3.16 Dacryocystorhinostomy showing the anastomosis between the lacrimal sac and the mucosa of the nose.

    opening of the common canaliculus and consists of anastomosis of the lacrimal sac to the mucosa of the middle nasal meatus (Fig. 3.16). The procedure is usually performed under hypotensive general anaesthesia. A vertical skin incision is made 10 mm medial to the inner canthus, the medial canthal tendon and lacrimal sac exposed and reflected and after removal of the intervening bone the sac is incised and attached to an opening created in the nasal mucosa (Fig. 3.17). The success rate is over 90%, but causes of failure include inadequate size and position of the ostium, unrecognized common canalicular obstruction, scarring and the 'sump syndrome', in which the surgical opening in the lacrimal bone is too small and too high. Complications include cutaneous scarring, injury to medial canthal structures, haemorrhage, infection and cerebrospinal fluid rhinorrhoea if the subarachnoid space is inadvertently entered.
  - Endoscopic DCR encompasses several techniques. A light pipe can be passed through the canalicular system into the lacrimal sac to guide an endoscopic approach from within the nose, or a microendoscopic transcanalicular procedure can be performed using a drill or laser to establish communication with the nasal cavity. Advantages over conventional DCR include less marked systemic disturbance with minimal blood loss and a lower risk of cerebrospinal fluid leakage, the avoidance of a skin incision and generally a shorter operating time. Disadvantages include generally a slightly lower success rate and visualization difficulties, meaning that additional procedures are sometimes needed.
  - Other procedures, often reserved for partial nasolacrimal duct obstruction, include probing and intubation, stent insertion and balloon dacryocystoplasty.

Dacryolithiasis

Dacryoliths (lacrimal stones) may occur in any part of the lacrimal system. They are more common in males. Although the

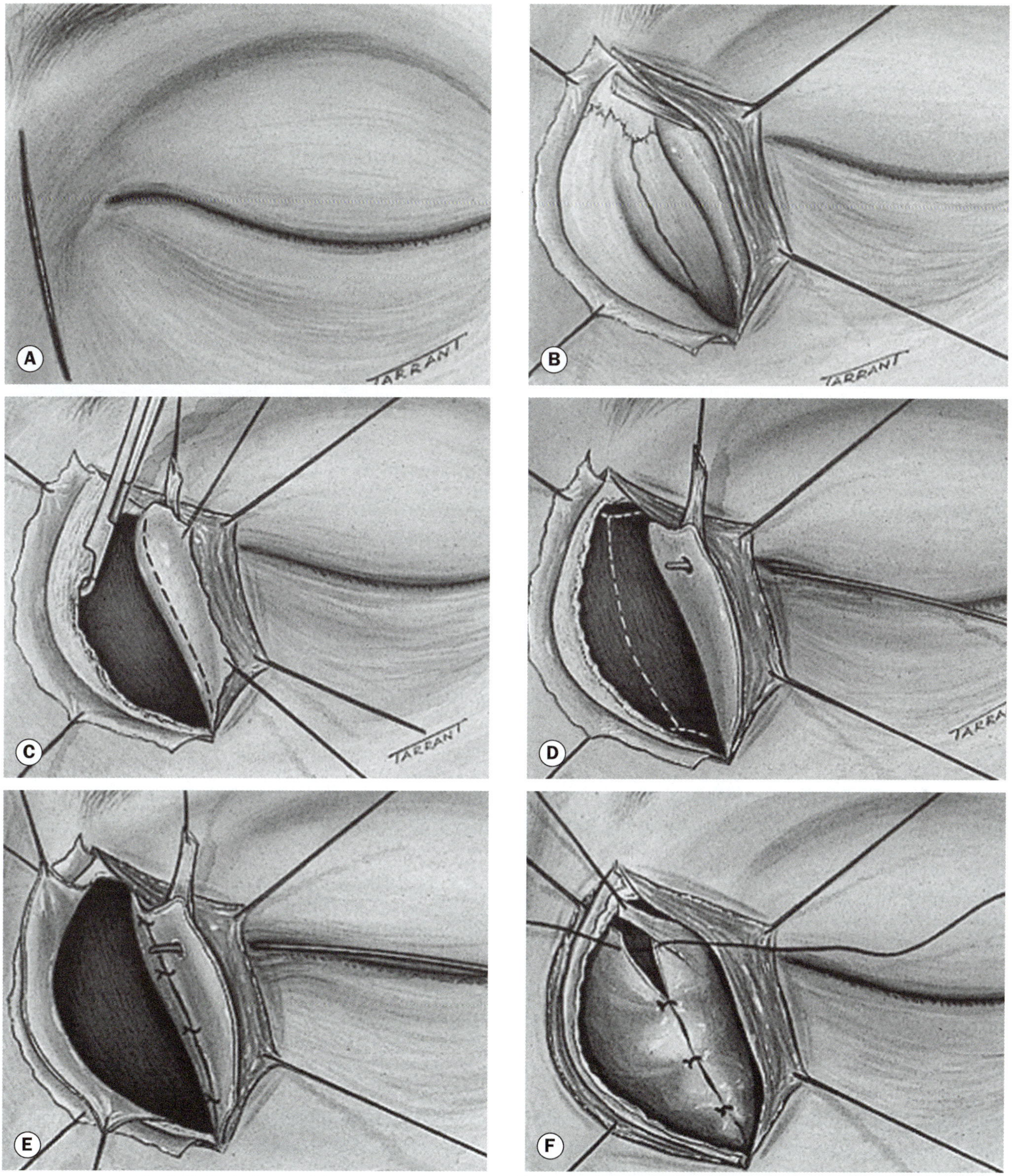

Fig. 3.17 Technique of dacryocystorhinostomy. **(A)** Vertical skin incision, made 10 mm medial to the inner canthus, avoiding the angular vein; **(B)** the anterior lacrimal crest is exposed and the periosteum is divided from the spine on the anterior lacrimal crest to the fundus of the sac and reflected forwards. The sac is reflected laterally from the lacrimal fossa; **(C)** the anterior lacrimal crest and the bone from the lacrimal fossa are removed; **(D)** the sac is incised in an 'H-shaped' manner to create two flaps. A vertical incision is made in the nasal mucosa to create anterior and posterior flaps; **(E)** the posterior flaps are sutured; **(F)** the anterior flaps are sutured.

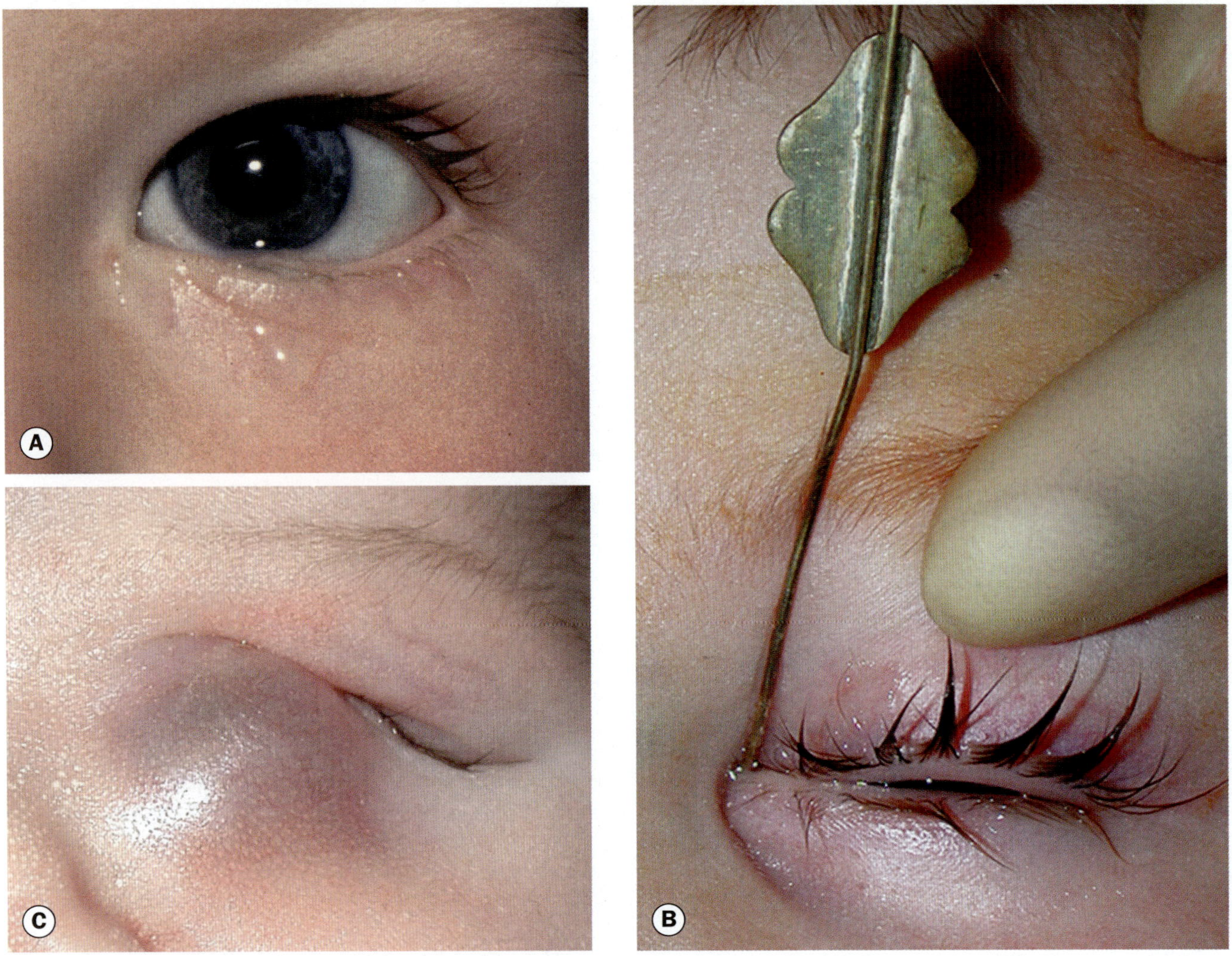

Fig. 3.18 Epiphora. **(A)** Child with a watering eye; **(B)** probing of the nasolacrimal duct; **(C)** congenital dacryocoele. *(Courtesy of Ken K Nischal – fig. B; A Pearson – fig. C.)*

pathogenesis is unclear, it has been proposed that tear stagnation secondary to inflammatory obstruction may precipitate stone formation, which tends to be associated with squamous metaplasia of the lacrimal sac epithelium. Presentation is often in late adulthood. Symptoms may include intermittent epiphora, recurrent attacks of acute dacryocystitis and lacrimal sac distension.

The lacrimal sac is distended and relatively firm, but is not inflamed and tender as in acute dacryocystitis.

Mucus reflux on pressure may or may not be present. Treatment involves a DCR.

CONGENITAL OBSTRUCTION

Nasolacrimal duct obstruction

The lower end of the nasolacrimal duct, in the region of the valve of Hasner, is the last portion of the lacrimal drainage system to canalize, with complete patency most commonly occurring soon after birth. Epiphora occurs in about 20 % of normal babies, but spontaneous resolution occurs in approximately 90% within the first year.

TIP Because congenital nasolacrimal obstruction with epiphora undergoes spontaneous resolution in 90% of babies by their first birthday, initial probing should be delayed until this age.

- **Signs**
  - Epiphora (Fig. 3.18A) and matting of eyelashes may be constant or intermittent and may be particularly noticeable when the child has an upper respiratory tract infection. Superimposed bacterial conjunctivitis may be treated with a broad-spectrum topical antibiotic.
  - Gentle pressure over the lacrimal sac may cause mucopurulent reflux.
  - Acute dacryocystitis is very rare.
  - Normal visual function should be confirmed as far as possible and an anterior segment examination with assessment of the red reflex performed.
  - The fluorescein disappearance test (see above) is highly specific in this setting. Only a fine line of dye, at most, should remain at 5–10 minutes under inspection with a blue light in a darkened room.

- **Differential diagnosis** includes other congenital causes of a watering eye, such as punctal atresia, congenital glaucoma, chronic conjunctivitis (e.g. chlamydial), keratitis and uveitis.
- **Treatment**
  - Massage of the lacrimal sac has been suggested as a means of rupturing a membranous obstruction by hydrostatic pressure. The index finger is initially placed over the common canaliculus to block reflux and then rolled over the sac, massaging downwards. The likelihood of success and the optimal regimen is undetermined.
  - Probing. Passage of a fine wire via the canalicular system and nasolacrimal duct (Fig. 3.18B) to disrupt the obstructive membrane at the valve of Hasner is usually regarded as the definitive treatment and may be preceded and followed by irrigation to confirm the site of obstruction and subsequent patency respectively. Probing can be repeated if a first procedure is unsuccessful. Nasal endoscopic guidance may enhance success and should be considered at least for repeat procedures. If symptoms are mild–moderate, probing may be delayed until the age of 12–18, or even 24, months and is carried out under general anaesthesia. For more marked symptoms, early probing may be appropriate and in young children is sometimes performed under topical anaesthesia in an outpatient setting. Risks include the induction of canalicular stenosis due to probe trauma, which may be relatively common. It should be noted that there is little evidence of a difference in final outcome at 24 months conferred by intervention versus non-intervention. Failure of probing may result from abnormal anatomy, which can usually be recognized by difficulty in passing the probe and subsequent non-patency of the drainage system on irrigation.
  - Options after probing failure include intubation with silicone tubing with or without balloon dilatation of the nasolacrimal duct, endoscopic procedures and dacryocystorhinostomy.

Congenital dacryocoele

A congenital dacryocoele (amniontocoele) is a collection of amniotic fluid or mucus in the lacrimal sac caused by an imperforate Hasner valve. Presentation is perinatal with a bluish cystic swelling at or below the medial canthus (Fig. 3.18C), accompanied by epiphora. If an intranasal component is large, it can cause respiratory distress. It should not be mistaken for an encephalocoele, the latter being characterized by a pulsatile swelling above the medial canthal tendon. Resolution is common with only conservative treatment, but if this fails, probing is usually adequate.

TIP A congenital dacryocoele should not be confused with an encephalocoele, which is characterized by a pulsatile swelling above the medial canthal ligament.

CHRONIC CANALICULITIS

Chronic canaliculitis is an uncommon condition, frequently caused by *Actinomyces israelii*, anaerobic Gram-positive bacteria

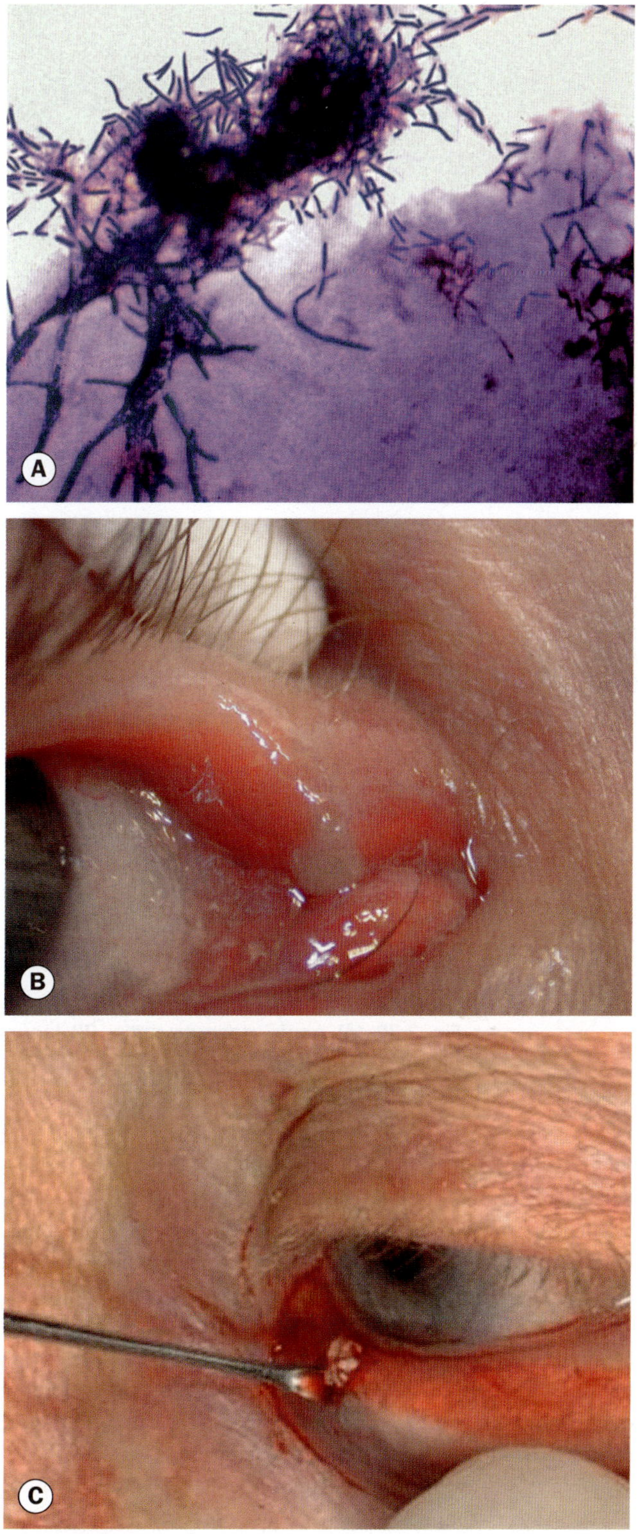

Fig. 3.19 Chronic canaliculitis. **(A)** Gram-stain of *Actinomyces israelii*; **(B)** mucopurulent discharge on pressure over an inflamed upper canaliculus; **(C)** sulfur concretions released by canaliculotomy.

(Fig. 3.19A). Occasionally scarring and canalicular obstruction may result. Presentation is with unilateral epiphora associated with chronic mucopurulent conjunctivitis refractory to conventional treatment. There is pericanalicular redness and oedema and mucopurulent discharge on pressure over the canaliculus

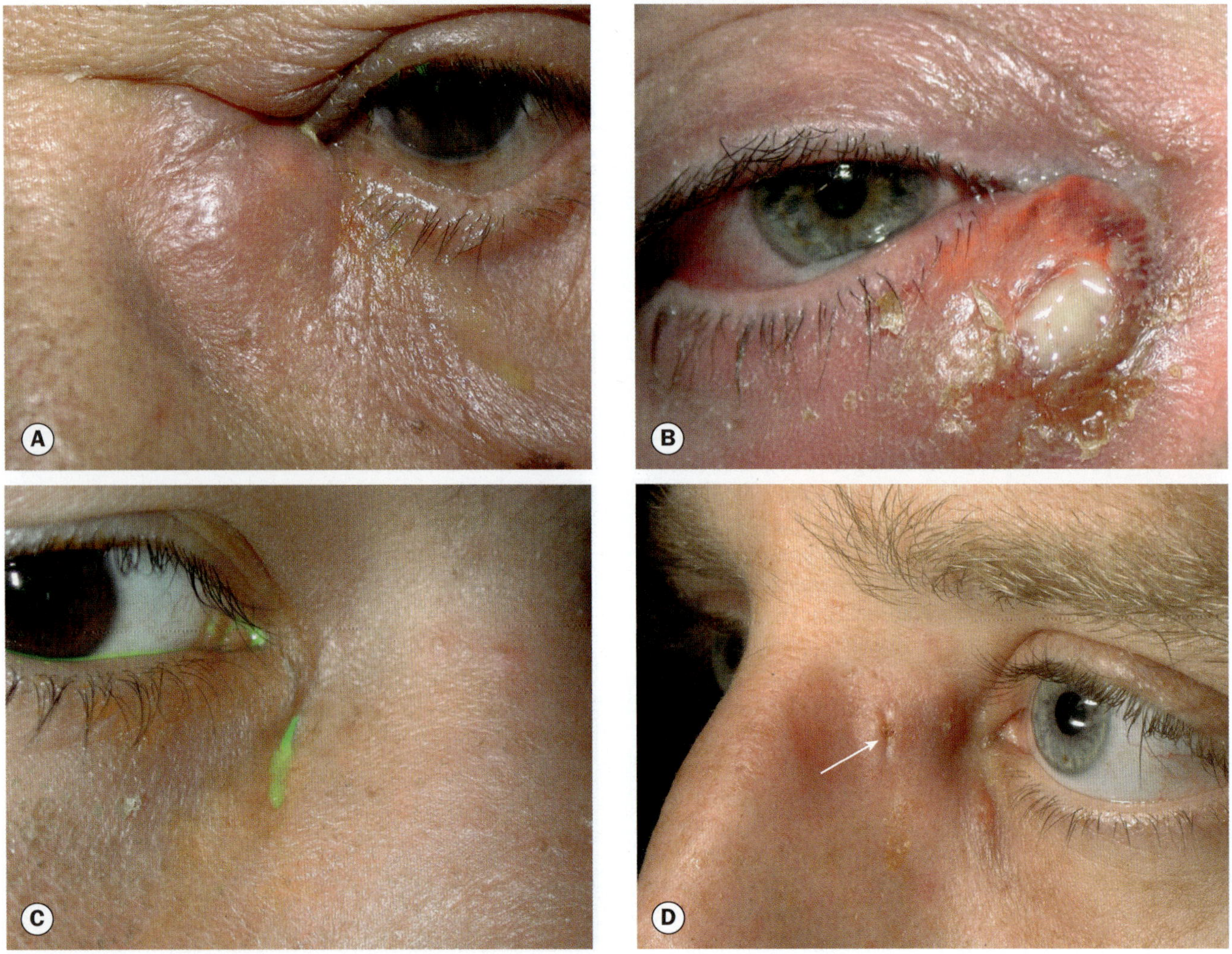

Fig. 3.20 (A) Acute dacryocystitis; **(B)** lacrimal abscess and preseptal cellulitis; **(C)** lacrimal fistula with fluorescein; **(D)** healed lacrimal fistula (arrow).

(Fig. 3.19B). A 'pouting' punctum (see Fig. 3.3F) may be a diagnostic clue in mild cases. In contrast to dacryocystitis, there is no lacrimal sac involvement. Concretions (sulfur granules) are metabolic products of *Actinomyces* and other hydrogen sulfide-utilizing bacteria and classically are expressed on canalicular compression or following canaliculotomy (Fig. 3.19C). A topical antibiotic such as a fluoroquinolone four times daily for 10 days may be tried initially, but is rarely curative unless combined with canaliculotomy (a linear incision into the conjunctival side of the canaliculus) and curettage of concretions. Giant fornix syndrome (see Ch. 6), dacryolithiasis and lacrimal diverticulum may give a similar clinical picture. Herpes simplex is a classic cause of acute – as opposed to chronic – canaliculitis.

TIP Chronic canaliculitis should be suspected in a patient with unilateral mucopurulent conjunctivitis that is refractory to conventional treatment.

DACRYOCYSTITIS

Infection of the lacrimal sac is usually secondary to obstruction of the nasolacrimal duct. It may be acute or chronic and is most commonly staphylococcal or streptococcal.

Acute dacryocystitis

Presentation is with the subacute onset of pain in the medial canthal area, associated with epiphora. A very tender, tense red swelling develops at the medial canthus (Fig. 3.20A), commonly progressing to abscess formation (Fig. 3.20B). There may be associated preseptal cellulitis.

- **Treatment**
  - Initial treatment involves the application of warm compresses and oral antibiotics such as flucloxacillin or co-amoxiclav. Irrigation and probing should not be performed.

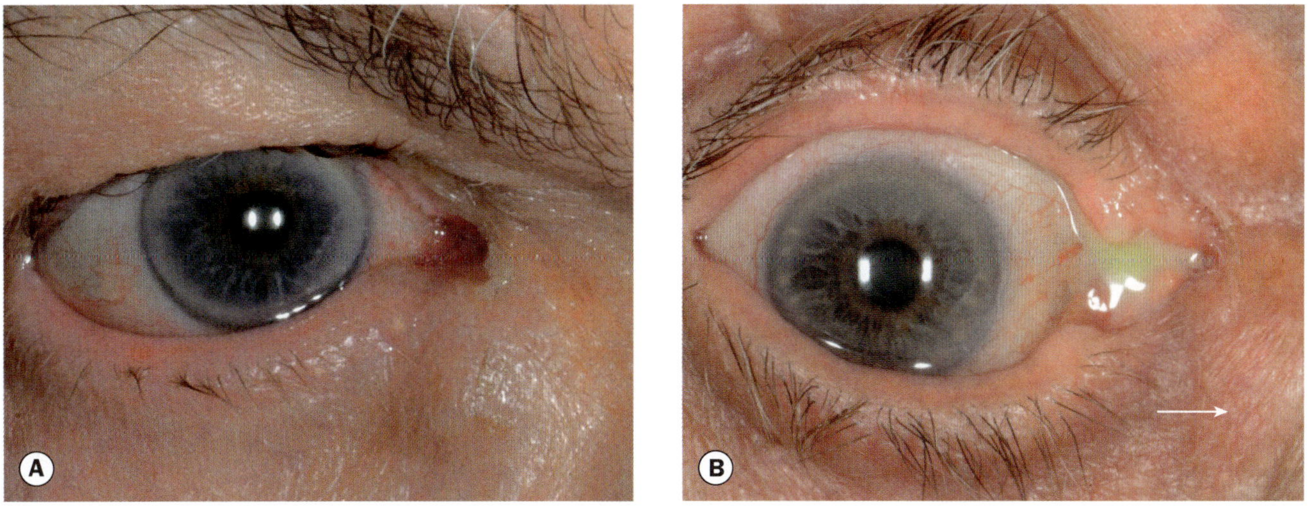

Fig. 3.21 **(A)** Mucocoele; **(B)** expression of mucopurulent material by applying pressure to the sac (arrow).

- Incision and drainage may be considered if pus points and an abscess is about to drain spontaneously. However, this carries the risk of a persistent sac–skin fistula (Fig. 3.20C).
- Dacryocystorhinostomy is commonly required after the acute infection has been controlled and may reduce the risk of recurrent infection and can result in closure of a fistula (Fig. 3.20D).

Chronic dacryocystitis

Presentation is with chronic epiphora, which may be associated with a chronic or recurrent unilateral conjunctivitis. A mucocoele is usually evident as a painless swelling at the inner canthus (Fig. 3.21A), but if an obvious swelling is absent pressure over the sac commonly still results in mucopurulent canalicular reflux (Fig. 3.21B). Treatment is with a dacryocystorhinostomy.

TIP To reduce the risk of endophthalmitis postpone intraocular surgery if there are any signs of lacrimal drainage system infection.

Chapter

Orbit 4

INTRODUCTION

Anatomy

The orbit is a pear-shaped cavity, the stalk of which is the optic canal (Fig. 4.1).

- **The roof** consists of two bones: the lesser wing of the sphenoid and the orbital plate of the frontal bone. It is located subjacent to the anterior cranial fossa and the frontal sinus. A defect in the orbital roof may cause pulsatile proptosis due to transmission of cerebrospinal fluid pulsation to the orbit.
- **The lateral wall** also consists of two bones: the greater wing of the sphenoid and the zygomatic. The anterior half of the globe is vulnerable to lateral trauma since it protrudes beyond the lateral orbital margin.
- **The floor** consists of three bones: the zygomatic, maxillary and palatine. The posteromedial portion of the maxillary bone is relatively weak and may be involved in a 'blowout' fracture (see Ch. 22). The orbital floor also forms the roof of the maxillary sinus so that maxillary carcinoma invading the orbit may displace the globe upwards.
- **The medial wall** consists of four bones: maxillary, lacrimal, ethmoid and sphenoid. The lamina papyracea, which forms part of the medial wall, is paper-thin and perforated by numerous foramina for nerves and blood vessels. Orbital cellulitis is therefore frequently secondary to ethmoidal sinusitis.
- **The superior orbital fissure** is a slit linking the cranium and the orbit, between the greater and lesser wings of the sphenoid bone. A number of important structures pass through it (Fig. 4.2).
  - The superior portion contains the lacrimal, frontal and trochlear nerves and the superior ophthalmic vein.
  - The inferior portion contains the superior and inferior divisions of the oculomotor nerve, the abducens and nasociliary nerves and sympathetic fibres from the cavernous plexus.
  - Inflammation of the superior orbital fissure and apex (Tolosa–Hunt syndrome) may therefore result in a multitude of signs including ophthalmoplegia and venous outflow obstruction.
- **The inferior orbital fissure** lies between the greater wing of the sphenoid and the maxilla, connecting the orbit to the pterygopalatine and infratemporal fossae. Through it run the maxillary nerve, the zygomatic nerve and branches of the pterygopalatine ganglion, as well as the inferior ophthalmic vein.
- **The sensory supply** of the eye and orbit is shown in Fig. 4.3.

Clinical features

Symptoms

Symptoms of orbital disease include eyelid and conjunctival swelling, redness, watering, pain (sometimes on, or exacerbated by, eye movement), increasing ocular prominence, displacement or a sunken impression of the eye, double vision and blurring and sometimes a pulsing sensation or audible bruit.

Soft tissue involvement

Eyelid and periocular oedema, skin discoloration, ptosis, chemosis (oedema of the conjunctiva, which may involve the plica and caruncle) and epibulbar injection (Fig. 4.4) may be seen. Causes include thyroid eye disease, orbital inflammatory diseases and obstruction to venous drainage.

Proptosis

Proptosis (Fig. 4.5) describes an abnormal protrusion of an organ, but is generally applied to the eyeball; exophthalmos refers specifically to the eyeball only. Proptosis may be caused by retrobulbar lesions or, less frequently, a shallow orbit. The intraorbital portion of the optic nerve is longer (25 mm) than the distance between the back of the globe and the optic canal (18 mm). This allows for

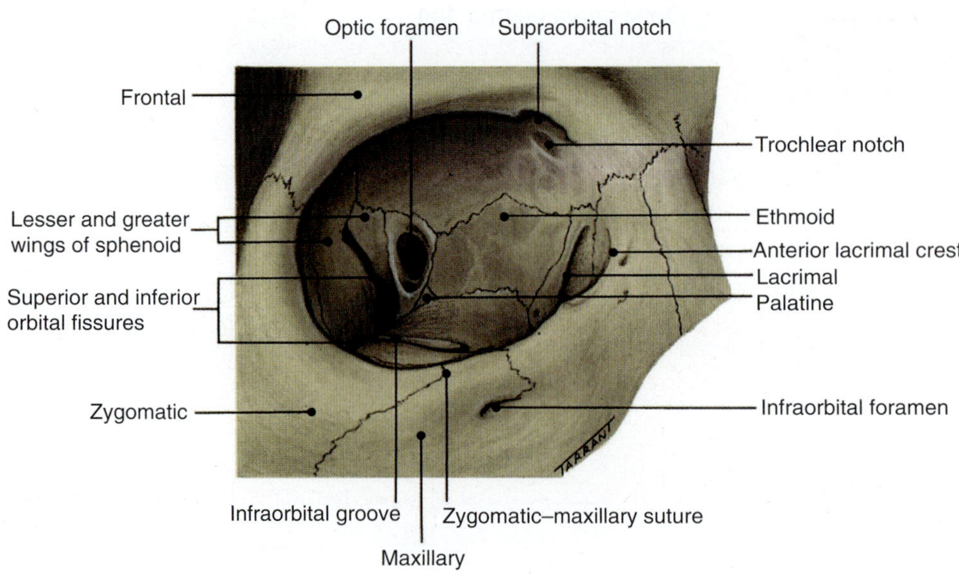

Fig. 4.1 Anatomy of the orbit.

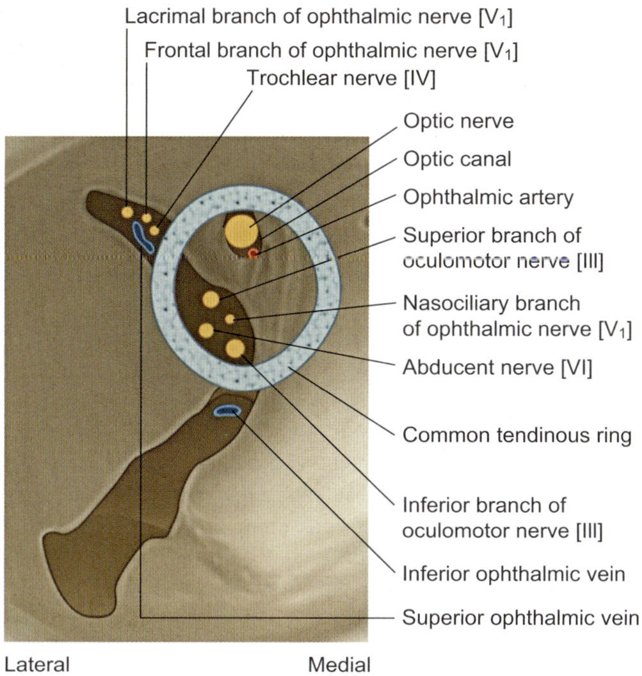

Fig. 4.2 Innervation of the orbit and eyeball.

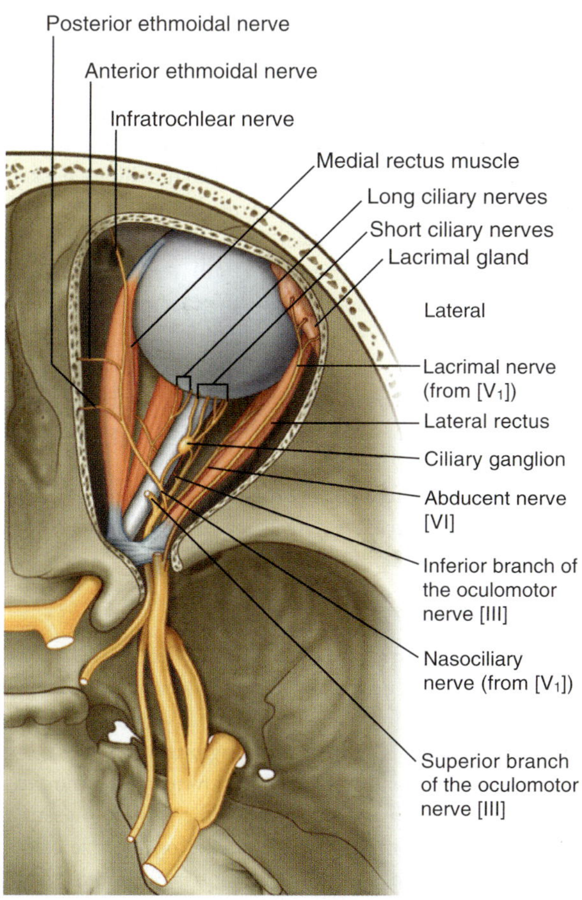

Fig. 4.3 Sensory nerve supply of the orbit.

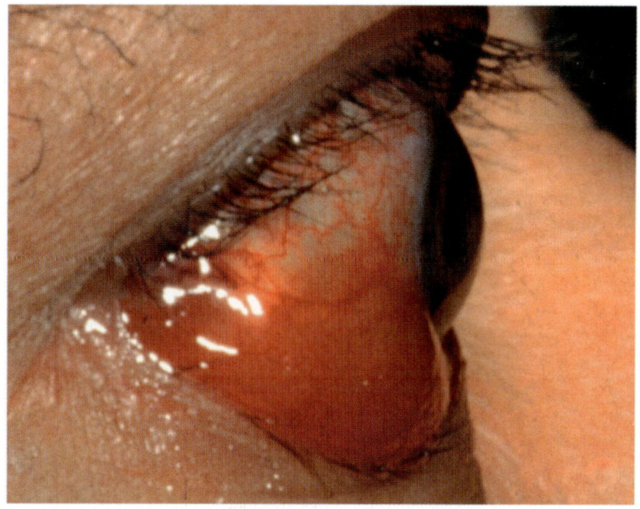

Fig. 4.4 Chemosis and injection in orbital disease.

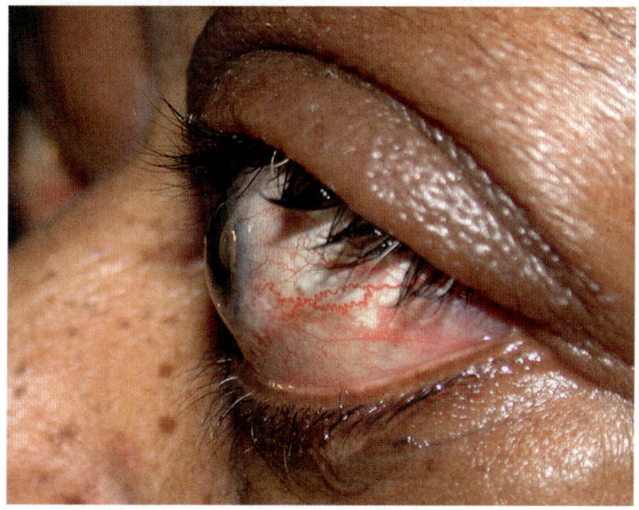

Fig. 4.5 Proptosis.

significant forward displacement of the globe (proptosis) without excessive stretching of the nerve.

- **Asymmetrical proptosis** is readily detected by looking down at the patient from above and behind (Fig. 4.6A).
- **The direction** of proptosis may indicate the likely pathology. For example, space-occupying lesions within the muscle cone such as a cavernous haemangioma or optic nerve tumours cause axial proptosis, whereas extraconal lesions usually give rise to combined proptosis and dystopia (see next).
- **Dystopia** implies displacement of the globe in the coronal plane, usually due to an extraconal orbital mass such as a lacrimal gland tumour (Fig. 4.6B). Horizontal displacement is measured from the midline (nose) to the centre of the pupil while vertical dystopia is read on a vertical scale perpendicular to a horizontal rule placed over the bridge of the nose. The measured eye should fixate straight ahead; if necessary, this can be facilitated by occluding the fellow eye.
- **The severity** of proptosis can be measured with a plastic rule resting on the lateral orbital margin, or with the

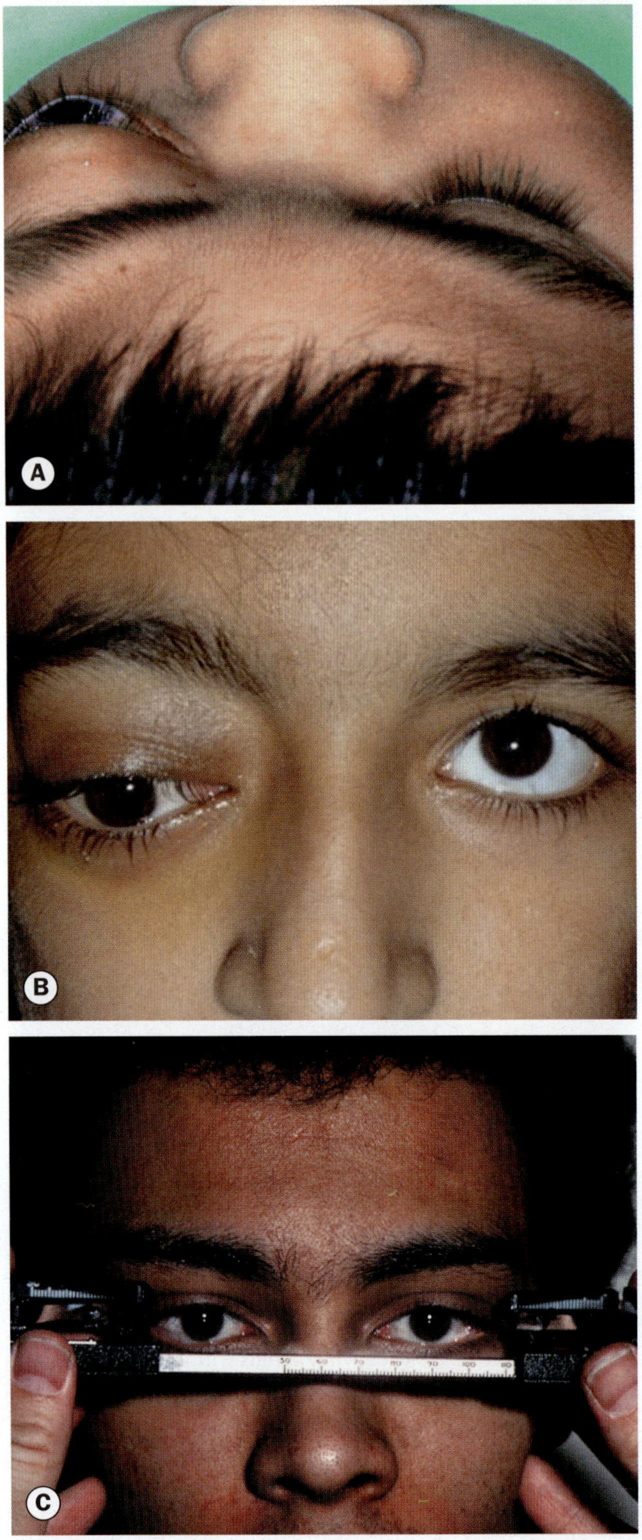

Fig. 4.6 General signs of orbital disease. **(A)** Left proptosis visualized from above; **(B)** right inferior dystopia; **(C)** measurement of proptosis with an exophthalmometer.

Luedde exophthalmometer using a similar principle. Commonly, a binocular exophthalmometer (e.g. Hertel Oculus) is employed, using visualization of the corneal apices to determine the degree of ocular protrusion from a scale (Fig. 4.6C). Measurements can be taken both relaxed and with the Valsalva manoeuvre. Readings greater than 20 mm are indicative of proptosis and a difference of 2–3 mm or more between the two eyes is suspicious regardless of the absolute values. The dimensions of the palpebral apertures and any lagophthalmos should also be noted.

- **Pseudoproptosis** (the false impression of proptosis) may be due to facial asymmetry, enlargement of the globe (e.g. high myopia or buphthalmos), lid retraction or contralateral enophthalmos.

Enophthalmos

Enophthalmos implies recession of the globe within the orbit. Causes include congenital and traumatic orbital wall abnormalities, atrophy of the orbital contents (e.g. radiotherapy, scleroderma, chronic eye poking in blind infants – the 'oculodigital' sign) or sclerosis (e.g. metastatic scirrhous carcinoma, sclerosing orbital inflammatory disease). Pseudoenophthalmos may be caused by a small or shrunken eye (microphthalmos or phthisis bulbi), by ptosis, or by contralateral proptosis or pseudoproptosis.

Ophthalmoplegia

Defective ocular motility is very common in orbital disease. Causes include an orbital mass, restrictive myopathy (e.g. thyroid eye disease – Fig. 4.7, orbital myositis, tethering of muscles or tissue after orbital wall fracture), ocular motor nerve involvement associated with lesions in the cavernous sinus, orbital fissures or posterior orbit (e.g. carotid–cavernous fistula, Tolosa–Hunt syndrome, malignant lacrimal gland tumours). The following tests may be used to differentiate a restrictive from a neurological motility defect:

- **Forced duction test.** Under topical anaesthesia, the insertion of the muscle in an involved eye is grasped with forceps and the globe rotated in the direction of reduced mobility. Checked movement of the globe indicates a restrictive problem. No resistance will be encountered with a neurological lesion.
- **Differential intraocular pressure (IOP) test** involves less discomfort than forced duction and an objective rather than subjective endpoint. The IOP is measured in the primary position of gaze and then with the patient attempting to look in the direction of limited mobility. An increase of 6 mmHg or more denotes resistance transmitted to the globe by muscle restriction (the Braley sign).
- **Saccadic eye movements** in neurological lesions are reduced in velocity, while restrictive defects manifest normal saccadic velocity with sudden halting of ocular movement.

Dynamic properties

- **Increasing venous pressure** by dependent head position, the Valsalva manoeuvre or jugular compression may induce or exacerbate proptosis in patients with orbital venous anomalies or infants with orbital capillary haemangioma.
- **Pulsation** is caused either by an arteriovenous communication or a defect in the orbital roof. In the former, pulsation may be associated with a bruit depending on the size of the communication. In the latter the pulsation is transmitted from the brain by the cerebrospinal fluid and there is no associated

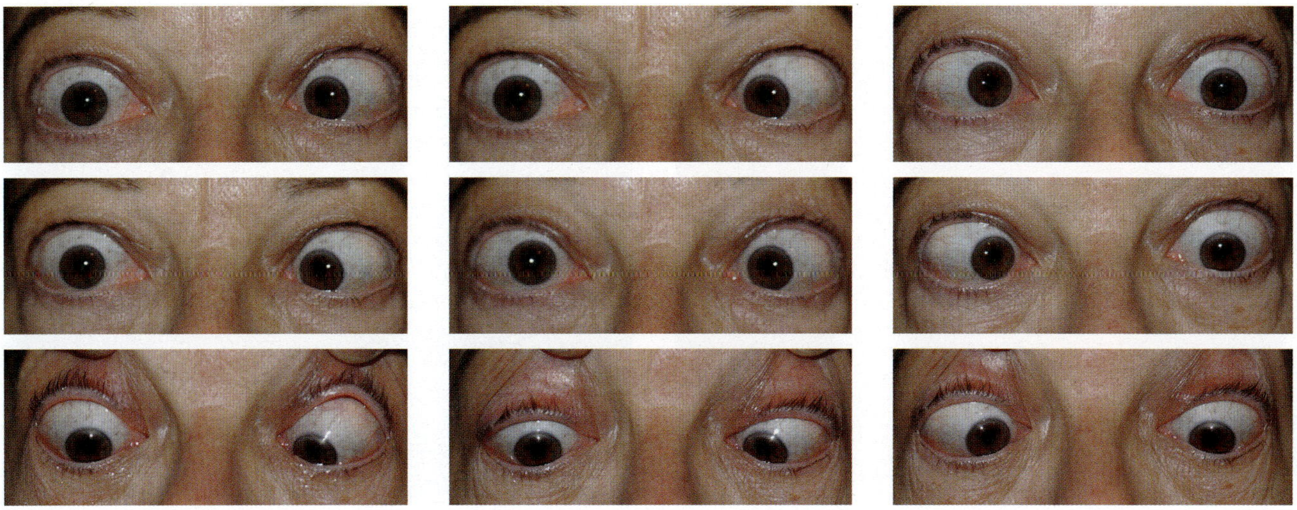

Fig. 4.7 Restrictive myopathy, bilateral lid retraction and proptosis in thyroid eye disease – nine positions of gaze. *(Courtesy of C Barry.)*

bruit. Mild pulsation is best detected on the slit lamp, particularly by applanation tonometry.

- **A bruit** is a sign found with a larger carotid–cavernous fistula. It is best heard with the bell of the stethoscope and is lessened or abolished by gently compressing the ipsilateral carotid artery in the neck.

Fundus changes

- **Optic disc swelling** may be the initial feature of compressive optic neuropathy (Fig. 4.8A).
- **Optic atrophy** (Fig. 4.8B), which may be preceded by swelling, is a feature of severe compressive optic neuropathy. Important causes include thyroid eye disease and optic nerve tumours.
- **Opticociliary collaterals** consist of enlarged pre-existing peripapillary capillaries that divert blood from the central retinal venous circulation to the peripapillary choroidal circulation when there is obstruction of the normal drainage channels. On ophthalmoscopy the vessels appear as large tortuous channels most frequently sited temporally, which disappear at the disc margin (Fig. 4.8C). The collaterals may be associated with any orbital or optic nerve tumour that compresses the intraorbital optic nerve and impairs blood flow through the central retinal vein. The most common tumour associated with shunts is an optic nerve sheath meningioma but they may also occur with optic nerve glioma, central retinal vein occlusion, idiopathic intracranial hypertension and glaucoma.
- **Choroidal folds** (Fig. 4.8B and D) are discussed in detail in Chapter 14. They may occur in a wide variety of orbital lesions. Although tending to be more common with greater amounts of proptosis and anteriorly located tumours, in some cases their presence can precede the onset of proptosis.

Investigation

- **Computed tomography (CT)** is useful for depicting bony structures and the location and size of space-occupying lesions. It is of particular value in patients with orbital trauma because it can detect small fractures, foreign bodies, blood, herniation of extraocular muscle and emphysema (see Ch. 22). It is, however, unable to distinguish different pathological soft tissue masses that are radiologically isodense. Confirmation of an orbital abscess in cellulitis is a relatively common indication.
- **Magnetic resonance imaging (MRI)** can demonstrate orbital apex lesions and intracranial extension of orbital tumours and is useful for imaging orbital inflammatory disease. Serial short T1 inversion recovery (STIR) scans are valuable in assessing inflammatory activity in thyroid eye disease (see Ch. 19).
- **Plain X-rays** are little used except for the initial diagnosis of traumatic bony injury.
- **Ultrasonography** can provide useful information, particularly with high-grade apparatus and an experienced operator, but does not image the orbital apex well.
- **Fine-needle biopsy** is sometimes performed, particularly in suspected neoplastic disease. Potential problems include haemorrhage and ocular penetration.

TIP The most common tumour associated with opticociliary shunt vessels on the disc is an optic nerve sheath meningioma.

THYROID EYE DISEASE

Introduction

Thyroid eye disease (TED), also known as thyroid-associated orbitopathy and Graves ophthalmopathy, is a common orbital disorder and is the most common cause of both bilateral and unilateral proptosis in an adult.

Thyrotoxicosis

Thyrotoxicosis (hyperthyroidism) is a condition involving excessive secretion of thyroid hormones. Graves disease, the most

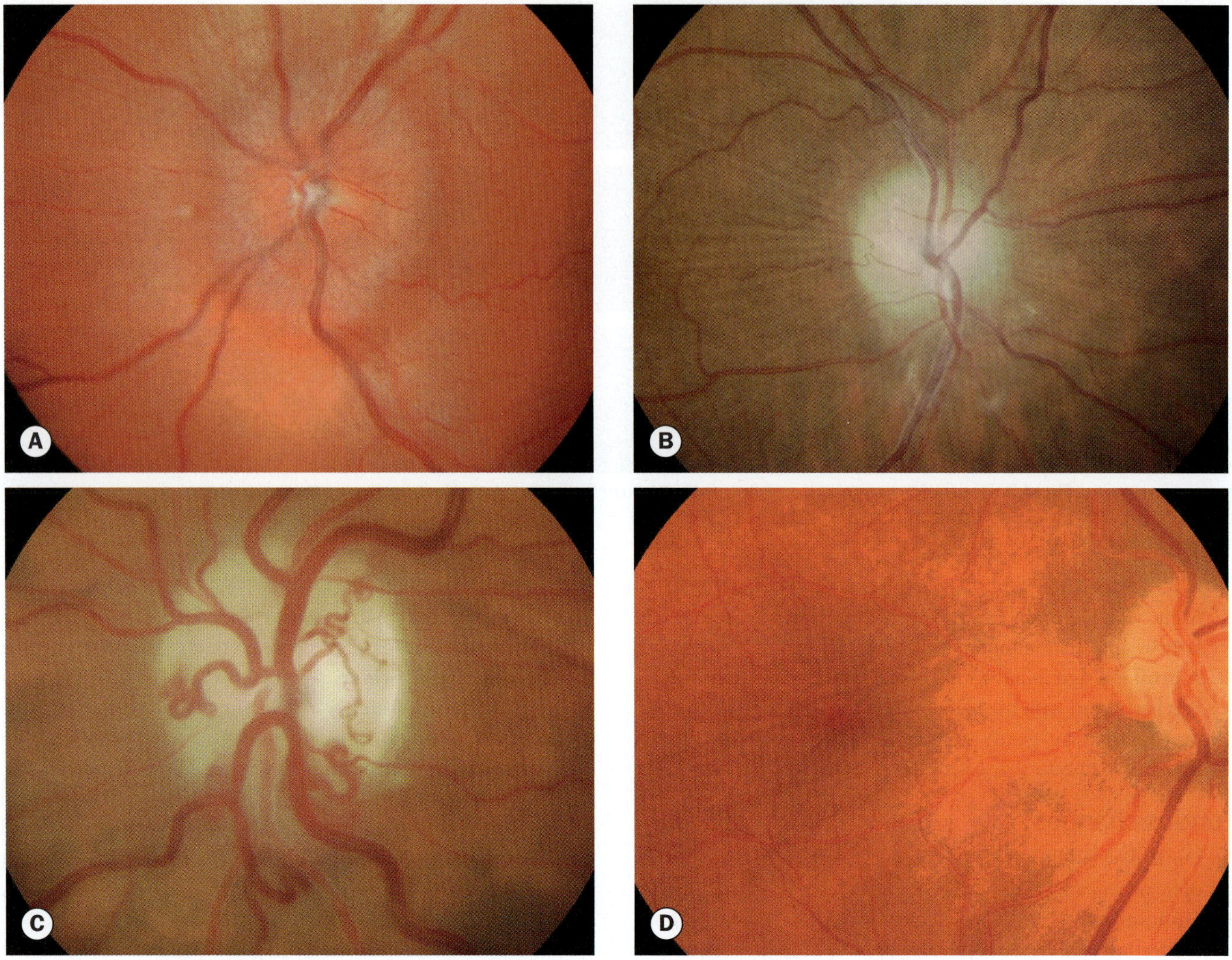

Fig. 4.8 Fundus changes in orbital disease. **(A)** Disc swelling; **(B)** optic atrophy with choroidal folds; **(C)** optociliary vessels in the presence of optic atrophy; **(D)** choroidal folds.

common form of hyperthyroidism, is an autoimmune disorder in which IgG antibodies bind to receptors in the thyroid gland and stimulate secretion of thyroid hormones. It is more common in females and may be associated with other autoimmune disorders. Presentation is often in the fourth or fifth decades with symptoms including weight loss despite good appetite, increased bowel frequency, sweating, heat intolerance, nervousness, irritability, palpitations, weakness and fatigue. There may be enlargement of the thyroid gland (Fig. 4.9A), tremor, palmar erythema and warm and sweaty skin. Thyroid acropachy is a phenomenon similar to clubbing of the fingers (Fig. 4.9B), occurring in 1%; pretibial myxoedema (1–5%) is indurated thickening of the skin of the shins. Cardiac manifestations may include sinus tachycardia and other arrhythmias. Other autoimmune disorders can be associated. Thyroid function is commonly tested initially with a TSH level. If this is low, or normal but thyroid disease is still suspected, a range of additional investigations can be carried out. Treatment options include carbimazole, propylthiouracil, propranolol, thyroid ablation with radioactive iodine and partial thyroidectomy.

Risk factors for ophthalmopathy

Once a patient has Graves disease, the major clinical risk factor for developing TED is smoking. The greater the number of cigarettes smoked per day, the greater the risk and giving up smoking seems to reduce the risk. Women are five times more likely to be affected by TED than men, but this largely reflects the increased incidence of Graves disease in women. Radioactive iodine used to treat hyperthyroidism can worsen TED. This condition can also, though less commonly, occur in euthyroid and hypothyroid (including treated hyperthyroid) patients. It can sometimes be the presenting manifestation of thyroid-related disease.

Pathogenesis of ophthalmopathy

Thyroid ophthalmopathy involves an organ-specific autoimmune reaction in which anti-thyrotropin-receptor antibody reacts against thyroid gland cells and orbital fibroblasts. Insulin-like growth factor 1 receptor (IGF-1R) and the thyroid-stimulating hormone receptor (TSHR) are upregulated in orbital and brow fat. This leads to inflammation of extraocular muscles, interstitial tissues, orbital fat and lacrimal glands. A pleomorphic cellular

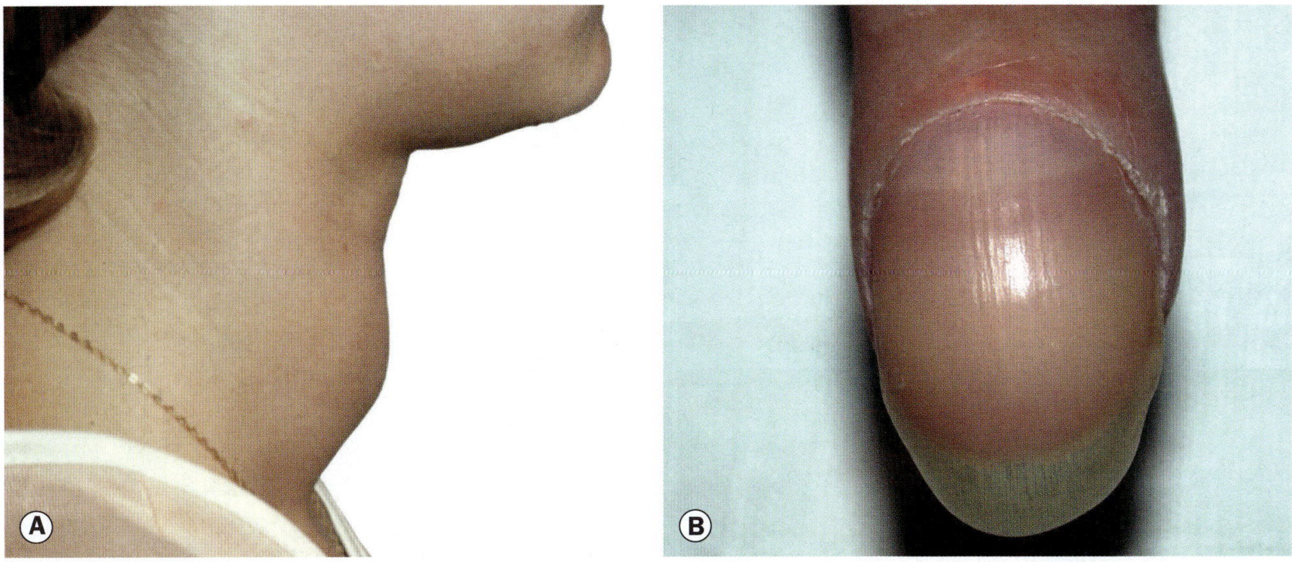

Fig. 4.9 Systemic signs in thyrotoxicosis. **(A)** Goitre; **(B)** acropachy.

infiltration and increased secretion of glycosaminoglycans leads to osmotic imbibition of water. The volume of the orbital contents increases and the muscles can swell up to eight times their normal size. There is also lipogenesis induced by fibroblasts and preadipocytes, which causes orbital fat enlargement. There may be a secondary elevation of intraorbital pressure and the optic nerve may be compressed. Subsequent degeneration of muscle fibres eventually leads to fibrosis, which exerts a tethering effect on the involved muscle, resulting in restrictive myopathy and diplopia.

Clinical features

Introduction

TED typically proceeds through a congestive (inflammatory) stage in which the eyes are red and painful. This tends to remit within 1–3 years and only about 10% of patients develop serious long-term ocular problems. A fibrotic (quiescent) stage follows in which the eyes are white, although a painless motility defect may be present. Clinical features broadly can be categorized into: (1) soft tissue involvement, (2) lid retraction, (3) proptosis, (4) optic neuropathy and (5) restrictive myopathy.

European Group on Graves Orbitopathy (EUGOGO) Classification (2021)

- **Activity**
  - Spontaneous retrobulbar pain.
  - Pain on attempted upward or downward gaze.
  - Redness of eyelids.
  - Redness of conjunctiva.
  - Swelling of conjunctiva or plica.
  - Swelling of eyelids.
  - Chemosis.
- **Severity**
  - Mild, with only a minor impact on daily life.
  - Moderate–severe, with one of moderate–severe soft tissue involvement, lid retraction of 2 mm or more, diplopia and proptosis of 3 mm or more.
  - Sight-threatening due to optic neuropathy or corneal breakdown.

Soft tissue involvement

- **Symptoms.** Grittiness, red eyes, lacrimation, photophobia, puffy lids and retrobulbar discomfort.
- **Signs** may include:
  - Epibulbar hyperaemia. This is a sensitive sign of inflammatory activity. Intense focal hyperaemia may outline the insertions of the horizontal recti (Fig. 4.10A).
  - Periorbital swelling is caused by oedema and infiltration behind the orbital septum. This may be associated with chemosis and prolapse of retroseptal fat into the eyelids (Fig. 4.10B).
  - Tear insufficiency and instability is common.
  - Corneal signs are exacerbated by lid retraction (see next) and can include punctate epithelial erosions, superior limbic keratoconjunctivitis (Fig. 4.10C and see Ch. 7) and occasionally bacterial keratitis, thinning and scarring.

Lid retraction

Retraction of upper and lower lids occurs in about 50% of patients with Graves disease. Overaction of Müller muscle is postulated to occur as a result of sympathetic overstimulation secondary to high levels of thyroid hormones. Fibrotic contracture of the levator palpebrae and inferior rectus muscles associated with adhesion to overlying orbital tissues is another probable mechanism, together with secondary overaction in response to hypo- or hypertropia produced by fibrosis.

- **Symptoms.** Patients may complain of a staring or bulging-eyed appearance, difficulty closing the eyes and ocular surface symptoms.

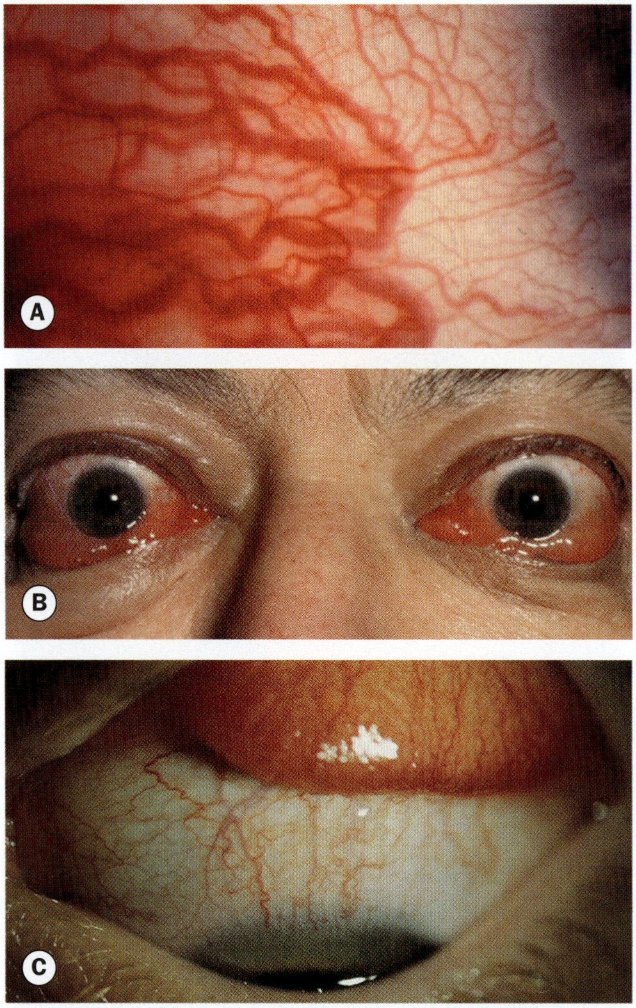

Fig. 4.10 Soft tissue involvement in thyroid eye disease. **(A)** Epibulbar hyperaemia overlying a horizontal rectus muscle; **(B)** periorbital oedema, chemosis and prolapse of fat into the eyelids; **(C)** superior limbic keratoconjunctivitis.

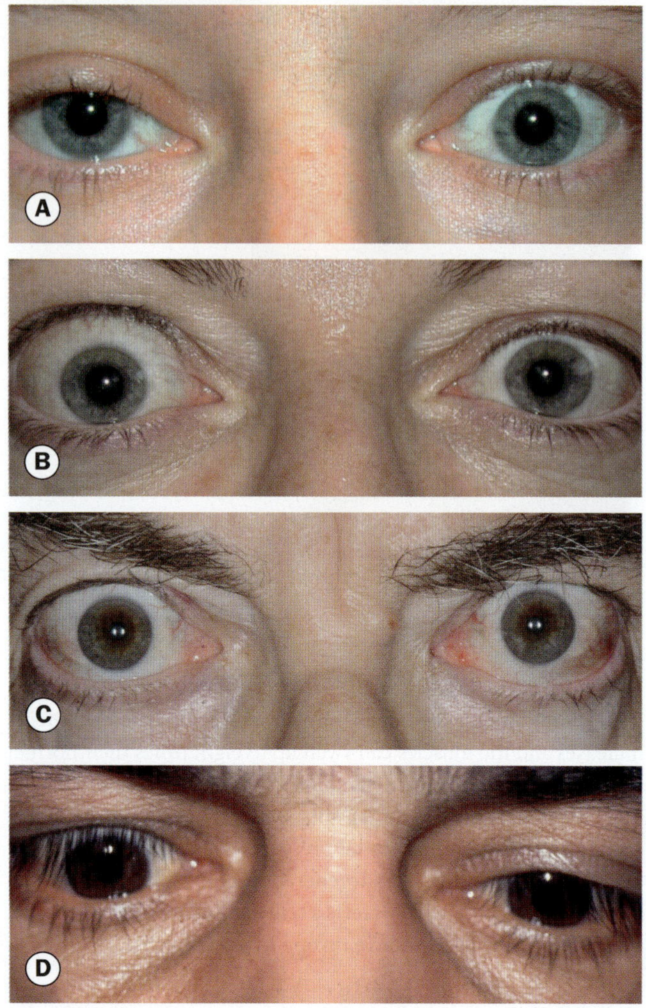

Fig. 4.11 Lid signs in thyroid eye disease. **(A)** Mild left lid retraction; **(B)** moderate bilateral asymmetrical lid retraction – Dalrymple sign; **(C)** severe bilateral lid retraction – Kocher sign; **(D)** right lid lag on downgaze – von Graefe sign.

- **Signs**
    - The upper lid margin normally rests 2 mm below the limbus (Fig. 4.11A, right eye). Lid retraction is suspected when the margin is either level with or above the superior limbus, allowing sclera to be visible ('scleral show'; Fig. 4.11A, left eye).
    - The lower eyelid margin normally rests at the inferior limbus. Retraction is suspected when sclera shows below the limbus. Lid retraction may occur in isolation or in association with proptosis, which exaggerates its severity.
    - The Dalrymple sign is lid retraction or lid spasm in primary gaze leading to a widened palpebral opening (Fig. 4.11B).
    - The Kocher sign describes a staring and frightened appearance of the eyes, which is particularly marked on attentive fixation (Fig. 4.11C).
    - The von Graefe sign signifies retarded descent of the upper lid on downgaze (lid lag – Fig. 4.11D).

Proptosis

- **Symptoms** are similar to those of lid retraction.
- **Signs.** Proptosis is axial, unilateral or bilateral, symmetrical (Fig. 4.12A) or asymmetrical (Fig. 4.12B) and frequently permanent. Severe proptosis may compromise lid closure and along with lid retraction and tear dysfunction can lead to exposure keratopathy, corneal ulceration and infection (Fig. 4.12C).

Restrictive myopathy

Between 30% and 50% of patients with TED develop ophthalmoplegia and this may be permanent. Ocular motility is restricted initially by inflammatory oedema and later by fibrosis.

- **Symptoms.** Double vision and often discomfort in some positions of gaze.
- **Signs,** in approximate order of frequency:
    - Elevation defect (Fig. 4.13A) caused by fibrotic contracture of the inferior rectus, may mimic superior rectus palsy and is the most common motility deficit.

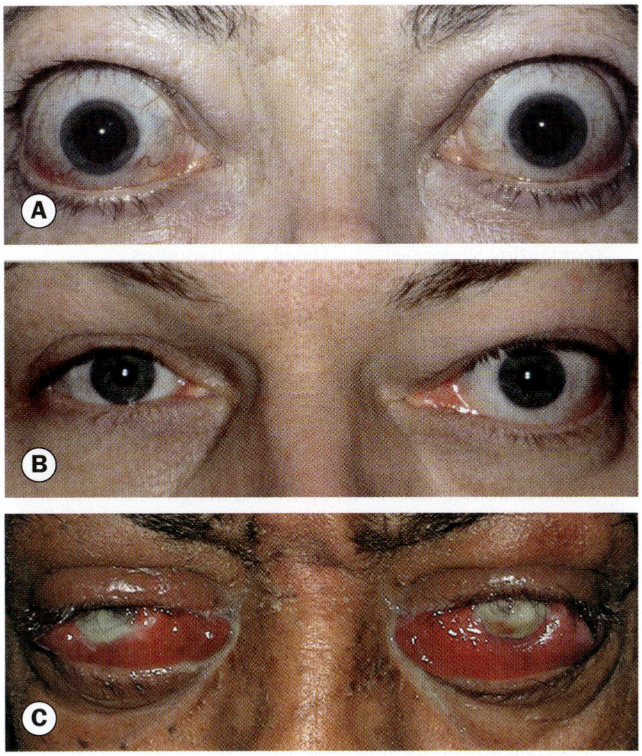

Fig. 4.12 Proptosis in thyroid eye disease. **(A)** Symmetrical; **(B)** asymmetrical; **(C)** bacterial keratitis due to severe exposure. *(Courtesy of ADN Murray – fig. C.)*

- ○ Abduction defect due to fibrosis of the medial rectus, which may simulate sixth nerve palsy (Fig. 4.13B).
- ○ Depression defect (Fig. 4.13C) secondary to fibrosis of the superior rectus.
- ○ Adduction defect caused by fibrosis of the lateral rectus.

Optic neuropathy

Optic neuropathy is a fairly common (up to 6%) serious complication caused by compression of the optic nerve or its blood supply at the orbital apex by the congested and enlarged recti (Fig. 4.14A and B) and swollen orbital tissue. Such compression, which may occur in the absence of significant proptosis, may lead to severe visual impairment if adequate and timely treatment is not instituted.

TIP In thyroid eye disease, compression of the optic nerve secondary to enlarged and congested rectus muscles may occur in the absence of proptosis.

- **Symptoms.** Impairment of central vision occurs in conjunction with other symptoms of TED. In order to detect early involvement, patients should be advised to monitor their own visual function by alternately occluding each eye, reading small print and assessing the intensity of colours, for example on a television screen.
- **Signs.** A high index of suspicion should be maintained for optic neuropathy and it is important not to mistakenly attribute disproportionate visual loss to minor disease.
  - ○ Visual acuity (VA) is usually reduced, but not invariably.

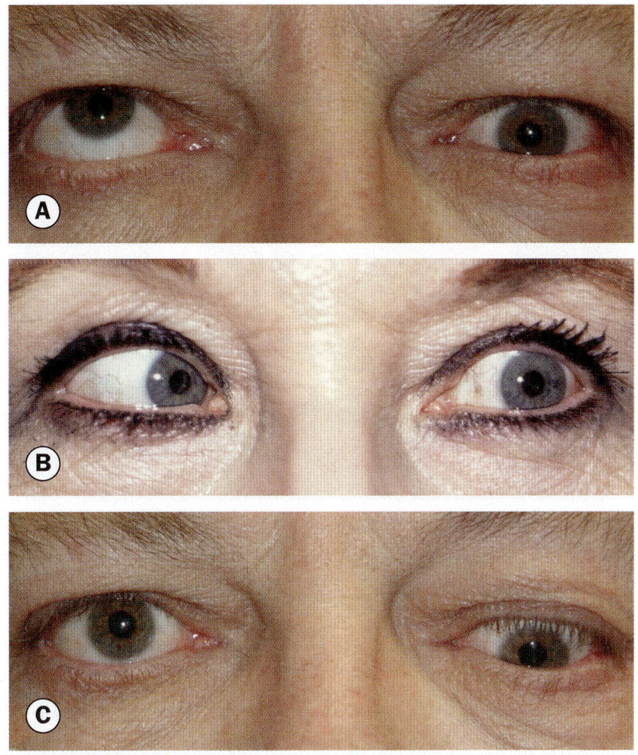

Fig. 4.13 Restrictive thyroid myopathy. **(A)** Defective elevation of the left eye secondary to fibrosis of the inferior rectus muscle; **(B)** reduced abduction of the left eye secondary to fibrosis of the left medial rectus muscle; **(C)** defective depression of the right eye secondary to fibrosis of the right superior rectus muscle.

  - ○ Colour desaturation is a sensitive feature.
  - ○ There may be diminished light brightness appreciation.
  - ○ A relative afferent pupillary defect, if present, should give cause for marked concern.
  - ○ Visual field defects can be central or paracentral and may be combined with nerve fibre bundle defects. These findings, in concert with elevated IOP, may be confused with primary open-angle glaucoma.
  - ○ The optic disc may be normal, swollen or, rarely, atrophic.

Investigation

Investigations other than blood tests for thyroid disease are not necessary if the diagnosis is evident clinically, but the exclusion of other conditions is sometimes indicated. Visual field testing is carried out if there is a suspicion of optic nerve compromise and may be performed as part of a baseline evaluation even if there is no apparent visual impairment. MRI, CT and ultrasonographic imaging of the orbits are indicated in some circumstances, such as helping to confirm an equivocal diagnosis by identification of the typical pattern of extraocular muscle involvement in TED, consisting of muscle belly enlargement with tendon sparing. Imaging is also used in the assessment of optic nerve compression and prior to orbital wall surgery. Visual evoked potentials are sometimes utilized in optic neuropathy.

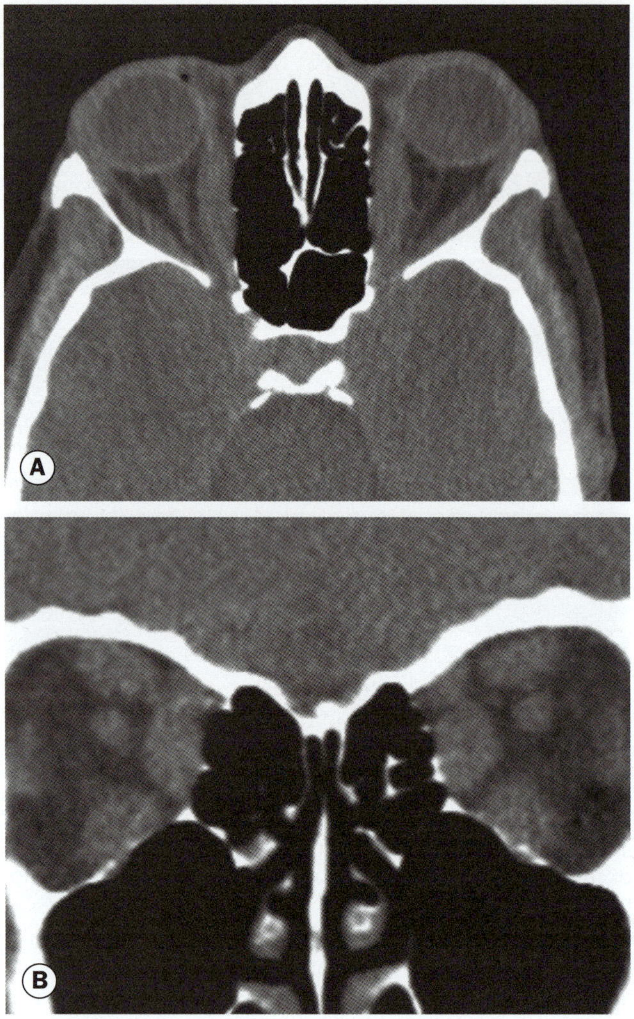

Fig. 4.14 CT scan showing muscle enlargement in thyroid eye disease. **(A)** Axial view showing fusiform enlargement of the medial rectus muscle; **(B)** coronal view showing symmetrical involvement of the medial, superior and inferior rectus muscles as well as the superior oblique muscles.

Treatment

- **The choice of treatment** depends on (a) clinical activity, (b) severity and (c) duration of the orbitopathy.
- **Anti-inflammatory/immunosuppressive treatment** is significantly less effective after 18 months of disease duration. Early referral to a specialized centre is fundamental for most patients with moderate–severe active orbitopathy. Counselling is needed to explain the aims and expectations, benefits and risks of different therapies.
- **Classification.** Treatment can be classified into that of: (a) mild disease (most patients), (b) moderate–severe active disease and (c) treatment of post-inflammatory complications.
- **Cessation of smoking** should be the first measure taken in all cases. Thyroid dysfunction should also be managed adequately.
- **If radioiodine treatment** is administered in patients with pre-existing TED, a short course of oral steroids should be given.

Mild and active disease

- **Lubricants** for superior limbic keratoconjunctivitis, corneal exposure and dryness.
- **Topical anti-inflammatory agents** (steroids, non-steroidal anti-inflammatory drugs (NSAIDs), ciclosporin) are advocated by some authorities.
- **Selenium** (in selenium deficient areas): sodium selenite 200 μg (containing 91.2 μg selenium) daily for 6 months.
- **Head elevation** with three pillows during sleep to reduce periorbital oedema.
- **Eyelid taping during sleep** may alleviate mild exposure keratopathy.

Moderate–severe active disease

- **'Clinical activity score'.** Using EUGOGO guidelines an activity score can be calculated to determine when immunosuppressives should be used. One point is assigned for each feature that is present, using the activity classification (see above). Treatment should be considered for a score of 3 or more out of 7. During subsequent review, a point is allocated for an increase in proptosis of 2 mm or more, a decrease in uniocular excursion in any one direction of 8° or more, or a decrease in Snellen acuity of one line (total 10).
- **Systemic steroids** are the mainstay of treatment for moderate–severe disease. Oral prednisolone 60–80 mg/day may be given initially and tapered depending on response. Intravenous methylprednisolone is often reserved for acute compressive optic neuropathy (see below), but tolerability is better, and outcomes are superior, when compared with oral treatment. Intravenous steroids should not be given to patients with co-existing significant hepatic dysfunction, significant cardiovascular disease, uncontrolled systemic hypertension or diabetes. A lower-intensity regimen of intravenous corticosteroids in the absence of acute sight-threatening disease should be used in most cases using the following regimen: 0.5 g once weekly for 6 weeks followed by 0.25 g once weekly for 6 weeks. A reduction in discomfort, chemosis and periorbital oedema usually occurs within 24 hours, with a maximal response within 2–8 weeks. Ideally, oral steroid therapy should be discontinued after several months, but long-term low-dose maintenance may be necessary.
- **Intravenous corticosteroids** weekly and mycophenolate sodium (0.72 g/day for 24 weeks) have been shown to be of greater benefit than intravenous corticosteroid monotherapy and is the regimen of choice in specialized centres.
- **Orbital steroid** (triamcinolone acetate) injections are occasionally used in selected cases to minimize systemic side effects, but are typically considerably less effective than systemic treatment.
- **Low-dose fractionated radiotherapy** is usually used as second-line therapy. It may be used in addition to steroids or when steroids are contraindicated or ineffective, but because of the delayed effect is not used as the sole treatment of acute optic nerve compression. A positive response is usually evident within 6 weeks, with maximal improvement by 4 months; around 40% will not respond. Adverse effects include cataract,

radiation retinopathy, optic neuropathy and an increased risk of local cancer. The threshold for its use should be higher in younger patients and diabetics, the latter because of a possibly increased risk of retinopathy.

- **Combined therapy** with irradiation, azathioprine and low-dose prednisolone may be more effective than steroids or radiotherapy alone.

TIP Immunosuppression in the active inflammatory phase of thyroid eye disease is important to reduce acute inflammation and to prevent long-term complications.

- **Optic neuropathy**, and less commonly intractable corneal exposure, requires aggressive treatment. Pulsed intravenous methylprednisolone is commonly used, regimens including 0.5–1 g on three successive days with conversion to oral treatment (e.g. 40 mg/day prednisolone) or 0.5–1 g on alternate days, 3–6 times, keeping the maximum dose below 8 g to reduce the risk of liver compromise, followed by oral prednisolone. Appropriate monitoring should be instituted, including liver function tests, as well as gastric protective treatment and osteoporosis prophylaxis if necessary. Orbital wall decompression (see below) and/or orbital apex decompression may be considered if steroids are ineffective (20% receiving intravenous treatment) or contraindicated. Orbital radiotherapy may also be administered, but is generally used only as an adjunct to other modalities.
- **Second-line management** for persistent, corticosteroid-resistant disease or non-response to first-line treatment includes the use of monoclonal antibody treatment with rituximab, tocilizumab or teprotumumab. Teprotumumab is an inhibitor of insulin-like growth factor 1 receptor (IGF-1R) and is effective in reducing proptosis and the Clinical Activity Score in patients with acute TED. In addition, teprotumumab appears to be effective in chronic non-inflammatory TED, resulting in a reduction of proptosis, diplopia and strabismus. This medication has been associated with mild to severe hearing loss in some individuals.
- **Post-inflammatory complications.** Eyelid surgery should be performed only after any necessary orbital and then strabismus procedures have been undertaken, as orbital decompression may impact both ocular motility and eyelid position, and extraocular muscle surgery may affect eyelid position.

TIP Surgical orbital decompression should be considered when there is sight-threatening compressive optic neuropathy in thyroid eye disease.

- **Proptosis.** After active inflammation has remitted, the patient can be left with cosmetically and functionally significant proptosis, the treatment of which is essentially surgical. Surgical decompression increases the volume of the orbit by removing the bony walls and may be combined with removal of orbital fat. Most surgery is undertaken via an external approach, though the medial wall and the medial part of the floor can be reached endoscopically. One-wall (deep lateral) decompression is effective (approximately 4–5 mm reduction in proptosis) and may reduce the risk of postoperative diplopia. Two-wall (balanced medial and lateral – Fig. 4.15) decompression provides a greater effect but with a significant risk of inducing diplopia. Three-wall decompression includes the floor with a reduction in proptosis of 6–10 mm but may lead to hypoglobus and carries a higher risk of infraorbital nerve damage and diplopia. Very severe proptosis may require removal of part of the orbital roof in addition (four-wall decompression).

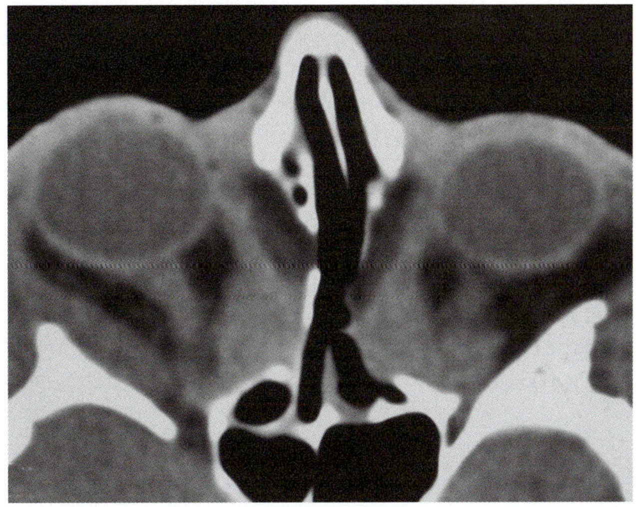

Fig. 4.15 Axial CT following bilateral lateral and medial wall decompression. *(Courtesy of A Pearson.)*

- **Restrictive myopathy.** Surgery is required in most cases experiencing persistent diplopia in the primary or reading positions of gaze, provided the inflammatory stage has subsided and the angle of deviation has been stable for at least 6–12 months. Until these criteria are met, diplopia may be alleviated, if possible, with prisms or sometimes botulinum toxin. The goal of operative treatment is to achieve binocular single vision in the primary and reading positions. Restrictive myopathy often precludes binocularity in all positions of gaze, though with time the field of binocular single vision may enlarge as a result of increasing fusional vergence. Recession of the inferior and/or medial recti is the most commonly indicated surgery (a rectus muscle is never resected, only recessed in TED), generally utilizing adjustable sutures (see Ch. 18). The suture is adjusted later the same day or on the first postoperative day to achieve optimal alignment.
- **Lid retraction.** Mild lid retraction frequently improves spontaneously so does not require treatment. Control of hyperthyroidism may also be beneficial. Botulinum toxin injection to the levator aponeurosis and Müller muscle may be used as a temporary measure in patients awaiting definitive correction. Müllerotomy (disinsertion of Müller muscle) is effective for mild lid retraction, but more severe cases may also require recession/disinsertion of the levator aponeurosis and the suspensory ligament of the superior conjunctival fornix. Recession of the lower lid retractors, with or without a hard palate graft, can be used when retraction of the lower lid is 2 mm or more (see also Ch. 2).

INFECTIONS

Chandler–Hubert classification of orbital complications of sinus infection

The classification helps to determine management and prognosis (Fig. 4.16).

- **Type I:** preseptal cellulitis
- **Type II:** post-septal cellulitis
- **Type III:** subperiosteal abscess
- **Type IV:** orbital abscess
- **Type V:** cavernous sinus thrombosis

Preseptal cellulitis

Introduction

Preseptal cellulitis is an infection of the subcutaneous tissues anterior to the orbital septum. It is considerably more common than orbital cellulitis and though regarded as less serious, can still be associated with severe complications such as abscess formation, meningitis and cavernous sinus thrombosis. Rapid progression to orbital cellulitis may occasionally occur. Organisms typically responsible are *Staphylococcus aureus* and *Streptococcus pyogenes*, with causes including skin trauma such as laceration or insect bites, spread from focal ocular or periocular infection such as an acute hordeolum, dacryocystitis, conjunctivitis or sinusitis and haematogenous spread from remote infection such as the upper respiratory tract or middle ear.

Diagnosis

The condition manifests with a swollen, often firm, tender red eyelid that may be very severe (Fig. 4.17A and B). However, in contrast to orbital cellulitis, proptosis and chemosis are absent and VA, pupillary reactions and ocular motility are unimpaired. The patient is often pyrexial. Imaging with MRI or CT is not indicated unless orbital cellulitis or a lid abscess is suspected, or if there is a failure to respond to therapy.

Treatment

Treatment is with oral antibiotics such as co-amoxiclav 250–500 mg/125 mg 2–3 times daily or 875/125 mg twice daily, depending

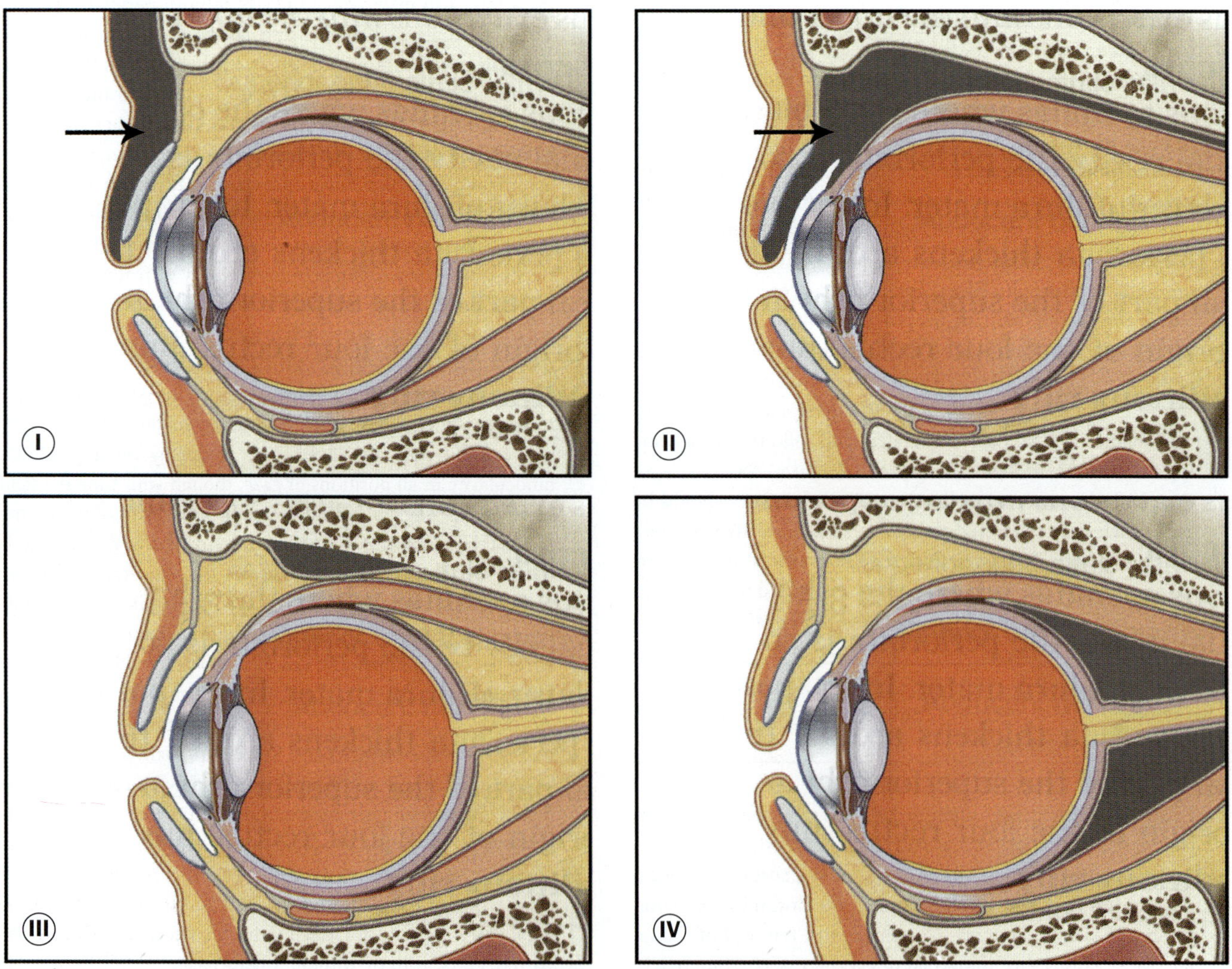

Fig. 4.16 Chandler–Hubert classification of orbital cellulitis secondary to sinus infection (see text; Type V is not illustrated).

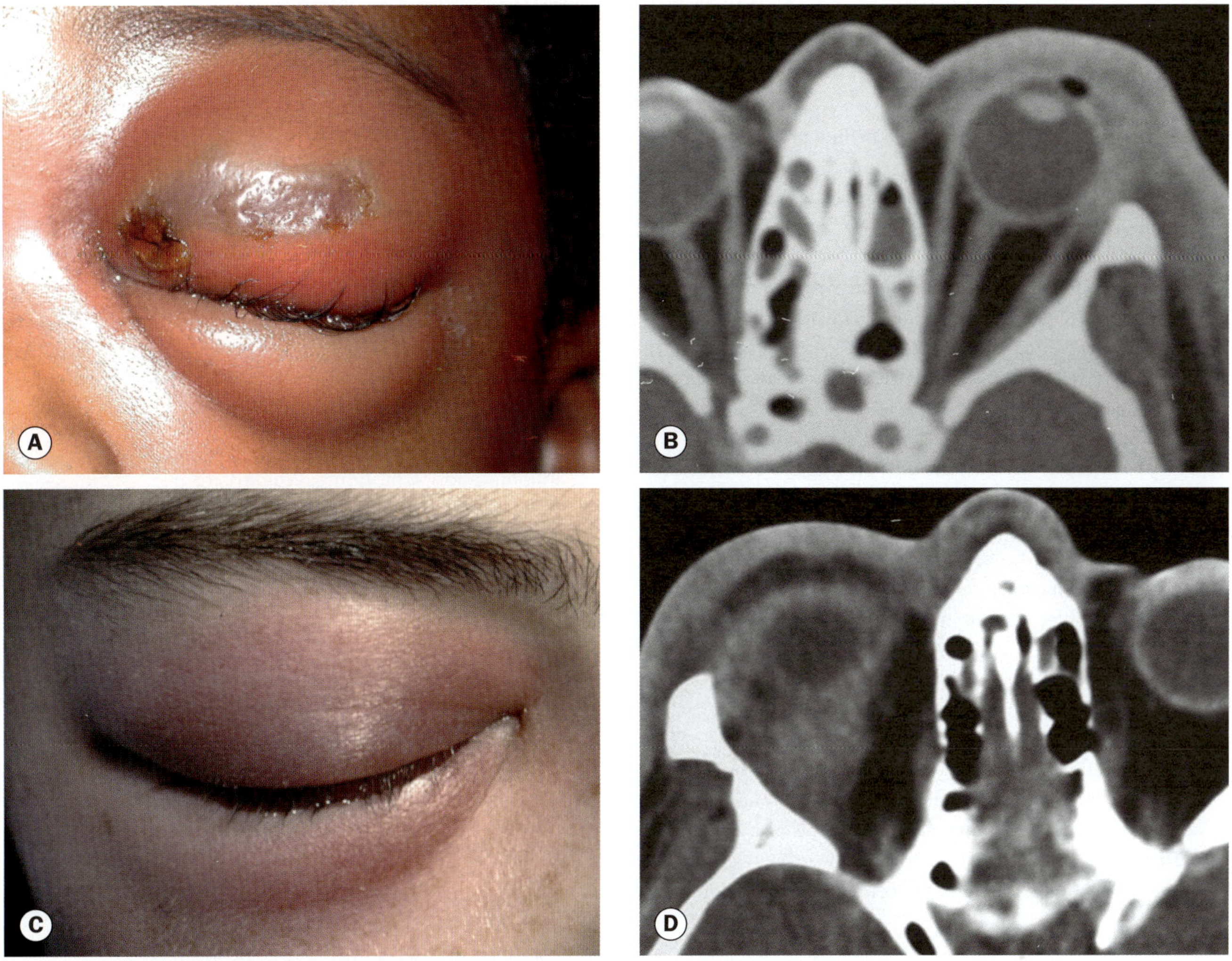

Fig. 4.17 Orbital cellulitis. **(A)** Left preseptal cellulitis resulting from an infected eyelid abrasion; **(B)** axial CT showing opacification anterior to the orbital septum; **(C)** right orbital cellulitis with ophthalmoplegia; **(D)** axial CT showing both preseptal and orbital opacification.

on severity. Severe infection may require intravenous antibiotics. The patient's tetanus status should be ascertained in cases following trauma.

TIP Visual acuity, pupillary responses, and ocular motility are unimpaired, and proptosis is absent in preseptal cellulitis.

Bacterial orbital cellulitis

Introduction

Bacterial orbital cellulitis is a serious infection of the soft tissues behind the orbital septum, which can be sight- and life-threatening. It can occur at any age but is more common in children. *Streptococcus pneumoniae*, *Staphylococcus aureus*, *Streptococcus pyogenes* and *Haemophilus influenzae* are common causative organisms, with infection originating typically from the paranasal (especially ethmoid) sinuses. Infection can also spread from preseptal cellulitis, dacryocystitis, midfacial skin or dental infection and can follow trauma, including any form of ocular surgery. Blood-borne spread from infection elsewhere in the body may occur.

Clinical features

- **Symptoms** consist of the rapid onset of pain exacerbated by eye movement, swelling of the eye, malaise and frequently visual impairment and double vision. There is commonly a recent history of nasal, sinus or respiratory symptoms.
- **Signs**
  - Pyrexia, often marked.
  - VA may be reduced and colour vision impaired, raising the possibility of optic nerve compression. The presence of a relative afferent pupillary defect in a previously normal eye makes this almost certain.
  - Tender, firm, erythematous and warm eyelids, with periocular and conjunctival (chemosis) oedema, conjunctival injection and sometimes subconjunctival haemorrhage. The signs are usually unilateral, though oedema may spread to the contralateral eyelids (Fig. 4.17C).

- Proptosis is common in established infection, but is often obscured by lid swelling. It may be non-axial (dystopia), particularly if an abscess is present.
- Painful ophthalmoplegia.
- Choroidal folds and optic disc swelling may be present on fundus examination.

- **Differential diagnosis.** Major diagnostic alternatives are listed in Table 4.1.
- **Complications**
  - Ocular complications include optic neuropathy, exposure keratopathy, raised IOP, endophthalmitis and occlusion of the central retinal artery or vein.
  - Subperiosteal abscess, most frequently located along the medial orbital wall.
  - Intracranial complications, which are uncommon (3–4%) but extremely serious, include meningitis, brain abscess and cavernous sinus thrombosis.

Investigation

Investigations may include:

- Ascertainment of tetanus immunization status in cases of trauma.
- White cell count.
- Blood cultures.
- Culture of nasal discharge.
- High-resolution CT of the orbit, sinuses and brain (Fig. 4.17B and D) is vital to confirm the diagnosis and exclude a subperiosteal or intracranial abscess. MRI is also sometimes performed.
- Lumbar puncture if meningeal or cerebral signs develop.

Treatment

- **Hospital admission** is mandatory, with urgent otolaryngological assessment and frequent ophthalmic review. Paediatric specialist advice should be sought in the management of a child and a low threshold should be adopted for infectious disease specialist consultation.
- **Delineation** of the extent of erythema on the skin using a surgical marker may help in judging progress.
- **Antibiotics** are given intravenously, with the specific drug depending on local sensitivities. Ceftazidime is a typical choice, supplemented by oral metronidazole to cover anaerobes. Intravenous antibiotics should be continued until the patient has been apyrexial for 4 days, followed by 1–3 weeks of oral treatment.
- **Monitoring of optic nerve function** is performed at least every 4 hours initially by testing VA, colour vision, light brightness appreciation and pupillary reactions. Deterioration should prompt the consideration of surgical intervention.
- **Surgery.** Drainage of an orbital abscess should be considered at an early stage. Drainage of infected sinuses should be considered if there is a lack of response to antibiotics, or if there is very severe sinus disease. Biopsy of inflammatory tissue may be performed for an atypical clinical picture. Severe optic nerve compression may warrant an emergency canthotomy/cantholysis (see Ch. 22).

Table 4.1 Differential Diagnosis of an Acutely Inflamed Orbit

Infection
• Bacterial orbital cellulitis • Fungal orbital infection • Dacryocystitis • Infective dacryoadenitis
Vascular lesions
• Acute orbital haemorrhage • Cavernous sinus thrombosis • Carotid–cavernous fistula
Neoplasia
• Rapidly progressive retinoblastoma • Lacrimal gland tumour • Other neoplasm, e.g. metastatic lesion with inflammation, lymphoma, Waldenström macroglobulinaemia • Rhabdomyosarcoma, leukaemia, lymphangioma or neuroblastoma in children
Endocrine
• Thyroid eye disease of rapid onset
Non-neoplastic inflammation
• Idiopathic orbital inflammatory disease • Tolosa–Hunt syndrome • Orbital myositis • Acute allergic conjunctivitis with lid swelling • Herpes zoster ophthalmicus • Herpes simplex skin rash • Sarcoidosis • Vasculitides: granulomatosis with polyangiitis, polyarteritis nodosa • Scleritis, including posterior scleritis • Ruptured dermoid cyst

TIP Because orbital cellulitis often occurs as a consequence of a sinus infection, urgent radiological investigation of the sinuses is mandatory.

Rhino-orbital mucormycosis

Introduction

Mucormycosis is a rare aggressive and often fatal infection caused by fungi of the family *Mucoraceae*. It typically affects patients with diabetic ketoacidosis or immunosuppression and is extremely rare in the immunocompetent. Infection is acquired by the inhalation of spores, which give rise to an upper respiratory infection. Spread then occurs to the contiguous sinuses and subsequently to the orbit and brain. Invasion of blood vessels by the hyphae results in occlusive vasculitis with infarction of orbital tissues.

Diagnosis

- **Symptoms.** Gradual onset facial and periorbital swelling, diplopia and visual loss.

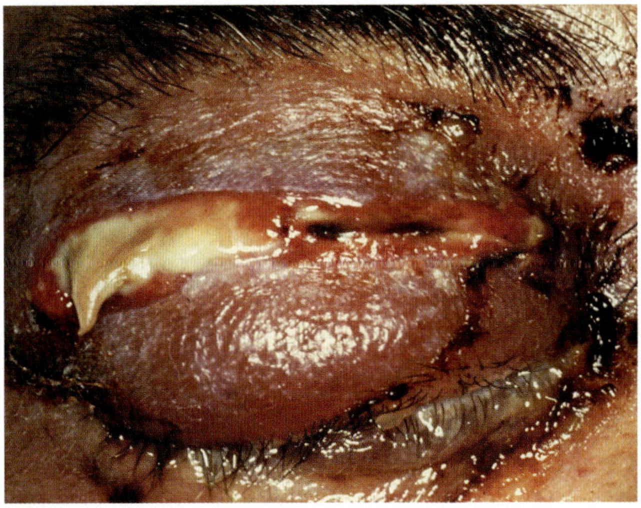

Fig. 4.18 Necrosis of the eyelid in rhino-orbital mucormycosis.

- **Signs** are similar to bacterial orbital cellulitis, but tend to be less acute and with slower progression. Infarction superimposed on septic necrosis is responsible for the classic black eschar that may develop on the palate, turbinates, nasal septum, skin and eyelids (Fig. 4.18).
- **Complications** include retinal vascular occlusion, multiple cranial nerve palsies and cerebrovascular occlusion.
- **Differential diagnosis** is listed in Table 4.1.
- **Investigation** is much the same as for bacterial orbital cellulitis.

Treatment

- Correction of the underlying metabolic defect should be instituted if possible.
- Intravenous antifungal treatment.
- Daily packing and irrigation of the involved areas with antifungal agent.
- Wide excision of devitalized and necrotic tissues. Exenteration may be required in unresponsive cases in order to reduce the risk of death.
- Adjunctive hyperbaric oxygen may be helpful.

NON-INFECTIVE INFLAMMATORY DISEASE

Idiopathic orbital inflammatory disease

Idiopathic orbital inflammatory disease (IOID), also called non-specific orbital inflammation or orbital pseudotumour, is an uncommon disorder characterized by non-neoplastic, non-infective, space-occupying orbital infiltration with inflammatory features. The process may preferentially involve any or all of the orbital soft tissues. Histopathological analysis reveals pleomorphic inflammatory cellular infiltration followed by reactive fibrosis. Unilateral disease is typical in adults, although in children bilateral involvement may occur. Intracranial extension is rare. Simultaneous orbital and sinus involvement is also rare and may be a distinct entity.

Diagnosis

- **Symptoms** typically consist of acute or subacute ocular and periocular redness, swelling and pain (Fig. 4.19A and B). Systemic symptoms are common in children.
- **Signs**
  - Pyrexia is present in up to 50% of children, but is rare in adults.
  - Congestive proptosis.
  - Mild to severe ophthalmoplegia may occur.
  - Features of optic nerve dysfunction, particularly if the inflammation involves the posterior orbit. There may be optic disc swelling.
  - Choroidal folds, if present, may be associated with reduced vision but optic neuropathy must always be suspected.
- **Course.** The natural history of the inflammatory process is very variable.
  - Spontaneous remission after a few weeks without sequelae.
  - Intermittent episodes of activity, usually with eventual remission.
  - Severe prolonged inflammation eventually leading to progressive fibrosis of orbital tissues, resulting in a 'frozen orbit' characterized by ophthalmoplegia, which may be associated with ptosis and visual impairment caused by optic nerve involvement.
- **Investigation**
  - CT shows ill-defined orbital opacification and loss of definition of contents (Fig. 4.19C and D).
  - Biopsy is generally required in persistent cases to confirm the diagnosis and particularly to rule out neoplasia and systemic inflammatory conditions.
  - A wide range of other investigations may be considered to aid in the exclusion of alternative diagnoses, particularly infection, lymphoma and non-neoplastic infiltrative disorders such as sarcoidosis and granulomatosis with polyangiitis.

Treatment

- **Observation**, for relatively mild disease, in anticipation of spontaneous remission.
- **NSAIDs** alone (e.g. ibuprofen) are often effective and may be tried in mild disease prior to steroid therapy. Co-prescription of a proton pump inhibitor should be considered.
- **Systemic steroids** should be administered only after the diagnosis has been confirmed, as they may mask other pathology such as infection and granulomatosis with polyangiitis. Oral prednisolone is initially given at a dose of 1.0–1.5 mg/kg daily, subsequently being tapered and discontinued over a number of weeks depending on clinical response. Further treatment may be needed in the event of recurrence.
- **Orbital depot steroid** injection may be useful in some cases.
- **Radiotherapy** may be considered if there has been no improvement after 2 weeks of adequate steroid therapy. Even low-dose treatment (e.g. 2 Gy fractionation daily up to 20 Gy total dose) may produce remission, though much higher total doses may be necessary (up to 36 Gy total dose).

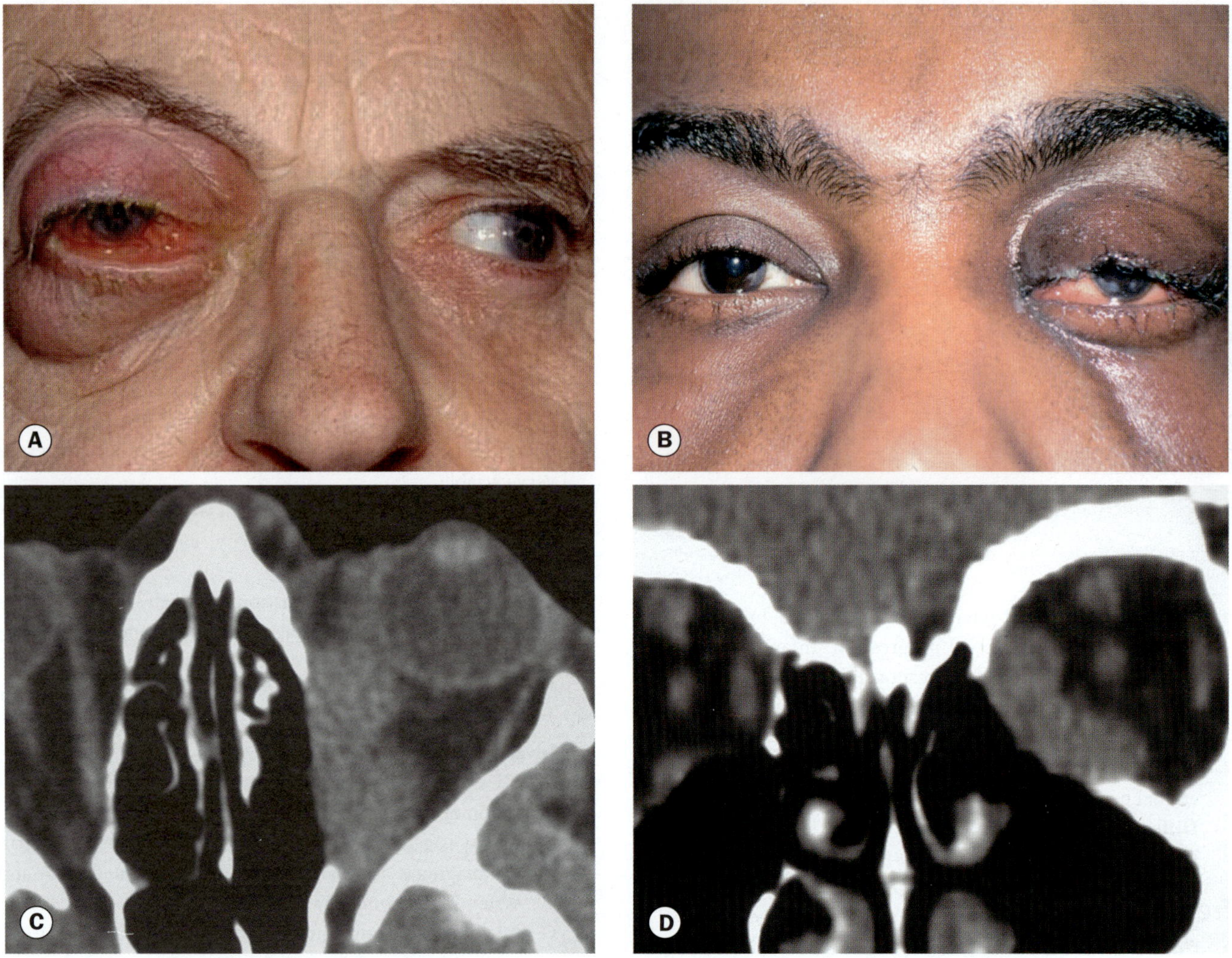

Fig. 4.19 Idiopathic orbital inflammation. **(A)** Idiopathic scirrhous inflammation showing an adduction weakness of the right eye, proptosis and ptosis; **(B)** left idiopathic inflammatory disease, showing lid swelling and ptosis; **(C)** CT axial view of left orbit showing ill-defined orbital opacification; **(D)** coronal view. *(Courtesy of G Rose – fig. A; R Bates – fig. B; A Pearson – figs C and D.)*

- **Other options**, usually as supplementary treatments or in resistant cases, include cytotoxic drugs (e.g. methotrexate, azathioprine), calcineurin inhibitors (e.g. ciclosporin, tacrolimus) and biological blockers.
- **Surgical resection** of an inflammatory focus may be contemplated in highly resistant cases.

Orbital myositis

Introduction

Orbital myositis is an idiopathic, non-specific inflammation of one or more extraocular muscles and is considered a subtype of IOID. Histology shows a chronic inflammatory cellular infiltrate associated with the muscle fibres (Fig. 4.20A).

Diagnosis

- **Symptoms.** Acute pain, exacerbated by eye movement and diplopia. Onset is usually in early adulthood.
- **Signs** are generally less obvious than IOID.
  - Lid oedema, ptosis and chemosis.
  - Pain and diplopia associated with eye movements (Fig. 4.20B).
  - Vascular injection over the involved muscle (Fig. 4.20C).
  - In chronic cases fibrosis of the affected muscle may occur with permanent restrictive myopathy.
- **Course**
  - Acute non-recurrent involvement that resolves spontaneously within 6 weeks.
  - Chronic disease characterized by either a single episode persisting for longer than 2 months (often for years) (Fig. 4.20D) or recurrent attacks.
- **Investigation** consists primarily of MRI or CT, which show enlargement of the affected muscles (Fig. 4.20E and F), with or without involvement of the tendons of insertion. This is in contrast to TED-related muscle enlargement, in which the tendon is always spared. Additional investigations may be required in some cases.

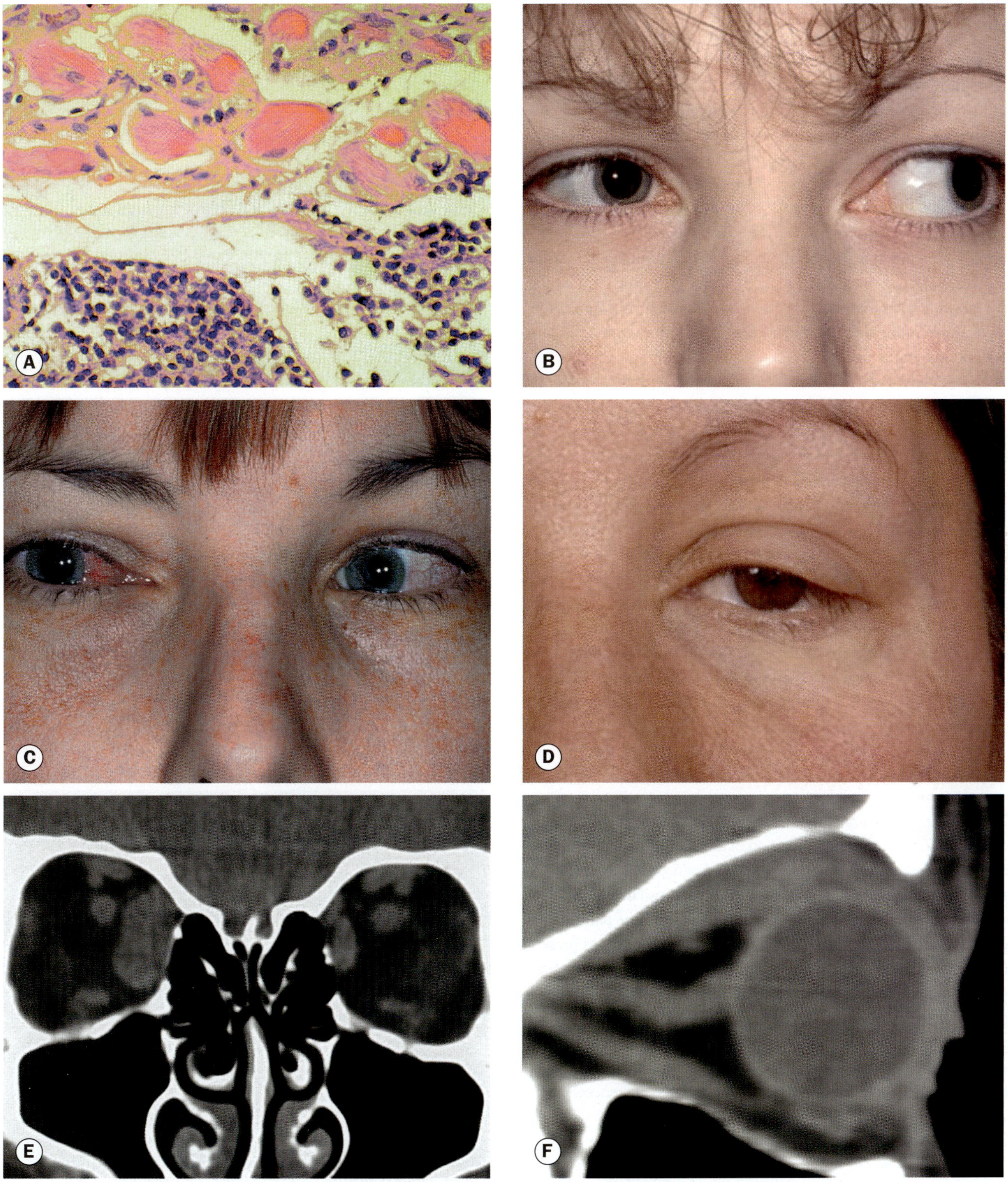

Fig. 4.20 Orbital myositis. **(A)** Histology showing a chronic inflammatory cellular infiltrate in relation to muscle fibres; **(B)** idiopathic myositis involving the right lateral rectus muscle with diplopia on left eye movement; **(C)** vascular injection over the insertion of the right medial rectus; **(D)** chronic myositis of superior rectus-levator complex; **(E)** coronal CT of **(C)**, showing enlargement of the right medial rectus **(F)** sagittal CT of **(D)** showing enlargement of superior rectus muscle. *(Courtesy of J Harry and G Misson, from* Clinical Ophthalmic Pathology, *Butterworth-Heinemann 2001 – fig. A; G Rose – figs B, D, F; J Nerad, K Carter and M Alford, from 'Oculoplastic and Reconstructive Surgery', in* Rapid Diagnosis in Ophthalmology, *Mosby 2008 – figs C and E.)*

Treatment

Treatment is aimed at relieving discomfort and dysfunction, shortening the course and preventing recurrences. NSAIDs may be adequate in mild disease, but systemic steroids are generally required and usually produce dramatic improvement, although recurrence is seen in 50%. Radiotherapy is also effective, particularly in limiting recurrence.

Acute dacryoadenitis

Acute dacryoadenitis may be idiopathic or due to viral (e.g. mumps, Epstein–Barr, cytomegalovirus) or – rarely – bacterial infection; the lacrimal gland is often involved in IOID. Chronic conditions such as sarcoidosis, Sjögren syndrome, thyroid disease and some chronic infections usually give a less acute onset and involvement can be bilateral. Presentation in acute disease is with the rapid onset of discomfort in the region of the gland. Lacrimal secretion may be reduced or increased and discharge may be reported. Swelling of the lateral aspect of the eyelid overlying the palpebral lobe leads to a characteristic S-shaped ptosis and enlargement of the orbital lobe may give a slight downward and inward dystopia (Fig. 4.21A) and occasionally proptosis and other signs of orbital disease. There is tenderness over the lacrimal gland and injection of the conjunctiva overlying the palpebral lobe may be seen on upper lid eversion (Fig. 4.21B). Chemosis may be present. There may be local (e.g. preauricular) lymph node enlargement. CT shows enlargement of the gland and involvement of adjacent tissues (Fig. 4.21C) without bony erosion; the latter suggests a tumour. Biopsy is sometimes indicated, particularly to exclude a tumour. Treatment varies according to the cause, but in many cases is not required.

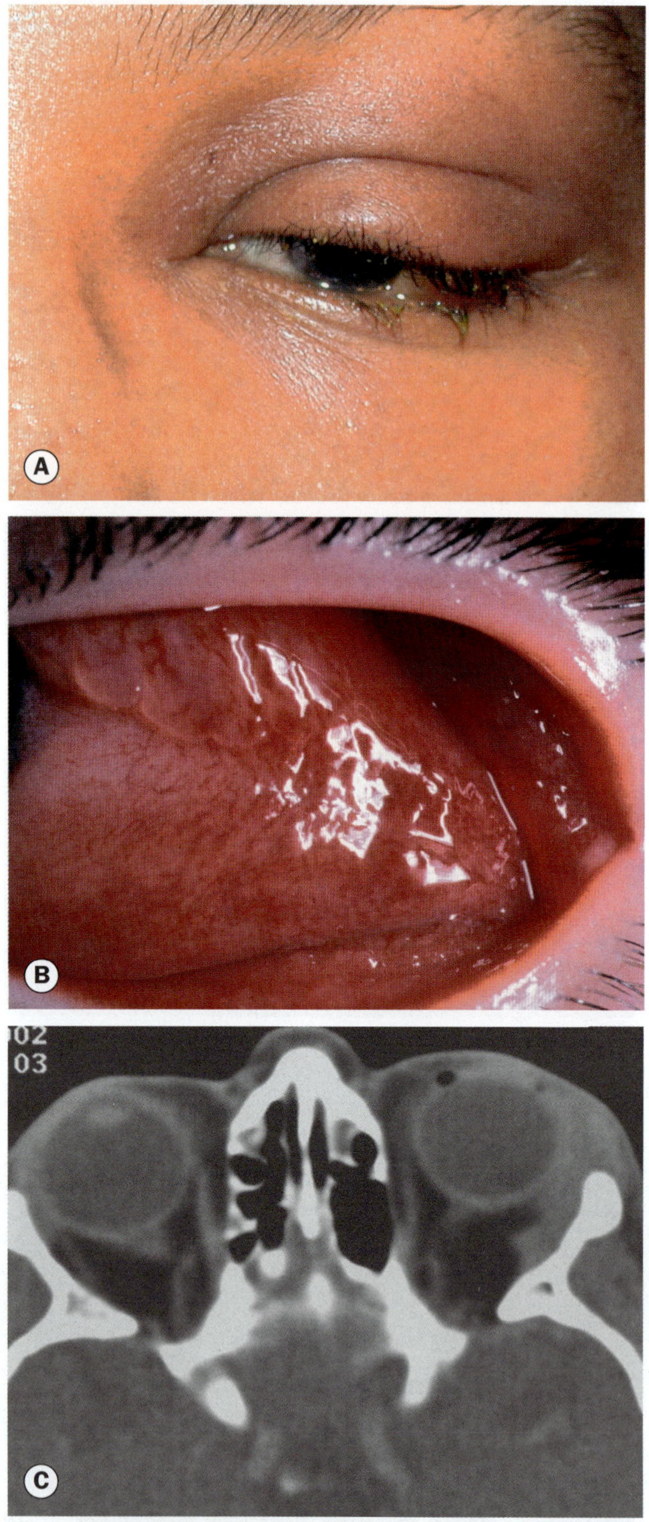

Fig. 4.21 Left acute dacryoadenitis. **(A)** Swelling on the lateral aspect of the eyelid and an S-shaped ptosis; **(B)** injection of the palpebral portion of the lacrimal gland and adjacent conjunctiva; **(C)** axial CT showing enlargement of the gland and opacification of adjacent tissues. *(Courtesy of R Bates – fig. B; A Pearson – fig. C.)*

Tolosa–Hunt syndrome

Tolosa–Hunt syndrome is a rare idiopathic condition caused by nonspecific granulomatous inflammation of the cavernous sinus, superior orbital fissure and/or orbital apex. It is a diagnosis of exclusion and should be investigated fully. Presentation is with ipsilateral periorbital or hemicranial pain and diplopia due to ocular motor paresis, with pupillary and eyelid involvement in many cases. Proptosis, if present, is usually mild. Sensory loss along the distribution of the first and second divisions of the trigeminal nerve is common. The patient may be pyrexial. Diagnosis is with imaging, together with other investigations to rule out identifiable causes, including neoplasia. Treatment is with systemic steroids and other immunosuppressants as necessary; the clinical course is characterized by remissions and recurrences.

Granulomatosis with polyangiitis

Granulomatosis with polyangiitis, previously called Wegener granulomatosis (see Ch. 9), is an idiopathic multisystem granulomatous disorder that may involve the orbit, often bilaterally, usually by contiguous spread from the paranasal sinuses or nasopharynx. Primary orbital involvement is less common. This condition should be considered in any patient with bilateral orbital inflammation, particularly if associated with sinus pathology. Antineutrophilic cytoplasmic antibody (cANCA variant) is a useful serological test. Other ocular features include scleritis, peripheral ulcerative keratitis, intraocular inflammation and retinal vascular occlusions. Treatment is with cyclophosphamide and steroids, which are usually effective. In resistant cases ciclosporin, azathioprine, antithymocyte globulin or plasmapheresis may be useful. Surgical decompression may be required for severe orbital involvement.

NON-NEOPLASTIC VASCULAR ABNORMALITIES

Cavernous sinus thrombosis

This refers to clotting within the cavernous sinus, usually resulting from infection such as sinusitis, orbital or preseptal cellulitis or otitis. There is a high mortality rate: 20% treated and up to 100% untreated die. Features are of rapid onset and may include severe headache, malaise, nausea and vomiting, unilateral or often bilateral proptosis, chemosis, congestion of the facial, conjunctival and retinal veins, reduced vision and signs resulting from compromised function of the third to sixth cranial nerves, which run through the cavernous sinus. Diagnosis is with imaging, especially MRI and MRI venography. Systemic investigation for infection is also performed, including lumbar puncture. Treatment consists of intravenous antibiotics and sometimes surgical drainage.

TIP Cavernous sinus thrombosis has a high mortality rate if the diagnosis is delayed and if intensive treatment is not instigated urgently.

Carotid–cavernous fistula

Introduction

A carotid–cavernous fistula involves the development of an arteriovenous fistula between the carotid artery and the venous cavernous sinus (see Fig. 19.64) with a rise in venous pressure in the sinus and structures draining to it. Ocular manifestations occur because of venous and arterial stasis around the eye and orbit, increased episcleral venous pressure and a decrease in arterial blood flow to the cranial nerves within the cavernous sinus. Carotid–cavernous fistulae are classified into 'direct' and 'indirect' forms.

- **Direct** fistulae are high-flow shunts in which carotid artery blood passes directly into the cavernous sinus through a defect in the wall of the intracavernous portion of the internal carotid artery as a result of trauma (75%), including surgery, spontaneous rupture of an intracavernous carotid aneurysm or an atherosclerotic artery, the latter frequently in a middle-aged hypertensive woman; spontaneous fistulae usually have lower flow.
- In an **indirect** fistula ('dural shunt'), the intracavernous portion of the internal carotid artery remains intact. Arterial blood flows through the meningeal branches of the external or internal carotid arteries indirectly into the cavernous sinus and the clinical features are subtler than in a direct fistula such that the condition may be overlooked. Spontaneous rupture of an atherosclerotic artery or of a congenital malformation is the usual cause and may be precipitated by minor trauma or straining. Connective tissue and collagen vascular disorders can be associated.

Diagnosis

- **Symptoms – direct.** Presentation may be days or weeks after head injury with a classic triad of pulsatile proptosis, conjunctival chemosis and a whooshing noise in the head.
- **Symptoms – indirect.** Gradual onset of redness of one or both eyes is a typical presentation, caused by conjunctival vascular engorgement.
- **Signs – direct**
  - Immediate visual loss may be due to ocular or optic nerve damage at the time of head trauma.
  - Delayed visual loss may occur as a result of exposure keratopathy, secondary glaucoma, central retinal vein occlusion, anterior segment ischaemia or ischaemic optic neuropathy.
  - Signs are usually ipsilateral to the fistula but may be bilateral, or even contralateral, because of midline connections between the two cavernous sinuses.
  - Marked epibulbar vascular dilatation (Fig. 4.22A).
  - Chemosis, commonly haemorrhagic, particularly in the early stages (Fig. 4.22B).
  - Pulsatile proptosis associated with a bruit and a thrill, both of which can be abolished by ipsilateral carotid compression in the neck.
  - Increased IOP due to elevated episcleral venous pressure and orbital congestion and sometimes angle-closure glaucoma.
  - Anterior segment ischaemia, characterized by corneal epithelial oedema, aqueous cells and flare and in severe cases iris atrophy, cataract and rubeosis iridis.
  - Ptosis due to third nerve involvement.
  - Ophthalmoplegia (60–70%) due to the ocular motor nerve damage from initial trauma, an intracavernous aneurysm or the fistula itself. The sixth cranial nerve is most frequently affected because of its free-floating location within the cavernous sinus. The third and fourth nerves, situated in the lateral wall of the sinus, are less frequently involved. Engorgement and swelling of extraocular muscles may also contribute to defective ocular motility.
  - Fundus examination may show optic disc swelling, venous dilatation and intraretinal haemorrhages from venous stasis and impaired retinal blood flow. Vitreous haemorrhage is rare.
- **Signs – indirect**
  - Milder epibulbar vascular dilatation than with a direct fistula (Fig. 4.22C).
  - Exaggerated ocular pulsation, which is readily detected on slit lamp applanation tonometry.
  - The presence of 'corkscrew' epibulbar vessels (Fig. 4.22D) is a common subtle later sign. These are not pathognomonic and can be found in normal eyes.
  - Raised IOP, often bilateral but higher on the side of the fistula.
  - Proptosis and bruit are mild if present.

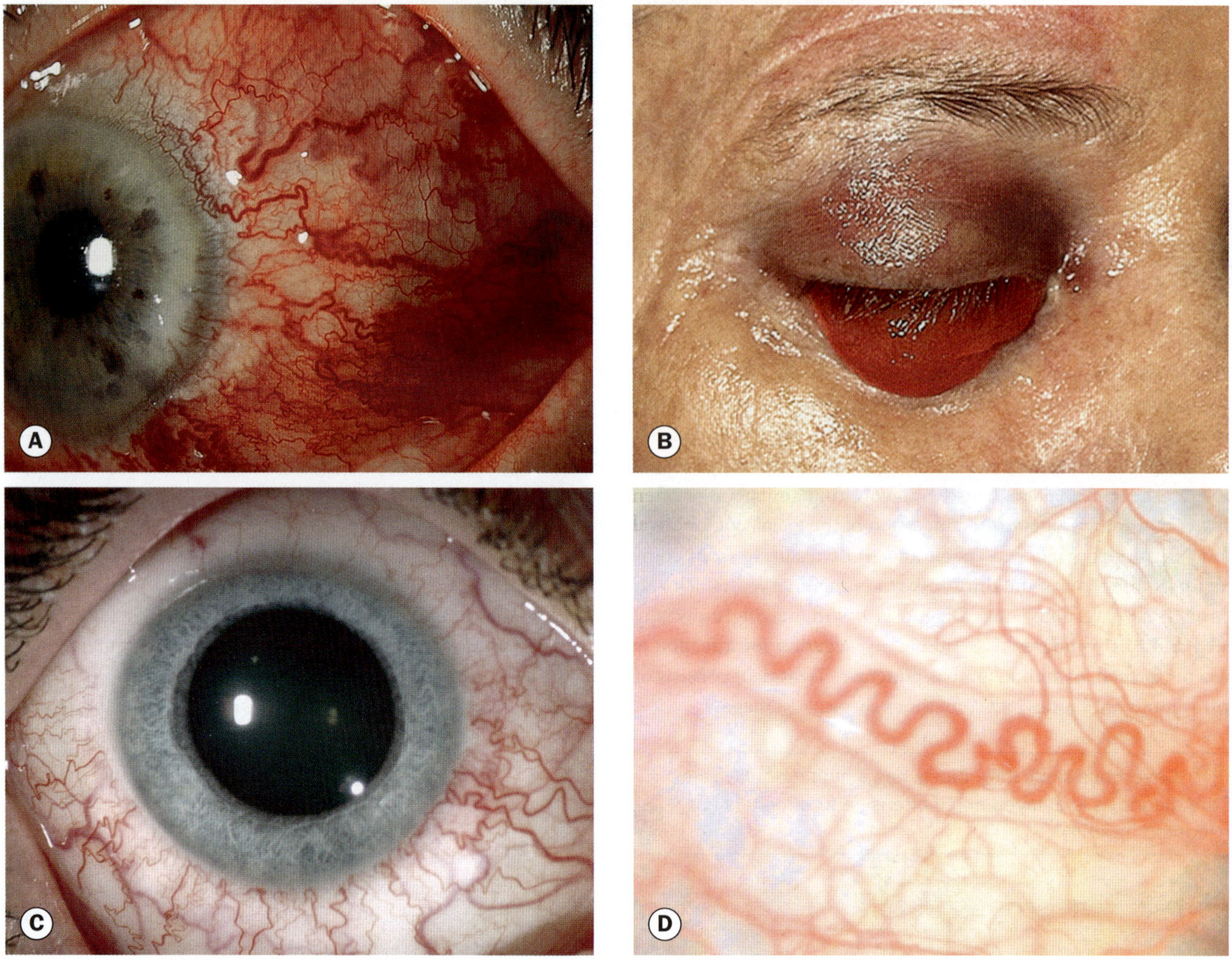

Fig. 4.22 Carotid–cavernous fistula. **(A)** Marked epibulbar vascular dilatation in an established direct fistula; **(B)** haemorrhagic chemosis in an acute direct fistula; **(C)** mild epibulbar vascular dilatation in an indirect fistula; **(D)** corkscrew conjunctival vessel. *(Courtesy of S Chen – fig. A; C Barry – figs C and D.)*

  - Ophthalmoplegia caused by sixth nerve palsy or swelling of extraocular muscles in marked cases.
  - Fundus may be normal or manifest moderate venous dilatation, with later tortuosity as with corkscrew conjunctival vessels, this is not pathognomonic (see Ch. 13).
- **Investigation.** CT and MRI may demonstrate prominence of the superior ophthalmic vein (Fig. 4.23A) and diffuse enlargement of extraocular muscles (Fig. 4.23B), though these may be visible only with a direct fistula. Orbital Doppler imaging may show abnormal flow patterns, particularly in the superior orbital vein. Definitive diagnosis may involve selective catheter digital subtraction angiography, especially in mild dural fistulae, though CT and MRI angiography can be useful.

Treatment

Ocular complications may require specific measures in addition to treatment of the fistula itself. Neurological subspecialist opinion should be sought at an early stage, even if features are mild, as some fistula patterns (e.g. cortical venous drainage) carry a high risk of stroke.

- **Direct.** Most carotid–cavernous fistulae are not life-threatening; the organ at major risk is the eye. Surgery is indicated if spontaneous closure does not occur. A post-traumatic fistula is much less likely to close on its own than a spontaneous fistula because of higher blood flow. Treatment is likely to consist of a transarterial approach to repair the artery (e.g. coil – Fig. 4.23C and D, other) or occlude the involved sinus (e.g. coil, balloon, other). Craniotomy for arterial repair is occasionally needed.
- **Indirect.** If required, treatment usually involves transvenous occlusion of the involved sinus. Spontaneous closure or occluding thrombosis sometimes (up to 50%) occurs. Intermittent carotid compression under specialist supervision has been reported to increase the likelihood that this will take place.

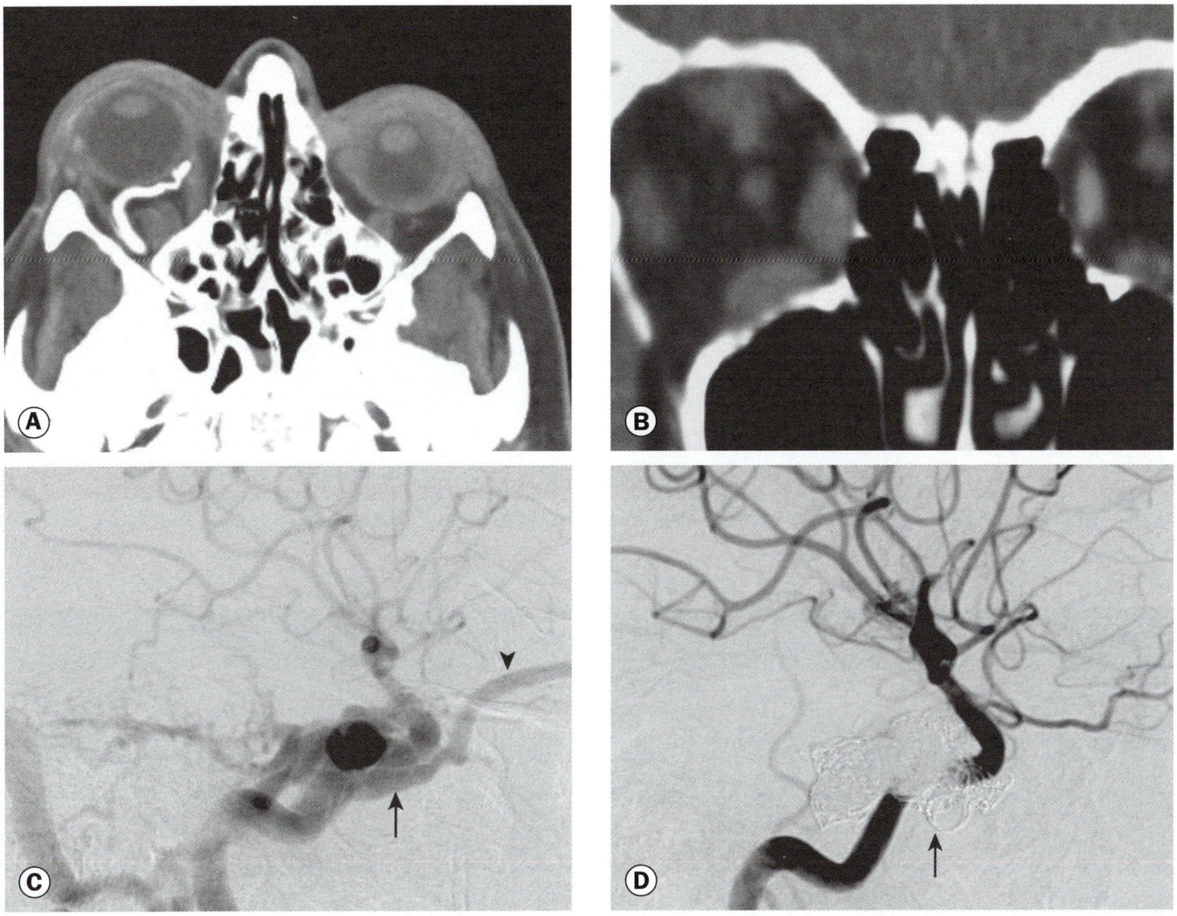

Fig. 4.23 CT in direct carotid–cavernous fistula. **(A)** Axial CT image showing enlargement of the right superior ophthalmic vein; **(B)** coronal view showing enlargement of extraocular muscles on the right; **(C)** early arterial phase catheter angiogram showing filling of the cavernous sinus (arrow) and superior ophthalmic vein (arrowhead); **(D)** following deposition of coils in the cavernous sinus – the fistula is closed and there is no retrograde flow in the superior ophthalmic vein. *(Courtesy of J Trobe, from 'Neuro-ophthalmology', in* Rapid Diagnosis in Ophthalmology, *Mosby 2008.)*

CYSTIC LESIONS

Dacryops

A dacryops is a frequently bilateral cyst of the lacrimal gland that is thought to develop from a dilated obstructed duct. A round cystic lesion protrudes into the superior fornix from the palpebral lobe of the gland (Fig. 4.24) and may present with inflammation. The possibility of a malignant tumour should always be considered. Treatment involves excision or marsupialization, with histopathological analysis.

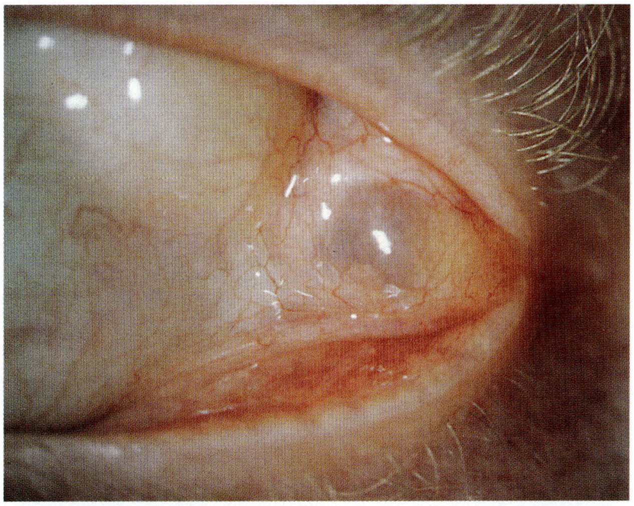

Fig. 4.24 Dacryops.

Dermoid cyst

Introduction

An orbital dermoid cyst is a choristoma (a mass of histologically normal tissue in an abnormal location) derived from displacement of ectoderm to a subcutaneous location along embryonic lines of closure. Dermoids are lined by keratinized stratified squamous epithelium (like skin), have a fibrous wall and contain dermal appendages such as sweat glands, sebaceous glands and hair follicles; epidermoid cysts do not contain adnexal structures. Dermoids may be 'superficial' or 'deep', located anterior or posterior to

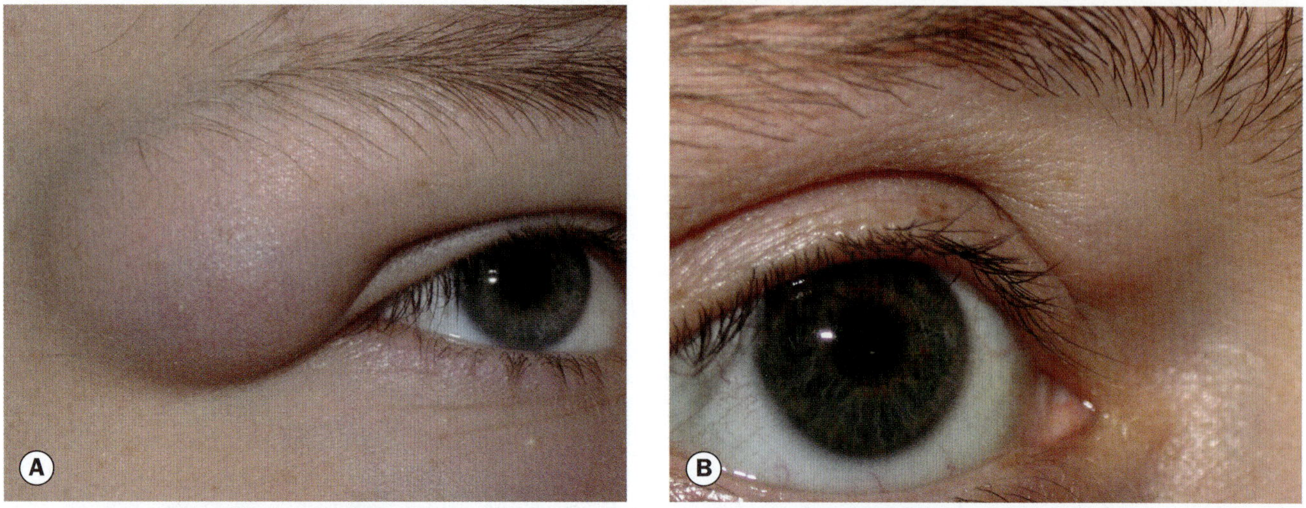

Fig. 4.25 Orbital dermoid cyst. **(A)** Superficial cyst right eye in a child; **(B)** superonasal deep cyst in a young adult.

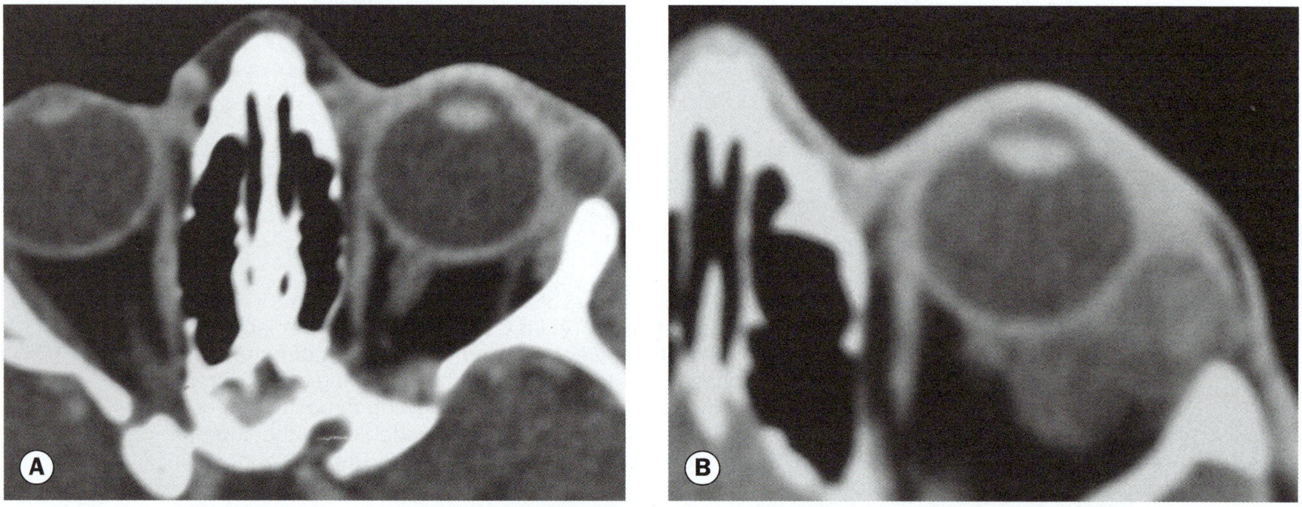

Fig. 4.26 Orbital dermoid cysts – imaging. **(A)** Axial CT image showing a well-circumscribed heterogeneous superficial lesion; **(B)** deep dermoid – CT showing a well-circumscribed cystic lesion. *(Courtesy of Ken K Nischal – fig. A.)*

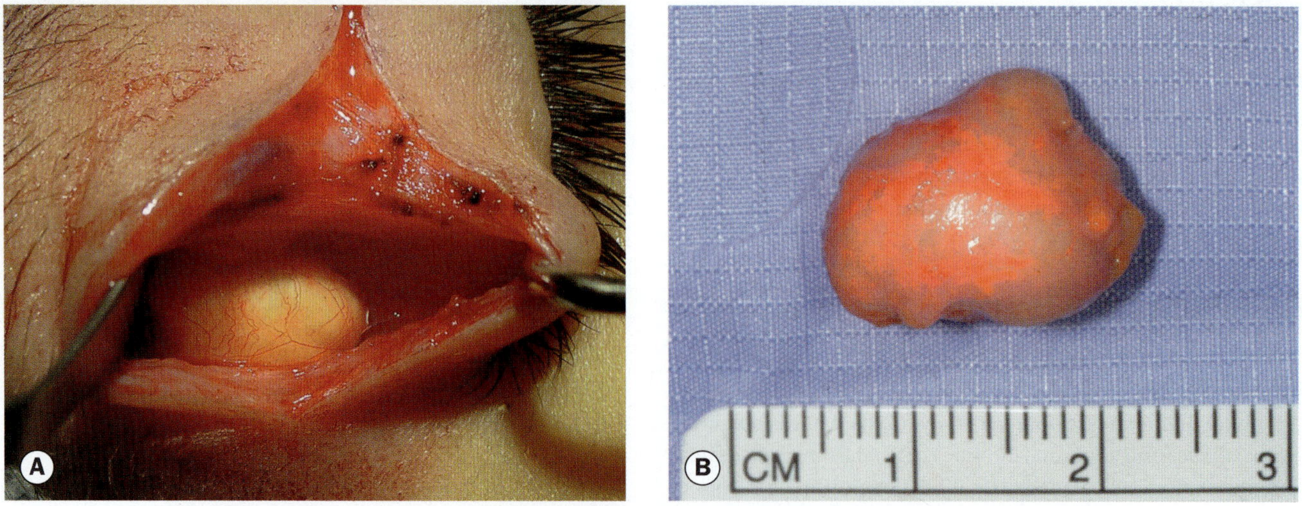

Fig. 4.27 Superficial orbital dermoid cyst. **(A)** Appearance at surgery; **(B)** excised specimen. *(Courtesy of JH Norris.)*

the orbital septum respectively. Epibulbar dermoids and dermolipomas are related lesions (see Ch. 20).

Diagnosis

Dermoid cysts are one of the most frequently encountered orbital tumours in children.

- **Symptoms**
  - A superficial orbital dermoid cyst presents in infancy with a painless nodule, most commonly located in the superotemporal and occasionally the superonasal part of the orbit.
  - A deep dermoid cyst presents in adolescence or adult life with a gradually increasingly protruding eye, or acutely with an inflamed orbit due to rupture.
- **Signs**
  - **Superficial:** a firm round smooth non-tender mass 1–2 cm in diameter (Fig. 4.25A), mobile under the skin but usually tethered to the adjacent periosteum. The posterior margins are easily palpable, denoting a lack of deeper origin or extension.
  - **Deep:** proptosis, dystopia or a mass lesion with indistinct posterior margins. (Fig. 4.25B).
- **Investigation**
  - Imaging is required in all cases to rule out dumb-bell or subperiosteal extension.
  - Superficial: imaging shows a well-circumscribed heterogeneous cystic lesion (Fig. 4.26A).
  - Deep: imaging shows a well-circumscribed lesion (Fig. 4.26B). Some deep dermoids, associated with bony defects, may extend into the inferotemporal fossa or intracranially.

TIP When removing an orbital dermoid cyst take care not to rupture the wall of the cyst, as this can cause a granulomatous inflammation in the surrounding tissue.

Treatment

- **Superficial dermoid.** Treatment is by excision *in toto* (Fig. 4.27), taking care not to rupture the lesion, since leaking of keratin into the surrounding tissue typically results in severe granulomatous inflammation.
- **Deep dermoid.** Excision *in toto* is advisable because deep dermoids enlarge and may leak into adjacent tissues inducing inflammation, often followed by fibrosis. If incompletely excised, dermoids may recur with persistent low-grade inflammation.

Sinus mucocoele

A mucocoele (US spelling – mucocele) develops when the drainage of normal paranasal sinus secretions is obstructed due to infection, allergy, trauma, tumour or congenital narrowing. A slowly expanding cystic accumulation of mucoid secretions and epithelial debris develops and gradually erodes the bony walls of the sinus, causing symptoms by encroachment upon surrounding tissues. Orbital invasion occurs usually from a frontal or ethmoidal mucocoele, but rarely from those arising in the maxillary sinus. Presentation is in adult life with proptosis or dystopia (Fig. 4.28A), diplopia or epiphora. Pain is uncommon unless secondary infection develops (mucopyocoele). CT shows a soft tissue mass with thinning or erosion of the bony walls of the sinus (Fig. 4.28B). Treatment involves complete excision.

Encephalocoele

An encephalocoele (US spelling – encephalocele) is formed by herniation of intracranial contents through a congenital defect of the base of the skull and can be located at the front or back of the head. A meningocoele contains only dura whilst a meningoencephalocoele also contains brain tissue. Presentation is usually during infancy. Anterior orbital encephalocoeles involve the superomedial part of the orbit and displace the globe forwards and laterally (Fig. 4.29A), whereas posterior orbital encephalocoeles (frequently associated with neurofibromatosis type 1) displace the globe forwards and downwards (Fig. 4.29B). The displacement increases on straining or crying and may be reduced

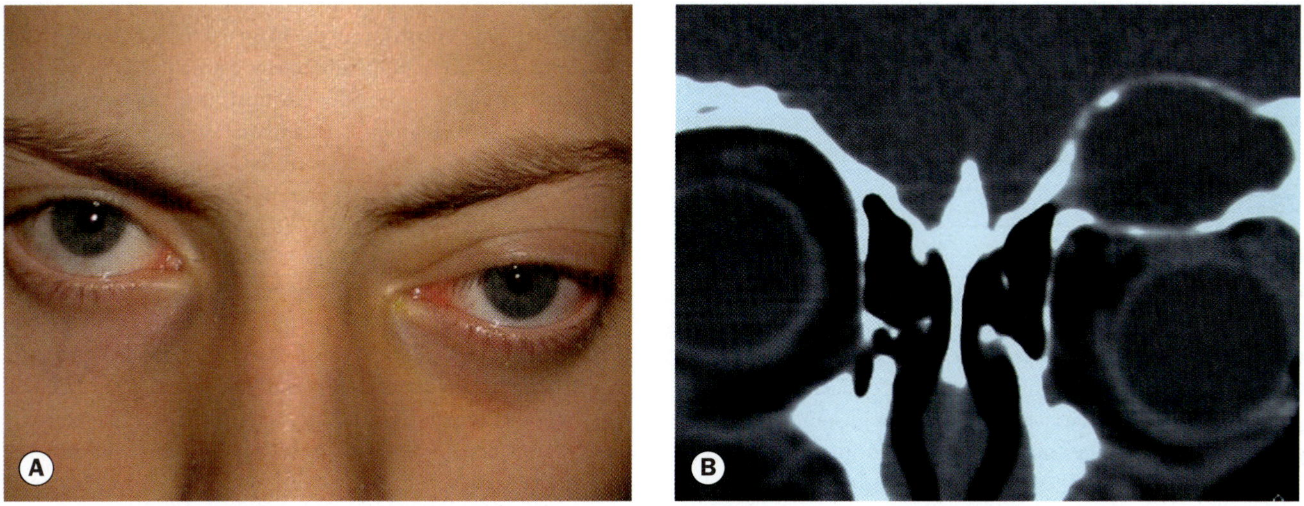

Fig. 4.28 **(A)** Left frontal sinus mucocoele causing globe displacement; **(B)** coronal CT showing mucocoele above the globe.

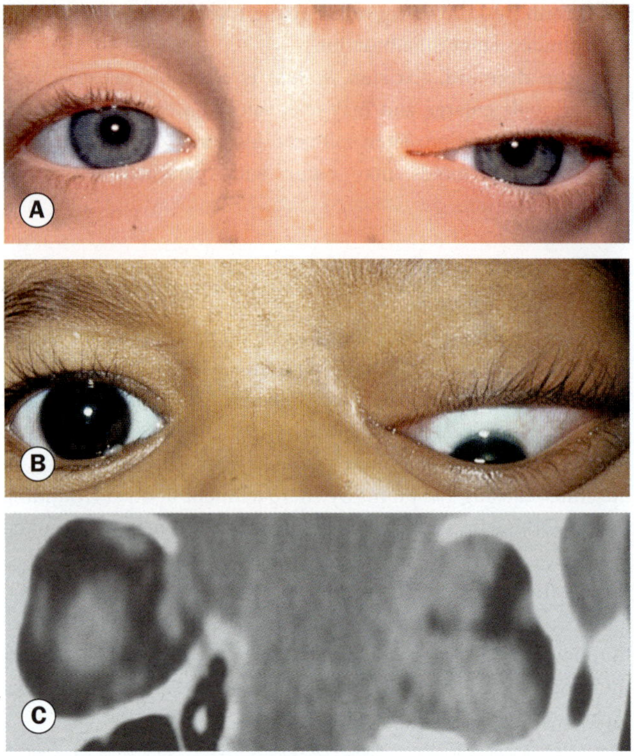

Fig. 4.29 Encephalocoele. **(A)** Anterior superomedial encephalocoele causing proptosis and down and out dystopia; **(B)** posterior encephalocoele causing proptosis and inferior dystopia; **(C)** coronal CT of posterior encephalocoele showing a large bony defect. *(Courtesy of A Pearson – fig. C.)*

by manual pressure. Pulsating proptosis may occur due to communication with the subarachnoid space but, because the communication is not vascular, there is neither a thrill nor a bruit. CT shows the bony defect responsible for the herniation (Fig. 4.29C). The differential diagnosis of anterior encephalocoele includes other causes of medial canthal swelling such as dermoid cyst and amniontocoele, and of posterior encephalocoele includes other orbital lesions that present during early life such as capillary haemangioma, juvenile xanthogranuloma, teratoma and microphthalmos with cyst.

VASCULAR TUMOURS

Varices

Introduction

Primary orbital varices (combined venous–lymphatic malformations of the orbit – see also next topic) consist of a plexus of thin-walled distensible low-flow vein-like vessels that are commonly, though not always, intrinsic to the normal circulation. They are probably hamartomatous (hamartoma – a disorganized overgrowth of mature tissues normally present in the involved area). Associations include varices of the eyelids (Fig. 4.30A and see Fig. 2.63) and conjunctiva (Fig. 4.30B). They commonly present at any time from early childhood to late middle age, but occasionally can be acquired later secondary to a local high-flow vascular lesion or trauma.

Diagnosis

Most cases are unilateral and the most frequent site is upper nasal. Intermittent non-pulsatile proptosis without a bruit is reported. If there is free communication with the normal circulation, reversible proptosis may be precipitated or accentuated by increasing venous pressure through coughing, straining, the Valsalva manoeuvre (Fig. 4.30C and D), assuming a head-down position or external compression of the jugular veins. Imaging (e.g. MRI and magnetic resonance venography [MRV], CT, ultrasound, venography) shows a lobulated mass with variable contrast enhancement and may demonstrate phleboliths (Fig. 4.30E) and sometimes orbital expansion (particularly in childhood) or an associated orbital wall defect. Complications include acute orbital haemorrhage, thrombosis (pain, proptosis, decreased vision) and optic nerve compression. Patients with long-standing lesions may develop atrophy of surrounding fat, giving enophthalmos with a deepened superior sulcus (Fig. 4.30F).

Treatment

Small lesions generally do not require treatment. Surgical excision is technically difficult and often incomplete because the lesions are friable and bleed easily. It can be complicated by severe orbital haemorrhage and vascular optic nerve compromise. Specialized techniques such as embolization and carbon dioxide laser surgery may be helpful adjuncts. Indications include recurrent thrombosis, pain, severe proptosis and optic nerve compression.

Lymphangioma

Introduction

Lymphangioma is a rare hamartomatous vascular tumour that tends to enlarge and infiltrate diffusely with time. Some authorities believe lymphangiomas to be a variant of venous orbital anomaly (varices) across a single spectrum and the term 'combined venous–lymphatic malformations of the orbit' has been suggested. Although usually isolated from the main circulation, bleeding into the lumen may occur with subsequent formation of blood-filled 'chocolate cysts' that regress spontaneously with time. Presentation is usually in early childhood. Differential diagnosis is principally from orbital venous anomalies and haemangiomas. Intracranial vascular malformations can be present in association.

Diagnosis

- **Anterior lesions** typically manifest as several soft bluish masses in the upper nasal quadrant (Fig. 4.31).
- **Posterior lesions** may cause slowly progressive proptosis, or initially may lie dormant and later present with the sudden onset of painful proptosis (Fig. 4.32A and B) secondary to spontaneous haemorrhage, which may be associated with optic nerve compression. Involvement of the lids, conjunctiva and oropharynx may be seen; intracranial lesions may also be present.

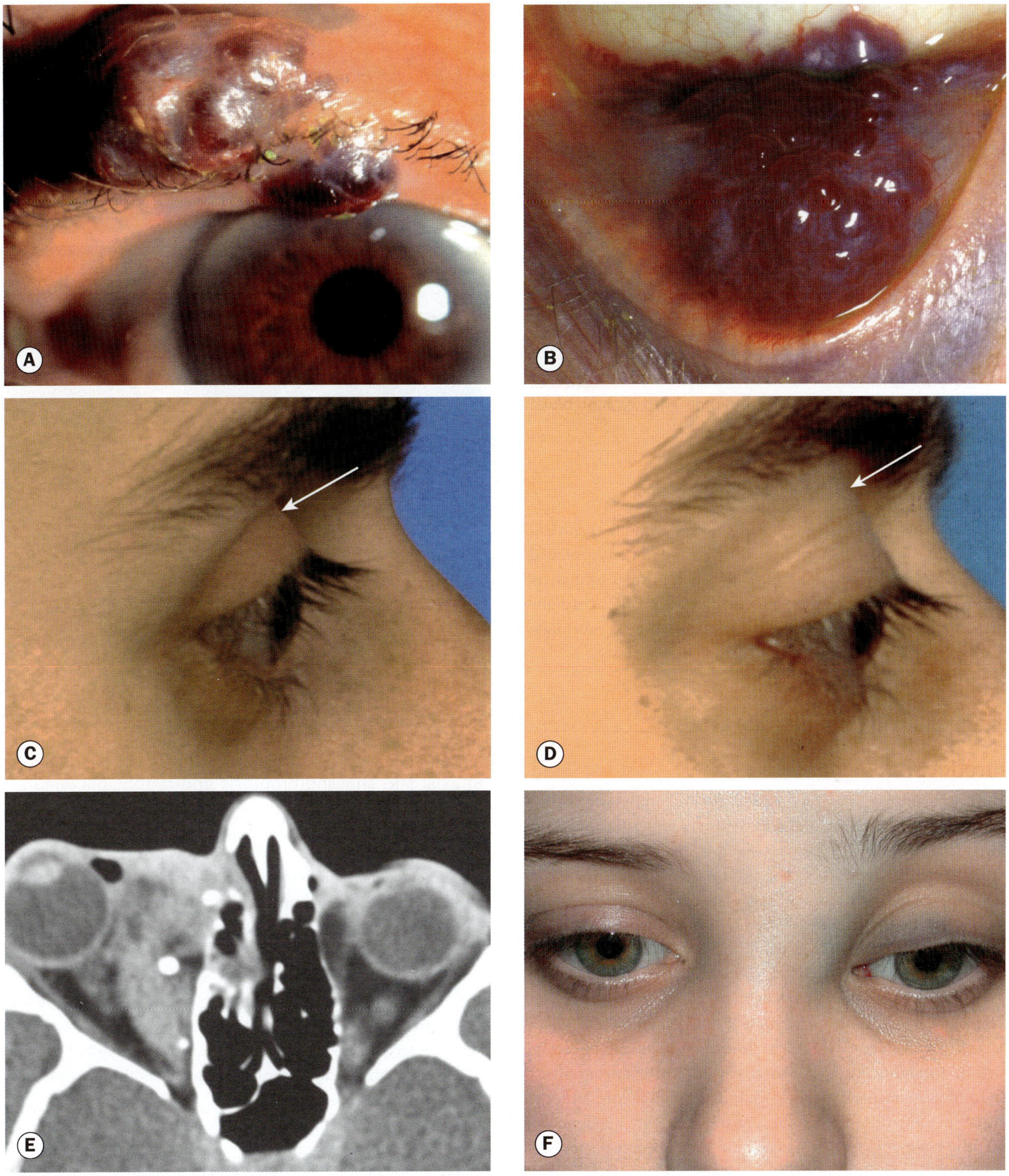

Fig. 4.30 **(A)** Substantial eyelid varices; **(B)** conjunctival varices; **(C)** orbital varices before Valsalva (arrow); and **(D)** with Valsalva showing forward movement of the eye and fullness of the upper lid (arrow); **(E)** axial CT showing medial opacification and phleboliths; **(F)** left fat atrophy resulting in enophthalmos and deep superior sulcus. *(Courtesy of G Rose – figs C and D; A Pearson – figs E and F.)*

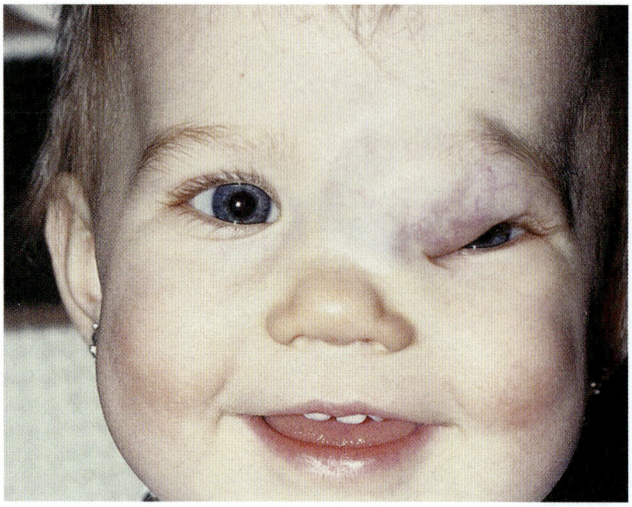

Fig. 4.31 Anterior orbital lymphangioma with typical bluish discoloration.

Treatment

In many cases the visual prognosis is good without treatment. Surgical excision is difficult because lesions are not encapsulated, friable, bleed easily and commonly infiltrate normal orbital tissues; repeated subtotal excision may be necessary. Persistent sight-threatening chocolate cysts can be drained or removed sub-totally by controlled vapourization using a carbon dioxide laser.

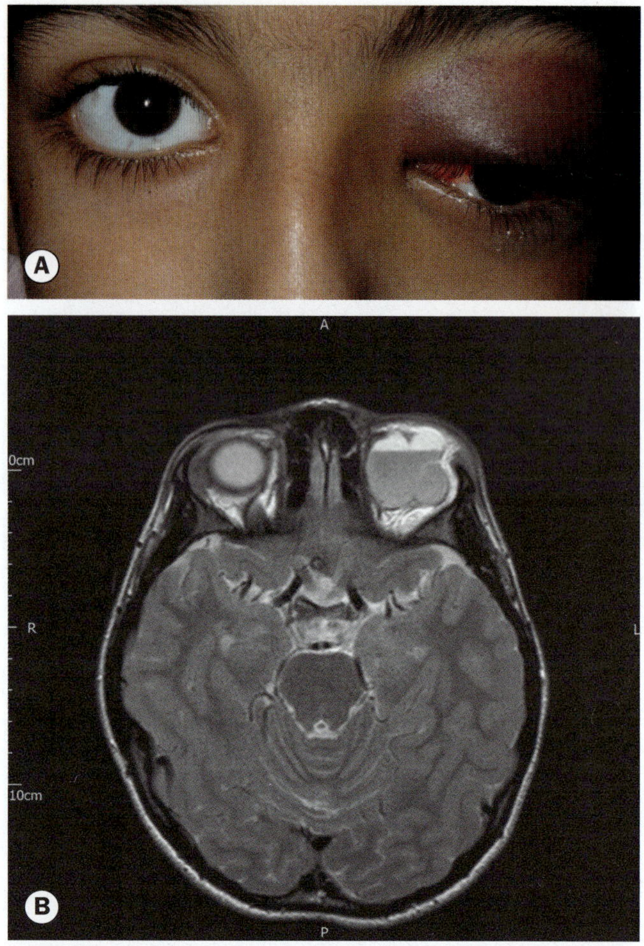

Fig. 4.32 Posterior orbital lymphangioma. **(A)** Left proptosis and inferior globe displacement with orbital haemorrhage; **(B)** axial MRI showing proptosis and retrobulbar lymphangioma.

Capillary haemangioma

Introduction

Capillary haemangioma is the most common tumour of the orbit and periorbital area in childhood. Girls are affected more commonly than boys (3:1). It may present as a small isolated lesion of minimal clinical significance, or as a large disfiguring mass that can cause visual impairment and systemic complications. An established tumour is composed of anastomosing small vascular channels without true encapsulation. It is a hamartoma – a disorganized overgrowth of mature tissues normally present in the involved area – and believed to be due principally to endothelial cell proliferation. Large or multiple lesions may have associated visceral involvement, which can lead to serious complications such as thrombocytopenia (Kasabach–Merritt syndrome, with up to 50% mortality) and high-output cardiac failure and systemic investigation should be considered. The incidence of infantile haemangioma in the general population is around 5% and a small proportion of these, especially if a large facial haemangioma is present, will have PHACE (PHACES) syndrome, which includes a range of possible systemic features including eye involvement.

Diagnosis

- **Symptoms.** The lesion is usually noticed by the parent, usually in the first few months of life. Approximately 30% are present at birth.
- **Signs.** Extensive underlying orbital involvement should always be ruled out in a seemingly purely superficial lesion.
  - A superficial cutaneous lesion ('strawberry naevus') is bright red (Fig. 4.33A and see Fig. 2.12A).
  - Preseptal (deeper) tumours appear dark blue or purple through the overlying skin (Fig. 4.33A and B) and are most frequently located superiorly.
  - A large tumour may enlarge and change in colour to a deep blue during crying or straining, but both pulsation and a bruit are absent.
  - Deep orbital tumours give rise to unilateral proptosis without skin discoloration.
  - Haemangiomatous involvement of the palpebral or forniceal conjunctiva is common (Fig. 4.33B).
  - Additional haemangiomas on the eyelids (see Ch. 2) or elsewhere are common.
- **Investigation.** Imaging is generally performed for other than very small lesions, mainly to rule out more extensive orbital disease. Ultrasound shows medium internal reflectivity and on MRI or CT the lesion appears as a soft tissue mass in the anterior orbit or as an extraconal mass with finger-like posterior

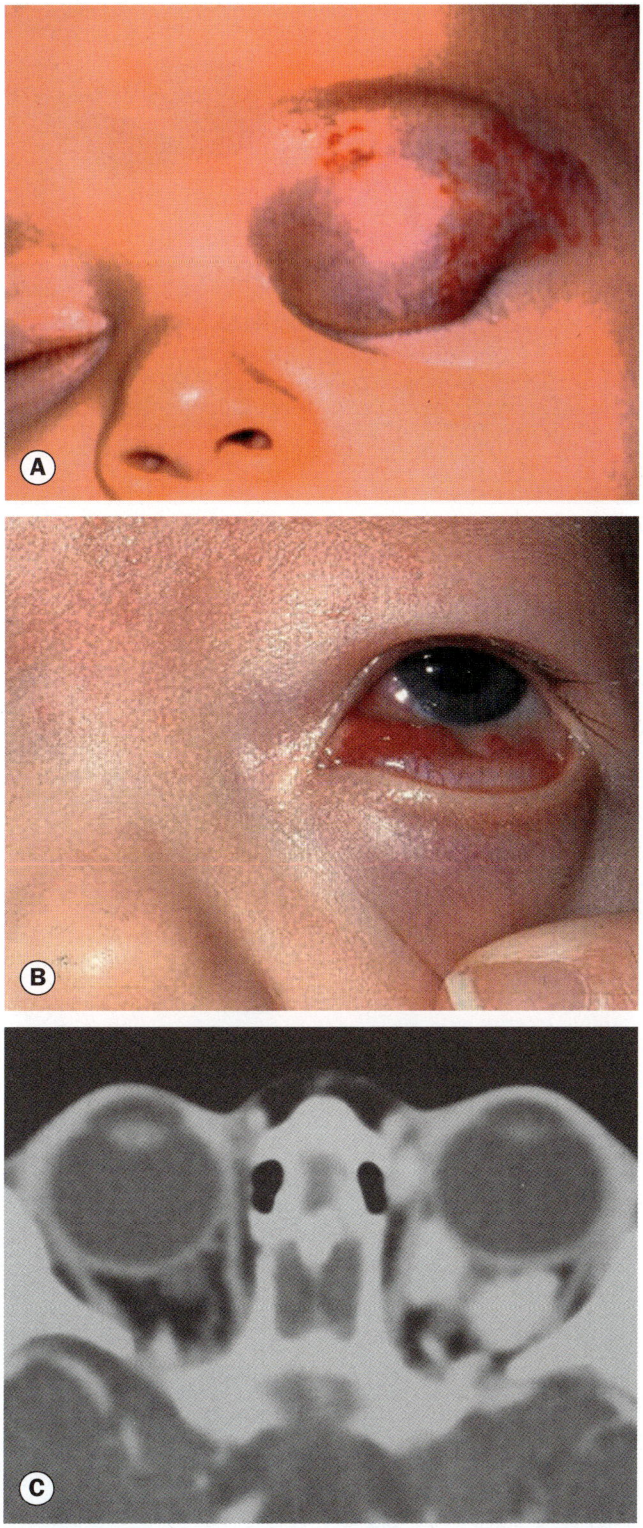

Fig. 4.33 Capillary haemangioma. **(A)** Large preseptal tumour causing ptosis and purple cutaneous discoloration, there is a superficial component (strawberry naevus); **(B)** involvement of forniceal conjunctiva; **(C)** axial enhanced CT showing a homogeneous intraconal orbital soft tissue mass. *(Courtesy of Ken K Nischal – fig. B; A Pearson – fig. C.)*

expansions (Fig. 4.33C). The orbital cavity may show enlargement but there is no bony erosion.

Treatment

The natural course is characterized by rapid growth (Fig. 4.34A and B) 3–6 months after diagnosis, followed by a slower phase of natural resolution in which 30% of lesions resolve by the age of 3 years and about 75% by the age of 7. Treatment is indicated principally for amblyopia secondary to induced astigmatism, anisometropia, occlusion or strabismus and less commonly for cosmesis, optic nerve compression or exposure keratopathy.

- **Beta-blockers.** Oral propranolol is now widely used. The prescription and monitoring should generally be carried out by a paediatrician. Topical preparations including timolol are equally effective, with excellent long-term results and no systemic side effects (Fig. 4.34C and D).
- **Steroids**
  - Injection of triamcinolone acetonide (1–2 ml total of 40 mg/ml over several injection sites) or betamethasone (4 mg/ml) into a cutaneous or preseptal tumour is usually effective in early lesions. Regression usually begins within 2 weeks but, if necessary, second and third injections can be given after about 2 months. It is advisable not to inject deeply into the orbit for fear of causing occlusion of the central retinal artery due to retrograde introduction of the suspension. Other complications include skin depigmentation and necrosis, fat atrophy and systemic effects such as adrenal suppression.
  - Topical high-potency steroids (e.g. clobetasol propionate cream) are sometimes appropriate but are slow to exert their effect.
  - Systemic steroids administered daily over several weeks may be used, particularly if there is a large orbital component or a rapid onset of action is required.
- **Laser** may be used to close blood vessels in superficial skin lesions less than 2 mm in thickness.
- **Interferon alfa-2a** and **vincristine** may be used for some steroid-resistant sight-threatening lesions.
- **Local resection** with cutting cautery or carbon dioxide laser may reduce the bulk of an anterior circumscribed tumour, but is usually reserved for the late inactive stage unless a resistant tumour is sight- or life-threatening.

Cavernous haemangioma

Introduction

Cavernous haemangioma occurs in middle-aged adults, with a female preponderance of 70%. The growth may be accelerated by pregnancy. It is the most common orbital tumour in adults and is probably a vascular malformation rather than a neoplastic lesion. Although it may develop anywhere in the orbit, it most frequently occurs within the lateral part of the muscle cone just behind the globe and behaves like a low-flow arteriovenous malformation. Histology shows endothelial-lined vascular channels of varying size separated by fibrous septa (Fig. 4.35A).

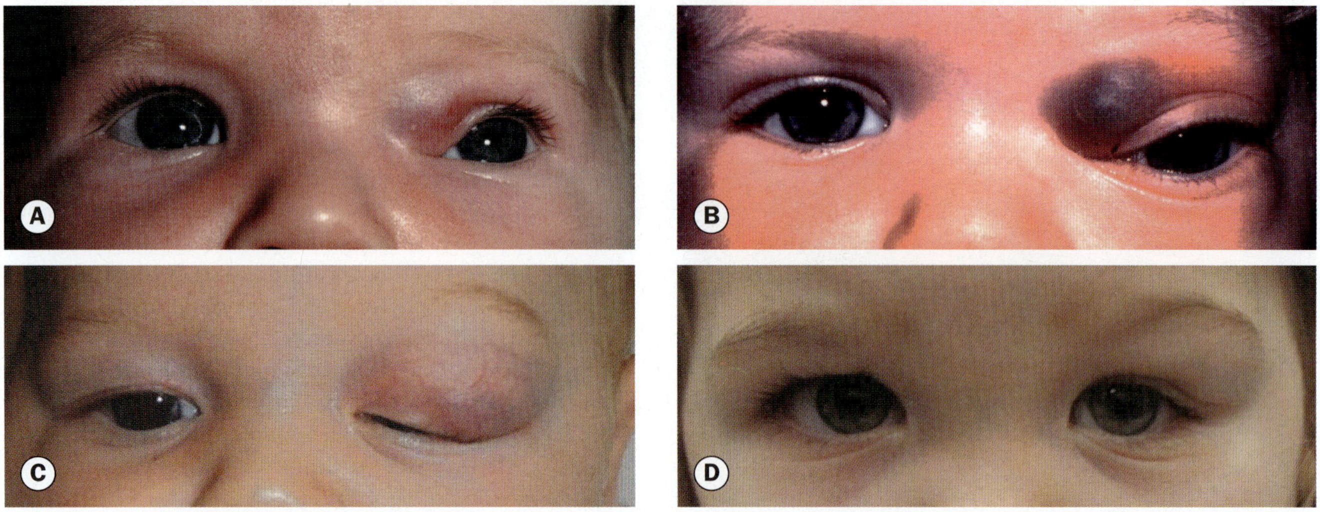

Fig. 4.34 Growth of capillary haemangioma. **(A)** At presentation; **(B)** several months later; **(C)** at presentation; **(D)** 6 months after treatment with topical beta-blocker. *(Courtesy of D Hildebrand – figs C and D.)*

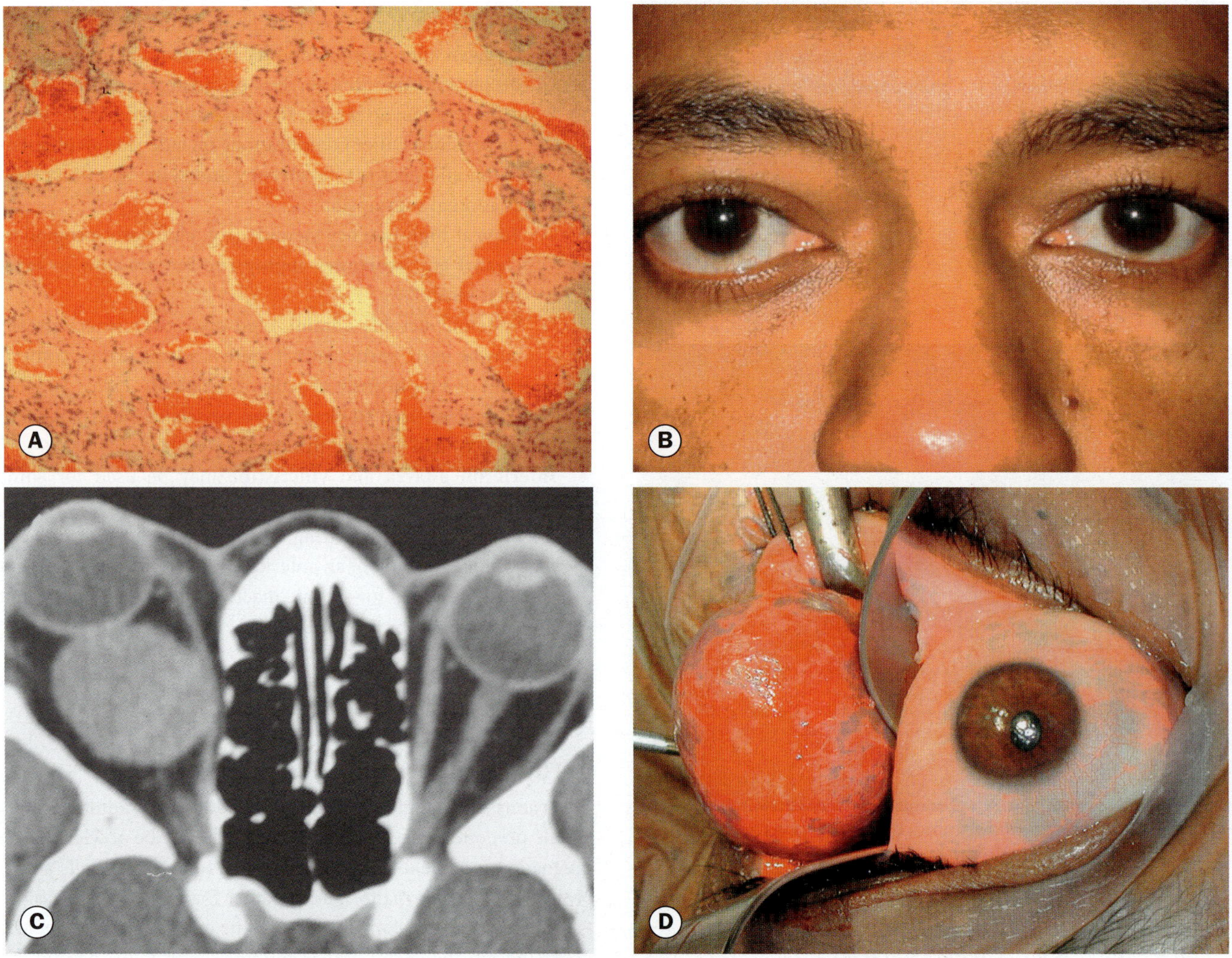

Fig. 4.35 Cavernous haemangioma. **(A)** Histology showing congested variably sized endothelial-lined vascular channels separated by fibrous septa; **(B)** right axial proptosis; **(C)** axial CT showing a well-circumscribed retrobulbar oval lesion and proptosis; **(D)** the tumour is encapsulated and relatively easy to remove. *(Courtesy of A Pearson.)*

Diagnosis

- **Symptoms.** Slowly progressive unilateral proptosis; bilateral cases are very rare.
- **Signs**
  - Axial proptosis (Fig. 4.35B), which may be associated with optic disc oedema and choroidal folds.
  - A lesion at the orbital apex may compress the optic nerve without causing significant proptosis. Gaze-evoked transient blurring of vision may occur.
  - There may be impairment of extraocular muscle excursion.
- **Investigation.** CT (Fig. 4.35C) and MRI show a well-circumscribed oval lesion, usually within the muscle cone. There is only slow contrast enhancement. Ultrasound is also useful.

Treatment

Many cavernous haemangiomas are detected by chance on scans performed for unrelated reasons and observation alone is often appropriate. Symptomatic lesions require surgical excision in most cases because they gradually enlarge. The cavernous haemangioma, unlike its capillary counterpart, is usually well-encapsulated and relatively easy to remove (Fig. 4.35D).

LACRIMAL GLAND TUMOURS

Pleomorphic lacrimal gland adenoma

Introduction

Pleomorphic adenoma (benign mixed-cell tumour) is the most common epithelial tumour of the lacrimal gland and is derived from the ducts and secretory elements including myoepithelial cells. On histopathology, the inner layer of cells forms glandular tissue that may be associated with squamous differentiation and keratin production (Fig. 4.36A). The outer cells undergo metaplastic change leading to the formation of myxoid tissue. Young to middle-aged adults are the predominantly affected group.

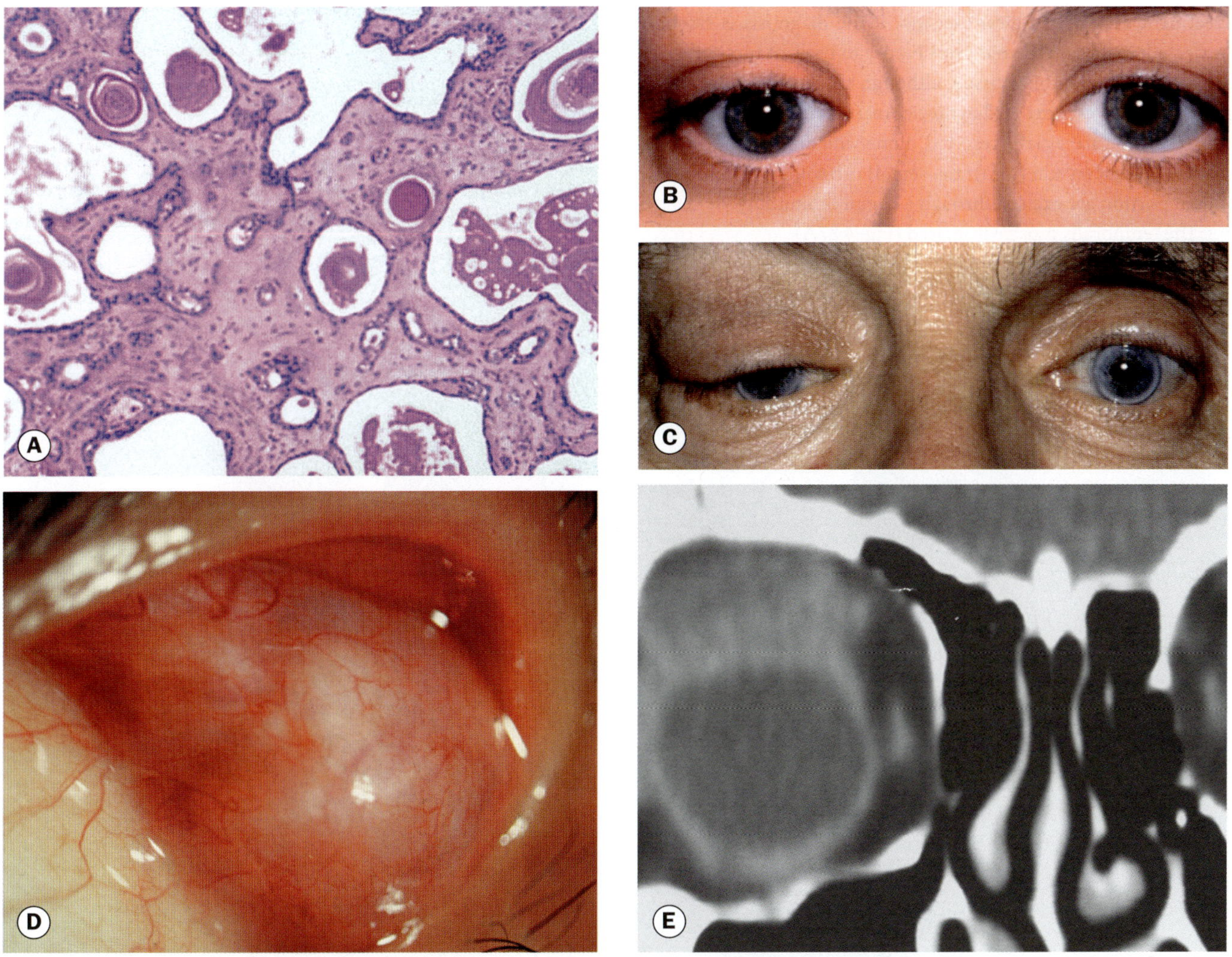

Fig. 4.36 Pleomorphic lacrimal gland adenoma. **(A)** Histology showing glandular tissue and squamous differentiation with keratin formation; **(B)** inferonasal dystopia due to a tumour arising from the orbital lobe; **(C)** eyelid swelling without dystopia; **(D)** eversion of the upper eyelid reveals the tumour; **(E)** coronal CT of **(B)** showing an orbital lobe lesion. *(Courtesy of J Harry and G Misson, from* Clinical Ophthalmic Pathology*, Butterworth-Heinemann 2001 – fig. A; A Pearson – figs B and E.)*

Diagnosis

- **Symptoms.** Painless slowly progressive proptosis or swelling in the superolateral eyelid, usually of more than a year's duration. Old photographs may reveal an abnormality many years prior to presentation.
- **Signs**
  - Orbital lobe tumour presents as a smooth, firm, non-tender mass in the lacrimal gland fossa with inferonasal dystopia (Fig. 4.36B). Posterior extension may cause proptosis, ophthalmoplegia and choroidal folds.
  - Palpebral lobe tumour is less common and tends to grow anteriorly causing upper lid swelling without dystopia (Fig. 4.36C), which may be visible to inspection (Fig. 4.36D).
- **Investigation.** CT shows a round or oval mass, with a smooth outline and indentation but not destruction of the lacrimal gland fossa (Fig. 4.36E). The lesion may indent the globe and calcification may be shown.

Treatment

Treatment involves surgical excision. If the diagnosis is strongly suspected, it is wise to avoid prior biopsy to prevent tumour seeding into adjacent orbital tissue, although this may not always be possible in the context of diagnostic uncertainty. Tumours of the palpebral lobe are usually resected, along with a margin of normal tissue, through an anterior (trans-septal) orbitotomy. Those of the orbital portion are excised through a lateral orbitotomy:

- The temporalis muscle is incised (Fig. 4.37A).
- The underlying bone is drilled for subsequent wiring (Fig. 4.37B).
- The lateral orbital wall is removed and the tumour excised, including a margin of adjacent tissue and periorbita (Fig. 4.37C).
- The lateral orbital wall (Fig. 4.37D) and temporalis are repaired.
- The prognosis is excellent provided excision is complete and without disruption of the capsule. Incomplete excision or preliminary incisional biopsy may result in seeding of the tumour into adjacent tissues, with recurrence and occasionally malignant change.

Lacrimal gland carcinoma

Lacrimal gland carcinoma is a rare tumour that carries a high morbidity and mortality. In order of frequency the main histological types are adenoid cystic (50%), pleomorphic adenocarcinoma, mucoepidermoid and squamous cell. Histopathology shows nests of basaloid cells with numerous mitoses (Fig. 4.38A). The peak incidence is in middle-aged adults.

Diagnosis

- **Symptoms.** A malignant mixed-cell tumour presents in three main clinical settings:
  - After incomplete or piecemeal excision of a benign pleomorphic adenoma, followed by one or more recurrences over a period of several years with eventual malignant transformation.

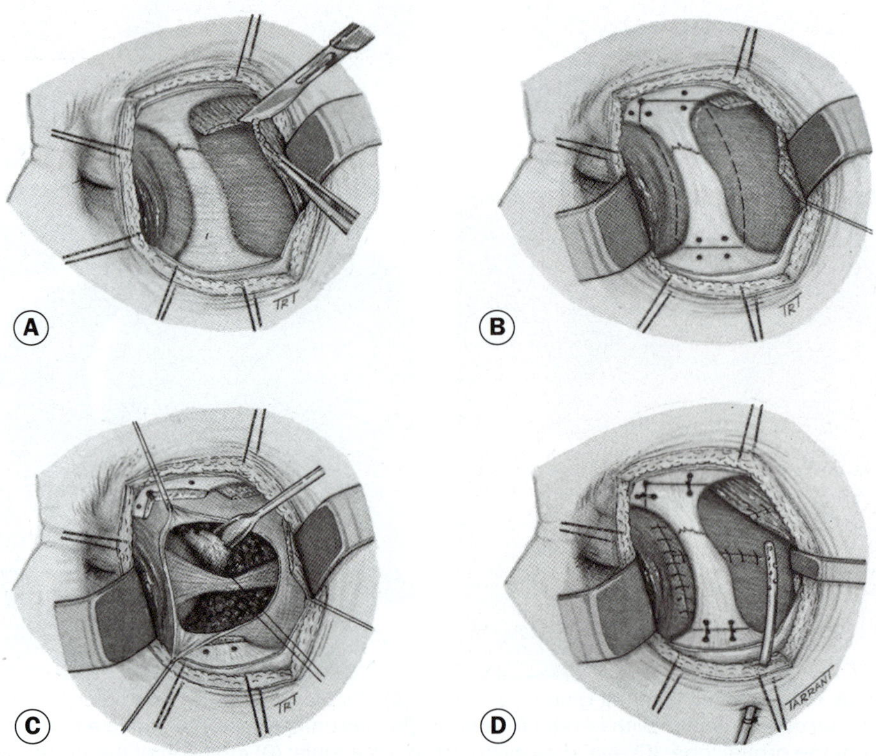

Fig. 4.37 Lateral orbitotomy. **(A)** Incision of temporalis muscle; **(B)** drilling of underlying bone for subsequent wiring; **(C)** removal of the lateral orbital wall and the tumour; **(D)** repair of the lateral orbital wall.

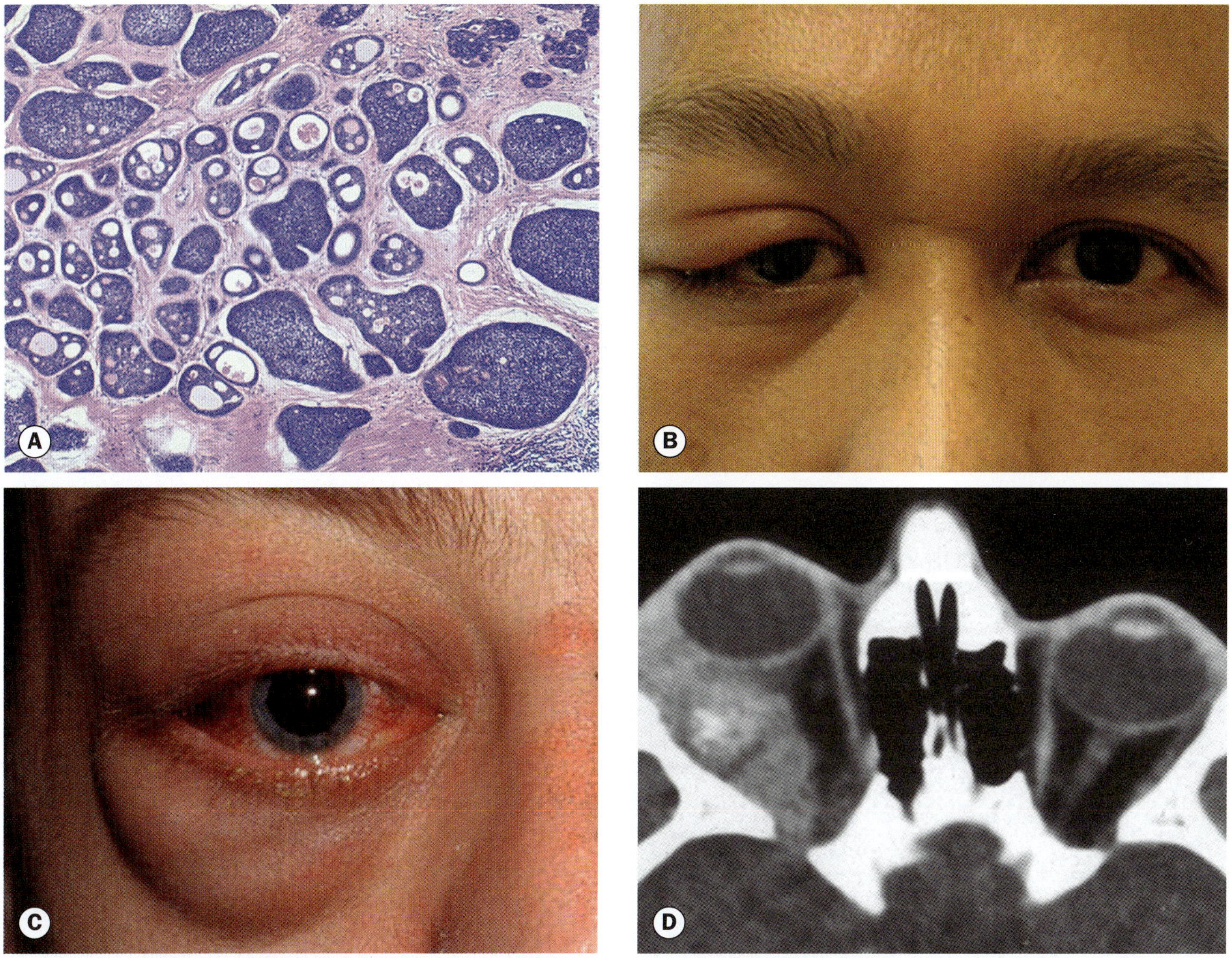

Fig. 4.38 Lacrimal gland carcinoma. **(A)** Histology of adenoid-cystic carcinoma showing nests of basaloid cells with solid and cribriform areas; **(B)** early changes showing lid swelling and ptosis; **(C)** proptosis, periorbital oedema and epibulbar congestion; **(D)** axial CT of **(C)** showing carcinoma surrounding the globe, extending along the lateral orbital wall and extending through the right superior orbital fissure. *(Courtesy of J Harry and G Misson, from* Clinical Ophthalmic Pathology, *Butterworth-Heinemann 2001 – fig. A; G Rose – figs C and D.)*

- As a long-standing proptosis or swollen upper lid that suddenly starts to increase.
- Without a previous history of a pleomorphic adenoma as a rapidly growing lacrimal gland mass, usually of several months' duration.
- The history is shorter than that of a benign tumour.
- Pain is a frequent feature of malignancy but may also occur with inflammatory lesions.

TIP Beware of an incomplete excision of a benign pleomorphic adenoma as this can result in malignant transformation.

- **Signs**
  - A mass in the lacrimal area causing swelling, ptosis and dystopia (Fig.4.38B).
  - Posterior extension, with involvement of the superior orbital fissure, may give rise to epibulbar congestion, proptosis, periorbital oedema and ophthalmoplegia (Fig. 4.38C).
  - Hypoaesthesia in the region supplied by the lacrimal nerve.
  - Optic disc swelling and choroidal folds.
- **Investigation**
  - CT shows a globular lesion with irregular serrated edges, often with contiguous erosion or invasion of bone (Fig. 4.38D). Calcification is commonly seen within the tumour.
  - Biopsy is necessary to establish the histological diagnosis. Subsequent management depends on the extent of tumour invasion of adjacent structures as seen on imaging.
  - Neurological assessment is mandatory because adenoid-cystic carcinoma exhibits perineural spread and may extend into the cavernous sinus.

Treatment

Treatment involves excision of the tumour and adjacent tissues. Extensive tumours may require orbital exenteration or midfacial resection, but the prognosis for life is frequently poor. Radiotherapy combined with local resection may prolong life and reduce pain. Adjuvant intra-arterial chemotherapy and/or brachytherapy may be utilized in some cases.

NEURAL TUMOURS

Optic nerve glioma

Introduction

Optic nerve glioma is a slowly growing, pilocytic astrocytoma that typically affects children (median age 6.5 years). Histopathology shows spindle-shaped pilocytic (hair-like) astrocytes and glial filaments (Fig. 4.39A). The prognosis is unpredictable; some have an indolent course with little growth, while others may extend intracranially and threaten life. Approximately 30% of patients have associated neurofibromatosis type 1 (NF1 – see Ch. 19) and in these patients the prognosis is superior. Malignant glioma (glioblastoma) is rare, has a very poor prognosis and usually occurs in adult males.

Diagnosis

- **Symptoms**
  - Slowly progressive visual loss followed later by proptosis, although this sequence may occasionally be reversed.
  - Acute loss of vision due to haemorrhage into the tumour can occur, but is uncommon.
- **Signs**
  - Proptosis is often non-axial, with temporal or inferior dystopia (Fig. 4.39B).
  - The optic nerve head, initially swollen, subsequently becomes atrophic (Fig. 4.39C).
  - Opticociliary collaterals (see Fig. 4.8C) and other fundus signs such as central retinal vein occlusion are occasionally seen.
  - Intracranial spread to the chiasm and hypothalamus may develop.

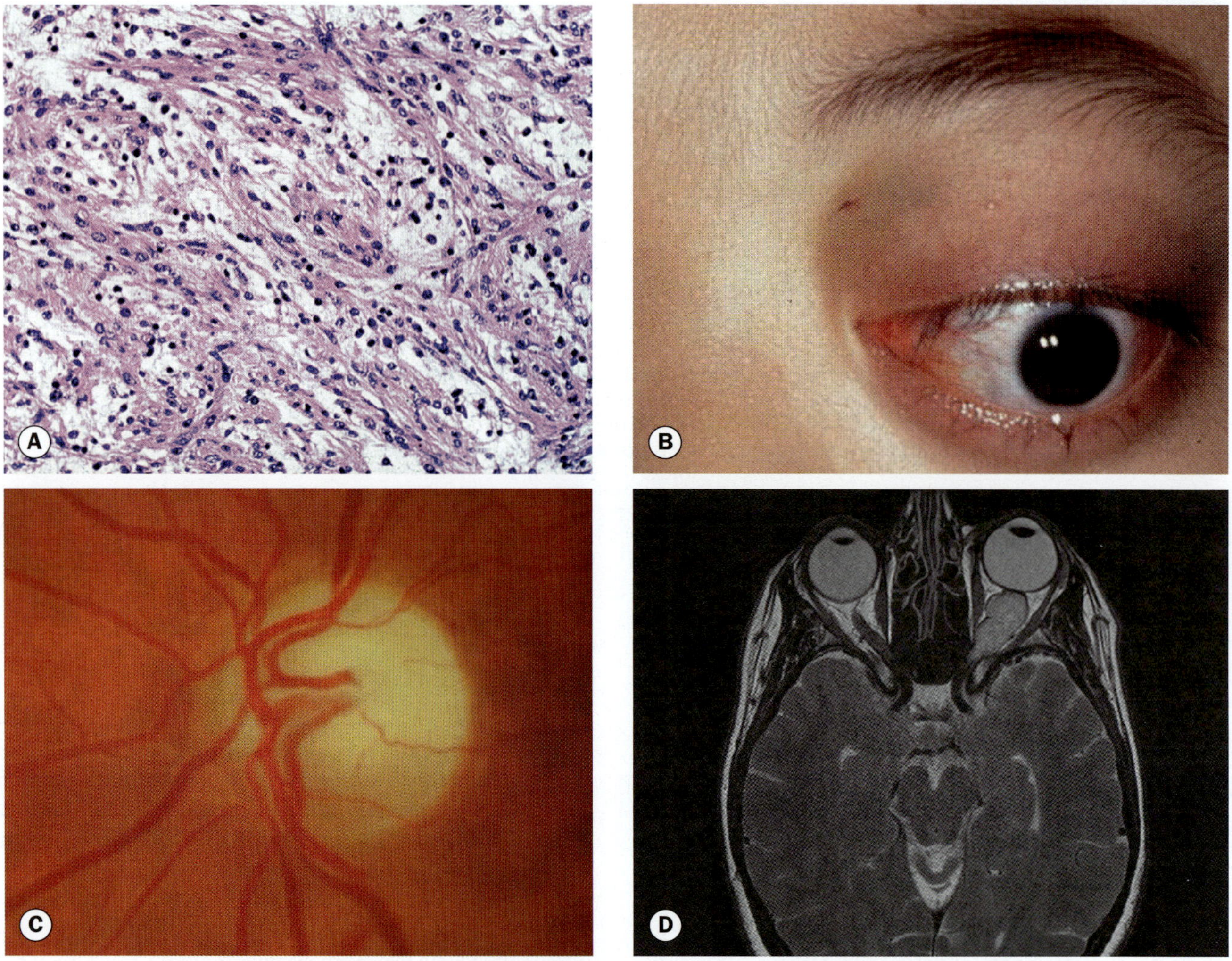

Fig. 4.39 Optic nerve glioma. **(A)** Histopathology – spindle-shaped pilocytic astrocytes and glial filaments; **(B)** proptosis with inferior dystopia; **(C)** optic disc atrophy; **(D)** axial T2-weighted MRI of **(C)** showing fusiform optic nerve enlargement. *(Courtesy of Ken K Nischal – fig. B.)*

- **Investigation**
  - MRI effectively demonstrates the tumour and may show intracranial extension if present (Fig. 4.39D).
  - CT in patients with associated NF1 shows a fusiform enlargement of the optic nerve with a clear-cut margin produced by the intact dural sheath. In patients without NF1 the nerve is more irregular and shows low-density areas.

Treatment

As the tumour is intrinsic to the optic nerve, resection means that all vision will be lost in the operated eye.

- **Observation** may be considered in patients with a typical pilocytic astrocytoma on imaging in whom the tumour is confined to the orbit, especially if there is good vision and no significant cosmetic impairment. Serial MRI is important if this option is chosen. Spontaneous regression has been reported, usually in NF1, but is very rare.
- **Surgical excision** with preservation of the globe is indicated in those with large or growing tumours where complete resection of the tumour can be achieved, particularly if vision is poor and proptosis significant. A key goal is to prevent chiasmal involvement and an intracranial approach may be necessary to achieve adequate resection.
- **Radiotherapy** may be combined with chemotherapy for tumours with extension that precludes complete surgical excision.

Optic nerve sheath meningioma

Introduction

Optic nerve sheath meningioma is a benign tumour arising from meningothelial cells of the arachnoid villi surrounding the intraorbital, or less commonly the intracanalicular, portion of the optic nerve. In some cases, the tumour merely encircles the optic nerve whilst in others it invades the nerve, growing along the fibrovascular pial septa. However, about two-thirds of all meningiomas affecting the optic nerve arise from extension of primarily intracranial lesions. Primary optic nerve sheath meningiomas are less common than optic nerve gliomas and, as with other meningiomas, typically affect middle-aged women. Histopathologically, meningothelial (irregular lobules of meningothelial cells separated by fibrovascular strands – Fig. 4.40A) and psammomatous (psammoma bodies among proliferating meningothelial cells – Fig. 4.40B) types are distinguished. The prognosis for life is good in adults, although the tumour may be more aggressive in children, in whom 25% occur. They are more common in neurofibromatosis type 2 (NF2).

TIP In optic nerve sheath meningioma, the onset of visual loss usually occurs before the onset of proptosis.

Diagnosis

- **Symptoms** typically consist of gradual visual impairment in one eye. Transient obscurations of vision may occur.
- **Signs.** The classic (Hoyt–Spencer) triad consists of progressive visual loss, optic atrophy and opticociliary shunt vessels, although the simultaneous occurrence of all three signs in one individual is actually uncommon. The usual sequence of involvement is the opposite of that seen in tumours that develop outside the dural sheath:
  - Optic nerve dysfunction and chronic disc swelling followed by atrophy.
  - Opticociliary collaterals (30%), which regress as optic atrophy supervenes.
  - Restrictive motility defects, particularly in upgaze (Fig. 4.40C).
  - Proptosis (Fig. 4.40D).
- **Investigation**
  - CT shows thickening and calcification of the optic nerve (Fig. 4.40E).
  - MRI is the investigation of choice (Fig. 4.40F).
  - Ultrasonography (especially coronal) may be useful.

Treatment

Treatment may not be indicated in a middle-aged patient with a slowly growing lesion, but excision is required for an aggressive tumour, particularly if the eye is blind or there is a risk of intracranial extension. Attempts at optic nerve-sparing surgery commonly fail but may be considered on a case basis. Fractionated stereotactic radiotherapy may be appropriate as a vision-sparing approach, or as adjunctive treatment following surgery.

Plexiform neurofibroma

Plexiform neurofibroma is the most common peripheral neural tumour of the orbit. It occurs almost exclusively in association with NF1. Presentation is in early childhood with periorbital swelling. Classically, involvement of the eyelids causes mechanical ptosis with a characteristic S-shaped deformity (see Fig. 2.14B), but diffuse involvement of the orbit with disfiguring hypertrophy of periocular tissues may occur. On palpation the involved tissues are said to resemble a 'bag of worms'. Malignant change can occur and should be suspected if there is rapid change; radiotherapy may promote this. Treatment is often unsatisfactory and complete surgical removal is extremely difficult. Orbital surgery should be avoided when possible, because of the intricate relationship between the tumour and important structures.

Isolated neurofibroma

Isolated (localized) neurofibroma is less common than plexiform neurofibroma; about 10% of patients have NF1. Presentation is in the third or fourth decades with insidious mildly painful proptosis, usually not associated with visual impairment or ocular motility dysfunction. Excision is commonly straightforward because the tumour is well circumscribed and relatively avascular.

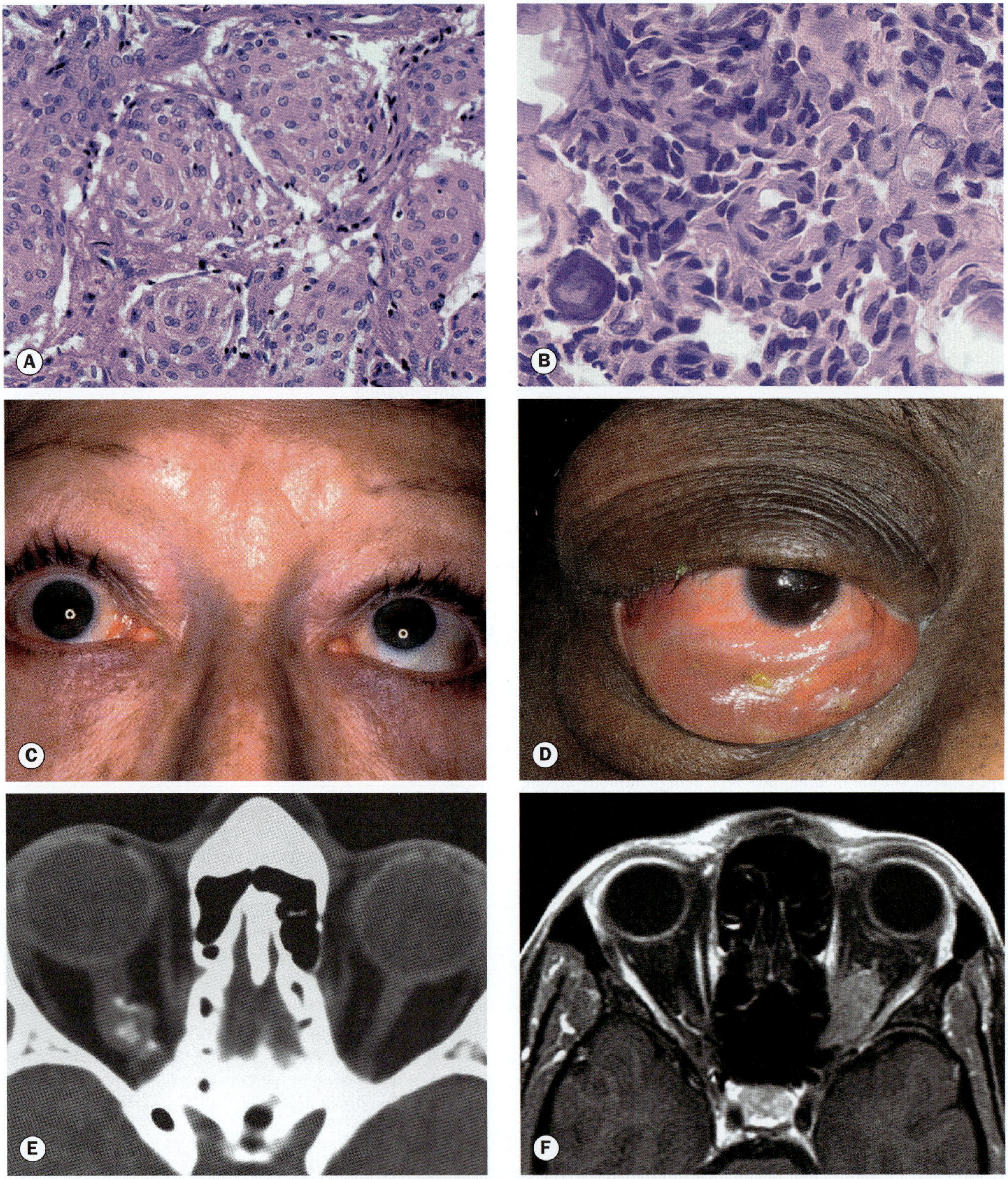

Fig. 4.40 Optic nerve meningioma. **(A)** Meningothelial histopathology; **(B)** psammomatous histopathology; **(C)** defective elevation of the right eye; **(D)** proptosis and severe chemosis; **(E)** axial CT of a small tumour showing calcification; **(F)** axial gadolinium-enhanced T1-weighted MRI showing lesion associated with left optic nerve. *(Courtesy of J Harry and G Misson, from* Clinical Ophthalmic Pathology, *Butterworth-Heinemann 2001 – figs A and B; A Pearson – fig. E.)*

LYMPHOMA

Introduction

Lymphomas of the ocular adnexa constitute approximately 8% of all extranodal lymphomas. The majority of orbital lymphomas are non-Hodgkin and most of these (80%) are of B-cell origin (Fig. 4.41A). Those affected are typically older individuals. The condition may be primary, involving one or both orbits only, or secondary if there are one or more identical foci elsewhere in the body. A substantial proportion of apparently primary lesions will develop disease elsewhere within a few years. The course is variable and relatively unpredictable. In some patients, histological features raise suspicion of malignancy and yet the lesion resolves spontaneously or with steroid treatment. Conversely, what appears to be reactive lymphoid hyperplasia may be followed by the development of lymphoma. Small lesions and those involving only the conjunctiva have the best prognosis. Conjunctival and intraocular lymphomas are discussed in Ch. 20.

Diagnosis

The onset is characteristically insidious.

- **Symptoms.** An absence of symptoms is common, but may include discomfort, double vision, a bulging eye or a visible mass.
- **Signs**
  - Any part of the orbit may be affected (Fig. 4.41B). Anterior lesions may be palpated and generally have a rubbery consistency (Fig. 4.41C).
  - Occasionally the lymphoma may be confined to the conjunctiva or lacrimal glands, sparing the orbit.
  - Local lymph nodes should be palpated, but systemic evaluation by an appropriate specialist is required.
- **Investigation**
  - Orbital imaging, usually with MRI (Fig. 4.41D).
  - Biopsy is usually performed to establish the diagnosis.
  - Systemic investigation to establish the extent of disease.

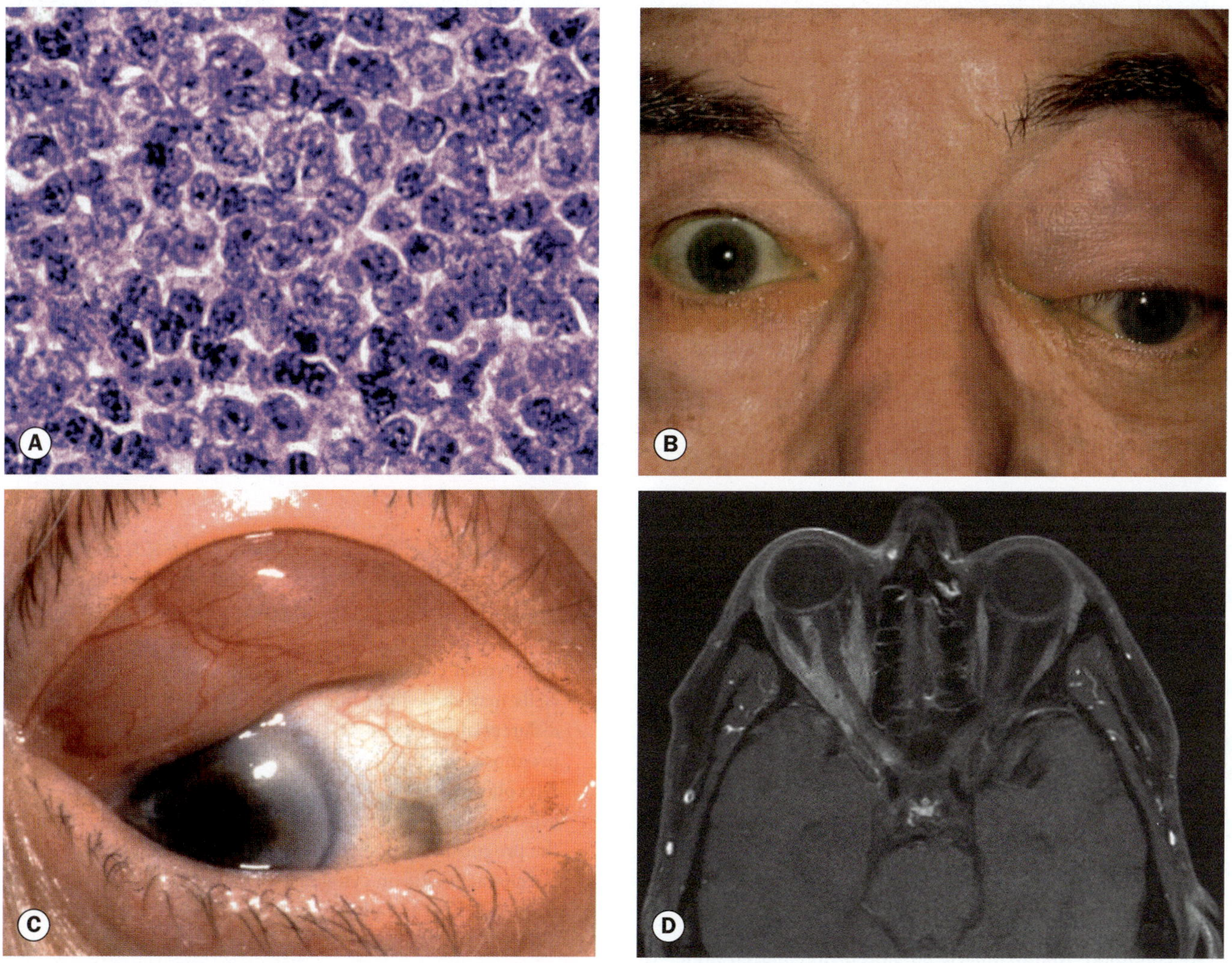

Fig. 4.41 Orbital lymphoma. **(A)** Histology showing neoplastic lymphoid cells; **(B)** involvement of the superior orbit causing proptosis and inferior dystopia; **(C)** anterior lesion; **(D)** axial, fat-saturated, gadolinium-enhanced T1-weighted MRI showing a tumour surrounding the right optic nerve sheath and extending to the orbital apex. *(Courtesy of J Harry and G Misson, from* Clinical Ophthalmic Pathology*, Butterworth-Heinemann 2001 – fig. A; A Pearson – fig. B.)*

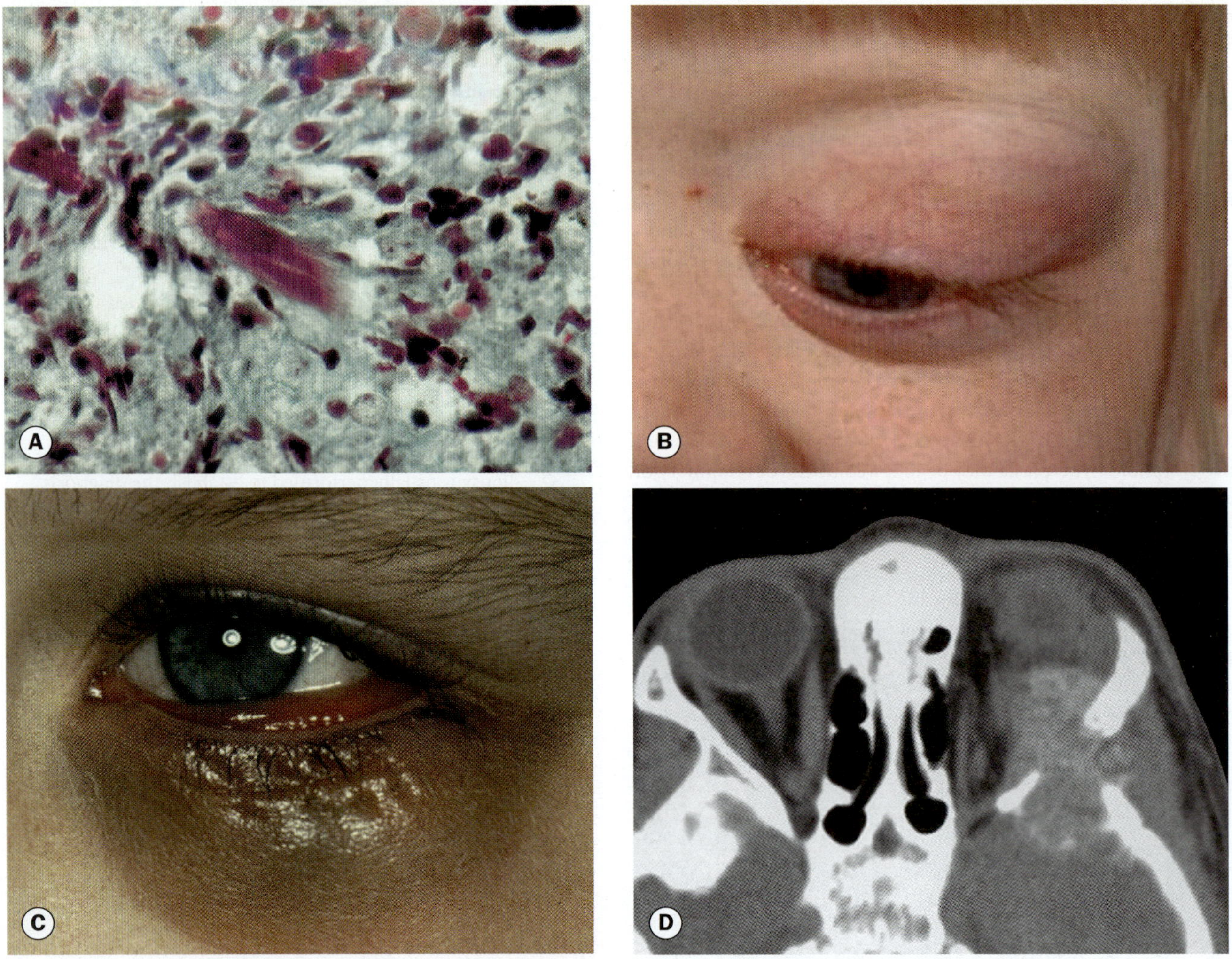

Fig. 4.42 Rhabdomyosarcoma. **(A)** Histology showing a differentiated tumour in which the rhabdomyoblast in the centre of the field has cross striations (Masson trichrome stain); **(B)** massive superiorly located lesion; **(C)** antero-inferiorly located lesion; **(D)** axial CT showing bony destruction and intracranial spread. *(Courtesy of J Harry and G Misson, from* Clinical Ophthalmic Pathology, *Butterworth-Heinemann 2001 – fig. A; G Rose – fig. B; S Chen – fig. D.)*

Treatment

Radiotherapy is used for localized lesions and chemotherapy for disseminated disease and some subtypes. Immunotherapy (e.g. rituximab) is a newer modality that may assume a dominant role in the future. Occasionally a well-defined orbital lesion may be resected.

RHABDOMYOSARCOMA

Introduction

Rhabdomyosarcoma (RMS) is the most common soft tissue sarcoma of childhood: 40% develop in the head and neck. It is the most common primary orbital malignancy in children but is still a rare condition. Approximately 90% occur in children under 16 years and the average age of onset is 7 years. The tumour is derived from undifferentiated mesenchymal cells that have the potential to differentiate into striated muscle. Various genetic predispositions have been identified, including variants of the *RB1* gene responsible for retinoblastoma. Emerging evidence supports the role of epigenetic dysregulation in rhabdomyosarcoma. Four subtypes are recognized:

- **Embryonal** constitutes the majority (85%) of orbital lesions. Cells may show light microscopic features of striated muscle differentiation (Fig. 4.42A). Embryonal usually carries a good prognosis.
- **Alveolar** makes up most of the balance of orbital RMS. Fewer cells show skeletal muscle differentiation than embryonal and the prognosis is worse. Particular chromosomal translocations are characteristic on cytogenetic analysis of biopsy material.
- **Botyroid** (4%) and **pleomorphic** RMS are much less common in the orbit.

TIP Rhabdomyosarcoma can mimic an orbital infection in a child.

Diagnosis

- **Symptoms.** Rapidly progressive unilateral proptosis is usual and may mimic an inflammatory condition such as orbital cellulitis.
- **Signs**
  - The tumour is most commonly superonasal or superior (Fig. 4.42B), but may arise anywhere in the orbit, including inferiorly (Fig. 4.42C). It can also arise in other tissues, such as conjunctiva and uvea.
  - Swelling and redness of overlying skin develop but the skin is not warm.
  - Diplopia is frequent, but pain is less common.
- **Investigation**
  - MRI shows a poorly defined mass.
  - CT shows a poorly defined mass of homogeneous density, often with adjacent bony destruction (Fig. 4.42D).
  - Incisional biopsy is performed to confirm the diagnosis and establish the histopathological subtype and cytogenetic characteristics.
  - Systemic investigation for metastasis should be performed, with lung and bone being the most common sites.

Treatment

Commonly used guidelines for staging and a corresponding treatment protocol were produced by the Intergroup Rhabdomyosarcoma Study Group (IRSG). Treatment encompasses a combination of radiotherapy, chemotherapy and sometimes surgical debulking. A single oncogenic fusion gene is associated with treatment resistance and a 40–45% decrease in overall survival. Entinostat with chemotherapy may improve the prognosis in selected cases of rhabdomyosarcoma, but has not yet been approved for clinical use. The prognosis for patients with disease confined to the orbit is good.

METASTATIC TUMOURS

Adult metastatic tumours

Introduction

Orbital metastases are an infrequent cause of proptosis and are much less common than metastases to the choroid. If the orbit is the site of initial manifestation of the tumour, the ophthalmologist may be the first specialist to see the patient. In approximate order of frequency, the most common primary sites are breast (up to 70%), bronchus, prostate, skin (melanoma), gastrointestinal tract and kidney.

Diagnosis

- **Signs.** Associated with the range of tumours that can spread to the orbit, presentation can take a variety of forms.
  - Dystopia and proptosis (Fig. 4.43A) are the most common features.
  - Infiltration of orbital tissues characterized by ptosis, diplopia, brawny indurated periorbital skin and a firm orbit, with resistance to manual retropulsion of the globe.
  - Enophthalmos with scirrhous tumours.
  - Chronic inflammation.
  - Primarily with cranial nerve involvement (II, III, IV, V, VI) and only mild proptosis with orbital apex lesions.
- **Investigation**
  - Imaging: CT (Fig. 4.43B) and MRI typically show a non-encapsulated mass.
  - Fine needle biopsy is useful for histological confirmation. If this fails, open biopsy may be required.
  - A search for a primary must be carried out if the patient was not previously known to have cancer.

Treatment

Treatment is aimed at preserving vision and relieving pain, because most patients die within a year (average 4 months). Radiotherapy

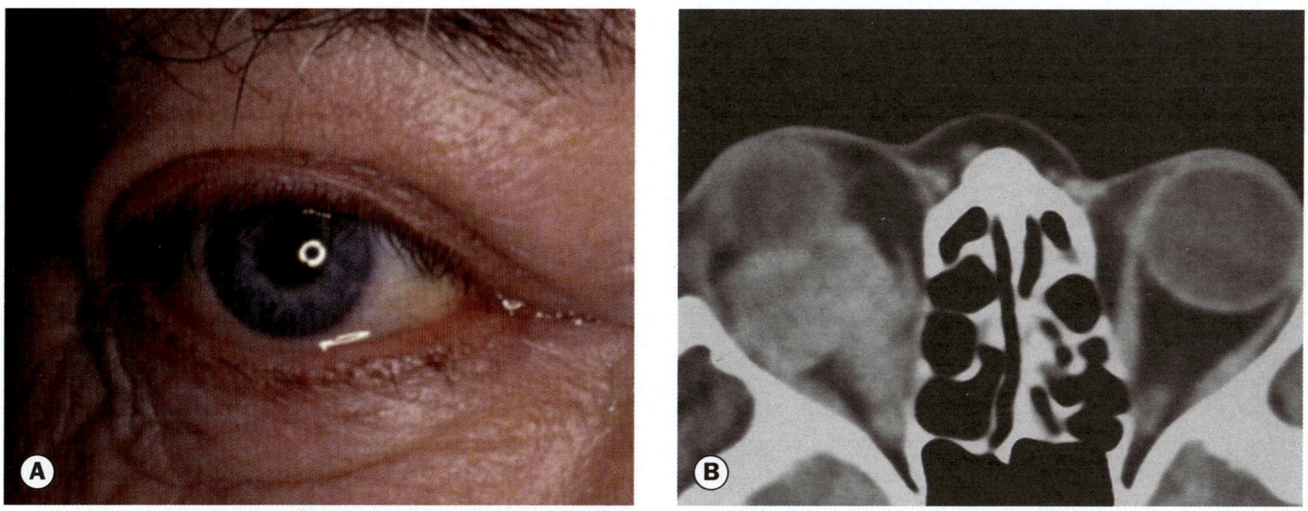

Fig. 4.43 Metastatic renal carcinoma. **(A)** Proptosis; **(B)** axial CT showing a non-encapsulated retrobulbar mass.

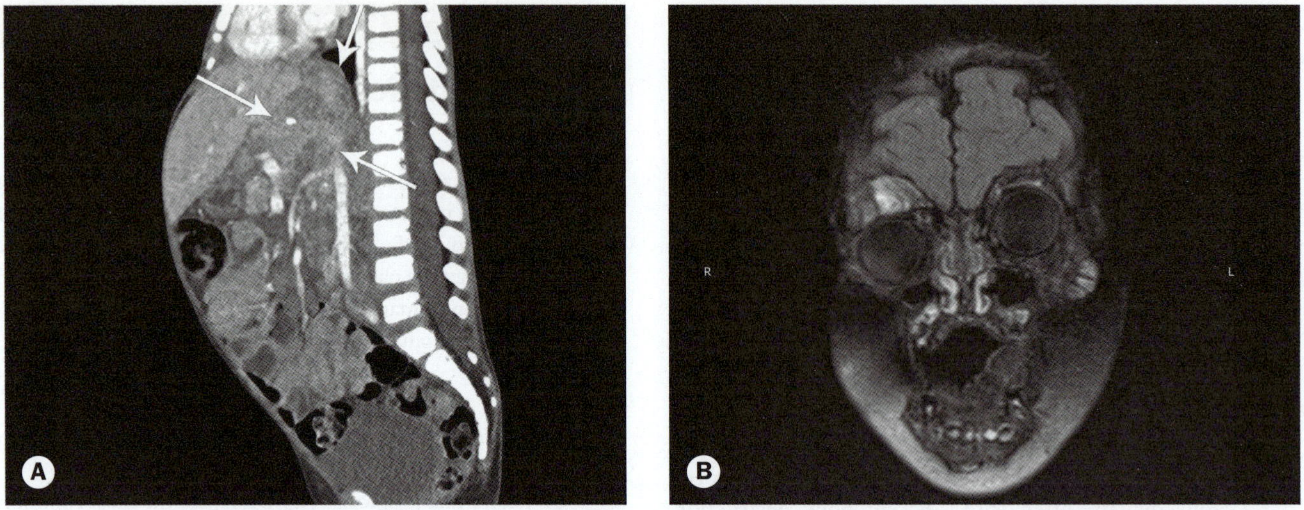

Fig. 4.44 Neuroblastoma in a child. **(A)** Abdominal CT scan showing a large retroperitoneal mass (arrows) with calcification, elevating the liver; **(B)** coronal MRI T2-weighted FLAIR sequence, showing a secondary tumour in the right upper orbit. *(Courtesy of E Blanco.)*

is the mainstay of local treatment, but systemic therapy may also be of benefit. Surgical excision of the focus is occasionally carried out. Orbital exenteration is usually only performed if other modalities fail to control intolerable symptoms.

Childhood metastatic tumours

Neuroblastoma

Neuroblastoma is one of the most common childhood malignancies. It arises from neural crest-derived tissue of the sympathetic nervous system, most commonly in the abdomen (Fig. 4.44A). Presentation is usually in early childhood. In almost half of all cases the tumour is disseminated at diagnosis, when it carries a very poor prognosis. Orbital metastases may be bilateral and typically present with the abrupt onset of proptosis accompanied by a superior orbital mass and lid ecchymosis. MRI shows the orbital tumour (Fig. 4.44B).

Myeloid sarcoma

Myeloid sarcoma (granulocytic sarcoma) is a solid tumour composed of malignant cells of myeloid origin. Because the tumour may exhibit a characteristic green colour it was formerly referred to as chloroma. Myeloid sarcoma may occur as a manifestation of established myeloid leukaemia, or it may precede the disease. Orbital involvement usually presents at about age 7 years with the rapid onset of proptosis, sometimes bilateral and can be associated with ecchymosis and lid oedema. When orbital involvement precedes systemic leukaemia, the diagnosis may be difficult.

Langerhans cell histiocytosis

Langerhans cell histiocytosis is a rare group of disorders due to clonal proliferations of histiocytes. Presentation ranges from localized disease, usually with bone destruction (eosinophilic granuloma), through multifocal bone involvement to a fulminant systemic disease. Soft tissues are less commonly involved, but cutaneous and visceral lesions may occur. Orbital involvement consists of unilateral or bilateral osteolytic lesions and soft tissue involvement, typically in the superotemporal quadrant. Patients with solitary lesions tend to have a more benign course and respond well to treatment with local curettage and intralesional steroid injection or radiotherapy. Systemic disease has a worse prognosis.

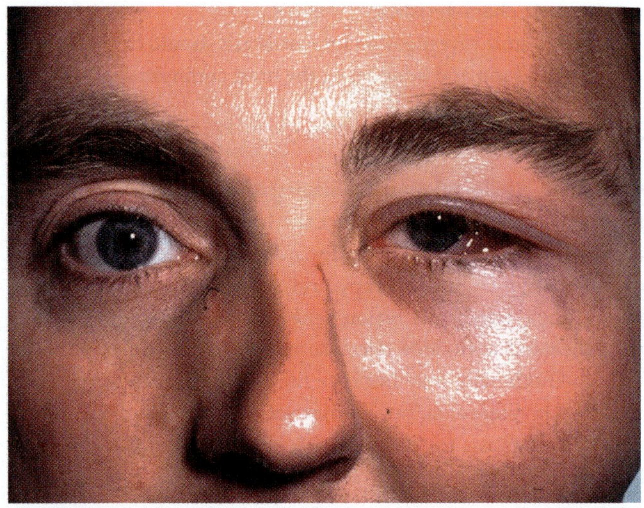

Fig. 4.45 Advanced maxillary carcinoma showing facial swelling and upward dystopia.

Orbital invasion from adjacent structures

Sinus tumours

Malignant tumours of the paranasal sinuses, although rare, may invade the orbit and carry a poor prognosis unless diagnosed early. It is therefore important to be aware of both their otorhinolaryngological and ophthalmic features.

- **Maxillary carcinoma** is by far the most common sinus tumour to invade the orbit (Fig. 4.45).

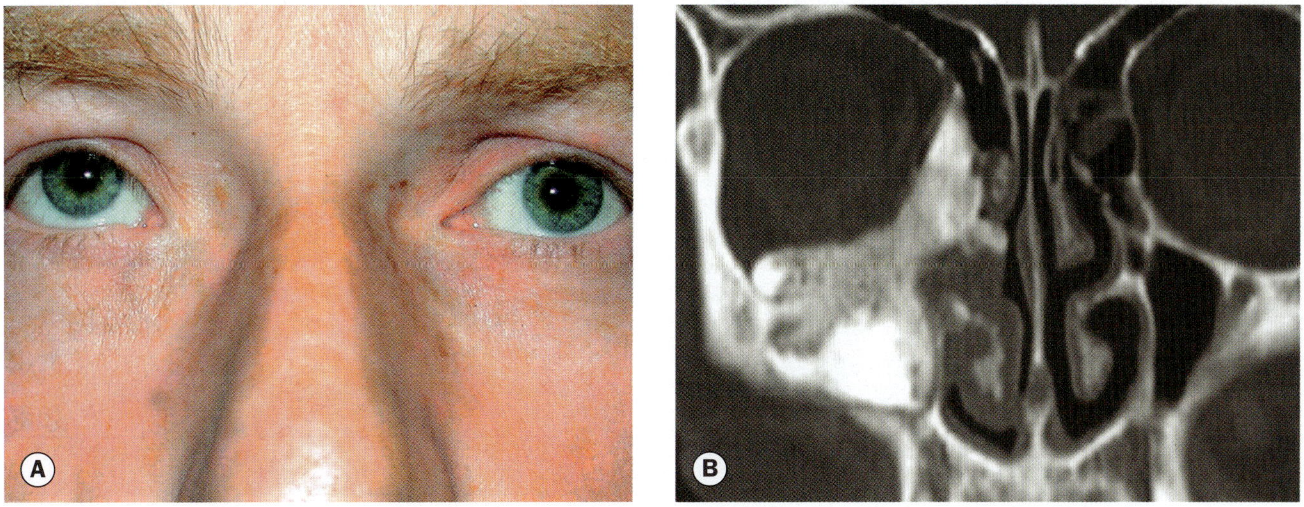

Fig. 4.46 Fibrous dysplasia of the orbit. **(A)** Upward displacement of the right eye; **(B)** coronal CT scan showing involvement of the floor and medial wall of the right orbit. *(Courtesy of A Pearson.)*

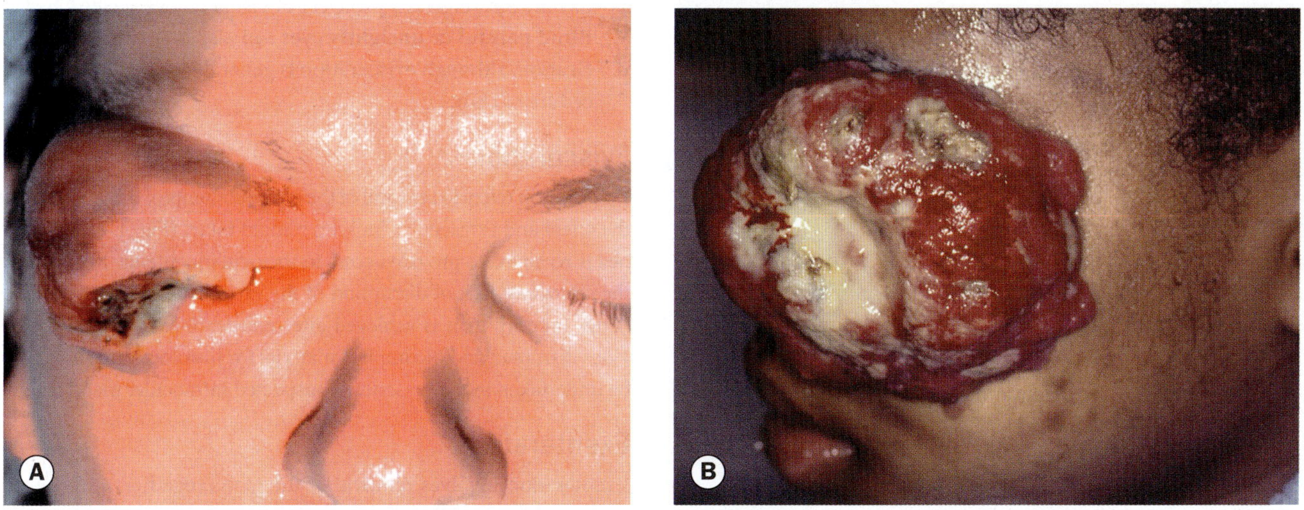

Fig. 4.47 **(A)** Orbital invasion by conjunctival melanoma; **(B)** orbital invasion by retinoblastoma.

  - Otorhinolaryngological manifestations include facial pain and swelling, epistaxis and nasal discharge.
  - Ophthalmic features include upward dystopia, diplopia and epiphora.
- **Ethmoidal carcinoma** may cause lateral dystopia.
- **Nasopharyngeal carcinoma** may spread to the orbit through the inferior orbital fissure; proptosis is a late finding.

Bony invasion

- **Intracranial meningioma** arising from the sphenoid ridge may invade the orbit by direct spread and cause proptosis (see Fig. 19.58). Occasionally tumours arising from the tuberculum sellae or olfactory groove may invade the orbit through the superior orbital fissure or optic canal.
- **Fibrous dysplasia** is a disorder in which fibrous tissue develops instead of normal bone, leading to weakening and a mass effect usually in childhood or early adulthood. Within the orbital region this may cause facial asymmetry, proptosis, dystopia (Fig. 4.46) and visual loss. Most orbital disease is due to the monostotic form. Polyostotic disease is associated with endocrine disorders and cutaneous pigmentation (McCune–Albright syndrome – 10% of cases).

Orbital invasion from eyelid, conjunctival and intraocular tumours

- Orbital invasion may occur from eyelid malignancies such as basal cell carcinoma, squamous cell carcinoma or sebaceous gland carcinoma, from conjunctival tumours (e.g. melanoma – Fig. 4.47A) and from intraocular tumours such as choroidal melanoma or retinoblastoma (Fig. 4.47B).

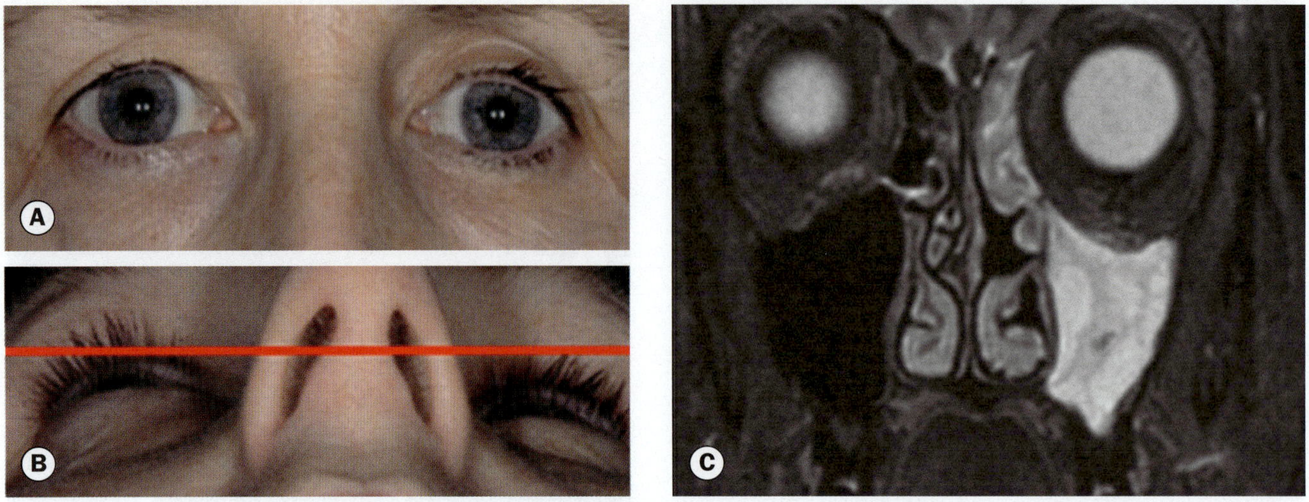

Fig. 4.48 Silent sinus syndrome. **(A)** Left enophthalmos and ptosis; **(B)** left enophthalmos; **(C)** coronal T2-weighted MRI showing opacification and volume loss of left maxillary sinus. *(Courtesy of JH Norris.)*

SILENT SINUS SYNDROME

In this rare condition, which usually affects middle-aged people, there is spontaneous asymptomatic collapse of the maxillary sinus and orbital floor secondary to a negative pressure in the sinus. The same problem may sometimes involve the frontal and ethmoidal sinuses. The diagnosis is confirmed by undertaking a CT scan.

Signs

- Facial asymmetry.
- Enophthalmos (Fig. 4.48A and B).
- Diplopia secondary to inferior oblique muscle entrapment may rarely occur.
- MRI shows maxillary sinus outlet obstruction, sinus opacification and sinus volume loss (Fig.4.48C).

Treatment

- **Early surgery** produces better results than delayed surgery.
- **Surgical treatment** involves restoring sinus function by improving the drainage from the sinus. Reconstruction of the orbital floor can be undertaken at the same time, but most authorities recommend waiting a further 6–8 months, as spontaneous remodeling of the orbital floor often occurs.

THE ANOPHTHALMIC SOCKET

Surgical procedures

Removal of an eye or the contents of the orbit may be indicated for intraocular or orbital malignancy or where the eye is blind and painful or unsightly. A number of different surgical and rehabilitation techniques are available.

Enucleation

Enucleation (removal of the globe) is indicated in the following circumstances:

- **Primary intraocular malignancies** where other treatment modalities are not appropriate. The tumour is left intact within the eye for histopathological examination.
- **After severe trauma** where the risk of sympathetic ophthalmitis may outweigh any prospect of visual recovery (see Ch. 22).
- **Blind painful or unsightly eyes** can also be managed by enucleation, although evisceration is generally considered the procedure of choice.

Evisceration

Evisceration refers to removal of the entire contents of the globe, whilst the sclera and extraocular muscles remain intact (Fig. 4.49). The cornea is removed to provide access to the ocular contents. Retention of the sclera and lack of disruption of the extraocular muscles provides better motility than is achieved after enucleation. Evisceration provides disrupted and incomplete material for histology and should not be undertaken in the presence of suspected intraocular malignancy.

Exenteration

Exenteration involves removal of the globe together with the soft tissues of the orbit (Fig. 4.50). Indications include:

- **Orbital malignancy**, either primary or where a tumour has invaded the orbit from the eyelids, conjunctiva, globe or adnexa, when other forms of treatment have a very poor chance of success. Anteriorly sited tumours may allow relative sparing of posterior orbital tissue and posterior tumours may allow sparing of eyelid skin to line the socket. Following exenteration, prostheses can be attached to the surrounding skin with adhesive, mounted on glasses (Fig. 4.51), or secured with osseo-integrated magnets mounted on the orbital rim bones. The socket may be lined with skin or a split-skin graft, or left to heal by secondary intention.
- **Non-malignant disease** such as orbital mucormycosis is a rare indication.

Rehabilitation

Cosmetic shell

A cosmetic shell is an ocular prosthesis that is used to cover a phthisical or unsightly eye. The shell can restore volume and often provides a good cosmetic appearance, with reasonable motility as a result of transmitted movements from the globe.

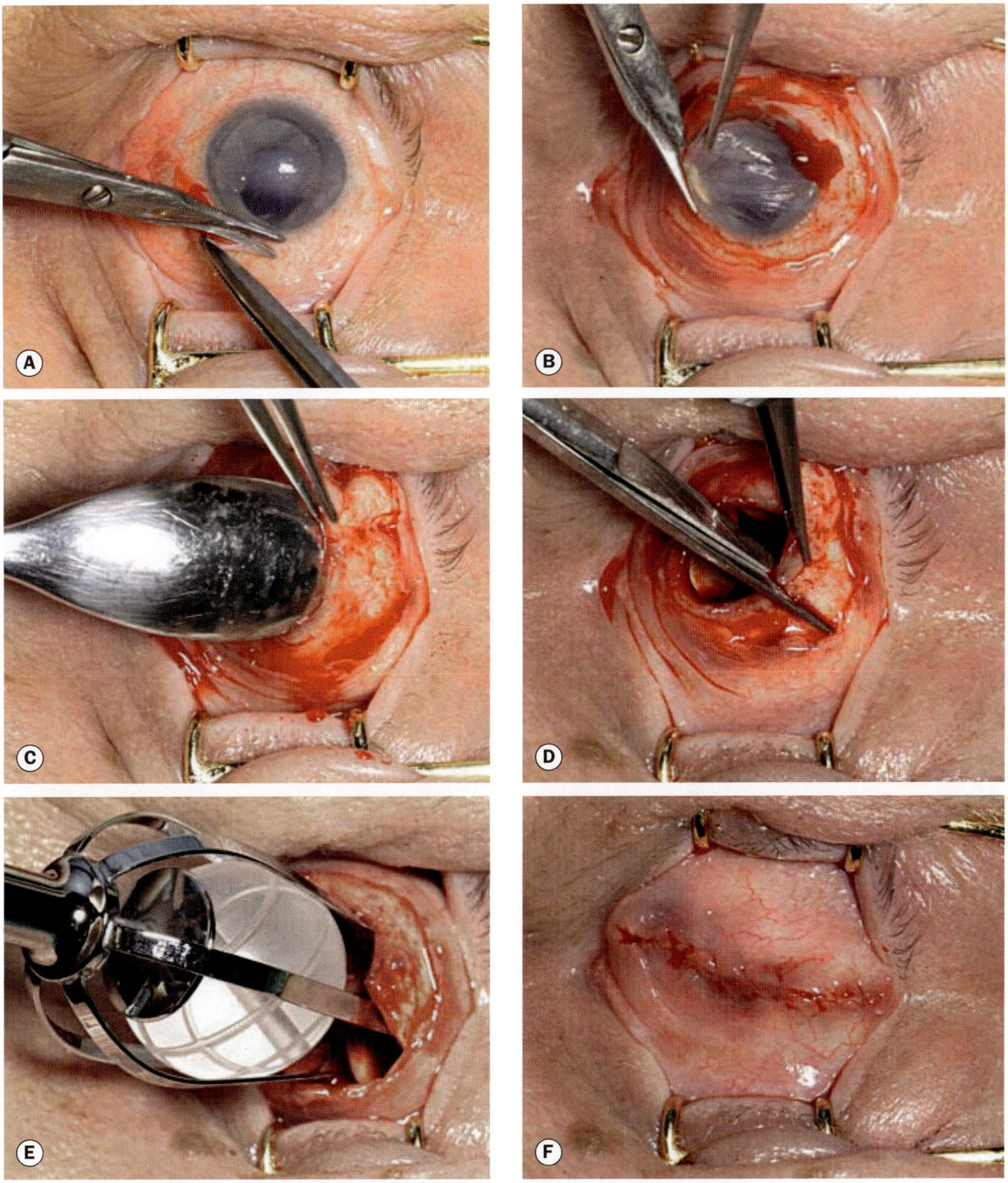

Fig. 4.49 Technique of evisceration. **(A)** Perilimbal conjunctival incision; **(B)** cornea removed with scissors; **(C)** evisceration spoon inserted between the uveal tract and sclera; **(D)** relieving incision in anterior sclera; **(E)** 22 mm ball is inserted with introducer; **(F)** anterior sclera closed with 6-0 absorbable sutures, followed by Tenon capsule and conjunctiva closed in two layers with 7-0 absorbable sutures. *(Courtesy of AG Tyers and JRO Collin, from* Colour Atlas of Ophthalmic Plastic Surgery, *Butterworth-Heinemann 2001.)*

Orbital implants

- **Orbital volume reduction.** Enucleation or evisceration leads to a reduction in volume of the orbital contents. A large prosthetic eye without an underlying orbital implant does not provide a satisfactory solution, due to stretching of the lower lid under its weight and to poor motility.

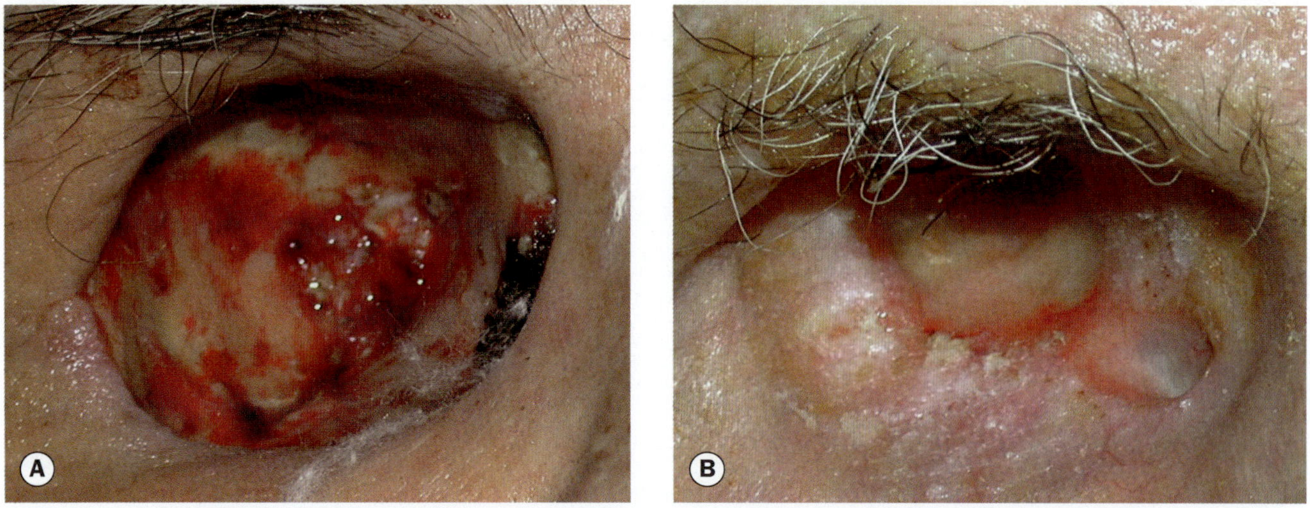

Fig. 4.50 Exenteration. **(A)** Including eyelid removal, 2 days postoperatively; **(B)** patient in **(A)** 6 months later. *(Courtesy of S Chen.)*

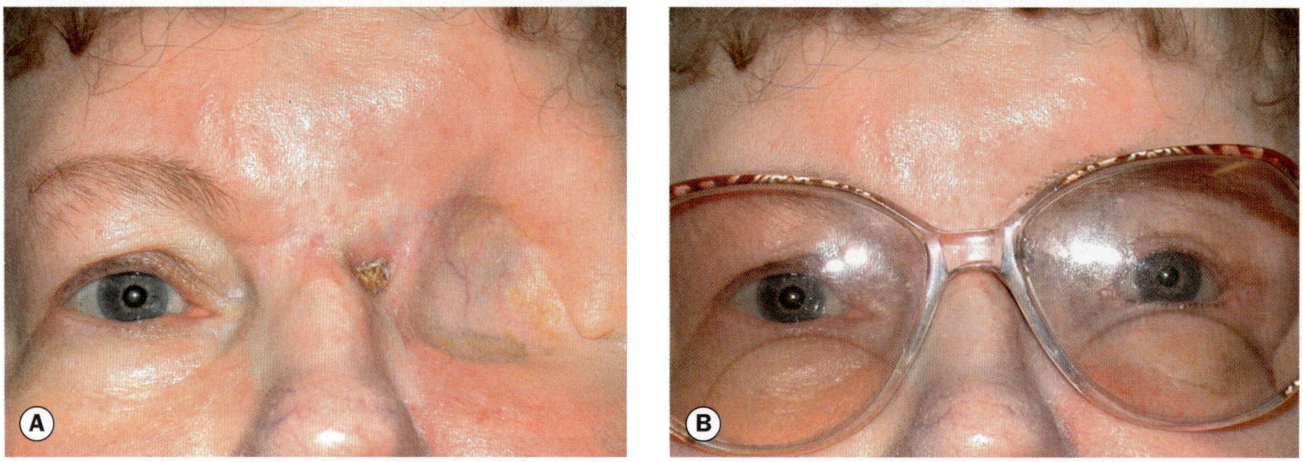

Fig. 4.51 **(A)** Healed exenteration; **(B)** prosthesis attached to glasses. *(Courtesy of A Pearson.)*

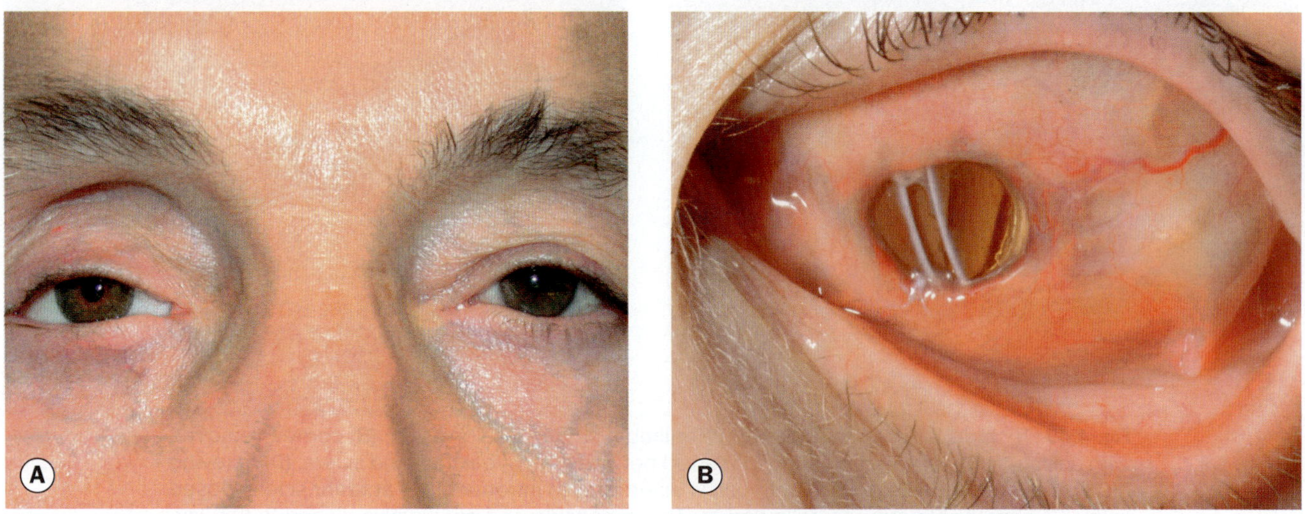

Fig. 4.52 **(A)** Right post-enucleation socket syndrome (PESS); **(B)** extruding ball implant.

- **An implant** is usually inserted during the surgery at which the eye is removed, though secondary placement can be performed later or a previously inserted implant exchanged. Implant materials may be solid ('non-integrated', e.g. silicone, acrylic) or porous ('integrated', e.g. polyethylene, hydroxyapatite). Fibrovascular ingrowth into the latter facilitates motility of an overlying prosthesis.
- **Post-enucleation socket syndrome** (PESS) describes a combination of signs that occur as a consequence of a volume deficit of

the orbital tissues. PESS is particularly common if an implant is not used. Some months after enucleation, the upper lid loses its support and drops down over the prosthesis. In time, the prosthesis tilts backwards and turns upwards, which puts forward pressure on the lower eyelid shallowing the fornix and causing drooping of the lower lid (Fig. 4.52A). The main features are:

  - Enophthalmos.
  - Upper lid ptosis.
  - Superior sulcus hollowing.
  - Sagging lower lid.
  - Surgical options include: (a) the insertion of a secondary implant if there is an absence of an implant; (b) the insertion of a silicone block into the inferior orbit if there is an implant; or (c) the implantation of a dermis-fat graft.

- **A peg** can also be inserted into porous implants to improve later motility, though the peg must be covered *in situ* by socket tissue and cannot attach directly to the overlying prosthesis. The motility of unpegged implants is also usually good, particularly if donor sclera or a mesh wrap is used and the extraocular muscles secured to the surface.
- **Extrusion** (Fig. 4.52B) is a significant concern with all implants. Careful placement of an implant, ensuring it is sufficiently deep and is well covered with vascularized tissue, is more important than the choice of implant material.

Ocular prosthesis

After enucleation or evisceration, a conformer (Fig. 4.53A) made of silicone or acrylic material is placed to support the conjunctival fornices and remains in place until the socket is fitted with an artificial eye (Fig. 4.53B). Initial socket impression moulds can usually be taken at around 6–8 weeks postoperatively and a temporary artificial eye placed whilst waiting for manufacture of a prosthesis shaped to fit the individual socket and matched to the fellow eye (Fig. 4.53C and D).

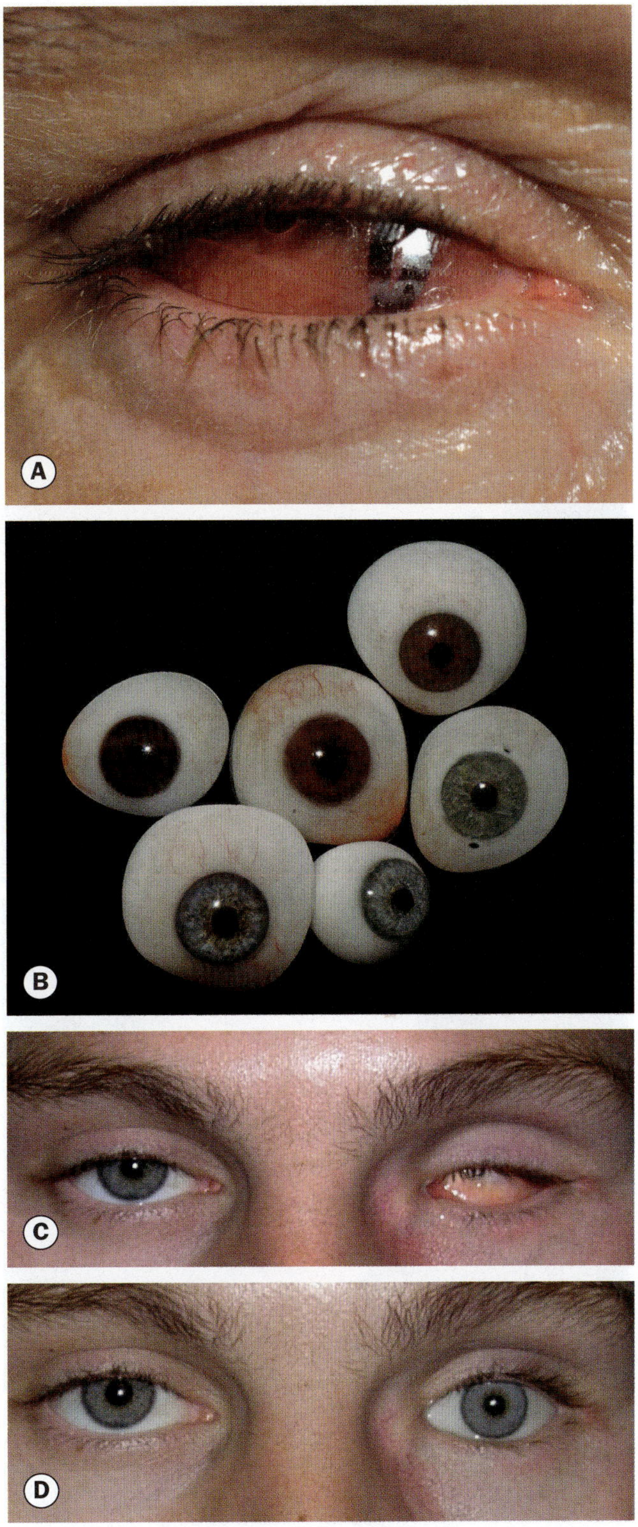

Fig. 4.53 **(A)** Conformer in place; **(B)** a selection of artificial eyes; **(C)** empty socket; **(D)** matching prosthesis in place. *(Courtesy of C Barry – fig. B; S Chen – figs C and D.)*

CRANIOSYNOSTOSES

The craniosynostoses are a group of rare congenital conditions in which an abnormally shaped skull results from premature closure of skull sutures.

- **Crouzon syndrome** features a short anteroposterior skull diameter, with midfacial hypoplasia giving a prominent lower jaw (Fig. 4.54A). Proptosis due to shallow orbits and hypertelorism (wide orbital separation) are the most conspicuous ocular features (Fig. 4.54B). Vision-threatening complications include exposure keratopathy and optic atrophy, mechanisms including chronic papilloedema and cerebral hypoperfusion secondary to sleep apnoea. Strabismus ('V' exotropia – see Fig. 4.54B), ametropia and amblyopia can occur and other ocular associations have been reported. Inheritance is usually autosomal dominant (AD); allelic variants in the gene *FGFR2* are responsible.
- **Apert syndrome** is the most severe of the craniosynostoses. Oxycephaly (conical skull), midfacial hypoplasia with a beaked nose and low-set ears (Fig. 4.54C), syndactyly (Fig. 4.54D) and developmental delay (30%) may be present. Shallow orbits, proptosis and hypertelorism are generally less pronounced than in Crouzon syndrome, but the same vision-threatening complications occur. Inheritance can be AD, but in the majority of cases the condition is sporadic and associated with older parental age. As with Crouzon syndrome, it is frequently the result of mutations in *FGFR2*.
- **Pfeiffer syndrome** features midfacial hypoplasia and down-slanting palpebral fissures (Fig. 4.54E and F). Ocular features are similar to Apert syndrome. Inheritance is AD with genetic heterogeneity.

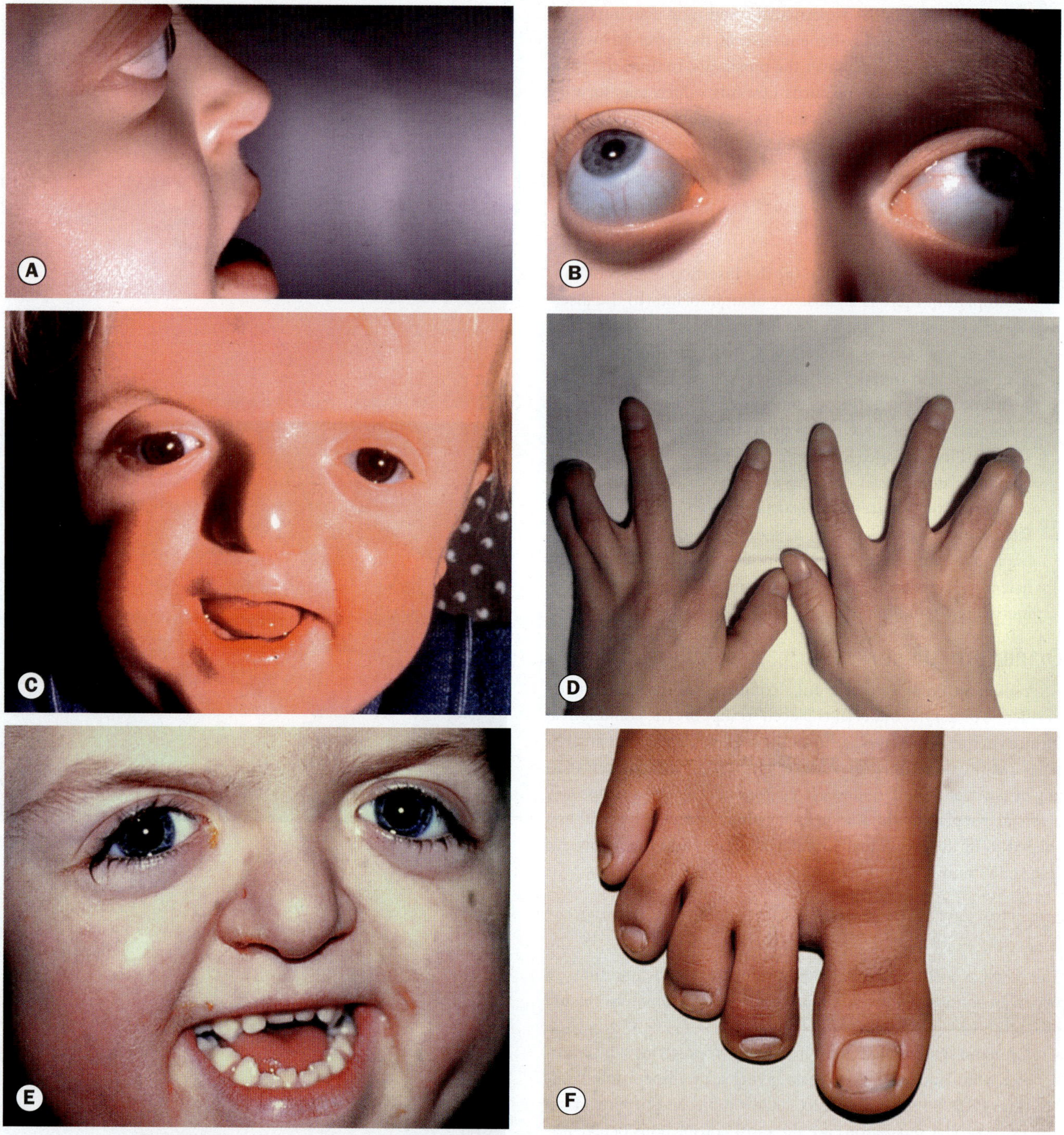

Fig. 4.54 Craniosynostosis. **(A)** Proptosis in Crouzon syndrome; **(B)** proptosis and hypertelorism – a 'V' exotropia is also shown; **(C)** Apert syndrome showing mild shallow orbits, midfacial hypoplasia and 'parrot-beak' nose and **(D)** syndactyly; **(E)** Pfeiffer syndrome showing midfacial hypoplasia and down-slanting palpebral fissures and **(F)** broad big toe. *(Courtesy of Ken K Nischal – figs E and F.)*

Chapter

Dry Eye 5

INTRODUCTION

Definitions

Dry eye occurs when there is inadequate tear volume or function, resulting in an unstable tear film and ocular surface disease. It is an extremely common condition, particularly in postmenopausal women and the elderly.

- **Dry eye disease** is a multifactorial disease of the ocular surface and tear film accompanied by increased osmolarity of the tear film and inflammation of the ocular surface.
- **Keratoconjunctivitis sicca** (KCS) refers to any eye with some degree of dryness.
- **Xerophthalmia** describes a dry eye associated with vitamin A deficiency.
- **Xerosis** refers to the extreme ocular dryness and keratinization that occurs in eyes with severe conjunctival cicatrization.
- **Sjögren syndrome** is an autoimmune inflammatory disease of which dry eyes is a feature.

Physiology

Tear film constituents

The tear film has three layers (Fig. 5.1):

- **Lipid** layer secreted by the meibomian glands.
- **Aqueous** layer secreted by the lacrimal glands.
- **Mucous** layer secreted principally by conjunctival goblet cells.

The constituents are complex, with as many as a hundred distinct proteins identified.

Spread of the tear film

The tear film is mechanically distributed over the ocular surface through a neuronally controlled blinking mechanism. Three factors are required for effective resurfacing of the tear film:

- Normal blink reflex.
- Contact between the external ocular surface and the eyelids.
- Normal corneal epithelium.

Lipid layer

- **Composition**
  - The outer lipid layer is composed of a polar phase containing phospholipids adjacent to the aqueous-mucin phase and a non-polar phase containing waxes, cholesterol esters and triglycerides.
  - The polar lipids are bound to lipocalins within the aqueous layer. These are small secreted proteins that have the ability to bind hydrophobic molecules and may also contribute to tear viscosity.
  - Lid movement during blinking is important in releasing lipids from glands. The thickness of the layer can be increased by forced blinking and conversely reduced by infrequent blinking.
- **Functions**
  - To prevent evaporation of the aqueous layer and maintain tear film thickness.
  - To act as a surfactant allowing spread of the tear film.
  - Deficiency results in evaporative dry eye.

Aqueous layer

- **Secretion**
  - The main lacrimal glands produce about 95% of the aqueous component of tears and the accessory lacrimal glands of Krause and Wolfring produce the remainder.
  - Secretion of tears has basic (resting) and much greater reflex components. The latter occurs in response to corneal and conjunctival sensory stimulation, tear break-up and ocular inflammation and is mediated via the fifth cranial nerve. It is reduced by topical anaesthesia and falls during sleep. Secretion can increase 500% in response to injury.
- **Composition**
  - Water, electrolytes, dissolved mucins and proteins.
  - Growth factors derived from the lacrimal gland, the production of which increases in response to injury.
  - Pro-inflammatory interleukin cytokines that accumulate during sleep when tear production is reduced.

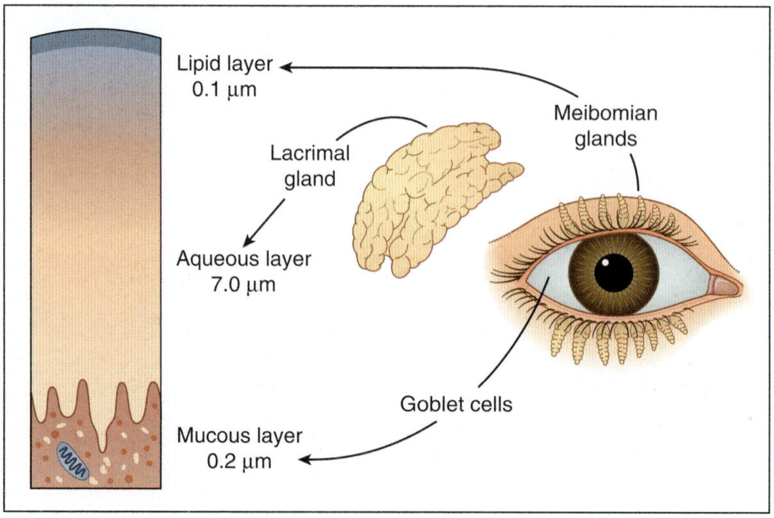

Fig. 5.1 The three layers of the tear film.

- **Functions**
  - To provide atmospheric oxygen to the corneal epithelium.
  - Antibacterial activity due to proteins such as IgA, lysozyme and lactoferrin.
  - To wash away debris and noxious stimuli and facilitate the transport of leukocytes after injury.
  - To optically enhance the corneal surface by abolishing minute irregularities.

Mucous layer

- **Composition**
  - Mucins are high-molecular-weight glycoproteins that may be transmembrane or secretory in type.
  - Secretory mucins are further classified as gel-forming or soluble. They are produced mainly by conjunctival goblet cells but also by the lacrimal glands.
  - The superficial epithelial cells of the cornea and conjunctiva produce transmembrane mucins that form their glycocalyx (extracellular coating).
  - Staining of diseased epithelium with rose Bengal indicates that the transmembrane and gel mucous layers are absent and the cell surface exposed. Damage to the epithelial cells will prevent normal tear film adherence.
- **Functions**
  - To permit wetting by converting the corneal epithelium from a hydrophobic to a hydrophilic surface.
  - Lubrication.
  - Deficiency of the mucous layer may be a feature of both aqueous deficiency and evaporative states. Goblet cell loss occurs with cicatrizing conjunctivitis, vitamin A deficiency, chemical burns and toxicity from medications.

Regulation of tear film components

- **Hormonal**
  - Androgens are the prime hormones responsible for regulation of lipid production.
  - Oestrogens and progesterone receptors in the conjunctiva and the lacrimal glands are essential for the normal function of these tissues.
- **Neural** via fibres adjacent to the lacrimal glands and goblet cells that stimulate aqueous and mucus secretion.

Mechanism of disease

The four core inter-related mechanisms thought to be responsible for the manifestations of dry eye are **tear instability**, **tear hyperosmolarity**, **inflammation** and **ocular surface damage**. Inflammation in the conjunctiva and accessory glands as well as the ocular surface is present in 80% of patients with KCS and may be both a cause and consequence of dry eye, amplifying and perpetuating disease. The presence of inflammation is the rationale for specific anti-inflammatory measures such as steroid therapy. There is a strong association between dry eye syndrome and reduced levels of systemic androsterone sulphate and epiandrosterone sulphate.

Classification

The classification of dry eye usually applied is that of the 2007 International Dry Eye Workshop (DEWS), with a basic division into aqueous-deficient and evaporative types. Most individuals have considerable overlap between mechanisms and it is important to be aware during patient assessment of the likely presence of multiple contributory factors.

Aqueous-deficient

- **Sjögren syndrome** dry eye (primary or secondary).
- **Non-Sjögren** syndrome dry eye.
  - Lacrimal deficiency: primary (e.g. age-related dry eye, congenital alacrima, familial dysautonomia) or secondary (e.g. inflammatory and neoplastic lacrimal gland infiltration, acquired immunodeficiency syndrome (AIDS), graft-versus-host disease, lacrimal gland or nerve ablation).
  - Lacrimal gland duct obstruction, e.g. trachoma, cicatricial pemphigoid, chemical injury, Stevens–Johnson syndrome.
  - Reflex hyposecretion: sensory (e.g. contact lens wear, diabetes, refractive surgery, neurotrophic keratitis) or motor block (e.g. seventh cranial nerve damage, systemic drugs).

Evaporative

- **Intrinsic**
  - Meibomian gland deficiency, e.g. posterior blepharitis, rosacea.
  - Disorders of lid aperture, e.g. excessive scleral show, lid retraction, proptosis, facial nerve palsy.
  - Low blink rate, e.g. Parkinson disease, prolonged computer monitor use, reading, watching television.
  - Drug action, e.g. antihistamines, beta-blockers, antispasmodics, diuretics.
- **Extrinsic**
  - Vitamin A deficiency.
  - Topical drugs including the effect of preservatives.
  - Contact lens wear.
  - Ocular surface disease, such as allergic conjunctivitis.

TIP Whether a patient has primary aqueous deficiency or evaporative dry eye, the end result is ocular surface inflammation and discomfort.

Effect of environmental factors

As well as the basic classification, DEWS draws attention to the effect of the environment on the type of dry eye with which a patient presents. These can be both internal factors, such as age, hormonal status and behaviour patterns, and external, such as the exacerbation of evaporative factors in an atmosphere with low relative humidity.

SJÖGREN SYNDROME

Sjögren syndrome (SS) is an autoimmune disorder characterized by lymphocytic inflammation and destruction of lacrimal and salivary glands (Fig. 5.2A) and other exocrine organs. The classic clinical triad consists of dry eyes, dry mouth (Fig. 5.2B) and parotid gland enlargement (Fig. 5.2C), but other features are common and can affect all organ systems. The condition is classified as primary when it exists in isolation and secondary when associated with another disease, commonly rheumatoid arthritis or systemic lupus erythematosus. Primary SS affects females more frequently than males. Although in clinical practice the diagnosis may be made on less stringent grounds, the American College of Rheumatology (ACR) criteria for diagnosis specify, in patients with a clinical picture suggestive of SS, the following:

- Positivity for anti-SSA or anti-SSB antibodies, or positive rheumatoid factor together with significantly positive antinuclear antibody.
- Ocular surface staining above a certain grade.
- Focal lymphocytic sialadenitis to a specified extent on salivary gland biopsy (see Fig. 5.2A).

Widely used but older American-European Consensus Group criteria are more extensive and include more clinical findings, but give results consistent with the ACR criteria.

Treatment options for SS include a range of symptomatic treatments for dry eye, as discussed below, dry mouth and other manifestations, salivary stimulants (e.g. oral pilocarpine) and, in some cases, immunosuppression and biological blockers such as rituximab.

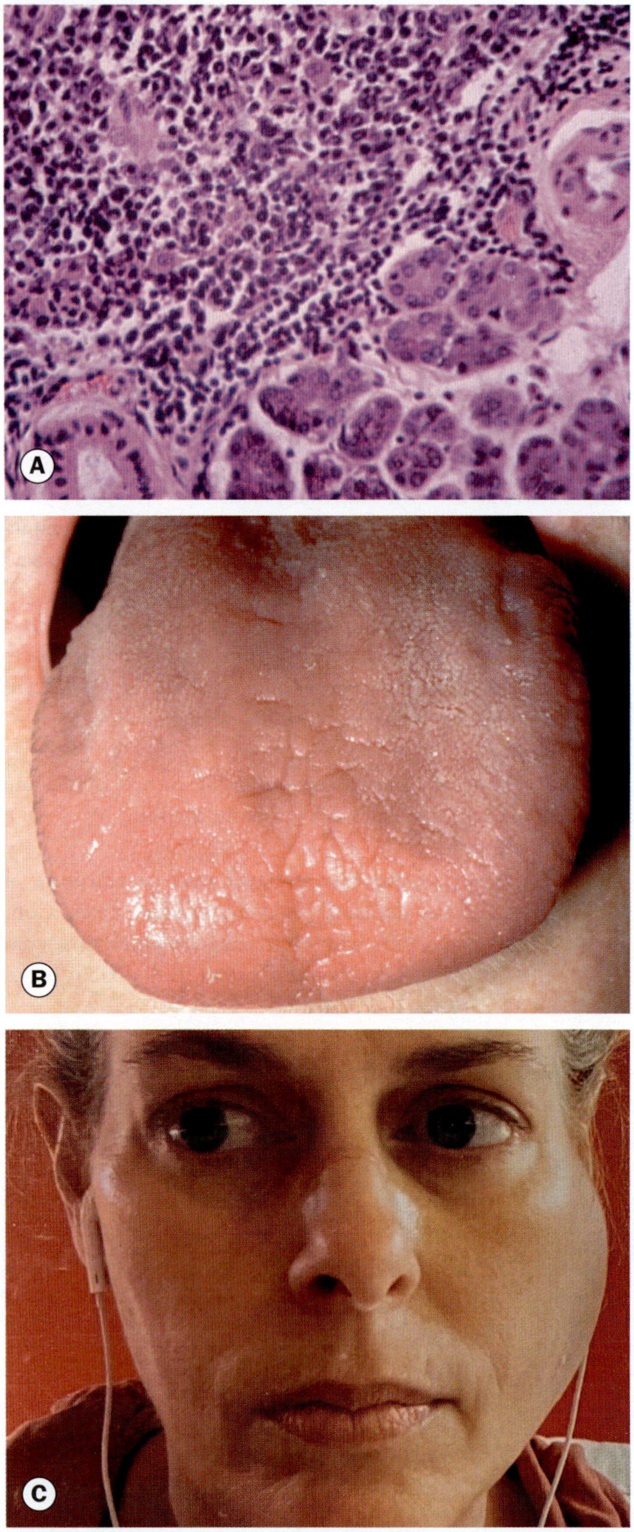

Fig. 5.2 Sjögren syndrome. **(A)** Histology of the lacrimal gland showing lymphocytic infiltration; **(B)** dry fissured tongue; **(C)** left parotid gland enlargement. *(Courtesy of J David – fig. C.)*

Clinical features

Symptoms

The most common ocular symptoms are feelings of dryness, grittiness and burning that characteristically worsen over the course of the day. Stringy discharge, transient blurring of vision, redness and crusting of the lids are also common. Lack of emotional or reflex tearing is unusual. The symptoms of KCS are frequently exacerbated on exposure to conditions associated with increased tear evaporation (e.g. air-conditioning, wind and central heating) or prolonged reading or video display unit use, when blink frequency is reduced.

TIP The symptoms associated with keratoconjunctivitis sicca are exacerbated by exposure to wind, air-conditioning and central heating.

Signs

- **Posterior (seborrhoeic) blepharitis** with meibomian gland dysfunction is often present (Fig. 5.3A and B).
- **Conjunctiva**
  - Redness.
  - Staining with rose Bengal (Fig. 5.4A) and lissamine green (Fig. 5.4B).
  - Keratinization.
  - Conjunctivochalasis is a common response to, and exacerbating factor for, the chronic irritation of dry eye, such that a self-sustaining cycle is maintained. It also commonly occurs in other ocular surface diseases (see Ch. 6).

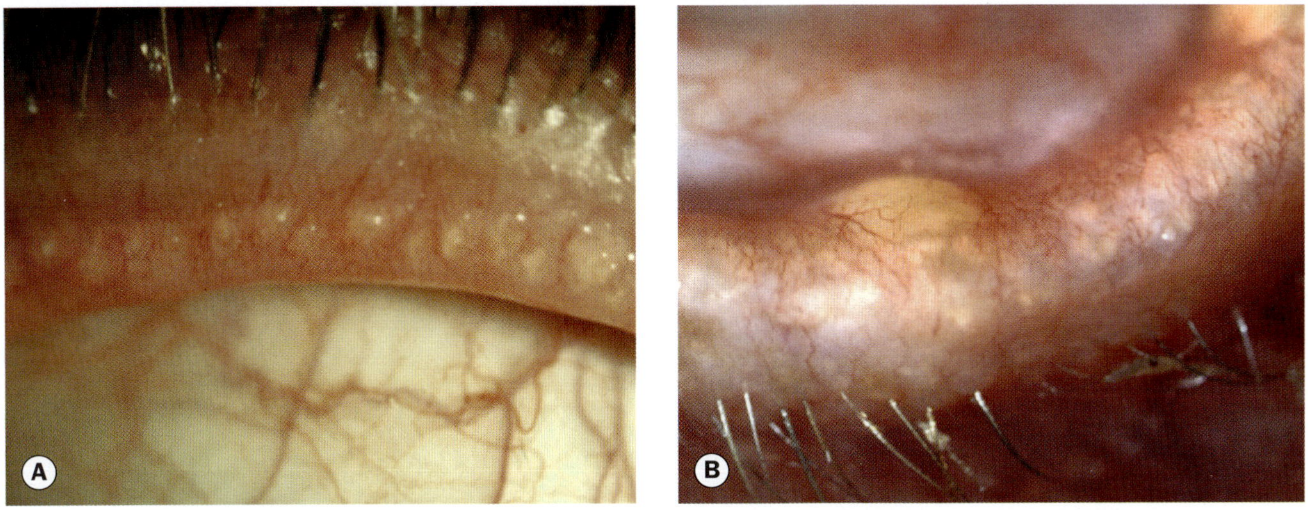

Fig. 5.3 Posterior blepharitis in dry eye. **(A)** Oil globules at meibomian gland orifices; **(B)** inflamed meibomian gland.

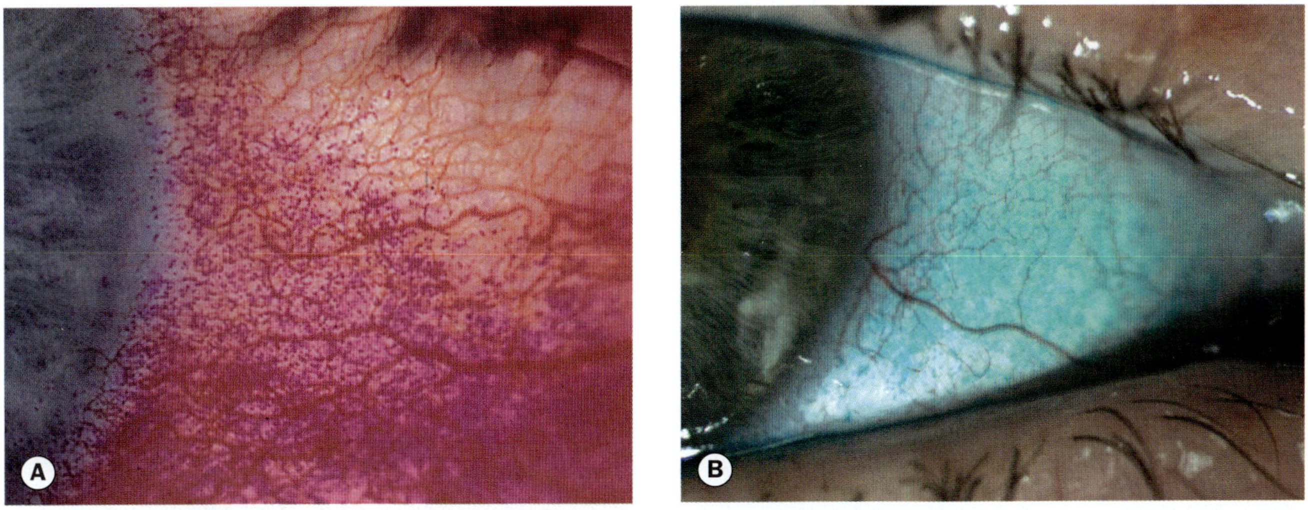

Fig. 5.4 Conjunctival staining in dry eye. **(A)** Rose Bengal; **(B)** lissamine green.

- **Tear film**
  - In the normal eye, as the tear film breaks down, the mucin layer becomes contaminated with lipid but is washed away.
  - In the dry eye, the lipid-contaminated mucin accumulates in the tear film as particles and debris that move with each blink (Fig. 5.5A).
  - The marginal tear meniscus (strip) is a crude measure of the volume of aqueous in the tear film. In the normal eye the meniscus is 0.2–0.4 mm in height, but in dry eye becomes thin (less than 0.25 mm) or absent (Fig. 5.5B).
- **Cornea**
- Punctate epithelial erosions that stain well with fluorescein (Fig. 5.6A).
- Filaments consist of strands of mucus and debris (such as shed epithelial cells) and are typically attached at one end to the corneal surface (Fig. 5.6B). The filaments stain well with rose Bengal (Fig. 5.6C), but less so with fluorescein.
- Mucous plaques with similar constituents may occur in severe dry eye. They consist of semi-transparent, white-to-grey, often slightly elevated lesions of varying size (Fig. 5.6D).
- **Complications** can be vision-threatening and include epithelial breakdown, melting (Fig. 5.7A), perforation (Fig. 5.7B) and occasionally bacterial keratitis (Fig. 5.7C).

TIP A patient with symptomatic dry eye syndrome may present with superficial punctate keratitis, which can be seen clinically with fluorescein staining.

INVESTIGATION

The aim of investigation is to confirm and quantify a clinical diagnosis of dry eye. Although the symptoms in a given patient do not change, objective signs can fluctuate. The correlation between symptoms and tests is poor. However, the reliability of tests improves as the severity of dry eye increases. The tests measure the following parameters:

- Stability of the tear film as related to its break-up time (BUT).

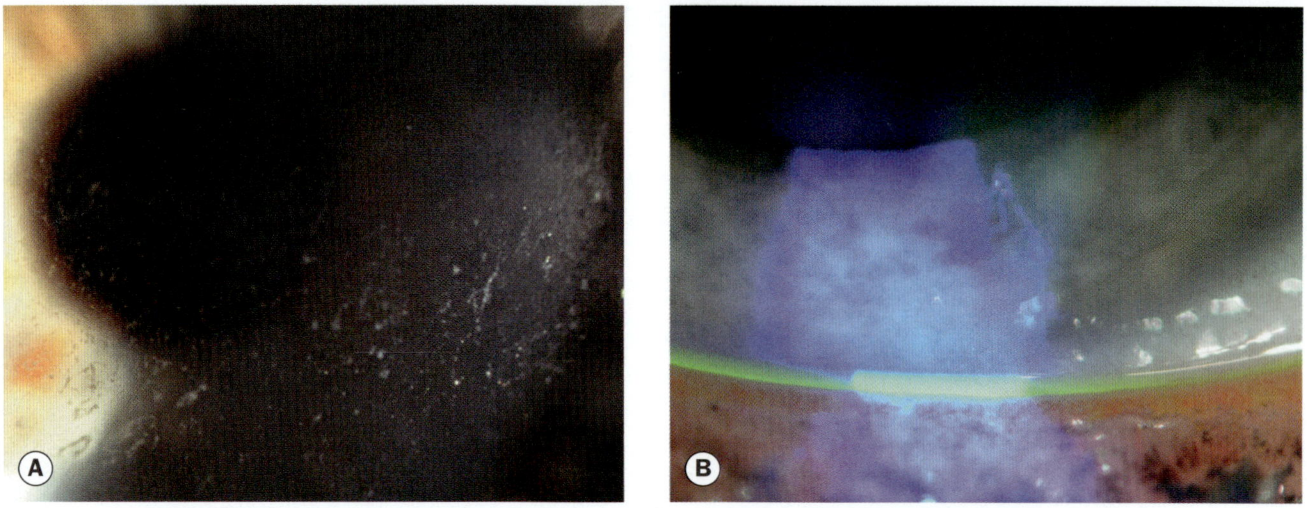

Fig. 5.5 Tear film abnormalities in dry eye. **(A)** Mucous debris; **(B)** thin marginal tear meniscus.

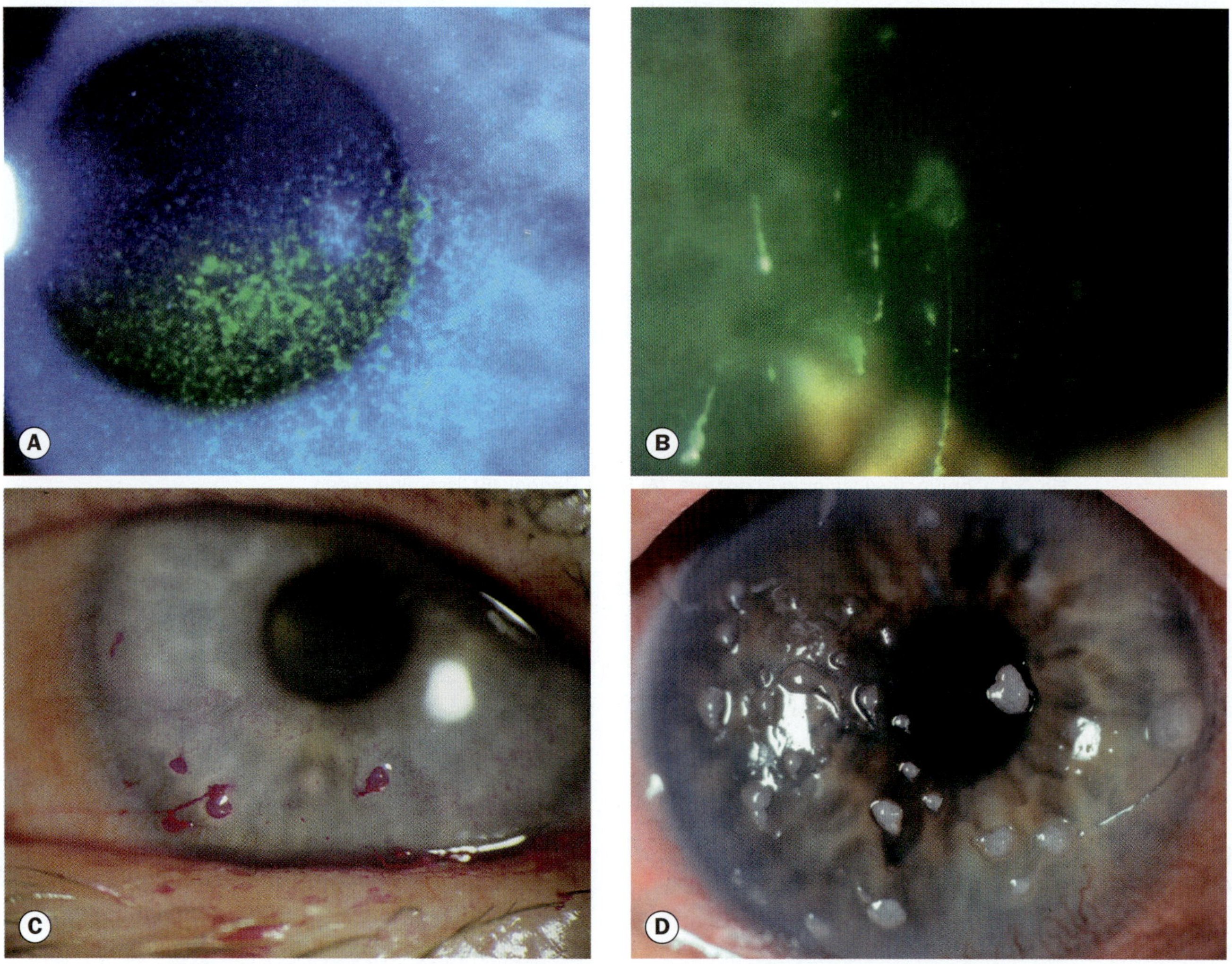

Fig. 5.6 Corneal signs in dry eye. **(A)** Punctate erosions stained with fluorescein; **(B)** corneal filaments; **(C)** mild (rose Bengal stain) and **(D)** severe mucous plaque formation. *(Courtesy of S Tuft – fig. B; R Bates – fig. D.)*

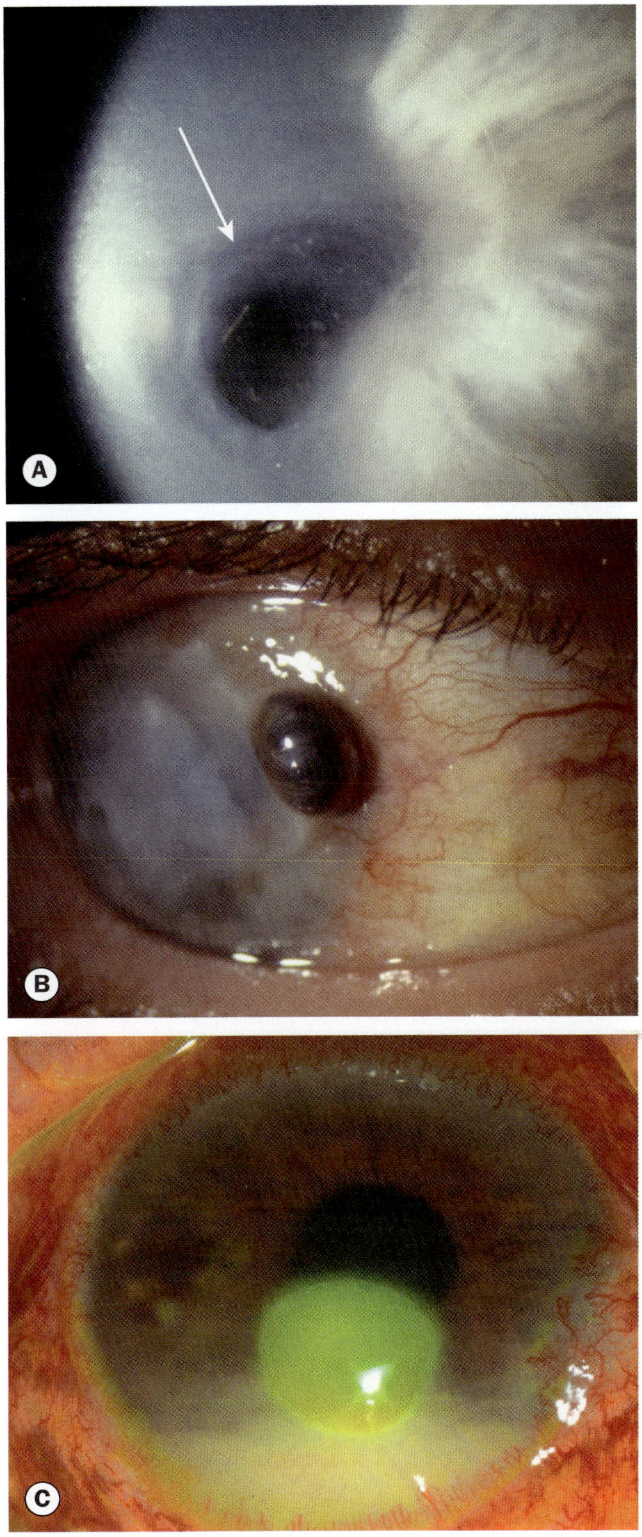

Fig. 5.7 Severe corneal complications of dry eye. **(A)** Melting (arrow); **(B)** perforation with iris plugging; **(C)** bacterial infection. *(Courtesy of S Tuft – fig. B; T Carmichael – fig. C.)*

TIP There is a poor correlation between symptoms and clinical tests in patients with dry eye syndrome. However, the reliability of tests improves as the severity increases.

- Tear production (Schirmer, fluorescein clearance and tear osmolarity).
- Ocular surface disease (corneal stains and impression cytology).

There is no clinical test that allows the diagnosis of evaporative dry eye to be definitively confirmed. It is therefore a presumptive diagnosis based on the presence of associated clinical findings. It is suggested the tests are performed in the following order because the Schirmer strip paper can damage the ocular surface and cause staining.

Tear film break-up time

The tear film BUT is abnormal in aqueous tear deficiency and meibomian gland disorders. It is measured as follows:

- Fluorescein 2% or an impregnated fluorescein strip moistened with non-preserved saline is instilled into the lower fornix.
- The patient is asked to blink several times.
- The tear film is examined at the slit lamp with a broad beam using the cobalt blue filter. After an interval, black spots or lines appear in the fluorescein-stained film (Fig. 5.8A), indicating the formation of dry areas.
- The BUT is the interval between the last blink and the appearance of the first randomly distributed dry spot. A BUT of less than 10 seconds is suspicious.

The development of dry spots always in the same location may indicate a local corneal surface abnormality (e.g. epithelial basement membrane disease) rather than an intrinsic instability of the tear film.

Schirmer test

The Schirmer test is a useful assessment of aqueous tear production. The test involves measuring the amount of wetting of a special (no. 41 Whatman) filter paper, 5 mm wide and 35 mm long. The test can be performed with or without topical anaesthesia. In theory, when performed with an anaesthetic (Schirmer 2) basic secretion is measured and without anaesthetic (Schirmer 1) it measures maximum basic plus reflex secretion. In practice, however, topical anaesthesia cannot abolish all sensory and psychological stimuli for reflex secretion. The test is performed as follows:

- Excess tears are delicately dried. If topical anaesthesia is applied the excess should be removed from the inferior fornix with filter paper.
- The filter paper is folded 5 mm from one end and inserted at the junction of the middle and outer third of the lower lid, taking care not to touch the cornea or lashes (Fig. 5.8B).
- The patient is asked to keep the eyes gently closed.
- After 5 minutes the filter paper is removed and the amount of wetting from the fold measured.
- Less than 10 mm of wetting after 5 minutes without anaesthesia or less than 6 mm with anaesthesia is considered abnormal.

Results can be variable and a single Schirmer test should not be used as the sole criterion for diagnosing dry eye, but repeatedly abnormal tests are highly supportive.

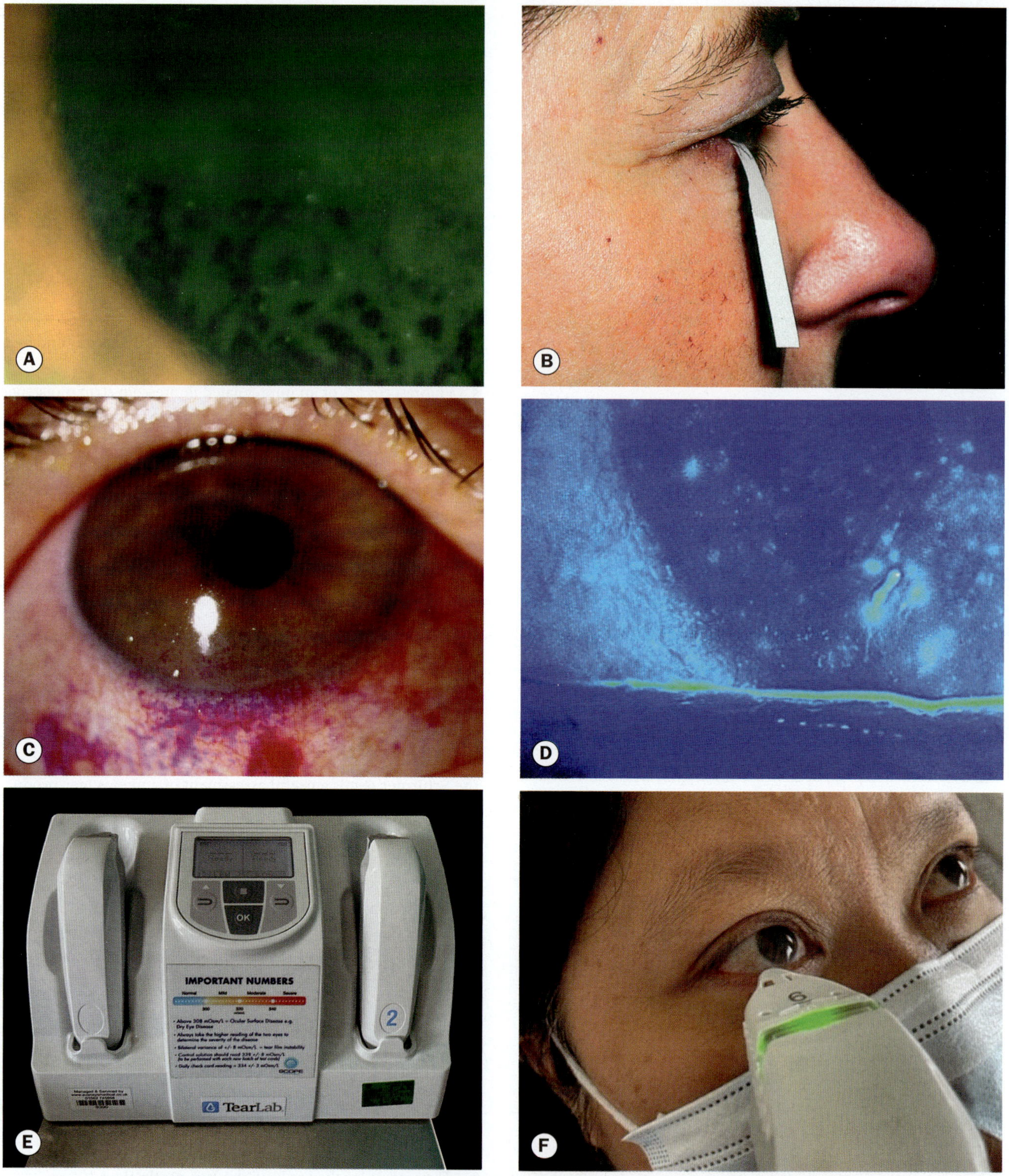

Fig. 5.8 Diagnostic tests in dry eye. **(A)** Tear film break-up time – numerous dry spots are present in a fluorescein-stained tear film; **(B)** Schirmer test; **(C)** corneal and conjunctival staining with rose Bengal and **(D)** with fluorescein; **(E)** TearLab instrument used to measure tear film osmolarity; **(F)** technique of obtaining a tear sample. *(Courtesy of G Ratnarajan – figs E and F.)*

Ocular surface staining

- **Fluorescein** stains corneal and conjunctival epithelium (see Fig. 5.6A) where there is sufficient damage to allow the dye to enter the tissues.
- **Rose Bengal** is a dye that has an affinity for dead or devitalized epithelial cells that have a lost or altered mucous layer (Fig. 5.8C). Corneal filaments and plaques (see Fig. 5.6B and D) are also shown up more clearly by the dye and the use of a red-free filter may help visualization. A 1% solution of rose Bengal or a moistened impregnated strip can be used. The dye may cause intense stinging that can last for up to a day, particularly in patients with severe KCS. To minimize irritation a very small drop should be used, immediately preceded by a drop of topical anaesthetic and the excess washed out with saline.
- **Lissamine green** stains in a similar fashion to rose Bengal but causes less irritation and may be preferred (see Fig. 5.4B).
- The **pattern** of staining may aid diagnosis:
  - Interpalpebral staining of the cornea and conjunctiva (see Fig. 5.4A and B) is common in aqueous tear deficiency.
  - Superior conjunctival stain may indicate superior limbic keratoconjunctivitis.
  - Inferior corneal and conjunctival stain is often present in patients with blepharitis or exposure (Fig. 5.8D).

TIP In dry eye syndrome lissamine green solution is preferable to 1% rose Bengal solution as it stains in a similar fashion, but causes less irritation.

Other investigations

The following tests are rarely performed in clinical practice.

- **Fluorescein clearance test** and the tear function index may be assessed by placing 5 µl of fluorescein on the ocular surface and measuring the residual dye in a Schirmer strip placed on the lower lateral lid margin at set intervals. Delayed clearance is observed in all dry eye states.
- **Tear film osmolarity** measurement techniques are available and are emerging as an accurate means of diagnosis (Fig. 5.8E and F). The threshold value that distinguishes between a healthy eye and an eye with dry eye syndrome varies from 305 mOsm/l and 316 mOsm/l, depending on the degree of tear film instability. A widely accepted threshold is 308 mOsm/l and a value of 316 mOsm/l appears to discriminate between mild and moderate/severe dry eye. Tear osmolarity may not correlate with ocular symptoms, but it does correlate with effective treatment when evaluated in the long term.
- **Tear constituent** measurement. Tear samples can be assayed for the presence of markers known to be elevated (e.g. matrix metalloproteinase-9) or decreased (e.g. lactoferrin) in dry eye.
- **Phenol red thread test** uses a thread impregnated with a pH-sensitive dye. The end of the thread is placed over the lower lid and the length wetted (the dye changes from yellow to red in tears) is measured after 15 seconds. A value of 6 mm is abnormal. It is comparable to the Schirmer test but takes less time to perform.
- **Tear meniscometry** is a technique to quantify the height and thus the volume of the lower lid meniscus.
- **Impression cytology** can determine goblet cell numbers.

TIP Measurement of tear film osmolarity is a useful tool when used to confirm the diagnosis and response to treatment in dry eye syndrome.

TREATMENT

Strategy

The underlying causative processes of dry eye are generally not reversible, and management is therefore structured around the control of symptoms and the prevention of surface damage. DEWS have produced guidelines based on earlier International Taskforce Guidelines for Dry Eye, in which suggested treatment options depend on the level of severity of disease graded from 1 to 4. The DEWS guidelines can also be applied in a graded approach, proceeding to the next level if the preceding measures are inadequate.

Level 1

- **Education and environmental/dietary modifications**
  - Establishment of realistic expectations and emphasis on the importance of compliance.
  - Lifestyle review, including the importance of blinking whilst reading, watching television or using a computer screen (which should be orientated below eye level to minimize palpebral aperture size) and the management of contact lens wear.
  - Environmental review, e.g. increasing humidity may be possible for some environments.
  - Instillation aids for eye drops (manufacturer-supplied or makeshift, such as nut-crackers to hold plastic bottles) should be advocated for patients with reduced dexterity (e.g. rheumatoid arthritis).
  - Caution the patient that laser refractive surgery can exacerbate dry eye.
- **Systemic medication review** to exclude contributory effects and eliminate offending agents. Discontinuation of toxic/preserved topical medication if possible.
- **Artificial tear substitutes, including gels and ointments** – see below. Some authorities advocate that use of preserved drops should fall within level 1 and categorize non-preserved drops as a level 2 measure. Mucolytic agents may be specifically indicated for some patients.
- **Eyelid therapy.** Basic measures such as warm compresses and lid hygiene for blepharitis. Reparative lid surgery (e.g. entropion, ectropion, excessive lid laxity or scleral show) may be considered as an early measure. Nocturnal lagophthalmos can be addressed by taping the lids closed at bedtime, wearing swimming goggles during sleep, or in extreme cases by lateral tarsorrhaphy.

Level 2

- **Non-preserved tear substitutes** are categorized as level 2 treatment by some authorities.
- **Anti-inflammatory agents** such as topical steroids, oral omega fatty acids and other agents such as topical ciclosporin.
- **Tetracyclines** (for meibomianitis, rosacea).
- **Punctal plugs.**
- **Secretagogues**, e.g. pilocarpine, cevimeline, rebamipide.
- **Moisture chamber spectacles and spectacle side shields.**

Level 3

- **Serum eye drops.** Autologous or umbilical cord serum.
- **Contact lenses.**
- **Permanent punctal occlusion.**

Level 4

- **Systemic anti-inflammatory agents.**
- **Surgery**
  - Eyelid surgery, such as tarsorrhaphy.
  - Salivary gland auto-transplantation.
  - Mucous membrane or amniotic membrane transplantation for corneal complications.

Tear substitutes

Tear substitutes have a relatively simple formulation that cannot approximate the complex components and structure of the normal tear film. Their delivery is also periodic rather than continuous. Almost all are based on replacement of the aqueous phase of the tear film. There are no mucus substitutes and paraffin is only an approximation to the action of tear lipids. The optimal frequency of instillation varies with agent and with severity.

- **Drops and gels.** A large range of preparations is available. One agent or category of preparation has not demonstrated superiority and particular agents are often preferred by individual patients with limited rationale.
  - Cellulose derivatives (e.g. hypromellose, methylcellulose) are appropriate for mild cases.
  - Carbomer gels adhere to the ocular surface and so are longer-lasting, but some patients are troubled by slight blurring.
  - Other agents include polyvinyl alcohol (PVA), which increases the persistence of the tear film and is useful in mucin deficiency, sodium hyaluronate, povidone, glycerine, propylene glycol, polysorbate and others.
  - Diquafosol is a newer agent that works as a topical secretagogue.
- **Ointments** containing petrolatum (paraffin) mineral oil can be used at bedtime to supplement daytime drops or gel instillation; daytime use is precluded by marked blurring. Some practitioners do not prescribe these for long-term use.
- **Eyelid sprays** are applied to the closed eye and typically contain a liposome-based agent that may stabilize the tear film and reduce evaporation.
- **Artificial tear inserts** emplaced once or twice daily offer extended duration treatment and are preferred by some patients.
- **Mucolytic agents.** Acetylcysteine 5% drops may be useful in patients with corneal filaments and mucous plaques, which acetylcysteine dissolves; it may cause stinging on instillation. Acetylcysteine is malodorous and has a limited shelf-life. Manual debridement of filaments may also be useful.
- **Preservatives** can be a potent source of toxicity, especially after punctal occlusion. Numerous non-preserved drops are now available, including some multi-dose products and in general should be used in preference to preservative-containing preparations in any more than mild disease or with instillation more than three or four times daily. If possible, preservative-free formulations should also be used for dry eye patients when other topical medication is required, for example in the treatment of glaucoma. Newer preservatives such as Polyquad and Purite seem to exhibit lower ocular surface toxicity than older agents such as benzalkonium chloride.
- **Haemoderivative treatment** has been used to manage severe ocular surface disease including graft-versus-host-related dry eye disease, Sjögren syndrome, post-LASIK dry eye persistent epithelial defects and recurrent erosions (see below).

TIP Excessive use of preserved lubricating eye drops can result in corneal toxicity.

Punctal occlusion

Punctal occlusion reduces drainage and thereby preserves natural tears and prolongs the effect of artificial tears. It is of greatest value in patients with moderate–severe KCS who have not responded to frequent instillation of topical agents.

- **Temporary** occlusion can be achieved by inserting collagen plugs into the canaliculi. These dissolve over a number of weeks. The main aim is to ensure that epiphora does not occur following permanent occlusion.
  - Initially the inferior puncta are occluded and the patient is reviewed after 1 or 2 weeks.
  - If the patient is now asymptomatic and without epiphora, the plugs can be removed and the inferior canaliculi permanently occluded (see below).
  - In severe KCS both the inferior and superior canaliculi can be plugged.
- **Reversible** prolonged occlusion can be achieved with silicone (Fig. 5.9) or long-acting (2–6 months) collagen plugs.
  - Problems include extrusion, granuloma formation and distal migration.
  - Plugs that pass into the horizontal portion of the canaliculus cannot be visualized and although they can usually be flushed out with saline, if they cause epiphora this is not always possible and surgical retrieval may be needed.
- **Permanent** occlusion should be undertaken only in patients with severe dry eye who have had a positive response to temporary plugs without epiphora. It should be avoided in

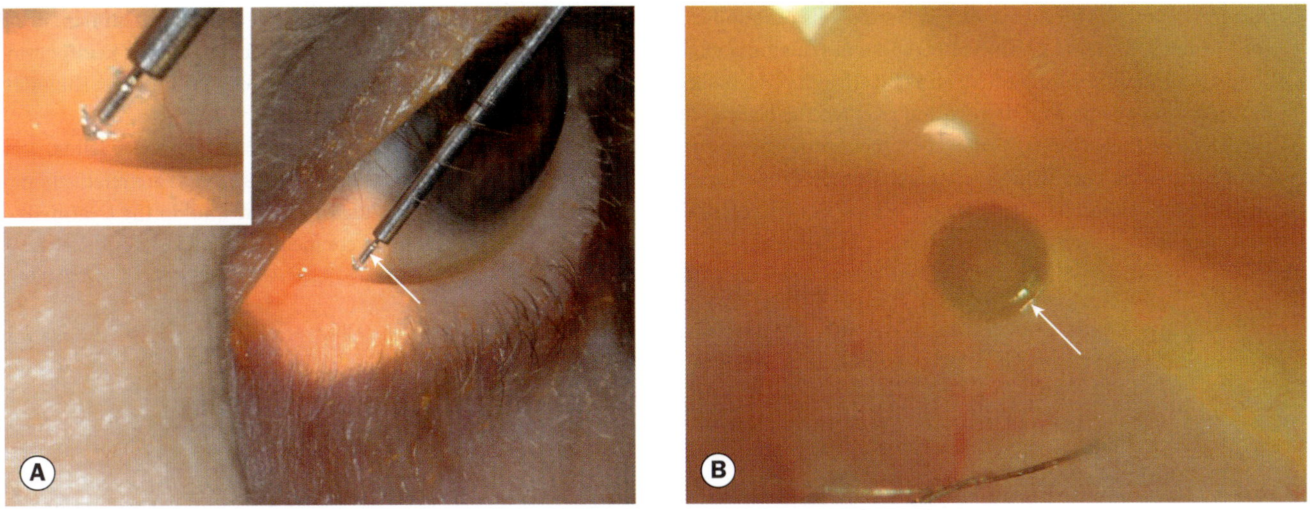

Fig. 5.9 **(A)** Insertion of a silicone plug (arrow); **(B)** plug in position (arrow).

patients, especially if young, who may have reversible pathology. All four puncta should not be occluded at the same time.

- Permanent occlusion is performed following punctal dilatation by coagulating the proximal canaliculus with cautery. Following successful occlusion, it is important to watch for signs of recanalization.
- Laser cautery seems to be less consistently effective than surgical thermal coagulation.

TIP Punctal occlusion with a silicone plug can be a useful therapeutic option in patients with moderate–severe keratoconjunctivitis sicca.

Anti-inflammatory agents

- **Topical steroids**, generally low-intensity preparations such as fluorometholone are effective supplementary treatment for acute exacerbations. The risks of longer-term treatment must be balanced against the potential benefits in each case.
- **Omega fatty acid supplements** (e.g. omega-3 fish oil, flax seed oil) can have a dramatic effect on symptoms and may facilitate the reduction of topical medication.
- **Oral tetracyclines** for an extended course, often 3 months at a relatively low dose, may control associated blepharitis, especially meibomianitis and reduce tear levels of inflammatory mediators. Doxycycline may be preferred to minocycline on the grounds of adverse effect profile.
- **Topical ciclosporin** (usually 0.05%) reduces T-cell-mediated inflammation of lacrimal tissue, resulting in an increase in the number of goblet cells and reversal of squamous metaplasia of the conjunctiva.

Contact lenses

Although contact lens wear can exacerbate dry eye, particularly due to inflammatory, sensory and evaporative effects, the symptoms can be outweighed by the reservoir effect of fluid trapped behind the lens. In addition, contact lenses are effective at relieving symptoms resulting from secondary corneal changes. However, patients should be cautioned that there is an increased risk of bacterial keratitis.

Several manufacturers have developed contact lenses specifically designed to reduce dry eye discomfort during lens wear. The materials used (silicone hydrogel) retain moisture for 12–16 hours and are single-use daily disposable. Occlusive gas-permeable scleral contact lenses provide a reservoir of saline over the cornea and are occasionally used in a patient with an extremely dry eye and exposure. Silicone rubber lenses, which were used in the past, are no longer available.

Optimization of environmental humidity

- **Reduction of room temperature** to minimize evaporation of tears.
- **Room humidifiers** may be tried but are frequently disappointing because much apparatus is incapable of significantly increasing the relative humidity of an average-sized room. A temporary local increase in humidity can be achieved with moist chamber goggles or side shields to glasses but may be cosmetically unacceptable.

Miscellaneous options

- **Botulinum toxin injection** to the orbicularis muscle may help control the blepharospasm that often occurs in severe dry eye. Injected at the medial canthus it can also reduce tear drainage, presumably by limiting lid movement.
- **Oral cholinergic agonists** such as pilocarpine (5 mg four times daily) and cevimeline may reduce the symptoms of dry eye and dry mouth in patients with Sjögren syndrome. Adverse effects including blurred vision and sweating may be less marked with cevimeline.
- **Submandibular gland transplantation** for extreme dry eye requires extensive surgery and may produce excessive levels of mucus in the tear film.

- **Serum/autologous blood eye drops.** Autologous or umbilical cord serum (20–100%), the blood component remaining after clotting, has produced subjective and objective improvements in studies in patients with dry eye and may aid the healing of persistent epithelial defects. However, their production and storage are associated with practical challenges. Finger prick autologous blood is a low cost, readily accessible and practical treatment that appears to be safe and effective.
- **Cenegermin 0.002%,** a topical recombinant human nerve growth factor (registered for use in neurotrophic keratopathy) may have a role to play in severe Sjögren disease. The safety and efficacy are being investigated.
- **Photobiomodulation therapy** applied to the eyelids. Low level light, red light and intense pulsed light are relatively new interventional options that may be helpful in the treatment of dry eye secondary to severe meibomian gland dysfunction.

Chapter 6

Conjunctiva

INTRODUCTION

Anatomy

The conjunctiva is a transparent mucous membrane that lines the inner surface of the eyelids and the anterior surface of the globe, terminating at the corneoscleral limbus. It is richly vascular, supplied by the anterior ciliary and palpebral arteries. There is a dense lymphatic network, with drainage to the preauricular and submandibular nodes corresponding to that of the eyelids. It has a key protective role, mediating both passive and active immunity. Anatomically, it is divided into the following:

- **The palpebral conjunctiva** starts at the mucocutaneous junction of the lid margins and is firmly attached to the posterior tarsal plates. The tarsal blood vessels are vertically orientated.
- **The forniceal conjunctiva is loose and redundant.**
- **The bulbar conjunctiva** covers the anterior sclera and is continuous with the corneal epithelium at the limbus. Radial ridges at the limbus form the palisades of Vogt, the likely reservoir of corneal stem cells. The stroma is loosely attached to the underlying Tenon capsule, except at the limbus, where the two layers fuse. The plica semilunaris (semilunar fold) is present nasally, medial to which lies a fleshy nodule (caruncle) consisting of modified cutaneous tissue.

Histology

- **The epithelium** is non-keratinizing and around five cell layers deep (Fig. 6.1). Basal cuboidal cells evolve into flattened polyhedral cells, subsequently being shed from the surface. Mucus-secreting goblet cells are located within the epithelium, being most dense inferonasally and in the fornices.
- **The stroma** (substantia propria) consists of richly vascularized loose connective tissue. The accessory lacrimal glands of Krause and Wolfring are located deep within the stroma. Secretions from the accessory lacrimal glands are essential components of the tear film.

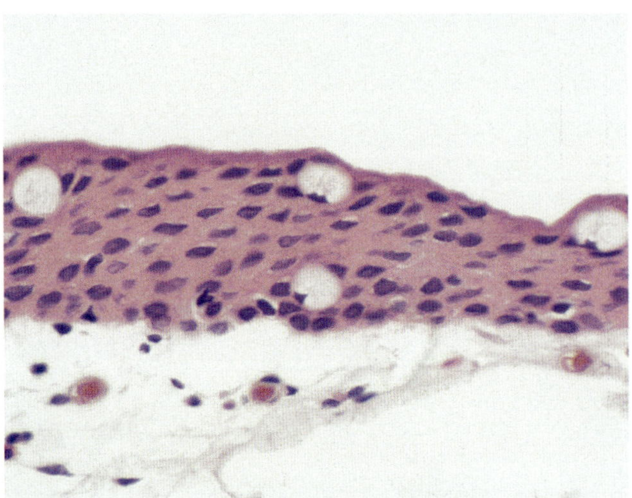

Fig. 6.1 Histology of the conjunctiva.

- **Conjunctiva-associated lymphoid tissue (CALT)** is critical in the initiation and regulation of ocular surface immune responses. It consists of lymphocytes within the epithelial layers, lymphatics and associated blood vessels, with a stromal component of lymphocytes and plasma cells, including follicular aggregates.

Clinical features of conjunctival inflammation

Symptoms

Non-specific symptoms include lacrimation, grittiness, stinging and burning. Itching is the hallmark of allergic disease, although it may also occur to a lesser extent in blepharitis and in patients with dry eye syndrome. The visual acuity is not usually affected. Significant pain, photophobia or a marked foreign body sensation suggest corneal involvement.

Discharge

- **Watery** discharge is composed of a serous exudate and tears and occurs in acute viral or acute allergic conjunctivitis.
- **Mucoid** discharge is typical of chronic allergic conjunctivitis and dry eye.
- **Mucopurulent** discharge typically occurs in chlamydial or acute bacterial infection.
- **Moderately purulent** discharge occurs in acute bacterial conjunctivitis.
- **Severe purulent** discharge is suggestive of gonococcal infection.

Conjunctival reaction

- **Hyperaemia** that is diffuse, beefy-red and more intense away from the limbus is usual in bacterial infection (Fig. 6.2A). This 'conjunctival injection' should be distinguished from the ciliary injection of iridocyclitis (see Ch. 12).
- **Haemorrhages** may occur in viral conjunctivitis, when they are often multiple, small and discrete ('petechial') and severe bacterial conjunctivitis, when they are larger and diffuse (Fig. 6.2B).
- **Chemosis** (conjunctival oedema) is seen as a translucent swelling (Fig. 6.2C), which may protrude through the eyelids. Acute chemosis usually indicates a hypersensitivity response (e.g. pollen), but can also occur in severe infective conjunctivitis. Subacute or chronic chemosis has numerous causes:
  - Local, e.g. thyroid eye disease, chronic allergic conjunctivitis, ocular or eyelid surgery, trauma.
  - Increased systemic vascular permeability, e.g. allergic conditions, infections including meningitis, vasculitis.
  - Increased venous pressure, e.g. superior vena cava syndrome, right-sided heart failure.
  - Decreased plasma oncotic pressure, e.g. nephrotic syndrome.
- **Membranes**
  - Pseudomembranes (Fig. 6.2D) consist of coagulated exudate adherent to the inflamed conjunctival epithelium. They can be peeled away leaving the underlying epithelium intact.

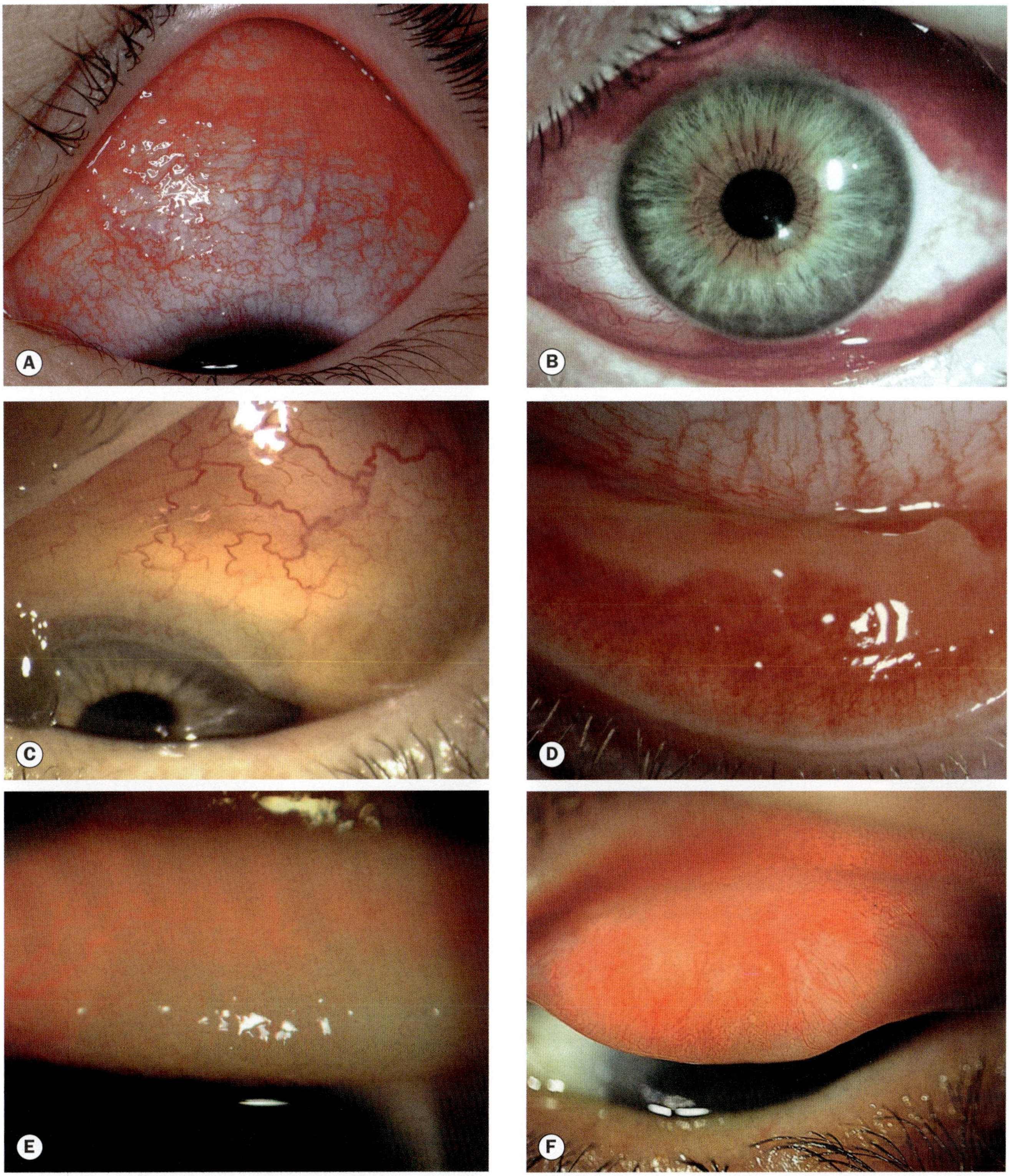

Fig. 6.2 Signs of conjunctival inflammation. **(A)** Hyperaemia (conjunctival injection); **(B)** subconjunctival haemorrhage in viral conjunctivitis; **(C)** chemosis; **(D)** pseudomembrane; **(E)** infiltration; **(F)** scarring. *(Courtesy of P Saine – fig. A.)*

- True membranes involve the superficial layers of the conjunctival epithelium so that attempted removal leads to tearing. The distinction between a true membrane and a pseudomembrane is rarely clinically helpful and both can leave scarring following resolution.
- Causes include severe adenoviral conjunctivitis, gonococcal and some other bacterial infections (*Streptococcus* spp., *Corynebacterium diphtheriae*), ligneous conjunctivitis and Stevens–Johnson syndrome.

- **Infiltration** represents cellular recruitment to the site of chronic inflammation and typically accompanies a papillary response. It is recognized by loss of detail of the normal tarsal conjunctival vessels, especially on the upper lid (Fig. 6.2E).
- **Subconjunctival cicatrization** (scarring) may occur in trachoma and other severe forms of conjunctivitis (Fig. 6.2F). Severe scarring is associated with loss of goblet cells and accessory lacrimal glands and can lead to cicatricial entropion.
- **Follicles**
  - Signs. Multiple, discrete, slightly elevated lesions resembling translucent grains of rice, most prominent in the fornices (Fig. 6.3A). Blood vessels run around or across rather than within the lesions.
  - Histology shows a subepithelial lymphoid germinal centre with central immature lymphocytes and mature cells peripherally (Fig. 6.3B).
  - Causes include viral and chlamydial conjunctivitis, Parinaud oculoglandular syndrome and hypersensitivity to topical medications. Small follicles are a normal finding in childhood (folliculosis), as are follicles in the fornices and at the margin of the upper tarsal plate in adults.
- **Papillae** can develop only in the palpebral conjunctiva and in the limbal bulbar conjunctiva where it is attached to the deeper fibrous layer.
  - Signs. In contrast to follicles, a vascular core is present. Micropapillae form a mosaic-like pattern of elevated red dots as a result of the central vascular channel, macropapillae (<1 mm – Fig. 6.3C) and giant papillae (>1 mm) develop with prolonged inflammation. Apical infiltrate or staining with fluorescein or the presence of mucus can be

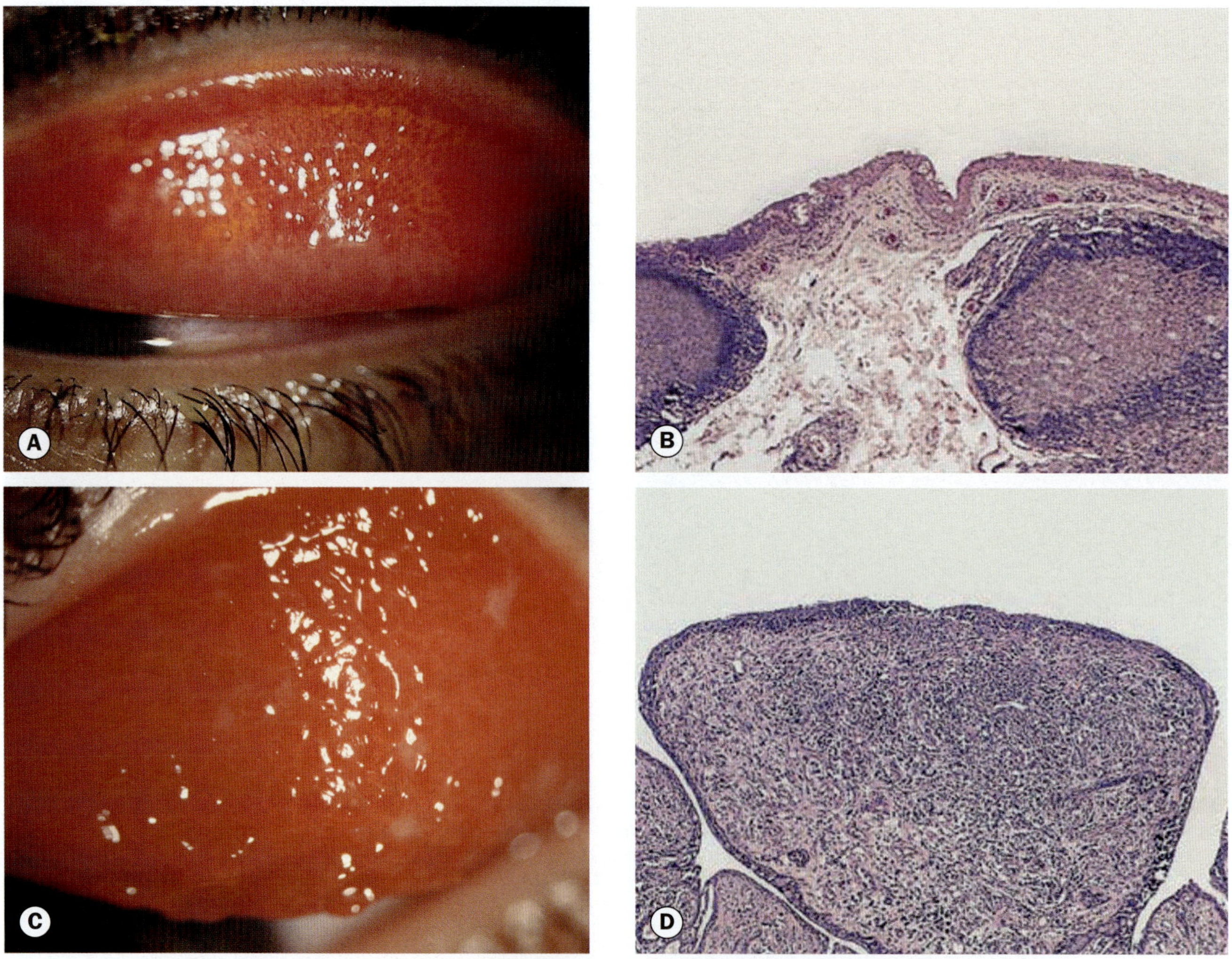

Fig. 6.3 **(A)** Conjunctival follicles; **(B)** histology of a follicle showing two subepithelial germinal centres with immature lymphocytes centrally and mature cells peripherally; **(C)** conjunctival macropapillae; **(D)** histology of a papilla showing folds of hyperplastic conjunctival epithelium with a fibrovascular core and subepithelial stromal infiltration with inflammatory cells.

present with marked activity. Limbal papillae have a gelatinous appearance.

- Histology shows folds of hyperplastic conjunctival epithelium with a fibrovascular core and subepithelial stromal infiltration with inflammatory cells (Fig. 6.3D). Late changes include superficial stromal hyalinization, scarring and the formation of crypts containing goblet cells.
- Causes include bacterial conjunctivitis, allergic conjunctivitis, chronic blepharitis, contact lens wear, superior limbic keratoconjunctivitis and floppy eyelid syndrome.

Lymphadenopathy

The most common cause of lymphadenopathy associated with conjunctivitis is viral infection. It may also occur in chlamydial and severe bacterial conjunctivitis (especially gonococcal) and Parinaud oculoglandular syndrome. The preauricular site is typically affected.

TIP Viral conjunctivitis tends to occur in epidemics and commonly causes preauricular lymphadenopathy.

BACTERIAL CONJUNCTIVITIS

Acute bacterial conjunctivitis

Acute bacterial conjunctivitis is a common and usually self-limiting condition caused by direct contact with infected secretions. The most common isolates are *Streptococcus pneumoniae*, *Staphylococcus aureus*, *Haemophilus influenzae* and *Moraxella catarrhalis*. A minority of severe cases are caused by the sexually transmitted organism *Neisseria gonorrhoeae*, which can readily invade the intact corneal epithelium. Meningococcal (*Neisseria meningitidis*) conjunctivitis is rare and usually affects children.

Diagnosis

- **Symptoms**
  - Acute onset of redness, grittiness, burning and discharge.
  - Involvement is usually bilateral although one eye may become affected 1–2 days before the other (Fig. 6.4A).
  - On waking, the eyelids are frequently stuck together and may be difficult to open.

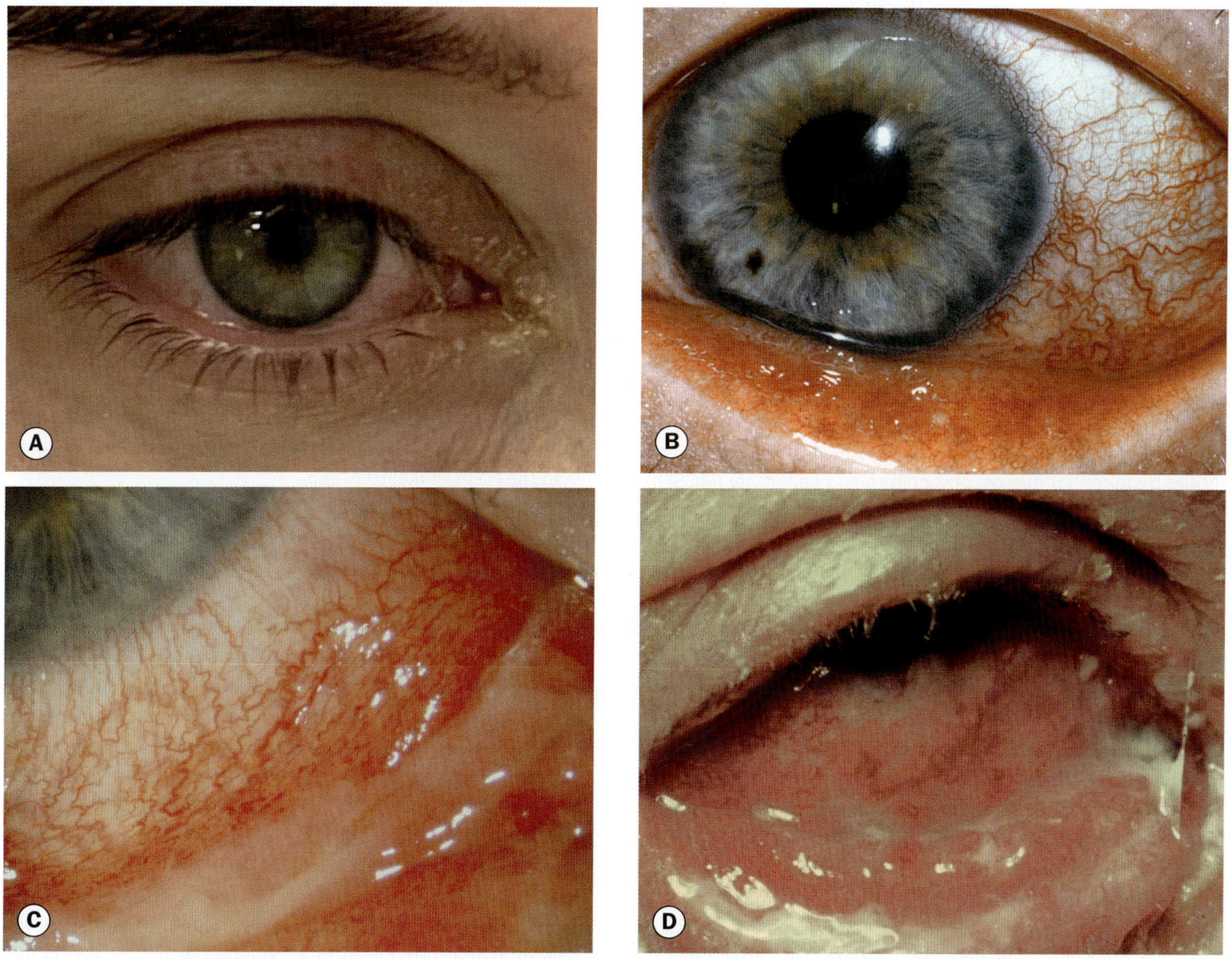

Fig. 6.4 Bacterial conjunctivitis. **(A)** Early infection with slight lid swelling and a sticky discharge; **(B)** diffuse tarsal and forniceal conjunctival hyperaemia (injection); **(C)** mucopurulent discharge; **(D)** profuse purulent discharge secondary to gonococcus.

- Systemic symptoms may occur in patients with severe conjunctivitis associated with gonococcus, meningococcus, *Chlamydia* and *H. influenzae.* In children, the possibility of progression to systemic involvement should always be borne in mind.
- **Signs** are variable and depend on the severity of infection.
  - The vision is usually normal.
  - Eyelid oedema and erythema may occur in severe infection, particularly gonococcal.
  - Conjunctival injection as previously described (Fig. 6.4B and see Fig. 6.2A).
  - The discharge can initially be watery, mimicking viral conjunctivitis, but rapidly becomes mucopurulent (Fig. 6.4C).
  - Hyperacute purulent discharge (Fig. 6.4D) may signify gonococcal or meningococcal conjunctivitis.
  - Superficial corneal punctate epithelial erosions are common.
  - Peripheral corneal ulceration may occur in gonococcal and meningococcal infection and may rapidly progress to perforation.
  - Lymphadenopathy is usually absent except in severe gonococcal and meningococcal infection.
- **Investigations** are not performed routinely but may be indicated in the following situations:
  - In severe cases, binocular conjunctival swabs and scrapings should be taken for urgent Gram staining, to exclude gonococcal and meningococcal infection (Gram-negative kidney-shaped intracellular diplococci).
  - Culture should include enriched media such as chocolate agar or Thayer–Martin for *N. gonorrhoeae* (see Fig. 7.8C).
  - Polymerase chain reaction (PCR) may be required for less severe cases that fail to respond to treatment, particularly to rule out the possibility of chlamydial and viral infection.

TIP A hyperacute purulent ocular discharge may be a sign of gonococcal or meningococcal conjunctivitis. A specimen should be taken for microscopy, culture and sensitivity (MCS) in order to prescribe an appropriate systemic antibiotic.

Treatment

About 60% resolve within 5 days without treatment.

- **Topical antibiotics**, usually four times daily for up to a week but sometimes more intensively, are frequently administered to speed recovery and prevent re-infection and transmission. There is no evidence that any particular antibiotic is more effective. Ointments and gels provide a higher concentration for longer periods than drops, but should be avoided during the day because blurred vision may follow. The following antibiotics are available:
  - Chloramphenicol, aminoglycosides (gentamicin, neomycin, tobramycin), quinolones (ciprofloxacin, ofloxacin, levofloxacin, lomefloxacin, gatifloxacin, moxifloxacin, besifloxacin), macrolides (erythromycin, azithromycin) polymyxin B, fusidic acid and bacitracin.
  - Some practitioners, particularly in the USA, believe that chloramphenicol should not be used for routine treatment because of a possible link with aplastic anaemia.
  - Gonococcal and meningococcal conjunctivitis should be treated with a quinolone, gentamicin, chloramphenicol or bacitracin 1–2 hourly as well as systemic therapy (see below).
- **Systemic antibiotics** are required in the following circumstances:
  - Gonococcal infection is usually treated with a third-generation cephalosporin such as ceftriaxone; quinolones and some macrolides are alternatives. It is essential to seek advice from a microbiologist and/or genitourinary specialist.
  - *H. influenzae* infection, particularly in children, is treated with oral amoxicillin with clavulanic acid. There is a 25% risk of developing otitis and other systemic problems.
  - Meningococcal conjunctivitis, particularly in children in whom early systemic prophylaxis may be life-saving, as up to 30% may develop systemic disease without treatment. The advice of paediatric and infectious disease specialists must be sought, but if in doubt treatment with intramuscular benzylpenicillin, ceftriaxone or cefotaxime, or oral ciprofloxacin should not be delayed.
  - Preseptal or orbital cellulitis (see Ch. 4).
- **Topical steroids** may reduce scarring in membranous and pseudomembranous conjunctivitis.
- **Irrigation** to remove excessive discharge may be useful in hyperpurulent cases.
- **Contact lens wear** should be discontinued until at least 48 hours after complete resolution of symptoms. Contact lenses should not be worn whilst topical antibiotic treatment continues.
- **Risk of transmission should be reduced** by hand-washing and the avoidance of towel sharing.
- **Review** is unnecessary for most mild/moderate adult cases, although patients should be cautioned to seek further advice in the event of deterioration.
- **Statutory notification of public health authorities** may be required locally for some causes.

Giant fornix syndrome

Giant fornix syndrome is an uncommon entity causing chronic relapsing pseudomembranous purulent conjunctivitis. It is believed to be due to retained debris in a voluminous upper fornix acting as a focus for persistent bacterial colonization (usually *S. aureus*) in an elderly patient with levator disinsertion. Large protein aggregations may be visualized in the upper fornix, though double eversion with a retractor may be necessary to identify these. Secondary corneal vascularization and lacrimal obstruction are common. It is frequently unilateral. Treatment involves repeated sweeping of the fornix with a cotton-tipped applicator and topical and systemic antibiotics; intensive topical steroid may be helpful. Surgical reconstruction of the fornix may be necessary in recalcitrant cases.

Adult chlamydial conjunctivitis

Pathogenesis

Chlamydia trachomatis (Fig. 6.5) is a species of *Chlamydiae*, a phylum of bacteria that cannot replicate extracellularly and hence depends on host cells. They exist in two principal forms: a robust infective extracellular 'elementary body' and a fragile intracellular replicating 'reticular body'. Adult chlamydial (inclusion) conjunctivitis is an oculogenital infection usually caused by serovars (serological variants) D–K of *C. trachomatis* and affects 5–20% of sexually active young adults in Western countries. Transmission is by autoinoculation from genital secretions, although eye-to-eye spread probably accounts for about 10%. The incubation period is approximately a week.

Urogenital infection

- **In males,** chlamydial infection is the most common cause of non-gonococcal urethritis (NGU), also termed non-specific urethritis (NSU). It should be noted that the latter term is also sometimes used to mean urethritis in which both gonococcal and chlamydial infection have been ruled out. Chlamydial urethritis is frequently asymptomatic in men. *C. trachomatis* may also cause epididymitis and can act as a trigger for Reiter syndrome.
- **In females,** chlamydial urethritis typically causes dysuria and discharge. It may progress to pelvic inflammatory disease (PID), carrying a risk of infertility. Approximately 5–10% of women with PID develop perihepatitis (Fitz-Hugh–Curtis syndrome).

Diagnosis

- **Symptoms** consist of the subacute onset of unilateral or bilateral redness, watering and discharge. Untreated, the conjunctivitis becomes chronic and though self-limiting may persist for several months. It is important to enquire about sexual exposure if chlamydial conjunctivitis is suspected.

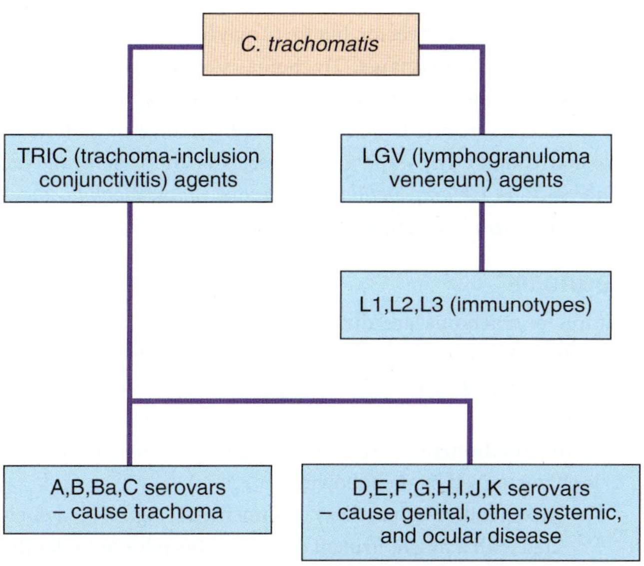

Fig. 6.5 Classification of *Chlamydia trachomatis*.

- **Signs**
  - Watery or mucopurulent discharge.
  - Tender preauricular lymphadenopathy.
  - Large follicles are often most prominent in the inferior fornix (Fig. 6.6A) and may also involve the upper tarsal conjunctiva (Fig. 6.6B).
  - Superficial punctate keratitis is common.
  - Perilimbal subepithelial corneal infiltrates (Fig. 6.6C) may appear after 2–3 weeks.
  - Chronic cases have less prominent follicles and commonly develop papillae.
  - Mild conjunctival scarring and superior corneal pannus (Fig. 6.6D) are not uncommon.
- **Investigations.** Tarsal conjunctival scrapings are obtained using a spatula or the blunt side of a scalpel blade.
  - Nucleic acid amplification tests such as PCR are likely to be the investigation of choice in time but validation for ocular specimens is limited at present.
  - Giemsa staining for basophilic intracytoplasmic bodies is performed by applying scrapings onto a glass slide.
  - Direct immunofluorescence detects free elementary bodies with approximately 90% sensitivity and specificity.
  - Enzyme immunoassay for direct antigen detection is also useful.
  - McCoy cell culture is highly specific.
  - Swabs taken for bacterial culture and serology may be helpful in selected cases.

Treatment

Empirical treatment may be given if the clinical picture is convincing pending investigation results.

- **Referral to a genitourinary specialist** is mandatory in confirmed cases, particularly for the exclusion of other sexually transmitted infections, contact tracing and pregnancy testing.
- **Systemic** therapy involves one of the following:
  - Azithromycin 1 g repeated after 1 week is generally the treatment of choice, although a second or a third course is required in up to 30% of cases. Some guidelines advocate only a single 1 g dose.
  - Doxycycline 100 mg twice daily for 10 days (tetracyclines are relatively contraindicated in pregnancy/breastfeeding and in children under 12 years of age).
  - Erythromycin, amoxicillin and ciprofloxacin are alternatives.
- **Topical** antibiotics such as erythromycin or tetracycline ointment are sometimes used to achieve rapid relief of ocular symptoms, but are insufficient alone.
- **Reduction of transmission risk** involves abstinence from sexual contact until completion of treatment (1 week after azithromycin), together with other precautions as for any infectious conjunctivitis.
- **Re-testing** for persistent infection should take place 6–12 weeks after treatment.
- It is important to be aware that symptoms commonly take weeks to settle and that follicles and corneal infiltrates can take

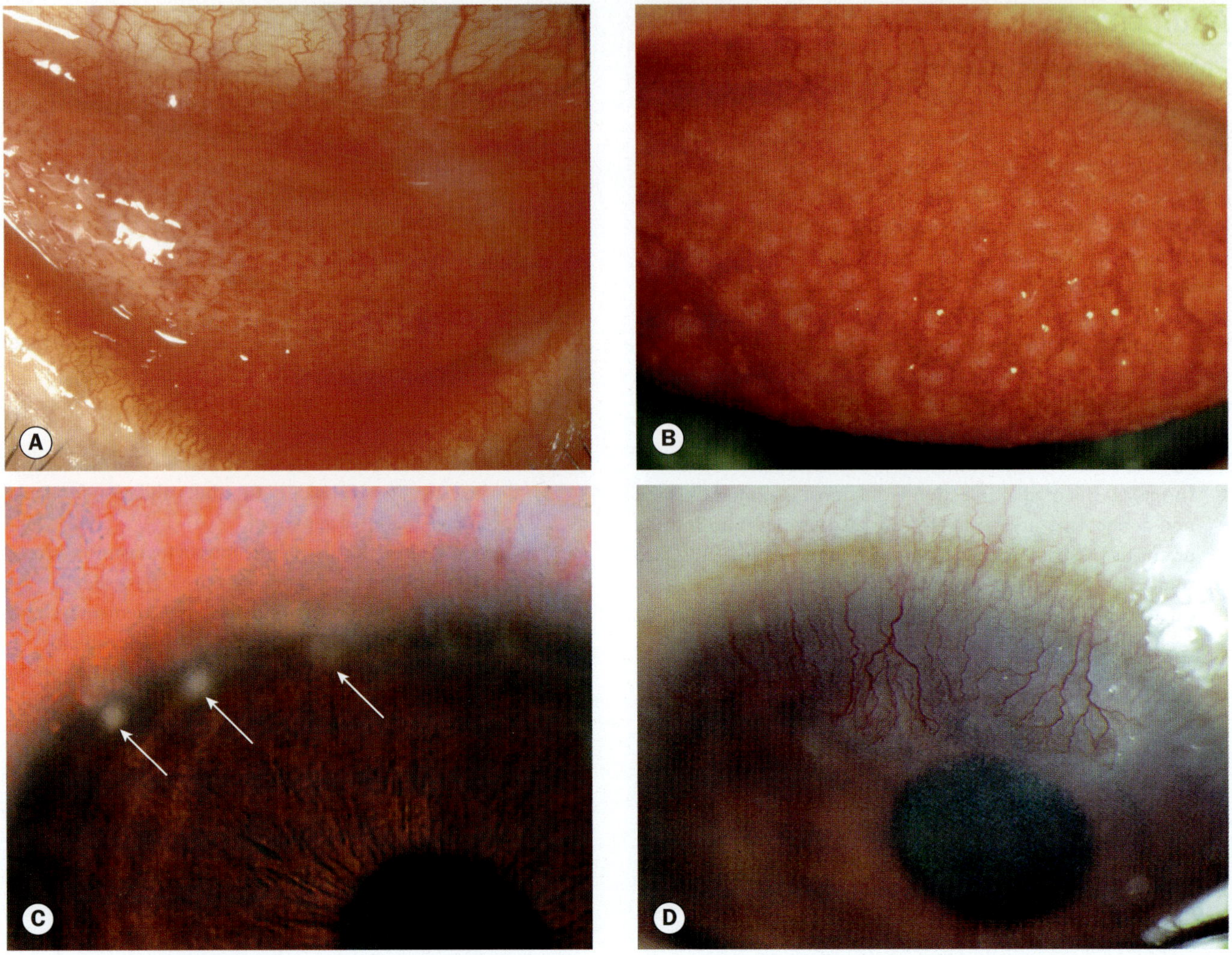

Fig. 6.6 Adult chlamydial conjunctivitis. **(A)** Large forniceal follicles; **(B)** superior tarsal follicles; **(C)** peripheral corneal infiltrates (arrows); **(D)** superior pannus.

months to resolve due to a prolonged hypersensitivity response to chlamydial antigen.

TIP In a patient with adult chlamydial conjunctivitis, other sexually transmitted infections should be excluded.

Trachoma

Pathogenesis

Trachoma is the world's leading cause of preventable irreversible blindness. It is related to poverty, overcrowding and poor hygiene, the morbidity being a consequence of the establishment of re-infection cycles within communities. Whereas an isolated episode of trachomatous conjunctivitis may be relatively innocuous, recurrent infection elicits a chronic immune response consisting of a cell-mediated delayed hypersensitivity (Type IV) reaction to the intermittent presence of chlamydial antigen and can lead to loss of sight. Prior contact with the organism confers short-term partial immunity but also leads to a heightened inflammatory reaction upon re-infection. Vaccination has an effect similar to primary infection in sensitizing the individual and as a consequence is not helpful. The family childcare group is the most important re-infection reservoir and young children are particularly vulnerable. The fly is an important vector, but there may be direct transmission from eye or nasal discharge. Trachoma is associated principally with infection by serovars A, B, Ba and C of *Chlamydia trachomatis*, but the serovars D–K conventionally associated with adult inclusion conjunctivitis and other species of the *Chlamydiaceae* family such as *Chlamydophila psittaci* and *Chlamydophila pneumoniae* have also been implicated.

Diagnosis

Features of trachoma are divided into an 'active' inflammatory stage and a 'cicatricial' chronic stage, with considerable overlap. A World Health Organization (WHO) grading system is in use (Table 6.1).

- **Active trachoma** is most common in pre-school children and is characterized by the following:
  - Mixed follicular/papillary conjunctivitis (Fig. 6.7A) associated with a mucopurulent discharge. In children under the age of 2 years the papillary component may predominate.

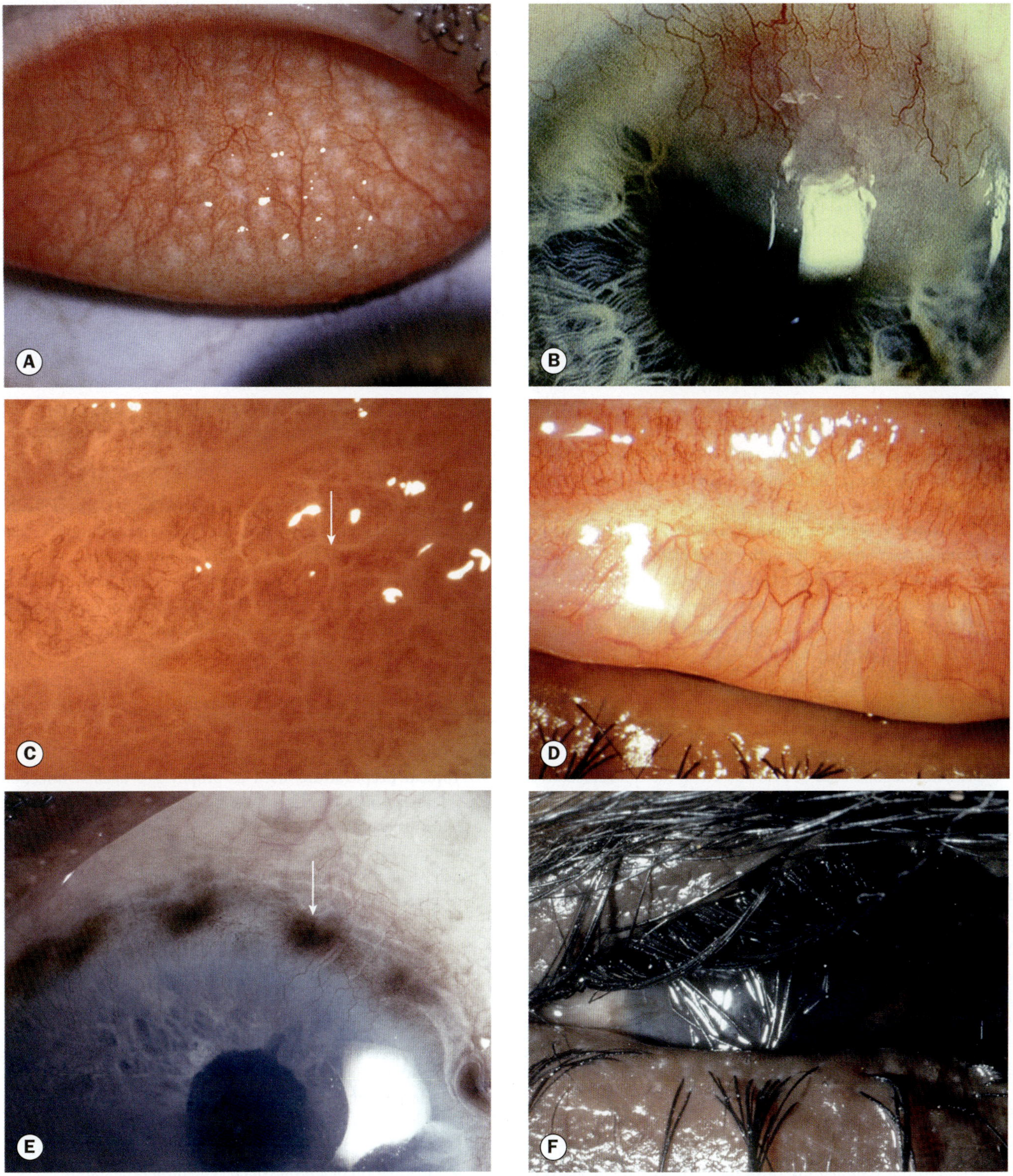

Fig. 6.7 Trachoma. **(A)** Typical white subtarsal follicles; **(B)** marked pannus; **(C)** stellate conjunctival scarring (arrow); **(D)** Arlt line and conjunctival follicles; **(E)** Herbert pit (arrow); **(F)** cicatricial entropion. *(Courtesy of C Barry – figs A, B, D–F.)*

Table 6.1 WHO Grading of Trachoma

TF = trachomatous inflammation (*follicular*): five or more follicles (>0.5mm) on the superior tarsal plate
TI = trachomatous inflammation (*intense*): diffuse involvement of the tarsal conjunctiva, obscuring 50% or more of the normal deep tarsal vessels; papillae are present
TS = trachomatous conjunctival scarring: easily visible fibrous white tarsal bands
TT = trachomatous trichiasis: at least one lash touching the globe
CO = corneal opacity sufficient to blur details of at least part of the pupillary margin

  - Superior epithelial keratitis and pannus formation (Fig. 6.7B).
- **Cicatricial trachoma** is prevalent in middle age.
  - Linear or stellate (Fig. 6.7C) conjunctival scars in mild cases, or broad confluent scars (Arlt line – Fig. 6.7D) in severe disease.
  - Although the entire conjunctiva is involved, the effects are most prominent on the upper tarsal plate.
  - Superior limbal follicles may resolve to leave a row of shallow depressions (Herbert pits – Fig. 6.7E).
  - Trichiasis, distichiasis, corneal vascularization and cicatricial entropion (Fig. 6.7F).
  - Severe corneal opacification.
  - Dry eye caused by destruction of goblet cells and the ductules of the lacrimal gland.
- **Investigations** are rarely used in the affected areas as in most cases the diagnosis can be made based on the clinical features. Various field techniques (e.g. dipstick enzyme immunoassay) are available and other investigations are similar to those for adult inclusion conjunctivitis.

Management

The SAFE strategy for trachoma management supported by the WHO and other agencies encompasses **S**urgery for trichiasis, **A**ntibiotics for active disease, **F**acial hygiene and **E**nvironmental improvement.

- **Antibiotics** should be administered to those affected and to all family members. A single antibiotic course is not always effective in eliminating infection in an individual and communities may need to receive annual treatment to suppress infection.
  - A single dose of azithromycin (20 mg/kg up to 1 g) is the treatment of choice.
  - Erythromycin 500 mg twice daily for 14 days or doxycycline 100 mg twice daily for 10 days (tetracyclines are relatively contraindicated in pregnancy/breastfeeding and in children under 12).
  - Topical 1% tetracycline ointment is less effective than oral treatment.
- **Facial cleanliness** is a critical preventative measure.
- **Environmental improvement**, such as access to adequate water and sanitation, as well as control of flies, is important.
- **Surgery** is aimed at relieving entropion and trichiasis and maintaining complete lid closure, principally with bilamellar tarsal rotation.

TIP Systemic tetracyclines should not be used in pregnancy and in children under 12 years of age because of the risk of tooth staining.

Neonatal conjunctivitis

Neonatal conjunctivitis (ophthalmia neonatorum) is defined as conjunctival inflammation developing within the first month of life. It is the most common infection of any kind in neonates, occurring in up to 10%. It is identified as a specific entity distinct from conjunctivitis in older infants because of its potentially serious nature (both ocular and systemic complications) and because it is often the result of infection transmitted from mother to infant during delivery.

Causes

- **Organisms acquired during vaginal delivery**: *C. trachomatis*, *N. gonorrhoeae* (now rare in wealthier countries, but previously responsible for 25% of childhood blindness) and herpes simplex virus (typically HSV-2). With all of these, conjunctivitis is not uncommonly associated with severe ocular or systemic complications. *C. trachomatis* is the most -common cause in cases involving moderate–severe conjunctival inflammation.
- **Staphylococci are usually responsible for mild conjunctivitis.** Other bacterial causes include streptococci, *H. influenzae* and various Gram-negative organisms.
- **Topical preparations** used as prophylaxis against infection (see below) may themselves cause conjunctival irritation (chemical conjunctivitis).
- **Congenital nasolacrimal obstruction.** Despite poor neonatal tear production, a persistently mildly watery eye with recurrent mild bacterial conjunctivitis may be secondary to a blocked tear duct.

Diagnosis

- **Timing of onset**
  - Chemical irritation: first few days.
  - Gonococcal: first week.
  - Staphylococci and other bacteria: end of the first week.
  - Herpes simplex virus (HSV): 1–2 weeks.
  - *Chlamydia*: 1–3 weeks.
- **History**
  - Instillation of a prophylactic chemical preparation.
  - Parental symptoms of sexually transmitted infection (STI).
  - Recent conjunctivitis in close contacts.
  - Features of systemic illness in the child: pneumonitis, rhinitis and otitis in chlamydial infection, skin vesicles and features of encephalitis in HSV. Disseminated gonococcal infection is relatively rare.
  - Prior persistent watering without inflammation may indicate a nasolacrimal duct that is not yet open.

- **Signs**
  - A mildly sticky eye may occur in staphylococcal infection, or with delayed nasolacrimal duct canalization (mucopurulent reflux on pressure over the lacrimal sac).
  - Discharge is characteristically watery in chemical and HSV infection, mucopurulent in chlamydial infection, purulent (Fig. 6.8) in bacterial infection and hyperpurulent in gonococcal conjunctivitis.
  - Severe eyelid oedema occurs in gonococcal infection. It may be difficult to distinguish severe conjunctivitis from preseptal or orbital infection. Signs of dacryocystitis should be excluded.
  - Eyelid and periocular vesicles may occur in HSV infection and can critically aid early diagnosis and treatment.
  - Corneal examination is mandatory and is particularly important if gonococcal infection is suspected, as ulceration with rapid progression is common. Use of a pen torch, insertion of an eyelid speculum and fluorescein drops may be helpful. The latter may facilitate identification of a dendritic or geographic epithelial lesion that may be present in HSV infection (in contrast to the punctate epitheliopathy seen in older children with primary herpetic conjunctivitis).
  - Pseudomembranes are not uncommon in chlamydial conjunctivitis.
  - Congenital glaucoma may masquerade as neonatal conjunctivitis and should always be considered, particularly in monocular cases.
- **Investigations** are tailored to the clinical picture:
  - The results of any parental prenatal testing for STI should be obtained.
  - Conjunctival scrapings are taken for nucleic acid amplification (PCR), particularly for *Chlamydia* and HSV.
  - Separate conjunctival scrapings are applied to a glass slide for Gram and Giemsa staining. Multinucleated giant cells may be present on Gram stain in HSV infection.
  - Conjunctival swabs are taken with a calcium alginate swab or a sterile cotton-tipped applicator, for standard bacterial culture and chocolate agar or Thayer–Martin (for *N. gonorrhoeae*).
  - Epithelial cells infected with HSV may show eosinophilic intranuclear inclusions on Papanicolaou smear.
  - Conjunctival scrapings or fluid from skin vesicles can be sent for viral culture for HSV.
  - Specimens should be taken prior to fluorescein instillation if immunofluorescent testing is planned.

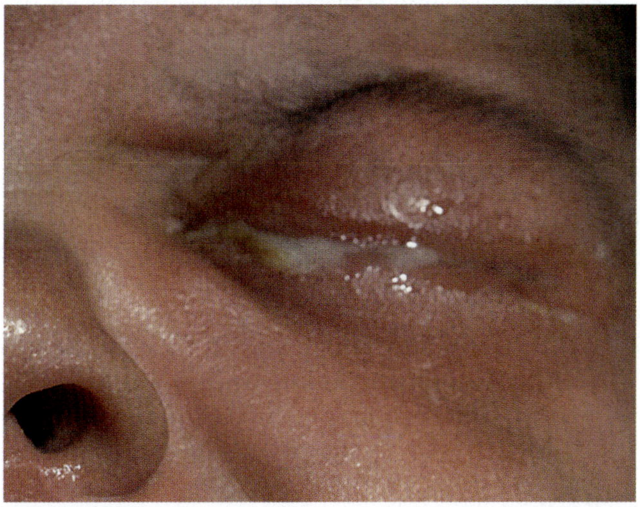

Fig. 6.8 Eyelid oedema and purulent discharge in neonatal conjunctivitis.

Treatment

- **Prophylaxis** is routinely performed but there is no standard protocol.
  - A single instillation of povidone-iodine 2.5% solution is effective against common pathogens.
  - Erythromycin 0.5% or tetracycline 1% ointment.
  - Silver nitrate 1% solution agglutinates gonococci and is still utilized in areas where gonococcal infection is common. It should be administered in conjunction with a single intramuscular dose of benzylpenicillin when maternal infection is present.
- **Chemical conjunctivitis** does not require treatment apart from artificial tears.
- **Mild conjunctivitis.** A mildly sticky eye is extremely common in neonates. Investigation is often unnecessary and a low-intensity regimen with a broad-spectrum topical antibiotic such as chloramphenicol, erythromycin or fusidic acid ointment is adequate in most cases. Further investigation and treatment can be instituted if the condition fails to settle.
- **Moderate–severe** cases should be investigated as above. Microscopy with Gram staining alone is highly sensitive and will often provide a working diagnosis.
  - If the diagnosis is uncertain but chlamydial infection is a reasonable possibility, oral erythromycin can be commenced on an empirical basis after samples have been collected.
  - If bacteria are evident on Gram stain, a broad-spectrum topical antibiotic (e.g. chloramphenicol, erythromycin or bacitracin for Gram-positive organisms, neomycin, ofloxacin or gentamicin for Gram-negatives) should be used until sensitivities are available. Additional systemic treatment should be considered in more severe cases.
- **Severe conjunctivitis**, or when systemic illness is suspected, requires hospital admission. Samples should be taken for a range of investigations, including urgent microscopy and a broad-spectrum topical antibiotic, such as erythromycin, commenced. The ocular risk is usually most acute from gonococcal infection, so empirical topical treatment should cover this and in most cases, consideration given to systemic treatment such as parenteral ceftriaxone.
- **Chlamydial infection** is treated with oral erythromycin for 2 weeks. A longer or supplementary course may be needed. Erythromycin or tetracycline ointment can be used in addition, but is probably unnecessary.
- **Gonococcal conjunctivitis** is treated systemically with a third-generation cephalosporin and often with supplementary topical treatment. Co-treatment for *Chlamydia* is prudent. Saline irrigation to remove excessive discharge should be considered.

- **Herpes simplex infection** should always be regarded as a systemic condition and is treated with high-dose intravenous aciclovir under paediatric specialist care. Early diagnosis and treatment of encephalitis (PCR of cerebrospinal fluid (CSF) is positive in 95%) may be life-saving or prevent serious neurological disability. Topical aciclovir may be considered in addition.
- **Microbiological** advice should be sought in severe cases, especially regarding local antibiotic sensitivities.
- **Paediatric** specialist involvement is mandatory when systemic disease may be present.
- **Genitourinary** referral for the mother and her sexual contacts is important when an STI is diagnosed. The neonate should be screened for other STIs.
- **Notification** of a case of neonatal conjunctivitis to the local public health authority is a statutory requirement in many countries.

VIRAL CONJUNCTIVITIS

Introduction

Viral conjunctivitis is a common external ocular infection, adenovirus (a non-enveloped double-stranded DNA virus) being the most frequent (90%) causative agent. It may be sporadic, or occur in epidemics in environments such as workplaces (including hospitals), schools and swimming pools. The spread of this highly contagious infection is facilitated by the ability of viral particles to survive on dry surfaces for weeks and by the fact that viral shedding may occur for many days before clinical features are apparent. Transmission is generally by contact with respiratory or ocular secretions, including via fomites such as contaminated towels.

TIP Viral conjunctivitis is highly contagious and great care should be taken to prevent transmission of the disease.

Presentation

The spectrum of viral conjunctivitis varies from mild subclinical disease to severe inflammation with significant morbidity. There will often be a history of a close contact with acute conjunctivitis.

- **Non-specific acute follicular conjunctivitis** is the most common clinical form of viral conjunctivitis and is typically due to adenoviral infection by a range of serological variants. Unilateral watering, redness, irritation and/or itching and mild photophobia occur, the contralateral eye generally being affected 1–2 days later, often less severely. The condition is usually milder than the other clinical forms of adenoviral conjunctivitis. Patients may have accompanying (usually mild) systemic symptoms, such as a sore throat or common cold.
- **Pharyngoconjunctival fever (PCF)** is caused mainly by adenovirus serovars 3, 4 and 7. It is spread by droplets within families with upper respiratory tract infection. Keratitis develops in about 30% of cases but is seldom severe. Symptoms are essentially as above, though sore throat is typically prominent.
- **Epidemic keratoconjunctivitis (EKC)** is caused mainly by adenovirus serovars 8, 19 and 37 and is the most severe ocular adenoviral infection. Keratitis, which may be marked, develops in about 80%. Photophobia may be correspondingly prominent.
- **Acute haemorrhagic conjunctivitis** usually occurs in tropical areas. It is typically caused by enterovirus and coxsackievirus, though other microorganisms may present similarly. It has a rapid onset and resolves within 1–2 weeks. Conjunctival haemorrhage is generally marked.
- **Chronic/relapsing adenoviral conjunctivitis** giving a chronic non-specific follicular/papillary clinical picture can persist over years, but is rare and eventually self-limiting.
- **Herpes simplex virus (HSV)** can cause a follicular conjunctivitis, particularly in primary infection. This is usually unilateral and there are often associated skin vesicles.
- **Systemic viral infections** such as those common in childhood, e.g. varicella, measles and mumps, can feature an associated follicular conjunctivitis. Varicella-zoster virus secondary infection commonly causes conjunctivitis as part of ophthalmic shingles. Conjunctivitis secondary to HIV infection is recognized.
- **Molluscum contagiosum** is a skin infection caused by a human specific double-stranded DNA poxvirus that typically affects otherwise healthy children, with a peak incidence between the ages of 2 and 4 years. Transmission is by contact, with subsequent autoinoculation. A chronic follicular conjunctivitis can be associated and is due to skin lesion shedding of viral particles. Chronic unilateral ocular irritation and mild discharge is typical. The eyelash line should be examined carefully in patients with chronic conjunctivitis so as not to overlook a molluscum lesion.
- **SARS-CoV-2 virus,** responsible for the COVID-19 pandemic, can lead to multi-organ involvement, including the eye. Viral RNA can be isolated in the tears of up to 25% of patients with laboratory-proven moderate or severe COVID-19 infection. Conjunctivitis is the most commonly reported ocular manifestation and results in hyperaemia, chemosis and epiphora. The infectious potential and risk of transmission from tears or ocular discharge is not known. Other ocular consequences of the virus include retinal microangiopathy (common) and optic neuritis (rare). COVID-19 vaccination generally does not increase the risk of ocular adverse events, except in some patients with preexisting uveitis where reactivation of ocular inflammation may follow.

Signs

- **Eyelid oedema** ranges from negligible to severe.
- **Lymphadenopathy** is common: tender preauricular.
- **Conjunctival** hyperaemia and follicles are typically prominent. Papillae may also be seen, particularly in the superior tarsal conjunctiva.
- **Severe inflammation** may be associated with conjunctival haemorrhages (Fig. 6.9A) (usually petechial in adenoviral infection), chemosis, membranes (rare) and pseudomembranes (Fig. 6.9B), sometimes with conjunctival scarring after resolution (Fig. 6.9C).
- **Keratitis** (adenoviral):
  - Epithelial microcysts (non-staining) are common at an early stage.

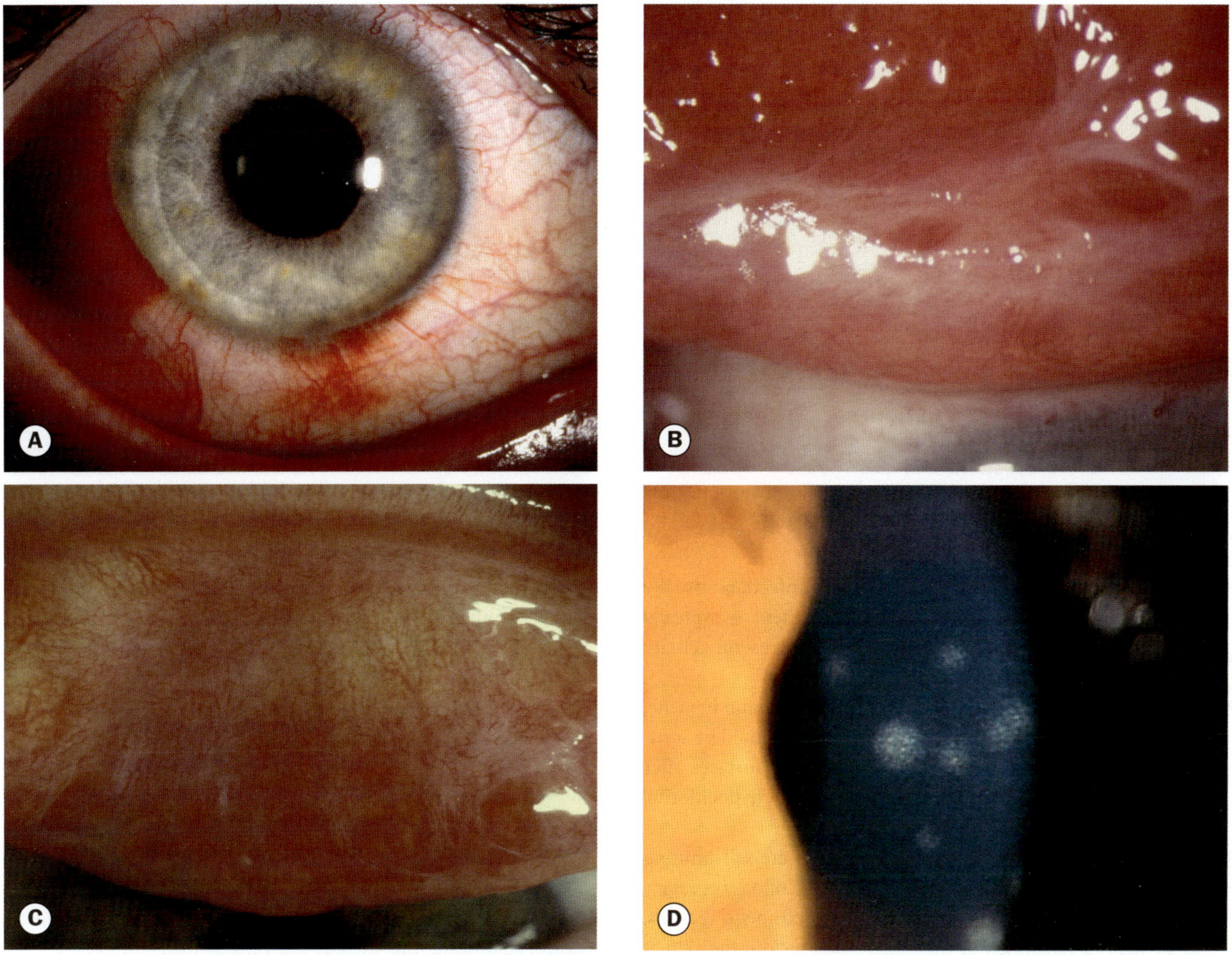

Fig. 6.9 Adenoviral keratoconjunctivitis. **(A)** Follicular conjunctivitis with sub-conjunctival haemorrhage; **(B)** pseudomembrane; **(C)** residual scarring; **(D)** subepithelial infiltrates. *(Courtesy of S Tuft – figs B and C.)*

  - Punctate epithelial keratitis (staining) may occur, usually within 7–10 days of the onset of symptoms, typically resolving within 2 weeks.
  - Focal white subepithelial/anterior stromal infiltrates (Fig. 6.9D) often develop beneath the fading epithelial lesions, probably as an immune response to the virus. They may persist or recur over months or years.
  - Small pseudodendritic epithelial formations sometimes occur.
- **Anterior uveitis** is sometimes present, but is mild.
- **Molluscum contagiosum**
  - A pale, waxy, umbilicated nodule on the lid margin (Fig. 6.10A) associated with follicular conjunctivitis (Fig. 6.10B) and mild watery and mucoid discharge.
  - Bulbar nodules and confluent cutaneous lesions may occur in immunocompromised patients.

Investigation

Investigation is generally unnecessary, but should be considered if the diagnosis is in doubt or there is failure of resolution.

- **Giemsa stain** shows predominantly mononuclear cells in adenoviral conjunctivitis and multinucleated giant cells in herpetic infection.
- **Nucleic acid amplification** techniques such as PCR are sensitive and specific for viral DNA.
- **Viral culture** with isolation is the reference standard but is expensive and fairly slow (days to weeks) and requires specific transport media. Sensitivity is variable but specificity is around 100%.
- **A 'point-of-care' immunochromatography** test takes 10 minutes to detect adenoviral antigen in tears; sensitivity and specificity are excellent.
- **Serology** for IgM or rising IgG antibody titres to adenovirus has limitations and is rarely used.
- **Investigation for other causes** such as chlamydial infection may be indicated in non-resolving cases.

Treatment

The treatment of herpetic ocular surface disease is addressed in Chapter 7.

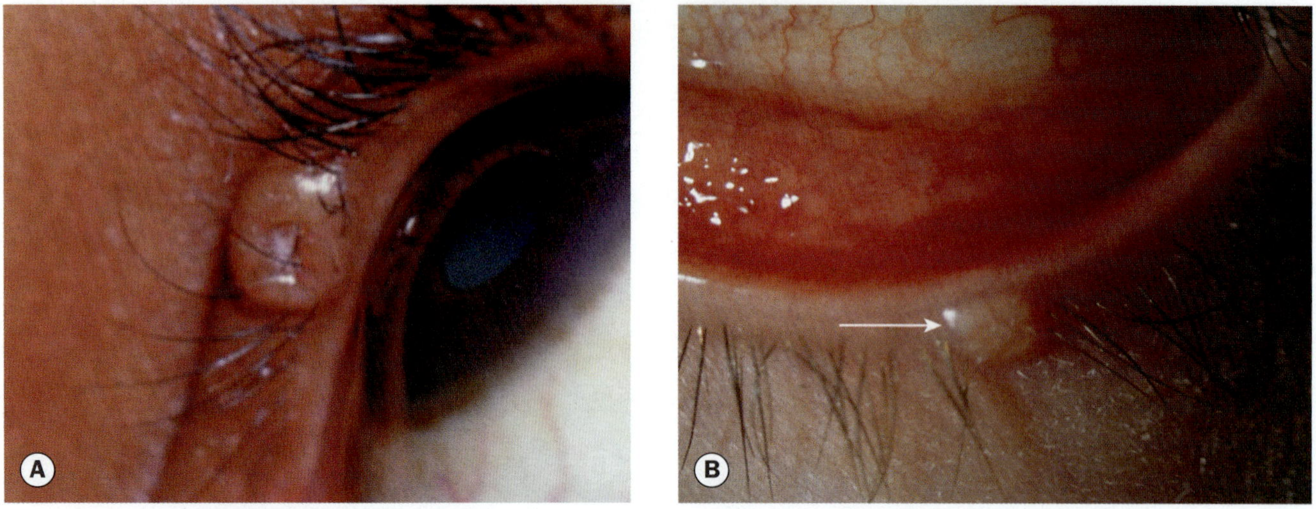

Fig. 6.10 (A) Molluscum eyelid lesion; **(B)** follicular conjunctivitis associated with a molluscum lesion (arrow).

- **Spontaneous resolution** of adenoviral infection usually occurs within 2–3 weeks, so specific treatment is typically unnecessary. No antiviral agent with clinically useful activity against adenovirus has yet been produced.
- **Reduction of transmission risk** by meticulous hand hygiene, avoiding eye rubbing and towel sharing. There should be scrupulous disinfection of instruments and clinical surfaces after examination of an infected patient (e.g. sodium hypochlorite, povidone-iodine).
- **Molluscum contagiosum.** Although lesions are self-limiting in immunocompetent patients, removal is often necessary to address secondary conjunctivitis or for cosmetic reasons. Expression is facilitated by making a small nick in the skin at the margin of the lesion with the tip of a needle.
- **Topical steroids** such as prednisolone 0.5% four times daily may be required for severe membranous or pseudomembranous adenoviral conjunctivitis. Symptomatic keratitis may require weak topical steroids but these should be used with caution as they do not speed resolution but only suppress inflammation and lesions commonly recur after premature discontinuation. Steroids may enhance viral replication and extend the period during which the patient remains infectious. Intraocular pressure should be monitored if treatment is prolonged.
- **Other measures**
  - Discontinuation of contact lens wear until resolution of symptoms.
  - Artificial tears four times daily may be useful for symptomatic relief. Preservative-free preparations may give superior comfort and if supplied in single-dose units may reduce transmission risk.
  - Cold (or warm) compresses for symptomatic relief.
  - Topical antihistamines and vasoconstrictors may improve symptoms, particularly itching.
  - The place of non-steroidal anti-inflammatory drops is not well established, but may be effective in some circumstances such as steroid weaning. They are not thought to promote viral replication.
  - Removal of symptomatic pseudomembranes or membranes.
  - Topical antibiotics if secondary bacterial infection is suspected.
  - Povidone-iodine is very effective against free (although less so against intracellular) adenovirus and has been proposed as a means of decreasing infectivity.

ALLERGIC CONJUNCTIVITIS

Atopy is a genetically determined predisposition to hypersensitivity reactions upon exposure to specific environmental antigens. Clinical manifestations include the various forms of allergic conjunctivitis, as well as hay fever (seasonal allergic rhinitis), asthma and eczema. Allergic conjunctivitis is a type I (immediate) hypersensitivity reaction, mediated by degranulation of mast cells in response to the action of IgE. There is evidence of an element of type IV hypersensitivity in at least some forms.

Acute allergic conjunctivitis

Acute allergic conjunctivitis is a common condition caused by an acute conjunctival reaction to an environmental allergen, usually pollen. It is typically seen in younger children after playing outside in spring or summer. Acute itching and watering are common, but the hallmark is chemosis (Fig. 6.11), which is frequently dramatic and worrying to the child and parents. Treatment is not usually required and the conjunctival swelling settles within hours as the acute increase in vascular permeability resolves. Cool compresses can be used and a single drop of adrenaline 0.1% may reduce extreme chemosis.

Seasonal and perennial allergic conjunctivitis

These common subacute conditions are distinguished from each other by the timing of exacerbations, thought to relate principally to differing stimulating allergens in each.

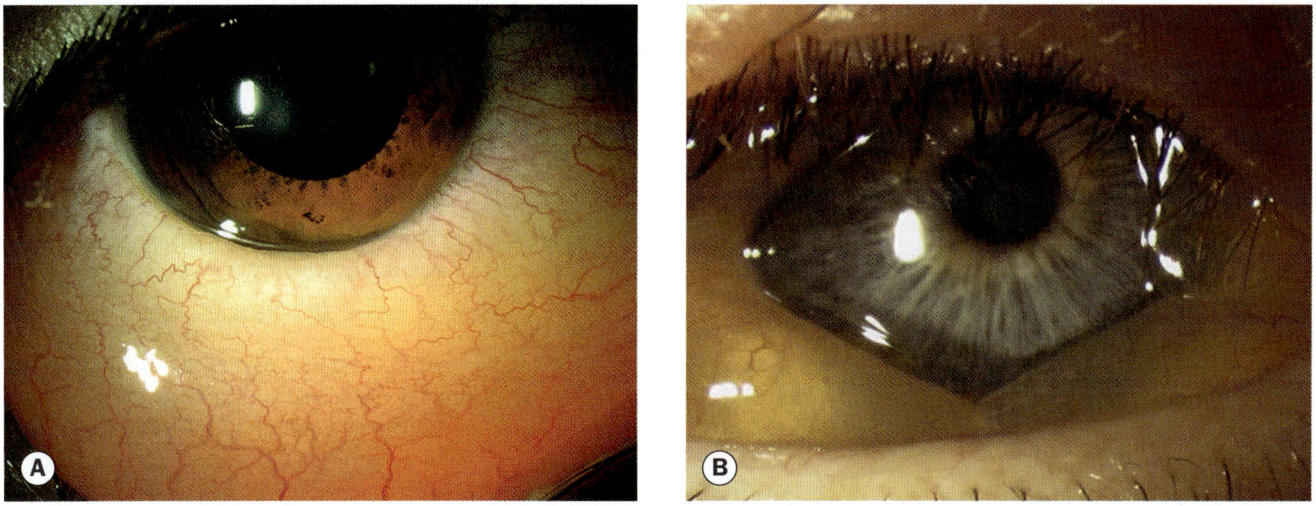

Fig. 6.11 **(A)** Moderate and **(B)** severe chemosis in acute allergic conjunctivitis.

- **Seasonal allergic conjunctivitis** ('hay fever eyes'), worse during the spring and summer, is the more common. The most frequent allergens are tree and grass pollens, although the specific allergen varies with geographic location.
- **Perennial allergic conjunctivitis** causes symptoms throughout the year, generally worse in the autumn when exposure to house dust mites, animal dander and fungal allergens is greatest. It is less common and tends to be milder than the seasonal form.

Diagnosis

- **Symptoms.** Transient acute or subacute attacks of redness, watering and itching, associated with sneezing and nasal discharge.
- **Signs.** Normal vision. Conjunctival hyperaemia with a relatively mild papillary reaction, variable chemosis and lid oedema.
- **Investigations** are generally not performed although conjunctival scraping in more active cases may demonstrate the presence of eosinophils. Skin testing for particular allergens is rarely required.

Treatment

- **Artificial tears** for mild symptoms.
- **Mast cell stabilizers** (e.g. sodium cromoglicate, nedocromil sodium, lodoxamide) must be used for a few days before exerting maximal effect, but are suitable (except lodoxamide) for long-term use if required.
- **Antihistamines** (e.g. emedastine, epinastine, levocabastine, bepotastine) can be used for symptomatic exacerbations and are as effective as mast cell stabilizers.
- **Dual action antihistamine and mast cell stabilizers** (e.g. azelastine, ketotifen, olopatadine) act rapidly and are often very effective for exacerbations.
- **Combined preparation** of an antihistamine and a vasoconstrictor (e.g. antazoline with xylometazoline).
- **Non-steroidal anti-inflammatory preparations** (e.g. diclofenac) can provide symptomatic relief but are rarely used.
- **Topical steroids** are effective but rarely necessary.
- **Oral antihistamines** may be indicated for severe symptoms. Some, such as diphenhydramine, cause significant drowsiness and may be useful in aiding sleep. Others, such as loratadine, have a far less marked sedative action.

Vernal keratoconjunctivitis

Pathogenesis

Vernal keratoconjunctivitis (VKC) is a recurrent bilateral disorder in which both IgE- and cell-mediated immune mechanisms play important roles. It primarily affects boys and onset is generally from about the age of 5 years onwards. There is remission by the late teens in 95% of cases, although many of the remainder develop atopic keratoconjunctivitis. VKC is rare in temperate regions, but relatively common in warm dry climates such as the Mediterranean, sub-Saharan Africa and the Middle East. In temperate regions over 90% of patients have other atopic conditions such as asthma and eczema and two-thirds have a family history of atopy. VKC often occurs on a seasonal basis, with a peak incidence over late spring and summer, although there may be mild perennial symptoms.

Classification

- **Palpebral VKC** primarily involves the upper tarsal conjunctiva. It may be associated with significant corneal disease as a result of the close apposition between the inflamed conjunctiva and the corneal epithelium.
- **Limbal** disease typically affects Black and Asian patients.
- **Mixed VKC** has features of both palpebral and limbal disease.

Diagnosis

The diagnosis is clinical and investigations are usually not required. Eosinophils may be abundant in conjunctival scrapings.

- **Symptoms** consist of intense itching, which may be associated with lacrimation, photophobia, a foreign body sensation, burning and thick mucoid discharge. Increased blinking is common.

- **Palpebral disease**
  - Early-mild disease is characterized by conjunctival hyperaemia and diffuse velvety papillary hypertrophy on the superior tarsal plate.
  - Macropapillae (<1 mm) have a flat-topped polygonal appearance reminiscent of cobblestones. Focal (Fig. 6.12A) or diffuse (Fig. 6.12B) whitish inflammatory infiltrates may be seen in intense disease.
  - Progression to giant papillae (>1 mm) can occur, as adjacent smaller lesions amalgamate when dividing septa rupture (Fig. 6.12C).
  - Mucus deposition between giant papillae (Fig. 6.12D).
  - Decreased disease activity is characterized by milder conjunctival injection and decreased mucus production.
- **Limbal disease**
  - Gelatinous limbal conjunctival papillae that may be associated with transient apically located white cellular collections (Horner–Trantas dots – Fig. 6.12E and F).
  - In tropical regions, limbal disease may be severe (Fig. 6.12 G and H).
- **Keratopathy** is more frequent in palpebral disease and may take the following forms:
  - Superior punctate epithelial erosions associated with layers of mucus on the superior cornea (Fig. 6.13A).
  - Epithelial macroerosions caused by a combination of epithelial toxicity from inflammatory mediators and a direct mechanical effect from papillae.
  - Plaques and 'shield' ulcers (Fig. 6.13B and C) may develop in palpebral or mixed disease when the exposed Bowman membrane becomes coated with mucus and calcium phosphate, leading to inadequate wetting and delayed re-epithelialization. This development is serious and warrants urgent attention to prevent secondary bacterial infection.
  - Subepithelial scars that are typically grey and oval and may affect vision.
  - Pseudogerontoxon can develop in recurrent limbal disease. It is characterized by a paralimbal band of superficial scarring resembling arcus senilis (Fig. 6.13D), adjacent to a previously inflamed segment of the limbus.
  - Vascularization does not tend to be prominent, though some peripheral superficial vessel ingrowth is common, especially superiorly.
  - Keratoconus and other forms of corneal ectasia are more common in VKC and are thought to be at least partly due to persistent eye rubbing.
  - Herpes simplex keratitis is more common than average, though less so than in atopic keratoconjunctivitis. It can be aggressive and is occasionally bilateral.
- **Eyelid disease** is usually mild, in contrast to atopic keratoconjunctivitis.

Atopic keratoconjunctivitis

Pathogenesis

Atopic keratoconjunctivitis (AKC) is a rare bilateral disease that typically develops in adulthood (peak incidence 30–50 years) following a long history of atopic dermatitis (eczema). Asthma is also extremely common in these patients. About 5% have suffered from childhood VKC. There is little or no gender preponderance. AKC tends to be chronic and unremitting, with a relatively low expectation of eventual resolution and is associated with significant visual morbidity. Whereas VKC is more frequently seasonal and generally worse in the spring, AKC tends to be perennial and is often worse in the winter. Patients are sensitive to a wide range of airborne environmental allergens.

Diagnosis

The distinction between AKC and VKC can be made clinically. Eosinophils tend to be less common in conjunctival scrapings than with VKC.

- **Symptoms** are similar to those of VKC, but are frequently more severe and unremitting.
- **Eyelids**
  - Skin changes (Fig. 6.14A) are more prominent than in VKC and are typically eczematoid: erythema, dryness, scaling and thickening, sometimes with disruption to epidermal integrity such as fissuring and scratches (excoriation), the latter due to intense itching.
  - Associated chronic staphylococcal blepharitis and madarosis are common.
  - There may be keratinization of the lid margin.
  - Hertoghe sign: absence of the lateral portion of the eyebrows.
  - Dennie–Morgan folds: lid skin folds caused by persistent rubbing.
  - Tightening of the facial skin may cause lower lid ectropion and epiphora.
  - Ptosis is not uncommon.
- **Conjunctival** involvement is preferentially inferior palpebral, whereas in VKC it is worse superiorly.
  - Discharge is generally more watery than the stringy mucoid discharge in VKC.
  - Hyperaemia; chemosis is not uncommon during active inflammation.
  - Papillae are initially smaller than in VKC although larger lesions may develop later.
  - Diffuse conjunctival infiltration and scarring may give a whitish, featureless appearance (Fig. 6.14B).
  - Cicatricial changes can lead to moderate symblepharon formation, forniceal shortening (Fig. 6.14C) and keratinization of the caruncle (Fig. 6.14D).
  - Limbal involvement similar to that of limbal VKC can be seen, including Horner–Trantas dots.
- **Keratopathy**
  - Punctate epithelial erosions over the inferior third of the cornea are common and can be marked.
  - Peripheral vascularization and stromal scarring are more common than in VKC (Fig. 6.14E).
  - Persistent epithelial defects (Fig. 6.14F), sometimes with associated focal thinning, can occasionally progress to perforation with descemetocoele (US spelling – descemetocele) formation.
  - Plaque formation may occur (see Fig. 6.13B and C).

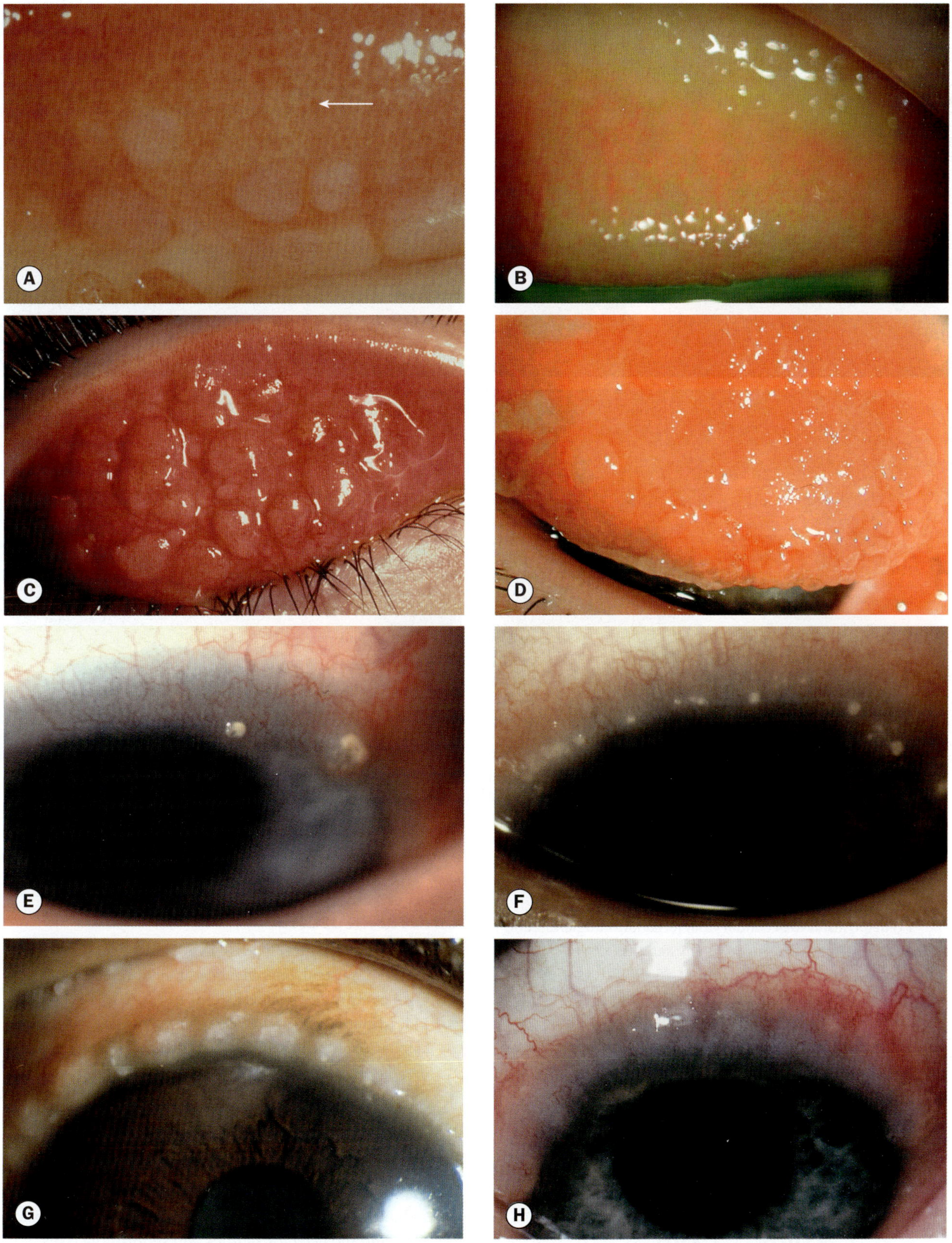

Fig. 6.12 Vernal disease. **(A)** Palpebral surface showing macropapillae with focal inflammatory infiltrates (arrow); **(B)** macropapillae with diffuse infiltrate; **(C)** giant papillae; **(D)** intense disease with mucus; **(E)** sparse limbal papillae; **(F)** limbal papillae with Horner–Trantas dots; **(G)** extensive limbal papillae; **(H)** severe limbal disease. *(Courtesy of S Tuft – fig. F.)*

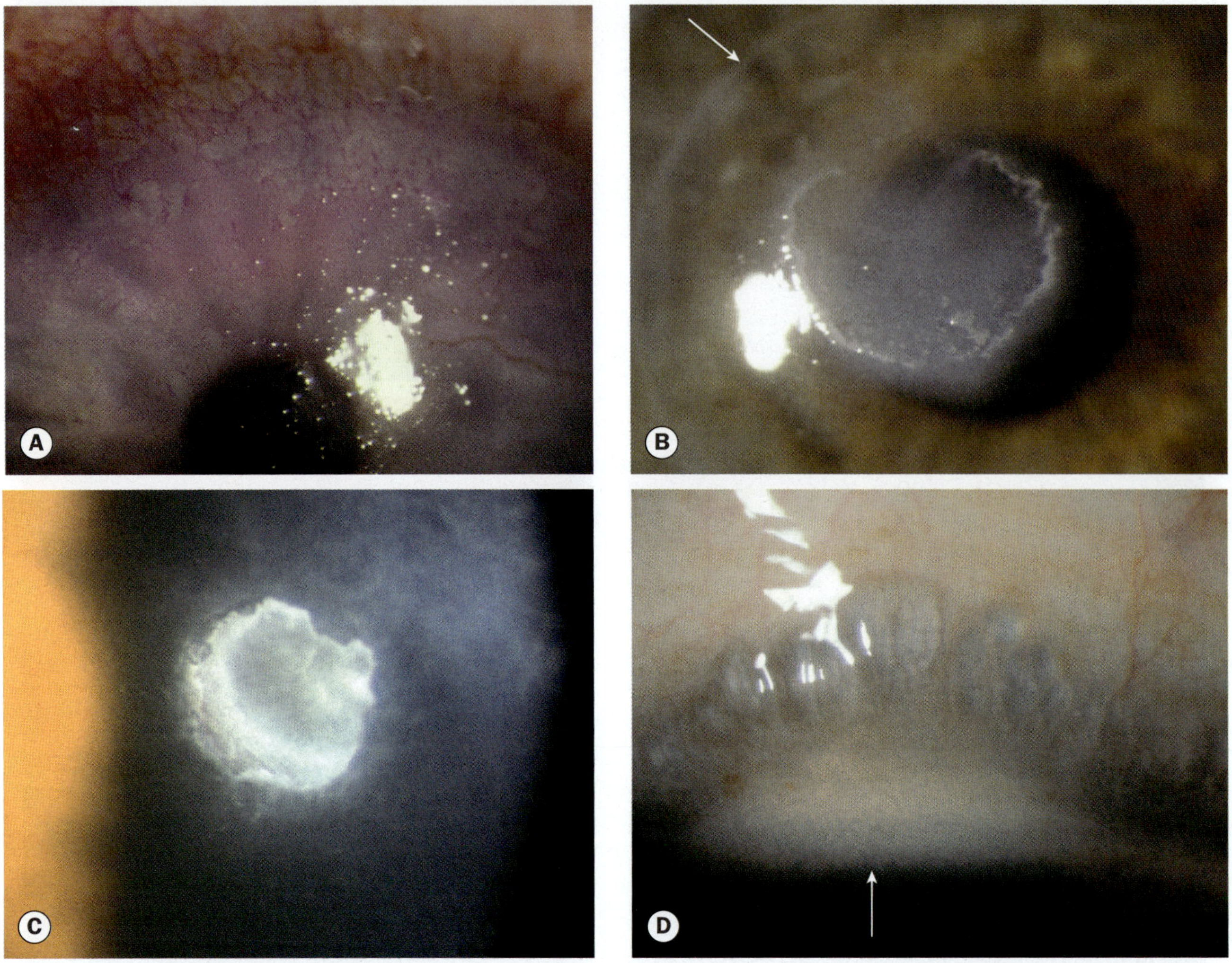

Fig. 6.13 Keratopathy in vernal disease. **(A)** Superior punctate erosions and mucus stained with rose Bengal; **(B)** early plaque in a corneal graft (arrow showing edge of graft); **(C)** plaque and shield ulcer; **(D)** pseudogerontoxon (arrow) and limbal papillae. *(Courtesy of S Tuft – fig. D.)*

  - Predisposition to secondary bacterial and fungal infection and to aggressive herpes simplex keratitis.
  - Keratoconus is common (about 15%) and as with VKC, may be secondary to chronic ocular rubbing.
- **Cataract**
  - Presenile shield-like anterior or posterior subcapsular cataracts are common and may be exacerbated by long-term steroid therapy.
  - Because of the high lid margin carriage of *S. aureus*, cataract surgery carries an increased risk of endophthalmitis.
  - Retinal detachment is more common than in the general population and is a particular risk following cataract surgery.

Treatment of VKC and AKC

The management of VKC does not differ substantially from that of AKC, although the latter is generally less responsive and requires more intensive and prolonged treatment.

General measures

- **Allergen avoidance**, if possible. Allergen (e.g. patch) testing is sometimes useful, but often gives non-specific results.
- **Cool compresses** may be helpful.
- **Lid hygiene** should be used for associated staphylococcal blepharitis. Moisturizing cream such as E45 can be applied to dry, fissured skin.
- **Bandage contact lens** wear to aid healing of persistent epithelial defects.

Local treatment

- **Mast cell stabilizers** (e.g. sodium cromoglicate, nedocromil sodium, lodoxamide) reduce the frequency of acute exacerbations and the need for steroids and so form the basis of many regimens, but are seldom effective in isolation. Several days to weeks of treatment are needed for a reasonable response and long-term therapy may be needed (lodoxamide is not licensed for long-term use).

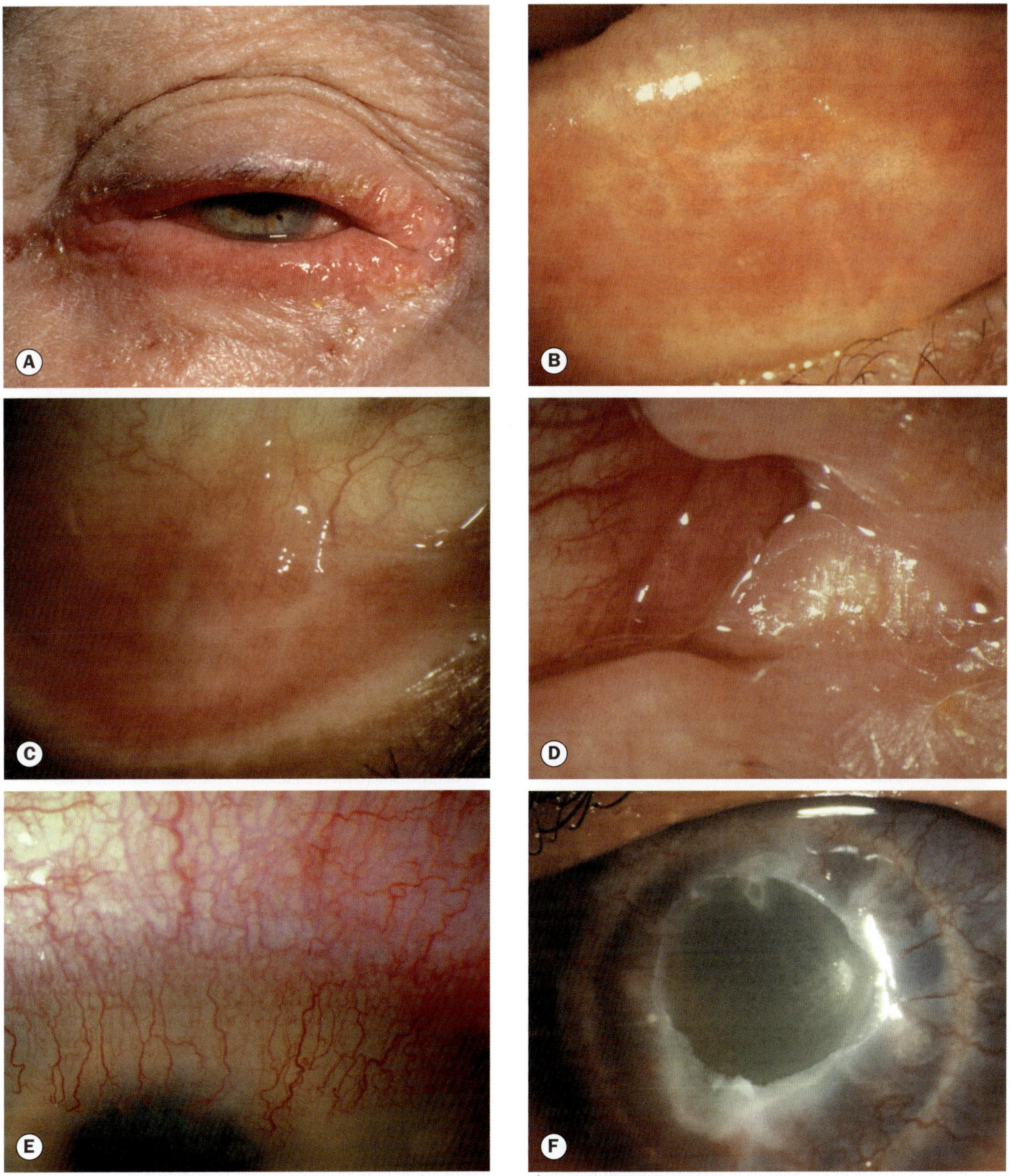

Fig. 6.14 Atopic disease. **(A)** Severe eyelid involvement; **(B)** infiltration and scarring of the tarsal conjunctiva; **(C)** forniceal shortening; **(D)** keratinization of the caruncle; **(E)** intense corneal vascularization; **(F)** persistent epithelial defect and peripheral corneal vascularization; a penetrating keratoplasty interface can be seen. *(Courtesy of S Tuft.)*

- **Topical antihistamines** (e.g. emedastine, epinastine, levocabastine, bepotastine) when used in isolation are about as effective as mast cell stabilizers. They are suitable for acute exacerbations but generally not for continuous long-term use and courses of several preparations are licensed for use only in courses of limited duration. A trial of several different agents may be worthwhile.
- **Combined antihistamine and vasoconstrictor** (e.g. antazoline with xylometazoline) may offer relief in some cases.
- **Combined action antihistamine/mast cell stabilizers** (e.g. azelastine, ketotifen, olopatadine) are helpful in many patients and have a relatively rapid onset of action.
- **Non-steroidal anti-inflammatory** preparations (e.g. ketorolac, diclofenac) may improve comfort by blocking non-histamine mediators. Combining one of these with a mast cell stabilizer is an effective regimen in some patients.
- **Topical steroids** (e.g. fluorometholone 0.1%, rimexolone 1%, prednisolone 0.5%, loteprednol etabonate 0.2% or 0.5%) are used for severe exacerbations of conjunctivitis and significant keratopathy. Reducing conjunctival activity generally leads to corneal improvement. They are usually prescribed in short but intensive (e.g. 2-hourly initially) courses, aiming for prompt tapering. Although the risk of elevation of intraocular pressure is low, monitoring is advisable if long-term treatment is necessary. Stronger preparations such as prednisolone 1% can be used, but carry a higher risk of steroid-induced glaucoma. Shield ulcers are often refractory to topical steroid treatment.
- **Steroid ointment** (e.g. hydrocortisone 0.5%) may be used to treat the eyelids in AKC, though as with eye drops, the duration of treatment should be minimized and the intraocular pressure (IOP) monitored.
- **Antibiotics** may be used in conjunction with steroids in severe keratopathy to prevent or treat bacterial infection.
- **Acetylcysteine** is a mucolytic agent that is useful in VKC for dissolving mucus filaments and deposits and addressing early plaque formation.
- **Immunomodulators**
  - **Ciclosporin** (0.05–2% between two and six times daily) may be indicated if steroids are ineffective, inadequate or poorly tolerated, or as a steroid-sparing agent in patients with severe disease. The effects typically take some weeks to be exerted and relapses may occur if treatment is stopped suddenly. Irritation and blurred vision are common.
  - **Calcineurin inhibitors** show increasing promise as an alternative to steroids in the treatment of allergic eye disease. Tacrolimus 0.03% ointment can be effective in AKC for severe eyelid disease. Instillation into the fornix has been effective in modulating conjunctival inflammation in refractory cases. Tacrolimus 0.1% ointment is particularly useful when applied topically in patients with shield ulcers and corneal epitheliopathy and can be used without topical steroids. Factors associated with a poor response to tacrolimus include the presence of a giant papillae and palpebral abnormality.
  - **Supratarsal steroid injection** may be considered in severe palpebral disease or for non-compliant patients. The injection is given into the conjunctival surface of the anaesthetized everted upper eyelid; 0.1 ml of betamethasone sodium phosphate 4 mg/ml, dexamethasone 4 mg/ml or triamcinolone 40 mg/ml is given.

TIP Topical steroids should not be used long term in a patient with allergic conjunctivitis without monitoring the IOP.

Systemic treatment

- **Oral antihistamines** help itching, promote sleep and reduce nocturnal eye rubbing. Because other inflammatory mediators are involved besides histamines, effectiveness is not assured. Some antihistamines (e.g. loratadine) cause relatively little drowsiness.
- **Antibiotics** (e.g. doxycycline 50–100 mg daily for 6 weeks, azithromycin 500 mg once daily for 3 days) may be given to reduce blepharitis-aggravated inflammation, usually in AKC.
- **Immunosuppressive agents** (e.g. steroids, ciclosporin, tacrolimus, azathioprine) may be effective at relatively low doses in AKC unresponsive to other measures. Short courses of high-dose steroids may be necessary to achieve rapid control in severe disease. Monoclonal antibodies against T cells have shown some promise in refractory cases.
- **Other treatments** that may be effective in some patients include aspirin in VKC (avoided in children and adolescents due to Reye syndrome risk), allergen desensitization and plasmapheresis in patients with high serum IgE levels.

Surgery

- **Superficial keratectomy** may be required to remove plaques or debride shield ulcers and allow epithelialization. Medical treatment must be maintained until the cornea has re-epithelialized in order to prevent recurrences. Excimer laser phototherapeutic keratectomy is an alternative.
- **Surface maintenance/restoration surgery** such as amniotic membrane overlay grafting or lamellar keratoplasty, or **eyelid procedures** such as botulinum toxin-induced ptosis or lateral tarsorrhaphy, may be required for severe persistent epithelial defects or ulceration. Gluing may be appropriate for focal ('punched-out') corneal perforations.

Non-allergic eosinophilic conjunctivitis

Non-allergic eosinophilic conjunctivitis (NAEC) is a recently proposed chronic non-atopic condition said to occur predominantly in middle-aged women in whom dry eye is also commonly present. It has been suggested that it is relatively common but under-diagnosed. It is thought to be of similar pathogenesis to non-allergic eosinophilic rhinitis. Conjunctival eosinophilia is present without significant IgE levels in the serum or tear film. Symptoms are similar to those of allergic conjunctivitis – itching, redness, foreign body sensation and mild watery discharge. Treatment is with a 1–2 week course of topical steroid for exacerbations followed by maintenance with topical mast cell stabilizers, non-steroidal anti-inflammatory agents or antihistamines.

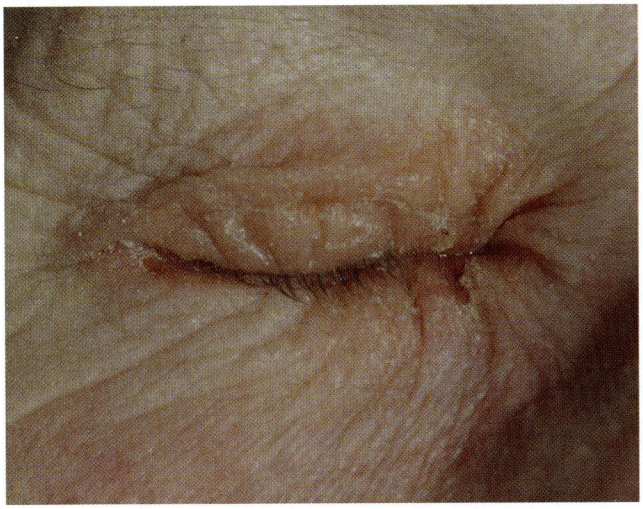

Fig. 6.15 Contact allergic blepharoconjunctivitis.

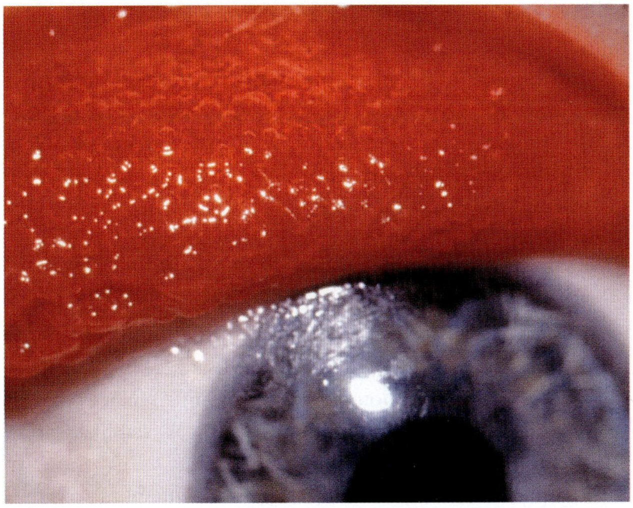

Fig. 6.16 Ocular prosthesis causing giant papillary conjunctivitis.

Contact allergic blepharoconjunctivitis

Analogous to contact dermatitis, this refers to the acute or subacute T-cell-mediated delayed hypersensitivity reaction seen most commonly by ophthalmologists as a reaction to eye drop constituents and by optometrists as a reaction to contact lens solutions. Mascara is a less common cause. There may be a conjunctival reaction, but signs predominantly involve the eyelid skin: erythema, thickening, induration and sometimes fissuring occur (Fig. 6.15). Treatment is by discontinuation of the precipitant. A mild topical steroid ointment can be helpful.

Giant (mechanically induced) papillary conjunctivitis

Pathogenesis

Mechanically induced papillary conjunctivitis, the severe form of which is known as giant papillary conjunctivitis (GPC), can occur secondary to a variety of mechanical stimuli of the tarsal conjunctiva. It is most frequently encountered with contact lens (CL) wear, when it is termed contact lens-associated papillary conjunctivitis (CLPC). The risk is increased by the build-up of proteinaceous deposits and cellular debris on the CL surface. Ocular prostheses (Fig. 6.16), exposed sutures and scleral buckles, corneal surface irregularity and filtering blebs can all be responsible. A related phenomenon is the so-called 'mucus fishing syndrome', when, in a variety of underlying anterior segment disorders, patients develop or exacerbate a chronic papillary reaction due to repetitive manual removal of mucus. Giant papillae can also be seen in other conditions, such as VKC and AKC.

Diagnosis

- **Symptoms** consist of a foreign body sensation, redness, itching, increased mucus production, blurring and loss of CL tolerance. Symptoms may be worse after lens removal. Patients should be questioned about CL cleaning and maintenance.
- **Signs**
  - Variable mucous discharge.
  - Substantial CL protein deposits may be present.
  - Excessive CL mobility due to upper lid capture.
  - Superior tarsal hyperaemia and papillae. By definition, 'giant' papillae are >1.0 mm in diameter, but the clinical syndrome of mechanically induced papillary conjunctivitis commonly features only fine/medium papillae, particularly in early or mild disease.
  - Focal apical ulceration and whitish scarring may develop on larger papillae.
  - Keratopathy is rare because of the relatively subdued secretion of inflammatory cytokines.
  - Ptosis may occur, mainly as a result of irritative spasm and tissue laxity secondary to chronic inflammation.

Treatment

Other causes of conjunctival papillae should be excluded, as well as CL intolerance due to other causes, such as a reaction to lens cleaning solutions and dry eyes.

- Removal of the stimulus
  - CL wear should be discontinued for several weeks and the current lenses replaced. For mild–moderate disease, this may be adequate for resolution, sometimes in conjunction with reduced wearing time. In severe CLPC a longer interval without lens wear may be needed.
  - Removal of other underlying causes, such as exposed sutures or a scleral buckle.
  - Assessment of the status and fit of an ocular prosthesis.
  - Filtering bleb: partial excision, revision with non-penetrating drainage surgery or glaucoma drainage device implantation.
- Ensure effective cleaning of CL or prosthesis
  - Changing the type of CL solution, particularly discontinuation of preservative-containing preparations.
  - Switching to monthly then daily disposable CL if the condition persists after renewing non-disposable lenses.

  - Rigid lenses carry a reduced risk of CLPC (5%), probably because they are easier to clean effectively.
  - Cessation of CL wear, substituting spectacles or refractive surgery, may be necessary for severe or refractory disease.
  - Regular (at least weekly) use of CL protein removal tablets.
  - Prosthesis: polishing, cleaning with detergent, coating.
- Topical
  - Mast cell stabilizers should be non-preserved in patients wearing soft contact lenses, or can be instilled when the lenses are not in the eye, with a delay of perhaps half an hour after drop instillation prior to lens insertion. Most can be continued long-term if necessary.
  - Antihistamines, non-steroidal anti-inflammatory agents and combined antihistamines/mast cell stabilizers may each be of benefit.
  - Topical steroids can be used for the acute phase of resistant cases, particularly those where effective removal of the stimulus is difficult, as in bleb-related disease.

CONJUNCTIVITIS IN BLISTERING MUCOCUTANEOUS DISEASE

Mucous membrane pemphigoid

Introduction

Mucous membrane pemphigoid (MMP), also known as ocular cicatricial pemphigoid (OCP), comprises a group of chronic autoimmune mucocutaneous blistering diseases. An unknown trigger leads to a type II (cytotoxic) hypersensitivity response resulting in antibodies binding at the basement membrane zone (BMZ), the activation of complement and the recruitment of inflammatory cells, with localized separation of the epidermis from the dermis at the BMZ and subsequent progression to scarring. Studies of HLA typing have found an increased susceptibility to the disease in patients with HLA-DR4. The HLA-DQB1 allele in particular shows a strong association with OCP and other forms of pemphigoid disease.

A wide range of epithelial tissues can be involved, including the skin and various mucous membranes. Particular clinical forms of MMP tend to involve specific target tissues: bullous pemphigoid (BP) shows a predilection for skin and ocular mucous membrane pemphigoid (OMMP, also known as ocular cicatricial pemphigoid – OCP) involves the conjunctiva in the majority of cases and causes progressive scarring (cicatrization). The disease typically presents in old age and affects females more commonly than males by a 2:1 ratio. Other causes of cicatrizing conjunctivitis include Stevens–Johnson syndrome, trachoma, drug-induced, trauma and severe or chronic conjunctivitis of many types. MMP should not be confused with pemphigus, a distinct group of disorders.

Ocular features

- **Diagnosis is principally clinical**, but biopsy of involved mucous membrane often shows supportive changes (linear antibody and complement BMZ deposition).
- **Michel's transport medium** should be used when taking a specimen for direct immunofluorescence and immunoelectron microscopy.

Progression of ocular disease has been divided into stages as follows:

- **Foster's classification system**
  - Stage I: early stage associated with chronic conjunctivitis, tear dysfunction and subepithelial fibrosis.
  - Stage II: forniceal shortening, particularly inferiorly.
  - Stage III: symblepharon formation.
  - Stage IV: surface keratinization and cicatricial ankyloblepharon.
- **Mondino's classification system** (based on inferior forniceal depth loss)
  - Stage I: up to 25%.
  - Stage II: 25–50%.
  - Stage III: 50–75%.
  - Stage IV: greater than 75%.
- **Symptoms.** Insidious or relapsing–remitting non-specific bilateral conjunctivitis; misdiagnosis (e.g. dry eye) is common.
- **Conjunctiva**
  - Papillary conjunctivitis, diffuse hyperaemia, oedema and subtle fibrosis (Fig. 6.17A).
  - Fine lines of subconjunctival fibrosis and shortening of the inferior fornices. Symblepharon (plural: symblephara) formation refers to adhesion between the bulbar and palpebral conjunctiva (Fig. 6.17B and C).
  - Necrosis in severe cases.
  - Flattening of the plica and keratinization of the caruncle.
  - Dry eye due to destruction of goblet cells and accessory lacrimal glands and occlusion of the main lacrimal ductules.
  - Monitoring should include the measurement of forniceal depth and noting the position of adhesions.
- **Eyelids**
  - Aberrant (trichiatic) lashes, chronic blepharitis and keratinization of the lid margin.
  - Ankyloblepharon is an adhesion at the outer canthus between the upper and lower lids (Fig. 6.17D).
- **Cornea**
  - Epithelial defects (Fig. 6.18A) associated with drying and exposure.
  - Infiltration and peripheral vascularization (Fig. 6.18B).
  - Keratinization and conjunctivalization of the corneal surface (Fig. 6.18C) due to epithelial stem cell failure.
  - End-stage disease is characterized by total symblepharon and corneal opacification (Fig. 6.18D).

Systemic features

- **Mucosal** involvement is very common and is characterized by subepidermal blisters, most frequently oral (Fig. 6.19A). Severe manifestations include oesophageal and laryngeal strictures.
- **Skin** lesions are less common (25%) and present as tense blisters and erosions of the head and neck, groin and extremities (Fig. 6.19B).

Systemic treatment

Systemic treatment is the mainstay of management. Any detectable inflammatory activity should be suppressed.

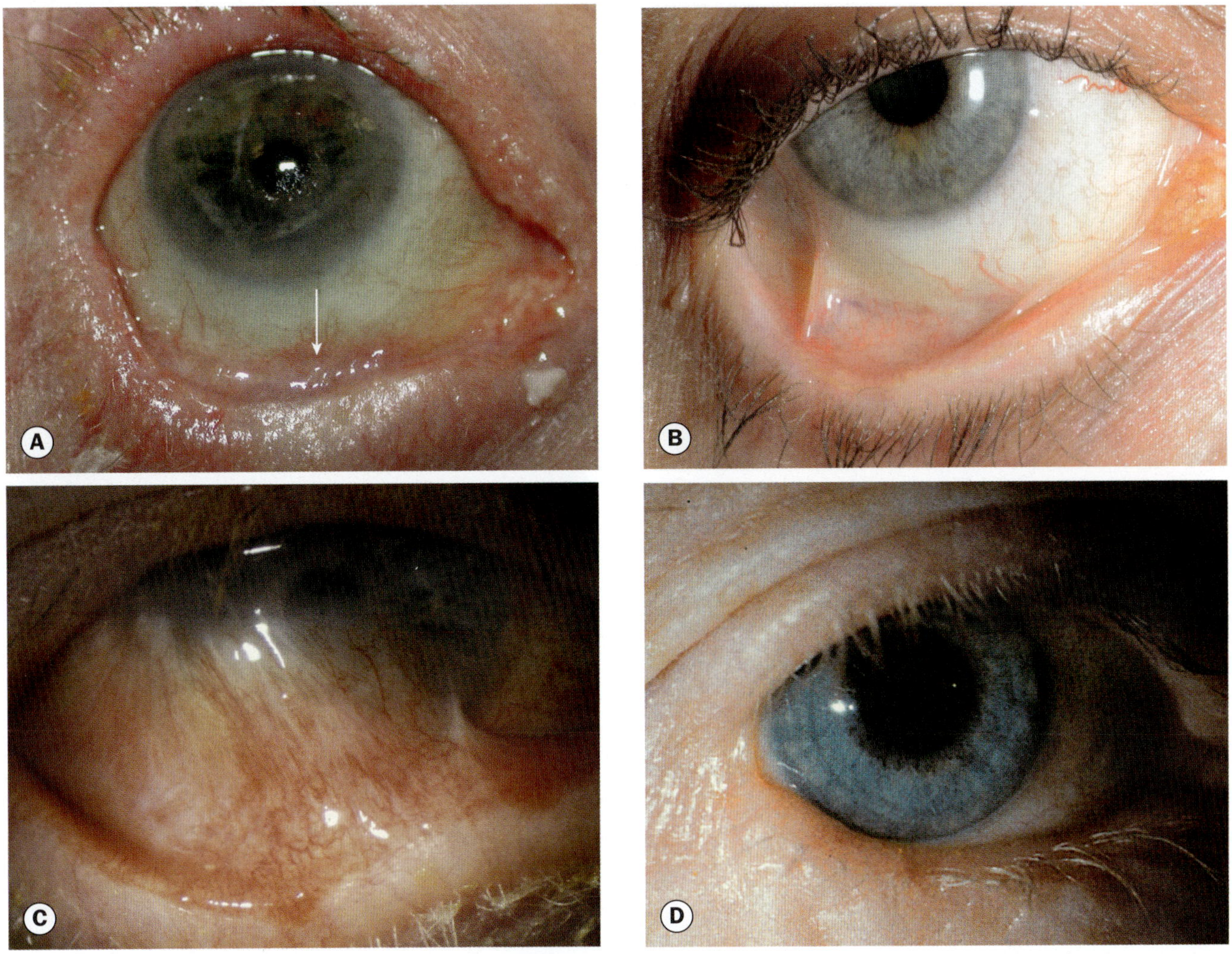

Fig. 6.17 Conjunctivitis in ocular cicatricial pemphigoid. **(A)** Early disease with hyperaemia and conjunctival fibrosis (arrow); **(B)** symblepharon formation; **(C)** severe fibrosis with forniceal shortening and symblepharon formation; **(D)** ankyloblepharon.

- **Dapsone** (diaminodiphenylsulfone) is a useful first-line treatment in patients with mild–moderate disease. Approximately 70% of patients respond favourably. It is contraindicated in glucose-6-phosphate dehydrogenase deficiency. Sulfasalazine is sometimes better tolerated.
- **Antimetabolites** (e.g. azathioprine, methotrexate, mycophenolate mofetil) are alternatives for mild–moderate disease if dapsone is contraindicated, ineffective or poorly tolerated and are suitable for long-term therapy. Dapsone can be used in conjunction if necessary. Cyclophosphamide may be reserved for severe or refractory disease.
- **Steroids** (prednisolone 1–1.5 mg/kg) are effective for rapid disease control, but adverse effects limit long-term use. IOP should be monitored.
- **Other measures** include intravenous immunoglobulin therapy and rituximab. Remission has been reported with a combination regimen.

Local treatment

- **Topical**
  - Artificial tears (preferably preservative-free) are an integral part of most regimens.
  - Topical steroids, ciclosporin or tacrolimus may be used as an adjunct to systemic immunosuppressive treatment.
  - Retinoic acid may reduce keratinization.
  - Antibiotics when indicated.
  - Lid hygiene and low-dose oral tetracycline for blepharitis.
- **Subconjunctival** mitomycin C and/or steroid injection may be used as a temporizing aid or if systemic immunosuppression is not possible.
- **Contact lenses** may be used with caution to protect the cornea from aberrant lashes and from dehydration.

Reconstructive surgery

Reconstructive surgery, preferably under systemic steroid cover, should be considered when active disease is controlled. Seemingly trivial surgical intervention can lead to exacerbation of disease.

- Aberrant eyelashes (see Ch. 2).
- Punctal occlusion to aid tear retention.

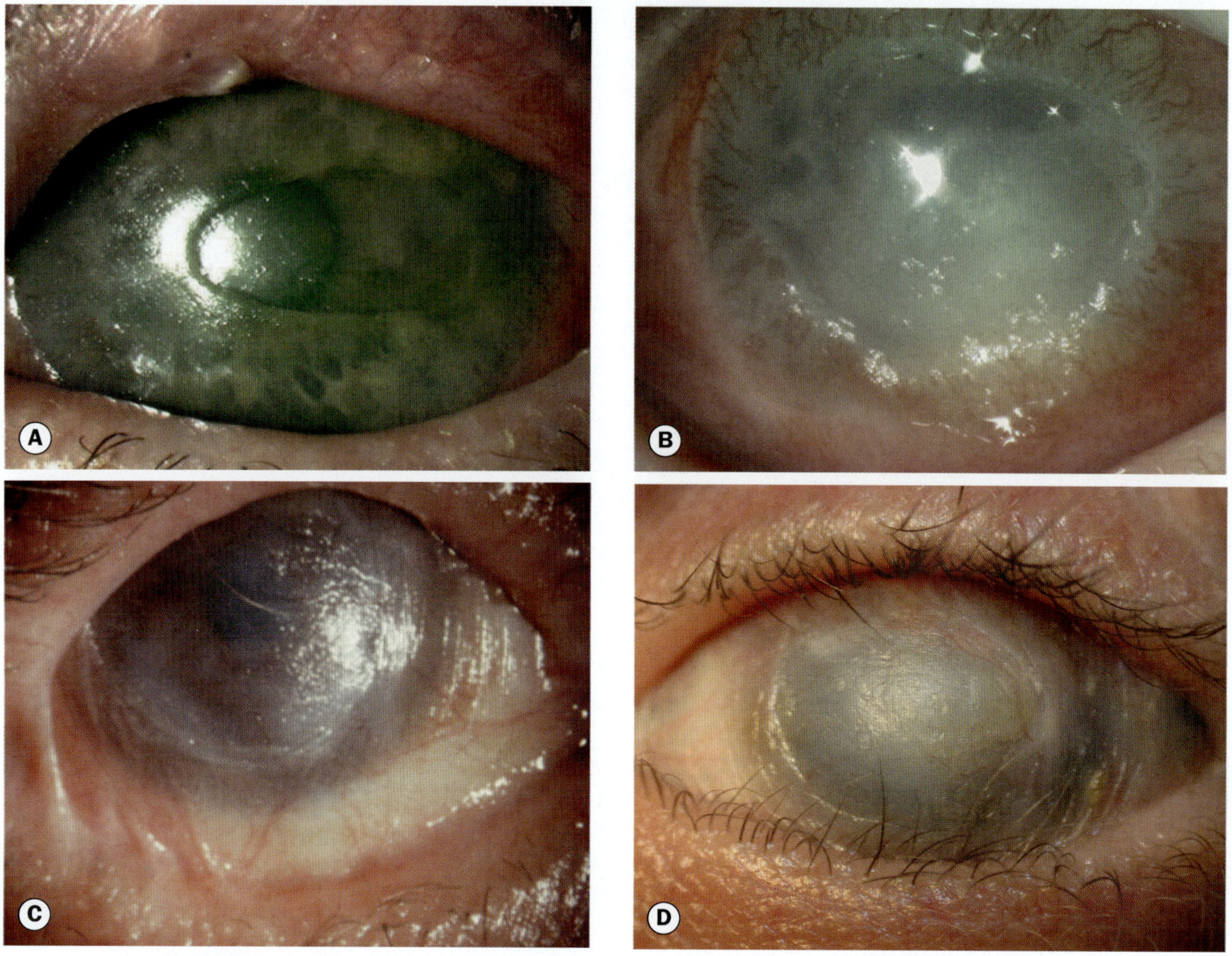

Fig. 6.18 Keratopathy in ocular cicatricial pemphigoid. **(A)** Epithelial defect; **(B)** peripheral vascularization and infiltration; **(C)** keratinization with ankyloblepharon; **(D)** end-stage disease. *(Courtesy of S Tuft – figs A–C.)*

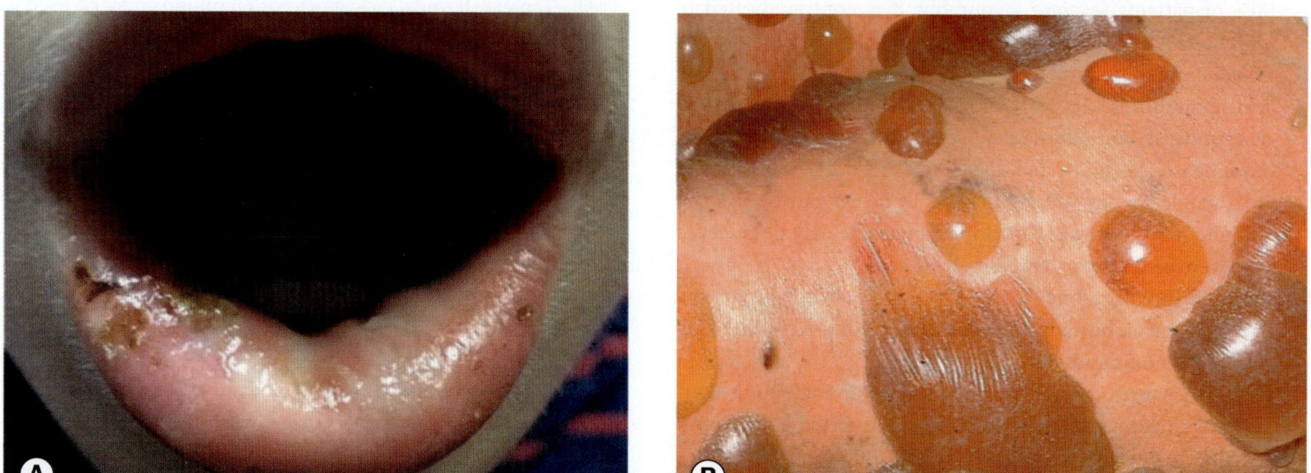

Fig. 6.19 Mucous membrane pemphigoid. **(A)** Oral blisters; **(B)** severe skin blistering. *(Courtesy of J David – fig. A.)*

- Lateral tarsorrhaphy or botulinum toxin-induced ptosis may be used to promote healing of corneal epithelial defects.
- Entropion repair: conjunctival incision is avoided if possible.
- Cataract surgery is commonly required.
- Mucous membrane autografting or amniotic membrane transplantation for conjunctival resurfacing and forniceal restoration.
- Limbal stem cell transfer may be attempted for corneal re-epithelialization.
- Keratoplasty carries a high risk of failure; lamellar grafts may be effective for perforation.
- Keratoprosthesis may be the only option in end-stage disease.

Stevens–Johnson syndrome/toxic epidermal necrolysis (Lyell syndrome)

Introduction

The terms 'Stevens–Johnson syndrome (SJS)' and 'erythema multiforme major' have historically been used synonymously. However, it is now believed that erythema multiforme (without the 'major') is a distinct disease, milder and recurrent, with somewhat dissimilar clinical features. Toxic epidermal necrolysis (TEN – Lyell syndrome) is a severe variant of SJS. SJS/TEN patients tend to be young adults, though other groups may be affected. The condition involves a cell-mediated delayed hypersensitivity reaction, usually related to drug exposure. A wide range of medications have been incriminated, including antibiotics (especially sulfonamides and trimethoprim), analgesics including paracetamol (acetaminophen), nevirapine (widely prescribed as a part of combination therapy for HIV infection), cold remedies and anticonvulsants. Infections due to microorganisms such as *Mycoplasma pneumoniae* and HSV and some cancers have also been implicated. Because symptoms often take weeks to develop, in many cases the precipitant cannot be identified. Mortality overall is around 5% in SJS (death is commonly due to infection), but is considerably higher in TEN.

Ocular features

In the acute stage there are often practical obstacles to standard slit lamp examination, as the patient may be bedridden and undergoing barrier nursing. A portable slit lamp may be helpful.

- **Symptoms.** Acute ocular symptoms may include redness, mild–severe grittiness, photophobia, watering and blurring.
- **Acute signs**
  - Haemorrhagic crusting of the lid margins (Fig. 6.20A) is characteristic. Skin lesions may be confluent and it is often difficult for an examiner to open the eyes without causing marked discomfort.
  - Papillary conjunctivitis, which can range from mild, transient and self-limiting to severe (Fig. 6.20B).
  - Conjunctival membranes and pseudomembranes (Fig. 6.20C), severe hyperaemia, haemorrhages, blisters and patchy infarction.
  - Keratopathy: a spectrum of lesions from punctate erosions to large epithelial defects, secondary bacterial keratitis and occasionally perforation.
  - Iritis is not infrequent and panophthalmitis has been reported.
- **Late signs**
  - Conjunctival cicatrization (Fig. 6.20D) with forniceal shortening and symblepharon formation.
  - Keratinization of the conjunctiva and lid margin (Fig. 6.20E), sometimes with abrasive plaque formation.
  - Eyelid complications include cicatricial entropion and ectropion, trichiasis, metaplastic lashes and ankyloblepharon.
  - Keratopathy including scarring, vascularization and keratinization (Fig. 6.20F) as a result of the primary inflammation and/or infection, as well as cicatricial entropion and aberrant lashes.
  - Watery eyes due to fibrosis of the lacrimal puncta. Dry eyes may also occur as a result of fibrosis of lacrimal gland ductules and conjunctival metaplasia with loss of goblet cells.

Systemic features

Skin biopsy may help to establish the diagnosis but is rarely necessary.

- **Symptoms.** Flu-like symptoms, which can be severe, may last up to 14 days before the appearance of lesions. In many cases the patient is very ill and hospitalization is required. Symptoms of systemic mucosal involvement include nasal pain and discharge, pain on micturition, diarrhoea, cough, shortness of breath and pain on eating and drinking.
- **Signs**
  - Mucosal involvement is characterized by blistering and haemorrhagic crusting of the lips (Fig. 6.21A). The blisters may also involve the tongue, oropharynx, nasal mucosa and occasionally the genitalia.
  - Small purpuric, vesicular, haemorrhagic or necrotic skin lesions involving the extremities, face and trunk (Fig. 6.21B). These are usually transient but may be widespread. Healing usually occurs within 1–4 weeks, leaving a pigmented scar.
  - Widespread sloughing of the epidermis is uncommon.
  - 'Target' lesions showing the classic three zones are now viewed as characteristic of erythema multiforme rather than SJS/TEN.

Systemic treatment

- **Removal of the precipitant** if possible, such as discontinuation of drugs and treatment of suspected infection.
- **General supportive measures** such as maintenance of adequate hydration, electrolyte balance and nutrition (especially protein replacement) are critical. Management in a specialist burns unit should reduce the chance of infection when the extent of skin involvement is substantial.
- **Systemic steroids** remain controversial. There are reports of increased mortality in older papers, but later research has raised the possibility that early short-term high-dose intravenous treatment may improve outcomes.
- **Other immunosuppressants** including ciclosporin, azathioprine, cyclophosphamide and intravenous immunoglobulin

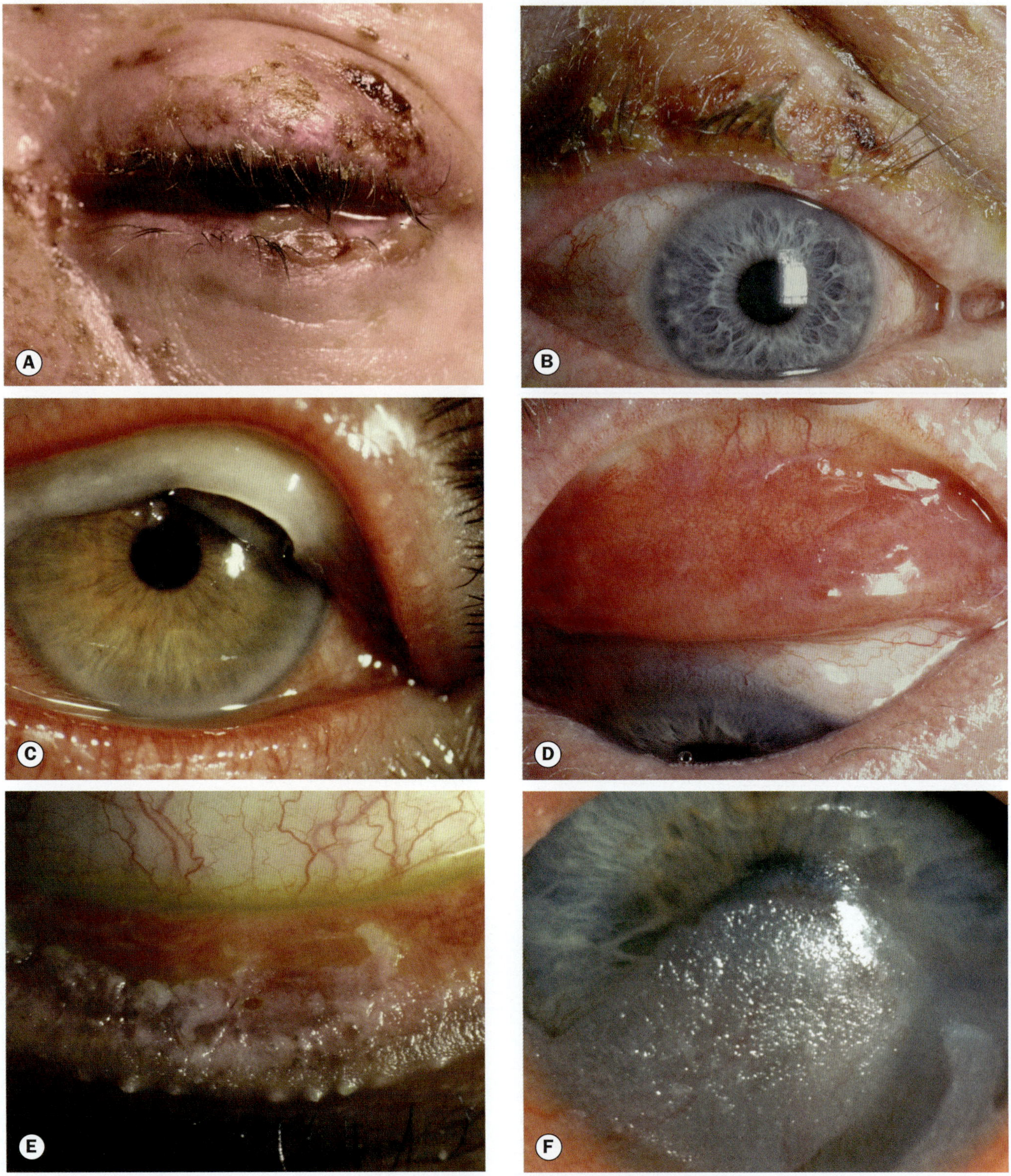

Fig. 6.20 Ocular features of Stevens–Johnson syndrome. **(A)** Haemorrhagic lid crusting; **(B)** acute conjunctivitis; **(C)** pseudomembrane; **(D)** conjunctival scarring; **(E)** keratinization with severe lid margin involvement; **(F)** corneal keratinization. *(Courtesy of R Bates – fig. A; S Tuft – figs E and F.)*

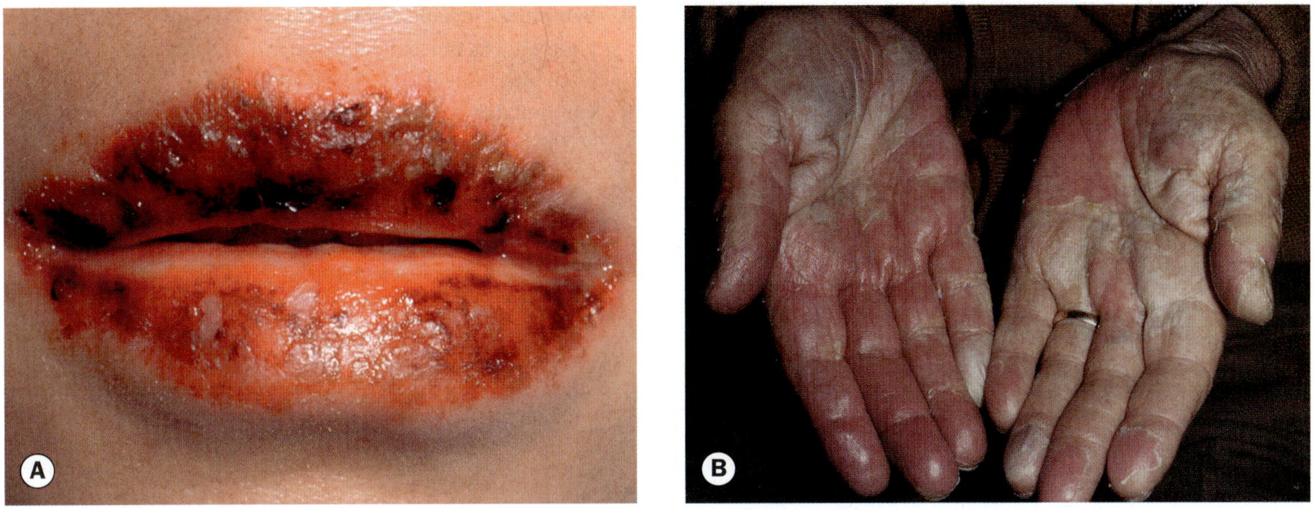

Fig. 6.21 Systemic features in Stevens–Johnson syndrome. **(A)** Haemorrhagic lip crusting; **(B)** excoriated skin.

may be considered in selected cases, but are controversial and controlled trials are lacking.

- **Systemic antibiotics** may be given as prophylaxis against skin or other systemic infection, avoiding those known to be at higher risk of precipitating SJS/TEN.

Ocular treatment

- **Acute disease.** Daily review is advisable initially in most patients to check the corneas and exclude symblepharon formation.
  - Topical lubricants are used as frequently as necessary, e.g. hypromellose 0.3% preservative-free up to hourly, high-viscosity ointment during sleep.
  - Prevention of corneal exposure, e.g. moisture chambers, gel pads if mechanically ventilated.
  - Topical steroids may be used for iritis and for conjunctival inflammation, though a benefit for the latter has not been demonstrated conclusively.
  - Topical cycloplegia (e.g. atropine 1% once or twice daily) may improve comfort.
  - Lysis of developing symblephara with a sterile glass rod or damp cotton bud.
  - A scleral ring, consisting of a large haptic lens, may help to prevent symblepharon formation (Fig. 6.22).
  - Pseudomembrane/membrane peeling can be considered, although the benefit is unproven.
  - Treatment of acute corneal problems such as bacterial keratitis.
  - Conjunctival swabs should be considered for prophylactic culture.
  - IOP monitoring may be prudent, using portable tonometry if necessary.
- **Chronic disease**
  - Adequate lubrication, including punctal occlusion if required.
  - Topical transretinoic acid 0.01% or 0.025% may reverse keratinization.
  - Treatment of aberrant lashes (see Ch. 2).

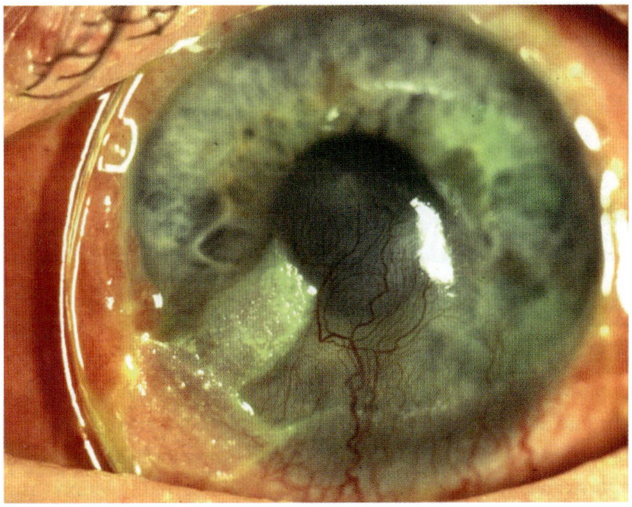

Fig. 6.22 Scleral ring used to prevent symblepharon formation in Stevens–Johnson syndrome. *(Courtesy of S Tuft.)*

  - Bandage contact lenses (typically gas permeable scleral lenses) to maintain surface moisture, protect the cornea from aberrant lashes and address irregular astigmatism.
  - Mucous membrane grafting (e.g. buccal mucosa autograft) for forniceal reconstruction.
  - Corneal rehabilitation may involve superficial keratectomy for keratinization, lamellar corneal grafting for superficial scarring (preferred to penetrating keratoplasty), amniotic membrane grafting, limbal stem cell transplantation and keratoprosthesis implantation in end-stage disease.

Graft-versus-host disease

Introduction

Ocular graft-versus-host disease (GVHD) occurs in patients who have undergone allogenic haematological stem cell transplantation, an operation that is undertaken on an estimated 25,000 people annually worldwide. It can occur in patients who have acute or chronic GVHD, although it is more frequently seen in the chronic form. Clinically it manifests in a similar fashion to Stevens–Johnson syndrome. Ocular manifestations develop in 40–60% of patients after stem cell transplantation and can lead to significant ocular surface consequences.

- **Ocular features**
  - Dry eye syndrome (keratoconjunctivitis sicca).
  - Conjunctival hyperaemia with pseudomembrane and membrane formation.
  - Chronic inflammation leading to cicatricial changes in the conjunctiva and occasionally entropion formation.
  - Superior limbic keratoconjunctivitis.
  - Corneal manifestations including punctate epithelial keratopathy, marginal keratitis and filamentary keratitis. Severe disease can lead to corneal erosion, thinning, ulceration and possible perforation.

Treatment

- **Artificial tears** can be helpful (see above).
- **Topical cyclosporine 0.5%** is the mainstay of treatment.
- **Systemic treatment** does not necessarily improve the ocular symptoms and signs. Oral steroids are often used.

MISCELLANEOUS DISORDERS OF THE CONJUNCTIVA

Superior limbic keratoconjunctivitis

Introduction

Superior limbic keratoconjunctivitis (SLK) is a relatively uncommon chronic disease of the superior limbus and the superior bulbar and tarsal conjunctiva. It affects one or both eyes of middle-aged women, approximately 50% of whom have abnormal thyroid function (usually hyperthyroidism). Approximately 3% of patients with thyroid eye disease have SLK. It can be associated with graft-versus-host disease. The condition is probably under-diagnosed because symptoms are typically more severe than signs. The course can be prolonged over years although remission eventually occurs spontaneously. There are similarities to mechanically induced papillary conjunctivitis and a comparable clinical picture has been described with CL wear and following upper lid surgery or trauma. It is unlikely to be caused by tight upper eyelids. The condition is believed to be the result of blink-related trauma between the upper lid and the superior bulbar conjunctiva, precipitated in many cases by tear film insufficiency and an excess of lax conjunctival tissue. With increased conjunctival movement there is mechanical damage to the tarsal and bulbar conjunctival surfaces, the resultant inflammatory response leading to increasing conjunctival oedema and redundancy, with the creation of a self-perpetuating cycle. It may be analogous to conjunctivochalasis affecting the lower bulbar conjunctiva (see Ch. 3).

Diagnosis

Enquiry should be made about contact lens wear and previous eyelid surgery or trauma.

- **Symptoms** include a foreign body sensation, burning, mild photophobia, mucoid discharge and frequent blinking, and are often intermittent.
- **Conjunctiva**
  - Hyperaemia of a radial band of the superior bulbar conjunctiva (Fig. 6.23A) that stains with rose Bengal and may be best seen macroscopically.
  - Limbal papillary hypertrophy (Fig. 6.23B). Limbal palisades may be lost superiorly.
  - Papillary hypertrophy of the superior tarsal plate, often having a diffuse velvety appearance (Fig. 6.23C).
  - Light downward pressure on the upper lid results in a fold of redundant conjunctiva crossing the upper limbus.
  - Petechial haemorrhages may be present.
  - Keratinization can be demonstrated on biopsy or impression cytology.
- **Cornea**
  - Superior punctate corneal epithelial erosions are common and are often separated from the limbus by a zone of normal epithelium.
  - Superior filamentary keratitis develops in about one-third of cases.
  - Mild superior pannus resembling arcus senilis may be seen in long-standing disease.
  - Keratoconjunctivitis sicca is present in only about 50%.
- **Investigation**
  - Thyroid function testing should be performed if the patient is not known to have thyroid disease.
  - Biopsy or impression cytology may reveal keratinization of the superior bulbar conjunctiva.

TIP Check thyroid function in patients with superior limbic keratoconjunctivitis.

Treatment

- **Topical**
  - Lubricants to reduce friction between the tarsal and bulbar conjunctiva should be used regularly and frequently.
  - Acetylcysteine 5% or 10% four times daily to break down filaments and provide lubrication.
  - Mast cell stabilizers and steroids to address any inflammatory component. Steroids may be best used in short intensive courses with rapid tapering and should be reserved for severe cases.
  - Promising results have been reported with topical rebamipide.
  - Ciclosporin 0.05% twice daily as primary or adjunctive therapy, particularly in the presence of coexisting keratoconjunctivitis sicca.
  - Retinoic acid to retard keratinization.
  - Autologous serum 20% drops can be beneficial but may require instillation up to 10 times a day.
- **Soft contact lenses**, which intervene between the lid and the superior conjunctiva, are effective in some cases. Interestingly, a unilateral lens may provide bilateral relief.

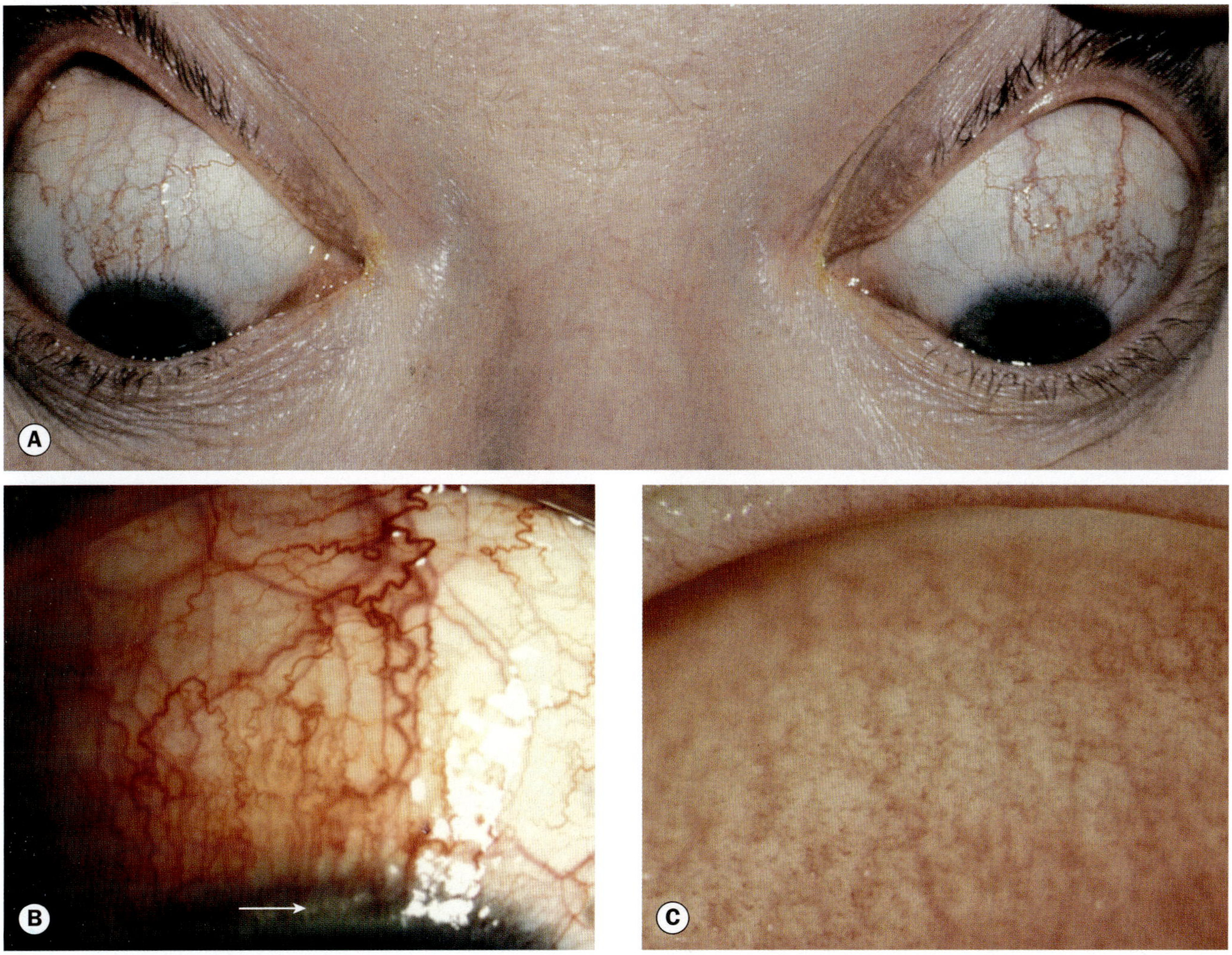

Fig. 6.23 Superior limbic keratoconjunctivitis. **(A)** Macroscopic appearance showing hyperaemia; **(B)** hyperaemic band of superior bulbar conjunctiva with limbal papillae (arrow); **(C)** diffuse velvety papillary hypertrophy.

- **Supratarsal steroid injection.** 0.1 ml of triamcinolone 40 mg/ml may break the inflammatory cycle.
- **Temporary superior and/or inferior punctal occlusion.**
- **Resection** of the superior limbal conjunctiva, either in a zone extending 2 mm from the superior limbus or of the area staining with rose Bengal, is often effective in resistant disease. Lax conjunctiva is removed, with regrowth tending to be firmly anchored. There is no consensus as to whether underlying Tenon capsule should be excised.
- **Conjunctival ablation** by applying silver nitrate 0.5% (not cautery sticks) or thermocautery to the affected area.
- **Treatment of associated thyroid dysfunction** may improve SLK.

Ligneous conjunctivitis

Introduction

Ligneous conjunctivitis is a very rare potentially sight- and even life-threatening disorder characterized by recurrent, often bilateral fibrin-rich pseudomembranous lesions of wood-like consistency that develop mainly on the tarsal conjunctiva. It is generally a systemic condition and may involve the periodontal tissue, the upper and lower respiratory tract, kidneys, middle ear and female genitalia. Death can occasionally occur from pulmonary involvement. In susceptible patients abnormal patterns of damage repair are found, particularly a failure of normal clearance of products of the acute stages of the healing process. This is manifested predominantly in mucosal tissue. A deficiency in plasmin-mediated fibrinolysis may be a key common factor in many patients. Episodes may be triggered by relatively minor trauma, or by systemic events such as fever and antifibrinolytic therapy.

Diagnosis

- **Histopathology** shows amorphous subepithelial deposits of eosinophilic material consisting predominantly of fibrin (Fig. 6.24A).
- **Presentation** is with non-specific conjunctivitis, usually in childhood (median age 5 years), although onset may be at any age. A conjunctival lesion is commonly noted by parents.

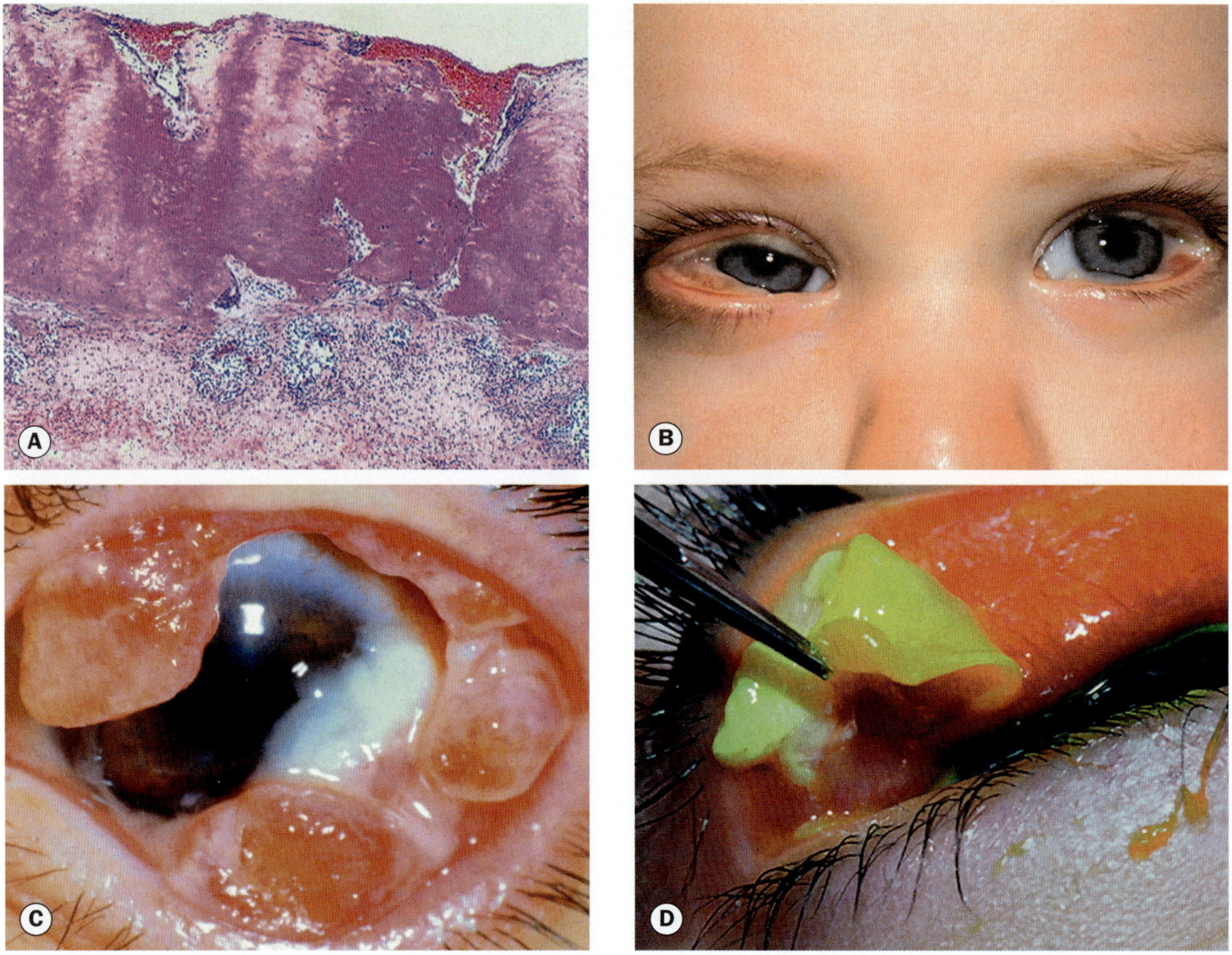

Fig. 6.24 Ligneous conjunctivitis. **(A)** Histology showing eosinophilic fibrinous coagulum on the conjunctival surface; **(B)** and **(C)** multiple ligneous lesions; **(D)** lesion removal. *(Courtesy of J Harry and G Misson, from* Clinical Ophthalmic Pathology, *Butterworth-Heinemann 2001 – fig. A; JH Krachmer, MJ Mannis and EJ Holland, from* Cornea, *Mosby 2005 – fig. C; J Dart – fig. D.)*

- **Signs**
  - Gradually enlarging red–white lobular conjunctival masses (Figs 6.24B and C) which may be covered by a thick yellow–white mucoid discharge.
  - Corneal scarring, vascularization, infection or melting.

Treatment

Treatment tends to be unsatisfactory and spontaneous resolution is rare. It is important to discontinue any antifibrinolytic drugs.

- **Surgical removal** (Fig. 6.24D) with meticulous diathermy of the base of the lesion. Preoperative topical plasminogen may soften pseudomembranes and facilitate removal.
- **Topical**
  - Following membrane removal, hourly heparin and steroids are commenced immediately and continued until the wound has re-epithelialized, with subsequent tapering over several weeks until all signs of inflammation have disappeared.
  - Recurrence may be retarded by long-term ciclosporin and steroid instillation.
- **Other modalities**
  - Intravenous or topical plasminogen.
  - Amniotic membrane transplantation to the conjunctiva following lesion removal.
  - Prophylactic heparin treatment may be of benefit prior to ocular surgery in at-risk patients.

Parinaud oculoglandular syndrome

Parinaud oculoglandular syndrome is a rare condition consisting of chronic low-grade fever, unilateral granulomatous conjunctivitis (Fig. 6.25) with surrounding follicles and ipsilateral regional (preauricular) lymphadenopathy. It is synonymous with cat-scratch disease (caused by *Bartonella henselae* – see Ch. 12), although several other causes have been implicated, including tularaemia, insect hairs (ophthalmia nodosum), *Treponema*

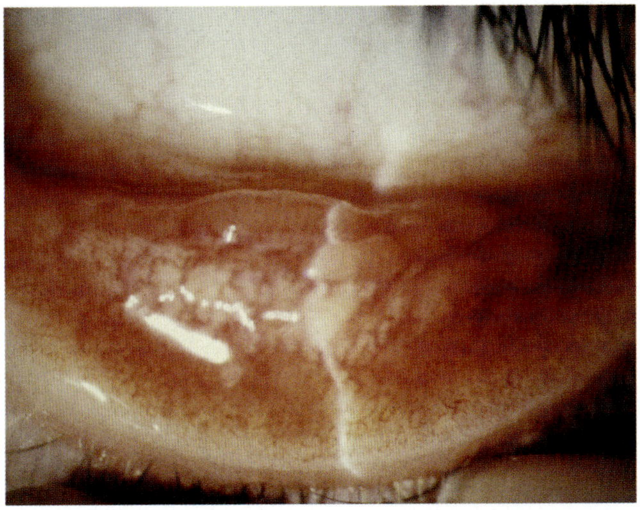

Fig. 6.25 Granulomatous conjunctivitis in Parinaud syndrome.

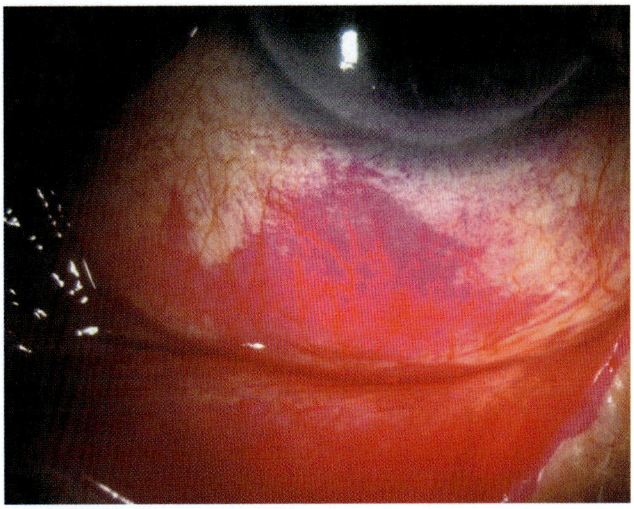

Fig. 6.26 Inferior conjunctival injection and staining with rose Bengal in factitious conjunctivitis. *(Courtesy of S Tuft.)*

pallidum, sporotrichosis, tuberculosis and acute *C. trachomatis* infection.

Factitious conjunctivitis

Introduction

Self-injury (factitious keratoconjunctivitis) is most often intentional, but can also occur inadvertently, as in mucus fishing syndrome and removal of contact lenses. Damage may be the result of either mechanical trauma or of the instillation of irritant but readily accessible household substances, such as soap. Occasionally over-instillation of prescribed ocular medication is responsible.

Diagnosis

- **Symptoms.** Reported symptoms may seem disproportionate to signs. The patient may have sought multiple medical opinions over an extended period, often from a range of specialists for different complaints.
- **Signs**
  - Inferior conjunctival injection and staining with rose Bengal (Fig. 6.26), with quiet superior bulbar conjunctiva.
  - Linear corneal abrasions, persistent epithelial defects and occasionally focal corneal perforation.
  - Secondary infection with *Candida* spp.
  - Sterile ring infiltrate and hypopyon.
  - Corneal scarring.

Management

- Exclude other diagnoses.
- Close observation may be required.
- Confrontation often leads to failure to return for review.
- A psychiatric opinion may be appropriate.

DEGENERATIONS

Pinguecula

Introduction

A pinguecula (plural pingueculae) is an innocuous but extremely common asymptomatic elastotic degeneration of the conjunctival stroma. A yellow–white mound or aggregation of smaller mounds is seen on the bulbar conjunctiva adjacent to the limbus (Fig. 6.27A). It is more frequently located at the nasal than the temporal limbus, but is frequently present at both. Calcification (Fig. 6.27B) is occasionally present. The cause is believed to be actinic damage, similar to the aetiology of pterygium (see below), which pinguecula resembles histologically. The distinction is that the limbal barrier to extension has remained intact with a pinguecula. Occasionally a pinguecula may become acutely inflamed (pingueculitis – Fig. 6.27C), particularly if the lesion is prominent or overlying calcification leads to epithelial breakdown. There is a small subgroup of patients with an inflamed nasal pinguecula and impaired ocular surface lubrication, who can progress to pterygium (Fig. 6.27D).

Treatment

Treatment is usually unnecessary because growth is absent or very slow.

- Irritation may be treated with topical lubrication.
- Pingueculitis can be treated with lubrication if mild or with a short course of topical steroid.
- Excision may be indicated for cosmetic reasons or for significant irritation. In contrast to pterygium (see next), the recurrence rate is low and simple excision is usually adequate.
- Thermal laser ablation can be effective. Gentian violet marking may be necessary to ensure adequate absorption in lighter-skinned individuals.

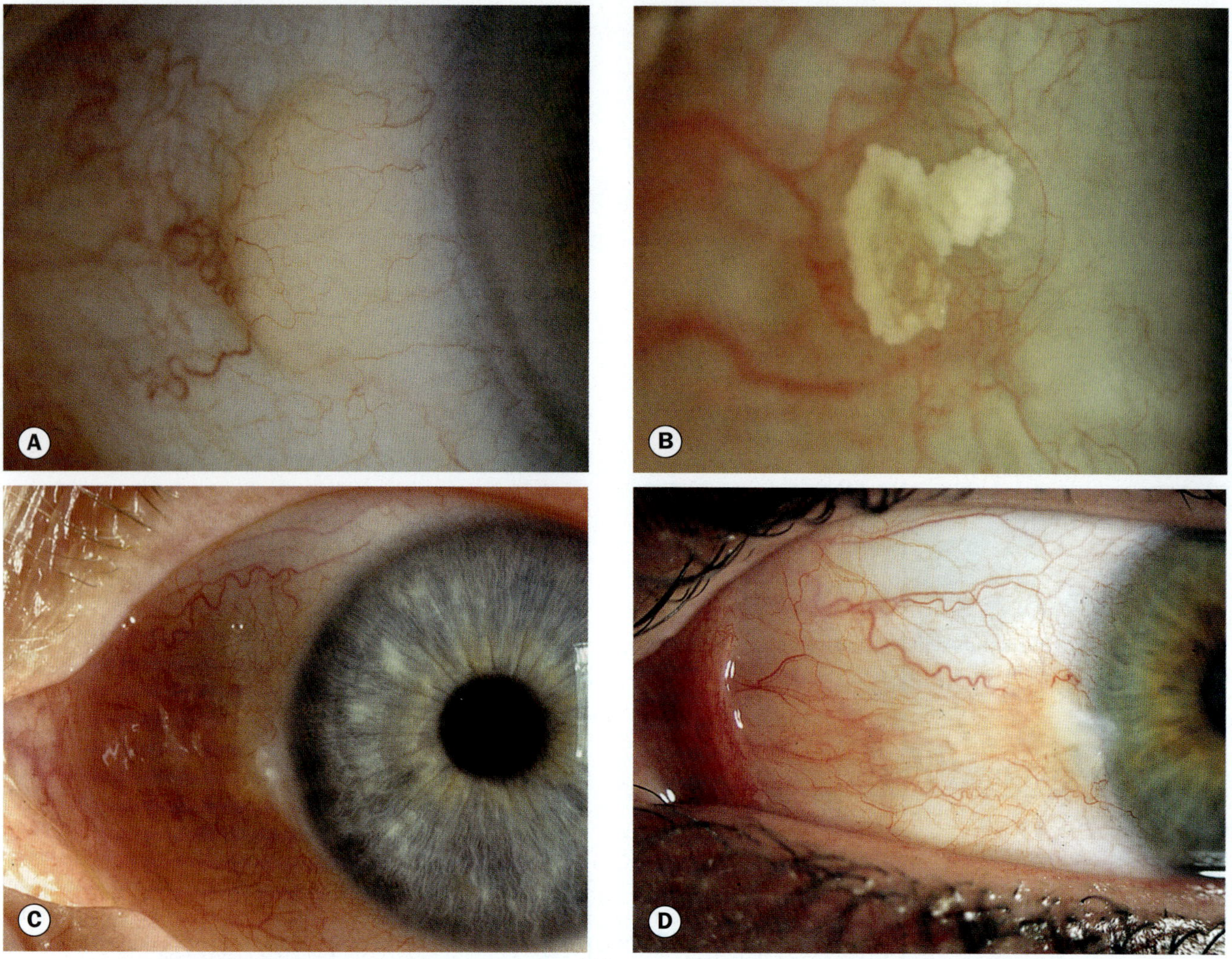

Fig. 6.27 **(A)** Pinguecula; **(B)** developing calcification; **(C)** pingueculitis; **(D)** early progression to pterygium.

Pterygium

Introduction

A pterygium (plural pterygia) is a triangular fibrovascular subepithelial ingrowth of degenerative bulbar conjunctival tissue over the limbus onto the cornea. It typically develops in patients who have been living in sunny countries and, as with pinguecula, may represent a response to ultraviolet exposure and to other factors such as chronic surface dryness. The condition tends to run in families. A pterygium is histologically similar to a pinguecula and shows elastotic degenerative changes in vascularized subepithelial stromal collagen (Fig. 6.28A). In contrast to pingueculae, pterygia encroach onto the cornea, invading the Bowman layer. Pseudopterygium appears similar clinically but is caused by a band of conjunctiva adhering to an area of compromised cornea at its apex. It forms as a response to an acute inflammatory episode such as a chemical burn, corneal ulcer (especially if marginal), trauma and cicatrizing conjunctivitis.

Clinical features

- **Symptoms.** Patients who present with a history of recent enlargement are more likely to require early excision for subsequent aggressive growth. Aggressive growth or an atypical appearance should prompt excision biopsy.
  - Most small lesions are asymptomatic.
  - Irritation and grittiness are caused by a dellen – localized drying – effect at the advancing edge due to interference with the precorneal tear film (more likely if the head of the pterygium is especially elevated).
  - Patients who wear contact lenses may develop symptoms of irritation at an earlier stage due to edge lift.
  - Lesions may interfere with vision by obscuring the visual axis or inducing astigmatism.
  - There may be intermittent inflammation similar to pingueculitis.
  - Cosmesis may be a significant problem.

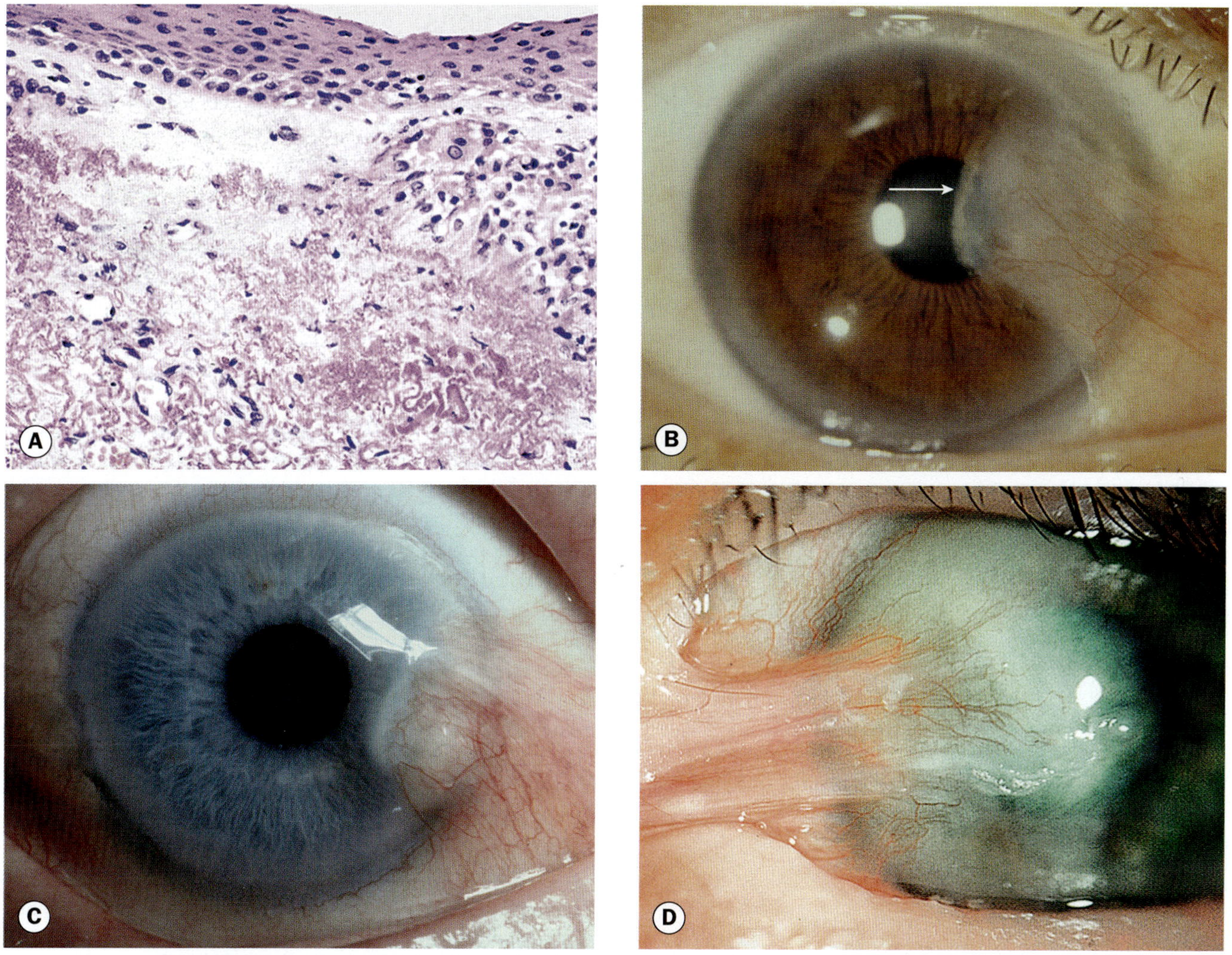

Fig. 6.28 Pterygium. **(A)** Histology showing collagenous degenerative changes in vascularized subepithelial stroma; **(B)** pterygium showing cap, head, body and Stocker line (arrow); **(C)** inflamed pterygium; **(D)** pseudopterygium secondary to a chemical burn.

  - Extensive lesions, particularly if recurrent, may be associated with subconjunctival fibrosis extending to the fornices that may cause restricted ocular excursion.
  - If pseudopterygium is suspected, there may be a history of a causative episode.
- **Signs**
  - A pterygium is made up of three parts: a 'cap' (an avascular halo-like zone at the advancing edge), a head and a body (Fig. 6.28B and C).
  - Linear epithelial iron deposition (Stocker line) may be seen in the corneal epithelium anterior to the head of the pterygium (Fig. 6.28B).
  - Fuchs islets are small discrete whitish flecks consisting of clusters of pterygial epithelial cells often present at the advancing edge.
  - A pseudopterygium (Fig. 6.28D) is classically distinguished by the fact that the location is away from the horizontal (though this may occasionally be seen with true pterygia) and that there is a firm attachment to the cornea only at its apex (head).

Treatment

- **Medical** treatment of symptomatic patients is as for pinguecula. The patient should be advised to wear sunglasses to reduce ultraviolet exposure.
- **Surgery.** Simple excision ('bare sclera' technique) is associated with a high rate of recurrence (around 80%), often with more aggressive behaviour than the original lesion.
  - The pterygium is excised from the cornea and conjunctiva leaving bare sclera (Fig. 6.29A).
  - Conjunctival autografting. The donor conjunctival patch is usually harvested from the superior or upper-temporal paralimbal region (Fig. 6.29B). The graft is sutured into position using 10-0 nylon sutures (Fig. 6.29C). The site heals rapidly. Conjunctival grafts can be secured with tissue glue (for example: TISSEEL fibrin glue) rather than sutures, thus shortening operating time and reducing postoperative irritation.
  - Adjunctive treatment with mitomycin C or beta-irradiation can be used in place of patching techniques.
  - Peripheral lamellar keratoplasty may be required for deep lesions.

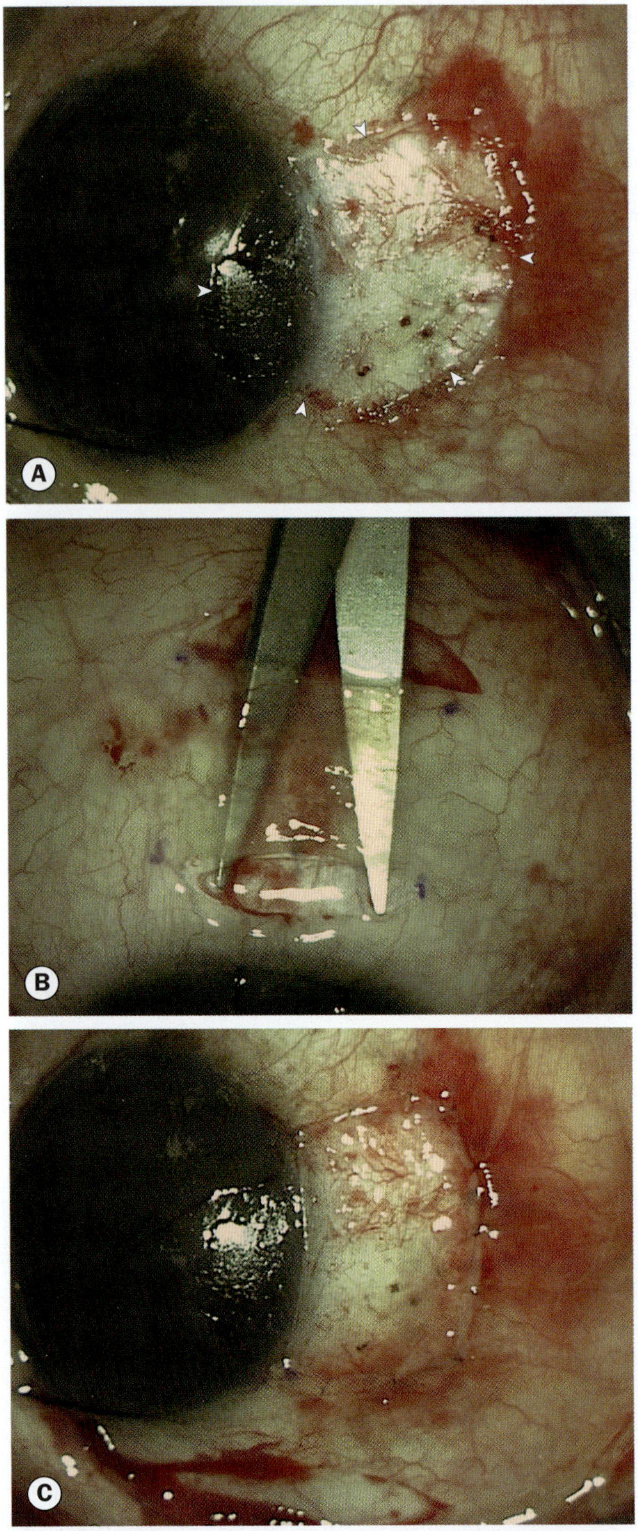

Fig. 6.29 Surgical treatment of pterygium. **(A)** Removal of pterygium head (arrowheads show edges of incision); **(B)** preparation of conjunctival autograft; **(C)** graft sutured into position. *(Courtesy of M Leyland.)*

TIP In a patient undergoing surgery for pterygium, the risk of recurrence can be reduced by using either a conjunctival autograft or by applying mitomycin C to the operation site.

Concretions

Concretions are extremely common and are usually associated with ageing, although they can also form in patients with chronic conjunctival inflammation such as trachoma. They appear as multiple tiny cysts containing yellowish-white deposits of epithelial debris including keratin, commonly located subepithelially in the inferior tarsal and forniceal conjunctiva (Fig. 6.30A). They can become calcified and, particularly if large, may erode through the overlying epithelium (Fig. 6.30B) and cause marked irritation. If symptomatic, treatment involves removal at the slit lamp with a needle under topical anaesthesia.

Conjunctivochalasis

Conjunctivochalasis usually appears as a fold of redundant conjunctiva interposed between the globe and lower eyelid, protruding over the lid margin (Fig. 6.31). It is probably a normal ageing change that may be exacerbated by inflammation and mechanical stress related to dry eye and lid margin disease. Symptoms include watering of the eye due to obstruction of the inferior punctum and interference with the marginal tear meniscus. Treatment consists of topical lubricants and treatment of any blepharitis. A short course of topical steroids or another anti-inflammatory agent may be helpful. Conjunctival resection can be performed in severe cases (see also Ch. 3).

Retention (primary epithelial inclusion) cyst

Conjunctival retention cysts are thin-walled lesions on the bulbar conjunctiva containing clear (Fig. 6.32A) or occasionally turbid fluid or blood (Fig. 6.32B). They do not usually cause discomfort, but may be a mild cosmetic blemish. Histology shows a fluid-filled internal cavity lined by a double epithelial layer. Treatment, if required, is initially by simple puncture with a needle under topical anaesthesia, but recurrence is common. Bleeding should be encouraged within the ruptured cyst as it may promote adhesion of the walls and reduce the chance of recurrence. Cyst wall excision under topical anaesthesia can be carried out for recurrent cyst formation. The differential diagnosis includes secondary inclusion cysts following conjunctival surgery and lymphangiectasia. The latter is characterized by strings of cystic or sausage-shaped clear-walled channels, which may become filled with blood (haemorrhagic lymphangiectasia – Fig. 6.33).

SUBCONJUNCTIVAL HAEMORRHAGE

Subconjunctival haemorrhage is a very common phenomenon that is often idiopathic and apparently spontaneous, occurring particularly in older people (Fig. 6.34A. It may result from surgery, conjunctivitis and trauma (Fig. 6.34B). The haemorrhage is usually asymptomatic but a momentary sharp pain or a snapping or popping sensation is sometimes felt. Coughing, sneezing and vomiting are common precipitants. In younger people contact

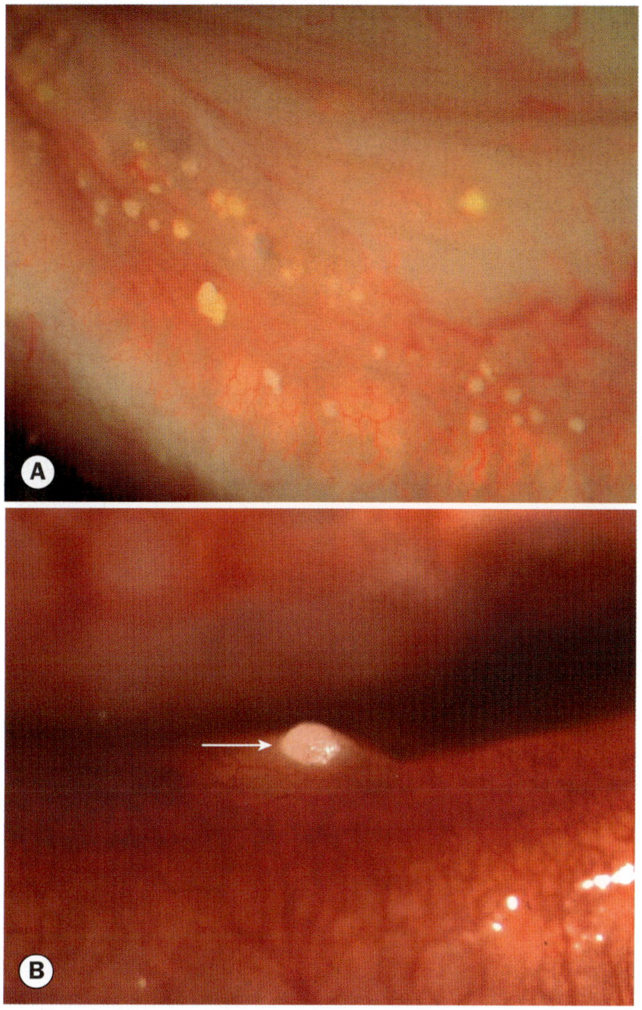

Fig. 6.30 (A) Multiple small concretions; **(B)** large concretion eroding through the conjunctival surface (arrow).

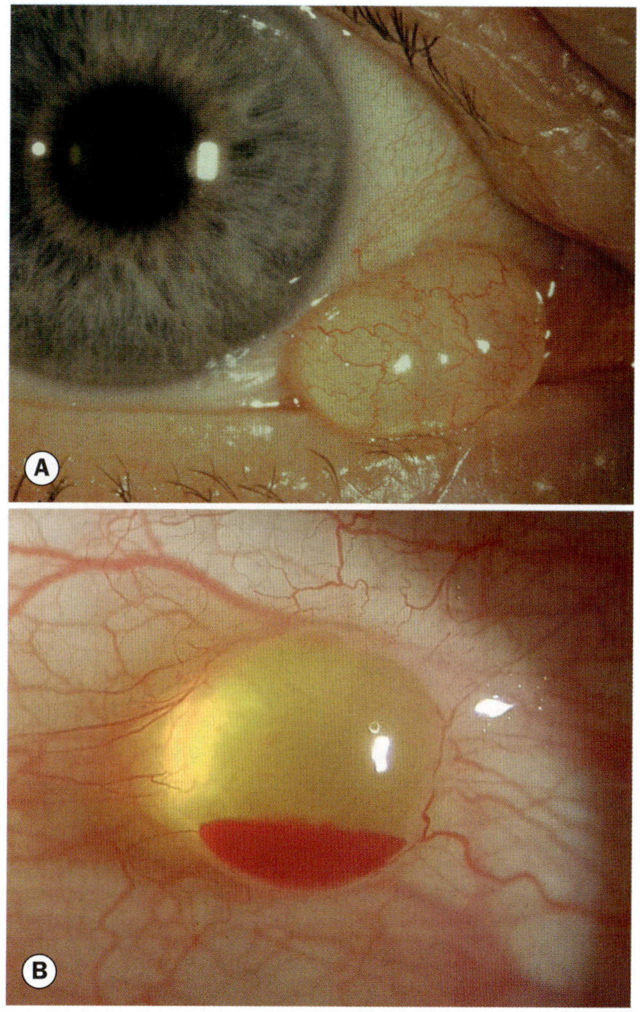

Fig. 6.32 Conjunctival cyst. **(A)** Clear fluid; **(B)** turbid fluid with blood. *(Courtesy of RSR Naik – fig. B.)*

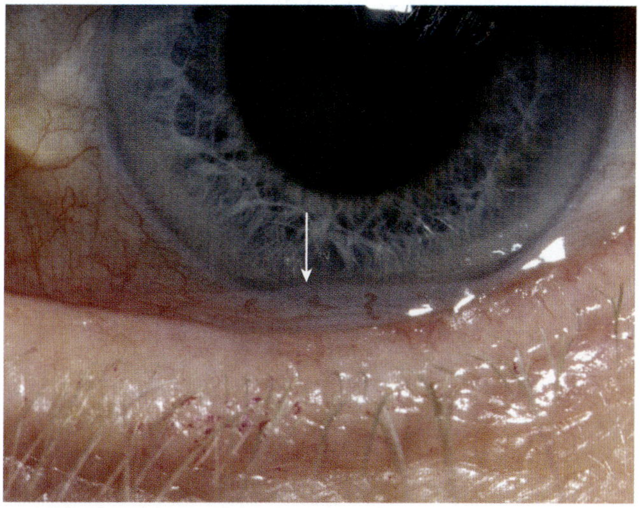

Fig. 6.31 Conjunctivochalasis (arrow).

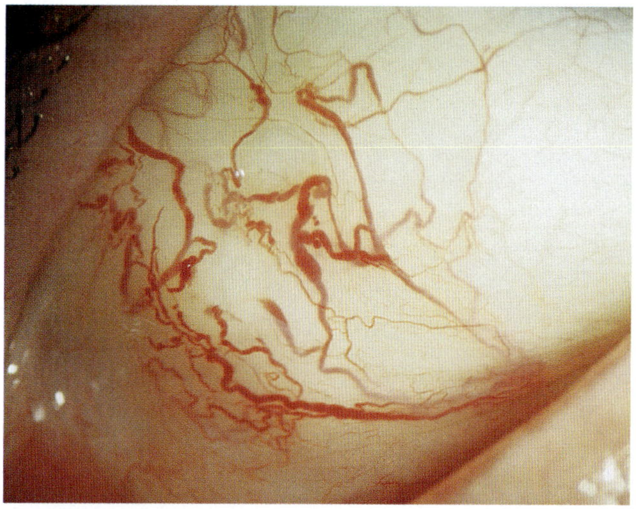

Fig. 6.33 Haemorrhagic lymphangiectasia.

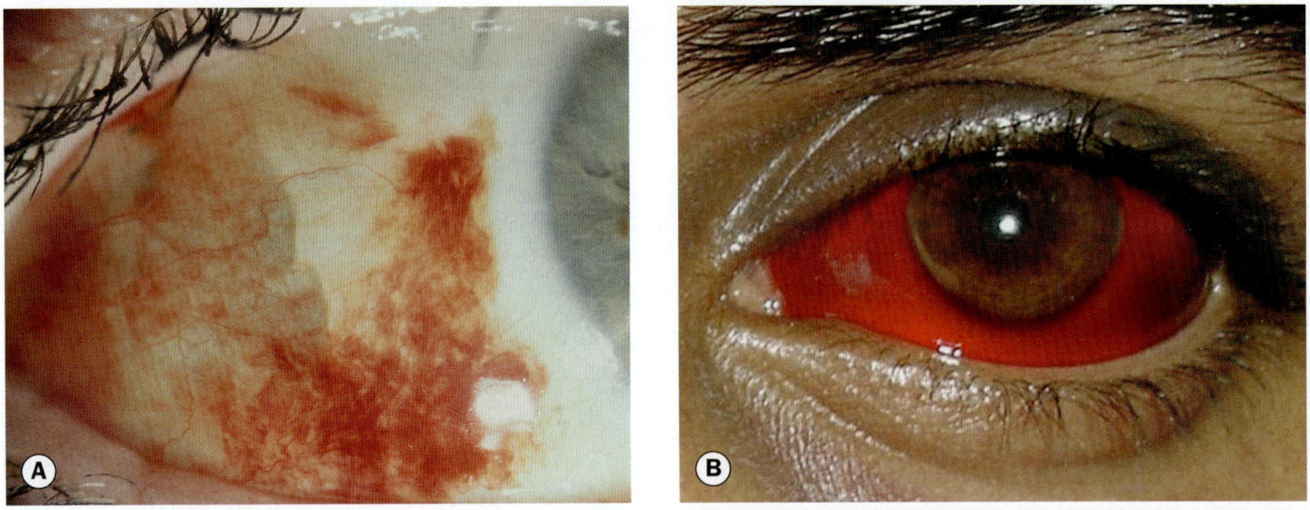

Fig. 6.34 Subconjunctival haemorrhage. (A) Spontaneous; (B) after blunt trauma.

lens wear is a common association and in older individuals systemic vascular disease (hypertension) is prevalent. A local ocular cause should be ruled out by slit lamp examination. Patients are often taking aspirin or similar products that have an effect on platelet function. Bleeding diatheses are a very rare association, but vitamin C deficiency and abusive trauma should always be considered in infants. The vision is usually unaffected unless a substantially elevated haemorrhage leads to a large localized corneal wetting deficit (dellen), which is often uncomfortable. A large bleed can track into the eyelids. Spontaneous resolution over a week or two is typical, but two or three narrowly spaced episodes are not uncommon.

Chapter 7 Cornea

INTRODUCTION

Anatomy and physiology

General

The cornea is a complex structure which, as well as having a protective role, is responsible for about three-quarters of the optical power of the eye. The normal hydration level is 78%. Nutrients are supplied and metabolic products removed via the aqueous humour posteriorly and the tears anteriorly. The cornea is the most densely innervated tissue in the body and conditions such as abrasion and bullous keratopathy are associated with marked pain, photophobia and reflex lacrimation. A subepithelial and a deeper stromal nerve plexus are supplied by the first division of the trigeminal nerve.

Dimensions

The average corneal diameter is 11.5 mm vertically and 12 mm horizontally. It is 540 μm thick centrally on average and thicker towards the periphery. The normal hydration level is 78%. Central corneal thickness does not differ between males and females, but varies between individuals and races. It is a key determinant of the intraocular pressure (IOP) measured with conventional techniques.

Structure

The cornea consists of the following layers (Fig. 7.1):

- **The epithelium** is stratified squamous and non-keratinized, and is composed of:
  - A single layer of columnar basal cells attached by hemidesmosomes to an underlying basement membrane.
  - Two to three strata of 'wing' cells.
  - Two layers of squamous surface cells.
  - The surface area of the outermost cells is increased by microplicae and microvilli that facilitate the attachment of the tear film and mucin. After a lifespan of a few days superficial cells are shed into the tear film.
  - Corneal stem cells are located at the corneoscleral limbus, possibly in the palisades of Vogt. Deficiency may result in chronic epithelial defects and 'conjunctivalization' (epithelial instability, vascularization and the appearance of goblet cells). They are thought to be critical in the maintenance of a physiological barrier, preventing conjunctival tissue from growing onto the cornea (e.g. pterygium). Deficiency may be addressed by stem cell auto- or allotransplantation.
- **Bowman layer** is the acellular superficial layer of the stroma and is formed from collagen fibres.
- **The stroma** makes up 90% of corneal thickness. It is arranged in regularly orientated layers of collagen fibrils whose spacing is maintained by proteoglycan ground substance (chondroitin sulphate and keratan sulphate) with interspersed modified fibroblasts (keratocytes). Maintenance of the regular arrangement and spacing of the collagen is critical to optical clarity. The stroma can scar, but cannot regenerate following damage.
- **Descemet membrane** is a discrete sheet composed of a fine latticework of collagen fibrils that are distinct from the collagen of the stroma. The membrane consists of an anterior banded zone that is deposited *in utero* and a posterior non-banded zone laid down throughout life by the endothelium, for which it serves as a modified basement membrane. It has regenerative potential.
- **The endothelium** consists of a monolayer of polygonal cells. Endothelial cells maintain corneal deturgescence throughout life by pumping excess fluid out of the stroma. The young adult cell density is about 3000 cells/mm^2. The number of cells decreases at about 0.6% per year and neighbouring cells enlarge to fill the space. The cells cannot regenerate. At a density of about 500 cells/mm^2 corneal oedema develops and transparency is impaired.
- The existence of a sixth corneal layer between the stroma and Descemet membrane **(Dua layer)** has been proposed, though some authorities believe this to be a previously described continuation of the posterior stroma.

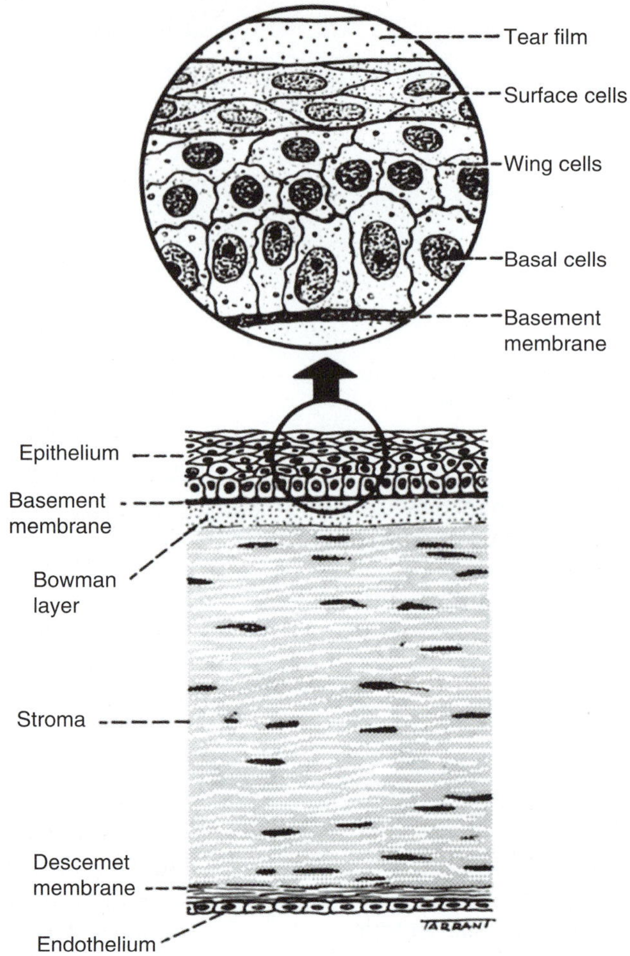

Fig. 7.1 Anatomy of the cornea.

TIP The cornea is densely innervated and a corneal abrasion is usually associated with intense pain, photophobia and reflex lacrimation.

Signs of corneal disease

Superficial

- **Punctate epithelial erosions (PEE)**, tiny epithelial defects that stain with fluorescein (Fig. 7.2A) and rose Bengal (Fig. 7.2B), are generally an early sign of epithelial compromise. Causes include a variety of stimuli. The location of the lesions may give an indication of aetiology:
  - Superior – vernal disease, chlamydial conjunctivitis, superior limbic keratoconjunctivitis, floppy eyelid syndrome and mechanically induced keratoconjunctivitis.
  - Interpalpebral – dry eye (can also be inferior), reduced corneal sensation and ultraviolet keratopathy.
  - Inferior – chronic blepharitis, lagophthalmos, eye drop toxicity, self-induced, aberrant eyelashes and entropion.
  - Diffuse – some cases of viral conjunctivitis and toxicity to drops.
  - Central – prolonged contact lens wear.
- **Punctate epithelial keratitis (PEK)** appears as granular, opalescent, swollen epithelial cells, with focal intraepithelial infiltrates. They are visible unstained but stain well with rose Bengal and variably with fluorescein. Causes include:
  - Infections: adenoviral, chlamydial, molluscum contagiosum, early herpes simplex and herpes zoster, microsporidial and systemic viral infections (e.g. measles, varicella, rubella).
  - Miscellaneous: Thygeson superficial punctate keratitis and eye drop toxicity.
- **Subepithelial infiltrates.** Tiny subsurface foci of non-staining inflammatory infiltrates (Fig. 7.2C). Causes include severe or prolonged adenoviral keratoconjunctivitis, herpes zoster keratitis, adult inclusion conjunctivitis, marginal keratitis, rosacea and Thygeson superficial punctate keratitis.
- **Superficial punctate keratitis** is a non-specific term describing any corneal epithelial disturbance of dot-like morphology.
- **Filaments.** Strands of mucus admixed with epithelium, attached at one end to the corneal surface, that stain well with rose Bengal (see Fig. 7.2B). The unattached end moves with each blink. Grey subepithelial opacities may be seen at the site of attachment. Dry eye is by far the most common cause. Other causes include superior limbic keratoconjunctivitis, neurotrophic keratopathy, long-term ocular patching and essential blepharospasm.
- **Epithelial oedema.** Subtle oedema may manifest with loss of normal corneal lustre, but more commonly, abundant tiny epithelial vesicles are seen. Bullae form in moderate–severe cases (Fig. 7.2D). The cause is usually endothelial decompensation, but it can follow acute elevation of IOP.
- **Superficial neovascularization** (Fig. 7.2E) is a feature of chronic ocular surface irritation or hypoxia, as in contact lens wear.
- **Pannus** describes superficial neovascularization accompanied by degenerative subepithelial change (Fig. 7.2F).

Deep

- **Infiltrates** are yellow– or grey–white opacities located initially within the anterior stroma (Fig. 7.3A), usually associated with limbal or conjunctival hyperaemia. They are stromal foci of acute inflammation composed of inflammatory cells, cellular and extracellular debris including necrosis. The key distinction is between sterile and infective lesions (Table 7.1); **'PEDAL'**: **P**ain, **E**pithelial defects, **D**ischarge, **A**nterior chamber reaction, **L**ocation is a useful mnemonic to distinguish these two types of lesions. Suppurative keratitis is caused by active infection with bacteria, fungi, protozoa and occasionally viruses. Non-infectious 'sterile keratitis' is due to an immune hypersensitivity response to antigen as in marginal keratitis and with contact lens wear.
- **Ulceration** refers to tissue excavation associated with an epithelial defect (Fig. 7.3B), usually with infiltration and necrosis.
- **'Melting'** describes tissue disintegration in response to enzymatic activity, often with mild or no infiltrate, e.g. peripheral ulcerative keratitis.
- **Vascularization** occurs in response to a wide variety of stimuli. Venous channels are easily seen, whereas arterial feeding vessels are smaller and require higher magnification. Non-perfused deep vessels appear as 'ghost vessels', best detected by retroillumination.
- **Lipid** deposition (Fig. 7.3C) may follow chronic inflammation with leakage from corneal new vessels.
- **Folds in Descemet membrane**, also known as striate keratopathy (Fig. 7.3D), may result from corneal oedema. Causes include inflammation, trauma (including surgery) and ocular hypotony.
- **Descemetocoele** (US spelling – descemetocele) is a bubble-like herniation of Descemet membrane into the cornea (Fig. 7.3E), plugging a defect that would otherwise be full-thickness.
- **Breaks in Descemet membrane** (Fig. 7.3F) may be due to corneal enlargement (Haab striae in infantile glaucoma) or deformation such as keratoconus and birth trauma. Acute influx of aqueous into the corneal stroma (acute hydrops) can follow.
- **The Seidel test** demonstrates aqueous leakage. A drop of 1% or 2% fluorescein is applied to the surface of the eye. Using a slit lamp, the cobalt blue filter is used to detect a change in colour from dark orange to bright yellow–green secondary to localized dilution at a site of leakage.

Documentation of clinical signs

Clinical signs should be illustrated with a colour-coded labelled diagram. Measuring lesion dimensions is particularly useful to facilitate monitoring (Fig. 7.4). Slit lamp photography is an increasingly used supplement or alternative, but must be of high quality.

- **Opacities** such as scars and degenerations are drawn in black.
- **Epithelial oedema** is represented by fine blue circles, stromal oedema as blue shading and folds in Descemet membrane as wavy blue lines.

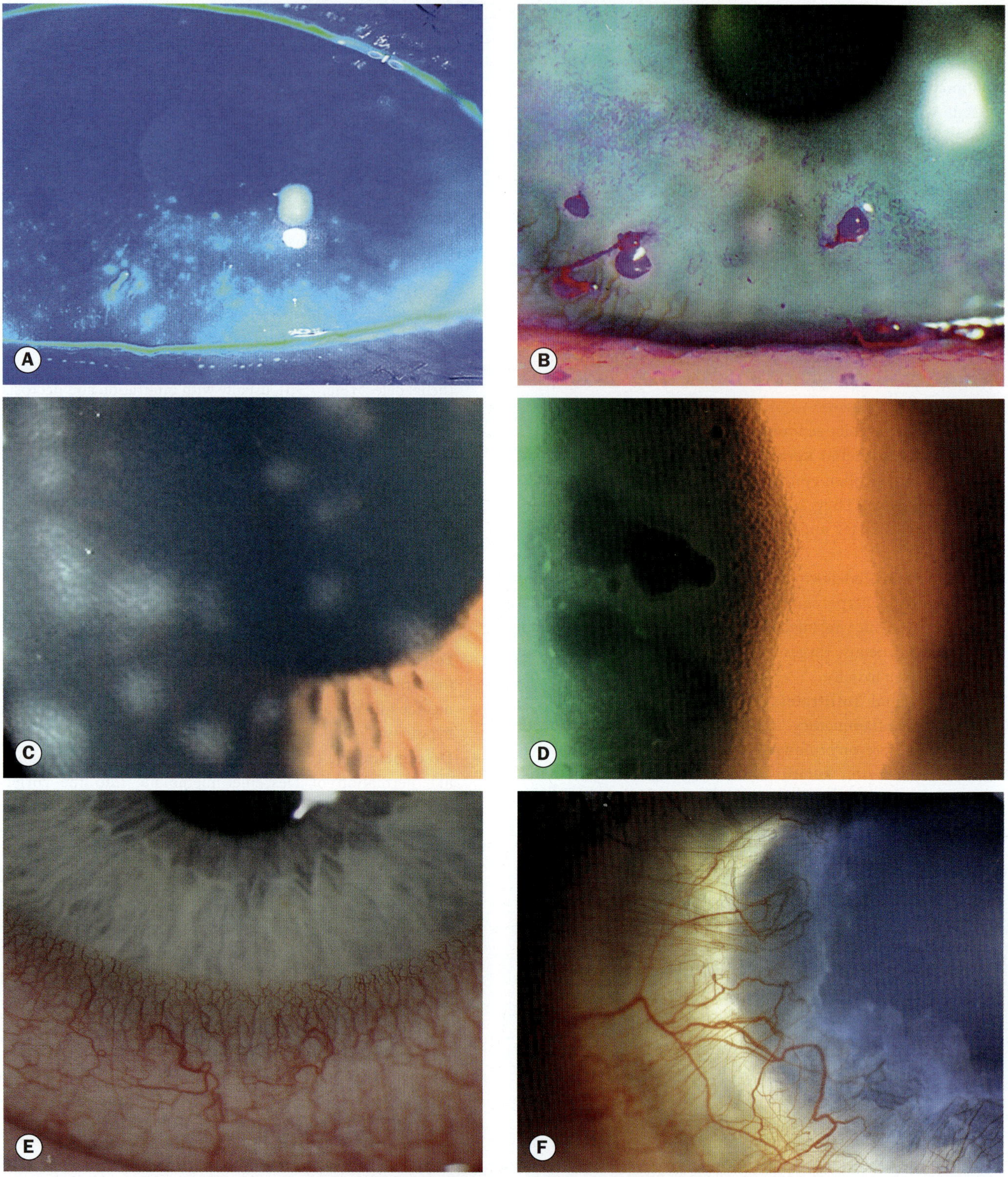

Fig. 7.2 Superficial corneal lesions. **(A)** Punctate epithelial erosions stained with fluorescein in dry eye; **(B)** filaments stained with rose Bengal; **(C)** subepithelial infiltrates; **(D)** corneal oedema with bullae; **(E)** superficial vascularization; **(F)** pannus. *(Courtesy of C Barry – fig. F.)*

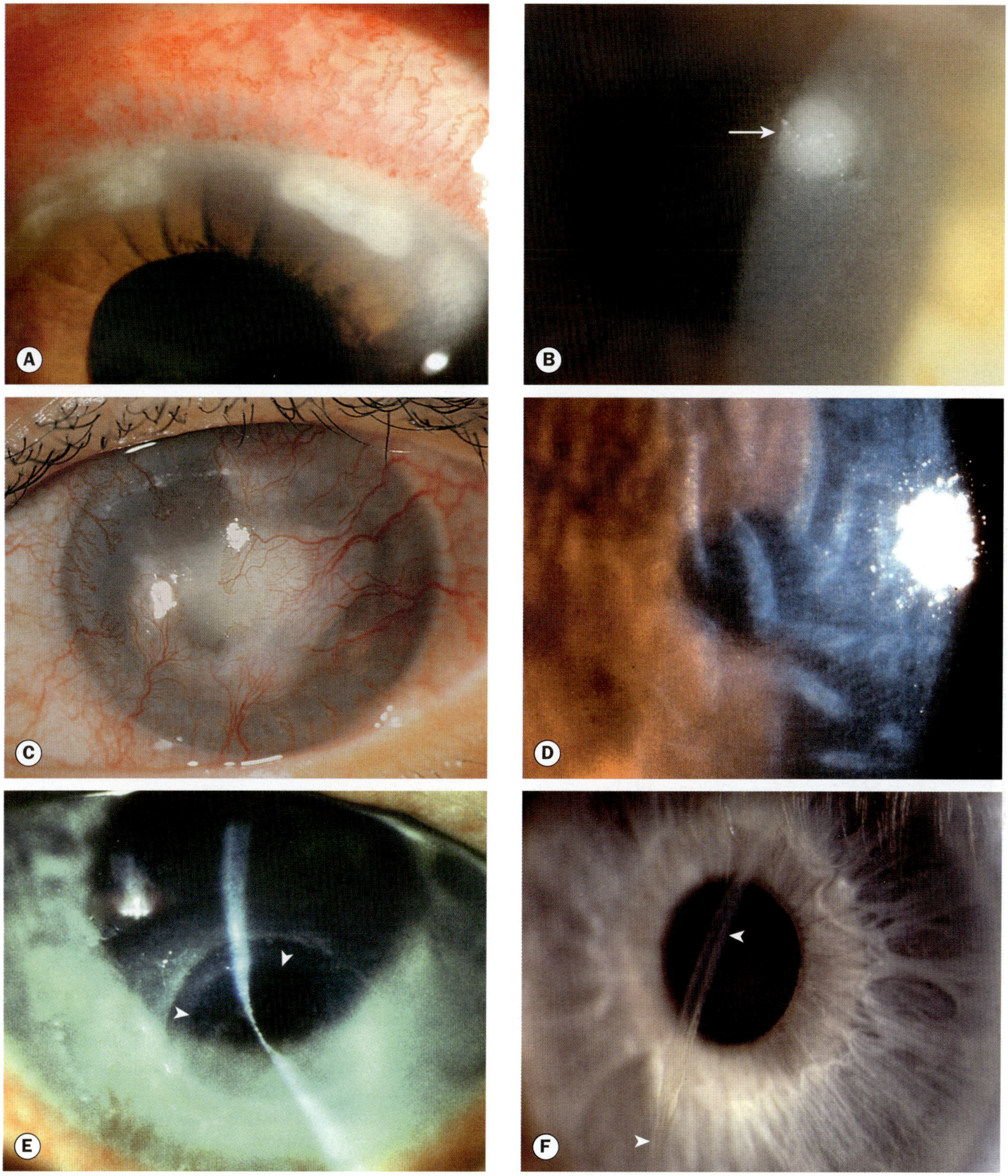

Fig. 7.3 Deeper corneal lesions. **(A)** Infiltration; **(B)** ulceration (arrow); **(C)** lipid deposition with vascularization; **(D)** folds in Descemet membrane; **(E)** descemetocoele (arrowheads); **(F)** traumatic break in Descemet membrane (arrowheads). *(Courtesy of C Barry – figs C and D.)*

Table 7.1 Characteristics of Infective Versus Sterile Corneal Infiltrates

	Infective	Sterile
Size	Tend to be larger	Tend to be smaller
Progression	Rapid	Slow
Epithelial defect	Very common and larger when present	Much less common and if present tends to be small
Pain	Moderate–severe	Mild
Discharge	Purulent	Mucopurulent
Single or multiple	Typically, single	Commonly multiple
Unilateral or bilateral	Unilateral	Often bilateral
Anterior chamber reaction	Severe	Mild
Location	Often central	Typically more peripheral
Adjacent corneal reaction	Extensive	Limited

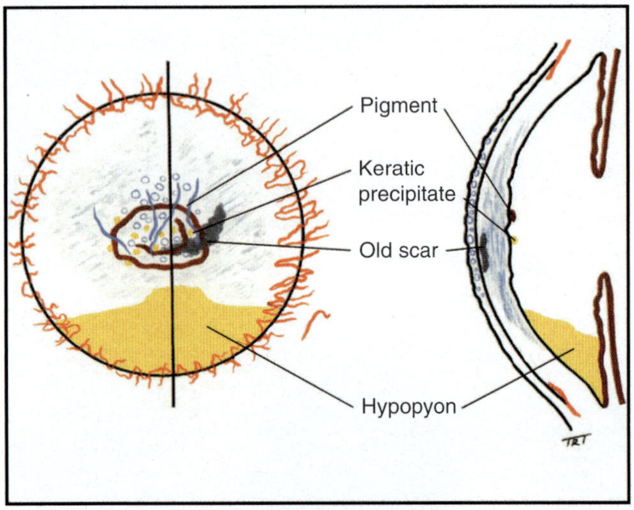

Fig. 7.4 Documentation of corneal lesions.

- **Hypopyon** is shown in yellow.
- **Blood vessels** are added in red. Superficial vessels are wavy lines that begin outside the limbus and deep vessels are straight lines that begin at the limbus.
- **Pigmented lesions** such as iron lines and Krukenberg spindles are shown in brown.

Specular microscopy

Specular microscopy is the study of corneal layers under very high magnification (100 times greater than slit lamp biomicroscopy). It is mainly used to assess the endothelium, which can be analysed for cellular size, shape, density and distribution. The healthy endothelial cell is a regular hexagon (Fig. 7.5A) and the normal cell density in a young adult is about 3000 cells/mm^2.

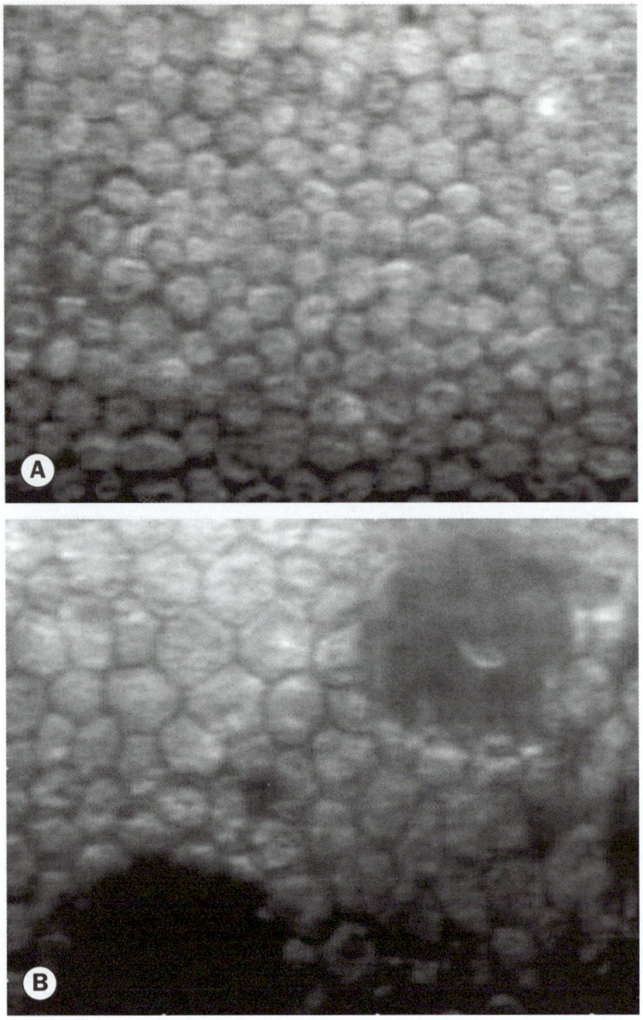

Fig. 7.5 Specular micrograph. **(A)** Normal corneal endothelium; **(B)** cornea guttata with marked loss of endothelial mosaic and greater size of the remaining cells. *(Courtesy of J Sharp.)*

- **Physics.** When a light beam of the specular photomicroscope passes through the cornea it encounters a series of interfaces between optically distinct regions. Some light is reflected specularly (i.e. like a mirror) back towards the photomicroscope and forms an image that can be photographed and analysed.
- **Indications**
  - Evaluation of the functional reserve of the corneal endothelium prior to intraocular surgery is the most common indication. A clear cornea with normal thickness on pachymetry is not necessarily associated with normal endothelial morphology or cell density. Corneal oedema is considerably more likely to occur with a cell density below 700 cells/mm^2 but unlikely above 1000 cells/mm^2.
  - Donor cornea evaluation.
  - To demonstrate pathology, particularly cornea guttata (Fig. 7.5B), Descemet membrane irregularities and posterior polymorphous dystrophy.

Corneal topography

Corneal topography is used to image the cornea by projecting a series of concentric rings of light on the anterior surface, constituting a Placido image. The reflected light is analysed using computer software to produce a detailed surface map. A major application is the detection and management of corneal ectasia, principally keratoconus. Screening for corneal ectasia is especially important prior to refractive surgery. It is used occasionally for contact lens fitting and to measure corneal thickness. Scheimpflug imaging is a new technology that may offer advantages in topographic imaging. Anterior segment optical coherence tomography (OCT) and ultrasound biomicroscopy can also be used to image the cornea.

Principles of treatment

Control of infection and inflammation

- **Antimicrobial agents** should be started as soon as preliminary investigations have been performed. The choice of agent is determined by the likely aetiology according to clinical findings. Broad-spectrum treatment is generally used initially, with more selective agents introduced if necessary, when the results of investigation are available.
- **Topical steroids** should be used with caution as they may promote replication of some microorganisms, notably herpes simplex virus and fungi, and retard reparative processes such as re-epithelialization. Nevertheless, they are vital in a range of conditions for the suppression of destructive vision-compromising inflammation.
- **Systemic immunosuppressive agents** are useful in some conditions, particularly autoimmune disease.

Promotion of epithelial healing

Re-epithelialization is of great importance in any corneal disease, as thinning seldom progresses if the epithelium is intact.

- **Reduction of exposure** to toxic medications and preservatives wherever possible.
- **Lubrication** with artificial tears (unpreserved if possible) and ointment. Taping the lids closed as a temporary measure is often used as a nocturnal adjunct.
- **Antibiotic ointment** prophylaxis should be considered.
- **Bandage soft contact lenses** should be carefully supervised to exclude superinfection and duration kept to a minimum. Indications include:
  - Promotion of healing by mechanically protecting regenerating corneal epithelium from the constant rubbing of the eyelids.
  - To improve comfort, particularly in the presence of a large corneal abrasion.
  - To seal a small perforation (Fig. 7.6A).
- **Surgical eyelid closure** is particularly useful in exposure and neurotrophic keratopathy, as well as in persistent epithelial defects. Lid closure may be used as a conservative method to heal an infective ulcer in selected cases, such as an eye with no visual potential in a patient with severe dementia.
  - Botulinum toxin injection into the levator muscle to induce a temporary (2–3 months) ptosis.
  - Temporary or permanent lateral tarsorrhaphy or medial canthoplasty and occasionally central tarsorrhaphy (Fig. 7.6B).
- **Conjunctival (Gundersen) flap** will protect and allow healing of a corneal epithelial defect. It is particularly suitable for chronic unilateral disease in which the prognosis for restoration of useful vision is poor. Buccal mucous membrane is an alternative.
- **Amniotic membrane patch grafting** (Fig. 7.6C) for persistent unresponsive epithelial defects.
- **Tissue adhesive** (cyanoacrylate glue) to seal small perforations. The glue can be applied to one side of a bespoke trimmed patch of sterile plastic drape, which is pressed over the defect after the edges are dried with a cellulose sponge. The patch remains in place to seal the defect and a bandage contact lens is inserted for comfort and to aid retention of the patch (Fig. 7.6D).
- **Corneal cross-linking** using ultraviolet light-A and riboflavin (photoactivated chromophore for infectious keratitis-corneal collagen cross-linking: PACK-CXL) can be used to treat resistant corneal infections, particularly if there is evidence of corneal melting. This treatment is usually used in combination with standard antimicrobial therapy, but has also been shown to have a microbicidal effect when used as first-line treatment in patients with early bacterial keratitis.
- **Limbal stem cell transplantation** may be used if there is stem cell deficiency as in chemical burns and cicatrizing conjunctivitis. The source of the donor tissue may be the fellow eye (autograft) in unilateral disease or a living or cadaver donor (allograft) when both eyes are affected. A newer technique involves the *in vitro* replication of the patient's own stem cells with subsequent re-implantation of the enhanced cell population.
- **Smoking** retards epithelialization and should be discontinued.

BACTERIAL KERATITIS

Pathogenesis

Pathogens

Bacterial keratitis usually develops only when ocular defences have been compromised (see below). However, some bacteria, including *Neisseria gonorrhoeae*, *Neisseria meningitidis*, *Corynebacterium diphtheriae* and *Haemophilus influenzae* are able to penetrate a healthy corneal epithelium, usually in association with severe conjunctivitis. It is important to remember that infections may be polymicrobial, including bacterial and fungal co-infection. Common pathogens include:

- ***Pseudomonas aeruginosa*** is a ubiquitous Gram-negative bacillus (rod) commensal of the gastrointestinal tract. The infection is typically aggressive and is responsible for over 60% of contact lens-related keratitis.
- ***Staphylococcus aureus*** is a common Gram-positive and coagulase-positive commensal of the nares, skin and

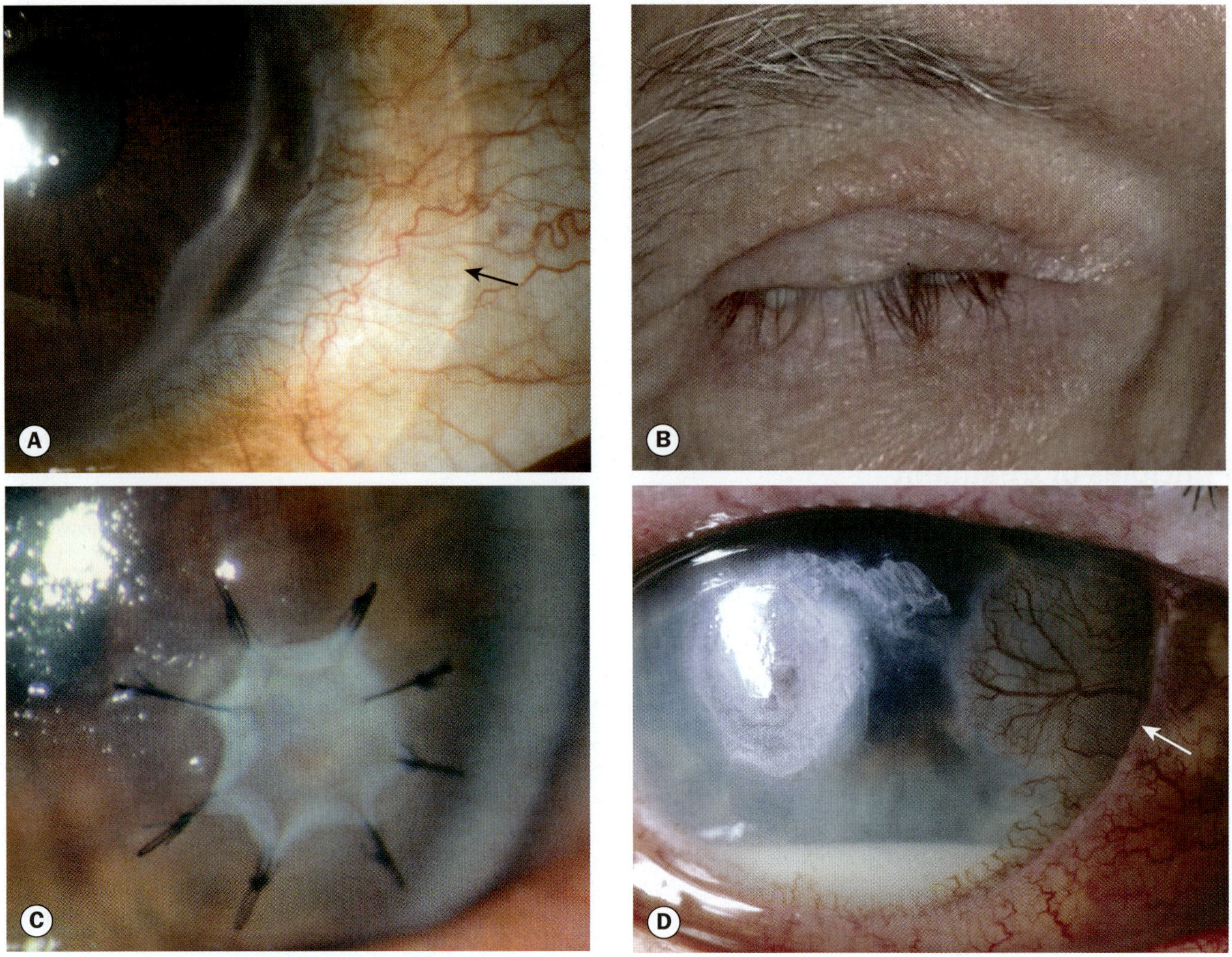

Fig. 7.6 Methods of promoting epithelial healing. **(A)** Bandage contact lens (arrow) in an eye with a small perforation; **(B)** central tarsorrhaphy; **(C)** amniotic membrane graft over a persistent epithelial defect; **(D)** tissue glue under a bandage contact lens (arrow) in an eye with severe thinning. *(Courtesy of S Tuft – figs A and C; S Chen – fig. B.)*

conjunctiva. Keratitis tends to present with a focal and fairly well-defined white or yellow–white infiltrate.

- **Streptococci.** *S. pyogenes* is a common Gram-positive commensal of the throat and vagina. *S. pneumoniae* (pneumococcus) is a Gram-positive commensal of the upper respiratory tract. Infections with streptococci are often aggressive.

Risk factors

- **Contact lens wear**, particularly if extended, is the most important risk factor. Corneal epithelial compromise secondary to hypoxia and minor trauma is thought to be important, as is bacterial adherence to the lens surface. Wearers of soft lenses are at higher risk than those wearing rigid gas permeable and other types. Infection is more likely if there is poor lens hygiene, but it can also occur even with apparently meticulous lens care and with daily disposable lenses.
- **Trauma**, including refractive surgery (particularly LASIK – laser-assisted *in situ* keratomileusis), has been linked to bacterial infection, including with atypical mycobacteria. In developing countries agricultural injury is the major risk factor, when fungal infection should be considered.
- **Ocular surface disease** such as herpetic keratitis, bullous keratopathy, dry eye, chronic blepharitis, trichiasis and entropion, exposure, severe allergic eye disease and corneal anaesthesia.
- **Other factors** include local or systemic immunosuppression, diabetes and vitamin A deficiency.

TIP Bacterial corneal ulceration should be excluded in a patient who wears contact lenses and presents with a painful red eye and blurred vision.

Clinical features

- **Presentation** is with unilateral pain, photophobia, blurred vision and mucopurulent or purulent discharge.

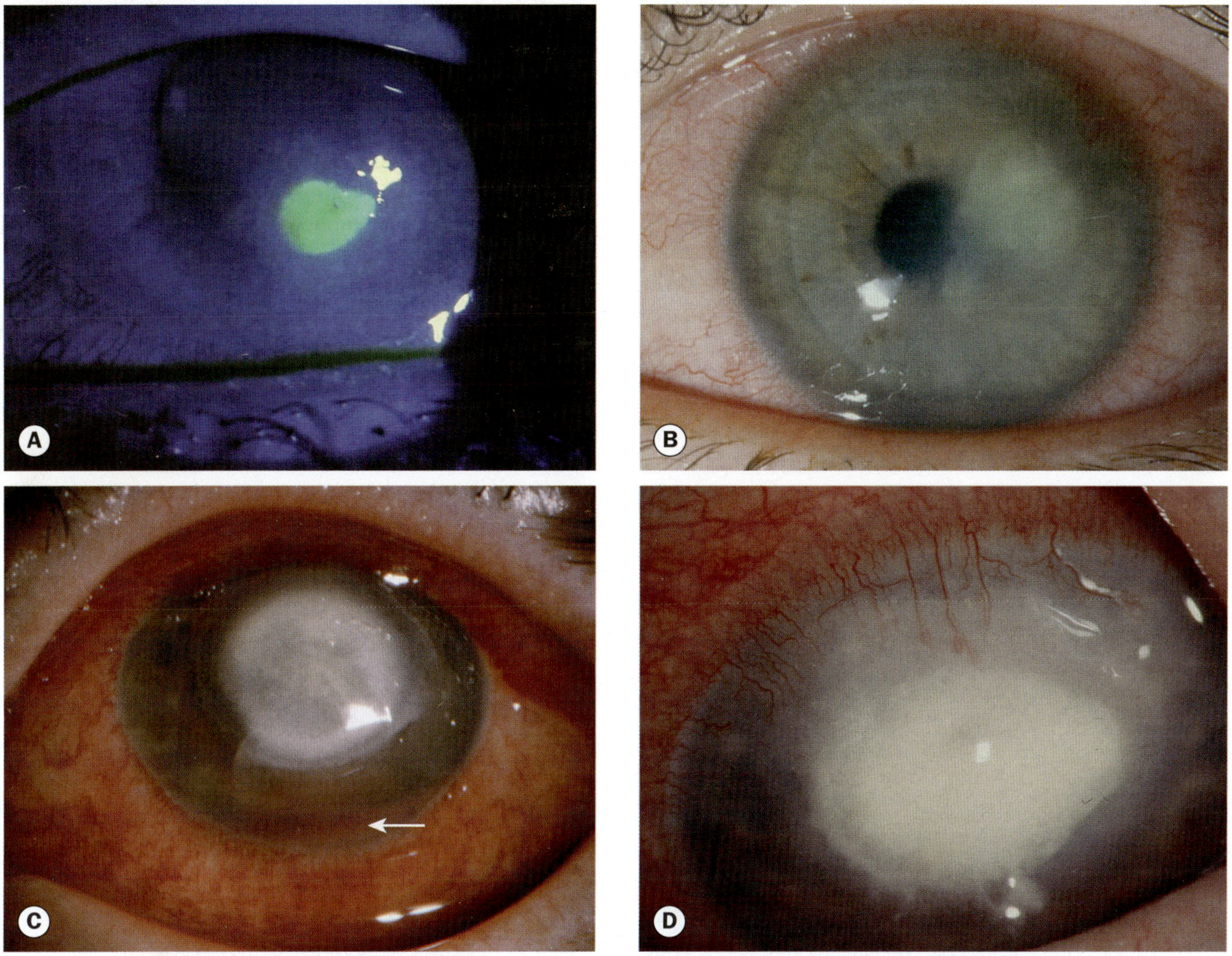

Fig. 7.7 Bacterial keratitis. **(A)** Corneal ulcer stained with fluorescein; **(B)** early contact lens-related ulcer; **(C)** ulcer with hypopyon (arrow); **(D)** large ulcer secondary to *Pseudomonas* infection. *(Courtesy of T Carmichael – fig. B; C Barry – fig. D.)*

- **Signs**
  - An epithelial defect with infiltrate involving a larger area and significant circumcorneal injection (Fig. 7.7A and B).
  - Stromal oedema, folds in Descemet membrane and anterior uveitis, commonly with a hypopyon (Fig. 7.7C) and posterior synechiae in moderate–severe keratitis. Plaque-like keratic precipitates can form on the endothelium contiguous with the affected stroma.
  - Chemosis and eyelid swelling in moderate–severe cases.
  - Severe ulceration (Fig. 7.7D) may lead to descemetocoele formation and perforation, particularly in *Pseudomonas* infection.
  - Scleritis can develop, particularly with severe perilimbal infection.
  - Endophthalmitis is rare in the absence of perforation.
  - Improvement is usually heralded by a reduction in eyelid oedema and chemosis, shrinking of the epithelial defect, decreasing infiltrate density and a reduction in anterior chamber signs.
  - Subsequent scarring may be severe, including vascularization. In addition to opacification, irregular astigmatism may limit vision.
- **Reduced corneal sensation** may suggest associated neurotrophic keratopathy, particularly where there is no other major risk factor. Sensation may also be reduced in chronic surface disease, herpetic keratitis and after long-term contact lens wear.
- **Differential diagnosis** includes keratitis due to other microorganisms (fungi, acanthamoeba, stromal herpes simplex keratitis and mycobacteria), marginal keratitis, sterile inflammatory corneal infiltrates associated with contact lens wear, peripheral ulcerative keratitis and toxic keratitis.

Investigations

- **Corneal scraping.** This may not be required for a small infiltrate, particularly one without an epithelial defect and away from the visual axis.

- Scrape all ulcers that are: (a) more than 2 mm in size, (b) involve the middle to deep stroma, (c) within the visual axis, (d) chronic in nature, (e) atypical in appearance.
- A non-preserved topical anaesthetic is instilled (preservatives may lower bacterial viability for culture). One drop of proxymetacaine 0.5% is usually sufficient but tetracaine may have a greater bacteriostatic effect.
- Scrapings are taken either with a disposable scalpel blade (e.g. No. 11 or Bard Parker), the bent tip of a larger diameter (e.g. 20- or 21-gauge) hypodermic needle, or a sterile spatula (e.g. Kimura).
- The easiest way to 'plate' scrapings without breaking the gel surface is with a spatula. If a fresh spatula is not available for each sample a single instrument should be flame-sterilized between scrapes (heat for 5 seconds, cool for 20–30 seconds). Alternatively, a fresh scalpel blade or needle can be used for each pass. Calcium alginate swabs may also be satisfactory.
- Loose mucus and necrotic tissue should be removed from the surface of the ulcer prior to scraping.
- The margins and base (except if very thin) of the lesion are scraped (Fig. 7.8A).
- A thin smear is placed on one or two glass slides for microscopy, including Gram stain (see below). A surface is provided on one side of one end of the slide (conventionally 'up') for pencil labelling. The sample is allowed to dry in air at room temperature for several minutes then placed in a slide carrier.
- Re-scraping is performed for each medium and samples are plated onto culture media (Table 7.2), taking care not to break the surface of the gel.
- Routinely, blood, chocolate and Sabouraud media (Fig. 7.8B and C) are used initially and the samples are placed in an incubator until transported to the laboratory. Refrigerated media should be gently warmed to room temperature prior to sample application.
- A blade or needle can be placed directly into bottled media such as brain–heart infusion (BHI). There is evidence that a single scrape, sent in BHI to the laboratory where it is homogenized and plated, provides similar results to the traditional multi-scrape method.

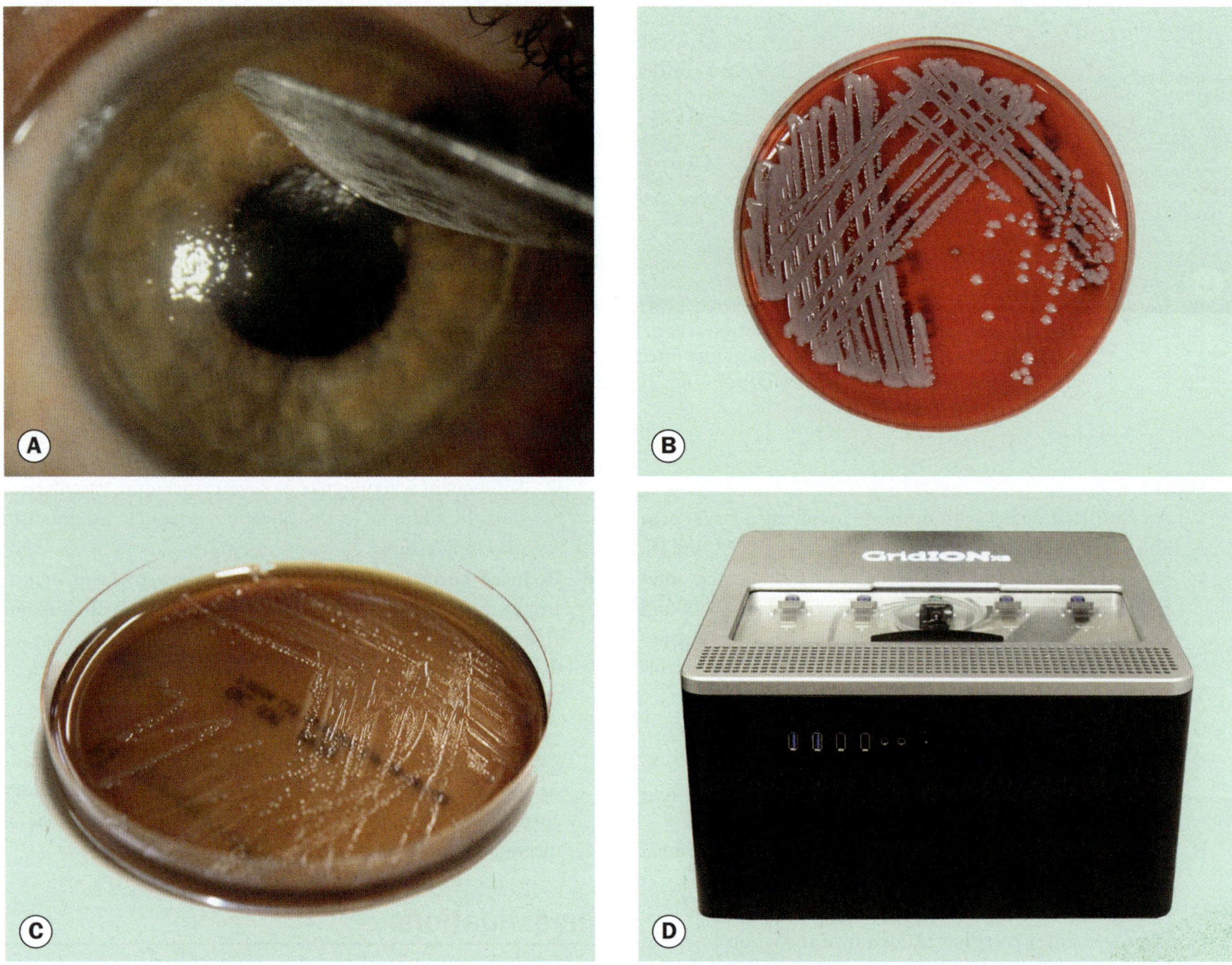

Fig. 7.8 Bacteriology. **(A)** Corneal scraping; **(B)** *S. aureus* grown on blood agar; **(C)** *N. gonorrhoeae* grown on chocolate agar; **(D)** the specimen can be amplified using PCR and then nanopore technology allows sequencing of the bacterial DNA.

Table 7.2 Culture Media for Corneal Scrapings

Medium	Notes	Specificity
Blood agar	5–10% sheep or horse blood	Most bacteria and fungi except *Neisseria*, *Haemophilus* and *Moraxella*
Chocolate agar	Blood agar in which the cells have been lysed by heating. Does not contain chocolate!	Fastidious bacteria, particularly *H. influenzae*, *Neisseria* and *Moraxella*
Sabouraud dextrose agar	Low pH and antibiotic (e.g. chloramphenicol) to deter bacterial growth	Fungi
Non-nutrient agar seeded with *Escherichia coli*	*E. coli* is a food source for *Acanthamoeba*	*Acanthamoeba*
Brain–heart infusion	Rich lightly buffered medium providing a wide range of substrates	Difficult-to-culture organisms; particularly suitable for streptococci and meningococci. Supports yeast and fungal growth
Cooked meat broth	Developed during the First World War for the growth of battlefield anaerobes	Anaerobic (e.g. *Propionibacterium acnes*) as well as fastidious bacteria
Löwenstein–Jensen	Contains various nutrients together with bacterial growth inhibitors	Mycobacteria, *Nocardia*

  - A small sample of DNA can be amplified using polymerase chain reaction (PCR) methodology. The bacterial DNA sequence can then be determined using modern nanopore technology (Fig. 7.8D). This establishes the exact species of bacterium and the antibiotic resistance of the organism. It is also important for epidemiologic studies (e.g. to trace the source of an infection).
  - Scraping may be delayed without treatment for 12 hours if antibiotics have previously been commenced.
- **Conjunctival swabs** may be worthwhile in addition to corneal scraping, particularly in severe cases, as occasionally an organism may be cultured when a corneal scrape is negative. Cotton wool, calcium alginate and synthetic swabs have all been found to have some bacteriostatic effect; calcium alginate may be the best option.
- **Contact lens cases**, as well as bottles of solution and lenses themselves, should be obtained when possible and sent to the laboratory for culture. The case should not be cleaned by the patient first!
- **Gram staining**
  - Differentiates bacterial species into 'Gram-positive' and 'Gram-negative' based on the ability of the dye (crystal violet) to penetrate the cell wall.
  - Bacteria that take up crystal violet are Gram-positive and those that allow the dye to wash off are Gram-negative.
  - Other stains, generally not requested at initial investigation, are listed in Table 7.3.
- **Culture and sensitivity reports** should be obtained as soon as possible. The type of bacteria will provide an indication of the antibiotic category to be used. An indication of resistance on standard sensitivity testing does not necessarily extrapolate to topical antibiotic instillation, where very high tissue levels can be achieved.

Table 7.3 Stains for Corneal and Conjunctival Scrapings

Stain	Organism
Gram	Bacteria, fungi, microsporidia
Giemsa	Bacteria, fungi, *Acanthamoeba*, microsporidia
Calcofluor white (fluorescent microscope)	*Acanthamoeba*, fungi, microsporidia
Acid-fast stain (AFB) e.g. Ziehl–Neelsen, auramine O (fluorescent)	*Mycobacterium*, *Nocardia* spp.
Grocott–Gömöri methenamine silver	Fungi, *Acanthamoeba*, microsporidia
Periodic acid–Schiff (PAS)	Fungi, *Acanthamoeba*

TIP Corneal scraping should be undertaken in most cases of corneal ulceration, so that the causative organism can be cultured and its sensitivity determined.

Treatment

General considerations

- **Hospital admission** should be considered for patients who are not likely to comply or are unable to self-administer treatment. It should also be considered for aggressive disease, particularly if involving an only eye.
- **Discontinuation of contact lens wear** is mandatory.
- **A clear plastic eye shield** should be worn between eye drop instillation if significant thinning (or perforation) is present.
- **Decision to treat**
  - Intensive treatment may not be required for small infiltrates that are clinically sterile and may be treated by

lower-frequency topical antibiotic and/or steroid and by temporary cessation of contact lens wear.
  - It is important to note that the causative organism cannot be defined reliably from the morphological appearance of the ulcer.
  - Empirical broad-spectrum treatment is usually initiated before microscopy results are available.
  - Daily follow-up is needed until a response to antibiotic treatment is noted.

Local therapy

Topical therapy (Table 7.4) can achieve high tissue concentration and initially should consist of broad-spectrum antibiotics that cover most common pathogens. Initially instillation is at hourly intervals day and night for 24–48 hours and then is tapered according to clinical progress.

- **Antibiotic monotherapy** has the major advantage over duotherapy of lower surface toxicity, as well as greater convenience.
  - A commercially available fluoroquinolone is the usual choice for empirical monotherapy and appears to be about as effective as duotherapy.
  - Ciprofloxacin or ofloxacin are used in countries where widespread resistance to earlier-generation fluoroquinolones has not been identified. Activity against some Gram-positive organisms, particularly some streptococci, may be limited.
  - Resistance to fluoroquinolones has been reported in some areas (e.g. *Staphylococcus* spp. in the USA and *Pseudomonas* in India). Moxifloxacin, gatifloxacin and besifloxacin are new generation fluoroquinolones that largely address this and also have better activity against Gram-positive pathogens. Moxifloxacin has superior ocular penetration. Novel drug preparations, with higher concentrations or modified vehicles, have been introduced to enhance antibacterial activity.
  - Ciprofloxacin instillation is associated with white corneal precipitates (Fig. 7.9) that may delay epithelial healing.
- **Antibiotic duotherapy** may be preferred as first-line empirical treatment in aggressive disease or if microscopy suggests streptococci or a specific microorganism that may be more effectively treated by a tailored regimen (see Table 7.4).
  - Empirical duotherapy usually involves a combination of two fortified antibiotics, typically a cephalosporin and an aminoglycoside, in order to cover common Gram-positive and Gram-negative pathogens.
  - The antibiotics are not commercially available and must be specially prepared (Table 7.5). A standard parenteral or lyophilized antibiotic preparation is combined with a compatible vehicle such that the antibiotic does not precipitate. Optimally, constitution should take place in the sterile preparation area of a pharmaceutical dispensary.
  - Disadvantages of fortified antibiotics include high cost, limited availability, contamination risk, short shelf-life and the need for refrigeration.
- **Subconjunctival antibiotics** are usually only indicated if there is poor compliance with topical treatment.
- **Mydriatics** (cyclopentolate 1%, homatropine 2% or atropine 1%) are used to prevent the formation of posterior synechiae and to reduce pain.
- **Steroids**
  - Steroids reduce host inflammation, improve comfort and minimize corneal scarring. However, they promote replication of some microorganisms, particularly fungi, herpes simplex and mycobacteria and are contraindicated if a fungal or mycobacterial agent is suspected (beware prior refractive surgery and trauma involving vegetation). By suppressing inflammation, they also retard the eye's response to bacteria and this can be clinically significant,

Table 7.4 Antibiotics for the Treatment of Keratitis

Isolate	Antibiotic	Concentration
Empirical treatment	Fluoroquinolone monotherapy or cefuroxime + 'fortified' gentamicin duotherapy	Varies with preparation 5% 1.5%
Gram-positive cocci	Cefuroxime vancomycin or teicoplanin	0.3% 5% 1%
Gram-negative rods	'Fortified' gentamicin or fluoroquinolone or ceftazidime	1.5% Varies with preparation 5%
Gram-negative cocci	Fluoroquinolone or ceftriaxone	Varies with preparation 5%
Mycobacteria	Amikacin or clarithromycin	2% 1%
Nocardia	Amikacin or trimethoprim + sulfamethoxazole	2% 1.6% 8%

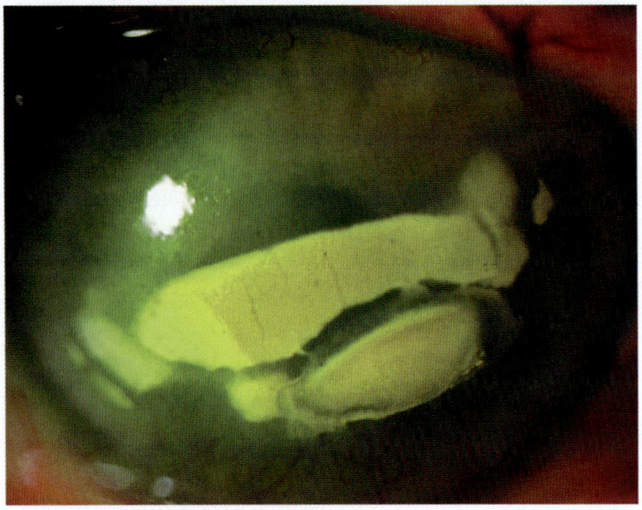

Fig. 7.9 Ciprofloxacin corneal precipitates.

Table 7.5 Preparation of Fortified Antibiotics

Antibiotic	Method	Concentration	Shelf-life
Cephalosporins: cefazolin, cefuroxime, or ceftazidime	500 mg parenteral antibiotic is diluted with 2.5 ml sterile water and added to 7.5 ml of preservative-free artificial tears	50 mg/ml (5%)	24 hours at room temperature; at least 4 days if refrigerated
Gentamicin	2 ml parenteral antibiotic (40 mg/ml) is added to 5 ml commercially available gentamicin ophthalmic solution (0.3%)	15 mg/ml (1.5%)	Up to 14 days if refrigerated

particularly if an antibiotic is of limited effect or bacteriostatic rather than bactericidal.

- Evidence that topical steroids improve the final visual outcome is mainly empirical. The Steroids for Corneal Ulcers Trial (SCUT) found no eventual benefit in most cases, but severe cases (counting fingers vision or large ulcers involving the central 4 mm of the cornea) tended to do better. A positive culture result was an inclusion criterion and steroids were introduced after 48 hours of moxifloxacin.
- Epithelialization may be retarded by steroids and they should be avoided if there is significant thinning or delayed epithelial healing. Corneal melting can occasionally be precipitated or worsened.
- Many authorities do not commence topical steroids until evidence of clinical improvement is seen with antibiotics alone, typically 24–48 hours after starting treatment. Others delay their use at least until the sensitivity of the isolate to antibiotics has been demonstrated, or do not use them at all.
- Regimens vary from minimal strength preparations at low frequency to dexamethasone 0.1% every 2 hours or prednisolone 0.5–1% four times daily.
- Early discontinuation may lead to a rebound recurrence of sterile inflammation.
- The threshold for topical steroid use may be lower in cases of corneal graft infection, as they may reduce the risk of rejection.

TIP Fluoroquinolone eyedrops have limited effectivity against Gram-positive organisms (particularly *Streptococcus*).

Systemic antibiotics

Systemic antibiotics are not usually given, but may be appropriate in the following circumstances:

- **Potential for systemic involvement**, when microbiological/infectious disease specialist advice should optimally be sought but should not delay treatment:
  - *N. meningitidis*, in which early systemic prophylaxis may be life-saving. Treatment is usually with intramuscular benzylpenicillin, ceftriaxone or cefotaxime, or oral ciprofloxacin.
  - *H. influenzae* infection should be treated with oral amoxicillin with clavulanic acid.
  - *N. gonorrhoeae* requires a third-generation cephalosporin such as ceftriaxone.
- **Severe corneal thinning** with threatened or actual perforation requires:
  - Ciprofloxacin for its antibacterial activity.
  - A tetracycline (e.g. doxycycline 100 mg twice daily) for its anticollagenase effect.
- **Scleral involvement** may respond to oral or intravenous treatment.

Management of apparent treatment failure

It is important not to confuse ongoing failure of re-epithelialization with continued infection. Drug toxicity, particularly following frequent instillation of fortified aminoglycosides, may give increasing discomfort, redness and discharge despite the eradication of infection.

- If no improvement is evident following 24–48 hours of intensive treatment, the antibiotic regimen should be reviewed, including contact with the microbiology laboratory to obtain the latest report.
- There is no need to change the initial therapy if this has induced a favourable response, even if cultures show a resistant organism.
- If there is still no improvement after a further 48 hours, suspension of treatment should be considered for 24 hours then re-scraping performed with inoculation on a broader range of media (see Table 7.2) and additional staining techniques requested (see Table 7.3). Consideration should be given to the possibility of a non-bacterial causative microorganism.
- If cultures remain negative, it may be necessary to perform a corneal biopsy for histology and culture.
- Consider collagen cross-linking treatment (PACK-CXL) if there is a suspicion of corneal melting or bacterial resistance.
- Excisional keratoplasty, penetrating or deep lamellar, may be considered in cases resistant to medical therapy, or for incipient or actual perforation (see below).

TIP Topical drug and preservative toxicity may cause a failure of corneal re-epithelialization, which can be confused with persistent infection.

Perforation

A small perforation in which infection is controlled may be manageable with a bandage contact lens. Tissue glue is often adequate for a slightly larger dehiscence. A penetrating keratoplasty or corneal patch graft may be necessary for larger perforations, or in those where infection is extensive or inadequately controlled. Occlusive surface repair techniques may be appropriate in some circumstances, such as an eye with no useful visual potential.

Endophthalmitis

No clear protocol exists for the management of this rare complication, but a similar approach to postoperative endophthalmitis should be considered, whilst continuing specific management of the corneal infection (see Ch. 10). Secondary sterile intraocular inflammation should not be mistaken for intraocular infection.

Visual rehabilitation

- **Keratoplasty** (lamellar may be adequate) may be required for residual dense corneal scarring.
- **Rigid contact lenses** may be required for irregular astigmatism but are generally only introduced at least 3 months after re-epithelialization.
- **Cataract surgery** may be required because secondary lens opacities are common following severe inflammation. Even in the absence of severe corneal opacification, surgery may be hampered by corneal haze, posterior synechiae and zonular fragility.
- **Prognosis** depends on the size, location, depth and aetiology of the corneal ulcer.

FUNGAL KERATITIS

Introduction

Pathogenesis

Fungi are a group of microorganisms that have rigid walls and a distinct nucleus with multiple chromosomes containing both DNA and RNA. Fungal keratitis is rare in temperate countries but is a major cause of visual loss in tropical and low-income countries. Though often evolving insidiously, fungal keratitis can elicit a severe inflammatory response – corneal perforation is common and the outlook for vision is frequently poor. Two main types of fungi cause keratitis:

- **Yeasts** (e.g. genus *Candida*), ovoid unicellular organisms that reproduce by budding, are responsible for most cases of fungal keratitis in temperate climates.
- **Filamentous fungi** (e.g. genera *Fusarium* and *Aspergillus*), multicellular organisms that produce tubular projections known as hyphae. They are the most common pathogens in tropical climates, but are not uncommon in cooler regions. The keratitis frequently follows an aggressive course.

Predisposing factors

Common predisposing factors include chronic ocular surface disease, the long-term use of topical steroids (often in conjunction with prior corneal transplantation), contact lens wear, systemic immunosuppression and diabetes. Filamentary keratitis may be associated with trauma, often relatively minor, involving plant matter or gardening/agricultural tools.

Candida and filamentous keratitis

Clinical features

The diagnosis is frequently delayed unless there is a high index of suspicion and often bacterial infection will initially have been presumed. Clinical signs are not a definitive means of distinguishing bacterial and fungal corneal infection. Signs such as satellite infiltrates (see below) can be caused by other microorganisms.

- **Symptoms.** Gradual onset of pain, grittiness, photophobia, blurred vision and watery or mucopurulent discharge.
- ***Candida* keratitis**
  - Yellow–white densely suppurative infiltrate is typical.
- **Filamentous keratitis**
  - Grey or yellow–white stromal infiltrate with indistinct fluffy margins (Fig. 7.10A).
  - Progressive infiltration, often with satellite lesions (Fig. 7.10B and C) or a ring-shaped infiltrate.
  - Feathery branch-like extensions may develop.
  - Rapid progression with necrosis and thinning can occur.
  - Penetration of an intact Descemet membrane may occur and lead to endophthalmitis without evident perforation.
- **An epithelial defect** is not invariable and is sometimes small when present.
- **Other features** include anterior uveitis, hypopyon, endothelial plaque, raised IOP, scleritis and sterile or infective endophthalmitis.
- **Differential diagnosis** includes bacterial, herpetic and acanthamoebal keratitis. Bacterial infection may sometimes present in a subacute fashion, particularly when atypical organisms are responsible. It is important to beware of co-infection, including with an additional fungal species.

Investigations

Samples for laboratory investigation should be acquired before commencing antifungal therapy.

- **Staining**
  - Potassium hydroxide (KOH) preparation with direct microscopic evaluation is a rapid diagnostic tool that can be highly sensitive.
  - Gram and Giemsa staining are both about 50% sensitive.
  - Other stains include periodic acid–Schiff, calcofluor white (Fig. 7.10D) and methenamine silver.
- **Culture.** Corneal scrapes should be plated on Sabouraud dextrose agar, although most fungi will also grow on blood agar or in enrichment media. It is important to obtain an effective scrape from the ulcer base. Sensitivity testing for antifungal agents can be performed in reference laboratories but the relevance of these results to clinical effectiveness is uncertain. If applicable, contact lenses and cases should be sent for culture.

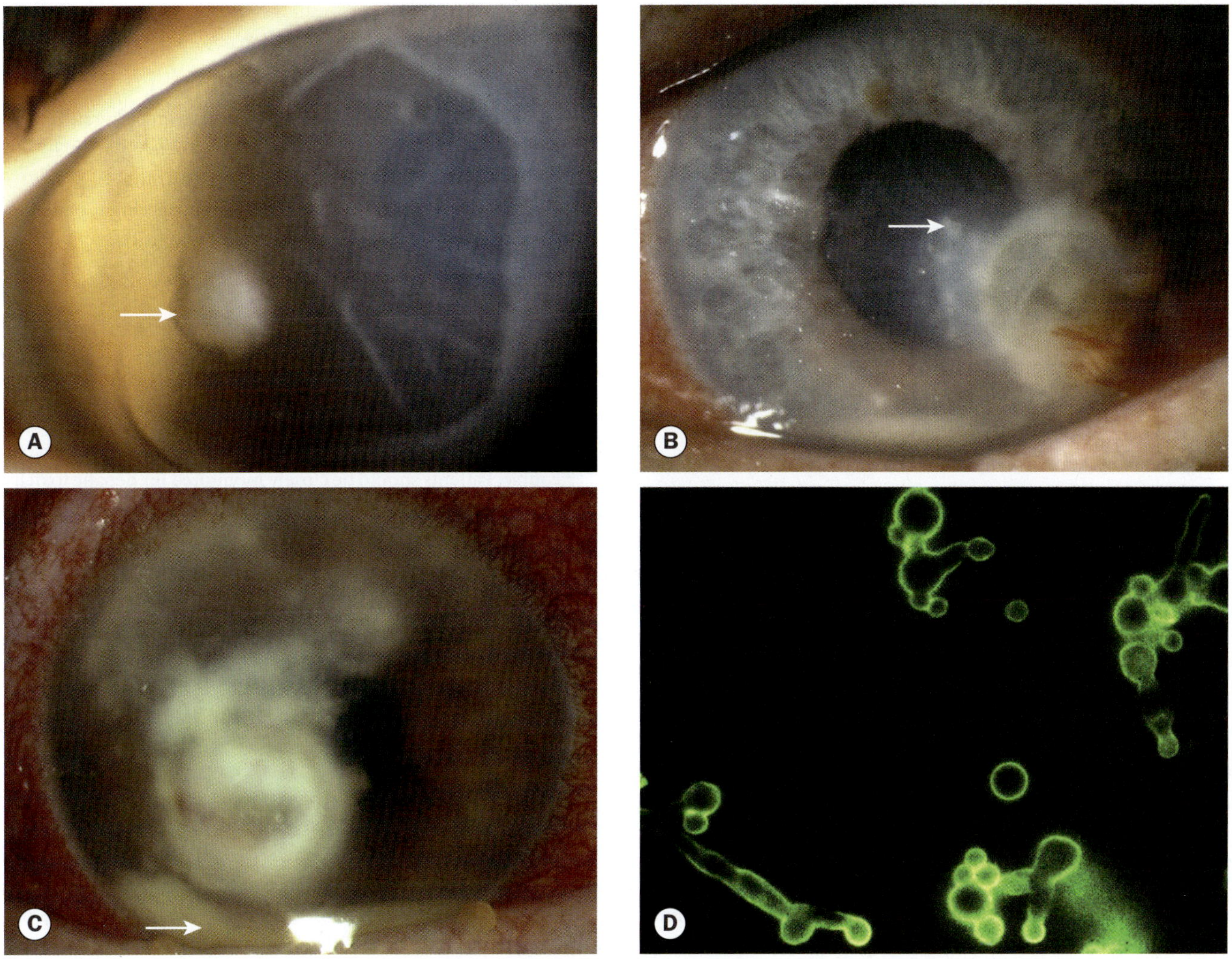

Fig. 7.10 Fungal keratitis. **(A)** Filamentous keratitis with fluffy edges (arrow). There is a large epithelial defect and folds in Descemet membrane; **(B)** ring infiltrate and satellite lesions (arrow); **(C)** large ulcer with satellite lesions and hypopyon (arrow); **(D)** *Candida* mycology stained with calcofluor white. *(Courtesy of S Tuft – fig. A.)*

- **Polymerase chain reaction (PCR) analysis** of specimens is rapid and highly sensitive (up to 90%) and may be the current investigation of choice. Calcium-containing swabs can inhibit polymerase activity and local collection protocols should be ascertained prior to specimen collection.
- **Corneal biopsy** is indicated in suspected fungal keratitis in the absence of clinical improvement after 3–4 days and if no growth develops from scrapings after a week. A 2–3 mm block should be taken, similar to scleral block excision during trabeculectomy. Filamentous fungi tend to proliferate just anterior to Descemet membrane and a deep stromal specimen may be required. The excised block is sent for culture and histopathological analysis.
- **Anterior chamber tap** has been advocated in resistant cases with endothelial exudate, because organisms may penetrate the endothelium.
- **Confocal microscopy** frequently permits identification of organisms *in vivo*, but is not widely available outside tertiary centres.

Treatment

Improvement may be slow in comparison to bacterial infection.

- **General measures** are as for bacterial keratitis although hospital admission is usually required.
- **Removal of the epithelium** over the lesion may enhance penetration of antifungal agents. It may also be helpful to regularly remove mucus and necrotic tissue with a spatula.
- **Topical antifungals** should initially be given hourly for 48 hours and then reduced as signs permit.
  - *Candida* infection is treated with amphotericin B 0.15% or econazole 1% (alternatives include natamycin 5%, fluconazole 2%, clotrimazole 1% and voriconazole 1 or 2%).
  - Filamentous infection is treated with natamycin 5% or econazole 1% (alternatives are amphotericin B 0.15%, miconazole 1% and voriconazole 1 or 2%).
  - Natamycin is the only topical drug approved by the FDA for use in mycotic keratitis.

- **A broad-spectrum antibiotic** might also be considered to address or prevent bacterial co-infection.
- **Cycloplegia** as for bacterial keratitis.
- **Subconjunctival** fluconazole may be used in severe cases.
- **Systemic antifungals** may be given in severe cases, when lesions are near the limbus and for suspected endophthalmitis. Options include voriconazole 400 mg twice daily for one day then 200 mg twice daily, itraconazole 200 mg once daily, reduced to 100 mg once daily, or fluconazole 200 mg twice daily.
- **Tetracycline** (e.g. doxycycline 100 mg twice daily) may be given for its anticollagenase effect when there is significant thinning.
- **Perforation** – actual or impending – is managed as for bacterial keratitis.
- **Superficial keratectomy** can be effective to debulk a lesion.
- **Therapeutic keratoplasty** (penetrating or deep anterior lamellar) is considered when medical therapy is ineffective or following perforation.
- **Anterior chamber washout** with intracameral antifungal injection may be considered for unresponsive cases in which there is a stable corneal infiltrate but enlarging endothelial exudation.

Microsporidial keratitis

Introduction

Microsporidia (phylum Microspora) are obligate intracellular single-celled parasites previously thought to be protozoa but now reclassified as fungi. They rarely cause disease in the immunocompetent and until the advent of acquired immunodeficiency syndrome (AIDS) were rarely pathogenic for humans. The most common general infection is enteritis and the most common ocular manifestation is keratoconjunctivitis.

Diagnosis

- **Signs**
  - Bilateral chronic diffuse PEK (Fig. 7.11A).
  - Unilateral slowly progressive deep stromal keratitis (Fig. 7.11B) may rarely affect immunocompetent patients.
  - Sclerokeratitis and endophthalmitis are rare.
- **Biopsy** shows characteristic spores and intracellular parasites.
- **PCR** of scrapings may have relatively low sensitivity.

Treatment

- **Medical** therapy of epithelial disease is with topical fumagillin. Highly active antiretroviral therapy (HAART) for associated AIDS may also help resolution. Stromal disease is treated with a combination of topical fumagillin and oral albendazole 400 mg once daily for 2 weeks, repeated 2 weeks later with a second course. Patients should be closely monitored for hepatic toxicity. Long-term fumagillin treatment may be required and it is difficult to eradicate the parasites in immunocompromised patients.
- **Keratoplasty** may be indicated although recurrence of disease can occur in the graft periphery. Cryotherapy to the residual tissue may reduce this risk.

HERPES SIMPLEX KERATITIS

Introduction

Herpetic eye disease is the most common infectious cause of corneal blindness in developed countries. As many as 60% of corneal ulcers in developing countries may be the result of herpes simplex virus and 10 million people worldwide may have herpetic eye disease. Approximately 10% of those who have any history of herpes simplex keratitis (HSK) will eventually have a final visual acuity of less than 6/60. Even in the patients who retain good vision, corneal opacities can result in aberrations, astigmatism and reduced

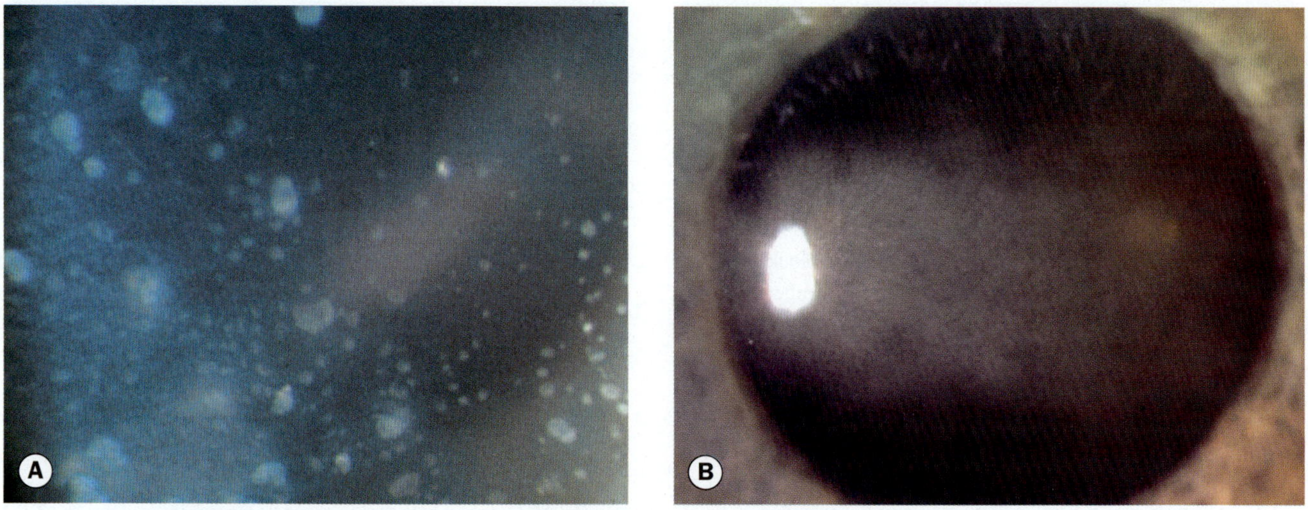

Fig. 7.11 Microsporidial keratitis. **(A)** Diffuse punctate epithelial keratitis; **(B)** deep stromal infiltrates. *(Courtesy of S Tuft.)*

quality of vision. In addition to visual loss, HSK also reduces the quality of life of those affected, even when the eye is not inflamed.

Herpes simplex virus (HSV)

HSV is enveloped with a cuboidal capsule and has a linear double-stranded DNA genome. The two subtypes are HSV-1 and HSV-2 and these reside in almost all neuronal ganglia. HSV-1 causes infection above the waist (principally the face, lips and eyes), whereas HSV-2 causes venereally acquired infection (genital herpes). Rarely HSV-2 may be transmitted to the eye through infected secretions, either venereally or at birth (neonatal conjunctivitis). HSV transmission is facilitated in conditions of crowding and poor hygiene.

Primary infection

Primary infection, without previous viral exposure, usually occurs in childhood and is spread by droplet transmission, or less frequently by direct inoculation. Due to protection by maternal antibodies, it is uncommon during the first 6 months of life. Occasionally severe neonatal systemic disease may occur in which early diagnosis and intravenous antiviral treatment are critical to reduce mortality and disability. The presence of maternal antibodies means that dendritic corneal ulcers may be seen. Most primary infections with HSV are subclinical or cause only mild fever, malaise and upper respiratory tract symptoms. Blepharitis and follicular conjunctivitis may develop but are usually mild and self-limited. Treatment, if necessary, involves topical aciclovir ointment for the eye and/or cream for skin lesions and occasionally oral antivirals. There is unfortunately no evidence that antiviral treatment at this stage reduces the likelihood of recurrent disease.

Recurrent infection

Recurrent disease (reactivation in the presence of cellular and humoral immunity) occurs as follows:

- **After primary infection** the virus is carried to the sensory ganglion for that dermatome (e.g. trigeminal ganglion) where latent infection is established. Latent virus is incorporated in host DNA and cannot be eradicated with presently available treatment.
- **Subclinical reactivation** can periodically occur, during which HSV is shed and patients are contagious.
- **Clinical reactivation.** A variety of stress factors such as fever, hormonal change, ultraviolet radiation, trauma, or trigeminal injury may cause clinical reactivation, when the virus replicates and is transported in the sensory axons to the periphery.
- **The pattern of disease** depends on the site of reactivation, which may be remote from the site of primary disease. Hundreds of reactivations can occur during a lifetime.
- **The rate of ocular recurrence** after one episode is about 10% at 1 year and 50% at 10 years. The higher the number of previous attacks the greater the risk of recurrence.
- **Risk factors for severe disease**, which may be frequently recurrent, include atopic eye disease, childhood, immunodeficiency or suppression, malnutrition, measles and malaria. Inappropriate use of topical steroids may enhance the development of geographic ulceration (see below).

TIP Herpes simplex is the commonest infectious cause of corneal disease in developed countries.

Epithelial keratitis

Clinical features

Epithelial (dendritic or geographic) keratitis is associated with active virus replication.

- **Symptoms.** Mild–moderate discomfort, redness, photophobia, watering and blurred vision.
- **Signs** in approximately chronological order:
  - Reduced visual acuity.
  - Swollen opaque epithelial cells arranged in a coarse punctate or stellate (Fig. 7.12A) pattern.
  - Central desquamation results in a linear-branching (dendritic) ulcer (Fig. 7.12B), most frequently located centrally. The branches of the ulcer have characteristic terminal buds and its bed stains well with fluorescein.
  - The virus-laden cells at the margin of the ulcer stain with rose Bengal (Fig. 7.12C). This may help distinction of herpetic ulceration from alternative conditions, particularly an atypical recurrent corneal abrasion.
  - Corneal sensation is reduced.
  - Inadvertent topical steroid treatment may promote progressive enlargement of the ulcer to a geographical or 'amoeboid' configuration (Fig. 7.12D).
  - Mild associated subepithelial haze is typical.
  - Anterior chamber activity may be present, but is usually mild.
  - Follicular conjunctivitis may be associated; topical antivirals can also cause this.
  - Vesicular eyelid lesions may coincide with epithelial ulceration.
  - Elevated IOP is not uncommon (tonometry should be performed on the unaffected eye first and a disposable prism used).
  - Following healing, there may be persistent PEE and irregular epithelium that settle spontaneously and should not be mistaken for persistent active infection. A whorled epithelial appearance commonly results from assiduous, especially prolonged, topical antiviral instillation.
  - Mild subepithelial haze (Fig. 7.12E) may persist for weeks after the epithelium heals. In some cases, mild scarring may develop, which tends to become more evident after each recurrence and may eventually threaten vision.
  - Recurrence may occur after a corneal graft, undertaken for stromal scarring (Fig. 7.12F).
- **Investigation** is usually unnecessary as the diagnosis can be made clinically. Pre-treatment scrapings can be sent in viral transport medium for culture. PCR and immunocytochemistry are also available. Giemsa staining shows multinucleated giant cells. HSV serological titres rise only on primary infection, but can be used to confirm previous viral

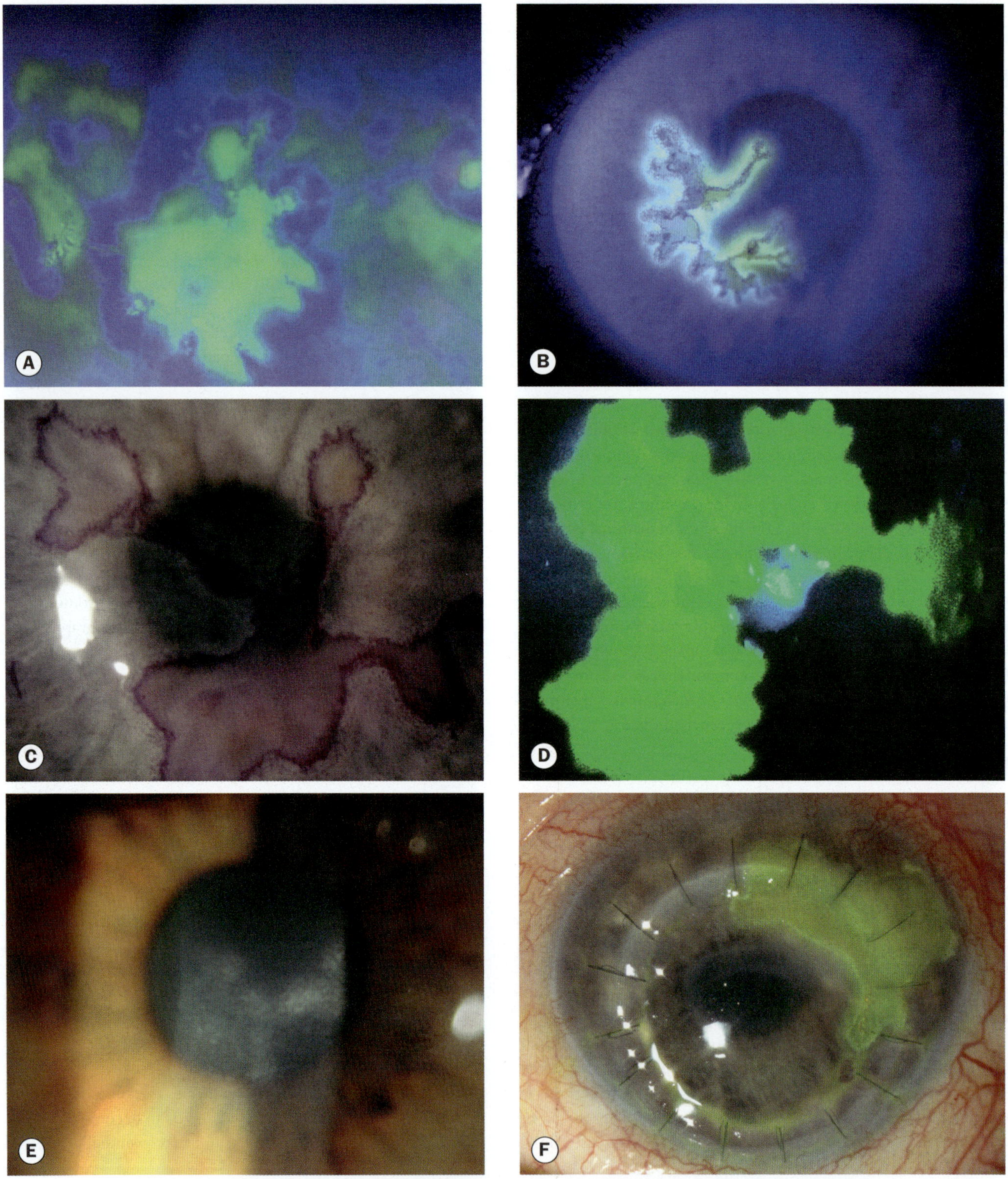

Fig. 7.12 Epithelial herpes simplex keratitis. **(A)** Stellate lesions; **(B)** bed of a dendritic ulcer stained with fluorescein; **(C)** margins of a dendritic ulcer stained with rose Bengal; **(D)** geographic ulcer; **(E)** residual subepithelial haze; **(F)** recurrent ulceration after a corneal graft. *(Courtesy of S Tuft – fig. C; T Carmichael – fig. F.)*

exposure, usually in cases of stromal disease when the diagnosis is in doubt.

- **Differential diagnosis** of dendritic ulceration includes herpes zoster keratitis, healing corneal abrasion (pseudodendrite), acanthamoeba keratitis, epithelial rejection in a corneal graft, tyrosinaemia type 2, the epithelial effects of soft contact lenses and toxic keratopathy secondary to topical medication. It has recently been reported that dendritiform keratopathy can be caused by polyquadernium-1, a common preservative in contact lens solutions and tear replacement products.

Treatment

Treatment of HSV disease is predominantly with nucleoside (purine or pyrimidine) analogues that disrupt viral DNA. The majority of dendritic ulcers will eventually heal spontaneously without treatment, though scarring and vascularization may be more significant.

- **Topical.** The most frequently used drugs are aciclovir 3% ointment or ganciclovir 0.15% gel, each administered five times daily. Trifluridine is an alternative, but requires instillation up to nine times daily until the epithelium closes and then five times daily. The drugs are relatively non-toxic, even when given for up to 60 days. They have approximately equivalent effect, acting preferentially on virus-laden epithelial cells and penetrating effectively into the stroma; 99% of ulcers heal within 2 weeks. Idoxuridine and vidarabine are older drugs that are less effective and are toxic to the corneal epithelium.
- **Debridement** may be used for resistant cases. The corneal surface is wiped with a sterile cellulose sponge or cotton-tipped applicator (cotton bud). Epithelium should be removed 2 mm beyond the edge of the ulcer, since involvement extends beyond the visible dendrite. The removal of the virus-containing cells protects adjacent healthy epithelium from infection and eliminates the antigenic stimulus to stromal inflammation. A topical antiviral agent should be used in conjunction.
- **Signs of treatment toxicity** include superficial punctate erosions, waves of whorled epithelium, follicular conjunctivitis and, rarely, punctal occlusion. Absence of epithelial whorling with a persistent epithelial lesion raises the possibility of poor or non-compliance.
- **Oral antiviral** therapy (e.g. aciclovir 200–400 mg five times a day for 5–10 days, famciclovir or valaciclovir) is indicated in most immunodeficient patients, in children and patients with marked ocular surface disease. It is an effective alternative to topical treatment when the latter is poorly tolerated, or in resistant cases. The newer oral agents may be better tolerated than aciclovir and require less frequent dosing, but optimal regimens are not yet defined.
- **Interferon monotherapy** does not seem to be more effective than antivirals, but the combination of a nucleoside antiviral with either interferon or debridement seems to speed healing.
- **Skin lesions** (see Ch. 2) may be treated with aciclovir cream five times daily, as for cold sores, and if extensive an oral antiviral may be given.
- **Cycloplegia**, e.g. homatropine 1% once or twice daily can be given to improve comfort if necessary.
- **Topical antibiotic prophylaxis** is recommended by some practitioners.
- **Prostaglandin derivatives** should be avoided if treatment is required to control the IOP, as these drops promote herpes virus activity.
- **Topical steroids** are not used unless significant disciform keratitis is also present (see below).
- **Slow healing or frequent recurrence** may indicate the presence of a resistant viral strain and an alternative topical agent or debridement may be tried. In especially refractory cases, a combination of two topical agents with oral valaciclovir or famciclovir may be effective. A significant minority of resistant cases are due to varicella-zoster virus.

TIP Topical steroids should not be used in epithelial herpes keratitis as this can result in worsening of the ulceration and may lead to corneal perforation.

Disciform keratitis

The aetiology of disciform keratitis (endotheliitis) is unclear. It may be the result of active HSV infection of keratocytes or endothelium, or a hypersensitivity reaction to viral antigen in the cornea.

Clinical features

- **Symptoms.** Blurred vision of gradual onset, which may be associated with haloes around lights. Discomfort and redness are common, but tend to be milder than in purely epithelial disease. A clear past history of epithelial ulceration is not always present and the possibility of a mimicking infection such as acanthamoeba or fungal keratitis should be borne in mind.
- **Signs**
  - A central zone of stromal oedema, often with overlying epithelial oedema (Fig. 7.13A and B). Occasionally the lesion is eccentric.
  - Large (granulomatous) keratic precipitates underlying the oedema.
  - Folds in Descemet membrane in severe cases.
  - A surrounding (Wessely) immune ring of deep stromal haze (Fig. 7.13C) signifies deposition of viral antigen and host antibody complexes.
  - The IOP may be elevated.
  - Reduced corneal sensation. This may aid in distinguishing other forms of infection.
  - Healed lesions often have a faint ring of stromal or subepithelial opacification and thinning.
  - Consecutive episodes may be associated with gradually worsening subepithelial and/or stromal scarring and superficial or deep vascularization (Fig. 7.13D).
  - Mid-stromal scarring from disciform keratitis is a cause of interstitial keratitis.

Treatment

A broad approach to management is set out below, but regimens should be tailored individually. Careful monitoring and adequate

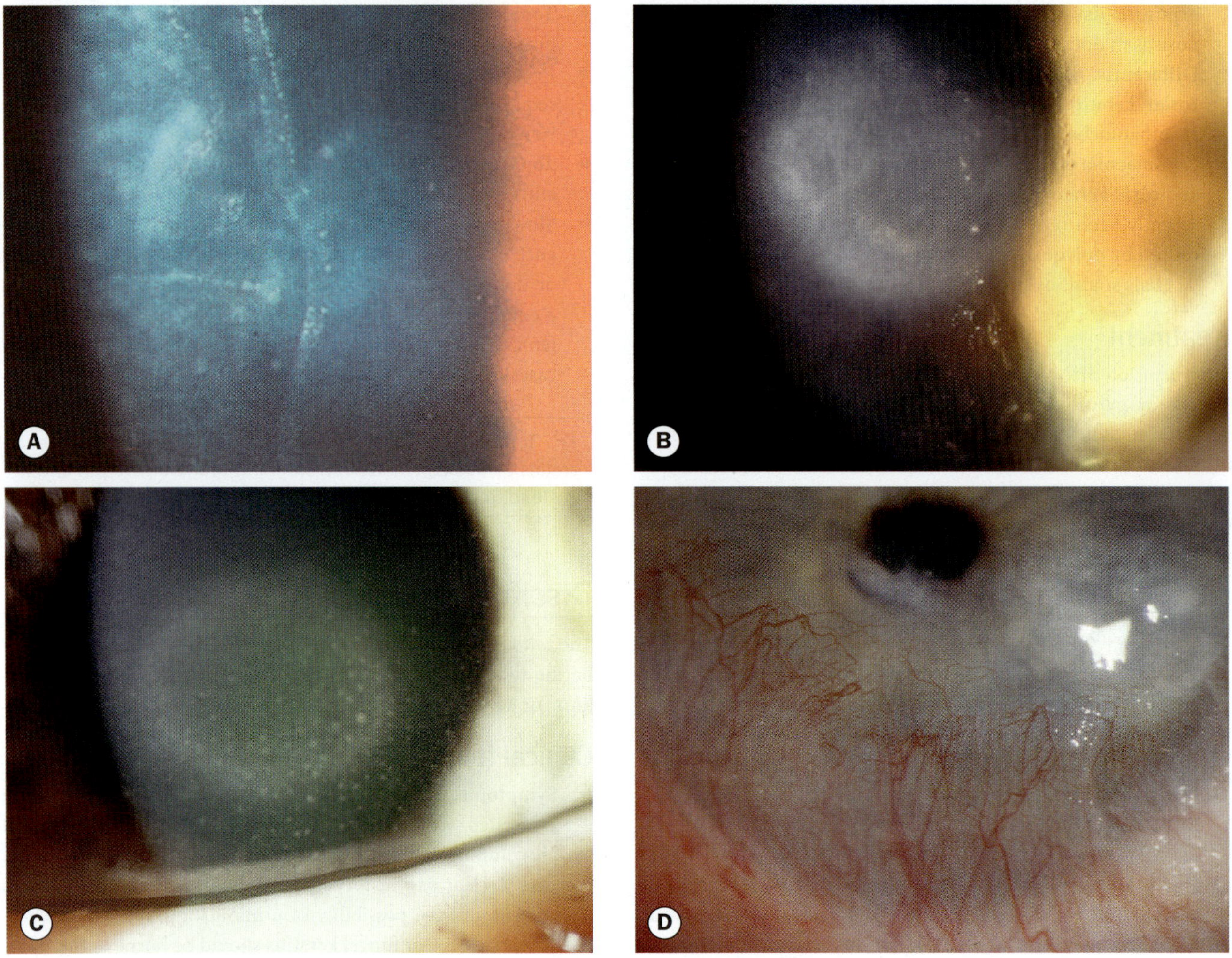

Fig. 7.13 Disciform herpes simplex keratitis. **(A)** Epithelial and stromal oedema, with Descemet membrane folds; **(B)** stromal oedema; **(C)** Wessely ring; **(D)** scarring with vascularization from recurrent disease

treatment, dependent on severity of inflammation, is critical to minimize progression of scarring. Patients should be cautioned to seek treatment at the first suggestion of recurrence, though some authorities feel that minimal inflammation may not warrant treatment or can be addressed with cycloplegia alone.

- **Initial** treatment is with topical steroids (prednisolone 1% or dexamethasone 0.1%) with antiviral cover, both four times daily. As improvement occurs, the frequency of administration of both is reduced in parallel over not less than 4 weeks. It is prudent to keep steroid intensity and duration to the minimum required for effective control of inflammation. IOP should be monitored. Cycloplegia can be used to improve comfort if necessary.
- **Subsequently** prednisolone 0.5% once daily is usually a safe dose at which to stop topical antiviral cover. Some patients require a weaker steroid such as fluorometholone 0.1% or loteprednol 0.2% on alternate days for many months. Periodic attempts should be made to stop the steroid altogether.
- With active epithelial ulceration it is reasonable to try to keep the steroid intensity as low as possible for adequate effect, with a more frequent antiviral regimen, e.g. initially topical antiviral five times daily, with steroid two or three times daily, titrated according to the signs of activity of both. Oral antiviral treatment may be helpful but its efficacy in this situation has not been established.
- Oral steroids are sometimes used in severe stromal inflammation as an adjunct.
- Topical ciclosporin 0.05% may be useful, particularly in the presence of epithelial ulceration and to facilitate tapering of topical steroids such as in steroid-related IOP elevation.
- Fine needle diathermy and laser techniques have been reported as successfully addressing established corneal neovascularization and improving vision.

Necrotizing stromal keratitis

This rare condition is thought to result from active viral replication within the stroma, though immune-mediated inflammation is likely to play a significant role. It may be difficult to distinguish from severe disciform keratitis and there may be a spectrum of disease, including overlap with neurotrophic keratopathy. As with disciform keratitis, a similar clinical picture may be caused by other infections.

- **Signs**
  - Stromal necrosis and melting, often with profound interstitial opacification (Fig. 7.14A).
  - Anterior uveitis with keratic precipitates underlying the area of active stromal infiltration.
  - An epithelial defect may be present.
  - Progression to scarring, vascularization (Fig. 7.14B) and lipid deposition is common (see Fig. 7.3C)
- **Treatment** is broadly similar to that of aggressive disciform keratitis, but oral antiviral supplementation, initially at the upper end of the dose range, is commonly used. The restoration of epithelial integrity is critical.

Neurotrophic keratopathy

Neurotrophic keratopathy (see also separate topic) is caused by failure of re-epithelialization resulting from corneal anaesthesia, often exacerbated by other factors such as drug toxicity.

- **Signs**
  - A non-healing epithelial defect is an early sign, sometimes after prolonged topical treatment (see Fig. 7.31A).
  - The stroma beneath the defect is grey and opaque and may become thin.
  - Secondary bacterial or fungal infection may occur.
- **Treatment** is that of persistent epithelial defects. Topical steroids to control any inflammatory component should be kept to a minimum.

Iridocyclitis

Herpetic iridocyclitis can occur without signs of active corneal inflammation and may be associated with direct viral activity. IOP elevation is common and is often presumed to be due to trabeculitis. However, steroid-induced IOP elevation may also be relatively common in herpetic iritis. The aetiology may be missed unless there is a history of previous herpes simplex keratitis. Patchy iris atrophy (Fig. 7.15A) may provide a clue and transillumination (Fig. 7.15B) may demonstrate subtle lesions. Aqueous sampling for PCR is diagnostic. Treatment is primarily with topical steroids, but adjunctive oral aciclovir may be given.

Other considerations

Prophylaxis

- **Long-term oral aciclovir** reduces the rate of recurrence of epithelial and stromal keratitis by about 50% and is usually tolerated well. Prophylaxis should be considered in patients with frequent debilitating recurrences, particularly if bilateral or involving an only eye. The standard daily dose of aciclovir is 400 mg twice daily for 12 months, but if necessary, a higher dose can be tried, based on practice in the management of systemic herpes simplex infection. Continual use for many years has been documented for systemic indications, but it can result in aciclovir-resistant HSV-1 viruses. The prophylactic effect decreases or disappears when the drug is stopped. Excretion is via the kidney, so renal function should be checked periodically during long-term treatment.
- **Oral valaciclovir** (500 mg once daily) or famciclovir are alternatives that are probably as effective as aciclovir, require less frequent dosing and may be better tolerated.
- **Topical.** Oral prophylaxis tends to be preferred to long-term topical administration as epithelial toxicity may occur, leading to mild blurring and persistent discomfort. Allergy and punctal stenosis are also potential problems.
- **Vaccination.** Therapeutic vaccination strategies are under investigation.

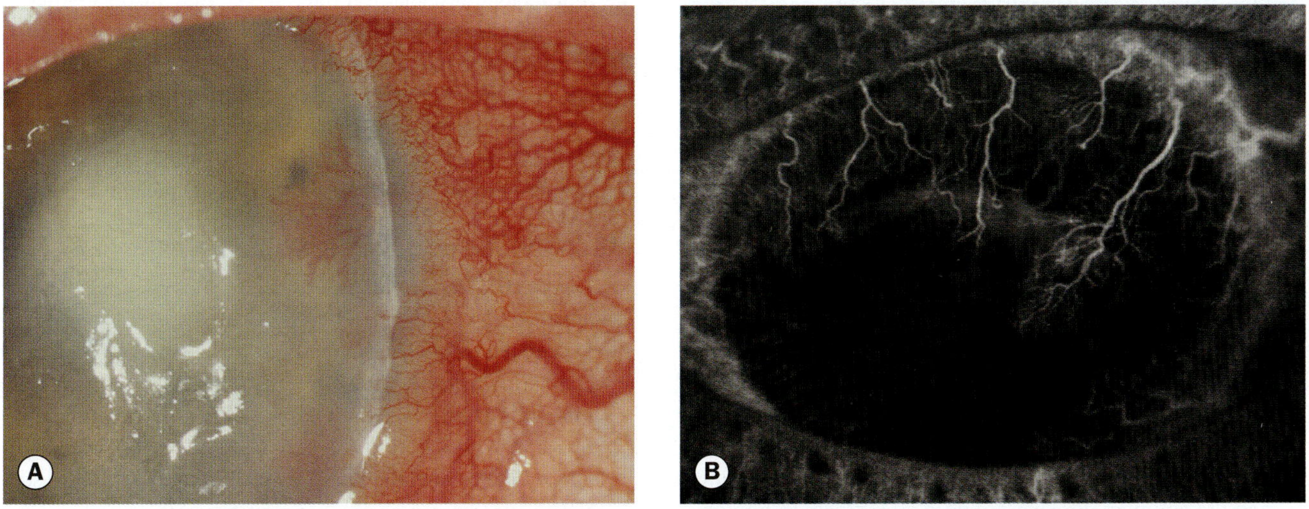

Fig. 7.14 Necrotizing stromal herpes simplex keratitis. **(A)** Stromal infection with peripheral vascularization; **(B)** ICG anterior segment image showing severe stromal vascularization. *(Courtesy of T Carmichael – fig. A.)*

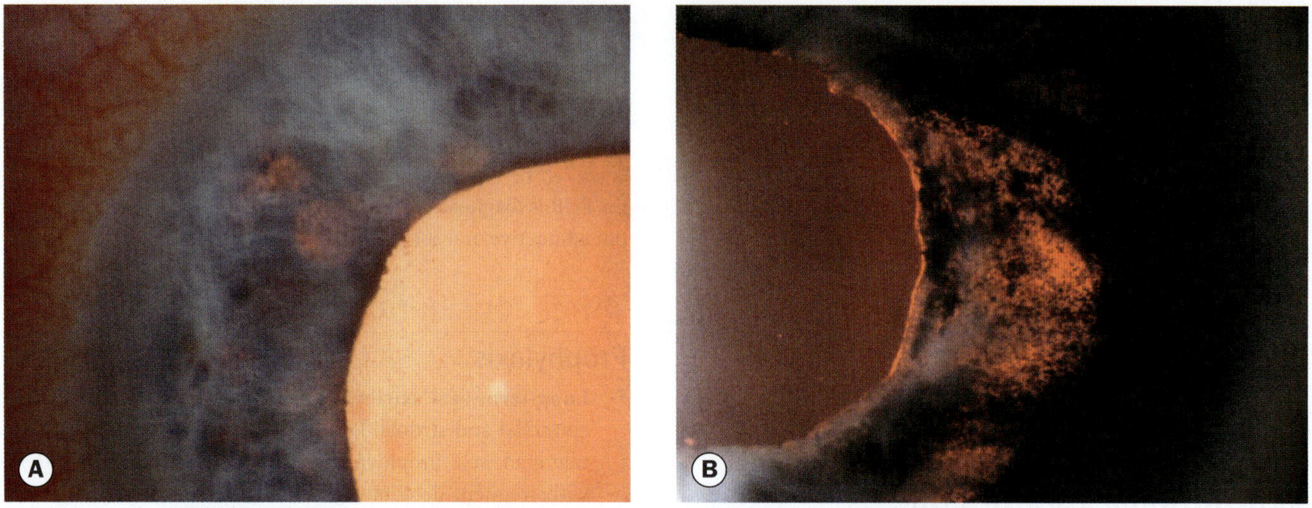

Fig. 7.15 Iris atrophy in herpetic iridocyclitis. (A) Characteristic patchy appearance; (B) trans-illumination. *(Courtesy of S Tuft – fig. A.)*

TIP Long-term use of oral aciclovir reduces the recurrence rate of epithelial and stromal herpes keratitis.

Complications

- **Secondary infection.** Herpetic eye disease is a major predisposing factor for microbial keratitis.
- **Glaucoma** secondary to inflammation or chronic steroid use may progress undetected, particularly if there is a poor view of the optic disc. Corneal thinning and distortion may give rise to an inaccurate reading on applanation and alternative forms of tonometry may be superior in these cases.
- **Stromal vascularization and lipid keratopathy.** Topical aganirsen results in a significant reduction in corneal vessels and an improvement in the quality of life, but no significant improvement in visual acuity is likely to follow.
- **Cataract** secondary to inflammation or prolonged steroid use.
- **Iris atrophy** secondary to kerato-uveitis (see Fig. 7.15).

Keratoplasty

A trial of a rigid contact lens is often worthwhile prior to committing to surgery. Recurrence of herpetic eye disease and rejection are common and threaten the survival of corneal grafts.

- **Topical** antivirals given during a rejection episode may reduce epithelial viral reactivation but toxicity may delay re-epithelialization.
- **Prophylactic oral aciclovir** (400 mg twice daily) improves graft survival and should be given to patients undergoing penetrating keratoplasty for herpetic eye disease. It should also be considered in patients with severe atopic eye disease but no history of ocular HSV involvement. The duration of treatment and the optimum dose has not been established. Immunohistochemistry should be performed on the excised tissue to confirm the presence of herpes antigen.

HERPES ZOSTER OPHTHALMICUS

Introduction

Herpes zoster is common, and it has been estimated that one in three people will develop the condition in their lifetime. Most patients are not immunocompromised.

Pathogenesis

Herpes zoster ophthalmicus (HZO) is the term used for shingles involving the dermatome supplied by the ophthalmic division of the fifth cranial (trigeminal) nerve. Ocular involvement can also occur (though is rarely clinically significant) when the disease affects the maxillary division alone. Varicella-zoster virus (VZV) causes both chickenpox (varicella) and shingles (herpes zoster). VZV belongs to the same subfamily of the herpes virus group as HSV – the viruses are morphologically identical, but antigenically distinct. After an episode of chickenpox, the virus travels in a retrograde manner to the dorsal root and cranial nerve sensory ganglia, where it may remain dormant for decades, with reactivation thought to occur after VZV-specific cell-mediated immunity has faded. Re-exposure to VZV via contact with chickenpox, or by vaccination, may reinforce immunity and protect against the development of shingles.

Mechanisms of ocular involvement

- **Direct viral invasion** may lead to conjunctivitis and epithelial keratitis.
- **Secondary inflammation** and occlusive vasculitis may cause episcleritis, scleritis, keratitis, uveitis (including segmental iris infarction), optic neuritis and cranial nerve palsies. Inflammation and destruction of the peripheral nerves or central ganglia, or altered signal processing in the central nervous system (CNS) may be responsible for post-herpetic neuralgia. Cicatrizing complications may arise following severe eyelid, periocular skin and conjunctival involvement.

- **Reactivation** causes necrosis and inflammation in the affected sensory ganglia, causing corneal anaesthesia that may result in neurotrophic keratopathy.

Risk of ocular involvement

- **Hutchinson sign** describes vesicles in the skin supplied by the external nasal nerve, a branch of the nasociliary nerve supplying the tip, side and root of the nose and ophthalmic herpes zoster (Fig. 7.16A). Contrary to previous teaching, Hutchinson's sign may not be predictive of ocular involvement, as both false-positive and false-negative findings are common. However, a rash in the distribution of the supratrochlear nerve (lower part of the forehead) is predictive. There is no apparent correlation between the severity of the rash and that of ocular complications.
- **Age.** HZO occurs most frequently in the sixth and seventh decades. In the elderly, signs and symptoms tend to be more severe than in the young and of longer duration.
- **AIDS** patients tend to have severe disease, and shingles can be an early indicator of human immunodeficiency virus (HIV) infection. A lower threshold for HIV testing should be adopted in populations at particular risk. The development of shingles in children or young adults classically has prompted a search for immunodeficiency or malignancy, though the requirement for this has been questioned as an abnormality will be found in only a small minority.

TIP All patients with herpes zoster involving the frontal nerve (V_1) should be fully evaluated for ocular involvement.

Acute shingles

General features

- **A prodromal phase** precedes the appearance of the rash. It lasts 3–5 days and is characterized by tiredness, fever, malaise and headache. Symptoms involving the affected dermatome vary from a superficial itching, tingling or burning sensation to a severe boring or lancing pain that is either constant or intermittent. Older patients with early severe pain and a larger area of involvement are at particular risk of post-herpetic neuralgia.
- **Skin lesions**
  - Painful erythematous areas with a maculopapular rash develop (Fig. 7.16B) and may be confused with cellulitis or contact dermatitis.
  - The rash respects the midline, which may aid in distinguishing shingles from HSV skin infection. Pain is also markedly worse in shingles. Bilateral disease is very rare.
  - Within 24 hours, groups of vesicles (Fig. 7.16C) appear and these become confluent over 2–4 days.
  - Although the rash itself does not affect the lower eyelid in HZO, boggy oedema of the upper and lower lids is common (see Fig. 7.16B) and often spreads to the contralateral side of the face (particularly if the patient sleeps on the side opposite to the infection).
  - The vesicles often pass through a pustular phase before they crust (Fig. 7.16D) and dry after 2–3 weeks.
  - Large, deep haemorrhagic lesions are more common in immunodeficient patients (Fig. 7.16E).
  - The lesions heal to leave residual skin destruction and depigmented scars (Fig. 7.16F).
  - Zoster sine herpete is shingles without a rash and may be more common than previously realized.
- **Disseminated zoster** involving multiple dermatomes and organ systems may develop in immunodeficiency or malignancy and with the advent of PCR testing, complications such as meningoencephalitis have increasingly been identified in immunocompetent individuals.
- **Investigation.** In the event that clinical diagnosis is uncertain, typically in immunodeficiency, vesicular fluid can be sent for PCR, or immunomicroscopy. A viraemia lasting a few days occurs in acute shingles. PCR of plasma for VZV DNA may be positive (40%), especially in immunosuppressed patients and can be particularly useful if zoster sine herpete is suspected. IgM antibodies to VZV are found in only a minority of early stage and convalescent patients.

Treatment

- **Oral antiviral treatment**, optimally given within 72 hours of rash onset, reduces the severity and duration of the acute episode and the risk of post-herpetic neuralgia. The incidence of late ophthalmic complications is also reduced by about 50%. Patients presenting later than 72 hours but still at the vesicular stage also derive benefit from treatment. Aciclovir (800 mg five times daily for 7–10 days) has been the mainstay of treatment, but newer agents such as valaciclovir 1 g three times daily or famciclovir 250–500 mg three times daily have more convenient regimens, are better tolerated and are at least as effective as aciclovir. Brivudine is available in some countries. Fatal interactions with 5-fluoropyrimidines have been reported and it should not be used in combination with even regional 5-fluorouracil.
- **Intravenous aciclovir** 5–10 mg/kg three times daily is generally indicated only for severe disease, particularly encephalitis and for moderate–severe immunocompromise.
- **Systemic steroids** (e.g. prednisolone 60 mg daily for 4 days, then 40 mg for 4 days, then 20 mg for 4 days) remain somewhat controversial but are commonly used in moderate–severe disease, particularly for neurological complications. They should be given only in conjunction with a systemic antiviral and should probably be avoided in immunodeficiency. A moderate reduction in acute pain and accelerated skin healing is conferred, but steroids have no effect on the incidence or severity of post-herpetic neuralgia.
- **Immunocompromised patients** require the input of an infectious disease specialist. Antiviral treatment should be extended and intravenous treatment may be optimal. Systemic steroids should probably be avoided.
- **Symptomatic** treatment of skin lesions is by drying, antisepsis and cold compresses. The benefit of topical antibiotic-steroid combinations is uncertain.

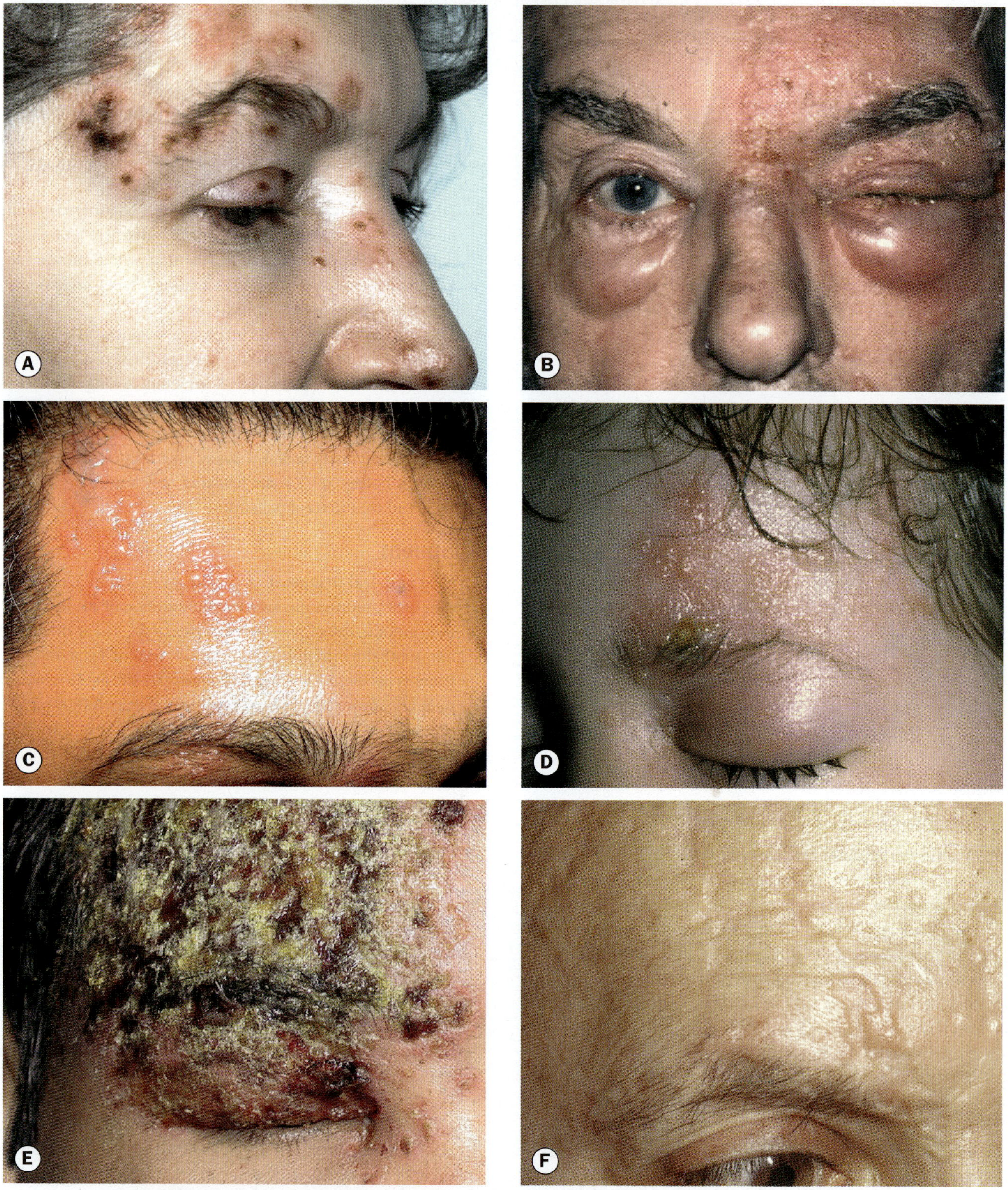

Fig. 7.16 Herpes zoster ophthalmicus. **(A)** Hutchinson sign – vesicles involving the side of the nose; **(B)** erythema and oedema (the swelling on the right is not a sign of infection on that side); **(C)** vesicular stage; **(D)** oedema with mixed vesicular and pustular rash beginning to show crusting in a child; **(E)** severe rash in a patient with AIDS; **(F)** typical healed appearance with mild–moderate scarring and depigmentation. *(Courtesy of R Bates – fig. D; S Chen – fig. E.)*

- **Patients with shingles can transmit chickenpox** so that contact with people not known to be immune (particularly pregnant women) and immunodeficient individuals should be avoided at least until crusting is complete.
- **VZV uveitis** is considered in depth in Chapter 12.

Prevention

Vaccination against herpes zoster reduces the incidence of HZO. Two vaccines are available and both are approved for individuals over the age of 50 years.

- **Zoster vaccine live** is an attenuated live virus with an important limitation that efficacy is lost within 10 years.
- **Recombinant zoster vaccine** requires two injections and has a 10% incidence of local or acute systemic reaction.

Eye disease

Acute eye disease

- **Acute epithelial keratitis** develops in over 50% of patients within 2 days of the onset of the rash and usually resolves spontaneously within a few days. It is characterized by dendritic lesions that are smaller and finer than herpes simplex dendrites and have tapered ends without terminal bulbs (Fig. 7.17A). The lesions stain better with rose Bengal than with fluorescein (Fig. 7.17B). Treatment, if required, is with a topical antiviral.
- **Conjunctivitis** (follicular and/or papillary) is common and often occurs in conjunction with lid margin vesicles. Treatment is not required in the absence of corneal disease, though some practitioners give topical antibiotic and/or antiviral prophylaxis.
- **Episcleritis** occurs at the onset of the rash and usually resolves spontaneously. A mild non-steroidal anti-inflammatory may be used if necessary.
- **Scleritis** and sclerokeratitis are uncommon but may develop at the end of the first week. Treatment of indolent lesions is with oral flurbiprofen 100 mg three times daily. Oral steroids with antiviral cover may be required for severe involvement.
- **Nummular keratitis** usually develops at the site of epithelial lesions about 10 days after the onset of the rash. It is

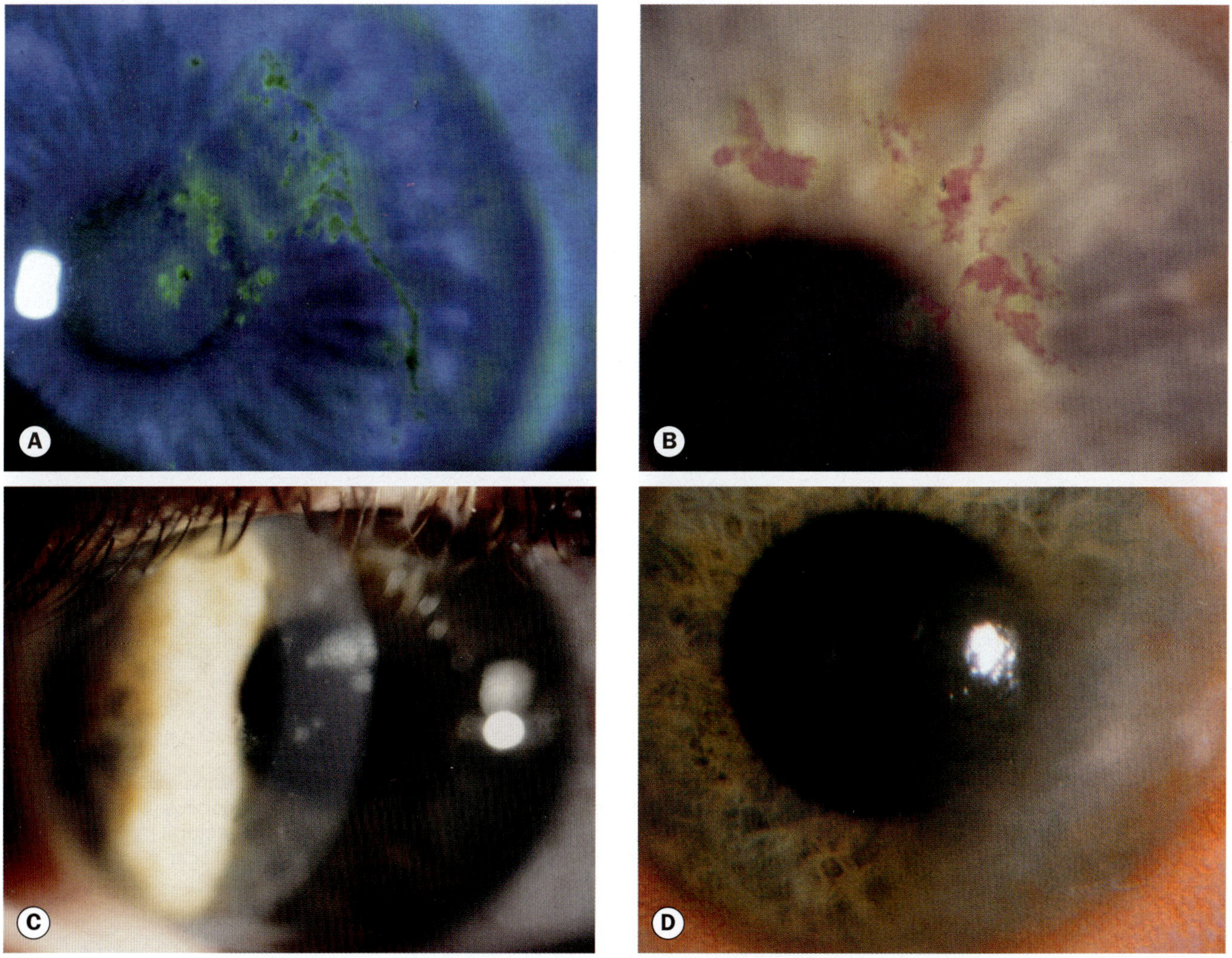

Fig. 7.17 Acute lesions in herpes zoster ophthalmicus. **(A)** Dendritic epithelial lesions with tapered ends stained with fluorescein; **(B)** dendritic epithelial lesions stained with rose Bengal; **(C)** nummular keratitis; **(D)** stromal keratitis. *(Courtesy of C Barry – fig. D.)*

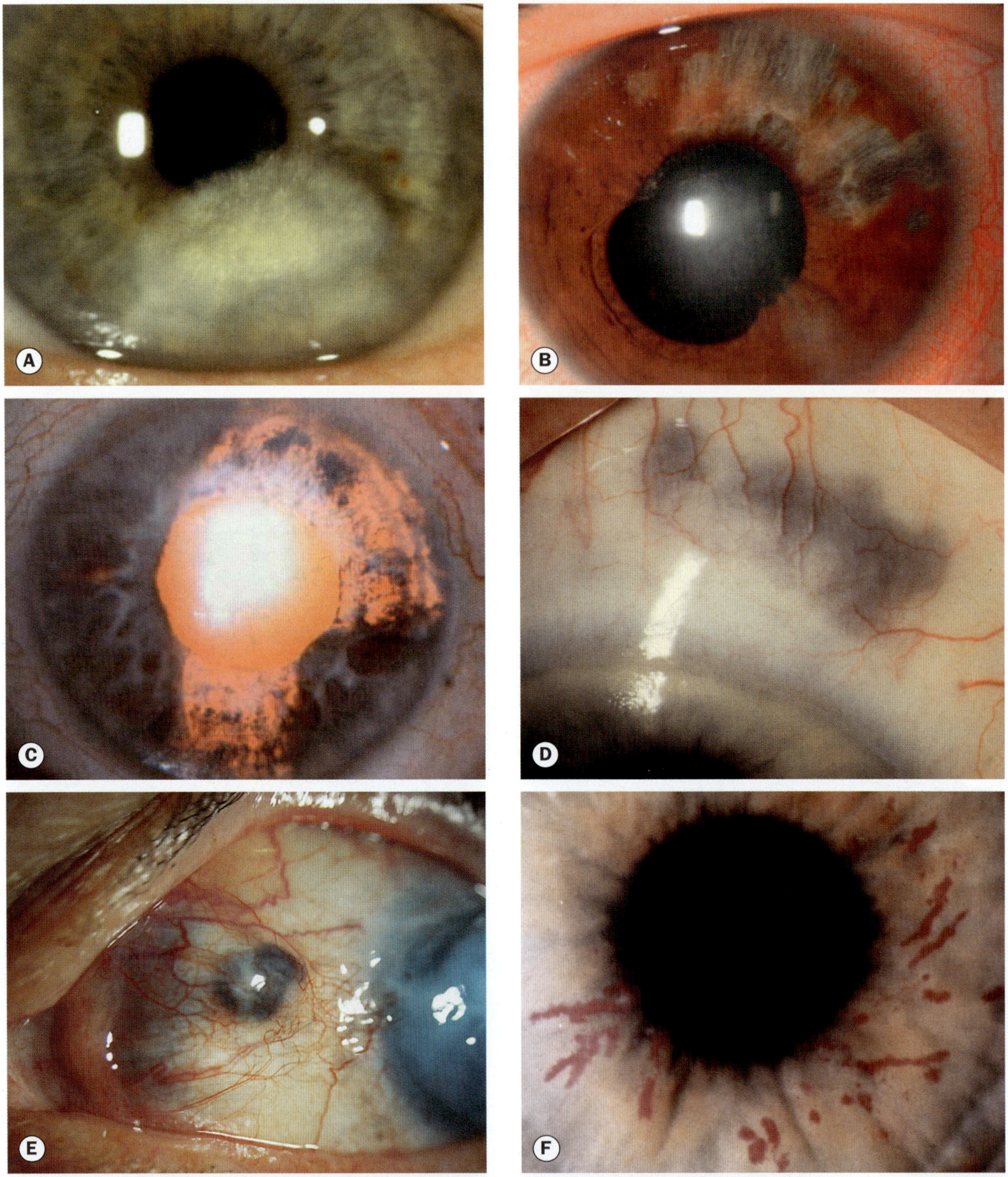

Fig. 7.18 Chronic lesions in herpes zoster ophthalmicus. **(A)** Scarring with lipid deposition following stromal keratitis; **(B)** iris atrophy in a typical sectoral pattern; **(C)** more severe sectoral iris atrophy on transillumination; **(D)** scleral atrophy; **(E)** staphyloma with severe corneal scarring; **(F)** mucous plaque keratitis

characterized by fine granular subepithelial deposits surrounded by a halo of stromal haze (Fig. 7.17C). The lesions fade in response to topical steroids but recur if treatment is discontinued prematurely.
- **Stromal (interstitial) keratitis** (Fig. 7.17D) develops in about 5% 3 weeks after the onset of the rash and significant scarring can occur (Fig. 7.18A). It usually responds to topical steroids but can become chronic and require slow tapering.
- **Disciform keratitis** (immune-mediated endotheliitis) is less common than with herpes simplex infection but may lead to corneal decompensation. Treatment is with topical steroids.
- **Anterior uveitis** affects at least a third of patients and can be associated with sectoral iris ischaemia and atrophy (Fig. 7.18B and C).
- **Posterior uveitis** (see Ch. 12). Progressive retinal necrosis is an aggressive retinitis usually occurring in immunodeficient individuals. Acute retinal necrosis can also be caused by VZV. Posterior segment examination should always be performed in patients with HZO as retinal vasculitis may occasionally occur.
- **IOP** should be monitored as elevation is common, including steroid-induced. Prostaglandin derivatives should be avoided if treatment is necessary.
- **Neurological complications** may require intravenous antivirals and systemic steroids.
  - Cranial nerve palsy affecting the third (most common), fourth and sixth nerves usually recovers within 6 months.
  - Optic neuritis is rare.
  - CNS manifestations are rare but include encephalitis, cranial arteritis and Guillain–Barré syndrome.

Chronic eye disease

- **Neurotrophic keratopathy** similar to that seen in HSV infection develops in up to 50%, but is usually relatively mild and settles over several months. Prolonged severe disease occurs in a minority (see also separate topic).
- **Scleritis** may become chronic and lead to patchy scleral atrophy (Fig. 7.18D). Staphyloma formation is rare (Fig. 7.18E).
- **Mucous plaque keratitis** develops in about 5%, most commonly between the third and sixth months. It is characterized by elevated mucous plaques staining with rose Bengal (Fig. 7.18F). Treatment involves a combination of topical steroid and acetylcysteine. Untreated, plaques resolve after a few months, leaving a faint diffuse corneal haze.
- **Lipid degeneration** may develop in eyes with persistent severe nummular or disciform keratitis (see Fig. 7.18A).
- **Lipid-filled granulomas** similar to those resulting from chronic irritation may develop in the tarsal conjunctiva and may progress to erosive calcified concretions.
- **Subconjunctival scarring** may occur.
- **Eyelid scarring** may result in ptosis, cicatricial entropion and occasionally ectropion, trichiasis, lid notching and madarosis.

Relapsing eye disease

In the relapsing phase lesions may reappear years after an acute episode, which may have been forgotten and eyelid scarring may be the only diagnostic clue. Reactivation of keratitis, episcleritis, scleritis or iritis can occur.

Post-herpetic neuralgia

Post-herpetic neuralgia is defined as pain that persists for more than one month after the rash has healed. It develops in up to 75% of patients over 70 years of age. Pain may be constant or intermittent, worse at night and aggravated by minor stimuli (allodynia), touch and heat. It generally improves slowly over time, with only 2% of patients affected after 5 years. Neuralgia can impair the quality of life and may lead to depression of sufficient severity to present a danger of suicide. Patients severely affected should be referred to a specialist pain clinic. Treatment may involve the following:
- **Local**
  - Cold compresses.
  - Topical capsaicin 0.075% or lidocaine 5% patches.
- **Systemic** treatment may be used in a staged fashion:
  - Simple analgesics such as paracetamol.
  - Stronger analgesics such as codeine.
  - Tricyclic antidepressants, e.g. nortriptyline, amitriptyline, initially 25 mg nightly adjusted up to 75 mg for several weeks if necessary.
  - Carbamazepine 400 mg daily for lancinating pain.
  - Gabapentin (300–600 mg up to three times daily), sustained-release oxycodone (10–30 mg twice daily), or both.

INTERSTITIAL KERATITIS

Introduction

Interstitial keratitis (IK) is an inflammation of the corneal stroma without primary involvement of the epithelium or endothelium. In most cases, the inflammation is thought to be an immune-mediated process triggered by an appropriate antigen. The term is most commonly used to refer to the late appearance of feathery mid-stromal scarring with ghost vessels rather than the acute presentation. The former is typically an incidental finding. Syphilitic IK is the archetype, but the relative frequency of causes varies markedly by geographic region. There is a wide range of causes, including herpes simplex, varicella zoster and other viral infections, tuberculosis, Lyme disease and other infections (parasitic diseases are an important cause in areas where these are endemic), sarcoidosis, Cogan syndrome and non-infectious inflammatory conditions.

Syphilitic IK

IK of syphilitic origin is usually the result of congenital infection, though acquired syphilis can also be responsible. All patients with acute IK, or with the incidental discovery of its chronic appearance, should be investigated to exclude congenital (and acquired) syphilis, irrespective of the presence of systemic clinical signs. There are numerous reported cases of congenital syphilis being identified for the first time in later life on this basis.

Congenital syphilis

Infection of the fetus can occur across the placenta, leading to stillbirth, subclinical infection, or a range of clinical features.

- **Early systemic features** include failure to thrive, a maculopapular rash, mucosal ulcers, characteristic fissures around the lips (rhagades) and a range of organ involvement.
- **Late systemic signs** include sensorineural deafness, saddle-shaped nasal deformity (Fig. 7.19A), sabre tibiae (Fig. 7.19B), bulldog jaw (mandibular prominence due to maxillary underdevelopment), Hutchinson teeth (notched, small, widely spaced teeth – Fig. 7.19C) and Clutton joints (painless effusions in large joints, especially the knees).
- **Ocular features** include anterior uveitis, IK (see below), dislocated/subluxated lens, cataract, optic atrophy, salt and pepper pigmentary retinopathy (Fig. 7.20) and Argyll Robertson pupils.

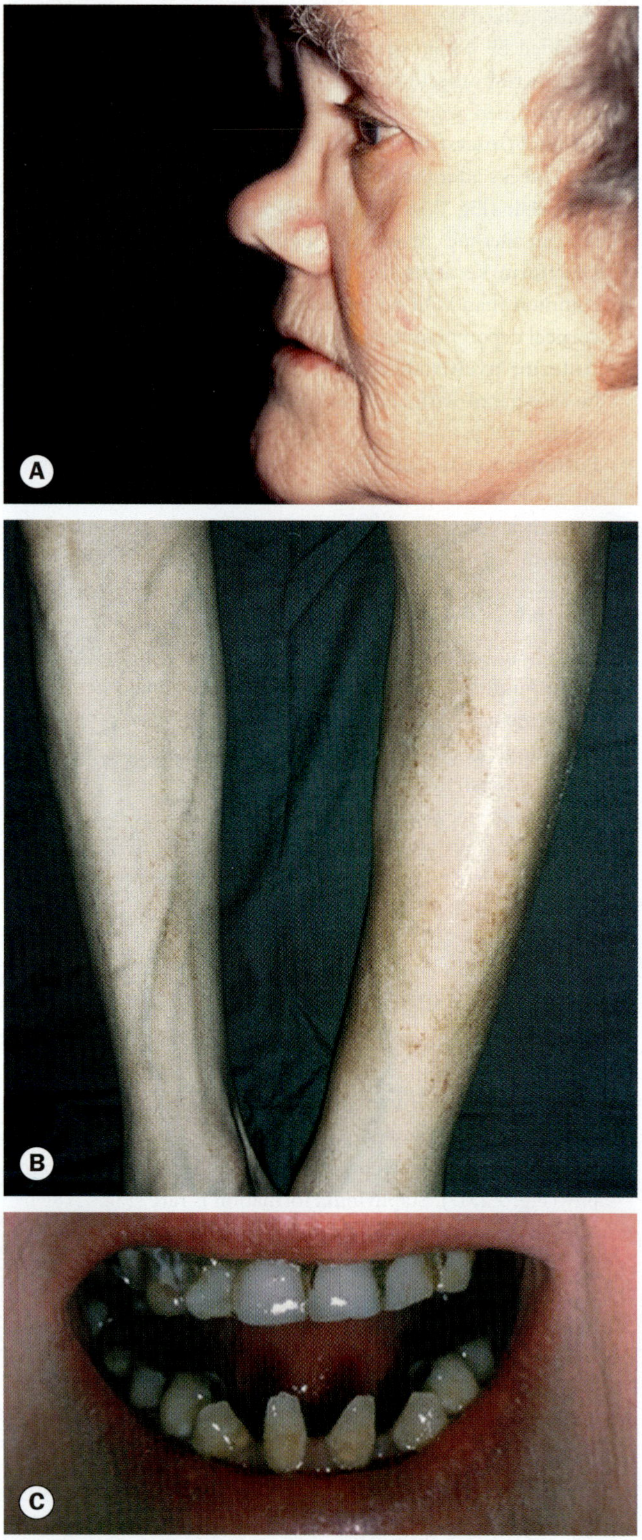

Fig. 7.19 Systemic signs of congenital syphilis. **(A)** Saddle-shaped nasal deformity; **(B)** sabre tibiae; **(C)** Hutchinson teeth.

Presentation of syphilitic IK

- **Symptoms.** The presentation of IK following congenital syphilitic infection is usually between the ages of 5 and 25 years. The initial symptoms are those of acute anterior uveitis with severe blurring. Involvement is bilateral in 80%, although usually not simultaneous. In acquired disease IK is less common and usually unilateral, typically occurring years after the age at which the disease was contracted, although it can occur as part of the syndrome of primary infection.
- **Signs**
  - Profoundly decreased visual acuity is typical in the active stage.
  - Limbitis associated with deep stromal vascularization, with cellular infiltration and clouding that may obscure the still-perfused vessels to give the characteristic pinkish 'salmon patch' appearance (Fig. 7.21A).
  - Granulomatous anterior uveitis.
  - After several months the cornea begins to clear and the vessels become non-perfused ('ghost vessels' – Fig. 7.21B).
  - If the cornea later becomes inflamed, the vessels may refill with blood and may rarely bleed into the stroma (Fig. 7.21C).
  - The healed stage is characterized by ghost vessels, feathery deep stromal scarring (Fig. 7.21D) and sometimes thinning, astigmatism and band keratopathy.
- **Treatment** of active syphilitic IK is with topical steroids and cycloplegics, as well as immediate systemic therapy under the care of a genitourinary or infectious diseases specialist.

Cogan syndrome

Introduction

Cogan syndrome is a rare systemic autoimmune vasculitis characterized by intraocular inflammation and vestibuloauditory dysfunction (particularly neurosensory) developing within months of each other. The disease primarily occurs in young adults, with both sexes affected equally; children can also be affected. Systemic features occur in 30% and may include multisystem vasculitis that can be life-threatening; multispecialty management is vital.

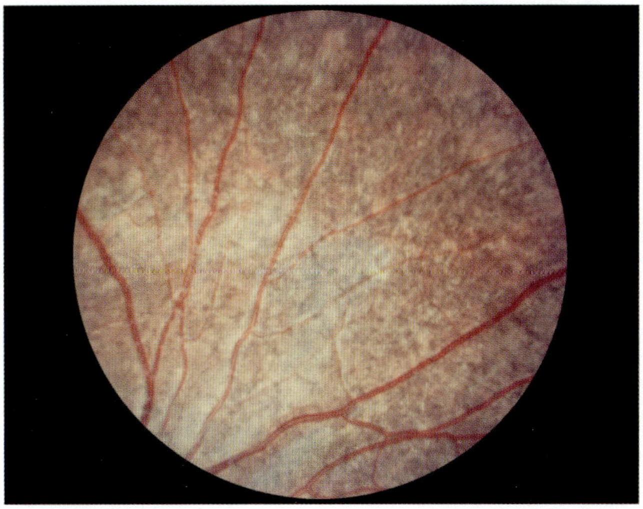

Fig. 7.20 Salt and pepper retinopathy following congenital syphilitic infection.

Diagnosis

Ocular and inner ear symptoms are often separated by a substantial period; the acute phase may last from months to years. Susac syndrome (retinocochleocerebral vasculopathy) should be considered in the differential diagnosis.

- **Vestibuloauditory symptoms.** Deafness, tinnitus and vertigo.
- **Ocular symptoms.** Redness, pain, photophobia and blurred vision.
- **Ocular signs.** Corneal involvement commences with faint bilateral peripheral anterior stromal opacities. Deeper opacities and corneal neovascularization (mid-stromal vascular loops) then ensue (Fig. 7.22A), often with central progression (Fig. 7.22B). Uveitis, scleritis and retinal vasculitis may develop.
- **Investigations**
  - Erythrocyte sedimentation rate (ESR) and C-reactive protein (CRP) may be elevated and the white cell count raised.
  - Antibodies to inner ear antigens may be detectable.
  - MRI may show inner ear and other abnormalities.

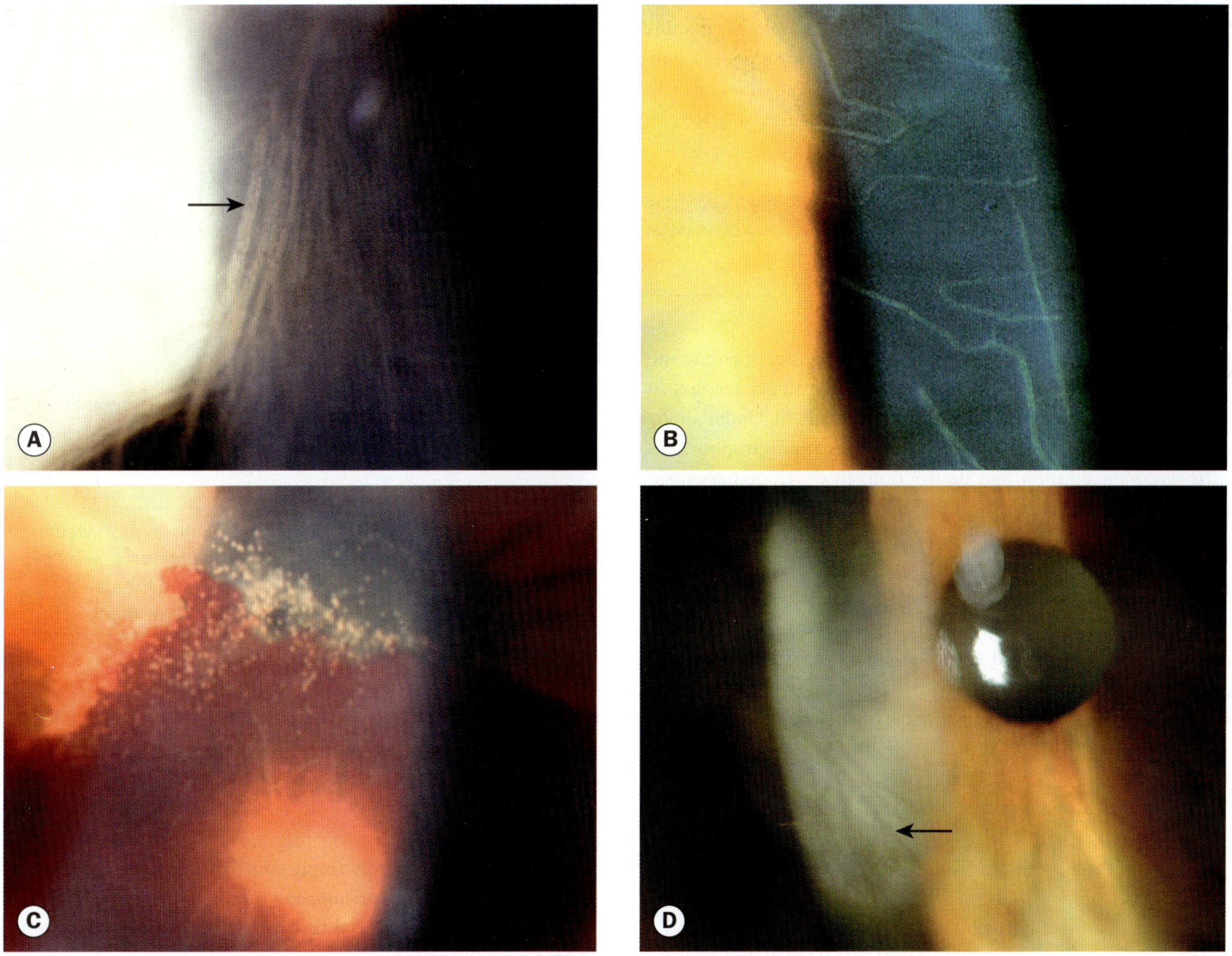

Fig. 7.21 Syphilitic interstitial keratitis. **(A)** Salmon patch showing deep stromal vascularization with clouding (arrow); **(B)** ghost vessels; **(C)** intrastromal corneal haemorrhage from re-perfused vessels; **(D)** typical feathery scarring, showing the tracks of ghost vessels (arrow).

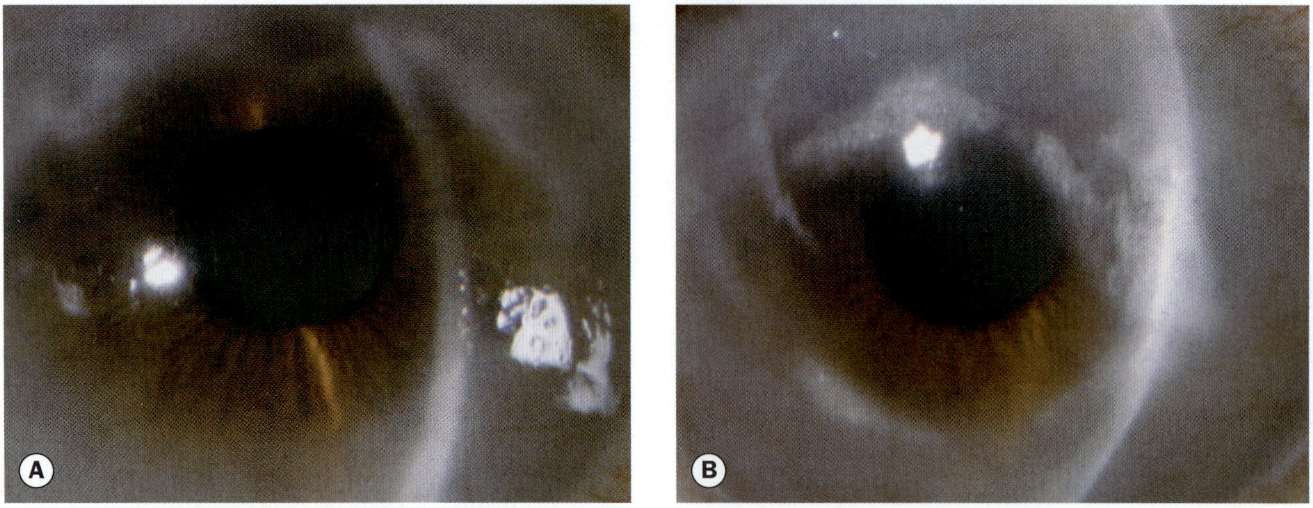

Fig. 7.22 Old interstitial keratitis in Cogan syndrome. **(A)** Peripheral; **(B)** more central scarring.

Treatment

- **Topical steroids** for keratitis, with additional measures as appropriate.
- **Systemic steroids.** Vestibuloauditory symptoms require immediate treatment with 1–2 g/kg prednisolone to prevent hearing loss. Immunosuppressive therapy may also be required. Systemic steroids may also be required for scleritis or retinal vasculitis.

PROTOZOAN KERATITIS

Acanthamoeba

Introduction

Acanthamoeba spp. are ubiquitous free-living protozoa commonly found in soil, fresh or brackish water and the upper respiratory tract. The cystic form (Fig. 7.23A) is highly resilient. Under appropriate environmental conditions, the cysts turn into trophozoites, with tissue penetration and destruction. In developed countries acanthamoeba keratitis is most frequently associated with contact lens wear, especially if tap water is used for rinsing.

Diagnosis

The condition is often diagnosed initially as herpes simplex keratitis. With more advanced signs the condition should be distinguished from fungal keratitis.

- **Symptoms.** Blurred vision and discomfort. Pain is often severe and characteristically disproportionate to the clinical signs.
- **Signs**
  - In early disease the epithelial surface is irregular and greyish (Fig. 7.23B).
  - Epithelial pseudodendrites resembling herpetic lesions may form.
  - Limbitis with diffuse or focal anterior stromal infiltrates.
  - Characteristic perineural infiltrates (radial keratoneuritis) are seen during the first few weeks and are virtually pathognomonic (Fig. 7.23C).
  - Gradual enlargement and coalescence of infiltrates to form a ring abscess (Fig. 7.23D and E) is typical.
  - Scleritis may develop and is generally reactive rather than an extension of infection.
  - Slowly progressive stromal opacification and vascularization.
  - Corneal melting may occur at any stage when there is stromal disease. The melt often develops at the periphery of the area of infiltrate (Fig. 7.23F).
- **Investigations**
  - Staining of corneal scrapings using periodic acid–Schiff or calcofluor white (a fluorescent dye with an affinity for amoebic cysts and fungi). Gram and Giemsa stains may also demonstrate cysts.
  - Culture. Non-nutrient agar seeded with dead *E. coli*, which trophozoites consume.
  - Other investigations include immunohistochemistry, PCR and *in vivo* confocal microscopy. Corneal biopsy may be necessary for diagnosis.

TIP In a patient with acanthamoeba keratitis a good visual outcome is achieved by making a speedy diagnosis, avoiding a misdiagnosis of herpes keratitis and avoiding the use of corticosteroids before commencing specific treatment.

Prevention

Teach contact lens wearers how to clean their contact lenses. Reduce their risk of contracting this disease by warning them that they should not use tap water to clean their lenses.

Treatment

- **Early treatment.** It is important to maintain a high index of suspicion for *Acanthamoeba* in any patient with a limited response to antibacterial therapy. The outcome is very much better if treatment is started early.
- **Debridement** of involved epithelium is believed to be helpful, as it may facilitate eye drop penetration.

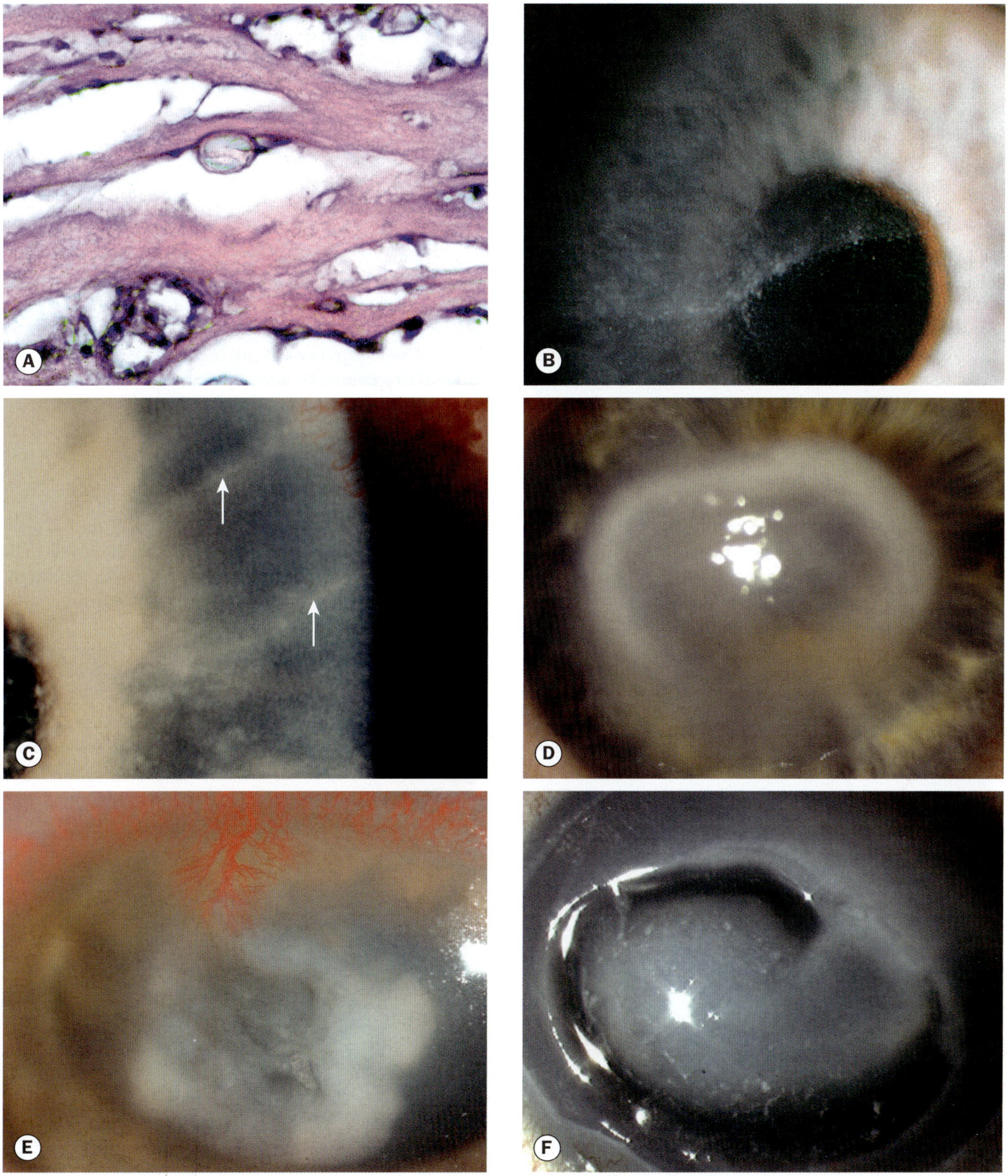

Fig. 7.23 Acanthamoeba keratitis. **(A)** Cysts in a corneal biopsy; **(B)** greyish early epithelial involvement; **(C)** radial perineuritis (arrows); **(D)** focal anterior stromal infiltrates; **(E)** progression of infiltration, with incipient formation of a ring abscess and early melting; **(F)** melting. *(Courtesy of S Tuft – fig. F.)*

- **Topical amoebicides.** *Acanthamoeba* cysts are resistant to most antimicrobial agents and although successful outcomes have been reported using a variety of topical preparations, it is likely that some of these are active only against the trophozoite stage.
    - Polyhexamethylene biguanide (PHMB) 0.02% and chlorhexidine (0.02%) kill trophozoites and are cysticidal.
    - Hexamidine or propamidine (Brolene); the former probably has greater activity.
    - Voriconazole and other azole antifungals are effective. Voriconazole is less toxic to the ocular surface than traditional therapy and has been used as a first-line treatment by some investigators.
    - An optimal regimen has not been established. Examples include PHMB as duotherapy with chlorhexidine, or either of these in combination with hexamidine or propamidine. Instillation is hourly at first and gradually reduced. A clear response may take 2 weeks.
    - Simultaneous antibacterial treatment for co-infection may be considered if the clinical picture suggests this.
    - Relapses are common as treatment is tapered and it may be necessary to continue treatment for many months.
    - Oral miltefosine can be considered in patients where there has been no resolution on topical treatment. Increased corneal inflammation, which often occurs on this treatment, responds to steroid eyedrops. It should not be used in pregnancy.
- **Topical steroids** should be avoided if possible although low-dose therapy delayed for at least 2 weeks after starting anti-amoebic treatment may be useful for persistent inflammation. Amoebicidal treatment should be continued in concert with and for several weeks after steroids.
- **Pain control** is with an oral non-steroidal anti-inflammatory agent.
- **Corneal cross-linking** treatment (PACK-CXL) can be considered in severe cases, but two sessions of treatment are often needed.
- **Therapeutic keratoplasty** may be necessary for resistant cases, including perforation. Late scarring may also require penetrating keratoplasty.

TIP Acanthamoeba infection of the cornea results in pain that is often severe and disproportionate to the clinical signs.

HELMINTHIC KERATITIS

Onchocerciasis

Onchocerciasis ('river blindness') is discussed in Chapter 12. Keratitis is a common feature.

BACTERIAL HYPERSENSITIVITY-MEDIATED CORNEAL DISEASE

Marginal keratitis

Introduction

Marginal keratitis is believed to be caused by a hypersensitivity reaction against staphylococcal exotoxins and cell wall proteins with deposition of antigen–antibody complexes in the peripheral cornea (antigen diffusing from the tear film, antibody from the blood vessels) with a secondary lymphocytic infiltration. The lesions are culture-negative but *S. aureus* can frequently be isolated from the lid margins.

Diagnosis

- **Symptoms.** Mild discomfort, redness and lacrimation. The inflammation may involve both eyes.
- **Signs**
    - Chronic blepharitis is typical.
    - Inferior punctate epitheliopathy is an early manifestation.
    - Subepithelial marginal infiltrates separated from the limbus by a clear zone, often associated with an adjacent area of conjunctival hyperaemia (Fig. 7.24A).
    - Characteristically, any epithelial defect will be considerably smaller than the area of infiltrate.
    - Coalescence and circumferential spread (Fig. 7.24B and C).
    - Usually little or no anterior chamber reaction, even with large infiltrates.
    - Without treatment, resolution generally occurs in 1–4 weeks, depending on severity. Occasionally there is residual superficial scarring and slight thinning with mild pannus (Fig. 7.24D). Iris new vessels may develop in the presence of persistent large lesions, but resolve when inflammation settles.

Treatment

A weak topical steroid such as fluorometholone or prednisolone 0.5% is instilled four times daily for 1–2 weeks, sometimes combined with a topical antibiotic. An oral tetracycline course (erythromycin in children, breastfeeding mothers and in pregnancy) may be required for recurrent disease. Blepharitis is treated as necessary.

Phlyctenulosis

Introduction

Phlyctenulosis is usually a self-limiting disease but may rarely be severe. Most cases in high-income countries are the result of a presumed delayed hypersensitivity reaction to staphylococcal antigen, sometimes associated with rosacea. In low-income countries, the majority are associated with tuberculosis or helminthic infestation, but causation may be uncertain and a range of other agents has been implicated.

Diagnosis

- **Symptoms.** Photophobia, lacrimation and blepharospasm, often in a child or young adult.
- **Signs**
    - A small white limbal (Fig. 7.25A) or conjunctival nodule (Fig. 7.25B) associated with intense local hyperaemia.
    - A limbal phlycten may extend onto the cornea (Fig. 7.25C and D).
    - Spontaneous resolution usually occurs within 2–3 weeks. A healed lesion often leaves a triangular limbal-based scar associated with superficial vascularization and thinning

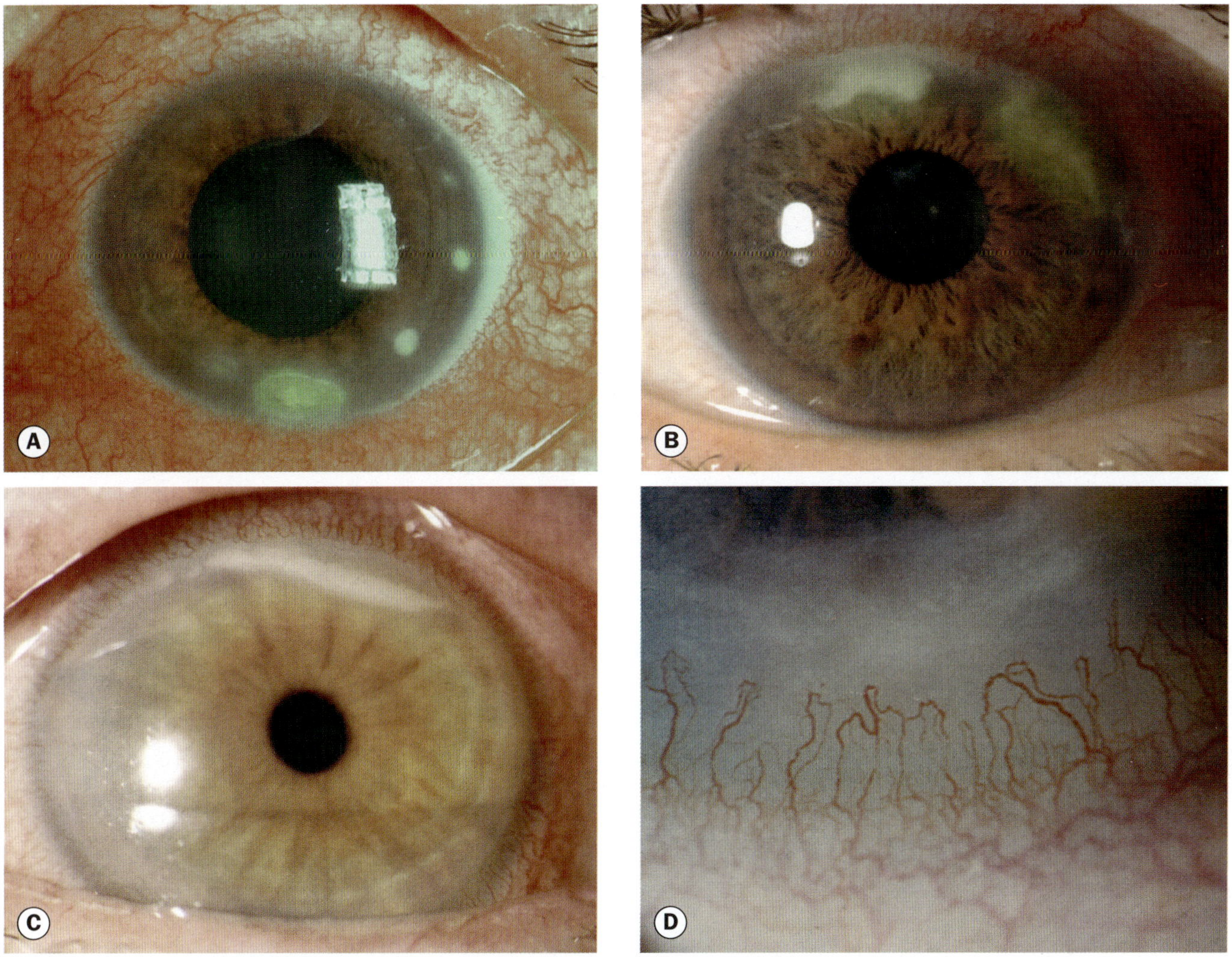

Fig. 7.24 Marginal keratitis. **(A)** Marginal infiltrates stained with fluorescein; **(B)** coalescing infiltrate; **(C)** circumferential coalescing infiltrate; **(D)** scarring with pannus.

but occasionally severe thinning and perforation can ensue.
    - Very large necrotizing or multiple (miliary) lesions may occur.
- **Investigation** for tuberculosis is generally indicated only in endemic areas or in the presence of specific risk factors.

Treatment

A short course of topical steroid accelerates healing and is often given with a topical antibiotic. Recurrent troublesome disease may require an oral tetracycline and it is important to treat associated blepharitis.

ROSACEA

Introduction

Rosacea (acne rosacea) is a common chronic idiopathic dermatosis involving the sun-exposed skin of the face and upper neck. Ocular complications develop in 6–18% of patients. Facial telangiectasia, papule and pustule formation, rhinophyma and facial flushing may occur (Fig. 7.26A). In contrast to acne vulgaris, comedones (blackheads or whiteheads) are absent.

The aetiology is probably multifactorial and may involve vascular factors, together with an abnormal response to commensal skin bacteria and *Demodex* follicular mites. Exacerbation by *H. pylori* infection has been suspected.

Ocular rosacea

- **Symptoms** include non-specific irritation and lacrimation.
- **Lid** signs include margin telangiectasia (Fig. 7.26B) and posterior blepharitis, often associated with recurrent meibomian cyst formation.
- **Conjunctival** hyperaemia, especially bulbar. Rarely, cicatricial conjunctivitis, conjunctival granulomas and phlyctenulosis may occur.
- **Cornea**
    - Inferior punctate epithelial erosions.
    - Peripheral vascularization in an inflamed eye (Fig. 7.26C).
    - Marginal keratitis.
    - Focal or diffuse corneal thinning in severe cases, usually in the inferior cornea.

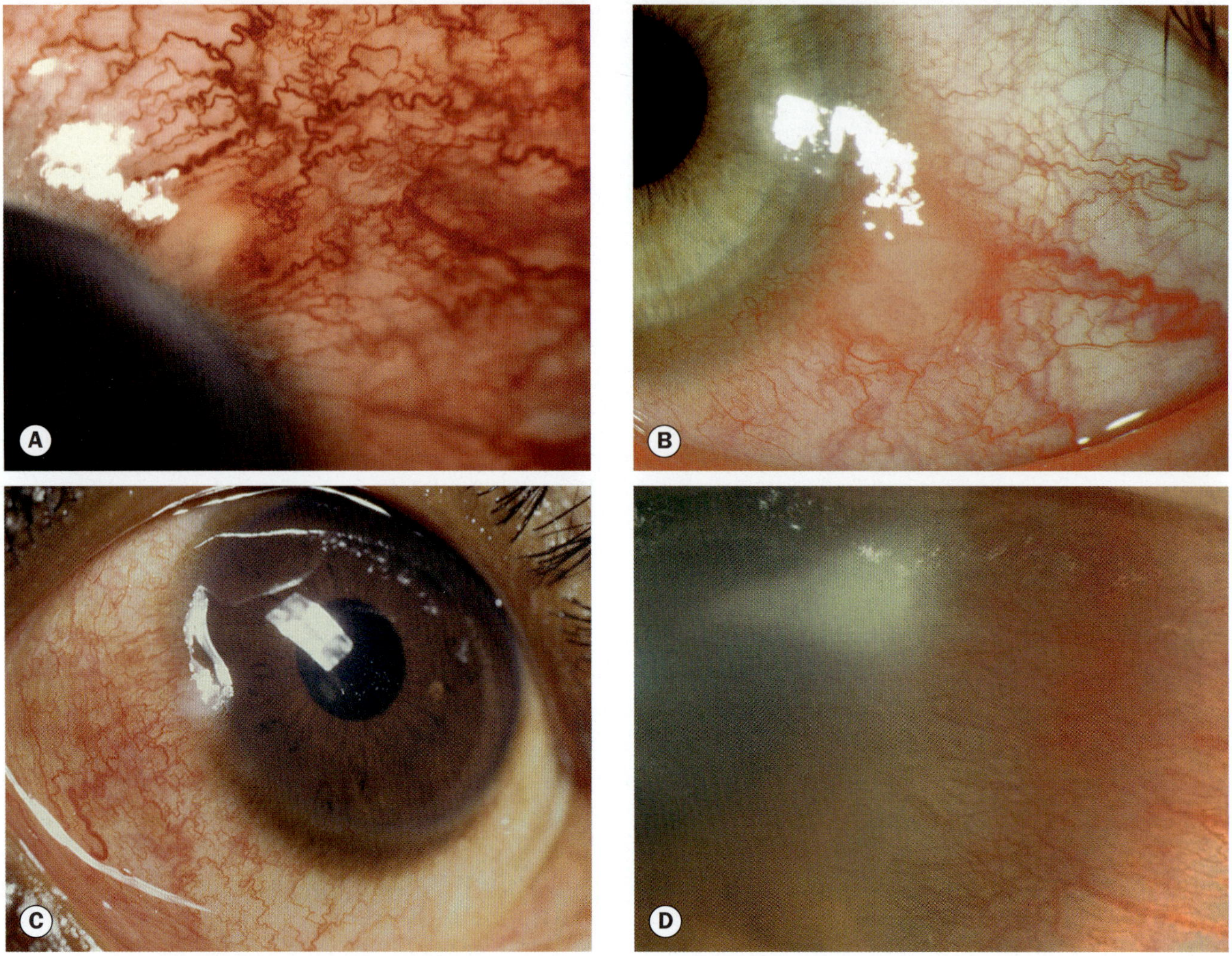

Fig. 7.25 Phlyctenulosis. **(A)** Limbal phlycten in an inflamed eye; **(B)** phlycten in a relatively quiet eye; **(C)** corneal phlycten; **(D)** corneal phlycten with intense vascularization. *(Courtesy of S Tuft – fig. D.)*

  - Perforation may occur as a result of severe peripheral or central melting and may be precipitated by secondary bacterial infection.
  - Corneal scarring and vascularization (Fig. 7.26D).
- **Topical treatment**
  - Lubricants (preferably unpreserved) for mild symptoms.
  - Hot compresses and lid hygiene.
  - Topical antibiotics (e.g. fusidic acid, erythromycin, azithromycin) to the lid margins at bedtime for 4 weeks.
  - Steroids are helpful for exacerbations. The lowest potency preparation compatible with improvement should be used in order to minimize the promotion of thinning.
- **Systemic therapy**
  - Tetracyclines may work by altering meibomian gland function to lower free fatty acid production in conjunction with a reduction in lid flora and probably by a direct anti-inflammatory effect. They also have an anticollagenase action and so may retard thinning. In relatively low dose but extended duration (e.g. doxycycline, which has a longer half-life than tetracycline, 100 mg once daily for 4 weeks then 50 mg daily if required) they may confer an improvement lasting several months but if necessary can be continued long term. Tetracyclines should not be used in children and pregnant or breastfeeding women, in whom erythromycin is an alternative. Efficacy has also been reported with other antibiotics.
  - Severe disease may require immunosuppression, e.g. azathioprine.
  - Retinoids can be helpful, but can worsen some features. They are absolutely contraindicated in pregnancy.

PERIPHERAL CORNEAL ULCERATION/ THINNING

Introduction

Peripheral corneal ulceration/thinning, known as 'peripheral ulcerative keratitis' (PUK) when inflammatory, refers to a presentation characterized by thinning and/or ulceration preferentially affecting the peripheral rather than central cornea and spreading

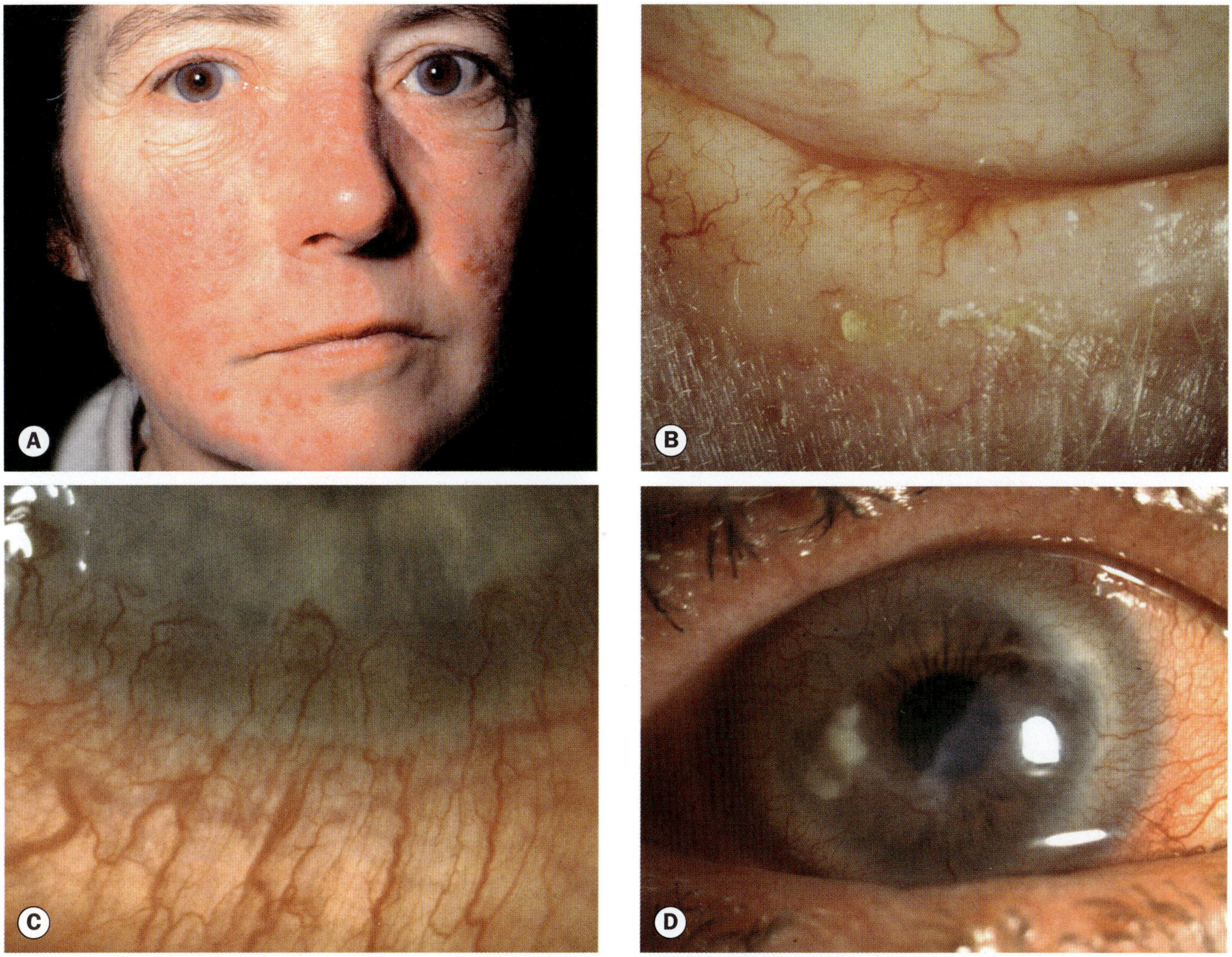

Fig. 7.26 Rosacea. **(A)** Papulopustular formation and facial flushing; **(B)** eyelid margin telangiectasia; **(C)** peripheral corneal vascularization; **(D)** severe scarring and vascularization.

around the margin. It should be noted that any cause of corneal ulceration can affect the periphery.

- **Marginal keratitis.** This is discussed above.
- **Mooren ulcer.**
- **Terrien marginal degeneration.**
- **Dellen.** Localized corneal disturbance associated with drying of a focal area, usually associated with an adjacent elevated lesion (e.g. pinguecula or a large subconjunctival haemorrhage – Fig. 7.27A) that impairs physiological lubrication. Generally mild though can occasionally be severe, including descemetocoele formation/corneal perforation.
- Associated with **systemic autoimmune disease.**
- **Others.** Ocular rosacea, furrow degeneration (mild peripheral thinning in the elderly, usually benign – Fig. 7.27B), pellucid marginal degeneration.

Mooren ulcer

Introduction

Mooren ulcer is a rare autoimmune disease characterized by progressive circumferential peripheral stromal ulceration with later central spread. It may represent a host reaction to calgranulin C, a normal hidden antigen in corneal keratocytes. There are two forms: the first affects mainly older patients, often in only one eye and usually responds well to medical therapy. The second is more aggressive and likely to need systemic immunosuppression, carries a poorer prognosis, may be bilateral and associated with severe pain and tends to occur in younger patients, including widespread reports in South Asian men. In at least some (usually milder) cases, there is a precipitating corneal insult such as surgery or infection. Associated systemic autoimmune disease and corneal infection should always be ruled out.

Diagnosis

- **Symptoms.** Pain is prominent and may be severe. There is photophobia and blurred vision.
- **Signs**
  - Peripheral ulceration involving the superficial one-third of the stroma, with variable epithelial loss. Several distinct foci may be present and subsequently coalesce.
  - An undermined and infiltrated leading edge is characteristic (Fig. 7.28A).

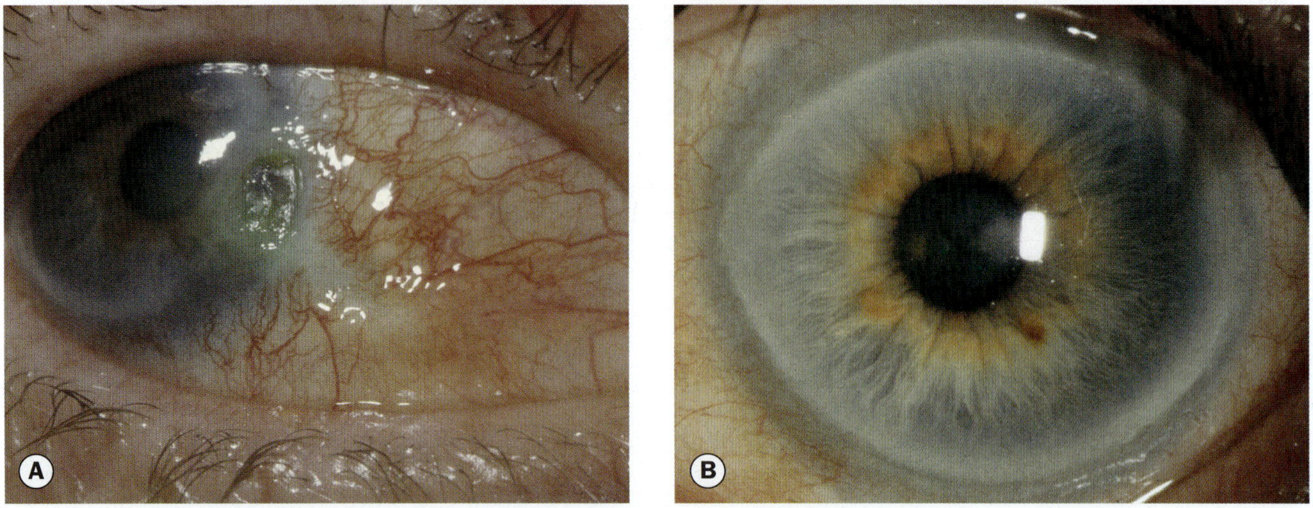

Fig. 7.27 Non-inflammatory peripheral corneal thinning. **(A)** Dellen secondary to pterygium surgery; **(B)** extensive furrow degeneration. *(Courtesy of S Tuft – fig. A.)*

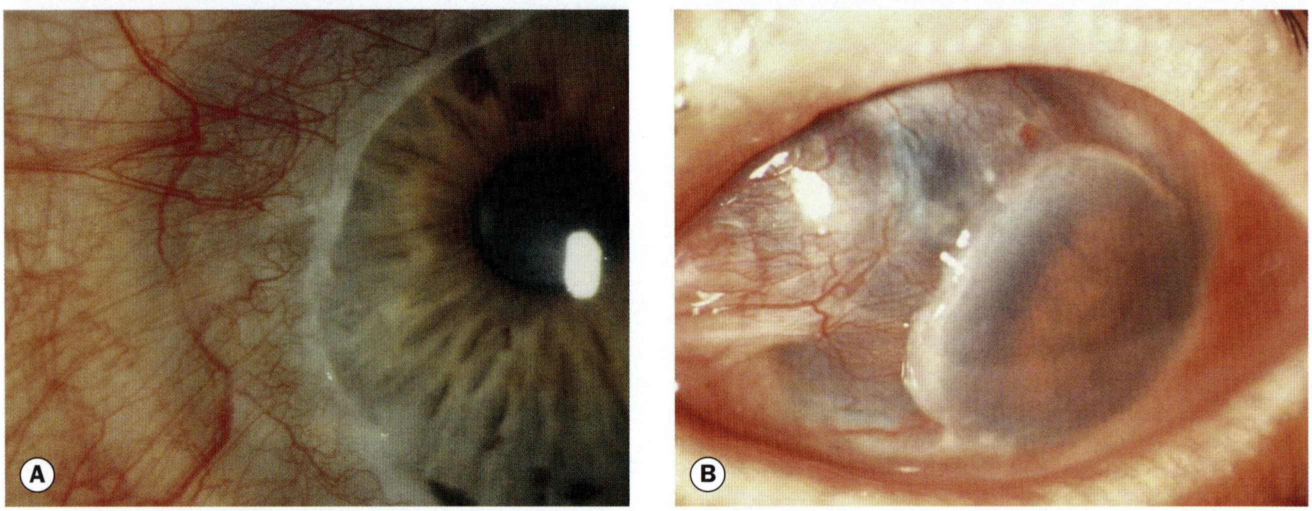

Fig. 7.28 Mooren ulcer. **(A)** Local peripheral ulceration; **(B)** undermined and infiltrated central edge in advanced disease.

    - Limbitis may be present, but not scleritis, which aids in distinguishing from systemic disease-associated PUK.
    - Progressive circumferential and central stromal thinning (Fig. 7.28B).
    - Vascularization involving the bed of the ulcer up to its leading edge but not beyond.
    - The healing stage is characterized by thinning, vascularization and scarring.
    - Iritis is not uncommon.
- **Complications** include severe astigmatism, perforation following minor trauma (spontaneous perforation is rare), secondary bacterial infection, cataract and glaucoma.

TIP Peripheral ulcerative keratitis is caused by an infection until proven otherwise. In the absence of an infection investigate for systemic autoimmune disease.

Treatment

- **Topical steroids** as frequently as hourly are combined with a low-frequency prophylactic topical antibiotic. If an effective response is seen, treatment is tapered over several months.
- **Topical ciclosporin** (up to 2%) may be effective, but can take weeks to exert a significant effect.
- **Tacrolimus 0.1% ointment** is effective in controlling refractory cases.
- **Adjunctive** topical therapy includes artificial tears and collagenase inhibitors such as acetylcysteine 10–20%.
- **Conjunctival resection**, which may be combined with excision of necrotic tissue, is performed if there is no response to topical steroids. The excised area should extend 4 mm back from the limbus and 2 mm beyond the circumferential margins. Keratoepithelioplasty (suturing of a donor corneal lenticule onto the scleral bed) may be combined to produce a

physical barrier against conjunctival regrowth and further melting. Steroids are continued postoperatively.

- **Systemic immunosuppression** may be needed, including steroids for rapid effect, and should be instituted earlier for bilateral disease, or if involvement is advanced at first examination. Biological blockers show some promise, e.g. rituximab
- **Systemic collagenase inhibitors** such as doxycycline may be beneficial.
- **Lamellar keratectomy** involving dissection of the residual central island in advanced disease may remove the stimulus for further inflammation.
- **Perforations.** Management is as discussed earlier in this chapter.
- **Visual rehabilitation.** Keratoplasty (with immunosuppressive cover) may be considered once inflammation has settled.

Peripheral ulcerative keratitis associated with systemic autoimmune disease

Introduction

PUK may precede or follow the onset of systemic features. Severe peripheral corneal infiltration (Fig.7.29A), ulceration (Fig. 7.29B) or thinning unexplained by evident ocular disease should prompt investigation for a (potentially life-threatening) systemic collagen vascular disorder. The mechanism includes immune complex deposition in peripheral cornea, episcleral and conjunctival capillary occlusion with secondary cytokine release and inflammatory cell recruitment, the upregulation of collagenases and reduced activity of their inhibitors. Systemic associations include:

- **Rheumatoid arthritis** (RA – the most common). PUK is bilateral in 30% and tends to occur in advanced RA (Fig.7.29B–D).
- **Granulomatosis with polyangiitis** (Wegener granulomatosis) is the second most common systemic association of PUK (Fig. 7.29 E and F). In contrast to RA, ocular complications are the initial presentation in 50%.
- **Other conditions** include polyarteritis nodosa, relapsing polychondritis, systemic lupus erythematosus and Crohn disease (see Fig. 7.29A).

TIP Peripheral ulcerative keratitis in the absence of other ocular disease should prompt investigation for a systemic autoimmune disease.

Clinical features

- **Crescentic ulceration** with an epithelial defect, thinning and stromal infiltration at the limbus. Spread is circumferential and occasionally central. In contrast to Mooren ulcer, extension into the sclera may occur.
- **Limbitis, episcleritis or scleritis** are usually present. As with a Mooren ulcer, there is no separation between the ulcerative process and the limbus.
- **Advanced disease** may result in a 'contact lens' cornea (see Fig. 7.29C) or perforation.
- **Rheumatoid paracentral ulcerative keratitis (PCUK)** is thought to be a distinct entity, with a punched-out more centrally located lesion with little infiltrate in a quiet eye (see Fig. 7.29D). Perforation can occur rapidly and there is usually a good response to topical ciclosporin, with bandage contact lens and tissue glue application, if necessary, rather than systemic treatment.

Treatment

Treatment is principally with systemic immunosuppression in collaboration with a rheumatologist.

- **Systemic steroids**, sometimes via pulsed intravenous administration, are used to control acute disease, with immunosuppressive therapy and biological blockers for longer-term management.
- **Topical lubricants** (preservative-free).
- **Topical antibiotics** as prophylaxis if an epithelial defect is present.
- **Oral tetracycline** (e.g. doxycycline 100 mg once or twice daily) for its anticollagenase effect.
- **Topical steroids** may worsen thinning so are generally avoided; relapsing polychondritis may be an exception.
- **Surgical management** is generally as for Mooren ulcer, including conjunctival excision if medical treatment is ineffective.

Terrien marginal degeneration

Terrien disease is an uncommon idiopathic thinning of the peripheral cornea occurring in young adult to elderly patients. Although usually categorized as a degeneration, some cases are associated with episodic episcleritis or scleritis. About 75% of affected patients are male and the condition is usually bilateral but may be asymmetrical.

Diagnosis

- **Symptoms.** The condition is commonly asymptomatic, but gradual visual deterioration can occur due to astigmatism. A few patients experience episodic pain and inflammation.
- **Signs**
  - Fine yellow–white refractile stromal opacities, frequently associated with mild superficial vascularization, usually start superiorly, spread circumferentially and are separated from the limbus by a clear zone. There is no epithelial defect and on cursory examination the condition may resemble arcus senilis.
  - Slowly progressive circumferential thinning results in a peripheral gutter, the outer slope of which shelves gradually, while the central part rises sharply (Fig. 7.30A). A band of lipid is commonly present at the central edge (Fig. 7.30B).
  - Perforation is rare but may be spontaneous or follow blunt trauma.
  - Pseudopterygia sometimes develop (Fig. 7.30C).

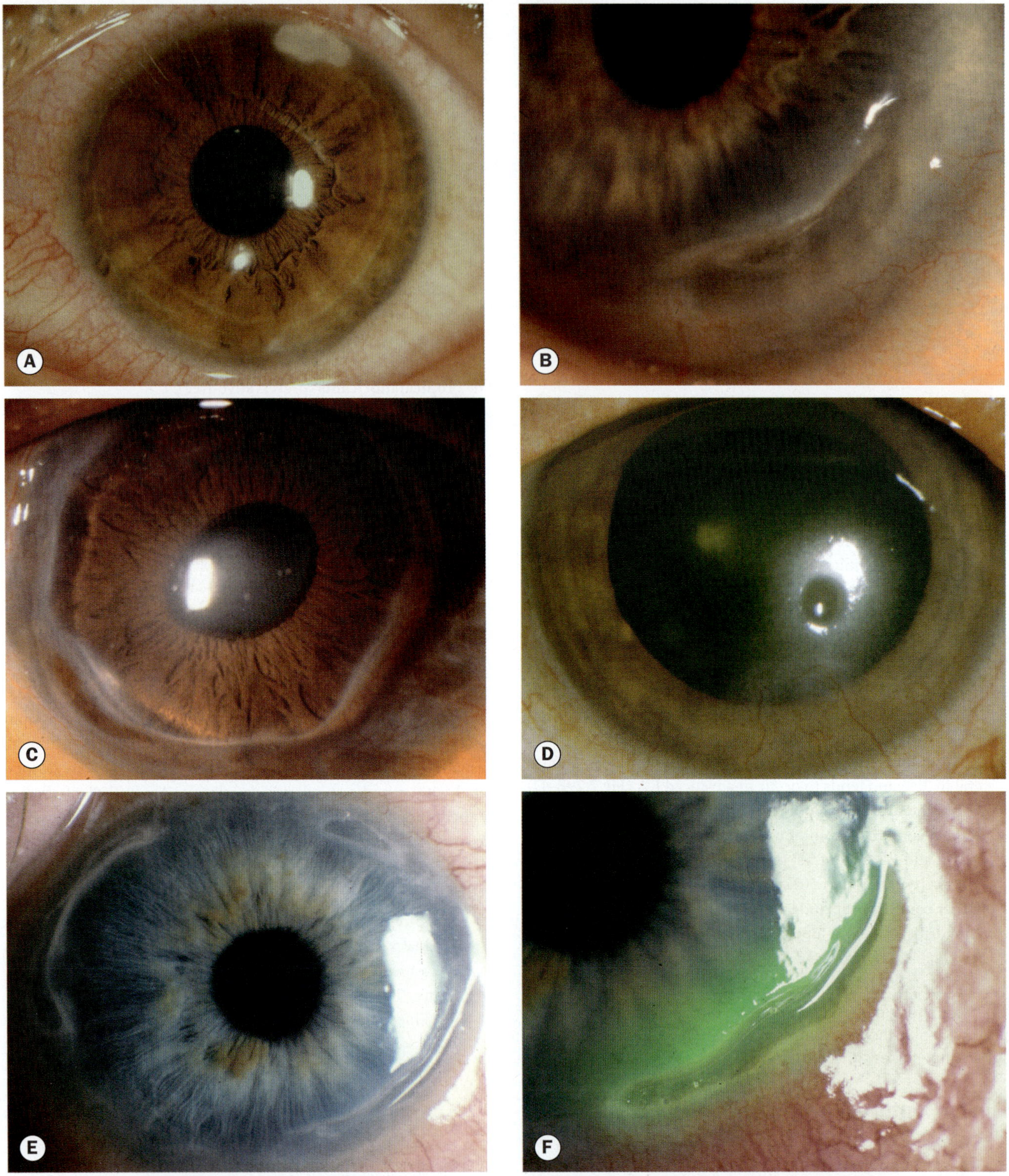

Fig. 7.29 Keratitis in systemic autoimmune disease. **(A)** Corneal infiltrate in Crohn disease; **(B)** early peripheral ulcerative keratitis in rheumatoid arthritis; **(C)** peripheral guttering in rheumatoid arthritis; 'contact lens' cornea; **(D)** rheumatoid paracentral ulcerative keratitis; **(E)** peripheral guttering and ulceration in granulomatosis with polyangiitis; **(F)** fluorescein staining of **(E)**.

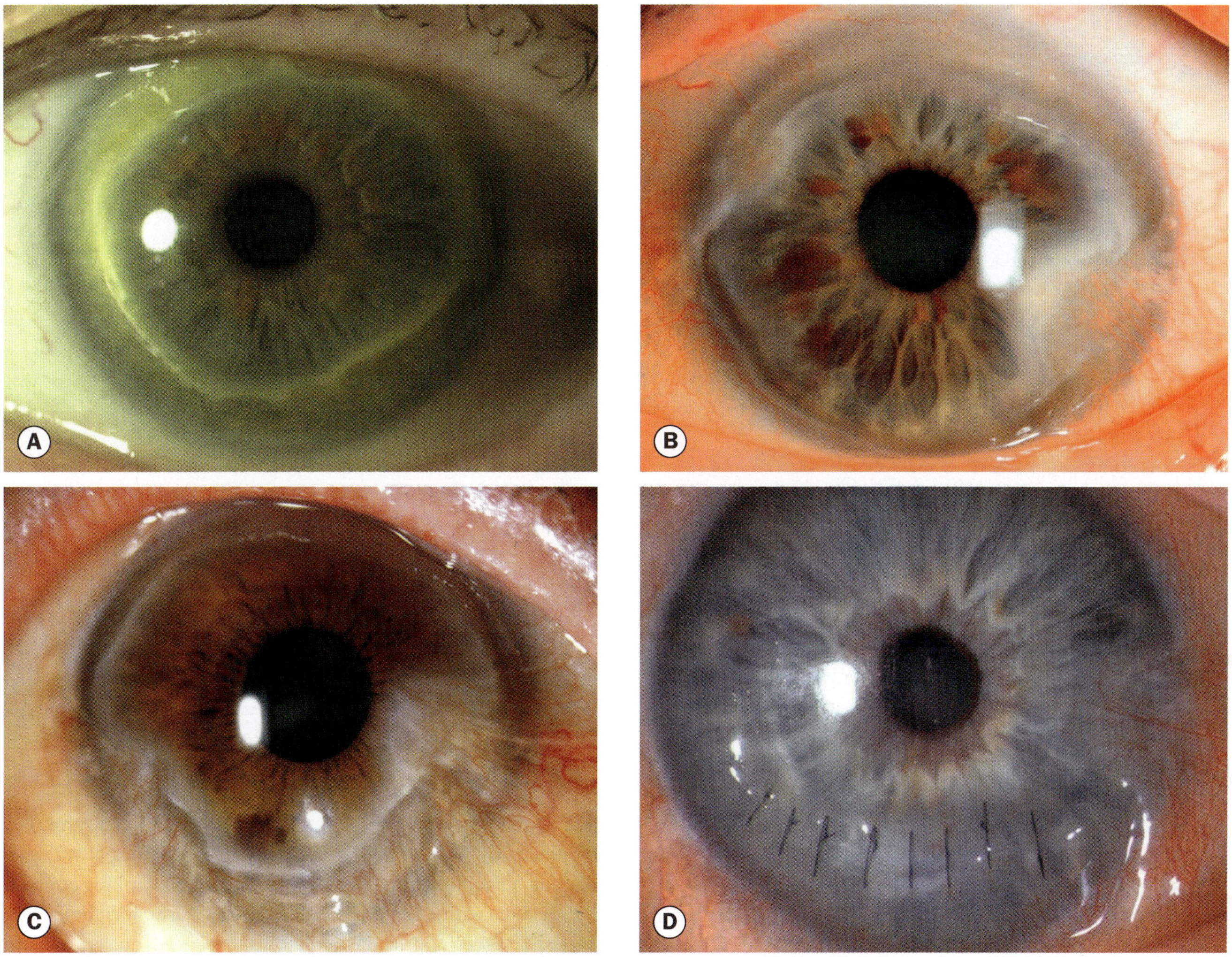

Fig. 7.30 Terrien marginal degeneration. **(A)** Circumferential thinning with peripheral guttering; **(B)** thinning, vascularization and lipid band at the central edge; **(C)** pseudopterygia; **(D)** gutter excision with lamellar graft repair. *(Courtesy of C Barry – figs C and D.)*

Treatment

- **Safety spectacles** (e.g. polycarbonate) if thinning is significant.
- **Contact lenses** for astigmatism. Scleral or soft lenses with rigid gas permeable 'piggybacking'.
- **Surgery** – crescentic or annular excision of the gutter with lamellar (Fig. 7.30D) or full-thickness transplantation – gives reasonable results and may arrest progression.

NEUROTROPHIC KERATOPATHY

Introduction

Neurotrophic keratopathy occurs when there is loss of trigeminal innervation to the cornea resulting in partial or complete anaesthesia. In addition to loss of the protective sensory stimulus, reduced innervation results in intracellular oedema, exfoliation, loss of goblet cells and epithelial breakdown with persistent ulceration. Causes include trigeminal ganglion surgical ablation for neuralgia, stroke, tumour, peripheral neuropathy (e.g. diabetes) and ocular disease such as herpes simplex and herpes zoster keratitis (when sensation loss may be sectoral).

Diagnosis

A full cranial nerve examination is mandatory.

- **Signs**
  - Corneal sensation is reduced.
  - Stage 1: interpalpebral epithelial irregularity and staining, with mild opacification, oedema and tiny focal defects.
  - Stage 2: larger persistent epithelial defect with rolled and thickened edges (Fig. 7.31A), subsequently assuming a punched-out configuration with underlying stromal oedema.
  - Stage 3: stromal melting, often with minimal discomfort. Secondary infection may occur.
  - Perforation is uncommon but may occur rapidly, especially with secondary infection (Fig. 7.31B).

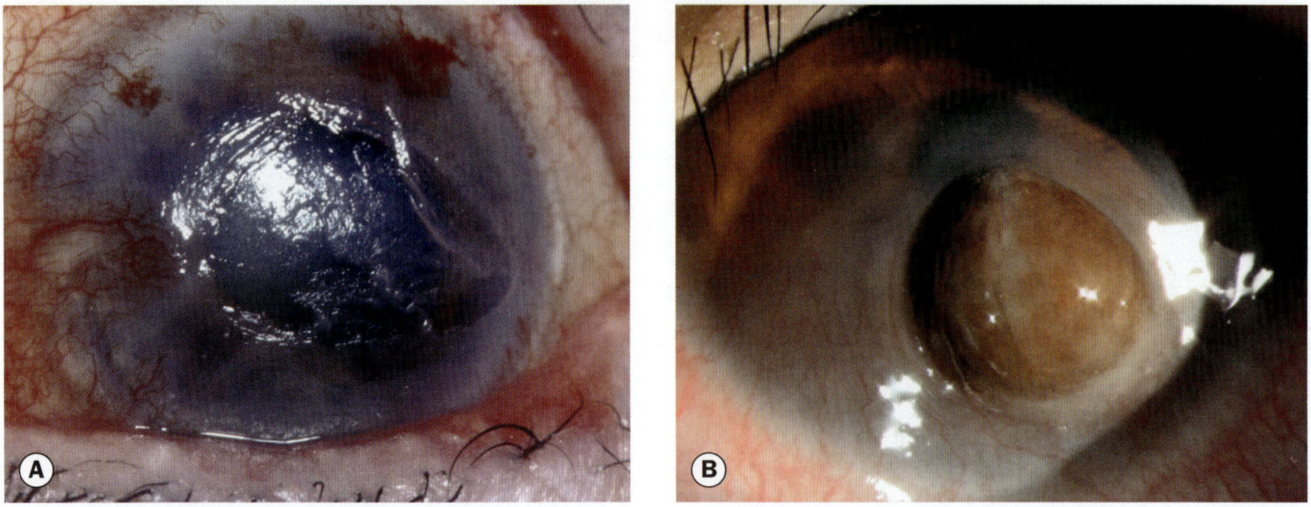

Fig. 7.31 Neurotrophic keratopathy. **(A)** Large epithelial defect; **(B)** perforation with iris prolapse. *(Courtesy of S Tuft – fig. A.)*

Treatment

- **Discontinuation**, if possible, of potentially toxic medications.
- **Topical lubricants** (non-preserved) for associated dry eye or corneal exposure. Topical insulin-like growth factor-1, substance P and neurogenic growth factor have been evaluated but are not commercially available.
- **Anticollagenase agents**: topical (e.g. acetylcysteine, tetracycline ointment) or systemic (e.g. tetracyclines).
- **Cenegermin 0.002%**, a topical recombinant human nerve growth factor, appears to be beneficial in moderate (persistent epithelial defect) or severe (corneal ulcer) neurotrophic ulcer in adults. Instilled six times daily for 2 months, this medication increases the corneal nerve density and facilitates healing. Diffuse lamellar keratitis has been reported as a late side effect in some patients. The long-term effectiveness is not known.
- **Protection of the ocular surface**
  - Simple taping of the lids, particularly at night, may provide modest protection.
  - Botulinum toxin-induced ptosis.
  - Tarsorrhaphy: temporary or permanent, lateral or central, according to the underlying pathology and visual potential.
  - Therapeutic silicone contact lenses may be fitted, provided the eye is carefully monitored for infection.
  - Amniotic membrane patching with temporary central tarsorrhaphy.
- **Perforation** is dealt with as discussed earlier in the chapter.
- **Corneal neurotization from the supratrochlear nerve using a sural nerve graft.** Corneal sensation can be restored using a multidisciplinary surgical approach. A segment of the medial cutaneous branches of the sural nerve is connected to the contralateral supratrochlear nerve (Fig. 7.32A and B). The grafted nerve is brought under the skin and into the opposite orbit (Fig. 7.32C and D). The nerve is divided and positioned under the conjunctiva and attached to the peripheral corneoscleral junction (Fig. 7.32E). The conjunctiva is closed over the branches (Fig. 7.32F). Sensation returns 6–8 months after the surgery.

EXPOSURE KERATOPATHY

Introduction

Exposure keratopathy is the result of incomplete lid closure (lagophthalmos), with drying of the cornea despite normal tear production. Lagophthalmos may only be present on blinking or gentle lid closure, with full forced lid closure. Causes include neuroparalytic, especially facial nerve palsy, reduced muscle tone as in parkinsonism, mechanical such as lid scarring, eczematous skin tightening and post-blepharoplasty and proptosis.

Diagnosis

- **Symptoms** are those of dry eye.
- **Signs**
  - Mild punctate epithelial changes involving the inferior third of the cornea, particularly with nocturnal lagophthalmos.
  - Epithelial breakdown (Fig. 7.33A).
  - Stromal melting (Fig. 7.33B), occasionally leading to perforation.
  - Inferior fibrovascular change with Salzmann degeneration may develop over time.
  - Secondary infection.

Treatment

Treatment depends on the severity of exposure and whether recovery is anticipated.

- **Reversible exposure**
  - Artificial tears (unpreserved) during the day and ointment at night.
  - Taping the lid closed at night may be an alternative to ointment.

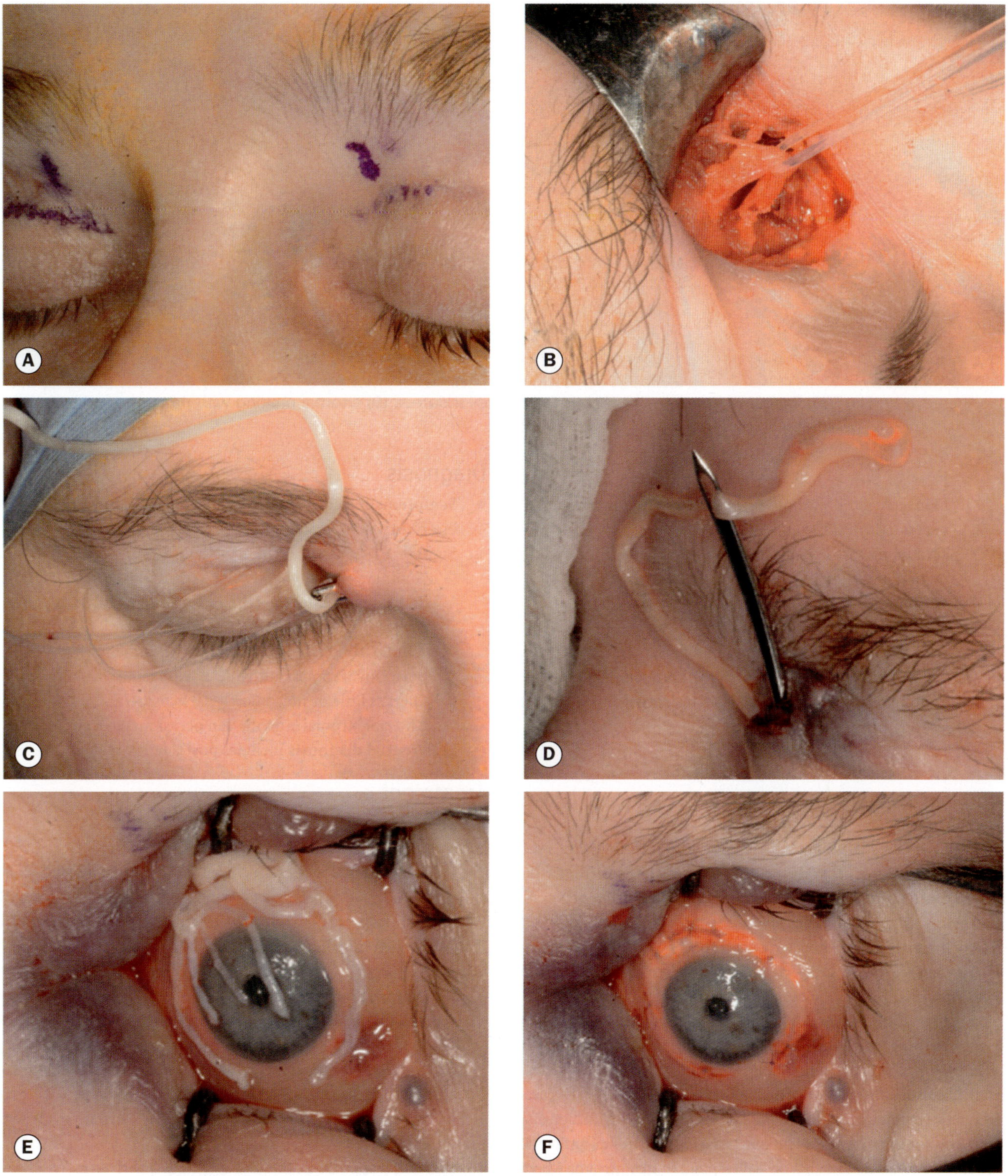

Fig. 7.32 Technique of corneal neurotization. **(A)** Left neurotrophic keratopathy showing skin incision sites; **(B)** isolation of contralateral supraorbital nerve; **(C)** and **(D)** the sural nerve graft is brought under the skin and into the opposite orbit; **(E)** the nerve is divided and the branches are sutured at the limbus; **(F)** the conjunctiva is closed over the branches. *(Courtesy of JH Norris.)*

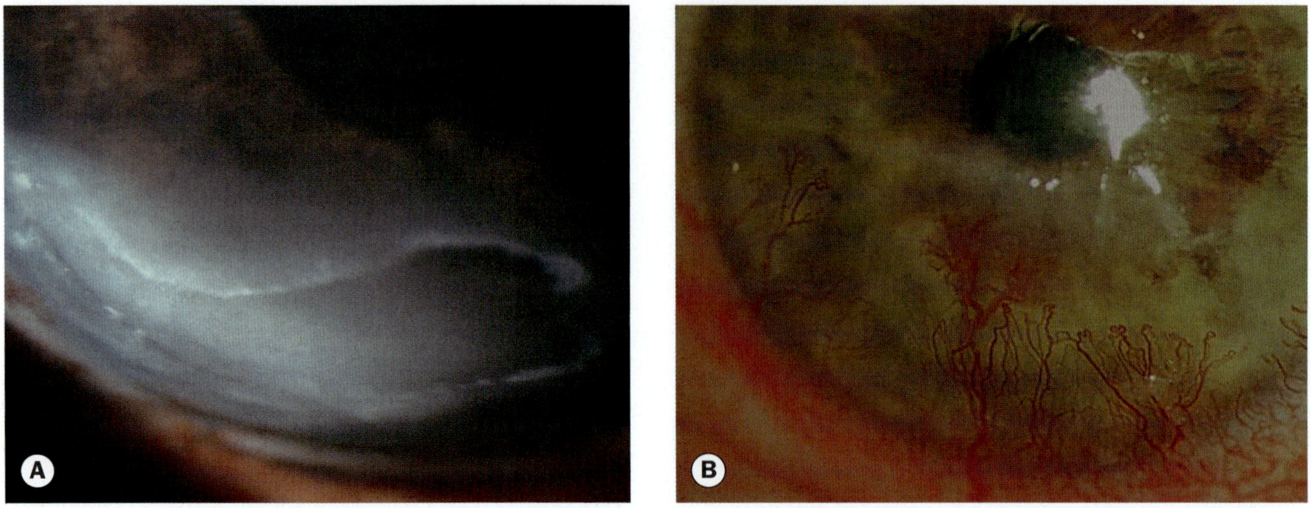

Fig. 7.33 Exposure keratopathy. (A) Inferior epithelial defect; (B) stromal melting with pannus formation.

- Bandage silicone hydrogel or scleral contact lenses.
- Management of proptosis by orbital decompression if necessary.
- Temporary tarsorrhaphy, Frost suture or overlay amniotic membrane grafting.

- **Permanent exposure**
  - Permanent tarsorrhaphy.
  - Gold weight upper lid insertion for facial nerve palsy.
  - Permanent central tarsorrhaphy, amniotic membrane grafting or conjunctival flap when vision is poor.

MISCELLANEOUS KERATOPATHIES

Infectious crystalline keratopathy

Infectious crystalline keratopathy is a rare indolent infection usually occurring in a patient on long-term topical steroid therapy with an associated epithelial defect, most frequently following penetrating keratoplasty. *Streptococcus viridans* is most commonly isolated, although numerous other bacteria and fungi have been implicated.

Slowly progressive, grey–white, branching stromal opacities are seen, associated with minimal inflammation and usually intact overlying epithelium (Fig. 7.34). A biofilm is present that allows survival of the microorganism, reduces antibiotic bioavailability and makes diagnostic detection difficult. Culture or biopsy is performed to determine the organism and topical antibiotics instilled for several weeks. Adjunctive therapies to enhance the efficacy of treatment include disruption of the microorganism biofilm by laser, intrastromal antibiotic and keratectomy. In cases that do not respond to treatment or where corneal scarring is present, corneal transplantation is required.

Thygeson superficial punctate keratitis

Thygeson superficial punctate keratitis is an uncommon idiopathic, usually bilateral, condition characterized by exacerbations and remissions. It is commonly of onset in young adulthood but can affect patients of any age and may recur over decades.

Diagnosis

- **Symptoms** consist of recurrent attacks of irritation, photophobia, blurred vision and watering.
- **Signs**
  - Granular, coarse, slightly elevated greyish epithelial lesions that stain with fluorescein and mainly involve the central cornea (Fig. 7.35A).
  - A mild subepithelial haze may be present (Fig. 7.35B), especially if topical antivirals have been used.
  - There is little or no conjunctival hyperaemia.
  - Anterior stromal scarring can occasionally occur.
- **Differential diagnosis** includes post-adenoviral keratitis.

Treatment

- **Topical**
  - Lubricants may suffice in mild cases.
  - Steroids. A low-potency preparation is used twice daily initially, with gradual tapering to as little as once-weekly instillation. High-intensity treatment may sometimes be needed initially.
  - Ciclosporin 0.05% is generally used if the response to steroids is inadequate, or as an alternative in longer-term therapy. However, some authorities recommend ciclosporin for initial treatment. Tacrolimus may also be effective.
  - Antivirals have not been found to be consistently helpful.
- **Contact lenses** (extended wear or daily disposable soft) may be considered if steroids are ineffective or contraindicated, as an alternative to ciclosporin.
- **Phototherapeutic keratectomy** brings short-term relief but recurrence is likely.

Filamentary keratopathy

Introduction

Filamentary keratopathy is a common condition that can cause considerable discomfort. It is thought that a loose area of

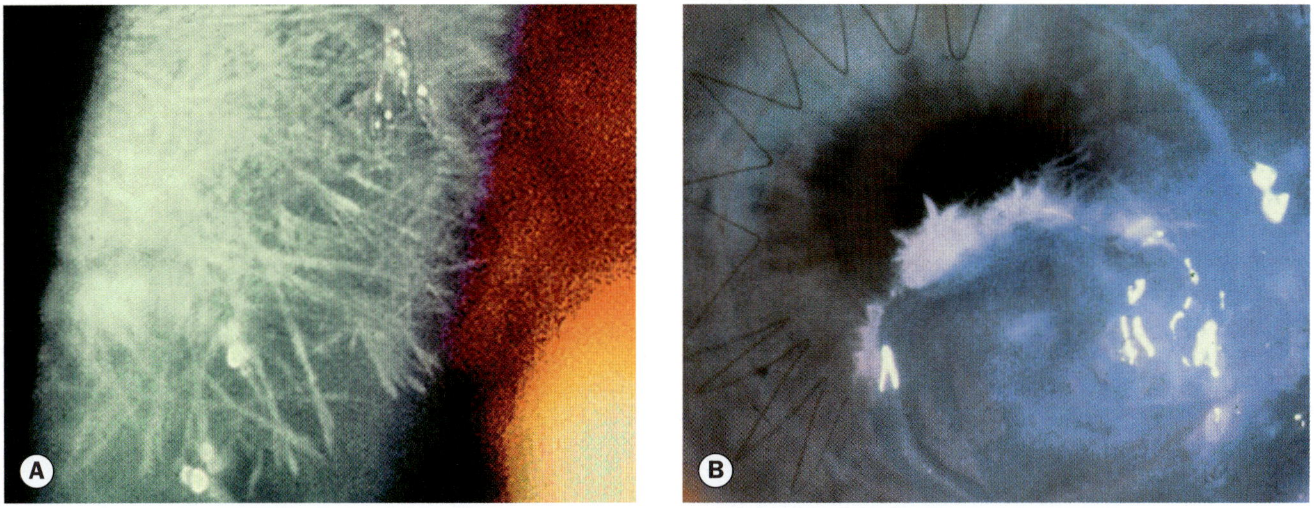

Fig. 7.34 **(A)** Infectious crystalline keratopathy; **(B)** crystalline keratopathy in a corneal graft.

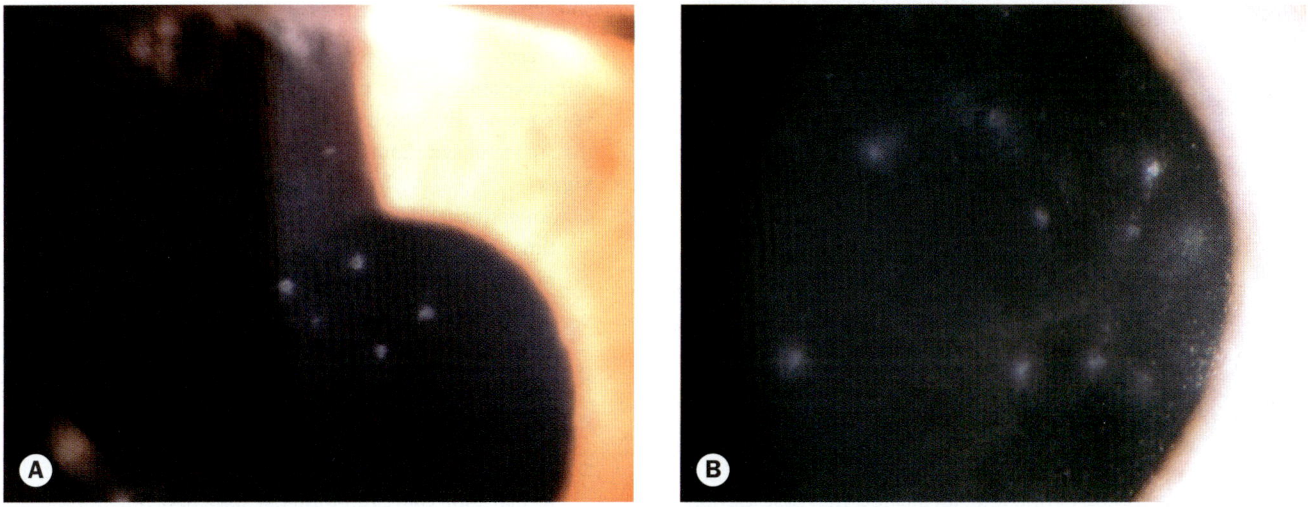

Fig. 7.35 **(A)** Thygeson superficial punctate keratitis; **(B)** associated subepithelial haze.

epithelium acts as a focus for deposition of mucus and cellular debris. The causes are shown in Table 7.6.

Diagnosis

- **Symptoms** consist of discomfort with foreign body sensation, redness and sometimes photophobia.
- **Signs**
  - Strands of degenerated epithelial cells and mucus that move with blinking and are typically attached to the cornea at one end (Fig. 7.36A).
  - Filaments stain well with rose Bengal (Fig. 7.36B) and to a lesser extent with fluorescein.
  - A small epithelial defect may be present at the base of a filament.
  - Chronic filaments may form plaques.

Treatment

- Any underlying cause should be treated.
- Topical medication should be changed if a toxic effect is suspected and unpreserved preparations used where possible.
- Mechanical removal of filaments gives short-term symptomatic relief.
- Mucolytics such as 5% or 10% acetylcysteine drops.
- Non-steroidal anti-inflammatory drops, e.g. diclofenac.
- Hypertonic saline (5% drops four times daily, ointment at bedtime) may encourage adhesion of loose epithelium.
- Bandage contact lenses may protect the cornea from the shearing action of the lids.

Table 7.6 Causes of Filamentary Keratopathy
Aqueous deficiency (keratoconjunctivitis sicca)
Excessive contact lens wear
Corneal epithelial instability (recurrent erosion syndrome, corneal graft, cataract surgery, refractive surgery and drug toxicity)
Superior limbic keratoconjunctivitis
Bullous keratopathy
Neurotrophic keratopathy
Prolonged or frequent eye closure

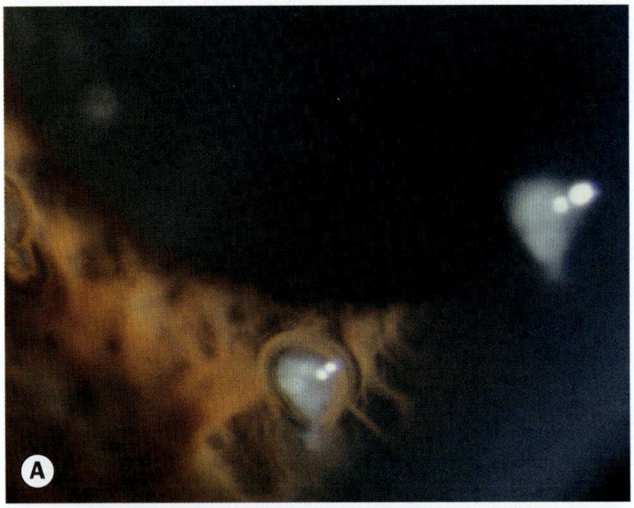

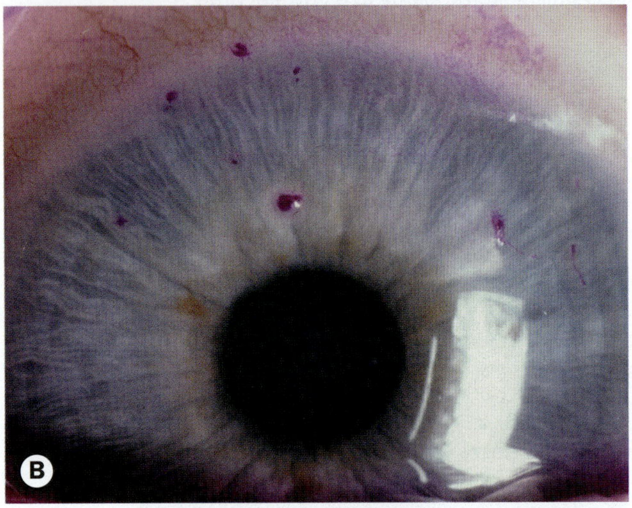

Fig. 7.36 Corneal filaments. **(A)** Comma-shaped lesions attached to the cornea at one end; **(B)** stained with rose Bengal. *(Courtesy of S Tuft – fig. A; R Bates – fig. B.)*

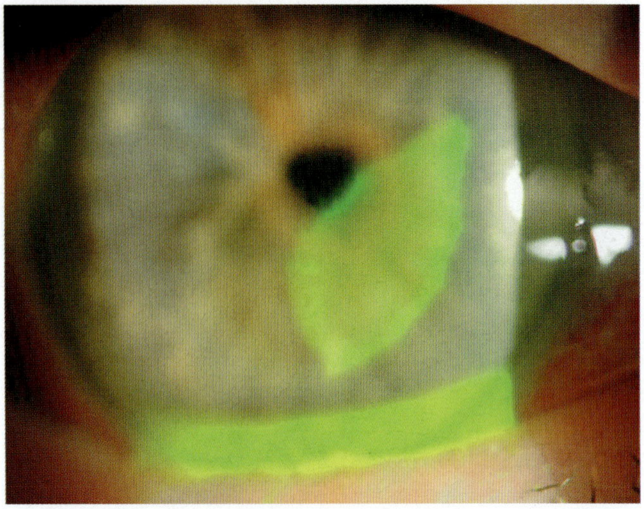

Fig. 7.37 Recurrent corneal erosion syndrome showing epithelial defect stained with fluorescein.

Recurrent corneal epithelial erosion

Introduction

Recurrent corneal epithelial erosion is caused by an abnormally weak attachment between the basal cells of the corneal epithelium and their basement membrane. Minor trauma, such as eyelid–cornea interaction during sleep, can be sufficient to precipitate detachment. Erosions may be associated with previous trauma or rarely corneal surgery and with some corneal dystrophies. Intervals between episodes can be very variable, even in the same patient, but may occur in spates over a short period.

Diagnosis

- **Symptoms.** Severe pain, photophobia, redness, blepharospasm and watering typically waken the patient during the night or are present on awaking in the morning. There is usually (but not invariably) a prior history of corneal abrasion, sometimes years previously, which may have been minor compared with the recurrent symptoms.
- **Signs**
  - An epithelial defect (Fig. 7.37) may not be present by the time the patient is examined, as healing can often be very rapid (hours), but the extent of loose epithelium may be highlighted by areas of pooling of fluorescein and rapid tear film breakup.
  - Infiltrate should not be present, though greyish sloughed and rolled epithelium may sometimes be reminiscent of this.
  - There may be no sign of abnormality once a defect has healed, but signs of epithelial basement membrane disturbance, such as microcysts, punctate or linear/fingerprint opacities, are often present. These will typically be bilateral in a stromal dystrophy and unilateral if injury is the cause.

Treatment

- **Acute symptoms**
  - Antibiotic ointment four times daily and cyclopentolate 1% twice daily.
  - Pressure patching should not be used as it may impair healing and does not improve comfort.
  - In severe cases a bandage contact lens alleviates pain but may not improve healing. Antibiotic drops rather than ointment should be used.
  - Debridement of heaped/scrolled areas of epithelium with a sterile cellulose sponge or cotton-tipped applicator (cotton bud) may improve comfort and allow healing from the edges of the defect.
  - Topical diclofenac 0.1% reduces pain.

- Topical anaesthetic dramatically relieves pain but should not be dispensed for patient use.
- Hypertonic sodium chloride 5% drops four times daily and ointment at bedtime may improve epithelial adhesion.
- Following resolution, some authorities advise using a prophylactic topical lubricant such as carbomer gel three or four times daily for several months.

- **Recurrent symptoms**
  - Topical lubricant gel or ointment, or hypertonic saline ointment, instilled at bedtime used long term may be sufficient.
  - A combination of oral doxycycline and topical steroid may be helpful. Both have been shown to inhibit metalloproteinase inhibitors important to disease pathogenesis.
  - Long-term extended-wear bandage contact lens.
  - Simple debridement of the epithelium in involved areas, which may be followed by smoothing of Bowman layer with a diamond burr or excimer laser. Most patients treated with excimer keratectomy do not get recurrences and the side effects are minimal.
  - Anterior stromal puncture for localized areas off the visual axis. It may not be necessary to remove the epithelium to facilitate this.

Xerophthalmia

Introduction

Vitamin A is essential for the maintenance of the body's epithelial surfaces, for immune function and for the synthesis of retinal photoreceptor proteins. Xerophthalmia refers to the spectrum of ocular disease caused by inadequate vitamin A intake and is a late manifestation of severe deficiency. Lack of vitamin A in the diet may be caused by malnutrition, malabsorption, chronic alcoholism or by highly selective dieting. The risk in infants is increased if their mothers are malnourished and by coexisting diarrhoea or measles.

Diagnosis

A World Health Organization (WHO) grading system is set out in Table 7.7.

- **Symptoms** are night blindness (nyctalopia), discomfort and loss of vision.
- **Conjunctiva**
  - Xerosis is characterized by dryness of the conjunctiva in the interpalpebral zone with loss of goblet cells, squamous metaplasia and keratinization.
  - Bitot spots are triangular patches of foamy keratinized epithelium (Fig. 7.38A) in the interpalpebral zone thought to be caused by *Corynebacterium xerosis.*
- **Cornea**
  - Lustreless appearance due to secondary xerosis.
  - Bilateral punctate corneal epithelial erosions in the interpalpebral zone can progress to epithelial defects but are reversible with treatment.
  - Keratinization.
  - Sterile corneal melting by liquefactive necrosis (keratomalacia), which may lead to perforation (Fig. 7.38B).
- **Retinopathy**, characterized by yellowish peripheral dots, may occur in advanced cases and is associated with decreased electroretinogram amplitude.

Treatment

Keratomalacia is an indicator of very severe vitamin A deficiency and should be treated as a medical emergency due to the risk of death, particularly in infants.

Table 7.7 WHO Grading of Xerophthalmia

XN = night blindness
X1 = conjunctival xerosis (X1A) with Bitot spots (X1B)
X2 = corneal xerosis
X3 = corneal ulceration, less than one-third (X3A); more than one-third (X3B)
XS = corneal scar
XF = xerophthalmic fundus

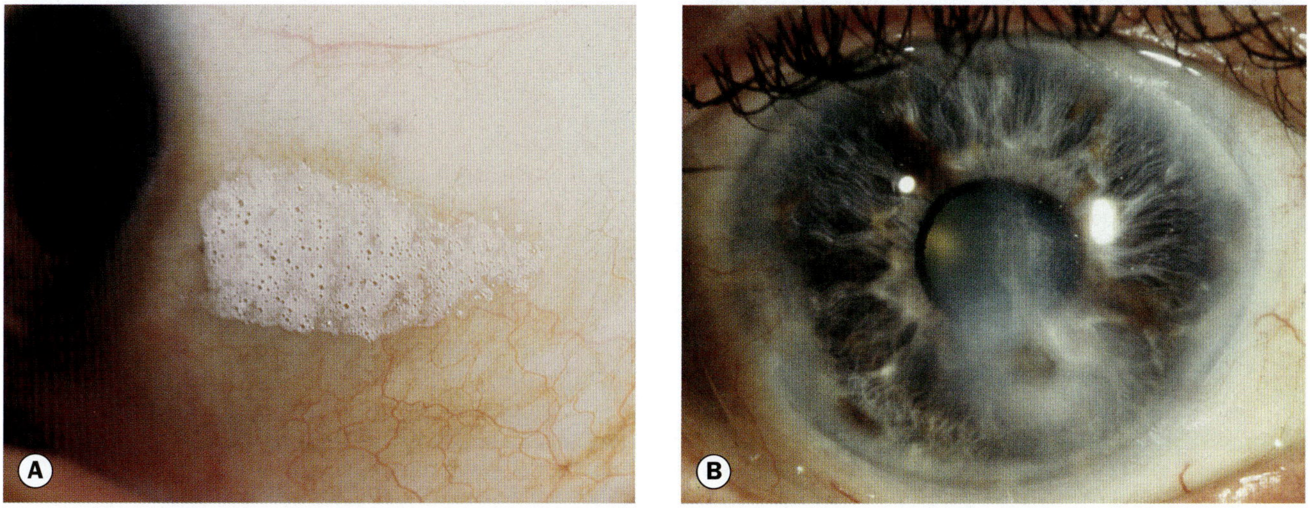

Fig. 7.38 Xerophthalmia. **(A)** Bitot spot; **(B)** keratomalacia with corneal melting.

- **Systemic** treatment involves oral (oil-based 200 000 IU) or intramuscular (aqueous-based 100 000 IU) vitamin A for keratomalacia. Multivitamin supplements and dietary sources of vitamin A are also administered.
- **Local** treatment consists of intense lubrication, topical retinoic acid and management of perforation.

CORNEAL ECTASIA

Keratoconus

Introduction

Keratoconus (KC) is a progressive disorder in which central or paracentral corneal stromal thinning occurs, accompanied by apical protrusion and irregular astigmatism. The prevalence is 0.1% to 0.2% and men are slightly more likely to be affected than women. Presentation is commonly during the teens or twenties, with features initially in only one eye. Approximately 50% of normal fellow eyes will progress to KC within 16 years. Both eyes are affected eventually, at least on topographical imaging, in almost all cases. It can be graded by the highest axis of corneal power on keratometry as mild (<48 D), moderate (48–54 D) or severe (>54 D). Most patients do not have a family history, with only about 10% of offspring developing KC; autosomal dominant transmission with incomplete penetrance has been proposed. Risk factors include allergy, asthma, eczema and persistent eye rubbing from any cause. Systemic associations include Down, Ehlers–Danlos and Marfan syndromes and osteogenesis imperfecta. Ocular associations include vernal keratoconjunctivitis, blue sclera, aniridia, Leber congenital amaurosis, retinitis pigmentosa.

Diagnosis

- **Symptoms.** Unilateral impairment of vision due to progressive myopia and astigmatism. Occasionally, initial presentation is with acute hydrops (see below).
- **Signs**
  - Direct ophthalmoscopy from a distance of half a metre shows a fairly well delineated 'oil droplet' reflex (Fig. 7.39A).
  - Retinoscopy shows an irregular 'scissoring' reflex.

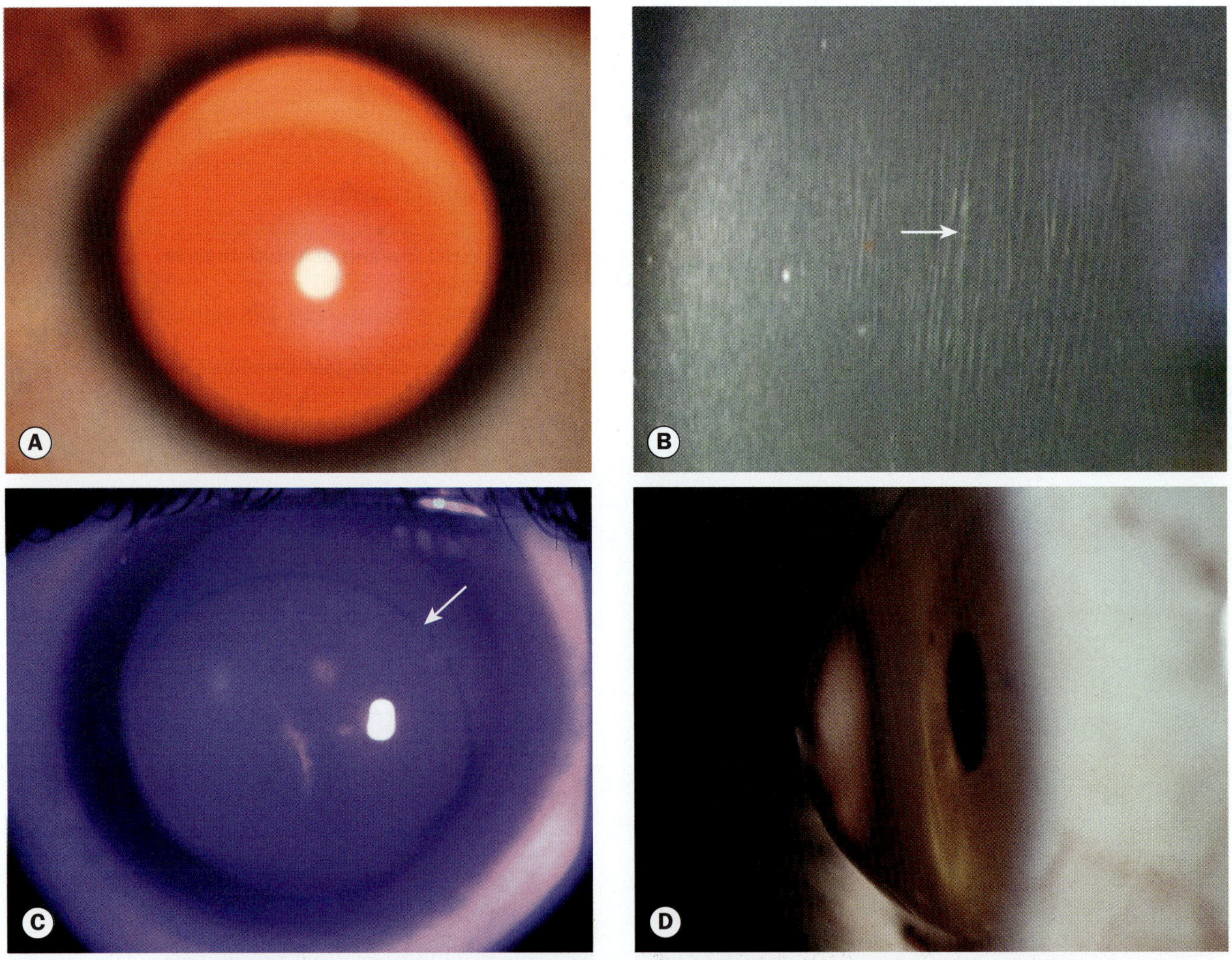

Fig. 7.39 Keratoconus. **(A)** 'Oil droplet' red reflex; **(B)** Vogt striae in the deep stroma (arrow); **(C)** Fleischer ring demonstrated by cobalt blue light as a blue circle (arrow); **(D)** typical cone. *(Courtesy of R Fogla – fig. C.)*

- Slit lamp biomicroscopy shows very fine, vertical, deep stromal stress lines (Vogt striae – Fig. 7.39B), which disappear with pressure on the globe.
- Epithelial iron deposits, best seen with a cobalt blue filter, may surround the base of the cone (Fleischer ring – Fig. 7.39C).
- Progressive corneal protrusion in a cone configuration (Fig. 7.39D), with thinning maximal at the apex.
- Bulging of the lower lid in downgaze (Munson sign) (Fig. 7.40A).
- Acute hydrops is caused by a rupture in the stretched Descemet membrane that allows a sudden influx of aqueous into the cornea (Fig. 7.40B and C), with accompanying pain, photophobia and decreased vision. Although the break usually heals within 6–10 weeks and the oedema clears, a variable amount of stromal scarring (Fig. 7.40D) may develop. This sometimes gives improved vision by flattening the cornea. Acute episodes are initially treated with cycloplegia, hypertonic (5%) saline ointment and patching or a soft bandage contact lens. Accelerated resolution has been reported with intracameral gas injection in the acute stage.

- **Keratometry** readings are steep.
- **Corneal topography** (video keratography) and various novel corneal profiling techniques are highly sensitive for detection and essential in monitoring. Characteristically, astigmatism progresses from a symmetrical bow-tie pattern, through an asymmetrical appearance to an inferotemporally displaced steep-sided cone (Fig. 7.41). Sometimes a central ('nipple') cone may develop. Contact lens warpage can sometimes appear similar to a cone on topography, but is generally more arcuate-shaped.

Treatment

- **Eye rubbing** should be avoided.
- **Spectacles** or soft contact lenses are generally sufficient in early cases. If thinning is marked, it may be prudent to consider wearing safety spectacles over contact lenses.
- **Rigid contact lenses,** sometimes scleral, are required for higher degrees of astigmatism to provide a regular refracting surface.
- **Corneal collagen cross-linking (CXL),** using riboflavin drops to photosensitize the eye followed by exposure to ultraviolet-A light, can stabilize the cornea if progression has been shown. CXL is successful in more than 90% of cases and in some cases

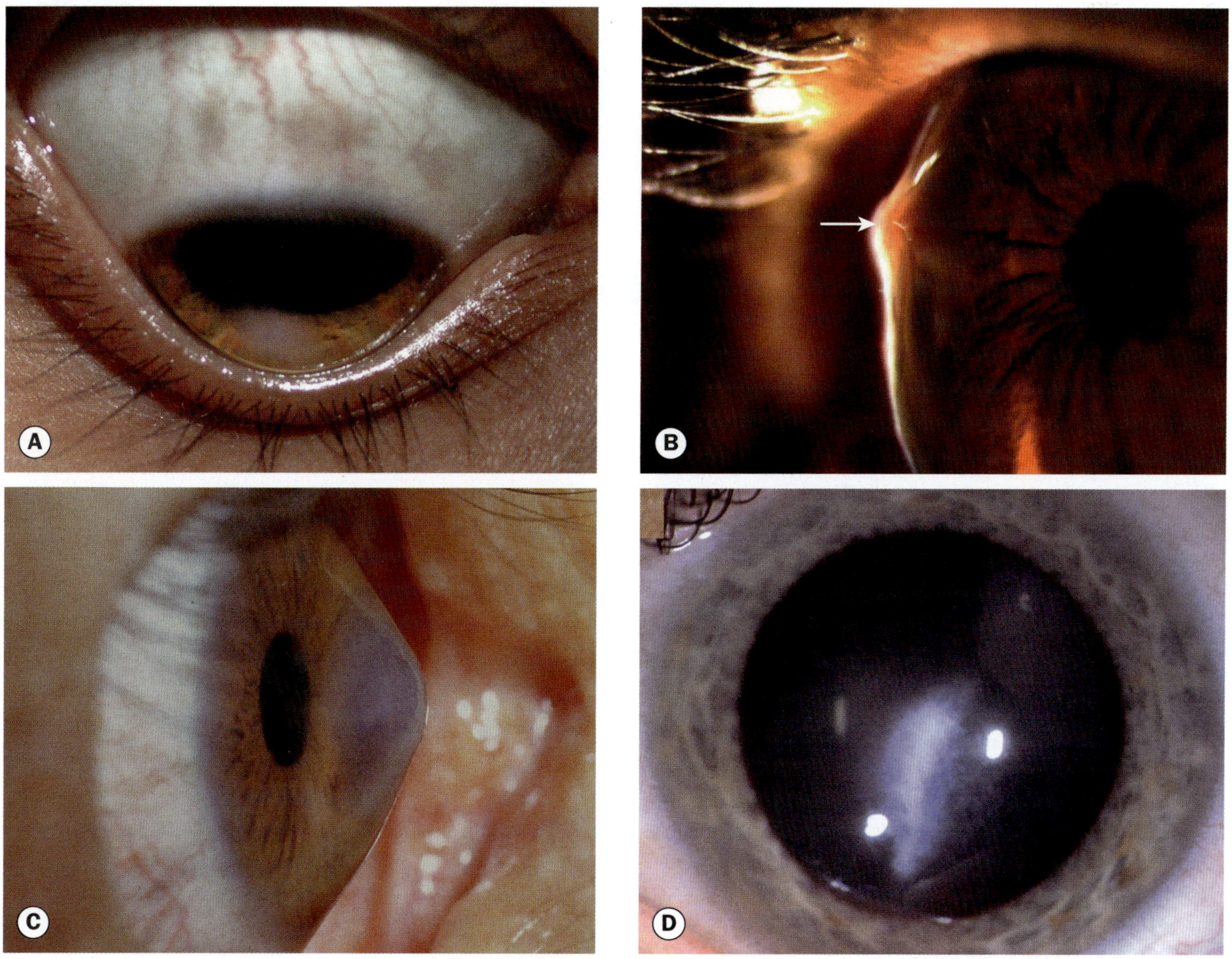

Fig. 7.40 Acute hydrops. **(A)** Munson sign with localized hydrops; **(B)** localized corneal oedema; 'nipple' cone (arrow); **(C)** severe diffuse oedema; **(D)** late scarring. *(Courtesy of C Barry – figs C and D.)*

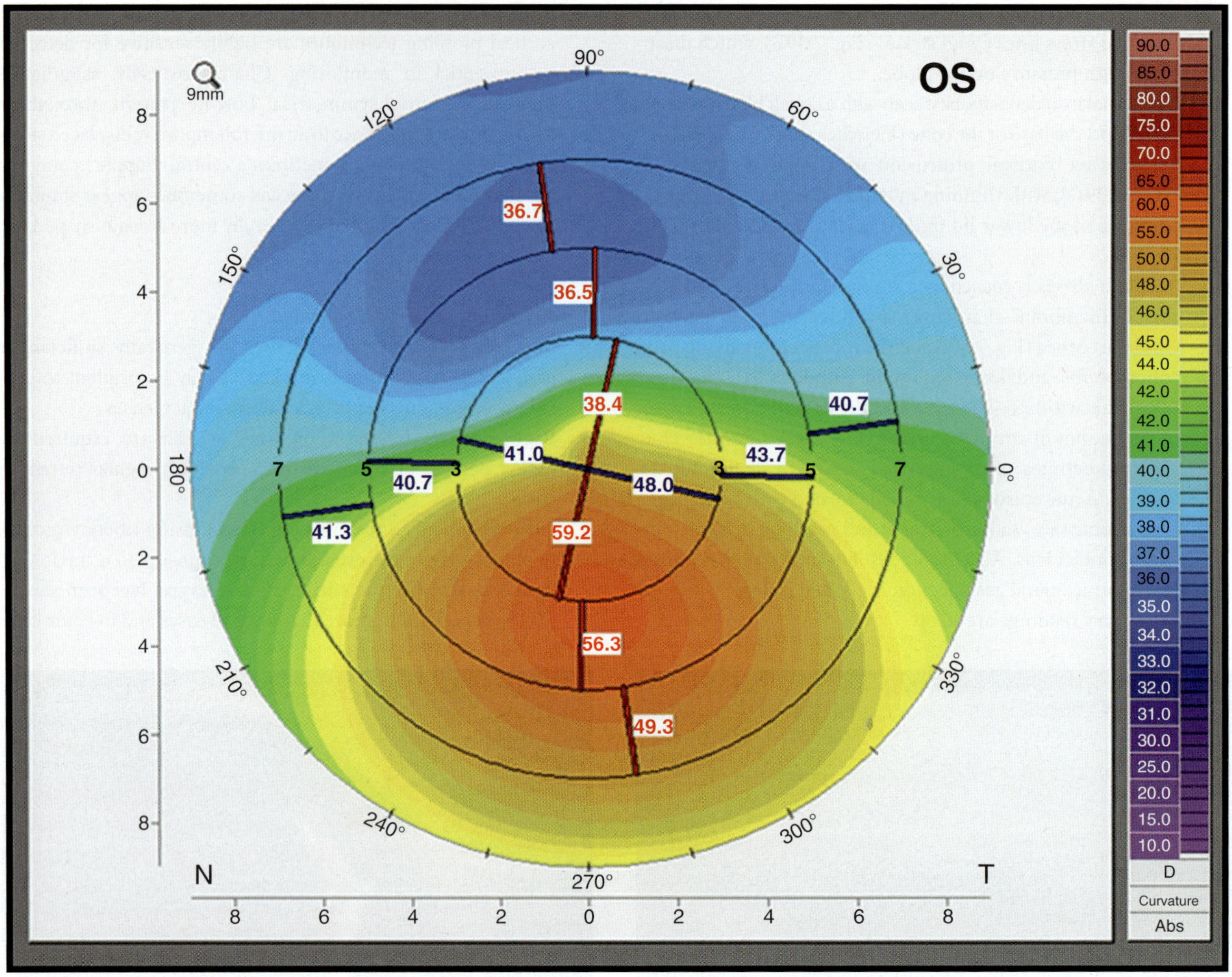

Fig. 7.41 Pentacam Scheimpflug topography showing keratoconus.

can even reverse the ectasia. The complication rate is low, but because the epithelium is removed at the time of surgery there is a small risk of infection or corneal scarring. A bandage contact lens should be used for 3 days after the procedure to reduce postoperative pain. It usually takes 1–2 weeks for the eye to settle.

- **Intracorneal ring segment implantation** (Fig. 7.42) using laser or mechanical channel creation is relatively safe and typically provides at least a moderate visual improvement, facilitating contact lens tolerance in advanced cases. It can be used at the same time as CXL.
- **Keratoplasty**, either penetrating or deep anterior lamellar (DALK), may be necessary in patients with severe disease. A history of hydrops is a contraindication to DALK due to the presence of a Descemet membrane discontinuity. Outcomes may be compromised by residual astigmatism and by anisometropia, necessitating contact lens correction for optimal acuity.
- **LASIK is contraindicated.** Patients should be screened for KC prior to corneal refractive surgery.

Pellucid marginal degeneration

Pellucid marginal degeneration is a rare progressive peripheral corneal thinning disorder, typically involving the inferior cornea in both eyes. Presentation is usually in adulthood.

Diagnosis

- **Symptoms.** Slowly progressive blurring due to astigmatism.
- **Signs**
  - Bilateral, slowly progressive, crescentic 1–2 mm band of inferior corneal thinning extending from 4 to 8 o'clock, 1 mm from the limbus (Fig. 7.43A).
  - The epithelium is intact and the cornea above the thinned area shows ectasia and appears flattened.
  - In contrast to keratoconus, Fleischer rings and Vogt striae do not occur and acute hydrops is rare.
- **Corneal topography** shows a 'butterfly' pattern, with severe astigmatism and diffuse steepening of the inferior cornea (Fig. 7.43B).

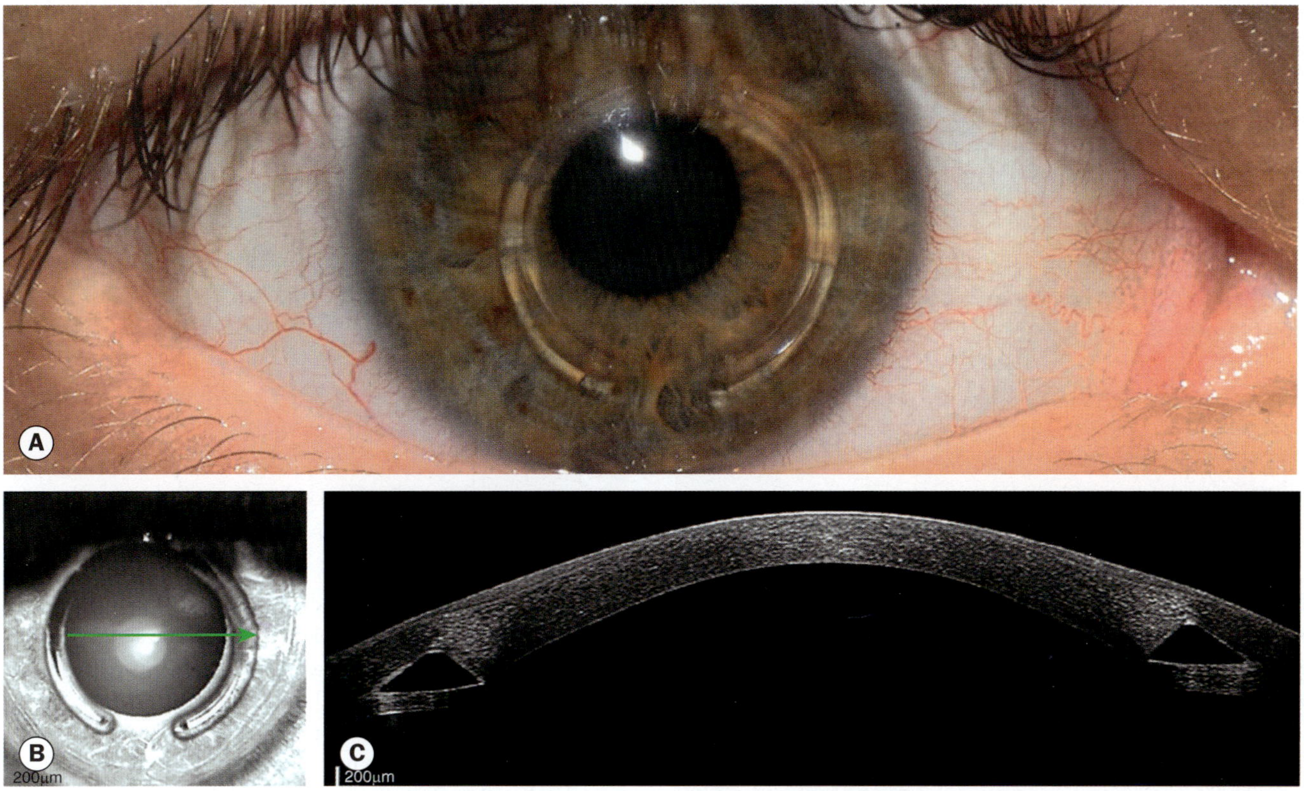

Fig. 7.42 (A–C) Intracorneal ring segments *in situ*. *(Courtesy of C Barry.)*

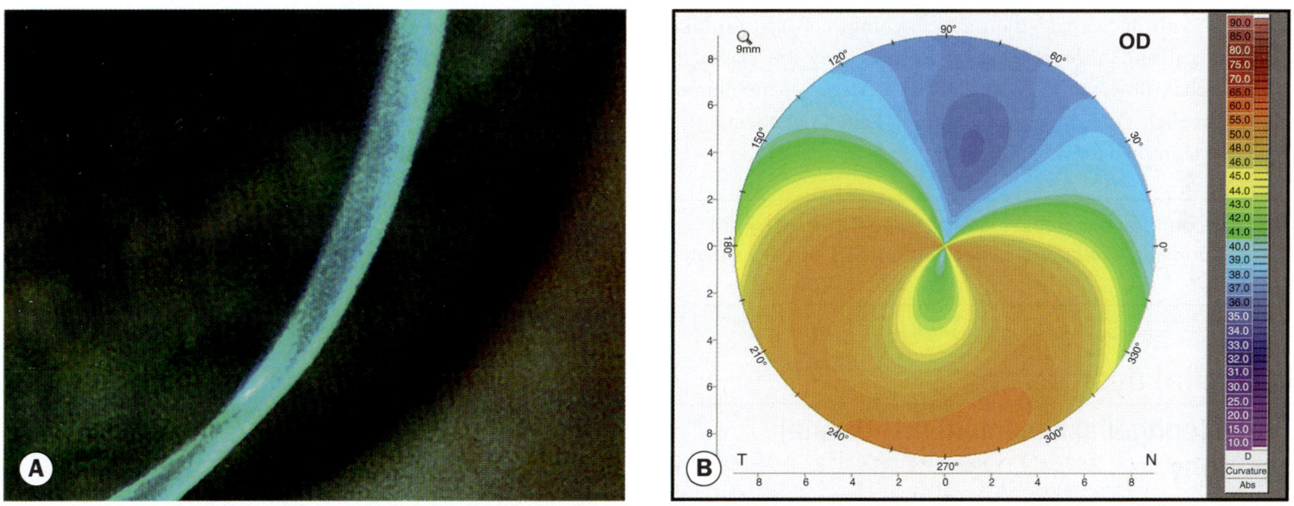

Fig. 7.43 (A) Pellucid marginal degeneration; **(B)** topography showing severe astigmatism and diffuse steepening of the inferior cornea.

Treatment

Early cases are managed with spectacles and contact lenses. Surgical options, none of which is ideal, in patients intolerant to contact lenses include large eccentric penetrating keratoplasty, thermocauterization, crescentic lamellar keratoplasty, wedge resection of diseased tissue, epikeratoplasty and intracorneal ring segment implantation. Results of collagen cross-linking are encouraging.

Keratoglobus

Keratoglobus is an extremely rare condition that can be present at birth when differential diagnosis is from congenital glaucoma and megalocornea and associations may be present, or acquired, with onset in adulthood. In contrast to keratoconus, the cornea develops globular rather than conical ectasia and is associated with generalized corneal thinning (Fig. 7.44). Acute hydrops is rare, but the cornea is more prone to rupture on relatively mild trauma. Corneal

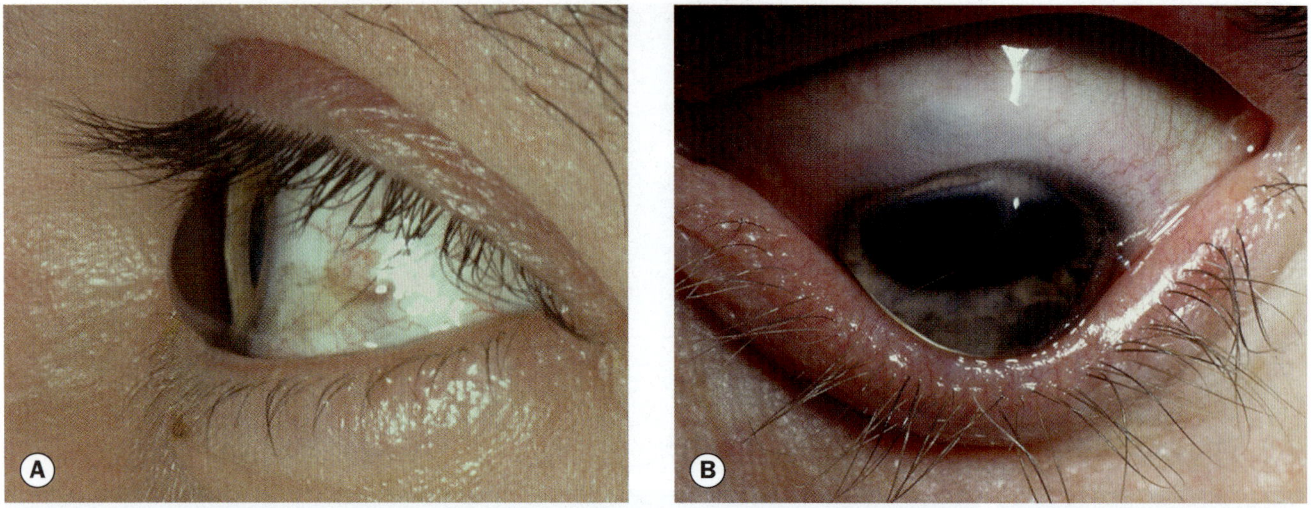

Fig. 7.44 **(A)** Keratoglobus; **(B)** Munson sign in keratoglobus.

topography shows generalized steepening. Surgery is difficult and contact lens wear is often unsatisfactory. Intrastromal ring segments and cross-linking may have utility. Special care should be taken to protect the eyes from trauma.

CORNEAL DYSTROPHY

The corneal dystrophies are a group of progressive, usually bilateral, variable corneal opacifying disorders, many of which are associated with decreased vision and discomfort. Based on biomicroscopical and histopathological features they are classified into epithelial, Bowman layer, stromal and Descemet membrane and endothelial. One or more underlying genetic abnormalities have been identified for most.

TIP As a general rule, most types of corneal dystrophy are bilateral, primarily affect one layer of the cornea and are slowly progressive.

Epithelial dystrophies

Cogan (epithelial basement membrane) dystrophy

Isolated familial cases of epithelial basement membrane (map-dot-fingerprint) corneal dystrophy have been reported. Since most patients seen in clinical practice have no documented family history of the condition, these corneal changes are now considered degenerative or secondary to trauma. The disease is often misdiagnosed, principally because of the variable appearance.

- **Inheritance.** The condition is usually sporadic and these cases may be degenerations rather than true dystrophies, in contrast to the rare familial (autosomal dominant – AD) cases.
- **Histology** shows thickening of the basement membrane with deposition of fibrillary protein between the basement membrane and the Bowman layer. Basal epithelial cell hemidesmosomes are deficient.
- **Onset** is in the second decade. About 10% of patients develop recurrent corneal erosions in the third decade and the remainder are asymptomatic throughout life. The occurrence of bilateral recurrent erosions with no history of trauma suggests basement membrane dystrophy.
- **Signs.** Lesions are often best visualized by retroillumination or scleral scatter. Over time pattern and distribution varies; they may be absent or subtle in a fellow eye. Similar features can be seen with recurrent erosions from any cause.
  - Dot-like and microcystic epithelial lesions (Fig. 7.45A).
  - Subepithelial map-like patterns surrounded by a faint haze (Fig. 7.45B).
  - Whorled fingerprint-like lines.
  - Bleb-like subepithelial pebbled glass pattern.
- **Treatment** is similar to that of recurrent corneal erosions.

Meesmann epithelial dystrophy

Meesmann dystrophy is a rare non-progressive abnormality of corneal epithelial metabolism, underlying which mutations in the genes encoding corneal epithelial keratins have been reported.

- **Inheritance** is AD.
- **Histology** shows irregular thickening of the epithelial basement membrane and intraepithelial cysts.
- **Symptoms.** Patients may be asymptomatic, or there may be recurrent erosions and blurring (usually mild).
- **Signs**
  - Myriad tiny intraepithelial cysts of uniform size but variable density are maximal centrally and extend towards but do not reach the limbus (Fig. 7.45C).
  - The cornea may be slightly thinned and sensation reduced.
- **Treatment** other than lubrication is not normally required.

Others

Other epithelial and subepithelial dystrophies are: gelatinous drop-like corneal dystrophy (Fig. 7.45D), Lisch epithelial corneal dystrophy (Figs 7.45E and F), subepithelial mucinous corneal dystrophy.

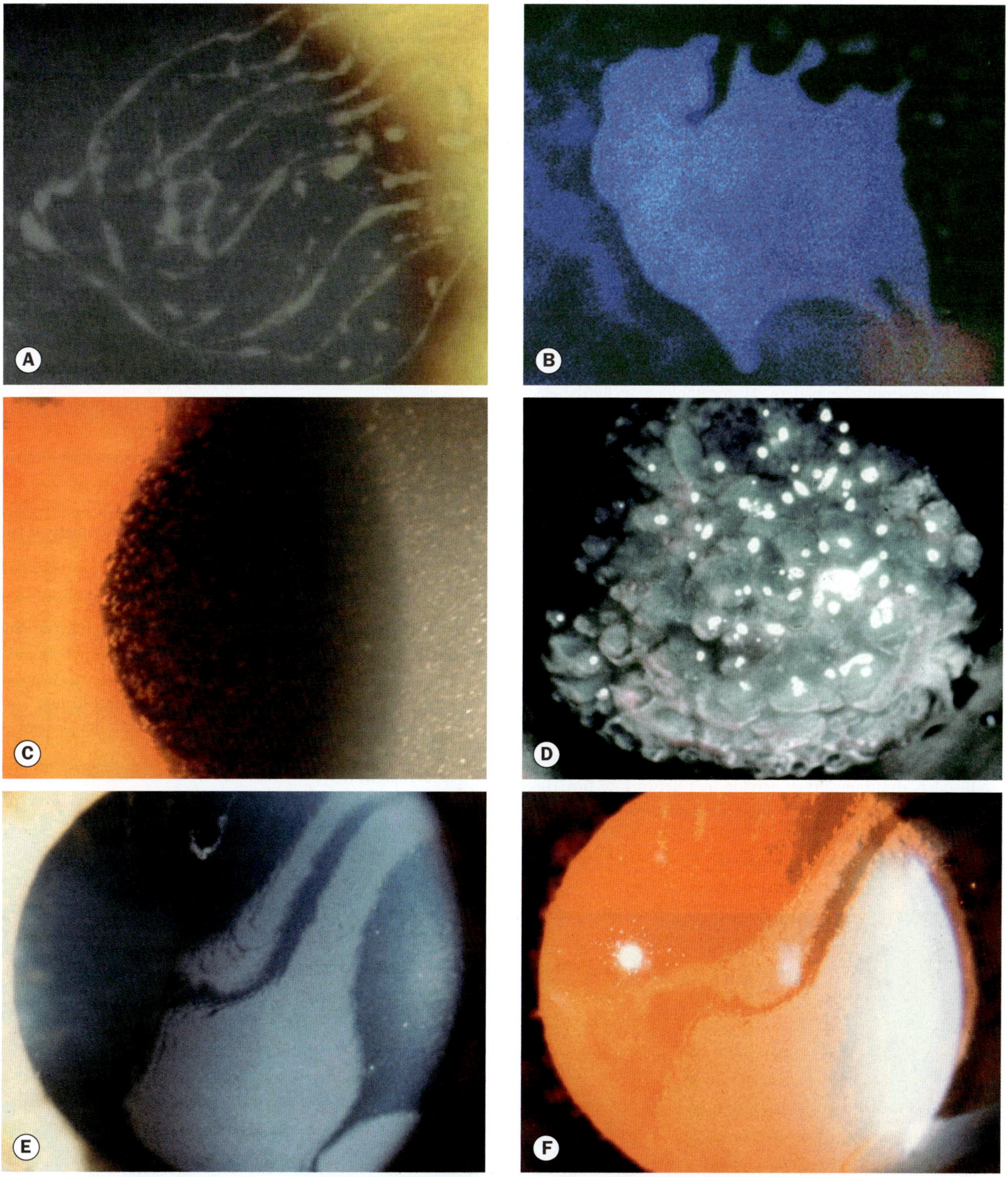

Fig. 7.45 Corneal epithelial and subepithelial dystrophies. **(A)** Cogan – dots and microcysts; **(B)** Cogan – map-like pattern; **(C)** Meesmann – myriad intraepithelial cysts; **(D)** gelatinous drop-like dystrophy; **(E)** Lisch – grey bands with a whorled configuration; **(F)** Lisch – retro-illumination showing densely crowded microcysts. *(Courtesy of D Palay, from J Krachmer, M Mannis and E Holland,* Cornea, *Mosby 2005 – fig. D; W Lisch – figs E and F.)*

Bowman layer/anterior stromal dystrophies

Reis–Bücklers corneal dystrophy

This may be categorized as an anterior variant of granular stromal dystrophy (GCD type 3 – see below) and is also known as corneal basement dystrophy type I (CBD1).

- **Inheritance** is AD; the affected gene is *TGFB1*.
- **Histology.** Replacement of the Bowman layer by connective tissue bands.
- **Symptoms.** Severe recurrent corneal erosions in childhood. Visual impairment may occur.
- **Signs**
    - Grey–white geographic subepithelial opacities, most dense centrally (Fig. 7.46A), increasing in density with age to form a reticular pattern. Histopathology, including electron microscopy, may be required for definitive distinction from Thiel–Behnke dystrophy in some cases.
    - Corneal sensation is reduced.
- **Treatment** is directed at the recurrent erosions. Excimer keratectomy achieves satisfactory control in some patients.

Thiel–Behnke corneal dystrophy

Also termed honeycomb-shaped corneal dystrophy and corneal basement dystrophy type II (CBD2); features are generally less severe than Reis–Bücklers.

- **Inheritance.** AD; gene *TGFB1* and at least one other.
- **Histology.** Bowman layer 'curly fibres' on electron microscopy.
- **Symptoms.** Recurrent erosions in childhood.
- **Signs.** Subepithelial opacities are less individually defined than the granular dystrophy-type lesions (see below) seen in Reis–Bücklers dystrophy. They develop in a network of tiny rings or honeycomb-like morphology, predominantly involving the central cornea (Fig. 7.46B).
- **Treatment** is not always necessary.

Stromal dystrophies

Lattice corneal dystrophy, *TGFB1* type

This is usually regarded as the classic form of lattice dystrophy. Clinical variants (e.g. IIIA – Fig. 7.47A and B) associated with more than 25 heterozygous mutations in *TGFB1* have been described.

- **Inheritance.** AD; gene *TGFB1*.
- **Histology.** Amyloid, staining with Congo red and exhibiting green birefringence with a polarizing filter (Fig. 7.47A).
- **Symptoms.** Recurrent erosions occur at the end of the first decade in the classic form, when typical stromal signs may not yet be present. Blurring may occur later.
- **Signs**
    - Refractile anterior stromal dots (Fig. 7.47C), coalescing into a relatively fine filamentous lattice that spreads gradually but spares the periphery (Fig. 7.47D).
    - A generalized stromal haze may progressively impair vision.
    - Corneal sensation is reduced.
- **Treatment** by penetrating or deep lamellar keratoplasty is frequently required. Recurrence is not uncommon.

Lattice corneal dystrophy, gelsolin type

Also known as LCD_2 and Meretoja syndrome, this is a systemic condition rather than a true corneal dystrophy.

- **Inheritance.** AD; gene *GSN*.
- **Histology** shows amyloid deposits in the corneal stroma.
- **Ocular symptoms.** Ocular irritation and late impairment of vision; erosions are rare.
- **Ocular signs**
    - Sparse stromal lattice lines spread centrally from the periphery.
    - Corneal sensation is impaired.

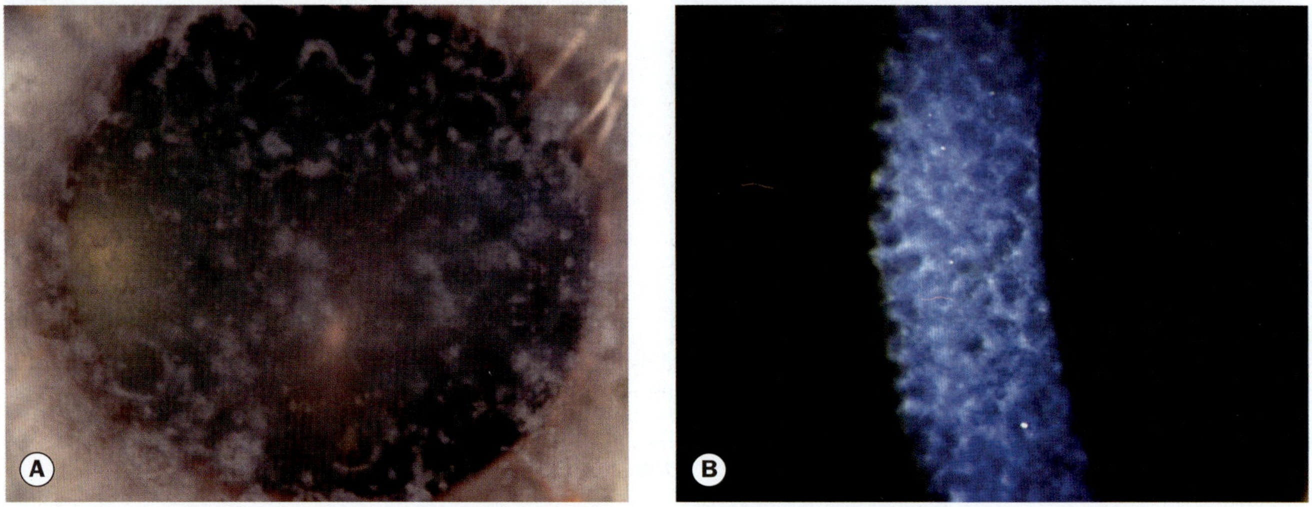

Fig. 7.46 Bowman layer/anterior stromal dystrophy. **(A)** Reis–Bücklers dystrophy showing typical moderately discrete geographical opacities; **(B)** Thiel–Behnke dystrophy. *(Courtesy of W Lisch – fig. A.)*

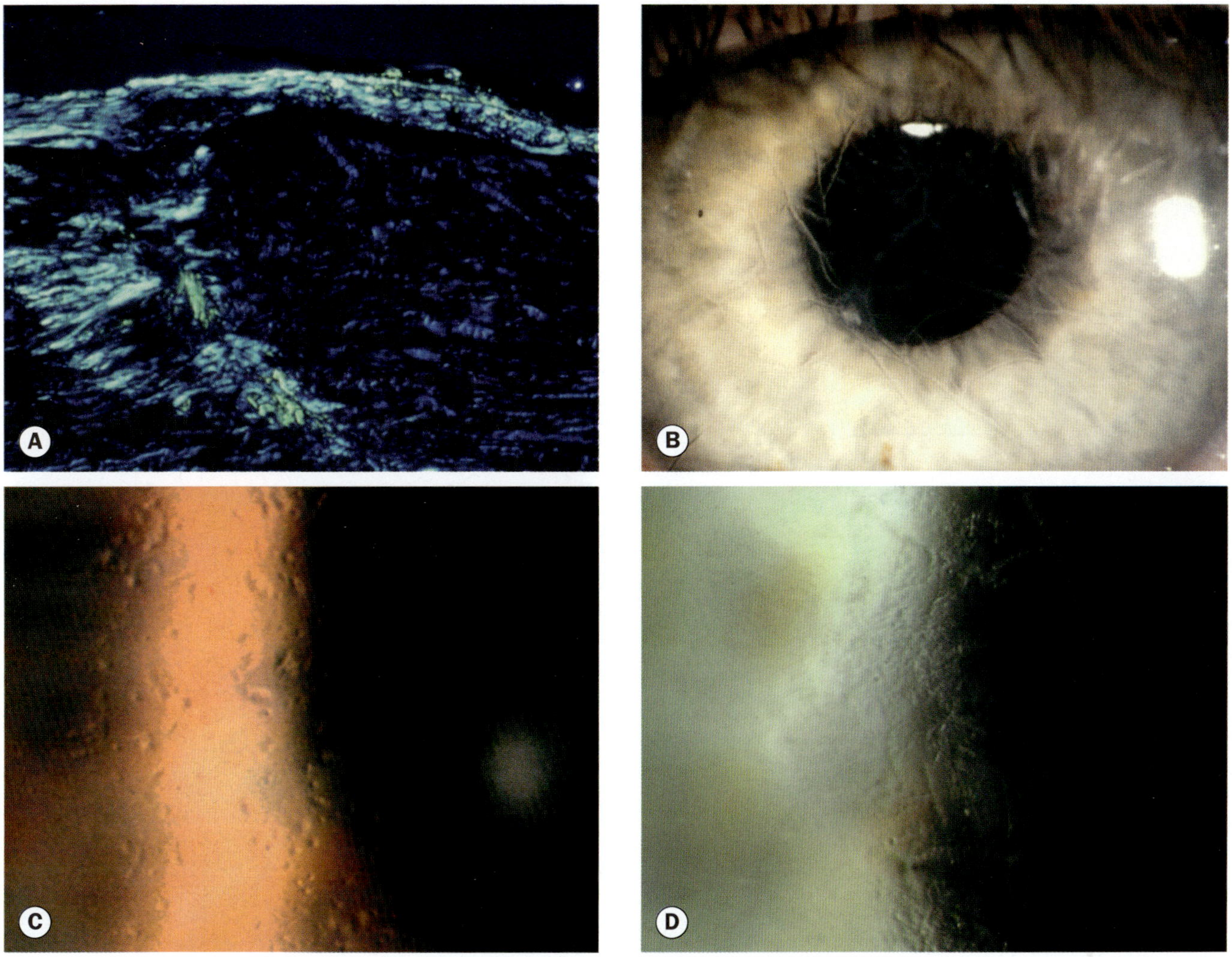

Fig. 7.47 Lattice dystrophy. **(A)** Histology showing green birefringence of amyloid when viewed through polarized light; **(B)** lattice dystrophy type IIIA; **(C)** glassy dots in the anterior stroma in type I; **(D)** fine lattice lines in type I. *(Courtesy of C Barry – fig. D.)*

- **Systemic features.** Progressive cranial and peripheral neuropathy, mask-like facies and autonomic features. Homozygous disease is rare but severe.
- **Treatment.** Keratoplasty may rarely be required in later life.

Granular corneal dystrophy, type 1 (classic)

- **Inheritance.** AD; gene *TGFB1*. Homozygous disease gives more severe features.
- **Histology.** Amorphous hyaline deposits staining bright red with Masson trichrome (Fig. 7.48A).
- **Symptoms.** Glare and photophobia, with blurring as progression occurs. Recurrent erosions are uncommon.
- **Signs**
  - Discrete white central anterior stromal deposits resembling sugar granules, breadcrumbs or glass splinters separated by clear stroma (Fig. 7.48B).
  - Gradual increase in number and size of the deposits with deeper and outward spread, sparing the limbus.
  - Gradual confluence and diffuse haze lead to visual impairment (Fig. 7.48C).
  - Corneal sensation is impaired.
- **Treatment** by penetrating or deep lamellar keratoplasty is usually required by the fifth decade. Superficial recurrences may require repeated excimer laser keratectomy.

Granular corneal dystrophy, type 2

Also known as Avellino and combined granular-lattice dystrophy.

- **Inheritance.** AD; gene *TGFB1*.
- **Histology** shows both hyaline and amyloid.
- **Symptoms.** Recurrent erosions tend to be mild. Visual impairment is a later feature.
- **Signs** are usually present by the end of the first decade in heterozygotes. Fine superficial opacities progress to form stellate or annular lesions (Fig. 7.48D), sometimes associated with deeper linear opacities.
- **Treatment** is usually not required. Corneal trauma accelerates progression; refractive surgery is contraindicated.

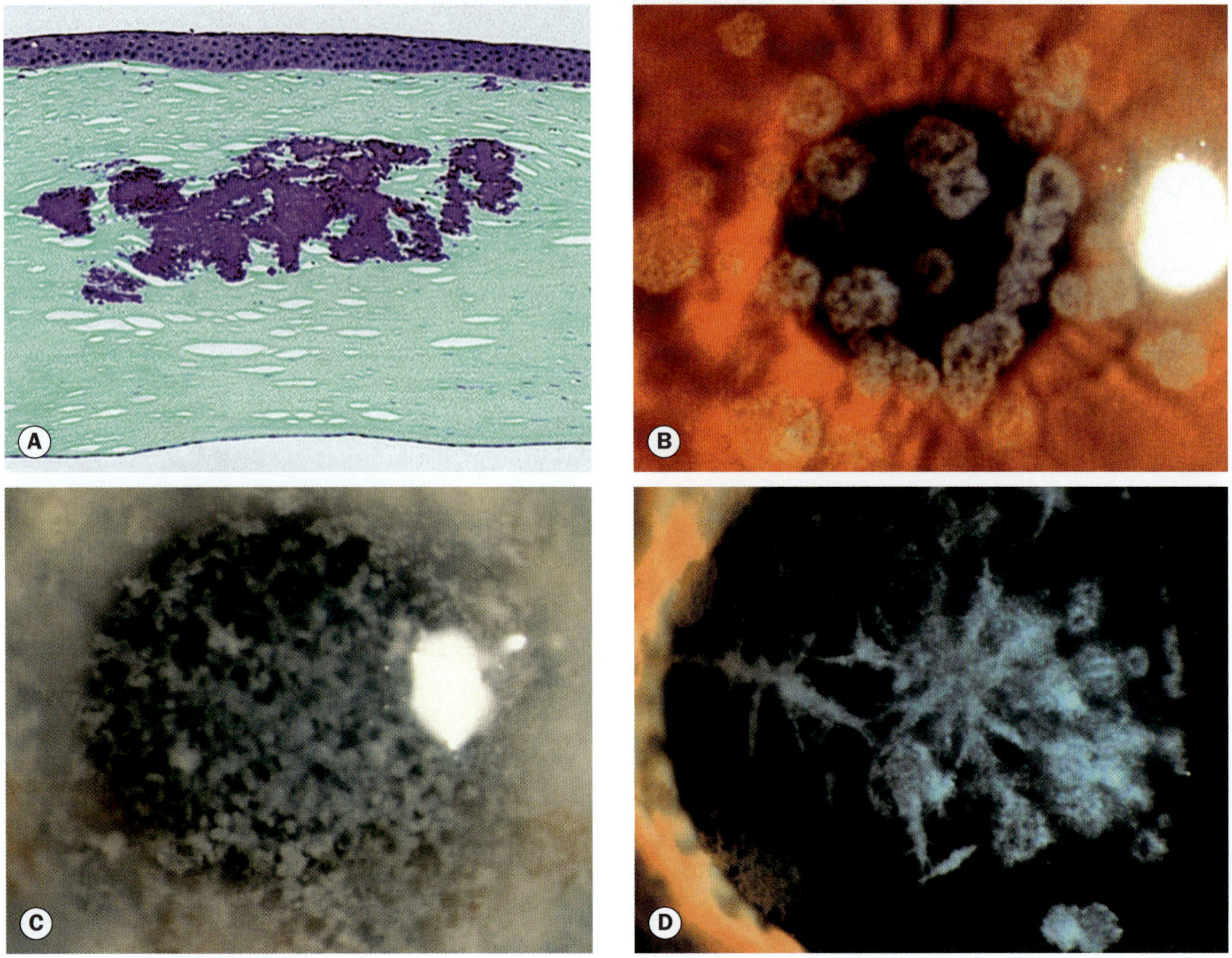

Fig. 7.48 Granular dystrophy type I. **(A)** Histology showing red-staining material with Masson trichrome; **(B)** sharply demarcated crumb-like opacities; **(C)** confluence with outward spread; **(D)** granular dystrophy type II (Avellino). *(Courtesy of W Lisch – fig. D.)*

Macular corneal dystrophy

- **Inheritance.** Autosomal recessive (AR); gene *CHST6*; the condition is relatively common in Iceland.
- **Histology.** Aggregations of glycosaminoglycans intra- and extracellularly; stain with Alcian blue and colloidal iron (Fig. 7.49A).
- **Symptoms.** Early (end of first decade) visual deterioration; recurrent erosions are very common.
- **Signs**
  - Dense but poorly delineated greyish-white spots centrally in the anterior stroma and peripherally in the posterior stroma (Fig. 7.49B and C). There is no clear delineation between opacities, which may be elevated.
  - Progression of the lesions occurs in conjunction with anterior stromal haze, initially involving the central cornea (Fig. 7.49D).
  - There is eventual involvement of full-thickness stroma, extending to the limbus with no clear zone.
  - Thinning is a fairly early feature, with late thickening from oedema due to endothelial dysfunction.
  - Sensation is reduced.
- **Treatment.** Penetrating keratoplasty. Recurrence is common.

Schnyder (crystalline) corneal dystrophy

This is a disorder of corneal lipid metabolism, associated in some patients with systemic dyslipidaemia. The use of crystalline in the name is no longer recommended as corneal crystals are not a ubiquitous feature.

- **Inheritance.** AD; gene *UBIAD1*.
- **Histology.** Phospholipid and cholesterol deposits.
- **Symptoms.** Visual impairment and glare.
- **Signs**
  - Central haze is an early feature (Fig. 7.50A), progressing to more widespread full-thickness involvement over time (Fig. 7.50B).

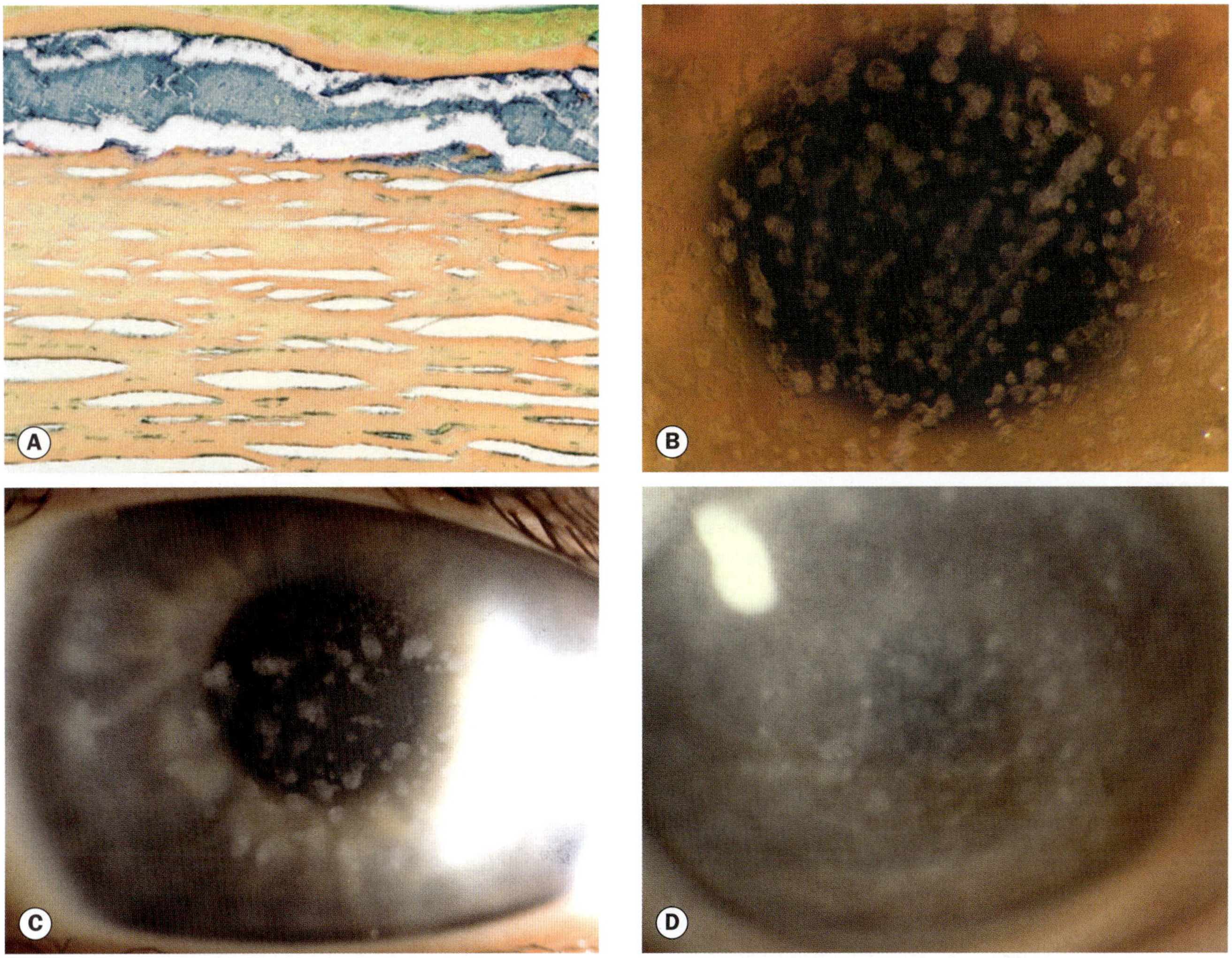

Fig. 7.49 Macular dystrophy. **(A)** Histology showing deposits of abnormal glycosaminoglycans that appear blue with colloidal iron stain; **(B)** and **(C)** poorly delineated deposits increase in number; **(D)** increase in size and confluence of lesions, with stromal haze.

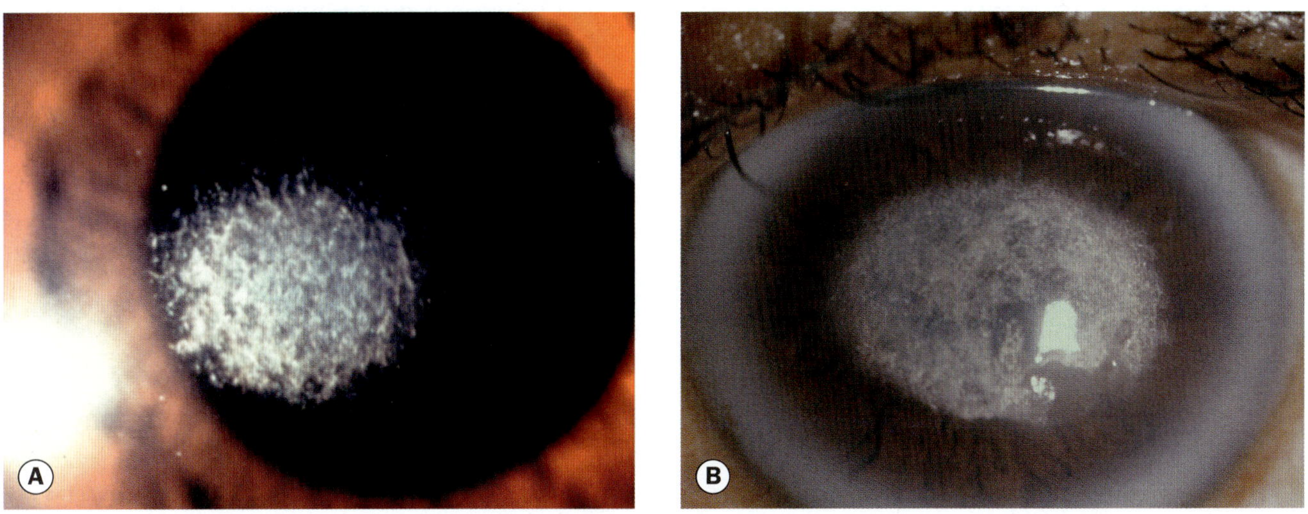

Fig. 7.50 Schnyder dystrophy. **(A)** Early lesion; **(B)** late appearance showing diffuse haze. *(Courtesy of K Nischal – fig. A; T Carmichael – fig. B.)*

- Subepithelial crystalline opacities are present in only around 50%.
- Prominent corneal arcus is typical and gradually progresses centrally leading to diffuse haze.

- **Treatment** is by excimer keratectomy or corneal transplantation.

François central cloudy dystrophy

It is not certain that this entity is a dystrophy; it may be clinically indistinguishable from the degeneration posterior crocodile shagreen.

- **Inheritance.** AD has been reported, but not clearly established.
- **Symptoms.** Almost always none.
- **Signs.** Cloudy greyish polygonal or rounded posterior stromal opacities, most prominent centrally (Fig. 7.51).
- **Treatment** is not required.

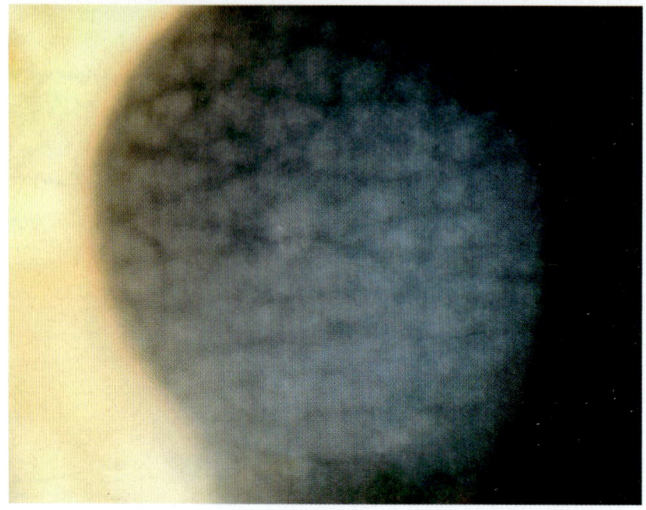

Fig. 7.51 Marked signs in François central cloudy dystrophy. *(Courtesy of W Lisch.)*

Others

Congenital stromal corneal dystrophy, fleck corneal dystrophy, posterior amorphous corneal dystrophy and pre-Descemet corneal dystrophy.

Descemet membrane and endothelial dystrophies

Fuchs endothelial corneal dystrophy

This disorder is characterized by bilateral accelerated endothelial cell loss. It is more common in women and is associated with a slightly increased prevalence of glaucoma.

- **Inheritance.** Most are sporadic, with occasional AD inheritance. Mutation in *COL8A2* has been identified in an early-onset variant and in the *TCF4* gene in most other cases.
- **Symptoms.** Gradually worsening blurring, particularly in the morning, due to corneal oedema. Onset is usually in middle age or later.
- **Signs**
  - Cornea guttata: the presence of irregular warts or 'excrescences' on Descemet membrane secreted by abnormal endothelial cells (Fig. 7.52A).
  - Subtle corneal endothelial radial lines which correlate with the peripheral cell arrangement that is seen microscopically.
  - Specular reflection shows tiny dark spots caused by disruption of the regular endothelial mosaic (Fig. 7.52B). Progression occurs to a 'beaten metal' appearance (Fig. 7.52C).
  - Endothelial decompensation gradually leads to central stromal oedema and blurred vision, worse in the morning.
  - Epithelial oedema develops in more advanced cases, with the formation of microcysts and bullae (bullous keratopathy – Fig. 7.52D) accompanied by discomfort. Rupture of bullae is associated with marked acute pain secondary to the exposure of nerve fibres. Subepithelial scarring and peripheral vascularization may be seen in longstanding cases.
- **Treatment**
  - Conservative options include topical sodium chloride 5% drops or ointment, reduction of IOP and use of a hair dryer for corneal dehydration.
  - Ruptured bullae can be made more comfortable by the use of bandage contact lenses, cycloplegia, antibiotic ointment and lubricants. Anterior stromal puncture may be helpful.
  - Posterior lamellar keratoplasty (e.g. Descemet membrane-stripping automated endothelial keratoplasty – DSAEK – or Descemet membrane endothelial keratoplasty – DMEK) and penetrating keratoplasty (see Ch. 7) have a high success rate.
  - Options in eyes with poor visual potential include conjunctival flaps and amniotic membrane transplantation.
  - A promising new treatment, topical Rho-kinase inhibitor with prior transcorneal endothelial cryotherapy, seems to stimulate endothelial cell proliferation and improve function.
- **Cataract surgery** may worsen the corneal status because of endothelial cell loss and protective steps should be taken to reduce this. Modern machines using torsional phacoemulsification use less ultrasound time than the older machines, which used longitudinal phacoemulsification and are therefore less likely to cause endothelial loss. A 'triple procedure' (combined cataract surgery, lens implantation and keratoplasty) may be considered in eyes with corneal oedema. Corneal oedema is less likely to occur after cataract surgery if the central corneal thickness is less than 630–640 μm.

TIP Persistent corneal oedema may follow cataract surgery in a patient with Fuchs endothelial dystrophy, particularly if the preoperative central corneal thickness is more than 630–640 μm.

Posterior polymorphous corneal dystrophy

There are three forms of posterior polymorphous dystrophy, PPCD1–3. Associations include iris abnormalities, glaucoma and Alport syndrome. The pathological basis involves metaplasia of endothelial cells.

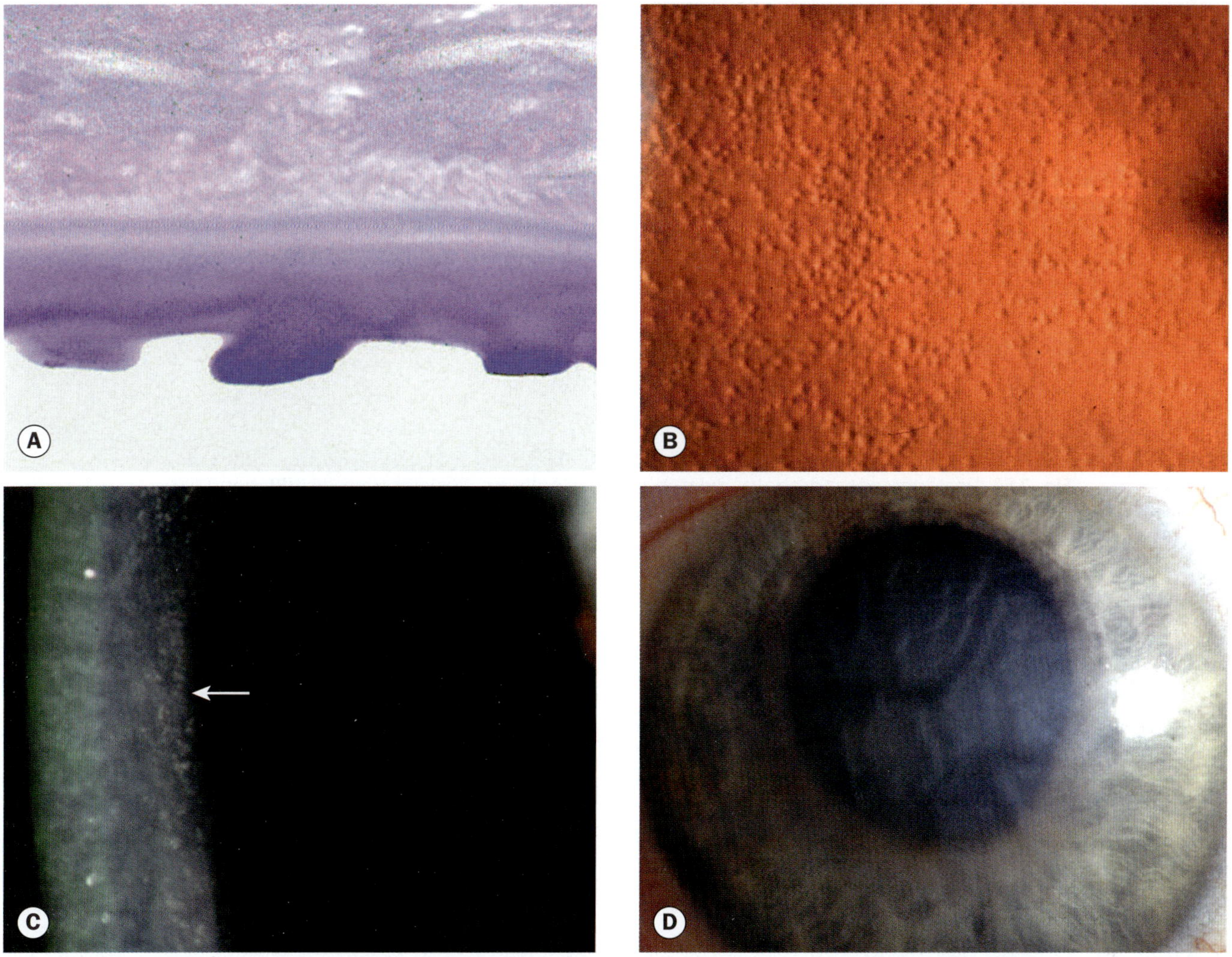

Fig. 7.52 Fuchs endothelial dystrophy. **(A)** Histology of cornea guttata showing irregular excrescences of Descemet membrane – PAS stain; **(B)** cornea guttata seen on specular reflection; **(C)** 'beaten-metal' endothelium (arrow); **(D)** corneal oedema.

- **Inheritance** is usually AD. The gene *VSX1* has been implicated in PPCD1, PPCD2 is caused by mutations in *COL8A2* and PPCD3 by *ZEB1* mutations.
- **Symptoms.** Usually absent, with incidental diagnosis.
- **Signs.** Subtle vesicular, band-like or diffuse endothelial lesions (Fig. 7.53A and B).
- **Treatment** is not required.

Congenital hereditary endothelial dystrophy

Congenital hereditary endothelial dystrophy (CHED) is a rare dystrophy in which there is focal or diffuse thickening of Descemet membrane and endothelial degeneration. CHED2 is a more common and more severe form than CHED1 and is occasionally associated with late-onset deafness (Harboyan syndrome).

- **Inheritance**
  - CHED1 is AD with the gene locus on chromosome 20. CHED1 may not be distinct from PPCD.
  - CHED2 is AR; gene *SLC4A11*.
- **Symptoms.** Photophobia and watering are common in CHED1, but not in CHED2.
- **Signs**
  - Corneal clouding and thickening (Fig. 7.54) are neonatal in CHED2 and develop during the first year or two in CHED1.
  - Visual impairment is variable and visual acuity may surpass that expected from the corneal appearance.
  - Nystagmus is more common in CHED2.
- **Treatment.** Lamellar or penetrating keratoplasty.

CORNEAL DEGENERATION

Age-related degeneration

Arcus senilis

Arcus senilis (gerontoxon, arcus lipoides) is the most common peripheral corneal opacity. It frequently occurs without any

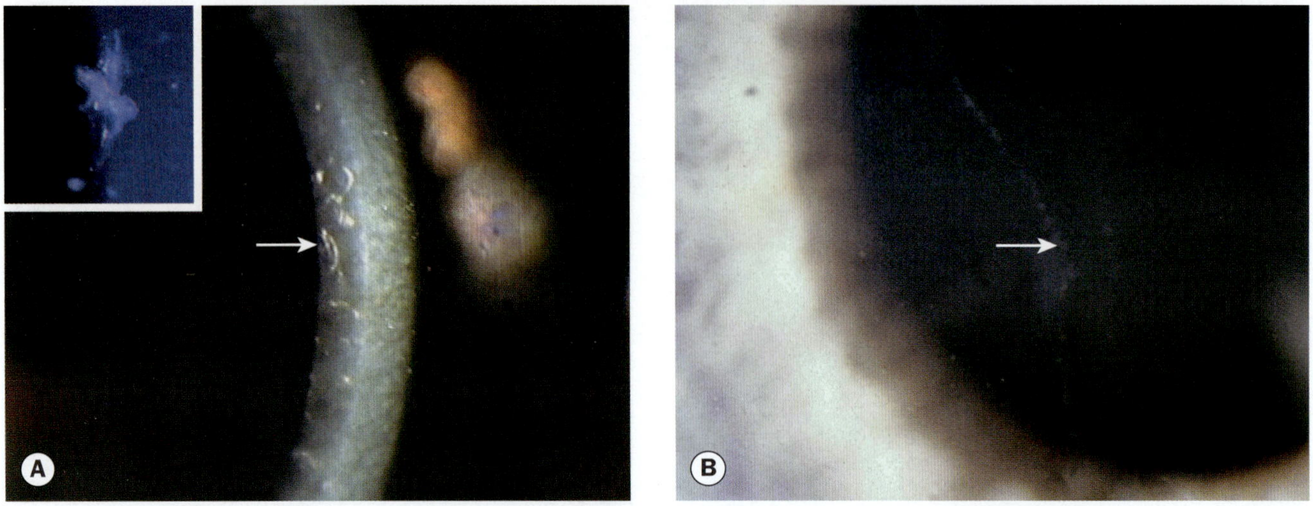

Fig. 7.53 Posterior polymorphous dystrophy. **(A)** Confluent vesicles (arrow); **(B)** band-like lesions (arrow). *(Courtesy of W Lisch – fig. A.)*

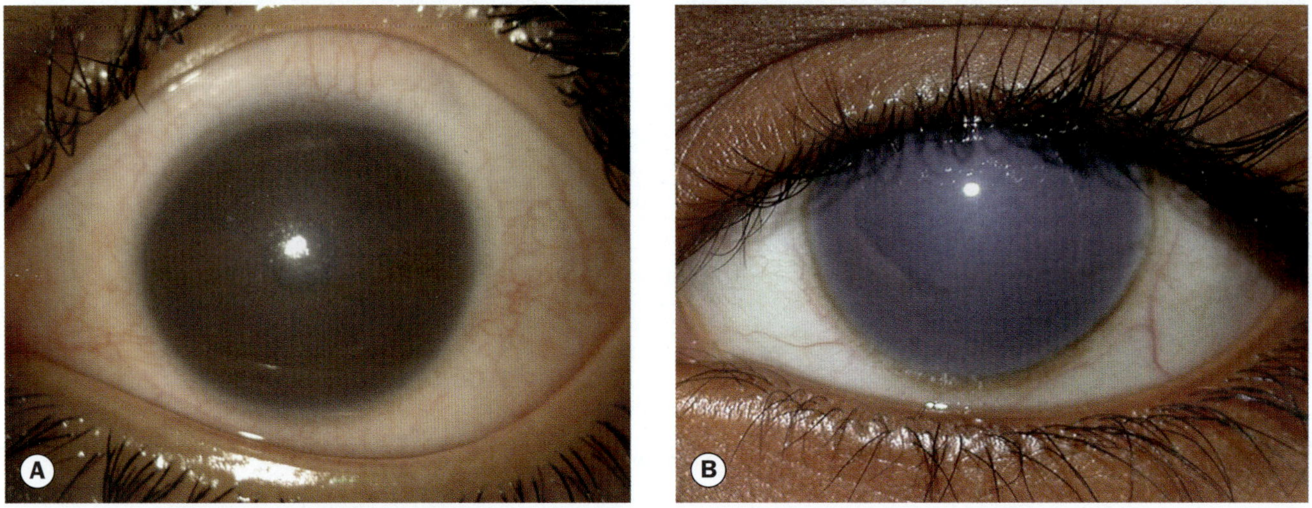

Fig. 7.54 Congenital hereditary endothelial dystrophy. **(A)** Mild corneal clouding; **(B)** moderate severity in an older child. Visual acuity may surpass that expected from the corneal appearance. *(Courtesy of R Fogla – fig. A.)*

predisposing systemic condition in elderly individuals, but may be associated with dyslipidaemia in younger patients (arcus juvenilis).

- **Signs**
  - Stromal lipid deposition, initially in the superior and inferior perilimbal cornea, progressing circumferentially to form a band about 1 mm wide (Fig. 7.55A).
  - The band is usually wider in the vertical than horizontal meridian.
  - The central border is diffuse, and the peripheral edge is sharp and separated from the limbus by a clear zone that may undergo mild thinning.

Vogt limbal girdle

Vogt limbal girdle is an innocuous condition that is present in up to 60% of individuals over 40 years of age, more commonly in women. It consists of whitish crescentic limbal bands composed of chalk-like flecks centred at 9 and/or 3 o'clock, more often nasally. There may be irregular central extension. **Type I** may be a variant of band keratopathy, featuring a 'Swiss cheese' hole pattern and a clear area separating the lesion from the scleral margin (Fig. 7.55B). **Type II** is more prevalent and is distinguished by the absence of holes and typically also of a juxtalimbal clear zone (Fig. 7.55C). Histologically the changes in both are similar to pinguecula and pterygium.

Cornea farinata

Cornea farinata is a visually insignificant condition characterized by bilateral, minute, flour-like deposits in the deep stroma, most prominent centrally (Fig. 7.55D).

Crocodile shagreen

Crocodile shagreen is characterized by asymptomatic, greyish-white, polygonal stromal opacities separated by relatively clear spaces (Fig. 7.55E). The opacities most frequently involve the anterior two-thirds of the stroma (anterior crocodile shagreen), but on occasion may be found more posteriorly (posterior

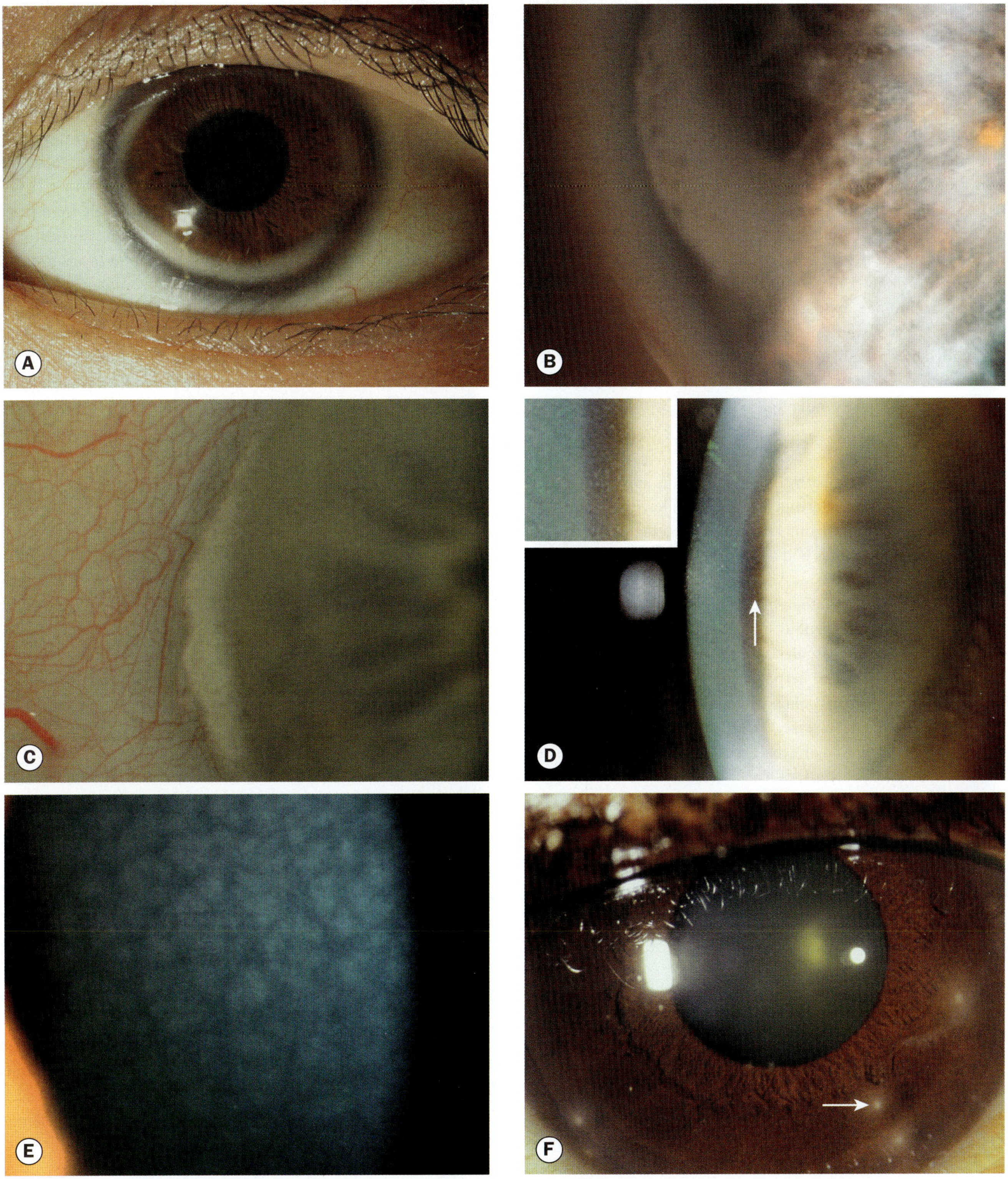

Fig. 7.55 Age-related degenerations. **(A)** Arcus senilis; **(B)** Vogt limbal girdle type I; **(C)** Vogt limbal girdle type II; **(D)** cornea farinata (arrow); **(E)** crocodile shagreen; **(F)** West Indian punctate keratopathy (arrow).

crocodile shagreen). It may be indistinguishable from François central cloudy dystrophy; conventionally the distinction is on the basis of François dystrophy being inherited, but this has been questioned.

West Indian punctate keratopathy

This is an unusual condition of unknown cause that is seen in elderly asymptomatic individuals, generally of West Indian origin. Males are more affected than females. It normally affects only one eye, but is occasionally bilateral, with one to four lesions found in the interpalpebral fissure outside the visual axis. The lesions are round, measuring 0.5 mm or less, and are located at the level of Bowman membrane, extending just into the superficial stroma. They usually have a central dot which is intensely white in colour, surrounded by a paler halo which merges with the adjacent cornea. The corneal epithelium appears normal and does not stain with fluorescein. Treatment is not required (Fig. 7.55F).

Lipid keratopathy

- **Primary** lipid keratopathy is rare and occurs apparently spontaneously. It is characterized by white or yellowish, often with a crystalline element, stromal deposits consisting of cholesterol, fats and phospholipids and is not associated with vascularization (Fig. 7.56A).
- **Secondary** lipid keratopathy is much more common and is associated with previous ocular injury or disease that has resulted in corneal vascularization. The most common causes are herpes simplex and herpes zoster keratitis (Fig. 7.56B).
- **Treatment** is primarily aimed at medical control of the underlying inflammatory disease. Other options include:
  - Photocoagulation or needle cautery (suture needle grasped with cautery forceps) of feeder vessels.
  - Penetrating keratoplasty may be required in advanced but quiescent disease, though vascularization, thinning and reduced sensation may affect the outcome.

Band keratopathy

Band keratopathy consists of the age-related deposition of calcium salts in the Bowman layer, epithelial basement membrane and anterior stroma.

- **Causes**
  - Ocular. Chronic anterior uveitis (particularly in children with juvenile idiopathic arthritis), glaucoma, phthisis bulbi, silicone oil in the anterior chamber, chronic corneal oedema and severe chronic keratitis.
  - Age-related affecting otherwise healthy individuals.
  - Metabolic (metastatic calcification) secondary to hypercalcaemia is uncommon and includes causes like hyperparathyroidism, vitamin D toxicity, milk-alkali syndrome, sarcoidosis, end-stage renal disease, Paget disease and multiple myeloma. Hyperuricaemia is a rare cause.
  - Hereditary causes include familial cases and ichthyosis.
- **Signs**
  - Peripheral interpalpebral calcification with clear cornea separating the sharp peripheral margins of the band from the limbus (Fig. 7.57A).
  - Gradual central spread to form a band-like chalky plaque containing transparent small holes (Fig. 7.57B) and occasionally clefts.
  - Advanced lesions may become nodular and elevated with considerable discomfort due to epithelial breakdown.
- **Treatment** is indicated if vision is threatened or if the eye is uncomfortable. It is important to recognize and treat any underlying condition.
  - Chelation is simple and effective for relatively mild cases and is performed using a microscope. The corneal epithelium overlying the opacity and a solid layer of calcification are first scraped off with forceps and a scalpel blade (e.g. No. 15). The cornea is then rubbed with a cotton-tipped applicator dipped in a solution of ethylenediaminetetraacetic acid (EDTA) 1.5–3.0% until all calcium has been removed. Adequate time (15–20 minutes) must be allowed for chelation to occur and more than one session may be necessary. Re-epithelialization can take many days.
  - Other modalities: diamond burr, excimer laser keratectomy and lamellar keratoplasty.

Spheroidal degeneration

Spheroidal degeneration (Labrador keratopathy, climatic droplet keratopathy) typically occurs in men whose working lives are spent outdoors. Ultraviolet exposure is likely to be an aetiological factor. The condition is relatively innocuous but visual impairment may occur. A secondary form can follow inflammation or injury.

- **Histology.** Irregular proteinaceous deposits in the anterior stroma that replace the Bowman layer.
- **Signs**
  - Amber-coloured granules in the superficial stroma of the peripheral interpalpebral cornea (Fig. 7.58A).
  - Increasing opacification, coalescence and central spread.
  - Advanced lesions commonly protrude above the corneal surface (Fig. 7.58B) and the surrounding stroma is often hazy. The conjunctiva can be involved.
- **Treatment.** Protection against ultraviolet damage with sunglasses and superficial keratectomy or lamellar keratoplasty in a minority.

Salzmann nodular degeneration

Salzmann nodular degeneration consists of nodules of hyaline tissue, usually located anterior to the Bowman layer. It can occur in any form of chronic corneal irritation or inflammation such as trachoma, dry eye, chronic blepharitis and chronic allergic keratoconjunctivitis.

- **Signs**
  - Superficial stromal opacities progressing to elevated whitish or blue–grey nodular lesions that may be round or elongated (Fig. 7.59).
  - The base of a nodule may be associated with pannus and epithelial iron deposition.
- **Treatment** consists mainly of lubrication together with control of the cause. Removal is via manual superficial keratectomy – the lesions can often be 'peeled' away and the surface flattened

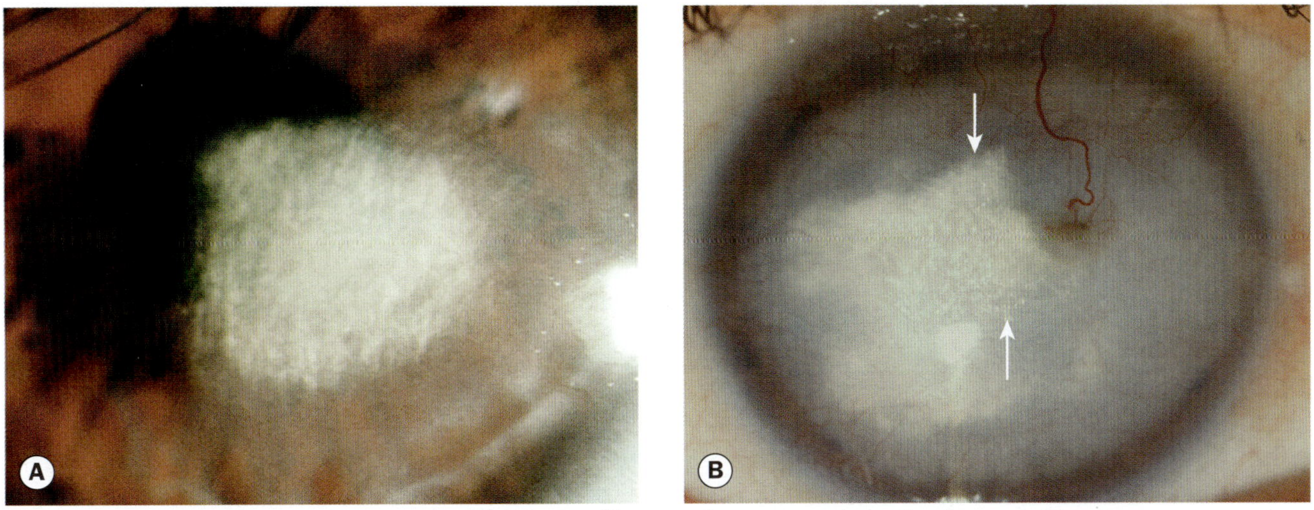

Fig. 7.56 Lipid keratopathy. **(A)** Primary; **(B)** secondary to vascularization (arrows). *(Courtesy T Carmichael – fig. B.)*

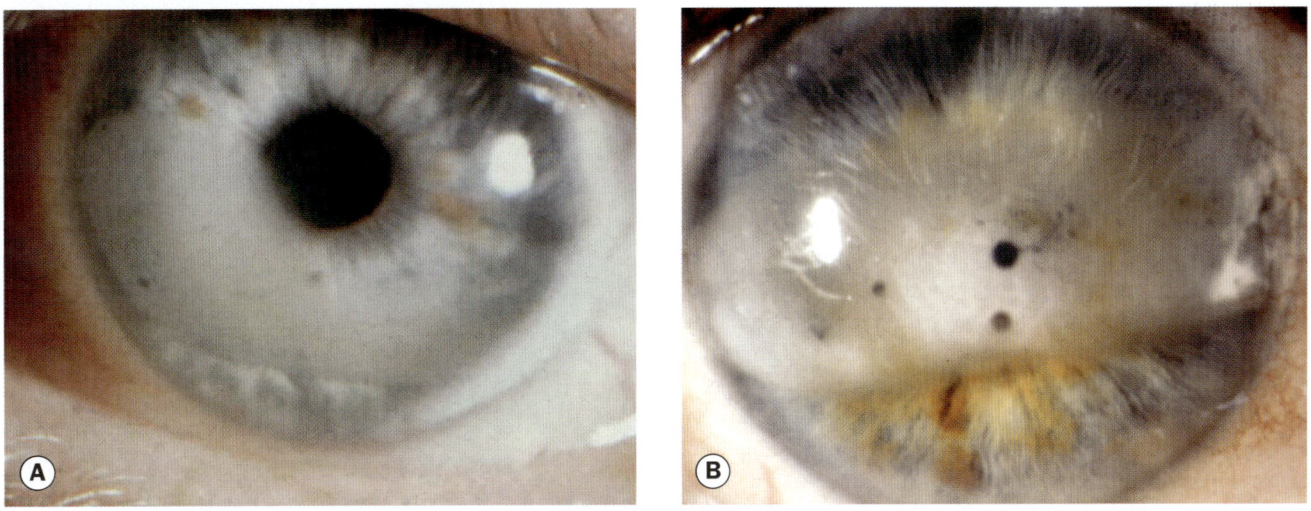

Fig. 7.57 Band keratopathy. **(A)** Typical appearance outside the visual axis; **(B)** advanced disease with small epithelial holes.

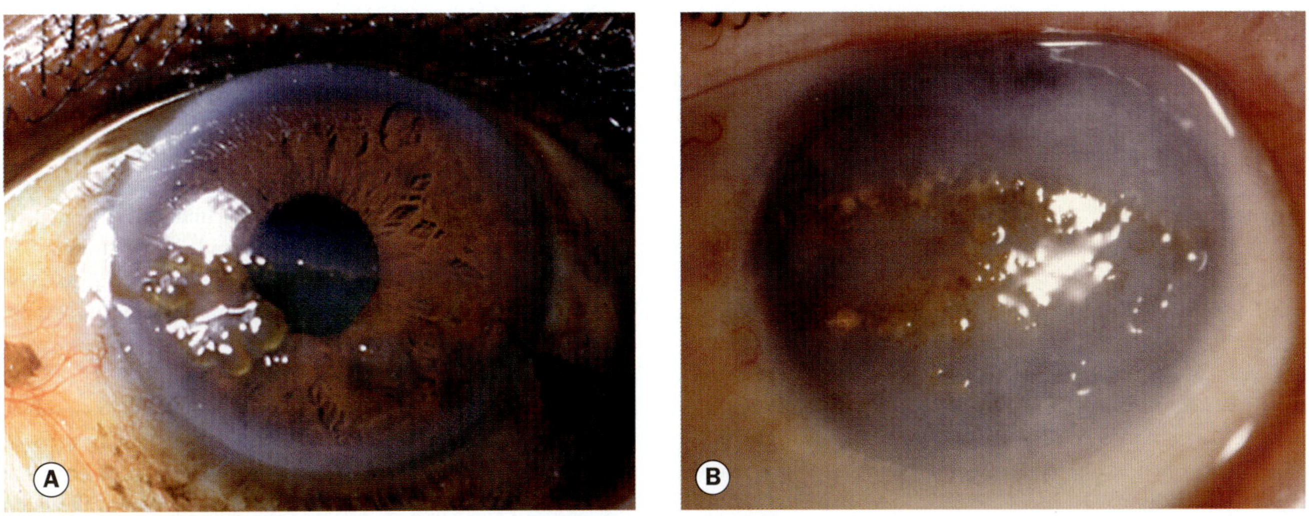

Fig. 7.58 Spheroidal degeneration. **(A)** Early; **(B)** advanced.

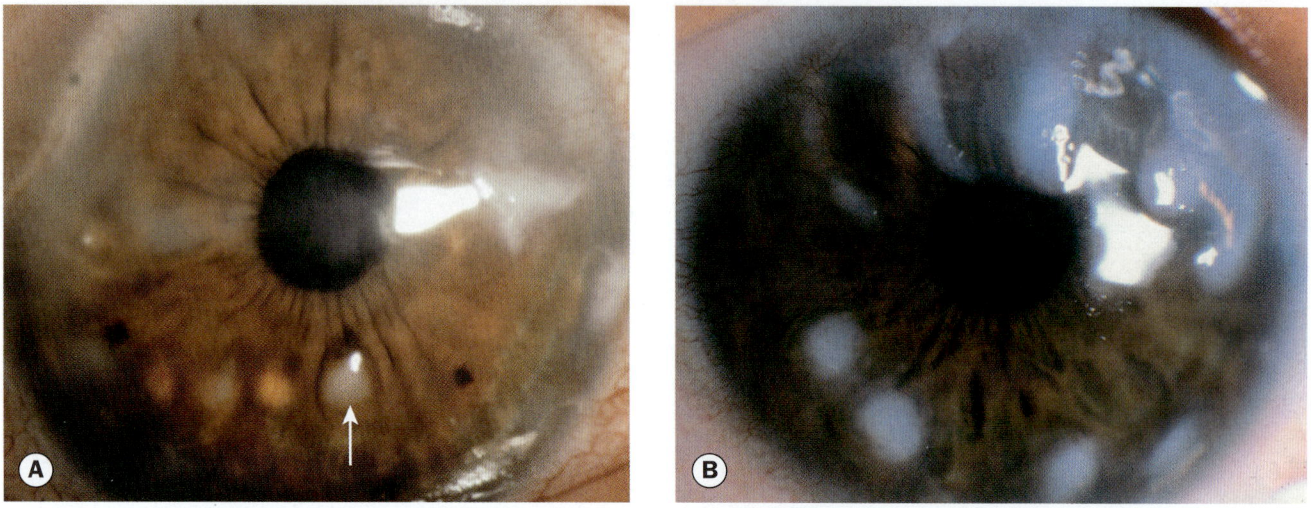

Fig. 7.59 Salzmann nodular degeneration. **(A)** Typical appearance (arrow); **(B)** multiple lesions. *(Courtesy of R Bates – fig. B.)*

with a diamond burr. Adjunctive mitomycin C applied for 10 seconds with a sponge may reduce the recurrence rate, though some authorities restrict its use to reoperations. Excimer laser phototherapeutic keratectomy or lamellar keratoplasty are occasionally required.

Advancing wave-like epitheliopathy

Advancing wave-like epitheliopathy (AWE) is characterized by an irregular advancing epithelial plaque encroaching gradually on the cornea, typically originating at the superior limbus (Fig. 7.60) and sometimes extending circumferentially from a pterygium. Topical fluorescein generally demonstrates the lesion well. Irritation and redness are common. The vision may be affected with central involvement. Reported risk factors include contact lens wear, certain contact lens solutions, topical glaucoma medication, prior ocular surgery and some skin conditions such as rosacea. Treatment of the cause may be curative, but otherwise is with 1% silver nitrate solution to the adjacent limbus or cryotherapy (1–2 seconds twice) to the limbus and abnormal tissue. Distinction from neoplasia may occasionally warrant impression cytology or excision biopsy.

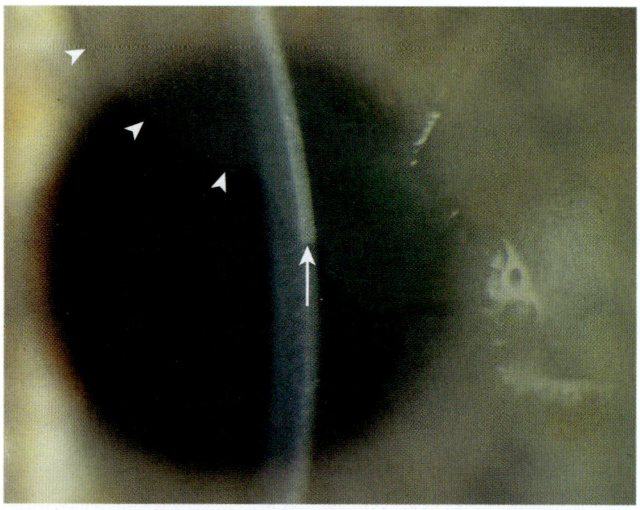

Fig. 7.60 Advancing wave-like epitheliopathy (arrowheads). Inferior extent illuminated in the slit beam (arrow).

METABOLIC KERATOPATHY

Cystinosis

Cystinosis is a rare AR (gene: *CTNS*) lysosomal storage disorder characterized by widespread tissue deposition of cystine crystals, leading to paediatric renal failure and a range of other severe systemic problems. Non-nephropathic (ocular), nephropathic and intermediate forms can occur. Keratopathy may develop in the first year, with progressive deposition of crystals in the cornea (Fig. 7.61A) and conjunctiva associated with photophobia, epithelial erosions and visual impairment. Systemic treatment is with cysteamine, which can be given in eye drop form to reverse corneal crystal formation.

Mucopolysaccharidoses

The mucopolysaccharidoses (MPS) are a group of lysosomal storage disorders involving enzyme dysfunction along the pathways for breakdown of glycosaminoglycans, long chain carbohydrates formerly known as mucopolysaccharides. Altered metabolites accumulate intracellularly in various tissues. Inheritance is mainly AR. Systemic features vary with the type of MPS, but can include facial coarseness, skeletal anomalies, heart disease and learning difficulties. Keratopathy comprises punctate corneal opacification and diffuse stromal haze (Fig. 7.61B) and occurs in all MPS except Hunter and Sanfilippo. Other ocular features may include pigmentary retinopathy and optic atrophy.

Wilson disease

Wilson disease (hepatolenticular degeneration) is a rare condition involving the widespread abnormal deposition of copper in tissues. It is caused by a deficiency of caeruloplasmin, the major

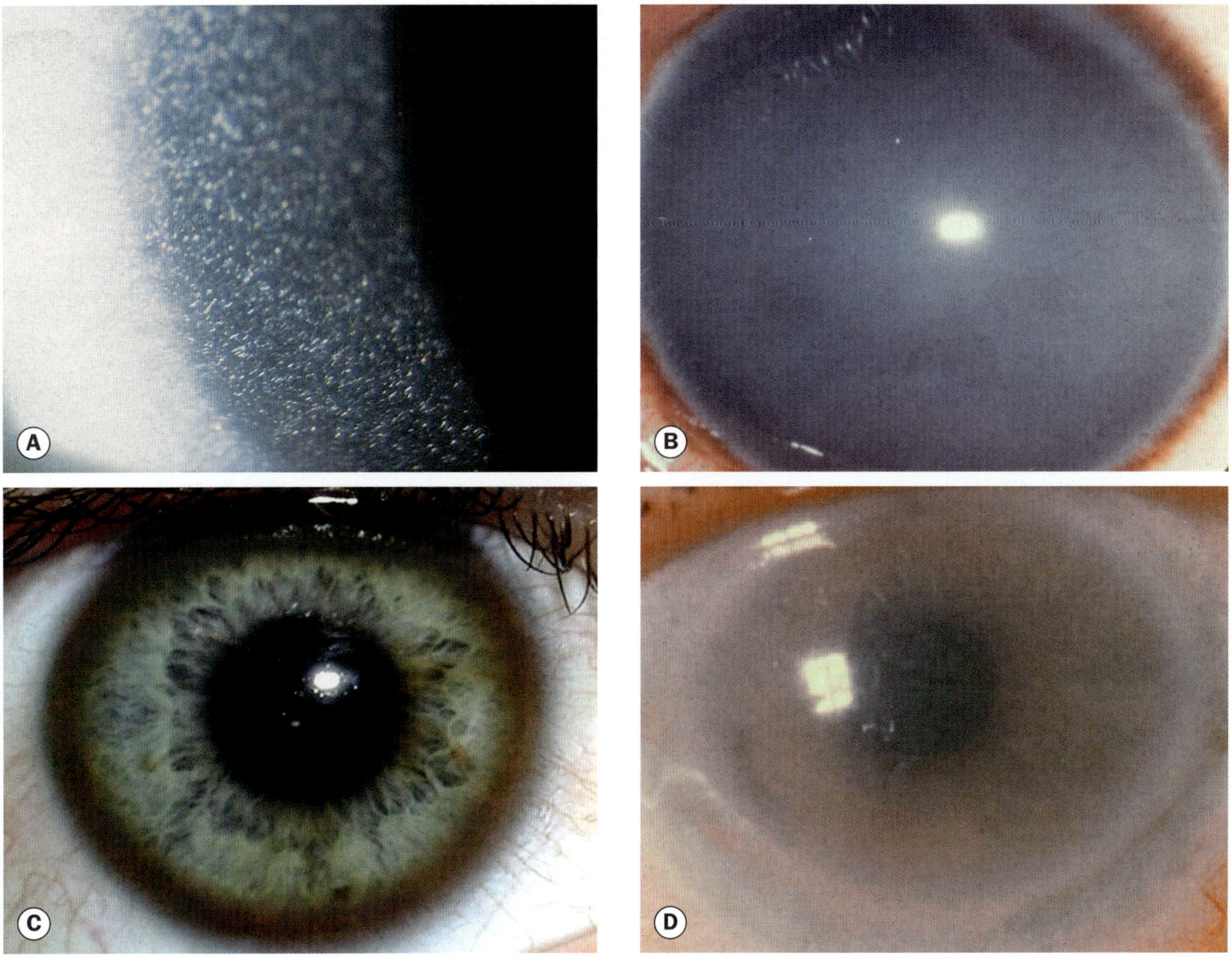

Fig. 7.61 Metabolic keratopathy. **(A)** Cystinosis; **(B)** typical appearance in a mucopolysaccharidosis; **(C)** Wilson disease; **(D)** LCAT (see text) deficiency. *(Courtesy of S Chen – fig. C; W Lisch – fig. D.)*

copper-carrying blood protein. Presentation is with liver disease, basal ganglia dysfunction or psychiatric disturbances. A Kayser–Fleischer ring is present in 95% of patients with neurological signs and consists of a brownish-yellow zone of fine copper dusting in peripheral Descemet membrane (Fig. 7.61C). This is best detected on gonioscopy when subtle. The deposits are preferentially distributed in the vertical meridian and may disappear with penicillamine therapy. Anterior capsular 'sunflower' cataract is seen in some patients.

Lecithin-cholesterol-acyltransferase deficiency

Lecithin-cholesterol-acyltransferase (LCAT) deficiency is a disorder of lipoprotein metabolism that has complete (Norum disease, with systemic manifestations including renal failure) and partial (fish eye disease, causing only corneal opacification) forms that are both AR (gene: *LCAT*). Keratopathy is characterized by numerous minute greyish dots throughout the stroma, often concentrated in the periphery in an arcus-like configuration (Fig. 7.61D).

Immunoprotein deposition

Diffuse or focal immunoprotein deposition is a relatively uncommon manifestation of several systemic diseases, including multiple myeloma, Waldenström macroglobulinaemia, monoclonal gammopathy of unknown cause, some lymphoproliferative disorders and leukaemia. Corneal involvement may be the earliest manifestation. Bands of punctate flake-like opacities are seen, mostly at the level of the posterior stroma. Treatment is that of the underlying disease. Severe corneal involvement may require corneal transplantation.

Tyrosinaemia type 2

Tyrosinaemia type 2 (oculocutaneous tyrosinaemia, Richner–Hanhart syndrome) is a very rare AR disease (gene: *TAT*) in which an enzyme deficiency leads to elevated plasma tyrosine levels. Ocular involvement may occasionally be the presenting feature. Painful palmar and plantar hyperkeratotic lesions and variable CNS involvement are seen. A bilateral pseudodendritic keratitis with crystalline edges often begins in childhood and causes photophobia, watering and redness.

Fabry disease

Fabry disease is an X-linked lysosomal storage disorder caused by a deficiency of the enzyme alpha-galactosidase A that leads to abnormal tissue accumulation of a glycolipid. All males with the gene develop the disease and some heterozygous females. Systemic features include periodic burning pain in the extremities (acroparaesthesia) and GI tract, angiokeratomas (Fig. 7.62A), cardiomyopathy and renal disease. Ocular manifestations include white to golden-brown corneal opacities in a vortex pattern (75%) that may be the first feature of the disease (Fig. 7.62B) facilitating early intervention, wedge- or spoke-shaped posterior cataract (Fabry cataract), conjunctival vascular tortuosity (corkscrew vessels) and aneurysm formation (Fig. 7.62C) and retinal vascular tortuosity.

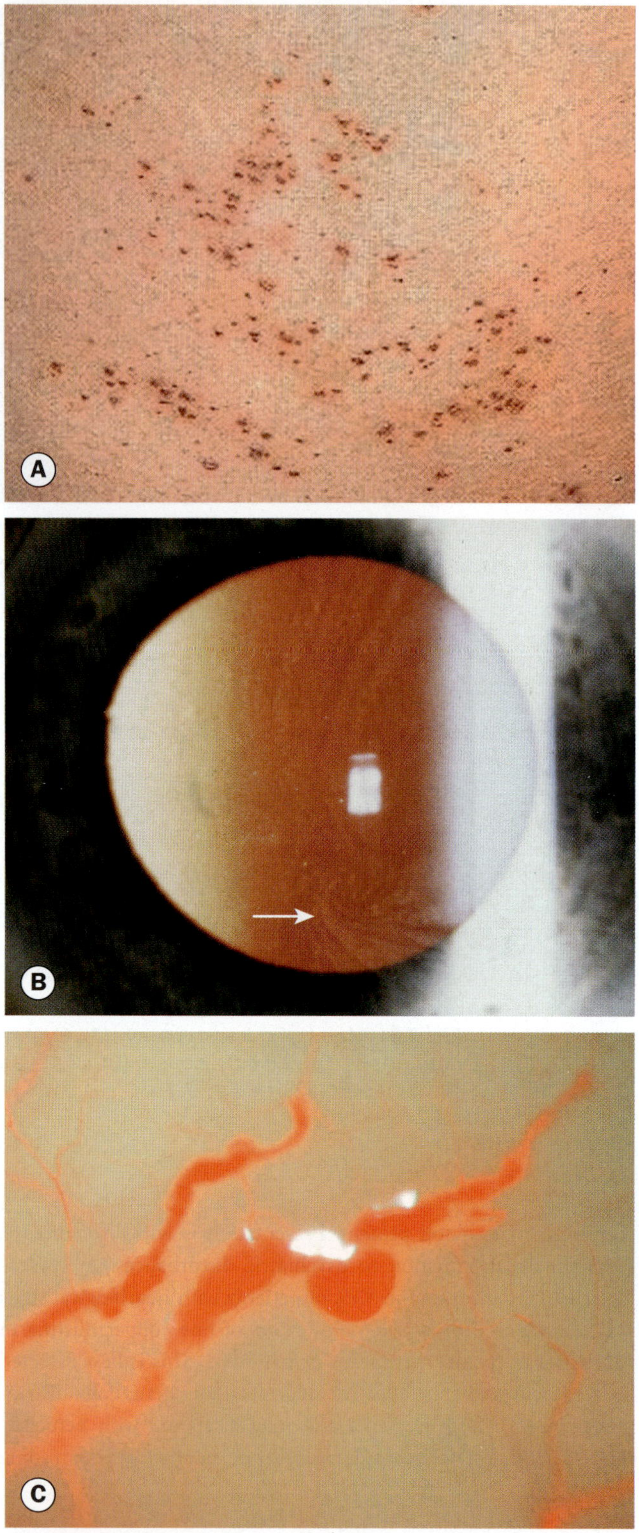

Fig. 7.62 Fabry disease. **(A)** Angiokeratomas; **(B)** vortex keratopathy (arrow); **(C)** conjunctival vessel tortuosity and aneurysms.

CONTACT LENSES

Therapeutic uses

The risks of fitting a contact lens to an already compromised eye are greater than with lens wear for cosmetic reasons. The benefit–risk balance should be considered in each case individually, with education and regular review to ensure early diagnosis and treatment of complications. The choice of lens type is dictated by the nature of the ocular pathology.

Optical

Optical indications are aimed at improving visual acuity when this cannot be achieved by spectacles in the following situations:

- **Irregular astigmatism** associated with keratoconus can be corrected with rigid contact lenses after spectacles have failed and before corneal grafting becomes necessary. Patients with astigmatism following corneal grafting may also benefit.
- **Superficial corneal irregularities** can be neutralized by rigid contact lenses, which provide a smoother and optically more regular surface. Visual acuity can only be substantially improved if irregularities are not too severe.
- **Anisometropia** in which binocular vision cannot be achieved by spectacles due to aniseikonia, such as may occur following monocular cataract surgery with high refractive error correction.

Promotion of epithelial healing

- **Persistent epithelial defects** often heal if the regenerating corneal epithelium is protected from the constant rubbing of the lids, allowing the development of hemidesmosomal attachments to the basement membrane.
- **Recurrent corneal erosions** associated with basement membrane dystrophy may require long-term contact lens wear to

reduce the recurrence rate. In post-traumatic cases, lens wear can usually be discontinued after a few weeks. Lens wear also improves comfort.

Pain relief

- **Bullous keratopathy** can be managed with soft bandage lenses that relieve pain by protecting the exposed corneal nerve endings from the shearing forces of the lids during blinking. The lens may also flatten bullae into diffuse fine epithelial cysts.
- **Filamentary keratopathy** resistant to topical treatment will usually achieve some relief from soft contact lens wear.
- **Other indications** include Thygeson superficial punctate keratitis and protection of the corneal epithelium from aberrant lashes in trichiasis. They can also be used as a temporizing measure in entropion prior to definitive surgery.

Preservation of corneal integrity

- **A descemetocoele** can be temporarily capped with a tight-fitting, large-diameter soft or scleral lens to prevent perforation and encourage healing.
- **Splinting** and apposition of the edges of a small corneal wound can be achieved by means of a contact lens. Slightly larger perforations may be sealed with glue followed by insertion of a bandage contact lens to both protect the glue and prevent irritation of the lids from the glue's irregular surface.

Miscellaneous indications

- **Ptosis props** to support the upper lids in patients with ocular myopathies.
- **Maintenance of the fornices** to prevent symblepharon formation in cicatrizing conjunctivitis.
- **Drug delivery** enhancement by a hydrogel lens imbued with topical medication is an occasional indication.

Complications

Mechanical and hypoxic keratitis

- **Pathogenesis.** Insufficient oxygen transmission through the lens. A tightly fitting contact lens that does not move with blinking will impair tear circulation under the lens. This is exacerbated by lid closure if the lens is worn during sleep. Hypoxia leads to anaerobic metabolism and lactic acidosis that inhibits the normal barrier and pump mechanisms of the cornea.
- **Superficial punctate keratitis** is the most common complication. The pattern may give a clue as to the aetiology. For example, staining at 3 and 9 o'clock is associated with incomplete blinking and drying in rigid lens wearers.
- **The tight lens syndrome** is characterized by indentation and staining of the conjunctival epithelium in a ring around the cornea.
- **Acute hypoxia** is characterized by epithelial microcysts (Fig. 7.63A) and necrosis and endothelial blebs. Very painful macroerosions may develop several hours after lenses are removed following a period of overwear.
- **Chronic hypoxia** may result in vascularization (Fig. 7.63B) and lipid deposition. Superficial peripheral neovascularization of <1.5 mm is common in myopic contact lens wearers and can be monitored.
- **Treatment** depends on the cause but may involve:
  - Increasing oxygen permeability by refitting with a thinner lens, a gas permeable rigid lens or a silicone hydrogel soft lens.
  - Modifying lens fit to increase movement.
  - Reducing lens wearing time.

Immune response (hypersensitivity) keratitis

A hypersensitivity response to bacterial antigen or the chemicals used in lens care can lead to the development of sterile marginal corneal infiltrates. The mechanism is thought to be similar to that of marginal keratitis.

- **Signs.** Mildly red eye associated with infiltrates, often marginally located, with no or minimal epithelial defects.
- **Treatment** involves cessation of lens wear until resolution occurs. Topical antibiotics and steroids may be used in some cases, but if the diagnosis is uncertain, treatment should be that of bacterial keratitis.

Toxic keratitis

- **Pathogenesis.** Acute chemical injury may be caused by inadvertently placing a contact lens on the eye without first neutralizing toxic cleaning agents such as hydrogen peroxide. Chronic toxicity can result from long-term exposure to disinfecting preservatives such as thiomersal or benzalkonium chloride.
- **Signs**
  - Acute pain, redness and chemosis on lens insertion, which may take 48 hours to resolve completely.
  - Vascularization and scarring of the cornea (Fig. 7.63C) and limbal conjunctiva in chronic cases.
- **Treatment** may involve switching to daily disposable lenses or using a non-preserved disinfectant such as hydrogen peroxide.

Suppurative keratitis

Contact lens wear is the greatest risk factor for the development of bacterial keratitis (Fig. 7.63D). The risk is probably least for rigid contact lenses. Bacteria in the tear film are normally unable to bind to the corneal epithelium, but following an abrasion and in association with hypoxia, they can attach and invade the epithelium. Microorganisms may also be introduced onto the corneal surface by poor lens hygiene or the use of tap water for rinsing.

Contact lens-associated giant papillary conjunctivitis

See Chapter 6.

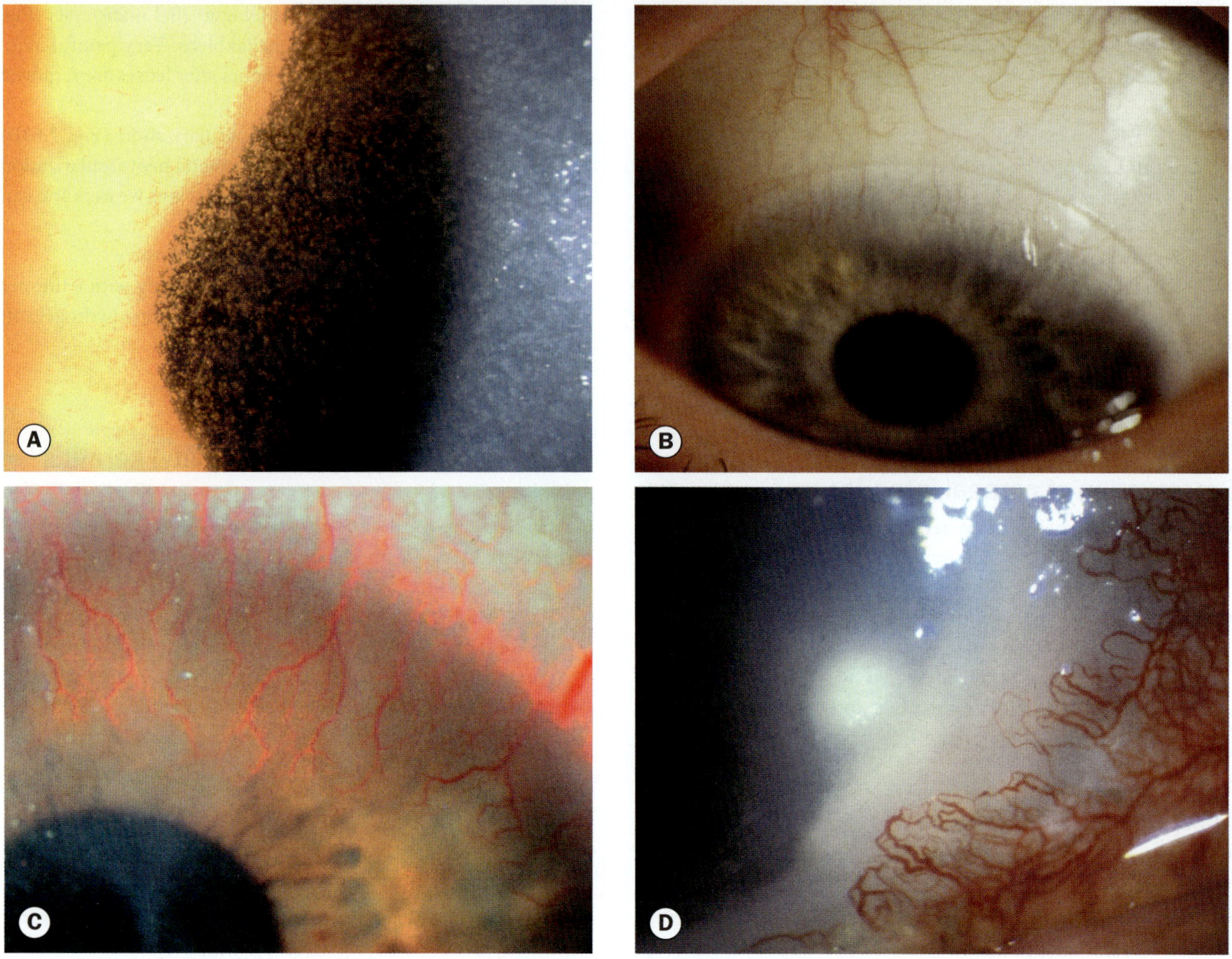

Fig. 7.63 Complications of contact lens wear. **(A)** Epithelial microcysts in acute hypoxia; **(B)** superior pannus from chronic hypoxia; **(C)** vascularization and scarring in chronic toxic keratitis; **(D)** acute bacterial keratitis with vascularization. *(Courtesy of S Tuft – fig. A; J Dart – fig. C.)*

CONGENITAL ANOMALIES OF THE CORNEA AND GLOBE

Microcornea

The normal neonatal corneal diameter is 10 mm and the adult diameter of 12 mm is usually reached by the age of 2 years. Microcornea is a rare autosomal dominant (sometimes sporadic) unilateral or bilateral condition in which the horizontal corneal diameter is 10 mm or less over 2 years of age (Fig. 7.64A), or less than 9 mm in the newborn. The cornea is steep on keratometry. There may be hypermetropia and a shallow anterior chamber but other dimensions are normal. Ocular associations include glaucoma (angle-closure and open angle), congenital cataract, leukoma (Fig. 7.64B), persistent fetal vasculature, coloboma, optic nerve hypoplasia, aniridia and nanophthalmos. Systemic associations have been reported. Refractive error and amblyopia should be managed appropriately.

Microphthalmos

Microphthalmos (microphthalmia – Fig. 7.65A) is a condition in which the entire eye is small, with an axial length at least two standard deviations below the mean for age. Simple or pure microphthalmos (nanophthalmos – see below) refers to an eye that is structurally normal apart from a short length and complex microphthalmos to eyes with other features of dysgenesis, for example a coloboma (Fig. 7.65B) or orbital cyst and a range of other ocular abnormalities. It may be unilateral or bilateral; when unilateral, abnormalities may be present in the fellow eye. Vision is variably affected, in conjunction with severity. It is typically sporadic but mutations in numerous genes have been implicated. Around 50% of cases may be associated with systemic abnormalities, including of the CNS. Potential environmental causes include fetal alcohol syndrome and intrauterine infections.

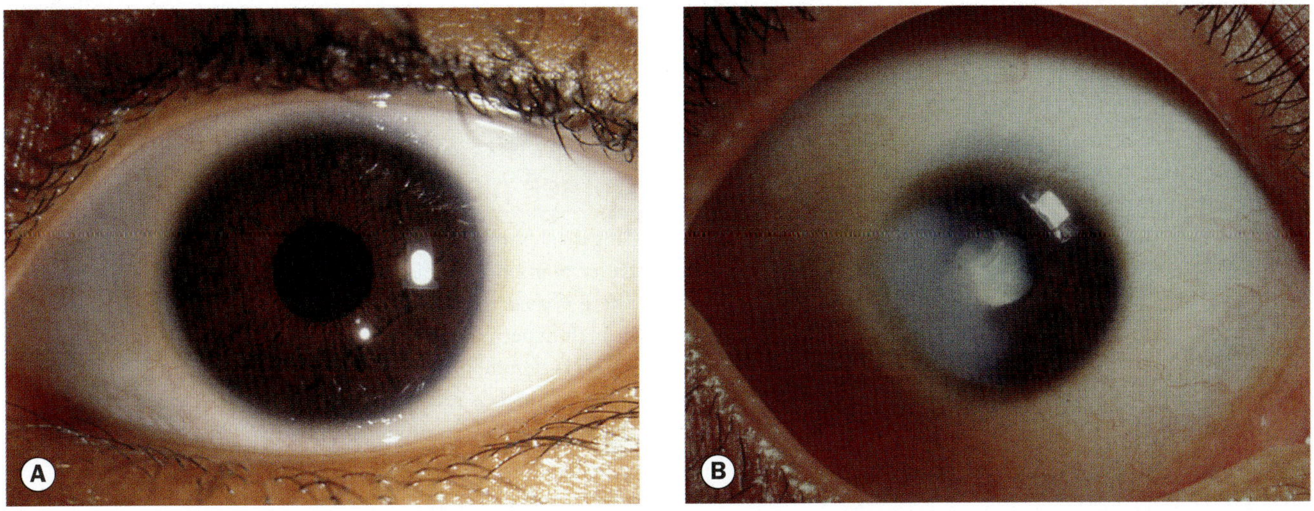

Fig. 7.64 Congenital anomalies of the cornea. **(A)** Microcornea; **(B)** microcornea and corneal opacity with dense cataract.

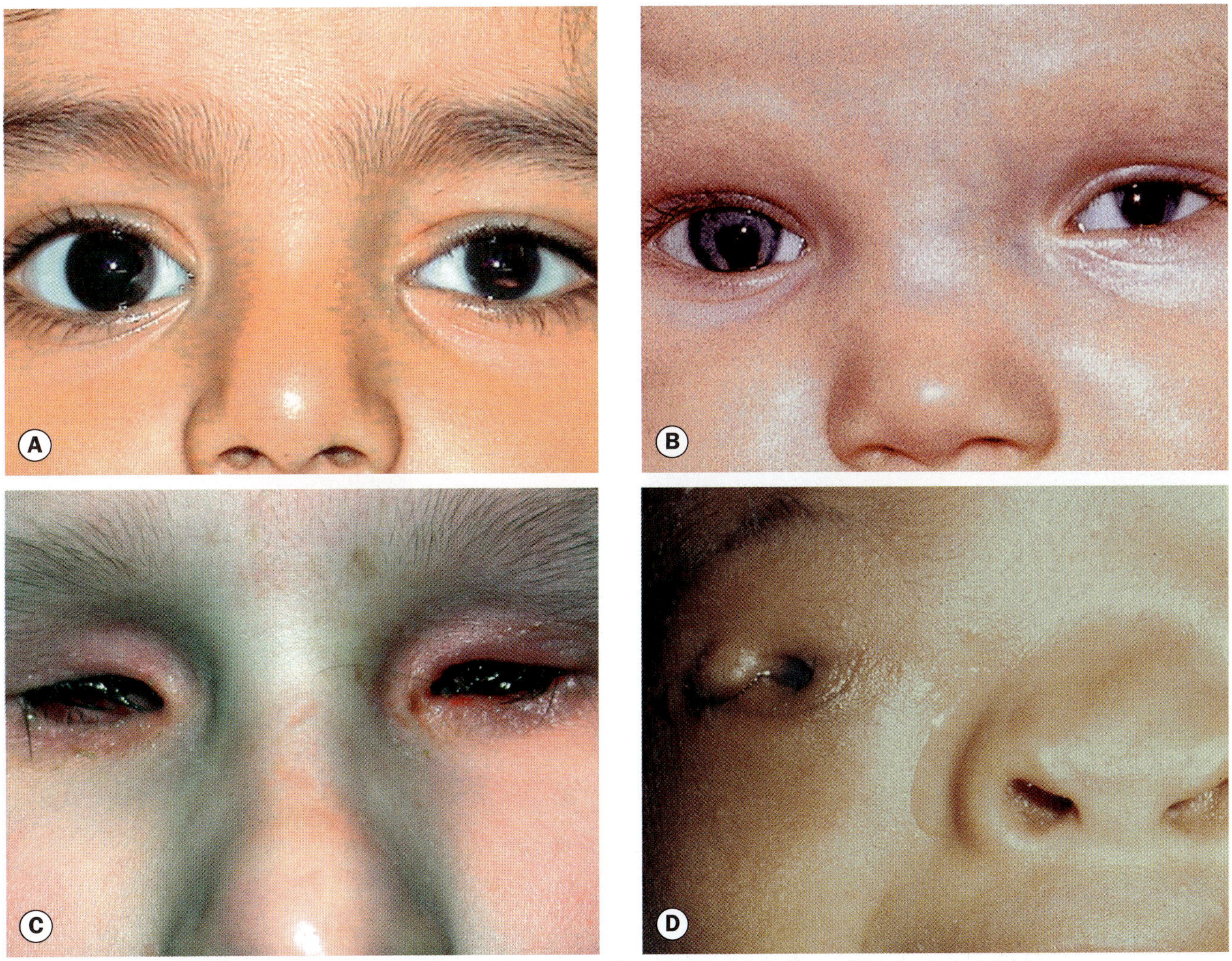

Fig. 7.65 Congenital anomalies of the globe: **(A)** Left microphthalmos; **(B)** left microphthalmos and bilateral iris colobomas; **(C)** bilateral simple anophthalmos; **(D)** monocular anophthalmos.

Nanophthalmos

In nanophthalmos the entire eye is small with an axial length of less than 20 mm. Both eyes are usually affected. Ocular associations include glaucoma (especially angle-closure as the lens is large relative to the size of the eye), hypermetropia, ametropia, amblyopia and strabismus. In childhood, management of refractive error and amblyopia are critical. Surgery for glaucoma is particularly hazardous and can result in aqueous misdirection and choroidal effusion ('small eye–big trouble'). The best option is lens extraction with IOL implantation. The surgery is technically challenging, but has the advantage of deepening the anterior chamber and reducing the refractive error if a suitable high-power lens implant is inserted.

Anophthalmos

Anophthalmos (anophthalmia) refers to the complete absence of any visible globe structure (Fig. 7.65C and D), though a microphthalmic remnant or cyst may be present. It is associated with other abnormalities such as absence of extraocular muscles, a short conjunctival sac and microblepharon. Causative factors are probably broadly similar to those of microphthalmos.

Megalocornea

Megalocornea is a rare, bilateral, non-progressive condition that is usually X-linked recessive. Approximately 90% of affected individuals are male. The adult horizontal corneal diameter is 13 mm or more, with a very deep anterior chamber (Fig. 7.66A). There is usually high myopia and astigmatism but normal corrected visual acuity. Lens subluxation may occur due to zonular stretching and pigment dispersion syndrome may occur (see Ch. 11). Numerous systemic associations have been reported.

Cornea plana

This is an extremely rare bilateral condition in which the cornea is flatter than normal (Fig. 7.66B) – the radius of curvature is larger. There is a corresponding reduction in refractive power resulting in high hypermetropia. Two forms are described, cornea plana 1, which is dominantly inherited (*CNA1*), being milder than cornea plana 2, which is recessively inherited (*CNA2*). Associated ocular abnormalities are common.

Sclerocornea

Sclerocornea is a very rare, usually bilateral, condition that may be associated with cornea plana (see below). Sporadic cases are common, but a milder form can be inherited as AD and a more severe form as AR. Peripheral corneal opacification, with no visible border between the sclera and cornea, confers the appearance of apparently reduced corneal diameter in mild–moderate disease (Fig. 7.67A). Occasionally the entire cornea is involved (Fig. 7.67B).

Keratectasia

Keratectasia is a very rare, usually unilateral, condition thought to be the result of intrauterine keratitis and perforation. It is characterized by protuberance between the eyelids of a severely opacified and sometimes vascularized cornea (Fig. 7.68). It is often associated with raised IOP.

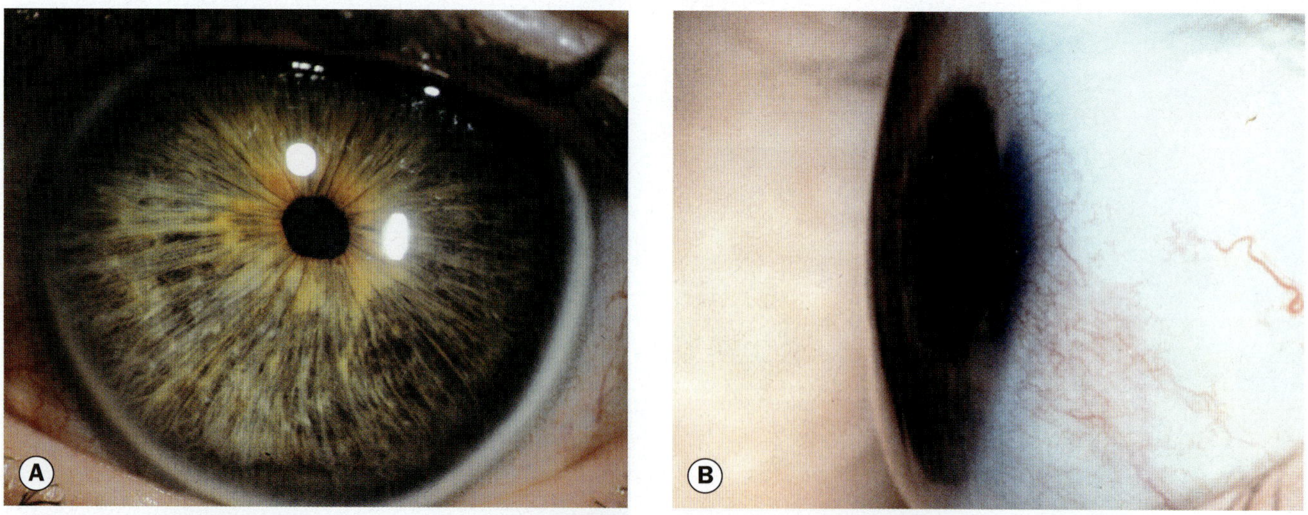

Fig. 7.66 (A) Clinical appearance of megalocornea; **(B)** cornea plana. *(Courtesy of R Visser – fig. B.)*

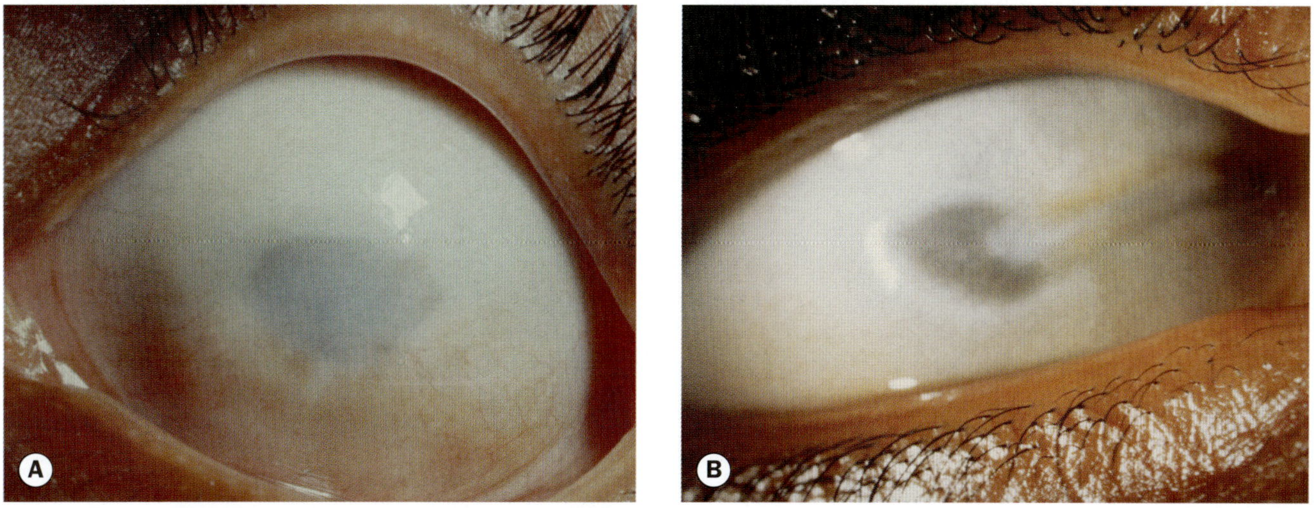

Fig. 7.67 Sclerocornea. **(A)** Moderate; **(B)** severe.

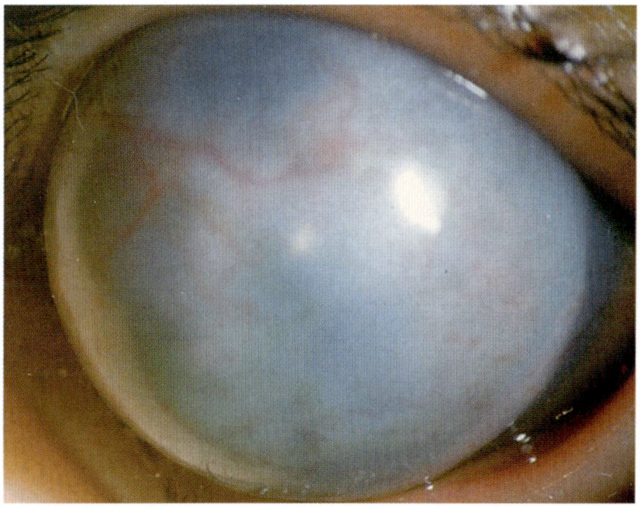

Fig. 7.68 Keratectasia.

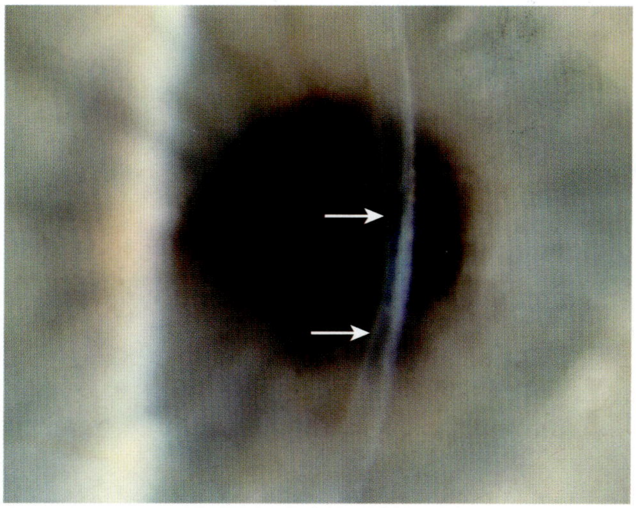

Fig. 7.69 Posterior keratoconus (arrows).

Posterior keratoconus

Posterior keratoconus is a sporadic condition in which there is unilateral non-progressive increase in curvature of the posterior corneal surface. The anterior surface is normal and visual acuity relatively unimpaired because of the similar refractive indices of the cornea and aqueous humour. Generalized (involvement of the entire posterior corneal surface) and localized types are described (paracentral or central posterior indentation – Fig. 7.69).

Chapter 8

Corneal and Refractive Surgery

KERATOPLASTY

Introduction

Corneal transplantation (grafting) refers to the replacement of diseased host corneal tissue by healthy donor cornea. A corneal graft (keratoplasty) may be partial-thickness (anterior or posterior lamellar) or full-thickness (penetrating).

General indications

- **Optical** keratoplasty is performed to improve vision. Important indications include keratoconus, scarring, corneal dystrophies (Fig. 8.1A), pseudophakic bullous keratopathy and corneal degenerations.
- **Tectonic** grafting may be carried out to restore or preserve corneal integrity in eyes with severe structural changes such as thinning with descemetocoele (US spelling – descemetocele) (Fig. 8.1B) and perforated corneal ulcer (Fig. 8.1C).
- **Therapeutic** corneal transplantation facilitates removal of infected corneal tissue in eyes unresponsive to antimicrobial therapy (Fig. 8.1D).
- **Cosmetic** grafting may be performed to improve the appearance of the eye, but is a rare indication.

Donor tissue

Donor tissue should be removed within 12–24 hours of death. There is an attempt to age-match donors and recipients. Corneas from infants (3 years and under) are used only very occasionally, even for paediatric transplants, as they are associated with surgical, refractive and rejection problems. Most corneas are stored in coordinating 'eye banks' prior to transplantation, where pre-release evaluation includes medical history review and donor blood screening to exclude contraindications and microscopic examination of the cornea including endothelial cell count determination. Corneas are preserved in hypothermic storage (up to 7–10 days) or organ culture medium (4 weeks) until needed. Culture allows

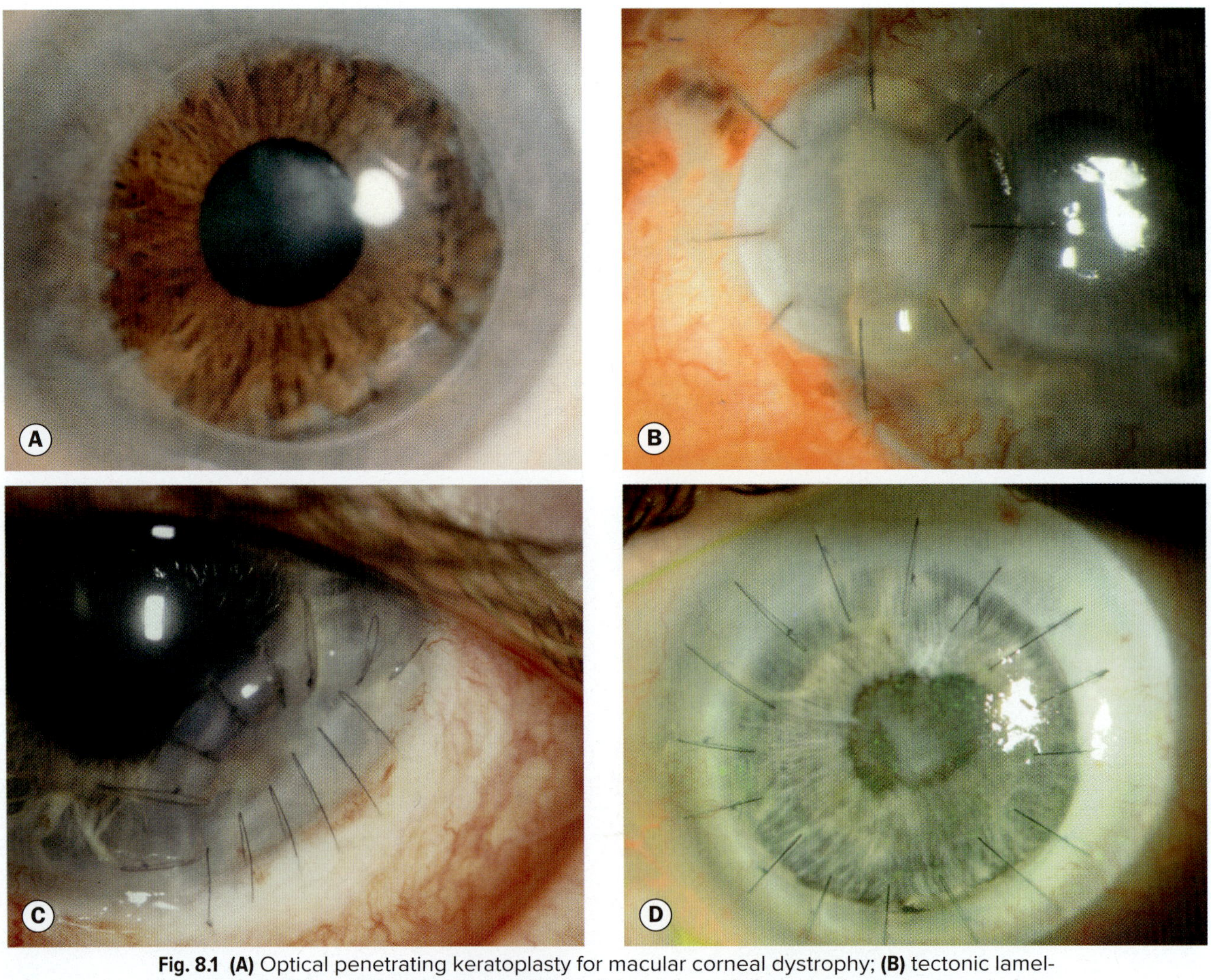

Fig. 8.1 **(A)** Optical penetrating keratoplasty for macular corneal dystrophy; **(B)** tectonic lamellar patch graft for descemetocoele; **(C)** lamellar patch graft for a perforated corneal ulcer; **(D)** penetrating keratoplasty for pseudomonas keratitis – a dense cataract and posterior synechiae are visible. *(Courtesy of S Tuft – fig. B.)*

extended testing for infective contamination. Contraindications to ocular tissue donation are set out below, though there is international variation and the list is not exhaustive:

- Death from unknown cause.
- Certain systemic infections such as human immunodeficiency virus (HIV), viral hepatitis, syphilis, congenital rubella, tuberculosis, septicaemia and active malaria.
- Prior high-risk behaviour for HIV and hepatitis such as sex with someone HIV-positive, men who have sex with men, intravenous drug abuse and prostitution.
- Within the last 12 months: sex with someone who has engaged in high-risk behaviour, who has received blood clotting factor concentrates or has undergone tattooing, acupuncture, ear/body piercing.
- Infectious and possibly infectious diseases of the central nervous system, such as Creutzfeldt–Jakob disease, systemic sclerosing panencephalitis, progressive multifocal leukoencephalopathy, encephalitis, Alzheimer disease and other dementias, Parkinson disease, multiple sclerosis and motor neurone disease.
- Receipt of a transplanted organ.
- Receipt of human pituitary-derived growth hormone.
- Brain or spinal surgery before 1992.
- Most haematological malignancies.
- Ocular disease such as inflammation and disease likely to compromise graft outcome, some malignant ocular tumours (e.g. retinoblastoma) and corneal refractive surgery.

Recipient prognostic factors

The following host factors may adversely affect the prognosis of a corneal graft and, if possible, should be optimized prior to surgery. In general, the most favourable cases are keratoconus, localized scars and dystrophies.

- Severe stromal vascularization (Fig. 8.2), absence of corneal sensation, extreme thinning at the proposed host–graft junction and active corneal inflammation.

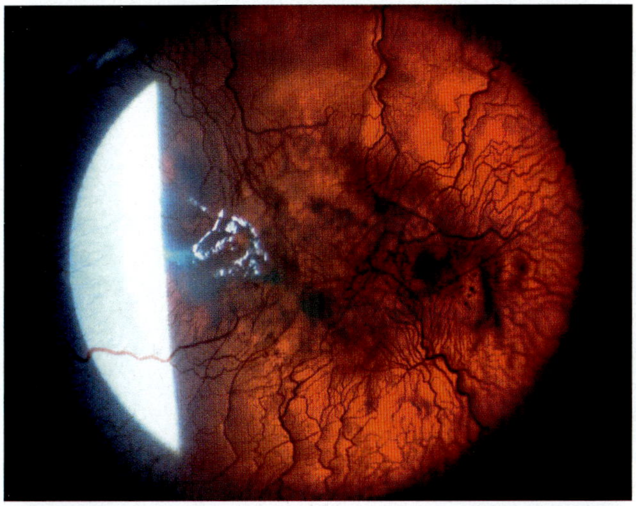

Fig. 8.2 Retroillumination of heavily vascularized cornea resulting from recurrent herpes simplex keratitis. *(Courtesy of C Barry.)*

- Abnormalities of the eyelids, such as blepharitis, ectropion, entropion and trichiasis. These conditions should be addressed before surgery.
- Recurrent or progressive forms of conjunctival inflammation, such as atopic conjunctivitis and ocular cicatricial pemphigoid.
- Tear film dysfunction.
- Anterior synechiae.
- Uncontrolled glaucoma.
- Uveitis.

Penetrating keratoplasty

Component layer grafting of the cornea is increasingly utilized, but full-thickness keratoplasty remains commonly performed and is the appropriate procedure for disease involving all layers of the cornea (Fig. 8.3). Key surgical points include:

- **A common graft size** is 7.5 mm. Small grafts may lead to high astigmatism and larger diameters are associated with an increasing tendency to peripheral anterior synechiae formation and raised intraocular pressure (IOP).
- **The donor button** is usually about 0.25 mm larger in diameter than the host site.
- **Preparation of donor cornea** should always precede excision of host tissue, in case a problem with the former means that the surgery cannot be completed.
- **Trephination.** Either mechanically guided manual or automated (including laser) trephination is commonly used.
- **Sutures.** The graft may be secured with either continuous (Fig. 8.4A) or interrupted (Fig. 8.4B) suture techniques, or a combination of both.

Postoperative management

- **Topical steroids** (e.g. prednisolone acetate 1%, dexamethasone phosphate 0.1%) are used to decrease the risk of immunological graft rejection. Initial administration is typically every 2 hours with gradual tapering depending on the likelihood of rejection and clinical progress. Long-term instillation at low intensity, such as once daily for a year or more, is usual.
- **Other immunosuppressants** such as oral azathioprine and topical and systemic ciclosporin are usually reserved for high-risk patients.
- **Cycloplegia** (e.g. homatropine 2% twice daily) is typically used for 1–2 weeks.
- **Oral aciclovir** may be used in the context of pre-existing herpes simplex keratitis to minimize the risk of recurrence.
- **Monitoring of IOP.** Applanation tonometry is relatively unreliable so measurement is commonly performed during the early postoperative period with a non-applanation method.
- **Monitoring endothelial function.** This can be done indirectly and quickly by measuring the central corneal thickness with a pachymeter.
- **Removal of sutures** is performed when the graft–host junction has healed. This is often after 12–18 months, although in elderly patients it may take much longer. Removal of broken or loose individual sutures should be performed as soon as identified, as this reduces the risk of graft rejection.

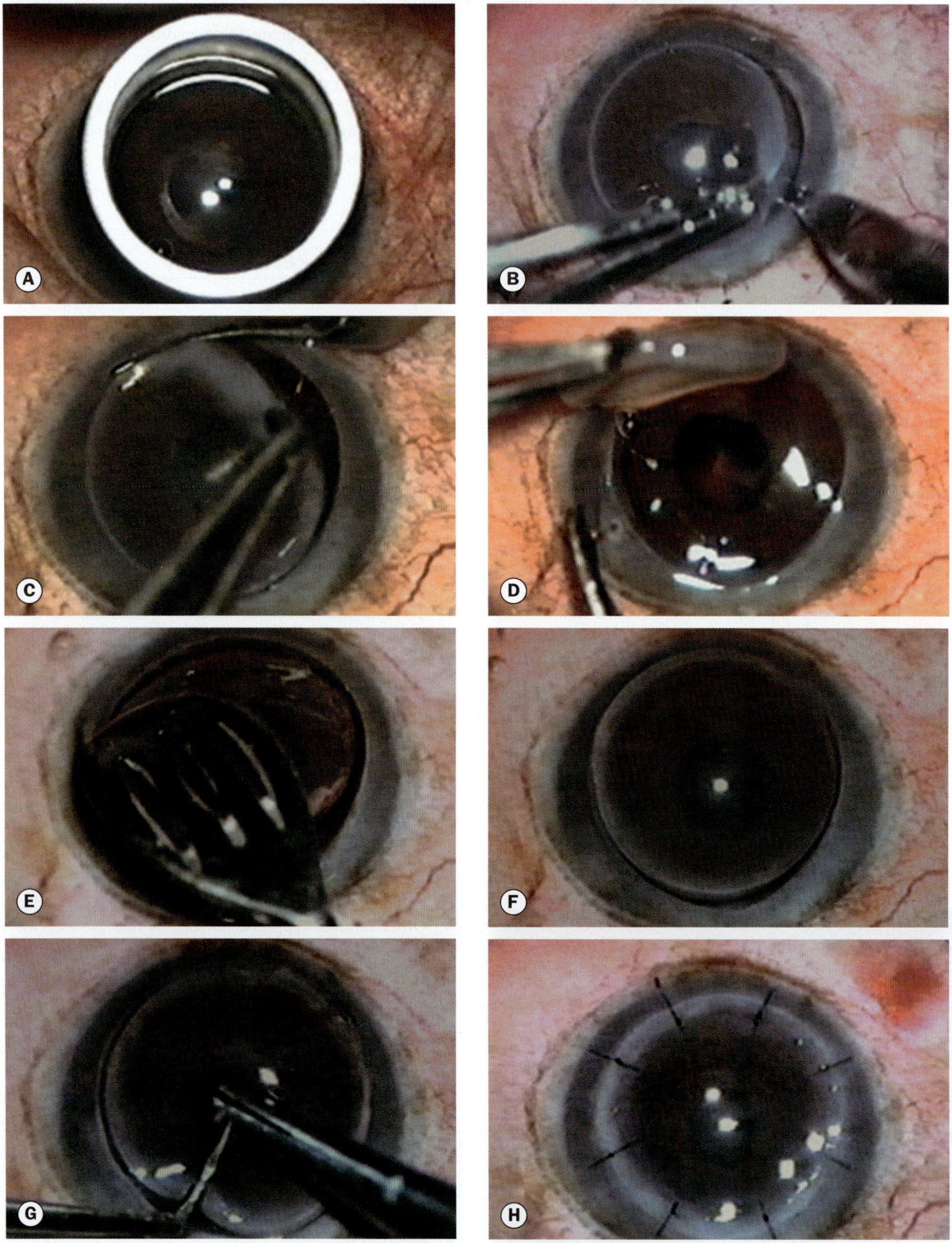

Fig. 8.3 Penetrating keratoplasty technique. **(A)** Partial-thickness trephination; **(B)** incision into the anterior chamber; **(C)** and **(D)** completion of excision; **(E** and **F)** donor button is placed onto the viscoelastic bed; **(G)** initial cardinal suture; **(H)** eight interrupted cardinal sutures in place. *(Courtesy of R Fogla.)*

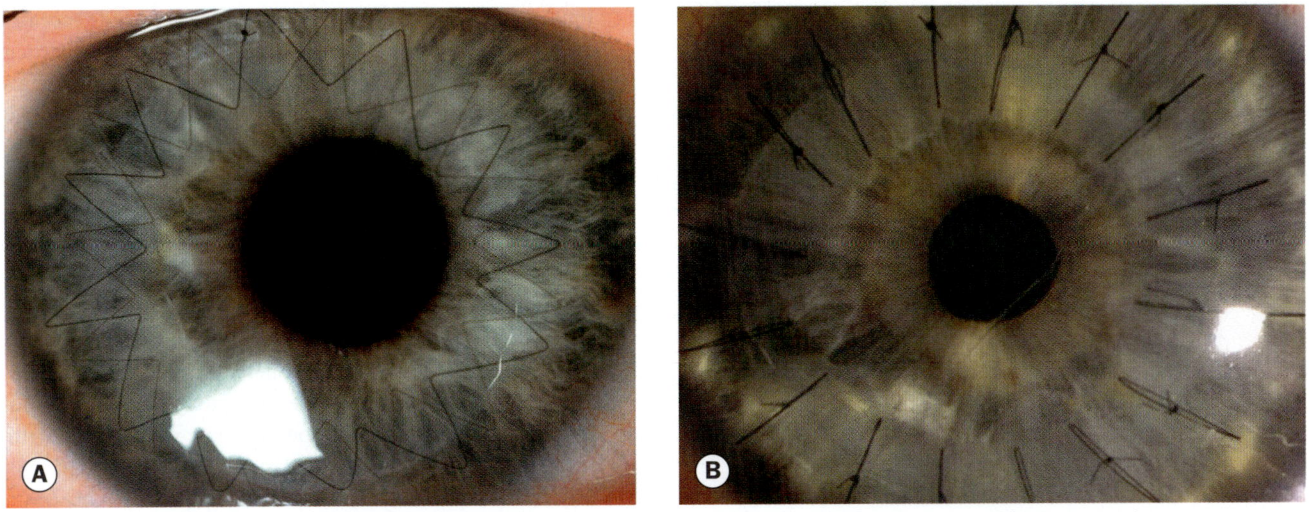

Fig. 8.4 Penetrating keratoplasty sutures. **(A)** Secured by continuous sutures; **(B)** interrupted sutures. *(Courtesy of C Barry.)*

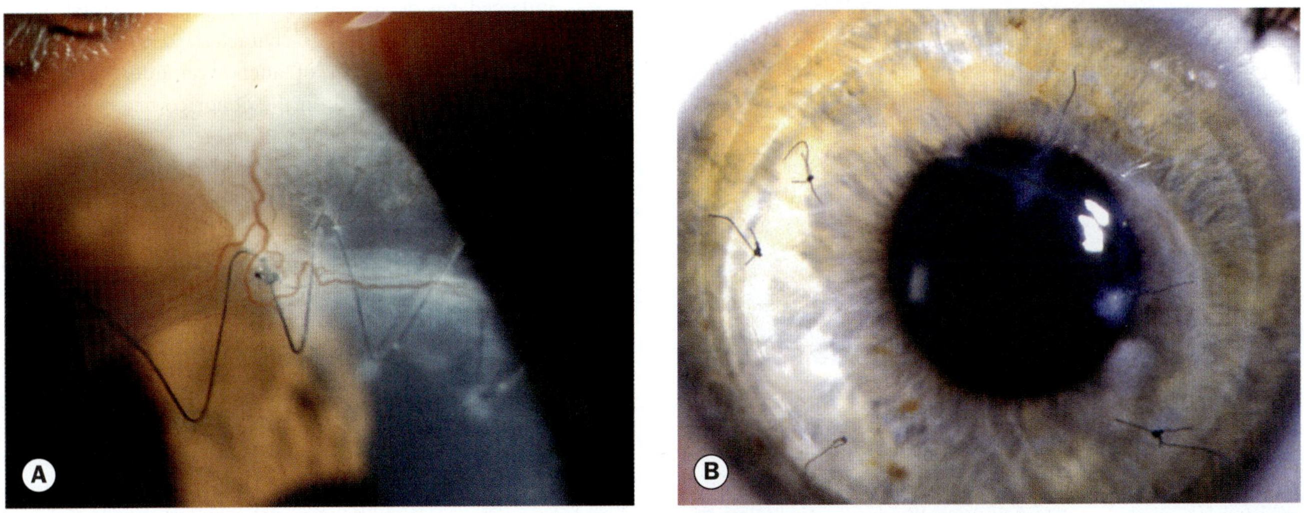

Fig. 8.5 **(A)** Protruding suture with vascular ingrowth; **(B)** broken sutures within stroma.

TIP In a patient with a corneal graft, broken or loose sutures should be removed as this reduces the risk of localized vascularization and graft rejection.

Postoperative complications

- **Early** complications include persistent epithelial defects, loose or protruding sutures (Fig. 8.5A and B) (risk of infection – marked sterile reaction, papillary hypertrophy), wound leak (sometimes with flat anterior chamber or iris prolapse), uveitis, elevation of intraocular pressure, traumatic graft rupture (Fig. 8.6A), cystoid macular oedema, microbial keratitis (Fig. 8.6B), endophthalmitis (Fig. 8.6C) and rejection (see below). A rare complication is a fixed dilated pupil (Urrets-Zavalia syndrome).
- **Late** complications include astigmatism, recurrence of underlying disease, late wound dehiscence, retro-corneal membrane formation, glaucoma, rejection (see below) and failure without rejection.

Corneal graft rejection

Immunological rejection of any layer of the cornea can occur. Rejection of separate layers (endothelial, stromal and epithelial) can occur in isolation, but typically a combination is present. Simple graft failure can occur in the absence of rejection, although rejection is a common contributory factor.

TIP The risk of corneal graft rejection is increased significantly by the presence of host stromal vascularization.

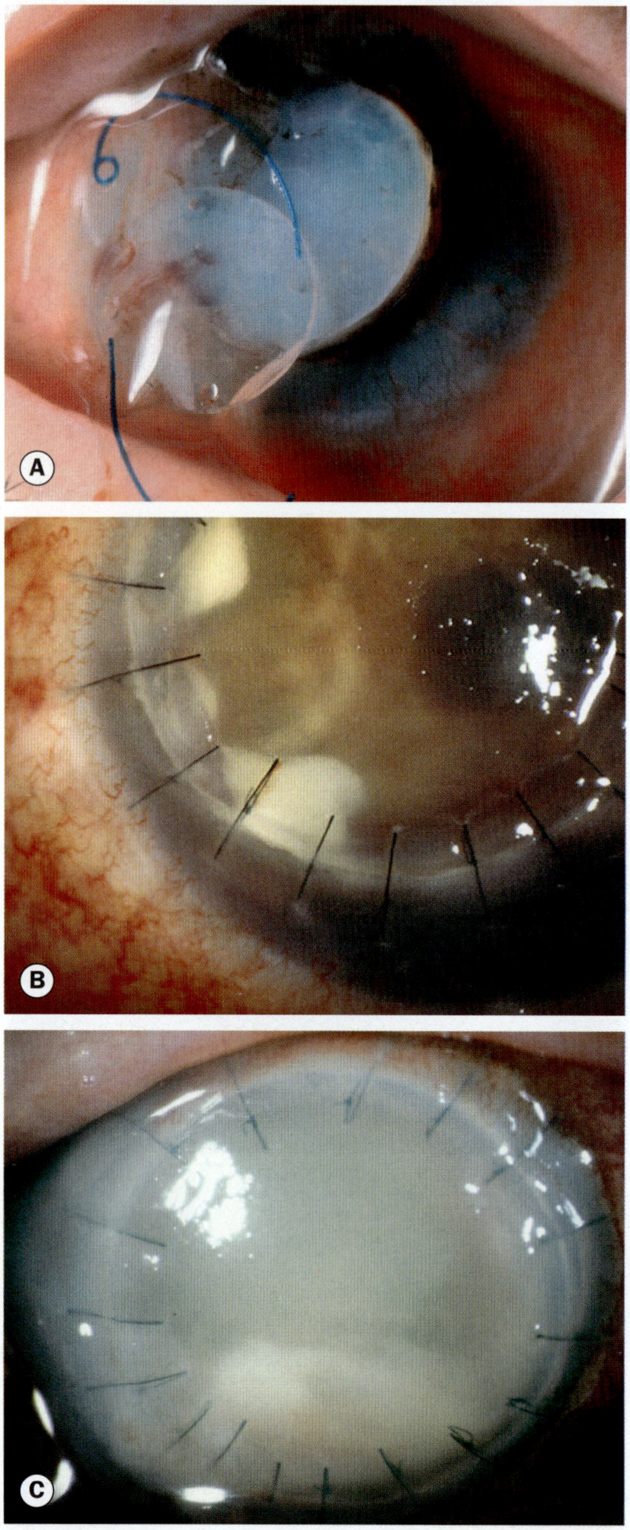

Fig. 8.6 Postoperative complications. **(A)** Traumatic graft rupture and extrusion of intraocular lens implant; **(B)** microbial keratitis; **(C)** endophthalmitis. *(R Bates – fig. A; S Tuft – fig. C.)*

- **Pathogenesis.** The corneal graft is immunologically privileged, with an absence of blood vessels and lymphatics and the presence of relatively few antigen-presenting cells. Inflammation and neovascularization contribute to loss of this privilege. Important predisposing factors for rejection include eccentric or larger grafts (over 8 mm in diameter), infection (particularly herpetic), glaucoma and previous keratoplasty. If the host becomes sensitized to histocompatibility antigens present in the donor cornea, rejection may result. Human leukocyte antigen (HLA) matching has a small beneficial effect on graft survival. Gender incompatibility has recently emerged as an important risk factor for graft rejection and failure. Whereas the cornea of a female donor can be used in either male or female recipients, the cornea of a male donor should not be allocated to a female recipient.
- **Symptoms.** Blurred vision, redness, photophobia and pain are typical, but many cases are asymptomatic until rejection is established. The timing of onset is very variable, occurring from days to years after keratoplasty.
- **Signs** vary depending on the type of graft.
  - Ciliary injection associated with anterior uveitis is an early manifestation (Fig. 8.7A).
  - Epithelial rejection may be accompanied by an elevated line of abnormal epithelium (Fig. 8.7B) in a quiet or mildly inflamed eye, occurring at an average of 3 months.
  - Subepithelial rejection is characterized by subepithelial infiltrates, reminiscent of adenoviral infection (Krachmer spots – Fig. 8.7C) on the donor cornea, with deeper oedema and infiltrative opacification.
  - Stromal rejection features deeper haze. It can be chronic or hyperacute, the latter in association with endothelial rejection.
  - Endothelial rejection is characterized by a linear pattern of keratic precipitates (Khodadoust line – Fig. 8.7D) associated with an area of inflammation at the graft margin.
  - Stromal oedema is indicative of endothelial failure.
- **Management.** Early intensive treatment greatly improves the likelihood of reversing the rejection. The most aggressive regimen is generally required for endothelial rejection, followed in order of severity by stromal, subepithelial and epithelial. Intraocular pressure monitoring is critical.
  - Preservative-free topical steroids hourly for 24 hours are the mainstay of therapy. The frequency is reduced gradually over several weeks. Steroid ointment can be used at bedtime as the regimen is tapered. High-risk patients can be maintained on the highest tolerated topical dose (e.g. prednisolone acetate 1% four times daily) for an extended period.
  - Topical cycloplegia (e.g. homatropine 2% or atropine 1% once or twice daily).
  - Topical ciclosporin 0.05% to 2% may be of benefit, but the onset of action is delayed.
  - Systemic steroids. Oral prednisolone 1 mg/kg daily for 1–2 weeks with subsequent tapering. If given within 8 days of onset, intravenous methylprednisolone 500 mg daily for up to 3 days may be particularly effective, suppressing rejection and reducing the risk of further episodes.
  - Subconjunctival steroid injection (e.g. 0.5 ml of 4 mg/ml dexamethasone) is sometimes used.
  - Other systemic immunosuppressants such as ciclosporin, tacrolimus or azathioprine can be considered.

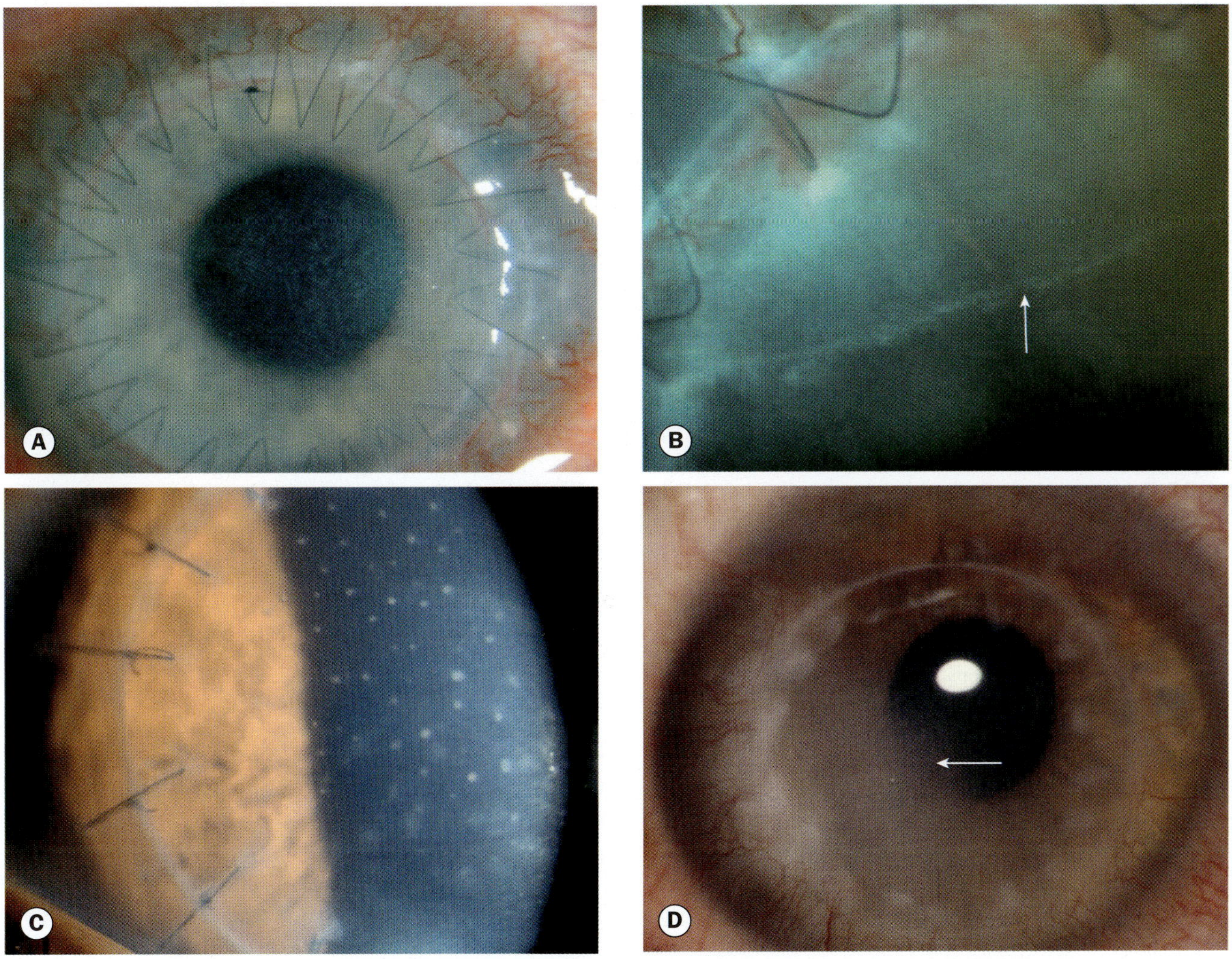

Fig. 8.7 Allograft rejection. **(A)** Ciliary injection; **(B)** elevated epithelial line in epithelial rejection (arrow); **(C)** Krachmer spots; **(D)** endothelial rejection with Khodadoust line (arrow). Note intense peripheral vascularization. *(Courtesy of S Tuft – figs A, B and C.)*

- **Differential diagnosis** includes graft failure (no inflammation), infective keratitis including fungal and herpetic, uveitis, sterile suture reaction, raised IOP and epithelial ingrowth.

TIP In a patient with acute corneal graft rejection, early intensive treatment greatly improves the likelihood of reversing the episode of rejection.

Superficial lamellar keratoplasty

This involves partial-thickness excision of the corneal epithelium and stroma so that the endothelium and part of the deep stroma are left behind as a bed for appropriately partial-thickness donor cornea. The area grafted depends on the extent of the disease process to be addressed.

- **Indications**
  - Opacification of the superficial one-third of the corneal stroma not caused by potentially recurrent disease.
  - Marginal corneal thinning or infiltration as in recurrent pterygium, Terrien marginal degeneration and limbal dermoid or other tumours.
  - Localized thinning or descemetocoele formation (see Fig. 8.1B).

Deep anterior lamellar keratoplasty

Deep anterior lamellar keratoplasty (DALK) is a technique in which corneal tissue is removed almost to the level of Descemet membrane. A theoretical advantage is the decreased risk of rejection because the endothelium, a major target for rejection, is not transplanted. The major technical difficulty lies in judging the depth of the corneal dissection as close as possible to Descemet membrane without perforation and if this is not achieved the visual outcome may be compromised.

- **Indications**
  - Disease involving the anterior 95% of corneal thickness with normal endothelium and the absence of breaks or

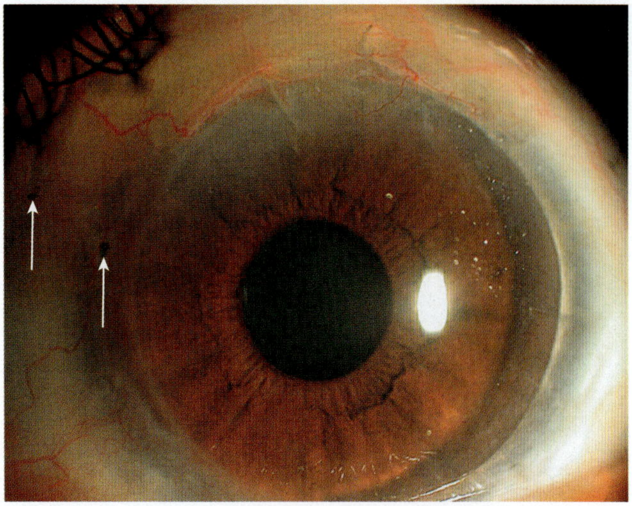

Fig. 8.8 Deep anterior lamellar keratoplasty for chemical injury. A superior conjunctival limbal autograft has also been performed (arrows indicate the edge of conjunctival graft).

scars in Descemet membrane (e.g. keratoconus without a history of acute hydrops, superficial trauma – Fig. 8.8).

- Chronic inflammatory disease such as atopic keratoconjunctivitis that carries an increased risk of graft rejection.

- **Advantages**
  - No risk of endothelial rejection, although epithelial/subepithelial/stromal rejection may occur.
  - Less astigmatism and a structurally stronger globe compared with penetrating keratoplasty.
  - Increased availability of graft material since endothelial quality is irrelevant.
- **Disadvantages**
  - Difficult and time-consuming with a high risk of perforation.
  - Interface haze may limit the best final visual acuity.
  - Postoperative management is similar to penetrating keratoplasty except that lower intensity topical steroids are needed and sutures can usually be removed after 6 months.

Endothelial keratoplasty

Endothelial keratoplasty involves removal of diseased endothelium along with Descemet membrane (DM) through a corneoscleral or corneal incision. Folded donor tissue is introduced through the same small (2.8–5.0 mm) incision. Descemet stripping (automated) endothelial keratoplasty (DSAEK) uses an automated microkeratome to prepare donor tissue and is currently the most commonly performed technique. A small amount of posterior stromal thickness is transplanted along with DM and endothelium (Fig. 8.9). In Descemet membrane endothelial keratoplasty (DMEK) only the DM and endothelium are transplanted.

Because the graft is only 5–10 µm thick it is difficult to handle. However, the grafts are able to attach to the host tissue with less unevenness, which leads to more rapid visual recovery. Visual outcomes and lower rejection rates are achieved, but intraoperative complication rates are higher than DSAEK.

- **Indications** include endothelial disease such as Fuchs endothelial corneal dystrophy and a localised tectonic graft for patching of a corneal perforation.
- **Advantages**
  - Relatively little refractive change and a structurally more intact globe.
  - Faster visual rehabilitation than penetrating keratoplasty.
  - Suturing is minimized.
- **Disadvantages**
  - Significant learning curve.
  - Specialized equipment is required.
  - The visual outcome is often suboptimal regardless of the graft clarity. Reasons include: (a) differences in graft thickness, (b) graft irregularities, (c) high order aberrations, (d) donor–recipient interface fibrosis.
  - Endothelial rejection can still occur (Fig. 8.10).

TIP Endothelial keratoplasty (DSAEK) results in more rapid visual improvement and less risk of rejection than penetrating keratoplasty.

Limbal stem cell grafting

Stem cells are undifferentiated cells that give rise to the differentiated cells that form tissues and organs. Tissue-specific stem cells are important for maintaining homeostasis and for tissue repair after injury. Corneal epithelium is constantly self-renewing and does so throughout life. Progeny of corneal stem cells divide and differentiate to form basal corneal epithelial cells (transient amplifying cells) that differentiate into wing cells (post-mitotic cells) and, finally, superficial squamous cells (terminally differentiated cells).

Various techniques have been described to replenish the limbal stem cell population in patients with severe ocular surface disease and associated stem cell deficiency. These include transplantation of a limbal area of limited size from a healthy fellow eye, complete limbal transplantation of a donor annulus and *ex vivo* expansion by culture of either host or donor stem cells with subsequent transplantation. In patients with unilateral ocular involvement in Stevens–Johnson syndrome and ocular cicatricial pemphigoid, donor tissue should not be taken from the unaffected eye (autologous).

- **Signs of limbal stem cell deficiency (LSCD)** include:
  - Conjunctivalization of cornea with goblet cells (confirmed with confocal microscopy, impression cytology with acid Schiff stain or monoclonal antibody against cytokeratin 19).
  - Superficial and deep corneal vascularization.
  - Fibrovascular pannus.
  - Persistent epithelial defects.
  - Scarring.
- **Algorithm for surgical interventions for LSCD**
  - All associated abnormalities (lids, conjunctiva, intraocular pressure) should be treated first.

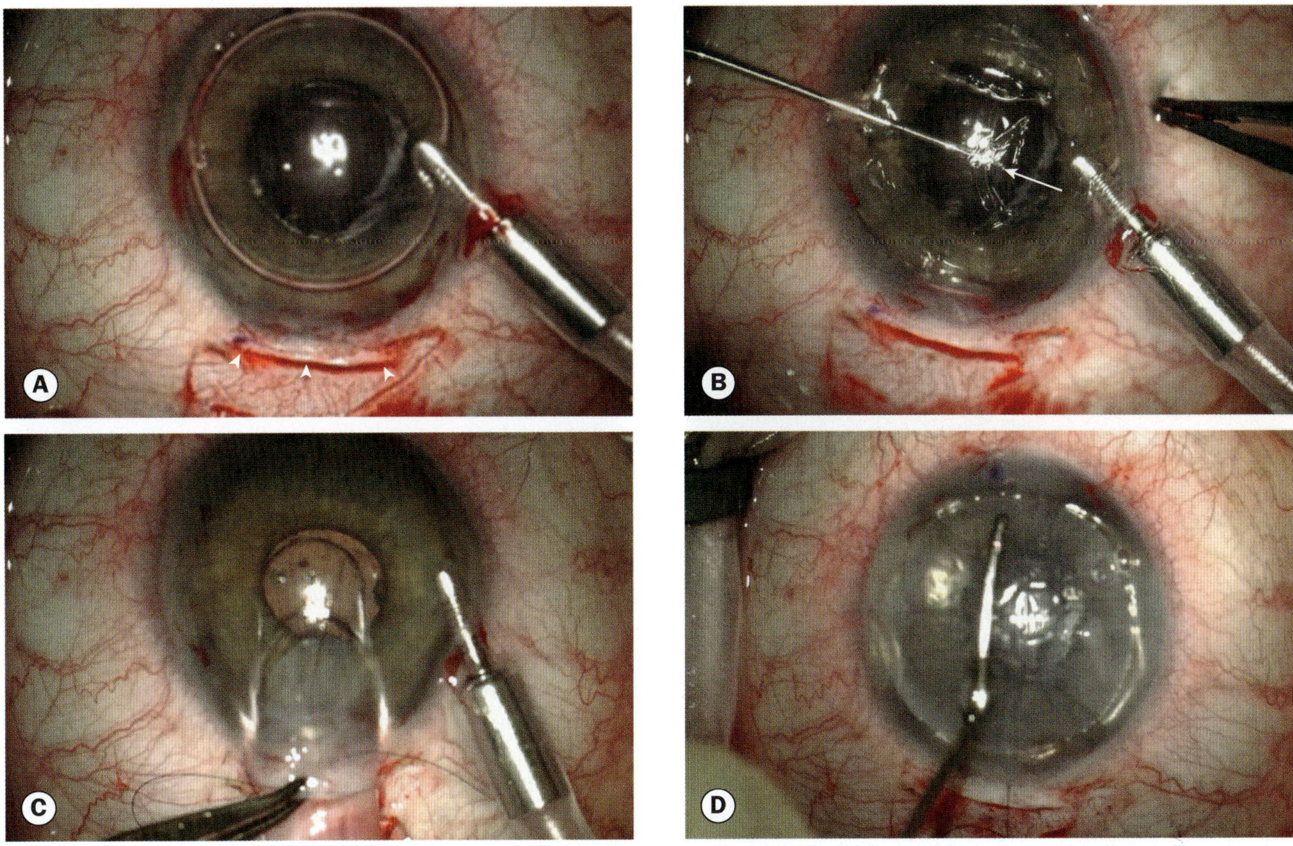

Fig. 8.9 DSAEK. **(A)** Scleral tunnel incision (arrowheads) with an air bubble in the anterior chamber to facilitate visualization of Descemet membrane; **(B)** the far edge of Descemet membrane is stripped using a reverse Sinskey hook (arrow); **(C)** the donor graft is inserted through the scleral tunnel using an endoglide system; **(D)** once the graft has unfolded and centred it can be gently stroked into position, making sure that there is no fluid in the donor/recipient interface. *(Courtesy of M Leyland.)*

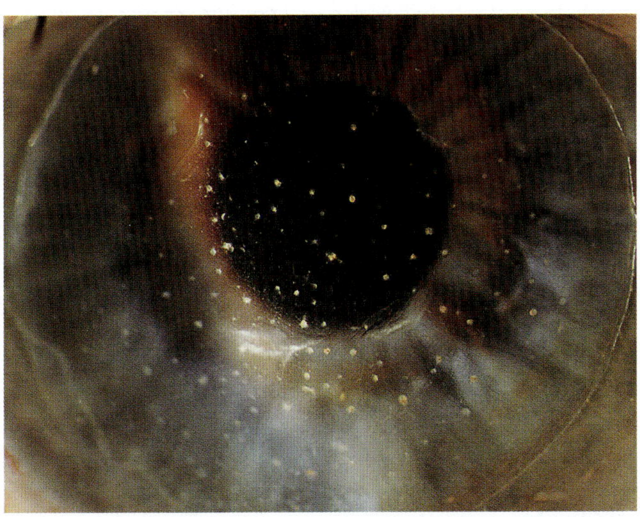

Fig. 8.10 Endothelial graft undergoing rejection. *(Courtesy of C Barry.)*

 - When the visual axis is involved, sequential sector conjunctival epitheliectomy should be considered with a sector limbal transplant.
 - In total unilateral stem cell deficiency, auto limbal transplantation is the procedure of choice.
 - In total bilateral stem cell deficiency, use of allografts from a living related donor or a cadaver donor is the only option.

- **Indications**
  - Congenital: for example, aniridia.
  - Traumatic: chemical and thermal burns.
  - Chronic inflammatory disease: Stevens–Johnson syndrome, ocular cicatricial pemphigoid.
  - Ocular surface malignancy.
  - Contact lens-related pathology.
- **Advantages**
  - Regeneration of corneal surface epithelium.
  - Visual improvement and improved comfort.
- **Disadvantages**
  - Autologous graft: conjunctivalization, filamentary keratitis, scarring of donor eye.
  - Allogenic graft: infection (especially in immunecompromised patients), rejection.

TIP An important sign of limbal stem cell deficiency is colonization of the cornea with goblet cells, detected with impression cytology.

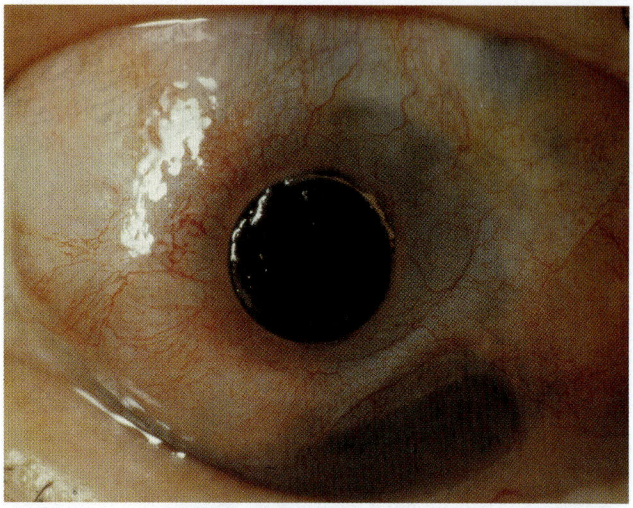

Fig. 8.11 Keratoprosthesis. *(Courtesy of R Bates.)*

KERATOPROSTHESES

Keratoprostheses (Fig. 8.11) are artificial corneal implants used in patients unsuitable for keratoplasty. The modern osteoodontokeratoprosthesis consists of the patient's own tooth root and alveolar bone supporting a central optical cylinder and is usually covered with a buccal mucous membrane graft. Surgery is difficult and time-consuming and is performed in two stages, 2–4 months apart. In experienced hands the retention rate is about 85% at 18 months. Approximately 80% of patients achieve visual acuity between counting fingers and 6/12 and occasionally even better. A poor outcome is usually associated with pre-existing optic nerve or retinal dysfunction. High patient motivation is a key factor to consider before proceeding to surgery.

- **Indications**
  - Bilateral blindness from severe, but inactive anterior segment disease with no realistic chance of success from conventional keratoplasty, e.g. Stevens–Johnson syndrome, ocular cicatricial pemphigoid, chemical burns and trachoma.
  - Vision of counting fingers or less in the better eye.
  - Intact optic nerve and retinal function, without marked glaucomatous optic neuropathy.
- **Complications**
  - Glaucoma in up to 40%. Management is inevitably extremely challenging and requires aggressive IOP-lowering medication and often the insertion of a drainage shunt.
  - Membrane formation behind the prosthesis (25%); usually managed with YAG-laser membranectomy.
  - Tilting or extrusion.
  - Retinal detachment and endophthalmitis (about 3% per patient year).

REFRACTIVE PROCEDURES

Introduction

- **Refractive surgery** encompasses a range of procedures aimed at changing the refraction of the eye by altering the cornea or lens, the principal refracting components. Myopia, hypermetropia (hyperopia) and astigmatism can all be addressed, though correction of presbyopia is yet to be achieved on a consistently satisfactory basis.
- **The patient population** consists of people with stable refractive error who desire an improvement in visual acuity or function after surgical correction.
- **A thorough preoperative assessment** is mandatory. Not everyone who requests this treatment is suitable. People who require a high level of quality vision, e.g, certain professions (pilot, air-traffic controller, truck-driver) and specific hobbies (contact sports, marksman, amateur astronomer) must understand the limitations of the surgery before proceeding.
- **Informed consent** is vitally important.
- **Contraindications** include: people with unacceptably high expectations, dry eye syndrome, non-stable refractive error, some systemic diseases (SLE, rheumatoid arthritis, immunocompromise) and those with ocular disease (chronic blepharitis, previous herpes simplex, glaucoma, macular degeneration).
- **The advantages and potential risks** should be discussed and the common adverse side effects such as under- and overcorrection, dry eye symptoms and eventual presbyopia should be emphasized. Care should be taken to discuss which adverse events are likely to be transient and which may be permanent.
- **Alternatives,** including new and emerging technology for treatment, should be discussed.
- **Patient satisfaction** depends on patient expectations and the surgical outcome. Most are satisfied after the surgery, but some may be unhappy because of induced ocular side effects and visual aberrations, even though the intended correction has been achieved.

TIP People who require a high level of quality vision because of their occupation or hobbies need to understand the limitations of refractive surgery and make an informed decision before proceeding to surgical correction.

Correction of myopia

- **Surface ablation procedures** (see below) can correct low-moderate degrees of myopia.
- **Laser *in situ* keratomileusis** (LASIK – see below) can correct moderate to high myopia depending on initial corneal thickness, but for very high refractive errors one of the intraocular procedures below is necessary.
- **Refractive lenticule extraction** (SMILE – see below) is a small incisional laser technique for the correction of myopia and myopic astigmatism.
- **Clear lens exchange** gives very good visual results but carries a small risk of the complications of cataract surgery (see Ch. 10), particularly retinal detachment in individuals with high myopia.
- **Iris clip** ('lobster claw') implant is attached to the iris (Fig. 8.12A). Complications include subluxation or dislocation due to dislodgement of one or both attachments, an oval pupil,

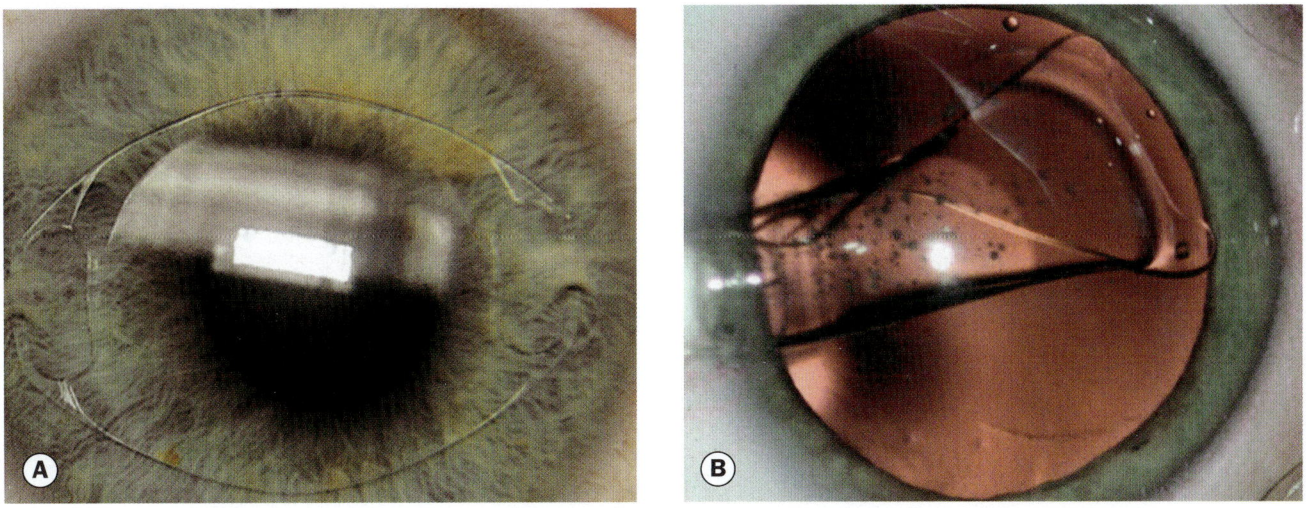

Fig. 8.12 Phakic intraocular implants for correction of myopia. **(A)** Anterior chamber iris claw implant with anterior iris attachment at 3 and 9 o'clock; **(B)** emplacement of a posterior chamber phakic implant between the iris and anterior lens surface. *(Courtesy of J Krachmer, M Mannis and E Holland from* Cornea, *Mosby 2005 – fig. B.)*

endothelial cell loss, cataract, pupillary-block glaucoma and retinal detachment.

- **Phakic posterior chamber implant** (implantable contact lens, ICL) is inserted behind the iris and in front of the lens (Fig. 8.12B) and supported in the ciliary sulcus. The lens is composed of material derived from collagen (Collamer) with a power of −3 D to −20.50 D. Visual results are usually good, but complications include uveitis, pupillary block, endothelial cell loss, cataract formation and retinal detachment.
- **Radial keratotomy** (Fig. 8.13) is now predominantly of historical interest.

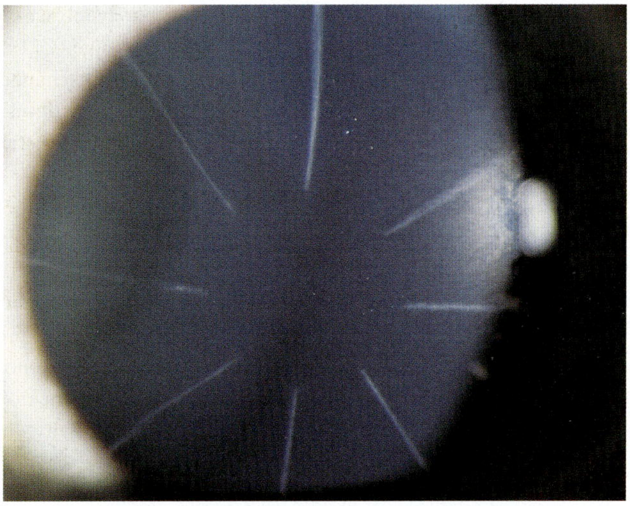

Fig. 8.13 Radial keratotomy. *(Courtesy of C Barry.)*

Correction of hypermetropia (hyperopia)

- **Surface ablation procedures** can correct low degrees of hypermetropia.
- **LASIK** can correct up to 4 D.
- **Conductive keratoplasty (CK)** involves the application of radiofrequency energy to the corneal stroma in order to correct low–moderate hypermetropia and hypermetropic astigmatism. Burns are placed in one or two rings in the corneal periphery using a micro-needle high-frequency probe. The resultant thermally induced stromal shrinkage is accompanied by an increase in central corneal curvature. Complications are infrequent, but the disadvantages include early overcorrection, significant regression and induced astigmatism. CK may also be helpful for presbyopia (see below). Laser thermal keratoplasty with a holmium laser is no longer used.
- **Other modalities** include clear lens extraction and phakic lens implants as described above for myopia. Intraocular surgical procedures are the only options for high degrees of refractive error.

Correction of astigmatism

- **Limbal relaxing incisions/arcuate keratotomy** involves making paired arcuate incisions on opposite sides of the cornea (Fig. 8.14A) in the axis of the correcting 'plus' cylinder (the steep meridian). The resultant flattening of the steep meridian coupled with a smaller steepening of the flat meridian at 90° to the incisions reduces astigmatism. The desired result can be controlled by varying the length and depth of the incisions and their distance from the optical centre of the cornea. Arcuate keratotomy may be combined with compression sutures placed in the perpendicular meridian, when treating large degrees of astigmatism such as can occur following penetrating keratoplasty.
- **PRK** and **LASEK** can correct up to 3 D.
- **LASIK** can correct up to 5 D.
- **Lens surgery** involves using a 'toric' intraocular implant incorporating an astigmatic correction (Fig. 8.14B). Postoperative rotation of the implant away from the desired axis occurs in a minority of cases.
- **Conductive keratoplasty** (see 'Correction of hypermetropia' above).

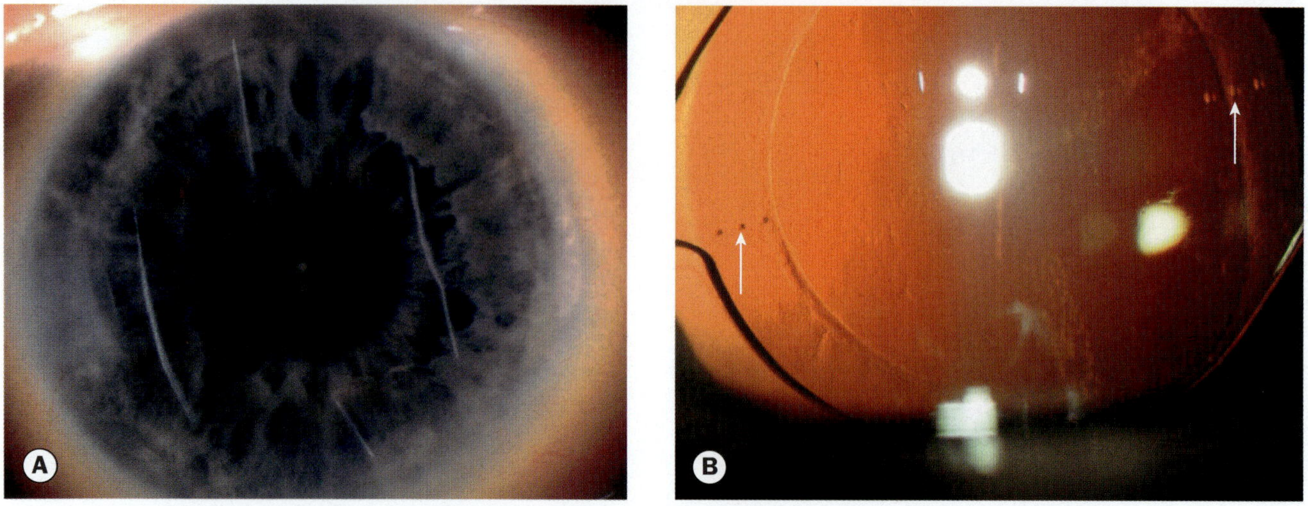

Fig. 8.14 Correction of astigmatism. **(A)** Arcuate keratotomies; **(B)** toric intraocular implant *in situ* – markings incorporated in the lens (arrows) facilitate correct orientation. *(Courtesy of C Barry – fig. A.)*

Correction of presbyopia

- **Lens extraction**, either to treat cataract or for purely refractive purposes. Acronyms used include clear lens exchange (CLE), refractive lens exchange (RLE) and presbyopic lens exchange (PreLEx). Much research effort is being applied to the development of effective accommodating and multifocal prosthetic lenses.
  - Implantation of a bifocal, trifocal diffractive, multifocal refractive, extended depth of focus or 'accommodating'/ pseudo-accommodative intraocular lens implant can optically restore reading vision, but glasses may still have to be used for some tasks. If appropriately screened, most recipients of multifocal IOLs are happy with the visual outcome. However, dissatisfaction may occur as a consequence of nocturnal glare, halo and reduced contrast sensitivity. In patients with intractable visual symptoms IOL exchange surgery should be undertaken. In some jurisdictions, implantation of a multifocal IOL is a contraindication to the holding of a private or commercial pilot's licence, or to military service.
  - 'Monovision' consists of the targeting of IOL-induced refractive outcomes so that one eye (usually the dominant) is optimized for clear uncorrected distance vision and the other for near or intermediate vision, in order to facilitate both good distance and near vision when the eyes are used together. Suppression of the blurred image and neuro-adaptation by the patient is required for this to be successful.
- **Conductive keratoplasty** (see 'Correction of hypermetropia' above). There is some evidence that CK can impart a degree of multifocal functionality to the cornea.
- **Laser-induced monovision** refers to the use of laser refractive surgery to optimize one eye for distance and the fellow for near or intermediate vision (see above under 'Lens extraction').
- **Corneal multifocality: presbyLASIK.** Several different approaches are under development utilizing a laser procedure to alter the shape of the cornea such that a bifocal or transitional effect is induced. Laser manufacturers have developed specific treatment algorithms based on the near-addition target (or planned according to the subject's age) to create a multifocal corneal profile. However, the effective change in refraction comes from the controlled change in the corneal asphericity from the centre to the periphery. The benefit of presbyLASIK over monofocal ablation is not yet clear.
- **Scleral expansion surgery.** Results have been inconsistent and unpredictable and this technique has not achieved sustained popularity.
- **Intracorneal inlays** provide substantial benefit in presbyopia, though in the past the biocompatibility of some materials has been relatively poor and complications such as corneal haze and extrusion can necessitate removal.
  - Types: (a) refractive corneal inlays (Fig. 8.15A and B), (b) corneal reshaping inlays and (c) small aperture inlays (Fig. 8.15C and D).
  - Inlay position. The inlay can be placed either in a stromal pocket or under a flap. Advantages of a stromal pocket include stable centration, minimal damage to corneal nerves and corneal striae. The advantage of placing the inlay under a flap is that the procedure can be combined with excimer laser ablation to correct refractive error.
  - Complications involve: (a) lens decentration, (b) dry eyes, (c) keratolysis, (d) vascularization, (e) opacification and (f) epithelial ingrowth. These complications are less likely to occur with modern implants as they are thin, have a small diameter and have high permeability with improved biocompatibility characteristics.
  - Late side effects include: (a) haloes, glare and disturbance of night vision, (b) loss of contrast sensitivity, (c) difficulty reading in dim light, (d) tear instability and (e) variable vision.

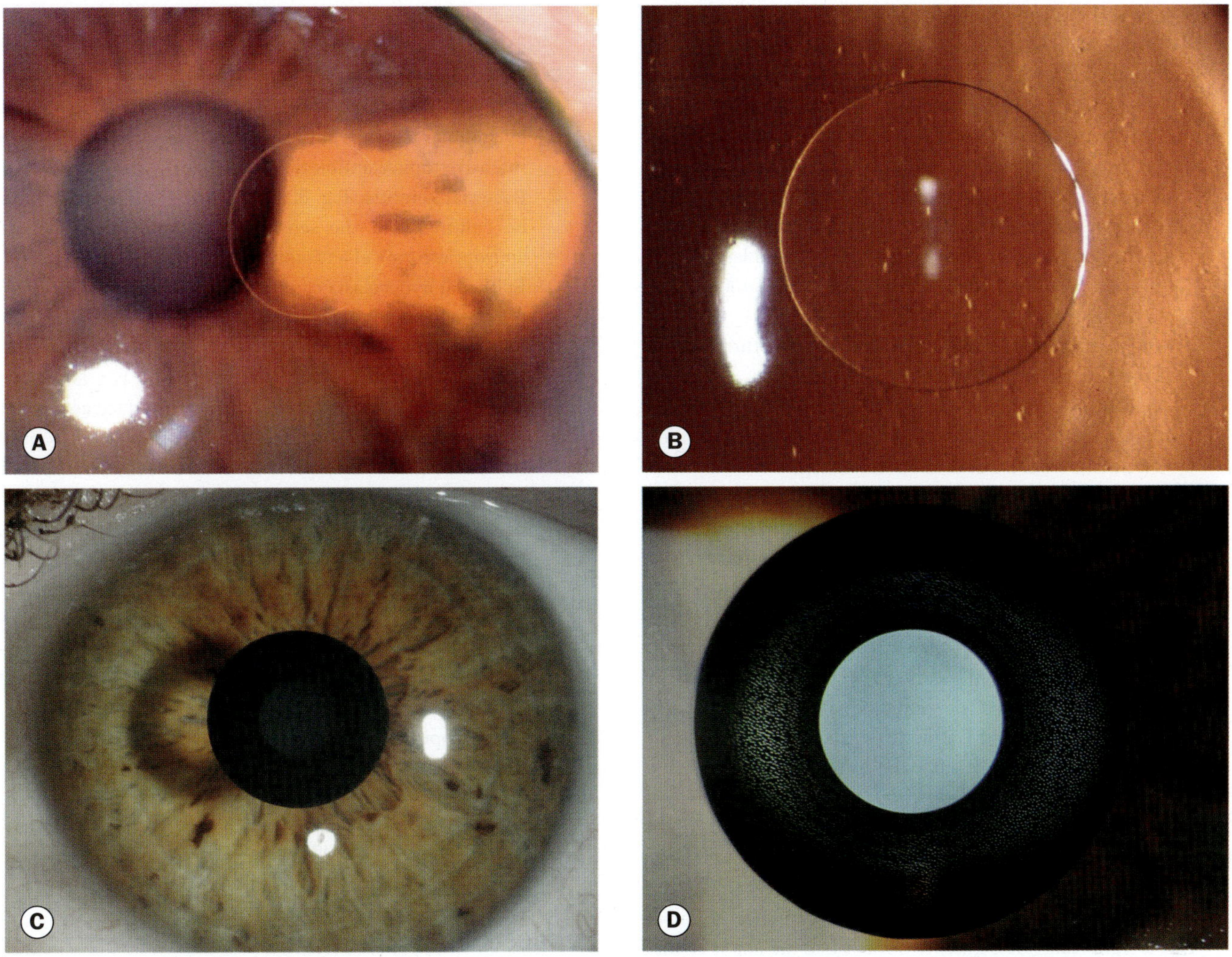

Fig. 8.15 Intracorneal inlays for presbyopia correction. **(A)** and **(B)** Refractive inlay; **(C)** and **(D)** small aperture inlay – utilizes the pinhole effect. *(Courtesy of C Barry.)*

Laser refractive procedures

To settle any contact lens-induced corneal distortion prior to definitive keratometry, soft contact lenses should probably be discontinued for 2 weeks and hard/rigid gas permeable lenses for at least 3 weeks (some surgeons suggest 1 week for each year of wear to date).

Laser *in situ* keratomileusis

Laser (or laser-assisted) *in situ* keratomileusis (LASIK) is a very common refractive procedure. Refraction should be stable for at least one year before LASIK surgery is undertaken. The excimer laser, which can ablate tissue to a precise depth with negligible disruption of surrounding areas, is used to reshape corneal stroma exposed by the creation of a superficial flap. The flap remains attached by a hinge to facilitate accurate and secure repositioning. Myopia is corrected by central ablative flattening and hypermetropia by ablation of the mid-periphery so that the centre becomes steeper. LASIK can generally be used to treat higher refractive errors than surface ablation techniques (see below): hypermetropia up to 3-4 D, astigmatism up to 5 D and myopia up to 6–8 D depending on initial corneal thickness. For refractive errors outside these parameters an alternative technique should be considered. To decrease the risk of subsequent ectasia, a residual corneal base at least 250 μm thickness must remain after ablation. The amount of tissue removed, and therefore the amount of refractive error correctable, is limited by the original corneal thickness. It follows that high refractive errors can be addressed only by an intraocular procedure. In addition to treatment of a wider range of refractive errors, advantages over surface ablation include greater postoperative comfort, faster visual rehabilitation, more rapid stabilization of refraction and milder stromal haze. The major disadvantage is the potential for serious flap-related complications.

- **Preoperative evaluation** includes:
  - Complete ocular examination.
  - Tear film osmolarity to exclude dry eye syndrome.
  - Corneal pachymetry to determine residual stromal bed thickness and to exclude mild keratoconus.
  - Corneal topography to exclude irregular astigmatism, keratoconus, and forme fruste keratoconus.

- Corneal OCT to produce an epithelial map of the cornea.
- Corneal and whole eye wavefront aberrometry.

- **Technique**
  - A suction ring centred on the cornea is applied to the globe which raises the intraocular pressure substantially.
  - The ring stabilizes the eye and provides the guide track for a mechanical microkeratome, which is advanced across the cornea to create a thin flap. In recent years, the creation of the flap is undertaken using a femtosecond laser, which allows a precise and uniform flap thickness of 100–120 μm to be made.
  - The flap is reflected and the bed reshaped by the laser, followed by flap repositioning (Fig. 8.16A).
  - Wavefront-guided LASIK is a variation of LASIK, where the excimer laser ablates a precise pattern based on measurements from a wavefront aberrometer.
  - 'Optomised' LASIK treatment refers to an ablation algorithm, patented by some lasers in standard mode to produce larger optical zones and better corneal asphericity, in order to reduce unwanted visual aberrations and postoperative glare.
  - LASIK Plus is a procedure where cross-linking is undertaken after the laser treatment. It might be considered in patients at risk of developing postoperative ectasia or refractive regression (refractive error greater than −7 D). A riboflavin solution is applied to the stromal bed while the flap is open, followed by irrigation of the stromal bed, replacement of the flap and application of ultraviolet light.
- **Intraoperative complications** include 'buttonholing' (penetration) or amputation of the flap, incomplete or irregular flap creation and, rarely, penetration into the anterior chamber. This is significantly less likely to occur when the flap is created with a femtosecond laser.
- **Early postoperative complications**
  - Flap decentration.
  - Wrinkling (Fig. 8.16B), distortion or dislocation of the flap.
  - Interface debris.
- **Late postoperative complications**
  - Refractive stability can take up to 3 months depending on the amount of treatment performed. Under-correction (primary treatment) and over-correction (retreatment) may occur.
  - Dry eye and tear film instability are the commonest side effects, occurring in up to 70%, but usually improve spontaneously in time.
  - Transient light sensitivity syndrome. This usually occurs between 2 and 8 weeks after surgery and is more likely to occur after hyperopic LASIK (9%) than myopic LASIK (5%) or SMILE (1%). Symptoms settle on topical steroids.
  - Subepithelial haze (Fig. 8.16C) leading to symptoms of glare, haloes and 'star bursts,' which are especially noticed at night. This usually settles within 3–6 months.
  - Epithelial ingrowth under the flap (1–2%) (Fig. 8.16D). Treatment is not always required, but when the vision is affected, repeat surgery should be considered. After lifting the flap the epithelial cells are scraped from the stromal bed and undersurface of the flap. Ethanol or mitomycin C can be applied, but this can result in adverse effects.
  - Diffuse lamellar keratitis ('sands of the Sahara' – Fig. 8.16E) may develop 1–7 days following LASIK. It is characterized by granular deposits at the flap interface. Treatment is with intensive topical antibiotic and steroid.
  - Bacterial keratitis (Fig. 8.16F) is rare. The organism must be cultured and the sensitivity determined so that an appropriate topical antibiotic can be prescribed.
  - Epithelial hyperplasia can result in regression and is diagnosed using an epithelial OCT map.
  - Persistent epithelial defects.
  - Pressure-induced stromal keratitis (PISK) is a late-onset visible fluid cleft which occurs in the interface as a result of elevated IOP, usually secondary to prolonged topical steroid use. This may present as an under-correction or regression.
  - Corneal ectasia (see Ch. 7). This is a devastating complication which is fortunately uncommon (0.2–0.6%). Ectasia is more likely to occur when there is: (a) abnormal preoperative topography (e.g. forme fruste keratoconus or pellucid marginal degeneration), (b) low preoperative central corneal thickness, (c) low post-ablation residual stromal bed thickness, (d) greater percentage corneal tissue altered, (e) high myopia, (f) young age. Careful pre-procedure screening should be performed to detect any predisposition.

TIP LASIK may cause transient symptoms of dry eye and glare secondary to subepithelial haze.

Surface ablation procedures

Like LASIK, photorefractive keratectomy (PRK) employs excimer laser ablation to reshape the cornea. PRK is able to correct myopia up to 6 D, astigmatism up to around 3 D and low–moderate hypermetropia. The main disadvantages compared with LASIK are the lower degrees of refractive error correctable and slower epithelial healing with unpredictable postoperative discomfort. However, as a flap is not created there is a lower risk of serious complications than with LASIK, including corneal ectasia and late flap dislocation and it may be the procedure of choice for patients at higher than average occupational or leisure-related risk of eye injury. It is also suitable for patients rendered ineligible for LASIK due to low corneal thickness. Other indications for surface ablation rather than LASIK include borderline dry eye syndrome, epithelial basement membrane disease, prior corneal transplantation or radial keratotomy and large pupil size.

- **Technique**
  - The corneal epithelium is removed prior to ablation. Methods used may include a sponge, an automated brush (Amoils epithelial scrubber) and alcohol.
  - Ablation of the Bowman layer and anterior stroma (Fig. 8.17) is performed, generally taking 30–60 seconds. In modern systems, sophisticated tracking mechanisms adjust laser targeting with eye movement and will pause the procedure if the eye is significantly decentred.

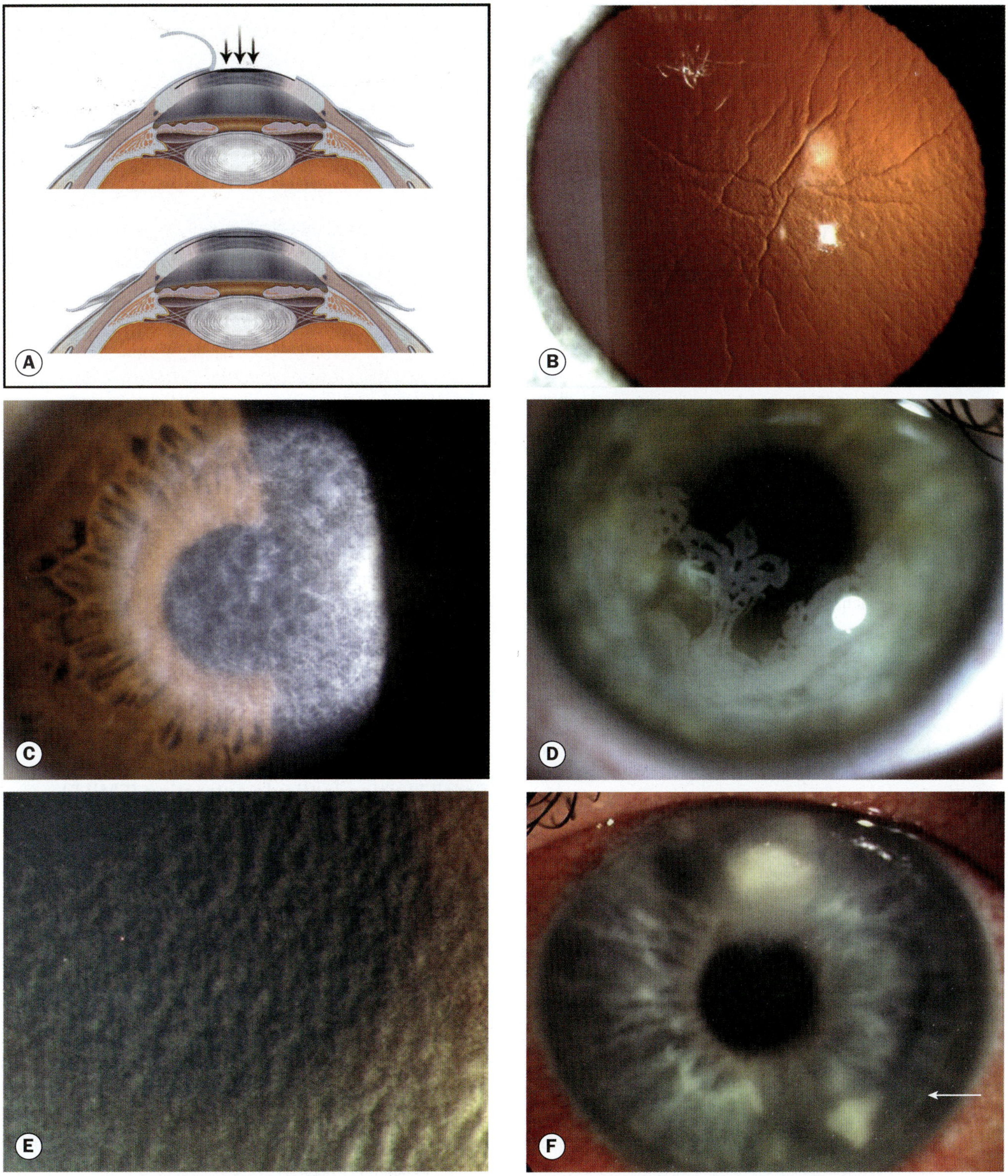

Fig. 8.16 Laser *in situ* keratomileusis (LASIK). **(A)** A flap is elevated either with a microkeratome or a femtosecond laser, the stromal bed is precisely reshaped with an excimer laser and the flap is repositioned; **(B)** retroillumination showing wrinkling of the flap; **(C)** subepithelial haze; **(D)** epithelial ingrowth; **(E)** diffuse lamellar keratitis ('sands of the Sahara'); **(F)** bacterial keratitis, with an arrow showing the edge of the flap. *(Courtesy of M Leyland – fig. D; S Tuft – fig. E; R Bates – fig. F.)*

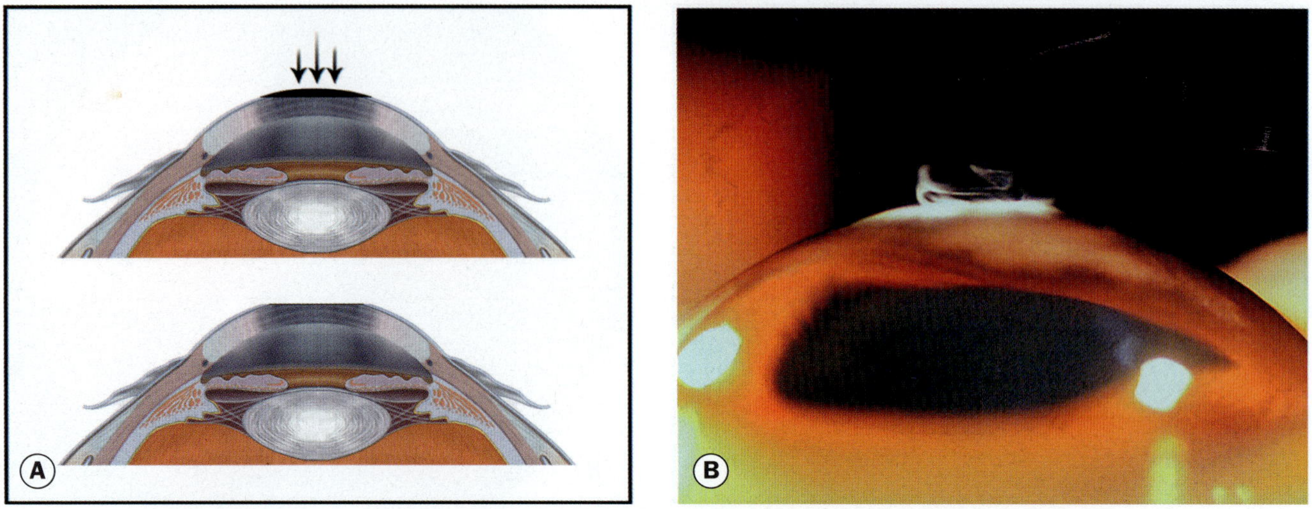

Fig. 8.17 Photorefractive keratectomy (PRK). **(A)** Laser ablation of Bowman layer and anterior stroma after removal of the epithelium. This results in reprofiling of the anterior curvature of the cornea and therefore changes its refractive power; **(B)** active laser ablation of the anterior surface of the cornea. *(Courtesy of C Barry – fig. B.)*

  - The epithelium usually heals within 48–72 hours. A bandage contact lens is generally used to minimize discomfort. Subepithelial haze invariably develops within 2 weeks and commonly persists for several weeks to months. Diminished final visual acuity is rare but there may be decreased contrast and nocturnal glare. Intraoperative application of mitomycin C (mitomycin-LASEK or M-LASEK) may reduce haze.
- **Complications** include slowly healing epithelial defects, corneal haze with blurring and haloes, poor night vision and regression of refractive correction. Uncommon problems include decentred ablation, scarring, abnormal epithelial healing, irregular astigmatism, reduced corneal sensation, sterile infiltrates, infection and acute corneal necrosis.
- **Variations of PRK.** A range of procedural variations with correspondingly varying terminology have been described. LASEK (laser epithelial keratomileusis or laser-assisted subepithelial keratectomy), Epi-LASIK (epipolis or epithelial LASIK; *epipolis* is a Greek word meaning superficial), modified PRK, advanced surface (laser) ablation (ASA or ASLA) and Trans-PRK (trans-epithelial PRK) are variations of PRK that utilize a variety of techniques to try to reduce discomfort and post-laser haze and to speed visual recovery. ASA and modified PRK are sometimes used generally to refer to all surface ablative procedures. In LASEK the epithelium is detached and peeled back after pre-treatment with dilute alcohol. Laser is then applied and the epithelium repositioned. Epi-LASIK employs a mechanical device, an epikeratome, to elevate a hinged sheet of epithelium with an oscillating blunt plastic blade and alcohol application is not usually required. Some recent reports suggest that healing occurs more rapidly if the epithelium is simply detached entirely without replacement (flap-off Epi-LASIK). In Trans-PRK, epithelial ablation is performed with the laser prior to the refractive ablation, reducing operative time and possibly conferring other benefits.

Small incision lenticule extraction (SMILE)

- **Small incision lenticule extraction** – SMILE is a technique that uses a femtosecond laser (Carl Zeiss VisuMax) to cut a lens-shaped piece of corneal tissue (a lenticule) within the intact cornea. This is then removed using a minimally invasive 4 mm incision. When the lenticle is removed via a LASIK-style flap the procedure is termed refractive lenticular extraction (ReLex).
- **Results** are similar to those obtained with LASIK.
- **Advantages**
  - Low risk of flap-related complications.
  - Biomechanical advantage.
  - Faster recovery of dry eye symptoms.
  - Quicker corneal reinnervation.
  - Surface disturbance is minimal in comparison to surface ablation procedures.

Chapter

9 Episclera and Sclera

ANATOMY

The scleral stroma is composed of collagen bundles of varying size and shape that are not uniformly orientated as in the cornea and so are not transparent. The inner layer of the sclera blends with the uveal tract. Anteriorly the episclera consists of a connective tissue layer between the superficial scleral stroma and Tenon capsule. There are three pre-equatorial vascular layers:

- **Conjunctival vessels** are the most superficial. Arteries are tortuous and veins straight.
- **Superficial episcleral plexus** vessels are straight with a radial configuration. In episcleritis, maximal congestion occurs at this level (Fig. 9.1A). Topical phenylephrine 2.5% will also constrict the conjunctival and 10% also the superficial episcleral vessels.
- **Deep vascular plexus** lies in the superficial part of the sclera and shows maximal congestion in scleritis (Fig. 9.1B). A purplish hue, best seen in daylight, is characteristic.

EPISCLERITIS

Episcleritis is a common, usually idiopathic and benign, recurrent and frequently bilateral condition. Females may be affected more commonly than males, except possibly in children, in whom episcleritis is rare. The average patient is middle-aged. It is typically self-limiting and tends to last from a few days up to 3 weeks, but rarely longer. Associated disease, either ocular (e.g. dry eye, rosacea, contact lens wear) or systemic (e.g. collagen vascular disorders such as rheumatoid arthritis, herpes zoster ophthalmicus, gout, Crohn disease and others), has been identified in tertiary referral centres. Infectious causes are very rare but a wide range has been reported. Investigation of recurrent cases is as for scleritis (see later).

TIP Acute episcleritis is common, usually idiopathic and has a good visual prognosis.

Simple episcleritis

Simple episcleritis accounts for 75% of cases. It tends to recur (60%), decreasing in frequency with time. Features often peak within 24 hours, gradually fading over the next few days.

- **Symptoms.** Discomfort ranges from absent (up to 50%) to moderate. Grittiness is common and photophobia may occur.
- **Signs.** More than half of cases are simultaneously bilateral.
  - Visual acuity is normal.
  - Redness may be sectoral (Fig. 9.2A) or diffuse (Fig. 9.2B). Often it has an interpalpebral distribution, in a triangular configuration with the base at the limbus.
  - Chemosis, ocular hypertension, anterior uveitis and keratitis are all rare.
- **Treatment**
  - If mild, no treatment is required. Cool compresses or refrigerated artificial tears may be helpful.

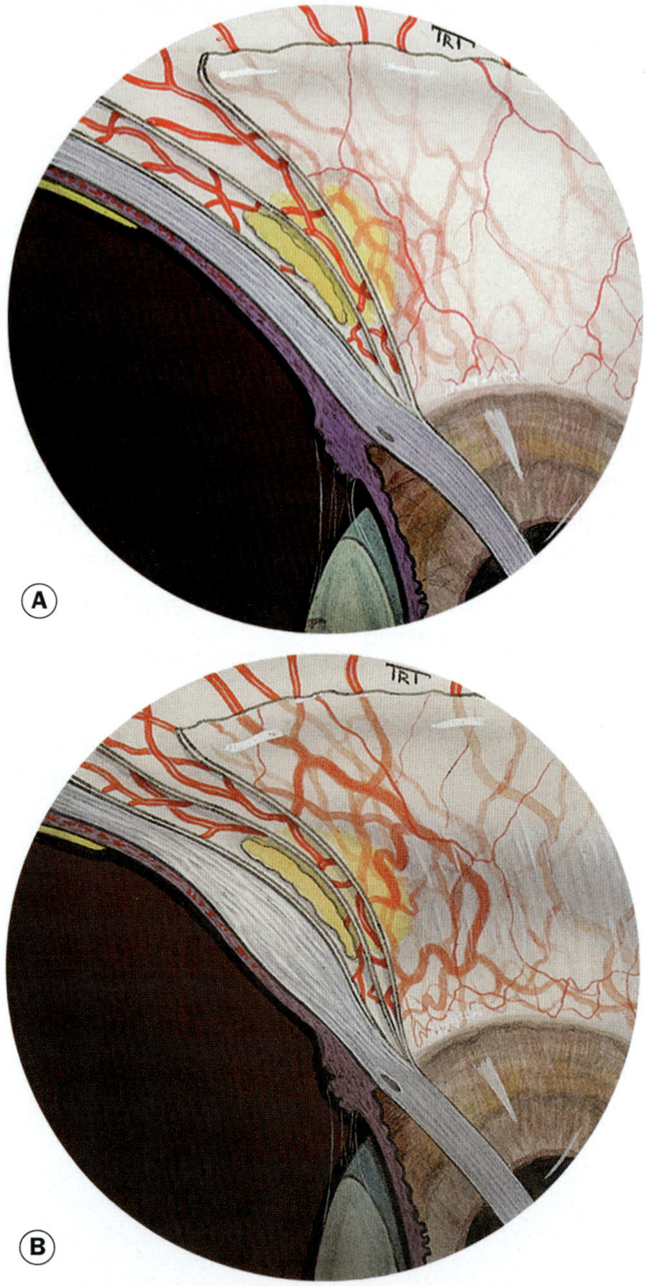

Fig. 9.1 (A) Episcleritis with maximal vascular congestion of the superficial episcleral plexus; **(B)** scleritis with scleral thickening and maximal vascular congestion of the deep vascular plexus.

  - A weak topical steroid four times daily for 1–2 weeks is usually sufficient, though occasionally more intensive instillation is needed initially or a more potent preparation can be used with rapid tapering. A topical non-steroidal anti-inflammatory (NSAID) is an alternative, though may be less effective.
  - An oral NSAID is occasionally required (e.g. ibuprofen 200 mg three times daily, or occasionally a more potent agent such as indomethacin).

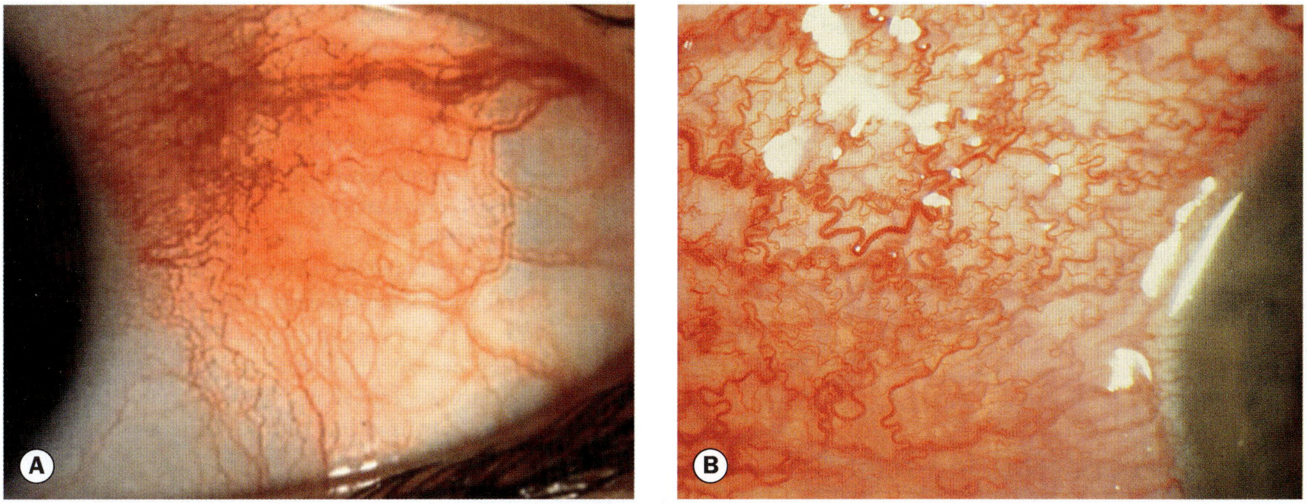

Fig. 9.2 Simple episcleritis. **(A)** Sectoral; **(B)** diffuse.

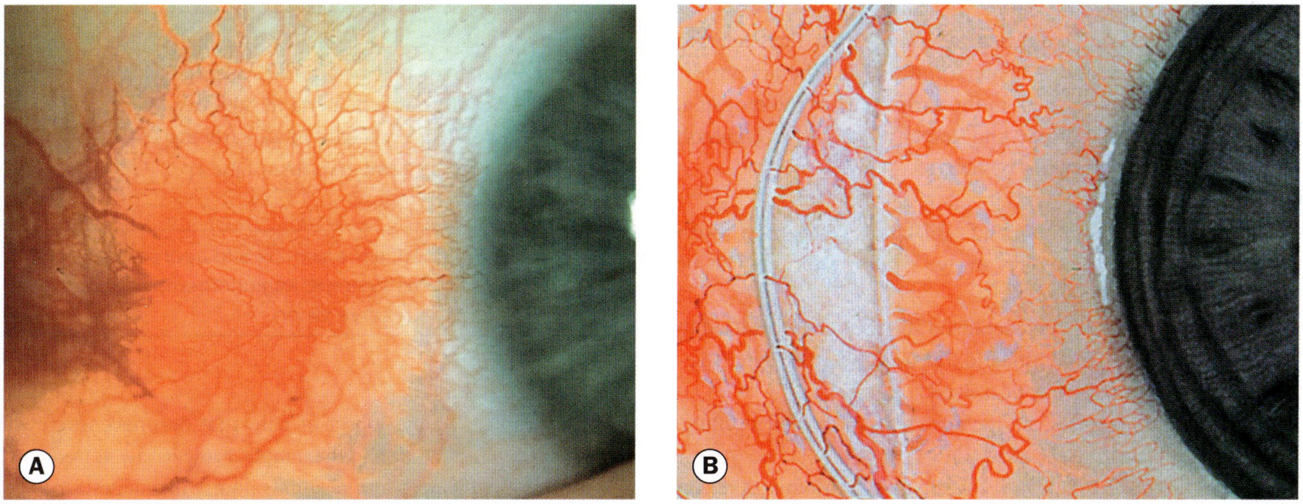

Fig. 9.3 **(A)** Nodular episcleritis; **(B)** slit illumination showing that the deep beam is not displaced above the scleral surface.

Nodular episcleritis

Nodular episcleritis also tends to affect females more than males but has a less acute onset and a more prolonged course than the simple variant.

- **Symptoms.** A red eye is typically first noted on waking. Over the next 2–3 days the area of redness enlarges and becomes more uncomfortable.
- **Signs.** Attacks usually clear without treatment, but tend to last longer than simple episcleritis.
  - A tender red vascular nodule, almost always within the interpalpebral fissure (Fig. 9.3A). Occasionally more than one focus is present.
  - A slit lamp section shows an underlying flat anterior scleral surface, indicating the absence of scleritis (Fig. 9.3B).
  - Intraocular pressure (IOP) is very occasionally elevated.
  - An anterior chamber reaction may be present but is uncommon (10%).
  - After several episodes, inflamed vessels may become permanently dilated.
  - It is important to exclude other causes of a nodule such as phlyctenulosis (a phlycten is within rather than beneath the conjunctiva) or a conjunctival granuloma.
- **Treatment** is similar to that of simple episcleritis.

IMMUNE-MEDIATED SCLERITIS

Scleritis is an uncommon condition characterized by oedema and cellular infiltration of the entire thickness of the sclera. Immune-mediated (non-infectious) scleritis is the most common type and is frequently associated with an underlying systemic inflammatory condition, of which it may be the first manifestation. Scleritis is much less common than episcleritis and comprises a spectrum from trivial and self-limiting disease to a necrotizing process that can involve adjacent tissues and threaten vision. A classification of non-infectious scleritis is shown in Table 9.1. Recurrences tend to be of the same type, though 10% progress to more aggressive disease.

Table 9.1 Classification of Immune-Mediated (Non-Infectious) Scleritis

Anterior
- Non-necrotizing
  - Diffuse
  - Nodular
- Necrotizing with inflammation
  - Vaso-occlusive
  - Granulomatous
  - Surgically induced (can also be infective)
- Scleromalacia perforans (necrotizing without inflammation)

Posterior

Anterior non-necrotizing scleritis

Diffuse

Diffuse disease is slightly more common in females and usually presents in the fifth decade.

- **Symptoms.** Ocular redness progressing a few days later to pain that may radiate to the face and temple. The discomfort typically wakes the patient in the early hours of the morning, improves later in the day and responds poorly to common analgesics. The vision may be blurred.
- **Signs**
  - Vascular congestion and dilatation associated with oedema. If treatment is started early the disease can be completely inhibited.
  - The redness may be generalized (Fig. 9.4A) or localized to one quadrant. If confined to the area under the upper eyelid the diagnosis may be missed.
  - Secondary features can include chemosis, eyelid swelling, anterior uveitis and raised IOP.
  - As the oedema resolves, the affected area often takes on a slight grey/blue appearance because of increased scleral translucency (Fig. 9.4B). This is due to rearrangement of scleral fibres rather than a decrease in scleral thickness.
  - Recurrences at the same location are common unless an underlying cause is treated.
- **Prognosis.** The average duration of disease is around 6 years, with the frequency of recurrences decreasing after the first 18 months. The long-term visual prognosis is good.

Nodular

The incidence of nodular and diffuse anterior scleritis is the same but a disproportionately large number of those with nodular disease have had a previous attack of herpes zoster ophthalmicus. The age of onset is similar to that of diffuse scleritis.

- **Symptoms.** The insidious onset of pain followed by increasing redness, tenderness of the globe and the appearance of a scleral nodule. The vision is often reduced.
- **Signs**
  - Scleral nodules may be single or multiple and most frequently develop in the interpalpebral region close to the limbus (Fig. 9.5A and B). They have a deeper blue–red colour than episcleral nodules and are immobile.
  - In contrast to episcleritis, a slit lamp beam shows an elevated anterior scleral surface.
  - Multiple nodules may expand and coalesce if treatment is delayed.
  - Instillation of 10% phenylephrine drops will constrict the conjunctival and superficial episcleral vasculature but not the deep plexus overlying the nodule.
  - As the inflammation in the nodule subsides, increased translucency of the sclera becomes apparent.
  - The duration of the disease is similar to diffuse scleritis.
  - More than 10% of patients with nodular scleritis develop necrotizing disease, but if treatment is instituted early superficial necrosis does not occur and the nodule heals from the centre leaving a small atrophic scar.

Anterior necrotizing scleritis with inflammation

Necrotizing disease is the aggressive form of scleritis. The age at onset is later than that of non-necrotizing scleritis, averaging 60 years. The condition is bilateral in 60% of patients and unless appropriately treated, especially in its early stages, may result in severe visual morbidity and even loss of the eye.

TIP Necrotizing scleritis is a serious and aggressive form of scleritis that requires systemic immunotherapy to control inflammation and to preserve vision.

Clinical features

- **Symptoms.** Gradual onset of pain that becomes severe and persistent and radiates to the temple, brow or jaw. It frequently interferes with sleep and responds poorly to analgesia.
- **Signs** vary according to the following three types of necrotizing disease.
  - Vaso-occlusive is commonly associated with rheumatoid arthritis. Isolated patches of scleral oedema with overlying non-perfused episclera and conjunctiva are seen (Fig. 9.6A). The patches coalesce and if unchecked rapidly proceed to scleral necrosis (Fig. 9.6B).
  - Granuloma formation may occur in conjunction with conditions such as granulomatosis with polyangiitis or polyarteritis nodosa. The disease typically starts with injection adjacent to the limbus and then extends posteriorly. Within 24 hours, the sclera, episclera, conjunctiva and adjacent cornea become irregularly raised and oedematous (Fig. 9.7).
  - Surgically induced scleritis typically starts within 3 weeks of a procedure, though much longer intervals have been reported. It may be induced by any type of surgery including strabismus repair, trabeculectomy with excessive exposure to mitomycin C (Fig. 9.8A), excision of pterygium (Fig. 9.8B) and scleral buckling. The necrotizing process starts at the site of surgery and extends outwards, but tends to remain localized to one sector.

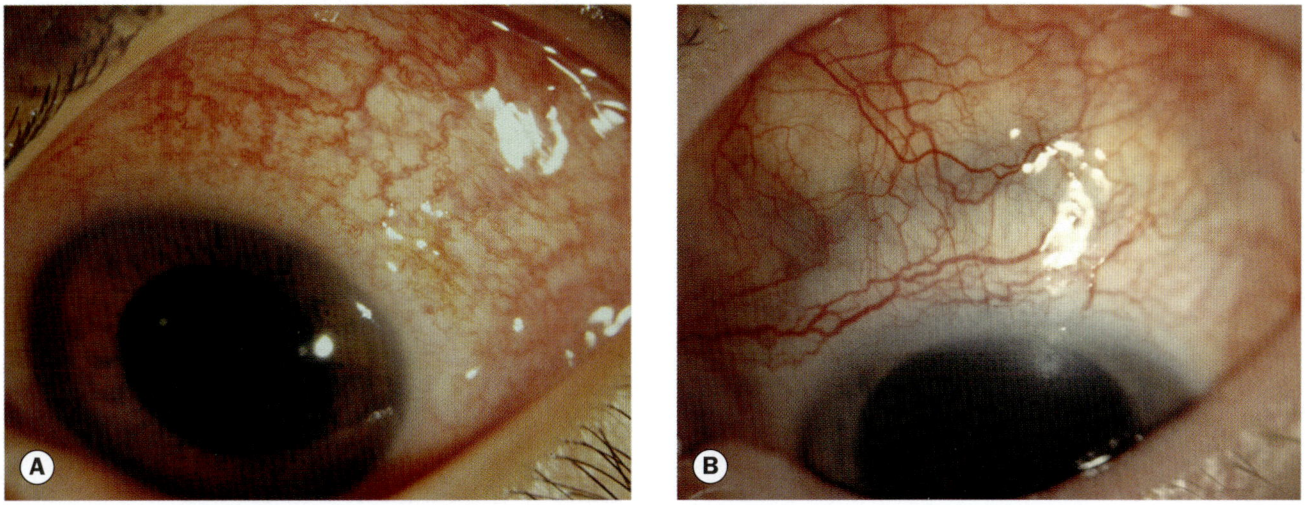

Fig. 9.4 **(A)** Diffuse non-necrotizing anterior scleritis; **(B)** scleral translucency following recurrent disease.

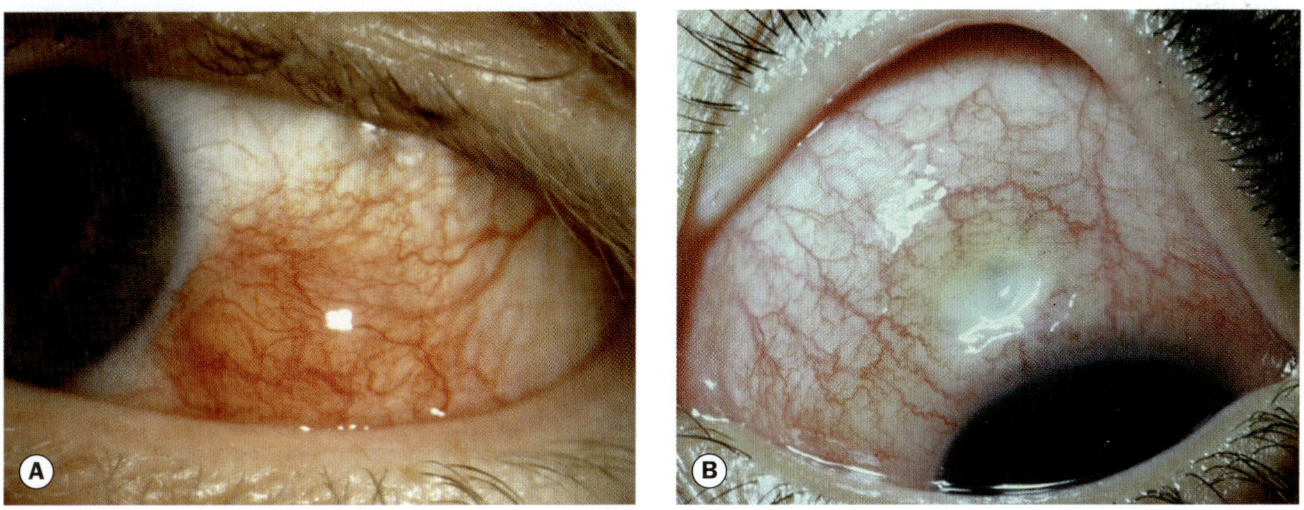

Fig. 9.5 Nodular non-necrotizing anterior scleritis. **(A)** Single scleral nodule with localized inflammation; **(B)** nodule with diffuse inflammation in Crohn disease.

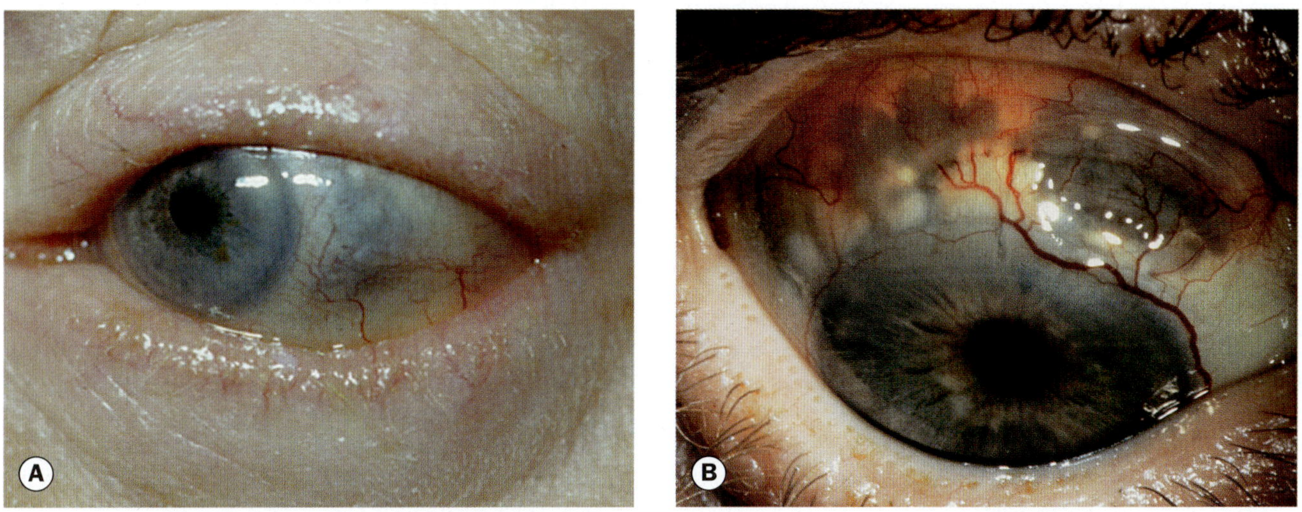

Fig. 9.6 Vaso-occlusive necrotizing scleritis. **(A)** Early stage; **(B)** severe late stage showing coalescence.

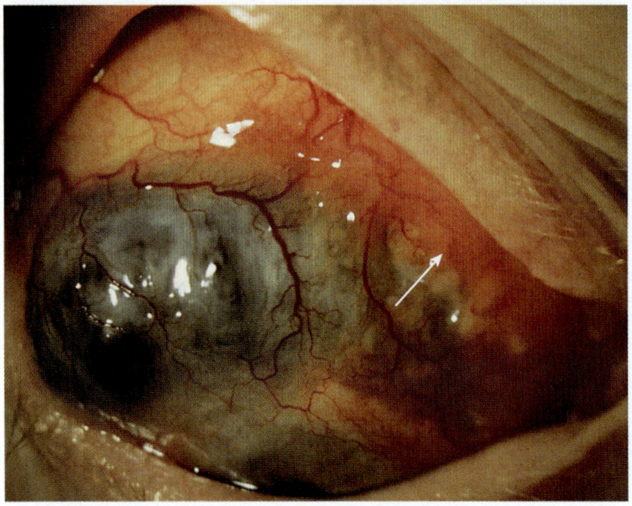

Fig. 9.7 Granulomatous necrotizing scleritis with inflammation (arrow).

Investigation

- **Laboratory.** Tests should be employed as adjuncts to clinical assessment and evaluation by a general physician or rheumatologist should be considered. Specific tests may include erythrocyte sedimentation rate (ESR), C-reactive protein (CRP), full blood count (e.g. anaemia related to inflammatory connective tissue disease, eosinophilia for polyarteritis nodosa, atopy or Churg–Strauss syndrome), rheumatoid factor, antinuclear antibodies (ANA), antineutrophil cytoplasmic antibodies (ANCA) and anti-cyclic citrullinated peptide (CCP) antibodies, serum uric acid, syphilis serology, Lyme serology, hepatitis B surface antigen (polyarteritis nodosa) and antiphospholipid antibodies. Investigation for tuberculosis, sarcoidosis or ankylosing spondylitis may be appropriate (see Ch. 12).
- **Radiological imaging.** Chest, sinus, joint and other imaging may be indicated in the investigation of a range of conditions such as tuberculosis, sarcoidosis, Churg–Strauss syndrome, granulomatosis with polyangiitis, ankylosing spondylitis and other conditions.
- **Angiography.** Fluorescein angiography of the anterior segment helps to distinguish necrotizing disease by the presence of non-perfusion and can be used for monitoring. Occlusion is predominantly venular in inflammatory disease and mainly arteriolar in scleromalacia perforans (see below). Indocyanine green is a more accurate indicator of disease activity.
- **Ultrasonography** can help to detect associated posterior scleritis (see below).
- **Biopsy.** This may be considered in resistant cases, especially if infection is suspected.

Complications of anterior scleritis

- **Acute infiltrative stromal keratitis** may be localized or diffuse (Fig. 9.9).
- **Sclerosing keratitis**, characterized by chronic thinning and opacification in which the peripheral cornea adjacent to the site of scleritis resembles sclera.

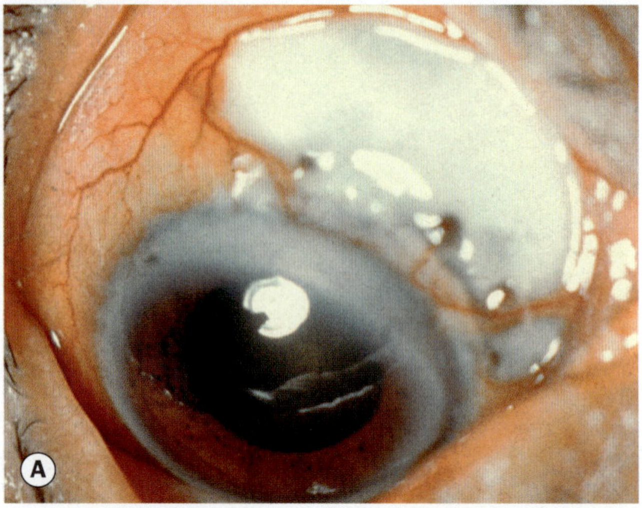

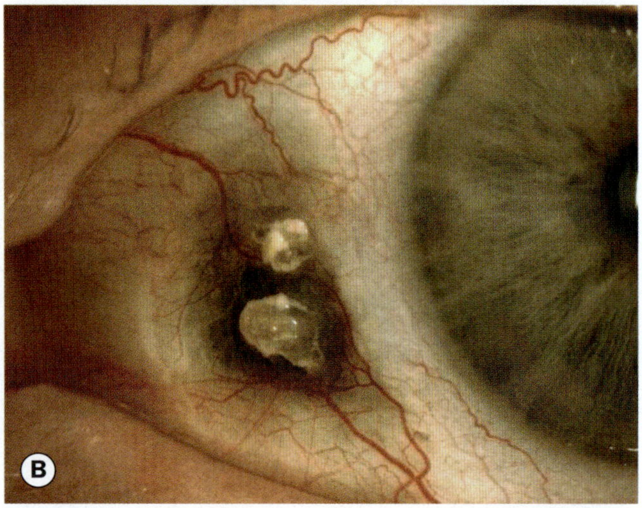

Fig. 9.8 Surgically induced necrotizing scleritis. **(A)** After trabeculectomy with mitomycin C; **(B)** many years after pterygium excision.

- **Peripheral ulcerative keratitis** is characterized by progressive melting and ulceration and may constitute a severe risk to the integrity of the eye. In granulomatous scleritis the destruction extends directly from the sclera into the limbus and cornea. This characteristic pattern is seen in granulomatosis with polyangiitis, polyarteritis nodosa and relapsing polychondritis. Peripheral corneal ulceration can occur at any stage of a necrotizing scleritis and, in rare cases, precede its onset. (See also Ch. 7.)
- **Uveitis**, if severe, may denote aggressive scleritis.
- **Glaucoma** is the most common cause of eventual loss of vision. The intraocular pressure can be very difficult to control in the presence of active scleritis.
- **Hypotony** (rarely phthisis) may be the result of ciliary body detachment, inflammatory damage or ischaemia.
- **Perforation** of the sclera as a result of the inflammatory process alone is extremely rare.

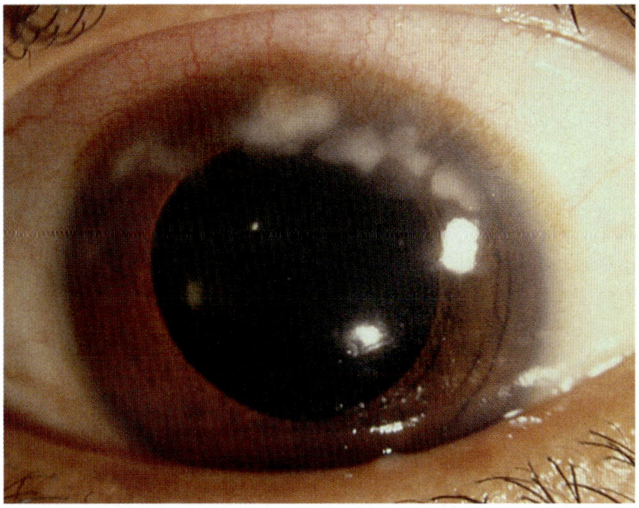

Fig. 9.9 Peripheral infiltrative stromal keratitis.

TIP Glaucoma is the commonest cause of visual loss in anterior scleritis, so control of the IOP is critically important.

Scleromalacia perforans

- Scleromalacia perforans (5% of scleritis) is a specific type of progressive scleral thinning without inflammation that typically affects elderly women with longstanding rheumatoid arthritis, but has also been described in association with other systemic disorders. Despite the nomenclature, perforation of the globe is rare as integrity is maintained by a thin layer of fibrous tissue. Differential diagnosis is from the innocuous scleral hyaline plaque and senile scleromalacia (see below).
- **Symptoms.** Mild non-specific irritation. Pain is absent and vision unaffected and keratoconjunctivitis sicca may be suspected.
- **Signs**
  - Necrotic scleral plaques near the limbus without vascular congestion (Fig. 9.10A).
  - Coalescence and enlargement of necrotic areas.
  - Slow progression of scleral thinning, with exposure of underlying uvea (Fig. 9.10B and C).
- **Treatment** may be effective in patients with early scleromalacia, but is less useful in advanced disease.
  - No consistent benefit from any specific agent has been demonstrated. Frequent lubricant instillation, local or systemic anticollagenase agents, immunosuppressives (including topical and oral, but not periocular injection of, steroids and topical ciclosporin) and biological blockers have been used. (See below.)
  - Underlying systemic disease should be treated.
  - Protection from trauma is important.
  - Surgical repair of scleral perforation (e.g. patch grafting) may be required to prevent phthisis bulbi.

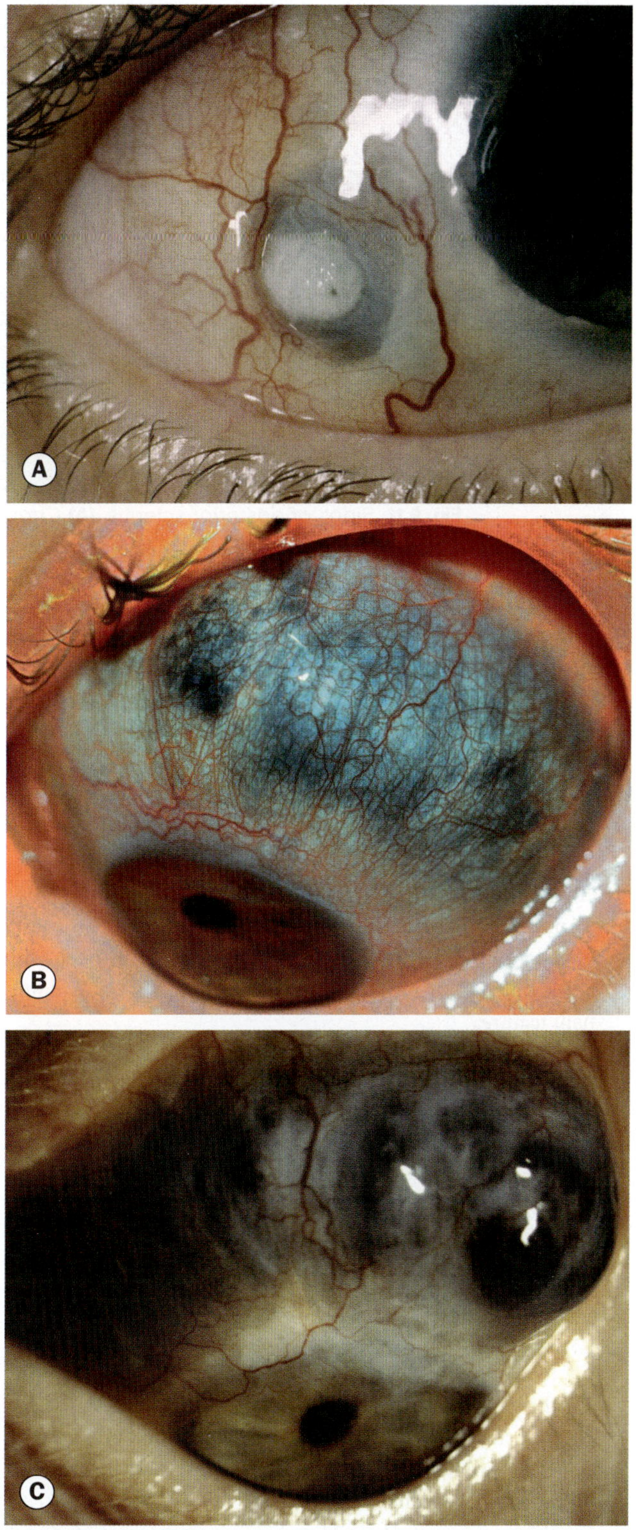

Fig. 9.10 Progression of scleromalacia perforans. **(A)** Asymptomatic necrotic patch; **(B)** moderate and **(C)** severe thinning and exposure of underlying uvea. *(Courtesy of R Bates – fig. A; C Barry – fig. B.)*

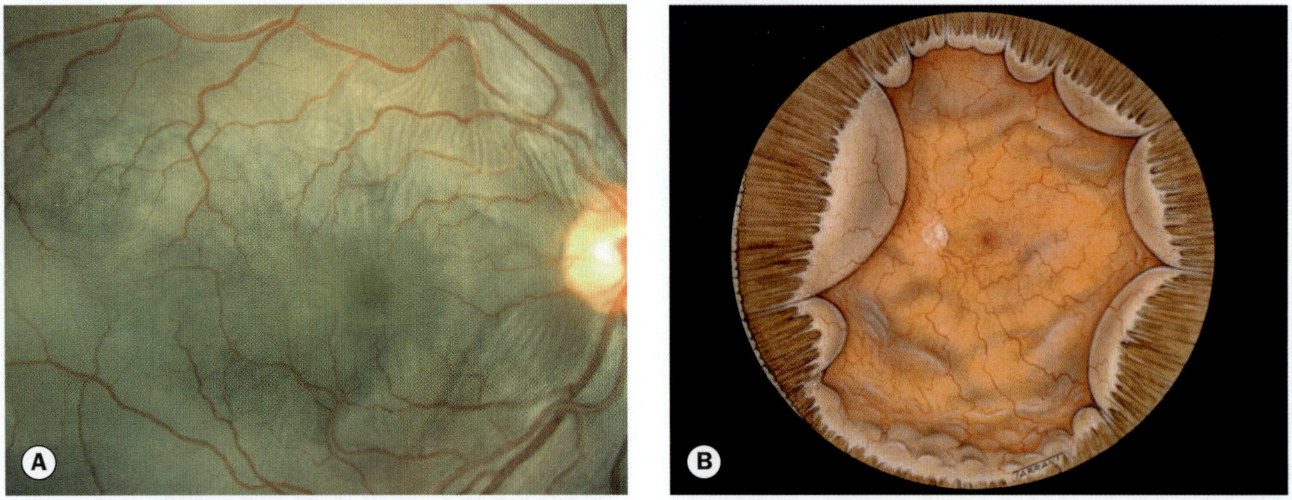

Fig. 9.11 Signs of posterior scleritis. (A) Choroidal folds; (B) uveal effusion.

Posterior scleritis

Posterior scleritis is a potentially blinding condition in which diagnosis is commonly delayed, with an adverse prognostic effect. The inflammatory changes in posterior and anterior scleral disease are identical and can arise in both segments simultaneously or separately. The age at onset is often less than 40 years. Young patients are usually otherwise healthy, but about a third over the age of 55 have associated systemic disease.

Diagnosis

- **Symptoms.** Pain does not correlate well with the severity of inflammation but tends to be more severe in those with accompanying orbital myositis. Photophobia is not a dominant feature.
- **Signs.** The disease is bilateral in 35%.
  - Choroidal folds (see Ch. 14) are usually confined to the posterior pole (Fig. 9.11A).
  - Exudative retinal detachment occurs in around 25%. The yellowish-brown subretinal exudative material can be mistaken for a choroidal tumour.
  - Uveal effusion with choroidal detachment may be present (Fig. 9.11B).
  - Disc oedema with accompanying reduction of vision is common and is caused by spread of inflammation into the orbital tissue and optic nerve. Treatment must not be delayed in these patients as permanent visual loss can rapidly ensue.
  - Myositis is common and gives rise to diplopia, pain on eye movement, tenderness to touch and redness around a muscle insertion.
  - Proptosis is usually mild and is frequently associated with ptosis.
  - Occasional features include raised IOP, periorbital oedema and chemosis. Associated anterior scleritis is a useful diagnostic aid but occurs only in a minority.
- **Ultrasonography** may show increased scleral thickness, scleral nodules, separation of Tenon capsule from sclera, disc oedema, choroidal folds and retinal detachment. Fluid in the Tenon space may give a characteristic 'T' sign, the stem of the T being formed by the optic nerve and the cross bar by the fluid-containing gap (Fig. 9.12).
- **MR** and **CT** may show scleral thickening and proptosis.

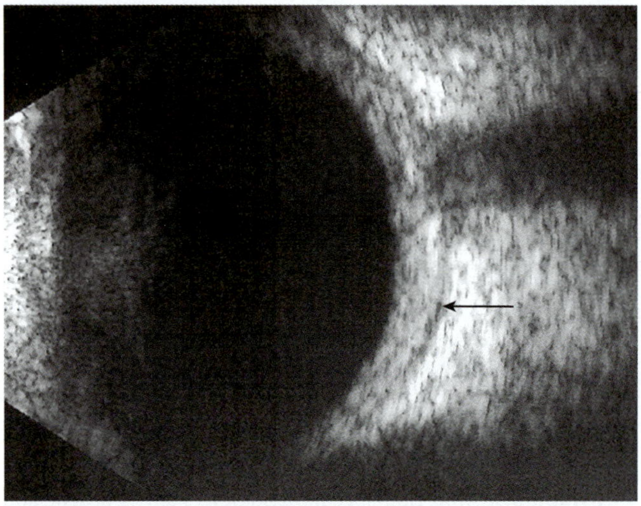

Fig. 9.12 B-scan ultrasonography in posterior scleritis showing scleral thickening and fluid in the sub-Tenon space (arrow), with the characteristic 'T' sign (see text).

Differential diagnosis

- **Subretinal mass.** Alternative lesions include miscellaneous granulomatous conditions and choroidal neoplasia.
- **Choroidal folds**, retinal striae and disc oedema may also occur in orbital tumours, orbital inflammatory disease, thyroid eye disease, papilloedema and hypotony.
- **Exudative retinal detachment.** Vogt–Koyanagi–Harada (VKH) syndrome and central serous retinopathy.
- **Orbital cellulitis** may cause proptosis and periocular oedema but is associated with marked pyrexia.

Important systemic associations of scleritis

Rheumatoid arthritis

- The autoimmune disease rheumatoid arthritis (RA) is the most common systemic association of scleritis and is characterized by a symmetrical deforming inflammatory polyarthropathy, with a spectrum of possible extra-articular manifestations.
- Presentation is commonly in the third decade with joint swelling, usually of the hands (Fig. 9.13A and B). It is much more common in females than males.
- Rheumatoid factor autoantibodies are present in 80–90%.
- All forms of immune-mediated scleritis have been described in RA and the clinical course is often more aggressive than when there is no systemic association. Other ocular manifestations of RA include keratoconjunctivitis sicca (secondary Sjögren syndrome), ulcerative keratitis (see Fig. 7.29B–D) and acquired superior oblique tendon sheath syndrome (very rare).

TIP Rheumatoid arthritis is the most common systemic association of scleritis and can manifest with any form of immune-mediated scleral inflammation.

Granulomatosis with polyangiitis

- Granulomatosis with polyangiitis (Wegener granulomatosis) is an idiopathic multisystem granulomatous disorder characterized by small vessel vasculitis typically affecting primarily the paranasal sinuses (Fig. 9.13C), lower respiratory tract, the kidneys and skin (Fig. 9.13D).
- There is a male predominance. Presentation is in the fifth decade on average, often with pulmonary symptoms.
- Antineutrophil cytoplasmic antibodies (cANCA) are found in over 90% of patients with active disease.
- Scleritis is often rapidly progressive, necrotizing and granulomatous. Other ocular manifestations include peripheral ulcerative keratitis (see Fig.7.29E), occlusive retinal vasculitis, orbital inflammatory disease, nasolacrimal obstruction, dacrocystitis and, rarely, tarsal–conjunctival disease.

Relapsing polychondritis

- Relapsing polychondritis is a rare idiopathic condition characterized by small vessel vasculitis involving cartilage resulting in recurrent, often progressive, inflammatory episodes involving multiple organ systems such as the ears (Fig. 9.13E), nasal cartilage (Fig. 9.13F), respiratory system, heart and joints.
- Presentation is frequently in middle age.
- Scleritis is often intractable and may be necrotizing or non-necrotizing. Isolated anterior uveitis may also occur.

Polyarteritis nodosa

- Polyarteritis nodosa (PAN) is an idiopathic aneurysmal vasculitis affecting medium-sized and small arteries, with a wide range of manifestations across multiple organ systems. Without treatment the 5-year survival is about 10%. The causes of death are kidney failure, myocardial infarction or stroke. Modern immuno-suppressive treatment improves the prognosis considerably.
- Presentation is in the third to sixth decades, often with constitutional symptoms. The male:female ratio is about 3:1.
- Ocular involvement may precede the systemic manifestations by several years. About one-third of patients have hepatitis B infection. Scleritis is often aggressive and necrotizing. Peripheral ulcerative keratitis, orbital pseudotumour and occlusive retinal periarteritis are other reported ocular features.

Systemic lupus erythematosus

- Systemic lupus erythematosus (SLE) is a chronic multisystem autoimmune inflammatory disease. There is often a family history, but no single causal gene has been identified.
- Females are affected far more often than males (ratio of 9:1).
- Antinuclear antibody testing is the key serological test in this condition. If the test is negative, SLE can be excluded (sensitivity: 99%; specificity: 49%).
- Up to 70% of patients with SLE have skin involvement, including the characteristic 'butterfly' rash on the cheeks, which is often induced by exposure to sunlight (Fig. 9.13G). Red scaly discoid patches can be seen elsewhere on the skin and hair loss may occur (Fig. 9.13H). Joint and muscle pain has been reported in up to 90%, but does not usually result in joint destruction. The heart, lungs, kidneys and brain may be affected.
- Ocular involvement is found in up to one-third of patients. The most common manifestation is dry eye syndrome and secondary Sjögren syndrome in 25%. Retinopathy occurs in up to 10% and is linked to the severity of the condition, indicating inadequate control of the systemic disease. Ischaemic optic neuropathy and bilateral optic neuritis are uncommon features of SLE. The incidence of episcleritis and scleritis is 1% and may be the presenting feature of the disease, usually manifesting with anterior diffuse or anterior nodular scleritis.
- Because of the long-term use of hydroxychloroquine treatment, maculopathy may follow in some patients (see Ch. 21).

Crohn disease

- Crohn disease is a chronic, relapsing inflammatory bowel disease of unknown cause.
- Extraintestinal complications occur frequently during the course of the disease. The commonest of these are peripheral arthritis and erythema nodosum.
- The eye is involved in 4% to 10% of patients and a wide spectrum of inflammatory conditions may be found. Acute episcleritis, acute anterior uveitis and marginal keratitis (see Fig. 9.9) are the commonest manifestation, although conjunctivitis, optic neuritis, orbital inflammatory disease and retinal vasculitis have been reported. Acute anterior scleritis is rare (see Fig. 9.5B) and may be complicated by the development of scleromalacia perforans. Acute episcleritis and increased bowel activity show a close correlation.

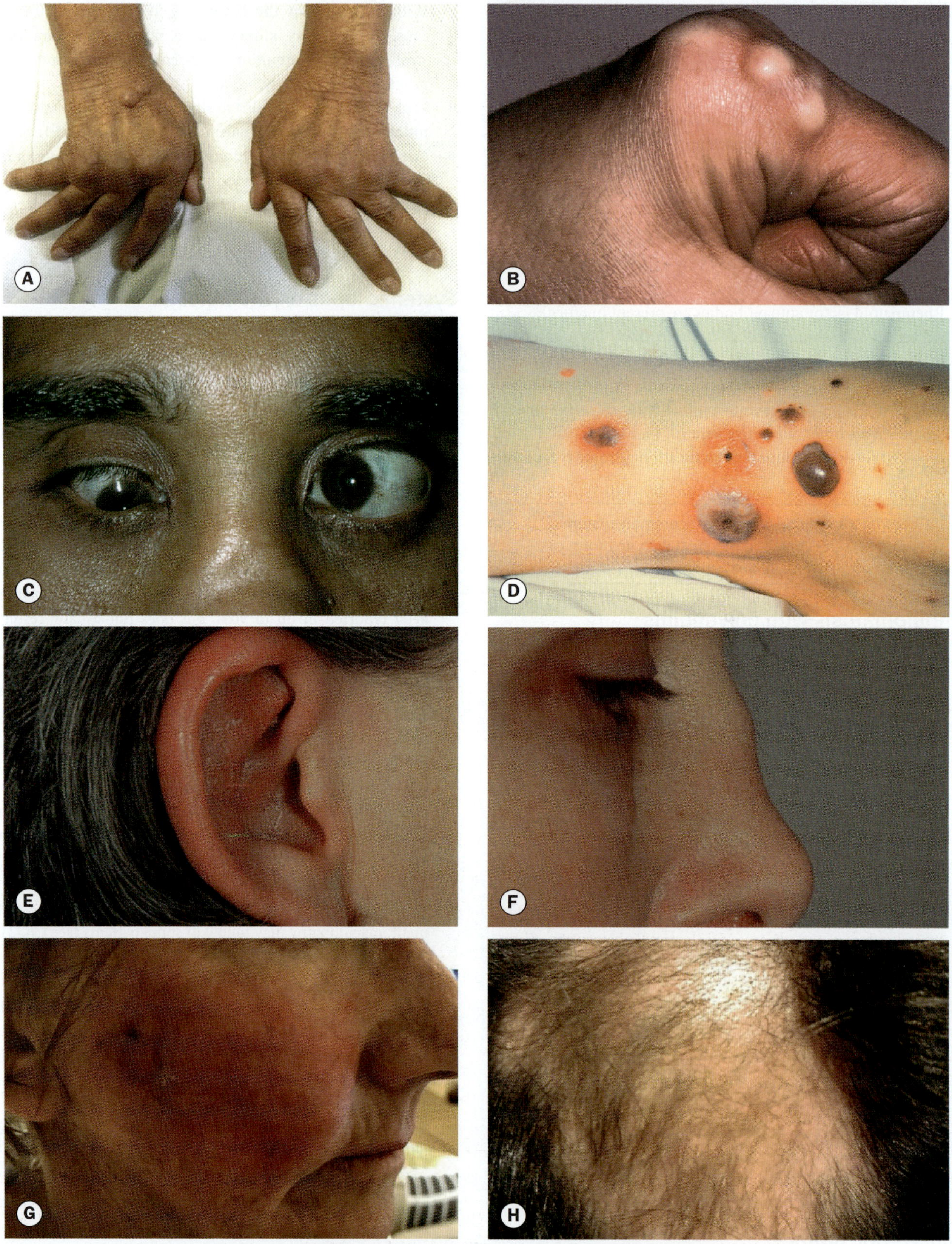

Fig. 9.13 Systemic associations of scleritis. **(A)** Rheumatoid arthritis showing ulnar deviation and arthritis in longstanding disease and **(B)** rheumatoid nodules; **(C)** granulomatosis with polyangiitis showing nasal collapse and a convergent squint secondary to extensive sinus disease and **(D)** erythematous papules and bullae typical of small vessel vasculitis; **(E)** relapsing polychondritis showing swelling of the pinna and **(F)** saddle-shaped nasal deformity; **(G)** systemic lupus erythromatosis, showing the typical malar rash and **(H)** alopecia. *(Courtesy of ADN Murray – fig. C; C Pavesio – figs E and F.)*

Treatment of immune-mediated scleritis

- **Topical steroids** do not affect the natural history of the scleral inflammation, but may relieve symptoms and oedema in non-necrotizing disease.
- **Systemic NSAIDs** should be used on their own only in non-necrotizing disease. It is often necessary to try a number of different drugs before finding one that provides adequate relief of symptoms. A cyclooxygenase (COX)-2 inhibitor may be preferred in elderly patients or if there is a history of peptic ulceration, but can result in cardiovascular side effects. Patients should be warned of the risk of gastrointestinal tract haemorrhage.
- **Periocular steroid injections** may be used in non-necrotizing disease but their effects are usually transient and should not be used in necrotizing scleritis.
- **Systemic steroids** (e.g. prednisolone is 1–1.5 mg/kg daily) are used when NSAIDs are inappropriate or inadequate (necrotizing disease). Intravenous methylprednisolone (0.5–1 g daily for 3 days) may be used initially for severe cases.
- **Immunosuppressives** and/or **immunomodulatory agents** should be considered if control is (a) incomplete with steroids alone, (b) as a steroid-sparing measure in long-term treatment, or (c) to treat underlying systemic disease. Patients with scleritis secondary to the following conditions: granulomatosis with polyangiitis, polyarteritis nodosa, RA (with necrotizing scleritis) and relapsing polychondritis, should be offered immediate treatment with immunomodulatory agents (see Ch. 12). A wide range of drugs are available, including cytostatics (e.g. cyclophosphamide, azathioprine, methotrexate), drugs acting on immunophilins (e.g. ciclosporin, tacrolimus) and biologicals. In necrotizing disease, rituximab is particularly effective.

TIP Rituximab is particularly effective in the treatment of necrotizing scleritis.

PORPHYRIA

Scleritis is a rare complication of congenital erythropoietic porphyria and two of the adult forms of porphyria: porphyria variegata and porphyria cutanea tarda. Overproduction and excessive storage of porphyrins occur in the liver. These highly photoactive chromophores are also deposited in the dermis and sclera, which are subsequently stimulated by exposure to the sun. The sclera becomes thin or excavated over a sharply demarcated area localized to the sun-exposed interpalpebral region adjacent to the cornea (Fig. 9.14). Acute diffuse anterior scleritis and posterior scleritis may occur. Patients should avoid sunlight and undergo phlebotomy.

INFECTIOUS SCLERITIS

Infectious scleritis is rare, but may present diagnostic difficulty as the initial clinical features are similar to those of immune-mediated disease. In some cases, infection may follow surgical or accidental trauma, endophthalmitis, or may occur as an extension of corneal infection.

Causes

- **Herpes zoster** is the most common infective cause. Necrotizing scleritis is extremely resistant to treatment and may result in a thinned or punched-out area (Fig. 9.15A and B).
- **Tuberculous** scleritis is rare and difficult to diagnose. The sclera may be infected by direct spread from a local conjunctival or choroidal lesion, or more commonly by haematogenous spread. Involvement may be nodular (Fig. 9.15C) or necrotizing.
- **Leprosy.** Recurrent necrotizing scleritis can occur, even after apparent systemic cure. Nodular disease may be seen in lepromatous leprosy.
- **Syphilis.** Diffuse anterior scleritis may occur in secondary syphilis and occasionally scleral nodules may be a feature of tertiary syphilis.
- **Lyme disease.** Scleritis (Fig. 9.15D) is common but typically occurs long after initial infection.
- **Other causes** include fungi, *Pseudomonas aeruginosa* and *Nocardia*.

Treatment

Once the infective agent has been identified, specific antimicrobial therapy should be initiated. Topical and systemic steroids may also be used to reduce the inflammatory reaction. If appropriate,

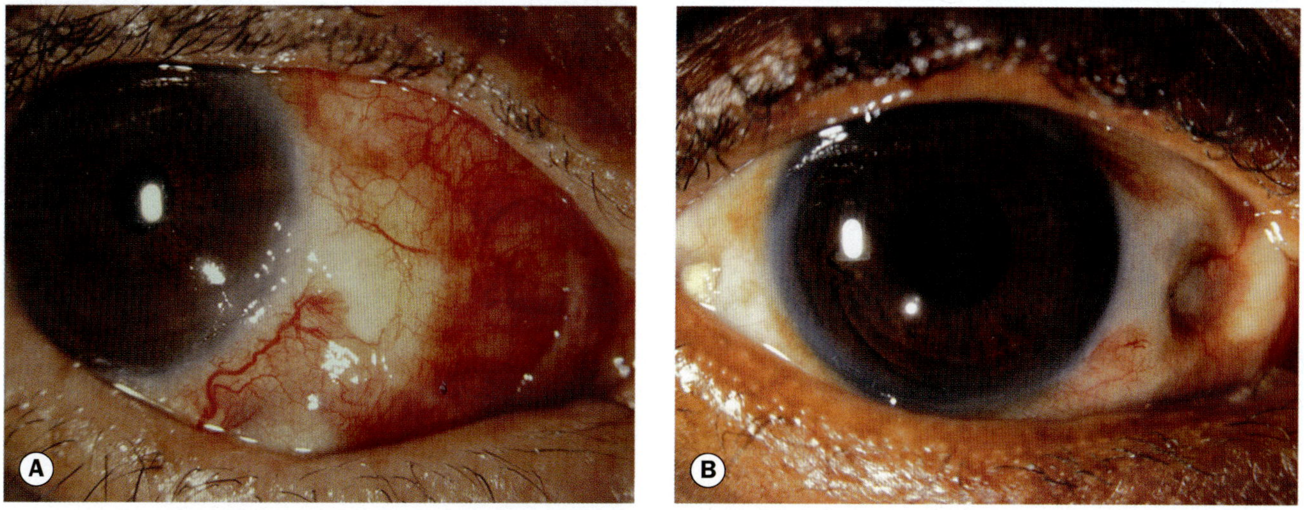

Fig. 9.14 Scleral involvement in porphyria. **(A)** Acute; **(B)** chronic scleral thinning.

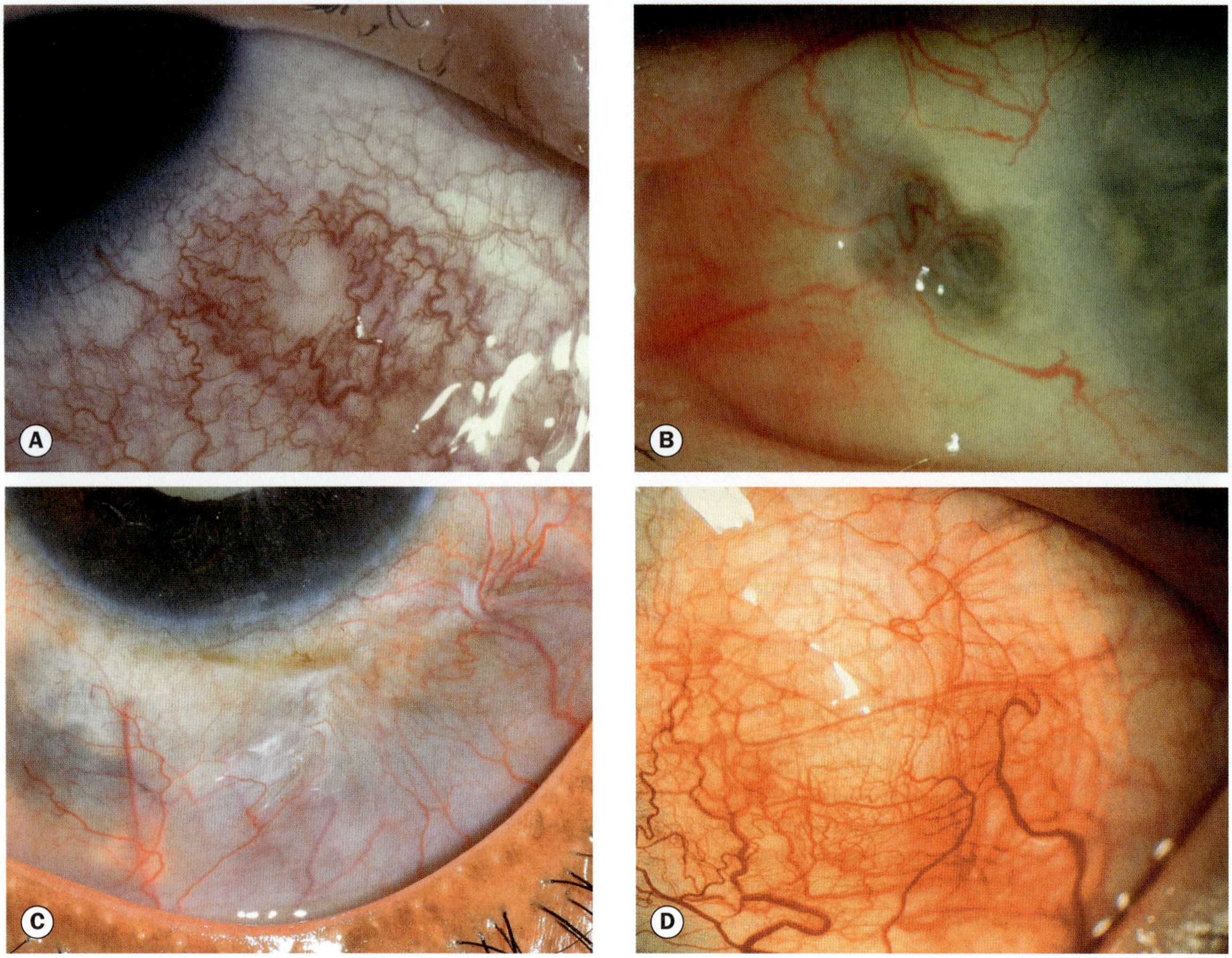

Fig. 9.15 Infectious scleritis. **(A)** Acute inflammation in herpes zoster; **(B)** focal necrosis secondary to herpes zoster; **(C)** nodular tuberculous disease; **(D)** nodular scleritis in Lyme disease. *(Courtesy of SR Rathinam – fig. C.)*

surgical debridement can be used to debulk a focus of infection and facilitates the penetration of antibiotics.

SCLERAL DISCOLORATION

Alkaptonuria

In this autosomal recessive condition, a defect in homogentisic acid oxidase results in the accumulation of homogentisic acid in collagenous tissues such as cartilage and tendon (ochronosis). Ocular manifestations include bluish-grey or black generalized pigmentation of the sclera and the tendons of horizontal recti associated with discrete pigmented globules (Fig. 9.16). Systemic features include dark urine and arthropathy.

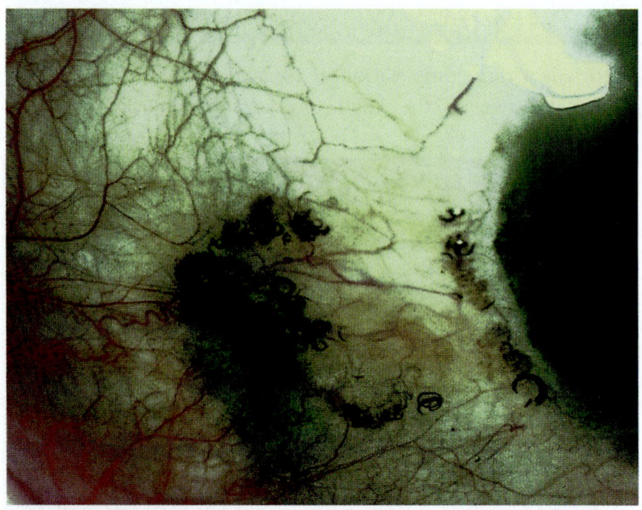

Fig. 9.16 Alkaptonuria: pigmentation (ochronosis) of the sclera and horizontal rectus tendons.

Haemochromatosis

The systemic features of haemochromatosis are caused by increased iron deposition in various tissues. Features may be more

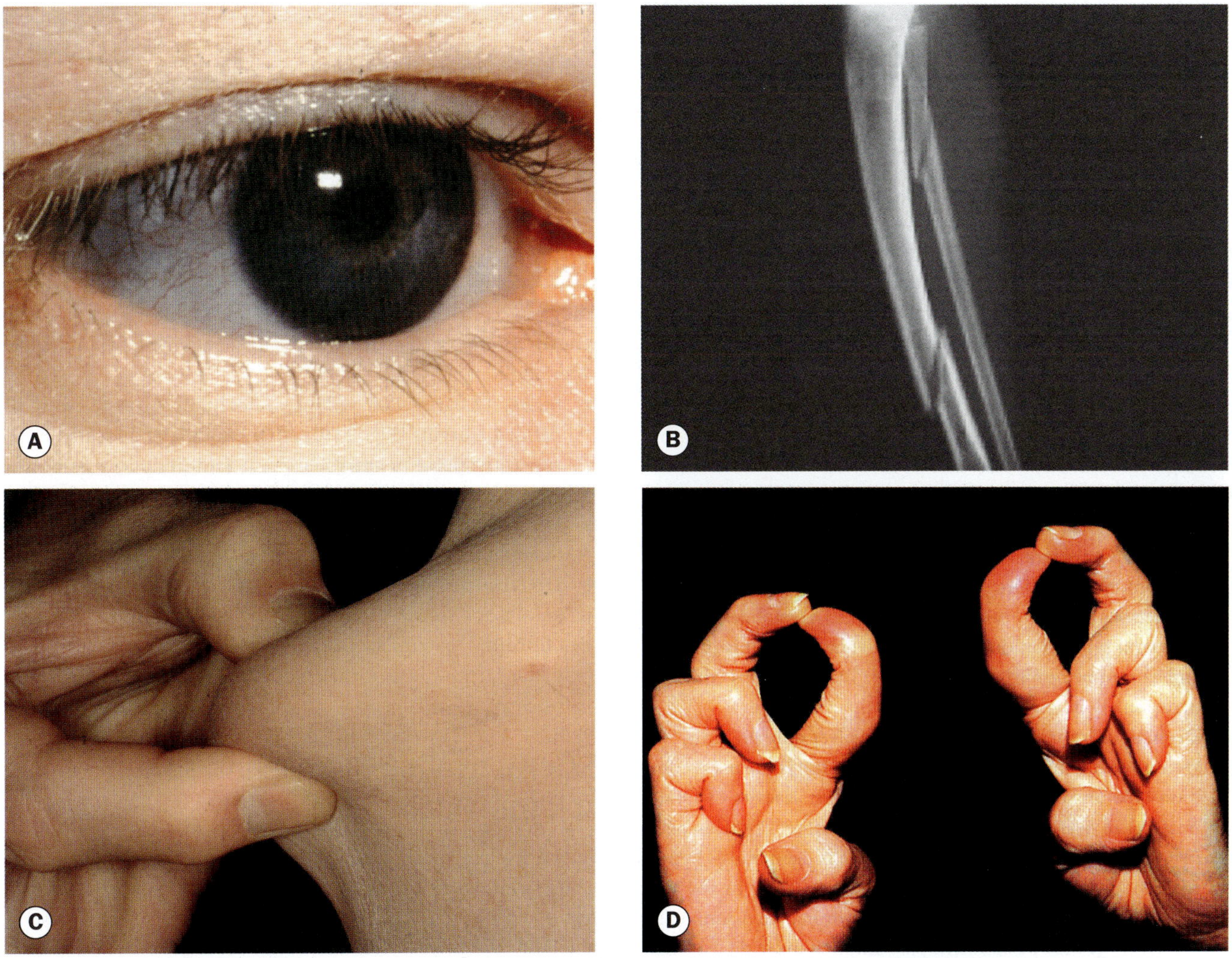

Fig. 9.17 Systemic associations of blue sclera. **(A)** Thin, translucent sclera; **(B)** leg fractures in osteogenesis imperfecta type IIA; **(C)** cutaneous hyperelasticity and **(D)** joint hypermobility in Ehlers–Danlos syndrome type VI.

subtle than the classic triad of a bronze complexion, hepatomegaly and diabetes. Inheritance is autosomal recessive. Dry eye and rusty-brown perilimbal conjunctival and scleral discoloration may develop.

BLUE SCLERA

Blue scleral discoloration is caused by thinning or transparency with resultant visualization of the underlying uvea (Fig. 9.17A). Major associations are discussed below. Rare associations include Marshall–Smith syndrome (accelerated prenatal skeletal maturation and growth), Russell–Silver syndrome (short stature and other features) and Hallermann–Streiff–François syndrome.

Osteogenesis imperfecta

Osteogenesis imperfecta is an inherited disease of connective tissue, usually caused by defects in the synthesis and structure of type 1 collagen. There are multiple types, at least two of which have ocular features.

- **Type I** is autosomal dominant. Patients suffer few fractures with little or no deformity, hyperextensible joints, dental hypoplasia, deafness and easy bruising. Possible ocular features include blue sclera, megalocornea and corneal arcus.
- **Type IIA** is either sporadic or inherited in an autosomal dominant manner. Systemic features include deafness, dental anomalies, multiple fractures (Fig. 9.17B) and short limbs, with death in infancy from respiratory infection. Ocular manifestations include blue sclera and shallow orbits.

Ehlers–Danlos syndrome type VI

Ehlers–Danlos syndrome VI (ocular sclerotic) is an inherited disorder of collagen formation. Patients have thin and hyper-elastic skin (Fig. 9.17C) that bruises easily and heals slowly. The joints are hypermobile (Fig. 9.17D), which may lead to recurrent dislocation and falls. Cardiovascular disease can be severe, including a bleeding diathesis, dissecting aneurysms, spontaneous rupture of large blood vessels and mitral valve prolapse. There are six major types but type VI and, rarely, type IV, are associated with ocular features. As well as blue sclera, other manifestations include scleral fragility (globe rupture may be caused by mild trauma), epicanthic folds, microcornea, keratoconus, keratoglobus, ectopia lentis, myopia and retinal detachment.

MISCELLANEOUS CONDITIONS

Congenital ocular melanocytosis

Congenital ocular melanocytosis is an uncommon condition characterized by an increase in number, size and pigmentation of melanocytes in the sclera and uvea. The periocular skin, orbit, meninges and soft palate may also be involved.

- **Ocular** melanocytosis, the least common, involves only the eye. Multifocal slate-grey pigmentation is seen within the sclera and episclera– the process does not involve the overlying conjunctival layers, unless there is incidental conjunctival pigmentation. The overlying conjunctiva is mobile over the episcleral pigmentation but the pigmentation itself is intrinsic and cannot be moved over the globe. The peripheral cornea is occasionally involved.
- **Dermal** melanocytosis (one-third) involves only the skin.
- **Oculodermal** melanocytosis (naevus of Ota) is the most common type and involves both skin and eye. Naevus of Ota is bilateral in 5%. It occurs frequently in darker-complexioned races but is rare in White people. There is deep bluish hyperpigmentation of the facial skin, most frequently in the distribution of the first and second trigeminal divisions (Fig. 9.18A–C). It may be subtle in pale-skinned individuals, when it is best detected under good lighting.
- **Ipsilateral associations**
  - Iris hyperchromia is common (see Fig. 9.18A).
  - Iris mammillations are uncommon, tiny, regularly spaced villiform lesions (Fig. 9.18D). They may also be found in neurofibromatosis type 1, Axenfeld–Rieger anomaly and Peters anomaly.
  - Fundus hyperpigmentation (Fig. 9.18E).
  - Trabecular hyperpigmentation (Fig. 9.18F). This is associated with glaucoma in about 10% of cases.
  - Uveal melanoma develops in a small minority of patients and long-term anterior and posterior segment review is required.

TIP Patients with oculodermal melanosis are at risk of developing glaucoma and occasionally uveal melanoma.

Idiopathic sclerochoroidal calcification

Idiopathic sclerochoroidal calcification is an innocuous, age-related condition that usually involves both eyes of an affected older adult.

- **Signs.** Geographical yellow–white fundus lesions with ill-defined margins (Fig. 9.19), often multiple and located in the superotemporal or inferotemporal mid-periphery associated with the vascular arcades.
- **Ultrasonography** shows highly reflective choroidal plaque-like lesions with orbital shadowing.
- **Differential diagnosis** is mainly from osseous metaplasia associated with a choroidal haemangioma and from choroidal osteoma, which is usually a single – though often large – lesion that usually (80–90%) involves only one eye.

Scleral hyaline plaque and senile scleromalacia

Scleral hyaline plaques are oval dark-greyish, generally sharply demarcated, areas located close to the insertion of the horizontal rectus muscles (Fig. 9.20). Senile scleromalacia refers to a spontaneously occurring irregular, oval or kidney-shaped partial-thickness scleral defect found at the same location, typically with one or more scleral hyaline plaques at the opposite location in the same eye or in the fellow eye. Separation of a scleral hyaline plaque to leave an area of scleromalacia has been described. Both these entities typically affect elderly patients, are innocuous and should not be confused with scleromalacia perforans (see above), which occurs in somewhat younger patients, may be located anywhere in the anterior sclera, is not associated with hyaline plaques elsewhere and can progress to a full-thickness scleral defect with uveal exposure.

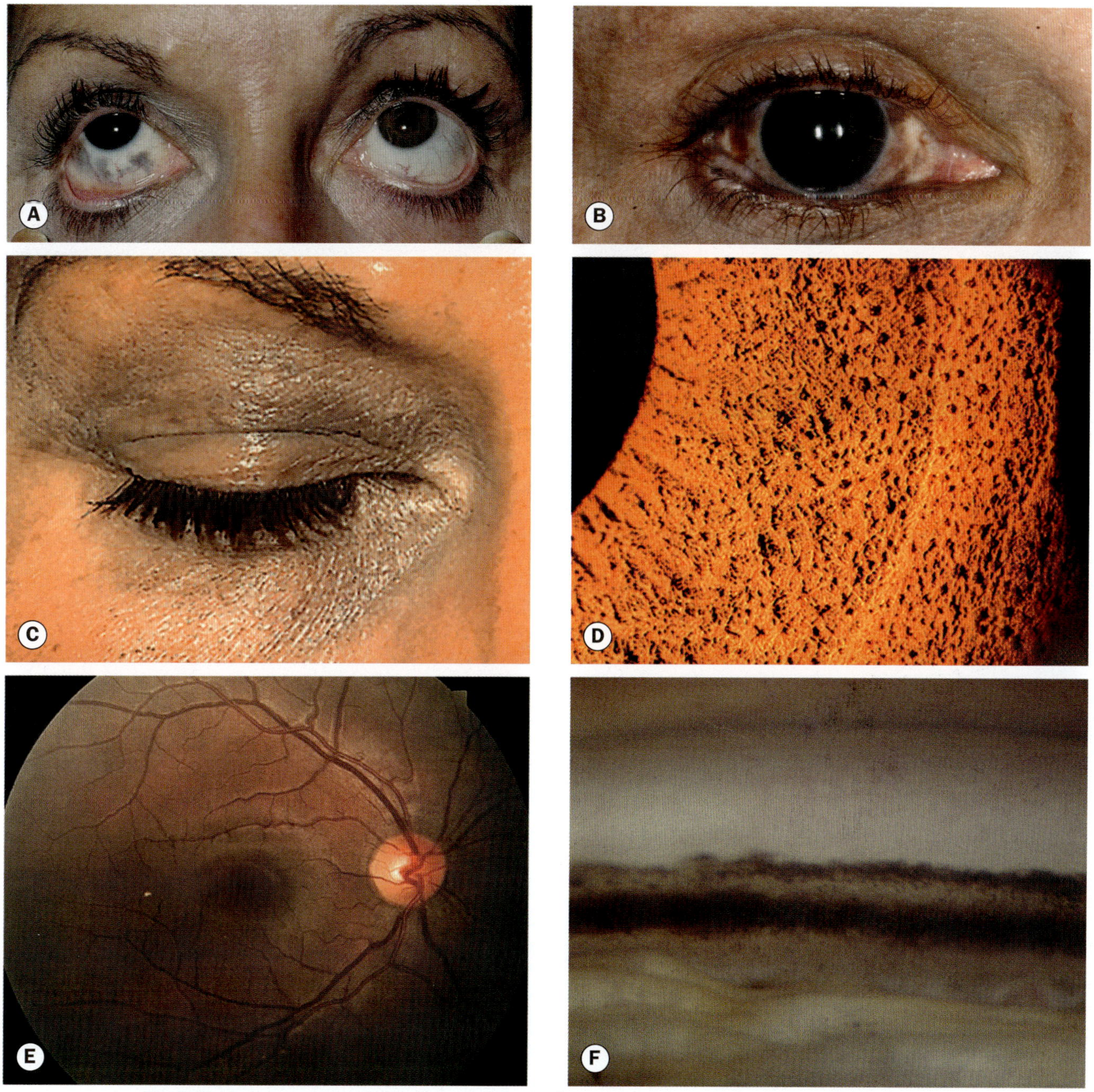

Fig. 9.18 Melanocytosis. **(A)** Iris heterochromia (hyperchromia in the right eye); **(B)** episcleral melanocytosis and **(C)** cutaneous melanocytosis in naevus of Ota; **(D)** iris mammillations; **(E)** fundus hyperpigmentation; **(F)** trabecular hyperpigmentation.

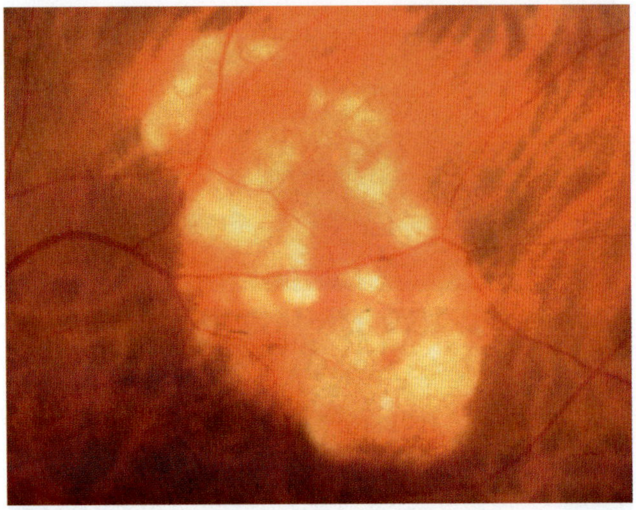

Fig. 9.19 Idiopathic sclerochoroidal calcification.

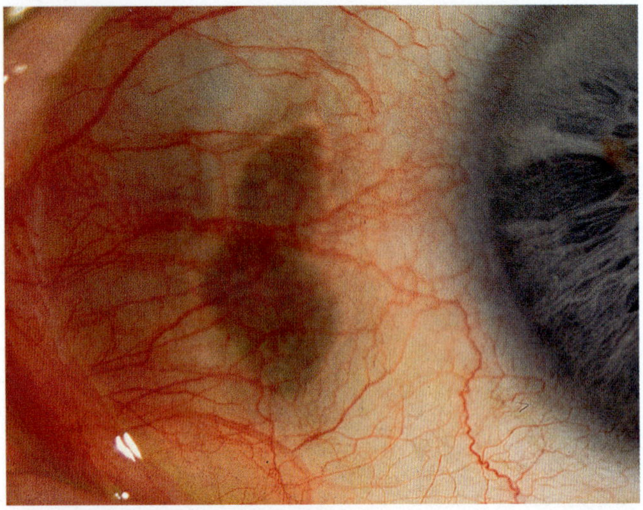

Fig. 9.20 Scleral hyaline plaque.

Chapter

Lens 10

INTRODUCTION

The primary function of the lens is to focus light on the retina.

- **Presbyopia** is the gradual loss of the ability of the lens to focus on near objects. It is an inevitable ageing phenomenon which occurs as a consequence of loss of accommodation secondary to reduced lens elasticity. Spectacles will usually correct the refractive error, but surgical treatment has become increasingly relevant in recent years.
- **Cataract (lens opacification)** is the commonest cause of reversible visual disability in the world. There is no medical treatment to prevent the development or progression of cataract. However, phacoemulsification with intraocular lens implantation is extremely successful in restoring vision and is the commonest surgical procedure undertaken in the world.

Anatomy

- **Zonules** hold the lens in position (Fig. 10.1A).
- **The capsule** is an acellular membrane that encloses the lens material.
- **Cuboid epithelial cells** are located beneath the anterior capsule and extend to the lens equator; cells in the germinative zone divide continuously and differentiate to form lens fibers (Fig. 10.1B).
- **The lens substance** is made up of a central nucleus surrounded by corticular material.

Effect on vision

Cataracts often develop slowly and in the early stages the vision alters subtly without the person being aware of the change. The effect on vision depends on: (a) the type of cataract, (b) the extent of opacification and (c) the position of the opacification. Symptoms include:

- **Reduced visual acuity**, which initially can be corrected with spectacles.
- **Loss of contrast sensitivity.**
- **Change in colour perception**, particularly an inability to accurately perceive blue colours.
- **Glare** secondary to light scattering, causing difficulty with night driving.
- **Monocular diplopia**, especially when looking at a point source of light.
- **Difficulty seeing in low-light situations**, including poor night vision.

ACQUIRED CATARACT

Age-related cataract

Subcapsular cataract

Anterior subcapsular cataract lies directly under the lens capsule and is associated with fibrous metaplasia of the lens epithelium. Posterior subcapsular opacity lies just in front of the posterior capsule and has a granular or plaque-like appearance on oblique slit lamp biomicroscopy (Fig. 10.2A), but typically appears black and vacuolated on retroillumination (Fig. 10.2B). The vacuoles are swollen migratory lens epithelial cells (bladder or Wedl), similar to those commonly seen postoperatively in posterior capsular opacification. Due to its location at the nodal point of the eye, a posterior subcapsular opacity often has a particularly profound effect on vision. Patients are characteristically troubled by glare, for instance from the headlights of oncoming cars, and symptoms are increased by miosis, such as occurs during near visual activity and in bright sunlight.

Nuclear sclerotic cataract

Nuclear cataract is an exaggeration of normal ageing change (Fig. 10.2C). It is often associated with myopia due to an increase in the refractive index of the nucleus, resulting in some elderly patients being able to read without spectacles again ('second sight of the aged'). In contrast, in the healthy ageing eye (and in occasional cases of cortical and subcapsular cataract) there is a mild hypermetropic shift. Nuclear sclerotic cataract is characterized by a yellowish hue due to the deposition of urochrome pigment and is best assessed with an oblique slit lamp beam. Retroillumination will show a good red reflex, but careful observation will reveal a subtle distinction between the nucleus and cortex (Fig. 10.2D). When advanced, the nucleus appears brown and, in rare cases, black.

Cortical cataract

Cortical cataract may involve the anterior, posterior or equatorial cortex. The opacities start as clefts and vacuoles between lens fibres due to cortical hydration. Subsequent opacification results in typical cuneiform (wedge-shaped) or radial spoke-like opacities (Fig. 10.2E and F), often found initially in the inferonasal quadrant. As with posterior subcapsular opacity, glare is a common symptom.

Christmas tree cataract

Christmas tree cataract, which is uncommon, is characterized by polychromatic needle-like formations in the deep cortex and nucleus (Fig. 10.2G and H).

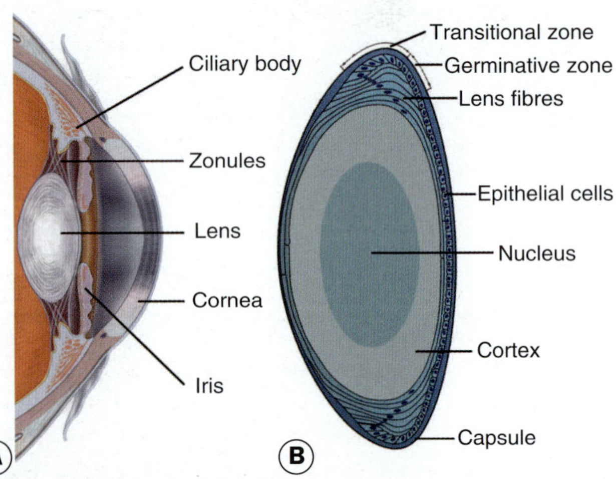

Fig. 10.1 (A) Cross-sectional anatomy of the anterior segment of the eye (see text); **(B)** histological features shown in cross section (epithelial cells are anterior; zones and magnification are not drawn to scale).

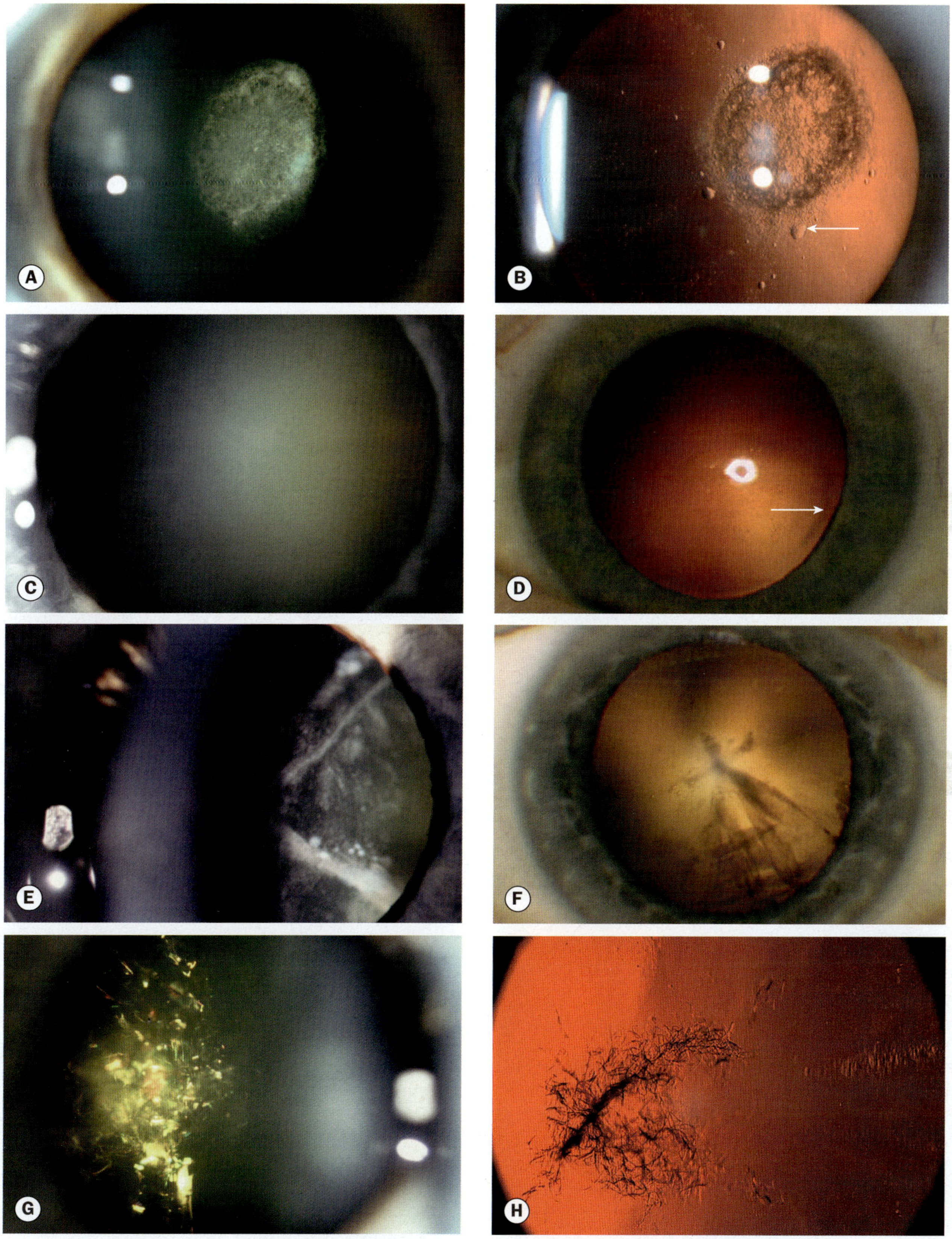

Fig. 10.2 Age-related cataract. **(A)** Posterior subcapsular; **(B)** posterior subcapsular on retroillumination, showing Wedl cells (arrow); **(C)** nuclear sclerosis; **(D)** nuclear sclerosis on retroillumination (arrow showing the demarcation between nucleus and cortex); **(E)** corticular; **(F)** corticular spokes on retroillumination; **(G)** Christmas tree; **(H)** Christmas tree on retroillumination.

Cataract maturity

- **Immature** cataract is one in which the lens is partially opaque.
- **Mature** cataract is one in which the lens is completely opaque (Fig. 10.3A and B).
- **Hypermature** cataract has a shrunken and wrinkled anterior capsule (Fig. 10.3C) due to leakage of water out of the lens.
- **Morgagnian** cataract is a hypermature cataract in which liquefaction of the cortex has allowed the nucleus to sink inferiorly (Fig. 10.3D).

Cataract in systemic disease

Diabetes mellitus

Hyperglycaemia is reflected in a high level of glucose in the aqueous humour, which diffuses into the lens. Here glucose is metabolized into sorbitol, which accumulates within the lens, resulting in secondary osmotic overhydration. In mild degree, this may affect the refractive index of the lens with consequent fluctuation of refraction in line with the plasma glucose level, hyperglycaemia resulting in myopia and vice versa. Cortical fluid vacuoles develop and later evolve into frank opacities. Classic diabetic cataract, which is rare, consists of snowflake cortical opacities (Fig. 10.4A) occurring in the young. It may mature within a few days or resolve spontaneously. Age-related cataract occurs sooner in people with diabetes mellitus. Nuclear sclerosis is common and tends to progress rapidly. Around one in five people who undergo cataract surgery have diabetes. The presence of diabetic macular oedema prior to cataract surgery is associated with worsening of the oedema, resulting in postoperative visual loss. The retina needs to be monitored before and after cataract surgery, even in patients with minimal oedema.

Myotonic dystrophy

About 90% of patients with myotonic dystrophy (see Ch. 19) develop fine iridescent cortical opacities in the third decade, sometimes resembling Christmas tree cataract. These evolve into visually disabling wedge-shaped cortical and subcapsular opacities, often star-like in conformation (Fig. 10.4B), by the fifth decade.

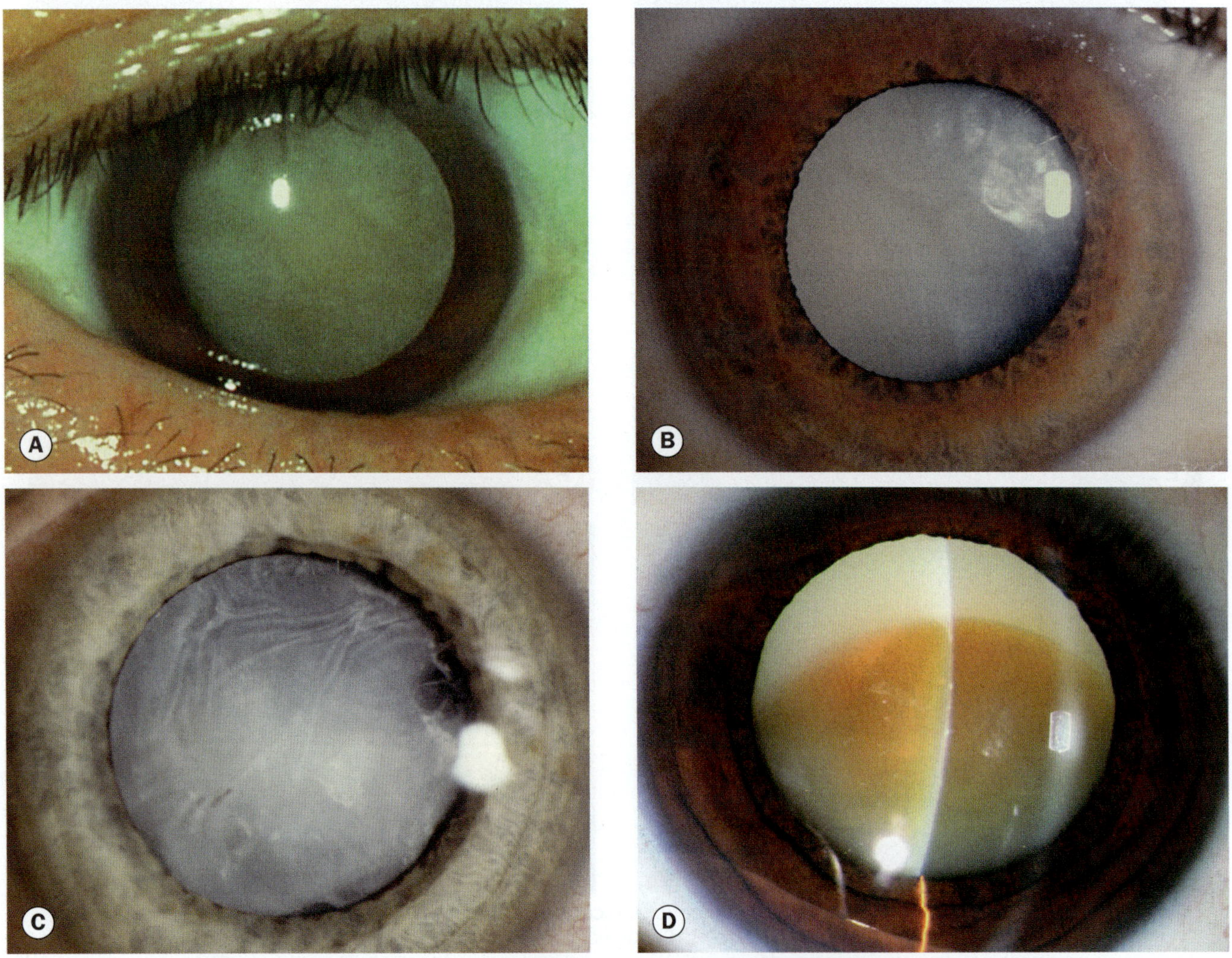

Fig. 10.3 Advanced cataract. **(A)** Mature nuclear sclerotic cataract; **(B)** dense corticular cataract; **(C)** hypermature cataract with wrinkling of the anterior capsule; **(D)** Morgagnian cataract with liquefaction of the cortex and inferior sinking of the nucleus.

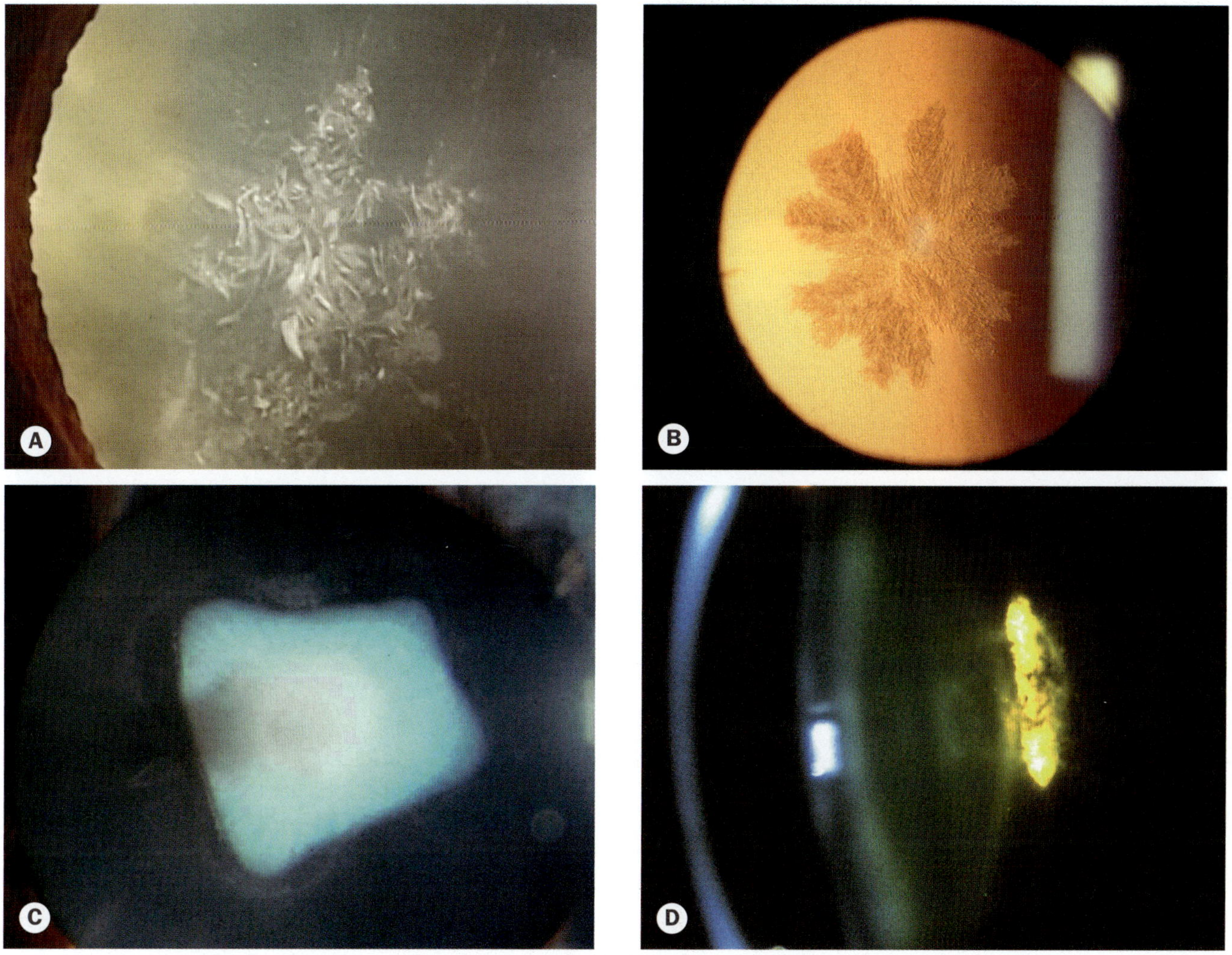

Fig. 10.4 Cataract in systemic disease. **(A)** Diabetic snowflake cataract; **(B)** posterior subcapsular cataract spokes assuming a stellate morphology in myotonic dystrophy; **(C)** shield-like anterior subcapsular cataract in atopic dermatitis; **(D)** posterior subcapsular cataract in neurofibromatosis type 2.

Later, the opacities may become indistinguishable from typical cortical cataract.

Atopic dermatitis

About 10% of patients with severe atopic dermatitis develop cataracts in the second to fourth decades. These are often bilateral and may mature quickly. Shield-like dense anterior subcapsular plaque that wrinkles the anterior capsule (Fig. 10.4C) is characteristic. Posterior subcapsular opacities may also occur.

Neurofibromatosis type 2

Neurofibromatosis type 2 (see Ch. 19) is associated with early cataract in more than 60% of patients. Opacities are posterior subcapsular (Fig. 10.4D) or capsular, cortical or mixed and tend to develop in early adulthood.

Secondary cataract

A secondary (complicated) cataract develops as a result of other primary ocular disease.

Chronic anterior uveitis

Chronic anterior uveitis is the most common cause of secondary cataract, the incidence being related to the duration and intensity of inflammation. Topical and systemic steroids used in treatment are also causative. The earliest finding is often a polychromatic lustre at the posterior pole of the lens. If inflammation persists, posterior and anterior opacities (Fig. 10.5A) develop. Cataract appears to progress more rapidly in the presence of posterior synechiae (Fig. 10.5B).

Acute congestive angle closure

Acute congestive angle closure may cause small anterior grey-white subcapsular or capsular opacities, glaukomflecken (Fig. 10.5C), to form within the pupillary area. These represent focal infarcts of the lens epithelium and are pathognomonic of previous acute congestive angle closure.

High myopia

High (pathological) myopia can be associated with posterior subcapsular lens opacity and early-onset nuclear sclerosis, which ironically may increase the myopic refractive error.

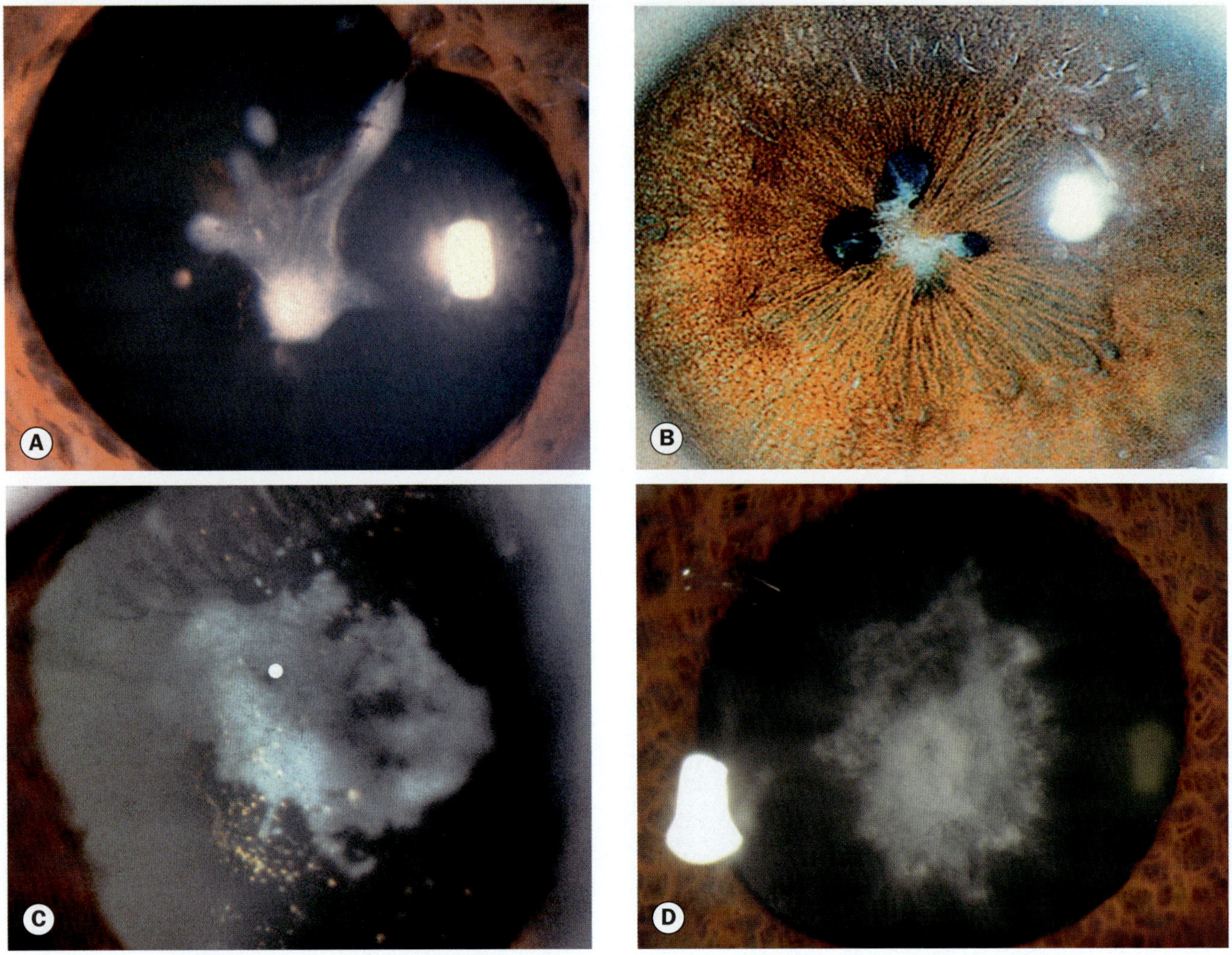

Fig. 10.5 Secondary cataract. **(A)** Uveitic anterior plaque opacities; **(B)** extensive posterior synechiae and anterior lens opacity; **(C)** glaukomflecken; **(D)** anterior subcapsular cataract in retinitis pigmentosa. *(Courtesy of S Chen – fig. D.)*

Hereditary fundus dystrophies

Hereditary fundus dystrophies (see Ch. 15) such as retinitis pigmentosa, Leber congenital amaurosis, gyrate atrophy and Stickler syndrome are usually associated with posterior subcapsular lens opacity. Anterior subcapsular lens opacity is rare (Fig. 10.5D) because surgery is usually undertaken at an early stage, when the opacification is limited to the posterior subcapsular region. Cataract surgery tends to improve visual function even in the presence of severe retinal changes.

Secondary to medication

Systemic and topical steroids can lead to cataract formation. These are usually posterior subcapsular in appearance and can be visually debilitating. Despite a good visual acuity, symptoms of glare and reduced near vision are pronounced (see Ch. 21). Long-term use of chlorpromazine leads to an anterior star-shaped lens opacity (see Fig. 21.2B).

Traumatic cataract

Trauma is the most common cause of unilateral cataract in young people.

- **Penetrating trauma** (Fig. 10.6A and B).
- **Blunt trauma** may cause a characteristic flower-shaped opacity (Fig. 10.6C).
- **Electric shock** is a rare cause of cataract, patterns including diffuse milky-white opacification and multiple snowflake-like opacities, sometimes in a stellate subcapsular distribution (Fig. 10.6D).
- **Infrared radiation**, if intense as in glassblowers, may rarely cause true exfoliation of the anterior lens capsule (Fig. 10.6E).
- **Ionizing radiation** exposure such as for ocular tumour treatment may cause posterior subcapsular opacities (Fig. 10.6F). These may not manifest for months or years.

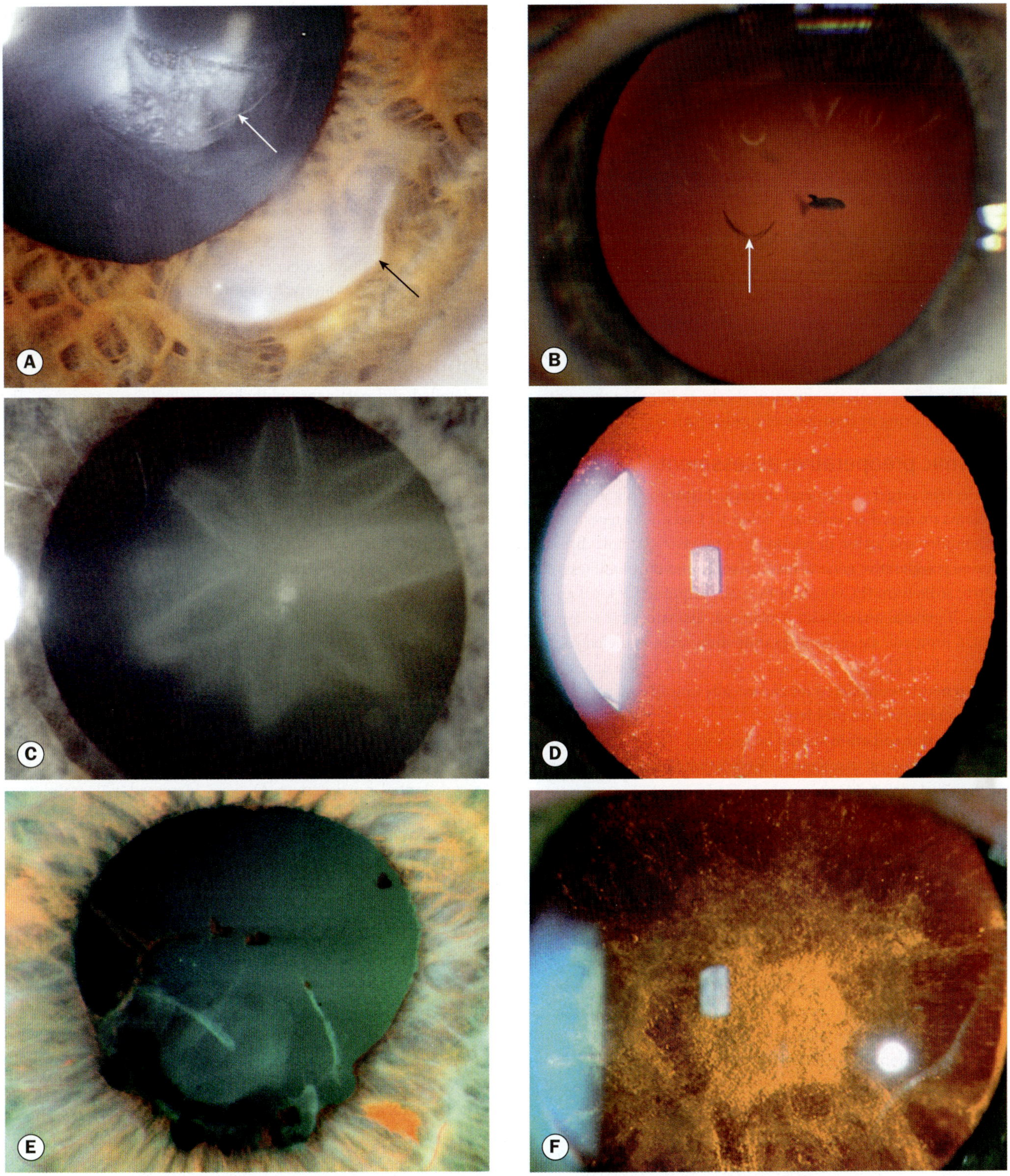

Fig. 10.6 Causes of traumatic cataract. **(A)** Penetrating trauma (black arrow indicates corneal penetration site and white arrow indicates a cut in the anterior capsule); **(B)** intralenticular metallic foreign body (arrow showing crescentic opening in capsule); **(C)** blunt trauma showing a flower-shaped opacity; **(D)** electric shock and lightning strike; **(E)** infrared radiation ('glassblower's cataract'); **(F)** ionizing radiation. *(Courtesy of J Schuman, V Christopoulos, D Dhaliwal, M Kahook and R Noecker, from 'Lens and Glaucoma', in* Rapid Diagnosis in Ophthalmology, *Mosby 2008 – figs D–F.)*

MANAGEMENT OF ACQUIRED CATARACT

Preoperative considerations

Indications for surgery

- **Visual improvement** is by far the most common indication for cataract surgery. An operation is indicated when the opacity develops to a degree sufficient to cause difficulty in performing daily activities. Clear lens exchange (replacement of the healthy lens with an artificial implant) is an option for the management of refractive error.
- **Medical** indications are those in which a cataract is adversely affecting the health of the eye. Examples include phacolytic or phacomorphic glaucoma. Cataract surgery to improve the clarity of the ocular media may also be required in the context of monitoring or treatment of fundus pathology.

Systemic preoperative assessment

For elective surgery, a general medical history is taken and any problems managed accordingly. Table 10.1 sets out suggested further enquiry and action in relation to a range of systemic diseases. Routine preoperative general medical examination, blood tests and electrocardiogram (ECG) are not usually required for local anaesthesia. If general anaesthesia is planned, assessment is according to local protocol, e.g. general examination, urea and electrolytes, random blood glucose, full blood count and ECG. An anaesthetic opinion may be considered for chronically unwell patients or those with complex medical problems.

- **Current medication** should be recorded. This will often guide general medical assessment. Medications relevant to eye surgery include:
  - Systemic alpha-blockers (e.g. tamsulosin) are commonly associated with intraoperative floppy iris syndrome (IFIS).
  - Management of anticoagulant therapy or an antiplatelet agent should follow local protocol. Most surgeons do not stop antiplatelet drugs for cataract surgery, though this may be preferred for oculoplastic procedures and glaucoma surgery. Anticoagulation status, usually expressed as the international normalized ratio (INR) level, should be within the therapeutic range appropriate for the individual indication (e.g. usually higher for heart valve thrombosis prophylaxis than following deep vein thrombosis). A common approach is to check the INR within the 24 hours prior to surgery in stable patients.
- **Allergy.** True allergy rather than intolerance should be confirmed.
  - Medication, including sulfonamides and antibiotics commonly used following cataract surgery.
  - Iodine or shellfish – the latter may indicate an iodine allergy. If allergy to iodine is present an alternative skin and conjunctival antiseptic such as chlorhexidine should be used.
  - Others: allergy to latex (latex-free gloves may be necessary), sticking plaster, local anaesthetics, insect bites (cross-reaction with hyaluronidase that is often used with local anaesthesia).
- **Methicillin-resistant *Staphylococcus aureus* (MRSA) carriage.** Relevant national and local protocols for the identification and management of patients at high risk for MRSA carriage should be followed.
- **Transport** (to hospital and to the operating theatre within hospital): special arrangements may be needed for patients with poor mobility or exceptionally high body mass.

TIP Systemic alpha-blockers (e.g. tamsulosin) are the main cause of intraocular floppy iris syndrome when undertaking phacoemulsification.

Ophthalmic preoperative assessment

A detailed and pertinent ophthalmic evaluation is required. The following should be considered:

- **Visual acuity** is usually tested using a Snellen chart.
- **Cover test.** A heterotropia may indicate amblyopia, which carries a guarded visual prognosis, or the possibility of diplopia if the vision is improved. A squint, usually a divergence, may develop in an eye with poor vision due to cataract and lens surgery alone may straighten the eye.
- **Pupillary responses.** Because cataract never produces an afferent pupillary defect, its presence implies substantial posterior pole pathology.
- **Ocular adnexa.** Dacryocystitis, blepharitis, chronic conjunctivitis, lagophthalmos, ectropion, entropion and tear film abnormalities may predispose to endophthalmitis. These conditions should be dealt with before intraocular surgery.
- **Cornea.** Eyes with decreased endothelial cell counts (e.g. substantial cornea guttata) have increased vulnerability to postoperative decompensation. Specular microscopy and pachymetry may be helpful in assessing risk and precautions should be taken to protect the endothelium (see below). A prominent arcus senilis is often associated with a surgical view of decreased clarity, as are stromal opacities.
- **Anterior chamber.** A shallow anterior chamber can render cataract surgery difficult. Recognition of a poorly dilating pupil allows intensive preoperative mydriatic drops, planned mechanical dilatation prior to capsulorhexis and/or intracameral injection of mydriatic. A poor red reflex compromises the creation of a capsulorhexis, but can be largely overcome by staining the capsule with trypan blue.
- **Lens.** Nuclear cataracts tend to be hard and may require more power for phacoemulsification, while cortical and subcapsular opacities tend to be softer. Black nuclear opacities are extremely dense and extracapsular cataract extraction rather than phacoemulsification may be the preferred option. Pseudoexfoliation indicates a likelihood of weak zonules (phakodonesis – lens wobble – may be present), a fragile capsule and poor mydriasis.
- **Fundus examination.** Pathology such as age-related macular degeneration may affect the visual outcome. Ultrasonography may be required, principally to exclude retinal detachment

Table 10.1 Management of General Medical Conditions Prior to Elective Surgery

Condition	Further questions/examination	Action
Diabetes mellitus	Well controlled? Will need blood test (finger-prick may be sufficient, consider additional tests if necessary)	If control poor, may need to defer surgery and contact patient's physician Medication and food and drink intake as usual on the day of surgery for local anaesthesia
Systemic hypertension	If systolic >170 mmHg or diastolic >100 mmHg may need physician opinion	Consider contacting physician for optimization and defer surgery if necessary
Actual or suspected myocardial infarction (MI) in the past	Date of MI?	Defer surgery for 3–6 months from date of MI. Contact physician/anaesthetist if concerns about current cardiovascular status
Angina	Stable/well controlled?	Bring glyceryl trinitrate (GTN) spray on day of surgery. If unstable, contact physician or anaesthetist
Respiratory disease	Is chest function currently optimal? Can the patient lie flat?	If the patient cannot lie flat, may need to discuss with operating surgeon. Trial of lying flat (at least half an hour) Chest function should be optimized as far as possible prior to surgery Remind patient to bring any inhalers to hospital
Leg ulcer or other skin wound	Acute or chronic? Evidence of active infection?	Surgery should be deferred until active infection has resolved. If healing is not possible (e.g. chronic leg ulcer) the lesion should be covered with a sterile dressing during the perioperative period. A preoperative wound swab for culture and prophylactic oral antibiotics may be considered
Rheumatic fever, transplanted or prosthetic heart valve, previous endocarditis	Does the patient usually require prophylactic antibiotic cover for operations?	Antibiotic prophylaxis only exceptionally required for ophthalmic surgery, e.g. removal of an infected eye
Stroke in the past	Date of stroke? Particular residual difficulties?	Defer surgery for at least 6 months from date of stroke Many have positional/other practical consequences
Rheumatoid arthritis	Does the patient have any problems lying flat or with neck position?	If in doubt about patient's ability to position appropriately, may need to discuss with operating surgeon; intubation for general anaesthesia may be more difficult in some patients
Jaundice or known viral hepatitis in the past	What was the underlying diagnosis?	If viral hepatitis suspected, note prominently as special precautions to avoid needlestick injury may be necessary
Human immunodeficiency virus (HIV) infection	If there are any high-risk factors, has the patient undergone an HIV test in the past?	Special precautions to avoid needlestick injury may be necessary
Sickle status	For patients of southern Asian and Afro-Caribbean ethnic origin, enquire about sickle status	Blood test if unknown and general anaesthesia planned
Parkinson disease or other cause of substantial tremor	Is the patient able to maintain head stability sufficiently to cooperate with local anaesthesia and surgery?	If not, may require general anaesthesia
Epilepsy	Is the condition well controlled?	General anaesthesia may be preferred
Myotonic dystrophy	Has the patient undergone surgery and anaesthesia in the past?	If general anaesthesia is planned, an anaesthetic opinion should be obtained well in advance of surgery

and staphyloma, in eyes with very dense opacity that precludes fundus examination.

- **Sclera.** If a prominent explant/encircling band has been placed during prior retinal detachment surgery, or if the eye is particularly large or the sclera thin (e.g. high myopia), peri- and retrobulbar local anaesthesia should be avoided.
- **Current refractive status.** It is critical to obtain details of the patient's preoperative refractive error in order to guide intraocular lens (IOL) implant selection. The keratometry readings (obtained during biometry – see below) should be noted in relation to the refraction, particularly if it is planned to address astigmatism by means of targeted wound placement, a toric

IOL or a specific adjunctive procedure. It is particularly important to obtain a postoperative refractive result from an eye previously operated upon so that any 'refractive surprise', even if minor, can be considered.

TIP Careful preoperative examination of the posterior pole is needed in a patient requiring cataract surgery to exclude unrelated pathology that may affect the final visual result.

General principles of informed consent

- **Consent** can be defined as 'the process of providing information that enables the patient to make an informed decision to undergo a specific treatment'. The process takes time, patience and clarity of explanation. It is important to establish whether the patient has the capacity to give consent and has the ability to understand, retain, weigh-up information and make a decision without duress. A 'competent' person has the right to refuse treatment, even if by refusing the proposed treatment it could result in visual disability, blindness or death.
- **Consent for cataract surgery.** It is essential that the patient arrives at a fully informed decision before proceeding to cataract surgery. It is useful to provide written information and a link to an online video of the surgery. As well as discussing the benefits, risks should be conveyed at a level appropriate to each patient's level of understanding, with an explanation of the more common and severe potential problems.
- **Risk.** Two legal principles are relevant in the United Kingdom:
  - Risk should be disclosed if a reasonable body of medical opinion would consider it important to disclose the risk.
  - If a reasonable person in the patient's position would attach significance to the risk, they should be told about it.
- **Points for discussion** with the patient may include:
  - Immediate sequential bilateral cataract surgery (ISBCS) versus delayed sequential bilateral cataract surgery. The option of ISBCS is subject to debate because of the potential risk of bilateral sight-threatening complications, especially endophthalmitis. However, large trials have shown no difference between the two alternatives in respect of visual acuity or complications at 1 month and 1 year postoperatively. Meticulous selection and preparation of appropriate cases is essential.
  - The merits and disadvantages of the various refractive options and in particular, the use of a multifocal or toric IOL.
  - Reassurance that most cataract operations are straightforward with good visual results.
  - Complications can be dealt with effectively and cause no long-term difficulties, but that some rare problems can be very serious and may mean that a second operation will be necessary.
  - A warning that in about 1 in 1000 cataract operations the eye will be left with little or no sight; in about 1 in 10,000 the patient will lose the eye.
  - Relatively mild and usually easily treatable but common complications include periocular ecchymosis, allergy to eye drops, intraocular pressure (IOP) spike, iridocyclitis, posterior capsular opacification.
  - Moderate–severe but less common complications: posterior capsular rupture/vitreous loss (1% or less for experienced surgeons, higher for trainees dependent on experience), zonular dehiscence, dropped nucleus (about 0.2%), leaking wound, cystoid macular oedema (CMO), corneal decompensation sufficient to need corneal graft, unexpected refractive outcome (may need contact lens wear, lens implant exchange or corneal surgery), retinal detachment (<1%), IOL dislocation, persistent ptosis and diplopia.
  - Rare but invariably very serious complications: endophthalmitis (0.1%) and suprachoroidal haemorrhage (0.04%).
  - The risks of anaesthesia should be conveyed by the person administering it. Local anaesthesia carries a low risk of problems. Some rare complications have the potential to be very serious including loss of the eye and even death: allergy to the anaesthetic agent, retrobulbar haemorrhage (see Ch. 22), perforation of the globe and inadvertent infusion of anaesthetic agent into the cerebrospinal fluid via the optic nerve sheath, causing brainstem anaesthesia.

Biometry

Biometry facilitates calculation of the lens power likely to result in the desired postoperative refractive outcome. In its basic form this involves the measurement of two ocular parameters, keratometry and axial (anteroposterior) length.

- **Keratometry** involves determination of the curvature of the anterior corneal surface (steepest and flattest meridians), expressed in dioptres or in millimetres of radius of curvature. This is commonly carried out with the interferometry apparatus used to determine axial length (see below), but if this is unavailable or unsuitable, manual keratometry (e.g. Javal–Schiøtz keratometer) or corneal topography can be performed.
- **Optical coherence biometry** (Fig. 10.7A) is a non-contact method of axial length measurement that utilizes two coaxial partially coherent low-energy laser beams to produce an interference pattern (partial coherence interferometry). Modern biometry devices also perform keratometry, anterior chamber depth and corneal white-to-white measurement and are able to calculate IOL power using a range of formulae. Measurements have high reproducibility and generally require less skill than ultrasonic biometry (see below).
- **A-scan ultrasonography** is a slightly less accurate method of determining the axial dimension and can be acquired either by direct contact (Fig. 10.7B) or more accurately (but with greater difficulty) by using a water bath over the eye (immersion ultrasonography). The sound beam must be aligned with the visual axis for maximal precision. Each reflecting surface is represented by a spike on an oscilloscope display monitor (Fig. 10.7C).
- **IOL power calculation formulae.** Numerous formulae have been developed that utilize keratometry and axial length to calculate the IOL power required to achieve a given refractive

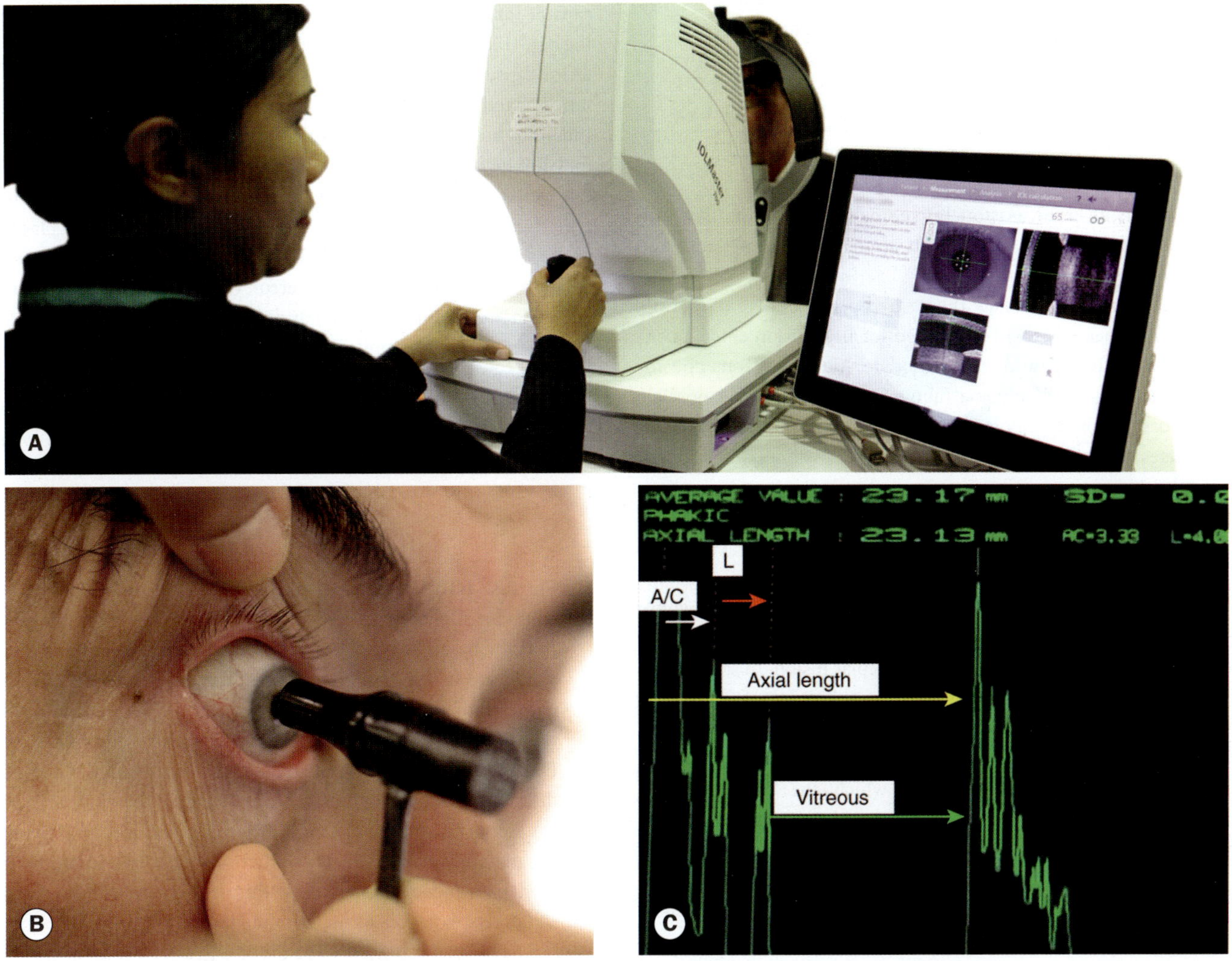

Fig. 10.7 Biometry. **(A)** Optical coherence biometry; **(B)** contact ultrasonic biometry; **(C)** ultrasonographic monitor display (A/C, anterior chamber depth; L, lens thickness).

outcome. Some formulae incorporate additional parameters such as anterior chamber depth and lens thickness to try to optimize accuracy. The SRK-T, Haigis, Hoffer Q and Holladay 1 and 2 are commonly used. Specific formulae may be superior for very short or long eyes, but opinions vary and it is always wise to plan individually for an unusual eye, consulting the latest research and recommendations. Short eyes in particular are prone to unexpected mean spherical error following surgery. Based on current literature, for shorter eyes (AL< 22 mm) Hoffer Q, Haigis, Hill-RBF and Kane formulae are recommended, whereas for long eyes (AL>26 mm) BU II, Holladay, Haigis (with optimized constant) and Kane formulae produce better outcomes. Factors that confound axial length measurements include:

- Poor patient fixation.
- Irregularities in globe contour.
- Silicone oil in the vitreous.

- **Previous refractive surgery.** Any form of corneal refractive surgery is likely to make a significant difference to the IOL power required and standard IOL calculations are unsuitable. Several different methods have been described to address this situation. Most involve the calculation of the post-refractive procedure 'true' corneal power using a special process (refractive history method, contact lens method) and insertion of this into a standard (e.g. Hoffer Q) or specific (e.g. Masket) formula, but the Haigis-L regression formula uses statistical data to facilitate calculation on post-refractive surgery eyes using only standard inputs. It may be prudent to utilize more than one method of IOL calculation. The patient needs to be warned that an under- or over-correction may follow the surgery.
- **Contact lenses.** If the patient wears soft contact lenses, these should not be worn for up to a week prior to biometry to allow corneal stabilization. Those patients who have a long history of wearing rigid gas permeable contact lenses require up to 6 weeks to achieve refractive stability before undertaking the measurements.
- **Personalized A-constant.** If a consistent postoperative refractive deviation is found in most of an individual surgeon's cases, it is assumed that some aspects of personal surgical (or possibly biometric) technique consistently and similarly influence outcome. A personalized A-constant can be programmed into biometry apparatus to take this into account.

TIP To achieve accurate preoperative biometry, soft contact lenses should not be worn for one week before the measurements are taken. Refractive stability takes up to 6 weeks for those wearing rigid gas-permeable contact lenses.

Postoperative refraction

- **Margins of error.** Postoperative unaided refraction is within 1.0 D of predicted outcome in almost 90% of patients and within 0.5 D in two-thirds.
- **Emmetropia** is typically the desired postoperative refraction, though spectacles will be needed for near vision since a conventional IOL cannot accommodate. Many surgeons aim for a small degree of myopia (about −0.25 D) to offset possible errors in biometry. Postoperative hypermetropia, which necessitates correction for clear vision at all distances, is less well tolerated than myopia.
- **Contralateral eye.** Postoperative refractive planning must consider the contralateral eye. If this has a significant refractive error but is unlikely to require cataract surgery within a few years, the postoperative target for the operated eye might be set for within less than 2.0 D of its fellow, to avoid problems with image size discrepancy and difficulty with binocular fusion. In some cases, such as when there is an early lens opacity in the fellow eye or when ametropia is extreme, the patient can be offered lens surgery to the other eye to facilitate targeting both at emmetropia.
- **'Monovision'** is a concept in which the (usually) non-dominant eye is left with between 1 and 2 dioptres of myopia to allow unaided vision for reading, whilst emmetropia is targeted in the dominant eye. This is attractive to some patients, generally those who have previously been using contact lenses or spectacles to achieve monovision.
- **Multifocal** lens options use a variety of optical means to achieve satisfactory near, distance and intermediate vision (see Ch. 8). Most patients are satisfied with the results, but a significant number are unhappy, complaining of phenomena such as glare and loss of contrast sensitivity. Highly accurate refractive outcomes, including limited astigmatism, are necessary for optimal function and a greater likelihood of tolerance.
- **Younger patients.** With a conventional monofocal IOL, patients younger than about 55 years need to be aware that they will experience a sudden loss of active focusing and that it will often take some time to adjust to the loss of unaided near vision.

TIP Patients younger than 55 years need to be warned that active focusing will be lost after the implantation of a conventional monofocal IOL.

Intraocular lenses

Positioning

An IOL (Fig. 10.8A) consists of an optic and haptics. The optic is the central refracting element and the haptics the arms or loops that sit in contact with peripheral ocular structures to centralize the optic. Modern cataract surgery, with preservation of the lens capsule, affords positioning of the IOL in the ideal location – 'in the bag' (Fig. 10.8B). Complicated surgery, with rupture of the posterior capsule, may necessitate alternative positioning in the posterior chamber with the haptics in the ciliary sulcus (a three-piece IOL only, not one-piece including those with plate haptics, as these may not be stable), or in the anterior chamber (AC) with the haptics supported in the angle – AC positioning requires a specific lens type. In some circumstances a supplementary IOL may be placed in the sulcus in addition to an IOL in the capsular bag, for instance to address a residual refractive error following primary surgery (secondary pseudopolyphakia) and thin-profile IOLs are available for this purpose. It is preferable to avoid a secondary sulcus IOL (primary pseudopolyphakia) in very short (e.g. nanophthalmic) eyes due to the risk of angle closure. Off-the-shelf IOLs of power up to 40 D are available and custom IOLs can be produced in even higher powers.

Design

- **Flexible IOLs** introduced into the eye via an injector and subsequently unrolled inside the eye are now in general use. Injector-based delivery utilizes a very small incision and also allows avoidance of implant contact with the ocular surface, so reducing the risk of bacterial contamination. Simple folding of the IOL is an alternative, but requires a slightly larger incision. Flexible materials are discussed below. There seems to be no distinct superiority of one material over another.
    - Acrylic IOLs. Hydrophobic (water content <1%) acrylic materials have a greater refractive index than hydrophilic lenses and are consequently thinner, though this can result in dysphotopsia (troublesome glare and reflections). They have been reported to produce a greater reaction in eyes with uveitis, but outcomes do not seem to be materially affected. Hydrophilic acrylic (hydrogel) in theory offers superior biocompatibility, but the image of hydrogel IOLs has been marred by the occurrence of calcification requiring IOL removal in some types and inflammation in others (these problems have been resolved by lens manufacturers). Posterior capsular opacification (PCO) rates may be higher with hydrogel IOLs than with other materials.
    - Silicone IOLs are available in both loop haptic (one- or three-piece) and plate haptic (one-piece) conformations, the latter consisting of a roughly rectangular leaf with the optic sited centrally. Silicone IOLs exhibit greater biocompatibility than hydrophobic acrylic IOLs, but may be prone to significant silicone deposition in silicone oil-filled eyes.
    - Collamer is composed of collagen, a poly-HEMA-based copolymer and an ultraviolet-absorbing chromophore. It is marketed principally on the basis of high biocompatibility and a favourable track record.
- **Rigid IOLs** are made entirely from polymethylmethacrylate (PMMA). They cannot be injected or folded so require an incision larger than the diameter of the optic, typically 5 or 6 mm, for insertion. For economic reasons, they continue to be widely used in developing countries. PCO rates are higher with PMMA lenses than silicone and acrylic. Some surgeons favour

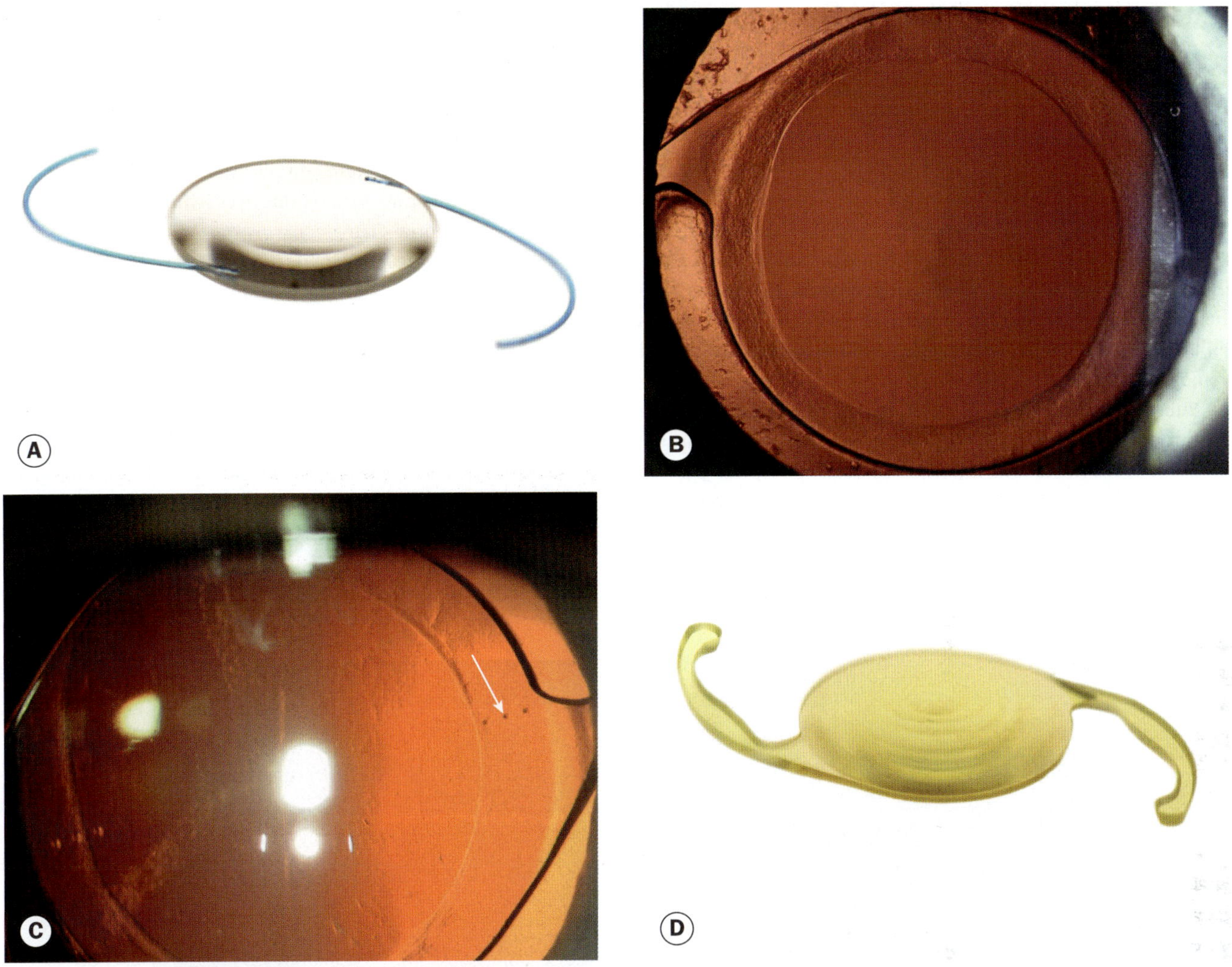

Fig. 10.8 Intraocular lens (IOL). **(A)** Three-piece acrylic foldable IOL – note the square-edged optic; **(B)** IOL *in situ* in the capsular bag; **(C)** implanted toric IOL showing diametrically opposite sets of three dots marking the lens axis (arrow); **(D)** one-piece, flexible, multifocal IOL (optic includes a blue light filter).

heparin-coated IOLs (see below) in eyes with previous uveitis, particularly in children.

- **Sharp/square-edged optics** (see Fig. 10.8A) are associated with a significantly lower rate of PCO compared with round-edged optics and the former is now the predominant design. However, square edges may be associated with a higher rate of dysphotopsia (see below).
- **Blue light filters.** Although all IOLs contain ultraviolet light filters, a number also include filters for blue wavelengths, in order to reduce the possibility of damage to the retina by this higher-energy visible light (see Fig. 10.8D). The blue filters impart a slight yellow tint to the IOL, though similar only to that of the physiological young adult lens. Some evidence suggests slightly poorer visual function in scotopic conditions of illumination.
- **Aspheric optics** to counteract corneal spherical aberration are widely available and have been shown to improve contrast, particularly in mesopic conditions. A potential drawback is that the aspheric element of the manufactured IOLs is set at a single standardized level (this differs between manufacturers), but the extent of spherical aberration varies between individuals; some will be over- and some under-compensated.
- **Heparin coating** reduces the attraction and adhesion of inflammatory cells and this may have particular application in eyes with uveitis. However, there is no clear evidence of the clinical benefit of heparin surface modification in these eyes.
- **Toric IOLs** (Fig. 10.8C) have an integral cylindrical refractive component to compensate for pre-existing corneal astigmatism. The main potential problem is rotation within the capsular bag, which occurs in a small percentage and may be corrected by early surgical repositioning.
- **Bifocal IOLs** (Fig. 10.8D) (see also Ch. 8) utilizing refractive or diffractive mechanisms aim to provide clear vision over a range of focal distances. So-called 'accommodative' IOLs attempt to flex and thereby alter focal length but in practice the amplitude of accommodation is slight.
- **Adjustable IOLs** allow the alteration of refractive power following implantation. One version uses low-level ultraviolet

irradiation at the slit lamp about a week after surgery to induce polymerization of its constituent molecules in specific patterns with precise spherical and cylindrical (astigmatism) correction.

Anaesthesia

Most cataract surgery is performed under local anaesthesia (LA), sometimes in conjunction with intravenous or oral sedation. General anaesthesia is required in some circumstances, such as children and many young adults, very anxious patients, some patients with learning difficulties, epilepsy, dementia and those with a head tremor.

- **Sub-Tenon block** involves insertion of a blunt-tipped cannula through an incision in the conjunctiva and Tenon capsule 5 mm from the limbus inferonasally (Fig. 10.9A) and passing it around the curve of the globe through the sub-Tenon space. The anaesthetic is injected beyond the equator of the globe (Fig. 10.9B). Although anaesthesia is good and complications minimal, akinesia is variable. Chemosis and subconjunctival haemorrhage are common but penetration of the globe is extremely rare.
- **Peribulbar block** is given through the skin (Fig. 10.9C and D) or conjunctiva with a 1-inch (25-mm) needle. It generally provides effective anaesthesia and akinesia. Penetration of the globe is a rare but severe complication. For this reason, peribulbar should be avoided in long eyes (which also tend to have a larger equatorial diameter).
- **Topical anaesthesia** involves drops or gel (proxymetacaine 0.5%, tetracaine 1% drops, lidocaine 2% gel), which can be augmented with intracameral preservative-free lidocaine 0.2–1%, often infused during hydrodissection. Patients receiving supplementary intracameral lidocaine have significantly less pain than those receiving topical anaesthesia alone. Intracameral Mydrane, a preservative-free combination of tropicamide 0.02%, phenylephrine 0.31% and lidocaine 1%, is commonly used for achieving mydriasis and anaesthesia during high-volume cataract surgery. Combined viscoelastic/lidocaine preparations are also commercially available. Despite the absence of akinesia, most patients can cooperate adequately.

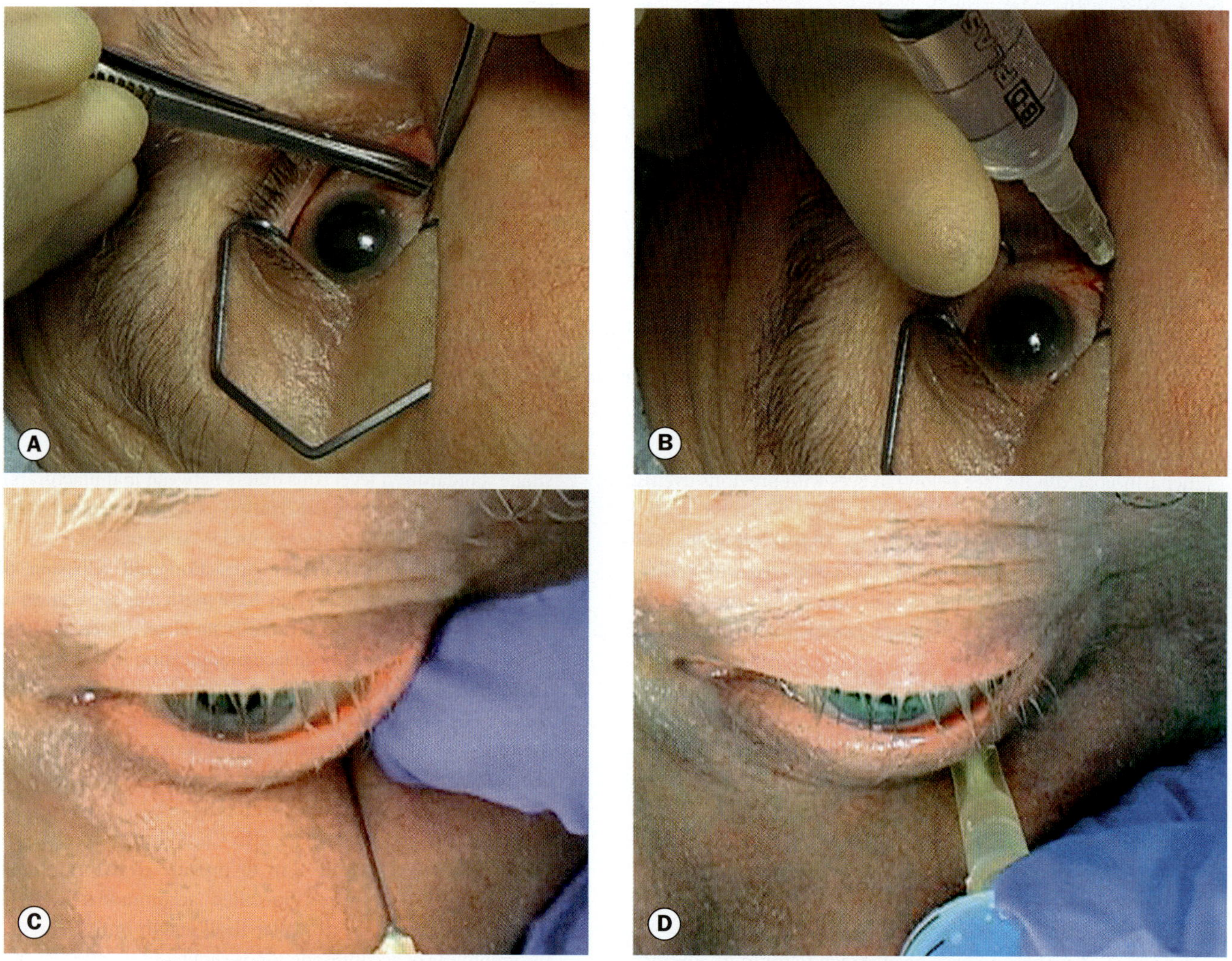

Fig. 10.9 Local anaesthesia for cataract surgery. **(A)** Conjunctival dissection for sub-Tenon anaesthesia; **(B)** sub-Tenon infiltration with a blunt cannula; **(C)** insertion of needle for peribulbar anaesthesia. **(D)** peribulbar infiltration of anaesthetic agent.

However, approximately 5% of patients experience pain when the surgery is undertaken with topical or intracameral anaesthesia.

Manual cataract surgery

When posterior chamber IOLs began to be widely used in the 1980s most surgeons adopted extracapsular cataract extraction (ECCE), abandoning the older intracapsular technique (ICCE). In ICCE, a cryoprobe is used to remove the lens complete with its capsule (Fig. 10.10A). In ECCE, after a large anterior capsulotomy is created, an extensive limbal incision (8–10 mm) is completed and the lens nucleus is expressed following hydrodissection to free its cortical attachments (Fig. 10.10B). Cortical matter is then aspirated, leaving behind a sufficiently intact capsular bag to support an IOL. Suturing of the incision is required, sometimes inducing considerable corneal astigmatism. Manual small-incision cataract surgery (MSICS) is a variant of ECCE used to address the requirement for high-volume surgical treatment of patients with dense cataracts in less affluent geographical regions. It involves the creation of a small self-sealing sclero-corneal tunnel (Fig. 10.11A), staining of the anterior capsule to facilitate capsulorhexis (Fig. 10.11B), manual one-piece expression of the nucleus (Fig. 10.11C), manual aspiration of the cortex (Fig. 10.11D) and IOL implantation. Visual rehabilitation is comparable to phacoemulsification but MSICS is faster and avoids the need for expensive technology.

Phacoemulsification

Introduction

Phacoemulsification ('phaco') is the standard method of cataract extraction in high-income countries and in regional centres in most lower-income countries.

Phacodynamics

Choosing appropriate settings makes surgery safer and easier.

- **Level of irrigating bottle** above the patient's eye is set to maintain AC stability with a reasonable IOP. Infusion flow is proportional to the height of the bottle.
- **Aspiration flow rate** (AFR) refers to the volume of fluid removed from the eye in millilitres per minute. For a higher AFR the irrigating bottle must be elevated to compensate for increased fluid loss. High AFR results in attraction of lens material towards the phaco tip, with faster vacuum build-up and swifter removal of lens matter but with less effective power. A high AFR should usually be avoided by trainee surgeons.
- **Vacuum**, measured in mmHg, is generated during occlusion when the pump is attempting to aspirate fluid. Vacuum level determines how tightly material is held by the phaco tip when occluded, providing the ability to manipulate lens fragments. High vacuum can decrease the total power required to remove the lens. As with AFR, a lower-vacuum setting slows down the speed of intraocular events, reduces the intensity of surge (see below) and makes inadvertent aspiration of iris or lens capsule less likely.
- **Post-occlusion surge.** When occlusion of the phaco tip by lens material is broken, pent-up energy results in a sudden temporary increase in outflow – 'surge'. This may result in complications such as capsular rupture and as far as possible is suppressed by modern phaco machines.

Pump type

The main implication of the type of pump employed by a particular phaco machine is the effect on vacuum behaviour.

- **Peristaltic (flow) pumps** pull fluid and lens material into the phaco tip by compressing tubing over variable speed rollers. Vacuum is generated only when occlusion of the tip occurs, following which the pump slows and stops when a set maximum is achieved.
- **Venturi (vacuum) pumps** create a negative pressure in a vessel by passing compressed gas across its entrance. This has the practical effect of synchronizing vacuum and AFR so there is generally no independent means of adjusting AFR. Depression

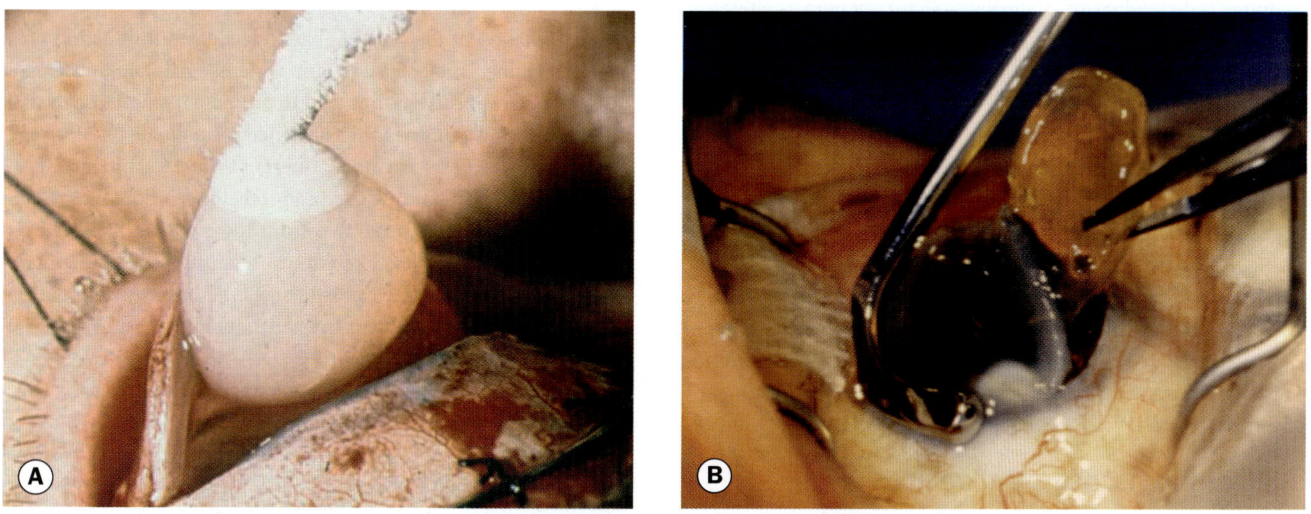

Fig. 10.10 Manual cataract surgery. **(A)** Intracapsular extraction; **(B)** extracapsular extraction. *(Courtesy of C Barry.)*

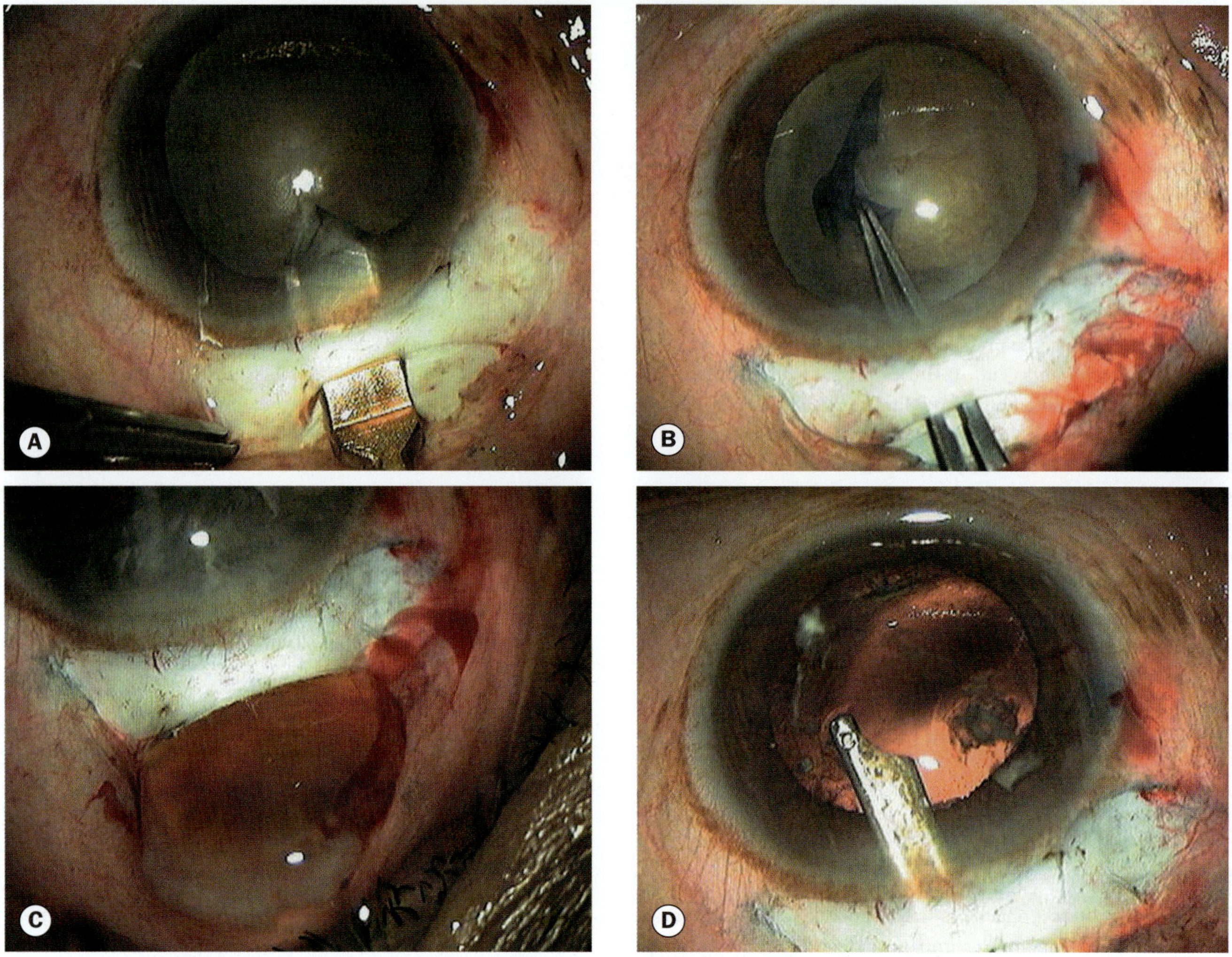

Fig. 10.11 Manual small-incision cataract surgery. **(A)** Scleral tunnel incision; **(B)** blue stain of the anterior capsule before capsulorhexis; **(C)** expression of the nucleus; **(D)** corticular aspiration with a Simcoe cannula. *(Courtesy of A Hennig.)*

of the foot pedal increases vacuum towards the pre-set maximum independent of occlusion and tip vacuum is therefore always available.

- **Hybrid pumps** are offered by some modern machines.

Handpiece

The phaco handpiece features a tip consisting of a hollow titanium needle with an enclosing fluid-cooling sleeve (Fig. 10.12) to protect the cornea from thermal and mechanical damage. Its emulsifying action is mediated by very high-frequency (ultrasonic) vibration leading to jackhammer, cavitation and other effects. Some machines offer variants such as a torsional phaco action or water jet-mediated phacoemulsification. Phaco tips of differing shapes and sizes are available, each having particular cutting and holding characteristics.

Ophthalmic viscosurgical devices

Ophthalmic viscosurgical devices (OVDs or viscoelastics) are biopolymers that play a critical role in modern cataract surgery.

- **Cohesive** OVDs are used to create and maintain intraocular spaces, for example to maintain the AC during capsulorhexis and inflation of the capsular bag to facilitate introduction of an IOL. Higher molecular weight variants maintain intraocular space more effectively, but tend to promote iris prolapse in shallow ACs and confer a more sustained postoperative IOP rise.
- **Dispersive** OVDs are more adherent to surfaces than cohesive OVDs and are typically used to protect the endothelium. They are more difficult to remove from the eye than cohesive viscoelastics, but are less likely to cause an IOP spike. The major practical disadvantage of dispersive OVDs is their tendency to retain air bubbles and lens fragments, compromising the surgical view.
- **Adaptive** OVDs display mixed characteristics.
- **'Soft shell'** technique involves the injection prior to the capsulotomy stage of an outer dispersive layer followed by an inner cohesive nucleus. Some surgeons use this routinely, others only for eyes at higher risk of corneal decompensation (e.g. cornea guttata).

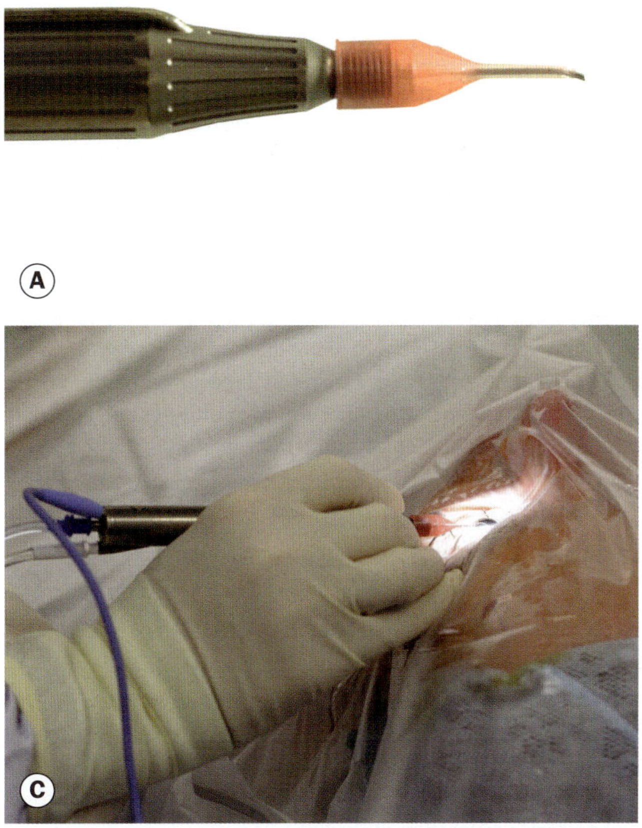

Fig. 10.12 Phaco handpiece. **(A)** With curved tip and sleeve; **(B)** in position during surgery.

- **Pupillary manipulation.** In an eye with a small pupil, a high molecular weight cohesive viscoelastic (e.g. Healon GV) will push the iris away from the lens and help to induce mydriasis. Adaptive OVDs' cohesive effect can be used to dilate a pupil intraoperatively and their dispersive effect to maintain the dilatation. OVDs can be used to break posterior synechiae with minimal trauma.
- **Cortical manipulation.** OVDs can be useful to dissect cortex away from the lens capsule to minimize traction on fragile zonular ligaments.
- **Capsulorhexis rescue.** If a capsulorhexis shows signs of running out to the periphery, injecting a cohesive viscoelastic will flatten the anterior capsule, aiding the exertion of a centrally directed vector and helping to expand the pupil.

TIP Trypan blue effectively stains the anterior capsule and facilitates accurate capsulorhexis in a patient with a poor 'red reflex' secondary to a dense cataract.

- **Capsular rupture.** In a small posterior capsular tear, a dispersive viscoelastic will push the vitreous back into the posterior chamber and maintain plugging of the capsular defect, facilitating completion of lens removal.

Technique

- **Preparation**
  - Topical anaesthetic is followed by povidone-iodine 5% (Fig. 10.13A) or chlorhexidine instillation into the conjunctival sac and cleaning of the eyelids (Fig. 10.13B), ensuring thorough eyelash application. The antiseptic should be left to work for a minimum of 3 minutes.
  - Careful draping (Fig. 10.13C) is performed, excluding the lashes and lid margins from the surgical field and a speculum is inserted.
- **Incisions**
  - A side port incision is made around 60° to the left (in right-handed surgeons) of the main incision. Some surgeons prefer two side ports approximately 180° apart.
  - Viscoelastic is injected into the AC.
  - Many surgeons locate the main corneal incision (Fig. 10.14A) on the steepest corneal axis, others prefer consistent siting. Temporal incisions can provide better access and less induced astigmatism but may be associated with a slightly higher risk of endophthalmitis.
- **Continuous curvilinear capsulorhexis** is performed with a cystotome, bent hypodermic needle and/or capsule forceps (Fig. 10.14B).
- **Hydrodissection** is performed to separate the nucleus and cortex from the capsule so that the nucleus can be manipulated. A blunt cannula is inserted just beneath the edge of the capsulorhexis and fluid injected gently under the capsule (Fig. 10.14C). A hydrodissection wave should be seen, provided there is an adequate red reflex.
- **'Divide and conquer'** is a widely used, safe technique for removal of the nucleus in which two perpendicular grooves are created (sculpting), the phaco tip and a second instrument engaged in opposite walls of the grooves and the nucleus cracked into quadrants by applying force in opposite directions (Fig. 10.14D). Each of the quadrants is then emulsified and aspirated in turn (Fig. 10.14E).
- **'Phaco chop'** has the advantage of slightly greater speed and a lower total phaco energy requirement, but takes longer to learn. In horizontal chopping, a blunt-tipped chopper is placed horizontally underneath the capsule and rotated vertically as the equator is reached. Vertical chopping is performed with a pointed-tip chopper that does not need to pass beyond the capsulorhexis. The nucleus is separated into several pieces for emulsification.
- **'Stop and chop'** is a combination technique.
- **Removal of lens cortex.** Cortical lens matter segments are carefully engaged by means of vacuum, peeled away centrally from the lens capsule and aspirated. Automated coaxial, bimanual automated (Fig. 10.14F) and manual aspiration (e.g. Simcoe cannula) methods are available.
- **IOL insertion.** The capsular bag is filled with cohesive viscoelastic. A loaded injector cartridge is introduced through the

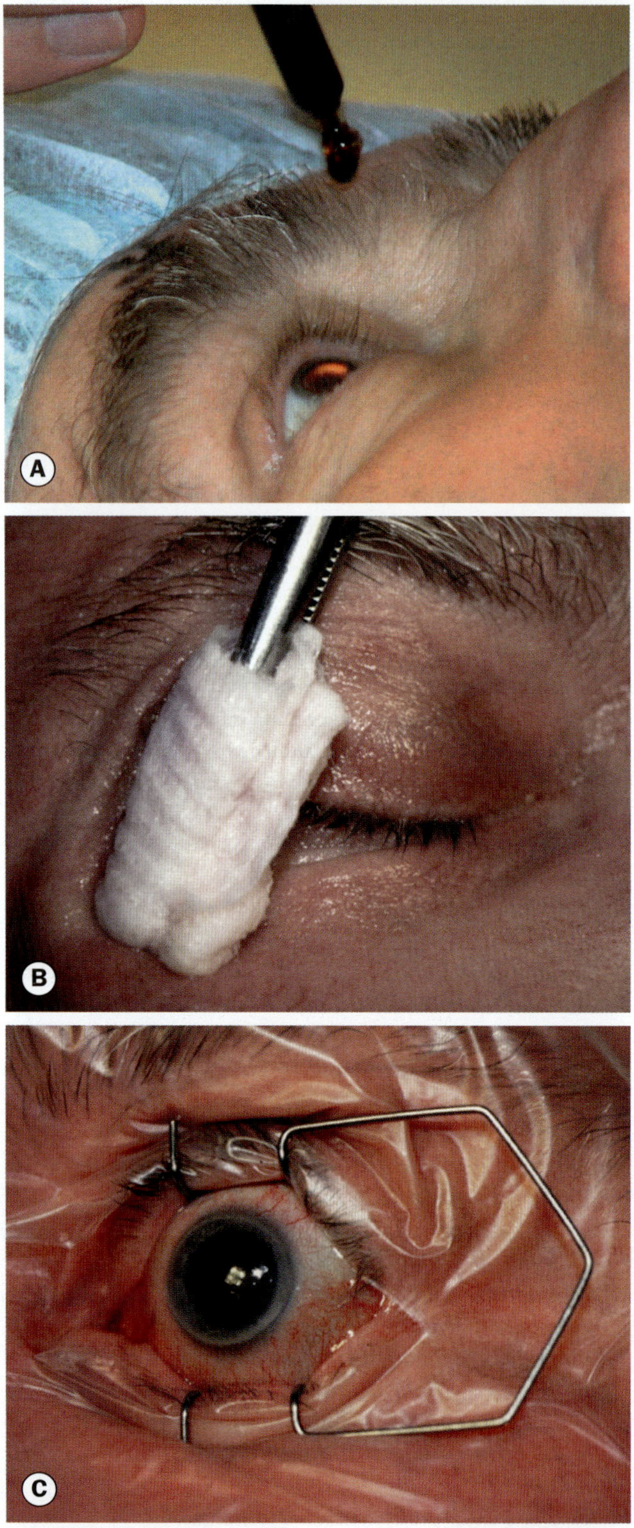

Fig. 10.13 Preparation. **(A)** Povidone-iodine 5% conjunctival fornix instillation; **(B)** cleaning the skin with povidone-iodine; **(C)** plastic drape and speculum isolating the operating field from the eyelids.

main section and the IOL slowly injected and unrolled inside the capsular bag (Fig. 10.15). A toric IOL (see Fig. 10.8C) should be rotated to the correct alignment. Viscoelastic may be aspirated prior to or following toric IOL rotation.

- **Completion.** Side port incisions and the main wound may be sealed with corneal stromal saline injection (hydrosealing). Prophylactic measures at the end of surgery may include intracameral (AC) antibiotic injection, subconjunctival injection of antibiotic and steroid and/or topical antibiotic.

Femtosecond lasers in cataract surgery

Femtosecond lasers, used in refractive surgery for several years, have recently been adopted by some surgeons, replacing several of the manual steps of phacoemulsification with an automated process. The corneal incisions, the capsulorhexis and initial fragmentation of the crystalline lens, as well as astigmatism-relieving incisions (Fig. 10.16), can be performed with laser. Potential advantages include greater precision and integrity of incisions, reduced phacoemulsification energy and possibly improved refractive outcomes due to more precise capsulorhexis placement. Disadvantages include substantially higher cost, longer total operating time and difficulties with technically challenging cases (e.g. small pupils). There is a substantial learning curve.

Operative complications

Rupture of the posterior lens capsule

Capsular rupture may be accompanied by vitreous loss, posterior migration of lens material and, rarely, expulsive haemorrhage. Sequelae to vitreous loss, particularly if inappropriately managed, include CMO, retinal detachment, endophthalmitis, updrawn pupil, uveitis, vitreous touch, vitreous wick syndrome, glaucoma and posterior dislocation of the IOL.

- **Signs**
  - Sudden deepening or shallowing of the AC and momentary pupillary dilatation.
  - The nucleus falls away and cannot be approached by the phaco tip.
  - Vitreous aspirated into the phaco tip often manifests with a marked slowing of aspiration.
  - The torn capsule or vitreous gel may be directly visible.

TIP Rupture of the posterior capsule manifests with a sudden change in the anterior chamber depth and momentary pupillary dilatation.

- **Management** depends on the magnitude of the tear, the size and type of any residual lens material and the presence or absence of vitreous prolapse.
  - Dispersive viscoelastic such as Viscoat may be injected (see above). If a complete or nearly complete nucleus remains, conversion to extracapsular extraction may be considered. A vitrector can be employed at this point (see below) to remove vitreous entangled with nuclear fragments.
  - The incision may be enlarged if necessary and a lens glide (Sheets glide) passed behind lens fragments to cover the

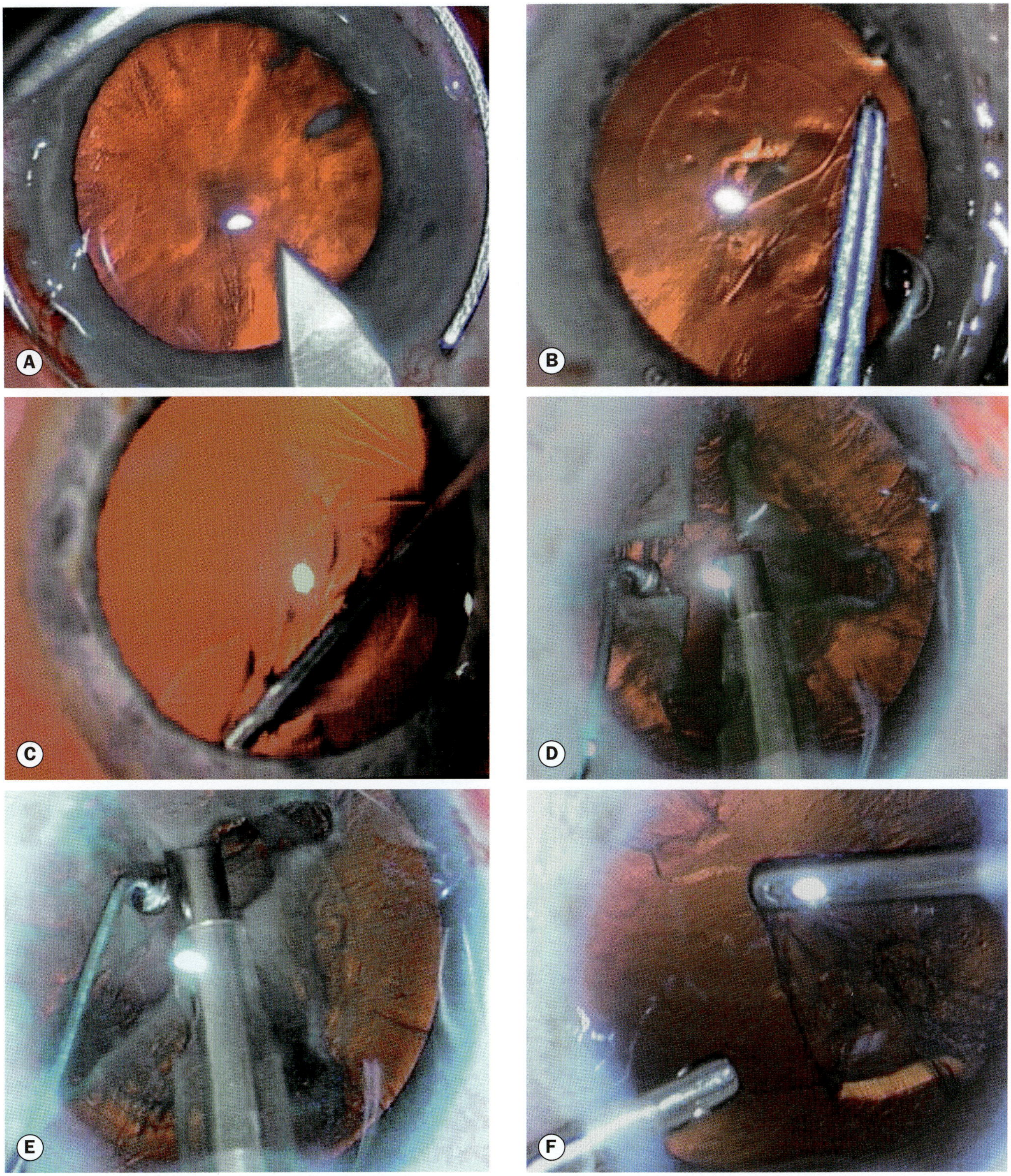

Fig. 10.14 Phacoemulsification. **(A)** Corneal incision; **(B)** capsulorhexis; **(C)** hydrodissection; **(D)** cracking of the nucleus; **(E)** phacoemulsification and aspiration of nuclear quadrants – 'divide and conquer' method; **(F)** cortical aspiration using a bimanual automated technique.

capsular defect, although it is important to confirm that vitreous has first been displaced or removed and will not be put under traction.

- Residual nuclear fragments are carefully removed by phaco using a low bottle height and low AFR, or, if large, by visco-expression after extending the main wound.
- Once nuclear remnants have been removed, a common approach is to re-plug the tear with dispersive OVD, gently filling the anterior chamber with a cohesive viscoelastic and using a manual aspiration cannula with the irrigation off to carefully aspirate residual cortex, topping up the AC with viscoelastic as necessary.

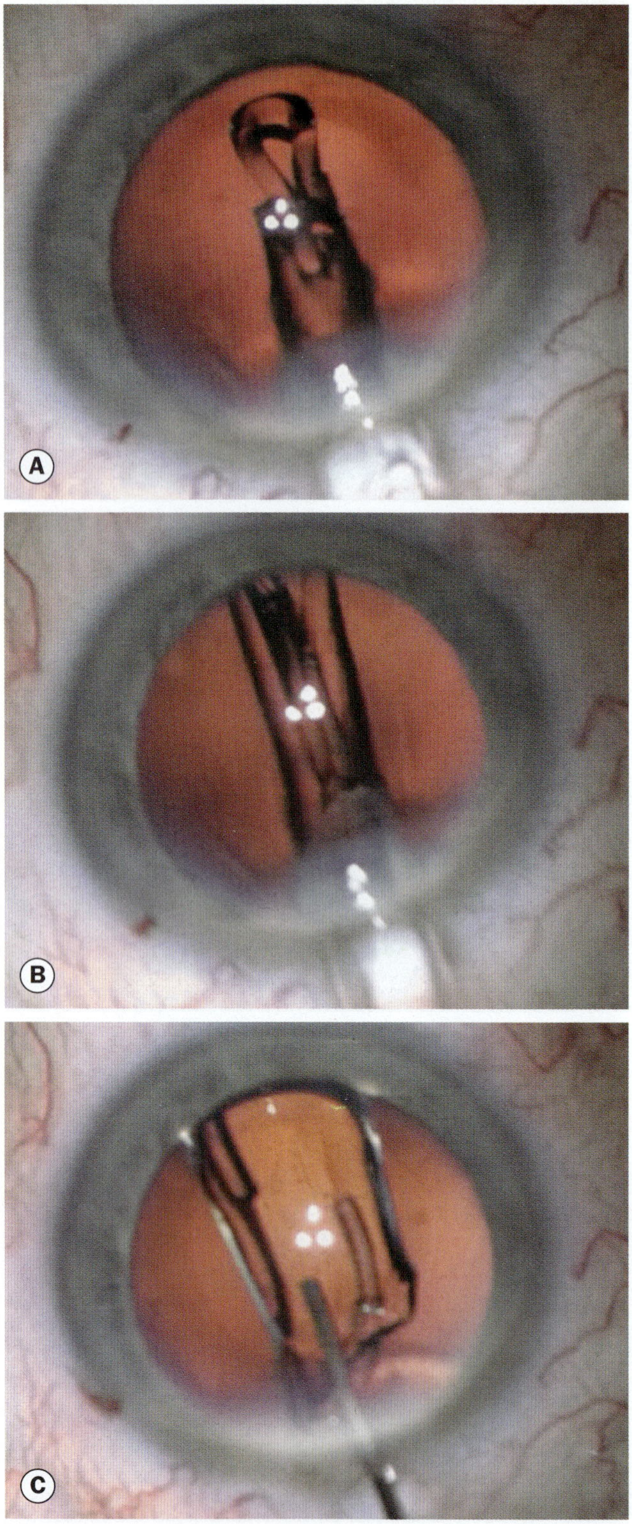

Fig. 10.15 Insertion of IOL. **(A)** Inferior loop inserted into the capsular bag; **(B)** slow unfolding of optic; **(C)** superior loop inserted into the capsular bag.

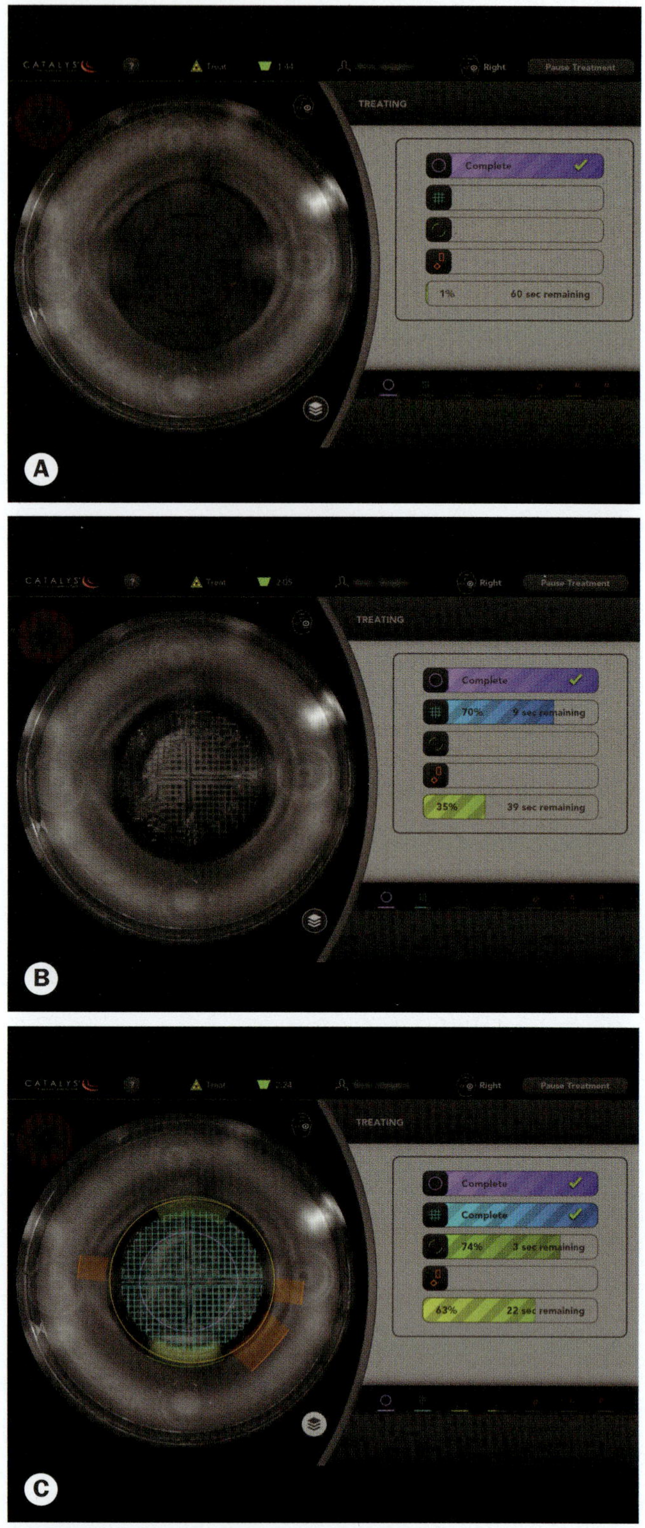

Fig. 10.16 Femtosecond laser for cataract surgery – graphical user interface. **(A)** Capsulotomy completed; **(B)** nuclear fragmentation; **(C)** limbal relaxing incisions for astigmatism.

- All vitreous is then removed from the AC and the wound with a vitrector, including deep to the capsular tear. A bimanual technique, with separate cutting and infusion instruments, is viewed as superior by many, as vitreous is not pushed away from the cutter. The position of the infusion cannula is kept high and that of the cutter low. The main practical difficulty is visualization of the vitreous gel. This can be enhanced by the instillation of trypan blue or 0.1 ml of 40 mg/ml triamcinolone (shaken well before use). The infusion bottle height should be sufficient to keep the AC maintained without intermittent shallowing.

TIP In the case of vitreous loss, visualization of residual vitreous strands can be enhanced by inserting triamcinolone into the anterior chamber.

- A small posterior capsular tear may allow careful in-the-bag implantation of a posterior chamber (PC) IOL.
- Even a large tear will usually allow ciliary sulcus placement of a three-piece (but not a one-piece) PC IOL. The centre of the haptic loops should be placed at 90° to a peripheral tear. If possible, after placing the IOL in the sulcus, the optic should be captured within an intact capsulorhexis of slightly smaller diameter by depressing each side of the optic beneath the capsulorhexis in turn. With capsulorhexis capture, the originally planned IOL power, or possibly 0.5 D less, can be used. Without capture, the power is reduced by 0.5–1.0 D.
- Acetylcholine solution is used to constrict the pupil following implantation of a PC IOL or prior to inserting an AC IOL.
- Insufficient capsular support may necessitate implantation of an AC IOL (Fig. 10.17). Importantly, an iridectomy is needed to prevent pupillary block. AC IOLs are associated with a higher risk than PC IOLs of complications including bullous keratopathy, hyphaema, iris tuck and pupillary irregularities. An iris-attached anterior (see Fig. 8.12A) or posterior chamber IOL or a scleral-secured posterior chamber IOL are alternatives.
- A suture should be used to secure the wound following capsular rupture, even if this seems adequately self-sealed.

Posterior loss of lens fragments

Dislocation of fragments of lens material into the vitreous cavity (Fig. 10.18A) after zonular dehiscence or posterior capsule rupture is rare but potentially serious as it may result in glaucoma, chronic uveitis, retinal detachment or chronic CMO. Initially, any uveitis or raised IOP must be treated. It may be reasonable to adopt a conservative approach for small fragments, but pars plana vitrectomy will usually be required for larger pieces.

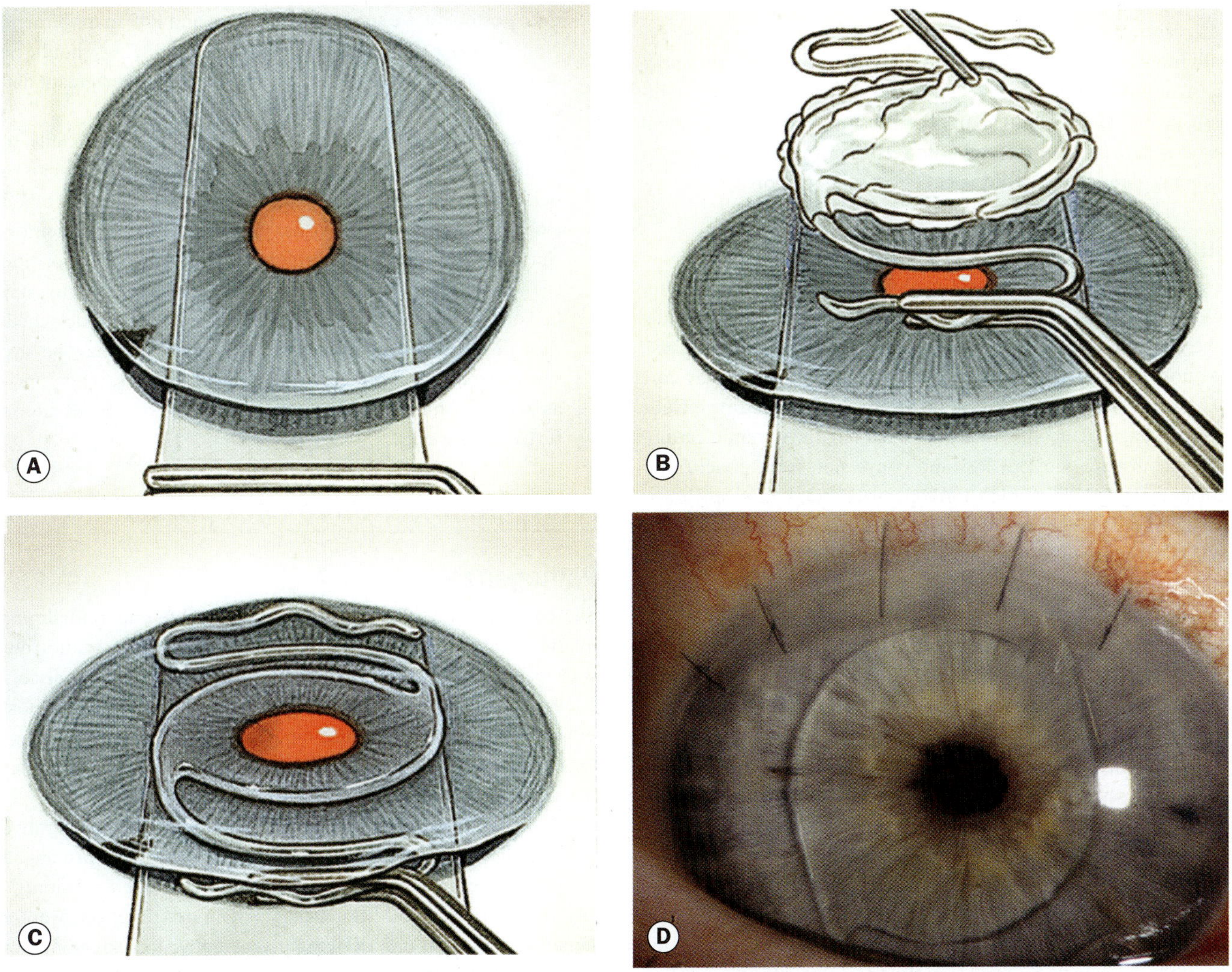

Fig. 10.17 Insertion of an anterior chamber IOL; note that an iridectomy has been created. **(A)** Insertion of a lens glide; **(B)** OVD (see text) coating the anterior surface of the IOL; **(C)** insertion of the IOL; **(D)** postoperative clinical appearance, showing sutures in position.

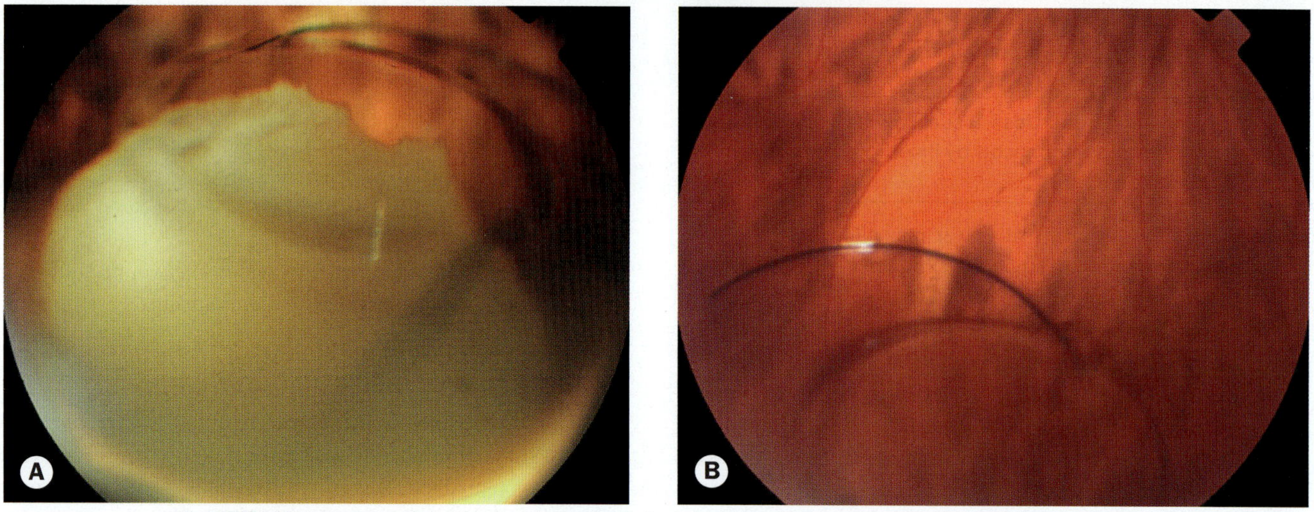

Fig. 10.18 (A) Large nuclear fragment in the inferior vitreous cavity – a dislocated IOL is also visible; **(B)** dislocated IOL.

Posterior dislocation of IOL

Dislocation of an IOL into the vitreous cavity (Fig. 10.18B) is rare. Loss can occur via a posterior capsular dehiscence, or in an eye with fragile zonular attachments (e.g. pseudoexfoliation) the entire capsular bag may dislocate. Complications include vitreous haemorrhage, retinal detachment, uveitis and chronic CMO. Treatment involves pars plana vitrectomy with IOL removal, repositioning or exchange depending on the extent of capsular support.

Suprachoroidal haemorrhage

A suprachoroidal haemorrhage involves a bleed into the suprachoroidal space from a ruptured posterior ciliary artery. If sufficiently severe it may result in extrusion of intraocular contents (expulsive haemorrhage). It is a dreaded complication, but extremely rare (0.04%) with phacoemulsification. Contributing factors include advanced age, glaucoma, increased axial length, systemic cardiovascular disease, vitreous loss and conversion from phacoemulsification to ECCE. A high intraoperative index of suspicion is critical and if there is any suggestion of a suprachoroidal haemorrhage the operation should be terminated and the incision sutured immediately.

- **Signs**
  - Progressive shallowing of the AC, increased IOP and prolapse of the iris.
  - Vitreous extrusion, loss or partial obscuration of the red reflex and the appearance of a dark mound behind the pupil.
  - In severe cases, posterior segment contents may be extruded into the AC and through the incision.
- **Immediate treatment** involves closure of the incision with a suture. Speed of closure is the key and residual viscoelastic can be left in the eye. Intraoperative posterior sclerostomy should not be undertaken. The diagnosis should be confirmed at the slit lamp as soon as possible. IOP-lowering medication such as oral acetazolamide is given to treat the pressure spike that often follows. Postoperatively, intensive topical and systemic steroids should be used to reduce intraocular inflammation, with standard postoperative antibiotic treatment and IOP management. Non-steroidal anti-inflammatory drugs (NSAIDs) should be avoided for analgesia and any antiplatelet or anticoagulant discontinued short-term, provided this is safe.
- **Subsequent treatment**, if spontaneous absorption fails to occur, consists of drainage of a large haemorrhage. This can be performed 7–14 days later, by which time liquefaction of blood clot has taken place. The visual prognosis for a large haemorrhage is highly variable. Prolonged chorioretinal apposition (>14 days) reduces the prognosis. Pars plana vitrectomy may be considered when the retina appears adherent or detached, though even apposed 'kissing' haemorrhages may resolve spontaneously without apparent retinal problems. If appropriate, completion of cataract surgery may be considered after a further 1–2 weeks.

Acute postoperative endophthalmitis

Pathogenesis

The contemporary reported incidence of acute endophthalmitis following cataract surgery varies substantially between studies, but is probably at least 0.1%. Acute intraocular infection is invariably a severe event. Toxins produced by infecting bacteria and the host inflammatory responses cause rapid and irreversible photoreceptor damage and ongoing effects can continue long after the ocular contents have been rendered sterile.

- **Risk factors** are difficult to establish but may include operative complications such as posterior capsule rupture, prolonged procedure time, combined procedure (e.g. with vitrectomy), clear corneal sutureless incision, temporal incision, wound leak on the first day, delaying postoperative topical antibiotics until the day after surgery, topical anaesthesia, adnexal disease and diabetes.

TIP In a one-eyed patient, make sure that the adjacent socket is free of infection before undertaking cataract surgery.

- **Pathogens.** About 90% of isolates are Gram-positive and 10% Gram-negative. *Staphylococcus epidermidis* is the most common and with early treatment carries a reasonable prognosis.
- **The source of infection** usually cannot be identified with certainty. It is thought that the flora of the eyelids and conjunctiva are the most frequent source, including contamination via incisions in the early postoperative stages. Other potential sources include contaminated solutions and instruments, environmental air and the surgeon, and other operating room personnel.

Prophylaxis

Because of the low rate of endophthalmitis it is very difficult to establish the effectiveness of any preventative measure.

- **Instillation of 5% povidone-iodine** into the conjunctival fornices and leaving this undisturbed for at least 3 minutes prior to surgery.
- **Scrupulous preparation** of the surgical site, with re-draping if eyelash coverage is inadequate.
- **Treatment of pre-existing infections** such as blepharitis, conjunctivitis, chronic dacryocystitis and infection in the contralateral eye or socket.
- **Antibiotic prophylaxis**
  - Intracameral cefuroxime (1 mg in 0.1 ml) injected into the AC at the end of surgery.
  - Alternatively, moxifloxacin (0.5 mg in 0.1 ml) injected into the AC at the end of surgery could be used if cefuroxime is not available.
  - Intracameral vancomycin has been reported to cause haemorrhagic occlusive retinal vasculitis in some patients and should be avoided as routine prophylaxis.
  - Postoperative subconjunctival injection can achieve bactericidal levels in the AC for at least 1–2 hours.
  - Preoperative topical fluoroquinolone antibiotics are frequently given in regimens from 1 hour to 3 days before surgery, but evidence for their efficacy is lacking.
- **Early resuturing** of leaking wounds rather than observation is likely to be prudent.
- **Reviewing personal surgical practice** to eliminate potentially risk-prone elements, particularly if a significant rate of endophthalmitis is encountered.

TIP Preoperative instillation of 5% povidone-iodine to the surface of the eye reduces the risk of endophthalmitis.

Clinical features

- **Symptoms.** Pain, redness and visual loss.
- **Signs** vary according to severity.
  - Eyelid swelling, chemosis, conjunctival injection and discharge.
  - A relative afferent pupillary defect is common.
  - Corneal haze.
  - Fibrinous exudate and hypopyon (Fig. 10.19A).
  - Vitritis with an impaired view of the fundus.
  - Severe vitreous inflammation and debris (Fig. 10.19B) with loss of the red reflex.

Differential diagnosis

If there is any doubt about the diagnosis, treatment should be that of infectious endophthalmitis, as early recognition leads to a better outcome.

- **Retained lens material** in the AC (Fig. 10.20) or vitreous may precipitate severe uveitis, corneal oedema and raised IOP.
- **Vitreous haemorrhage**, especially if blood in the vitreous is depigmented.

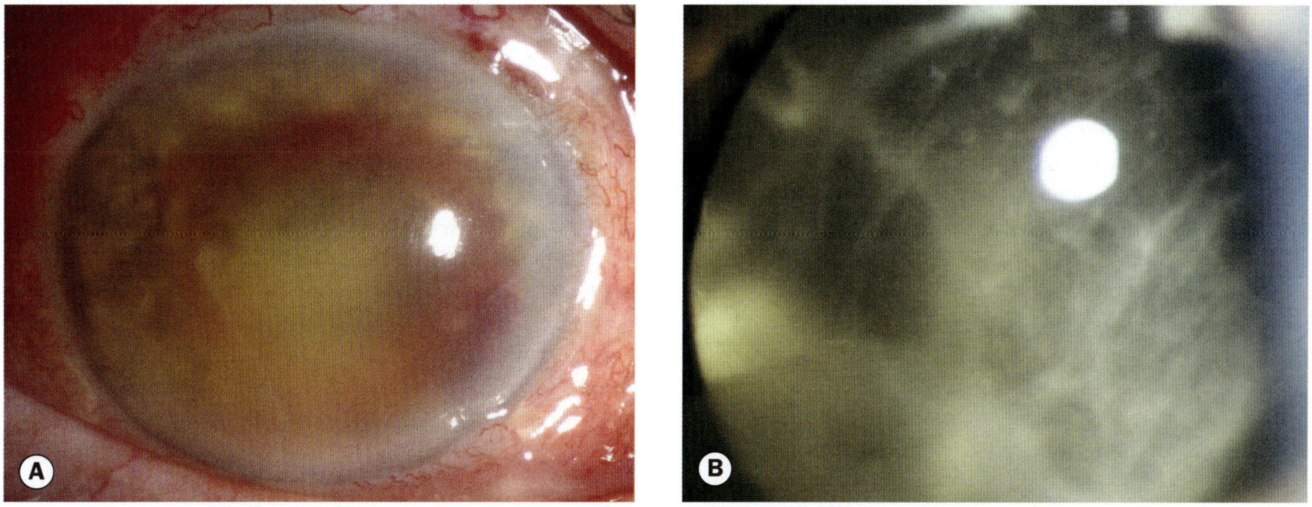

Fig. 10.19 Acute postoperative bacterial endophthalmitis. **(A)** Severe anterior chamber infection with fibrinous exudate; **(B)** severe vitreous involvement. *(Courtesy of S Tuft – fig. B.)*

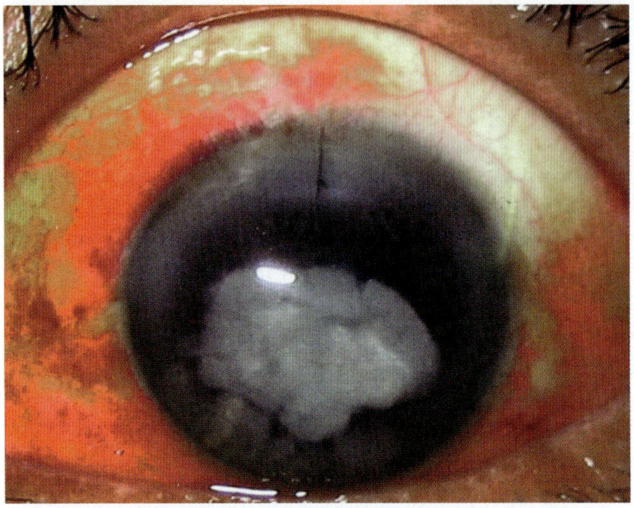

Fig. 10.20 Retained lens fragment in the anterior chamber following cataract surgery. *(Courtesy of S Chen.)*

- **Postoperative uveitis.** A confident diagnosis of infection is not always straightforward. If signs of inflammation are mild a trial of topical steroid therapy and early review (6–24 hours) is appropriate. If there is no substantial improvement, management should be that of endophthalmitis.
- **Toxic reaction** to the use of inappropriate or contaminated irrigating fluid or viscoelastic. An intense fibrinous reaction with corneal oedema may develop although other signs of infectious endophthalmitis are absent. Treatment is with intensive topical steroids and a cycloplegic.
- **Complicated or prolonged surgery** may result in corneal oedema and uveitis.

Identification of pathogens

Samples for culture should be obtained from aqueous and vitreous to confirm the diagnosis. Negative culture does not necessarily rule out infection and treatment should be continued. An operating theatre with experienced staff is the best setting, but samples can be taken in a minor procedure room to avoid delay.

- **B-scan ultrasound** should be performed prior to vitreous sampling if there is no clinical view, to exclude retinal detachment.
- **Preparation**
  - Povidone-iodine 5% is instilled.
  - Topical and subconjunctival, sub-Tenon or peribulbar anaesthesia is administered. The inflamed eye is often resistant to LA and sedation or general anaesthesia may be necessary.
  - The eye is draped as for cataract surgery, with insertion of a speculum.
- **Aqueous sampling** – 0.1–0.2 ml of aqueous is aspirated via a limbal paracentesis using a 25-gauge needle on a tuberculin syringe. The syringe is then capped and labelled.
- **Vitreous sampling** is more likely to yield a positive culture than aqueous. A 1- or 2-ml syringe and 23-gauge needle may be used, or optimally a disposable vitrector. The vitreous cavity is entered 3.5 mm from the limbus (pseudophakic eye), measured with a caliper. 0.2–0.4 ml is aspirated from the mid-vitreous cavity. If using a disposable vitrector, the tubing is capped and both the vitrector and tubing sent for analysis.
- **Conjunctival swabs** may be taken in addition, as significant culture may be helpful in the absence of a positive result from intraocular samples.
- **Microbiology.** Specimens should be sent to the microbiology laboratory immediately. Most laboratories prefer to receive a sample in the acquiring apparatus and will divide the specimen for microscopy and culture. Polymerase chain reaction (PCR) can be helpful in identifying unusual organisms and if culture results have been negative. However, its high sensitivity means that contamination can lead to false-positive results.

Treatment

- **Intravitreal antibiotics** are the key to management because levels above the minimum inhibitory concentration of most pathogens are achieved and are maintained for days. They should be administered immediately after culture specimens have been obtained. Antibiotics commonly used in combination are ceftazidime, which will kill most Gram-negative organisms (including *Pseudomonas aeruginosa*) and vancomycin to address Gram-positive cocci (including MRSA).
  - The concentrations are ceftazidime 2 mg in 0.1 ml and vancomycin 2 mg in 0.1 ml. Amikacin 0.4 mg in 0.1 ml is an alternative to ceftazidime in patients with a definite penicillin allergy, but is more toxic to the retina. Table 10.2 provides details of preparation.
  - The antibiotics are injected slowly into the mid-vitreous cavity using a 25-gauge needle.
  - After the first injection has been given, the syringe may be disconnected but the needle left inside the vitreous cavity so that the second injection can be given through the same needle. Alternatively, a second needle can be used.
- **Subconjunctival antibiotic injections** are often given but are of doubtful additional benefit if intravitreal antibiotics have been used. Suggested doses are vancomycin 50 mg and ceftazidime 125 mg (or amikacin 50 mg if penicillin-allergic).
- **Topical antibiotics** are of limited benefit and are often used only 4–6 times daily in order to protect the fresh wounds from contamination. Vancomycin 5% (50 mg/ml) or ceftazidime 5% (50 mg/ml) applied intensively may penetrate the cornea in therapeutic levels. Third or fourth generation fluoroquinolones achieve effective levels in the aqueous and vitreous, even in uninflamed eyes and may be considered.
- **Oral antibiotics.** Fluoroquinolones penetrate the eye well and moxifloxacin 400 mg daily for 10 days is recommended. Clarithromycin 500 mg twice daily may be helpful for culture-negative infections. Evidence suggests these may attack bacterial biofilm.
- **Oral steroids.** The rationale for the use of steroids is to limit destructive complications of the inflammatory process. Prednisolone 1 mg/kg daily may be considered in severe cases after 12–24 hours provided fungal infection has been excluded from examination of smears. Contraindications must be excluded and gastric protection (e.g. lansoprazole 30 mg once daily)

Table 10.2 Preparation of Antibiotics for Intravitreal Injection

Ceftazidime (broad spectrum, including *Pseudomonas*)
A. Begin with a 500mg ampoule B. Add 10 ml water for injection (WFI) or saline and dissolve thoroughly (for a 250 mg vial add 5 ml WFI or saline, for a 1 g vial add 20 ml WFI or saline) C. Draw up 1 ml of the solution, containing 50 mg of antibiotic D. Add 1.5 ml WFI or saline giving 50 mg in 2.5 ml E. Draw up about 0.2 ml (excess to facilitate priming) into a 1 ml syringe. When ready to inject, fit the Rycroft cannula or the needle to be used and discard all but 0.1 ml (contains 2 mg of antibiotic) for injection
Vancomycin (action primarily against Gram-positive organisms)
Only saline, not WFI, should be used with vancomycin As A–E above, again preferably starting with a 500 mg ampoule
Amikacin
Alternative to ceftazidime; as it carries a higher risk of retinal infarction, use only if well-defined penicillin or cephalosporin allergy is present; note the lower intravitreal dose than ceftazidime and vancomycin Note different dilution procedure to ceftazidime and vancomycin A. Presentation: vial contains 500 mg of amikacin in 2 ml of solution B. Use a 2.5 ml syringe to draw up 1 ml of amikacin solution then 1.5 ml of WFI C. Inject 0.4 ml of the solution, containing 40 mg of antibiotic, into a 10 ml syringe and dilute to 10 ml (giving 4 mg per ml) D. Draw up about 0.2 ml (excess to facilitate priming) into a 1 ml syringe. When ready to inject, fit the needle to be used and discard all but 0.1 ml (contains 0.4 mg of antibiotic) for injection

prescribed with appropriate monitoring including baseline blood tests. If necessary, general medical advice should be requested prior to commencement.

- **Periocular steroids.** Dexamethasone or triamcinolone should be considered if systemic therapy is contraindicated.
- **Topical dexamethasone** 0.1% 2-hourly initially for anterior uveitis.
- **Topical mydriatic** such as atropine 1% twice daily.
- **Intravitreal steroids** may reduce inflammation in the short term but do not influence the final visual outcome; some studies even suggest a detrimental effect. Conversely, improvement in outcome in some bacterial sub-groups has been reported.
- **Pars plana vitrectomy.** The Endophthalmitis Vitrectomy Study (EVS) showed a benefit for immediate pars plana vitrectomy in eyes with a visual acuity (VA) of perception of light (*not* hand movements vision or better) at presentation, with a 50% reduction in severe visual loss. If vitrectomy is not immediately available, it is prudent to take samples as above and give intravitreal antibiotics as a temporizing measure. The conclusions of the EVS in post-cataract surgery eyes cannot necessarily be extrapolated to other forms of endophthalmitis.

Subsequent management

Subsequent management should proceed according to culture results and clinical response.

- **Signs of improvement** include contraction of fibrinous exudate and reduction of AC cellular activity and hypopyon. In this situation treatment is not modified irrespective of culture results. Ultrasonography may be useful in vitreous assessment.
- **If the clinical signs are worsening** after 48 hours antibiotic sensitivities should be reviewed and therapy modified accordingly. Pars plana vitrectomy should be considered if not previously performed. Intravitreal antibiotics can be repeated after 2 days. If amikacin has previously been used, repeated administration should probably be avoided to reduce the risk of retinal toxicity.
- **Outcome** is related to the duration of the infection prior to treatment and the virulence of organisms.
  - If VA at presentation is perception of light, 30% of eyes achieve 6/12 following treatment. If VA is better than light perception, this figure increases to 60%.
  - Infection with *Bacillus cereus* or streptococci often has a poor visual outcome despite aggressive and appropriate therapy, with 70% and 55% respectively achieving a final VA of 6/60 or less. This poor visual outcome may be related to early retinopathy from exotoxins.
- **Late problems**
  - Persistent vitreous opacification. Aggressive and extended topical, periocular and if necessary oral steroid treatment will often lead to resolution. Vitrectomy can be considered if the opacification is persistent.
  - Maculopathy in the form of epiretinal membrane, cystoid oedema and ischaemia.
  - Hypotony. Wound leak should be excluded and persistent inflammation addressed. Choroidal effusion should be identified and drained if necessary. Retinal detachment and anterior vitreous membranes may require vitrectomy.
  - Other problems include chronic uveitis, secondary glaucoma, retinal detachment and phthisis.

Delayed-onset postoperative endophthalmitis

Pathogenesis

Delayed-onset endophthalmitis following cataract surgery develops when an organism of low virulence, such as *P. acnes*, becomes trapped within the capsular bag (saccular endophthalmitis). Organisms can become sequestered within macrophages, protected from eradication but with continued expression of bacterial antigen. Onset ranges from 4 weeks to years (mean 9 months) postoperatively and typically follows uneventful cataract surgery. It may rarely be precipitated by laser capsulotomy release of the organism.

Diagnosis

- **Symptoms.** Painless mild progressive visual deterioration is typical and floaters may be present.

- **Signs**
  - Low-grade anterior uveitis, sometimes with medium-large keratic precipitates (Fig. 10.21A). A degree of vitritis is common.
  - The inflammation initially responds well to topical steroids, but recurs when treatment is stopped and may eventually become steroid-resistant.
  - An enlarging capsular plaque composed of organisms sequestrated in residual cortex within the peripheral capsular bag is common (Fig. 10.21B).
- **Differential diagnosis** is principally from other causes of anterior uveitis, particularly idiopathic, sterile post-surgical and chronic/recurrent viral infection (see Ch. 12).
- **Initial management.** Later-generation fluoroquinolones, such as moxifloxacin, penetrate the eye well and are concentrated within macrophages. An empirical 10–14-day course of moxifloxacin (alternatives include clarithromycin) may be worthwhile prior to more invasive options.
- **Investigation.** Sampling of aqueous and vitreous should be considered if oral antibiotics are ineffective. Anaerobic culture should be requested if *P. acnes* infection is suspected and isolates may take 10–14 days to grow. The detection rate can be greatly improved with the use of PCR, which should also screen for the common causes of viral anterior uveitis.
- **Treatment if persistent**
  - Intravitreal antibiotics alone are usually unsuccessful in resolving the infection.
  - Removal of the capsular bag, residual cortex and IOL, requiring pars plana vitrectomy. Secondary IOL implantation may be considered at a later date. Intravitreal antibiotics are combined: vancomycin (1–2 mg in 0.1 ml) is the antibiotic of choice and can also be irrigated into any capsular remnant. *P. acnes* is also sensitive to methicillin, cefazolin and clindamycin.

Posterior capsular opacification

Visually significant PCO, also known as 'after cataract', is the most common late complication of uncomplicated cataract surgery, occurring in 20–25% of patients. It is caused by the proliferation of lens epithelial cells that have remained within the capsular bag following cataract extraction. The incidence of PCO is reduced when the capsulorhexis opening is in complete contact with the anterior surface of the IOL. PMMA (and probably to a lesser extent hydrogel) IOLs are particularly prone to PCO. Implant design is more important than material. A square optic edge appears to inhibit PCO (though may have a higher rate of dysphotopsia – see below).

TIP Posterior capsular thickening is the commonest cause of late visual deterioration after small incisional cataract surgery and is easily treated with a Nd:YAG laser.

Diagnosis

- **Symptoms** include persistent slowly worsening blurring, glare and sometimes monocular diplopia.
- **VA** is variably reduced, though dysfunction may be more marked on contrast sensitivity testing.
- **Signs** typically include more than one pattern of opacification.
  - Vacuolated (pearl-type) PCO (Fig. 10.22A) consists of proliferating swollen lens epithelial cells, similar to the bladder (Wedl) cells seen in posterior subcapsular cataract (see Fig. 10.2A). They are commonly termed 'Elschnig pearls', particularly when grouped into clusters at the edge of a capsulotomy (Fig. 10.22B), though strictly Hirschberg–Elschnig pearls refers to globular or grape-like collections of swollen cells seen following traumatic or surgical anterior capsular rupture.

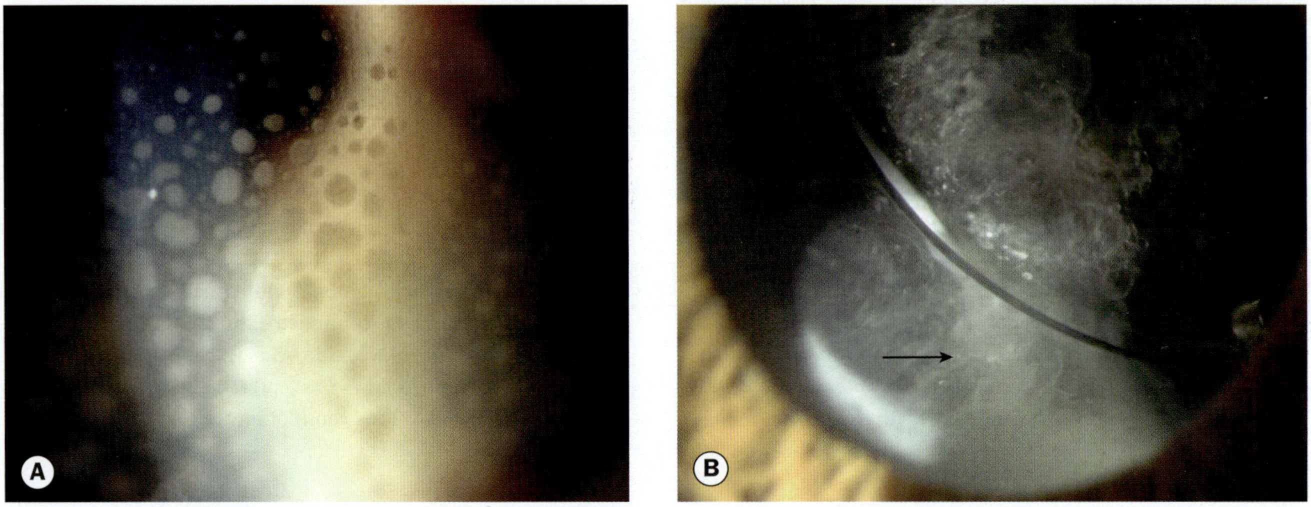

Fig. 10.21 Delayed-onset postoperative endophthalmitis. **(A)** Anterior uveitis with large keratic precipitates; **(B)** white capsular plaque in chronic postoperative endophthalmitis (arrow).

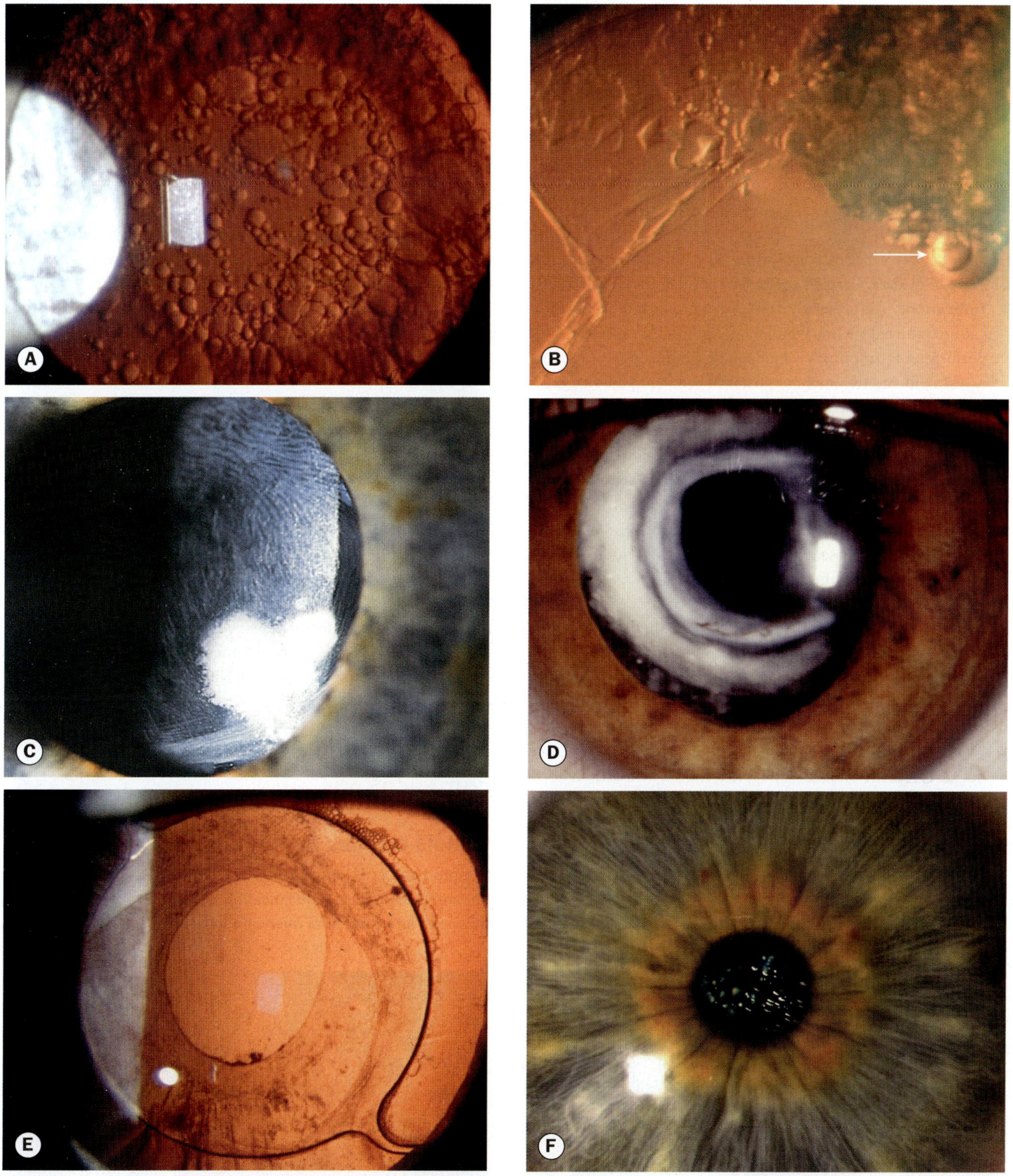

Fig. 10.22 Posterior capsular opacification. **(A)** Vacuolated or pearl-type on retroillumination; **(B)** Elschnig pearl formation (arrow) on edge of capsulotomy; **(C)** slit-lamp appearance of fibrotic capsule; **(D)** Soemmering ring following congenital cataract surgery; **(E)** appearance following laser capsulotomy; **(F)** laser pitting of an IOL.

- Fibrosis-type PCO (Fig. 10.22C) is thought to be due to fibroblastic metaplasia of epithelial cells, which develop contractile qualities.
- A Soemmering ring (Fig. 10.22D) is a whitish annular or doughnut-shaped proliferation of residual cells that classically formed almost in the periphery of the capsular bag following older methods of cataract surgery, but is uncommon now. It may form at the edge of a capsulorhexis or capsulotomy.

Treatment

Treatment involves the creation of an opening in the posterior capsule using a Nd:YAG laser (termed a posterior capsulotomy) (Fig. 10.22E).

- **Indications.** The presence of visual symptoms is the main indication (reduced VA and glare). Less commonly, capsulotomy is performed to improve an inadequate fundus view impairing assessment and treatment of posterior segment pathology.
- **Technique.** Safe and successful laser capsulotomy involves accurate focusing and use of the minimum energy required. Laser power is initially set at 1 mJ/pulse and may be increased if necessary. A series of punctures is applied in a cruciate or circumferential pattern using single-pulse shots. The opening should equate approximately to the size of the physiologically dilated pupil under scotopic conditions – this should average around 4–5 mm in the pseudophakic eye. A larger capsulotomy may be necessary if glare persists, or for retinal examination or treatment, but the capsulotomy should not extend beyond the edge of the optic in case vitreous prolapses around its edge. It may be prudent to adopt a higher threshold for treatment, and minimizing its extent, in eyes at risk of retinal detachment (e.g. high myopia), CMO (e.g. history of uveitis) or lens displacement (e.g. pseudoexfoliation). Some research suggests that the total energy applied should be less than 80 mJ in order to reduce the risk of a significant IOP spike.
- **Complications** include pitting of the IOL (Fig. 10.22F) that is usually visually inconsequential. The IOP may rise, particularly in patients with glaucoma, but is typically mild and transient. A retinal tear or detachment may follow the treatment and myopic individuals should be warned to return if they develop symptoms compatible with a posterior vitreous detachment (PVD). CMO may occur, but is less common when the capsulotomy is delayed for 6 months or more after cataract surgery. IOL subluxation or dislocation is rare.

Anterior capsular fibrosis and contraction

Since the advent of continuous curvilinear capsulorhexis, significant contraction of the anterior capsular opening is sometimes seen (capsulophimosis – Fig. 10.23). It typically progresses over months and if severe, Nd:YAG laser anterior capsulotomy may be required. Risk factors include a small capsulorhexis, pseudoexfoliation syndrome (where the capsulorhexis contracts postoperatively by up to 25%), retinitis pigmentosa and plate-haptic silicone IOL.

Capsular bag distension syndrome

In this rare complication of phacoemulsification and IOL implantation fluid accumulates between the IOL and the posterior capsule leading to distension of the posterior capsule, slight anterior displacement of the IOL and a myopic shift (Fig. 10.24). The trapped fluid becomes turbid in time, which results in a reduction of vision. Most cases have an axial length that is greater than 25 mm and a small capsulorhexis, with adhesion between the lens optic and the anterior capsular rim. Anterior segment OCT can be helpful to confirm the diagnosis. A rapid improvement in vision follows the application of Nd:YAG laser to the posterior capsule.

Miscellaneous postoperative complications

Cystoid macular oedema

Symptomatic CMO (see Ch. 14) is relatively uncommon following uncomplicated phacoemulsification and in most cases is mild and transient. It occurs more often after complicated surgery and has a

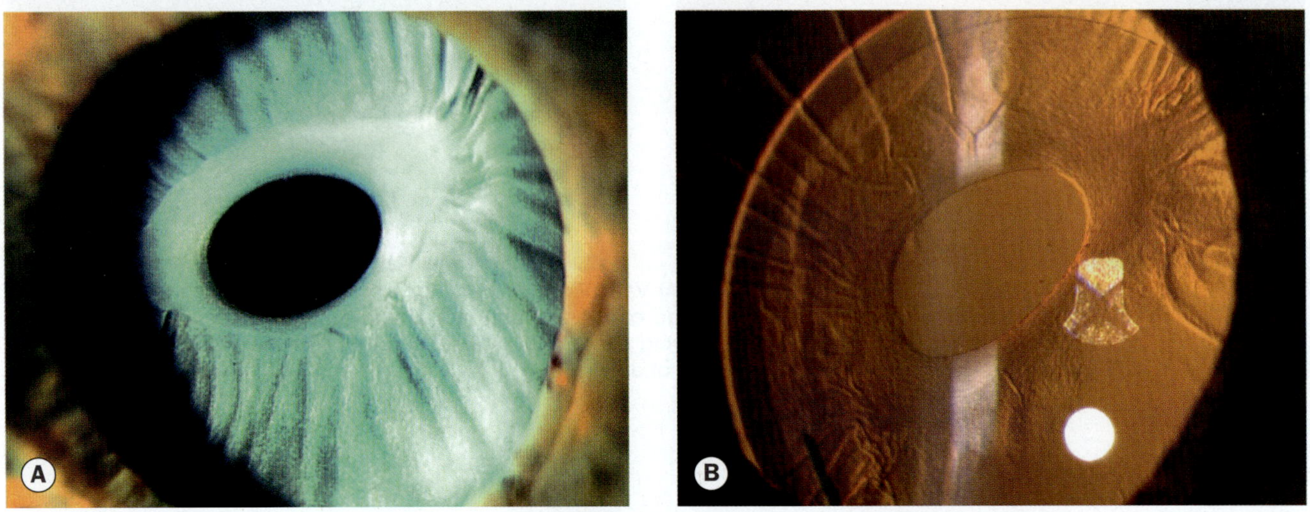

Fig. 10.23 Anterior capsular contraction and fibrosis. **(A)** Clinical appearance; **(B)** retroillumination.

peak incidence at 6–10 weeks, although the interval to onset may be much longer.

- **Risk factors** include epiretinal membrane, a history of CMO in the other eye, operative complications such as posterior capsular rupture with vitreous loss, particularly with vitreous incarceration into the incision site (Fig. 10.25A), anterior chamber IOL (Fig. 10.25B), secondary IOL implantation, diabetes (approximately ten times greater risk), uveitis and topical prostaglandin treatment.
- **Symptoms.** Blurring, especially for near tasks, and sometimes distortion. Subtle CMO may not be readily visible clinically, but is demonstrated well on OCT.

TIP In the event of vitreous loss and raised IOP, avoid prostaglandin drops as this increases the risk of cystoid macular oedema.

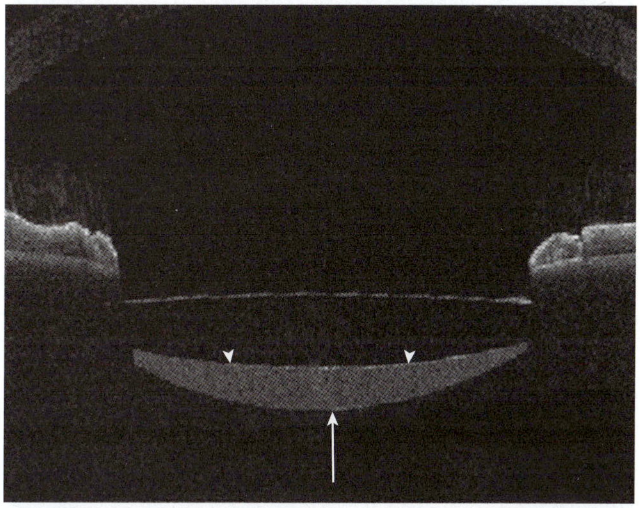

Fig. 10.24 Capsular bag distension syndrome. OCT showing turbid fluid between the posterior surface of the lens (arrow heads) and the posterior capsule (arrow). *(Courtesy of J Wesierski.)*

- **Treatment.** One or a combination of the following modalities may be used.
  - Anterior vitrectomy or YAG laser applied to a vitreous wick if present.
  - Topical NSAIDs (e.g. ketorolac four times daily, bromfenac twice daily, nepafenac three times daily) reduce the risk of developing CMO in non-diabetic and diabetic patients. In addition, these drops may be beneficial even in long-standing cases. Treatment may be necessary for several months.
  - Steroids. Topically, by periocular or intravitreal (triamcinolone acetate 0.05–0.1 ml of 40 mg/ml) injection.
  - Carbonic anhydrase inhibitors given systemically or topically.
  - Intravitreal anti-VEGF agents.
  - Pars plana vitrectomy may be useful for CMO refractory to medical therapy, even in eyes without apparent vitreous disturbance.

Dysphotopsia

Up to 1 in 10 patients complain of annoying visual phenomena following uncomplicated cataract surgery with monofocal IOL implantation. Multifocal IOLs have particular issues that are discussed separately above. Improvement in and adaptation to the symptoms typically occurs over several months and the number of monofocal IOL patients actually requiring further surgery for the symptoms is very small. Rounded-edged IOLs may be less prone to negative photopsia and silicone IOLs may be less liable to result in dysphotopsia than acrylic IOLs. Optic and capsulorhexis size may also be important.

- **Symptoms.** A dark shadow in the temporal periphery (negative dysphotopsia – often the most troublesome), scintillations, haloes, peripheral or central flaring or flashes (positive dysphotopsia) and possibly monocular diplopia.
- **Treatment**
  - Encouraging the patient that the symptoms usually improve over time, both because of anatomical changes

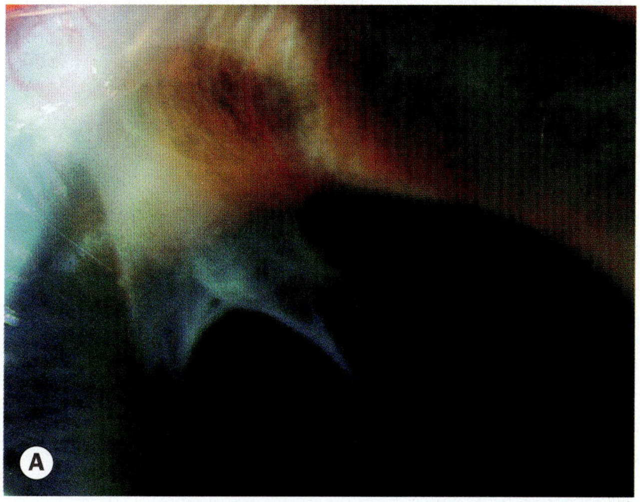

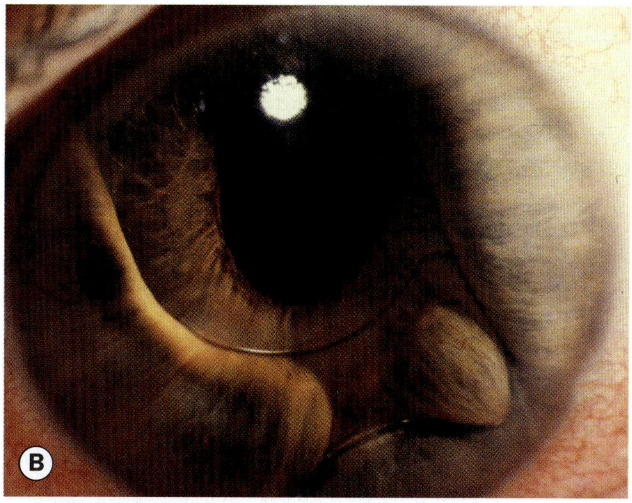

Fig. 10.25 Factors predisposing to cystoid macular oedema. **(A)** Vitreous incarceration in the incision; **(B)** secondary anterior chamber IOL with pupil block after previous vitreous loss.

(e.g. capsulorhexis edge thickening) and because the brain is able to ignore unwanted images.

- Positive nocturnal symptoms can be helped with gentle pupillary constriction (e.g. brimonidine), but dilatation may help negative dysphotopsia.
- Successful alleviation of symptoms has been reported with a variety of techniques, including reverse optic capture (vaulting the optic forward out of the capsular bag, leaving the haptics in place), ciliary sulcus IOL re-implantation and piggyback IOL implantation in the sulcus.
- IOL exchange (round-edged) may be considered.
- Laser capsulotomy is best avoided as it markedly complicates IOL exchange. However, in some eyes, Nd:YAG laser removal of a sector of capsulorhexis edge has resulted in reduced symptoms.

Corneal decompensation

Corneal oedema (see Ch. 7) may occur postoperatively, but is usually mild and transient. Eyes with pre-existing corneal endothelial pathology, particularly low cell counts, are at increased risk. Causes of significant oedema include a dense nucleus, which requires high phacoemulsification energy, complicated or prolonged surgery, pseudoexfoliation, intraoperative endothelial trauma and elevated postoperative IOP. Use of a dispersive viscoelastic may help to protect the corneal endothelium during surgery in high-risk eyes.

Ptosis

Mild ptosis secondary to a variety of mechanisms (especially the use of postoperative topical steroids), is not uncommon after cataract surgery, but usually improves without intervention. Corrective lid surgery should not be undertaken for at least a year postoperatively.

Malposition of the IOL

Although uncommon, malposition (Fig. 10.26A–C) may be associated with both optical and structural problems. Significant malposition may require repositioning or replacement, occasionally with an iris or scleral-fixated lens.

Retinal detachment

Rhegmatogenous retinal detachment (RRD) is uncommon after uncomplicated phacoemulsification with IOL implantation. Preoperative risk factors include lattice degeneration, retinal breaks and high myopia. The key intraoperative risk is vitreous loss. Pars plana vitrectomy is usually the surgical modality employed for pseudophakic RRD.

Refractive 'surprise'

Small under- or over-corrections are not uncommon after this surgery. The risk of this happening can be reduced by preoperatively checking that the difference in axial length between eyes is less than 0.7 mm and that the difference in average keratometry between eyes is less than 0.9 D. If there is a significant residual refractive error as a consequence of a failure to achieve the intended postoperative refractive target, patient dissatisfaction may ensue.

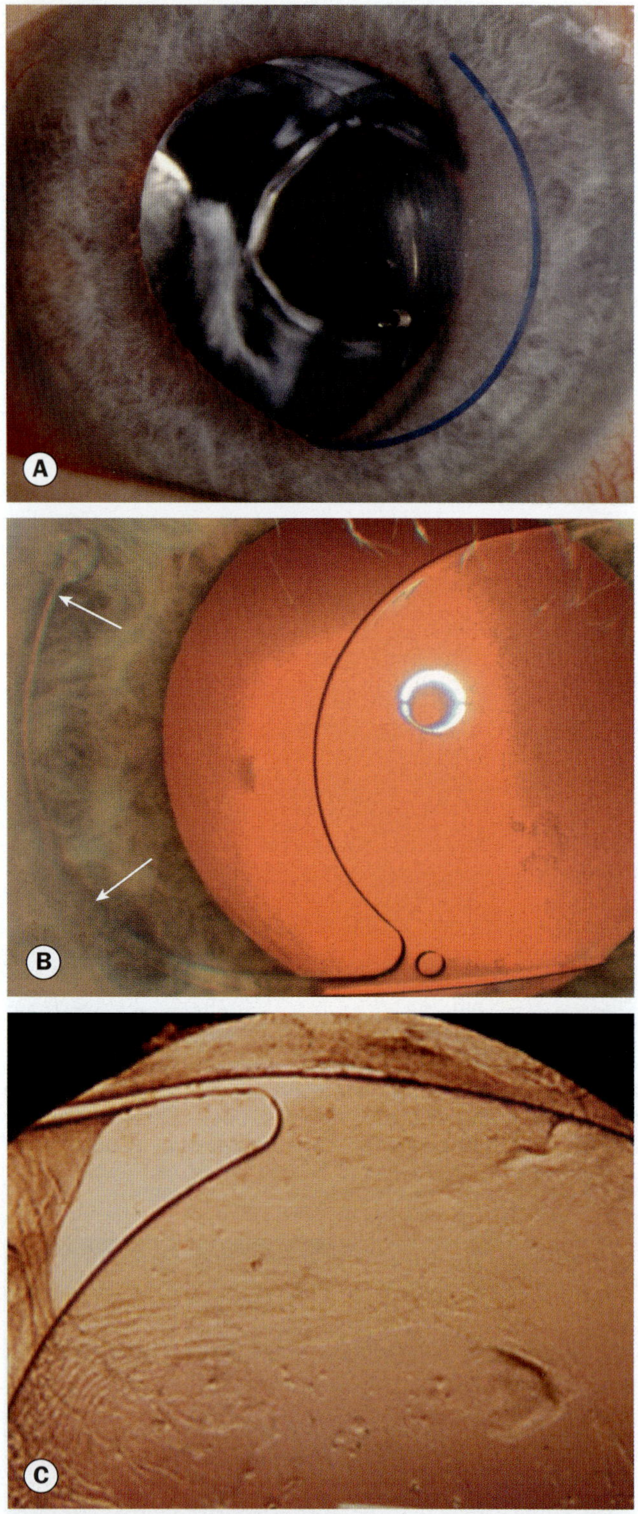

Fig. 10.26 IOL malposition. **(A)** Decentered optic in the ciliary sulcus, with an acrylic haptic anterior to the iris; **(B)** decentred optic with one haptic in the angle (arrows) and the other in the bag; **(C)** red reflex showing slight inferior decentration of an IOL.

TIP Inaccurate biometry is the commonest cause of a refractive surprise. Make sure the biometry is in keeping with the previous refraction.

- **Management**
  - Identify the cause.
  - Obtain a subjective refraction.
  - Examine the eye to exclude conditions like a distended capsular bag (myopic shift) and CMO (hyperopic shift).
  - Check the biometry and the strength of the implanted IOL.
  - Repeat the biometry, keratometry (undiagnosed keratoconus) and measure corneal thickness (undiagnosed previous laser refractive surgery).
- **Treatment**
  - If no obvious cause can be identified and the patient is happy to use spectacles or wear a contact lens to correct the refractive error, no further treatment is needed.
  - If the patient remains dissatisfied and once the refraction is stable, undertake further surgery.
  - IOL exchange is a good early option, but should be undertaken before capsular fibrosis occurs.
  - Corneal refractive surgery could be considered, as this can deal with a range of refractive errors.
  - 'Piggy back' sulcus IOL implantation is a reasonable option for high degrees of uncorrected refractive error, but is less accurate than laser refractive surgery.

Postoperative dry eye syndrome

Cataract surgery is a risk factor for the induction or exacerbation of dry eye symptoms in up to one-third of patients. Switching to preservative-free postoperative medication and prescribing preservative-free artificial tears is key to the management. Additional treatment options are detailed in Chapter 5.

CONGENITAL CATARACT

Aetiology

Congenital cataract occurs in about 3 in 10,000 live births. In general, one-third are associated with systemic disease, one-third are inherited and one-third are of unknown cause. Two-thirds are bilateral and a cause can be identified in about half of these. Autosomal dominant (AD) inheritance is the most common aetiological factor. Others include chromosomal abnormalities, metabolic disorders and intrauterine infections. Isolated inherited congenital cataracts carry a better visual prognosis than those with coexisting ocular and systemic abnormality. Unilateral cataracts are usually sporadic, without a family history or systemic disease and affected infants are usually otherwise healthy.

Associated metabolic disorders

Galactosaemia

Galactosaemia is an autosomal recessive (AR) condition characterized by impairment of galactose utilization caused by absence of the enzyme galactose-1-phosphate uridyl transferase (GALT). Unless galactose (milk and milk products) is withheld from the diet, severe systemic complications culminate in early death. 'Oil droplet' lens opacity (see Fig. 10.27E) develops within the first few days or weeks of life in a large percentage of patients. Exclusion of galactose may reverse early lens changes.

Lowe syndrome

Lowe (oculo-cerebro-renal) syndrome is an X-linked recessive (gene: *OCRL1*) inborn error of amino acid metabolism with neuromuscular, renal and other manifestations. Cataract is universal and microphakia may also be present. Congenital glaucoma is present in about half of patients. Female carriers may have visually insignificant cortical lens opacities.

Mannosidosis

Mannosidosis is an AR disorder with deficiency of α-mannosidase. Infantile and juvenile-adult forms are seen, both of which feature progressive mental deterioration, musculoskeletal and other abnormalities. Punctate lens opacities arranged in a spoke-like pattern in the posterior lens cortex are frequent. Corneal clouding can also occur but is less common.

Other metabolic disorders

Potential causes include hypo- and pseudohypoparathyroidism and hypo- and hyperglycaemia.

Associated intrauterine infections

Rubella

Congenital rubella results from transplacental transmission of virus from an infected mother and may lead to severe fetal malformations. Pearly nuclear or more diffuse unilateral or bilateral cataract occurs in around 15%. (See also Ch. 12.)

Toxoplasmosis

Ophthalmic features of congenital toxoplasmosis include cataract, chorioretinitis, microphthalmos and optic atrophy. (See also Ch. 12.)

Cytomegalovirus infection

Systemic features of congenital cytomegalovirus (CMV) infection include jaundice, hepatosplenomegaly, microcephaly and intracranial calcification. Ocular features apart from cataract include chorioretinitis, microphthalmos, keratitis and optic atrophy.

Varicella

Systemic features include learning disability, cortical cerebral atrophy, cutaneous scarring and limb deformities. Death in early infancy is common. Ocular features may include cataract, microphthalmos, chorioretinitis, optic disc hypoplasia and optic atrophy.

Others

Measles, syphilis, herpes simplex and human immunodeficiency virus (HIV). (See also Ch. 12.)

Other systemic associations

Down syndrome (trisomy 21)

- **Systemic features** include learning difficulties, stunted growth, distinctive facial and peripheral features, thyroid dysfunction, cardiorespiratory disease and reduced life span.
- **Ocular features.** Cataract of varied morphology (75%). The opacities are usually symmetrical and often develop in late childhood. Other features include iris Brushfield spots (see Fig. 20.15B) and hypoplasia, chronic blepharitis, myopia, strabismus and keratoconus.

Edwards syndrome (trisomy 18)

- **Systemic features.** Characteristic facial and peripheral features, deafness, cardiac anomalies, learning disability and early death.
- **Ocular features** apart from cataract include ptosis, microphthalmos, corneal opacity, uveal and disc coloboma and vitreoretinal dysplasia.

Miscellaneous

Hallermann–Streiff syndrome features impaired growth and other features, with cataract in 90%. Nance–Horan syndrome is an X-linked condition comprising distinctive dental and facial anomalies together with congenital cataract and microcornea. Female carriers may show Y suture opacities (see Fig. 10.27F).

Management

Ocular assessment

In the neonate, determining the visual significance of lens opacity is based principally on the appearance of the red reflex and the quality of the fundus view. There are three possibilities:

- **A very dense catarac**t with no red reflex.
- **A less dense** but still visually significant cataract (e.g. central or posterior opacities over 3 mm in diameter) will permit visualization of the retinal vasculature with the indirect but not with the direct ophthalmoscope.
- **A visually insignificant opacity** will allow clear visualization of the retinal vasculature with both the indirect and direct ophthalmoscope.
- **Other indicators of severe visual impairment** include absence of central fixation, nystagmus and strabismus.
- **Morphology**
    - Blue dot opacities (Fig. 10.27A) are common and innocuous.
    - Nuclear opacities (Fig. 10.27B) are confined to the embryonic or fetal nucleus. The cataract may be dense or composed of fine dust-like (pulverulent) opacities.
    - Coronary (supranuclear) cataract lies in the deep cortex, surrounding the nucleus like a crown. It is usually sporadic but occasionally hereditary (Fig. 10.27C).
    - Lamellar opacities affect a particular lamella of the lens both anteriorly and posteriorly and may be associated with radial extensions ('riders' – Fig. 10.27D). Lamellar opacities may be AD or occur in isolation as well as in association with metabolic disorders and intrauterine infections.
    - Central 'oil droplet' opacities (Fig. 10.27E) are characteristic of galactosaemia.
    - Sutural, in which the opacity follows the anterior or posterior Y suture (Fig. 10.27F). This may be seen in female Nance–Horan carriers.
    - Anterior polar cataract may be flat or project into the AC (Fig. 10.27G). Occasional associations include persistent pupillary membrane, aniridia, Peters anomaly and anterior lenticonus.
    - Posterior polar cataract (Fig. 10.27H) may be associated with posterior lenticonus or fetal vascular remnants including a Mittendorf dot. This form of opacity is often closely integrated with the lens capsule and/or a pre-existing defect, with a very high risk of dehiscence during surgery.
- **Associated ocular pathology** may involve the anterior (e.g. corneal clouding, microphthalmos, glaucoma, persistent fetal vasculature) or posterior segments (e.g. chorioretinitis, Leber amaurosis, rubella retinopathy, foveal or optic nerve hypoplasia). Its presence may give an additional indication of visual prognosis. The differential diagnosis of leukocoria may apply (see Ch. 20).
- **Assessment of family members** for subclinical familial cataract is prudent.
- **Ultrasonography** should be performed if the fundus is not visible and may reveal a definitive cause such as persistent fetal vasculature.
- **Special tests** such as forced-choice preferential looking and visual evoked potentials may provide useful supporting information.

Systemic investigations

Investigation of familial cataract is unnecessary, but otherwise the following should be considered. Assessment beyond a search for infection and possibly urinary reducing substance is probably unnecessary in unilateral cases.

- **Screening** for intrauterine infections should usually be performed in all unilateral and bilateral cases.
- **Urine.** Urinalysis for reducing substance after drinking milk (galactosaemia) and chromatography for amino acids (Lowe syndrome).
- **Other investigations** may include fasting blood glucose, serum calcium and phosphorus, red blood cell GALT and galactokinase levels. Children who have calcium and phosphorus anomalies severe enough to cause cataract are likely to be unwell.
- **Referral to a paediatrician** may be warranted for dysmorphic features or suspicion of other systemic diseases. Chromosome analysis may be useful in this context.

Treatment

The requirement for urgent surgery is balanced by the fact that the earlier this takes place, particularly before 4 weeks of age, the higher the chance of glaucoma developing during the juvenile years.

- **Bilateral dense** cataracts require surgery between 4 and 10 weeks of age to prevent the development of stimulus

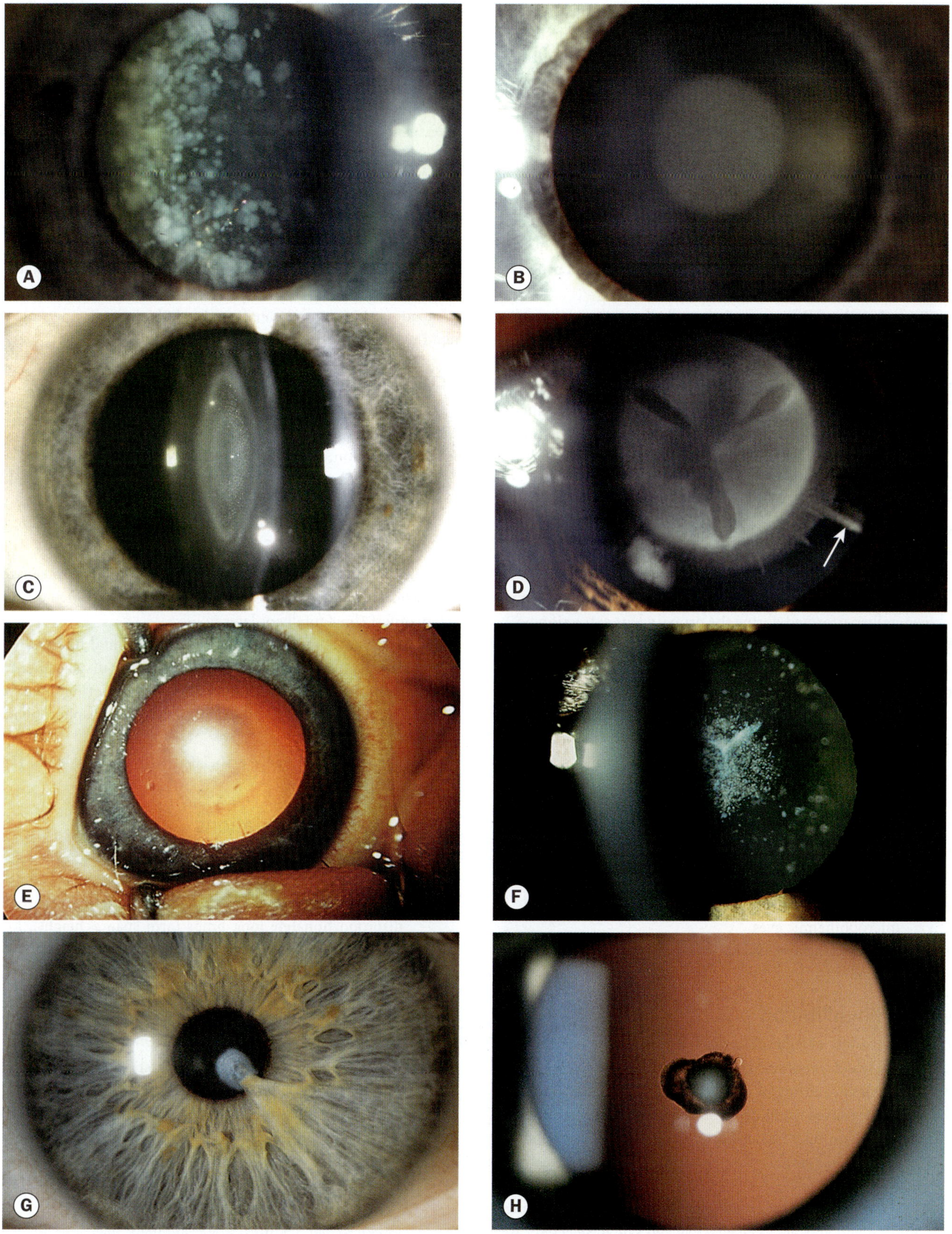

Fig. 10.27 Congenital cataracts. **(A)** Extensive blue dot; **(B)** nuclear; **(C)** coronary; **(D)** lamellar with riders (arrow); **(E)** 'oil droplet'; **(F)** sutural with blue dots; **(G)** anterior polar; **(H)** posterior polar. *(Courtesy of Ken K Nischal – fig. E.)*

deprivation amblyopia. If severity is asymmetrical, the eye with the more marked opacity should be addressed first.

- **Bilateral partial** cataracts may not require surgery until later, or indeed at any stage. In case of doubt, it may be prudent to defer surgery in favour of careful monitoring.
- **Unilateral dense** cataract merits more urgent surgery. However, there is no consensus regarding timing, except that 6 weeks is the latest point at which elective surgery should be performed. Many authorities would advocate surgery between 4 and 6 weeks, followed by aggressive anti-amblyopia therapy. Despite this, the VA results are often disappointing. If the cataract is detected after 16 weeks of age, then the visual prognosis is particularly poor.
- **Partial unilateral** cataract can usually be observed or treated non-surgically with pupillary dilatation and possibly part-time contralateral occlusion.
- **Surgery** involves anterior capsulorhexis, aspiration of lens matter, capsulorhexis of the posterior capsule, limited anterior vitrectomy and IOL implantation, if appropriate. It is important to correct associated refractive errors.

Postoperative complications

Surgery carries a higher incidence of complications than in adults.

- **Posterior capsular opacification** is nearly universal if the posterior capsule is retained and can have a substantial amblyogenic effect. Posterior capsulorhexis with vitrectomy is generally performed during the primary lens extraction.
- **Secondary membranes** may form across the pupil, particularly if postoperative uveitis is not treated aggressively.
- **Proliferation of lens epithelium** is universal, often forming a Soemmering ring (see Fig. 10.22D). It is usually visually inconsequential.
- **Glaucoma**
  - The younger the age at which the surgery is undertaken the greater the risk of developing glaucoma.
  - Secondary open-angle glaucoma may develop in up to 20% of eyes by 5 years after surgery.
  - Angle closure may occur in the immediate postoperative period secondary to pupillary block, especially in microphthalmic eyes.
- **Retinal detachment** is an uncommon and usually late complication.

Visual rehabilitation

The visual results of cataract surgery in infants are hampered by amblyopia, which should be treated aggressively (see Ch. 18).

- **Spectacles** are useful for older children with bilateral aphakia.
- **Contact lenses** provide a superior optical solution for unilateral or bilateral aphakia. After the age of about 2 years compliance may worsen as the child becomes more independent.
- **IOL implantation** is increasingly being performed in younger children and appears to be effective and safe in selected cases. Hypermetropia (correctable with spectacles) is initially targeted and as the child ages slow change towards emmetropia and then myopia is usually found.

TIP After cataract surgery in a child, measures need to be taken to prevent amblyopia.

ECTOPIA LENTIS

Introduction

Ectopia lentis refers to a hereditary or acquired displacement of the lens from its normal position. The lens may be completely dislocated, rendering the eye functionally aphakic (luxated), or partially displaced, remaining partly within the pupillary area (subluxated). The early stages of subluxation may manifest with a tremulous lens (phacodonesis), demonstrated on the slit lamp by lens wobble on rapid return of the eye to the primary position.

Acquired causes

- Trauma.
- Pseudoexfoliation.
- Inflammation, e.g. chronic cyclitis, syphilis.
- Hypermature cataract.
- Large eye, e.g. high myopia, buphthalmos.

Without systemic associations

- **Familial ectopia lentis.** This is an AD condition characterized by bilateral symmetrical superotemporal displacement. It may manifest congenitally or later in life.
- **Ectopia lentis et pupillae** is a rare congenital bilateral disorder with AR inheritance characterized by displacement of the pupil and the lens in opposite directions (Fig. 10.28A). The pupils are small and dilate poorly. Microspherophakia may be present.
- **Aniridia** is occasionally associated with ectopia lentis (Fig. 10.28B).

With systemic associations

- **Marfan syndrome**
  - AD inheritance (gene: *FBN1*) with variable expressivity.
  - Musculoskeletal features include a tall, thin stature with disproportionately long limbs (arm span > height), long fingers (Fig. 10.29A) and toes (arachnodactyly), a narrow high-arched ('gothic') palate (Fig. 10.29B).
  - Kyphoscoliosis, sternal abnormalities, mild joint laxity, muscular underdevelopment and predisposition to hernias.
  - Cardiovascular lesions include dilatation of the aortic root, mitral valve prolapse and aortic aneurysm formation.
  - Bilateral ectopia lentis (80%); subluxation is most frequently superotemporal (Fig. 10.29C). The zonules are frequently intact so that accommodation is retained, although rarely the lens may dislocate into the AC or vitreous (Fig. 10.29D).
  - Other ocular features: angle anomaly may lead to glaucoma and lattice retinal degeneration to retinal detachment. There may be hypoplasia of the dilator pupillae, microspherophakia and strabismus.

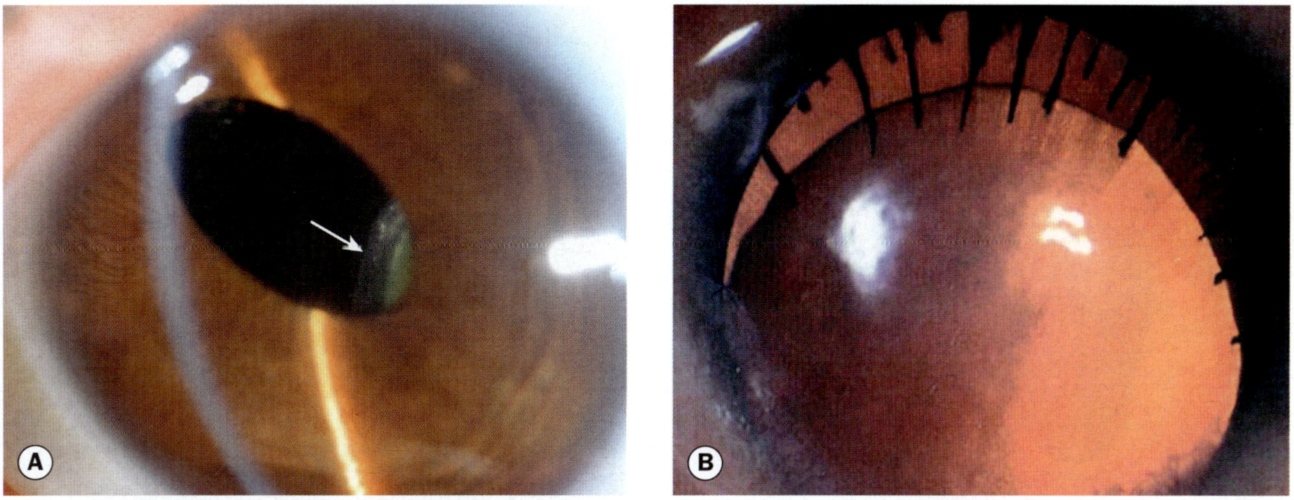

Fig. 10.28 Ectopia lentis without systemic associations. **(A)** Ectopia lentis (arrow) et pupillae; **(B)** inferior subluxation in aniridia.

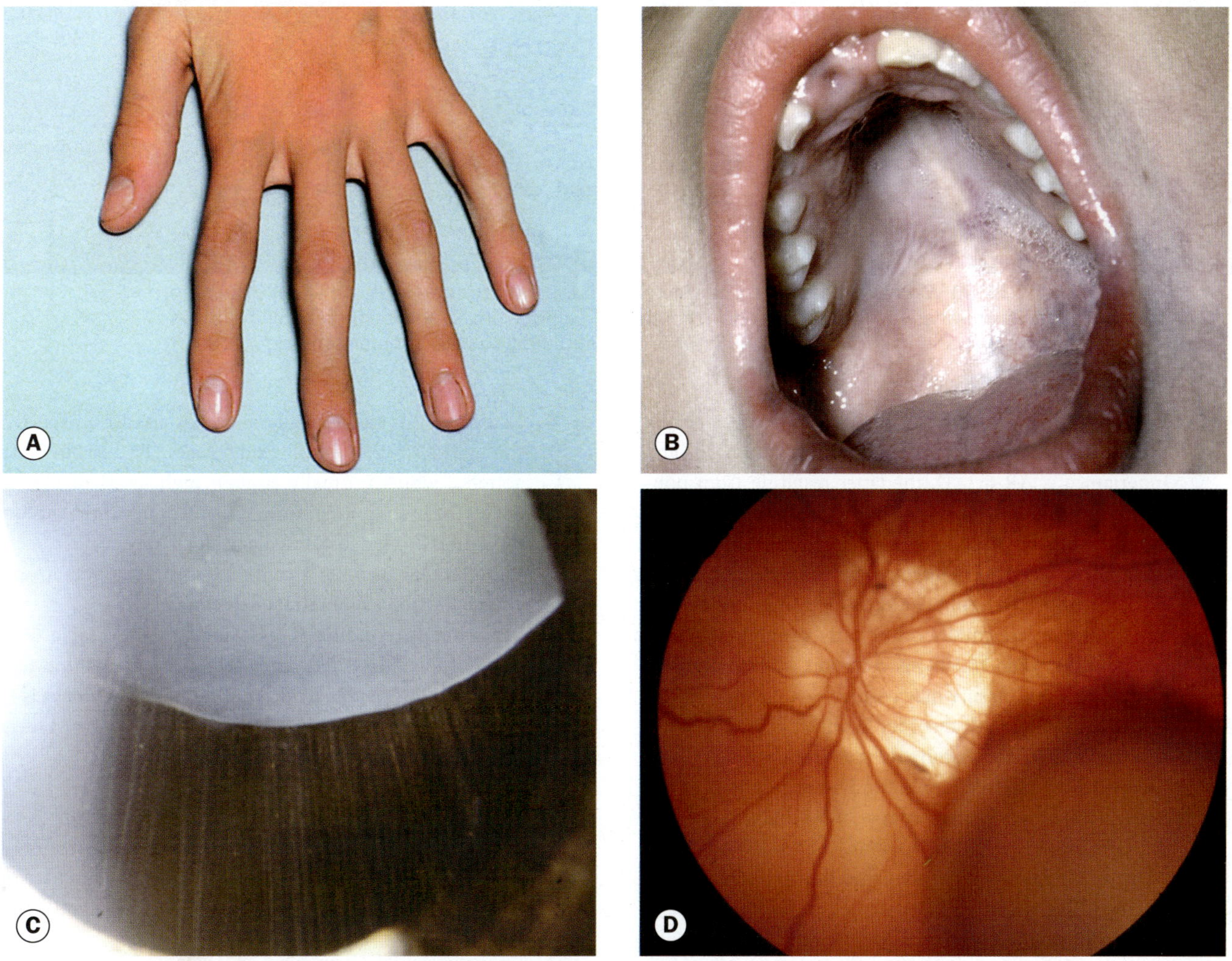

Fig. 10.29 Marfan syndrome. **(A)** Arachnodactyly; **(B)** high-arched palate; **(C)** superotemporal subluxation with intact zonules; **(D)** dislocation into the vitreous (rare)

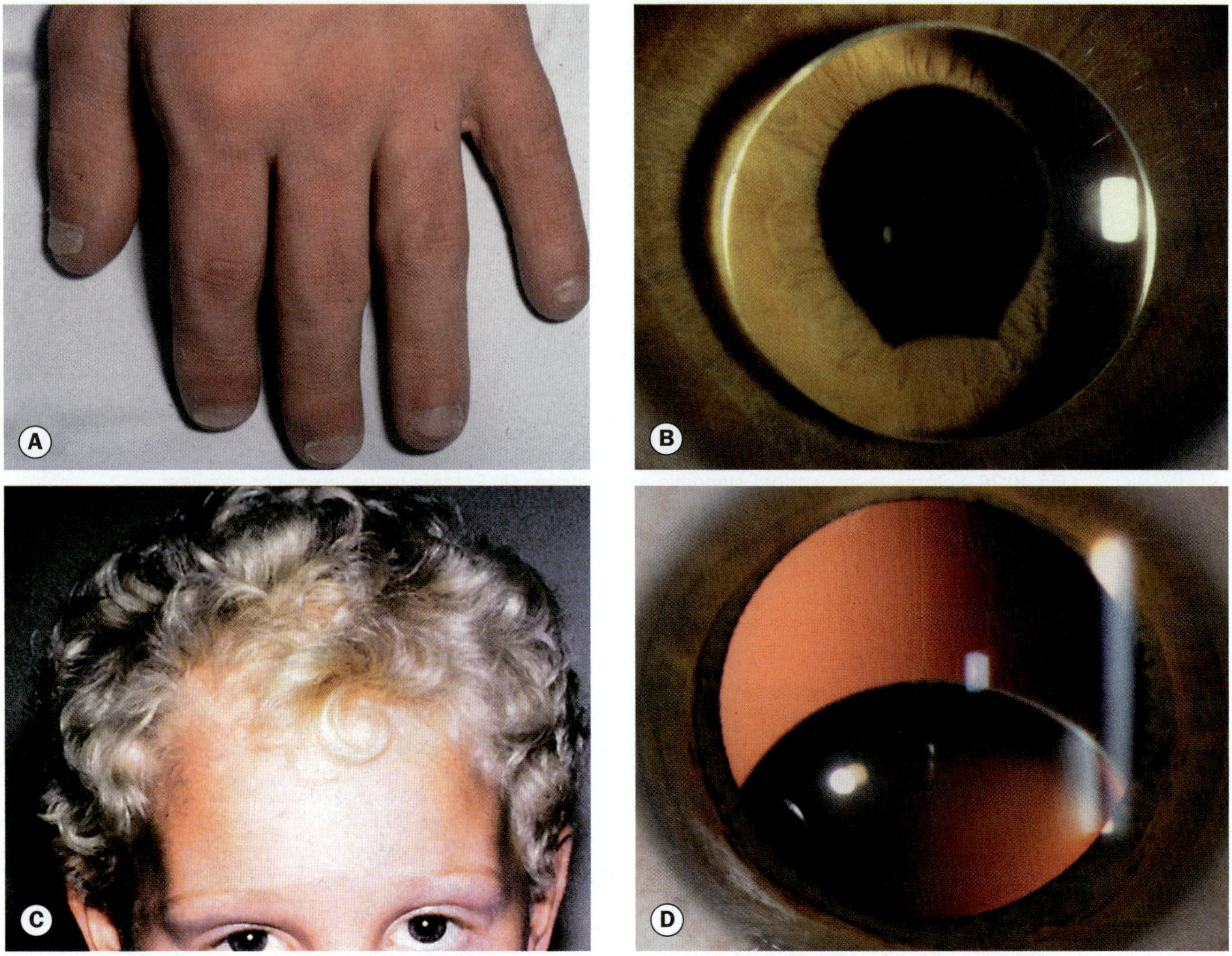

Fig. 10.30 **(A)** Weill–Marchesani syndrome associated with brachydactyly and **(B)** dislocation of microspheric lens into the anterior chamber; **(C)** child with homocystinuria showing coarse blonde hair and associated with **(D)** inferior lens subluxation with zonular disintegration.

- **Weill–Marchesani syndrome** is a rare systemic connective tissue disease, conceptually the converse of Marfan syndrome.
  - Inheritance is AR or AD, the latter resulting from polymorphisms in *FBN1*, the same gene as Marfan syndrome.
  - Systemic features include short stature, short fingers and toes (brachydactyly) and learning difficulties (Fig. 10.30A).
  - Ectopia lentis (50%). Subluxation is in an inferior direction and occurs in late childhood or early adulthood. Microspherophakia (Fig. 10.30B) is common, so that pupillary block with angle closure may ensue.
- **Homocystinuria** is an AR disorder in which decreased enzymatic metabolism of the amino acid methionine results in systemic accumulation of methionine and homocysteine.
  - Systemic features include coarse blond hair, blue irises, malar flush, Marfanoid habitus, neurodevelopmental delay, marked thrombotic predisposition and early atherosclerosis (Fig. 10.30C).
  - Treatment involves oral pyridoxine, folic acid and vitamin B_{12} to reduce plasma homocysteine and methionine levels.
  - Ectopia lentis, typically inferonasal, is almost universal by the age of 25 years in untreated cases (Fig. 10.30D). The zonules, which normally contain high levels of cysteine (deficient in homocystinuria), disintegrate so that accommodation is often lost. Pupillary block may occur.
  - Other ocular features include iris atrophy, optic atrophy, cataract, myopia and retinal detachment.
- **Other systemic conditions** associated with ectopia lentis include sulfite oxidase deficiency (ectopia lentis is universal) and occasionally Stickler syndrome (retinal detachment is the most common ocular manifestation – see Ch. 16), Ehlers–Danlos syndrome and hyperlysinaemia.

Management

The main complications of ectopia lentis are refractive error of any type depending on lens position, optical distortion due to astigmatism and/or lens edge effect, glaucoma (see Ch. 11) and, rarely, lens-induced uveitis.

- **Spectacle correction** may correct astigmatism induced by lens tilt or edge effect in eyes with mild subluxation. Aphakic correction may also afford good visual results if a significant portion of the visual axis is clear in the undilated state.

- **Surgical removal** of the lens is indicated for intractable ametropia, meridional amblyopia, cataract, lens-induced glaucoma or uveitis, or endothelial touch.

ABNORMALITIES OF LENS SHAPE

Anterior lenticonus

Anterior lenticonus consists of a bilateral axial projection of the anterior surface of the lens into the AC (Fig. 10.31A and B). The 'oil droplet' sign can be seen on retroillumination (Fig. 10.31C). Almost all patients have Alport syndrome, a hereditary condition characterized by progressive sensorineural deafness and renal disease associated with abnormal glomerular basement membrane (see Fig. 15.22). Retinal flecks and posterior polymorphous corneal dystrophy may also occur.

Posterior lenticonus

Bulging of the posterior axial lens (Fig. 10.31D) is associated with local thinning or absence of the capsule in posterior lenticonus. Most cases are unilateral, sporadic and not associated with systemic disease. With age, bulging progressively increases and the lens cortex may opacify. Posterior subcapsular opacification is common (Fig. 10.31E). Progression of cataract is variable, but an acutely opacified lens is sometimes seen in early childhood.

Lentiglobus

Lentiglobus is a very rare, usually unilateral, generalized hemispherical deformity of the lens. It may be associated with posterior polar opacity.

Microspherophakia and microphakia

The lens is small and spherical in microspherophakia (Fig. 10.31F), which may be seen as an isolated familial (dominant) abnormality, or in association with a number of systemic conditions including Marfan and Weill–Marchesani syndromes, hyperlysinaemia and congenital rubella. Ocular associations include Peters anomaly and familial ectopia lentis et pupillae. Complications can include lenticular myopia, subluxation and dislocation. Microphakia (Fig. 10.31G) is the term used for a lens with a smaller than normal diameter. It may be found in isolation, but may also occur in patients with Lowe syndrome.

Coloboma

This is characterized by congenital indentation of the lens periphery (Fig. 10.31H) and occurs as a result of localized zonular deficiency. It is not a true coloboma, as there is no focal absence of a tissue layer due to failure of closure of the optic fissure. Occasionally a lens coloboma is associated with a coloboma of the iris or fundus.

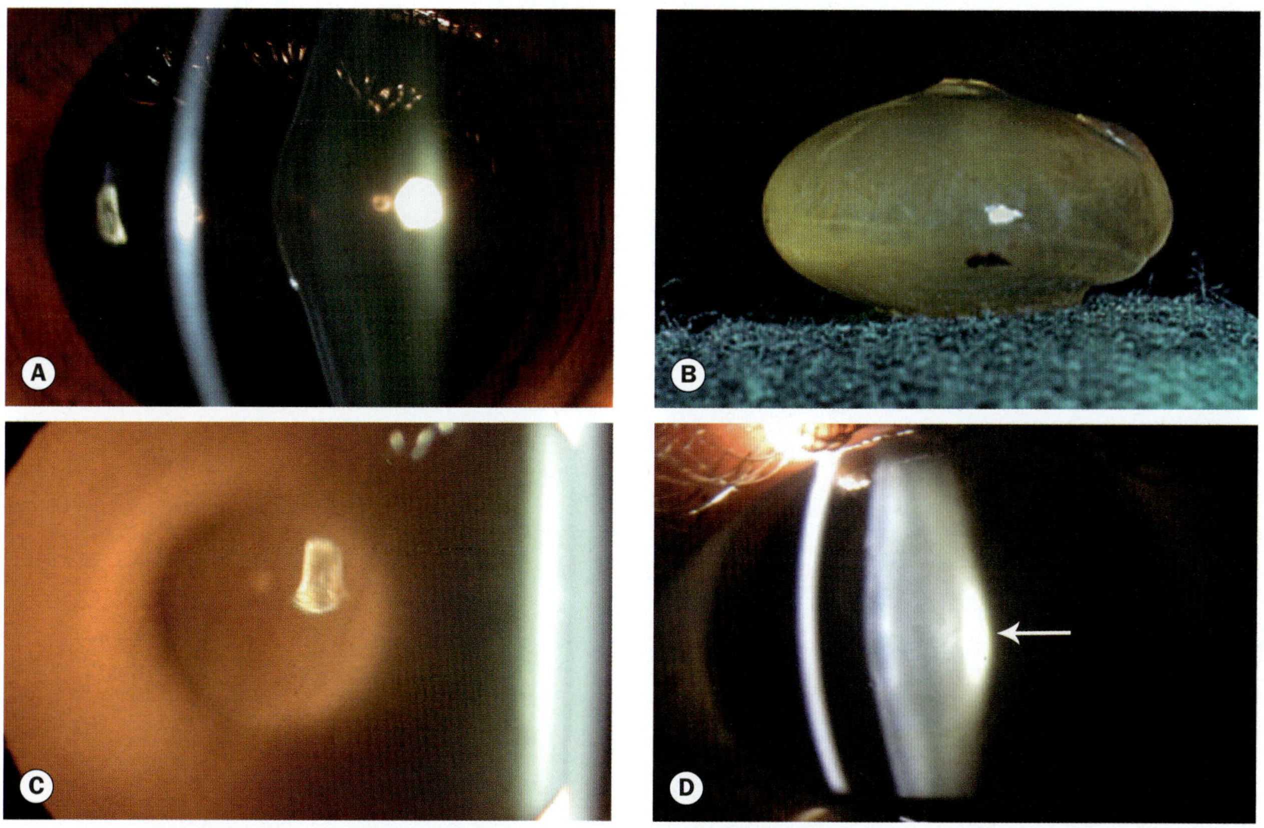

Fig. 10.31 Abnormalities of lens shape. **(A)** Anterior lenticonus; **(B)** anterior lenticonus after intracapsular lens extraction; **(C)** 'oil droplet' sign; **(D)** posterior lenticonus (arrow); *(cont'd)*

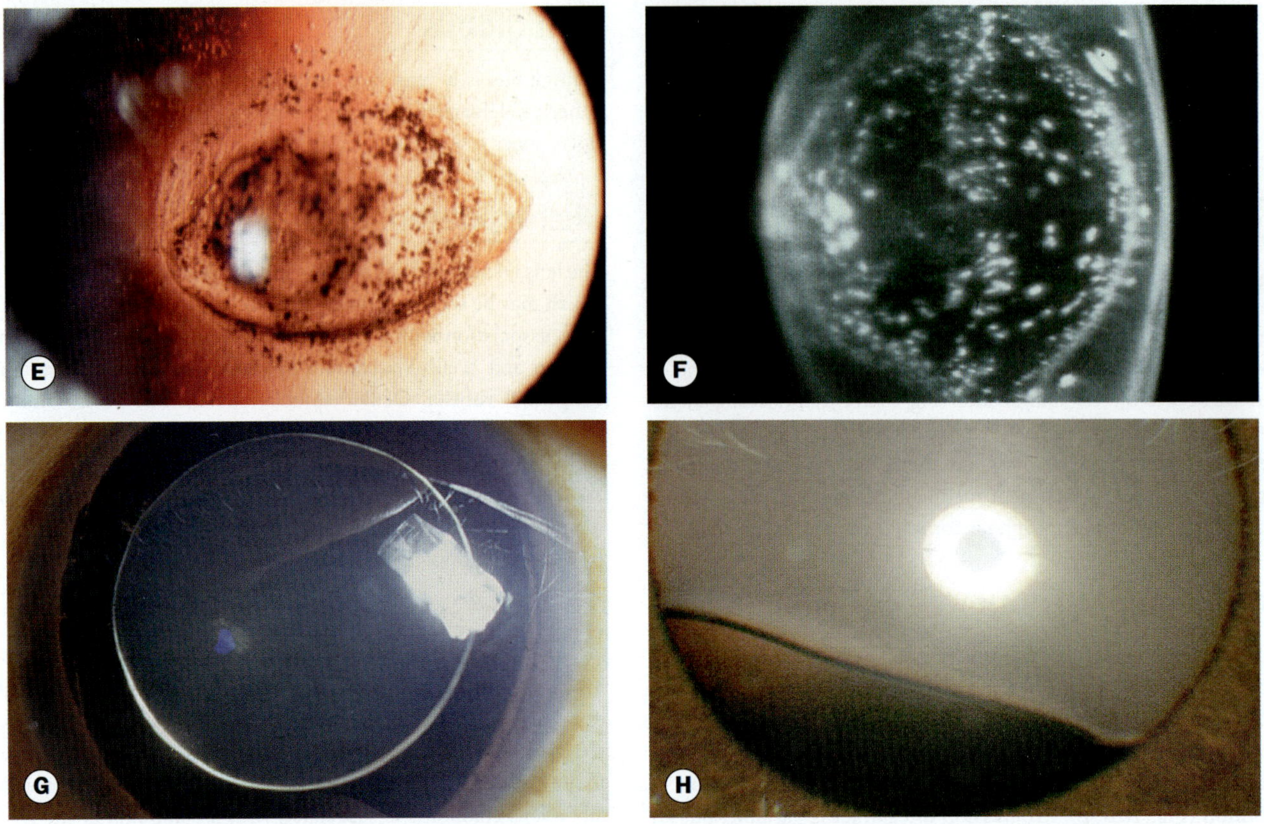

Fig. 10.31—cont'd (E) retroillumination showing opacification of the posterior capsule; **(F)** microspherophakia; **(G)** microphakia; **(H)** lens coloboma. *(Courtesy of R Bates – fig. A, ADN Murray – fig. B.)*

Chapter 11 Glaucoma

INTRODUCTION

Aqueous production

Aqueous humour is produced from plasma by the ciliary epithelium of the ciliary body pars plicata, using a combination of active and passive secretion. A high-protein filtrate passes out of fenestrated capillaries (ultrafiltration) into the stroma of the ciliary processes, from which active transport of solutes occurs across the dual-layered ciliary epithelium. The osmotic gradient thereby established facilitates the passive flow of water into the posterior chamber. Secretion is subject to the influence of the sympathetic nervous system, with opposing actions mediated by beta-2 receptors (increased secretion) and alpha-2 receptors (decreased secretion). Enzymatic action is also critical – carbonic anhydrase is among those playing a key role.

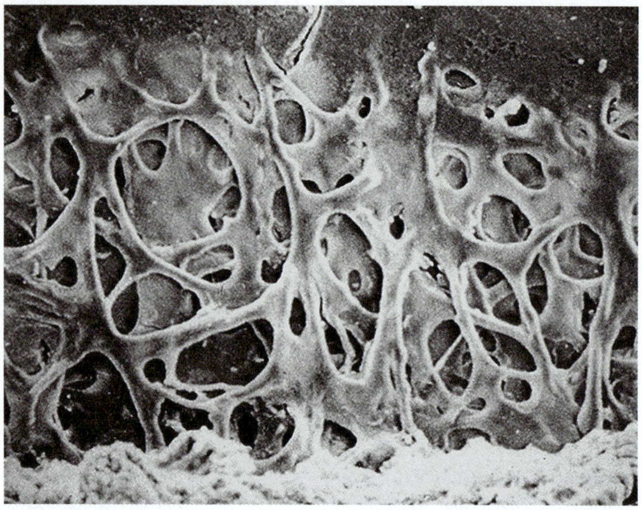

Fig. 11.1 Scanning electron micrograph of the trabecular meshwork.

Aqueous outflow

Anatomy

- **The trabecular meshwork** (trabeculum) is a sieve-like structure (Fig. 11.1) at the angle of the anterior chamber (AC) through which 90% of aqueous humour leaves the eye. It has three components (Fig. 11.2).
  - The uveal meshwork is the innermost portion, consisting of cord-like endothelial cell-covered strands arising from the iris and ciliary body stroma. The intertrabecular spaces are relatively large and offer little resistance to the passage of aqueous.
  - The corneoscleral meshwork lies external to the uveal meshwork to form the thickest portion of the trabeculum. It is composed of layers of connective tissue strands with overlying endothelial-like cells. The intertrabecular spaces are smaller than those of the uveal meshwork, conferring greater resistance to flow.
  - The juxtacanalicular (cribriform) meshwork is the outer part of the trabeculum and links the corneoscleral meshwork with the endothelium of the inner wall of the Schlemm canal. It consists of cells embedded in a dense extracellular matrix with narrow intercellular spaces and offers the major proportion of normal resistance to aqueous outflow.
- The **Schlemm canal** is a circumferential channel within the perilimbal sclera. The inner wall is lined by irregular spindle-shaped endothelial cells containing infoldings (giant vacuoles) that are thought to convey aqueous via the formation of transcellular pores. The outer wall is lined by smooth flat cells and contains the openings of collector channels, which leave the canal at oblique angles and connect directly or indirectly with episcleral veins. Septa commonly divide the lumen into 2–4 channels.

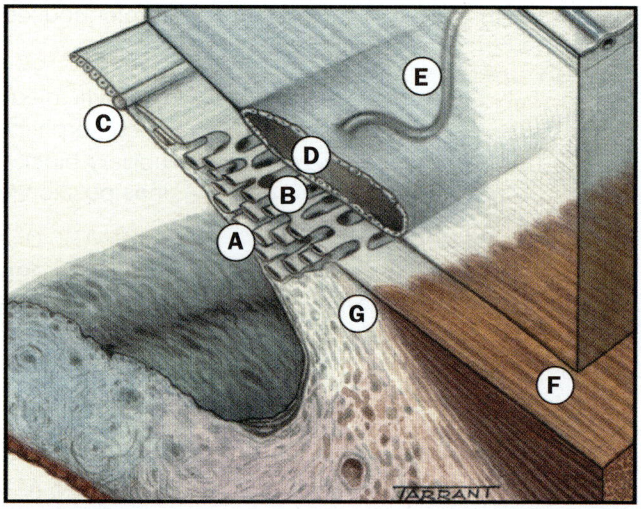

Fig. 11.2 Anatomy of outflow channels. **(A)** Uveal meshwork; **(B)** corneoscleral meshwork; **(C)** Schwalbe line; **(D)** Schlemm canal; **(E)** connector channels; **(F)** longitudinal muscle of the ciliary body; **(G)** scleral spur.

Physiology

Aqueous flows from the posterior chamber via the pupil into the AC, from where it exits the eye via three routes (Fig. 11.3).

- **Trabecular** outflow (90%): aqueous flows through the trabeculum into the Schlemm canal and then the episcleral veins. This is a bulk flow pressure-sensitive route so that increasing intraocular pressure will increase outflow.
- **Uveoscleral** drainage (10%): aqueous passes across the face of the ciliary body into the suprachoroidal space and is drained by the venous circulation in the ciliary body, choroid and sclera.
- **Iris**: some aqueous also drains via the iris.

Intraocular pressure

Intraocular pressure (IOP) is determined by the balance between the rate of aqueous production and the rate of aqueous outflow. The latter is related to factors that include the resistance encountered in the trabeculum and the level of episcleral venous pressure.

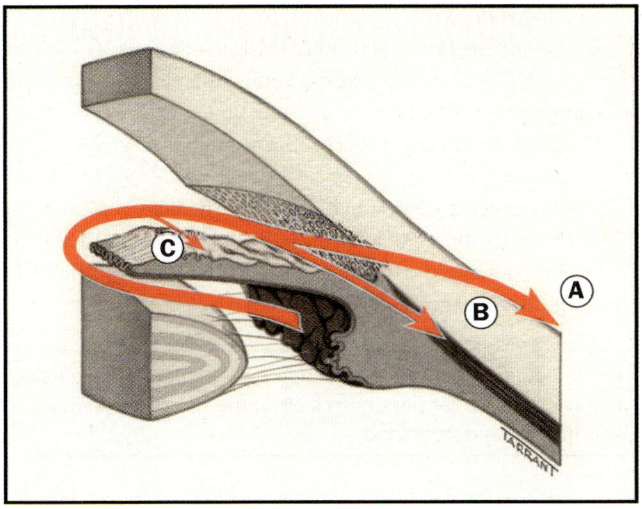

Fig. 11.3 Routes of aqueous outflow. **(A)** Trabecular; **(B)** uveoscleral; **(C)** iris.

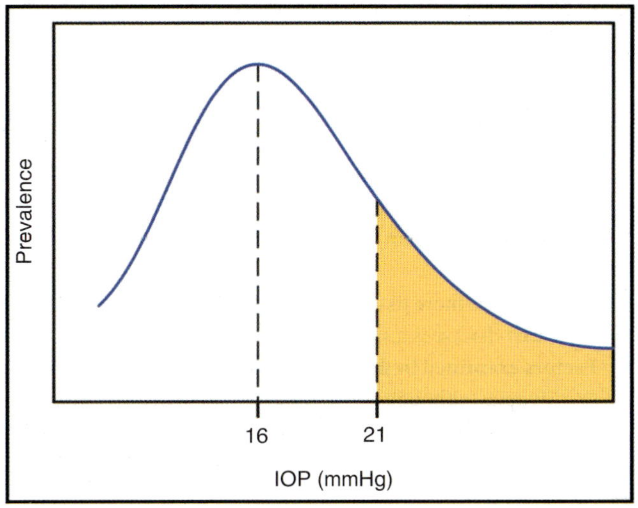

Fig. 11.4 Distribution of IOP in the general population.

Concept of normal intraocular pressure

The upper range of normal for adults is 21 mmHg on applanation tonometry (see below). Some individuals develop glaucomatous damage with IOP less than 21 mmHg, but others remain unscathed with IOP well above this level. Whilst reduction of IOP is a key modifiable element in all types of glaucoma, additional incompletely understood factors are critical in determining whether a particular individual or eye develops glaucomatous damage. These include factors affecting the susceptibility of the optic nerve to damage, such as the integrity of its blood supply and structural vulnerability to mechanical stress at the optic nerve head.

Fluctuation

Normal IOP varies with time of day (diurnal variation), heartbeat, blood pressure and respiration. The diurnal pattern varies, with a tendency to be higher in the morning and lower in the afternoon and evening. This is at least partially due to a diurnal pattern in aqueous production, which is lower at night. Glaucomatous eyes exhibit greater than normal fluctuation, the extent of which is directly proportional to the likelihood of progressive visual field damage and a single reading may therefore be misleading. It is good practice to note the time of day in conjunction with a recorded IOP.

Measurement of IOP

See Chapter 1.

OCULAR HYPERTENSION

Definition

In the general population the mean IOP is 16 mmHg. Two standard deviations on either side of this provides a 'normal' IOP range for individuals over the age of 40 years of 11–21 mmHg. The distribution is Gaussian with the curve skewed to the right (Fig. 11.4). The upper range of normal in individuals over 70 years is 23 mmHg. It is estimated that 4–7% of the population over the age of 40 have an IOP >21 mmHg with open filtration angles and without detectable glaucomatous damage. These individuals are referred to as having 'ocular hypertension' (OHT).

Approximately 1 in 10 will develop glaucoma over a 10-year period and the majority will not develop glaucoma in their lifetime.

Risk factors for developing glaucoma in OHT

The **Ocular Hypertension Treatment Study (OHTS)** was a multicentre longitudinal trial. In addition to looking at the effect of treatment of individuals with ocular hypertension (IOP in one eye between 24 mmHg and 32 mmHg), invaluable information was gained about the effect of a range of putative risks for conversion from OHT to glaucoma. The percentage of OHT patients likely to develop glaucoma at 6 years taking key factors into account is set out in Tables 11.1 and 11.2.

- **Limitations** include the following: the study goal was an IOP reduction of 20%, which may not be sufficient in some individuals, compliance with medication was not measured and there is a possibility that early glaucomatous damage was already present in some patients.
- **Conclusions based on factors that were significant on multivariate analysis**
  - Intraocular pressure. The risk of developing glaucoma increases with increasing IOP.
  - Age. Older age is associated with greater risk.
  - Central corneal thickness (CCT). The risk is greater in eyes with OHT and CCT <555 μm and lower in eyes with high CCT (>588 μm). This may be due to under- and overestimation of IOP, although it is more likely that associated structural factors, perhaps at the lamina cribrosa, might be involved. CCT can be determined using optical imaging (for example: Orbscan) or ultrasonography (for example: Pachmate) (Fig. 11.5).
  - Cup/disc (C/D) ratio. The greater the C/D ratio the higher the risk. This may be because an optic nerve head with a large cup is structurally more vulnerable, or it may be that early damage is already present.

  - Pattern standard deviation (PSD). The higher the PSD value the greater the risk. (This possibly signifies early glaucomatous field change.)
- **Conclusions based on factors that were significant on univariate analysis only** (these were over-ridden when the factors discussed above were considered)
  - African racial background (including Afro-Caribbean, African-American) is associated with a higher glaucoma risk.
  - Males are more likely to convert.
  - Heart disease is a significant risk factor.
- **Factors examined in the OHTS but found to be insignificant**
  - Myopia (although it is suspected that myopic discs are more susceptible to glaucomatous damage at a lower IOP than emmetropic discs).
  - Diabetes.
  - Family history of glaucoma (which is curious, as patients with glaucoma often have a family history of the disease).
- **Conclusions of OHTS**
  - Early treatment reduces the cumulative incidence of glaucoma.
  - The effect is greatest in high-risk individuals.
  - Early treatment of low-risk individuals is not needed.
  - Individualized assessment of risk is useful and helps to guide management.

TIP In ocular hypertension, validated prediction models using an individual's ocular parameters allow the risk of developing glaucoma to be determined.

Table 11.1 Risk of Developing Glaucoma According to IOP (Intraocular Pressure) and CCT (Central Corneal Thickness)

Mean IOP >25.75mmHg	36%	13%	6%
Mean IOP >23.75 to ≤25.75mmHg	12%	10%	7%
Mean IOP <23.75mmHg	17%	9%	2%
	CCT ≤555μm	CCT >555 to ≤588μm	CCT >588μm

Table 11.2 Risk of Developing Glaucoma According to Vertical C/D Ratio and CCT

C/D ratio ≥0.50	22%	16%	8%
C/D ratio >0.30 to <0.50	26%	16%	4%
C/D ratio ≤0.30	15%	1%	4%
	CCT ≤555μm	CCT >555 to ≤588μm	CCT >588μm

Genetics of ocular hypertension

A single nucleotide polymorphism in *TMC01* appears to be significantly associated with conversion to glaucoma in White people with ocular hypertension (three-fold risk in individuals with two risk alleles compared with those with no risk alleles). A recent meta-analysis has identified 112 genetic loci associated with IOP and suggests a major role for angiopoietin-receptor tyrosine kinase signalling, lipid metabolism, mitochondrial function and developmental processes as risk factors for elevated IOP.

Clinical evaluation

History and examination should be carried out as for glaucoma (see below). Consideration should be given to whether any systemic medication is being taken that might be influencing IOP, either upwards (e.g. steroids) or downwards (e.g. beta-blockers).

Pre-perimetric glaucoma

This concept refers to glaucomatous damage, usually manifested by a suspicious optic disc and/or the presence of retinal nerve fibre layer defects, in which no visual field abnormality has developed. The field-testing modality for this purpose is usually taken as standard achromatic automated perimetry.

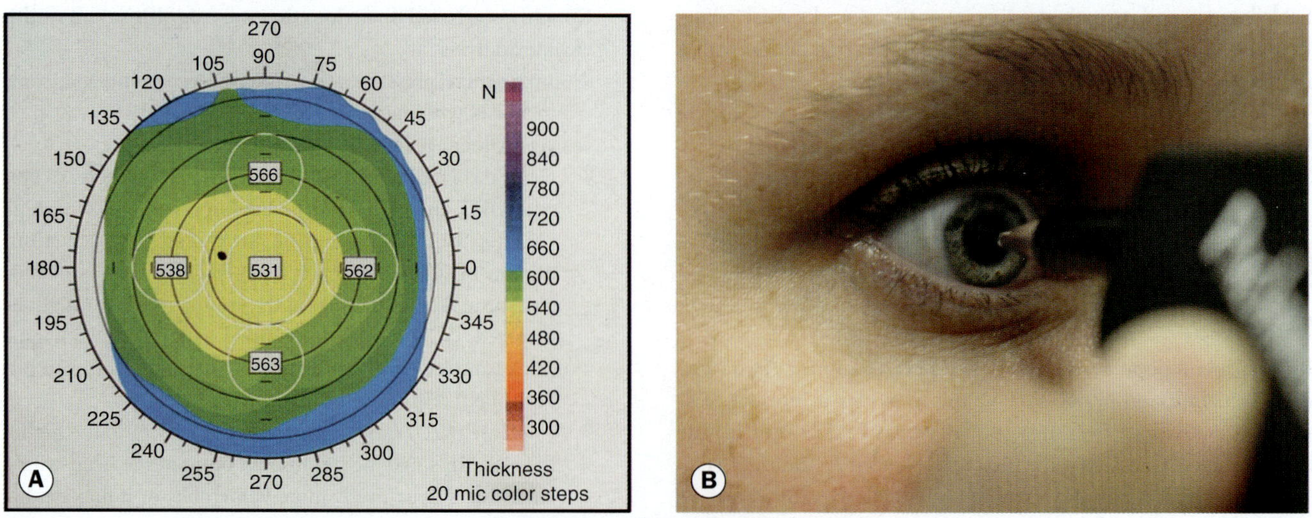

Fig. 11.5 Measurement of CCT. **(A)** Orbscan; **(B)** Pachmate.

Management

Raised IOP is an important risk factor in the development of glaucoma and can be modified with treatment. However, it is difficult to justify the treatment of all individuals with raised IOP because of the high prevalence of ocular hypertension, the low conversion rate to glaucoma and the cost and side effects of treatment. In the OHTS, untreated patients with ocular hypertension had a 9.5% cumulative risk of developing primary open-angle glaucoma (POAG) after 5 years. Treatment (which aimed to reduce IOP by 20% or more and to reach 24 mmHg or less) reduced this to 4.4%.

- Validated prediction models using the ocular parameters of a given individual with ocular hypertension allow the 5-year risk of developing glaucoma to be estimated and expressed as a percentage. This helps in deciding on the frequency of testing and whether to start treatment.
- In general, only those at high risk should be treated, although patient preference may be a decisive factor.
- Age, and therefore life expectancy, is a key point to consider.
- Most practitioners would treat every patient with an IOP of 30 mmHg or more (>40% 5-year risk of glaucoma). The decision to treat in patients with varying risk profiles is not straightforward and has to be made on an individual basis.
- OHT increases the risk of retinal venous occlusion, an additional point to consider when deciding whether to start treatment.
- Treatment options are the same as for POAG, although a less aggressive pressure-lowering approach is frequently taken.
- Careful monitoring is a reasonable alternative in many circumstances: baseline visual fields and retinal nerve fibre layer (RNFL)/disc imaging should be performed.

OVERVIEW OF GLAUCOMA

Definition

Glaucoma is the term that is used to describe a group of conditions that have in common a chronic progressive optic neuropathy that results in characteristic morphological changes at the optic nerve head and in the retinal nerve fibre layer. Progressive retinal ganglion cell death and visual field loss are associated with these changes. Intraocular pressure is a key modifiable factor.

Goal of treatment

The goal of glaucoma treatment is to slow the rate of progression throughout a patient's lifetime in order to maintain visual function and related quality of life, at a sustainable cost.

Classification

Glaucoma may be congenital (developmental) or acquired. Open-angle and angle-closure types are distinguished based on the mechanism by which aqueous outflow is impaired with respect to the AC angle configuration. Distinction is also made between primary and secondary glaucoma. In the latter a recognizable ocular or non-ocular disorder contributes to elevation of IOP.

Epidemiology

Glaucoma affects 2–3% of people over the age of 40 years, but up to 50% may be undiagnosed. It is the second leading cause of blindness in the world. POAG is the most common form in White, Hispanic/Latino and Black individuals (with the prevalence especially high in the latter). On a worldwide basis, primary angle closure (PAC) constitutes up to half of cases and has a particularly high prevalence in people of Asian descent. With improved assessment such as the routine performance of gonioscopy in a darkened rather than a bright environment, PAC is more prevalent in White people than previously realized.

Natural history of open-angle glaucoma

The **Early Manifest Glaucoma Trial (EMGT)** provides prospective natural history data on progression of glaucoma in three common glaucoma types: high tension glaucoma (HTG), normal-tension glaucoma (NTG) and pseudoexfoliation glaucoma (PXEG), using change in the visual field and optic disc as end-points. Without treatment to reduce the IOP the mean rate of change in each group is as follows: HTG −1.31 dB/year, NTG −0.36 dB/year, PXEG −3.13 dB/year. Large differences exist among individuals and different glaucoma types, but based on the mean rate of change in those untreated, visual function in an average glaucoma patient appears to deteriorate from normal to blindness over a period of approximately 25 years. This is influenced significantly by using treatment to reduce IOP. In patients with glaucoma under routine care, approximately 1 in 8 eyes exhibit a change of mean deviation (MD) of more than 1 dB/year and the same proportion also show this in the central 10° region. When seeking to prevent functional disability it is important to also assess progressive central visual field loss in patients with glaucoma.

PRIMARY OPEN-ANGLE GLAUCOMA

Introduction

Definition

Primary open-angle glaucoma (POAG) is a chronic, progressive optic neuropathy of adult onset. It is characterized by:

- Retinal nerve fibre layer thinning.
- Glaucomatous optic nerve damage.
- Characteristic visual field loss as damage progresses.
- An open anterior chamber angle.
- Absence of signs of secondary glaucoma or a non-glaucomatous cause for the optic neuropathy.
- IOP is a key modifiable risk factor.

POAG is the most prevalent type of glaucoma in people of European and African ethnic origin. In those older than 70 years of age the prevalence of POAG has been reported to be approximately 6% in White populations, 16% in Black populations and around 3% in Asian populations. It affects both genders equally.

Risk factors

- **IOP.** The higher the IOP, the greater the likelihood of glaucoma. Asymmetry of IOP of 4 mmHg or more is also significant.
- **Age.** POAG is more common in older individuals.

- **Race.** It is significantly (perhaps four times) more common, develops at an earlier age and may be more difficult to control in Black people than in White people.
- **Family history of POAG.** First-degree relatives of patients with POAG are at increased risk. An approximate risk to siblings is four times and to offspring twice the normal population risk, though surveyed figures vary.
- **Diabetes mellitus.** Longitudinal studies show no increased risk of glaucoma. Selection bias probably explains why clinic-based studies report a higher prevalence of glaucoma in people with diabetes.
- **Myopia** is associated with an increased incidence of POAG and myopic eyes may be more susceptible to glaucomatous damage.
- **Anti-VEGF (vascular endothelial growth factor) therapy.** Patients undergoing anti-VEGF therapy for age-related macular degeneration or diabetic macular oedema are at risk of sustained IOP elevation. This is more likely to occur after recurrent injections with bevacizumab than with ranibizumab. The risk is significantly greater for patients with glaucoma than for normal individuals. The risk that glaucoma surgery will be needed increases after six injections.
- **Systemic calcium-channel blockers.** Meta-analysis of large population-based studies shows a higher prevalence of glaucoma in people using this medication as monotherapy.
- **Vascular disease.** A range of systemic conditions linked to vascular compromise may be associated, though clear-cut relationships have proved difficult to demonstrate consistently. Systemic hypertension, cardiovascular disease, diabetes and vasospastic conditions such as migraine have all been implicated. Poor ocular perfusion may be a risk factor for glaucoma progression.
- **Translaminar pressure gradient.** Studies suggest that a difference in the levels of IOP and orbital CSF pressure may increase the likelihood of the development and progression of glaucomatous damage, perhaps due to associated deformation of the lamina cribrosa.
- **Optic disc area.** Large discs are more vulnerable to damage.
- **Ocular perfusion pressure** is the difference between the arterial BP and the IOP and has been shown in population studies to be linked to increased risk for the development and progression of glaucoma. A low ocular perfusion pressure increases the risk.

Genetics

- **Loci.** POAG has been associated with at least 127 loci in the human genome (Nature Communications 2021). Most loci have broadly consistent effects in all races.
- **Mutations** in only the *MYOC* gene, coding for the protein myocilin that is found in the trabecular meshwork and the *OPTN* gene, which codes for optineurin, are broadly accepted as causing glaucoma. A number of different mutations have been described in the *MYOC* gene, though the normal function of myocilin and its role in glaucoma is as yet undetermined.
- **Family history.** If a single family member develops glaucoma prior to age 35 years, the chances of a mutation in the myocilin gene may be as high as 33%.Genetic investigation of a patient and family may be considered if three or more first-degree relatives from two generations are affected, or for research purposes.
- **A polygenetic risk score** (PRS) has been developed that can predict glaucoma susceptibility and the risk of developing advanced disease. It is possible that in time the PRS will result in a personalized approach for earlier treatment of high-risk individuals, with less intensive monitoring and treatment being possible for those at low risk.

Pathogenesis of glaucomatous optic neuropathy

Retinal ganglion cell death in glaucoma occurs predominantly through apoptosis (programmed cell death) rather than necrosis. The preterminal event is calcium ion influx into the cell body and an increase in intracellular nitric oxide. Glutamine metabolism is intrinsically involved. After initial injury, a cascade of events results in astrocyte and glial cell proliferation and alterations in the extracellular matrix of the lamina cribrosa, with subsequent optic nerve head remodelling. The process of glaucomatous damage and the relationship with IOP and other potential influences is still poorly understood. One or both of the following mechanisms may be involved:

- **Direct mechanical** damage to retinal nerve fibres at the optic nerve head, perhaps as they pass through the lamina cribrosa. Accumulating evidence of the influence of mechanical deformability in the region of the lamina cribrosa supports this.
- **Ischaemic damage**, possibly due to compression of blood vessels supplying the optic nerve head. This may relate to ocular perfusion pressure as a possible risk factor for glaucoma.
- **Common pathways of damage.** Both mechanisms might lead to a reduction in axoplasmic flow, interference with the delivery of nutrients or removal of metabolic products, deprivation of neuronal growth factors, oxidative injury and the initiation of immune-mediated damage.

Screening

Universal population screening for glaucoma has not been demonstrated to be cost-effective and current practice restricts case-finding to high-risk groups, such as: (a) older individuals, (b) those over the age of 40 with a history of POAG in a close family member and (c) people of African racial background. In these groups, screening tends to be performed sporadically via routes such as commercial optometric eye examinations, which may lead to the relative exclusion of underprivileged economic groups. Population screening with tonometry alone is unsatisfactory, since it will label as normal a significant number of cases with other features of POAG such as cupping and visual field loss, and routine screening eye examinations should include visual field assessment as well as tonometry and ophthalmoscopy.

Diagnosis

History

- **Visual symptoms** will usually be absent, unless damage is advanced. Sometimes symptomatic central field defects may occur at an early stage, in the presence of a relatively normal peripheral field.
- **Previous ophthalmic history.** Specific enquiry should be made about:
  - Refractive status, as myopia carries an increased risk of POAG and hypermetropia of primary angle-closure glaucoma (PACG).
  - Causes of secondary glaucoma such as ocular trauma or inflammation. Previous eye surgery, including refractive surgery which may affect IOP readings.
- **Family history**
  - POAG or related conditions such as OHT.
  - Other ocular disease in family members.
- **Past medical history**
  - Asthma, heart failure or block, peripheral vascular disease, which are contraindications to the use of beta-blockers.
  - Head injury, intracranial pathology including stroke, as these conditions may cause optic atrophy or visual field defects.
  - Vasospasm: migraine and Raynaud phenomenon.
  - Diabetes, systemic hypertension and cardiovascular disease may increase the risk of POAG.
  - Oral contraceptive pill for several years may be associated with an increased risk of glaucoma.
- **Current medication**
  - Steroids, including skin cream and inhalants.
  - Oral beta-blockers may lower IOP.
  - Social history, including smoking and alcohol intake, especially if toxic/nutritional optic neuropathy is suspected.
  - Allergies, particularly to any drugs likely to be used in glaucoma treatment, e.g. acetazolamide is contraindicated if there is a history of sulfonamide allergy.

Examination

- **Visual acuity (VA)** is likely to be normal except in advanced glaucoma.
- **Pupils.** Exclude a relative afferent pupillary defect (RAPD). If initially absent but develops later, this constitutes an indicator of substantial progression.
- **Colour vision assessment** such as Ishihara chart testing if there is any suggestion of an optic neuropathy other than glaucoma.
- **Slit lamp examination.** Exclude features of secondary glaucoma such as pigmentary and pseudoexfoliation.
- **Tonometry** prior to pachymetry, noting the time of day.
- **Gonioscopy.**
- **Optic disc examination** for glaucomatous changes (see below) should be performed with the pupils dilated, provided gonioscopy does not show critically narrow angles. Red-free light can be used to detect RNFL defects.

Evaluation of the optic nerve head

Normal optic nerve head

- **Neuroretinal rim.** The neuroretinal rim (NRR) is the orange-pink tissue between the outer edge of the cup and the optic disc margin. The inferior rim is the broadest followed by the superior, nasal and temporal (the 'ISNT' rule). This has high sensitivity (81%) for glaucoma but is not specific (32%), i.e. eyes without glaucoma often do not respect the rule.
- **Cup/disc (C/D) ratio.** The C/D ratio indicates the diameter of the cup expressed as a fraction of the diameter of the disc. The vertical rather than the horizontal ratio is generally taken (Fig. 11.6A). It is difficult to estimate the C/D ratio accurately without imaging. As a basic principle, small diameter optic discs have small cups (Fig. 11.6B) and large diameter discs have large cups (Fig. 11.6C). Only 2% of the population have a C/D ratio greater than 0.7. In any individual, asymmetry of 0.2 or more between the eyes should also be regarded with suspicion, though it is critical to exclude a corresponding difference in overall disc diameter (Fig. 11.7A and B).
- **Optic disc size.** Optic disc size is important in deciding if a C/D ratio is normal and is also a prognostic indicator. Large discs are believed to be more likely to sustain damage, particularly in NTG. This may be the result of the larger diameter conferring relative mechanical weakness and hence greater vulnerability to IOP-induced displacement of the lamina cribrosa, which has been found to be thinner in eyes with NTG. Disc size varies on average between racial groups and is largest in those of African descent. Imaging can objectively measure disc area, but vertical diameter is the parameter most frequently used clinically. Normal median vertical diameter (for non-glaucomatous discs) is 1.5–1.7 mm in a white population.
  - A narrow slit beam is focused on the disc using a fundus lens.
  - The height of the beam is adjusted until it matches the distance between the superior and inferior limits of the NRR (not the scleral rim surrounding the neural tissue) and the diameter in millimetres is read from the slit lamp graticule.
  - A correction factor may be necessary, depending on the lens used (Table 11.3). Refractive error affects measurement only minimally, although myopia above −8 dioptres may distort the result.
- **Inter-eye disc asymmetry.** A vertical cup/disc ratio asymmetry of 0.2 or more is found in about 5% of normal individuals and in about 25% of those with glaucoma. However, asymmetry of the vertical cup/disc ratio alone is not useful in identifying patients with glaucoma. When comparing the two discs, a difference in the appearance of the neuroretinal rim is a good sign of early glaucoma (Fig. 11.7 C–F).

TIP A large disc has a large cup and may be entirely healthy, while any cupping in a small disc may be abnormal.

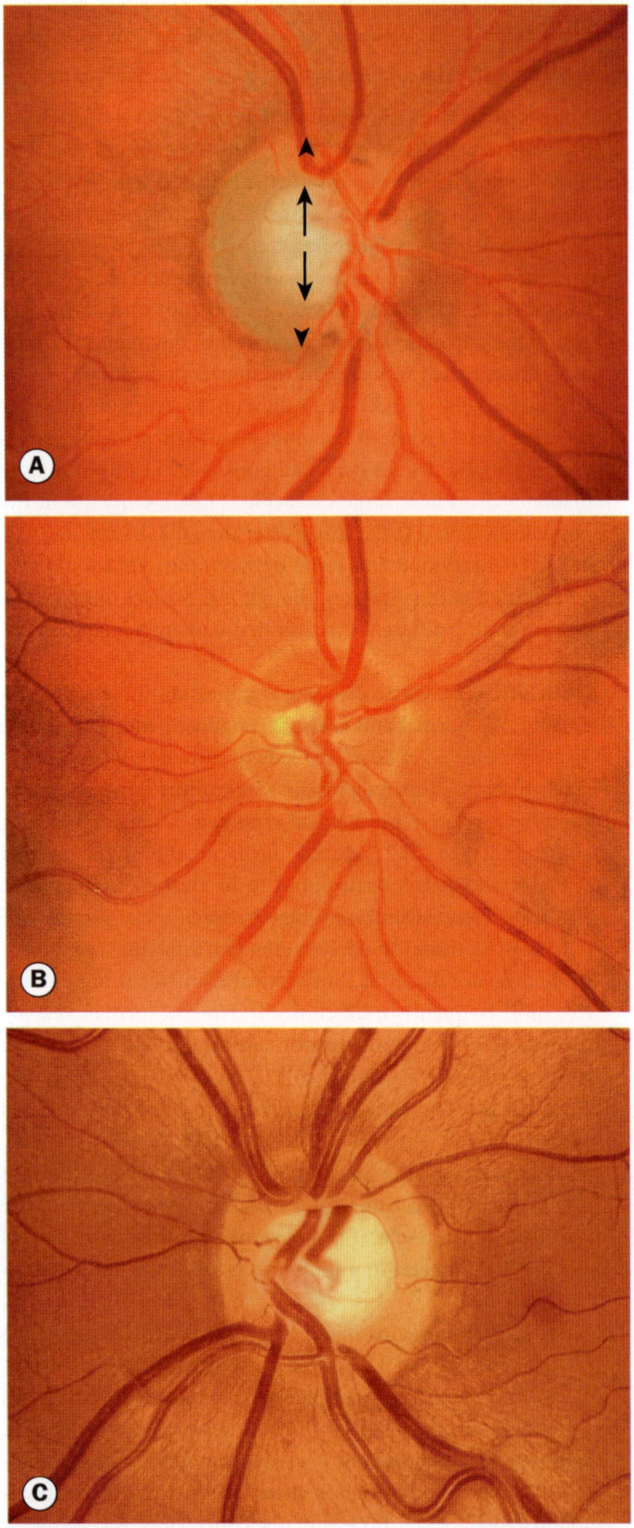

Fig. 11.6 Normal optic disc. **(A)** Cup/disc ratio (arrows show cup and arrow heads show edge of optic disc); **(B)** small disc with a low cup/disc ratio; **(C)** large disc with a proportionally larger cup.

Changes in glaucoma

In some cases, it is not possible to be certain whether an individual optic disc is glaucomatous. The clinical findings and results of investigation should be considered together to guide management.

Glaucomatous damage results in characteristic signs involving (a) the optic nerve head, (b) the peripapillary area and (c) the retinal nerve fibre layer.

- **Optic nerve head.** Pathological cupping is caused by an irreversible decrease in the number of nerve fibres, glial cells and blood vessels. A documented increase in cup size is always significant (Fig. 11.8). If an eye with a small optic disc and correspondingly small cup develops glaucoma, the cup will increase in size, but even in the presence of substantial damage may still be smaller than that of a large physiological cup.
- **Subtypes of glaucomatous damage.** Four morphological glaucomatous disc appearances have been described and although the majority of discs are unclassifiable the descriptions encompass a useful overview of patterns of glaucomatous damage and may provide clues to underlying pathological processes.
  - Focal ischaemic discs (Fig. 11.9A) are characterized by localized superior and/or inferior notching and are associated with localized field defects with early threat to fixation.
  - Myopic disc with glaucoma (Fig. 11.9B) refers to a tilted (obliquely inserted), shallow disc with a temporal crescent of parapapillary atrophy, together with features of glaucomatous damage. Dense superior or inferior scotomas threatening fixation are common. This morphology is most common in younger male patients.
  - Sclerotic discs (Fig. 11.9C) are characterized by a shallow, saucerized cup and a gently sloping NRR, variable peripapillary atrophy and peripheral visual field loss. The peripapillary choroid is thinner than in other disc types. Patients are older, of either gender and there is an association with systemic vascular disease.
  - Concentrically enlarging discs (verified by serial monitoring) are characterized by fairly uniform NRR thinning (Fig. 11.9D) and are frequently associated with diffuse visual field loss. IOP is usually significantly elevated at presentation.
- **Non-specific signs of glaucomatous damage.** Other disc signs of glaucomatous damage include:
  - Disc haemorrhages (Fig. 11.10A and B) often extend from the NRR onto the retina, most commonly inferotemporally. Their presence is a risk factor for the development and progression of glaucoma. They are more common in NTG but can also occur in healthy individuals as well as patients with systemic vascular disease. When screening for glaucoma, approximately three out of four people with a disc haemorrhage will not have glaucoma.

Table 11.3 Correction Factors for Estimating Optic Disc Diameter

Lens	Correction factor
Volk 60D	×0.88–1.0
Nikon 60D	Around 1.0
Volk 90D	×1.3
Volk 78D	×1.1
Goldmann 3-mirror	×1.27

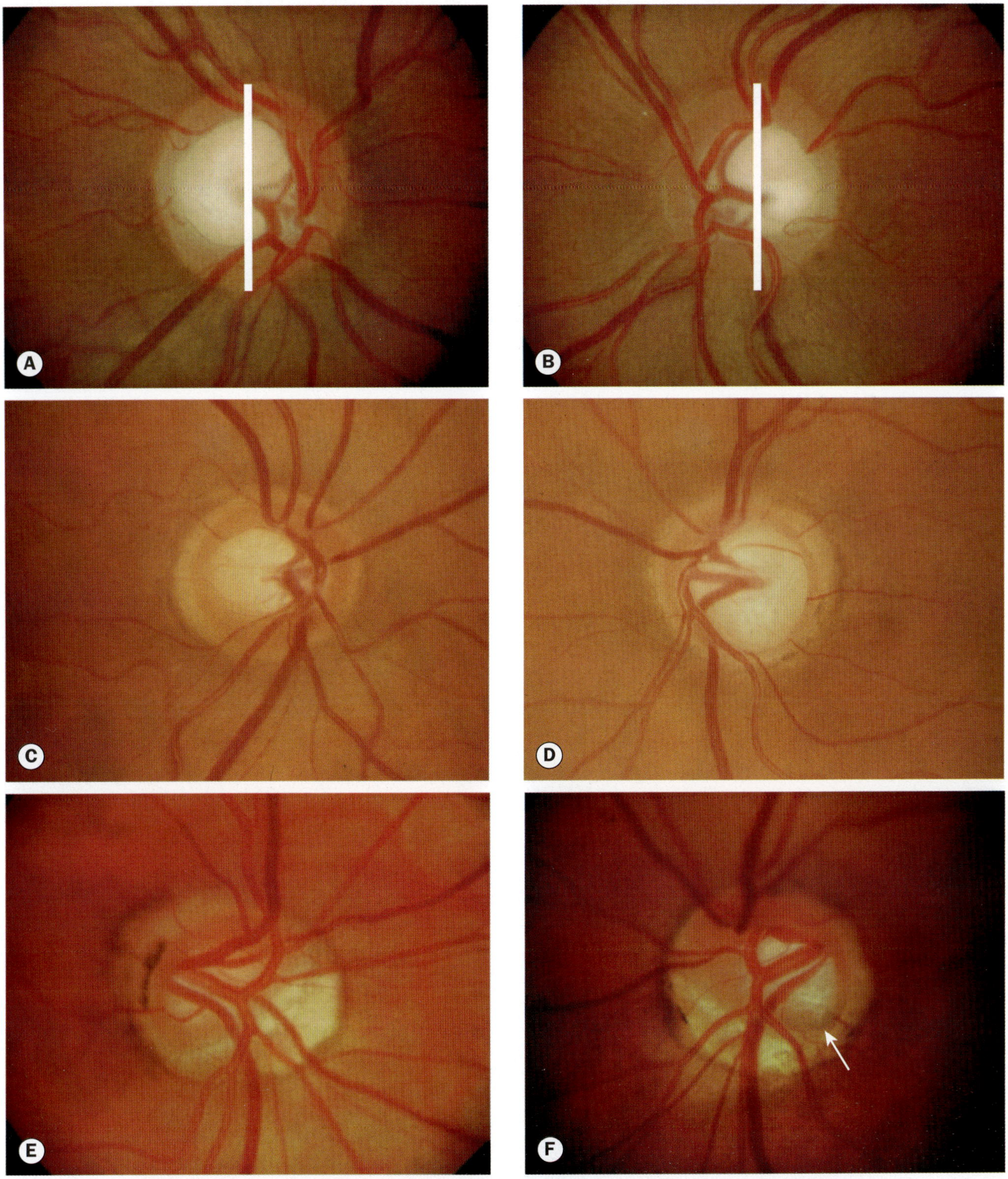

Fig. 11.7 Optic disc asymmetry. **(A)** and **(B)** Physiological cupping in a normal individual, showing a larger optic disc in the right eye than in the left eye. The white bar shows the difference in vertical size; **(C)** showing a normal optic disc in the right eye and **(D)** a glaucomatous optic disc in the left eye; **(E)** showing a tilted but normal optic disc in the right eye and **(F)** a tilted disc with superimposed inferior neuroretinal rim glaucomatous defect (arrow) in the left eye.

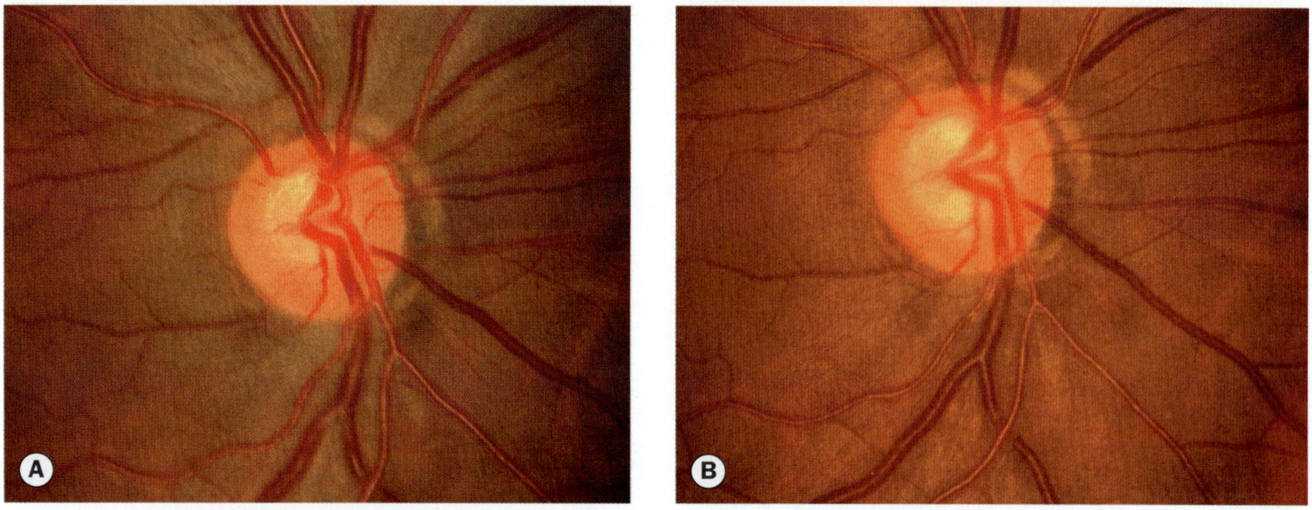

Fig. 11.8 **(A)** Normal optic disc with a small cup; **(B)** same disc 2 years later showing concentric glaucomatous enlargement.

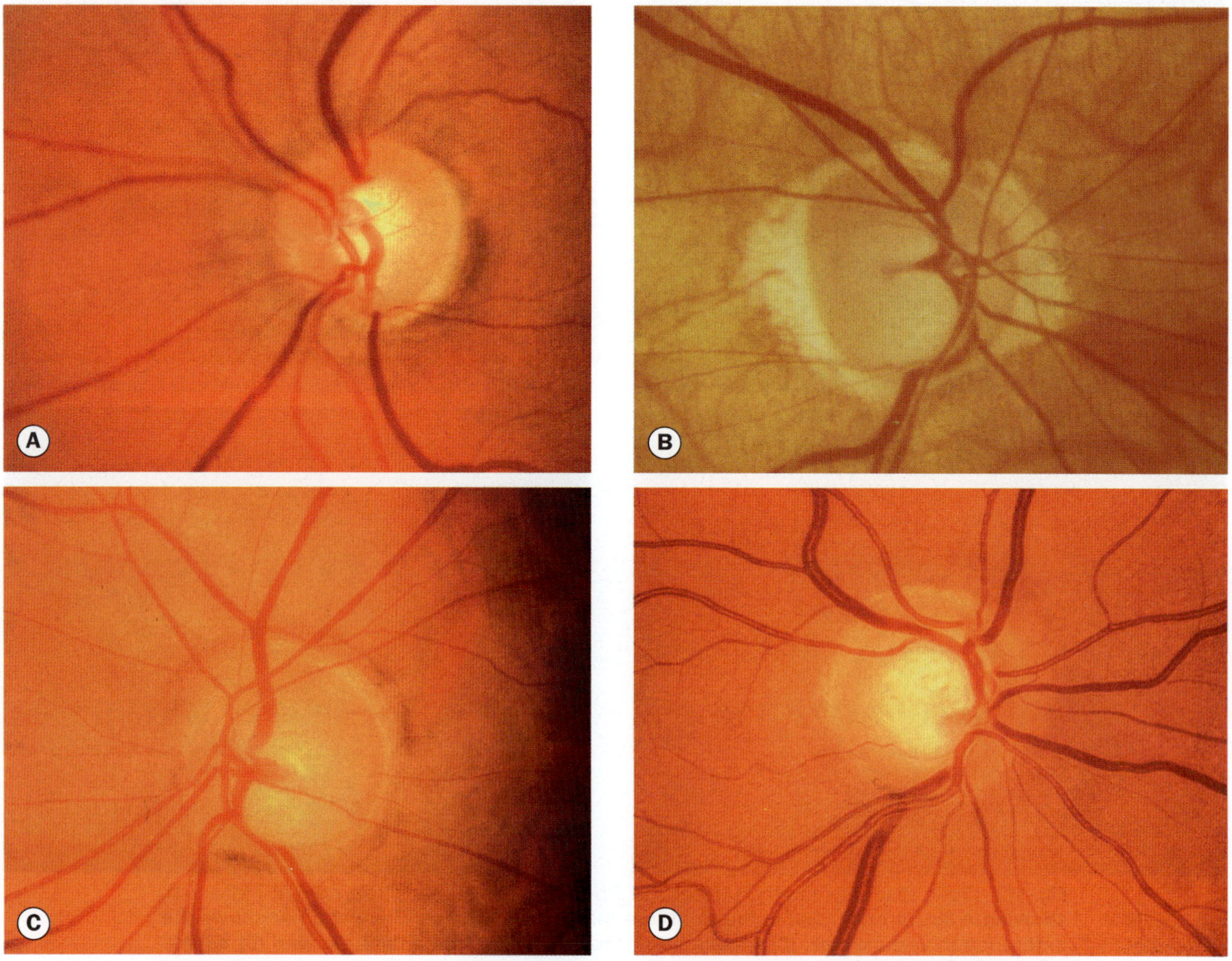

Fig. 11.9 Classic subtypes of glaucomatous damage. **(A)** Focal ischaemic – inferior notch; **(B)** myopic with a temporal crescent and loss of the inferior neuroretinal rim; **(C)** sclerotic with superior shelving and inferior notching; **(D)** concentrically enlarged with deep uniform enlargement of the optic cup

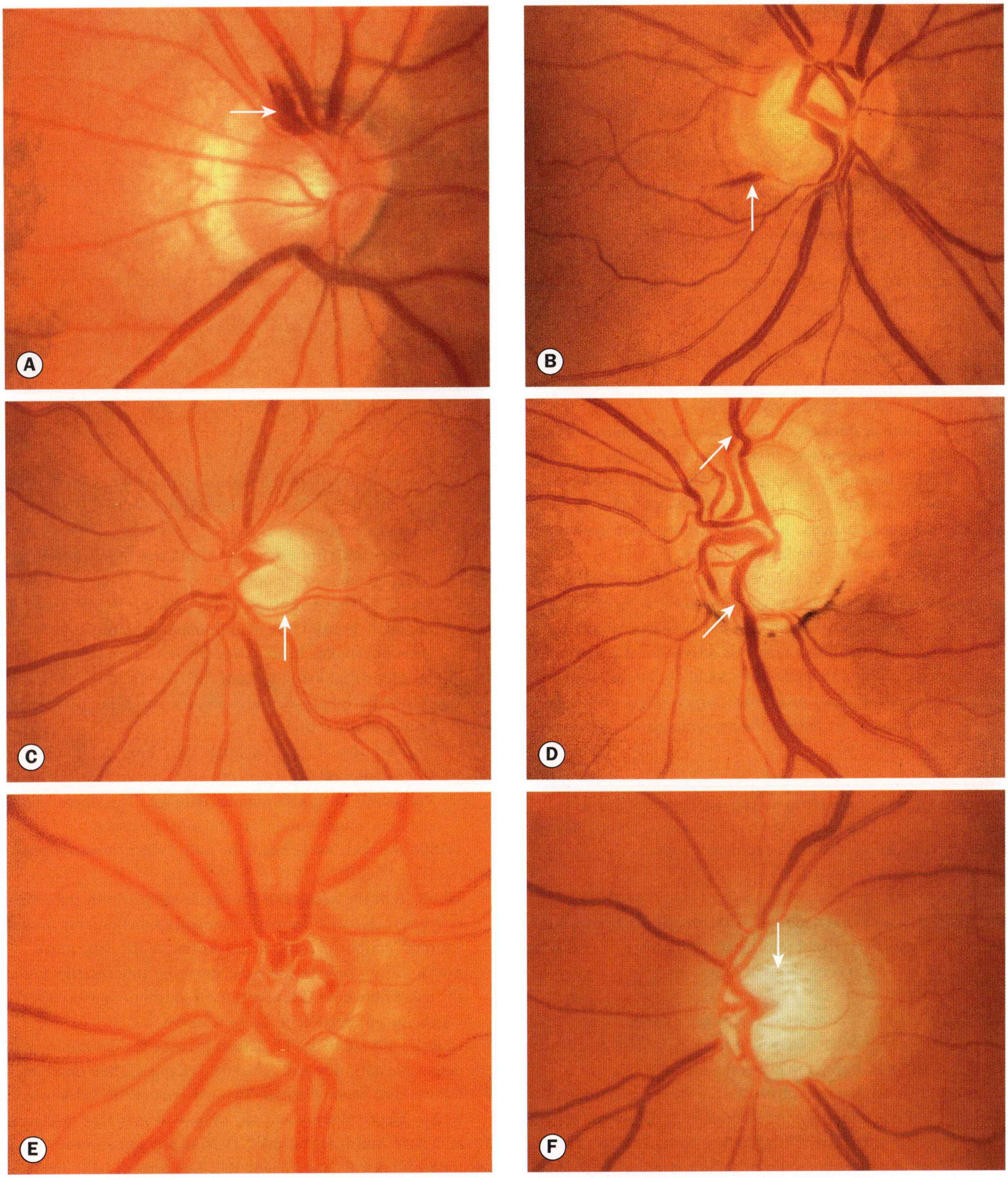

Fig. 11.10 Non-specific signs of glaucomatous damage. **(A)** and **(B)** Disc haemorrhage (arrow); **(C)** baring of inferior circumlinear blood vessel (arrow); **(D)** bayoneting of superior and inferior blood vessels (arrows) associated with advanced glaucomatous damage; **(E)** collateral vessels; **(F)** laminar dot sign (arrow) and nasal cupping associated with advanced glaucomatous damage.

- Baring of circumlinear blood vessels is a sign of early thinning of the NRR. It is characterized by a space between the neuroretinal rim and a superficial blood vessel (Fig. 11.10C).
- Bayoneting is characterized by double angulation of a blood vessel. With NRR loss, a vessel entering the disc from the retina may angle sharply backwards into the disc and then turn towards its original direction to run across the lamina cribrosa (Fig. 11.10D).
- Collaterals between two veins at the disc (Fig. 11.10E), similar to those following central retinal vein occlusion (CRVO), are relatively uncommon. They are probably caused by chronic low-grade circulatory obstruction. Retinal vascular tortuosity may also occur.
- Loss of nasal NRR (Fig. 11.10F) is a sign of moderately advanced damage. A space may develop between the NRR and the central retinal vasculature.
- The laminar dot sign occurs in advancing glaucoma. Grey dot-like fenestrations in the lamina cribrosa (see Fig. 11.10F) become exposed as the NRR recedes. The fenestrations sometimes appear linear and this itself may be a sign of advanced damage, indicating distortion of the lamina. The dots may be seen in normal eyes.
- 'Sharpened edge' or 'sharpened rim' is a sign of advancing damage. As NRR is lost adjacent to the edge of the disc, the disc margin contour assumes a sharper angle backwards. Bayoneting of vessels is often seen at a sharpened edge (see Fig. 11.10 D). This should not be confused with a 'sharpened nasal polar edge', which refers to the sharp angulation of the NRR at the nasal margin of a focal vertical polar notch.

TIP An optic disc haemorrhage is a risk factor for the development and progression of glaucoma and can be missed unless magnification is used to examine the disc.

- **Peripapillary changes.** Peripapillary atrophy (PPA) surrounding the optic nerve head may be of significance in glaucoma (Fig. 11.11) and may be a sign of early damage in patients with ocular hypertension.
  - Alpha (outer) zone is characterized by superficial retinal pigment epithelial changes. It tends to be larger and possibly more common in glaucomatous eyes.
  - Beta (inner) zone is characterized by chorioretinal atrophy. It is distinct from the scleral rim, the white band of exposed sclera central to the beta zone. The beta zone is larger and more common in glaucoma and is a risk factor for progression. The location of beta-zone PPA seems to indicate the orientation of likely visual field loss.
- **Retinal nerve fibre layer.** An understanding of the distribution of the 1.2 million ganglion cell axons as they pass across the retina to enter the scleral canal to form the optic nerve head (optic disc) is key to the interpretation of visual field loss in relation to optic nerve cupping in glaucoma. Within the retina the arrangement is as follows (Fig. 11.12A):

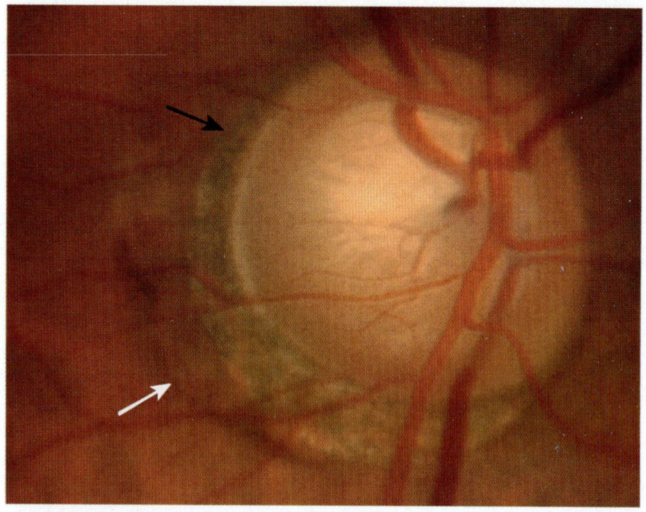

Fig. 11.11 Peripapillary changes. Alpha zone (white arrow) and beta zone (black arrow).

  - Fibres arising from the macula follow a straight course to the optic nerve head, forming a spindle-shaped area (papillomacular bundle).
  - Fibres arising from the nasal retina also follow a relatively straight course to the optic nerve.
  - Fibres arising temporal to the macula follow an arcuate path around the papillomacular bundle to reach the optic nerve head. They do not cross the horizontal raphe that extends from the foveola to the temporal retinal periphery, demarcating the superior and inferior halves of the retina.
  - The arcuate fibres reaching the superotemporal and inferotemporal aspect of the optic nerve head are most vulnerable to glaucomatous damage. The fibres in the papillomacular bundle are the most resistant.

  Within the optic nerve head, the retinal fibres are arranged as follows (Fig. 11.12B):
- Fibres from the peripheral fundus lie deep within the retinal nerve fibre layer (i.e. nearer the pigment epithelium) but occupy the most peripheral (superficial) portion of the optic nerve.
- Fibres arising near to the optic nerve lie superficially within the nerve fibre layer (i.e. near the vitreous) but they occupy the central (deep) portion of the optic nerve.
- In glaucoma subtle RNFL defects precede the development of detectable optic disc and visual field changes. Their onset often follows disc haemorrhages. Two patterns occur: (a) localized wedge-shaped defects and (b) diffuse defects that are larger and have indistinct borders. Defects are sometimes evident following disc haemorrhages. Red-free (green) light increases the contrast between normal retina and defects on slit lamp biomicroscopy or fundus photography and typically makes identification easier (Fig.11.13). Optical coherence tomography (OCT) and scanning laser polarimetry are highly effective means of quantifying the RNFL (see Fig. 11.16 and 11.17). It should be noted that RNFL defects are not specific to glaucoma and can be seen in a range of neurological disease, as well as in apparently normal individuals.

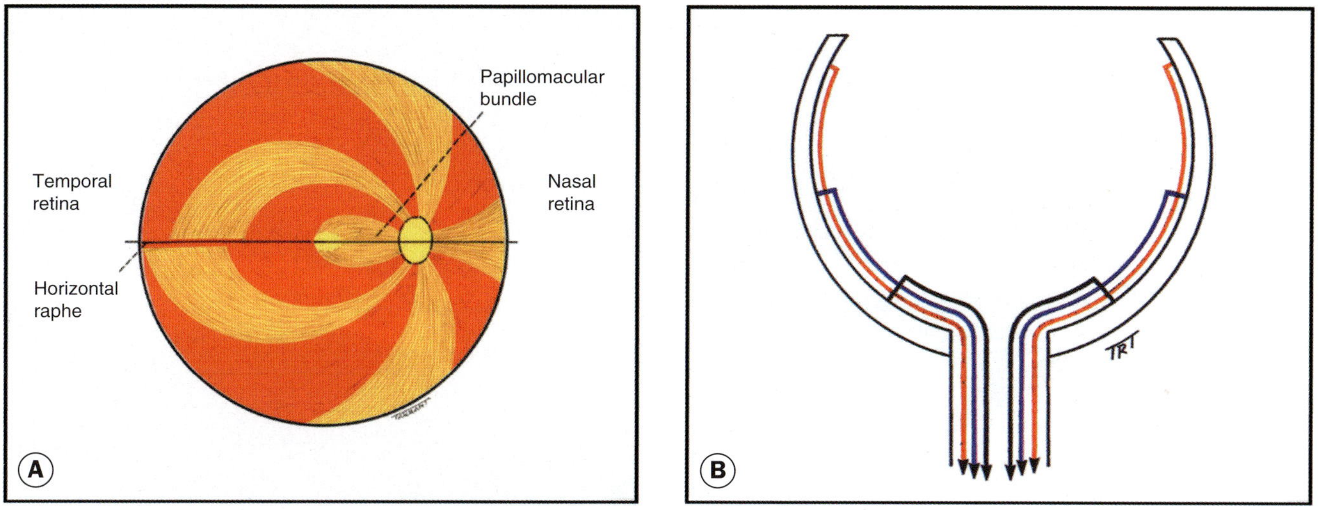

Fig. 11.12 (A) Anatomy of retinal nerve fibres; **(B)** relative positions of retinal nerve fibres. Red = peripheral, blue = equatorial, black = central.

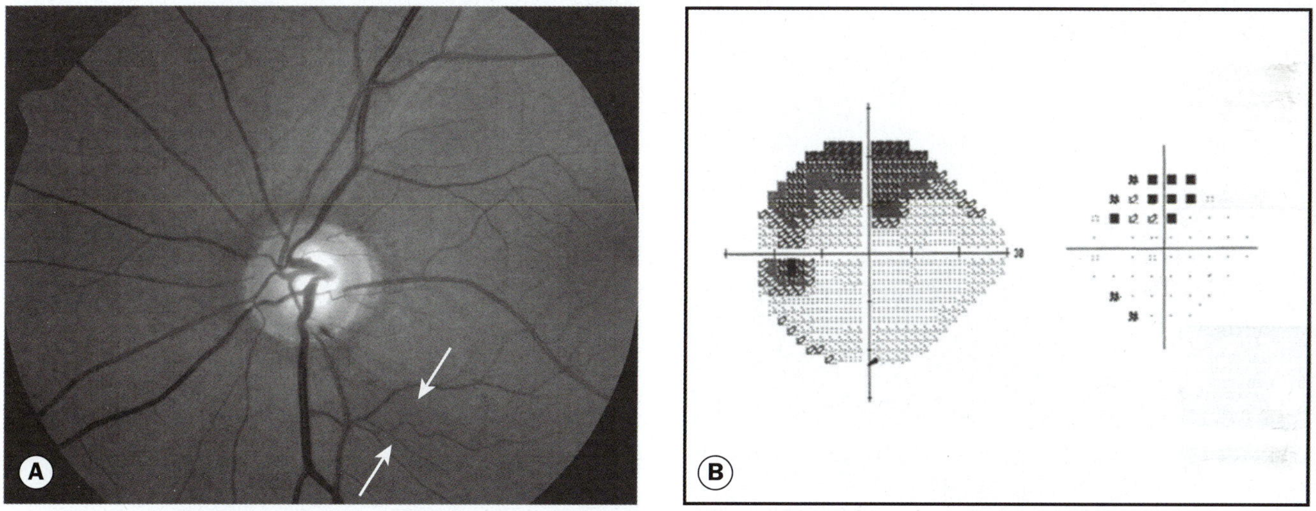

Fig. 11.13 Retinal nerve fibre layer defect. **(A)** Red-free photograph (arrows show wedge-shaped defect) and a disc margin haemorrhage); **(B)** corresponding superior arcuate defect in the visual field (grey scale and pattern deviation).

TIP Retinal nerve fibre layer defects precede the development of optic disc and visual field change in glaucoma.

Imaging in glaucoma

Imaging has become an indispensable tool in the management of patients with glaucoma. However, it is important to remember that in order to determine a diagnosis or to assess change, imaging should always be used to supplement clinical examination and visual field results, rather than as the sole investigation.

- **Pachymetry,** the measurement of corneal thickness, is an essential part of the assessment of glaucoma patients (see Fig. 11.5).
- **Stereo disc photography.** Stereo photography has historically been regarded as the reference standard in optic disc imaging and remains a valuable option. The images are taken by repositioning slightly between shots, either manually or using a stereo separator built into the camera.
- **Ultrasound biomicroscopy (UBM).** This is a type of ultrasound that creates a more detailed image than regular ultrasound and is used for imaging the anterior segment of the eye. This results in resolutions up to 25 μm axially and 50 μm laterally, but the depth of tissue penetration is less than this. It is particularly useful to show the anatomy in patients with primary angle-closure glaucoma (Fig. 11.14). In comparison to anterior segment OCT, the main strength of UBM is its ability to demonstrate structures behind the iris, particularly the ciliary body and lens.
- **Optical coherence tomography of the anterior segment.** Anterior segment optical coherence tomography has an expanding range of clinical applications primarily in the evaluation of angle-closure glaucoma. It is useful when demonstrating the relationship of the peripheral iris to the filtration angle (Fig. 11.15).

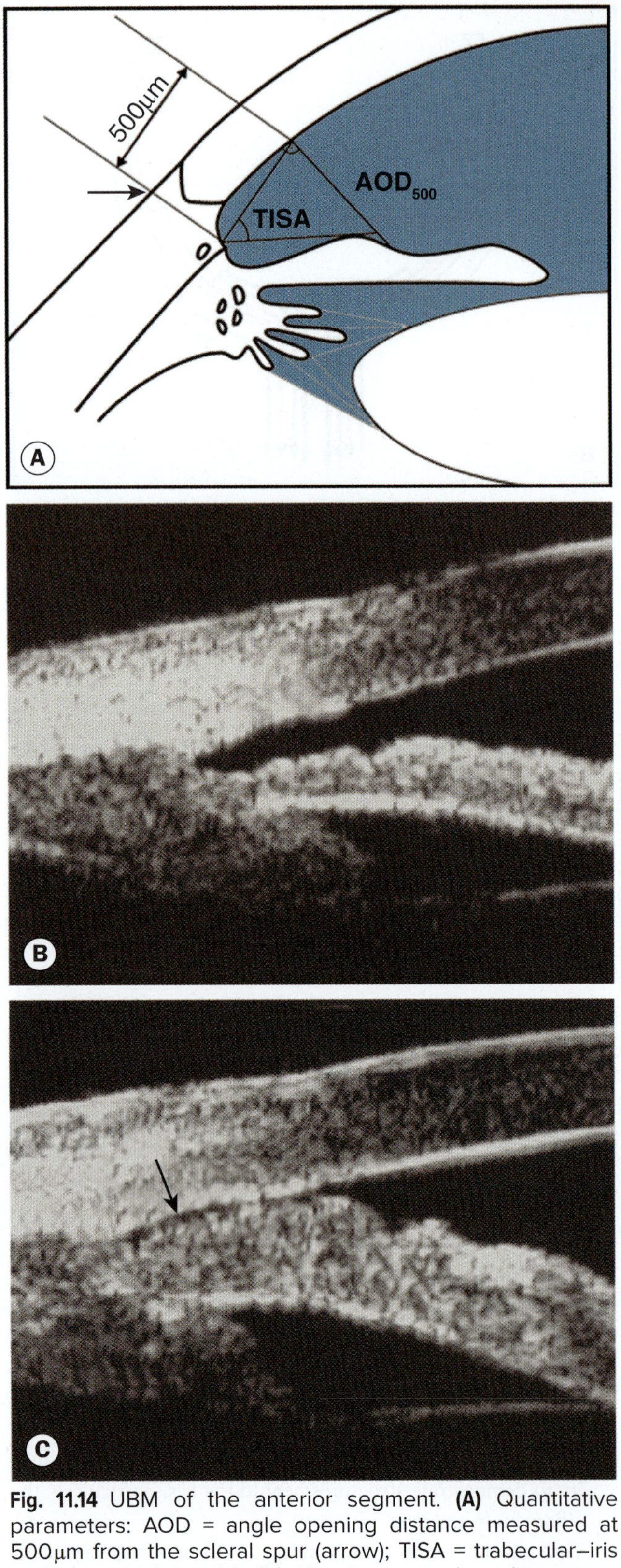

Fig. 11.14 UBM of the anterior segment. **(A)** Quantitative parameters: AOD = angle opening distance measured at 500μm from the scleral spur (arrow); TISA = trabecular–iris surface area (triangle); **(B)** showing normal angle appearance; **(C)** showing closed angle (arrow).

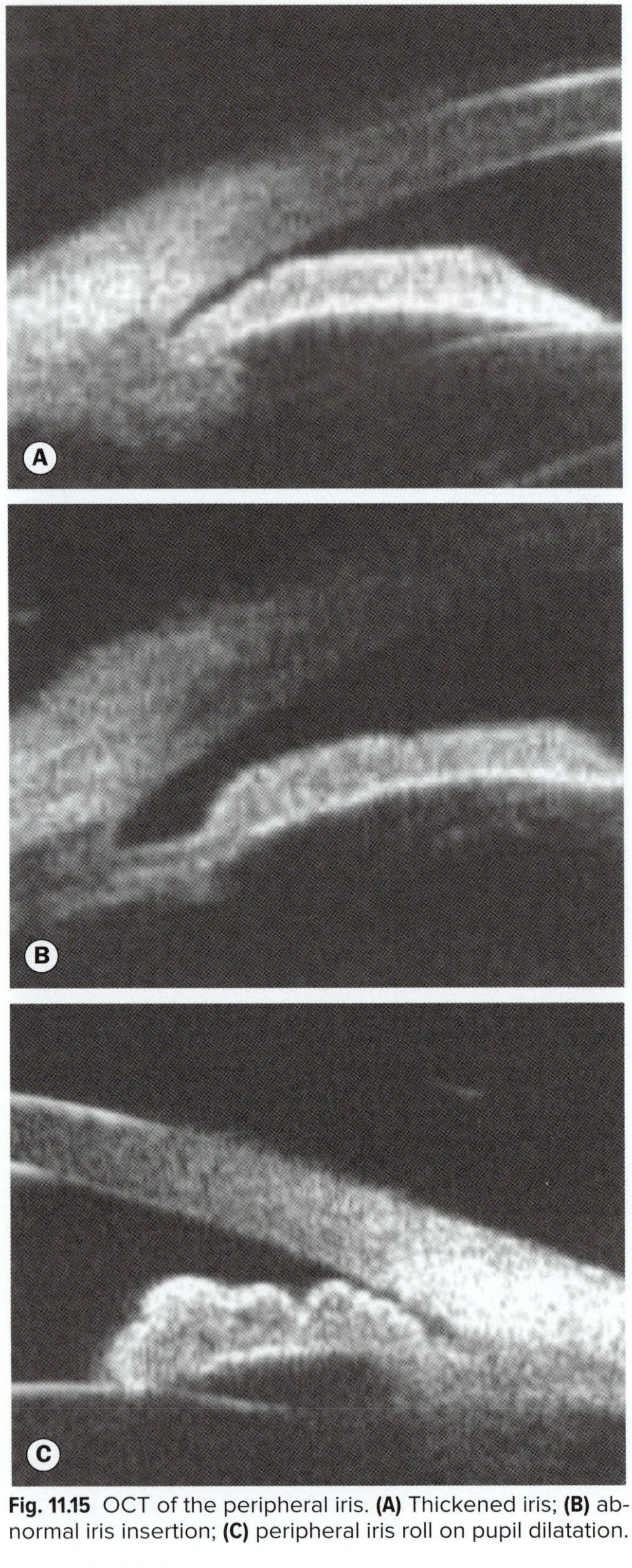

Fig. 11.15 OCT of the peripheral iris. **(A)** Thickened iris; **(B)** abnormal iris insertion; **(C)** peripheral iris roll on pupil dilatation.

- **Anterior chamber depth measurement.** Objective measurement of the depth of the AC is often clinically useful in glaucoma management. Indications include assessment of PAC risk and monitoring of progression in conditions where the AC is shallow, such as post-trabeculectomy hypotony and ciliolenticular block. Older methods used a slit lamp with or without a special attachment, but an accurate and repeatable measurement can be obtained using OCT, ultrasonographic or optical interferometric methods (e.g. Zeiss IOLMaster).
- **Optical coherence tomography of the posterior pole.** OCT is most useful when the patient is either a glaucoma suspect or has early–moderate disease (Fig. 11.16). It can be used to detect damage and progression (Fig. 11.17). In advanced glaucoma it is less helpful because of the 'floor' effect (i.e. when the retinal nerve fibre layer reaches 45–50 µm it does not decrease any further even though progressive damage may be occurring). Macular thickness measurements may be more helpful in these circumstances. Sensitivity and specificity utilizing comparison with a normative database is as high as 90%.
  - Peripapillary RNFL. This involves the acquisition of a circular scan of the retina around the optic nerve head. Because different OCT devices use different scanning protocols, caution should be taken when comparing RNFL thickness between machines. By using the Bruch membrane opening rather than the optic disc margin, centration of the image can be enhanced. The results are compared to a colour-coded normative database. When assessing structural changes over time, it is often difficult to distinguish between glaucomatous change and measurement variability or age-related structural loss. Up to 4 µm inter-test fluctuation has been reported. A new defect, widening of an established defect or deepening of a defect are important features of glaucomatous change.
  - Optic nerve head. Radial cross-sectional scans permit an objective and repeatable assessment of disc morphology, with reasonable discriminatory value. This function is less commonly used than RNFL.
  - Ganglion cell complex (GCC) analysis involves measurement of the thickness of the RNFL, the ganglion cell layer and the inner plexiform layer at the macula in order to detect early glaucomatous damage and avoids the confounding effect of optic disc anatomical variation. This is as effective for diagnosing glaucoma and assessing progression as analysis of the RNFL. OCT signal quality is good, particularly in the elderly and diseased eye. It should be considered supplementary to RNFL assessment (Figs 11.18 and 11.19).
  - Progression analysis software has been introduced on several machines and provides a computed assessment of the extent of damage over time. Trend-based analysis using a number of scans, measures the shape of change and is particularly useful when confirming that progressive change has occurred.

TIP OCT imaging of the optic disc should not be used in isolation but rather to supplement the findings of clinical examination.

- **Confocal scanning laser ophthalmoscopy.** This employs a scanning laser ophthalmoscope (SLO) to build a three-dimensional image of the optic nerve head and retina.
  - The Heidelberg Retinal Tomograph (HRT) is still in widespread clinical practice, but has been superseded by optical coherence tomography. As with the OCT, it is used to distinguish normal from glaucomatous eyes by comparison against a normative database (Moorfields regression analysis) and to monitor disease progression.
  - Keratometry values must be entered and significant (>1.0 dioptre) astigmatism corrected by means of a cylindrical lens. High-quality images can usually be acquired without pupillary dilatation and through mild–moderate lens opacity. After image capture, for greatest accuracy the operator should manually mark the contour line that defines the edge of the neuroretinal rim.
  - Images, data and analysis can be examined on a computer screen or print-out (Fig. 11.20).
  - Detailed stereometric data are presented, with abnormal readings identified.
- **Scanning laser polarimetry.** The GDx (Glaucoma Diagnosis) VCC (variable corneal compensation) RNFL analyser assesses the nerve fibre layer thickness by using its 'birefringent' (resolving or splitting a light wave into two unequally reflected or transmitted waves) nature to change the polarization of incident polarized diode laser light. The amount of alteration is directly related to the thickness of the layer.
  - A display provides colour images of the optic nerve head, together with RNFL maps in four quadrants. Deviation maps show the location and magnitude of RNFL defects as tiny colour-coded squares and parameters for each eye are displayed in a table (Fig. 11.21).
  - A global value based on the entire thickness map is the optimal parameter for discriminating normal from glaucoma.
  - This technology has been superseded in recent years by OCT.

TIP Imaging has become an indispensable tool in the management of patients with glaucoma.

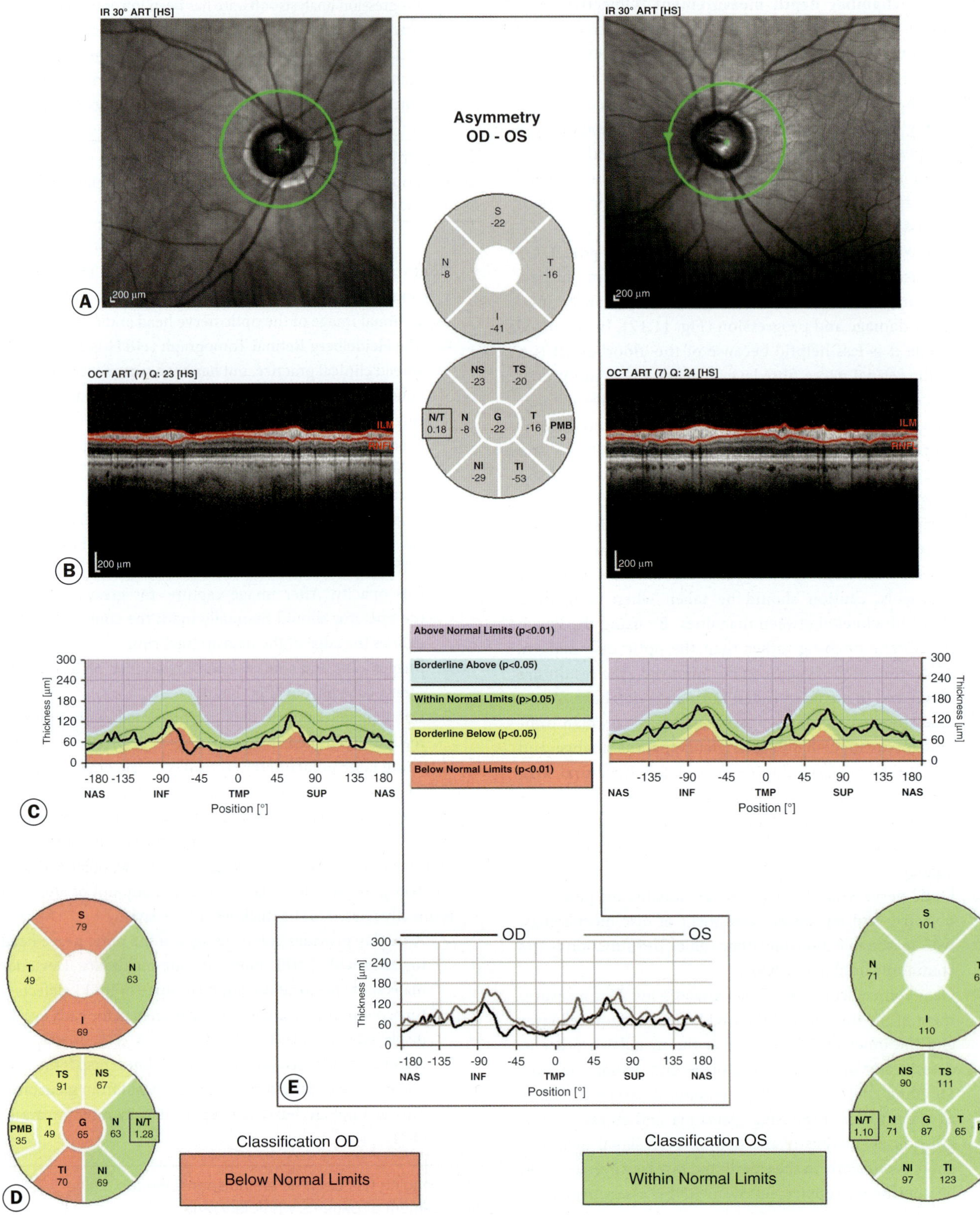

Fig. 11.16 Heidelberg spectralis OCT of the optic disc showing retinal nerve fibre layer thinning above and below the disc on the right. The left optic disc shows no abnormality. **(A)** Disc morphology, showing the green circle of 3.46 mm in diameter which is used as the reference point for the evaluation of the RNFL thickness; **(B)** internal/external limits of the RNFL; **(C)** cross-sectional graph of RNFL thickness in quadrants: Temporal, Superior, Nasal, Inferior, Temporal measurements (TSNIT graph); **(D)** thickness values in micrometres; **(E)** right versus left measurements in micrometres (μm).

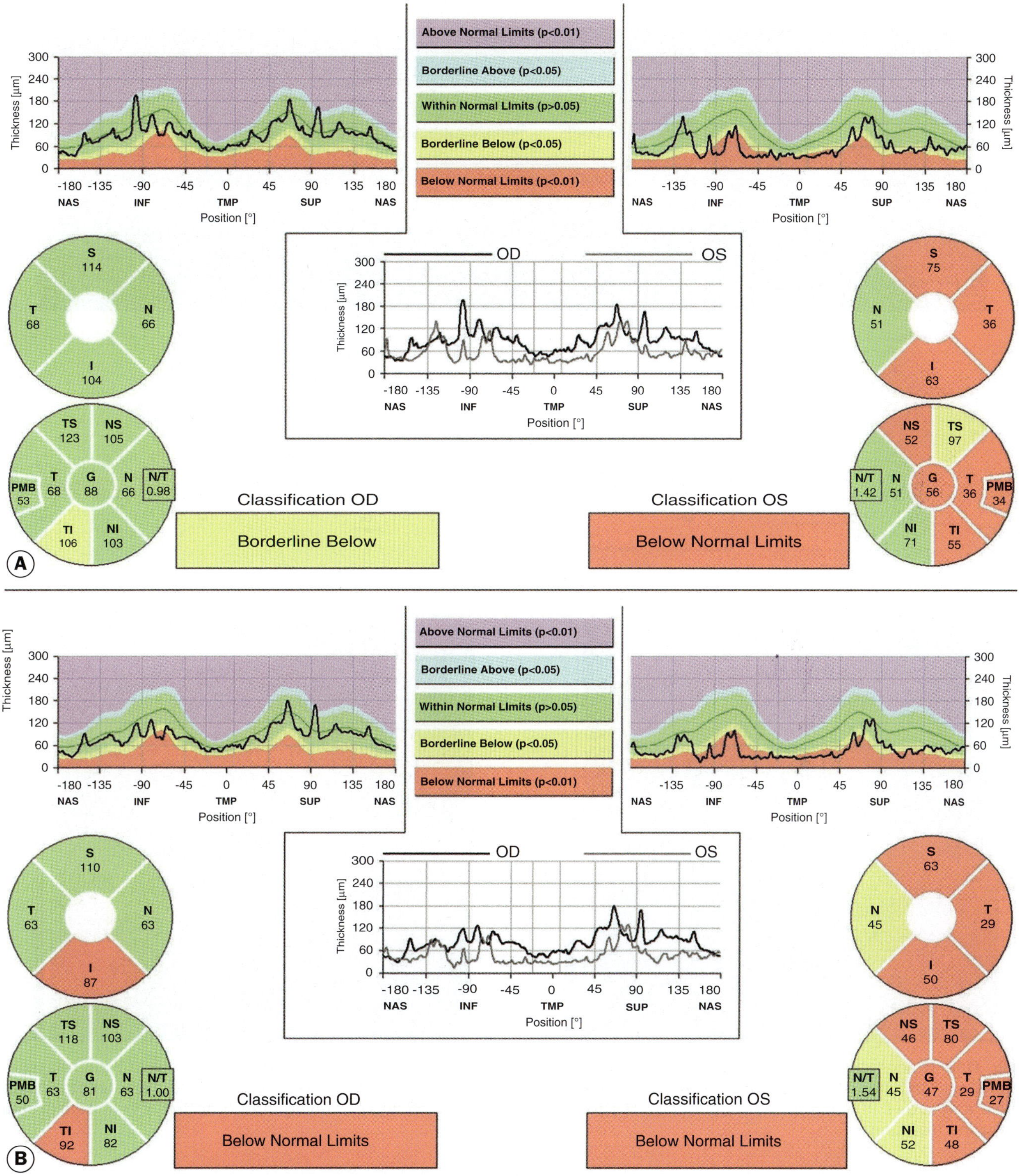

Fig. 11.17 Heidelberg spectralis OCT of the optic disc. **(A)** At presentation; **(B)** after 2 years showing progressive RNFL thinning.

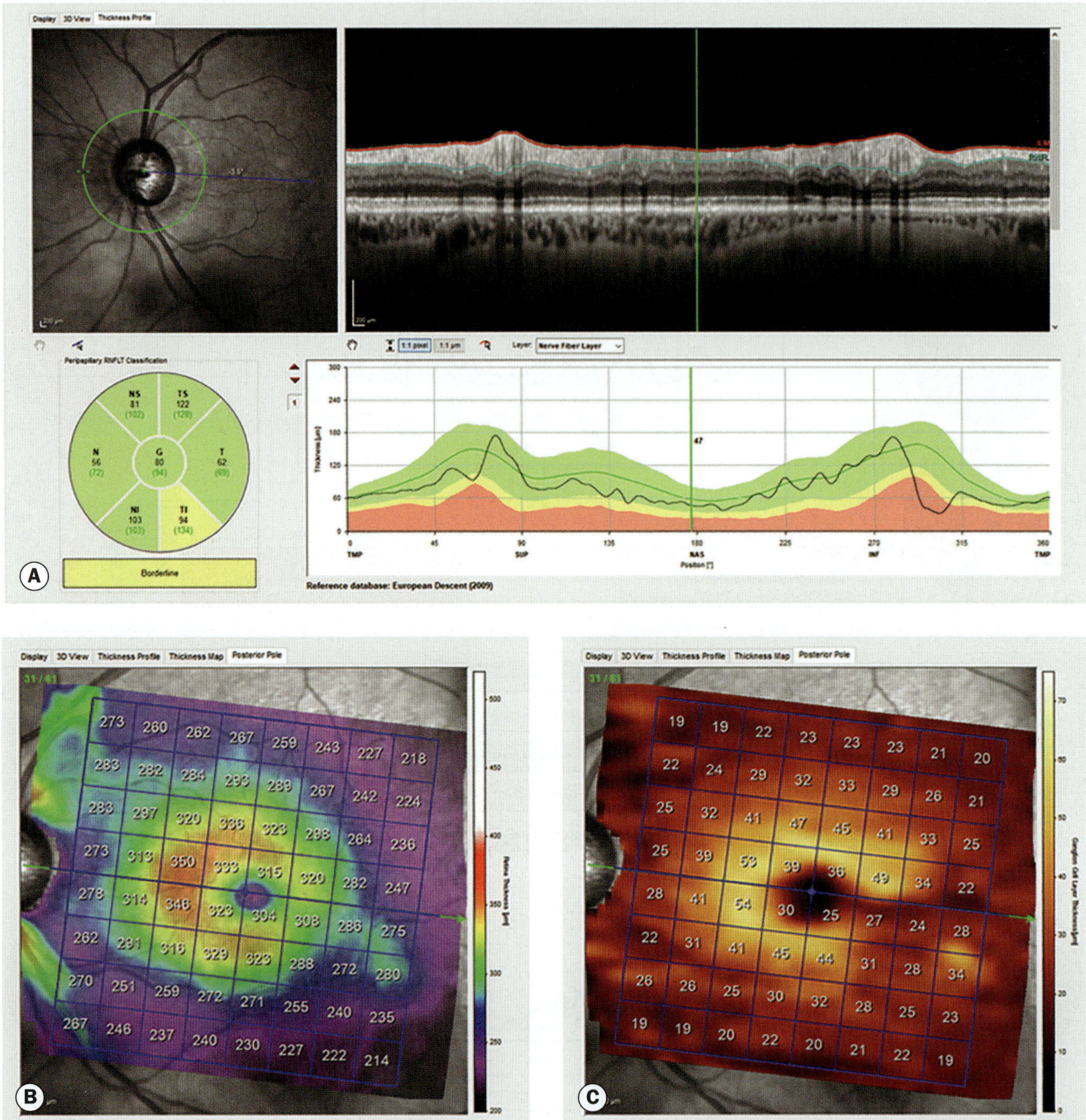

Fig. 11.18 Heidelberg spectralis OCT of the optic disc and macula in early glaucoma. **(A)** Infero-temporal retinal nerve fibre layer thinning; **(B)** the scanned area (containing 65 individual square cells) corresponds to 200 of the central visual field and shows thinning of the retina below the fovea; **(C)** ganglion cell layer thinning inferior to the fovea measured in micrometres (μm).

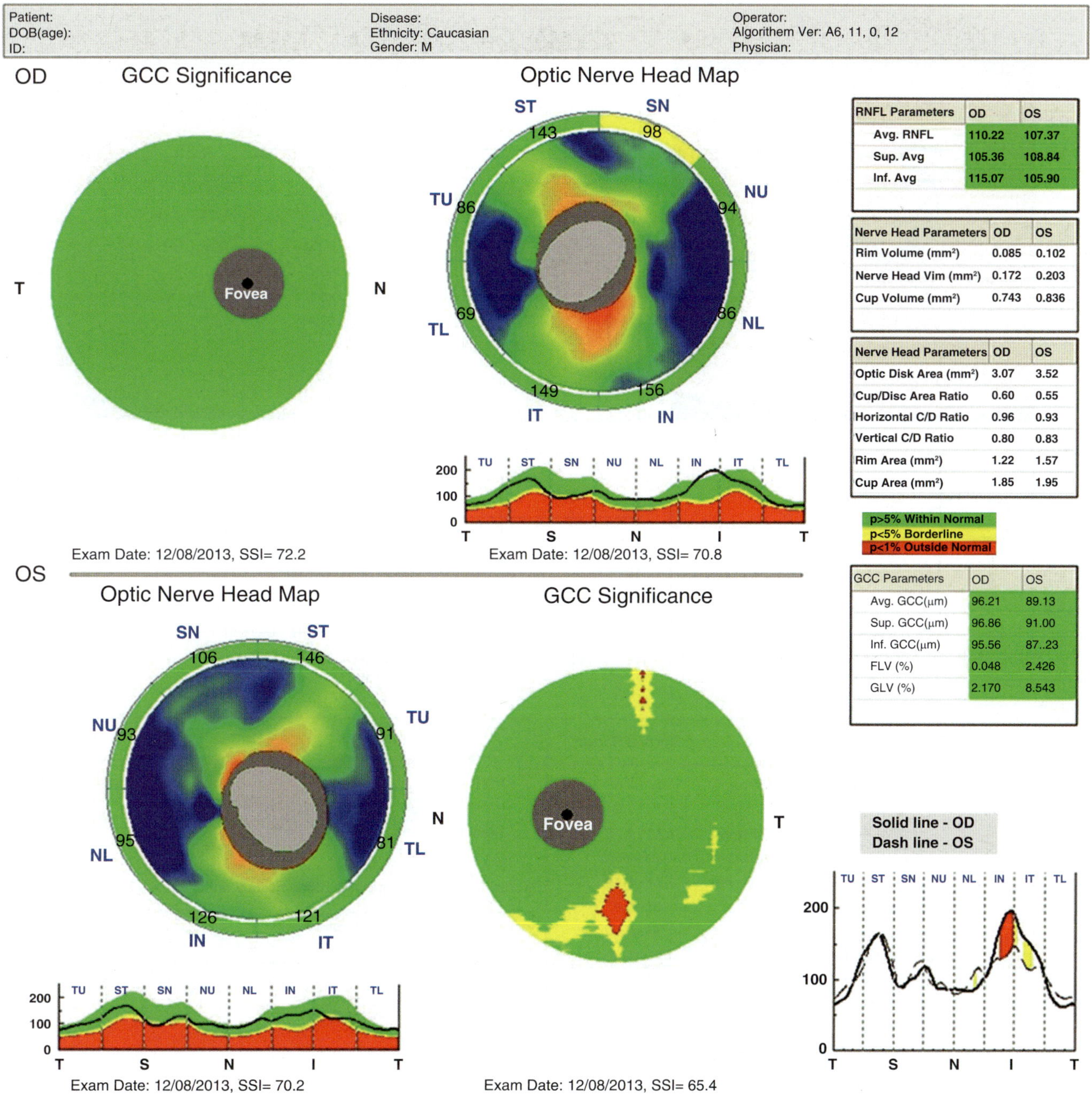

Fig. 11.19 XR Avanti spectral domain glaucoma-protocol OCT showing optic nerve head, peripapillary retinal nerve fibre layer and ganglion cell complex analysis. FLV = focal loss volume (%); GLV = global loss volume (%).

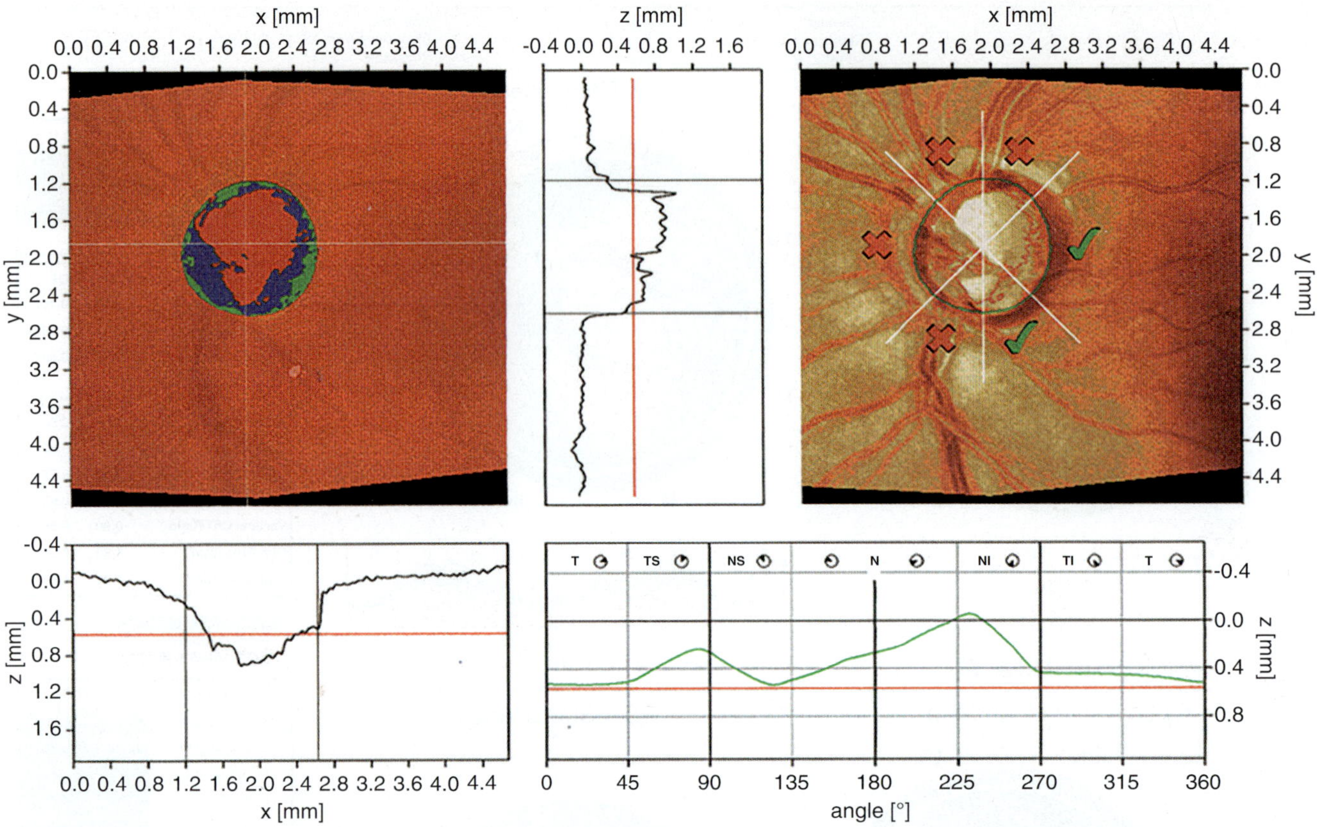

Stereometric Analysis ONH		Normal Range
Disk Area	1.658 mm²	1.69 - 2.82
Cup Area	0.883 mm²	0.26 - 1.27
Rim Area	**0.775 mm²**	**1.20 - 1.78**
Cup Volume	0.146 cmm	-0.01 - 0.49
Rim Volume	**0.129 cmm**	**0.24 - 0.49**
Cup/Disk Area Ratio	0.532	0.16 - 0.47
Linear Cup/Disk Rstio	0.730	0.36 - 0.80
Mean Cup Depth	0.257 mm	0.14- 0.38
Maximum Cup Depth	0.567 mm	0.46- 0.90
Cup Shape Measure	**-0.059**	**-0.27 - -0.09**
Height Variation Contour	**0.591 mm**	**0.30 - 0.47**
Mean RNFL Thickness	**0.202 mm**	**0.18 - 0.31**
RNFL Cross Sectional Area	0.924 mm²	0.95 - 1.61
Reference Height	0.562 mm	
Topography Std Dev.	35 μm	

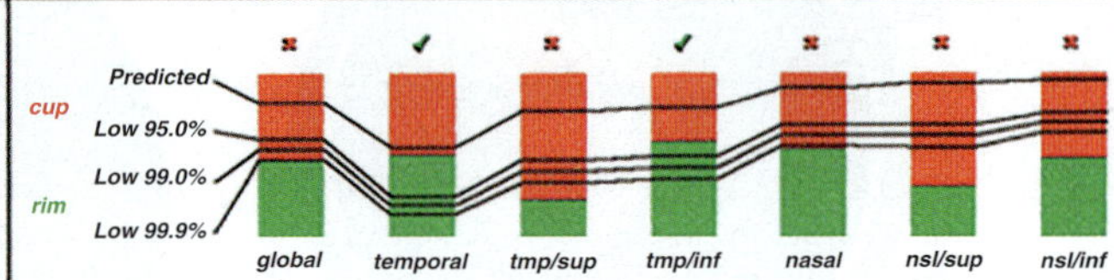

Moorfields Classification: Outside normal limits (*)

(*) Moorfields regression classification (Ophthalmology 1998:105:1557-1563), Classification based on statistics. Diagnosis is physician's responsibility.

Comments:

Date: **Signature:**

Software: IR1-V1.7/2641

Fig. 11.20 Heidelberg Retinal Tomograph of the disc of a glaucomatous eye.

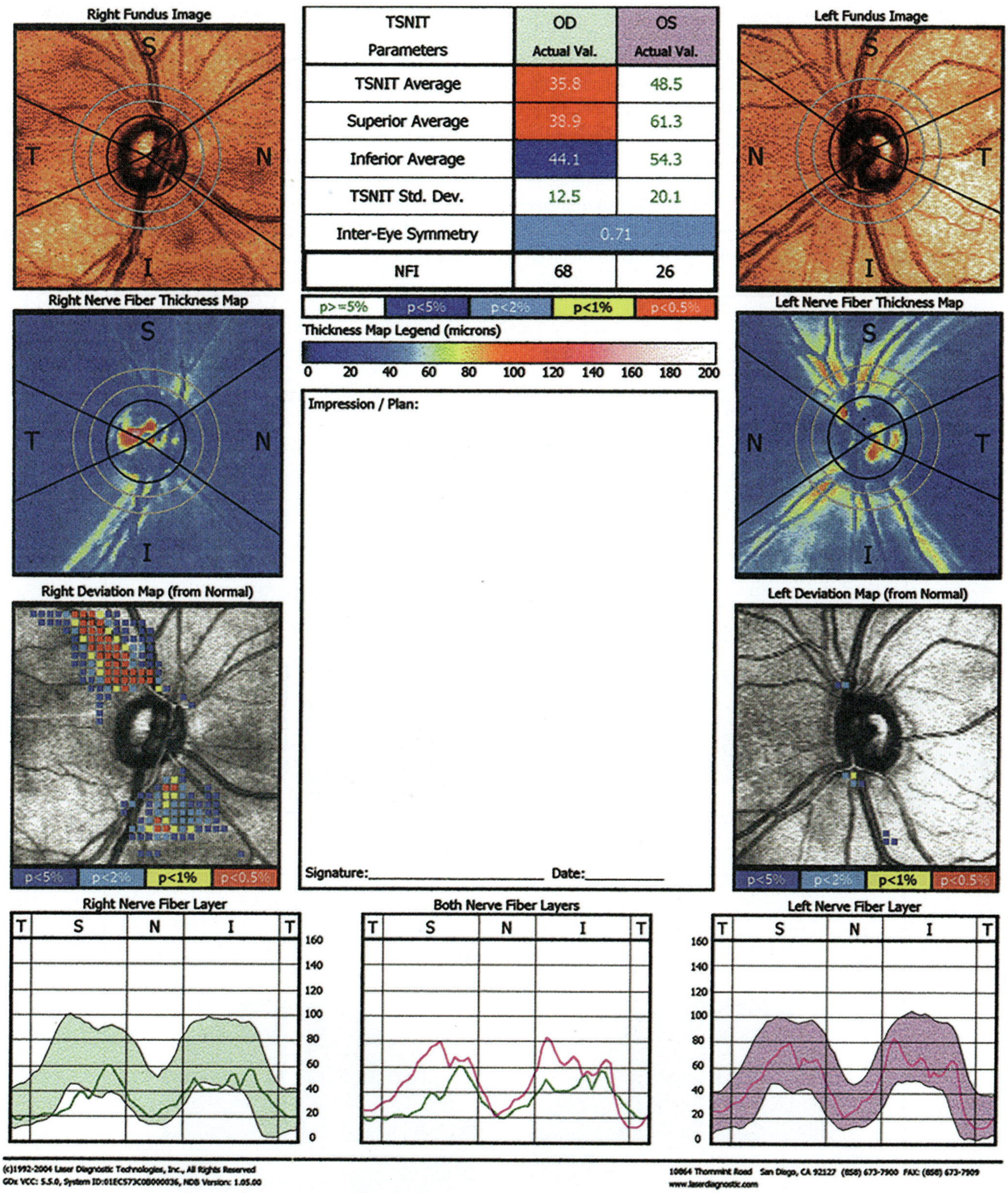

Fig. 11.21 GDx VCC (variable corneal compensation) showing reduction in retinal nerve fibre density in the right eye and abnormal parameters.

Visual field defects (see Ch. 1, perimetry)

Nerve damage in glaucoma is believed to be inflicted at the optic nerve head and the resultant visual field defect corresponds to the pattern of fibres in the retinal area served. Standard automated perimetry (SAP) is relatively insensitive in the early stages of the disease.

- **Early changes** include increased variability of responses in areas that subsequently develop defects and slight asymmetry between the two eyes. Special modalities such as frequency doubling technology (FDT) and short wavelength automated perimetry (SWAP) may demonstrate defects at an earlier stage.
- **Small paracentral depressions** (Fig. 11.22A) can form at a relatively early stage, often superonasally. They are more commonly seen in NTG.
- **Nasal step** represents a difference in sensitivity above and below the horizontal midline in the nasal field. The defect is bounded by the horizontal midline, corresponding to the retinal nerve fibre layer horizontal raphe. Inferior optic disc and OCT changes with a corresponding superior nasal step are shown in Fig. 11.22B.

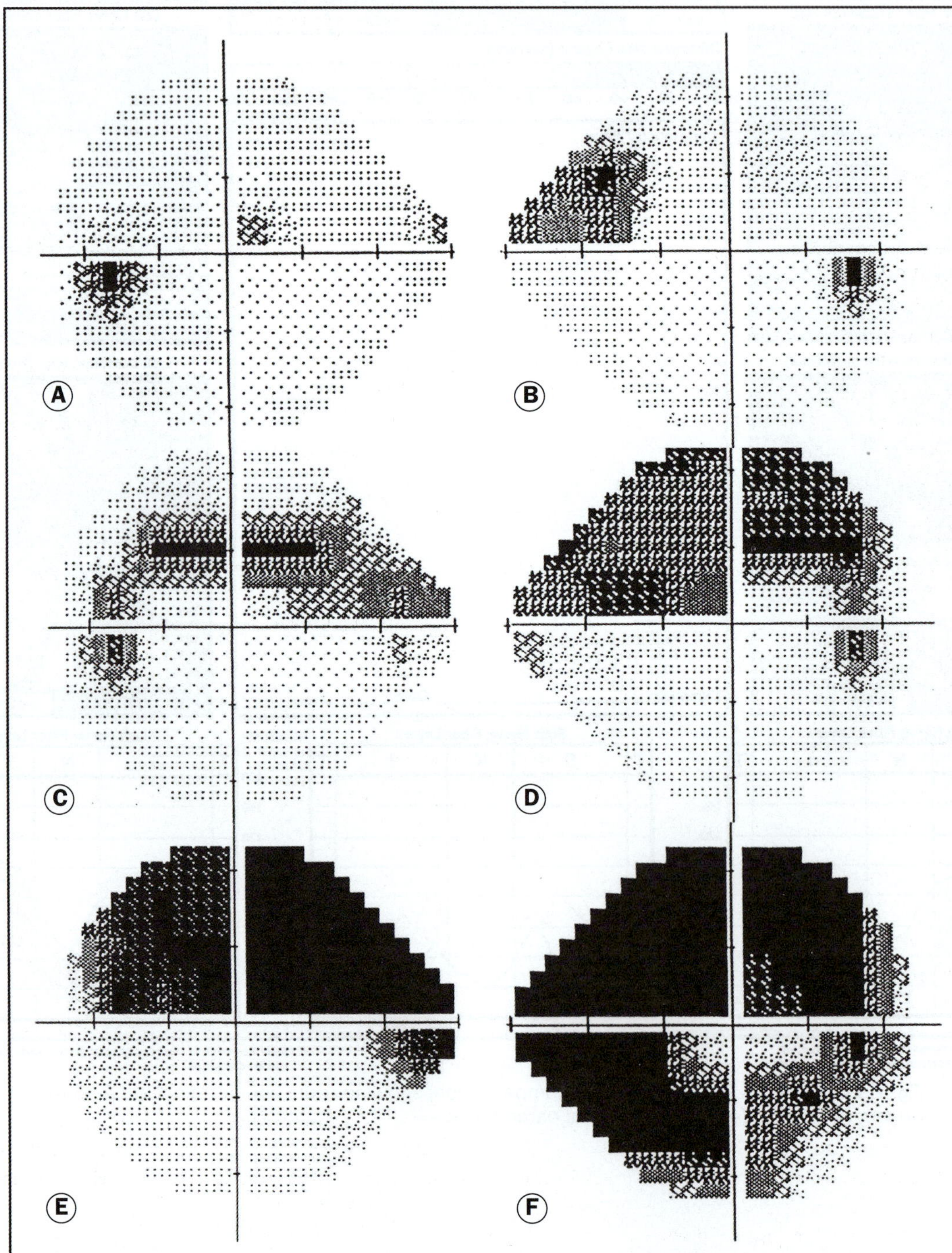

Fig. 11.22 (A–F) Grey-scale display showing progression of glaucomatous damage in different patients (see text).

- **Temporal wedge** is less common than a nasal step but has similar implications.
- **Arcuate defects** (Fig. 11.22C) develop as a result of coalescence of paracentral scotomas. They typically develop between 10° and 20° of fixation as downward or upward extensions from the blind spot around fixation. With time, they tend to elongate circumferentially along the distribution of arcuate nerve fibres (Fig. 11.22D and E).
- **A ring scotoma** develops when superior and inferior arcuate defects become continuous, usually in advanced glaucoma (Fig. 11.22F).
- **End-stage** changes are characterized by a small island of central vision, typically accompanied by a temporal island. The 10-2 perimetry pattern facilitates monitoring of the residual central field.
- **Minimal criteria for glaucomatous damage on SAP.** One of the following defects on Humphrey visual field testing (Hodapp, Parrish and Anderson's criteria)
  - Glaucoma hemifield test outside normal limits on at least two consecutive occasions. This provides information concerning differences between superior and inferior halves of the visual field by evaluating threshold at mirror-image points above and below the horizontal meridian. This program also compares the overall height of the hill of vision with age-adjusted normal values.
  - A cluster of three or more non-edge points in a location typical for glaucoma, all of which are depressed on PSD at P <5% level and one which is depressed at P <1% level, on two consecutive occasions (Fig. 11.23).
  - Corrected PSD that occurs in less than 5% of normal individuals on two consecutive fields.
- **Summary measures** should always be considered. On average, an annual deterioration in mean total deviation of just over 1.0 dB can be expected in untreated patients, but there is significant individual variation (see 'Natural history of open-angle glaucoma' above) (Fig. 11.24).
- **Staging.** A discrete-levels staging system can be used to determine the stage of damage. Early glaucomatous loss is a MD of < −6 dB (Fig. 11.25), moderate glaucomatous loss −6 to −12 dB (Fig. 11.26) and severe glaucomatous loss > −12 dB (Fig. 11.27). Any absolute defect (0 dB) in the central 5 degrees is considered 'severe'.

Pattern ERG (pERG)

The electroretinogram (ERG) measures the electrical activity of the retina in response to a light stimulus (see Ch.15). Pattern ERG (pERG) uses a similar stimulus to that used when measuring visual evoked potential (pattern reversal) and targets macular ganglion cell function. It is an objective measure of retinal function that can be recorded non-invasively under physiological conditions.

- **Accurate refraction** and a clear ocular media are important for pERG measurements.
- **The pERG waveform** consists of a small negative deflection near 35 ms (N35 component), a positive deflection near 50 ms (P50 component) and a positive deflection near 95 ms (N95 component). The amplitude and implicit time of each of these components can be measured. The M95 component is reduced in glaucoma.
- **Clinical uses.** This technology detects subtle optic neuropathy and may have a role to play in the follow-up of some patients with glaucoma. It is not a substitute for clinical examination, visual field testing and OCT examination of the RNFL. Steady state pattern ERG may demonstrate: (a) decline of ganglion cell function, (b) treatment response, (c) recovery of ganglion cell function (Fig. 11.28).

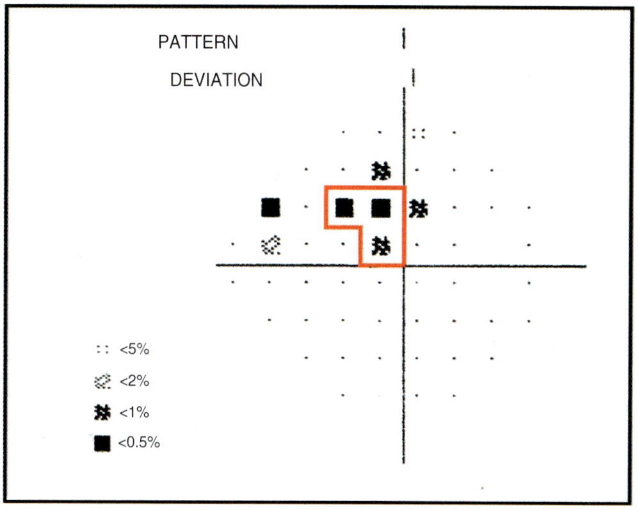

Fig. 11.23 Positive diagnostic criterion for glaucoma showing a cluster of three non-edged points.

Management

The primary aim of treatment is to prevent functional impairment of vision within the patient's lifetime and to maintain a good quality of life by slowing the rate of ganglion cell loss. Currently the only proven method of achieving this is to reduce IOP. Both higher mean IOP and substantial variation in IOP are predictive of progressive visual field loss in patients with glaucoma, whether newly diagnosed or advanced.

Patient instruction

An explanation should be offered concerning the nature of the disease and relevant literature provided. The timing of medication use should be specified, and the patient educated in the technique of eye drop instillation. At follow-up visits the patient's proficiency at instilling drops should be checked. In order to maximize drug contact time with the anterior segment and to minimize systemic absorption, the patient should be instructed either to perform lacrimal sac occlusion by applying fingertip pressure at the medial canthus or to close the eyes for about 3 minutes after instillation. Common or severe potential adverse effects should be explained at the commencement of treatment and their occurrence enquired about at review visits.

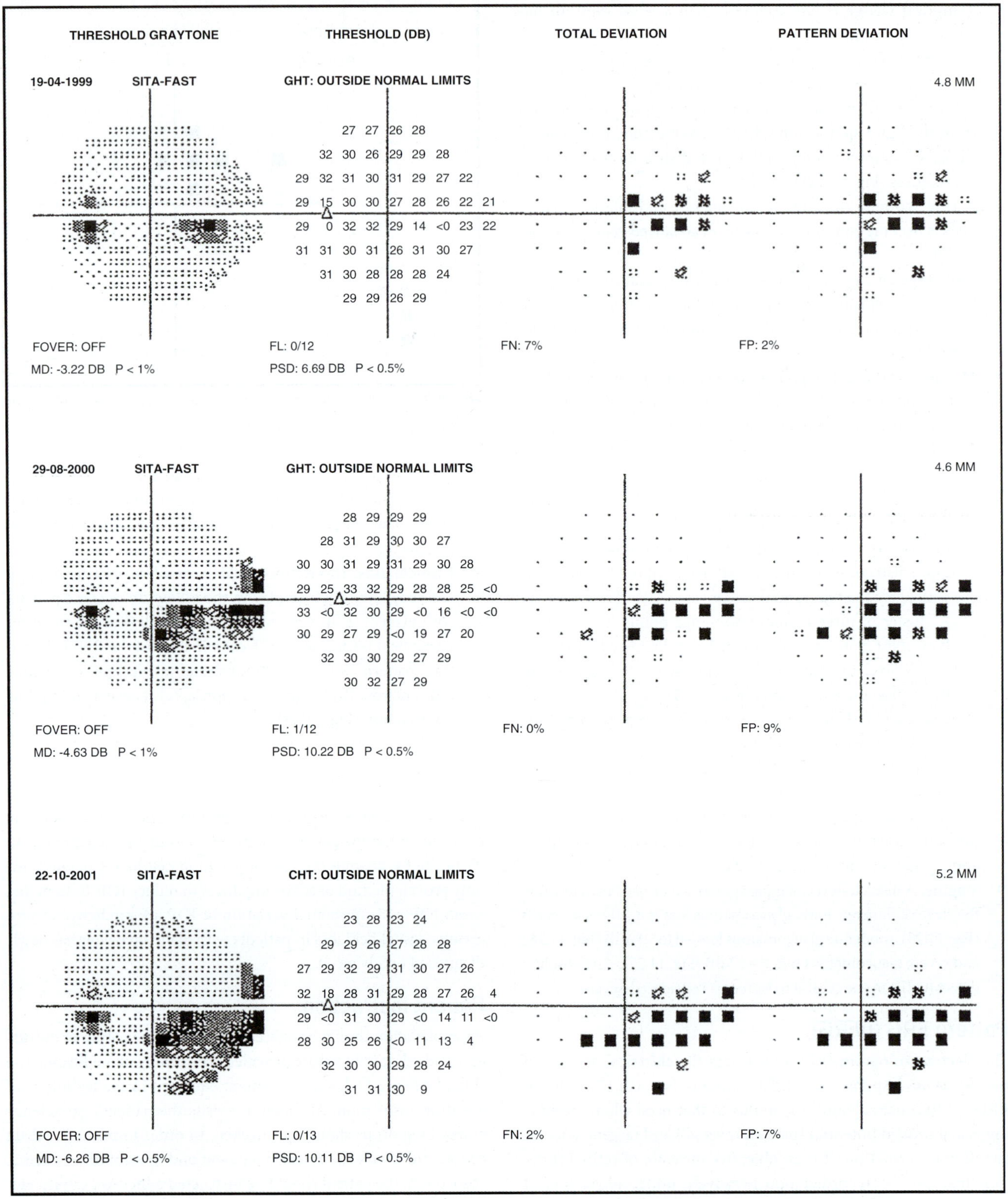

Fig. 11.24 Progression of visual field defect and deterioration of global indices over a period of 30 months.

Treatment goals

- **Target pressure.** It is assumed that the pre-treatment level of IOP has damaged the optic nerve and will continue to do so. An IOP level is identified below which further damage is considered unlikely: the target pressure. This is identified considering the severity of existing damage (particularly a greater vertical C/D ratio and a higher mean deviation on visual fields), the level of IOP, CCT, the rapidity with which damage occurred if known and the age and general health of the patient. Greater age is associated with a higher likelihood of rapid progression, but a shorter life expectancy may also influence management. Therapy should maintain the IOP at or below the target level. If not achievable by conservative measures, a decision is made on whether to proceed to surgery or to continue monitoring with an above-target IOP.
- A **reasonable initial goal** is to reduce the IOP to less than 18 mmHg. This is based on the results of the Advanced Glaucoma Intervention Study (AGIS), which found that significant visual field progression is unlikely to occur in most patients in the medium term if IOP can be kept below 18 mmHg at all times.
- **Progression risk,** as found by the EMGT, is influenced by: (a) magnitude of initial IOP reduction, (b) height of the baseline IOP, (c) presence of pseudoexfoliation syndrome, (d) presence of bilateral disease, (e) worse mean deviation, (f) older age.
- **Response to progression.** If damage progresses despite a target pressure having been reached consistently, the target IOP is set to a lower level. As damage progresses, the loss of each remaining ganglion cell has a greater proportional impact on visual function and there is less reserve capacity. If further visual loss occurs despite apparently good IOP control, surgery should be considered.

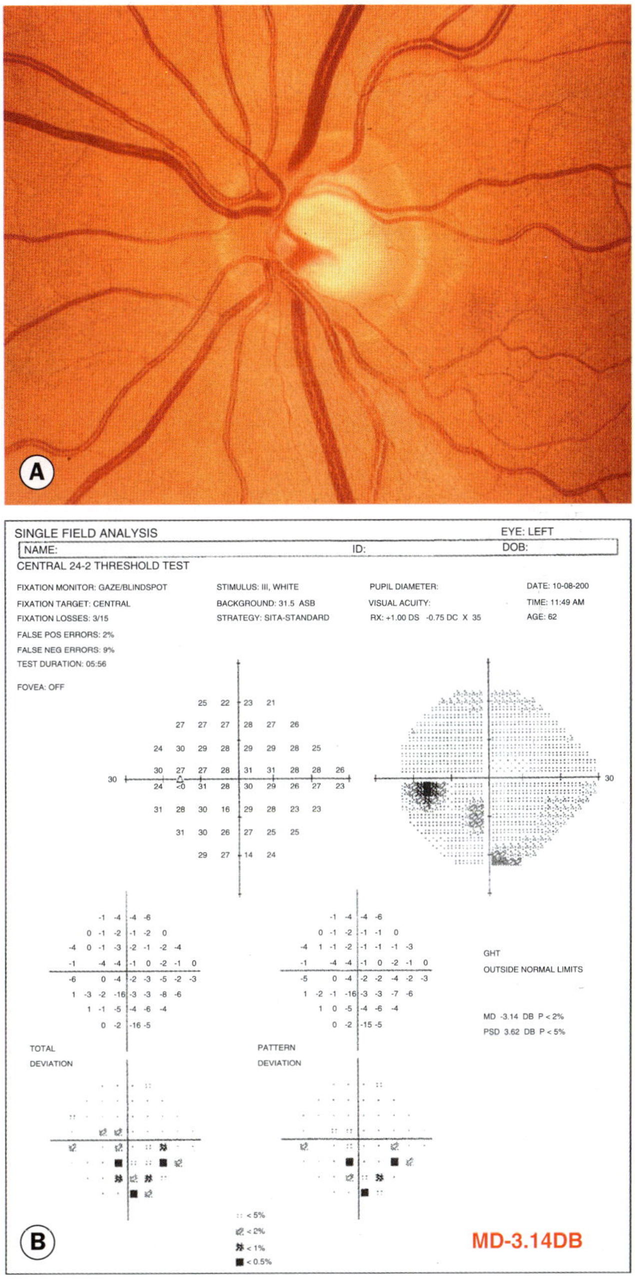

Fig. 11.25 Mild glaucomatous damage. **(A)** Minimal cupping; **(B)** paracentral scotoma.

Medical therapy

See later in this chapter.

- **Commencing medical therapy**
  - Any drug chosen should be prescribed in the lowest concentration consistent with the desired therapeutic effect and administered as infrequently as possible.
  - Ideally the drug with the fewest potential side effects should be used.
  - Initial treatment is usually with one type of medication, typically a prostaglandin analogue or beta-blocker.
- **Review**
  - The interval to review after starting medication is set according to the individual patient, but is usually 4–8 weeks.
  - Response to the drug is assessed against the target IOP.
  - If the response is satisfactory, subsequent assessment is generally set for a further 3–6 months.
  - If there has been little or no response the initial drug is withdrawn and another substituted.
  - If there has been an apparently incomplete response another drug may be added or a fixed combination substituted.
  - When two separate drugs are used the patient should be instructed to wait 5 minutes before instilling the second drug to prevent washout of the first.
  - Sometimes it may be worthwhile to allow a further month or two of treatment before altering a regimen, as response may improve over time.
  - Inadequate drop instillation technique should be considered as a cause of unsatisfactory IOP response.
  - Poor adherence should always be borne in mind, e.g. if progression occurs despite excellent IOP readings at review assessments.

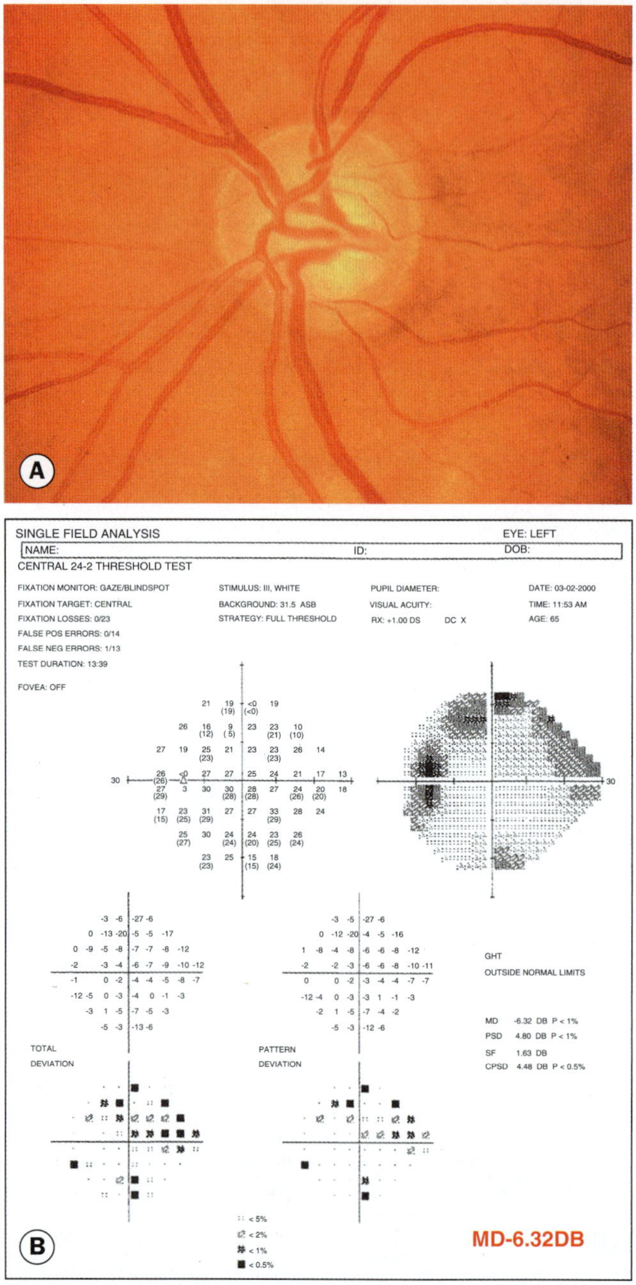

Fig. 11.26 Moderate glaucomatous damage. **(A)** Moderate cupping; **(B)** arcuate scotoma.

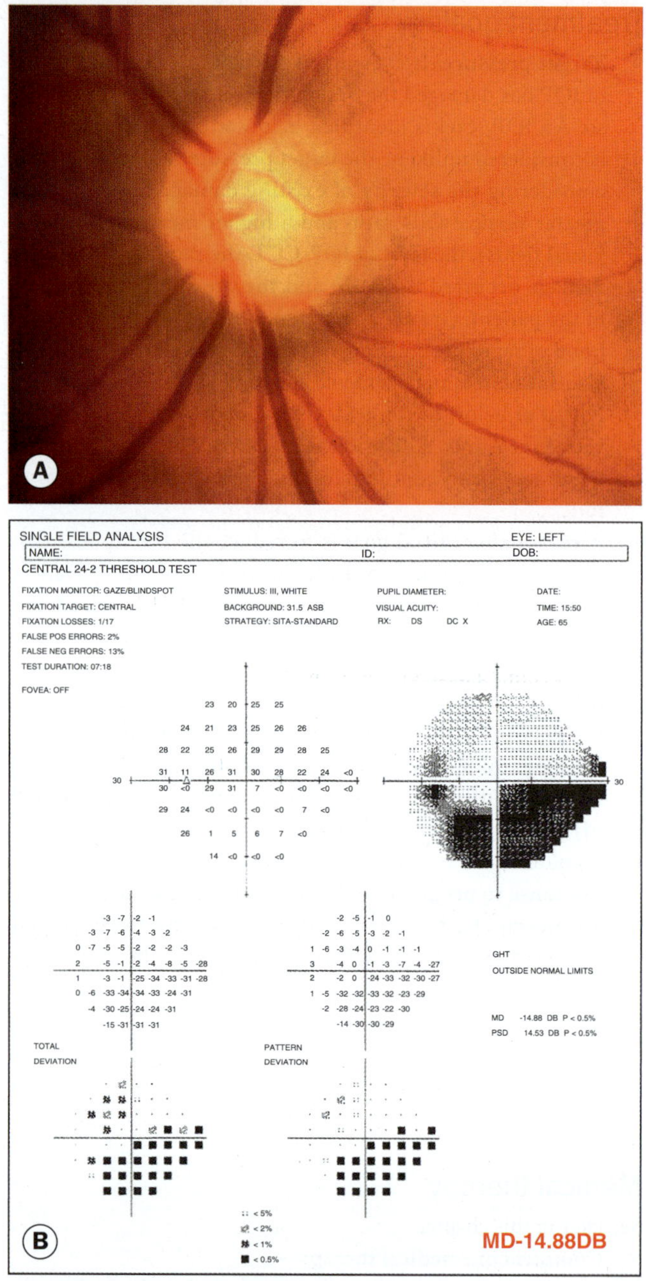

Fig. 11.27 Severe glaucomatous damage. **(A)** Marked cupping; **(B)** extensive visual field loss.

- When drops are administered in the morning, it is good practice always to ask whether that day's dose has been used prior to attendance.

- **Perimetry.** If IOP control is good and glaucomatous damage mild or moderate with no substantial threat to central vision, perimetry every 6–12 months is generally sufficient.
- **Gonioscopy** should be performed annually in most patients because the anterior chamber angle tends to narrow with age.
- **Optic disc examination** should be performed at each visit, as a disc haemorrhage may indicate ongoing damage. A new haemorrhage should be recorded pictorially, optimally by photography.
- **Serial imaging** is increasingly viewed as standard care.
- **Causes of treatment failure**
  - Inappropriate target pressure. If the IOP is maintained in the upper part of the statistically normal range, progressive field loss is relatively common.
  - Poor adherence to the therapeutic regimen occurs in at least 25% of patients.
  - Wide fluctuations in IOP are not uncommon in patients treated medically and are associated with a tendency to progression.
  - Patients may deteriorate despite apparently good IOP control. Causes include occult adherence failure, undetected diurnal variation and possibly other mechanisms not

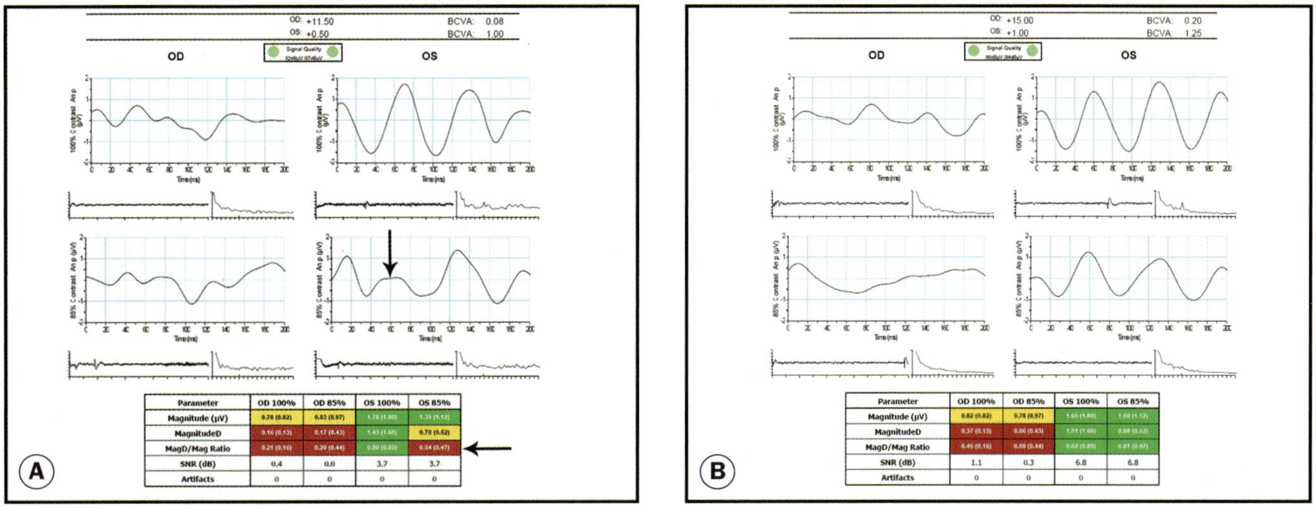

Fig. 11.28 Pattern ERG in glaucoma. **(A)** Previous injury right eye and primary angle-closure left eye with a full visual field, showing steady state pERG responses before treatment (arrows indicate abnormality); **(B)** 4 months after successful treatment, showing recovery of responses, presumably secondary to improvement of ganglion cell function in the left eye. *(Courtesy of T Devogelaere.)*

readily detectable clinically such as impaired optic nerve perfusion. The possibility of an alternative pathology, particularly a compressive lesion, should always be considered in these circumstances.

- **Laser trabeculoplasty** (see later in this chapter). Selective laser trabeculoplasty (SLT) is as effective as medical monotherapy in reducing the IOP. Based on the 6-year results of the LiGHT trial (which shows that SLT results in reduced progression rates, cost-saving and improved quality of life compared to topical medication) SLT has recently been recommended as first-line treatment in patients with newly diagnosed ocular hypertension and chronic open-angle glaucoma.
- **Surgery** (see later in this chapter). Trabeculectomy is the surgical procedure most commonly performed for POAG. In recent years the threshold for glaucoma drainage device implantation has been lowered by many surgeons. Non-penetrating surgery (e.g. deep sclerectomy, viscocanalostomy) is utilized extensively in POAG by some specialists. There is a role for micro-invasive glaucoma surgery (MIGS) in selected cases of glaucoma. Phacoemulsification alone is frequently associated with a 15% fall in IOP, but is generally only offered to patients in whom significant lens opacity is present. It can be combined with a filtration or a MIGS procedure. Progressive damage is more likely to be slowed after surgery, probably because the resultant IOP is often lower than the preoperative level, is less likely to fluctuate and because adherence is no longer a factor.
- **Prognosis.** Most patients with POAG will not go blind in their lifetime, but the incidence of blindness varies considerably depending on multiple factors such as the presence of advanced damage at diagnosis and non-compliance with treatment. In a White population with POAG the lifetime chance of blindness in both eyes has historically been 5–10%. Given the long-term nature of progression in glaucoma, the prognosis appears to have significantly improved with new treatment strategies. The average period from diagnosis to death has been estimated at around 16 years and only about a third will still be alive 20 years after diagnosis.

NORMAL-TENSION GLAUCOMA

Introduction

NTG, also referred to as low-tension or normal-pressure glaucoma, is usually regarded as a variant of POAG. The distinction between NTG and POAG is based on an epidemiologically derived range of normal IOP. It is an arbitrary division that may not have significant clinical value, though it is possible that a spectrum exists in which, towards the NTG end, IOP-independent factors are of increasing relative importance. Depending on ethnic background, 30–65% of patients with open-angle glaucoma may have an IOP that is within the normal range on initial assessment.

NTG is characterized by:

- IOP consistently equal to or less than 21 mmHg on diurnal testing.
- Signs of optic nerve damage in a characteristic glaucomatous pattern.
- Visual field loss as damage progresses, consistent in pattern with the nerve appearance.
- An open anterior chamber angle.
- No features of secondary glaucoma or a non-glaucomatous cause for the neuropathy.

Pathogenesis

Any aetiological factors distinct from those in POAG have not been conclusively determined, although various mechanisms have been postulated including anomalies of local and systemic vascular function, structural optic nerve anomalies and autoimmune disease. With the introduction of widespread CCT assessment, NTG in some patients can be explained by very low CCT.

Overall CCT in patients with NTG is lower than in POAG. A small proportion of NTG patients have been found to have marked nocturnal IOP spikes, sometimes only detected on testing in the supine position.

Risk factors

- **Age.** Patients tend to be older than those with POAG, though this may be due to delayed diagnosis.
- **Gender.** Some studies have found a higher prevalence in females.
- **Race.** NTG occurs more frequently in Japanese people.
- **Family history.** The prevalence of POAG is greater in families of patients with NTG than in the normal population. Mutations in the *OPTN* gene coding for optineurin have been identified in some patients with NTG, though also in patients with POAG.
- **CCT** is lower in patients with NTG than POAG.
- **Abnormal vasoregulation**, particularly migraine and Raynaud phenomenon, has been found more commonly in NTG than POAG by some investigators. However, others have found abnormalities just as commonly in POAG. Systemic diseases associated with vascular risk, such as diabetes, carotid insufficiency, hypertension and hypercoagulability may also be important.
- **Systemic hypotension** including nocturnal blood pressure dips of >20%, particularly in those on oral hypotensive medication (Fig. 11.29). The EMGT confirms that low blood pressure is a risk factor in patients with NTG. The duration and magnitude of decrease in nocturnal blood pressure below the daytime mean blood pressure predicts progression in NTG.
- **Obstructive sleep apnoea syndrome** may be associated, perhaps via an effect on ocular perfusion.
- **Autoantibody levels** have been found to be higher in some groups of NTG patients by some investigators.
- **Low serum retinol levels** are more likely to be present in NTG patients.
- **Translaminar pressure gradient.** This may on average be larger than in POAG.
- **Ocular perfusion pressure** may be relatively lower than in POAG.
- **Myopia** is associated with a greater likelihood of glaucoma and of its progression.
- **Thyroid disease** may be more common.

Differential diagnosis

- **Angle closure** should always be ruled out by meticulous dark-room gonioscopy.
- **Low CCT** leading to underestimation of IOP. It is possible that a thin posterior ocular wall may increase mechanical stress in the region of the lamina cribrosa. Prior refractive surgery and corneal ectasia also lead to falsely low IOP readings.
- **POAG** presenting with apparently normal IOP because of wide diurnal fluctuation. Plotting a diurnal IOP curve over an 8-hour period (phasing) during office hours may detect daytime elevation, but detection of nocturnal IOP spikes requires substantial resource commitment.
- **Previous episodes of raised IOP** may have occurred as a result of ocular trauma, uveitis or local or systemic steroid therapy.
- **Masking by systemic treatment** such as an oral beta-blocker, commenced after glaucomatous damage has already been sustained.
- **Spontaneously resolved pigmentary glaucoma.** The typical examination features of pigmentary glaucoma tend to become less evident with increasing age. The IOP in some cases of POAG may also spontaneously normalize over time.
- **Progressive retinal nerve fibre defects not due to glaucoma** such as may occur in myopic degeneration and optic disc drusen.
- **Congenital disc anomalies** simulating glaucomatous cupping, such as a disc pit or coloboma (see Fig. 19.24).
- **Neurological** lesions causing optic nerve or chiasmal compression can produce visual field defects that may be misinterpreted as glaucomatous and neuroimaging should be performed if there is any suspicion, particularly in young patients.
- **Previous anterior ischaemic optic neuropathy (AION), particularly secondary to temporal arteritis** may give rise to a disc appearance and visual field defect consistent with glaucoma (see Fig. 19.14D). Non-arteritic AION often occurs in a 'crowded' disc and the fellow eye should be examined for this. Previous retinal vascular occlusion should also be considered.
- **Previous acute optic nerve insult** such as hypovolaemic or septicaemic shock, or head injury.
- **Miscellaneous optic neuropathies** including inflammatory, infiltrative and drug-induced pathology will often be clinically obvious, but can occasionally masquerade as NTG.

Clinical features

History and examination are essentially the same as for POAG but specific points warrant attention.

- **History**
  - Migraine and Raynaud phenomenon.
  - Episodes of shock.
  - Head or eye injury.
  - Headache and other neurological symptoms (intracranial lesion).
  - Medication, e.g. systemic steroids, beta-blockers.
- **IOP** is usually in the high teens, but may rarely be in the low teens. In asymmetrical disease the more damaged disc typically corresponds to the eye with the higher IOP.
- **Optic nerve head**
  - The optic nerve head tends to be larger on average in NTG than in POAG (Fig. 11.30).
  - The pattern of cupping is similar, but acquired optic disc pits and focal nerve fibre layer defects are more common.
  - Peripapillary atrophic changes may be more prevalent.
  - Splinter haemorrhages on the disc margin are more frequent than in POAG and are associated with a greater likelihood of progression. These are often missed if the disc is

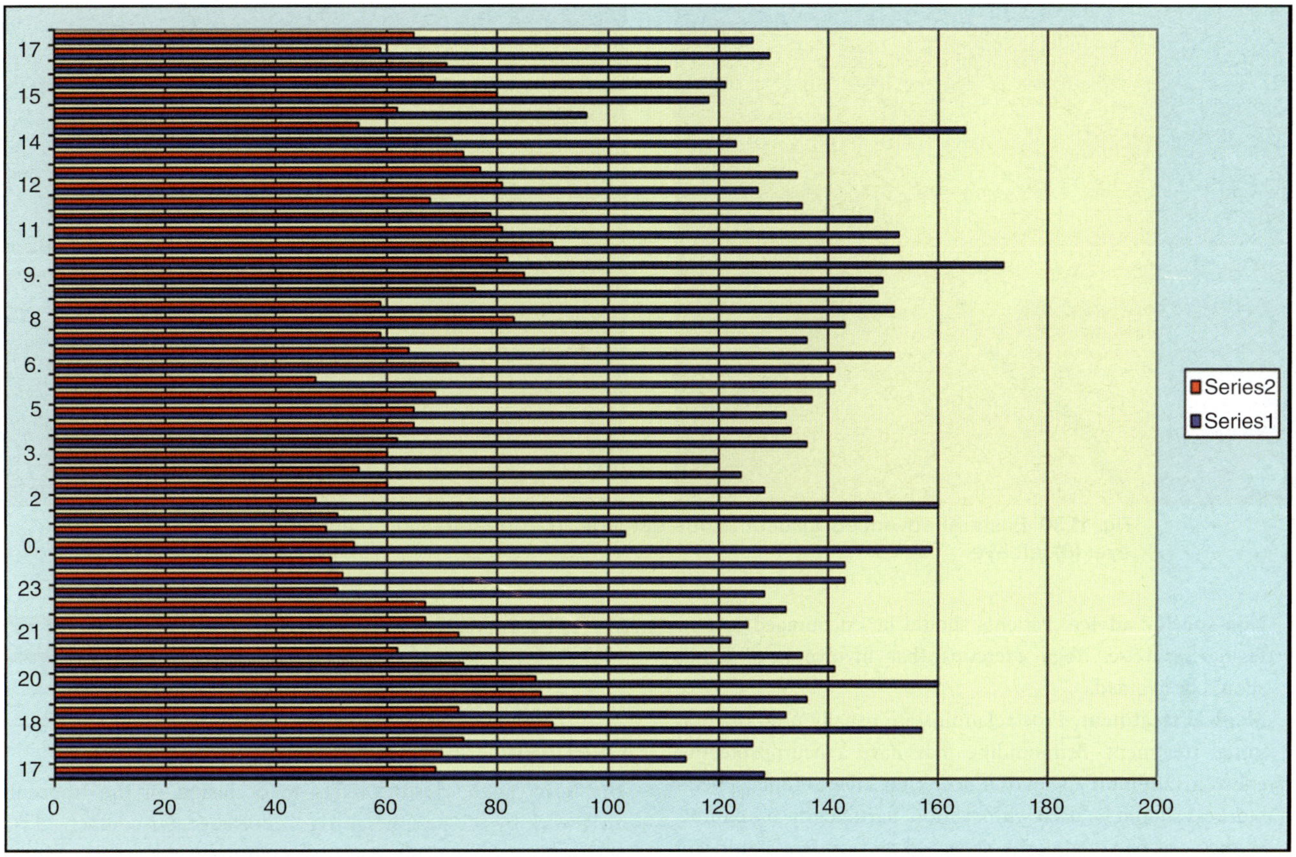

Fig. 11.29 24-hour blood pressure chart showing a nocturnal dip.

not photographed or is examined without magnification (see Fig. 11.10A and B).

- Pallor disproportionate to cupping should prompt a suspicion of an alternative diagnosis.

- **Visual field defects** are the same as in POAG although there is some evidence that they tend to be closer to fixation, deeper, steeper and more localized. In more than half of patients, field changes are non-progressive over a period of 5 years or more without treatment. However, perhaps because of delayed diagnosis, patients tend to present with more advanced damage than in POAG. A high level of suspicion for a deficit pattern suggesting a lesion posterior to the optic nerve is important.
- **Other investigations** are as for POAG although in selected patients the following can be considered:
  - Assessment of systemic vascular risk factors.
  - Blood pressure measurement can be used to calculate ocular perfusion pressure. 24-hour ambulatory monitoring will exclude nocturnal systemic hypotension in selected patients.
  - Blood tests for other causes of non-glaucomatous optic neuropathy such as vitamin B_{12}, red cell folate, full blood count, erythrocyte sedimentation rate/C-reactive protein, treponemal serology including Lyme disease, serum angiotensin-converting enzyme level, plasma protein electrophoresis and autoantibody screen.
  - Indications for neuroimaging in a patient with NTG:
    - Loss of VA out of proportion to cupping
    - Loss of colour vision on Ishihara testing
    - Visual field loss not consistent with retinal nerve fibre layer drop-out
    - Pallor of the neuroretinal rim of the disc
    - Rapid progression despite normal pressure
  - Carotid duplex imaging.
  - Ocular blood flow assessment (e.g. laser flowmetry) may have useful clinical potential.

TIP In a patient with glaucoma undertake neuroimaging if there is deterioration of colour vision or if the visual field defect is not consistent with retinal nerve fibre layer loss.

Treatment

As a large proportion of untreated patients will not deteriorate (approximately 50% at 5–7 years), progression should be demonstrated before commencing treatment in most patients. Some cases of NTG progress more rapidly than others and because further lowering of IOP is effective in reducing progression, treatment should be considered in patients with advanced glaucomatous damage, particularly if central vision is threatened and in those with a long life expectancy. Regular assessment including perimetry should be performed at 6-monthly intervals initially.

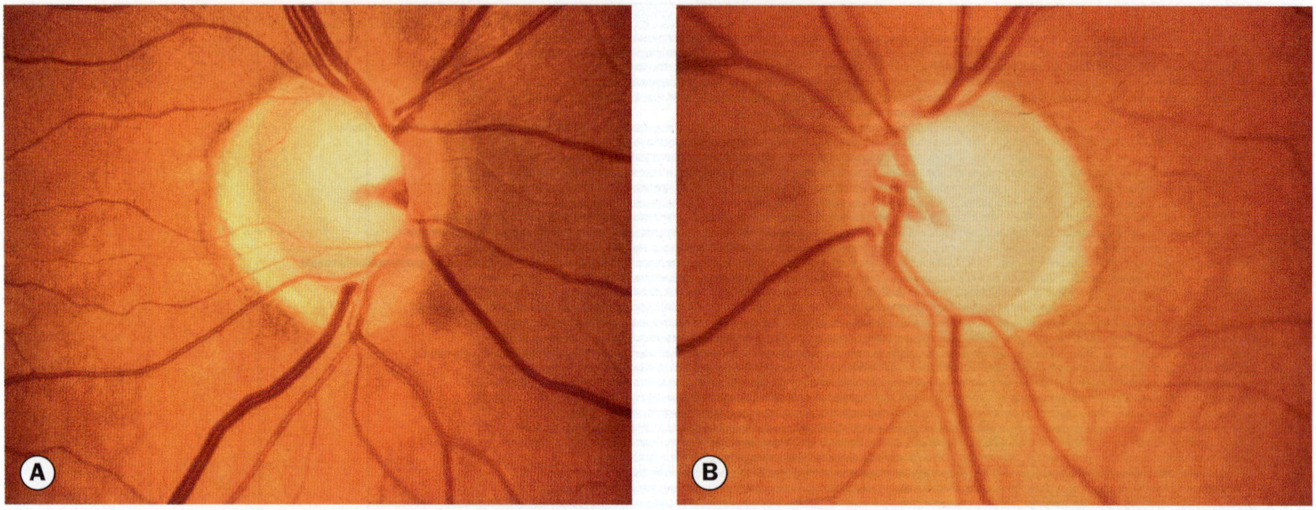

Fig. 11.30 Bilateral advanced glaucomatous damage in normal-tension glaucoma. **(A)** Right eye; **(B)** left eye.

- **Non-specific advice.** Patients should be encouraged to take regular exercise. Yoga exercises that involve head-stands should be avoided.
- **Medical treatment.** Prostaglandins are usually prescribed as initial treatment. Brimonidine may have a neuroprotective effect in addition to an IOP-lowering effect. Topical beta-blockers should be used with caution, particularly at bedtime, as they can be systemically absorbed and cause a significant dip in nocturnal blood pressure. Betaxolol is the beta-blocker of choice in these circumstances.
- **Selective laser trabeculoplasty** is a reasonable initial option to achieve IOP targets.
- **Surgery** should be considered if progression occurs despite IOP in the low teens. Antimetabolite enhancement of trabeculectomy is likely to be indicated in order to achieve a satisfactorily low pressure and to prevent IOP spikes.
- **Control of systemic vascular disease** such as diabetes, hypertension and hyperlipidaemia may be important, in order to optimize optic nerve perfusion.
- **Systemic calcium-channel blockers** to address vasospasm have been advocated by some authorities.
- **Antihypotensive measures.** If significant nocturnal dips in BP are detected, it may be necessary to reduce antihypertensive medication, especially if taken at bedtime. Selected patients might be encouraged to increase their salted food intake, in consultation with the patient's cardiovascular physician.
- **Effects of sleeping in a head-up position.** The IOP is higher in a flat position than in a 30° head-up position. Although this effect differs between individuals, patients with progressive disease should be encouraged to sleep in a head-up position, as the mean IOP is 20% lower in this position than in a flat position in at least a third of individuals.
- **Neuroprotective agents** of proven benefit are not yet available. Memantine is used to retard neuronal death in some central nervous system (CNS) disorders, but has not been shown to be beneficial in glaucoma. Ginkgo biloba (40 mg three times daily) may confer some benefit in selected cases.

PRIMARY ANGLE-CLOSURE GLAUCOMA

Introduction

Overview

The term 'angle closure' refers to occlusion of the trabecular meshwork by the peripheral iris (iridotrabecular contact – ITC), obstructing aqueous outflow. Angle closure can be primary, when it occurs in an anatomically predisposed eye, or secondary to another ocular or systemic factor. PACG may be responsible for up to half of all cases of glaucoma globally and is particularly common in Asia. It progresses rapidly and is more likely to result in visual loss than POAG.

Gonioscopy

See Chapter 1.

Grading of angle width

In practice, the angle is graded by many practitioners simply according to the number of structures visible (Fig. 11.31), together with qualifying comments relating to the width of the iris approach. The angle is usually narrowest superiorly. The main aims are to evaluate the functional status of the angle, the degree of closure and the risk of future closure.

Shaffer system. The Shaffer system records the angle in degrees between two imaginary lines tangential to the inner surface of the trabeculum and the anterior surface of the iris about one-third of the distance from its periphery. The system assigns a numerical grade to each quadrant of the angle.

- **Grade 4** (35–45°) is the widest angle, characteristic of myopia and pseudophakia. The ciliary body can be visualized without tilting the lens.
- **Grade 3** (25–35°) is an open angle in which the scleral spur is visible.
- **Grade 2** (20°) is an angle in which the trabeculum but not the scleral spur can be seen.

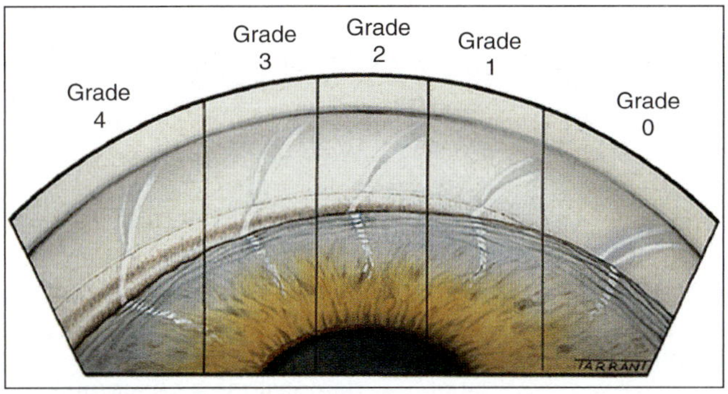

Fig. 11.31 Grading of angle width according to number of visible structures.

- **Grade 1** (10°) is a very narrow angle in which only the Schwalbe line and perhaps the top of the trabeculum can be identified.
- **Slit angle** is one in which there is no obvious iridocorneal contact but no angle structures can be identified.
- **Grade 0** (0°) is closed due to iridocorneal contact.
- **Indentation** will distinguish appositional from synechial angle closure.

Other systems

- The **Spaeth** system is detailed but underused. It allows formal description of the position of iris insertion, the angular approach and peripheral iris curvature.
- The **Scheie** classification refers to the angle structures visible and allocates a Roman numeral accordingly. In contrast to common clinical use, in the original system a higher numeral (e.g. IV) actually signifies a narrower angle.
- The **van Herick** method (Table 11.4) uses the slit lamp alone to estimate the AC angle width:
  - A thin but bright slit beam is set approximately perpendicularly to the corneal surface (offset from the optics by about 60°) to the patient's temporal side for each eye.
  - The beam is used to estimate the ratio of the corneal thickness to the most peripheral part of the AC.
  - It is useful as a screening tool, but overestimates angle width in a proportion of patients, particularly those with plateau iris configuration.

TIP Evaluation of the filtration angle using gonioscopy is key to the diagnosis and treatment of primary angle-closure glaucoma.

Classification

As knowledge about the epidemiology and mechanisms of angle closure has increased, classification has moved away from a symptom-based approach (acute, subacute and chronic) to reflect the stages in the natural history of the disease. The scheme below has been suggested by a consensus group of the Association of International Glaucoma Societies:

- **Primary angle closure suspect (PACS)**
  - Axial anterior chamber depth is less than normal (Fig. 11.32A). Because of the convexity of the iris–lens diaphragm, a crescentic shadow forms over the nasal iris when a light is projected across the anterior chamber from the temporal side (the 'eclipse' sign) (Fig. 11.32B).
  - Gonioscopy shows posterior meshwork ITC in three or more quadrants but no peripheral anterior synechiae (PAS).
  - A lower threshold for diagnosis is used if gonioscopy reveals two quadrants of ITC and signs of intermittent closure, like pigment smudging (Fig. 11.32C).
  - Normal IOP, optic disc and visual field.
  - No PAS.
  - Anterior segment OCT shows an occludable angle (Fig. 11.32D).
  - The risk of developing angle-closure disease in individuals classified as PAC suspects is low.
- **Primary angle closure (PAC)**
  - Gonioscopy shows three or more quadrants of ITC associated with raised IOP and/or PAS, best evaluated using indentation gonioscopy (Fig. 11.33).
  - Normal optic disc and field.
  - Some authorities further classify PAC into non-ischaemic and ischaemic, the latter showing anterior segment evidence of prior substantial IOP elevation such as iris changes or glaukomflecken (see below).
- **Primary angle-closure glaucoma (PACG)**
  - ITC in three or more quadrants, associated with glaucomatous optic neuropathy.
  - Optic nerve damage from an episode of severe IOP elevation, such as acute angle closure, may not appear as typical glaucomatous cupping.

Mechanism

The mechanisms involved in angle closure can be categorized according to the anatomical level (anterior to posterior) at which causative forces act. In many patients more than one level is contributory.

- **Relative pupillary block**
  - Failure of physiological aqueous flow through the pupil leads to a pressure differential between the anterior and posterior chambers, with resultant anterior bowing of the iris (Fig. 11.34).
  - Usually anatomically relieved by peripheral iridotomy, which equalizes anterior and posterior chamber pressure. Reduction of IOP will follow provided the angle has opened adequately. This may not occur if there are substantial PAS or an additional mechanism of angle closure is in effect. Trabecular meshwork damage can prevent normalization of IOP even with an anatomically open angle.
  - The lens vault quantifies the portion of the lens located anterior to the anterior chamber angle. A common definition is the distance between the anterior pole of the lens and a horizontal line joining the scleral spur at diametrically opposite locations. A large lens vault is independently associated with angle closure, though it is not clear whether this is entirely via a pupillary block or non-pupillary block mechanism, or both.

Table 11.4 Van Herick Method for Anterior Chamber Angle Assessment

Anterior chamber depth as a proportion of corneal thickness	Description	Grade	Comment
≥1	Peripheral AC space equal to full corneal thickness or larger	4	Wide open
¼–½	Space between one-fourth and one-half corneal thickness	3	Incapable of closure
¼	Space equal to one-fourth corneal thickness	2	Should undergo gonioscopy
<¼	Space less than one-fourth corneal thickness	1	Gonioscopy will usually demonstrate a dangerously narrowed angle

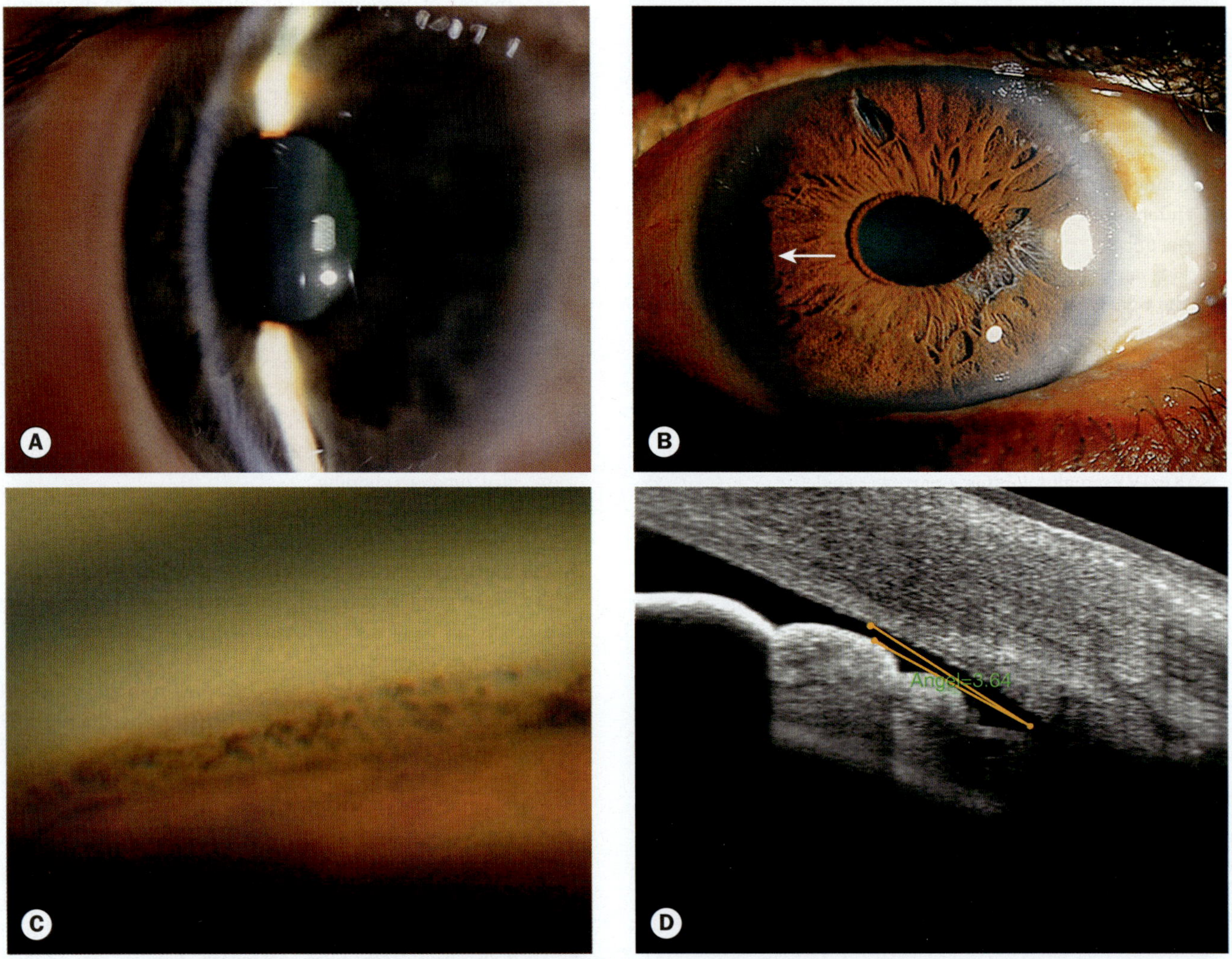

Fig. 11.32 Primary angle closure suspect. **(A)** Shallow anterior chamber and a convex-shaped iris–lens diaphragm; **(B)** 'eclipse' sign (arrow) in an eye with a shallow anterior chamber – note the oval pupil; **(C)** on gonioscopy Schwalbe line and part of the non-pigmented trabecular meshwork are visible; **(D)** very narrow angle on dark-room anterior segment OCT.

- **Non-pupillary block**
  - This is an important mechanism in many Asian patients.
  - Associated with a deeper AC than found in those with pure pupillary block.
  - Patients with non-pupillary block, particularly those with plateau iris, tend to be younger than those with pure pupillary block.
  - An element of pupillary block is invariably present, but angle closure is not fully relieved by iridotomy. The term

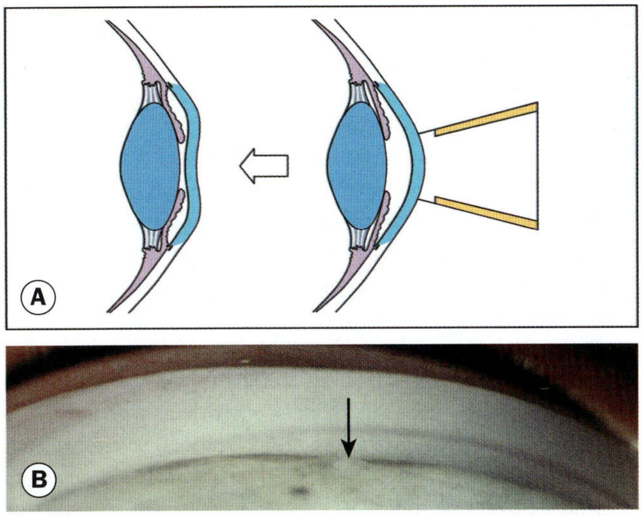

Fig. 11.33 Primary angle closure on indentation gonioscopy. **(A)** Diagrammatic representation; **(B)** in a narrow angle showing inferior PAS (arrow).

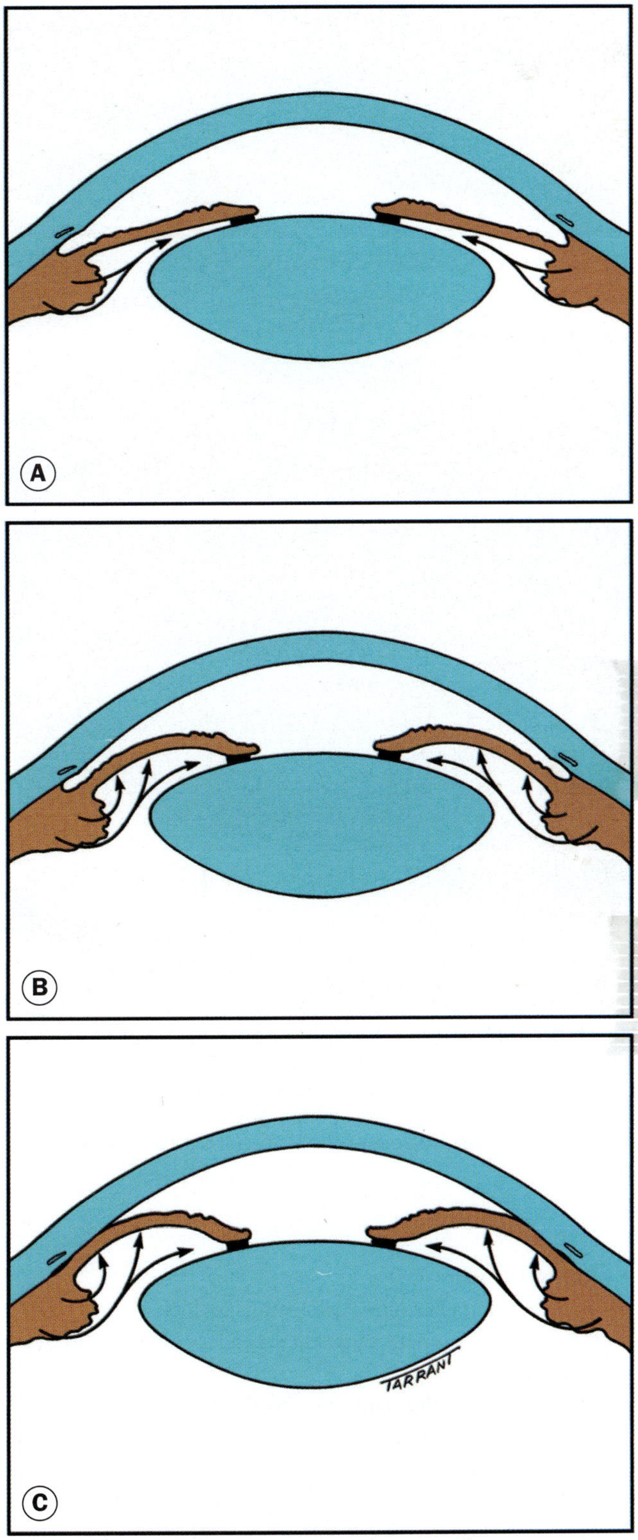

Fig. 11.34 Mechanism of angle closure. **(A)** Relative pupil block; **(B)** iris bombé; **(C)** iridocorneal contact.

'mixed mechanism' has been suggested to describe glaucoma in which both significant pupillary block and non-pupillary block mechanisms co-exist.

- Specific anatomical causative factors include plateau iris secondary to anteriorly positioned/rotated ciliary processes (Fig. 11.35A) and a thicker or more anteriorly positioned iris. The concept of a 'thick peripheral iris roll' has been introduced by some authorities. A thick peripheral iris may be relatively important in Asians (see Fig. 11.15C).
- Plateau iris *configuration* is characterized by a flat or only slightly convex central iris plane, often in association with normal or only slightly shallow central anterior chamber depth (Fig. 11.35B). The angle recess is typically very narrow, with a sharp backward iris angulation over anteriorly positioned and/or oriented ciliary processes. A characteristic 'double hump' sign is seen on indentation gonioscopy, the central hump being due to the underlying central lens supporting the iris and the peripheral hump resulting from the underlying ciliary processes.
- Plateau iris *syndrome* describes the persistence of gonioscopic angle closure despite a patent iridotomy in a patient with morphological plateau iris. Factors such as a dark environment or pharmacological pupillary dilatation may be necessary to demonstrate the angle closure. It is divided into a complete form in which occlusion of the functional trabecular meshwork (TM) is present and the IOP is elevated and an incomplete form with occlusion to a lesser extent and normal IOP.

- **Lens-induced angle closure.** Angle closure that is predominantly lens-induced or due to a retrolenticular cause is often categorized as secondary (see below).
  - This includes those cases in which a sudden change in lens volume and/or position leads to an acute or subacute IOP rise.
  - Usually rapid progression of lens intumescence (phacomorphic glaucoma) or anterior lens subluxation.
  - All cases of pupillary block have a phacomorphic element that increases with age as the lens thickens.

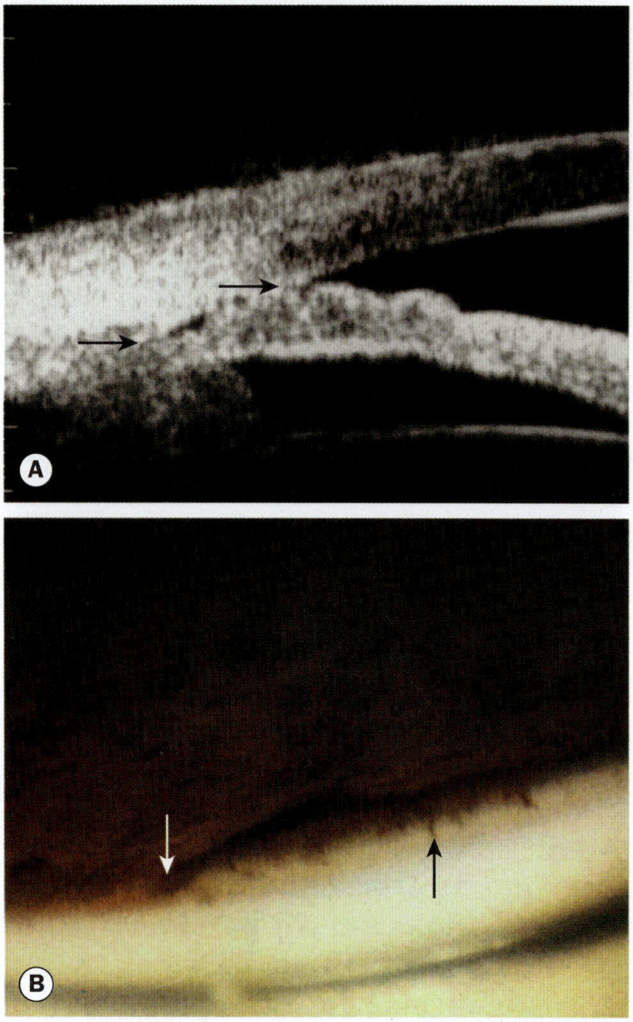

Fig. 11.35 Plateau iris configuration. **(A)** High-resolution ultrasound showing anteriorly rotated ciliary processes and slit-like angle (arrows); **(B)** gonioscopic appearance showing chronic closure (white arrow showing the border between closed and open angle); note iris processes (black arrow).

- **Retrolenticular**
  - Malignant glaucoma ('ciliolenticular block').
  - Posterior segment causes of secondary angle closure (see below).
- **'Combined mechanism'** has been proposed as a formal label for the combination of angle-closure and open-angle elements.
- **Reduced aqueous outflow** in angle closure has been postulated to be caused by the following mechanisms in varying degree:
  - Appositional obstruction by the iris.
  - Degeneration of the TM itself due to chronic or intermittent contact with the iris or damage sustained due to elevated IOP.
  - Permanent occlusion of the TM by PAS. The prognosis for IOP control correlates well with the extent of PAS.

Risk factors

- **Age.** The average age of relative pupillary block is about 62 years at presentation. Non-pupillary block forms of primary angle closure tend to occur at a younger age.
- **Gender.** Females are more commonly affected than males.
- **Race.** Particularly prevalent in Far Eastern and Indian Asians, where non-pupillary block is relatively more significant.
- **Family history.** Genetic factors are important but poorly defined, with an increased prevalence of angle closure in family members.
- **Refraction.** Eyes with 'pure' pupillary block are usually hypermetropic. Non-pupillary block mechanism can occasionally occur in myopic eyes. Up to one in six patients with hypermetropia of one dioptre or more are primary angle closure suspects, so routine gonioscopy should be considered in all adults who are hypermetropic.
- **Axial length.** Short eyes tend to have a shallow AC secondary to a relatively anterior lens position. Eyes with nanophthalmos (axial length less than 20 mm) have a very short eye and are at particular risk.

Diagnosis

Symptoms

- **Unilateral painful red eye.** Most patients with acute congestive angle closure present with a unilateral painful red eye. In about 5% the symptoms occur simultaneously in both eyes.
- **Precipitating factors** include watching television in a darkened room, pharmacological mydriasis or, rarely, miosis, adoption of a semi-prone position (e.g. reading), acute emotional stress and occasionally systemic medication: parasympathetic antagonists or sympathetic agonists including inhalers, motion sickness patches and cold/flu remedies (mydriatic effect), topiramate and other sulfa derivatives (ciliary body effusion).
- **Presentation** can be with intermittent symptoms of blurring ('smoke-filled room') and haloes ('rainbow around lights') due to corneal epithelial oedema, or acutely with markedly decreased vision, redness and ocular/periocular pain and headache.
- **Systemic symptoms** include abdominal pain, nausea and vomiting.

Signs

- **Acute primary angle closure (APAC)**, previously called 'acute glaucoma'
  - VA is usually 6/60 to HM.
  - The IOP is usually very high (50–80 mmHg).
  - Conjunctival hyperaemia with violaceous circumcorneal injection.
  - Corneal epithelial oedema.
  - The AC is shallow and aqueous flare is usually present.
  - A non-reactive mid-dilated vertically oval pupil is classic (Fig. 11.36).

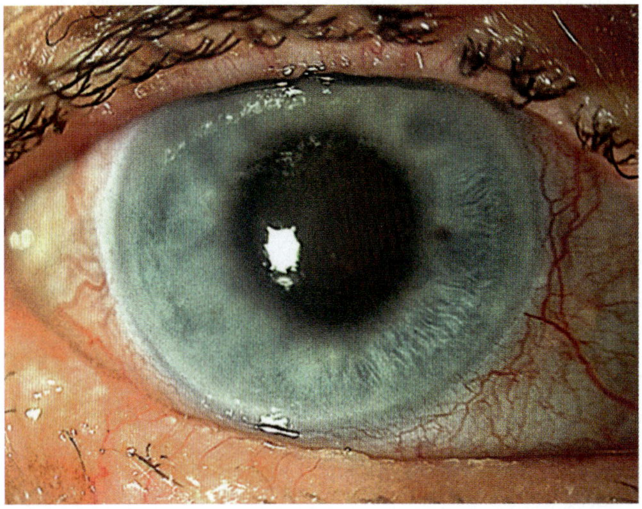

Fig. 11.36 Acute (congestive) primary angle closure showing a mid-dilated vertically oval pupil.

   - The fellow eye typically shows an occludable angle. If this is not present, secondary causes of angle closure should be considered.
- **Resolved APAC**
   - Early: low IOP (ciliary body shutdown and effect of intensive treatment), folds in Descemet membrane if IOP has reduced rapidly (Fig. 11.37A), optic nerve head congestion, choroidal folds.
   - Late: iris atrophy with a spiral-like configuration, glaukomflecken (Fig. 11.37B) (white foci of necrosis in the superficial lens) and other forms of cataract and irregular pupil due to iris sphincter/dilator damage and posterior synechiae (Fig. 11.37C). The optic nerve may be normal or exhibit varying signs of damage, including pallor and/or cupping (Fig. 11.37D).
   - The greater the duration of an attack of APAC and the extent of post-APAC PAS, the lower the likelihood of IOP control with medical treatment alone.
- **Subacute angle closure** is used to describe the clinical scenario of intermittent episodes of spontaneously resolving mild/moderate APAC, usually in patients with pupillary block. The clinical course may be chronic, or may culminate in a more severe/unresolving episode of APAC.
- **Chronic presentation**
   - These patients are usually asymptomatic.
   - VA is normal unless damage is advanced.
   - The AC is usually shallower in relative pupillary block than non-pupillary block.
   - IOP elevation may be only intermittent.
   - 'Creeping' angle closure is characterized by a gradual band-like anterior advance of the apparent insertion of the iris. It starts in the deepest part of the angle superiorly and spreads circumferentially.
   - Intermittent ITC may be associated with the formation of discrete PAS, individual lesions having a pyramidal ('saw-tooth') appearance (see Fig. 11.33B).
   - Optic nerve signs depend on the severity of damage.

Investigation

- **Anterior segment OCT** (AS-OCT – see Fig. 11.15), ultrasound biomicroscopy or Scheimpflug photography may be useful to supplement gonioscopic findings and for patient education.
- **Anterior chamber depth measurement** is helpful in some cases.
- **Biometry** if lens extraction is considered.
- **Posterior segment ultrasonography** in atypical cases to exclude causes of secondary angle closure.
- **Provocative testing.** This may aid decision-making in some circumstances, particularly when plateau iris syndrome is suspected.
   - Pharmacological mydriasis is a poor discriminator and carries a small risk of precipitating APAC in susceptible patients without a patent iridotomy.
   - Dark room/prone provocative test (DRPPT): the patient sits in a dark room, face down for 1 hour without sleeping (sleep induces miosis). The IOP is checked before and immediately after the test, as IOP can normalize very rapidly. An IOP rise of 8 mmHg or more is considered significant. Gonioscopy without indentation should be used to confirm closure of the angle. If the test is positive in a patient with a patent laser iridotomy, the underlying anatomical cause is usually plateau iris, which can be confirmed with ultrasound biomicroscopy (see Fig. 11.14). A positive response is abolished after lens extraction.

Differential diagnosis of acute IOP elevation

- **Lens-induced angle closure** due to a swollen or subluxated lens.
- **Malignant glaucoma** (aqueous misdirection), especially if the patient has recently undergone intraocular surgery.
- **Other causes of secondary angle closure**, with or without pupillary block.
- **Neovascular glaucoma** may occasionally cause the sudden onset of pain and congestion.
- **Hypertensive uveitis**, e.g. iridocyclitis with trabeculitis (particularly herpetic including cytomegalovirus), glaucomatocyclitic crisis (Posner–Schlossman syndrome).
- **Scleritis** with or without angle closure.
- **Pigment dispersion.**
- **Pseudoexfoliation.**
- **Orbital/retro-orbital lesions** including orbital inflammation, retrobulbar haemorrhage and carotid-cavernous fistula.

Treatment

APAC

- **Patients with acute and subacute angle closure should receive urgent treatment.**
- **Initial treatment**
   - The patient should lie down in a supine position to encourage the lens to shift posteriorly under the influence of gravity.

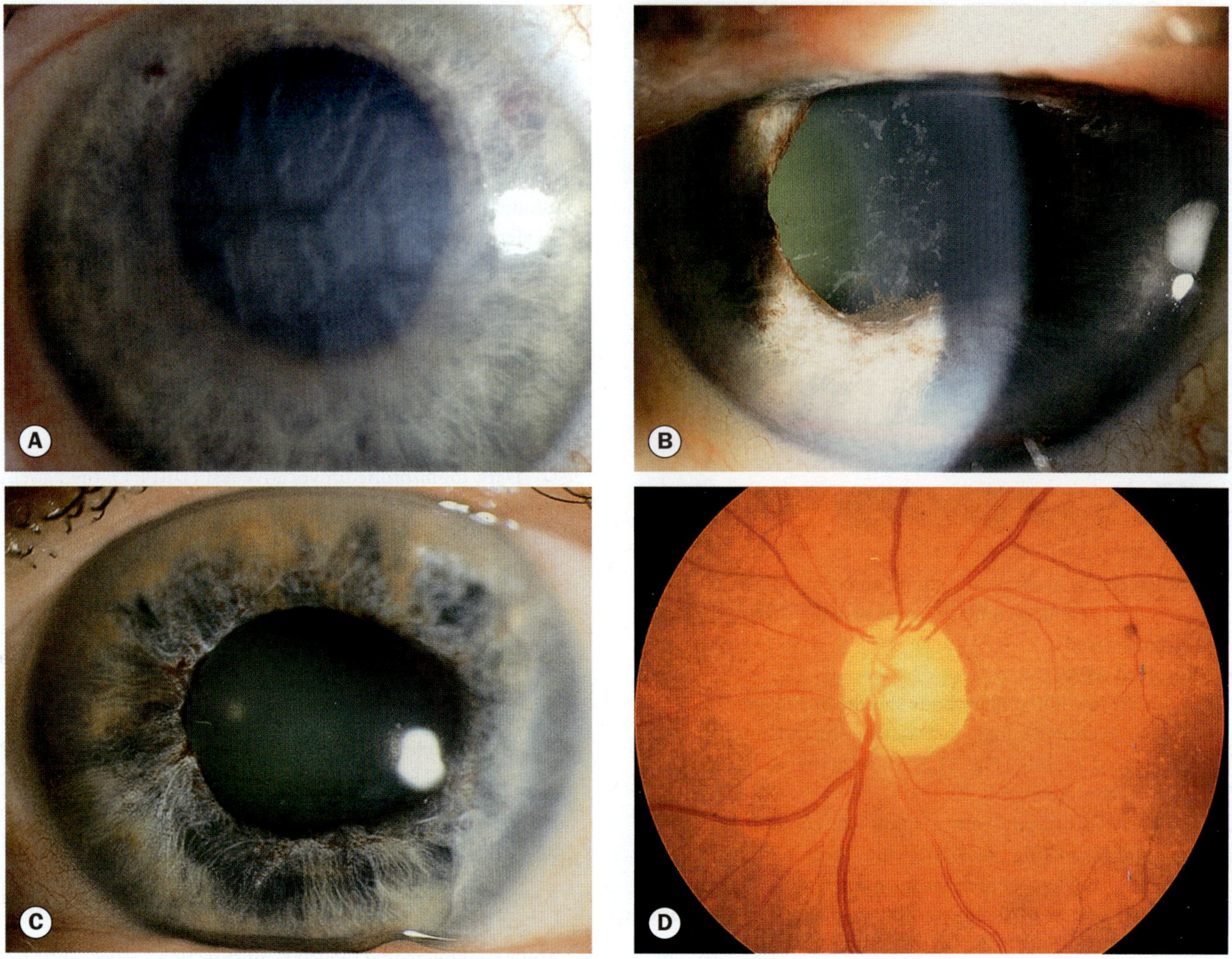

Fig. 11.37 Resolved acute primary angle closure. **(A)** Residual corneal oedema and folds in Descemet membrane in post-congestive angle closure; **(B)** glaukomflecken, spiral-shaped atrophic iris, dilated pupil and posterior synechiae; **(C)** iris atrophy in post-congestive angle closure; **(D)** optic atrophy – combined pallor and cupping.

- Acetazolamide 500 mg is given intravenously if IOP is >50 mmHg and orally (not slow-release) if IOP <50 mmHg.
- Contraindications include sulfonamide allergy and angle closure secondary to topiramate or other sulfonamide derivatives.
- A single dose of apraclonidine 0.5% or 1%, timolol 0.5% and prednisolone 1% or dexamethasone 0.1% is instilled into the affected eye, leaving 3–5 minutes between each.
- Pilocarpine 2% one drop to the affected eye, repeated after half an hour and one drop of 1% into the fellow eye. This should not be repeated if the IOP remains >40 mmHg as ischaemia may compromise its action, may exert a forward vector and excessive dosing carries a systemic toxicity risk.
- Analgesia and an antiemetic may be required.

- **Resistant cases**
  - Central corneal indentation with a squint hook or indentation goniolens to force aqueous into the angle. Epithelial oedema can be cleared first with topical 50% glycerol to improve visualization and to avoid abrasion.
  - Mannitol 20% 1–2 g/kg intravenously over 1-hour, oral glycerol 50% 1 g/kg, or oral isosorbide 1–1.5 g/kg, having checked for contraindications.
  - Early laser iridotomy or iridoplasty after clearing corneal oedema with glycerol.
  - Paracentesis is effective, but carries a small risk of lens damage.
  - Surgical options: peripheral iridectomy, lens extraction, goniosynechialysis, trabeculectomy and cyclodiode laser treatment.
- **Subsequent medical treatment**
  - Pilocarpine 2% four times daily to the affected eye and 1% four times daily to the fellow eye.
  - Topical steroid (prednisolone 1% or dexamethasone 0.1%) four times daily if the eye is acutely inflamed.
  - Any or all of the following should be continued according to response: timolol 0.5% twice daily, apraclonidine 1% three times daily and oral acetazolamide 250 mg four times daily.

- **Bilateral laser iridotomy** is performed once an attack has been broken, signified by a clear cornea and preferably normal IOP. Topical steroids are continued for at least a week.
- **Gonioscopy** needs to be repeated to ensure that the angle is open.
- **Subsequent management** is as for post-iridotomy chronic PAC/PACG. A low threshold may be adopted for cataract surgery, particularly if a significant phacomorphic element is suspected. Trabeculectomy is occasionally necessary for persistent IOP elevation despite a successfully opened angle.

PACS

- **Laser iridotomy** (Fig. 11.38). The ZAP (Zhongshan Angle Closure Prevention) trial concludes that laser peripheral iridotomy (PI) has a small prophylactic effect over a 6-year period and should therefore only be offered to those with the highest risk of developing acute congestive angle closure or chronic angle-closure glaucoma.
- **Factors** that may influence the decision to perform a prophylactic laser iridotomy include:
  - Symptoms suggestive of previous intermittent angle closure.
  - Systemic medication with an atropine-like structure that potentially may provoke pupillary block.
  - Where there is a need for frequent dilated eye examination (e.g. diabetes, AMD).
  - When the health or occupation of the person makes it difficult to immediately access ophthalmic care.
- If significant ITC persists after iridotomy, options include observation (most), laser iridoplasty and long-term pilocarpine prophylaxis, e.g. 1% twice daily. If symptomatic cataract is present, lens extraction usually opens the angle (Fig. 11.39). If IOP is elevated, then by definition PAC is present.

PAC and PACG

- **Management** is the same as that recommended for PACS, but with a lower threshold for further intervention if angle widening is inadequate after iridotomy, particularly if IOP remains elevated.
- **Review.** Urgency and intensity of treatment and frequency of review is tailored to the individual patient, considering IOP, extent of angle closure and glaucomatous damage, if present.
- **Medical treatment** as for POAG may be required for eyes with substantial synechial closure or with persistently elevated IOP despite an opened angle.
- **Trabeculectomy with mitomycin C** is an option, but may result in malignant glaucoma.
- **Phacoemulsification with intraocular lens implantation** is highly effective as it corrects hypermetropia, deepens the anterior chamber and opens the filtration angle. IOP control is achieved in almost all patients whose IOP is within the normal range prior to surgery and in up to 80% of those whose IOP is higher than normal preoperatively. The EAGLE study (Effectiveness of early lens extraction for the treatment of primary angle-closure glaucoma) concludes that clear lens extraction with IOL implantation shows greater efficacy and is more cost-effective than laser peripheral iridotomy in patients with primary angle closure and IOP >29 mmHg or in patients with primary angle-closure glaucoma.

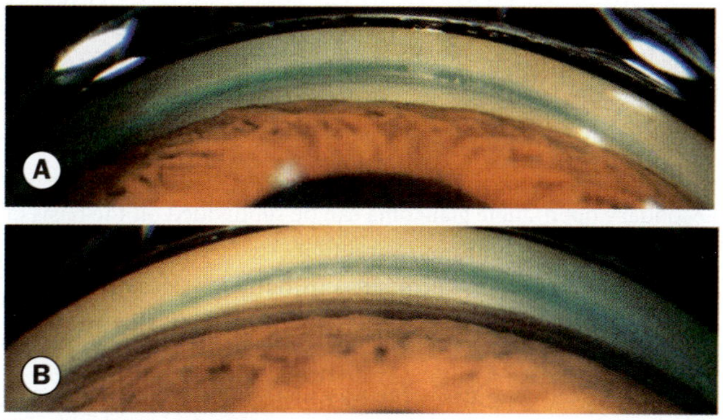

Fig. 11.38 **(A)** Gonioscopy showing total angle closure; **(B)** open angle following laser iridotomy.

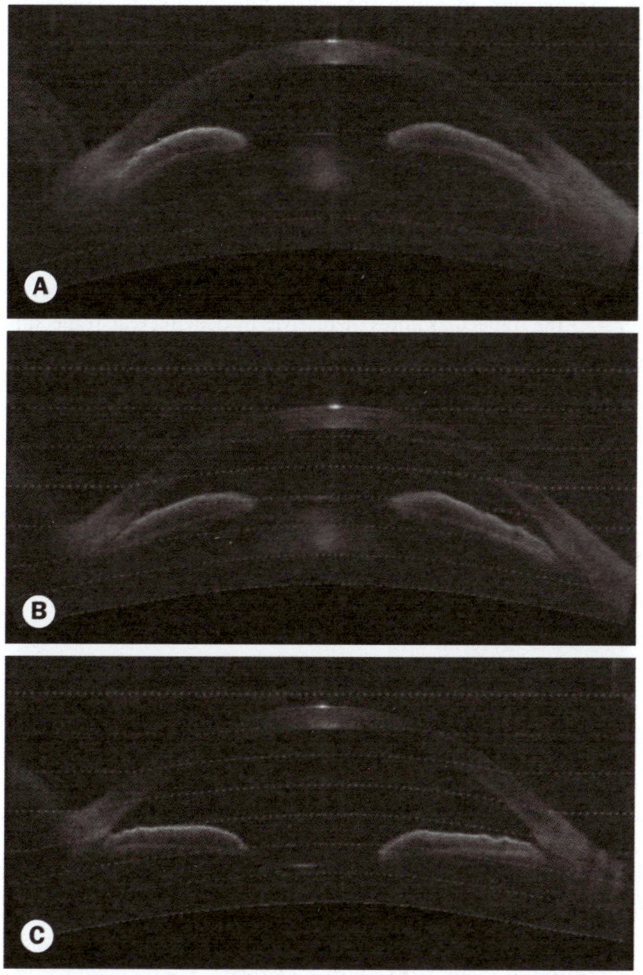

Fig. 11.39 OCT showing **(A)** configuration of iris before laser PI; **(B)** after laser PI showing no change in central anterior chamber depth; **(C)** after lens extraction showing a deep anterior chamber and open angle.

CLASSIFICATION OF SECONDARY GLAUCOMA

Open-angle

Secondary open-angle glaucoma can be subdivided on the basis of the site of aqueous outflow obstruction.

- **Pre-trabecular**, in which aqueous outflow is obstructed by a membrane covering the trabeculum (Fig. 11.40A), which may consist of:
  - Fibrovascular tissue (neovascular glaucoma).
  - Endothelial cellular membranous proliferation (iridocorneal endothelial syndrome).
  - Epithelial cellular membranous proliferation (epithelial ingrowth).
- **Trabecular**, in which the obstruction occurs as a result of 'clogging up' of the meshwork (Fig. 11.40B) and secondary degenerative changes.
  - Pigment particles (pigmentary glaucoma).
  - Red blood cells (red cell glaucoma).
  - Degenerate red cells (ghost cell glaucoma).
  - Macrophages and lens proteins (phacolytic glaucoma).
  - Proteins (probably an element in hypertensive uveitis).
  - Pseudoexfoliative material (pseudoexfoliation glaucoma).
  - Trabecular glaucoma may also be caused by alteration of the trabecular fibres themselves by oedema (e.g. trabeculitis in hypertensive uveitis) or scarring (e.g. post-traumatic angle recession).
- **Post-trabecular** in which the trabeculum itself is normal but aqueous outflow is impaired as a result of elevated episcleral venous pressure.
  - Carotid-cavernous fistula.
  - Sturge–Weber syndrome.
  - Obstruction of the superior vena cava.

Closed angle

- **With pupillary block** (Fig. 11.40C)
  - Seclusio pupillae (360° posterior synechiae), usually secondary to recurrent iridocyclitis.
  - Subluxated lens.
  - Phacomorphic glaucoma.
  - Capsular block syndrome with 360° iris–capsule adhesion in a pseudophakic eye.
  - Aphakic pupillary block.
  - Anterior chamber lens implant without a patent iridotomy.
- **Without pupillary block** (Fig. 11.40D)
  - Secondary causes of PAS such as advanced neovascular glaucoma and chronic anterior uveitis.
  - Cilio-choroidal effusion.
  - Capsular block syndrome without iris–capsule adhesion.
  - Ciliary body/iris cyst or other ciliary body or posterior segment tumour.
  - Contraction of retrolenticular fibrovascular tissue such as in proliferative vitreoretinopathy and retinopathy of prematurity.
  - Malignant glaucoma (ciliolenticular block).

PSEUDOEXFOLIATION SYNDROME AND GLAUCOMA

Introduction

Pseudoexfoliation syndrome (PXS) is an important ocular manifestation of a systemic disorder and is the commonest cause of secondary open-angle glaucoma. It is easily overlooked in the early stages, as the signs are not always obvious. It is rare before the age of 50 years, but the prevalence increases rapidly after the sixth decade of life, with a prevalence of 5% at age 75–85 years. It is more common in women than men and although the condition is found worldwide, the prevalence is highest in Scandinavia. Not all patients with PXS will develop glaucoma and there is no reliable method of determining which patients with the condition will subsequently develop optic disc damage. The incidence of glaucoma (PXG) at diagnosis of PXS is 15–30% and the cumulative risk of eyes with PXS requiring glaucoma treatment may be as high as 60% at 5 years. It should be distinguished from true capsular exfoliation, which occurs secondary to chronic infrared exposure ('glassblower's cataract' – see Fig. 10.6E).

TIP Pseudoexfoliation glaucoma progresses more rapidly than primary open-angle glaucoma and is more likely to result in significant visual loss.

Pathogenesis

Pseudoexfoliative material is a grey-white fibrillary substance deriving from abnormal extracellular matrix metabolism in ocular and other tissues. The material is deposited on various ocular structures, including the lens capsule (Fig. 11.41), zonular fibres, iris, trabeculum and conjunctiva. Pseudoexfoliative material has been found in skin and visceral organs, leading to the concept that PXS is the ocular manifestation of a systemic disorder. PXS is associated with an increased prevalence of high-tone hearing loss and cardiovascular disorders. The pathogenesis is multifactorial, but in some populations almost all patients with PXS have single nucleotide polymorphisms (SNPs) in the *LOXL1* gene on chromosome 15, which codes for an enzyme that is involved in cross-linking of tropoelastin and collagen and is therefore important for the formation and maintenance of elastic fibres and extracellular matrix. However, these SNPs are common in the general population and most individuals with the SNPs do not develop PXS. Plasma and aqueous humour homocysteine levels tend to be higher than controls and inadequate dietary folate intake (folate reduces homocysteine) may be a risk factor. Open-angle glaucoma (sometimes termed 'capsular glaucoma') is usually due to elevated IOP secondary to trabecular obstruction by pseudoexfoliative material and liberated iris pigment leading to secondary degenerative outflow dysfunction. Curiously, despite the systemic nature of the condition and the fact that biopsy reveals subclinical pseudoexfoliative material in the apparently unaffected eye, glaucoma remains confined to one eye in about two-thirds of patients.

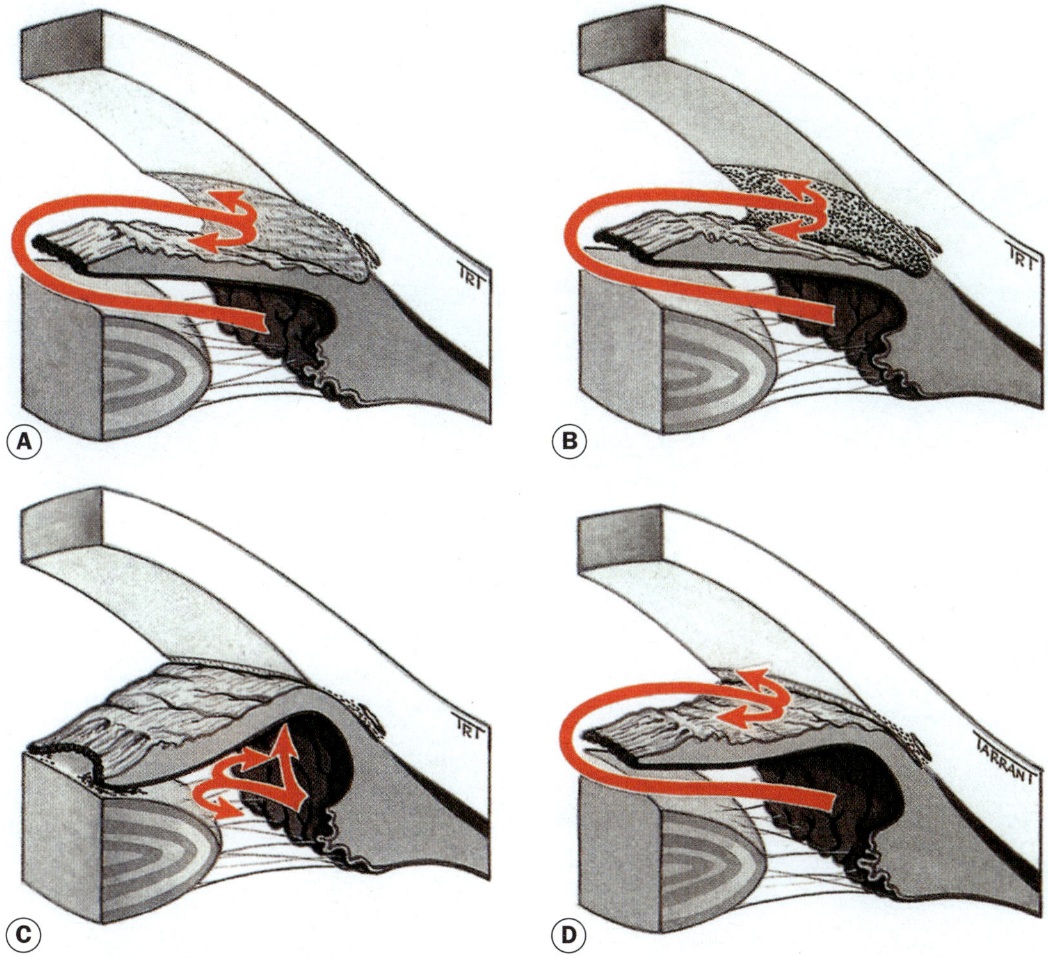

Fig. 11.40 Pathogenesis of secondary glaucoma. **(A)** Pre-trabecular obstruction; **(B)** trabecular obstruction; **(C)** angle closure with pupillary block; **(D)** angle closure without pupillary block.

Clinical features

Diagnosis is usually incidental but can follow vision loss from advanced glaucoma.

- **Cornea.** Pseudoexfoliative material may be deposited on the endothelium and scattered pigment deposits are common. A vertical (Krukenberg) spindle may rarely form, similar to that seen in pigment dispersion syndrome. Endothelial cell abnormality, such as low density, is more common than average.
- **Anterior chamber.** Pseudoexfoliative material particles are sometimes seen. Mild aqueous flare from an impaired blood–aqueous barrier is common.
- **Iris.** Granular pseudoexfoliative material deposits, pupillary ruff loss and patchy transillumination defects at the pupillary margin (Fig. 11.42A).
- **Lens.** The anterior lens capsule typically shows a central disc and a radially indented peripheral layer of pseudoexfoliative material, separated by a clear zone maintained by pupillary abrasion (Fig. 11.42B). Peripheral capsular deposition is often visible only with pupillary dilatation (Fig. 11.42B and C).

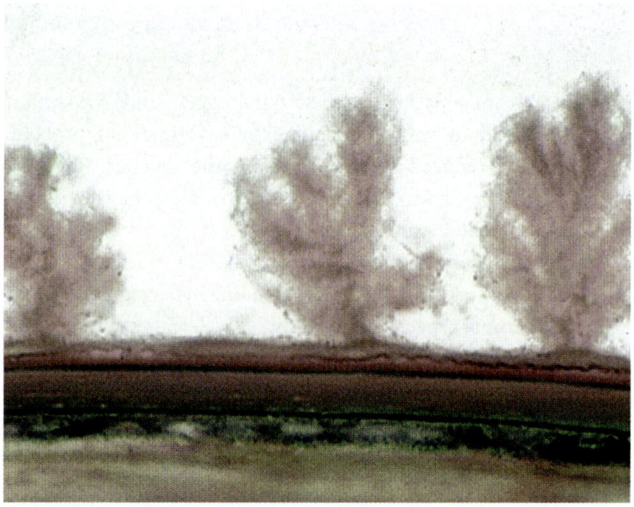

Fig. 11.41 Christmas tree-like deposits of pseudoexfoliative material on the lens capsule. *(Courtesy of J Harry and G Misson, from* Clinical Ophthalmic Pathology, *Butterworth-Heinemann 2001.)*

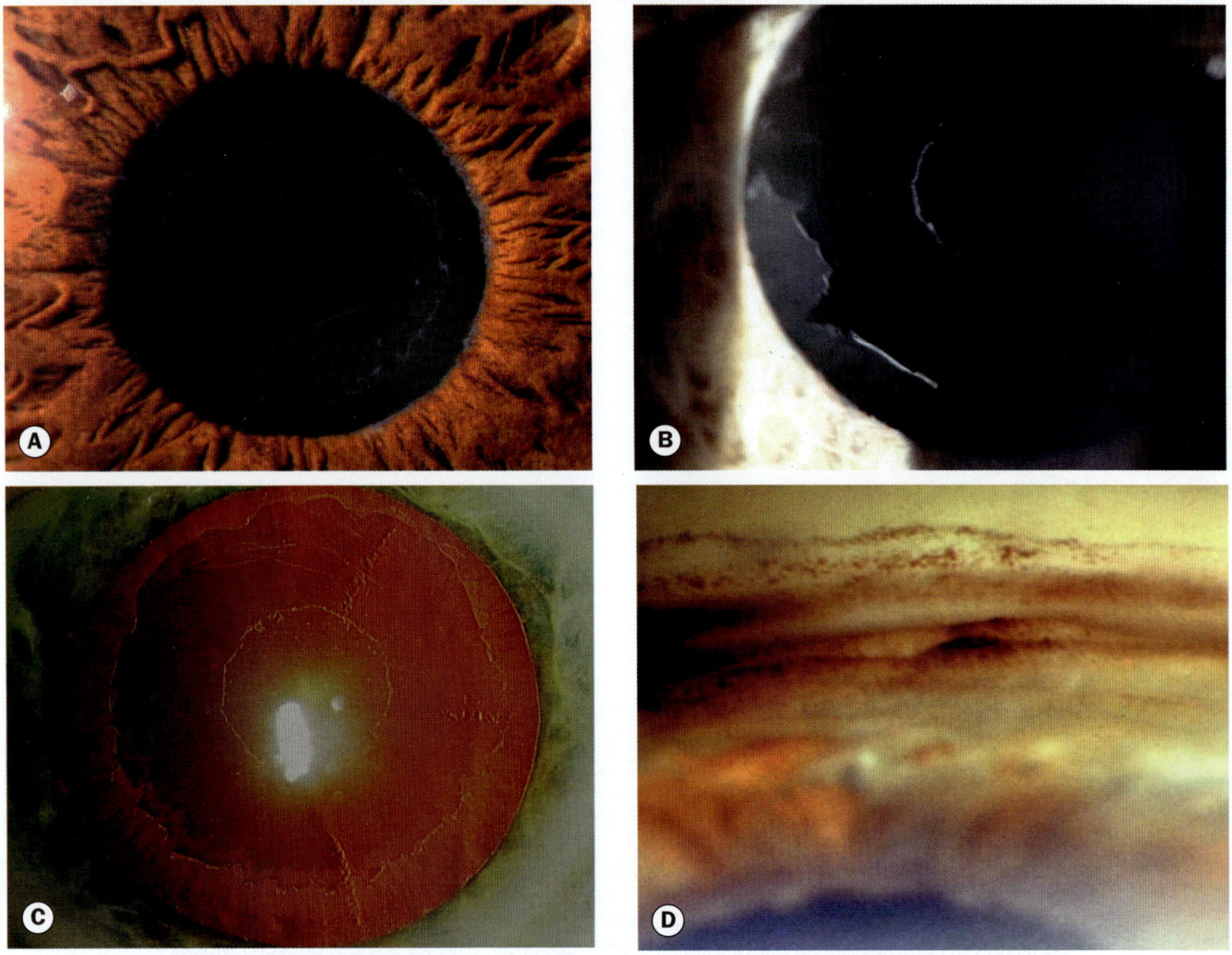

Fig. 11.42 Anterior segment signs in pseudoexfoliation syndrome. **(A)** Loss of the pupillary ruff and pseudoexfoliative material on the pupillary margin; **(B)** peripheral pseudoexfoliative material on the lens more obvious with pupil dilatation; **(C)** retroillumination; **(D)** gonioscopy showing patchy trabecular hyperpigmentation and a markedly irregular Sampaolesi line.

Deposits may be flaky, with scrolled edges. Cataract is more common in an eye with pseudoexfoliative material, probably because of reduced ascorbate levels in the aqueous. Phacodonesis (lens instability) due to zonular weakness may be present, but spontaneous subluxation is rare.

- **Anterior chamber angle.**
  - Patchy trabecular and Schwalbe line hyperpigmentation is common, especially inferiorly.
  - A Sampaolesi line, which is an irregular band of pigment running on or anterior to the Schwalbe line, is commonly seen (Fig. 11.42D). It is not pathognomonic and can be found in pigment dispersion syndrome.
  - Dandruff-like pseudoexfoliative material deposits may be seen.
  - There is an increased risk of angle closure probably because of zonular laxity.
- **IOP.** In most eyes the presence of glaucomatous damage is associated with elevated IOP. The majority of patients have a chronic open-angle glaucoma that is usually unilateral at first. Occasionally the IOP may rise acutely despite a wide angle, mimicking acute angle closure.
- **Prognosis.** This is worse than POAG as the IOP is usually higher and may exhibit marked fluctuation. Severe damage may be present at diagnosis and can develop rapidly. In the long term, these patients are at significant risk of visual loss and blindness. It is therefore important to monitor patients closely and it may be prudent for review in patients with PXS to take place at intervals of no more than 6 months.
- **Systemic manifestations.** These include: high-tone hearing loss, ischaemic cardiovascular/cerebrovascular disease and an increased risk of pelvic organ prolapse in older women.

Treatment

- **Medical** treatment is similar to that of POAG, but failure is more common.
- **Laser trabeculoplasty** is more effective than in POAG, with mean IOP reduction around 30% following SLT. Care should be taken not to apply excessive energy, as trabecular

pigmentation may confer higher absorption resulting in transient IOP spikes. A significant rise in IOP may occur approximately 2 years after SLT.

- **Phacoemulsification** alone may significantly lower IOP, though it may give better control combined with trabeculectomy. There is a high risk of complications, due to poor mydriasis, increased fragility of the zonules and lens capsule and endothelial deficiency. There is also an increased risk of a postoperative IOP spike, postoperative corneal oedema, inflammation, capsular opacification, capsulorhexis contraction (capsular phimosis) and late IOL decentration or dislocation.
- **Filtration surgery** in PXG has a similar success rate to POAG.
- **Trabecular aspiration** alone seems to confer at least a short-term benefit and can be performed at the same time as other intraocular procedures.

PIGMENT DISPERSION SYNDROME AND PIGMENTARY GLAUCOMA

Introduction

Pigment dispersion syndrome (PDS) is characterized by the liberation of pigment granules from iris pigment epithelium and their deposition throughout the anterior segment. Secondary pigmentary glaucoma (PG) is common. PDS and PG are more common in males, particularly young myopic White men. In African people, where it is rare, the condition tends to affect older hypermetropic women. About 15% of patients with PDS will develop elevated IOP or glaucoma after 15 years. AD inheritance with incomplete penetrance seems to be present in at least some families and a range of genetic loci have been linked. Myopia is a risk factor for clinical manifestation, higher degrees of myopia being associated with earlier and more severe glaucoma. Secondary pigment dispersion can occur as a consequence of trauma, intraocular tumour and rubbing of a malpositioned IOL on the iris pigment epithelium.

Pathogenesis

In primary PDS/PG, pigment shedding is precipitated by rubbing of the posterior pigment layer of the iris against the zonules as a result of excessive posterior bowing of the mid-peripheral portion of the iris (Fig. 11.43A). It is believed that an increase in anterior chamber pressure relative to the posterior chamber occurs due to reverse pupillary block, supported by the observation that peripheral iridotomy flattens the iris and decreases iridozonular contact (Fig. 11.43B). The pigment epithelium itself may be abnormally susceptible to shedding in affected individuals. Pigment shedding decreases from middle age onwards due to physiological changes resulting in decreased iridozonular contact. Acute IOP elevation can occur due to direct trabecular obstruction by released melanin granules. Chronic elevation appears to be caused by pigmentary obstruction of the intertrabecular spaces and damage to the trabeculum secondary to denudation, collapse and sclerosis. Patients with pigmentary glaucoma have an increased incidence of steroid responsiveness.

Diagnosis

- **Presentation.** PDS and PG are typically detected at a routine eye examination. The myopic individuals who tend to develop the condition are likely to be under regular optometric review. Occasionally symptoms from glaucomatous visual loss lead to attendance, or from corneal oedema due to an acute IOP rise following the release of pigment granules (particularly after physical exercise). Signs of PDS are usually bilateral but may be subtle and go undetected.
- **Cornea.** Pigment is deposited on the endothelium in a vertical spindle shape (Krukenberg spindle; Fig. 11.44A) The spindle is not always present, tends to become less obvious in longstanding cases and is not pathognomonic.
- **Anterior chamber (AC).** The AC is deep and melanin granules may be seen in the aqueous.
- **Iris.** Characteristic radial spoke-like transillumination defects (Fig. 11.44B) are seen in lighter, but often not in dark, irides. To best demonstrate these, the room should be minimally illuminated and a short, narrow but intense slit beam directed through the pupil. Visualization may be aided by asking the patient to look up. Melanin granules may be present on the surface of the iris, usually inferiorly, which become less obvious with age. There may be partial loss of the pupillary ruff (Fig. 11.44C).
- **Gonioscopy.** The angle is wide open and there is often a characteristic mid-peripheral iris concavity where the iris bows backwards. The trabecular meshwork is heavily pigmented in all four quadrants, with a dense homogeneous circumferential posterior meshwork band (Fig. 11.44D). Pigment may also be seen on or anterior to the Schwalbe line. Pigmentation of the angle typically reduces with increasing age.
- **Lens.** Pigment granules may be deposited on the anterior surface. There may be a line (Scheie stripe) or a (Zentmayer) ring of pigment on the peripheral/equatorial surface around the zonular insertions.
- **IOP.** This may be volatile, some patients exhibiting higher levels and wider fluctuations of IOP than in POAG. Over time the control of IOP may become easier as pigment liberation decreases and occasionally the IOP may revert to normal. NTG can be erroneously diagnosed if the IOP has normalized spontaneously and the PDS signs resolved.
- **Posterior segment.** Peripheral retinal pigmentation may be seen and lattice degeneration is more common than in myopic patients without PDS or PG. The incidence of retinal detachment may also be higher. Glaucomatous optic neuropathy is dependent on disease stage and extent and may be markedly asymmetrical. It is common to find advanced disease in one eye and relatively mild damage in the other.

Treatment

Individuals with PDS should be reviewed annually to exclude the development of raised IOP and/or glaucomatous damage. If

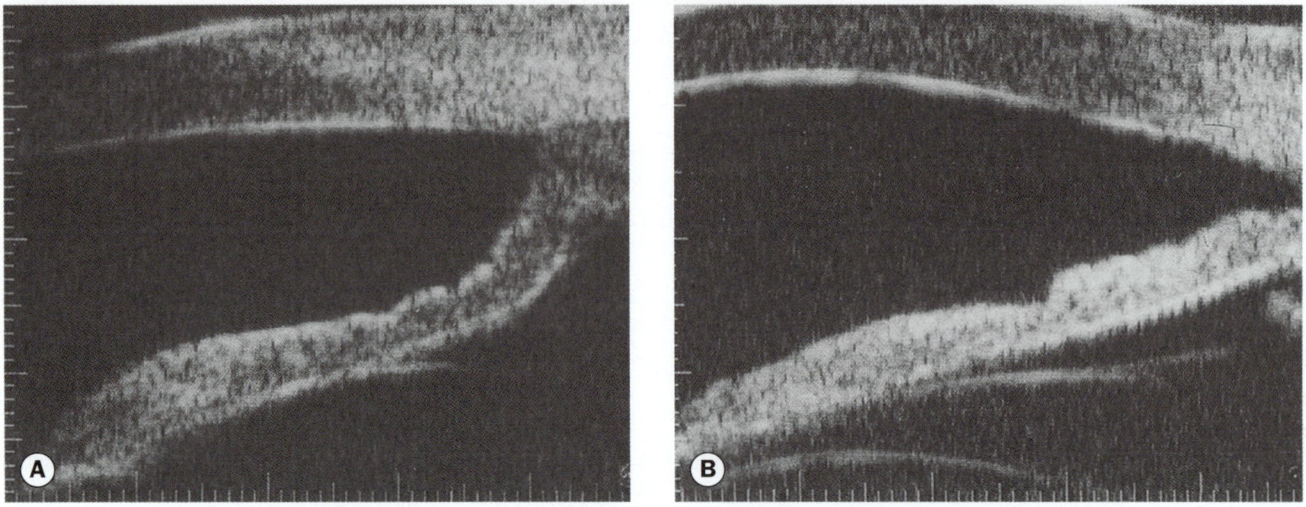

Fig. 11.43 Ultrasound biomicroscopy in pigment dispersion syndrome. **(A)** Deep anterior chamber and posterior bowing of the peripheral iris; **(B)** flattening of the peripheral iris following laser iridotomy.

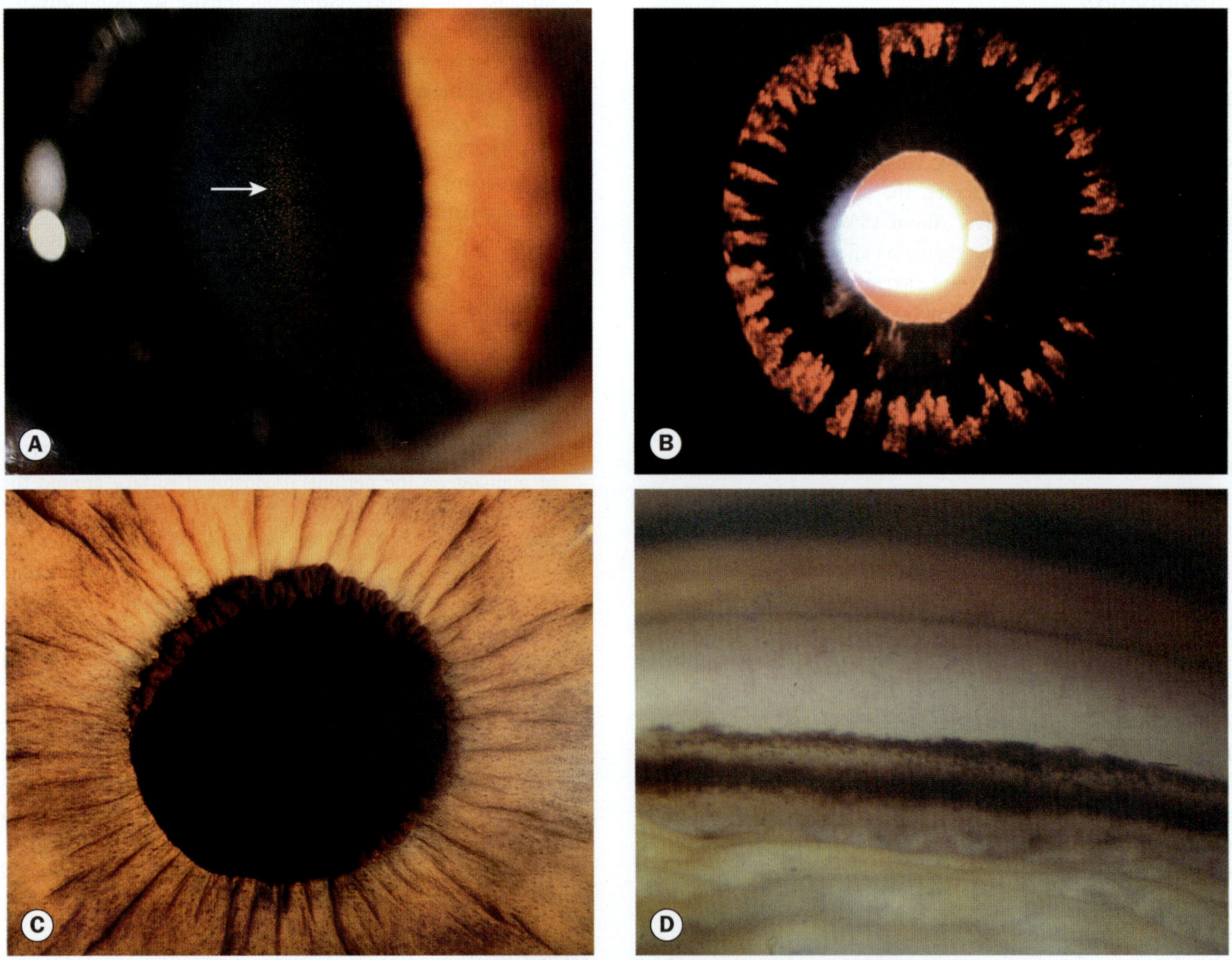

Fig. 11.44 Pigment dispersion syndrome. **(A)** Krukenberg spindle (arrow); **(B)** radial spoke-like iris transillumination defects; **(C)** pigment granules on the iris surface and inferior loss of the pupillary ruff; **(D)** homogeneous band of trabecular hyperpigmentation.

glaucomatous atrophy is present the patient should be monitored at 4–6-monthly intervals as the combination of myopia and PDS can result in rapid deterioration of visual function.

- **Lifestyle measures.** Excessive exercising can be associated with increased iris pigment dispersion with acute symptoms in some cases. If the history confirms this, appropriate advice should be given to alter exercise behaviour.
- **Medical** treatment is similar to that of POAG. Miotics are theoretically of benefit because they decrease iridozonular contact in addition to facilitating aqueous outflow but are poorly tolerated by younger patients. This medication has the disadvantage of exacerbating myopia and also carries a risk of precipitating retinal detachment in short-sighted eyes. Topical thymoxamine, a selective alpha-adrenergic antagonist, induces miosis without causing spasm of accommodation, but is also poorly tolerated as it causes irritation.
- **Laser trabeculoplasty** is often effective. It is important not to over-treat eyes with heavily pigmented angles. To reduce the risk of an IOP spike, use the lowest laser setting and treat only two quadrants.
- **Laser iridotomy** has been proposed to retard pigment liberation by reversing iris concavity and eliminating iridozonular contact. It can reduce the risk of intermittent IOP spikes, especially in patients under the age of 40 years, but does not reduce the risk of developing glaucoma.
- **Filtration surgery** is indicated more commonly than in POAG. The use of adjunctive antimetabolites improves surgical outcome, particularly in younger patients in whom there is a risk of failure. Postsurgical hypotony and suprachoroidal haemorrhage are more common in young patients with myopia.

Acute bilateral iris pigment loss with raised IOP

Bilateral acute depigmentation of the iris (BADI) and bilateral acute iris transillumination (BAIT) have recently been proposed as distinct idiopathic clinical syndromes involving pigment dispersal from the iris into the anterior chamber. They are said to be more common in young to middle-aged women, occurring spontaneously or following a flu-like illness and possibly after oral antibiotic treatment, especially moxifloxacin. It is possible that the primary process is inflammation, but there is evidence that the mechanism is phototoxicity following sensitization in predisposed individuals. Presentation is usually with acute bilateral ocular redness and photophobia. Both may be associated with an IOP rise, but this has been reported to be more severe and resistant in BAIT. Findings described in the two differ in that pigment is lost from the iris stroma in BADI and the iris pigment epithelium in BAIT, with marked iris transillumination defects and irregular mydriasis in the latter. It is possible that BADI and BAIT represent different points on a common disease spectrum. Differential diagnosis is principally from viral anterior uveitis and pigment dispersion syndrome.

NEOVASCULAR GLAUCOMA

Pathogenesis

Neovascular glaucoma (NVG) occurs as a result of aggressive iris neovascularization (rubeosis iridis), which leads to progressive angle closure and rapid glaucomatous atrophy (Fig. 11.45A and B). The common aetiological factor is severe, diffuse and chronic retinal ischaemia. It is postulated that hypoxic retinal tissue produces angiogenic factors in an attempt to revascularize hypoxic areas. The most important of these is VEGF.

Causes

- **Ischaemic central retinal vein occlusion** accounts for 35–50% of cases. A VA of less than 6/60, a relative afferent pupillary defect and extensive peripheral retinal capillary non-perfusion on fluorescein angiography are useful predictors of the risk of subsequent NVG. Glaucoma typically occurs 3 months after the occlusive event ('100-day glaucoma'), but intervals from 4 weeks to 2 years have been documented.
- **Diabetes mellitus** accounts for a smaller proportion. Whereas diabetes was the cause in 30% of cases in the past, this has dropped to 10–15% of cases in communities where yearly screening of diabetic retinopathy occurs. The risk of glaucoma is decreased by panretinal photocoagulation and by anti-VEGF treatment. Pars plana vitrectomy in diabetics may precipitate NVG (7% overall in a large study), especially if angle neovascularization is present preoperatively.
- **Arterial retinal vascular disease** such as central retinal artery occlusion and ocular ischaemic syndrome are less common causes.
- **Miscellaneous** causes include intraocular tumours, long-standing retinal detachment (RD) and chronic intraocular inflammation.

Clinical features

- **Symptoms** vary from none to severe pain, decreased vision, redness and photophobia.
- **Cornea.** Elevated IOP, particularly when substantial and acute, leads to corneal oedema.
- **IOP** may be normal early in the disease process, but is frequently extremely high later on. The anterior segment will often be congested once progression to elevated IOP has occurred. In advanced disease hypotony may supervene.
- **Anterior chamber.** Flare, cells and posterior synechiae may be present, depending on severity and stage. Presentation is sometimes with anterior chamber haemorrhage.
- **Pupillary margin.** Subtle vessels at the pupillary margin are often an early sign (Fig. 11.45C), but may be missed unless the iris is examined carefully under high magnification. Diagnosis at this stage is likely to substantially improve the prognosis.
- **Iris surface.** New vessels grow radially over the surface of the iris towards the angle (Fig. 11.45D), sometimes joining dilated blood vessels at the collarette. At this stage the IOP may still be normal, but elevation can occur fairly acutely.

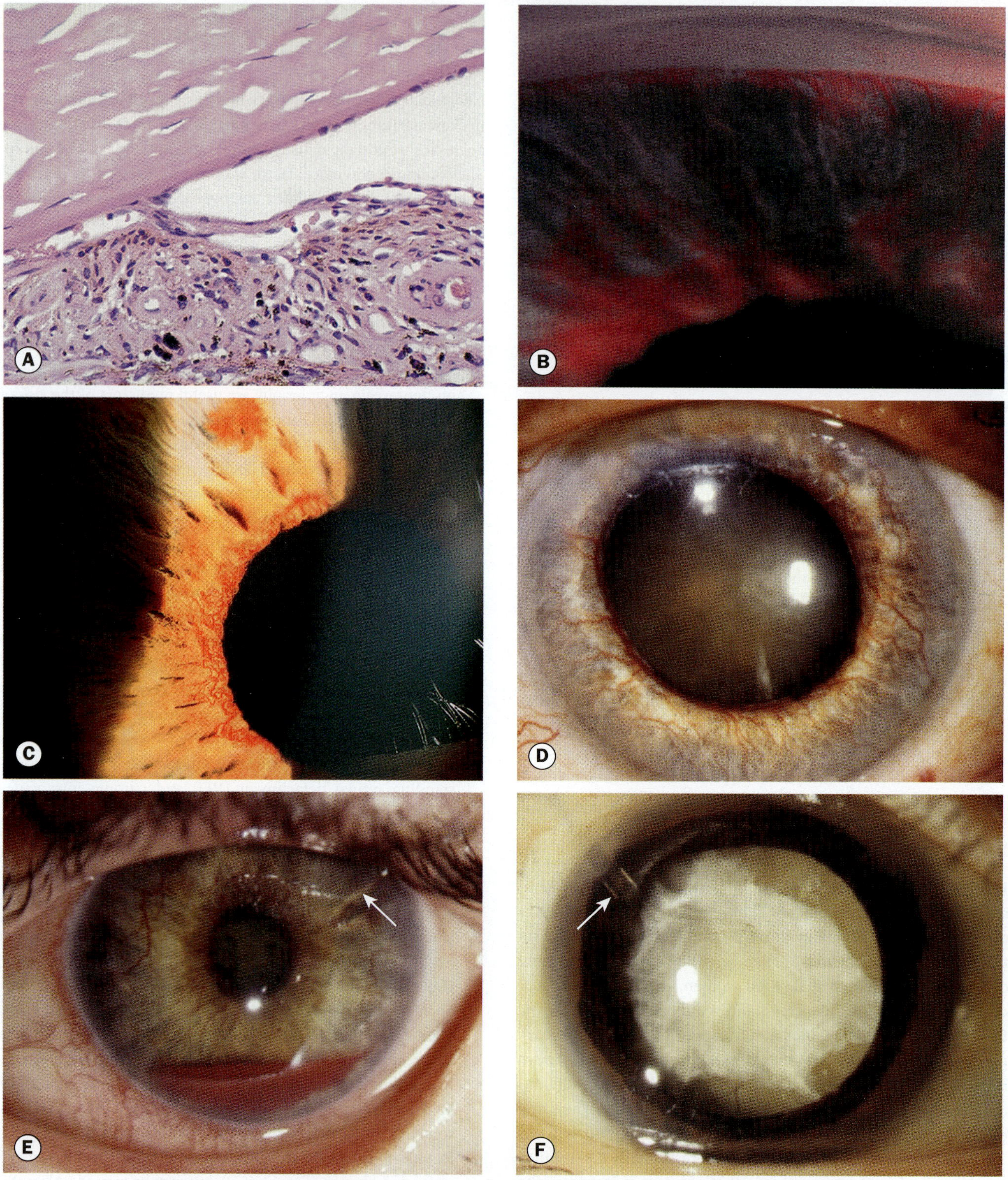

Fig. 11.45 Neovascular glaucoma. **(A)** Rubeosis and angle closure by PAS; **(B)** progressive synechial angle closure; **(C)** mild rubeosis iridis at pupil margin; **(D)** severe rubeosis iridis; **(E)** tube (arrow) with hyphaema; **(F)** blind eye showing dilated pupil, ectropion uvea and cataract in the presence of a tube (arrow). *(Courtesy of J Harry and G Misson, from* Clinical Ophthalmic Pathology, *Butterworth-Heinemann 2001 – fig. A.)*

- **Gonioscopy.** Angle neovascularization may commonly occur without other signs, particularly after CRVO and it is important to perform careful non-mydriatic gonioscopy in eyes at risk. Early signs may be very subtle, even in the presence of moderate IOP elevation. Neovascular tissue proliferates across the face of the angle, forming an obstructing fibrovascular membrane that subsequently contracts to close the angle. The angle closes circumferentially leading to very high IOP, severe visual impairment, congestion of the globe and pain. The visual prognosis is generally poor by this stage, but aggressive management can achieve comfort and retain useful sight in some cases.
- **Cataract** is common once ischaemia is established.
- **Posterior segment.** Signs correspond to aetiology. Glaucomatous optic neuropathy may be present.
- **Investigations.** Fluorescein angiography may be helpful in confirming aetiology and delineating ischaemia. B-scan ultrasonography will help to exclude potential causes such as RD or a tumour when the posterior segment view is impaired. Anterior segment OCT has been proposed as a useful tool for angle assessment.

Treatment

It is critical to address the cause of the neovascularization as well as the elevated IOP. Appropriate management of systemic disease is also of key importance in order to reduce the risk to the fellow eye, to reduce the risk of stroke and to prolong life expectancy. Factors that predict a poor visual outcome include: young age, VA less than 6/60 and IOP >35 mmHg on presentation.

- **Review.** Frequent review during high-risk periods is critical: the first few months following an ischaemic CRVO and the first few weeks following diabetic vitrectomy.
- **Medical treatment of elevated IOP** is as for POAG but miotics should be avoided. Topical atropine 1% twice daily will resist synechiae formation, and increase the outflow of aqueous through the uveoscleral route. Topical steroids are beneficial in the acute stage. Topical apraclonidine and oral acetazolamide may be useful temporizing measures. Acetazolamide can be associated with renal dysfunction in diabetes, especially type 1 and should be used with caution in these patients.
- **Panretinal photocoagulation (PRP)** is usually effective in inducing regression of neovascularization and, if performed early, preventing progression to glaucoma. It will not reverse an established fibrovascular membrane. The timing of PRP in CRVO is discussed in Chapter 13. If the retinal view is poor, indirect ophthalmoscopic application may provide better access; if necessary, performed in the operating room with iris hooks to open a small pupil caused by posterior synechiae. Trans-scleral cryotherapy may be used in eyes with opaque media or as an adjunct for increasing peripheral retinal coverage.
- **Intraocular VEGF inhibitors**, e.g. bevacizumab (Avastin) at a dose of 1.25 mg in 0.05 ml, is an effective adjunctive measure whilst waiting for PRP to take effect, particularly if fibrovascular angle closure has not yet supervened and usually leads to rapid pain relief. Intracameral (AC) injection is an alternative to the intravitreal route. The duration of control from a single injection is limited and most patients require ongoing injections. In patients with ischaemic CRVO treated in this manner, the onset of NVG can be delayed by up to 18 months. There is a small risk of central retinal artery occlusion in patients with ocular ischaemic syndrome.
- **Retinal detachment repair** should be performed once the IOP is controlled, particularly if there is a tractional detachment involving the macula.
- **Ciliary body ablation.** Cyclodiode should be considered if medical IOP control is not possible. These have conventionally been used only in eyes with poor visual potential, but can be employed if there is reasonable vision in order to prevent severe glaucomatous damage occurring whilst neovascularization is brought under control. Lowering a substantially raised IOP generally improves comfort and clearing corneal oedema may facilitate an adequate retinal view for PRP. Care should be taken not to use excessive treatment, which can lead to hypotony. Endoscopic cyclophotocoagulation is an alternative to trans-scleral treatment.
- **Filtration surgery** may be considered if VA is HM or better. Options include an artificial filtering shunt (glaucoma drainage device) (Fig. 11.45E) and trabeculectomy with mini-shunt implantation, adjunctive mitomycin C and postoperative subconjunctival 5-fluorouracil. Active neovascularization and inflammation should be controlled preoperatively (including preoperative anti-VEGF treatment) to improve the chances of surgical success. Even with treatment there is a relatively high risk of hypotony. Postoperative anti-inflammatory treatment should be aggressive and may include systemic steroids.
- **Pars plana vitrectomy** with peroperative endolaser at an early stage may improve the prognosis in eyes with vitreous haemorrhage, especially in CRVO. Preoperative intravitreal anti-VEGF may be of benefit.
- **Retrobulbar alcohol injection** is useful in relieving pain but may cause permanent ptosis and does not relieve congestion.
- **Enucleation or evisceration** may be considered if all else fails.

TIP The underlying cause of neovascular glaucoma needs to be determined and treated in order to reduce the risk of visual loss in the fellow eye and to increase life expectancy.

Prognosis

Patient expectations need to be realistic and the best outcome is often a blind but comfortable eye. The prevalence of blindness in the affected eye varies from 25% to 50% depending on the length of follow-up (Fig. 11.45F). Life expectancy is reduced significantly in these patients (approximately 50% of expected lifespan). A good presenting VA in the affected eye is a useful predictor of longer life expectancy.

INFLAMMATORY GLAUCOMA

Introduction

Overview

Elevation of IOP secondary to intraocular inflammation frequently presents a diagnostic and therapeutic challenge. The elevation of IOP may be transient and innocuous, or persistent and severely damaging. The prevalence of secondary glaucoma increases with chronicity and severity of disease. Secondary glaucoma is particularly common in Fuchs uveitis syndrome and chronic anterior uveitis associated with juvenile idiopathic arthritis. Posterior uveitis is less likely to affect the aqueous outflow pathway and consequently less likely to lead to IOP elevation.

Diagnostic dilemmas

Assessment of glaucomatous damage may be hampered by a small pupil or opacities in the media. Poor VA may also compromise accurate perimetry.

- **IOP fluctuation** may be dramatic in uveitic glaucoma and phasing may be helpful in patients with borderline IOP.
- **Ciliary body shutdown** caused by acute exacerbation of chronic anterior uveitis is frequently associated with lowering of IOP that may mask the underlying tendency to glaucoma. Even eyes with considerably elevated IOP (30–35 mmHg) may become hypotonous during acute exacerbations of uveitis. Return of ciliary body function with subsidence of uveitis may be associated with a rise in IOP in the presence of permanently compromised outflow facility.
- **Topical steroids**, when used intermittently, can cause a fluctuating IOP.
- **Iris vessels** may give rise to diagnostic confusion with neovascular glaucoma.

Angle-closure glaucoma with pupillary block

Pathogenesis

Secondary angle closure is caused by posterior synechiae extending for 360° (seclusio pupillae), which obstruct aqueous flow from the posterior to the anterior chamber. The resultant increased pressure in the posterior chamber produces anterior bowing of the peripheral iris (iris bombé – Fig. 11.46A) resulting in shallowing of the anterior chamber and apposition of the iris to the trabeculum and peripheral cornea (Fig. 11.46B). Such an inflamed iris easily sticks to the trabeculum and the iridocorneal contact may become permanent, with the development of PAS.

Diagnosis

- **Slit lamp biomicroscopy** shows seclusio pupillae, iris bombé and a shallow anterior chamber.
- **Gonioscopy** shows angle closure from iridotrabecular contact. Indentation may be used to assess the extent of appositional as opposed to synechial angle closure.

Angle-closure glaucoma without pupillary block

- **Pathogenesis.** Chronic anterior uveitis causes the deposition of inflammatory cells and debris in the angle (Fig. 11.47A and B). Subsequent organization and contraction pull the peripheral iris over the trabeculum, causing gradual and progressive synechial angle closure (Fig. 11.47C) and eventual elevation of IOP. The eye with a pre-existing narrow angle may be at higher risk.
- **Diagnosis.** The anterior chamber is deep but gonioscopy shows extensive angle closure by PAS.

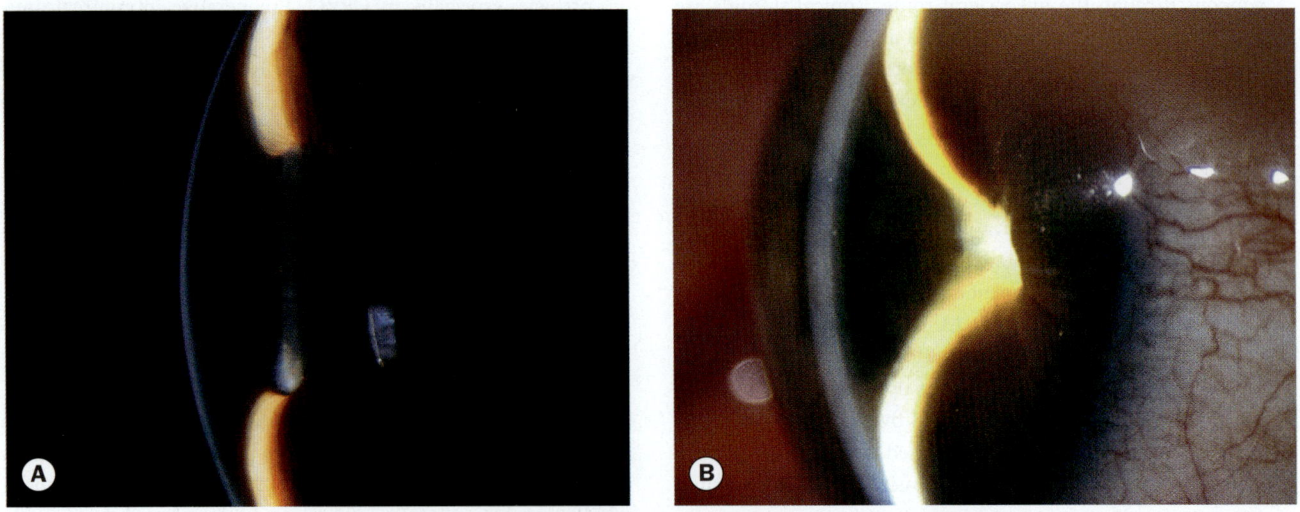

Fig. 11.46 Secondary angle closure with pupillary block. **(A)** Iris bombé; **(B)** iridocorneal contact.

Open-angle glaucoma

In acute anterior uveitis

In acute anterior uveitis the IOP is usually normal or subnormal due to concomitant ciliary shutdown. Occasionally, however, secondary open-angle glaucoma develops due to obstruction of aqueous outflow, most commonly as acute inflammation is subsiding and ciliary body function returning (Fig. 11.47D). This effect, which is often transient and innocuous, may be steroid-induced or caused by a combination of the following mechanisms:

- **Trabecular obstruction** by inflammatory cells and debris, which may be associated with increased aqueous viscosity due to leakage of protein from inflamed iris blood vessels.
- **Acute trabeculitis** involving inflammation and oedema of the trabecular meshwork with secondary diminution of intertrabecular porosity may result in a reduction in outflow facility. It is thought that this is especially relevant in anterior uveitis associated with herpes zoster, herpes simplex, other viral anterior uveitides and toxoplasma retinitis.

In chronic anterior uveitis

In chronic anterior uveitis the main mechanism for reduced outflow facility is thought to be trabecular scarring and/or sclerosis secondary to chronic trabeculitis. The importance of this mechanism is, however, difficult to determine as most eyes also have some degree of synechial angle closure. Because of the variable appearance of the angle on gonioscopy, definitive diagnosis of trabecular damage is difficult. In some eyes, a gelatinous exudate is seen on the trabeculum.

Treatment

Medical

- Medical control of IOP is more likely to be achieved if the angle is completely open.

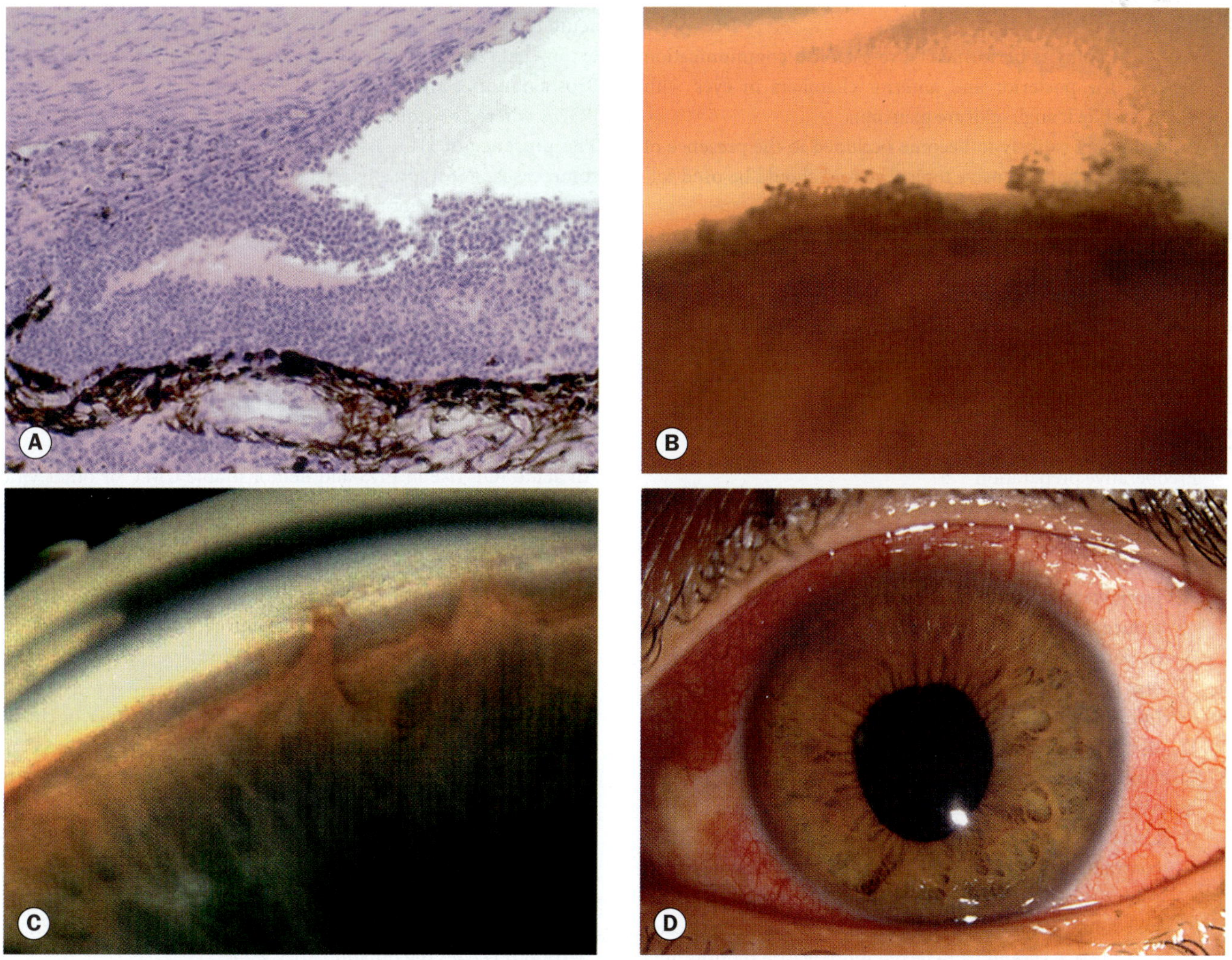

Fig. 11.47 Secondary angle closure without pupillary block. **(A)** Deposition of inflammatory cells in the angle; **(B)** gonioscopy showing inflammatory debris; **(C)** synechial angle closure (saw-toothed PAS); **(D)** acute anterior uveitis with secondary raised IOP. *(Courtesy of J Harry and G Misson, from* Clinical Ophthalmic Pathology, *Butterworth-Heinemann 2001 – fig. A.)*

- If there are a number of possible mechanisms causing the rise in IOP and the patient is using a topical steroid, stop the topical steroid for 2 days and remeasure the IOP.
- Long-acting depot steroid preparations should not be used in known or suspected steroid-responders.
- The effect of ocular hypotensive drugs is less predictable in uveitis, e.g. some cases may be unexpectedly sensitive to topical carbonic anhydrase inhibitors (CAI).
- A beta-blocker is usually the drug of first choice.
- Prostaglandin derivatives should be avoided if possible as they may promote inflammation.
- The choice of additional agents often depends on the IOP level. If this is very high, oral acetazolamide may be required. For moderate elevation (e.g. less than 35 mmHg on a beta-blocker) in the absence of significant glaucomatous damage, an alpha-adrenergic agonist or topical CAI might be adequate.
- Miotics are contraindicated as they increase vascular permeability and as miosis promotes the formation of posterior synechiae.

Laser iridotomy

- Laser iridotomy is performed to re-establish communication between the posterior and anterior chambers in eyes with pupillary-block angle-closure glaucoma.
- An iridotomy is likely to become occluded in the presence of active uveitis and intensive topical steroid should be used following the laser.
- Correction of pupillary block alone may not control the IOP if there is insufficient exposed functional angle, though a patent iridotomy may retard progressive PAS formation.
- Surgical iridectomy is the definitive method of preventing further pupil block and may be required if laser fails to maintain a viable iridotomy.

Surgery

- Preoperative preparation
  - Control of chronic uveitis for a minimum of 3 months before surgery is ideal.
  - Preoperative topical steroids should be used, not only as prophylaxis against recurrent inflammation but also to reduce the conjunctival inflammatory cell population.
  - In patients with particularly labile inflammatory disease oral prednisolone should be considered (0.5 mg/kg daily). Immunosuppressive treatment has improved the prognosis in recent years.
- Trabeculectomy with mitomycin C or the implantation of a long-tube implant can be used in these circumstances.
  - Combined cataract and glaucoma surgery is relatively contraindicated, but may sometimes be performed in conjunction with goniosynechialysis; occasionally cataract surgery alone can be appropriate. In most cases cataract surgery should be deferred for at least 6 months after trabeculectomy.
  - Postoperative hypotony is a particular risk as a delicate balance may exist between reduced aqueous production and restricted outflow. This is particularly likely to occur if there has been a pronounced reduction in the IOP when acetazolamide is introduced.
  - Following surgery, steroids are tapered more slowly than in non-inflammatory glaucoma.
- **Cyclodestructive** procedures should be used with caution as they may exacerbate inflammation. Possible underlying ciliary body insufficiency also carries the risk of profound hypotony that may progress to phthisis bulbi.

TIP Inappropriate use of topical steroids is a significant risk factor for the development of raised IOP and glaucoma.

Posner–Schlossman syndrome (PSS)

Introduction

PSS (glaucomatocyclitic crisis) is a rare condition characterized by recurrent attacks of unilateral acute raised IOP associated with mild anterior uveitis. The mechanism is speculated to be acute trabeculitis and there is evidence that infection, possibly cytomegalovirus (CMV) or *Helicobacter pylori*, may play a role. Prostaglandins are involved in the pathogenesis, particularly PGE_2, where the aqueous levels positively correlate with IOP. The presence of HLA-Bw54 haplotype has been implicated in some cases. PSS typically affects young to middle-aged adults. Males are affected more frequently than females. Episodes are unilateral, although 50% of patients have involvement of the other eye at different times. The intervals between attacks vary, but usually become longer with time. Patients should be followed even after the attacks have completely subsided, because a significant proportion will develop chronic IOP elevation, with the fellow eye also at risk.

Diagnosis

An acute IOP rise in PDS and demonstrable CMV or other viral anterior uveitis can present in an almost identical manner. The signs of the former may be atypical in older patients and those with dark irides. Simple IOP volatility in POAG, especially the juvenile variant, must also be distinguished.

- **Presentation** is with mild discomfort, haloes around lights and slight blurring of vision in one eye and sometimes redness.
- **Slit lamp biomicroscopy** typically shows a few anterior chamber cells and one to several fine white central keratic precipitates. Injection is likely to be absent or minimal. Mild corneal epithelial oedema is frequent.
- **Mydriasis** is common. Posterior synechiae are not a feature.
- **IOP** is typically raised to over 40 mmHg, out of proportion to iritis severity and untreated persists for hours to weeks. Elevation precedes the inflammatory signs.
- **Gonioscopy** shows an open angle without PAS.
- **Glaucomatous optic neuropathy** is relatively uncommon in most cases. Reversible cupping has been described.

Treatment

Topical steroids are used to control inflammation, with aqueous suppressants to lower the IOP. Topical steroids should only be used while there is active inflammation and should not be used prophylactically. Topical or oral non-steroidal anti-inflammatory agents may also be beneficial. The benefit of antiviral treatment is unclear. Trabeculectomy with mitomycin C may occasionally be needed, especially when there are signs of glaucomatous nerve damage or progressive visual field loss.

Steroid-induced glaucoma

Introduction

Around one in three individuals develop some degree of elevation of IOP in response to a course of potent topical steroid, dividing the population into steroid 'responders' and 'non-responders'. Responders are more likely than non-responders to develop POAG and a majority of patients with POAG are responders. Steroid-induced glaucoma is a form of secondary glaucoma, which is typically associated with the use of topical, periocular, intraocular or steroid therapy, although it can occur with any type of corticosteroid administration. The rise in IOP is a consequence of increased resistance to the outflow of aqueous secondary to altered function of the extracellular matrix or endothelial cells of the trabecular meshwork. The IOP elevation is dependent on the steroid type, potency, dose, duration and route of administration and usually occurs 2–4 weeks after commencement of treatment. The rise in IOP after intravitreal triamcinolone typically lasts 2–4 months and after dexamethasone intravitreal implant (Ozurdex) up to 6 months. The clinical picture resembles that of chronic open-angle glaucoma with a normal-appearing anterior chamber angle and an absence of symptoms. Much less often the condition may result in an acute presentation with pain and a significant IOP rise.

Risk factors

- Established glaucoma/ocular hypertension.
- Family history of glaucoma.
- High myopia.
- Young age, especially childhood.
- Connective tissue disease, especially rheumatoid arthritis.

Treatment

- Discontinuation of the topical steroid is usually all that is required to reduce the IOP back to normal. In the acute form this occurs within days and in the chronic form within 1–4 weeks.
- A less potent steroid drop can be prescribed, for example fluorometholone 0.1%, rimexolone 1% or loteprednol etabonate.
- In 3% of patients, elevated IOP may persist despite stopping all steroids. The duration of steroid therapy influences the reversibility of IOP elevation. This is usually seen in patients with a family history of glaucoma.
- Persistent IOP elevation should be managed with medication or glaucoma surgery. Steroid-induced raised IOP is unlikely to occur in the presence of an established bleb.

TIP In any patient with raised IOP who is using topical steroids, simply discontinuing the steroids will often result in a rapid reduction of IOP (thus identifying the patient as a 'steroid responder').

LENS-RELATED GLAUCOMA

Phacolytic glaucoma

Introduction

Phacolytic glaucoma is a secondary open-angle glaucoma occurring in association with a hypermature cataract. Trabecular obstruction is caused by high molecular-weight lens proteins that leak through the intact capsule into the aqueous humour leading to trabecular obstruction. Macrophages containing lens proteins may also contribute (Fig. 11.48A). Phacolytic glaucoma should not be confused with phacogenic (previously phacoanaphylactic) uveitis, an autoimmune granulomatous reaction to exposed lens proteins occurring with a compromised lens capsule (see Ch. 12).

Diagnosis

- **Presentation** is with pain. Vision is poor due to cataract.
- **Slit lamp biomicroscopy** shows corneal oedema, a hypermature cataract and a deep anterior chamber. There may be large floating white particles in the AC, consisting of lens protein and protein-containing macrophages (Fig. 11.48B), which may impart a milky appearance to the aqueous if very dense (Fig. 11.48C) and can form a pseudohypopyon (Fig. 11.48C and D).
- **Gonioscopy**, if a reasonable view can be obtained, shows an open angle with lens-derived material and inflammatory cells that are most substantial inferiorly.

Treatment

After IOP is controlled medically, proteinaceous material is washed out from the anterior chamber and the cataract is removed. Care should be taken not to rupture the zonule, which is likely to be more fragile than usual.

Phacomorphic glaucoma

Pathogenesis

Phacomorphic glaucoma is an acute secondary angle-closure glaucoma precipitated by an intumescent cataractous lens. Equatorial age-related growth of the lens slackens the suspensory ligament and allows the lens to move anteriorly. Associated anteroposterior growth leads to increased iridolenticular contact and potentiates pupillary block and iris bombé.

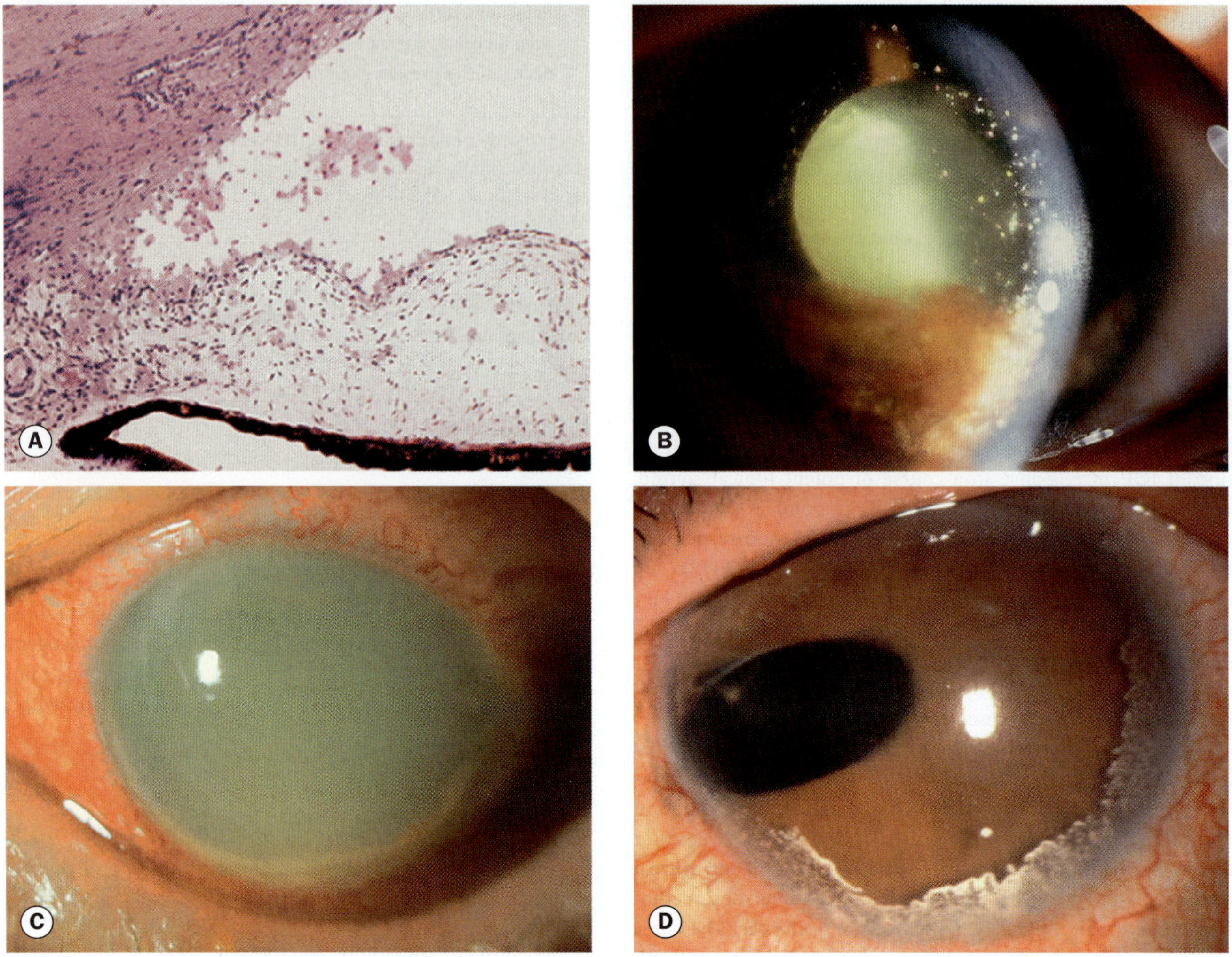

Fig. 11.48 Phacolytic glaucoma. **(A)** Lens protein-containing macrophages in the angle; **(B)** hypermature cataract, lens protein-containing macrophages floating in the aqueous; **(C)** dense milky aqueous with pseudohypopyon; **(D)** residual particles in the anterior chamber following incomplete irrigation after complicated surgery. *(Courtesy of J Harry and G Misson, from* Clinical Ophthalmic Pathology, *Butterworth-Heinemann 2001 – fig. A.)*

Diagnosis

- **Presentation** is similar to acute PACG with a shallow AC and mid-dilated pupil. A dense white cataract is evident (Fig. 11.49).
- **The fellow eye.** Phacomorphic glaucoma is more likely in eyes with a shorter axial length and shallower AC, but the fellow eye may demonstrate a deep AC and an open angle.
- **Anterior segment OCT** or US biomicroscopy may be useful.

Treatment

- **Medical** treatment is initially similar to that of acute PACG.
- **Miotics** are omitted as they tend to increase iris–lens apposition and shift the lens anteriorly. Dilatation is sometimes helpful but should be implemented with caution.
- **Systemic hyperosmotic agents** may be required more commonly than in PACG.
- **Laser iridotomy** may be worthwhile but is often not possible (due to corneal oedema or lens–cornea proximity) or ineffective. A similar procedure should be considered for the fellow eye.
- **Laser iridoplasty** may be a useful temporizing measure.
- **Cataract extraction** constitutes the definitive treatment, ideally once the IOP has been normalized and the eye is quiet. The surgery can be difficult and carries a higher risk of complications.

Pupillary block from disruption of lens position

Causes

- **Blunt ocular trauma**, even if relatively trivial, may result in lens dislocation in eyes with a weak zonule as in pseudoexfoliation and homocystinuria.
- **Congenitally small lens** (microspherophakia), e.g. Weill–Marchesani syndrome.

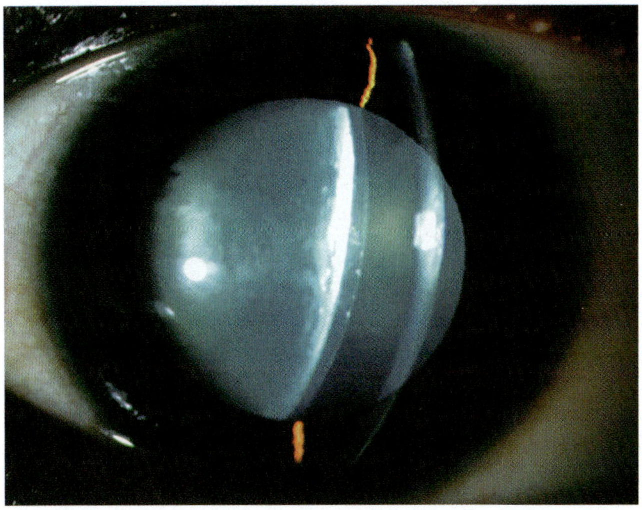

Fig. 11.49 Intumescent cataract, shallow anterior chamber, dilated pupil and corneal oedema in phacomorphic glaucoma.

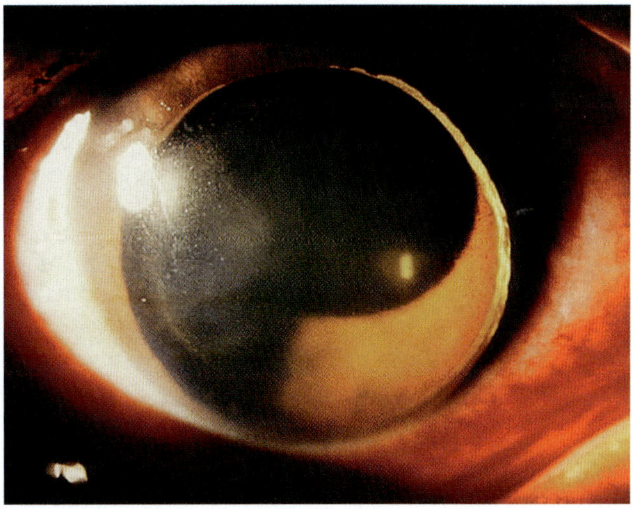

Fig. 11.50 Traumatic dislocation into the anterior chamber of a normal-size lens.

Dislocation may be into the AC, the zonules may be stretched or only part of the attachments may be disrupted so that the intact part acts as a hinge and the lens may remain fully or partially in the posterior chamber. Vitreous herniation may be contributory.

Diagnosis

A lens fully or partially dislocated into the anterior chamber will usually be evident (Fig. 11.50). Acute pupillary block will cause a sudden severe elevation of IOP with associated visual impairment. Imaging such as ultrasound biomicroscopy may be diagnostic.

Treatment

The IOP is initially reduced with osmotic agents, which reduce vitreous volume. Treatment should be urgent as prolonged lenticulocorneal contact, particularly in the presence of high IOP, may cause permanent endothelial damage.

- **Initial treatment.** The patient should adopt a supine posture with the pupil dilated, to attempt to reposition the lens in the posterior chamber, following which a miotic can be used with caution. Bilateral laser iridotomy may provide extended control in some cases, but lens extraction may be necessary.
- **Definitive treatment** consists of surgical lens extraction. An anterior chamber IOL, iris- or sclera-fixated IOL will be necessary.

TRAUMATIC GLAUCOMA

Hyphaema

Introduction

In a patient with a small traumatic hyphaema, which is usually innocuous and transient, IOP elevation may still result from trabecular obstruction by red blood cells. The size of a hyphaema is a useful indicator of visual prognosis and risk of complications. A hyphaema involving less than half the anterior chamber is associated with a 20% incidence of complications and a final VA of better than 6/18 in 80% of eyes (Fig. 11.51A). However, a hyphaema involving more than half the anterior chamber is associated with an 80% incidence of complications and a final VA of better than 6/18 in only one-third (Fig. 11.51B). The visual prognosis is determined mainly by the extent of injury to the retina sustained at the time of the original injury. Severe and prolonged elevation of IOP may cause corneal blood staining and damage to the optic nerve. The optic nerve is endangered by IOP of greater than 50 mmHg. Secondary haemorrhage, often more severe than the primary bleed, may develop within 3–5 days of the initial injury and is associated with a reduced visual outcome. Patients with sickle-cell haemoglobinopathy are at increased risk of complications, especially IOP elevation due to trabecular meshwork obstruction by deformed red cells and vascular occlusion.

Treatment

- **General**
  - A coagulation abnormality, particularly a haemoglobinopathy, should be excluded.
  - Any current anticoagulant medication should be discontinued after liaison with a general physician to assess the risk. NSAIDs should not be used for analgesia. Likewise, specialist advice should be sought regarding the management of a patient with a haemoglobinopathy, particularly before administering high-risk medication (see below).
  - Hospital admission may be required for a large hyphaema.
  - Strict bed rest is probably unnecessary, but substantially limiting activity is prudent and the patient should remain in a sitting or semi-upright posture, including during sleep.
  - A protective eye shield should be worn.

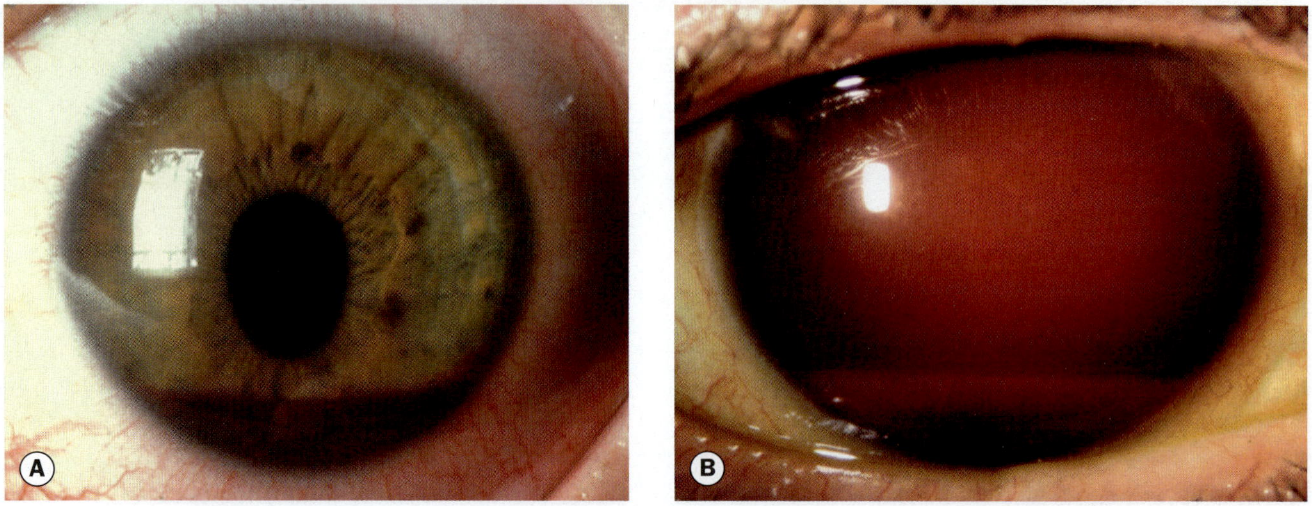

Fig. 11.51 Hyphaema. **(A)** Small with low risk of raised IOP; **(B)** secondary haemorrhage with raised IOP and increased risk of glaucoma and corneal blood staining.

- **Medical**
  - Topical prostaglandins, beta-blockers and/or a topical or systemic CAI is administered, depending on the IOP. CAI should not be used in sickle haemoglobinopathies. Miotics should also be avoided as they may increase pupillary block and disrupt the blood–aqueous barrier.
  - Occasionally a hyperosmotic agent is needed, though as with CAI and alpha-agonists a high threshold is adopted in sickle patients.
  - Topical steroids should be used since they reduce the risk of secondary haemorrhage and suppress inflammation.
  - Atropine is often recommended in patients with a large hyphaema to achieve constant mydriasis and to reduce the chance of secondary haemorrhage.
  - Antifibrinolysis with systemic tranexamic acid or aminocaproic acid (ACA) may be considered under higher-risk circumstances such as recurrent bleeding.
- **Laser photocoagulation** of angle bleeding points via a gonioprism has been described, though gonioscopy should probably be deferred for 5–6 days post-injury.
- **Anterior chamber paracentesis or surgical evacuation** of blood is required in around 5%. Indications for surgery include a total hyphaema, an IOP of >50 mmHg for 2 days or an IOP >35 mmHg for 5 days. Surgical intervention reduces the risk of permanent corneal staining and optic atrophy and prevents the occult development of peripheral anterior synechiae and chronic secondary glaucoma. Particular vigilance is required in patients with sickle-cell anaemia (even moderate pressure elevation can lead to optic atrophy), patients with prior glaucomatous optic neuropathy and in young children with a risk of amblyopia. A glaucoma filtration procedure may be necessary in some cases.
- **On discharge** the patient should be advised to avoid any activity with a risk of even minor eye trauma for several weeks. Symptoms of a rebleed should prompt immediate review.

Angle recession glaucoma

Introduction

Angle recession involves rupture of the face of the ciliary body, the portion between the iris root and the scleral spur, due to blunt trauma. Although a large percentage of eyes with traumatic hyphaema exhibit some degree of angle recession, glaucoma develops in less than 10% after 10 years. The rise in IOP is secondary to associated trabecular damage rather than from angle recession itself. However, the risk of glaucoma is directly related to the extent of angle recession and is unlikely to follow if less than three quadrants are recessed.

Diagnosis

- **Presentation** is with unilateral chronic glaucoma.
- **Slit lamp examination** may show signs of previous blunt trauma. These may be mild, such as a small sphincter rupture.
- **Gonioscopy** may initially reveal irregular widening of the ciliary body band (Fig. 11.52). In longstanding cases, the recession may become obscured by fibrosis and the angle may show hyperpigmentation.

Treatment

- **Follow-up**: Individuals with more than two quadrants of angle recession should have their IOP checked on a yearly basis. They should be reassured that their risk of developing secondary glaucoma is low.
- **Medical treatment** is as for other types of secondary open-angle glaucoma but is frequently unsatisfactory. Laser trabeculoplasty is of no benefit.
- **Trabeculectomy** with adjunctive antimetabolite is generally effective.
- **An artificial filtering shunt or cyclodiode** should be considered if trabeculectomy fails.

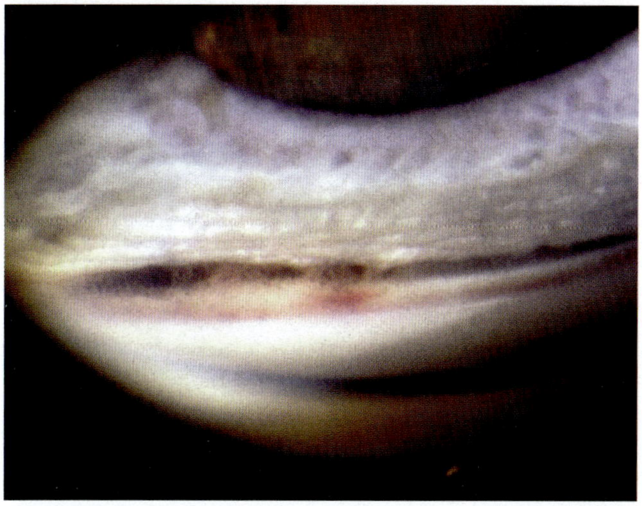

Fig. 11.52 Gonioscopy of angle recession showing irregular widening of the ciliary body band.

GHOST CELL 'GLAUCOMA'

Pathogenesis

Ghost cell 'glaucoma' is due to trabecular obstruction by degenerate erythrocytes, which causes raised IOP and, rarely, glaucoma. Approximately 2 weeks after a vitreous haemorrhage, haemoglobin leaks from the erythrocytes, which evolve into ghost cells. These then pass through a defect in the anterior hyaloid face and pass into the anterior chamber. Because their pliability is lost, the cells become entrapped within the pores of the trabecular meshwork and obstruct aqueous outflow. The condition may occur in the following settings:

- **Cataract surgery** in the context of pre-existing vitreous haemorrhage.
- **Vitreous haemorrhage in an already aphakic or pseudophakic eye.**
- **When cataract surgery is complicated** by a vitreous haemorrhage and hyphaema. The hyphaema clears but the red cells in the vitreous persist and evolve into ghost cells.

Clinical features

- The cornea may be oedematous due to elevated IOP.
- The anterior chamber exhibits ghost cells, which may be recognized as reddish-brown or khaki particles in the aqueous. They should not be confused with leucocytes, since this may result in unwarranted treatment for uveitis.

Treatment

- **Medical treatment** with aqueous suppressants.
- **Irrigation of the anterior chamber** with washing out of the ghost cells if medical therapy fails.
- **Pars plana vitrectomy** may occasionally be required for persistent vitreous haemorrhage.

IRIDOCORNEAL ENDOTHELIAL SYNDROME

Introduction

Iridocorneal endothelial (ICE) syndrome typically affects one eye of a middle-aged woman. It consists of the following three clinical presentations: Chandler syndrome, progressive (also termed essential) iris atrophy and iris naevus (Cogan–Reese) syndrome. The pathological basis in all three is an abnormal corneal endothelial cell layer with a predilection for proliferation and migration across the anterior chamber angle and onto the surface of the iris, with subsequent progression to glaucoma (50%) and corneal decompensation in a substantial proportion of involved eyes. Glaucoma is due to trabecular obstruction by proliferating tissue followed by angle closure secondary to contraction. Polymerase chain reaction (PCR) testing shows the presence of herpes simplex virus DNA in a substantial percentage of ICE syndrome corneal and trabecular meshwork specimens, suggesting a possible viral aetiology.

Diagnosis

Clear differentiation between the three presentations may be difficult. Apparent transition from one to another has been reported. Differentiation depends primarily on iris appearance, but there is often substantial overlap. Gonioscopically visible changes in some patients may be subtle despite elevated IOP, particularly in early disease. The specular microscopic appearance is characteristic.

- **Chandler syndrome** is the most common clinical presentation and is characterized by an abnormal corneal endothelial appearance said to resemble hammered silver (Fig. 11.53A). It frequently presents with blurred vision and haloes due to corneal oedema. Iris atrophy is absent in about 60% and in the remainder is variable in severity. Corectopia is mild–moderate when present. When glaucoma occurs, it is usually less severe than in the other two presentations.
- **Progressive (essential) iris atrophy** is characterized by iris changes including corectopia (pupil malposition – Fig. 11.53B), iris atrophy in the early stage, pseudopolycoria (supernumerary false pupil) (Fig. 11.53C), and broad-based PAS that often extend anterior to the Schwalbe line (Fig. 11.53D). Severe iris atrophy occurs in the late stage and is associated with ectropion uveae and severe glaucoma (Fig. 11.53E).
- **Iris naevus (Cogan–Reese) syndrome** is characterized by either a diffuse naevus that covers the anterior iris, or by iris nodules (Fig. 11.53F). Iris atrophy is absent in 50% of cases and in the remainder, it is usually mild–moderate, although corectopia may be severe. The appearance may be mimicked by a diffuse iris melanoma.

Treatment

- **Medical** treatment of glaucoma is usually ineffective.
- **Trabeculectomy** with mitomycin C can be tried, but the long-term results are poor.

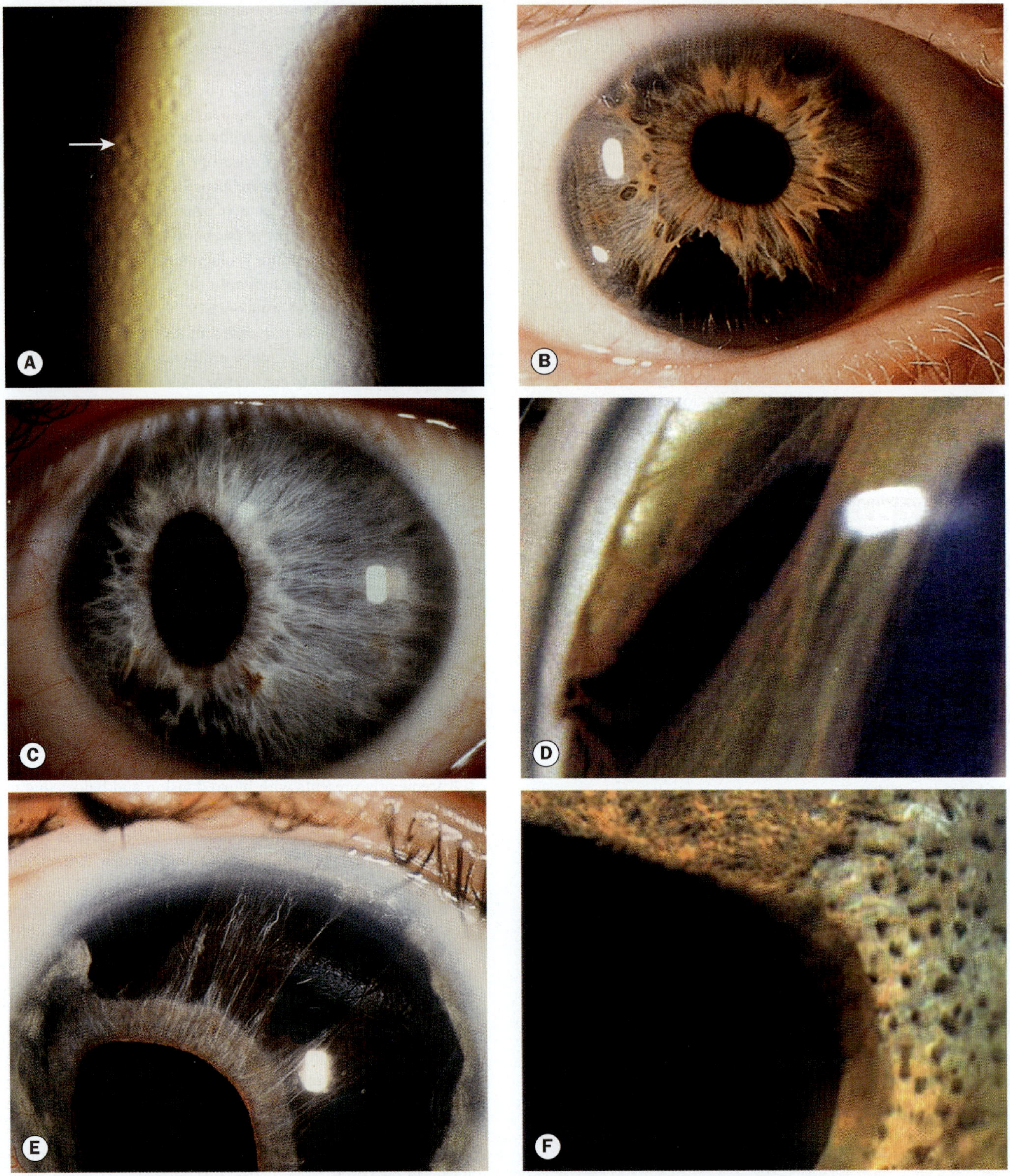

Fig. 11.53 Iridocorneal endothelial syndrome. **(A)** Chandler syndrome showing 'hammered silver' endothelial changes (arrow); **(B)** iris atrophy; **(C)** corectopia with pseudopolycoria; **(D)** gonioscopy showing broad peripheral synechiae; **(E)** progressive iris atrophy with polycoria; **(F)** iris nodules in Cogan–Reese syndrome.

- **Glaucoma drainage device or cyclodiode laser** may be required.
- **Corneal treatment.** Oedema can be treated with topical hypertonic saline in early disease and transplantation later on.
- **Prognosis.** The long-term prognosis is poor.

GLAUCOMA ASSOCIATED WITH INTRAOCULAR TUMOURS

Approximately 5% of eyes with intraocular tumours develop a secondary elevation of IOP. Potential mechanisms are set out below:

- **Trabecular block.** Distinction between different mechanisms may not be possible clinically.
  - Angle invasion by a solid iris melanoma (see Fig. 20.16F)
  - Trabecular infiltration by neoplastic cells originating from an iris melanoma (Fig. 11.54A). Rarely, tumour seeding from a retinoblastoma may also invade the trabeculum.
  - Melanomalytic glaucoma may occur in some eyes with iris melanoma. It is due to trabecular blockage by macrophages that have ingested pigment and tumour cells, similar to phacolytic glaucoma.
- **Secondary angle closure**
  - Neovascular glaucoma is the most common mechanism in eyes with choroidal melanoma or retinoblastoma.
  - Anterior displacement of iris–lens diaphragm may occur in an eye with a ciliary body melanoma or a large tumour of the posterior segment (Fig. 11.54B).

GLAUCOMA SECONDARY TO EPITHELIAL INGROWTH

Introduction

Epithelial ingrowth (downgrowth) is a rare but potentially blinding complication of anterior segment surgery or trauma, occurring when conjunctival or corneal epithelial cells migrate through a wound and proliferate in the anterior segment (Fig. 11.55A). Elevation of IOP is due to trabecular obstruction by one or more of an epithelial membrane, secondary synechial angle closure and desquamated epithelial and inflammatory cells. The associated glaucoma can be particularly intractable and the prognosis poor.

Diagnosis

- Persistent postoperative anterior uveitis.
- Diffuse epithelialization characterized by a greyish translucent membrane with a scalloped border that involves the posterior corneal surface in the area of a surgical or traumatic wound.
- Cystic and fibrous proliferative patterns sometimes occur and tend to have a better prognosis (Fig. 11.55B).
- Pupillary distortion.

Treatment

The aim of treatment is the eradication of all invading epithelium to avoid recurrence.

- **Block excision** involves the simultaneous excision of adjacent iris and pars plicata of the ciliary body, together with all layers of the sclera and cornea in contact with the lesion. The resultant defect is covered with a tectonic corneoscleral graft. The

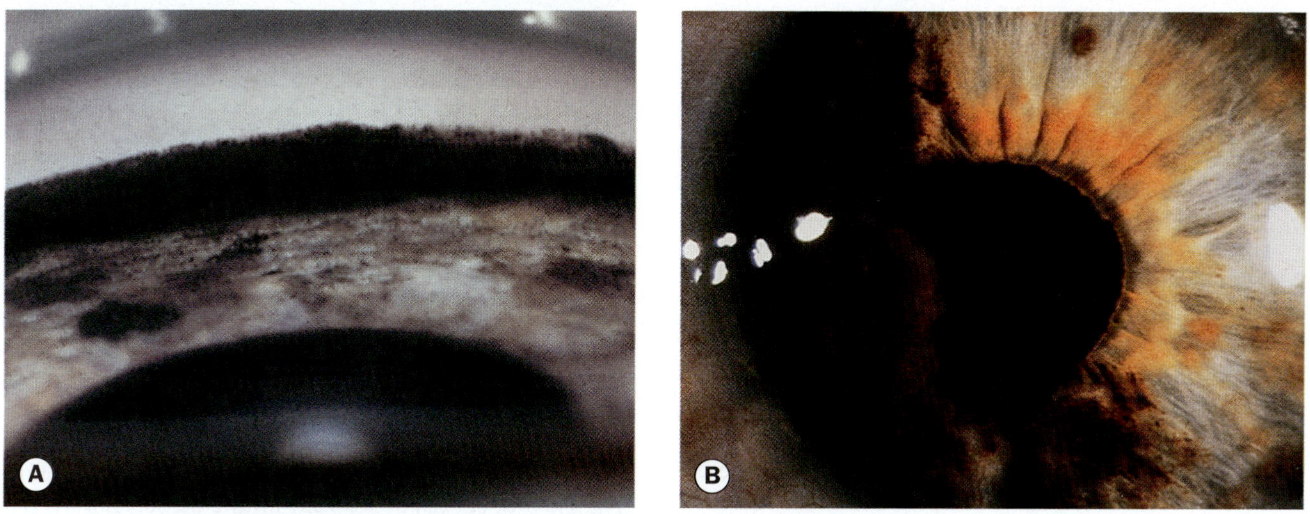

Fig. 11.54 Glaucoma secondary to intraocular melanoma. **(A)** Melanoma cells infiltrating the trabeculum; **(B)** anterior displacement of the iris by a ciliary body melanoma.

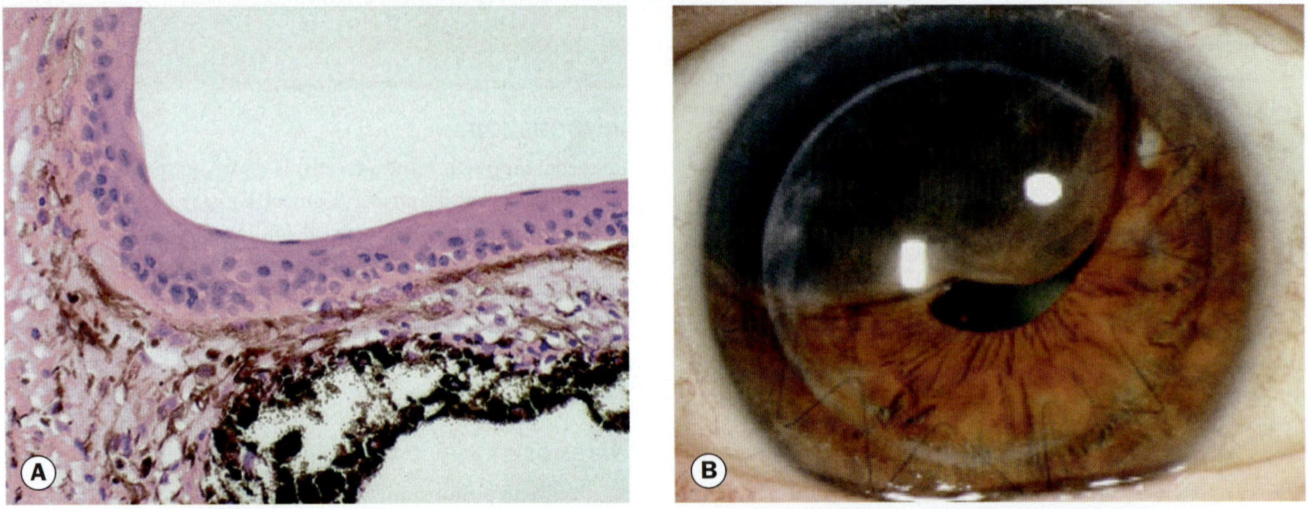

Fig. 11.55 Diffuse epithelial ingrowth. **(A)** Stratified squamous epithelium lining the anterior iris surface and filtration angle; **(B)** cystic epithelial ingrowth after penetrating keratoplasty. *(Courtesy of J Harry and G Misson, from* Clinical Ophthalmic Pathology, *Butterworth-Heinemann 2001 – fig. A.)*

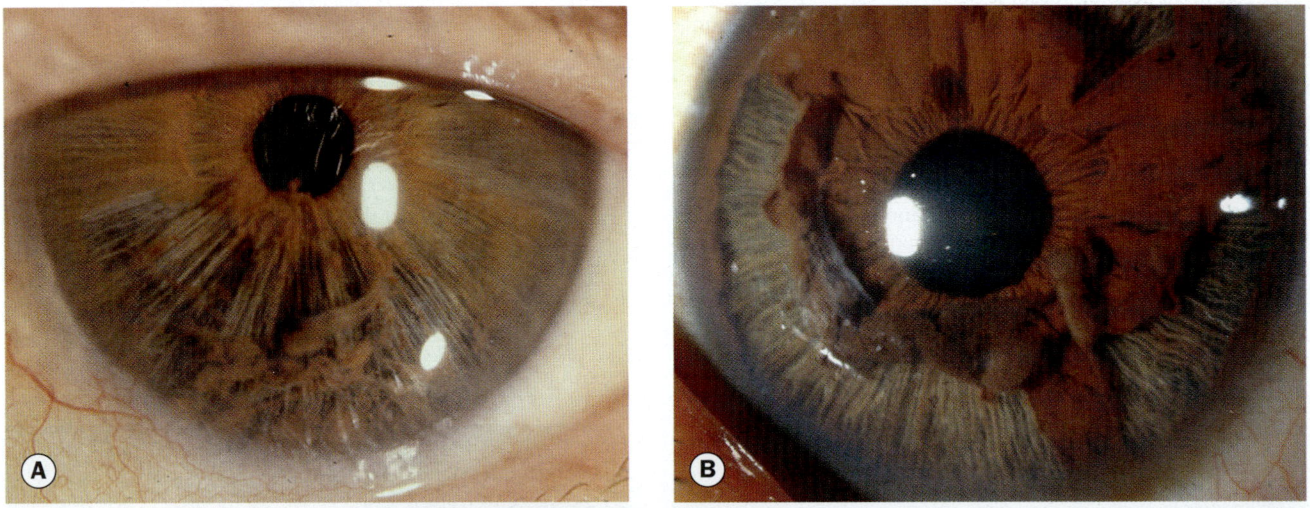

Fig. 11.56 Iridoschisis. **(A)** Mild; **(B)** severe.

area of iris involvement may be delineated by applying argon laser burns, which will cause whitening of the affected area.

- **Cryotherapy** may be applied to devitalize the epithelium remaining on the posterior surface of the cornea, in the angle and on the ciliary body. Intraocular air is used to insulate other tissues from the effects of the cryotherapy.
- **Intracameral 5-fluorouracil** has been tried with variable results.
- **Intravitreal injection of methotrexate** (400 mg/0.1 ml every 2 weeks for six cycles) has been reported to lead to successful resolution of the ingrowth.
- **Glaucoma drainage devices** are of value for medically uncontrolled glaucoma associated with extensive epithelial ingrowth unsuitable for surgical excision.

IRIDOSCHISIS

Iridoschisis is a rare condition typically affecting both eyes of an older patient. Primary angle closure and PACG is associated in up to 90%. This appearance may rarely occur after trauma. The mechanism is incompletely understood, but it has been proposed that intermittent substantial elevation of IOP results in iris atrophy, with severity ranging from stromal atrophy to fibrillar disintegration of the anterior layer. Changes are more marked inferiorly (Fig. 11.56A), but can occasionally involve the superior iris (Fig. 11.56B). The pupil is usually normal and the anterior chamber is typically shallow. Gonioscopy commonly shows an occludable angle, often with PAS. Angle closure should be treated with a laser iridotomy.

PRIMARY CONGENITAL GLAUCOMA

Introduction

Primary congenital glaucoma (PCG) is rare, with an incidence of 1:10 000 live births, in many populations. Boys are more commonly affected than girls in most surveys. The rate is 5–10 times higher in children from consanguineous relationships. Involvement is more often bilateral, but frequently asymmetrical. The condition can be classified as follows:

- **True congenital glaucoma** (40%), in which IOP is elevated during intrauterine life.
- **Infantile glaucoma** (55%), which manifests prior to age 3.
- **Juvenile glaucoma**, the least common, in which IOP rises between 3 and 16 years of age.

Primary congenital glaucoma is, by definition, not associated with other major ocular abnormalities. It is thought to be caused by impaired aqueous outflow due to maldevelopment of the anterior chamber angle (trabeculodysgenesis). It is usually sporadic, but approximately 10% are inherited in an autosomal recessive fashion with variable penetrance. Angiopoietin receptor *TEK* mutations play a role in the aetiology of some cases of primary congenital glaucoma and are transmitted as an autosomal dominant pattern with variable expressivity. Other gene mutations have been implicated in autosomal recessive congenital glaucoma, prominently *CYP1B-1*coding for cytochrome P450 and *LTBP2*. Currently, the chance of identifying a genetic cause is 40% when genetic testing is done. The prognosis is dependent on severity and age at onset/diagnosis. Secondary infantile glaucoma can be caused by a range of conditions including tumours such as retinoblastoma, persistent fetal vasculature (persistent hyperplastic primary vitreous) and uveitis.

TIP Primary congenital glaucoma is always treated surgically as soon as the diagnosis has been confirmed.

Diagnosis

- **Presentation** usually occurs when watering, photophobia or blepharospasm is noticed by parents or a health-care professional, or when an abnormality is found, such as corneal haze, large (Fig. 11.57A) or asymmetrical eye size (Fig. 11.57B).
- **Corneal haze** is due to diffuse oedema secondary to raised IOP, or localized oedema due to breaks in Descemet membrane (Fig. 11.57C).
- **Buphthalmos** is a large eye (see Fig. 11.57A–C) as a result of stretching due to elevated IOP prior to the age of 3 years. A corneal diameter of more than 12 mm before the age of 1 should be treated with suspicion, especially if there is asymmetry. The thinned sclera often appears blue due to increased visualization of the underlying uvea. Complications include myopia and lens subluxation.
- **Haab striae** (Fig. 11.57D) are curvilinear healed breaks in Descemet membrane.
- **Corneal scarring** and vascularization.
- **Optic disc cupping** in infants may regress once IOP is normalized. Most normal infants exhibit no apparent cup.
- **Evaluation under general anaesthesia** is generally required. Intravenous ketamine lowers IOP less than other agents.
  - IOP measurement should be performed first, optimally with more than one method (e.g. Perkins, Tono-Pen, iCare). It is preferable where possible for this to be measured in a conscious or sedated child; 10–12 mmHg is normal.
  - Anterior chamber examination with an operating microscope and/or portable slit lamp.
  - Optic disc examination; asymmetry or a cup/disc ratio of >0.3 is suspicious.
  - Corneal diameter measurement; >12 mm prior to the age of 1 year is highly suspicious.
  - Increased axial length measurement using ultrasound: a measurement of more than 20.25 mm at 1 month is usually abnormal, particularly if there is inter-eye asymmetry. One of the most reliable signs of IOP control after surgery is stabilization of the axial length measurements.
  - Gonioscopy using a direct goniolens may be normal or reveal trabeculodysgenesis (Fig. 11.58), vaguely characterized by an anteriorly located iris insertion and a hypoplastic-appearing peripheral iris. The old concept of a discrete (Barkan) membrane has not been definitively confirmed.
  - Refraction.

Treatment

Surgery is always required and is successful in 80–90%. Medication may be used as temporary or supplementary therapy. Caution is required with selection of medication in young children, as most are relatively contraindicated.

- **Goniotomy.** Under direct gonioscopic visualization, an incision is made at the midpoint of the trabecular meshwork (Fig. 11.59A).
- **Trabeculotomy** may be necessary if corneal clouding prevents an adequate view of the angle and is also an option when repeated goniotomy has failed. A partial-thickness scleral flap is created (Fig. 11.59B) and a Harms trabeculotome (Fig. 11.59C) is inserted into the Schlemm canal and rotated into the anterior chamber.
- **A modification of trabeculotomy** is used in some centres. An illuminated canaloplasty device is threaded into the Schlemm canal followed by a 6-0 Prolene suture, which is then pulled into the anterior chamber thus opening 360% of the trabecular meshwork (Fig. 11.59D). The postoperative IOP using this technique is approximately 5 mmHg lower at 2 years than that obtained with the traditional approach.
- **Other procedures** when angle surgery fails include trabeculectomy, tube shunt implantation and ciliary body ablative procedures.
- **Monitoring** of IOP, corneal diameter, axial length and other parameters is required long term.
- **Amblyopia and refractive error** should be managed aggressively.

Differential diagnosis

- **Cloudy cornea**
  - Birth trauma.
  - Rubella keratitis (congenital rubella is also associated with congenital glaucoma).

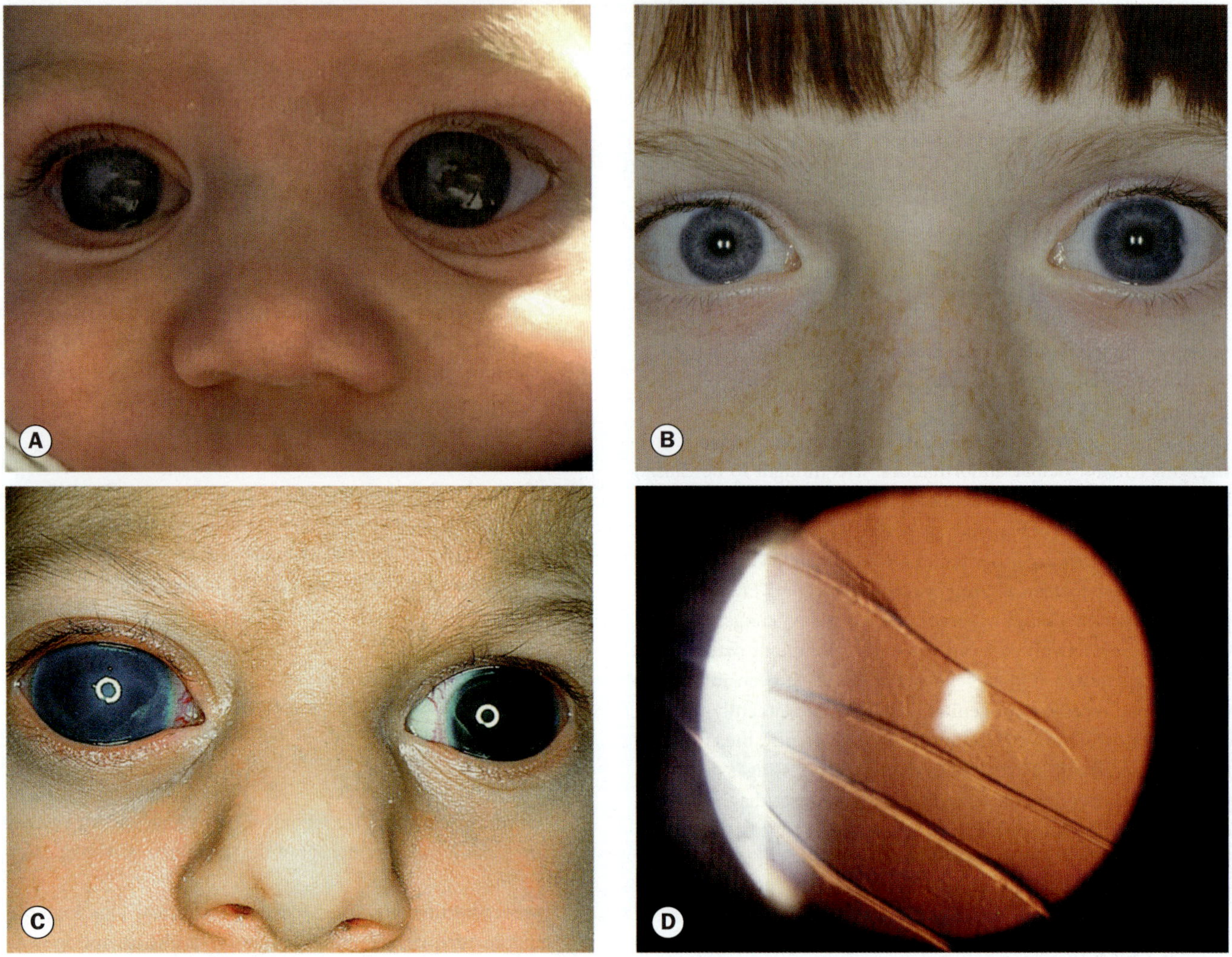

Fig. 11.57 Congenital glaucoma. **(A)** Bilateral buphthalmos; **(B)** buphthalmos in the left eye; **(C)** severe buphthalmos, worse in the right eye, which exhibits marked diffuse corneal oedema; **(D)** Haab striae on retroillumination.

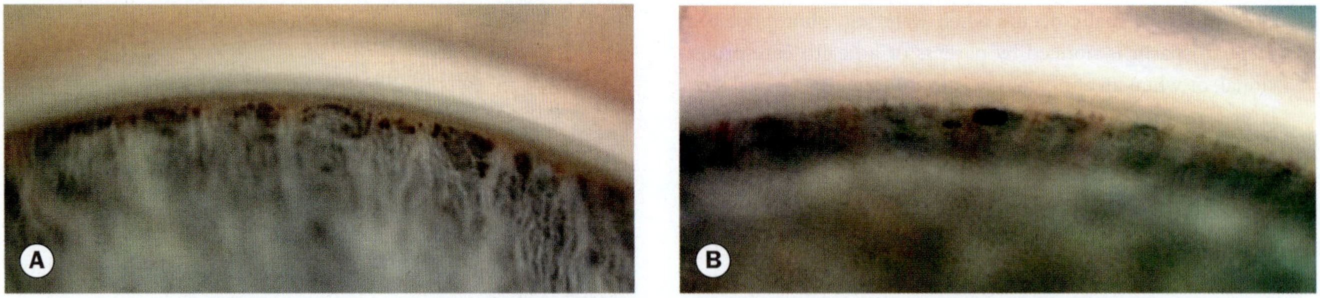

Fig. 11.58 **(A)** Normal infant angle showing the iris root, prominent ciliary body band but no discernible scleral spur and trabeculum; **(B)** one angle variant in congenital glaucoma showing the iris root but not the ciliary body band due to translucent amorphous tissue that obscures the trabeculum. *(Courtesy of Ken K Nischal.)*

  - Metabolic disorders such as mucopolysaccharidoses and mucolipidoses.
  - Congenital hereditary endothelial dystrophy.
  - Sclerocornea.
- **Large cornea**
  - Megalocornea.
  - High myopia.
- **Epiphora**
  - Delayed/failed canalization of the nasolacrimal duct.
  - Lacrimation secondary to ocular irritation, e.g. conjunctivitis, aberrant eyelashes, entropion.

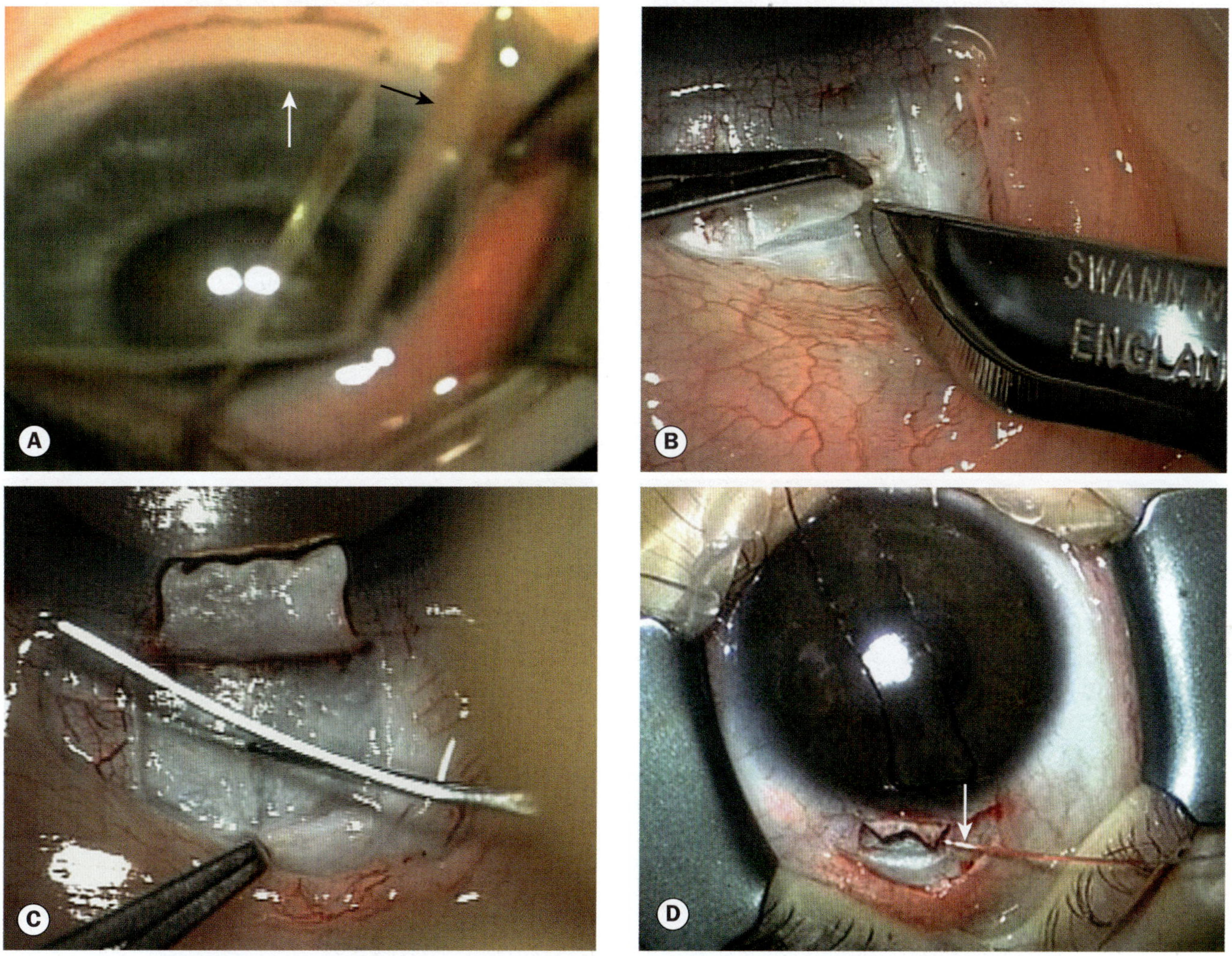

Fig. 11.59 Surgery for congenital glaucoma. **(A)** Goniotomy (white arrow shows the cleft; black arrow shows direction of needle); **(B** and **C)** trabeculotomy (see text); **(D)** modification of trabeculotomy using illuminated microcatheter (arrow). *(Courtesy of M Papadopoulos – figs A and D; Ken K Nischal – figs B and C.)*

IRIDOCORNEAL DYSGENESIS

Posterior embryotoxon

Posterior embryotoxon refers to a prominent and anteriorly displaced Schwalbe line, seen as a thin grey-white arcuate ridge adjacent to the limbus on the inner surface of the cornea (Fig. 11.60A). It is an innocuous isolated finding in up to 15% of the general population, but is one of the features of Axenfeld–Rieger anomaly. It is also seen in the multisystem genetic disorder Alagille syndrome, in which optic disc drusen are also common.

Axenfeld–Rieger syndrome

Introduction

Axenfeld–Rieger syndrome is the umbrella term for a spectrum of disorders featuring bilateral developmental ocular anomalies: Axenfeld anomaly, Rieger anomaly and Rieger syndrome. It is caused by defective neural crest cell-related processes during fetal development. This can lead to incomplete development of the trabecular meshwork or Schlemm canal. An abnormal endothelial cell membrane has been identified on anterior segment structures in some patients. The key implication of the syndrome is a 50% risk of glaucoma. Associated variants in several different genes have been found, including *PITX2, PAX6, FOXC1* and *RIEG2*. Different genetic abnormalities can give a similar clinical picture (genetic heterogeneity). Cases may be sporadic, but a family history is common, when inheritance is autosomal dominant with variable expressivity but very high penetrance. There is no gender predilection.

Clinical features

- **Axenfeld anomaly** is characterized by posterior embryotoxon (Fig. 11.60A) with attached strands of peripheral iris, the latter best viewed with gonioscopy.

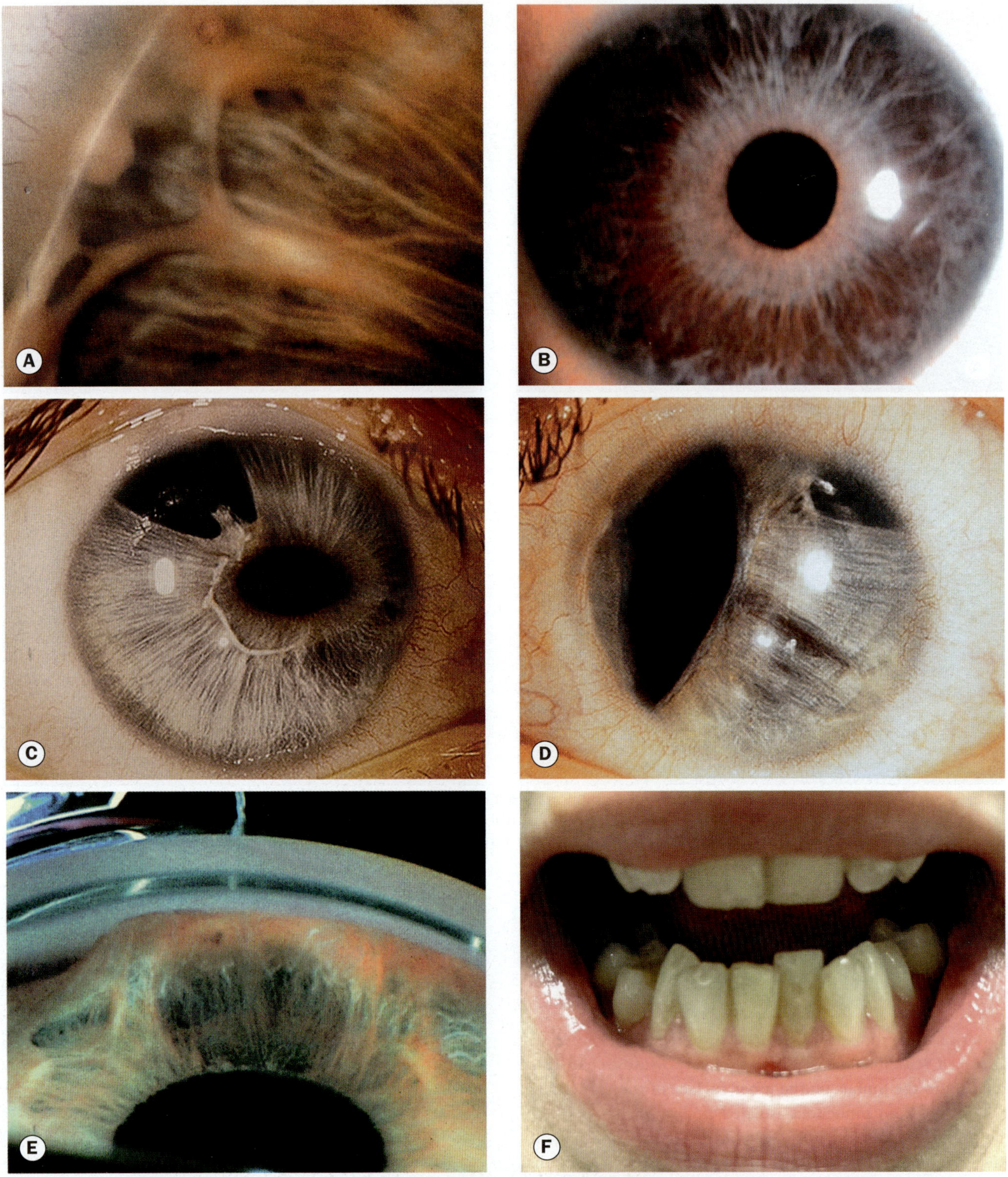

Fig. 11.60 Axenfeld–Rieger syndrome. **(A)** Posterior embryotoxon; **(B)** severe iris stromal hypoplasia; **(C)** full-thickness iris hole with corectopia (in the right eye); **(D)** severe corectopia (in the left eye of the same patient shown in **(C)**); **(E)** gonioscopy showing peripheral anterior synechiae; **(F)** dental anomalies.

- **Rieger anomaly** often manifests with an anterior segment appearance similar to that of iridocorneal endothelial (ICE) syndrome.
  - Posterior embryotoxon.
  - Iris stromal hypoplasia (Fig. 11.60B).
  - Ectropion uveae.
  - Corectopia and full-thickness iris defects (Fig. 11.60C and D).
- **Gonioscopy** in mild cases shows the Axenfeld anomaly. In severe cases, broad leaves of iris adhere to the cornea anterior to the Schwalbe line (Fig. 11.60E).
- **Glaucoma** develops in about 50%, usually during childhood or early adulthood. Surgical management is often necessary.
- **Rieger syndrome** is characterized by the Rieger anomaly together with extraocular malformations that, as with the ocular features, are caused by defective neural crest cell-related tissue development:
  - Dental anomalies (Fig. 11.60F), including hypodontia (few teeth) and microdontia (small teeth).
  - Facial anomalies: maxillary hypoplasia, broad nasal bridge, telecanthus and hypertelorism.
  - Other anomalies include redundant paraumbilical skin and hypospadias. Hearing loss, hydrocephalus, cardiac and renal anomalies and congenital hip dislocation are rare.

Peters anomaly

Introduction

Peters anomaly is a rare but often severe condition that is bilateral in more than half of cases. It is the result of defective neural crest cell migration during fetal development. Manifestations range from mild to severe. Most cases are sporadic, although autosomal recessive inheritance has been described.

Clinical features

Peters type I affects the cornea alone, type II shows both corneal and lens abnormalities.

- **Central corneal opacity** of variable density (Fig. 11.61A and B).
- **Posterior corneal defect** involving the posterior stroma, Descemet membrane and endothelium with or without iridocorneal or lenticulocorneal (Fig. 11.61C) adhesions.
- **Glaucoma** occurs in about 50% due to associated angle anomaly. Onset is usually in infancy but occasionally in childhood or later. The prognosis tends to be worse than in primary congenital glaucoma.
- **Systemic associations** including craniofacial and central nervous system anomalies have been reported. 'Peters plus' syndrome includes a particular constellation of systemic abnormalities.

Aniridia

Genetics

Aniridia is a rare bilateral condition that may have life-threatening associations. It occurs as a result of abnormal neuroectodermal development secondary to a mutation in the *PAX6* gene. *PAX6* is adjacent to gene *WT1*, mutation of which predisposes to Wilms tumour.

- **Autosomal dominant** aniridia accounts for about two-thirds of cases and has no systemic implications. Penetrance is complete (all patients with the genotype will have the phenotype) but expressivity (severity) is variable.
- **Sporadic**, including WARG, previously known as Miller syndrome (Wilms tumour, Aniridia, mental Retardation, Genitourinary abnormalities), includes about a third of patients. Children with sporadic aniridia have about a 30% chance of developing Wilms tumour.
- **Gillespie syndrome** accounts for only about 1% of cases. Inheritance is AR but is not caused by *PAX6* mutations. Cerebellar ataxia and learning disabilities are features.

Diagnosis

All patients with sporadic aniridia should have abdominal ultrasonography every 3 months until 5 years of age, every 6 months until 10 years of age and annually until 16 years of age to detect the development of Wilms tumour or until molecular genetic analysis confirms the absence of a *WT1* mutation.

- **Presentation** is typically at birth with nystagmus and photophobia. The parents may have noticed the absence of irides or apparently large pupils.
- **Aniridia** is variable in severity, ranging from minimal, detectable only by retroillumination, to total absence (Fig. 11.62A and B).
- **Lids** often show meibomian gland dysfunction.
- **Cornea**
  - Tear film instability, dry eye and epithelial defects are common.
  - Limbal stem cell deficiency may result in 'conjunctivalization' of the peripheral cornea.
  - Total corneal central stromal scarring and vascularization may occur in end-stage disease.
- **Fundus.** Possible abnormalities include foveal and/or optic nerve hypoplasia and choroidal coloboma.
- **Gonioscopy** even in eyes with apparently total aniridia usually shows a hypoplastic or rudimentary frill of iris tissue (Fig. 11.62C).
- **Lens** changes can include cataract and subluxation.
- **Glaucoma** (75%) usually presents in late childhood or adolescence. It is caused by synechial angle closure secondary to the contraction of rudimentary iris tissue. Treatment is difficult and the prognosis guarded.

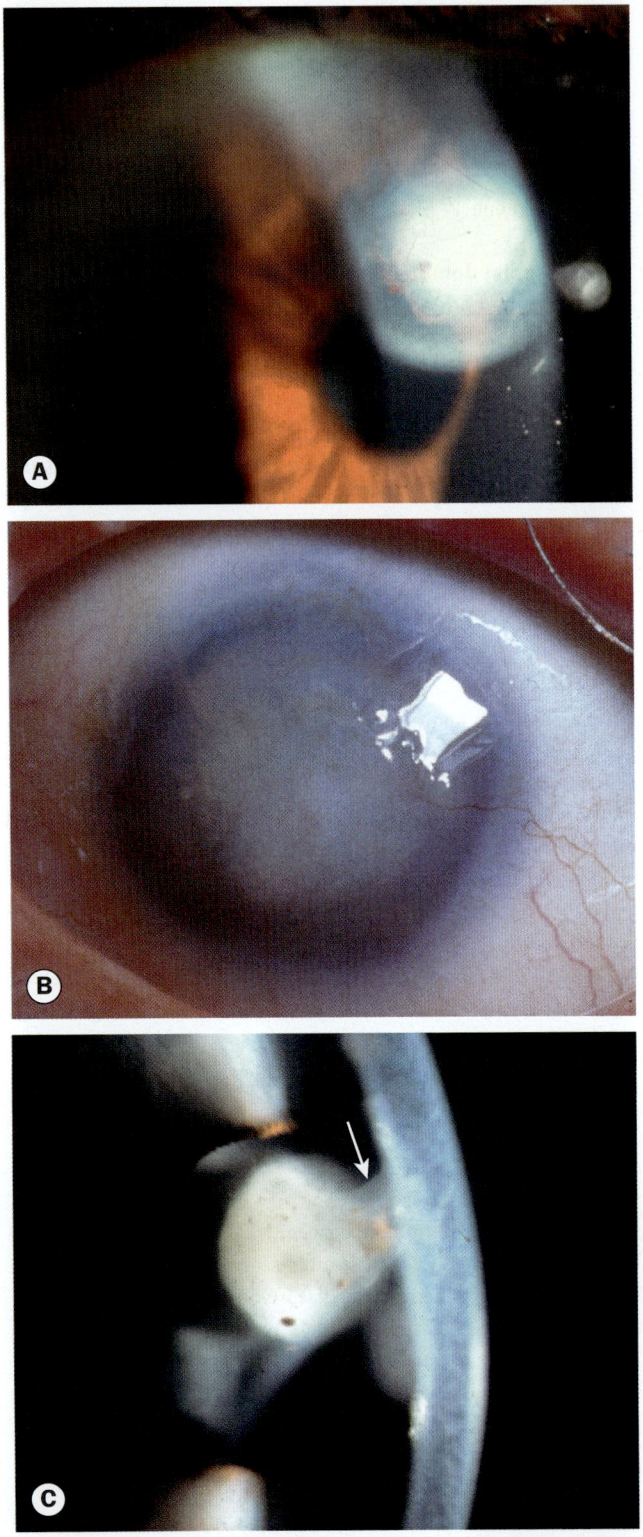

Fig. 11.61 Peters anomaly. **(A)** Corneal opacity; **(B)** large central opacity; **(C)** lenticulocorneal adhesion (arrow).

Treatment

- **Glaucoma**
  - Medical treatment is usually inadequate.
  - Trabeculectomy with mitomycin C or combined trabeculectomy–trabeculotomy have been tried in the past but usually fail to control the IOP.
  - Glaucoma drainage devices offer the best chance of long-term successful control of IOP.
  - Diode laser cycloablation may be necessary if other modalities fail.
- **Painted contact lenses** may be used to create an artificial pupil and improve both vision and cosmesis. Simple tinted lenses are an alternative. Both may improve nystagmus.
- **Lubricants** are frequently required for associated keratopathy.
- **Cataract surgery** is often required. (Fig. 11.62D). A tinted artificial lens implant may be used to try to reduce photophobia. Trauma to the corneal limbus should be minimized in order to preserve stem cell function.
- **Prosthetic iris implantation** has been described in pseudophakic aniridic eyes, but may be complicated by, or worsen, glaucoma.
- **Limbal stem cell transplantation** with or without keratoplasty may be required.
- **Refractive errors, amblyopia and squint** should be managed aggressively.

GLAUCOMA IN PHACOMATOSES

Sturge–Weber syndrome

Introduction

Sturge–Weber syndrome (encephalotrigeminal angiomatosis) is a congenital, sporadic phacomatosis (see Ch. 2). Glaucoma ipsilateral to the facial haemangioma develops in about 30% and in 60% of these IOP elevation occurs before the age of 2 years and may result in buphthalmos (Fig. 11.63A). In the remainder, glaucoma may develop at any time from infancy to adulthood. The pathogenesis is uncertain but putative mechanisms include trabeculodysgenesis in infants and raised episcleral venous pressure associated with arteriovenous communication in an episcleral haemangioma (Fig. 11.63B) in older patients.

Treatment

- **Medical** treatment alone may be adequate.
- **Goniotomy** may be successful in eyes with angle anomalies.
- **Combined trabeculotomy–trabeculectomy** gives good results in early-onset cases, but carries a relatively high risk of choroidal effusion and suprachoroidal haemorrhage. Other surgical options may be utilized.

Neurofibromatosis type 1

Neurofibromatosis is a disorder that primarily affects cell growth of neural tissues. Inheritance is AD with irregular penetrance and variable expressivity (see Ch. 19). Glaucoma is relatively rare and, when present, usually unilateral and congenital. About 50% of patients with glaucoma have an ipsilateral plexiform neurofibroma of the upper eyelid, or facial hemiatrophy (Fig. 11.64A). Various mechanisms have been identified, including congenital angle anomaly, which may be associated with ectropion uveae (Fig. 11.64B and see Fig. 19.103).

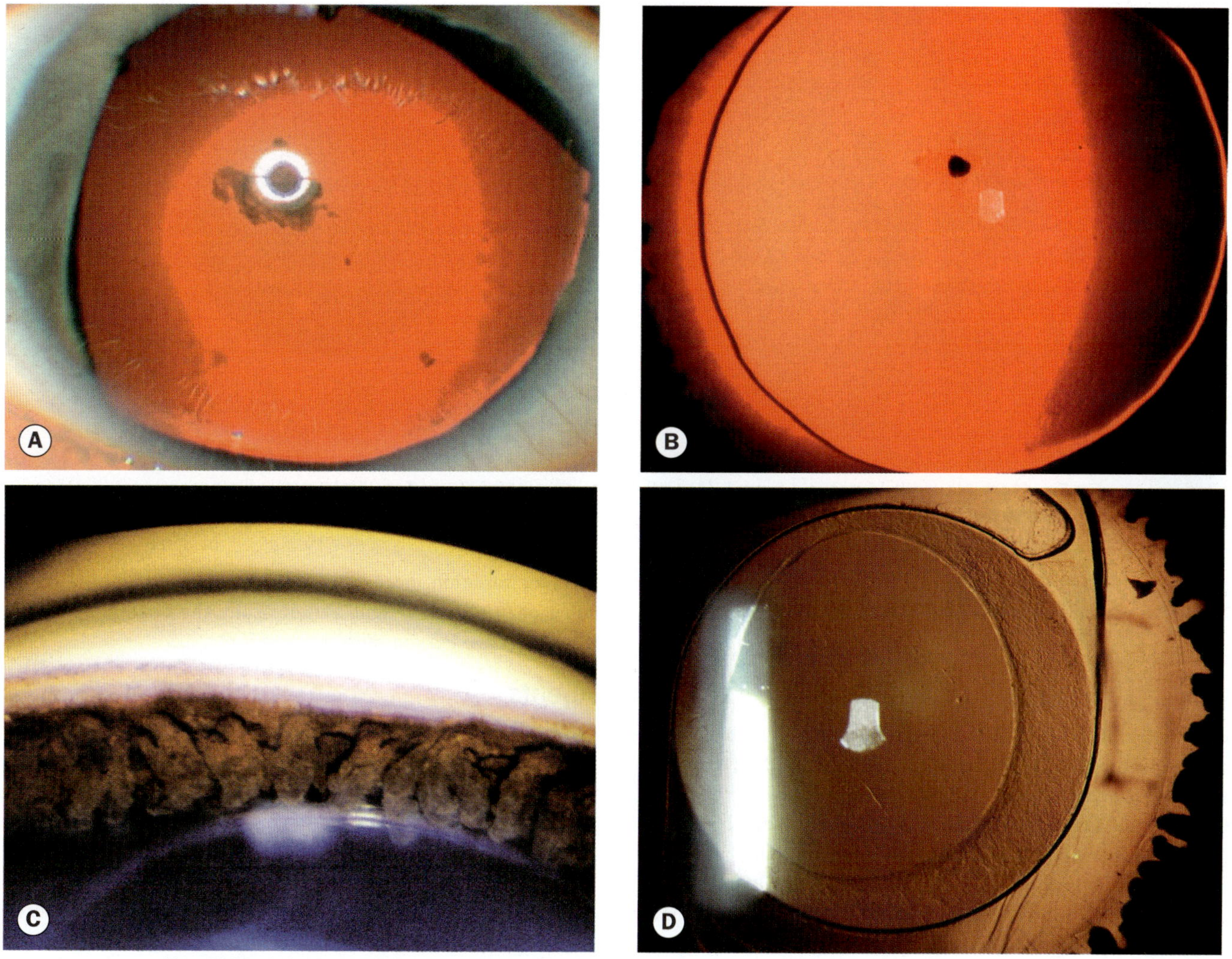

Fig. 11.62 Aniridia. **(A)** Partial; **(B)** total; **(C)** gonioscopy in aniridia: open angle showing remnants of the iris root; **(D)** transillumination of pseudophakic eye showing silhouetted ciliary processes.

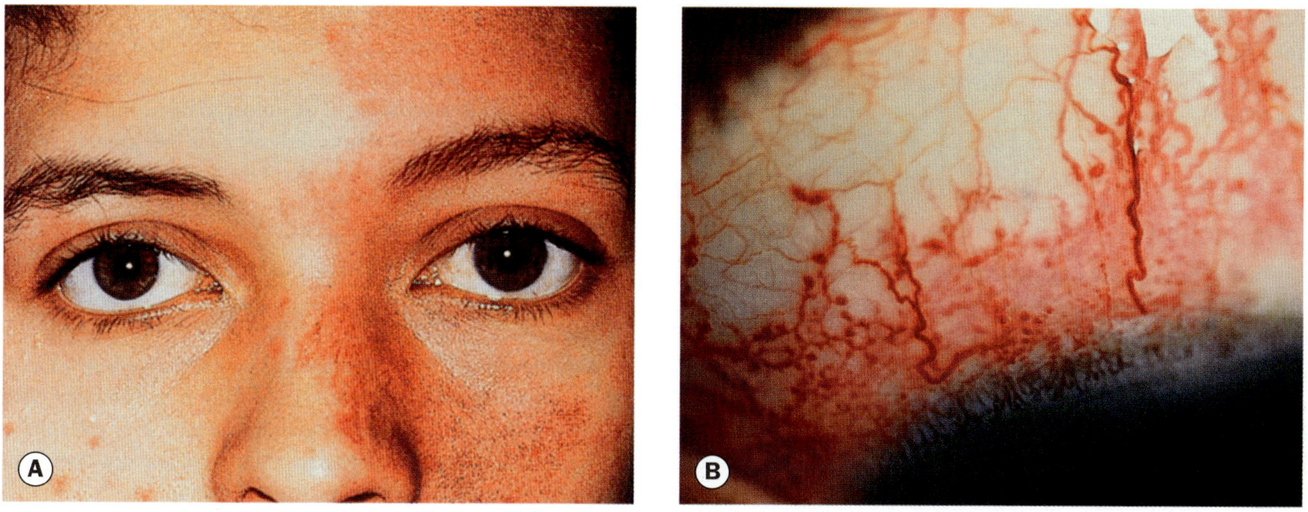

Fig. 11.63 Glaucoma in Sturge–Weber syndrome. **(A)** Left buphthalmos; **(B)** episcleral haemangioma.

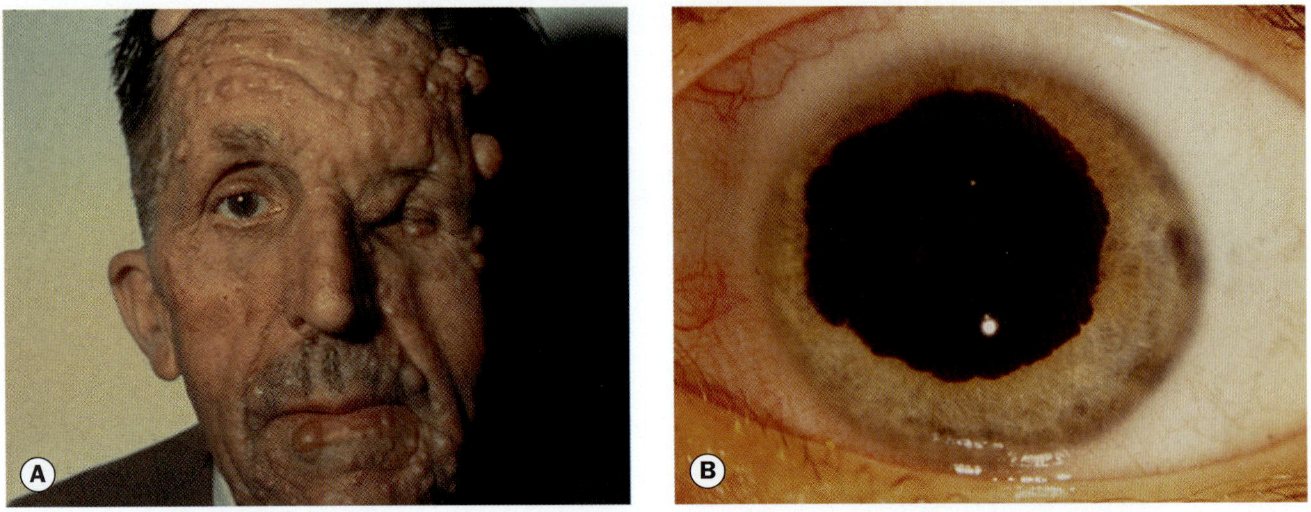

Fig. 11.64 Neurofibromatosis type 1. (A) Left facial hemiatrophy and multiple neurofibromas; (B) congenital ectropion uveae.

MEDICAL TREATMENT OF GLAUCOMA

Introduction

It is important to attempt to maximize adherence by providing an explanation of the disease and the rationale for treatment. A discussion of the medication being prescribed, including technique and timing of administration and its potential adverse effects, is also essential. The provision of written information may be helpful. Most glaucoma medications are administered topically, but significant systemic absorption can still occur, with resultant systemic adverse effects. Systemic absorption may be minimized by lacrimal occlusion following instillation: simply closing the eyes for 3 minutes will reduce systemic absorption by about 50% and this can be enhanced by applying digital pressure over the lacrimal sac – these measures also prolong eye–drug contact. Effects on the periocular skin may be reduced by blotting overflow from the eyelids with a clean dry tissue immediately after instillation. Glaucoma medications should be avoided in pregnancy, if possible, with systemic carbonic anhydrase inhibitors perhaps carrying the greatest risk due to teratogenicity concerns.

Prostaglandin derivatives

Introduction

The major mode of prostaglandin (PG) action is the enhancement of uveoscleral aqueous outflow, although increased trabecular outflow facility and other mechanisms have been identified. Their IOP-lowering effect is typically greater than alternatives and a reduction of 27–35% from baseline can be expected. A prostaglandin derivative is typically preferred to a beta-blocker as first-line treatment for glaucoma because of the latter's potential for systemic side effects. Duration of action may extend for several days, though administration once every day (at bedtime) is generally recommended. Systemic side effects are few. The most commonly troublesome ocular side effect is conjunctival hyperaemia. If one prostaglandin fails to show adequate efficacy, inter-individual receptor variation means that an alternative preparation may be superior in a given patient. Paradoxically, the concomitant use of more than one PG can cause a rise in IOP.

Agents

- **Latanoprost** may cause fewer ocular adverse events than other PG agents and so is often used first line. Approximately 5–10% of patients show no response (IOP reduction of less than 10%) to latanoprost, but may respond to one of the other prostaglandins.
- **Travoprost** is similar to latanoprost but fewer patients tend to be non-responders. Polyquad is a novel proprietary preservative introduced by a major pharmaceutical manufacturer in its travoprost formulation that may reduce ocular surface-related adverse effects.
- **Bimatoprost** 0.03% has a slightly greater IOP-lowering effect than latanoprost, but is more likely to cause conjunctival hyperaemia. A new 0.01% preparation has a comparable IOP-lowering effect to latanoprost with less hyperaemia. Preservative-free bimatoprost is available. Sustained-release intra-cameral bimatoprost is undergoing clinical evaluation and preliminary results indicate that IOP control can be achieved in up to 70% of subjects for 6 months with a single injection.
- **Tafluprost** is a preservative-free drop. Its IOP-lowering efficacy may be slightly less than that of other PG agents, but it is well tolerated and seems to cause less disruption of the ocular surface.
- **Omidenepag** 0.002% solution is a new selective E-prostanoid sub-type 2 agonist that is used once daily. It has a similar effect on the IOP as other prostaglandin agents. It is effective in patients who do not respond to latanoprost and does not cause periorbitopathy. Hyperaemia occurs in about 5%.

Side effects

- **Ocular**
  - Conjunctival hyperaemia is very common.

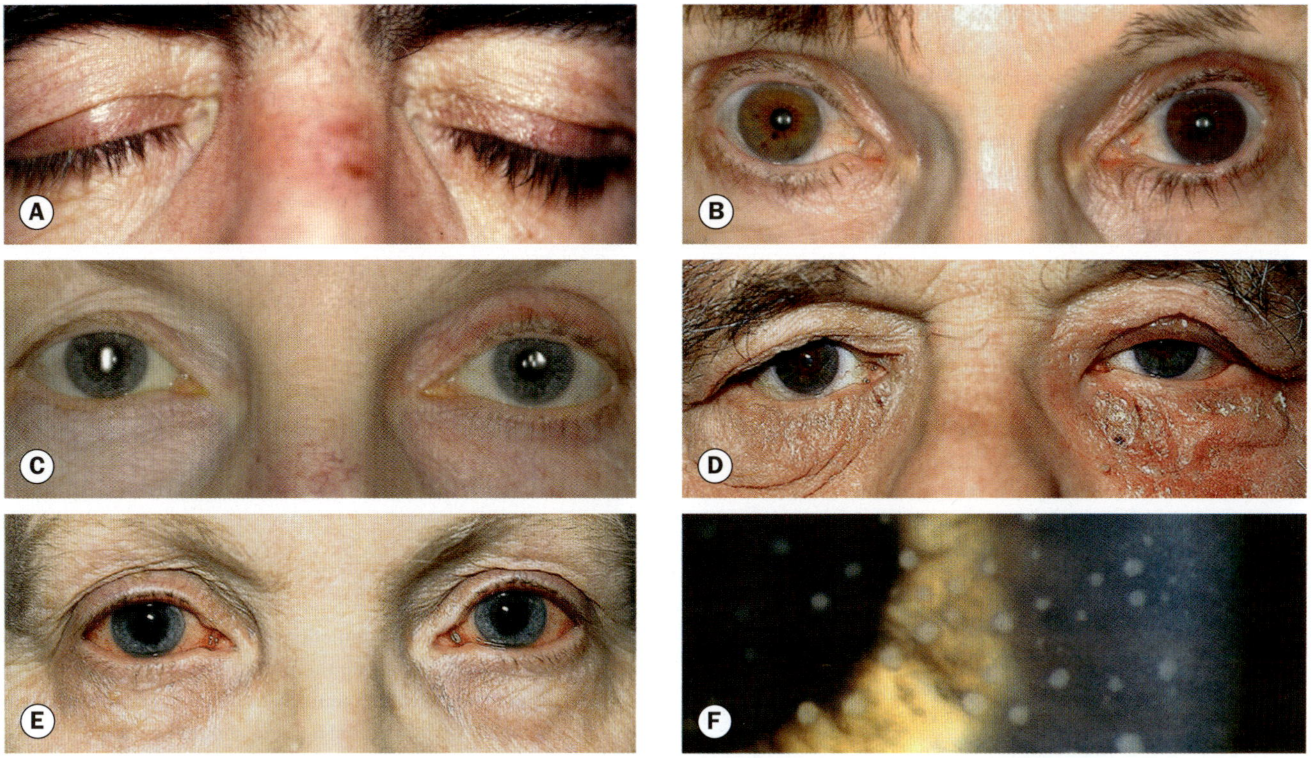

Fig. 11.65 Side effects of topical medication. **(A)** Lengthening and hyperpigmentation of lashes with prostaglandin analogue treatment; **(B)** monocular prostaglandin analogue treatment – darkening of left iris and eyelid skin; **(C)** periocular atrophy on the left; **(D)** blepharoconjunctivitis due to topical carbonic anhydrase inhibitors; **(E)** allergic conjunctivitis due to brimonidine; **(F)** iritis secondary to brimonidine, showing keratic precipitates.

    ○ Eyelash lengthening, thickening, hyperpigmentation (Fig. 11.65A) and occasionally an increase in number.
    ○ Irreversible iris hyperpigmentation (Fig. 11.65B) occurs in up to a quarter of patients after 6 months. The highest incidence is in green–brown irides, less in yellow-brown irides and least in blue-grey/brown irides. It is caused by an increase in the number of pigmented granules within the superficial stroma rather than an increase in the number of melanocytes. Iris naevi and freckles are not affected.
    ○ Hyperpigmentation of periocular skin is common but reversible.
    ○ Periocular atrophy (Fig. 11.65C).
    ○ Preoperative use of PG agents may increase the likelihood of cystoid macular oedema following cataract surgery. This is more likely to occur if PG agents are used in the postoperative period, particularly if there has been vitreous loss at the time of the surgery.
    ○ Anterior uveitis is rare, but prostaglandins should be used with caution in inflamed eyes.
    ○ Promotion of herpetic keratitis can occur, so prostaglandins should be used with caution in patients with a history of the condition.
- **Systemic** side effects include occasional headache, precipitation of migraine in susceptible individuals, malaise, myalgia, skin rash and mild upper respiratory tract symptoms.

Beta-blockers

Introduction

Beta-blockers reduce IOP by decreasing aqueous production, mediated by an effect on the ciliary epithelium. A reduction of 21–27% from baseline can be expected in most patients. In approximately 10% of cases the response decreases with time (tachyphylaxis), sometimes within only a few days. There may be limited supplementary effect if a topical beta-blocker is prescribed for a patient who is already on a systemic beta-blocker. The combination may also increase the risk of systemic side effects. Beta-blockers should not be instilled at bedtime as this medication may cause a significant drop in blood pressure while the individual is asleep, thus reducing optic disc perfusion and potentially causing visual field deterioration. The IOP-lowering effect is also believed to be less marked during sleep, as nocturnal aqueous production is normally less than half the daytime rate. However, a beta-blocker may be preferred under some circumstances, such as monocular treatment to avoid the cosmetic disadvantage of the asymmetrical periocular skin darkening and/or conjunctival hyperaemia with prostaglandins. Beta-blockers are also preferred in conditions such as ocular inflammation and cystoid macular oedema, or where there is a history of herpes simplex keratitis.

Side effects

- **Ocular.** Ocular side effects are few but include allergy and punctate keratitis. Granulomatous uveitis has been reported with metipranolol.

- **Systemic.** Though severe problems are rare, deaths have been associated with topical beta-blocker use.
  - **Bronchospasm.** This may be fatal in asthma or other reversible airways disease and it is critical to exclude a history of asthma before prescribing a beta-blocker. About 1 in 50 patients without asthma will develop reversible airways disease requiring treatment within 12 months of commencing a topical beta-blocker.
  - **Cardiovascular.** There is a strong suggestion that cardiovascular mortality is higher in patients taking a topical beta-blocker. Effects include heart block, bradycardia, worsening of heart failure and hypotension, induction of the latter by topical beta-blocker having been reported as a common cause of falls in elderly patients. The pulse should be assessed before prescription. A peripheral vasoconstrictive effect means that they should be avoided or used with caution in patients with peripheral vascular disease, including Raynaud phenomenon.
  - **Unpleasant but less severe side effects** include sleep disorders, reduced exercise tolerance, hallucinations, confusion, depression, fatigue, headache, nausea, dizziness, decreased libido and dyslipidaemia.
  - **Alopecia** is uncommon but is reversible on stopping the beta-blocker medication.

Agents

- **Timolol** is available in various forms, including 0.25% and 0.5% solutions used twice daily. There is no evidence of a clinically significant difference in efficacy between the two solution concentrations. Gel-forming preparations of 0.1%, 0.25% and 0.5% are used once daily in the morning.
- **Betaxolol** 0.25% and 0.5% twice daily has a lower hypotensive effect than timolol. However, optic nerve blood flow may be increased due to a calcium-channel blocking effect. Betaxolol is relatively cardioselective (beta-1 receptors) and is therefore less likely to cause bronchoconstriction.
- **Levobunolol** is a long-acting beta-blocker and is used once or twice daily with a similar profile to timolol.
- **Carteolol** twice daily is similar to timolol and also exhibits intrinsic sympathomimetic activity. It has a more selective action on the eye than on the cardiopulmonary system and so may have a lower systemic side effect incidence.
- **Metipranolol** twice daily is similar to timolol but has been linked with granulomatous anterior uveitis.

Topical carbonic anhydrase inhibitors

Introduction

The carbonic anhydrase inhibitors (CAI) are chemically related to sulfonamide antibiotics. They lower IOP by inhibiting aqueous secretion and via the topical route are used three times daily as monotherapy or twice daily as adjunctive treatment. In general, they are slightly less effective than beta-blockers but may have a supplementary neuroprotective effect. They precipitate corneal decompensation in patients with corneal endothelial dysfunction. Idiosyncratic bone marrow suppression can occur. Though cross-reaction is uncommon, topical (and systemic) CAI are relatively contraindicated in patients allergic to sulfonamide antibiotics. Research suggests that concomitant treatment with a topical and systemic CAI does not usually give an additive effect.

Agents

- **Dorzolamide.** The main adverse effects are stinging and a transient bitter taste following administration. Allergic blepharoconjunctivitis may occur, but is uncommon (Fig. 11.65D).
- **Brinzolamide** is similar to dorzolamide, but is less likely to cause stinging and local allergy. It is a suspension and a white residue may be left on the eyelids after instillation if excess is not wiped away.

Alpha-2 agonists

Introduction

Ocular alpha-2 receptor stimulation decreases aqueous synthesis via an effect on the ciliary epithelium and increases uveoscleral outflow. There is probably a neuroprotective effect. This medication crosses the blood–brain barrier and should be used with great caution in young children, in whom severe CNS depression and hypotension have been reported (contraindicated under the age of 2 years). They may potentiate vascular insufficiency. They should not be given with oral monoamine oxidase inhibitor antidepressants due to the risk of hypertensive crisis.

Agents

- **Brimonidine** 0.2% twice daily as a single agent generally has a slightly less marked IOP-lowering effect than timolol. Allergic conjunctivitis (Fig. 11.65E) is common, but the onset may be delayed for up to 18 months after commencement of therapy. Granulomatous anterior uveitis can occur, but is rare (Fig. 11.65F). Systemic side effects include xerostomia and fatigue, the latter sometimes being severe. A brimonidine preparation, Alphagan P, containing a proprietary preservative, Purite, has been introduced as an alternative to the more common benzalkonium-containing forms and may have greater ocular surface tolerability.
- **Apraclonidine** 1% (or 0.5%) is used principally to prevent or treat an acute rise in IOP following laser surgery on the anterior segment. The 0.5% concentration is typically used as a temporizing measure over the course of several weeks, such as whilst a patient is awaiting glaucoma surgery. It is not suitable for long-term use because of a loss of therapeutic effect over weeks to months and a high incidence of topical side effects.

Miotics

Introduction

Miotics are cholinergic agonists that are predominantly used in the treatment of angle closure, though they were formerly a mainstay of the treatment of open-angle glaucoma. They can be useful in patients with pseudophakic or aphakic glaucoma. In angle-closure glaucoma, miotic-induced contraction of the sphincter pupillae pulls the peripheral iris away from the trabecular meshwork, opening the angle. Miotics also reduce IOP by contraction of the ciliary muscle, which increases the facility of aqueous outflow through the trabecular meshwork. Local side effects include miosis, brow ache, myopic shift and exacerbation of the symptoms of cataract. Visual field defects appear denser and larger. Systemic side effects are rare, but include confusion, bradycardia, bronchospasm, gastrointestinal symptoms and urinary frequency.

Agents

- **Pilocarpine** 0.5%, 1%, 2%, or 4% solution as four times daily monotherapy is equal in efficacy to beta-blockers. Pilocarpine gel (Pilogel) 4% (discontinued in the UK in 2011) is instilled once daily at bedtime so that induced myopia and miosis are predominantly confined to sleep. Gel, or drops twice daily, may be used to prevent angle closure following laser iridotomy in the presence of a substantial non-pupillary block element.
- **Carbachol** is an alternative to pilocarpine.

Combined preparations

Combined preparations with similar ocular hypotensive effects to the sum of the individual components improve convenience and patient adherence. They are also more cost effective. Proprietary examples include:

- **Cosopt**: timolol and dorzolamide, administered twice daily.
- **Xalacom**: timolol and latanoprost, once daily.
- **Timpilo**: timolol and pilocarpine, twice daily.
- **Combigan**: timolol and brimonidine, twice daily.
- **DuoTrav**: timolol and travoprost, once daily.
- **Ganfort**: timolol and bimatoprost, once daily.
- **Taptiqom**: timolol and tafluprost, once daily.
- **Azarga**: timolol and brinzolamide, twice daily.
- **Simbrinza**: brimonidine and brinzolamide: the only combination that does not contain the beta-blocker timolol, administered twice daily.

New topical medications

- **Latanoprostene bunod 0.024%** (Vyzulta) is a new FDA-approved topical medication that reduces IOP significantly. It has a dual mechanism of action: the latanoprost component increases outflow through the uveoscleral route and the butanediol mononitrate component undergoes further metabolism in the anterior chamber to produce nitric oxide, which has an effect on the trabecular meshwork leading to enhanced aqueous outflow. It is used once daily and reduces the IOP more effectively than latanoprost alone. It has similar side effects to other prostaglandins.
- **Rho-kinase (ROCK) inhibitors** are a novel class of topical medication that increase outflow of aqueous through the trabecular meshwork. The drops are instilled once daily and are effective in combination with latanoprost (Rocklatan). Rho-kinase inhibitors are slightly more effective than latanoprost in reducing the IOP.

Systemic carbonic anhydrase inhibitors

Introduction

Systemically administered CAI are generally used for short-term treatment, particularly in patients with acute glaucoma. Because of their systemic side effects, long-term use is reserved for patients at high risk of visual loss. Sulfonamide ('sulfa') allergy is a relative contraindication.

Agents

- **Acetazolamide** is available as 250 mg tablets (250–1000 mg daily in divided doses), sustained-release 250 mg capsules (250–500 mg daily) and 500 mg powder vials for injection (single dose, typically used in acute angle-closure glaucoma).
- **Dichlorphenamide** 50 mg tablets (50–100 mg two or three times daily).
- **Methazolamide** 50 mg tablets (50–100 mg two or three times daily). This has a longer duration of action than acetazolamide but is less widely available.

Side effects

- **Ocular.** Choroidal effusion, particularly after cataract surgery. Angle closure may result.
- **Systemic.** Paraesthesia ('pins and needles' sensation in the extremities), hypokalaemia (reduced blood potassium level – common), malaise and lowered mood, gastrointestinal symptoms, renal stones, Stevens–Johnson syndrome (very rare), dose-related bone marrow suppression, idiosyncratic aplastic anaemia (exceptionally rare but with 50% mortality).

Osmotic agents

Introduction

Osmotic agents lower IOP by creating an osmotic gradient so that water is 'drawn out' from the vitreous into the blood. They are employed when a short-term reduction in IOP is required that cannot be achieved by other means, such as in resistant acute angle-closure glaucoma or when the IOP is very high prior to intraocular surgery. They are of limited value in inflammatory glaucoma, in which the integrity of the blood–aqueous barrier is compromised. Side effects include cardiovascular overload as a result of increased extracellular volume (caution in patients with cardiac or renal disease), urinary retention (especially elderly men), headache, backache, nausea and confusion.

Agents

- **Mannitol** is given intravenously (1 g/kg body weight or 5 ml/kg body weight of a 20% solution in water) over 30–60 minutes, with a peak action within 30 minutes.
- **Glycerol** is an oral agent (1 g/kg body weight or 2 ml/kg body weight of a 50% solution) with a sweet and sickly taste and can be given with lemon (not orange) juice to avoid nausea. Peak action occurs within 1 hour. Glycerol is metabolized to glucose and careful monitoring with insulin cover may be required if administered to a (well-controlled only) diabetic patient.
- **Isosorbide** is a metabolically inert oral agent with a minty taste, using the same dose as glycerol. It may be safer for diabetic patients.

Other systemic therapeutic options

- Trials have commenced to determine whether regular supplementary nicotinamide (also known as niacinamide, the water-soluble active form of vitamin B3) is helpful in patients with glaucoma.
- Losartan, an angiotensin-receptor blocker, may have a neuroprotective role.

LASER TREATMENT OF GLAUCOMA

Laser trabeculoplasty

Introduction

Laser trabeculoplasty (LTP) involves the delivery of laser to the trabecular meshwork with the aim of enhancing aqueous outflow and thereby lowering IOP.

- **Selective laser trabeculoplasty (SLT)** has increased in popularity over recent years and is now widely performed. Based on the results of the LiGHT trial, SLT has been recommended as first-line treatment in patients with ocular hypertension and primary open angle glaucoma. Individuals in this trial who underwent SLT first (rather than drops first) were less likely to show disease progression and less likely to require trabeculectomy or phacoemulsification with IOL implantation 6 years after diagnosis. A 532 nm frequency-doubled, Q-switched Nd:YAG laser is used to selectively target melanin pigment in TM cells, leaving non-pigmented structures unscathed. It is probably similar in efficacy to medical monotherapy and argon laser trabeculoplasty (see below). The mechanism is incompletely understood, but possibly includes stimulation of TM cell division, macrophage and extracellular matrix recruitment. Laser application is made easier by a broad targeted and treated area (Fig. 11.66, left), which may lead to more consistent results. Reported protocols (e.g. 180° or 360° TM treatment) and results vary markedly, but IOP reductions of 10–40% can be expected after 6 months in responsive patients, with 25% being common. Probably around two-thirds of patients will achieve a reasonable IOP fall within 6 months of 180° TM treatment. In patients with ocular hypertension and early glaucoma approximately 80% will be drop free and at target pressure at 3 years. The effects generally wane over time, but because there is no thermal tissue damage, treatment can be repeated with a successful outcome, even if initial treatment has been unsuccessful. The prior use of topical glaucoma medication does not seem to affect results. Energy delivered to the TM is much lower than with argon laser and complications are relatively mild but include transient mild inflammation with mild discomfort, PAS formation and IOP elevation. The latter is usually mild but substantial rises have been reported, especially in heavily pigmented angles, for which overtreatment should be avoided. The concern has been raised that the extensive treated area causes damage to corneal endothelial cells, with rare reports of endothelial decompensation. Herpes simplex keratitis reactivation has been reported, as has macular oedema.

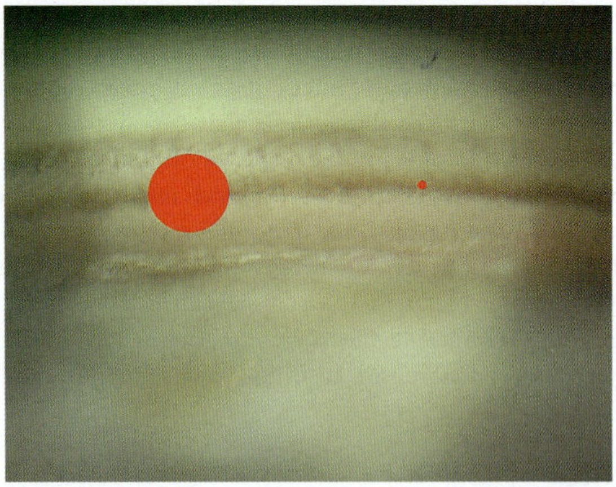

Fig. 11.66 Targeted area in selective (left) and conventional argon (right) and subthreshold (micropulse) laser trabeculoplasty.

- **Argon laser trabeculoplasty (ALT)** is a long-established procedure that uses laser burns to achieve IOP reduction comparable to SLT. There is an extensive body of published research reporting good outcomes. Mechanisms are likely to overlap with those of SLT and there may also be a mechanical opening of the trabecular spaces. As the TM sustains thermal damage, repeat treatment is of limited benefit and is infrequently performed. Complications include peripheral anterior synechiae, acute elevation of IOP (should be monitored carefully over subsequent weeks in patients with severe glaucomatous damage), cystoid macular oedema and anterior uveitis (usually mild). There is concern that there may be an adverse effect on the outcome of subsequent filtration surgery.
- **Micropulse laser trabeculoplasty (MLT)** is a relatively new modality that uses extremely short duration pulses of laser to deliver thermal energy to the TM to stimulate cells without damage. Unlike SLT and ALT, there is no visible tissue reaction. A smaller area is targeted than in SLT (Fig. 11.66, right), limiting potential collateral effects on adjacent tissue. Initial results suggest a benign safety profile with results comparable to other LTP forms.

Indications

- **Type of glaucoma.** LTP can be used in primary and secondary open-angle glaucoma (including primary, pseudoexfoliative and pigmentary) and can also be used in ocular hypertension.
- **Primary therapy.** As SLT has increasingly demonstrated a favourable safety profile, its use as a primary alternative to topical medication has increasingly been recommended.
- **Failure of adherence** to the medical regimen.
- **Adjunctive treatment** to avoid polypharmacy.
- **Intolerance** of topical medication including allergy.
- **Failure of medical therapy**, as a less aggressive treatment measure than surgery.

Technique

- LTP is performed under topical anaesthesia.
- A drop of apraclonidine or brimonidine is instilled 30–60 minutes pre-procedure with the aim of preventing or minimizing an early post-laser IOP rise. A similar drop is instilled post-procedure.
- Some practitioners instil a drop of pilocarpine prior to the procedure, particularly if the angle is not wide. There is likely to be greater potential for PAS formation in narrow angles, particularly with ALT, and this should be borne in mind when considering a particular patient's suitability for LTP.
- A goniolens is inserted with the mirror at the 12 o'clock position and the inferior angle is visualized.
- ALT: initial settings are commonly 50 μm spot size, 0.1 s duration and 700 mW power (range of 400–1200 mW, largely dependent on angle pigmentation). The aiming beam is focused at the junction of the pigmented and non-pigmented TM ensuring that the spot is round and has a clear edge. The optimal reaction is a very light blanching or the appearance of a minute gas bubble. If the reaction is inadequate, the power is increased by 50–200 mW. Fifty burns are applied at regularly spaced intervals over 180° of the angle. Many practitioners apply initial treatment of 180° of the angle, treating the other 180° if the initial response is unsatisfactory. Primary treatment of the entire circumference is associated with a higher risk of IOP spikes. Topical fluorometholone or prednisolone 0.5% four times daily for 1 week is prescribed post-laser.
- SLT: a common initial power setting is 0.8 mJ. As with ALT, this should be varied depending on angle pigmentation (range 0.3–1.0 mJ). The spot size and duration are fixed at 400 μm and 3 ns respectively. The TM is brought into focus rather than the aiming beam. The beam is centred on the pigmented TM and then fired, an optimal reaction consisting of a few tiny ('champagne') bubbles with adjustment of the power higher or lower as required to achieve this. The number of burns applied is as for ALT. The total energy used for SLT is considerably less than for ALT and it is common not to prescribe any post-laser anti-inflammatory drops, though non-steroidal or weak steroid drops can be used if significant inflammation occurs.
- With practice it is possible to perform LTP by continually rotating the goniolens and applying each burn through the centre of the mirror. Using this technique, treatment of the entire inferior half of the angle is accomplished by first rotating the lens to one side (e.g. anticlockwise) by 90° whilst applying 25 shots, then returning to the 12 o'clock position before applying an additional 25 shots whilst rotating the lens to the opposite side (clockwise in this example).
- An IOP check should be performed 30–60 minutes after the laser to exclude a substantial early spike, with further IOP measurement, treatment and review as appropriate if this occurs, depending on each patient's risk profile.
- Medical glaucoma therapy is generally continued.
- Follow-up is dependent on the perceived level of risk (usually 1–2 weeks).

Laser iridotomy

Introduction

Laser iridotomy is used principally in the treatment of primary angle closure, but may also be indicated in secondary angle closure with pupillary block. It is also sometimes performed in pigment dispersion syndrome, though its effectiveness in this scenario remains under investigation.

Technique

- A topical anaesthetic agent is instilled.
- Apraclonidine or brimonidine is given prophylactically as for LTP.
- The pupil is constricted with topical pilocarpine (e.g. one drop of 2%).
- A special iridotomy contact lens (e.g. Abraham [Fig. 11.67A], Volk MagPlus) is inserted.
- Many practitioners target a site under the upper eyelid between 11 and 1 o'clock (Fig. 11.67B), though some prefer 3 or 9 o'clock (Fig. 11.67C). The highest risk of monocular dysphotopsia or glare (see below) occurs when an iridotomy is half-covered by the lid margin. Radially, the iridotomy should be located within the outer third in order to reduce the risk of damage to the crystalline lens. Targeting an iris crypt, if present, is usually associated with much easier achievement of an adequate opening.
- It is important to remember that effective power settings vary somewhat between machines. The spot size and duration are fixed. Most iridotomies are made with power settings of 4–5 mJ. For a thin blue iris, the typical required energy level is 2–4 mJ. The risk of crystalline lens damage increases with settings of more than 5 mJ. Some practitioners prefer single pulse shots, others shots of up to three pulses.
- Pre-treatment with thermal (argon or diode) laser is often required in thick dark irides. Suitable parameters include power of 600–900 mW using a small spot size of 50 μm and relatively short duration of 0.03–0.05 s, though larger, lower power, longer duration settings can be equally effective.
- The beam is focused precisely, and the laser fired. Successful penetration is characterized by a gush of pigment debris. The number of shots required to produce an adequate iridotomy is very variable. The optimal size is 150–200 μm.

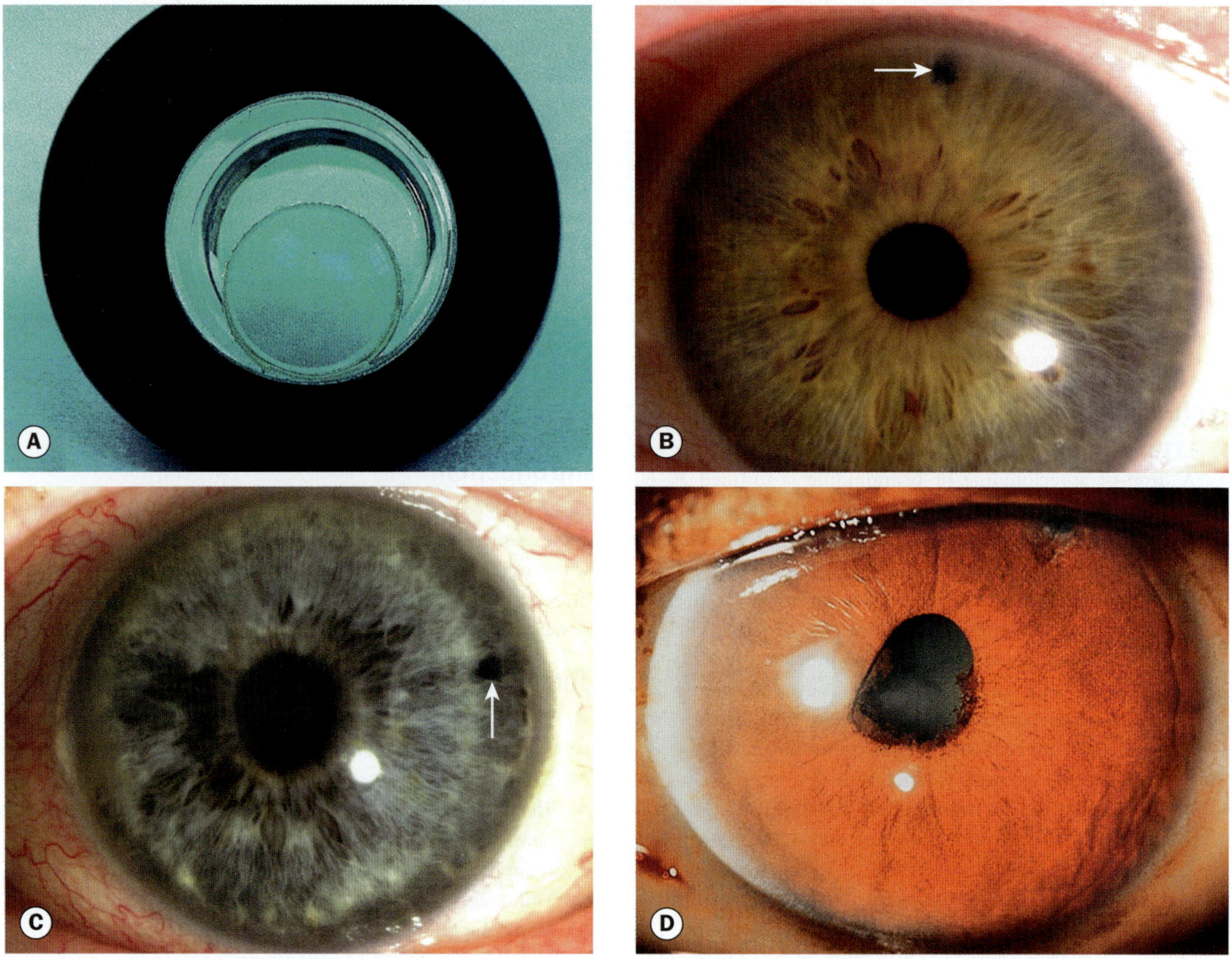

Fig. 11.67 Nd:YAG iridotomy. **(A)** Abraham lens; **(B)** appropriate iridotomy size in upper quadrant (arrow); **(C)** temporal iridotomy (arrow); **(D)** posterior synechiae due to laser-induced iritis.

- Overtreatment should be avoided due to the risk of substantial postoperative inflammation and a pressure spike. Further treatment can be applied after a few days if the iridotomy is not patent. In urgent circumstances moving to a different site is a reasonable alternative.
- A second drop of apraclonidine is instilled following the procedure. Oral acetazolamide may also be given in patients at high risk, such as those with advanced glaucomatous damage or high IOP pre-treatment.
- A potent topical steroid (e.g. dexamethasone 0.1%) is prescribed post-procedure. Varying regimens have been described, with a limited evidence base for the optimal approach. Instillation every 10 minutes for a half hour followed by hourly for 6–8 hours immediately post-laser is commonly used and significantly reduces the risk of inflammation and posterior synechiae. Four times daily for 1 week is a reasonable subsequent regimen, particularly in patients with a lightly pigmented iris.
- The IOP should be checked 1–2 hours after the procedure to exclude an early spike. Routine review is usually at 1 or 2 weeks, with subsequent monitoring according to individual circumstances. Patients with marked glaucomatous damage may require extended ocular hypotensive cover and earlier review.

Complications

- **Bleeding** occurs in around 50% but is usually mild and stops after only a few seconds. Persistent bleeding can be terminated by increasing contact lens pressure.
- **IOP elevation.** Usually early and transient but occasionally persistent.
- **Iritis.** Especially if excessive laser is applied or post-laser steroid therapy is inadequate, or in darker irides (including those due to prostaglandin derivative treatment) (Fig. 11.67D).
- **Corneal burns** may occur if a contact lens is not used or if the AC is shallow, but these usually heal rapidly without sequelae.
- **Cataract.** Localized lens opacities occasionally develop at the treatment site. There is some evidence that age-related cataract formation may be accelerated by iridotomy.
- **Linear dysphotopsia** (unwanted optical images) may occur regardless of the location, size of the iridotomy or the amount of laser energy used, but usually settles without intervention.

Diode laser cycloablation

Diode laser ablation (cyclodiode) lowers IOP by destroying part of the secretory ciliary epithelium, thereby reducing aqueous secretion. More than one treatment session is commonly required for adequate IOP control because ciliary epithelium can regenerate. Diode laser (810 nm wavelength) is applied to the ciliary processes using either a trans-scleral technique (trans-scleral cyclophotocoagulation; TS-CPC) or using an endoscope (ECP). In the past it was used mainly in uncontrolled end-stage secondary glaucoma with minimal visual potential, mainly to control pain. However, its use in eyes with good vision, especially those with a poor prognosis for penetrating drainage surgery, has been well described over recent years. More than one treatment session is commonly required for adequate pressure control. Moderate post-procedure pain and anterior segment inflammation are common. A temporary IOP rise is not uncommon during the first few weeks. Serious complications are rare but include chronic hypotony, phthisis bulbi, suprachoroidal haemorrhage, corneal decompensation and retinal detachment.

Indications

- Raised IOP in patients with poor vision.
- Pain relief in a blind eye with raised IOP.
- In patients with uncontrolled secondary glaucoma (e.g. neovascular glaucoma or malignant glaucoma).
- In patients where glaucoma filtration surgery or drainage implantation is unlikely to be successful or technically difficult (e.g. in the presence of conjunctival scarring).

Technique of trans-scleral cyclophotocoagulation

- A sub-Tenon or peribulbar anaesthetic is administered.
- Laser settings are 1.5–2 s and 1500–2000 mW; the spot size is fixed.
- The power is adjusted over sequential shots until a 'popping' sound is heard and then reduced to just below that level.
- Approximately 12–24 burns are placed posteriorly to the limbus over 360°, avoiding the neurovascular bundles at 3 and 9 o'clock (Fig. 11.68). Fewer shots (e.g. treatment of only one or two quadrants) can be used for eyes with good vision, in order to reduce the risk of complications. However, more treatment sessions are likely to be required using this approach.
- A strong topical steroid is prescribed hourly on the day of treatment and then 2-hourly for 2 days and four times daily for at least 2 weeks. A topical antibiotic and a cycloplegic (e.g. cyclopentolate 1% twice daily) are used for 3 days.
- Pre-laser glaucoma treatment may be continued, or reduced slightly.
- Oral non-steroidal anti-inflammatory agents may be prescribed for 2 days.
- Review is generally after 1–4 days, depending on risk, to exclude significant reactive inflammation and/or an IOP spike.

Technique of endo-cyclophotocoagulation

- A sub-Tenon or peribulbar anaesthetic is administered.
- Laser settings: 0.2 W, continuous wave.
- The probe can be inserted either at the limbus or through the pars plana. In the limbal approach a cohesive viscoelastic is placed behind the iris and anterior to the lens to deepen the ciliary sulcus space. In a pseudophakic eye a pars plana approach is preferable.
- Three to four quadrants are treated.
- The power is titrated to achieve whitening and shrinkage of the ciliary processes by positioning the probe either closer or further from the processes (Fig. 11.69).
- Post-procedural management as above.

Complications

- Moderate post-procedural pain and anterior segment inflammation is common.
- A temporary IOP rise may occur during the first few weeks.
- Visual reduction in 6–13% of patients.

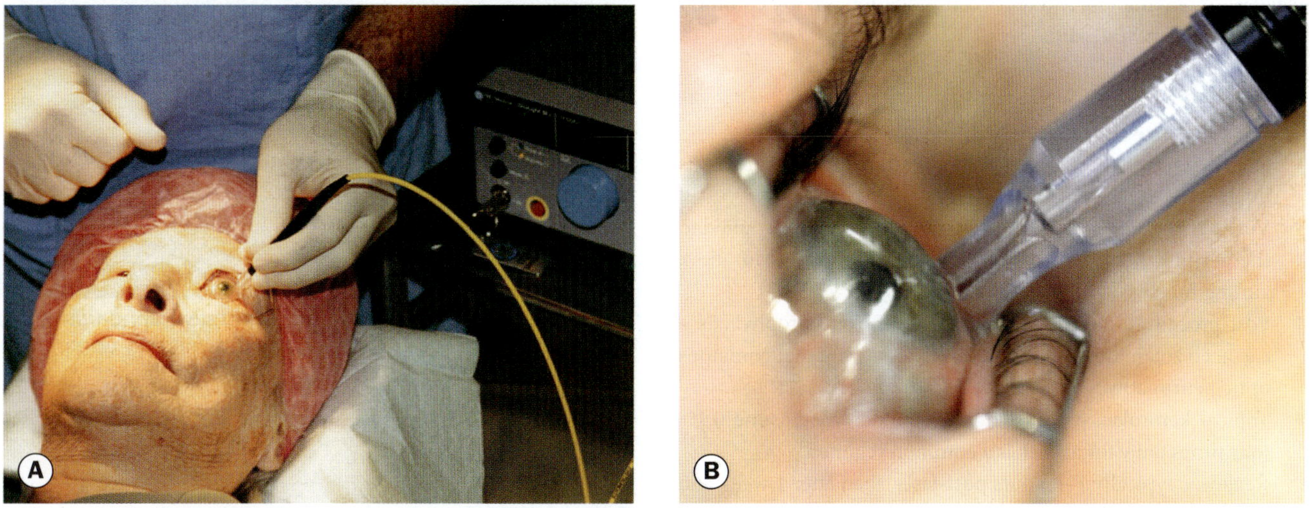

Fig. 11.68 (A) Diode laser cycloablation; **(B)** close-up of cyclodiode probe during laser application.

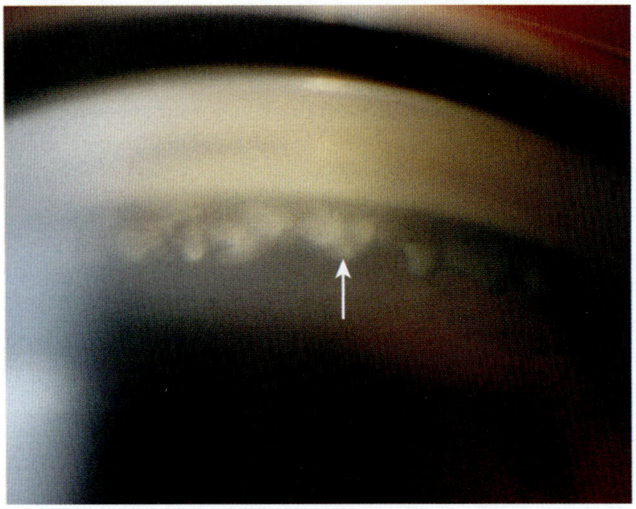

Fig. 11.69 Direct cycloablation of ciliary body (arrow).

- Conjunctival burn may rarely be a consequence of TS-CPC if the eye becomes dry during the procedure or in the presence of subconjunctival blood.
- Fibrinous uveitis, hyphaema and cystoid macular oedema may follow ECP in approximately 5% of cases.
- Serious complications are rare and include chronic hypotony, phthisis bulbi, suprachoroidal haemorrhage and serous retinal detachment.
- There are single reports of scleritis and sympathetic ophthalmitis following this treatment.

Laser iridoplasty

Laser iridoplasty is performed to widen the anterior chamber angle by contraction of the peripheral iris away from the angle recess (Fig. 11.70A). It can be used to attempt to break an episode of acute angle closure, but is more commonly applied on an elective basis, for example in plateau iris syndrome (Fig. 11.70B and C). Complications tend to be mild, but heavy treatment can be associated with a substantial and persistent IOP spike that may be potentiated by heavy iris pigmentation. Altered accommodation is fairly common but almost always transient.

Technique

- A topical anaesthetic is instilled.
- One drop each of 1% pilocarpine and 1% apraclonidine is instilled.
- Via an iridotomy lens, 1–2 burns per clock hour are applied to the periphery, 500 µm size, 100–400 mW, 0.2–0.5 s duration, aiming for slight visible iris contraction.
- Post-procedure 1% apraclonidine is given (oral prophylaxis – e.g. acetazolamide – may be given if significant glaucomatous optic neuropathy is present).
- Topical ketorolac, prednisolone 1% or dexamethasone 0.1% four times daily for a week is a common regimen.
- Review is typically 1–2 hours post-laser, then after 1 week and subsequently depending on progress and glaucomatous damage – patients with significant glaucomatous neuropathy may need frequent review for the first few weeks to exclude an IOP spike.

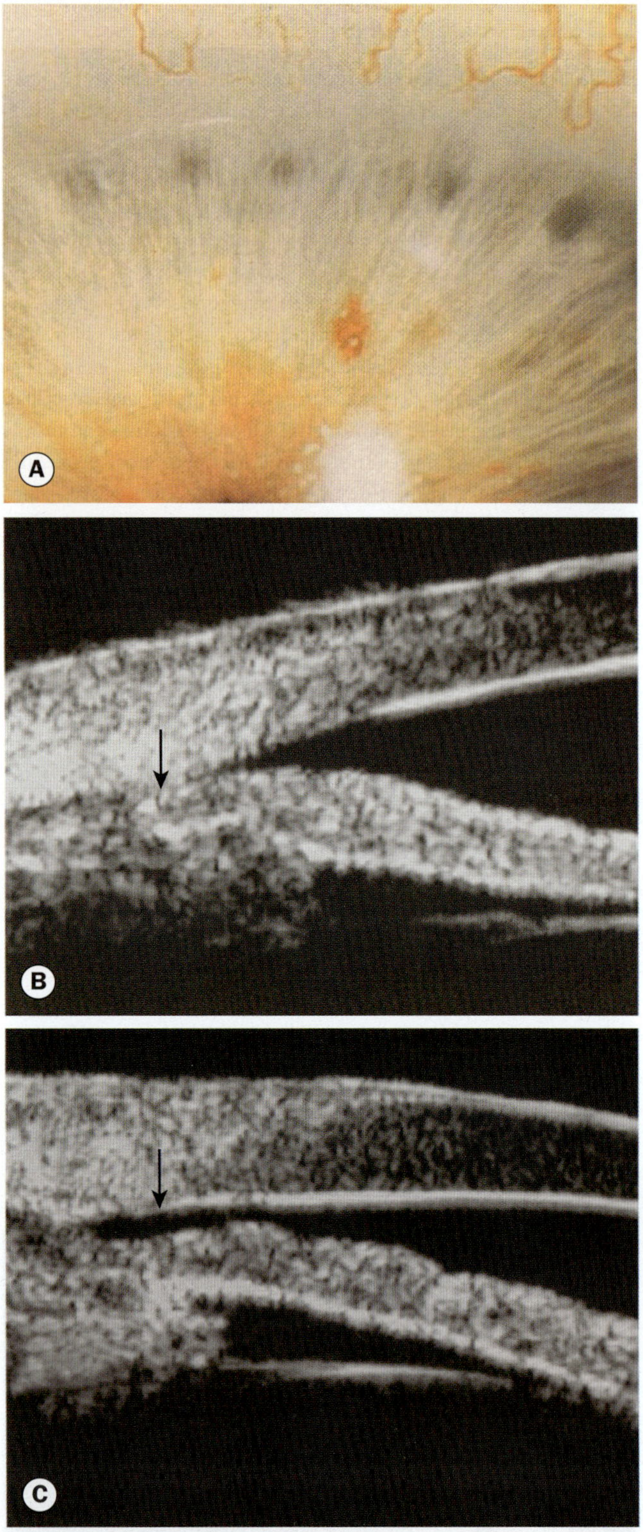

Fig. 11.70 Laser iridoplasty. **(A)** Postoperative appearance; **(B)** UBM before and **(C)** after treatment showing an open angle (arrow).

TRABECULECTOMY

Trabeculectomy is glaucoma filtration surgery that lowers IOP by creating a fistula, protected by a superficial scleral flap, to allow aqueous outflow from the anterior chamber to the sub-Tenon space (Fig. 11.71).

Indications

- **Failure of conservative therapy** to achieve adequate IOP control.
- **Progressive deterioration despite seemingly adequate IOP control** (including poor adherence to the recommended medical regimen).
- **Primary therapy.** Advanced disease requiring a very low target pressure may achieve a superior long-term outcome from early surgery, particularly in younger patients.
- **Patient preference.** Occasionally patients express a strong desire to be free of the commitment to chronic medical treatment.

Technique

Numerous modifications are in use. The following description relates predominantly to the classical procedure. By placing the incisions at 12 o'clock there is less likelihood of bleb dysaesthesia.

- The pupil is constricted preoperatively (e.g. pilocarpine 2%).
- A bridle suture is inserted (commonly superior cornea or superior rectus muscle).
- A limbal or fornix-based flap of conjunctiva and Tenon capsule is fashioned superiorly.
- Episcleral tissue is cleared and major vessels cauterized.
- Incisions are made through about 50% of scleral thickness, to create a 'trapdoor' lamellar scleral flap (Fig. 11.72A). This flap may be rectangular (3 × 3–4 mm), trapezoidal or triangular, according to preference.
- The superficial flap is dissected forwards until clear cornea is reached (Fig. 11.72B).
- A paracentesis is made in temporal peripheral clear cornea.
- The AC is entered along most of the width of the trapdoor base.
- A block of deep sclera is excised, usually using a punch (e.g. Kelly – Fig. 11.72C).
- A peripheral iridectomy is created to prevent blockage of the internal sclerostomy (Fig. 11.72D). Some surgeons omit this step in pseudophakic eyes, but there remains a small risk of iris prolapse into the sclerostomy site if that option is adopted.
- The superficial scleral flap is sutured at its posterior corners, either so that it is lightly opposed to the underlying bed or tightly closed with releasable or lysable sutures to reduce the risk of postoperative leakage. Some surgeons insert a suture into each of the radial edges to reduce the risk of a substantial lateral leak (Fig. 11.72E).
- Balanced salt solution is injected through the paracentesis to deepen the anterior chamber and to test the patency of the fistula (see Fig. 11.72E).
- Conjunctiva/Tenon capsule flap is sutured (Fig. 11.72F). Irrigation through the paracentesis is repeated to produce a bleb, which is checked for leakage.
- A drop of atropine 1% is instilled. When no iridectomy has been performed, pilocarpine 2% may be used instead.
- Steroid and antibiotic are injected under the inferior conjunctiva.
- Steroid and antibiotic drops are used four times daily for 2 weeks and then changed to steroid alone for a further 8–12 weeks.

Ex-Press mini-shunt

This is a valveless titanium MRI-compatible stent inserted under a scleral flap during a modified trabeculectomy, with a principal aim of standardization of drainage (Fig. 11.73). Following creation of the scleral flap as for a standard trabeculectomy, a needle is used to enter the anterior chamber instead of creating a punch sclerostomy. A peripheral iridectomy is not performed. The rate of complications such as hypotony and hyphaema is lower than with standard trabeculectomy, but IOP control is equivalent. It is not viewed as suitable in primary angle-closure glaucoma without prior or contemporaneous cataract surgery.

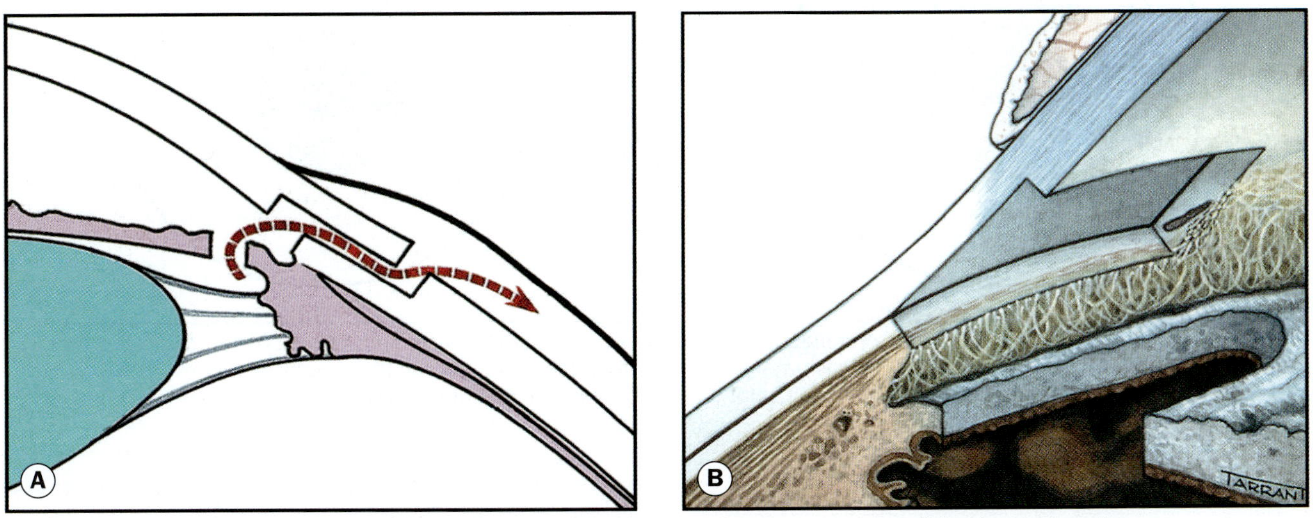

Fig. 11.71 Trabeculectomy principles. **(A)** Pathway of aqueous egress following trabeculectomy; **(B)** schematic representation of appearance from inside the eye following completion.

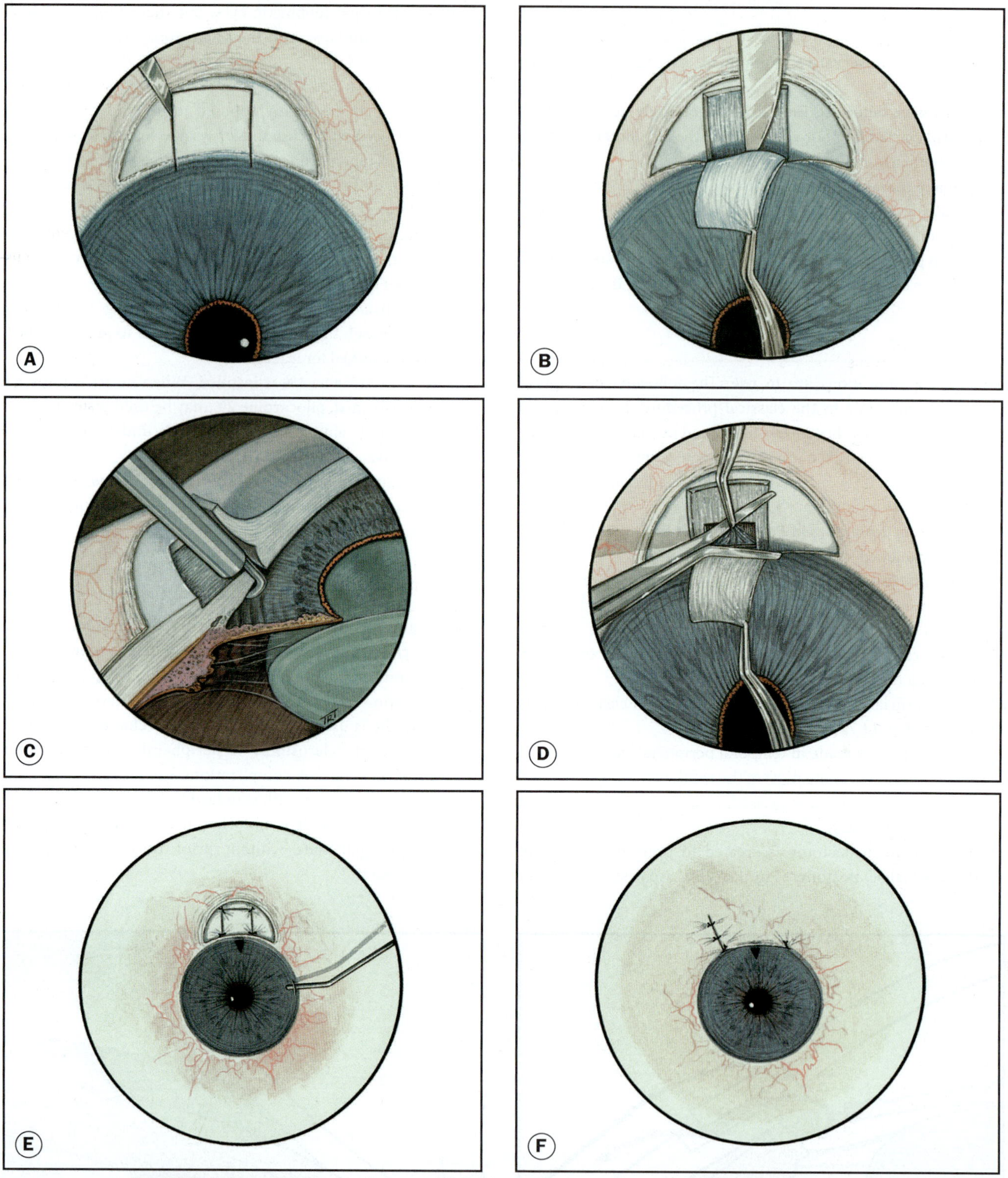

Fig. 11.72 Trabeculectomy technique. **(A)** Outline of superficial scleral flap; **(B)** dissection of superficial scleral flap; **(C)** excision of deep scleral tissue with a punch; **(D)** peripheral iridectomy; **(E)** injection of balanced salt solution into the anterior chamber; **(F)** appearance following suturing of a fornix-based flap.

Antimetabolites in filtration surgery

Indications

Adjunctive antimetabolites inhibit the natural healing response that may preclude successful filtration surgery. They should be used with caution because of potential complications and are usually considered in the presence of risk factors for surgical failure. In uncomplicated glaucoma the use of low-dose antimetabolites may improve long-term control of IOP.

- **Risk factors** for surgical failure:

- Previous failed trabeculectomy or MIGS.
- Previous conjunctival or cataract surgery.
- Secondary glaucoma (e.g. inflammatory, neovascular, post-traumatic).
- Demographic: Black race, age under 65 years.
- Patients on topical medication (particularly sympathomimetics) for over 3 years.

5-fluorouracil

5-fluorouracil (5-FU) inhibits fibroblast proliferation by retarding DNA synthesis. It is a less aggressive antimetabolite than mitomycin C (see below), but substantial complications can still occur, notably persistent corneal epithelial defects and bleb leakage.

- **Intraoperative** use involves the application of one or more small cellulose sponges soaked in a 50 mg/ml solution, placed under the dissected flap of Tenon's capsule at the site of filtration for 5 minutes prior to creation of the scleral trapdoor.

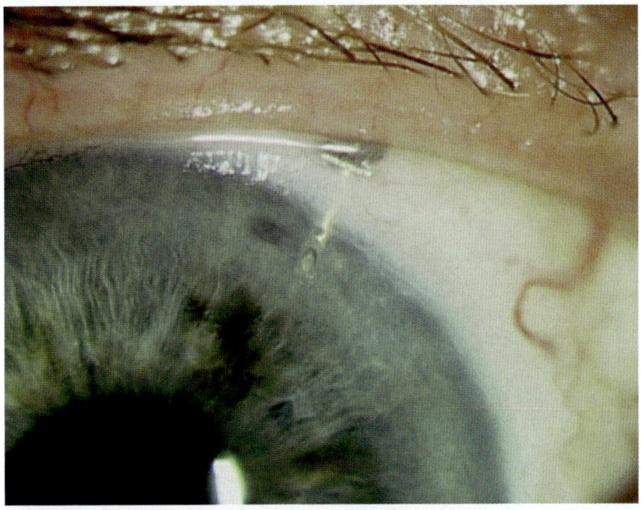

Fig. 11.73 Ex-Press mini-shunt in place.

- **Postoperative** subconjunctival injection of 0.1 ml of 25 mg/ml or 50 mg/ml solution can be used. Placement may be away from the fistula, even at the opposite limbus. Various regimens are described, including daily injections for several postoperative days and ad hoc use if a drainage bleb appears to be unduly vascularized or fibrotic. It is also often used as an adjunct to a limited 'needling' revision of a trabeculectomy (see below).

Mitomycin C

Mitomycin C (MMC) is an alkylating agent that inhibits proliferation of fibroblasts and suppresses vascular ingrowth. It is more potent than 5-FU. It is generally used intraoperatively in the manner described above for 5-FU, a typical exposure protocol being 0.2 mg/ml for 2 minutes, though a higher concentration (e.g. 0.4 mg/ml) may be used for particularly high-risk patients. Higher concentrations and extended exposure times are associated with an increased risk of complications. A cystic thin-walled bleb is common following the use of mitomycin C and may predispose to chronic hypotony, late-onset bleb leak and endophthalmitis. The bleb profile can be considerably improved by placing the MMC-soaked sponges well away from the limbus.

Bevacizumab

Bevacizumab is a monoclonal antibody against VEGF that can be used at the time of trabeculectomy. Intracameral or subconjunctival bevacizumab is more effective than placebo in these circumstances, but it appears to increase the risk of bleb encapsulation. It is not more effective than mitomycin C and combining it with MMC does not appear to improve the success rate.

Shallow anterior chamber

A shallow anterior chamber (Fig. 11.74A) following trabeculectomy may be due to pupillary block, overfiltration or malignant glaucoma. Severe and sustained shallowing is uncommon, the chamber re-forming spontaneously in most cases. However, those

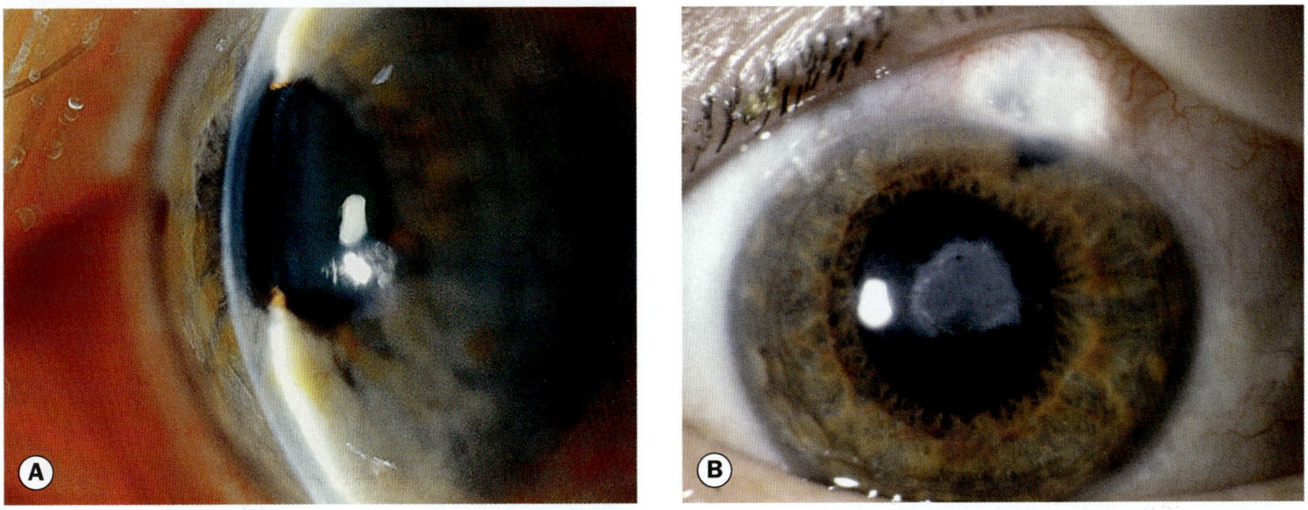

Fig. 11.74 Shallow anterior chamber. **(A)** With pupillary border – corneal apposition; **(B)** cataract following a flat anterior chamber.

that do not may develop severe complications such as peripheral anterior synechiae, corneal endothelial damage and cataract (Fig. 11.74B).

Pupillary block

Pupillary block may occur with a non-patent peripheral iridectomy.

- **Signs**
  - High IOP and flat bleb.
  - Negative Seidel test.
  - Iris bombé with a non-patent iridectomy.
- **Treatment** involves Nd:YAG laser to the pigment epithelium at the iridectomy site if the anterior iris stroma appears to have been largely removed (common), or the creation of a new laser iridotomy.

Overfiltration

Overfiltration may be caused by insufficient resistance to outflow at the lamellar scleral flap, but bleb leakage through an inadvertent buttonhole or due to inadequate closure of the conjunctiva and Tenon capsule is more common.

- **Signs**
  - Low IOP with a well-formed bleb in a scleral flap leak and flat in a bleb leak.
  - The Seidel test is negative in a scleral flap leak but positive (Fig. 11.75A) in a bleb leak.
  - The cornea may show signs of hypotony such as folds in Descemet membrane.
  - Choroidal detachment (Fig. 11.75B and C) may be present.
- **Treatment** depends on the cause and degree of shallowing.
  - Initial management in eyes with mild overfiltration such as may be caused by a small bleb leak, may consist simply of observation, with atropine to prevent PAS formation.
  - Subsequent treatment if the above measures are ineffective involves temporary tamponade of the conjunctiva to enhance spontaneous healing by simple pressure patching, a large diameter soft bandage contact lens, a collagen shield or a Simmons shell designed for the purpose.
  - Definitive treatment often consists of the insertion of additional conjunctival sutures and if necessary, placement of a transconjunctival scleral flap suture. If potentially serious shallowing is present, the anterior chamber can be reformed with a viscoelastic. A choroidal detachment rarely requires drainage.

Malignant glaucoma

Malignant glaucoma is a rare but serious complication of trabeculectomy in patients with primary angle closure and primary angle-closure glaucoma. It is caused by anterior rotation of the ciliary processes and iris root (ciliolenticular block) leading to a posterior misdirection of aqueous.

- **Signs**
  - Shallow anterior chamber with myopic shift. Patients will usually notice an improvement in their unaided near vision.
  - High IOP and absent bleb.
  - Negative Seidel test.
- **Treatment**
  - Initial treatment is with mydriatics (atropine 1% and phenylephrine 10%) to dilate the ciliary ring and to increase the distance between the ciliary processes and the equator of

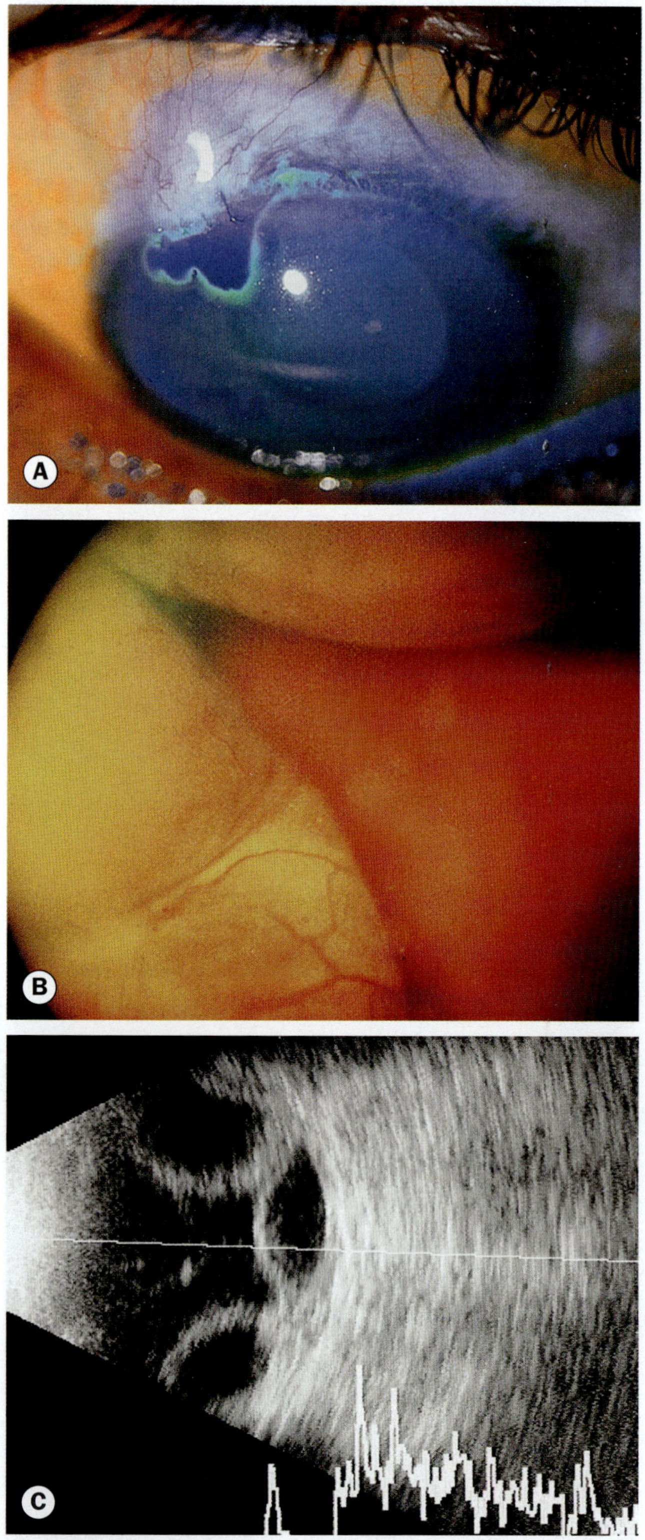

Fig. 11.75 Complications of surgery. **(A)** Positive Seidel test; **(B)** wide-field image of choroidal detachment; **(C)** ultrasound of choroidal detachment in a hypotonous eye.

the lens, thereby tightening the zonules and pulling the lens posteriorly into its normal position. Intravenous mannitol may be used if mydriatics are ineffective, allowing shrinkage of the vitreous gel and causing the lens to move posteriorly.

- Subsequent treatment if medical therapy fails is with Nd:YAG laser fired through the iridectomy in order to disrupt the anterior hyaloid face. In pseudophakic eyes, laser posterior capsulotomy and disruption of the anterior hyaloid face should be performed. Cyclodiode laser may also be effective.
- Pars plana vitrectomy is performed if laser therapy fails. The key is to remove sufficient anterior vitreous gel to allow free flow of aqueous to the anterior chamber.

Failure of filtration

Diagnosis

A normally functioning bleb should be slightly elevated, relatively avascular (Fig. 11.76A) and show superficial microcysts, which are distended conjunctival goblet cells. A cystic thin-walled bleb is not uncommon after the use of mitomycin C (Fig. 11.76B). Poor filtration is indicated by increasing IOP and a bleb with one of the following appearances:

- **Flat** without vascularization.
- **Vascularized** bleb (Fig. 11.76C) due to episcleral fibrosis.
- **Encapsulated** bleb (Tenon cyst) (Fig. 11.76D), characterized by a localized, highly elevated, dome-shaped, fluid-filled cavity of hypertrophied Tenon capsule, often with engorged surface blood vessels.

Causes

Causes of failure can be classified according to the site of obstruction:

- **Extrascleral** causes include subconjunctival and episcleral fibrosis, sometimes with bleb encapsulation.
- **Scleral** causes include over-tight suturing of the scleral flap and gradual scarring in the scleral bed.
- **Intraocular** causes are uncommon and include blockage of the sclerostomy by vitreous, blood or uveal tissue or by a variety of thin membranes derived from surrounding cornea or sclera.

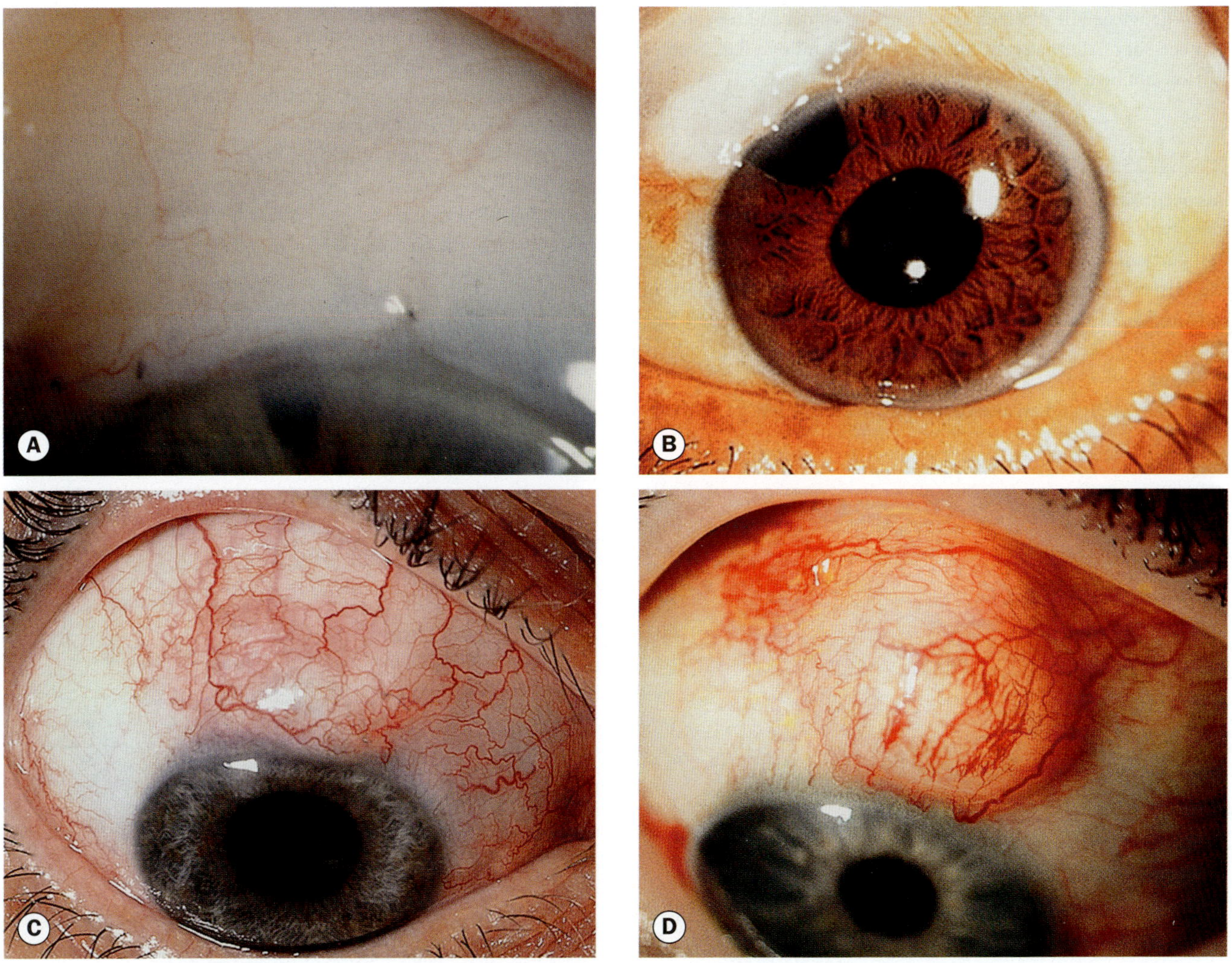

Fig. 11.76 Filtering blebs. **(A)** Diffuse shallow; **(B)** thin polycystic; **(C)** vascularized poorly filtering; **(D)** encapsulated – Tenon cyst.

Management

Management of filtration failure depends on the cause and may involve one or more of the following:

- **Ocular 'digital massage'** in an effort to force outflow through the surgical fistula may be performed by digital compression through the upper lid whilst looking downwards. This can be carried out by the patient 4–8 times a day for up to several weeks until the bleb is deemed stable.
- **Suture manipulation** may be considered 7–14 days postoperatively if the eye has high IOP, a flat bleb and a deep anterior chamber. Releasable sutures can be cut or released according to the technique of initial placement. Argon or diode laser suture lysis is useful if releasable sutures have not been used. It may be performed through a suture lysis lens or a Zeiss four-mirror goniolens.
- **Needling** of an encysted bleb may be performed at the slit lamp or using an operating microscope under topical anaesthesia. It can be augmented with 5-fluorouracil or mitomycin C to enhance the success rate.
- **Subconjunctival injection of 5-fluorouracil** may be used in the first 7–14 days to suppress episcleral fibrosis. An injection of 2.5–5 mg (0.1 ml of 25–50 mg/ml solution) is given using a 30-gauge needle directed away from the fistula and repeated as necessary. Alternatively, mitomycin C 0.1 ml of a 0.02% solution can be used.

Late bleb leakage

This occurs due to disintegration of conjunctiva overlying a sclerostomy, typically following peroperative application of antimetabolites, particularly mitomycin C. Necrosis of the surface epithelium results in transconjunctival drainage of aqueous. Complications of untreated leaks include infection and hypotony maculopathy (see Ch. 14).

- **Signs**
  - Low IOP and an avascular cystic bleb (see Fig. 11.76B).
  - Seidel testing may initially be negative with only multiple punctate staining areas ('sweating'), though this alone may well be sufficient to cause hypotony. The formation of a hole may result in gross leakage with a positive test and a very low IOP.
  - A shallow anterior chamber and choroidal detachments may be present in severe cases.
- **Treatment** can be difficult. The following are options:
  - Treatment depends on whether the leakage involves merely 'sweating' or is due to a hole. Sweating blebs may be treated by injection of autologous blood into the bleb, 'compression' sutures or a transconjunctival scleral flap suture, or sometimes surgery.
  - A full-thickness hole always requires surgical revision. The easiest option is to remove the existing bleb dissecting backwards from the limbus, followed by conjunctival advancement and resuturing. A fornix relieving incision may occasionally be needed and a scleral or donor pericardium graft can be used to limit flow through the sclerostomy.

Bleb dysaesthesia

Postoperative ocular discomfort secondary to tear film disturbance adjacent to the bleb occurs in approximately 5% of patients undergoing trabeculectomy. It is more likely to arise in young patients and in those with a thin-walled nasal-positioned bleb (Fig. 11.77A). The key sign is a number of small bubbles adjacent to the bleb, which are best visualized with fluorescein (Fig. 11.77B). The symptoms can often be relieved with topical lubricants, but surgical revision of the bleb may be needed if symptoms persist.

Bleb-associated bacterial infection and endophthalmitis

Glaucoma filtration-associated infection is classified as limited to the bleb (blebitis) or endophthalmitis, although there is some

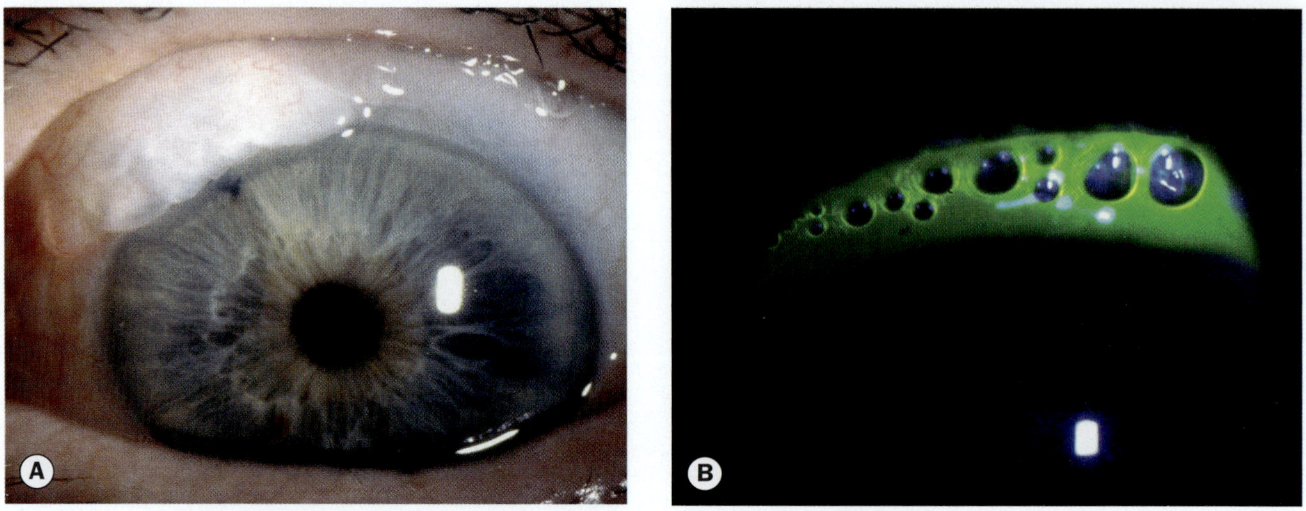

Fig. 11.77 Bleb dysaesthesia. **(A)** Large nasal bleb; **(B)** fluorescein-stained bubbles adjacent to the bleb, visible after blinking.

overlap. The incidence of blebitis following trabeculectomy with mitomycin has been estimated to be up to 5% per year, though many studies show a far lower rate. Patients who have undergone trabeculectomy should be warned of the possibility of late infection and strongly advised to report immediately should they develop a red and sticky eye, or blurred vision. Preserved lubricating drops tend to get contaminated in time and should be avoided.

- **Risk factors** include (a) antimetabolite use, (b) an inferior-placed bleb and (c) bleb leak. Blepharitis and conjunctivitis are also risk factors. Late bleb leaks should be treated aggressively to reduce the risk of infection.
- **Pathogens.** The most frequent are *Haemophilus influenzae*, *Streptococcus* spp. and *Staphylococcus* spp. and Gram-negative organisms. The poor visual prognosis is related to the virulence of these organisms.

Blebitis

Blebitis describes infection without vitreous involvement.

- **Symptoms** consist of a painful, red, photophobic and typically sticky eye.
- **Signs**
  - A white bleb that appears to contain inflammatory material (Fig. 11.78A).
  - Anterior uveitis may be absent or mild, but may be moderate and a hypopyon may be present.
  - The red reflex is normal.
- **Treatment**
  - Bleb-related infection is an urgent condition that needs immediate and intensive treatment.
  - A conjunctival swab should be taken. A sample should not be aspirated from within the bleb.
  - Broad-spectrum topical antibiotics instilled every hour, e.g. ofloxacin and a cephalosporin. The latter may be prepared from an intravenous ampoule.
  - Oral co-amoxiclav 500/125 mg three times daily and ciprofloxacin 750 mg twice daily for at least 5 days. Alternatively, azithromycin 500 mg daily can be used.
  - The role of topical steroids is undefined. Their introduction may be considered after a definite response to antibiotics.

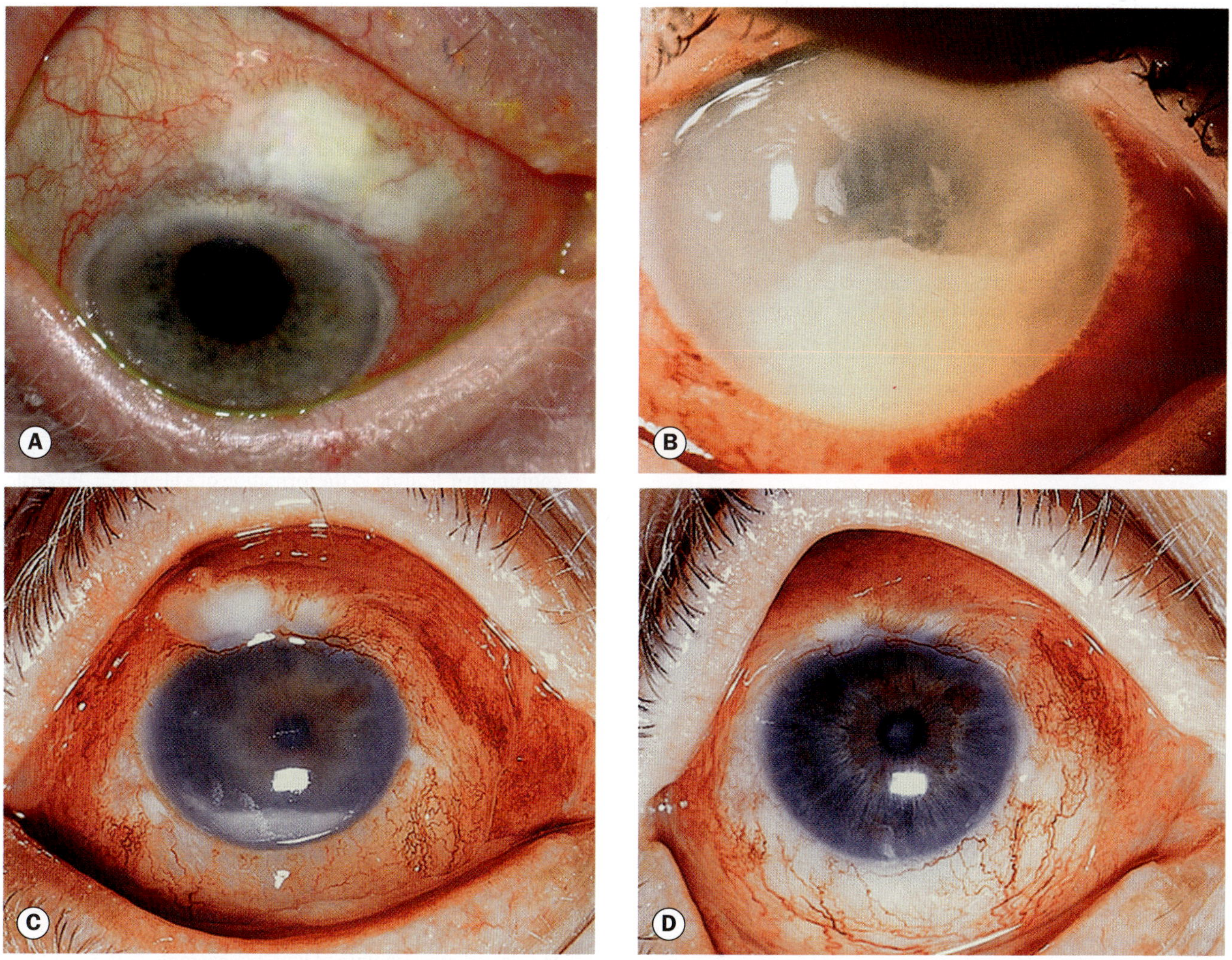

Fig. 11.78 Bacterial infection of a trabeculectomy site. **(A)** Blebitis; **(B)** severe bleb-associated endophthalmitis; **(C)** bleb-associated endophthalmitis on presentation; **(D)** appearance following successful treatment.

TIP Bleb-related infection is an urgent condition that needs immediate and intensive treatment.

Endophthalmitis

Fistula-related endophthalmitis, even with early treatment, can be associated with a very poor outcome, including blindness or even loss of the eye, mainly because the organisms that are isolated are significantly more virulent than those found in infections that follow cataract surgery (Fig. 11.78B). An aggressive treatment regimen should be instituted as soon as possible.

- **Symptoms** are generally much more severe than those of blebitis.
- **Signs**
  - White milky bleb, as in blebitis but of greater severity.
  - Severe injection.
  - Severe anterior uveitis; a substantial hypopyon is typical.
  - Vitritis and impairment of the red reflex.
- **Treatment**
  - Vitreous and aqueous samples should be obtained immediately on presentation and ceftazidime 2 mg in 0.1 ml and vancomycin 2 mg in 0.1 ml should be injected into the vitreous cavity. After 48 hours repeat intravitreal antibiotics and consider undertaking a posterior vitrectomy. Start topical steroids after 48 hours. Oral fluoroquinolones should be used for 10–14 days.
  - Topical and systemic therapy as for blebitis (Fig. 11.78C and D).

TIP The organisms involved in fistula-related endophthalmitis tend to be more virulent than after cataract surgery. Vitreous and aqueous samples should be obtained immediately on presentation.

NON-PENETRATING GLAUCOMA SURGERY

Overview

In non-penetrating filtration surgery, the anterior chamber is not entered and the internal trabecular meshwork is preserved, thus reducing the incidence of postoperative overfiltration with hypotony and its potential sequelae. Two concentric lamellar scleral flaps are fashioned and the deep flap excised leaving behind a thin membrane consisting of trabeculum/Descemet membrane through which aqueous diffuses from the AC to the subconjunctival space. The surgery is technically challenging and requires meticulous dissection of a deep scleral flap to avoid entering the anterior chamber through the delicate Descemet membrane.

Indications

The main indication for non-penetrating surgery is POAG, although other open-angle glaucomas may also be amenable. In general, the IOP reduction is less than that achieved by trabeculectomy, so that topical medication often needs to be recommenced. Conventional filtration is therefore still the procedure of choice when the target IOP is in the low teens though non-penetrating surgery is probably associated with a lower risk of 'snuffing out' central vision when advanced damage is present.

Technique

- **Deep sclerectomy** (Fig. 11.79). A Descemet window is created to allow aqueous migration from the AC. Subsequent egress is subconjunctival, resulting in a shallow filtration bleb, as well as along deeper suprachoroidal routes. The long-term results can be enhanced by using a collagen implant at the time of surgery and postoperative application of Nd:YAG laser to the meshwork at the surgical site using a gonioscopy lens (goniopuncture).
- **Viscocanalostomy** involves the creation of a filtering window, with identification and dilatation of the Schlemm canal with high density viscoelastic. The superficial scleral flap is sutured tightly so that subconjunctival fluid outflow and bleb formation are minimized. The procedure probably causes inadvertent microscopic ruptures in the juxtacanalicular tissue and meshwork.

MINIMALLY INVASIVE GLAUCOMA SURGERY (MIGS)

MIGS is the term applied to the various implants and techniques that aim to lower IOP with less surgical risk than traditional glaucoma surgery. MIGS is commonly combined with cataract surgery and is not suitable for all forms of glaucoma.

Current procedures can be classified into three groups:

- **Surgery that avoids the formation of a bleb** by manipulating the Schlemm canal, either by excision of trabecular meshwork (Trabectome, Kahook Dual Blade) or by bypassing the trabecular meshwork (iStent inject or Hydrus Microstent) (Fig. 11.80A and B), or by dilation of the canal (ab-interno canaloplasty with iTrack).
- **Implants that result in drainage under Tenon capsule and conjunctiva**, leading to the formation of a bleb (Xen, Preserflo, InnFocus MicroShunt) (Fig. 11.80C). Mitomycin C (0.02% 0.1 ml) is usually injected under the conjunctiva adjacent to the implant to reduce the risk of bleb fibrosis. Bleb needling is often required postoperatively.
- **Surgery that increases aqueous outflow from the anterior chamber into the supraciliary space.** (MINIject). An ab-interno approach is used and a 5-mm long silicone implant consisting of thousands of interconnected hollow spheres is placed into the supraciliary space, protruding 0.5 mm into the anterior chamber. No bleb is created and an anti-metabolite is not used.

Indications

- Mild to moderate glaucoma, where the rate of visual field loss is slow and the target pressure goal is modest (aiming for 15–17 mmHg).
- In selected cases combined with phacoemulsification and IOL implantation, to reduce the need for topical medication.

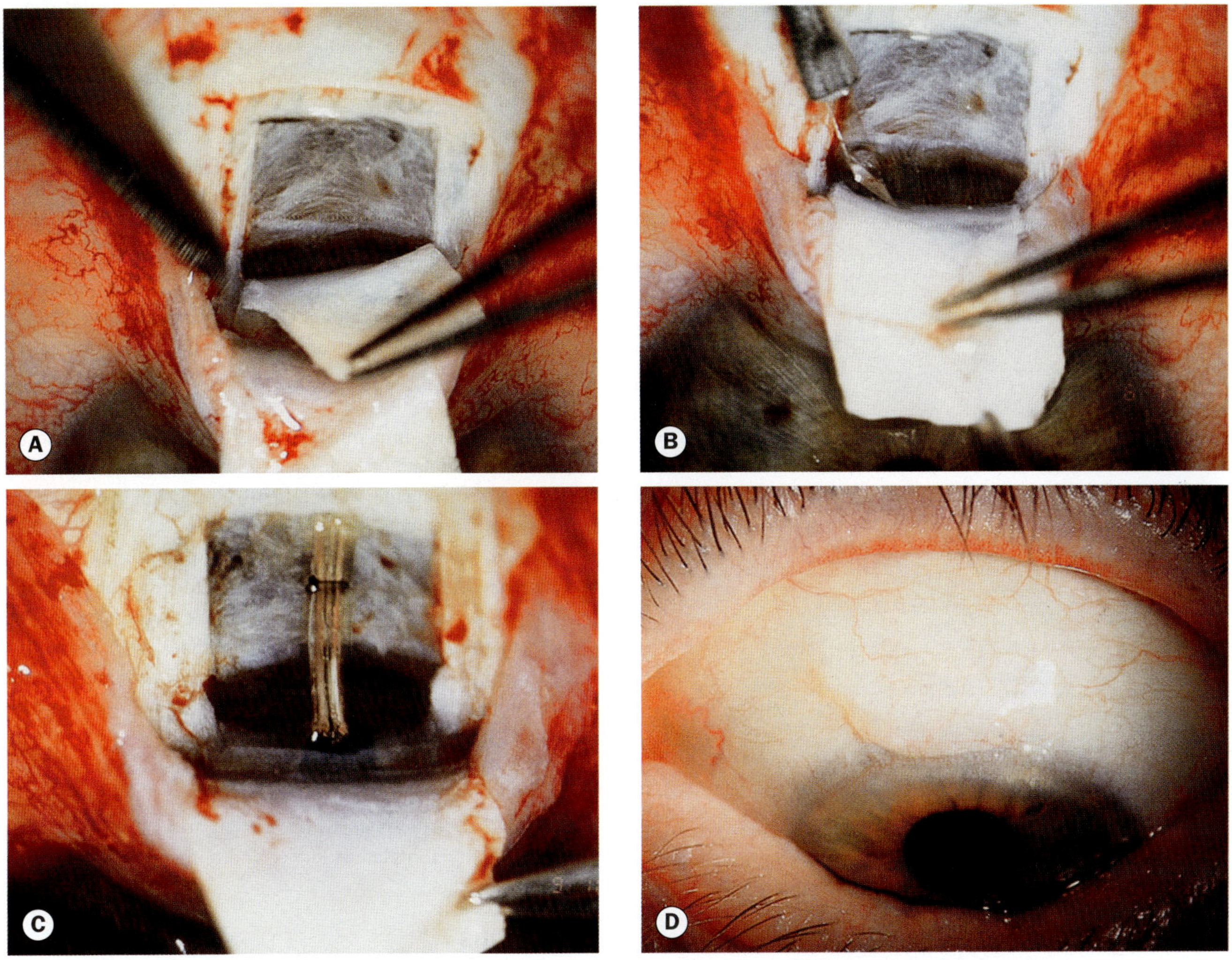

Fig. 11.79 Non-penetrating filtration surgery: deep sclerectomy. **(A)** Dissection of deep scleral flap; **(B)** dissection into clear cornea exposing the Schlemm canal; **(C)** collagen implant; **(D)** shallow diffuse avascular bleb. *(Courtesy of A Mermoud.)*

Complications

- In those procedures that involve manipulation of the Schlemm canal there is a risk of implant malposition, haemorrhage, infection and late corneal decompensation.
- In the procedures that depend on the formation of a bleb, the complications that follow trabeculectomy may occur. Because insertion of a micro-stent is involved, malposition and erosion of the stent can occasionally be seen.
- In procedures involving the placement of an implant into the supraciliary space there is a small risk of late corneal endothelial cell loss.
- Late failure of MIGS increases the risk of bleb fibrosis should trabeculectomy be subsequently required to control the IOP.

Results of surgery

- The results of MIGS are biased by the fact that this surgery is often undertaken at the same time as cataract surgery, which independently reduces the IOP by about 15%.
- Meta-analysis of 'stand-alone' iStent implantation results reveals an overall IOP reduction of about 30% from baseline for up to 5 years after surgery.
- Two years after 'stand-alone' MIGS (Xen implant or goniotomy/canaloplasty) one in four patients need further surgery to control the IOP.
- The Horizon study of the Hydrus Microstent concludes that the stent is safe, less likely to result in visual field loss and is more effective at lowering the IOP with fewer medications than phacoemulsification and IOL implantation alone, at 5 years.

DRAINAGE SHUNTS

Shunts using episcleral explants

Introduction

Glaucoma drainage devices (GDD) create a communication between the anterior chamber and the sub-Tenon space via a

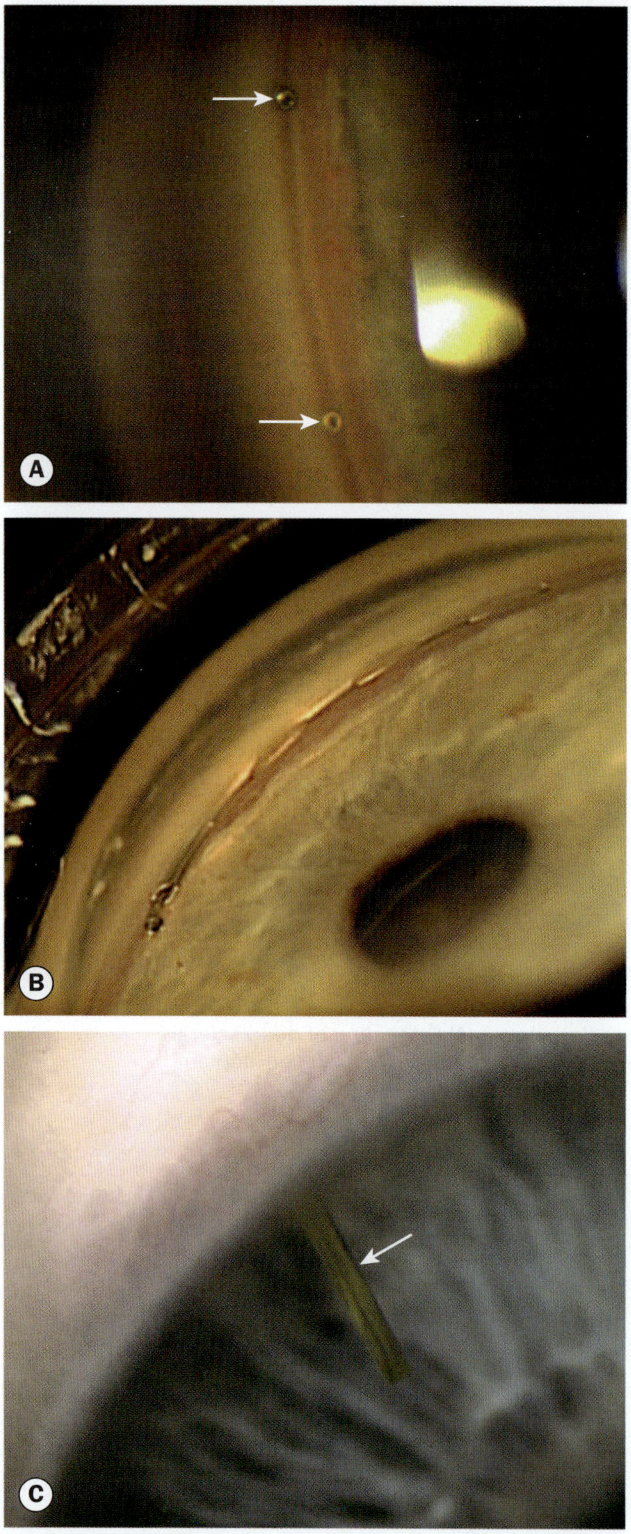

Fig. 11.80 MIGS. **(A)** iStent (arrows); **(B)** Hydrus; **(C)** Xen (arrow). *(Courtesy of G Ratnarajan – fig. A.)*

tube attached to a posteriorly explanted episcleral reservoir (Fig. 11.81). Some contain pressure-sensitive valves for the regulation of aqueous flow. Reduction of IOP is due to passive, pressure-dependent flow of aqueous, limited by the wall of a tissue capsule that forms around the explant over the course of several weeks postoperatively. In recent years the use of GDD has increased, with a large trial, the Tube Versus Trabeculectomy Study, providing good-quality evidence of their safety and comparability to mitomycin C-enhanced trabeculectomy. Five years after tube surgery the IOP reduction, rates of surgical failure and visual loss are similar to those found after MMC-enhanced trabeculectomy, but more postoperative medication is needed to control the IOP in those receiving a tube. In practice the threshold for GDD implantation has been lowered, though the number of patients undergoing trabeculectomy remains significantly higher than those undergoing GDD implantation. Examples of GDD implants include:

- **Molteno3.** This consists of a silicone tube connected to one (137 mm^2) or two (274 mm^2) polypropylene plates 13 mm in diameter.
- **Baerveldt.** This implant consists of a silicone tube connected to a silicone plate of large area (250 mm^2 or 350 mm^2) (Fig. 11.81A). Silicone may elicit little tissue reaction in comparison with polypropylene.
- **Ahmed.** This is a valved implant consisting of a silicone tube connected to a silicone sheet valve held in a polypropylene body (184 mm^2) (Fig. 11.81B). The valve mechanism consists of two thin silicone elastomer membranes, with the aim of reducing early postoperative hypotony and its complications. The implant needs to be primed by injecting saline through the valve before the surgery is undertaken.
- **PAUL.** This is a new valveless GDD. A silicone tube (with a significantly smaller tube diameter than other devices), is attached to a footplate which has an area of 344 mm^2 (Fig. 11.81C). The footplate is longer and not as wide as the Baerveldt footplate.

Indications

The circumstances under which GDD may be superior to trabeculectomy are incompletely defined and many factors must be considered, including an individual surgeon's experience and expertise. GDD may be considered in the following situations:

- **Severe conjunctival scarring** precluding accurate dissection of the conjunctiva.
- **Uncontrolled glaucoma despite previous trabeculectomy** with adjunctive antimetabolite therapy.
- **Secondary glaucoma** where routine trabeculectomy, with or without adjunctive antimetabolites, is less likely to be successful. Examples include aniridia, neovascular glaucoma, ICE syndrome and glaucoma following traumatic anterior segment disruption.
- **Certain types of congenital glaucoma** where conventional procedures have failed.

Complications

The rate of serious complications is similar to that of mitomycin trabeculectomy.

- **Excessive drainage**, resulting in hypotony and a shallow anterior chamber.
- **Bleb encapsulation.** This is characterized by raised IOP 1–6 weeks after aqueous enters the area of the footplate. Clinically an inflamed thick-walled bleb can be seen over the footplate.

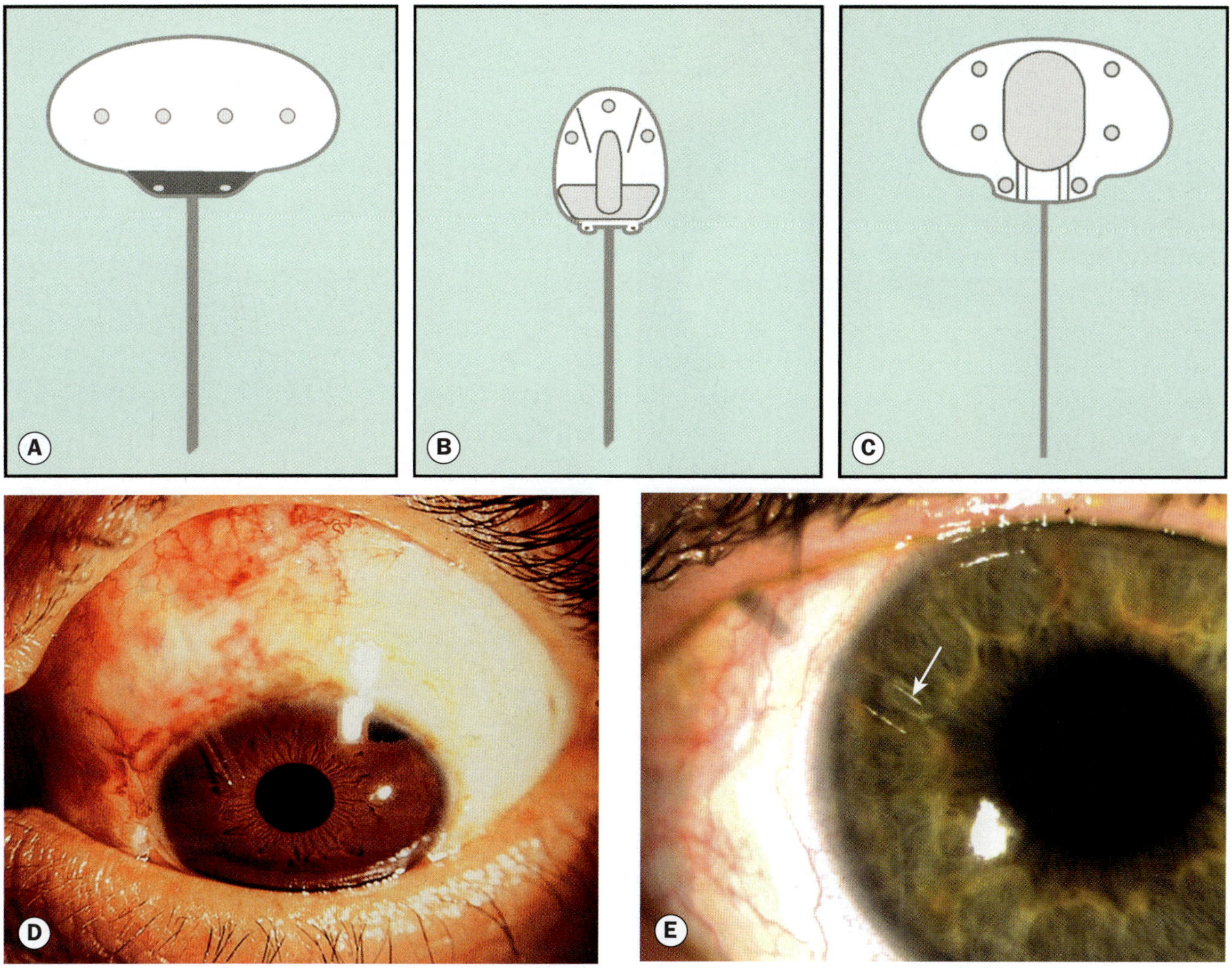

Fig. 11.81 Long-tube implant. (A) Baerveldt tube; (B) Ahmed valve; (C) PAUL tube; (D) immediate postoperative appearance; (E) 3 months after surgery in a different patient (arrow).

It is more common after the insertion of an Ahmed valve than a non-valved tube.

- **Malposition** (Fig. 11.82A) may result in endothelial or lenticular touch with corneal decompensation and cataract, respectively. Ciliary sulcus or pars plana tube placement can be used in some eyes to negate the possibility of corneal touch.
- **Tube erosion** through the sclera and conjunctiva (Fig. 11.82B).
- **Corneal decompensation** due to endothelial cell loss.
- **Early drainage failure** may occur as a result of blockage of the end of the tube by vitreous, blood or iris.
- **Late drainage failure** occurs in about 10% of cases per year and is comparable to, or perhaps slightly better than, that following trabeculectomy (Fig. 11.82C).
- **Double vision** due to extraocular muscle interference (Fig. 11.82D). This is more likely to occur if the footplate is placed in the upper nasal quadrant and is less likely to occur with the PAUL GDD because it is not placed under the rectus muscles.

Results

The results depend on the type of glaucoma. In general, an IOP in the mid-teens is achieved, but topical medication is frequently required in the medium and longer term. The Ahmed Baerveldt Comparison (ABC) study (where the average preoperative IOP was 30 mmHg) showed an average postoperative IOP of 14.7 mmHg in the Ahmed group and 12.7 mmHg in the Baerveldt group at 5 years. The long-term success rate in some conditions such as neovascular glaucoma and ICE syndrome is poor. Adjunctive mitomycin C may enhance the success rate of drainage shunt surgery.

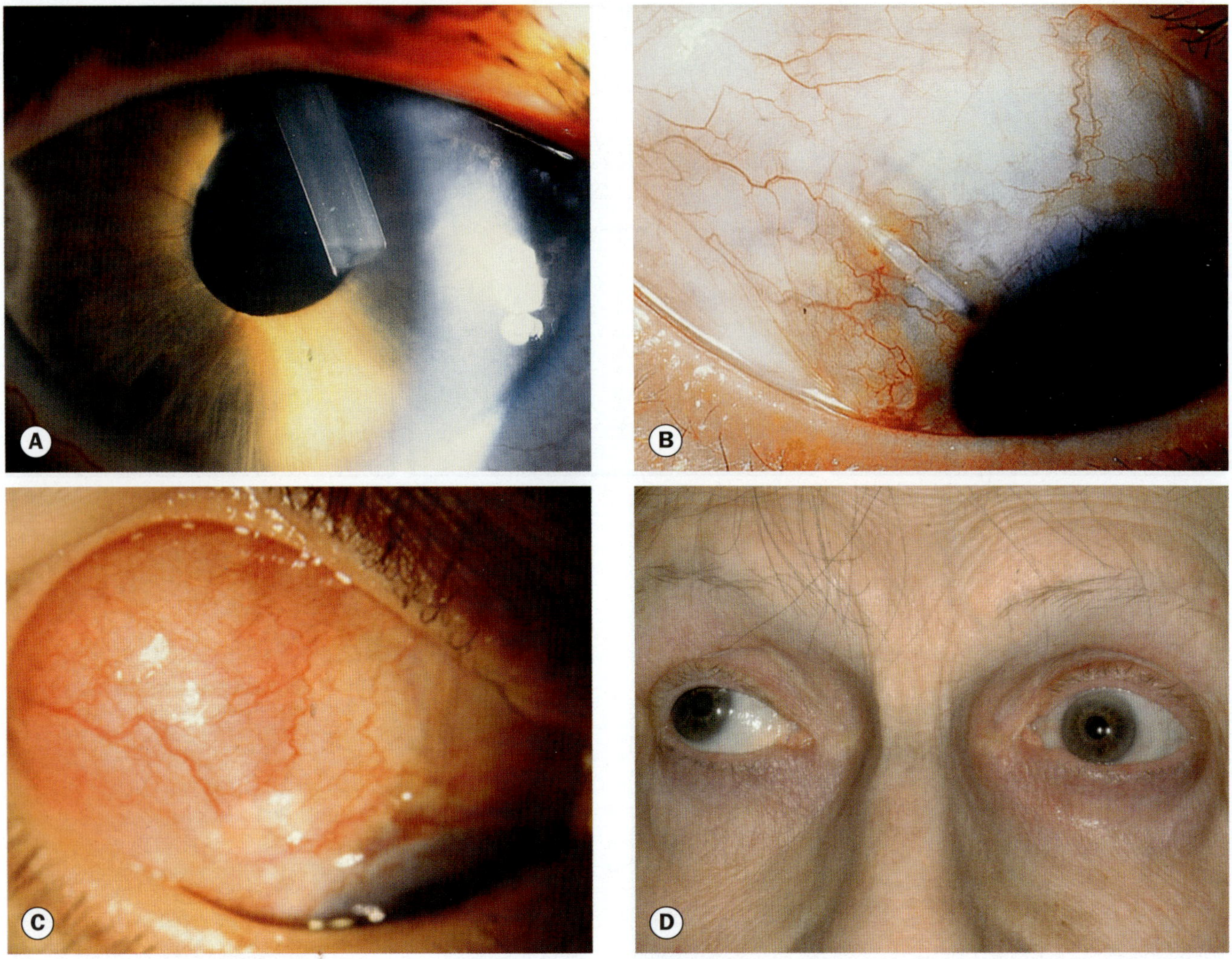

Fig. 11.82 Complications of drainage implants. **(A)** Malposition; **(B)** tube erosion; **(C)** bleb encapsulation and vascularization over the footplate associated with failure of drainage; **(D)** acquired Brown syndrome (left eye).

Chapter 12 Uveitis

CLASSIFICATION

The Standardization of Uveitis Nomenclature (SUN) Working Group guidance on uveitis terminology, endorsed by the International Uveitis Study Group (IUSG), categorizes uveitis anatomically (Fig. 12.1):

- **Anterior**: the anterior chamber is the primary site of inflammation.
- **Intermediate**: primarily vitreous inflammation including pars planitis.
- **Posterior**: retina and/or choroid.
- **Panuveitis**: all uveal structures are involved.

An IUSG clinical classification based on aetiology is also in use:

- **Infectious**: bacterial, viral, fungal, parasitic, others.
- **Non-infectious**: with and without a known systemic association.
- **Masquerade**: neoplastic and non-neoplastic.

The SUN Working Group guidance includes the following descriptions relating to the timing of inflammatory activity:

- **Onset**: sudden or insidious.
- **Duration**: limited (3 months or less) or persistent.
- **Clinical course**: acute (of sudden onset and limited duration), recurrent (repeated episodes separated by untreated inactive periods), or chronic (persistent duration, with relapse less than 3 months after discontinuation of treatment). Remission is defined as inactivity (no visible cells) for 3 months or longer.

CLINICAL FEATURES

Anterior uveitis

Introduction

Anterior uveitis is inflammation involving the anterior uveal tract – the iris and the anterior part (pars plicata) of the ciliary body – and is the most common form of uveitis. Iritis refers to inflammation primarily involving the iris and iridocyclitis to involvement of both the iris and anterior ciliary body. In practice these are interchangeable as they cannot be distinguished clinically.

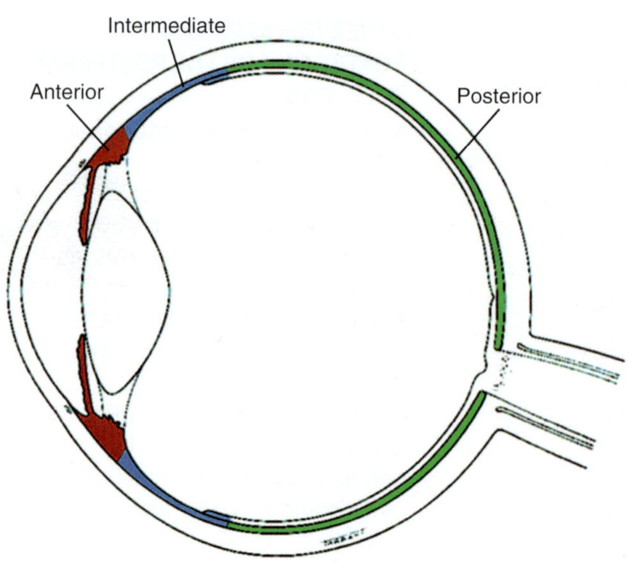

Fig. 12.1 Anatomical classification of uveitis.

Acute anterior uveitis (AAU) is the most common presentation, of which HLA-B27-related and idiopathic forms make up the largest proportion. Aetiology in these cases is uncertain, but may involve cross-reactivity with particular microbial antigens in genetically predisposed individuals. Interleukin-6, which is released by monocytes and macrophages in response to other inflammatory cytokines, plays a key role in the aberrant immune response that drives uveitis. AAU can be a feature of a wide variety of ocular conditions such as trauma (including surgery), lens-related inflammation and herpes simplex infection, or can be secondary to inflammation elsewhere in the eye, such as bacterial keratitis and scleritis. AAU can also be the presenting clinical scenario, without accompanying intermediate or posterior uveitis, in a range of systemic conditions including chronic inflammatory disorders such as sarcoidosis.

Chronic anterior uveitis (CAU) is less common than AAU. It is more commonly bilateral and associated systemic disease is more likely. Granulomatous inflammatory signs (see below) are often present.

Surveys of systemic associations of anterior uveitis vary in their findings. Table 12.1 lists important possibilities, but is not exhaustive.

The prognosis is usually good in most idiopathic and HLA-B27-related AAU provided management is adequate. Outcomes are more variable in CAU and in cases where there is an underlying ocular or systemic disorder.

Clinical features

- **Symptoms** in AAU consist of the rapid onset of unilateral pain, visual loss, photophobia, redness and watery discharge,

Table 12.1 Systemic Associations of Anterior Uveitis

Idiopathic	No detectable systemic association – around 50%
Infectious	Varicella zoster – usually current or past ophthalmic shingles Tuberculosis Syphilis Lyme disease Miscellaneous systemic viral infections
Non-infectious	HLA-B27 positivity – around 20% of AAU – with or without manifestations of HLA-B27-related systemic disease (see text) Juvenile idiopathic arthritis Sarcoidosis Behçet disease Tubulointerstitial nephritis and uveitis syndrome Systemic lupus erythematosus Multiple sclerosis Drug-induced (see Ch. 21)
Masquerade	Neoplastic, e.g. lymphoma, anterior segment melanoma Non-neoplastic, e.g. juvenile xanthogranuloma

sometimes preceded by mild ocular discomfort for a few days. As recurrent disease is common, especially with the idiopathic and HLA-B27-related types, there will often be a history of previous similar episodes. CAU may be of insidious or acute onset and can be asymptomatic until the development of complications such as cataract.

- **Visual acuity** is variably impaired depending on the severity of inflammation and the presence of complications. It is frequently only mildly reduced in AAU.
- **'Ciliary injection'** (perilimbal injection, ciliary flush or just 'injection') is circumcorneal conjunctival hyperaemia with a violaceous (purplish) hue due to involvement of deeper blood vessels (Fig. 12.2A) and is typically seen in anterior uveitis of acute onset. Ciliary injection is characteristically absent in some forms of CAU and occasionally AAU.
- **Miosis** due to pupillary sphincter spasm (Fig. 12.2B) predisposes to the formation of posterior synechiae (see below).
- **Anterior chamber cells** are a dependable indicator of inflammatory activity. Grading (SUN Working Group) is performed by estimating the number of cells in a 1 mm by 1 mm slit beam field, employing adequate light intensity and magnification (Table 12.2). This must be performed before pupillary dilatation, which can lead to shedding of pigment cells into the aqueous. Swept-source anterior segment optical coherence tomography is a sensitive method of showing individual inflammatory cells (Fig. 12.2C). Cells are commonly also seen in the anterior vitreous.
- **Aqueous flare** is haziness of the normally clear fluid in the anterior chamber, reflecting the presence of protein due to breakdown of the blood–aqueous barrier. Based on work in children with juvenile idiopathic arthritis-associated CAU, it is now thought that in most or all patients the presence of flare indicates active inflammation with a resultant higher risk of complications over the longer term. Flare may be graded clinically using a slit lamp to assess the degree of interference with visualization of iris and lens (Table 12.3). When available, laser flare photometry gives greater objectivity.
- **Hypopyon** (Fig. 12.2D) refers to a whitish purulent exudate composed of myriad inflammatory cells in the inferior part of the anterior chamber (AC), forming a horizontal level under the influence of gravity. Hypopyon is common in HLA-B27-associated AAU (see below), when a high fibrin content makes it immobile and slow to absorb. In patients with Behçet disease the hypopyon contains minimal fibrin and so characteristically shifts according to the patient's head position.
- **Keratic precipitates (KP)** are deposits on the corneal endothelium composed of inflammatory cells such as lymphocytes, plasma cells and macrophages (Fig. 12.3A and B). They are usually concentrated inferiorly, often in a triangular pattern with the apex pointing up (Arlt triangle) under the influence of gravity and aqueous convection currents. A notable exception is Fuchs uveitis syndrome, in which they are diffusely distributed. Their characteristics indicate the probable type of uveitis: smaller in the non-granulomatous inflammation typical of AAU and medium to large in (classically chronic) granulomatous inflammation in which cell types may include epithelioid and multinucleated cells. Large greasy-appearing granulomatous KP are said to have a 'mutton fat' appearance (Fig. 12.3C). KP are small to medium and adopt a star-shaped ('stellate' – Fig. 12.3D) or filamentous morphology in Fuchs uveitis syndrome. KP usually resolve as acute inflammation subsides: longstanding non-granulomatous KP may become pigmented. Granulomatous KP may become pigmented (Fig. 12.3E) and/or assume a 'ground glass' appearance. Endothelial dusting by numerous individual cells precedes the formation of true KP aggregates (Fig. 12.3F).
- **Fibrinous exudate** in the AC (Fig. 12.4A and B) is common in severe AAU and as with hypopyon is often seen with HLA-B27-related inflammation.
- **Iris nodules** can occur in both granulomatous and non-granulomatous anterior uveitis (Fig. 12.5A). Busacca nodules involve the iris stroma (Fig. 12.5B) and are a feature of granulomatous uveitis. Koeppe nodules are located on the pupillary margin and may be the site of posterior synechiae formation (see below) (Fig. 12.5B and C). Yellowish nodules can develop from dilated iris vessels (roseolae) in syphilitic uveitis. Iris 'pearls' may be seen in lepromatous CAU. Iris crystals (Russell bodies), thought to consist of immunoglobulin deposits, are a rare finding in some cases of chronic uveitis (Fig. 12.5D), including Fuchs uveitis syndrome.
- **Posterior synechiae (PS)** are inflammatory adhesions between the pupil margin and the anterior lens capsule (Fig. 12.6A and B) and may be particularly likely to form at the location of a Koeppe nodule. They can develop rapidly and to prevent their formation initial prophylaxis with a mydriatic agent is routine in all but very mild AAU. Once established, every attempt must be made to break PS before they become permanent (Fig. 12.6C and D).
- **Iris atrophy** may offer useful diagnostic clues. Diffuse stromal atrophy is seen in Fuchs uveitis syndrome and patchy or sectoral atrophy can occur in herpetic uveitis (Fig. 12.7). Both patterns may be seen in both simplex and zoster-related inflammation, though the latter is said to more commonly give a sectoral pattern.
- **Heterochromia iridis** refers to a difference in colour between the iris of the two eyes, best seen in daylight. In the context of uveitis, heterochromia characteristically occurs in Fuchs uveitis syndrome (see also Table 12.7).
- **Iris neovascularization (rubeosis iridis)** can occur, particularly in chronic inflammation. The process tends to be less acute than with a primary vascular cause such as central retinal vein occlusion. Abnormal iris vessels are very common in Fuchs uveitis syndrome, but do not cause synechial angle closure. Iris neovascularization may also occur in posterior uveitis, particularly when retinal perfusion is compromised. New iris vessels may be difficult to differentiate from dilated normal vessels (sometimes called 'pseudo-rubeosis'); normal vessels course radially in contrast to the irregular distribution of neovascularization. Fluorescein angiography may show leakage from new vessels, though this can also be seen with dilated normal vessels, particularly in the presence of active inflammation.

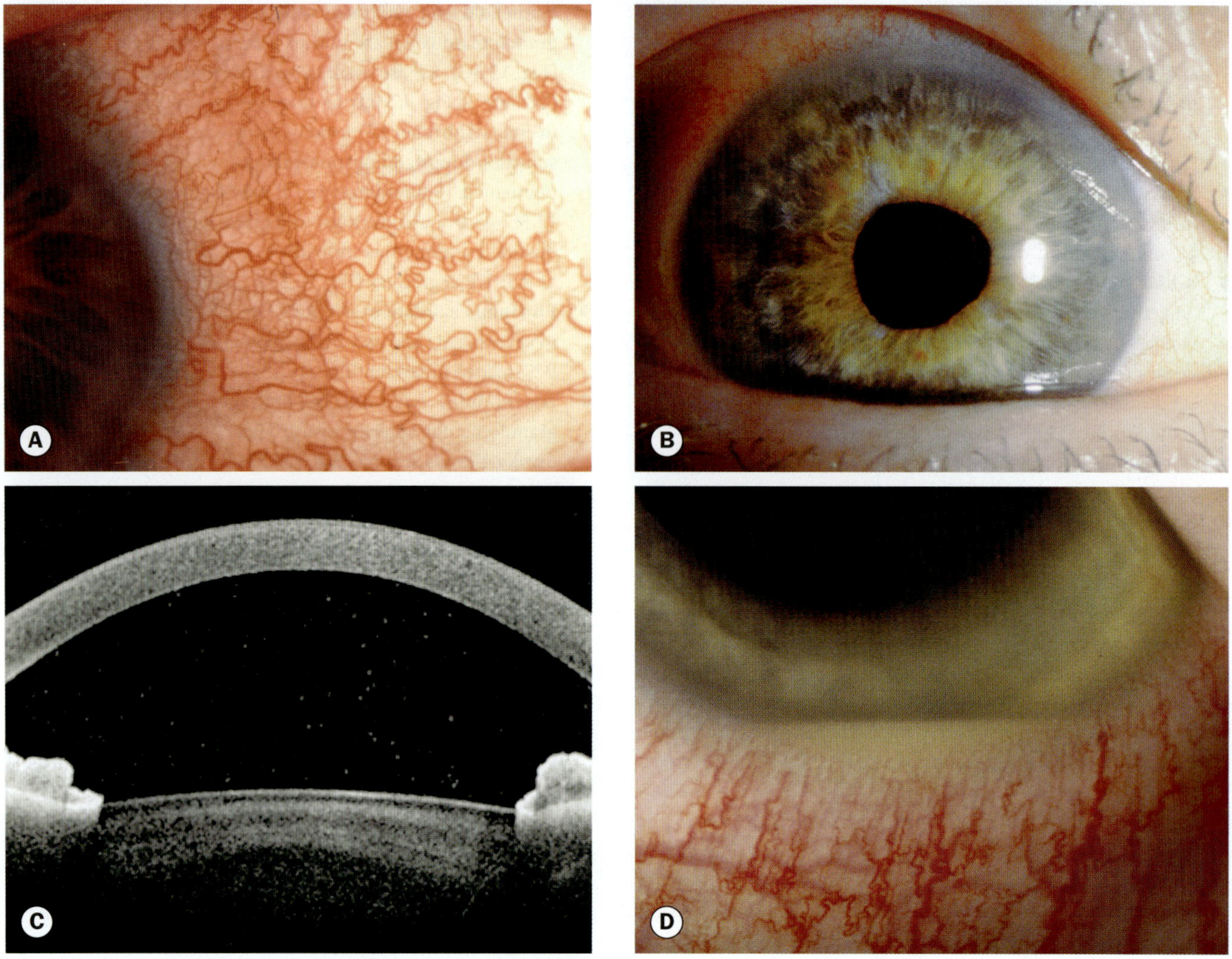

Fig. 12.2 Signs of acute anterior uveitis. **(A)** Ciliary injection; **(B)** miosis; **(C)** anterior chamber cells using the Tomey Casia2 swept-source OCT; **(D)** hypopyon. *(Courtesy of L. Solebo – fig. C.)*

Table 12.2 Standardization of Uveitis Nomenclature (SUN) Working Group Grading of Anterior Chamber Cells (1 mm by 1 mm Slit Beam)

Grade	Cells in field
0	<1
0.5+	1–5
1+	6–15
2+	16–25
3+	26–50
4+	>50

Table 12.3 SUN Working Group Slit Lamp Grading Scheme for Anterior Chamber Flare

Grade	Description
0	None
1+	Faint
2+	Moderate (iris and lens details clear)
3+	Marked (iris and lens details hazy)
4+	Intense (fibrin or plastic aqueous)

- **Intraocular pressure (IOP)** may be reduced as the result of impairment of aqueous secretion by the ciliary epithelium, or elevated due to a variety of mechanisms (see 'Inflammatory glaucoma' in Ch. 11), including the use of topical steroids.
- **Posterior segment examination** should always be performed to detect a masquerading cause of anterior uveitis (e.g. retinal detachment, tumour), primary intermediate or posterior segment inflammation and complications of anterior uveitis such as cystoid macular oedema.

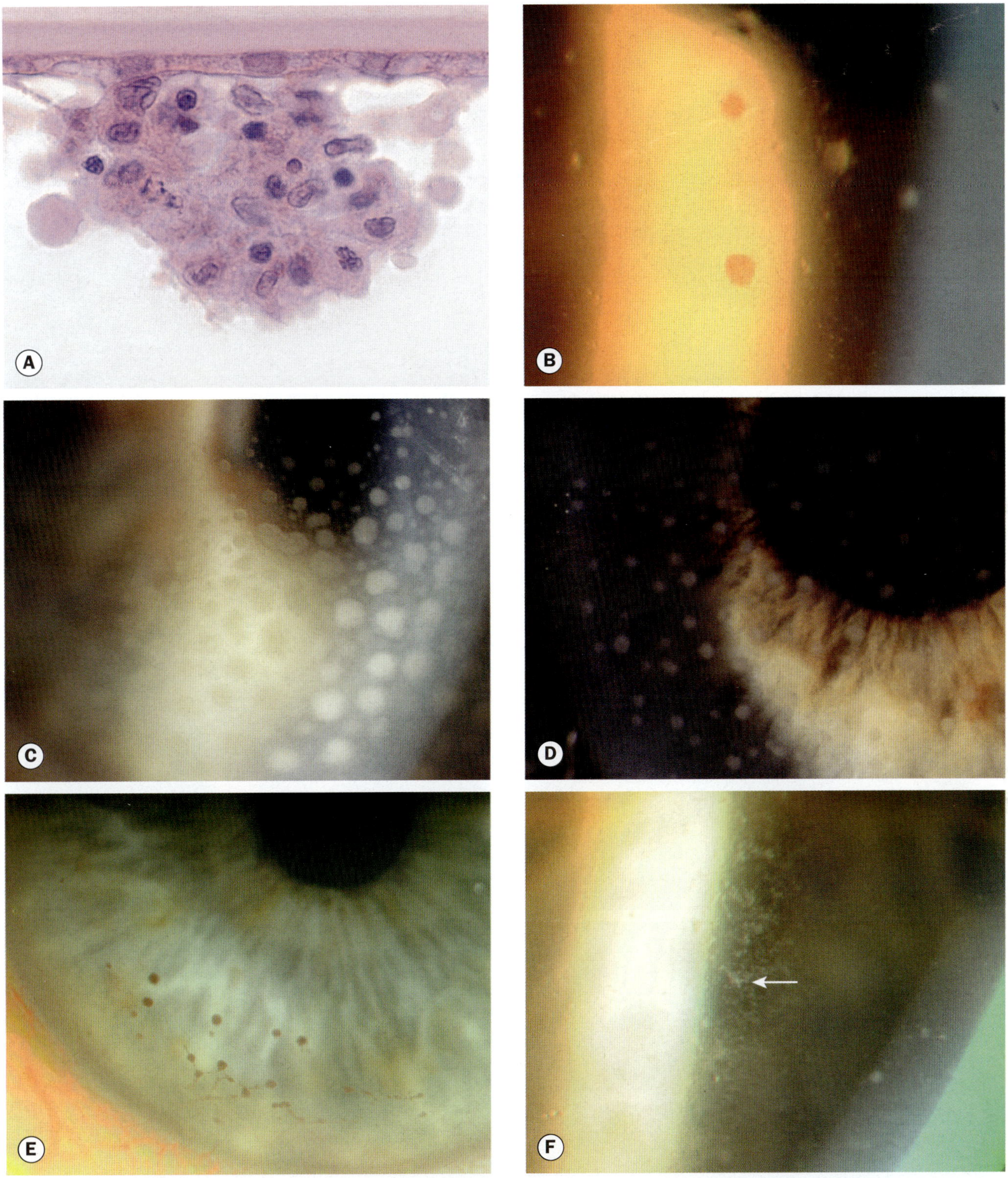

Fig. 12.3 Keratic precipitates (KP). **(A)** Histology showing typical aggregate of inflammatory cells on the corneal endothelium; **(B)** highly magnified view of fresh KP in early anterior uveitis; **(C)** large 'mutton fat' keratic precipitates; **(D)** stellate KP in Fuchs uveitis syndrome; **(E)** old pigmented granulomatous KP; **(F)** endothelial cellular 'dusting' (arrow) and early KP formation. *(Courtesy of J Harry and G Misson, from* Clinical Ophthalmic Pathology, *Butterworth-Heinemann 2001 – fig. A.)*

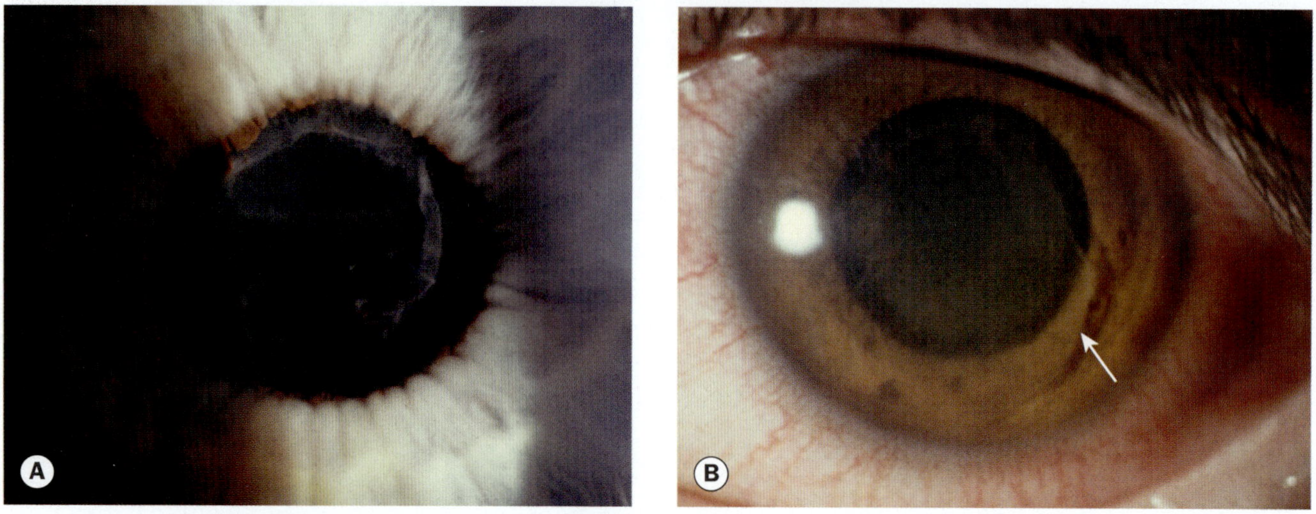

Fig. 12.4 Fibrinous exudate. **(A)** Mild; **(B)** severe (arrow).

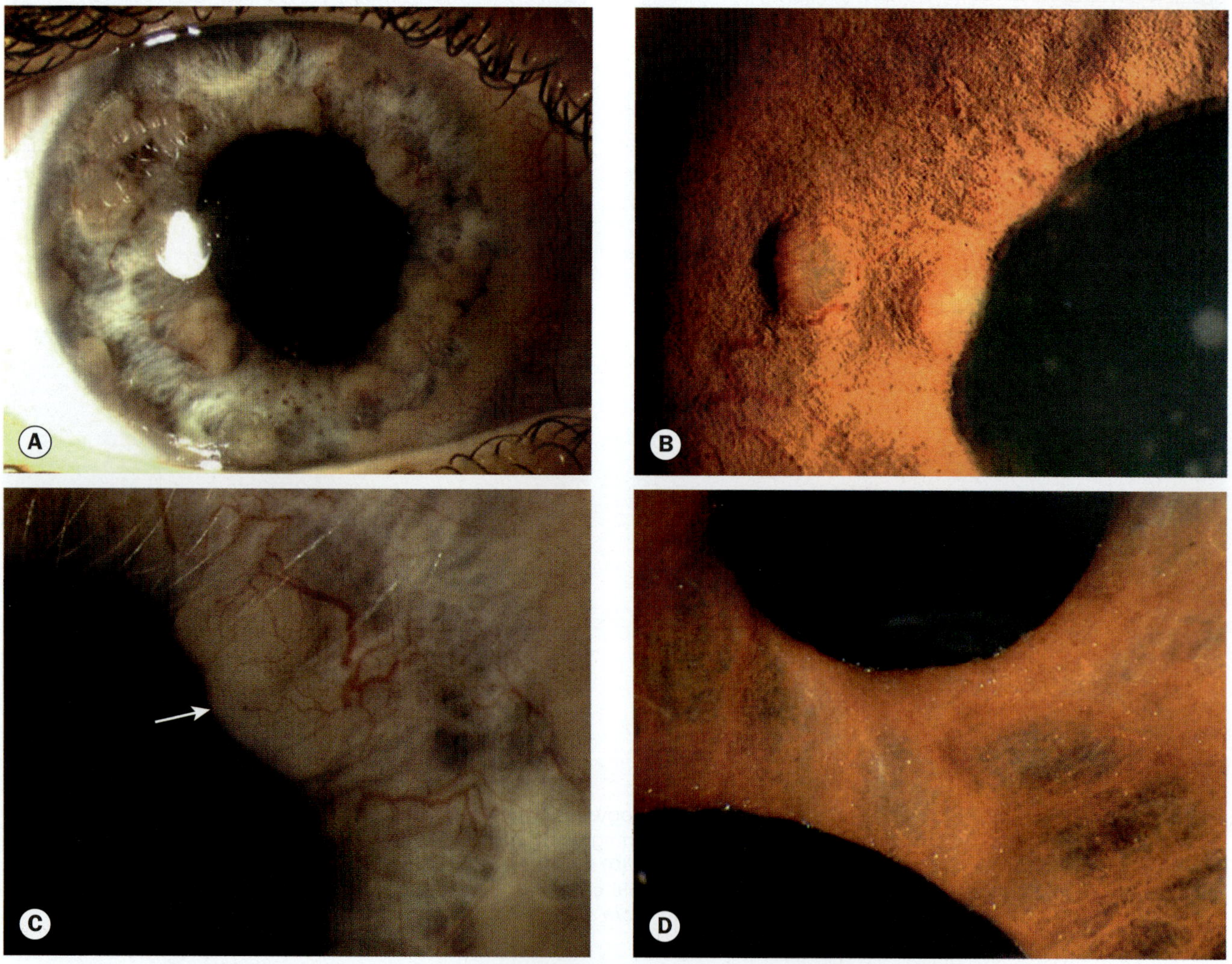

Fig. 12.5 Iris nodules in anterior uveitis. **(A)** Large nodules in sarcoid uveitis; **(B)** Busacca and Koeppe nodules; **(C)** Koeppe nodule (arrow); **(D)** iris crystals (Russell bodies) in chronic syphilitic uveitis. *(Courtesy of C Pavesio – fig. B; S Chen – fig. D.)*

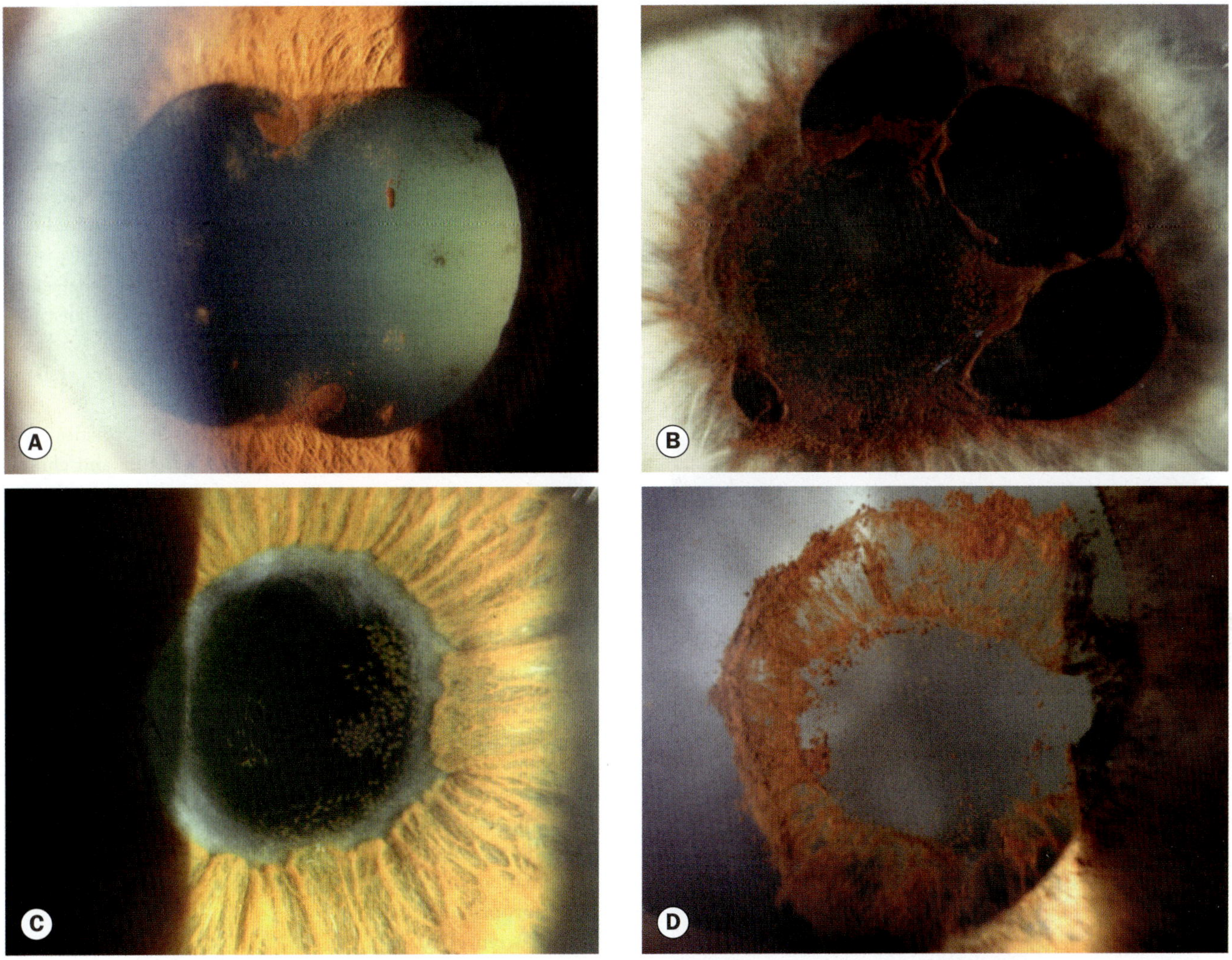

Fig. 12.6 Posterior synechiae. **(A)** Adhesions in active acute anterior uveitis; **(B)** extensive synechiae and pigment on the lens following severe acute anterior uveitis; **(C)** bound-down pupil; **(D)** after dilatation showing pigment on the lens

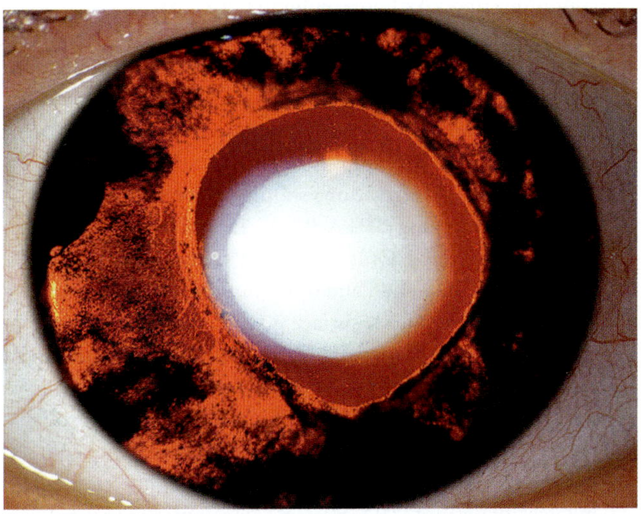

Fig. 12.7 Extensive iris atrophy following herpes zoster ophthalmicus – predominantly sectoral pattern. *(Courtesy of C Barry.)*

Posterior uveitis

Posterior uveitis encompasses the clinical entities of retinitis, choroiditis and retinal vasculitis. Some lesions may originate primarily in the retina or choroid but often there is involvement of both (retinochoroiditis and chorioretinitis). Specific conditions will be discussed later in the chapter.

- **Presentation** varies according to the location of the inflammatory focus and the presence of vitritis. For example, a patient with a peripheral lesion may complain of floaters, whereas a patient with a lesion involving the macula will predominantly complain of impaired central vision.
- **Retinitis** may be focal (solitary), multifocal, geographic or diffuse. Active lesions are characterized by whitish retinal opacities with indistinct borders due to surrounding oedema (Fig. 12.8A). As the lesion resolves, the borders become better defined.
- **Choroiditis** may also be focal, multifocal, geographic or diffuse. It does not usually induce vitritis in the absence of

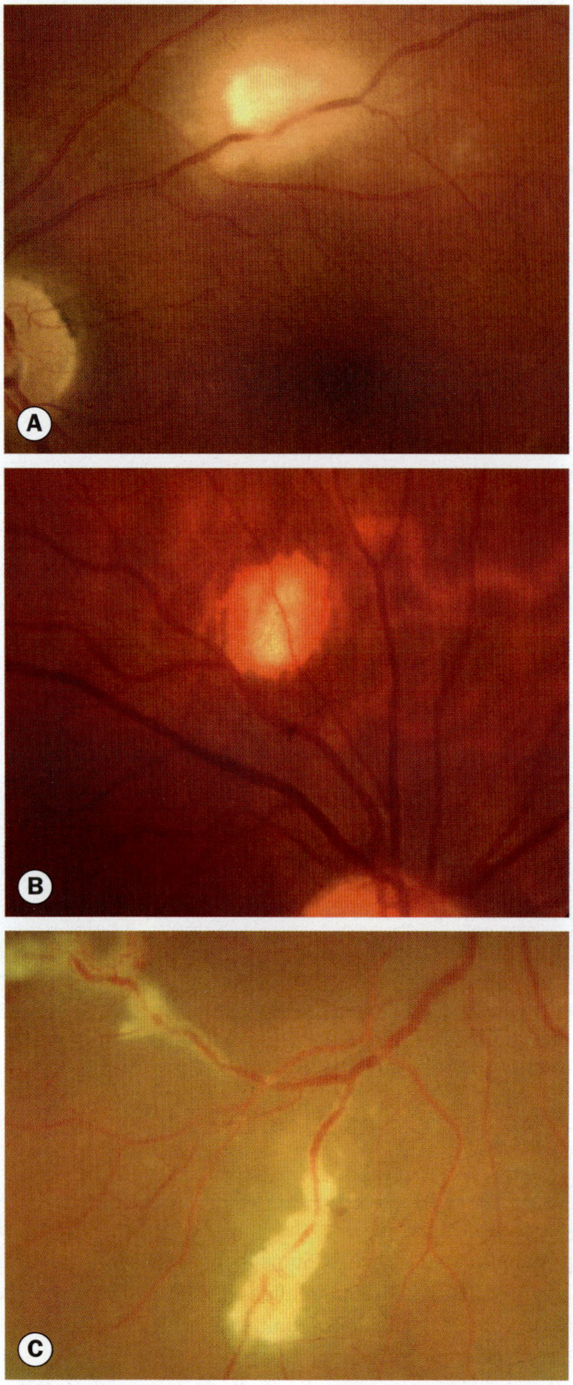

Fig. 12.8 Signs of posterior uveitis. **(A)** Retinitis; **(B)** choroiditis; **(C)** vasculitis.

concomitant retinal involvement. Active choroiditis is characterized by a round, yellow nodule (Fig. 12.8B).

- **Vasculitis** may occur as a primary condition or as a secondary phenomenon adjacent to a focus of retinitis. Both arteries (periarteritis) and veins (periphlebitis) may be affected, although venous involvement is more common. Active vasculitis is characterized by yellowish or grey-white, patchy, perivascular cuffing (Fig. 12.8C) sometimes associated with haemorrhage. Quiescent vasculitis may leave perivascular scarring, which should not be mistaken for active disease.

INVESTIGATIONS

- **Tailor the investigations.** Investigations are often negative, with no clear underlying cause determined in many patients. Rather than performing a battery of screening tests, investigation is tailored to each patient, directed by clinical features. Sometimes a likely cause may be obvious, such as severe anterior uveitis following intraocular surgery when endophthalmitis will lead the differential diagnosis list. In most cases, a careful review for systemic symptoms is essential to detect any clues to underlying disease, with referral to a specialist physician for further assessment where appropriate. Many associations of uveitis can present with a wide range of systemic features.
- **Multimodal imaging** of the posterior segment provides rapid, objective and accurate assessment of the retina and choroid and has become important in the management and follow-up of patients with posterior uveitis. Widespread use of this technology is improving standards of care in clinical practice, as well as defining outcome measures in uveitis research.

Investigation is generally not required in the following circumstances:

- **A single episode** of unilateral mild/moderate (no hypopyon) non-granulomatous AAU with no ocular or systemic suggestion of underlying disease.
- **A systemic diagnosis** compatible with the clinical features (e.g. sarcoidosis) has already been confirmed.
- **Typical clinical features** of a specific entity for which investigation is not usually indicated (e.g. Fuchs uveitis syndrome).

Situations in which **investigation of anterior uveitis is generally appropriate** include:

- Recurrent AAU.
- Severe AAU.
- Bilateral AAU.
- Anterior uveitis that is persistent, chronic or resistant to treatment.
- Granulomatous inflammatory signs (note that granulomatous conditions may give non-granulomatous AAU).
- Associated intermediate or posterior uveitis.
- Ocular or systemic clinical features suggesting underlying disease.

Repeating targeted previously negative investigations several years later is sometimes helpful.

The following investigations should be considered:

- **HLA tissue typing (HLA-B27).** The major histocompatibility complex (MHC) is a group of genes involved in white cell–antigen interaction and other immune functions, including the encoding of cell surface glycoproteins. In humans the MHC, found on chromosome 6, is called the human leukocyte antigen (HLA) system. HLA typing is used to determine organ transplantation compatibility and can also indicate predisposition to particular diseases. It has conventionally been performed by serological antigen identification, but increasingly involves analysis of DNA. HLA-B27 is a common (e.g. 6–8% of the White population in the USA, 0.5% of patients of Japanese ethnic origin) cell surface protein that presents peptides to T cells. The phenotype has a very strong association with AAU, ankylosing spondylitis and some other inflammatory conditions such as reactive arthritis (Reiter syndrome), psoriatic arthritis and arthritis in inflammatory bowel disease. It is present in 50% of patients with AAU who are otherwise fit and well and 90% of patients with AAU who have an associated spondyloarthropathy, notably ankylosing spondylitis. Many HLA-B27 subtypes have been identified and their significance is subject to ongoing investigation. HLA types associated with ocular inflammatory disease are listed in Table 12.4. HLA-B27 testing should be performed in any adult or child with recurrent or chronic non-granulomatous anterior uveitis.

- **Syphilis serology**
  - Treponemal antibody tests such as the ELISA (enzyme-linked immunosorbent assay) are highly sensitive and specific, but take around 3 months to become positive.
  - Non-specific titratable cardiolipin antibody tests such as the rapid plasma reagin (RPR) or venereal disease research laboratory (VDRL) are more commonly positive in early infection and are used to help monitor disease activity. These tests become negative over time, typically in treated disease. False-positive results can occur.
  - Both categories of test should be performed when screening for ocular syphilis.
  - Clinical features suggesting a diagnosis of syphilis should prompt urgent referral to a physician specializing in infectious or sexually transmitted diseases.
- **Serum angiotensin-converting enzyme (ACE)**: a non-specific test that indicates the presence of a granulomatous disease such as sarcoidosis, tuberculosis and leprosy. Elevation occurs in up to 80% of patients with acute sarcoidosis but may be normal during remissions. In normal children serum ACE levels tend to be higher and diagnostically less useful. Vigorous exercise can elevate ACE.
- **Lysozyme** is a group of enzymes found in polymorphonuclear neutrophils and numerous secretions including tears. It has a strong antibacterial action, mediating breakdown of the bacterial cell wall. Serum lysozyme assay is generally slightly less sensitive and specific than serum ACE in the diagnosis of sarcoidosis, but performing both tests may increase sensitivity and specificity.

Table 12.4 Examples of HLA Associations with Uveitis

HLA type	Associated disease
HLA-B27	Recurrent acute anterior uveitis
HLA-A29	Birdshot retinochoroidopathy
HLA-B51 and HLA B5	Behçet syndrome
HLA-B7 and HLA-DR2	(Presumed) ocular histoplasmosis syndrome
HLA-DR4	Sympathetic ophthalmia
HLA-DR4	Vogt–Koyanagi–Harada syndrome

- **Erythrocyte sedimentation rate (ESR) and C-reactive protein (CRP)**: acute-phase reactants that are probably of limited value, but may be elevated in a range of systemic inflammatory disorders.
- **Complete blood count**: leukocytosis may raise suspicion of infection and, exceptionally, haematological malignancy. Eosinophilia may occur in parasitic infection.
- **Lyme disease**: serology may be considered, particularly in endemic areas. Serology for other infectious diseases such as **brucellosis** and **leptospirosis** can be requested if relevant risk factors are present (e.g. endemic region).
- **Antinuclear antibody (ANA)**: limited use, except in children. In those with juvenile idiopathic arthritis (JIA) its presence is associated with a higher risk of CAU. Cases of possible subclinical JIA have been reported in ANA-positive children with CAU.
- **Antineutrophil cytoplasmic antibody (ANCA)**: limited use in anterior uveitis unless associated with scleritis and/or peripheral ulcerative keratitis, when cytoplasmic ANCA (c-ANCA) testing should be considered as evidence of granulomatosis with polyangiitis (Wegener granulomatosis).
- **Interferon-gamma release assay** (e.g. QuantiFERON-TB Gold) blood test for tuberculosis.
- **HIV serology**: indicated for selected patients, usually those in whom an opportunistic infection has been diagnosed or is suspected.
- **Sacroiliac joint X-ray** may show evidence of sacroiliitis in ankylosing spondylitis and other seronegative spondyloarthropathies.
- **Chest X-ray** may show evidence of sarcoidosis or tuberculosis. A high level of suspicion for both of these treatable conditions should always be adopted, particularly if the inflammation is granulomatous.
- **Fundus autofluorescence (FAF)** is a non-invasive technique that detects lipofuscin and melanin in retinal pigment epithelium (RPE) cells. This provides information on RPE function and the integrity of the chorioretinal interface and is extremely helpful when assessing inflammatory conditions of the choriocapillaris. Pronounced autofluorescence can be detected in patients with multiple evanescent white dot syndrome (MEWDS) (see Fig. 12.60C), serpiginous choroidopathy (see Fig. 12.62D) and acute zonal occult outer retinopathy (AZOOR) (see Fig. 12.68A).
- **Optical coherence tomography (OCT).** This technique obtains precise, reproducible, high-resolution images that correlate well with the histopathology. OCT can be used to detect and monitor macular oedema, vitreomacular surface disease and structural damage to the macula (see Fig. 14.49). Inner retinal infiltrates that show hyperreflective focal retinal thickening are seen in Behçet disease and some viral infections. Outer retina changes are seen in punctate inner choroidopathy (PIC), MEWDS, acute posterior multifocal placoid pigment epitheliopathy (APMPPE), serpiginous choroiditis, AZOOR and acute macular neuroretinopathy (AMN) (see Fig. 12.67B). OCT can be used to visualize choroidal granulomas (e.g. sarcoidosis and tuberculosis) and primary choroidal inflammatory diseases

like acute Vogt–Koyanagi–Harada (VKH) syndrome (see Fig. 12.18E and F) and sympathetic ophthalmia.

- **Fluorescein angiography** (FA; see Ch. 14). The fluorescein molecule diffuses easily out of minimally inflamed vessels (retinal vasculitis; see Fig. 12.32B) and can also be used to demonstrate occlusive vasculopathy (see Fig. 12.54B). In inflammatory eye disease FA is used to assess optic disc swelling and subretinal fluid accumulation (see Fig. 12.32D). FA is the investigation of choice when imaging inflammatory retinal foci, showing early hypofluorescence and late hyperfluorescence. Loss of the RPE shows up as a 'window defect' and pigment clumping gives a masking effect, as seen for example in APMPPE (see Fig. 12.61B). Chorioretinal atrophy is shown as a hyperfluorescent area.
- **Indocyanine green angiography** (ICGA; see Ch. 14). Indocyanine green angiography (ICGA) is rarely indicated in anterior uveitis, but is the investigation of choice in patients with predominantly choroidal inflammation. Because the ICG molecule is almost completely protein-bound, retinal leakage only occurs when there is major inflammation in these vessels (e.g. in Behçet disease). However, in the choroid the protein-bound ICG leaks slowly, but unimpaired. After recirculation, more and more ICG is entrapped and gradual impregnation of the choroid occurs. In the late phases active absorption of ICG by the RPE results in diffuse background hyperfluorescence. Alteration of choroidal impregnation is the main parameter studied by ICGA in inflammatory eye disease. Two broad categories of inflammation are seen: (a) choriocapillaris inflammation, where there is patchy hypofluorescent areas of different sizes, especially in the late images, e.g., APMPPE (see Fig. 12.61E) and serpiginous chorioretinopathy (see Fig. 12.62F) and (b) stromal choroiditis, where there are foci of hypofluorescence, followed by late diffuse hyperfluorescence as a consequence of leakage from large choroidal vessels. This can be a consequence of primary choroidal inflammation (e.g. VKH, sympathetic ophthalmia) or secondary choroidal inflammation (e.g. sarcoidosis, tuberculosis and syphilis).
- **Ultrasound biomicroscopy (UBM)** is particularly indicated in cases of hypotony and may demonstrate pathology such as subtle choroidal effusion, cyclodialysis cleft and cyclitic membrane. B-scan ultrasonography can be helpful if the posterior segment view is compromised by a very small pupil or opaque media.
- **Aqueous tap**: historically rarely performed in anterior uveitis, but viral causes are now recognized as being more frequent than previously realized. Herpesviruses (including cytomegalovirus) and rubella should be considered in clinically suspicious cases, especially unexplained hypertensive uveitis and cases relatively unresponsive to topical steroids. An aqueous humour sample can be sent for: (a) polymerase chain reaction (PCR) analysis, to check for evidence of viral genetic material and (b) for microscopy, culture and antibody assay. PCR may also help to exclude *Propionibacterium* infection in a chronically inflamed pseudophakic eye.
- **Iris biopsy** is rarely performed.
- **Vitreous biopsy** tends to be confined to the investigation of obscure posterior segment inflammation and suspected infectious endophthalmitis.
- **Chorioretinal biopsy.** To determine the cause of a persistent and severe posterior uveitis of unknown aetiology for which all workup is negative, consider undertaking a retinochoroidal biopsy.

TIP Multimodal imaging using OCT and indocyanine green angiography is indispensable in the investigation of patients with predominantly choroidal inflammation.

- **Conjunctival biopsy**: sampling of tissue such as a suspected granuloma or infiltrative lesion is occasionally indicated.
- **Referral to a specialist physician with resultant further investigation.** This is vital when systemic disease is suspected. For instance, if respiratory symptoms are present, a chest physician may arrange additional testing such as a high-resolution computed tomography (CT) chest scan, a whole-body gallium scan (sarcoidosis), a purified protein derivative skin test for tuberculosis (negative test is a diagnostic indicator in sarcoidosis) and bronchoscopy with lavage/biopsy. Similarly, neurological referral may lead to cranial magnetic resonance imaging (MRI) and lumbar puncture, and gastroenterological referral to endoscopy.

TREATMENT

For patients with a treatable cause of inflammation such as an infection, specific treatment (see individual topics) is given either instead of or in addition to the general anti-inflammatory measures discussed below. Review frequency is set according to the severity and chronicity of inflammation. Patients with severe inflammation may need to be seen within a day or two of initiating treatment. Those with mild recurrent idiopathic AAU may not need to be seen for several weeks after treatment is commenced.

- **Topical steroids**
    - Prednisolone 1% or dexamethasone 0.1% is commonly utilized as a first choice. Other preparations, of varying availability geographically, include difluprednate 0.05% (may be administered at a lower frequency), loteprednol etabonate 0.2% and 0.5% (moderate to marked potency but a lower tendency to elevate IOP), betamethasone, prednisolone 0.5%, fluorometholone and rimexolone (the latter three are of moderate to lower potency). The selection of topical steroid preparation can be modified according to severity and other factors such as a known tendency to IOP elevation. Steroid ointment (e.g. betamethasone) may be instilled at bedtime to supplement the drops. Additional anti-inflammatory treatment (see below) is necessary in some cases.
    - Treatment of AAU initially involves instillation at a frequency appropriate to the severity of inflammation, typically starting with one drop hourly in moderate–severe cases. Once the inflammation is controlled the instillation

frequency should be carefully tapered. A commonly adopted regimen might consist of:

- one drop hourly for 3 days, then
- every 2 hours for 3 days, then
- four times a day for 1 week, then
- three times a day for 1 week, then
- twice a day for 1 week, then
- once a day for 1 week and stop. Treatment is often discontinued by 5–6 weeks.

Periodic review is undertaken as appropriate during the treatment course, with further assessment a week or two after cessation, following which the patient can be discharged but cautioned to re-attend urgently should symptoms recur.

  - Treatment of CAU is generally targeted at complete suppression of inflammation, with no AC cellular activity or flare – the latter is now thought to be an indicator of active inflammation in most or all cases. Even low-grade ongoing activity is associated with a greater incidence of complications that outweighs the risk of complications from treatment. Exacerbations are initially treated in the same way as AAU, though with more gradual tapering and typically a maintenance regimen. Fuchs uveitis syndrome is an exception to this approach.
  - Common complications of topical steroids include transient elevation of IOP in susceptible individuals ('steroid responders'). Long-term treatment may lead to permanent IOP elevation with glaucomatous damage. Cataract can be induced, but is less common than with systemic steroid administration. The risk increases with dose and duration of therapy. Corneal complications are uncommon and include secondary infection with bacteria and fungi, recrudescence of herpes simplex keratitis and corneal melting. Systemic side effects are rare with topical steroids, but may occur following prolonged administration, particularly in children, in whom measures to reduce systemic absorption such as medial canthal pressure and blotting away of overspill from the eyelids following instillation should be discussed.

- **Cycloplegic agents.** These are used in AAU and in exacerbations of CAU to prevent the formation of PS, to break down recently formed synechiae and to promote comfort by relieving spasm of the pupillary and ciliary muscle. Commonly used anticholinergic agents in order of increasing potency and duration of action include cyclopentolate (duration 12–24 hours), homatropine (3 days) and atropine (7–10 days). In the acute stage, phenylephrine 2.5% or 10% may be used to supplement anticholinergics and break PS. In mild or CAU, a cycloplegic can be instilled at bedtime to prevent difficulties with accommodation during the day. In children, care should be taken to avoid systemic toxicity, as a range of systemic adverse effects have occurred including seizures. Prolonged uniocular cycloplegia may induce amblyopia in the susceptible age group.
- **Mydricaine No. 2.** This is a preparation containing adrenaline and atropine that is used to try to break fresh PS when drops are ineffective. It also contains local anaesthetic to improve comfort. Constituent quantities vary according to manufacturer but 0.3 ml containing 0.12 mg adrenaline, 1 mg atropine and 6 mg procaine is typical. It is usually administered by subconjunctival injection. An alternative to injection is insertion of a cotton pledget soaked in Mydricaine into the superior and inferior fornices for 5 minutes. Serious cardiovascular events have been reported following injection (a transient sinus tachycardia is common) and the patient should be monitored after injection. Mydricaine No. 1 is a paediatric version that may also be effective in adults.
- **Tissue plasminogen activator (TPA).** In severe fibrinous anterior uveitis 12.5–25 µg of TPA in 0.1 ml injected into the AC (intracamerally) with a 30-gauge needle under topical anaesthesia will dissolve dense fibrinous exudate and may break down recently formed PS. Antiseptic precautions similar to those for intravitreal injection should be taken.
- **Subconjunctival steroid** can be administered in severe cases or to patients in whom poor compliance is likely. For example, betamethasone sodium phosphate solution (4 mg in 1 ml) can be given alone or in a combined preparation with betamethasone acetate suspension for a sustained effect (e.g. Celestone, 6 mg in 1 ml).
- **Regional steroid injection.** The use of an inferior approach ('orbital floor') or posterior sub-Tenon (Fig. 12.9) injection of depot steroid preparations (e.g. triamcinolone acetonide, methylprednisolone acetate) is common in the treatment of posterior segment inflammation, but is generally reserved in anterior uveitis patients for the treatment of cases complicated by cystoid macular oedema (CMO) and for patients non-compliant with topical administration. Periocular injections may also be administered at the time of surgery and may rarely be used to supplement systemic therapy or when systemic steroids are contraindicated. The peak action is at about 4 weeks, with a maximum duration of action of around 3 months. Complications include subconjunctival haemorrhage, globe penetration, refractory elevation of IOP (up to 25%), cataract, ptosis, eyelid haemorrhage, eyelid ischaemic necrosis, retrobulbar haemorrhage, subdermal fat atrophy, extraocular muscle paresis, optic nerve injury, retinal and choroidal vascular occlusion and cutaneous hypopigmentation. Systemic adverse effects are rare but can occur. Table 12.5 gives injection procedures; there is no clear evidence of the superiority of one route over the other, but there may be a lower risk of ocular perforation, of raised IOP and of ptosis with the orbital floor approach. Utilizing a plastic intravenous cannula via a superior sub-Tenon route has been described and is thought to offer a lower risk of perforation.
- **Intraocular steroids.** Intravitreal triamcinolone acetonide (4 mg in 0.1 ml, i.e. one-tenth of the orbital dose) is occasionally used in anterior uveitis for CMO unresponsive to other forms of therapy and rarely may be considered at the time of intraocular surgery in high-risk anterior uveitis patients. Complications include elevation of IOP, cataract, endophthalmitis (sterile or infectious), haemorrhage, retinal detachment and pseudohypopyon. Slow-release intravitreal implants may occasionally be indicated.

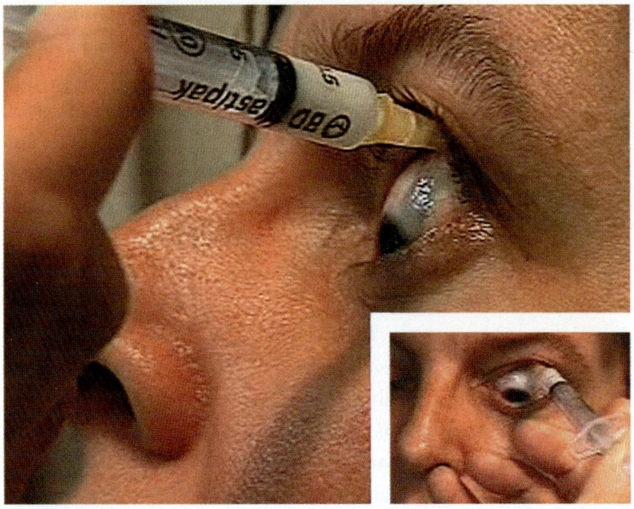

Fig. 12.9 Posterior sub-Tenon steroid injection. *(Courtesy of C Pavesio.)*

- **Systemic steroids** are very rarely required for anterior uveitis, but may be needed where the response to topical treatment is inadequate. They are sometimes given as a short course prior to intraocular surgery as prophylaxis against worsening inflammation, having the advantage of rapid cessation of effect in comparison with depot peri- or intraocular steroid injection, but have major potential adverse effects (Table 12.6).
- **Non-steroidal anti-inflammatory drugs (NSAIDs)** such as naproxen and tolmetin may be effective in CAU and can be used long-term under appropriate specialist physician supervision.
- **Antimetabolites** such as methotrexate and mycophenolate mofetil are generally not required in the treatment of anterior uveitis, though may be necessary in exceptional patients such as juvenile idiopathic arthritis-associated CAU when other measures fail to control inflammation, or as a steroid-sparing measure.

Table 12.5 Procedure for Inferior Transseptal and Posterior Sub-Tenon Regional Steroid Injection

Route	Technique
Inferior transseptal ('orbital floor') injection	A topical anaesthetic such as tetracaine (amethocaine) is instilled to prevent stinging by the antiseptic agents The skin of the lower eyelid and maxillary area is cleaned with an antiseptic agent such as an alcohol swab or povidone-iodine 5% The vial containing the steroid is shaken 1 ml steroid (triamcinolone acetonide or methylprednisolone acetate 40 mg/ml) is drawn up into a 2 ml syringe and the drawing-up needle replaced with a 25-gauge 5/8 inch (16 mm) needle The patient is asked to maintain gaze straight ahead The needle is inserted through the skin (some practitioners inject via the conjunctiva) at approximately the junction of the outer third and inner two-thirds of the lower orbital rim, entering close to the bony margin whilst clearing the margin itself The needle is slowly advanced tangentially to (or, anatomy permitting, away from) the globe in similar fashion to a peribulbar local anaesthetic block up to the needle hub The skin may be indented to ensure the needle tip is sufficiently posterior to deposit the steroid away from the anterior subconjunctival area The tip may be felt to engage the bony orbital floor and/or to pierce the orbital septum; as with the superior injection technique, the needle can be moved from side to side to ensure the sclera has not been engaged The plunger is slightly withdrawn and, if no blood enters the syringe, the full 1 ml is slowly injected, and the needle carefully withdrawn Special care is required in a patient with a large eye (e.g. myopia) to avoid penetration of the globe
Posterior sub-Tenon approach	A topical anaesthetic such as tetracaine (amethocaine) is instilled A small cotton pledget impregnated with tetracaine, lidocaine (lignocaine) 2% gel or an alternative is placed into the superior fornix at the site of injection for 2 minutes The vial containing the steroid is shaken 1 ml steroid (triamcinolone acetonide methylprednisolone acetate or 40 mg/ml) is drawn up into a 2 ml syringe and the drawing-up needle replaced with a 25-gauge 5/8 inch (16 mm) needle The patient is asked to look in the direction opposite to the superotemporal injection site The bulbar conjunctiva is penetrated with the tip of the needle, bevel towards the globe, slightly on the bulbar side of the fornix The needle is slowly inserted posteriorly, following the contour of the globe, keeping it as close to the globe as possible. In order not to penetrate the globe accidentally, wide side-to-side motions are made as the needle is being inserted and the limbus watched; movement of the limbus means that the sclera has been engaged When the needle has been advanced to the hub the plunger is slightly withdrawn and, if no blood enters the syringe, the full 1 ml is slowly injected A method utilizing a plastic intravenous cannula introduced via the same route following conjunctival incision and limited blunt dissection has been described

Table 12.6 Side Effects of Oral Corticosteroids Dependent on: Duration of Treatment and Dose

Common short-term
Weight gain Indigestion Insomnia Mood changes (behavioural change, cognitive dysfunction) Excessive sweating
Serious
Infections (varicella zoster, tuberculosis) Stomach ulceration/pancreatitis Hyperglycaemia/hypokalemia Mental health problems (depression, psychotic reactions) Anaphylaxis (rare)
Long-term
Cushing syndrome Osteoporosis/myopathy Hypertension Diabetes Adrenal gland suppression Visual change (cataract, glaucoma)

TIP In a patient with uveitis, it is important to ensure that there is no potentially life-threatening systemic disease present or an infectious cause for the inflammation.

IMMUNOMODULATORY THERAPY FOR NON-INFECTIOUS UVEITIS

Introduction

This therapy plays an important role in modifying the immune response and should be supervised by a multidisciplinary team that includes an ocular inflammatory disease specialist. Shared decisions should be made on when to start treatment and subsequently, on whether to modify or withdraw treatment. The specific medication to be used should be based on the type of uveitis and the known efficacy and safety profiles of the proposed agents. Before starting treatment, careful informed consent should be taken, detailing the advantages and potential side effects of the medication and emphasizing the need for regular follow-up. Active infections (especially tuberculosis) should be excluded and haematological, renal and hepatic function should be checked. The aim of treatment is to obtain steroid-free remission of the disease.

Indications

- **Immediate treatment**
  - Systemic lupus erythematosus with retinal vasculitis.
  - Behçet disease with retinal vasculitis.
- **Early treatment** should be considered for:
  - Sympathetic ophthalmia.
  - Vogt–Koyanagi–Harada syndrome.
  - Birdshot retinochoroidopathy.
  - Serpiginous choroidopathy.
  - Multifocal choroiditis and panuveitis.
  - Juvenile inflammatory arthritis.
- **As an alternative to steroids**
  - Therapeutic: inadequate response to topical and periocular steroids or to an oral dose >0.5 mg/kg/day prednisolone; intolerance of systemic steroids or as a steroid-sparing measure.
  - Ocular: acute disease that is sight-threatening or chronic and persistent, exudative retinal detachment or disease involving the macula.

Side effects of medication

- These need to be discussed with the patient and regular monitoring should be undertaken.
- In the doses used, the commonly prescribed immunosuppressives (steroids, azathioprine, methotrexate, mycophenolate mofetil, cyclosporin A) do not increase cancer mortality. The use of azathioprine monotherapy or anti-tumour necrosis factor (TNF) monotherapy is associated with a small but statistically significant risk of lymphoma. The risk is higher with combination treatment.
- As a general rule most of these medications are well tolerated, but side effects like headache, tiredness, gastrointestinal upset, bone marrow suppression and increased risk of opportunistic infections have been reported.
- Individual agents have complications that are specific to that particular medication.

Classes of medication

- **Antimetabolites**
  - Methotrexate, mycophenolate mofetil and azathioprine inhibit purine metabolism.
- **Inhibitors of calcineurin signalling in T cells**
  - Cyclosporin A, tacrolimus, voclosporin and sirolimus.
- **Alkylating agents**
  - Cyclophosphamide and chlorambucil.
- **Biopharmacologicals**
  - This is a rapidly changing field and new agents are constantly evolving that are effective in suppressing ocular inflammation.
  - Infliximab, adalimumab, etanercept, golimumab and certolizumab are anti-TNF α monoclonal antibodies that are registered for use in non-infectious uveitis.
  - Tocilizumab is a recombinant monoclonal antibody that binds to interleukin-6 receptors thereby inhibiting the activity of pro-inflammatory cytokines.
  - These agents take time to suppress inflammation (2 weeks to 3 months). Topical and systemic steroids may be needed initially to control acute inflammation.
- **An approach to severe uveitis** when systemic immunosuppression is needed (based on the underlying immunology and aligning with clinical experience) is as follows:
  - Steroids and antimetabolites are expected to work for all forms of severe uveitis.

- In T-cell critical uveitis (e.g. VKH, birdshot retinochoroidopathy) consider the use of calcineurin inhibitors.
- In neutrophil and macrophage critical uveitis (e.g. Behçet disease, sarcoidosis) consider the use of anti-TNF agents.
- In B-cell critical inflammation (e.g. scleritis, particularly ANCA+) treat with rituximab.

UVEITIS IN SPONDYLOARTHROPATHIES

The spondyloarthropathies are a group of disorders featuring HLA-B27 positivity and enthesitis as common factors. There is often a family history of one or more of the group, which comprises ankylosing spondylitis, undifferentiated spondyloarthropathy, psoriatic arthritis, reactive arthritis (Reiter syndrome) and spondyloarthropathy with inflammatory bowel disease (ulcerative colitis and Crohn disease). They are often referred to as seronegative spondyloarthropathies, in that rheumatoid factor is not present and the pathophysiological basis differs. The American Uveitis Society has recently endorsed the use of biological blockers such as infliximab for second-line systemic immunosuppression in vision-threatening chronic uveitis.

TIP Monoclonal antibody treatment (adalimumab/infliximab) has improved the prognosis in patients with vision-threatening chronic uveitis.

Ankylosing spondylitis

Introduction

Ankylosing spondylitis (AS) is characterized by inflammation, calcification and finally ossification of ligaments and capsules of joints with resultant bony ankylosis of the axial skeleton. It more commonly affects males, of whom 90% are HLA-B27-positive.

Systemic features

- **Presentation** is commonly in the third to fourth decades with the insidious onset of pain and stiffness in the lower back or buttocks.
- **Spondyloarthritis** causes progressive limitation of spinal movements and eventually the spine may become fixed in flexion (Fig. 12.10A). Spinal stenosis and fractures may occur.
- **Enthesitis** is characterized clinically by inflammation and pain at ligamentous attachments to bone.
- **Cardiac complications** are rare.
- **Radiology** of the sacroiliac joints shows juxta-articular osteoporosis in the early stages, followed by sclerosis and bony obliteration of the joint (Fig. 12.10B). Calcification of spinal ligaments gives rise to a 'bamboo spine'. Radiological changes often predate clinical symptoms.

Ocular features

- **AAU** is by far the most common ocular association and occurs in about 25% of patients with AS. Approximately 25% of males with AAU will have AS. Either eye is frequently affected at different times but bilateral simultaneous involvement is rare. There is often no correlation between the severity and activity of eye and joint involvement. Chronicity occurs in a few patients. HLA-B27-positive AS patients tend to have worse disease across a range of parameters, including earlier onset and greater intensity of inflammation with an increased frequency of complications.
- **Other ocular features** include scleritis, episcleritis, keratitis and mechanical ptosis.

Reactive arthritis

Introduction

Reactive arthritis (ReA, also known as Reiter syndrome) is characterized by a triad of non-specific urethritis, conjunctivitis and arthritis.

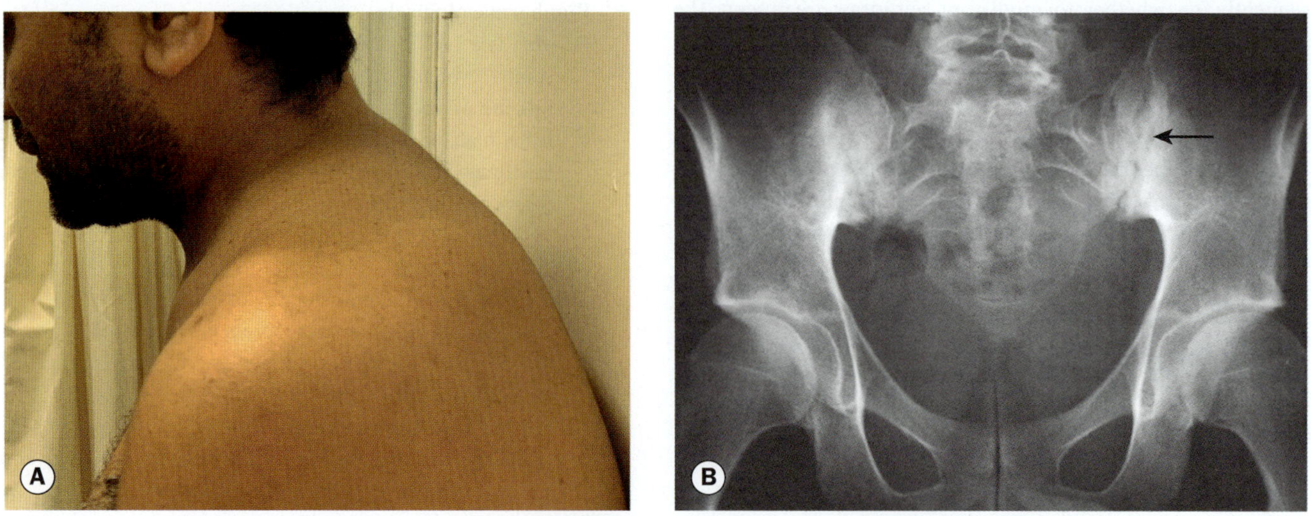

Fig. 12.10 Ankylosing spondylitis. **(A)** Fixed flexion deformity of the cervical spine; **(B)** sclerosis and bony obliteration of the sacroiliac joints (arrow). *(Courtesy of P Beckwith – fig. A.)*

Around 75% of patients are positive for HLA-B27. A range of infective agents can trigger the syndrome, which develops in 1–3% of men after non-specific urethritis and around 4% of individuals after enteric infections caused by a range of organisms including *Shigella*, *Salmonella* and *Campylobacter*. *Chlamydia trachomatis* is the most common cause of reactive arthritis following urethritis. *Chlamydia pneumoniae* respiratory infection and others may also precede ReA.

TIP Patients with uveitis secondary to the various spondyloarthropathies are often HLA-B27-positive.

Systemic features

- **Presentation** is with the acute onset of malaise, with fever and dysuria 1–4 weeks after a linked infection in a patient aged between 20 and 40, with arthritis that may be preceded by conjunctivitis. A variety of other features may be present, though not always the defining triad.
- **Peripheral oligoarthritis** is acute, asymmetrical and migratory. Two to four joints tend to be involved, most commonly the knees, ankles and toes.
- **Spondyloarthritis** affects about 50% of patients, manifesting with low back pain. This sometimes becomes chronic.
- **Enthesitis** manifests with plantar fasciitis, Achilles tenosynovitis, bursitis and calcaneal periostitis. Reactive bone formation in the latter may result in a calcaneal spur.
- **Mucocutaneous lesions** include painless mouth ulceration, circinate balanitis and keratoderma blennorrhagica – skin lesions resembling psoriasis – involving the palms and soles (Fig. 12.11A).
- **Genitourinary involvement** includes cervicitis, prostatitis and epididymitis.
- **Aortitis** occurs in 1–2%.

Ocular features

The eye is involved in 50% of cases with a urogenital inciting infection and 75% of enteric ReA syndrome.

- **Conjunctivitis** is very common and classically follows urethritis, but precedes arthritis. The inflammation is usually mild, bilateral and mucopurulent with a papillary and/or follicular reaction (Fig. 12.11B). Spontaneous resolution occurs within 7–10 days and treatment is not required. Some patients develop peripheral corneal infiltrates.
- **AAU** occurs in 20%.
- **Episcleritis** sometimes occurs.

Treatment

- **The main goal** is to identify the causative organism and treat with appropriate antibiotics if the organism is still present.
- **Non-specific urethritis** should be treated with oral tetracycline.
- **Steroids and immunosuppressants** may be needed for severe symptoms that do not respond to simple treatment.

Psoriatic arthritis

Introduction

Up to 40% of patients with psoriasis develop arthritis. The arthritis is more common in White populations than other racial groups and affects both sexes equally. There is a first-degree family history in 40% or more and many genetic markers have been identified.

Systemic features

- **Presentation** of psoriatic arthritis is usually in middle age – later than skin features.
- **Skin.** There are multiple types of psoriasis. Plaque-type, the most common form, is characterized by well-demarcated raised silvery inflamed plaques (Fig. 12.12A) on the scalp, trunk, arms and legs. Psoriatic erythroderma features widespread exfoliative skin changes with associated inflammation and pustular psoriasis inflamed but non-infectious pustules limited or generalized in distribution.
- **Nail changes (dystrophy)** include pitting, transverse depression and onycholysis (Fig. 12.12B).

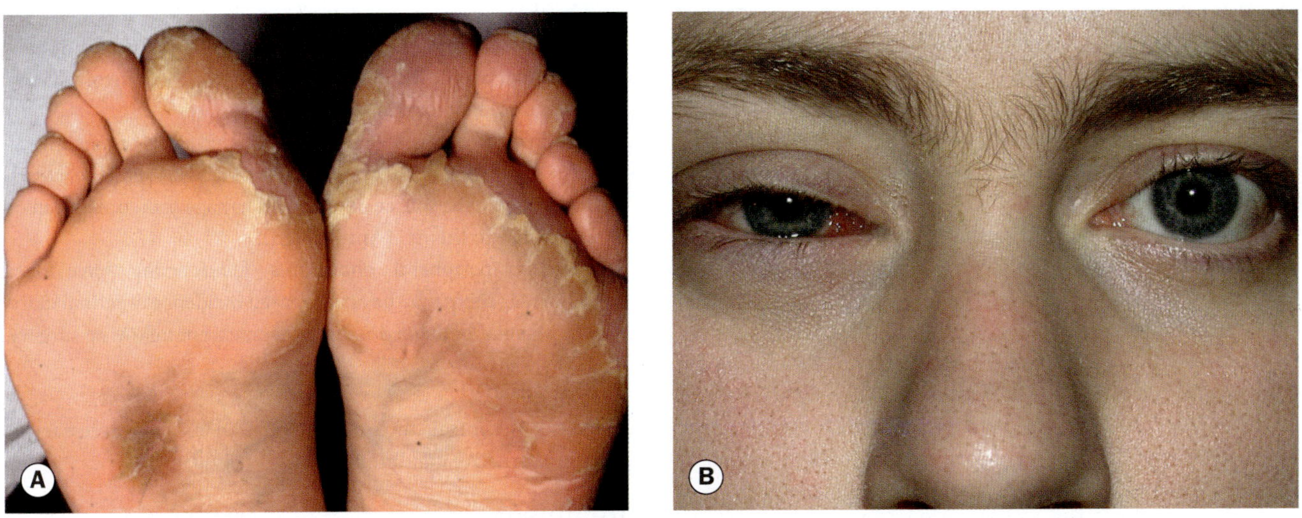

Fig. 12.11 Reiter syndrome. **(A)** Keratoderma blennorrhagica in reactive arthritis; **(B)** acute conjunctivitis.

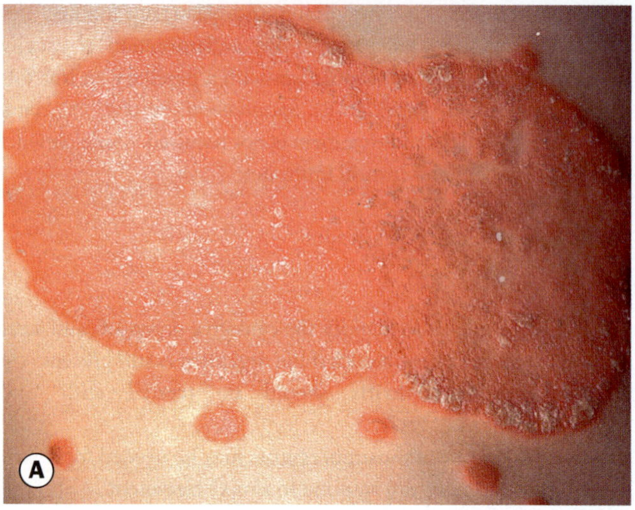

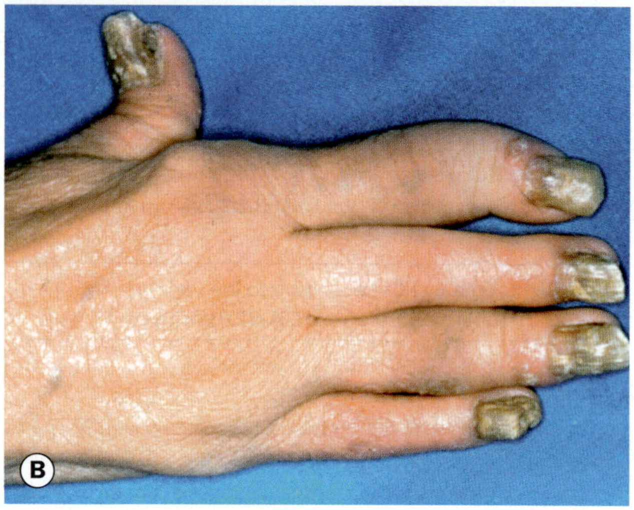

Fig. 12.12 Psoriasis. **(A)** Skin plaques; **(B)** arthritis and severe nail dystrophy.

- **Arthritis** is typically asymmetrical and involves the distal interphalangeal joints (sausage digits). Some patients develop enthesitis.

Ocular features

AAU occurs in approximately 7%. Conjunctivitis, marginal corneal infiltrates and secondary Sjögren syndrome may occur but are uncommon.

FUCHS UVEITIS SYNDROME

Introduction

Fuchs uveitis syndrome (FUS), also known as Fuchs heterochromic iridocyclitis or cyclitis (FHC), is a chronic non-granulomatous condition diagnosed at an average of 40 years of age. There is no gender or racial predilection. The cause is uncertain, but there is evidence that implicates the rubella virus. Signs in toxoplasmosis can be similar and *T. gondii* has also been suspected as a cause. It is possible that most of the anterior chamber (AC) activity is due to blood–aqueous barrier breakdown rather than inflammation.

Clinical features

Detection is often incidental. Findings are usually unilateral (90–95%).

- **Symptoms.** Gradual blurring due to cataract is a common presentation, as are persistent floaters. Heterochromia (see next) may be noted.
- **Heterochromia iridis** (Table 12.7) is demonstrated most effectively in daylight and in most patients the affected eye is hypochromic (Fig. 12.13A). Its quality is determined by the relative degrees of atrophy of the stroma and posterior pigment epithelium. It may be absent or subtle, particularly in brown eyes. In blue eyes, stromal atrophy allows the posterior pigmented layer to show through and become the dominant pigmentation, so that the eye sometimes becomes hyperchromic.
- **Posterior synechiae (PS)** are absent, except occasionally following cataract surgery.
- **AC** shows faint flare and usually only mild cellular activity, though exacerbations can sometimes be marked. The eye is virtually always white, even during exacerbations.
- **Keratic precipitates** are characteristically stellate and grey-white in colour and are located diffusely over the entire corneal endothelium (Fig. 12.13B).
- **Iris nodules** (30%) on the pupillary border (Koeppe – Fig. 12.13C). Tiny crystals (Russell bodies) may be present on the iris surface.
- **Iris atrophy** is diffuse with loss of crypts. The iris appears smooth, with a prominent sphincter pupillae and sometimes blood vessels (see Fig. 12.13C). Pigment epithelial atrophy can be demonstrated by retroillumination (Fig. 12.13D).
- **Iris vessels.** Fine irregular iris surface vessels are commonly present.
- **Vitritis.** Opacities in the anterior gel may be dense.
- **Posterior subcapsular cataract** is extremely common (Fig. 12.13E).
- **Glaucoma** is typically a later manifestation but is occasionally present at diagnosis. It develops in up to 60% of involved eyes. Several mechanisms are suspected.
- **Gonioscopy** may show fine radial angle vessels or small irregular peripheral anterior synechiae (Fig. 12.13F). The vessels are typically the source of the haemorrhage sometimes seen on incision into the AC (Amsler sign).
- **Fundus**: peripheral choroiditis foci/scarring have been reported. There may be an increased incidence of retinal dialysis. Macular oedema does not occur, except following surgery.

Investigation

Diagnosis is clinical, though investigation may be necessary to exclude alternative conditions.

Treatment

- **Long-term monitoring** is indicated to detect glaucoma and other complications.

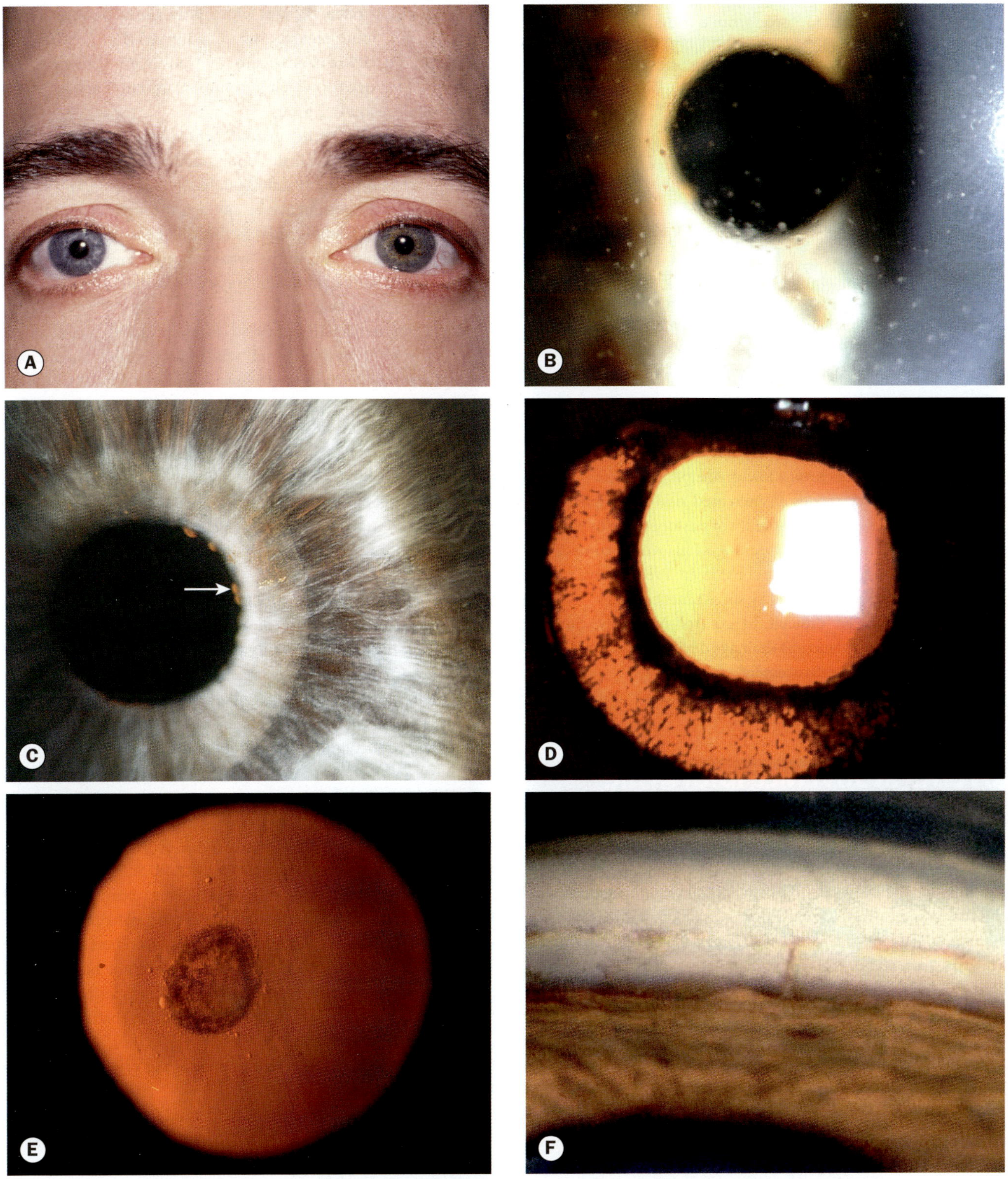

Fig. 12.13 Fuchs uveitis syndrome. **(A)** Right eye involvement showing hypochromia; **(B)** diffuse stellate keratic precipitates; **(C)** Koeppe nodules (arrow) with iris atrophy and loss of stromal architecture; **(D)** band-like posterior pigment layer atrophy seen on retroillumination; **(E)** posterior subcapsular cataract seen on retroillumination; **(F)** angle vessels and small peripheral anterior synechiae

Table 12.7 Causes of Heterochromia Iridis

Hypochromic
Idiopathic congenital Horner syndrome, particularly if congenital Waardenburg syndrome
Hyperchromic
Unilateral use of a topical prostaglandin analogue for glaucoma Oculodermal melanocytosis (naevus of Ota) Ocular siderosis Diffuse iris naevus or melanoma Sturge–Weber syndrome
Hypo- or hyperchromic
Fuchs uveitis syndrome Other chronic anterior uveitides

- **Topical steroids** may be used short-term for moderate/severe exacerbations, but are generally not thought to be helpful in the management of chronic low-grade inflammation.
- **Cataract surgery** carries an increased risk of complications. Poor mydriasis and the possibility of postoperative hyphaema, increased inflammation, worsening of glaucoma control and zonular dehiscence should be considered. Preoperative topical or systemic steroids are used by some practitioners.
- **Glaucoma** can be difficult to control medically. Surgical options include a glaucoma drainage device or trabeculectomy with mitomycin-C enhancement.
- **Pars plana vitrectomy** may be considered for visually problematic vitreous opacification.

UVEITIS IN JUVENILE IDIOPATHIC ARTHRITIS (JIA)

Introduction

JIA is by far the most common systemic disease associated with childhood anterior uveitis with a prevalence of about 1:1000. It is defined as arthritis of unknown aetiology that begins before the age of 16 years and persists for at least 6 weeks. Up to 50% of children affected have persistently active disease after 10 years. It may result from exposure to one or more unknown antigens in genetically predisposed individuals.

TIP Immunomodulatory treatment should be considered early in the course of JIA, which is the commonest systemic disease associated with childhood anterior uveitis.

Clinical features

- **Arthritis.** JIA is classified by the International League of Associations for Rheumatology (ILAR, 2004 revision), according to the extent of joint involvement during the first 6 months.
  - Oligoarticular is the most common form. Four or fewer joints are involved, the knees most commonly, followed by the ankles and wrists (Fig. 12.14A). Girls are affected five times as often as boys, with a peak age of onset around 2 years. Some patients subsequently develop polyarthritis. About 75% of children are ANA-positive, a strong risk factor for uveitis, which is common, affecting about 20% of children in this group.
  - Polyarticular (rheumatoid factor-negative) affects five or more joints, typically both small and large joints symmetrically. The female: male ratio is about 3: 1. The disease may commence at any age throughout childhood. Systemic features such as fever and rash may occur but are milder than in the systemic onset form (see below). About 40% of children are ANA-positive. Uveitis occurs in 5–10% of cases.
  - Polyarticular (rheumatoid factor-positive) again affects five or more joints and may resemble adult rheumatoid arthritis. There is a very low risk of uveitis.
  - Systemic, also known as Still (Still's) disease. Systemic features such as fever, episodic erythematous maculopapular rash, lymphadenopathy and hepatosplenomegaly may precede arthritis. The disease occurs with equal frequency in boys and girls and may occur at any age throughout childhood. The majority are negative for ANA and uveitis is rare.
  - Enthesitis-related (inflammation of the connective tissue where tendons/ligaments attach to bone), psoriatic and undifferentiated are three other forms under the ILAR classification. The first two have a relatively high risk of uveitis, but risk in the latter is usually low.
- **Anterior uveitis** is a key cause of morbidity in JIA. It is particularly common in oligoarticular JIA and relatively frequent in several other types. Progression to blindness has been high in the past, but shows a declining trend in recent years associated with improved screening and management. Arthritis usually antedates the diagnosis of uveitis.
  - Presentation. The uveitis of JIA is particularly dangerous because it is invariably asymptomatic and must generally be detected by screening with slit lamp examination. Even during acute exacerbations with +4 aqueous cells, it is rare for patients to complain, although a few report an increase in vitreous floaters. Often uveitis may not be suspected until the parents recognize complications such as strabismus, or an abnormal appearance of the eyeball due to band keratopathy or cataract.
  - Injection is usually absent even in the presence of severe uveitis.
  - Inflammation is chronic and non-granulomatous. Both eyes are affected in 70% and there is symmetrical severity of inflammation. During acute exacerbations, the entire endothelium shows 'dusting' by many hundreds of cells, but hypopyon is absent.
  - PS are common in longstanding undetected cases.
  - Band keratopathy and cataract (Fig. 12.14B) are common in severe cases.
  - Other serious complications include glaucoma (common), amblyopia, maculopathy (cystoid macular oedema, epiretinal membrane), cyclitic membrane and phthisis.

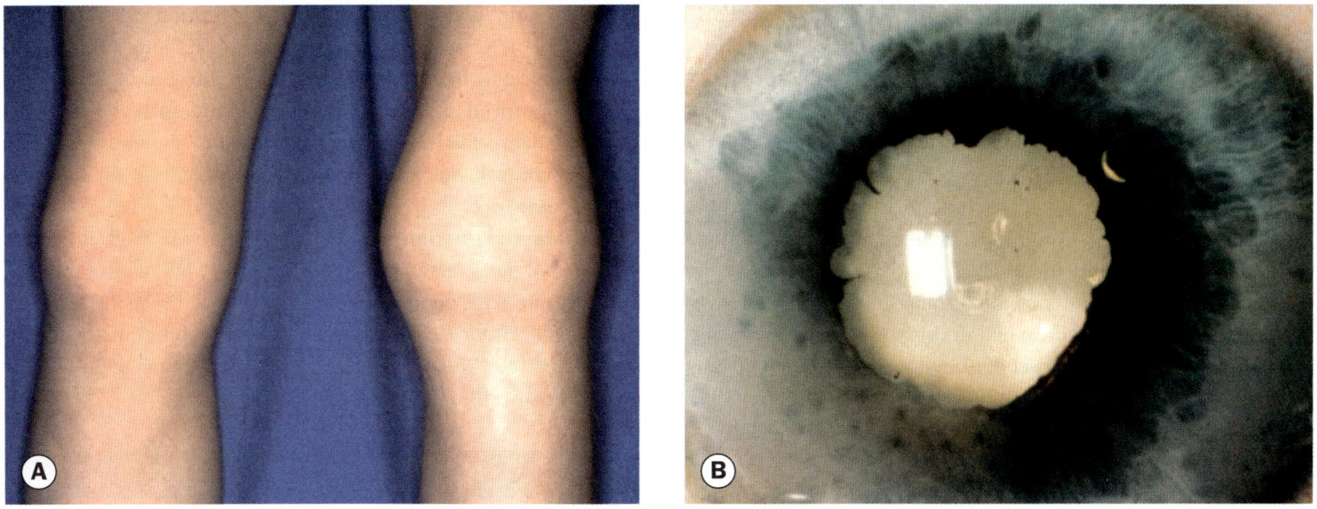

Fig. 12.14 Juvenile idiopathic arthritis. **(A)** Inflammation of the knee in a child; **(B)** band keratopathy, posterior synechiae and mature cataract in chronic anterior uveitis.

- Prognosis. In about 10% the uveitis is mild, with never more than +1 aqueous cells and persists for less than 12 months. About 15% of patients have one attack lasting less than 4 months, the severity of inflammation varying from +2 to +4 aqueous cells. In 50% of cases, the uveitis is moderate to severe and persists for more than 4 months and in 25%, the uveitis is very severe, lasts for several years and responds poorly to conventional treatment. The presence of complications at initial examination appears to be an important risk factor for the development of subsequent complications, regardless of therapy. Good visual outcomes can be achieved by early case recognition and rapid referral to a specialist for immunomodulatory therapy.

Investigation

- **Systemic diagnosis and management** should be performed by a physician familiar with the management of JIA, typically a paediatric rheumatologist.
- **Antinuclear antibody (ANA).** Positivity denotes an increased risk of uveitis.
- **HLA-B27 testing** is useful in differential diagnosis (see above) and if present may indicate an increased risk of uveitis.
- **Rheumatoid factor** is also useful in differential diagnosis.
- **Screening.** There has been a shift in recommendation towards long-term 3- to 4-monthly review intervals in all higher-risk categories. Review should continue in most cases until the age of 12 years.
  - Initial examination within 6 weeks of first diagnosis of JIA. Delayed early examination is an important cause of morbidity.
  - Visual symptoms or a suspicion of ocular signs (synechiae, cataract, band keratopathy) should lead to urgent ophthalmological referral and slit lamp examination within a week.
  - Initial 2-monthly examinations for 6 months may be considered for all newly diagnosed oligoarticular, psoriatic, polyarticular and enthesitis-related patients, regardless of ANA status, followed by 3- to 4-monthly intervals.
  - Polyarticular: every 3–4 months, but some guidelines reduce the interval to 6-monthly after a number of years. Higher-risk factors that might be considered in deciding whether to alter the interval include the presence of ANA, onset before 7 years of age and female gender.
  - Systemic onset and polyarticular RF-positive patients: most authorities recommend at least an initial screening examination, with some guidelines suggesting annual review.
  - Missed appointments must be effectively detected and patients rebooked.
  - Information for parents should include an emphasis on the importance of compliance with screening, as well as the need to seek urgent advice should there be any cause for concern such as visual symptoms, ocular redness or clouding, or abnormal pupils.
  - Self-monitoring. At eventual discharge from screening, patients should be warned to self-monitor by checking the monocular vision at least once a week because the risk of uveitis has not entirely disappeared by this age. They should also attend an optometrist annually for an eye examination. Selected patients such as those with learning difficulties may require ongoing ophthalmological screening.
- **Differential diagnosis**: Particular considerations in children include:
  - Idiopathic juvenile chronic iridocyclitis: otherwise healthy patients with juvenile CAU.
  - Other types of juvenile arthritis and uveitis including juvenile reactive arthritis, juvenile inflammatory bowel disease-associated arthritis.
  - Juvenile sarcoidosis is rare. Pulmonary involvement is less common than in adults, may be granulomatous and involve the posterior segment.
  - Lyme disease usually presents with intermediate uveitis in conjunction with significant anterior uveitis.

- Intermediate uveitis: 20% of all cases of paediatric uveitis.
- Neonatal-onset multisystem inflammatory disease is a rare, idiopathic, chronic relapsing disease that predominantly involves the skin, joints and the central nervous system. About 50% of children develop recurrent anterior uveitis. The absence of PS and no tendency to glaucoma and cataract formation are characteristic.
- Masquerade syndromes such as anterior segment involvement by retinoblastoma.
- Familial juvenile systemic granulomatosis (Blau syndrome) is a rare autosomal dominant disorder characterized by childhood onset of granulomatous disease of skin, eyes (panuveitis and multifocal choroiditis) and joints.

Treatment

The aim of treatment should be the suppression of all active inflammation. These children should be referred as soon as possible to a uveitis specialist.

- **Topical steroids** are initially effective in 80% of cases.
- **Mydriatic agents** can be used to prevent synechiae formation. A relatively short-acting preparation such as cyclopentolate should be prescribed and discontinued as early as possible, particularly in monocular treatment of younger children susceptible to the development of amblyopia.
- **Periocular steroids.**
- **Oral steroids.**
- **NSAIDs.**
- **Systemic immunosuppressive agents** (e.g. methotrexate, infliximab and adalimumab) should be considered at an early stage, as this has improved the overall visual prognosis in recent years. These children are usually under the management of a uveitis specialist, typically working in collaboration with a paediatric rheumatologist. Etanercept should be avoided as it can result in severe worsening of inflammation. Tocilizumab, an interleukin-6 blocking agent, has recently been shown to be effective in the treatment of some children with refractory uveitis secondary to JIA.
- **Secondary glaucoma.** If topical medication does not control the IOP, surgery may be needed. The long-term results of trabeculectomy with mitomycin C in children with JIA are improved if they are using systemic anti-TNF medication. Baerveldt implantation also results in good long-term IOP control, but is associated with a 5% risk of hypotony maculopathy.
- **Cataract extraction** is often needed. Primary IOL implantation was a controversial issue in the past, but a low complication rate with good visual results has been recently reported with this approach in children on immunomodulatory treatment. Posterior capsular thickening requiring treatment occurs in approximately half.

UVEITIS IN BOWEL DISEASE

Ulcerative colitis

Introduction

Ulcerative colitis (UC) is an idiopathic chronic relapsing inflammatory disease, involving the rectum and extending proximally to involve part or all of the large intestine. The disease is characterized by contiguous surface ulceration of the bowel mucosa with the development of crypt abscesses and pseudopolyps (Fig. 12.15A). Longstanding disease carries an increased risk of carcinoma of the colon. A genetic predisposition is thought to be important as inflammatory bowel disease is more common in patients with other autoimmune diseases such as ankylosing spondylitis, psoriasis and multiple sclerosis.

Systemic features

- **Presentation** is in the second to third decades with bloody diarrhoea, lower abdominal cramps, urgency and tenesmus. Constitutional symptoms include tiredness, weight loss, malaise and fever.
- **Cutaneous lesions** include oral aphthous ulceration, erythema nodosum and pyoderma gangrenosum (Fig. 12.15B).

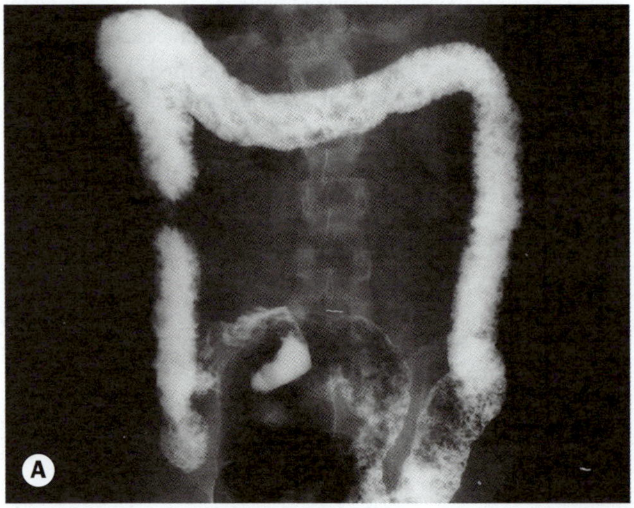

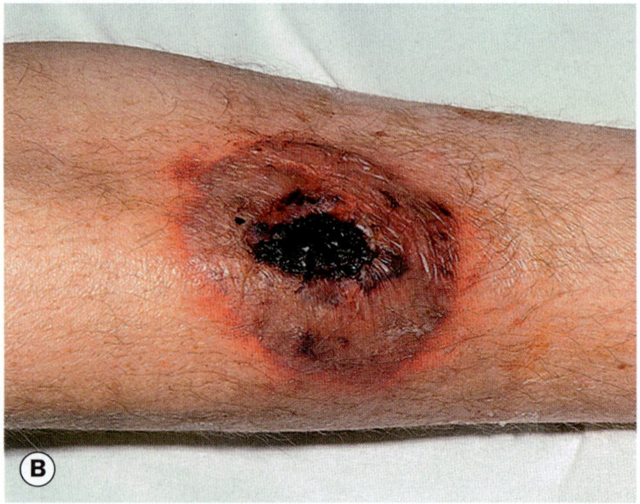

Fig. 12.15 Ulcerative colitis. **(A)** Barium enema showing pseudopolyposis, lack of haustral markings and straightening of the ascending colon; **(B)** pyoderma gangrenosum.

- **Arthritis** is typically asymmetrical and involves large joints of the legs. Sacroiliitis and ankylosing spondylitis (AS) may develop in HLA-B27-positive patients.
- **Hepatic disease** may be in the form of autoimmune hepatitis, sclerosing cholangitis and cholangiocarcinoma.
- **Thrombosis** may affect both arteries and veins.

Ocular features

- **AAU** occurs in about 5% and may coincide with exacerbations of colitis. As expected, uveitis is more common in patients with associated arthritis, AS and HLA-B27 positivity.
- **Other ocular features**: conjunctivitis, episcleritis and scleritis may all be more common than in the general population.

Crohn disease

Introduction

Crohn disease (CD) is an idiopathic chronic relapsing disease characterized by multifocal full-thickness granulomatous inflammation of the intestinal wall. It most frequently involves the terminal ileum and colon but in contrast to UC any area of the gastrointestinal tract, including the mouth, may be affected. There is strong evidence for a genetic aetiological component such as mutations in the *CARD15* (previously *NOD2*) gene. Infective agents almost certainly play a role.

Systemic features

- **Presentation** is typically in the second–third decades with abdominal pain and diarrhoea. Weight loss, fever, vomiting, oral aphthous ulceration and perirectal lesions such as abscesses and fistulae may occur.
- **Cutaneous lesions** include erythema nodosum and pyoderma gangrenosum (see Fig. 12.15B).
- **Anaemia** is common.
- **Hepatic disease** may occur.
- **Skeletal** features include finger clubbing, acute peripheral arthritis, sacroiliitis and AS (especially if HLA-B27-positive).

Ocular features

Approximately 12% of patients with CD experience some form of ocular inflammation. AAU occurs in 3%. Other manifestations include episcleritis, scleritis, follicular conjunctivitis, myositis and optic neuritis (see Ch. 9).

Whipple disease

Introduction

Whipple disease (intestinal lipodystrophy) is a rare chronic gastrointestinal inflammatory condition caused by infection with the bacterium *Tropheryma whipplei*. It occurs mainly in White middle-aged men and when diagnosed (duodenal biopsy; DNA detection in blood, ocular and other fluids) can be cured with antibiotics.

Systemic features

Inflammatory bowel disease with malabsorption. Joint, cardiac and central nervous system (CNS) involvement is common.

Ocular features

- **Uveitis.** Keratitis, anterior uveitis, vitritis, retinitis with retinal haemorrhages, cotton-wool spots and potentially vascular occlusion and multifocal choroiditis.
- **Neuro-ophthalmic** manifestations can be varied, e.g. gaze palsy, nystagmus, ophthalmoplegia, papilloedema and optic atrophy. Oculomasticatory myorhythmia is characteristic.

UVEITIS IN RENAL DISEASE

Tubulointerstitial nephritis and uveitis

Introduction

Tubulointerstitial nephritis and uveitis (TINU) is an uncommon disorder of immune origin characterized by a combination of acute tubulointerstitial nephritis and uveitis. It typically occurs in adolescent girls. Renal disease usually precedes uveitis.

Systemic features

Presentation is with constitutional symptoms, proteinuria, anaemia, hypertension and renal failure. The response to systemic steroid therapy is good and renal function usually returns to normal within a few months without complication.

Ocular features

- **Bilateral non-granulomatous (occasionally granulomatous) anterior uveitis** that usually responds well to topical steroids. Disc and macular oedema may occur. Many cases are relapsing and some require systemic steroids or immunosuppressive therapy.
- **Intermediate, posterior or panuveitis** may occur.

TIP In a patient with ocular and renal inflammation, consider the following in the differential diagnosis: sarcoidosis, tuberculosis, SLE, tubulointerstitial nephritis and IgA nephropathy.

IgA nephropathy

IgA nephropathy (Berger disease) is a relatively common kidney disease in which immunoglobulin A is deposited in the glomerular mesangium. Presentation is usually at age 16–35 with recurrent haematuria, often associated with an upper respiratory tract infection, but may be asymptomatic. AAU and other ocular inflammatory phenomena may occur but are uncommon.

INTERMEDIATE UVEITIS

Introduction

Intermediate uveitis (IU) is a chronic, relapsing disease of insidious onset in which the vitreous is the primary site of inflammation. It incorporates the following entities: pars planitis, posterior cyclitis and hyalitis. The diagnosis is made clinically. IU may be idiopathic (at least half) or associated with a systemic disease. Pars planitis

(PP) is the term used for a subset of IU in which there is snowbanking and/or snowball formation, but only if the inflammation is idiopathic – that is, with no identifiable underlying infection or systemic disease – otherwise the term intermediate uveitis is used. IU accounts for up to 15% of all uveitis cases and about 20% of paediatric uveitis. A minority of patients have a benign course, with spontaneous resolution within several years. In other patients the disease is more severe and prolonged with episodic exacerbations. IU associated with systemic disease has a variable course.

Clinical features

- **Symptoms.** Presentation is with the insidious onset of blurred vision, often accompanied by vitreous floaters. There is usually no pain or redness. Though initial symptoms are often unilateral, objective findings are typically present asymmetrically in both eyes.
- **Visual acuity** is variably affected depending on inflammatory activity and complications, particularly CMO. The disease may last as long as 15 years and preservation of vision will depend largely on control of macular disease. In follow-up of up to 4 years, 75% of patients maintain a visual acuity of 6/12 or better.
- **Anterior uveitis.** In PP there may be a few cells and small scattered KP which occasionally have an inferior linear distribution. In other forms of IU, anterior uveitis and its associated findings, such as PS, can be more prominent, especially in children and in sarcoidosis and Lyme disease.
- **Vitreous.** Vitreous cells with anterior predominance are universal. Vitreous condensation and haze (Table 12.8) is found in severe cases (Fig. 12.16A). Snowballs are whitish focal collections of inflammatory cells and exudate, usually most numerous in the inferior vitreous (Fig. 12.16B).
- **Peripheral periphlebitis** (Fig. 12.16C) is common, particularly in multiple sclerosis. Careful examination of a normal fellow eye in apparently unilateral disease may reveal mild vascular sheathing.
- **Snowbanking** (Fig. 12.16D) is characterized by a grey–white fibrovascular and/or exudative plaque that may occur in any or all quadrants, but is most frequently found inferiorly.
- **Neovascularization** may occur, particularly in the retinal periphery (often associated with snowbanks) and on the optic nerve head. The latter usually resolves when activity is controlled. This can sometimes lead to vitreous haemorrhage, retinal detachment and cyclitic membrane formation. Focal peripheral retinal vasoproliferative tumours (see Ch. 20) are uncommon. Vitreous haemorrhage is more common in children.

Table 12.8 Grading of Vitreous Haze

Haze severity	Grading
Good view of nerve fibre layer (NFL)	0
Clear disc and vessels but hazy NFL	+1
Disc and vessels hazy	+2
Only disc visible	+3
Disc not visible	+4

- **Optic disc swelling** is common, especially in younger patients.
- **CMO** occurs in up to half of patients and is the major cause of impaired visual acuity.
- **Macular epiretinal membrane** formation is common.
- **Cataract** can be caused by steroid treatment or by the inflammation itself.
- **Glaucoma** may occur in eyes with prolonged inflammation, particularly if receiving long-term steroid therapy.
- **Retinal detachment** is generally uncommon, but as it can progress to hypotony and phthisis in advanced cases, prevention should be a major goal of management. The aetiology may be tractional, rhegmatogenous and occasionally exudative. Retinoschisis has also been described.

TIP An insidious onset of blurred vision accompanied by vitreous floaters without pain or redness suggests a possible diagnosis of intermediate uveitis.

Investigation

Inflammatory markers such as ESR and/or CRP should be checked, together with a complete blood count, as they may raise suspicion of a systemic inflammatory process. OCT is key to excluding subtle CMO and FA will help in assessing severity. Other investigations are targeted at the exclusion of an underlying cause as below.

- **Multiple sclerosis.** Enquiry should be made in all patients about neurological symptoms, noting that IU may precede other symptoms of demyelination. MS should be suspected in patients aged 20–50 and is twice as common in women. Granulomatous AAU may occur. Cranial MRI imaging should be performed if any suspicion is raised.
- **Sarcoidosis.** Sarcoid-associated IU is relatively uncommon and as with MS may antedate the onset of systemic disease. The presence of associated granulomatous anterior uveitis should arouse suspicion. A serum ACE level and chest X-ray should be performed in all adult patients.
- **Lyme disease-associated** IU is often associated with severe anterior uveitis. Serology should be performed in individuals from an endemic area.
- **Syphilis serology** – treponemal and cardiolipin antibody tests – should be performed.
- **Tuberculosis** is an uncommon association that may give respiratory symptoms and be demonstrated on chest X-ray. Tuberculin skin and/or blood (e.g. QuantiFERON) testing should be performed prior to steroid treatment in the presence of any suspicion.
- **Other conditions** that may give vitritis mimicking IU include FUS, intraocular lymphoma (older patients), *Toxocara* granuloma, Whipple disease, endogenous *Candida* endophthalmitis (risk factors such as intravenous drug use) and toxoplasmosis. These will commonly be suspected on the basis of the history and specific clinical findings.

Treatment

An identified infection or other underlying disease should be treated specifically, supplemented by anti-inflammatory measures. Many authorities aim to abolish all active inflammation regardless

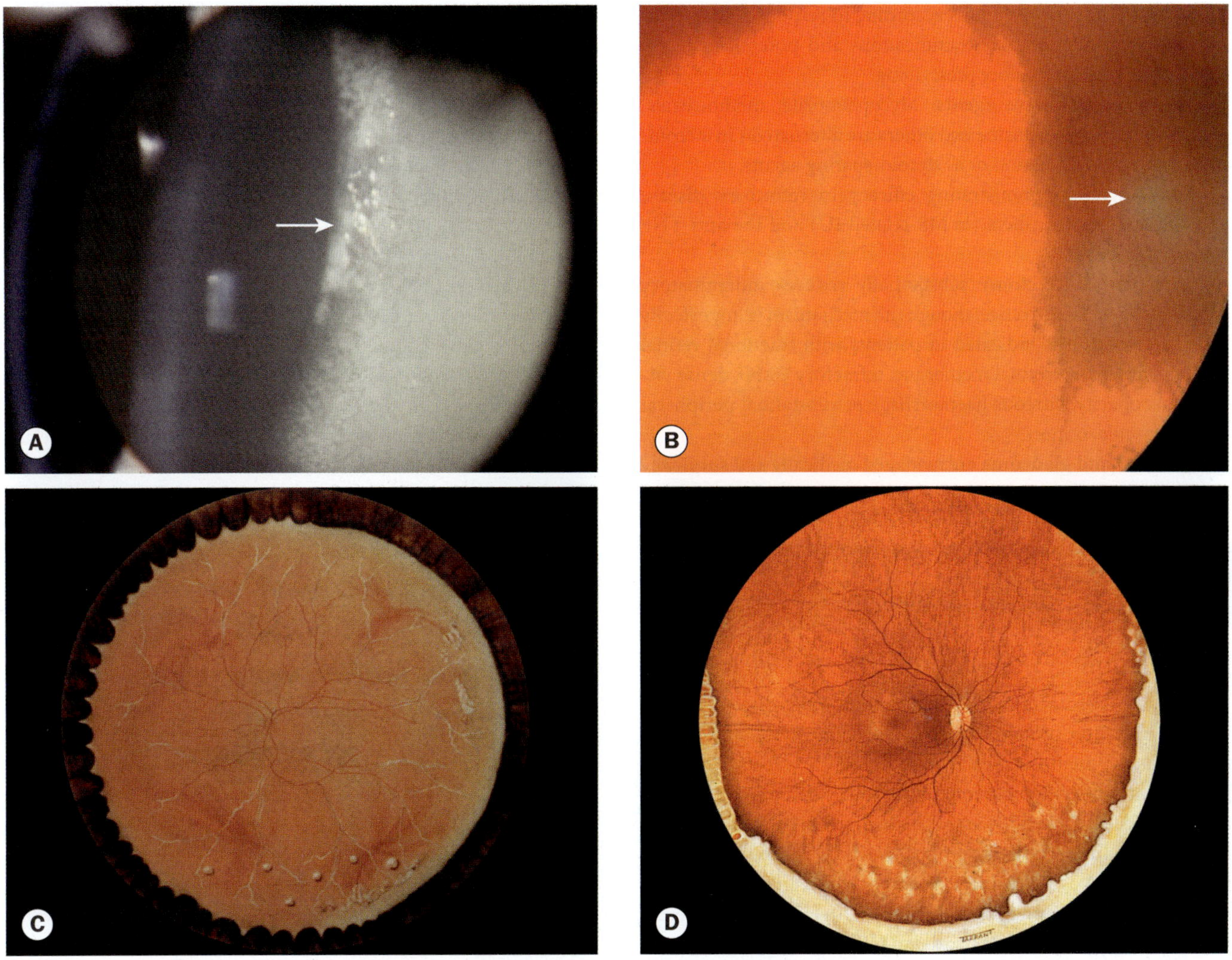

Fig. 12.16 Intermediate uveitis. **(A)** Vitreous inflammatory activity showing vitreous condensation and haze visible in the slit beam (arrow); **(B)** snowballs (arrow); **(C)** peripheral periphlebitis and snowballs; **(D)** inferior snowbanking and snowballs. *(Courtesy of CL Schepens, ME Hartnett and T Hirose, from* Schepens' Retinal Detachment and Allied Diseases, *Butterworth-Heinemann 2000 – fig. C.)*

of whether vision has been affected. Factors such as the presence of peripheral neovascularization may prompt earlier intervention.

- **Topical steroids** do not reach the posterior segment in high concentrations and therefore have a limited role. This medication is used mainly to treat any anterior segment inflammation. It has been proposed that in mild IU a course of frequent topical steroid of a few weeks' duration may exert some benefit and identify individuals at high risk of IOP elevation without committing to the extended action of depot injection.
- **Regional steroid injection.** Orbital floor or posterior sub-Tenon injection as described for anterior uveitis. Depending on severity, injection is performed 4–6 times at intervals of 2–4 weeks, accompanied by IOP monitoring.
- **NSAID.** If inflammation persists after regional injection, an agent such as naproxen 500 mg twice daily can be commenced.
- **Cryotherapy** (double freeze–thaw) to the pars plana and retinal periphery under peribulbar anaesthesia can be highly effective if inflammation is steroid-resistant and may be appropriate prior to systemic steroids. It can be associated with transiently increased vitritis and other complications including retinal detachment, cataract, vitreous and AC haemorrhage, epiretinal membrane formation and hypotony. A repeat application may be needed after several months. Some authorities reserve cryotherapy for peripheral neovascularization with haemorrhage.
- **Peripheral retinal laser** adjacent to snowbanking and/or to ischaemic areas on FA is an alternative to cryotherapy and may be as effective with a lower rate of complications.
- **Intraocular steroid.** Intravitreal triamcinolone has shown benefit, but the effect is of relatively short duration. Slow-release implants have demonstrated promising results.
- **Systemic steroids.** This modality is preferred over regional steroid by some practitioners if symptomatic inflammation is bilateral. Others prefer to avoid systemic steroids in most cases, proceeding directly to immunosuppressive chemotherapeutic agents. A large dose of 1–2 mg/kg daily is commenced,

tapered slowly over months according to response. It is essential to consider the contraindications and potential adverse effects of steroids before prescribing.

- **Immunosuppressive agents.** Mycophenolate, methotrexate, tacrolimus, cyclosporine and others are alternatives in steroid-resistant inflammation or as steroid-sparing agents.
- **Other agents** demonstrating efficacy in refractory disease include interferon-beta (in MS-related IU) and the anti-TNF infliximab.
- **Pars plana vitrectomy** substantially reduces inflammatory intensity and recurrence, though the mechanism is imperfectly understood. It is indicated in patients with tractional retinal detachment, epiretinal membrane, refractory CMO, dense vitreous opacity, vitreous haemorrhage or substantial peripheral neovascularization.
- **Cataract and glaucoma** are managed medically and surgically if necessary.

VOGT–KOYANAGI–HARADA (VKH) SYNDROME

Introduction

VKH is an idiopathic multisystem autoimmune disease featuring inflammation of melanocyte-containing tissues such as the uvea, ear and meninges. VKH predominantly affects Hispanic, Japanese and heavily pigmented individuals, usually in the 2nd and 5th decade of life. It is associated with HLA-DR1 and HLA-DR4 across different racial groups. VKH is sometimes subdivided into (a) Vogt–Koyanagi disease, characterized mainly by skin changes and anterior uveitis and (b) Harada disease, in which neurological features and exudative retinal detachments predominate.

Clinical features

- **Prodromal phase** lasting a few days: neurological (meningitis and rarely encephalopathy with cranial nerve paresis and other focal lesions) and auditory manifestations (tinnitus, vertigo and deafness). Cranial nerve palsies and optic neuritis may occur.
- **Acute uveitic phase.** Bilateral granulomatous anterior and multifocal posterior uveitis with diffuse choroidal infiltration, Dalen–Fuchs nodules (see also sympathetic ophthalmia below), vitritis, papillitis and exudative retinal detachments (Fig. 12.17A and Fig. 12.18A). Ciliary effusion with iris–lens diaphragm rotation can occur.
- **Convalescent phase** follows several weeks later: localized alopecia, poliosis and vitiligo, depigmented fundus appearance ('sunset glow' fundus – Fig. 12.17B) and depigmented limbal lesions (Sugiura sign) in pigmented, especially Japanese, patients.
- **Chronic recurrent phase** is characterized by smouldering anterior uveitis with exacerbations. Recurrent posterior uveitis is much less common.
- **Diagnostic criteria** for VKH are set out in Table 12.9. In complete VKH, criteria 1–5 must be present, in incomplete VKH, criteria 1–3 and either 4 or 5 must be present, and in probable VKH (isolated ocular disease), criteria 1–3 must be present.
- **Ocular complications** include macular neovascularization, subretinal fibrosis, preretinal and disc new vessels and vitreous haemorrhage, cataract and glaucoma.
- **Prognosis** is variable and is partly dependent on achieving control in the early stages. Neurological and auditory manifestations tend to resolve but skin, lash and hair changes usually persist.

Investigation

Systemic manifestations should be investigated and managed by an appropriate specialist.

- **Lumbar puncture** if diagnosis uncertain. CSF shows a transient lymphocytic pleocytosis and melanin-containing macrophages.
- **FAF** demonstrates hyperautofluorescence in areas of serous detachment (Fig. 12.18B).

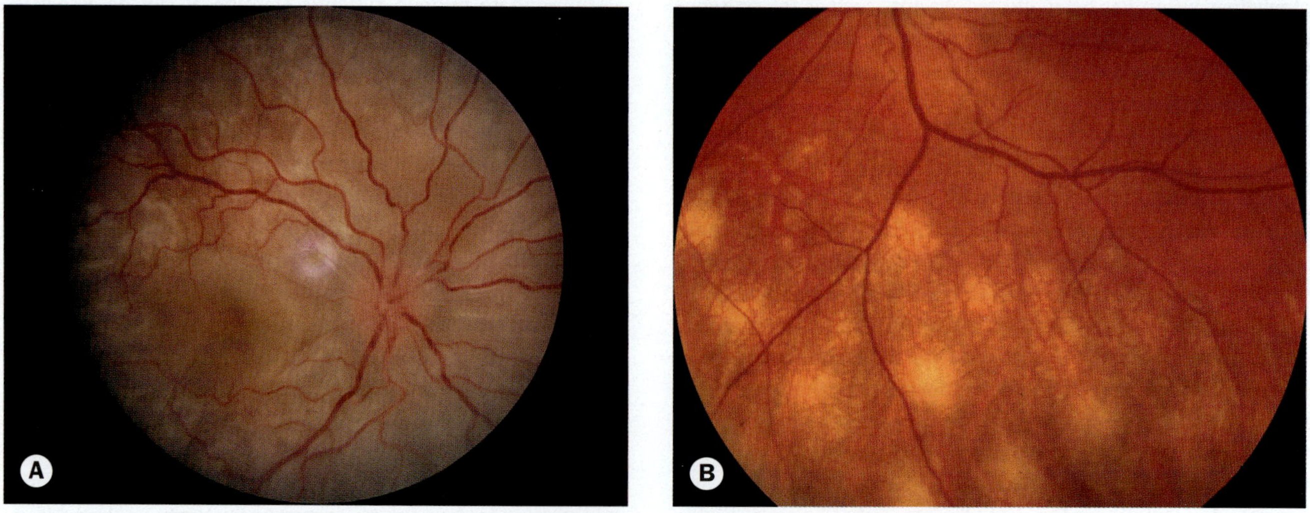

Fig. 12.17 Vogt–Koyanagi–Harada syndrome. **(A)** Multifocal exudative retinal detachments in the acute uveitic phase; **(B)** 'sunset glow' fundus in late stage.

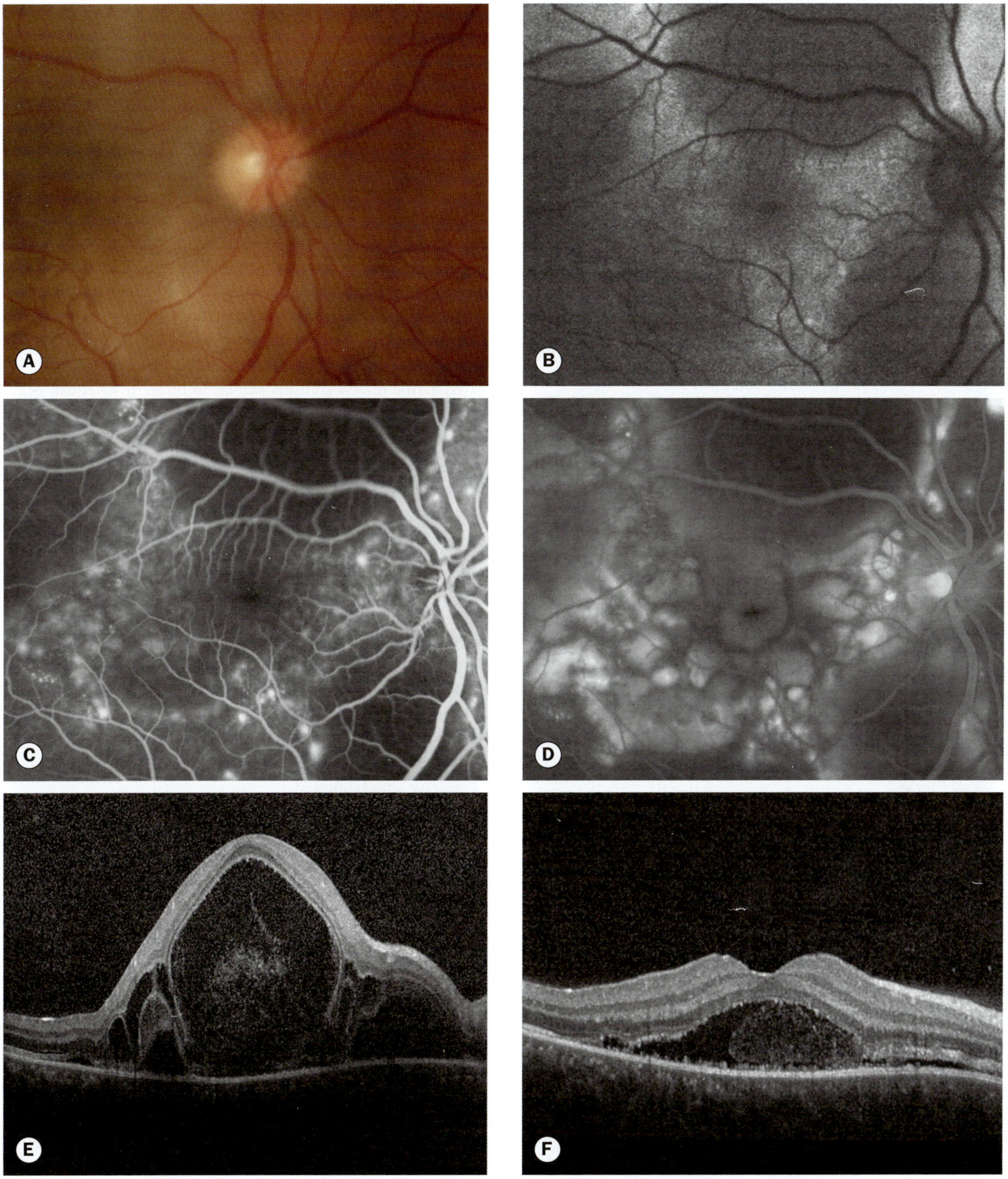

Fig. 12.18 Imaging in ocular Vogt–Koyanagi–Harada syndrome. **(A)** Multifocal exudative retinal detachment in the acute uveitic phase; **(B)** FAF of the eye demonstrating multiple exudative detachments; **(C)** FA – multiple hyperfluorescent leaking spots in venous phase; **(D)** pooling of dye within detached areas in late FA images; **(E)** OCT of a different patient on presentation showing subretinal septae – the height of subretinal fluid correlates with disease activity; **(F)** 5 days after systemic steroid showing subretinal fluid with hyperreflective material. *(Courtesy of C Barry – figs A–D; P Charbel Issa – figs E and F.)*

Table 12.9 Modified Diagnostic Criteria for Vogt–Koyanagi–Harada Syndrome

1. Absence of a history of penetrating ocular trauma
2. Absence of other ocular disease entities
3. Bilateral uveitis
4. Neurological and auditory manifestations
5. Integumentary findings, not preceding onset of central nervous system or ocular disease, such as alopecia, poliosis and vitiligo

- **Ultrasonography** shows diffuse choroidal thickening and excludes posterior scleritis. UBM can be used to demonstrate a ciliary effusion.
- **FA** of the acute phase shows multifocal hyperfluorescent dots at the level of the retinal pigment epithelium (RPE – Fig. 12.18C) followed by subretinal pooling (Fig. 12.18D). The chronic phase shows RPE window defects.
- **OCT** allows quantification of subretinal fluid. The subretinal septae are typical (Fig. 12.18E and F).
- **ICGA** during the acute phase of the disease shows regularly distributed hypofluorescent spots, most of which remain hypofluorescent during the late phase, when diffuse hyperfluorescence over the posterior pole is also shown. ICGA is useful for monitoring.

Treatment

High-dose (1–2 mg/kg daily) oral prednisolone, tapered over 3–6 months. This may be preceded by intravenous methylprednisolone pulse therapy (500–1000 mg/day). Topical steroids and cycloplegics are used for anterior uveitis. Steroid-resistant patients may require immunosuppressives. Biological blockers such as infliximab should be used early in the course of the disease if there is no response to steroids.

SYMPATHETIC OPHTHALMIA

Introduction

Sympathetic ophthalmia (SO) is a bilateral granulomatous panuveitis occurring after penetrating trauma where uveal prolapse may have been a feature of the trauma. Less frequently the condition occurs following intraocular surgery, usually multiple vitreoretinal procedures. The condition has been associated with specific HLA haplotypes, which would suggest that in some patients there is a genetic predisposition. Presentation in trauma-induced cases is between 2 weeks and 3 months after initial injury in 65%. The incidence is probably 0.2–0.5% after injury and 0.01% following intraocular surgery. A recent meta-analysis of sympathetic ophthalmia following open globe injury found an incidence of 0.19%. Histopathology shows a diffuse lymphocytic infiltration of the choroid. Scattered aggregates of epithelioid cells are seen, many of which contain fine granules of melanin (Fig. 12.19A). Dalen–Fuchs nodules, which also occur in Vogt–Koyanagi–Harada syndrome (see above), are granulomas located between Bruch membrane and the RPE (Fig. 12.19B).

Clinical features

- **Symptoms.** There is a history of causative trauma. The exciting eye is frequently red and irritable. The sympathizing eye develops irritation, blurred vision, photophobia and loss of accommodation.
- **Anterior uveitis** develops in both eyes, which may be mild or severe and is usually granulomatous (Fig. 12.20A). The severity of inflammation may be markedly asymmetrical.
- **Fundus**: multifocal choroidal infiltrates develop in the mid periphery (Fig. 12.20B), with sub-RPE infiltrates corresponding to Dalen–Fuchs nodules. Exudative retinal detachment, vasculitis and optic disc swelling may all manifest. As inflammation settles, residual chorioretinal scarring may confer a 'sunset glow' appearance similar to VKH (see Fig. 12.17B). Extensive chorioretinal scarring may follow (Fig. 12.20C).
- **Systemic manifestations** similar to those in VKH can occur but are uncommon.
- **Prognosis** depends on the severity and location of disease and the response to treatment. With aggressive therapy 75% of sympathizing eyes retain a visual acuity of better than 6/60. Long-term follow-up is mandatory because relapses occur in 50% of cases and may be delayed for several years.

Investigation

- **OCT** is useful for quantifying and monitoring change.
- **B-scan ultrasonography** may demonstrate choroidal thickening.
- **FA** shows multiple foci of leakage at the level of the RPE, with subretinal pooling in the presence of exudative retinal detachment.
- **ICGA** shows hypofluorescent spots in active disease, which resolve with treatment.
- **FAF** is helpful when following these patients, as it provides a non-invasive and objective method of monitoring disease progression and response to treatment (Fig. 12.20D).
- **Ultrasound** may show choroidal thickening and exudative retinal detachment in the acute stage.

Treatment

- **Enucleation** of a severely injured eye within 10–14 days of the injury has historically been considered effective in preventing or reducing the severity of SO and should be considered for an injured eye with a hopeless visual prognosis. Evisceration is an acceptable option provided all uveal tissue is removed.
- **Steroids** are the basis of initial treatment. High-dose oral prednisolone is given for several months and gradually tapered according to response. Initiation with intravenous methylprednisolone may be used in some cases. Supplementary topical steroids and cycloplegics may be given to target anterior uveitis and peri- and intraocular steroids, including slow-release intravitreal implants, may facilitate reduced systemic treatment.
- **Immunomodulatory treatment** should be considered early in the course of the disease (see above).

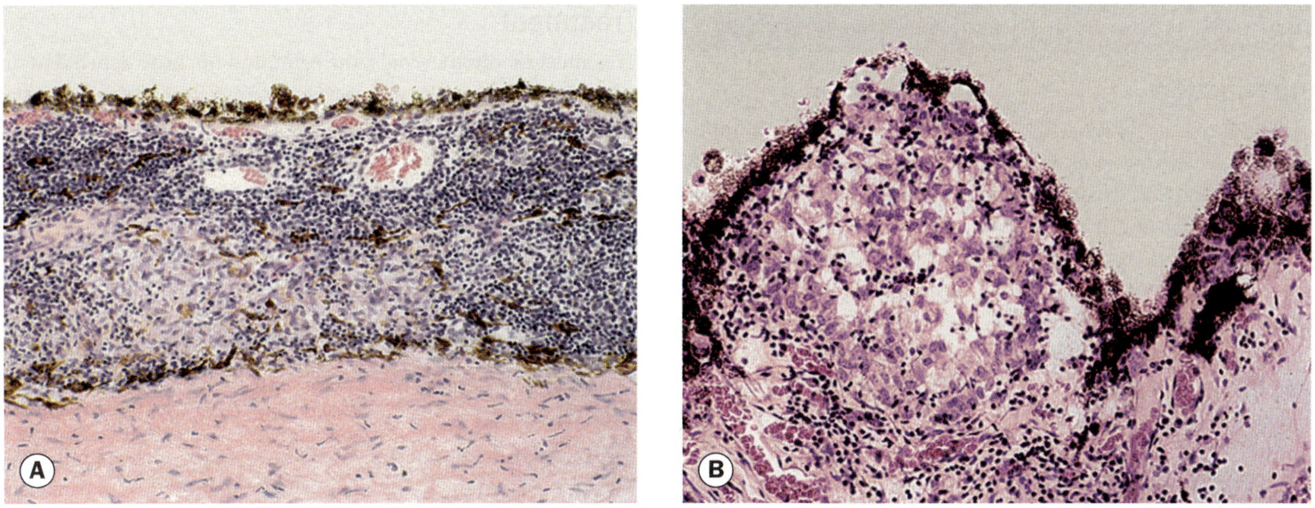

Fig. 12.19 Histology of sympathetic ophthalmia. **(A)** Infiltration of the choroid by lymphocytes and scattered aggregations of epithelioid cells, many of which contain fine granules of melanin; **(B)** Dalen–Fuchs nodule – a granuloma situated between Bruch membrane and the retinal pigment epithelium.

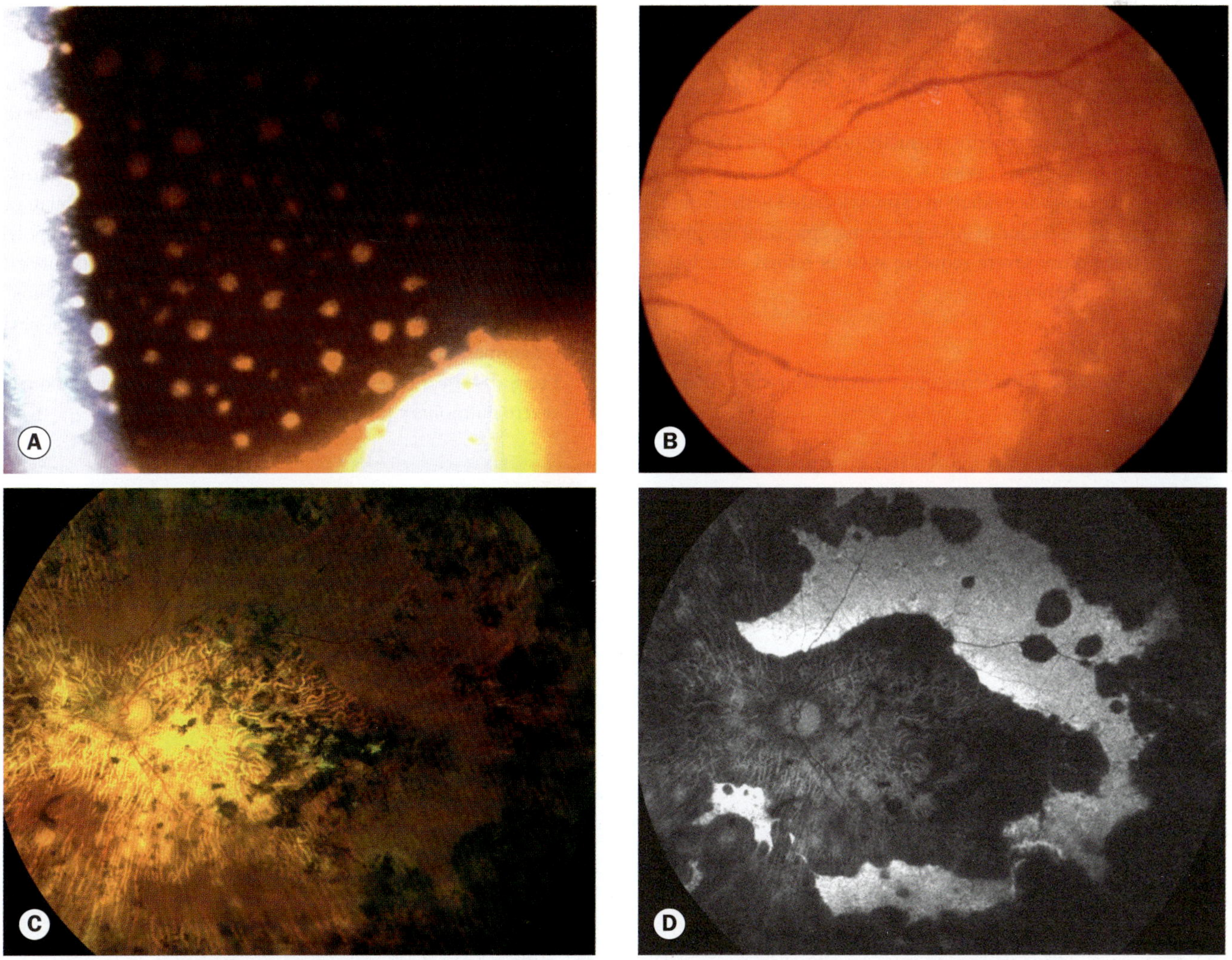

Fig. 12.20 Sympathetic ophthalmia. **(A)** Large keratic precipitates in the sympathizing eye; **(B)** multifocal choroidal infiltrates; **(C)** chorioretinal scarring in a sympathizing eye after aggressive immunosuppressive treatment; **(D)** FAF image of **(C)** showing hyperautofluorescence, which can be used to monitor disease progression. *(Courtesy of S Sharma – figs C and D.)*

LENS-INDUCED UVEITIS

Introduction

Lens-induced or phacogenic uveitis results from an immune response to lens proteins following exposure due to incomplete cataract extraction, trauma or rarely capsular degeneration in a mature cataract (Fig. 12.21A). The most commonly encountered modern scenario is that of retained lens fragments following phacoemulsification, either in the posterior segment after posterior capsular rupture or zonular dehiscence, or an overlooked piece of nucleus or soft lens matter settling in the AC (see also Ch. 10). This must be differentiated from bacterial endophthalmitis, which is usually more severe.

Clinical features

- **Symptoms.** Variable pain, photophobia, redness and blurring, usually with a history of recent (complicated or uncomplicated) cataract surgery and uncommonly of injury.
- **Anterior uveitis** may be mild, moderate or severe (Fig. 12.21B).
- **Corneal oedema** is common adjacent to an AC lens fragment.
- **IOP** is frequently elevated.
- **Lens fragments** may be visible in the anterior or posterior segment.
- **Vitritis** of variable severity is usually present if lens fragments lie within the vitreous cavity.
- **Lens injury** may be evident in cases associated with trauma.
- **Complications** include CMO, glaucoma, epiretinal membrane and, rarely, more severe sequelae such as retinal detachment and cyclitic membrane.

Investigation

OCT, B-scan and biomicroscopic ultrasonography may be indicated.

Treatment

Treatment involves steroids, the route and intensity dependent on clinical circumstances, with surgical removal of all lens material from the AC or via pars plana vitrectomy as required. Small lens fragments in the posterior segment can often be managed conservatively and will absorb slowly over months. Cycloplegia and IOP-lowering treatment are commonly indicated. Penetrating or (uncommonly) blunt ocular injury should be managed concomitantly as appropriate, including removal of the damaged lens.

SARCOIDOSIS

Introduction

Sarcoidosis is a chronic disorder of unknown cause, manifesting with non-caseating granulomatous inflammatory foci. It can affect any organ system, but the lungs and lymph nodes are the most commonly involved. It affects Black people significantly more often than White people by a margin of 10: 1 and is more common in colder climates. It is one of the most common systemic associations of uveitis.

Systemic features

- **Presentation.** Respiratory symptoms (cough, shortness of breath on exertion) and constitutional symptoms (malaise, arthralgia) each occur in about 50% of patients. Löfgren syndrome is an acute presentation carrying a good prognosis, characterized by the triad of erythema nodosum, bilateral hilar lymphadenopathy (Fig. 12.22A) on chest X-ray and polyarthralgia, usually seen in women. A minority of patients are asymptomatic (incidentally abnormal chest X-ray). Diagnosis may be made as the result of investigation of extrapulmonary inflammation such as uveitis.
- **Lung** disease ranges from mild parenchymal infiltration to severe pulmonary fibrosis.

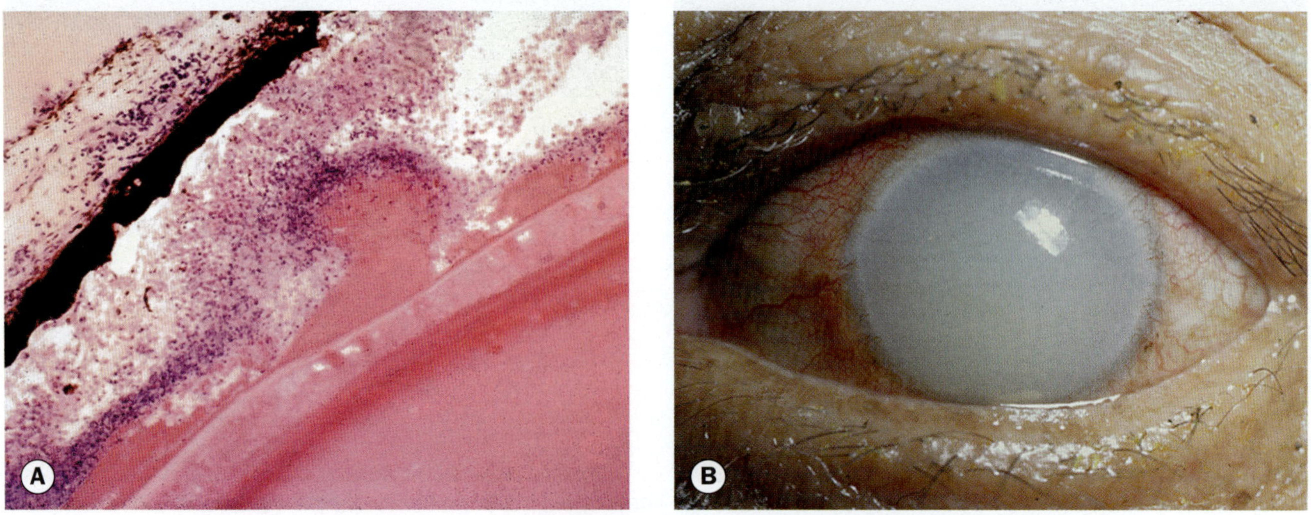

Fig. 12.21 Lens-induced uveitis. **(A)** Histology showing exposed lens material producing an inflammatory reaction; **(B)** clinical appearance *(Courtesy of J Harry and G Misson, from* Clinical Ophthalmic Pathology, *Butterworth-Heinemann 2001 – fig. A; ADN Murray – fig. B.)*

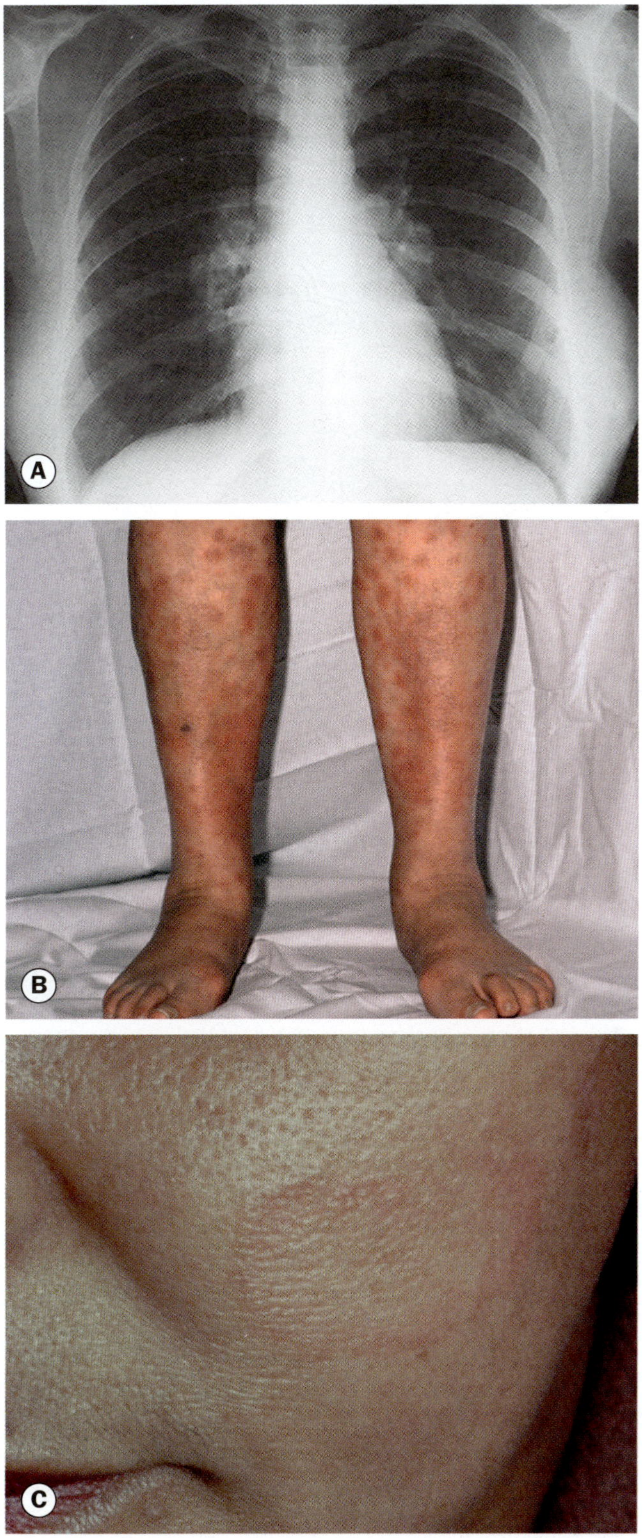

Fig. 12.22 Sarcoidosis. **(A)** Bilateral hilar lymphadenopathy; **(B)** erythema nodosum; **(C)** lupus pernio of the cheek.

- **Skin** lesions are seen in about 25% of patients and can include erythema nodosum (tender erythematous plaques typically involving the shins – Fig. 12.22B), lupus pernio (indurated violaceous lesions involving exposed parts of the body such as the nose, cheeks, fingers and ears – Fig. 12.22C) and granulomatous papules or macules.
- **Neurological** disease is rare, but meningitis and cranial nerve palsies may occur. Pituitary involvement can lead to hormonal abnormalities.
- **Cardiac involvement** is relatively uncommon (5% clinically), but is critically important as it may lead to arrhythmia and sudden death.
- **Lymphadenopathy.** Enlargement of superficial nodes is sometimes the initial clinical manifestation.

Ocular features

Ocular inflammation occurs in 25–70% of sarcoid patients depending on ethnicity. Granulomatous anterior uveitis is the most common manifestation. Blindness can occur if not adequately managed. AAU typically affects patients with acute-onset sarcoidosis. CAU, typically granulomatous, tends to affect older patients with chronic pulmonary disease. The International Workshop on Ocular Sarcoidosis (IWOS), reporting in 2009, identified seven key signs in the diagnosis of intraocular sarcoidosis:

- **'Mutton fat' KPs** (Fig. 12.23A) and/or small granulomatous KPs and/or iris nodules (Koeppe and/or Busacca – Fig. 12.23B).
- **Trabecular meshwork nodules** (Fig. 12.23C) and/or tent-shaped PAS.
- **Vitreous opacities:** snowballs (Fig. 12.23D) and/or 'strings of pearls'.
- **Multiple chorioretinal peripheral lesions** (active and/or atrophic). Choroidal lesions are uncommon and vary in appearance: multiple small pale-yellow infiltrates, sometimes with a punched-out appearance (Fig. 12.24A and B) are the commonest and are often most numerous inferiorly. Multiple large confluent infiltrates are less common (Fig. 12.24C). Multifocal choroiditis carries a poor visual prognosis even after resolution of activity, as a result of secondary macular neovascularization associated with macular or peripapillary chorioretinal scarring. Retinal granulomas may also occur, seen as discrete small yellow–white lesions (Fig. 12.24D).
- **Nodular and/or segmental periphlebitis (± 'candle wax drippings') and/or retinal macroaneurysm in an inflamed eye.** Periphlebitis appears as yellowish or grey-white perivenous sheathing. Perivenous exudates referred to as 'candle wax drippings' ('en taches de bougie') are typical of severe sarcoid periphlebitis (Fig. 12.25A). Occlusive periphlebitis (Fig. 12.25B) is uncommon, but peripheral retinal neovascularization may develop secondary to retinal capillary dropout. In Black patients it may be mistaken for proliferative sickle-cell retinopathy.
- **Optic disc nodule(s)/granuloma(s) and/or solitary choroidal nodule.** Solitary choroidal nodules are less common than multiple lesions in sarcoidosis. Focal optic nerve granulomas do not usually affect vision (see Fig. 19.11). Persistent disc oedema is a frequent finding in patients with retinal or vitreous involvement (Fig. 12.25C and D) and papilloedema due to CNS involvement may occur in the absence of other ocular manifestations.
- **Other ocular manifestations** include conjunctival nodules resembling those of follicular conjunctivitis, lacrimal gland

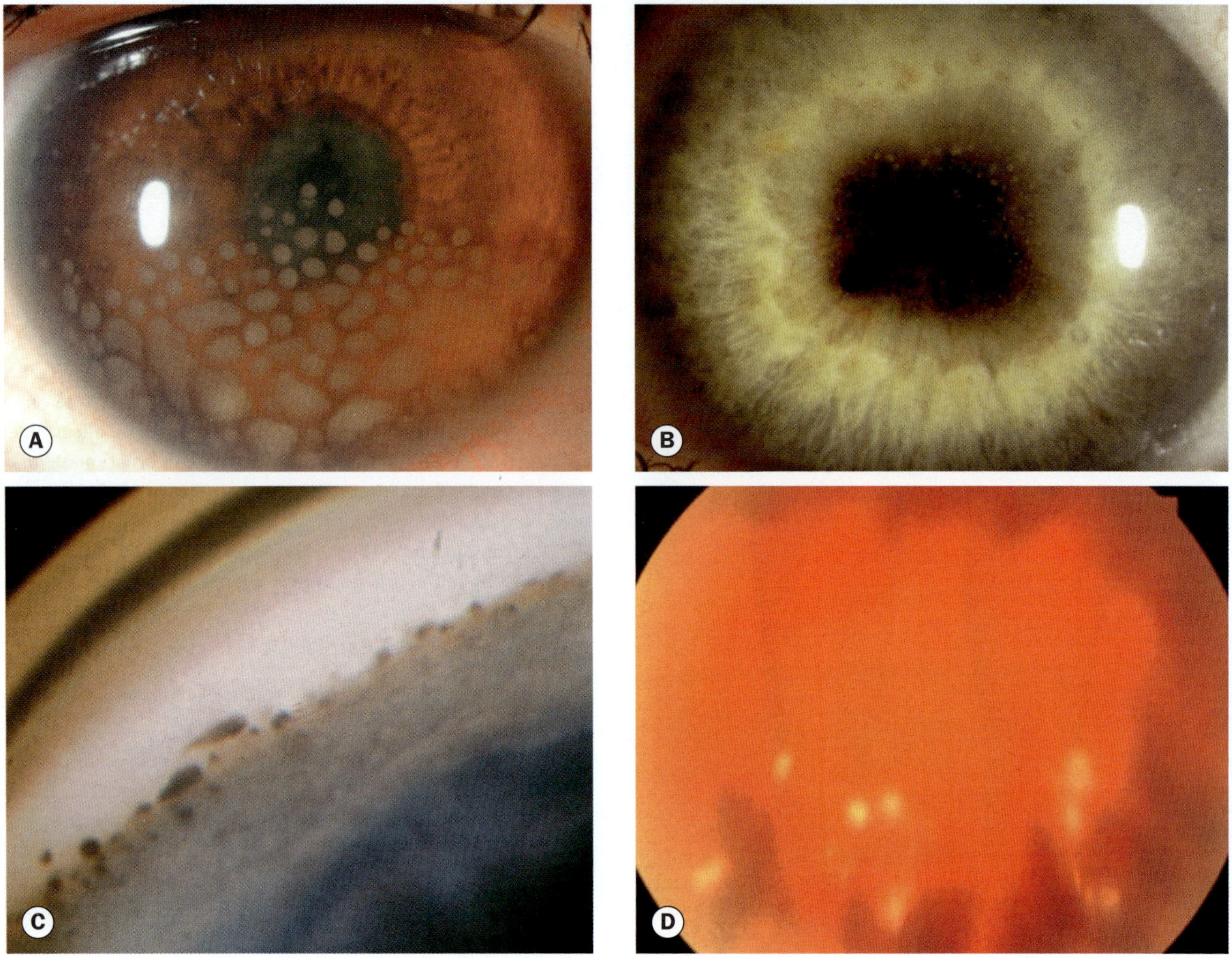

Fig. 12.23 Ocular sarcoidosis. **(A)** Very large granulomatous 'mutton fat' keratic precipitates; **(B)** large iris nodules; **(C)** nodular involvement of the trabecular meshwork; **(D)** snowballs.

infiltration (Fig. 12.26A), dry eye, eyelid nodules (Fig. 12.26B), orbital and scleral lesions. Complications are those typically seen in idiopathic uveitis, including cataract, glaucoma, posterior and peripheral anterior synechiae, band keratopathy, vitreous haemorrhage, maculopathy (CMO, epiretinal membrane, macular neovascularization), retinal detachment and phthisis.

Investigation

In addition to the acquisition of histopathological evidence, IWOS judged the following five investigations to be of significant value in the diagnosis of ocular sarcoidosis in patients having a compatible uveitis:

- **Negative tuberculin skin test** in a BCG-vaccinated patient or in a patient having had a positive tuberculin skin test previously. A tuberculin skin test is negative in most sarcoid patients. A strongly positive reaction to one tuberculin unit makes a diagnosis of sarcoidosis highly unlikely.
- **Elevated serum ACE levels** and/or elevated serum lysozyme as described for investigation of AAU.
- **Chest X-ray** showing bilateral hilar lymphadenopathy (BHL). Chest radiography is abnormal in 90%.
- **Abnormal liver enzyme tests.**
- **Chest CT scan** in patients with a negative chest X-ray result. High-resolution CT scanning is of considerably greater value than standard resolution imaging.

Other investigations are discussed below:

- **Fibreoptic bronchoscopy** with biopsy. Histopathological confirmation of sarcoidosis is almost always required before starting treatment. The lung is a common site from which to establish this in the presence of clinical or investigational evidence of pulmonary disease. However, a more easily accessible superficial lesion should be chosen if available.
- **Thoracic endosonography** (endobronchial or oesophageal) with needle aspiration has been shown in a large trial to be a more sensitive technique than bronchoscopic biopsy.
- **Miscellaneous biopsy sites** include superficial lymph nodes or skin lesions, conjunctival nodules and lacrimal glands (up to 75% of enlarged glands are positive). If the eye is involved, vitreous biopsy is very useful (e.g. CD4/CD8 ratio).

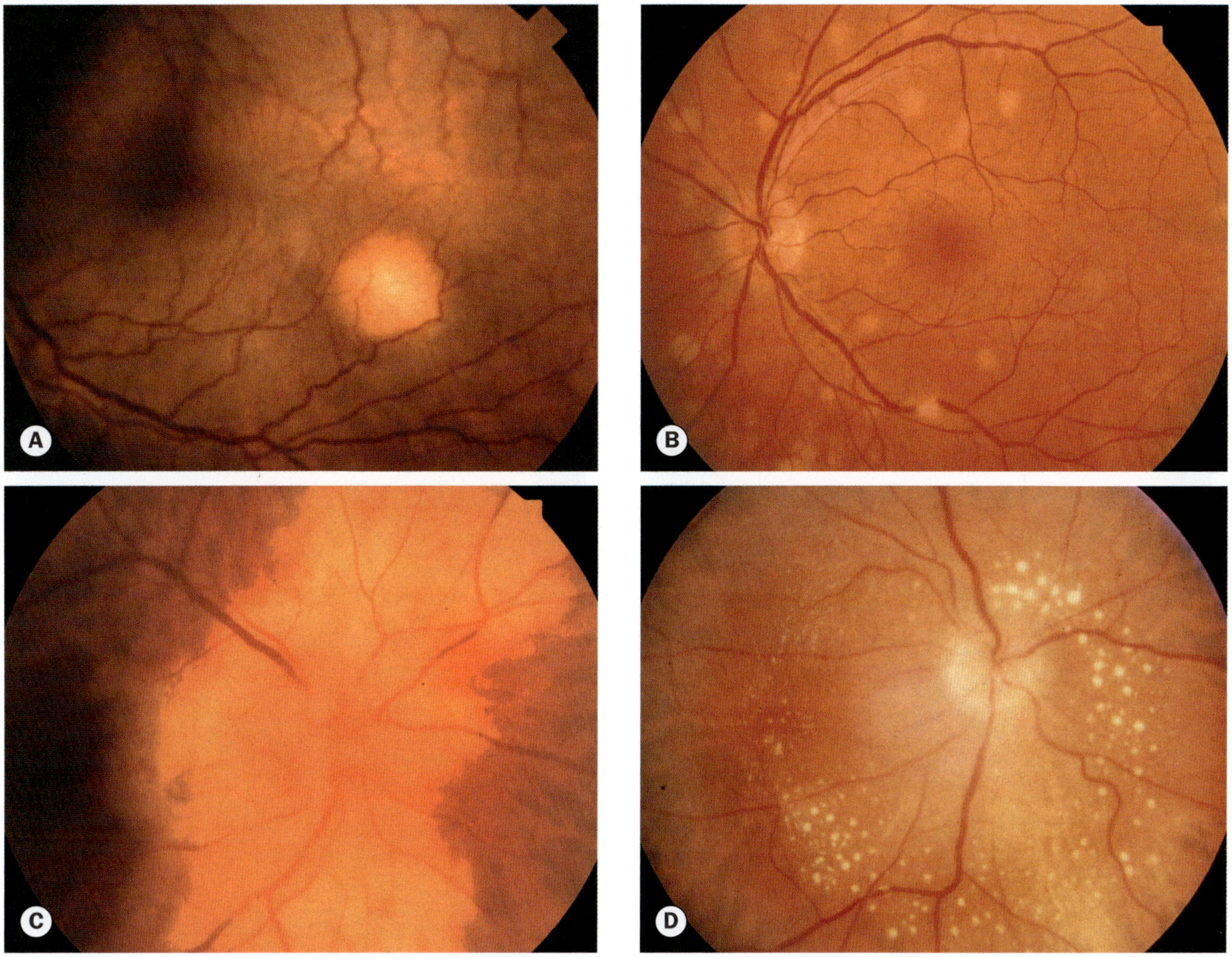

Fig. 12.24 Choroidal and retinal involvement in sarcoidosis. **(A)** Choroidal granuloma; **(B)** multifocal granulomas; **(C)** confluent choroidal infiltration; **(D)** multiple small retinal granulomas.

- **Other imaging modalities** include MRI cardiac and CNS imaging (MRI is less useful than CT for thoracic evaluation), PET scanning and occasionally whole-body gallium scanning.
- **Calcium and vitamin D** levels may be abnormal depending on disease pattern and level of activity.
- **Hypercalciuria** is common.
- **Pulmonary function testing.**
- **Bronchoalveolar lavage fluid (BALF)** shows characteristic changes. CD4/CD8 T cell ratios are a key indicator.
- **Induced sputum analysis** correlates strongly with BALF and is a non-invasive technique.
- **Four diagnostic levels** were defined by the IWOS for ocular sarcoidosis:
  - Definite ocular sarcoidosis: biopsy-supported diagnosis in the presence of a compatible uveitis.
  - Presumed ocular sarcoidosis: biopsy not done but chest X-ray shows BHL with a compatible uveitis.
  - Probable ocular sarcoidosis: biopsy not done, no BHL on chest X-ray but >3/7 of the intraocular signs above and >2/5 positive laboratory tests.
  - Possible ocular sarcoidosis: lung biopsy negative but >4/7 signs and >2/5 positive laboratory tests.

It is critical that alternative causes of uveitis are adequately excluded by appropriate assessment and investigation.

Treatment

Corticosteroids have conventionally been the major treatment modality in ocular and systemic sarcoidosis, though immunosuppressives are being used more commonly, particularly as steroid-sparing agents and in refractory disease. Treatment should be initiated aggressively to prevent sight-threatening complications.

- **Treatment of anterior and intermediate uveitis** is approached in a stepwise fashion as for idiopathic inflammation.
- **Posterior uveitis** generally requires systemic steroids and occasionally immunosuppressive agents such as methotrexate, azathioprine, ciclosporin and TNF inhibitors (e.g. adalimumab).
- **Peripheral retinal neovascularization** can be treated with scatter photocoagulation to ischaemic areas demonstrated by FA.
- **Cystoid macular oedema** may respond to a topical NSAID.

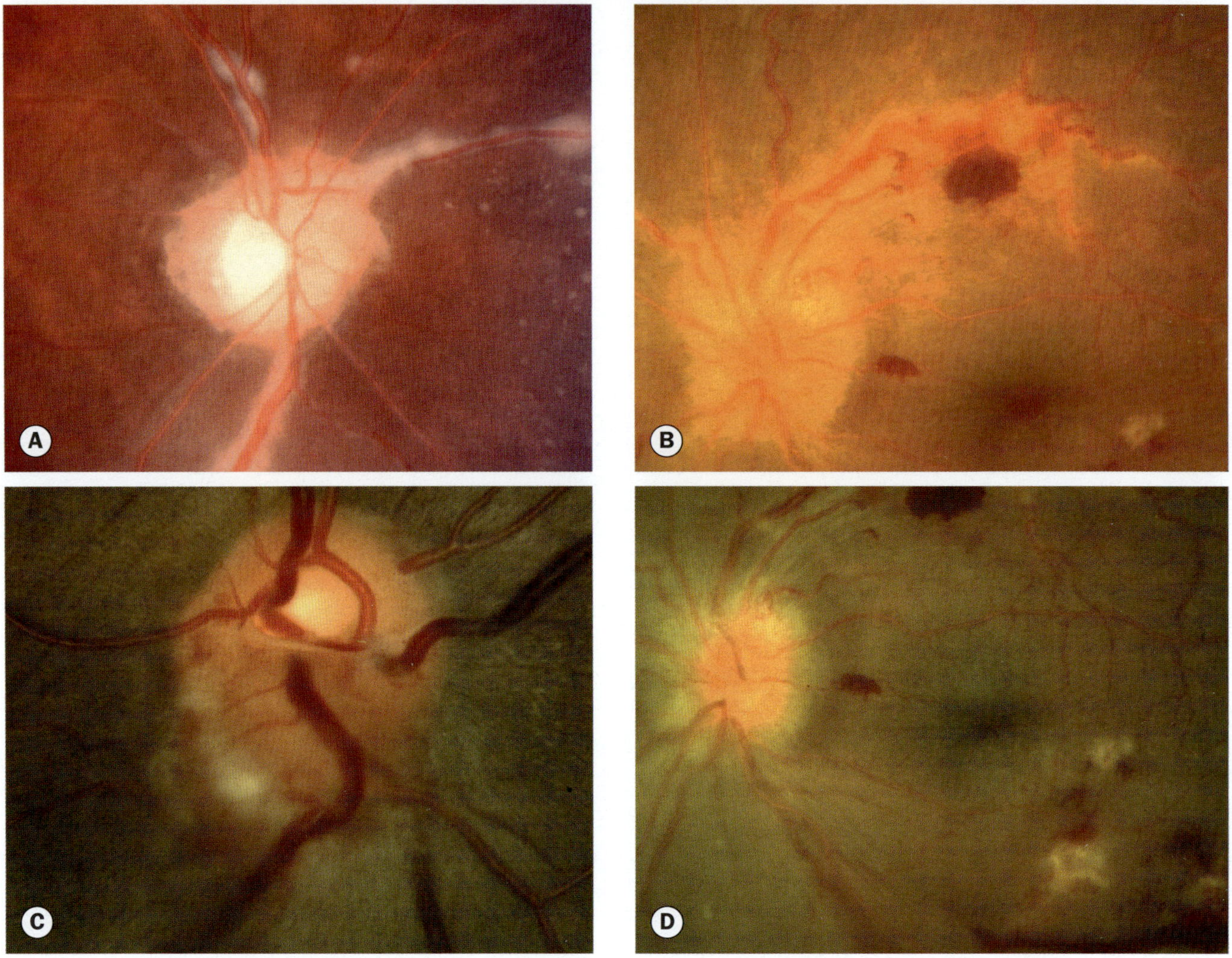

Fig. 12.25 Periphlebitis and optic disc involvement in sarcoidosis. **(A)** 'Candle wax drippings'; **(B)** occlusive periphlebitis and disc oedema; **(C)** disc swelling; **(D)** persistent disc oedema with periphlebitis and macular oedema. *(Courtesy of C Pavesio – fig. B.)*

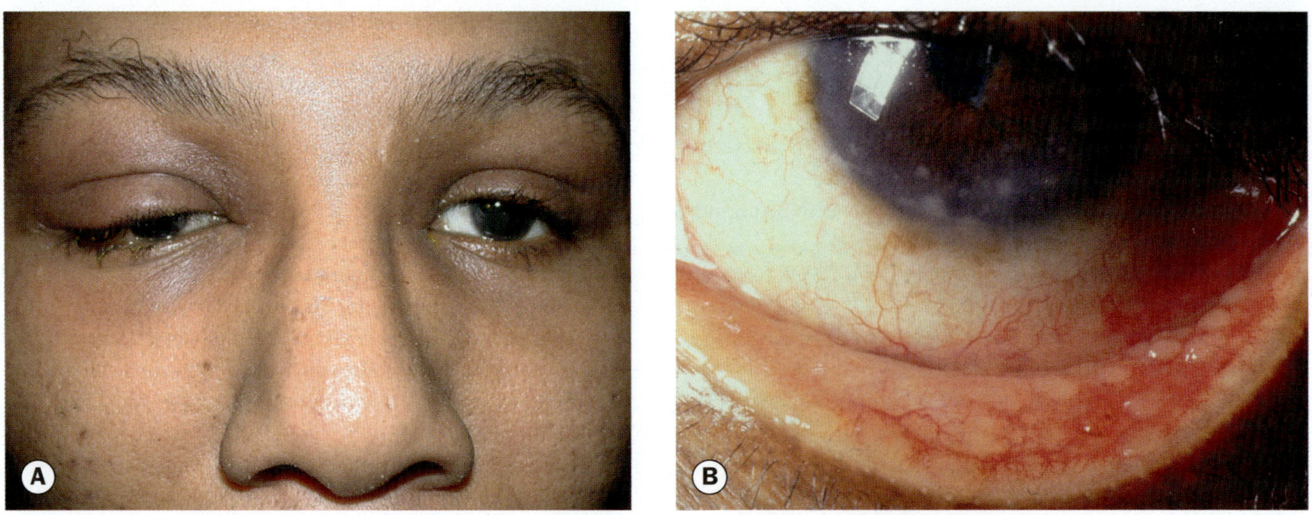

Fig. 12.26 Sarcoidosis. **(A)** Lacrimal gland enlargement; **(B)** lower lid granulomas.

- **Cataract and glaucoma** may require treatment. Inflammation should be suppressed prior to surgery, preferably for at least 3 months in the case of cataract surgery.

BEHÇET DISEASE

Introduction

Behçet disease (BD) is an idiopathic, multisystem syndrome characterized by recurrent aphthous oral ulcers, genital ulceration and uveitis. Vasculitis is a key pathogenetic component and may involve small, medium and large veins and arteries. Mortality is around 5% at 5–10 years, typically due to cardiovascular or CNS complications. The condition probably has an autoimmune basis and may be precipitated by exposure to an infectious agent with subsequent cross-reaction. It typically affects patients from Turkey, the Middle and Far East (the ancient 'Silk Road' route), with a lower prevalence in Europe and North America. It is strongly associated with HLA-B51; the ethnic groups with a higher prevalence of Behçet disease also have a higher rate of HLA-B51 positivity. The peak age of onset is the third decade. Reported gender prevalence varies with ethnicity.

TIP A transient hypopyon in a relatively white eye is typical of Behçet disease and JIA-associated uveitis.

Systemic features

The International Study Group for Behçet Disease (ISGBD), reporting in 1990, established **criteria for diagnosis**: (a) recurrent oral ulceration (Fig. 12.27A) characterized by oral ulcers at least three times in a 12-month period, plus at least two of: (b) genital ulceration, (c) ocular inflammation, (d) characteristic skin lesions (erythema nodosum – see Fig. 12.22B, pseudofolliculitis, acneiform nodules, papulopustular lesions) and (e) a pathergy reaction: pustule 24–48 hours after a sterile needle prick (>95% specific, but often negative in European and North American patients).

Presentation does not always conform to the criteria above. Additional features include:

- **Vascular lesions.** Aneurysms, including pulmonary and coronary and venous thrombosis/thrombophlebitis.
- **Arthritis** occurs in 30%, though arthralgia is more common.
- **Dermatographia** (Fig. 12.27B), similar to the pathergy reaction, indicates skin hypersensitivity and consists of the formation of erythematous lines following stroking or scratching.
- **Neurological manifestations** (5%) such as meningoencephalitis of the brainstem, dural sinus thrombosis and cerebral aneurysms.
- **Gastrointestinal inflammation**, especially ileocecal.
- **Hepatic and renal lesions** are relatively uncommon.

Ocular features

Ocular inflammation occurs in about 70%, tends to be more severe in men and is the presenting manifestation in about 10%. Signs are virtually always bilateral eventually. Relapsing/remitting acute onset panuveitis with retinal vasculitis and often spontaneous resolution even without treatment is the classical pattern of eye involvement. Retinal vascular disease (vasculitis and occlusion) is the main cause of visual impairment.

- **AAU**, often bilateral, is typical. It is not granulomatous. A transient mobile hypopyon in a relatively white eye (Fig. 12.28A) is characteristic.
- **Vitritis** may be severe and is universal in eyes with active posterior segment disease.
- **Retinitis.** Transient superficial white infiltrates (Fig. 12.28B) that heal without scarring may be seen during acute systemic disease. There may be deeper more diffuse retinitis similar in appearance to viral inflammation. Exudative detachments can also occur. Inflammatory deposits analogous to KPs may be seen on the inferior peripheral retina.
- **Retinal vasculitis** – arteritis as well as phlebitis, in contrast to pure venous involvement in sarcoidosis – can manifest with sheathing, perivascular haemorrhages and occlusion (Fig. 12.28C). Vascular leakage may give rise to diffuse retinal oedema and CMO.

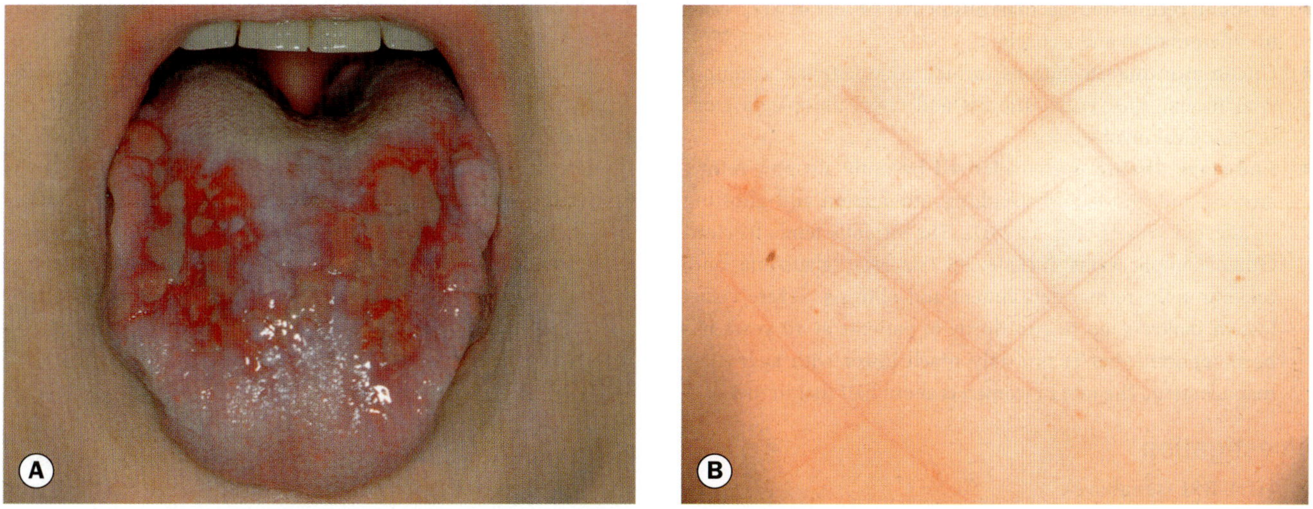

Fig. 12.27 Behçet disease. **(A)** Major aphthous ulceration; **(B)** dermatographia.

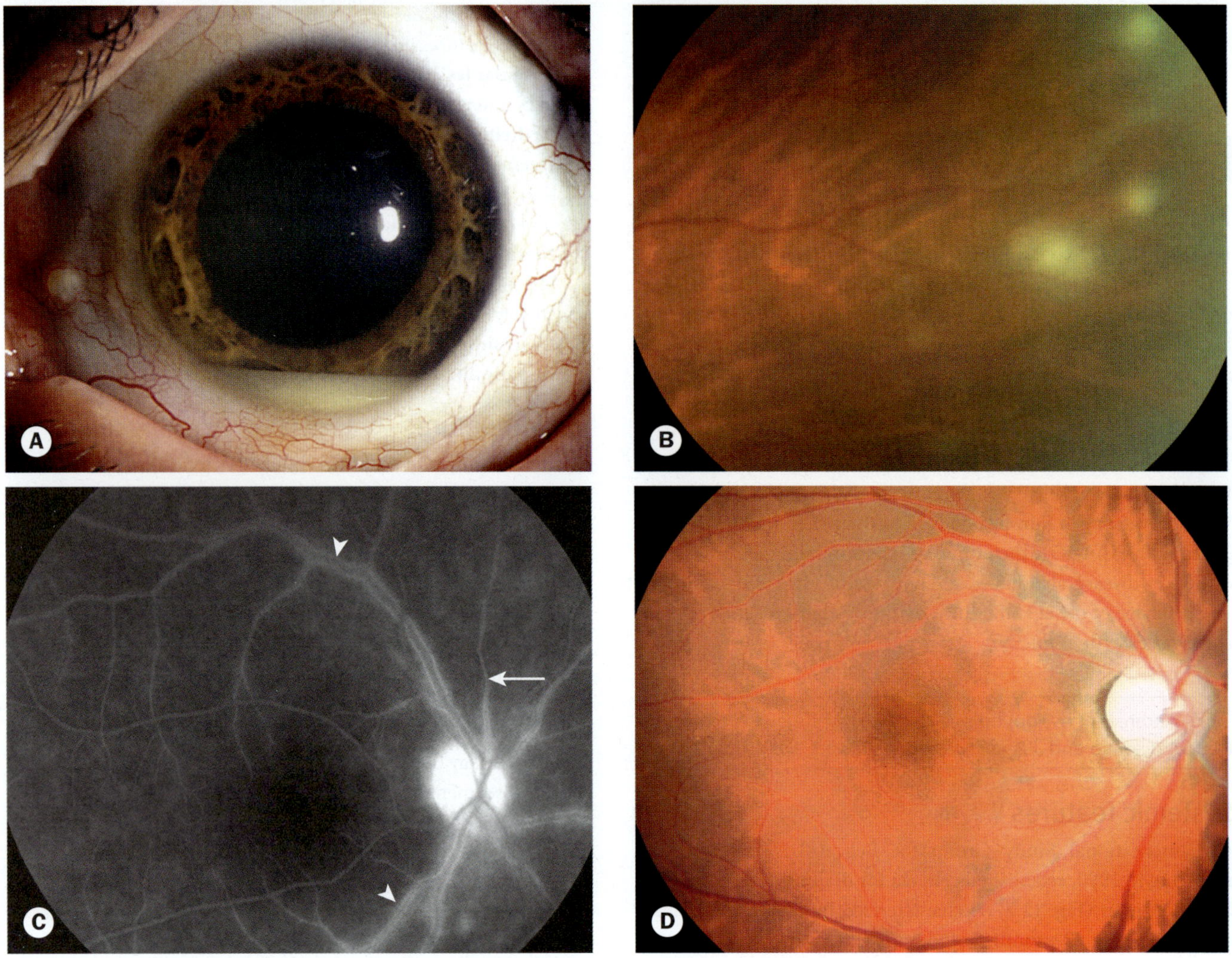

Fig. 12.28 Ocular manifestations of Behçet disease. **(A)** Hypopyon in a white eye; **(B)** retinal infiltrates; **(C)** FA showing periphlebitis (arrow heads) and arterial attenuation (arrow); **(D)** end-stage disease.

- **Optic disc hyperaemia and oedema.** Raised intracranial pressure can also cause optic disc swelling and optic atrophy in BD.
- **Disc and retinal neovascularization** may be seen as a response to inflammation and ischaemia.
- **Uncommon manifestations** include conjunctivitis, conjunctival ulcers, episcleritis, scleritis and ophthalmoplegia from neurological involvement.
- **End-stage disease** is characterized by optic atrophy, retinal atrophy and gliosis and sheathing, attenuation and ghosting of affected vessels (Fig. 12.28D). The vitreous tends to clear. Other complications include PS, cataract, glaucoma and, uncommonly, retinal detachment and phthisis. Severe visual loss in males of up to two-thirds of patients at 10 years has been reported, but is probably much lower with aggressive management. The rate in women is about half that in men.

Investigation

- **HLA-B51** (see above).
- **Pathergy test** (see above).
- **Inflammatory markers** (e.g. ESR, CRP, complement levels, white cell count) may be elevated.
- **Thrombophilia screening** is appropriate in some patients to exclude other causes of thrombosis.
- **FA** delineates ischaemic areas and aids detection of posterior segment inflammation and monitoring of disease activity.
- **Laser flare photometry** of the AC correlates well with FA in determining the level of inflammatory activity.
- **Superficial lesion biopsy**, synovial fluid aspiration and lumbar puncture may be used to help rule out alternative diagnoses.
- **Systemic imaging** may include brain MRI/magnetic resonance angiography (MRA), CT/computed tomography angiography (CTA) and conventional angiography to identify ischaemia.

Treatment

Immunosuppressants are the mainstay of treatment, but availability and expense may limit therapeutic options in many regions.

- **Topical steroids** alone may be adequate if – rarely – there is no trace of posterior segment involvement.

- **Systemic steroids and azathioprine** (2.5 mg/kg daily) in combination are recommended for the initial management of posterior uveitis in European League Against Rheumatism (EULAR) 2008 BD guidelines. Steroids should be tapered slowly. Topical and/or regional steroids may also be used. There may be a high rate of ocular hypertension with intravitreal steroid injection. Azathioprine may have a role in prophylaxis.
- **Cyclosporine** (2–5 mg/kg daily) or infliximab, in combination with azathioprine and systemic steroids, is recommended by EULAR for severe eye disease (>2 lines reduction in visual acuity and/or retinal vasculitis or macular involvement). A recent study recommended a single infliximab infusion as initial treatment of posterior uveitis. Hypertension, nephrotoxicity and neurotoxicity are concerns with cyclosporine, which should be avoided in patients with CNS involvement unless it is determined that severe eye disease warrants the risk. Infliximab may lead to activation of tuberculosis and screening-positive patients should receive prophylactic treatment (e.g. isoniazid). Intravitreal administration is a novel alternative route of administration for infliximab.
- **Infliximab** or **adalimumab** should be considered early for vision-threatening BD (American Uveitis Society recommendation).
- **Interferon-alfa** (6 million IU per day subcutaneously initially, gradually tapered) with or without steroids is a EULAR-recommended alternative to the ciclosporin/infliximab/azathioprine/steroid regimen above for severe disease. It should not be used in combination with azathioprine (risk of myelosuppression).
- **Anticoagulants** are not recommended.

PARASITIC UVEITIS

Toxoplasmosis

Introduction

Toxoplasmosis is caused by *Toxoplasma gondii*, an obligate intracellular protozoan. It is estimated to infest at least 10% of adults in northern temperate countries and more than half of adults in Mediterranean and tropical countries. The cat is the definitive host, with intermediate hosts including mice, livestock, birds and humans. Oocysts are excreted in cat faeces and then ingested by intermediate hosts (Fig. 12.29), including via contaminated water supplies. Cat litter disposal with subsequent transfer to food is a well-known potential mode of infection in humans (though indoor cats have a low rate of toxoplasmosis infestation). The bradyzoite is an inactive stage lying dormant within cysts in tissues such as the eye, brain and skeletal muscle and consumption of undercooked meat (or eggs) from an intermediate host can lead to infestation. Bradyzoite cysts can rupture to release tachyzoites, the proliferating active form, stimulating an inflammatory reaction. Conceptually it may be helpful to think of an acute phase and a long-term chronic phase of infection. During the latter, new retinochoroidal scars may form asymptomatically over the course of years or decades. A critical mode of human infection is transplacental haematogenous spread to the fetus in a pregnant woman with active (not inactive latent) toxoplasmosis – this is usually primary infection in an immunocompetent host but occasionally reactivation of latent infection, the latter predominantly in the immunocompromised. Occasionally

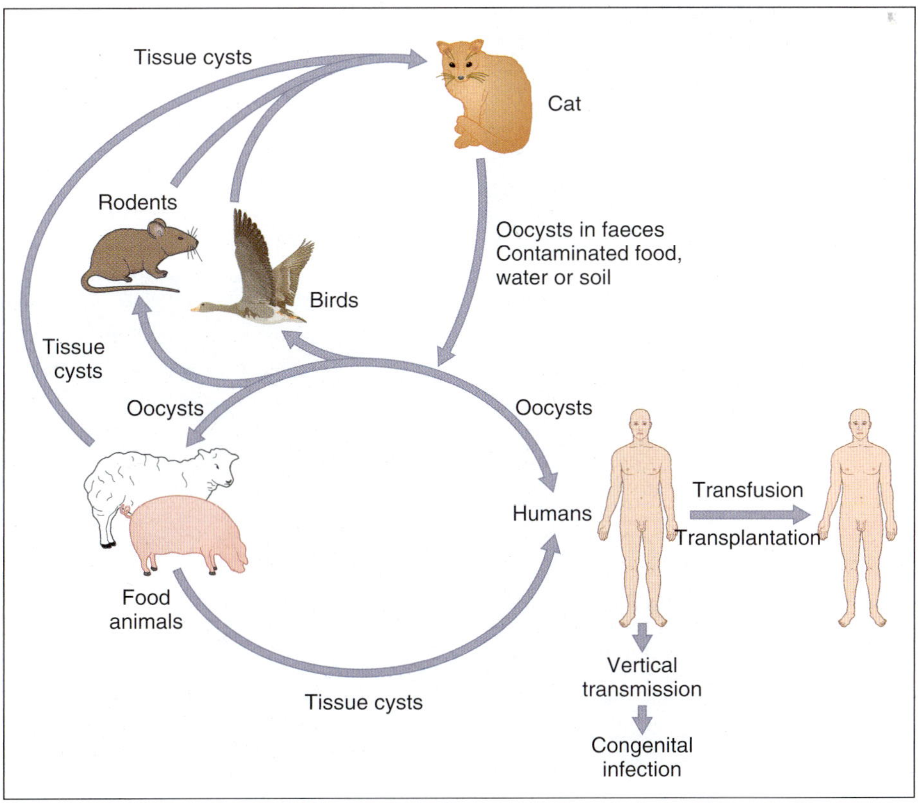

Fig. 12.29 Life cycle of *Toxoplasma gondii*.

infection may be transmitted via organ transplantation or blood transfusion.

TIP Toxoplasmosis is the most common identifiable cause for focal retinitis, which typically causes inflammation adjacent to a chorioretinal scar.

Systemic features

- **Congenital toxoplasmosis.** The mother is often symptom-free or has only mild constitutional manifestations. The severity of fetal involvement is related to the duration of gestation at the time of maternal infection, tending to be more severe in early pregnancy, when fetal death may result (10% of all congenital toxoplasmosis). Neurological and visceral involvement may be very severe, but many cases are subclinical, especially in later pregnancy. Retinochoroiditis may occur in over 75%, leaving scars that are commonly a later incidental finding (Fig. 12.30).
- **Postnatal childhood acquisition** probably accounts for over 50% of cases of childhood toxoplasmosis. As with adults, in immunocompetent individuals this is usually subclinical. Ocular lesions are probably common but may not develop for years after the initial infection.
- **Acquired toxoplasmosis in immunocompetent adults** is subclinical in 80–90%. Cervical lymphadenopathy, fever, malaise and pharyngitis are common features in symptomatic patients, but more serious systemic manifestations are rare. Early retinitis may occur in up to 20%.
- **Toxoplasmosis in immunocompromised patients** may be acquired or result from reactivation of pre-existing disease. As well as the constitutional symptoms occurring in the immunocompetent, meningoencephalitis, pneumonitis, retinochoroiditis and a range of other features can occur.

Ocular features

Toxoplasmosis is responsible for 20–60% of all cases of posterior uveitis depending on the country surveyed (85% in Brazil). Reactivation at previously inactive cyst-containing scars is the rule in the immunocompetent, although many represent new infection. More than half of quiescent retinal lesions will have been acquired from postnatal infection. Recurrent episodes of inflammation are

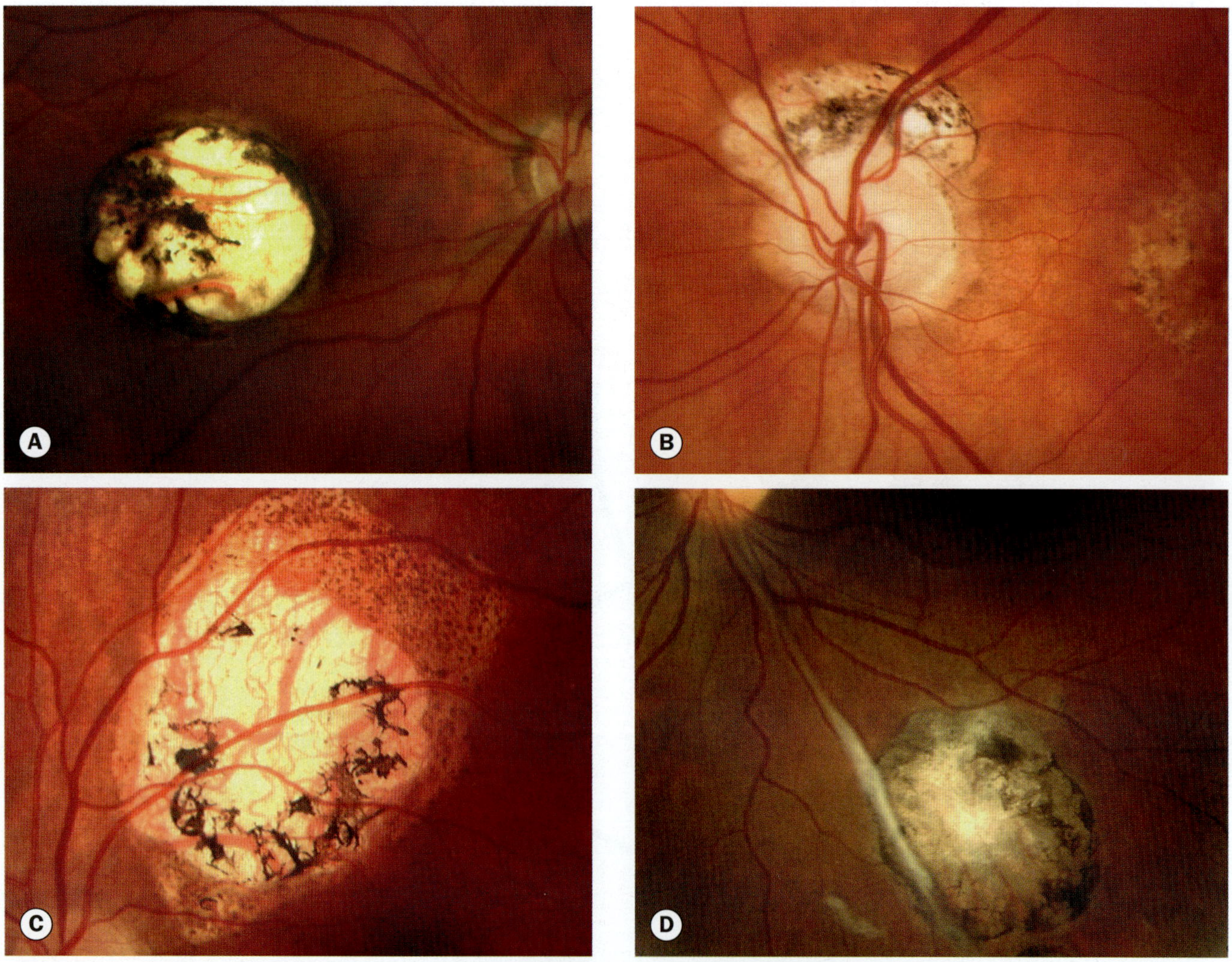

Fig. 12.30 Retinochoroidal scars in congenital toxoplasmosis. **(A)** Macular lesion; **(B)** peripapillary scarring; **(C)** large upper temporal scar; **(D)** inferonasal peripheral scar.

common, especially in the year after the initial episode and occur when the cysts rupture and release hundreds of tachyzoites into normal retinal cells. First presentation with symptomatic ocular infection occurs at an average age of 29 years, perhaps due to decreasing specific immunity. Ocular involvement from congenital infection may only be detected later in life with the incidental discovery of typical retinochoroidal scars, though occasionally macular or optic nerve damage may impair vision in childhood.

- **Symptoms.** Unilateral acute or subacute onset of floaters, blurring and photophobia.
- **'Spill-over' anterior uveitis** is common. It may be granulomatous or resemble FUS. Elevated IOP may follow.
- **A single inflammatory focus** of fluffy white retinitis or retinochoroiditis associated with a pigmented scar ('satellite lesion') is typical (Fig. 12.31A and B). Lesions tend to involve the posterior pole.
- ***De novo* foci** not associated with an old scar and multiple lesions (Fig. 12.31C) are relatively uncommon in the immunocompetent but occur more frequently in the immunocompromised.
- **Vitritis** may be severe and impair fundus visualization. 'Headlight in the fog' is the classic description of a white retinal inflammatory nidus viewed through vitritis (Fig. 12.31D).
- **Vasculitis** may be arterial but is more commonly venous.
- **Optic disc oedema** is common.
- **Extensive and fulminant retinal involvement** is generally confined to the immunocompromised, in whom it may be bilateral and difficult to distinguish from viral retinitis.
- **Retinochoroiditis may be absent** in the acute phase of acquired disease, with activity consisting of anterior uveitis, vitritis and retinal vasculitis. Typical retinal scars may form later.
- **Neuroretinitis** similar to that seen in cat-scratch disease is rare and may be a marker of acutely acquired rather than reactivated infection.
- **Punctate outer retinal toxoplasmosis** is an atypical manifestation featuring clusters of small (25–75 μm diameter) grey–white lesions and tends to occur in younger patients.
- **Visual loss.** Causes of permanently reduced vision (around 25% of eyes) include macular inflammatory lesions and oedema, optic nerve involvement, vascular occlusion (Fig. 12.32A and B), serous, rhegmatogenous and tractional retinal detachment (Fig. 12.32C and D) and late secondary macular neovascularization (Fig. 12.32E and F).
- **Healing** in immunocompetent hosts usually occurs spontaneously within 6–8 weeks, although vitreous opacities take longer to clear. The inflammatory focus is replaced by a sharply demarcated atrophic scar that develops a pigmented border (Fig. 12.33).
- **Recurrence.** The average number of recurrent attacks per patient is 2.7. The frequency of recurrences does not differ in geographic areas and is about 12–15% in the first 2 years. Within 5 years more than half may experience a further episode.

Investigation

Diagnosis is usually based on clinical examination findings.

- **Serology.** *Toxoplasma* IgG antibodies are detectable in the serum within 1–2 weeks of initial infection and indicate exposure to the organism at some point in the past, providing circumstantial evidence to support clinical suspicion. However, community seroprevalence is high – at least a third of individuals in most communities. Positivity to IgM antibodies usually means that infection has been acquired within the last year and helps to distinguish between acute (newly acquired) and chronic infection. It is a critical test if newly acquired infection is suspected during pregnancy. Occasionally IgM is positive due to persistence or reactivation following earlier infection.
- **PCR testing** of intraocular fluid is variably sensitive (16–67%) but highly specific and can be diagnostic in clinically uncertain cases. Aqueous and vitreous probably give similar yields.
- **Ocular fluid antibody assessment.** Calculating the ratio (Goldmann–Witmer coefficient) of specific IgG in aqueous humour to that in serum seems to be a reasonably sensitive (48–90%) investigation.
- **Imaging.** OCT will demonstrate macular oedema. B-scan ultrasonic imaging can be used to exclude retinal detachment in the presence of severe vitritis and FAF may facilitate monitoring of inflammatory activity.

Treatment

- **Active ocular toxoplasmosis** is treated with antibiotics, but none of the current approaches has been shown to be better than another in respect of the final visual outcome, lesion size or recurrence rate.
- **Eradication of the parasite** is difficult to determine, but parasite activity and multiplication may be reduced leading to a decrease in size of the eventual retinochoroidal scar.
- **Treatment is not needed in every case.** The agents that are used have the potential for significant morbidity and spontaneous resolution often occurs, even without treatment.
- **Clear indications** include:
  - A sight-threatening lesion involving the macula, papillomacular bundle, optic nerve head or a major blood vessel.
  - Severe vitritis.
  - Active ocular toxoplasmosis in the immunocompromised.
- **Treatment duration:** typically, 4–6 weeks with complete healing of active lesions over 4–6 months.
- **Treatment of congenital toxoplasmosis** in neonates with antimicrobials for 1 year may reduce the frequency of subsequent development of retinochoroidal scars.
- **Prednisolone** (1 mg/kg) is given initially and tapered according to clinical response, but should always be used in conjunction with a specific anti-*Toxoplasma* agent, most frequently pyrimethamine combined with sulfadiazine ('classic' or 'triple' therapy, sometimes supplemented with clindamycin). Some authorities start steroids only after 24–48 hours of antimicrobial therapy. Systemic steroids should be used with extreme caution in immunocompromised patients and children should undergo varicella zoster vaccination if they have not had chickenpox.
- **Pyrimethamine** is a folic acid antagonist that is believed to be highly effective. It is administered as a loading dose of 75–100 mg for 1–2 days followed by 25–50 mg daily

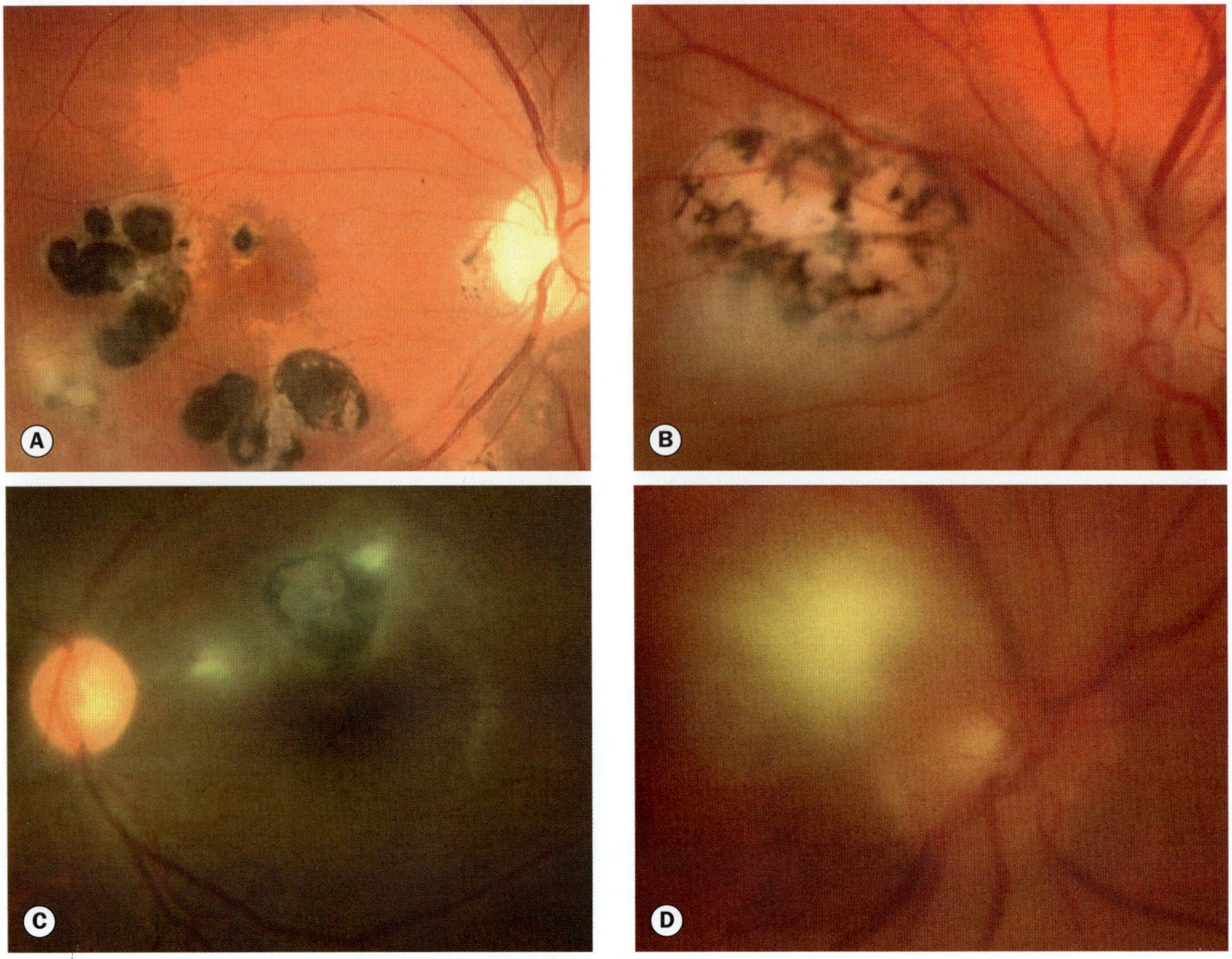

Fig. 12.31 Active *Toxoplasma* retinitis. **(A)** and **(B)** Typical 'satellite' lesion adjacent to an old scar; **(C)** two small active foci; **(D)** vitreous haze and 'headlight in the fog' appearance of lesion. *(Courtesy of S Chen – fig. A; C Pavesio – fig. C.)*

for 4 weeks in combination with oral folinic (not folic) acid 5 mg three times a week to retard thrombocytopenia, leukopenia and folate deficiency. Weekly blood counts should be performed. In acquired immunodeficiency syndrome (AIDS) pyrimethamine is avoided or used at a lower dosage because of possible pre-existing bone marrow suppression and the antagonistic effect of zidovudine when the drugs are combined.

- **Sulfadiazine** 1 g four times daily for 3–4 weeks is usually given in combination with pyrimethamine. Side effects of sulfonamides include renal stones, allergic reactions and Stevens–Johnson syndrome.
- **Intravitreal therapy** with clindamycin (1 mg) and dexamethasone (400 μg) may be as effective as triple therapy in reactivated infection. Two to three injections (at 2-weekly intervals) may be required. It may be preferred in recurrent infection in pregnancy, but would not generally be used in isolation in the immunocompromised, and in newly acquired (IgM-positive) infection systemic therapy has superior efficacy. Depot steroid intra- and periocular preparations such as triamcinolone should be avoided as uncontrolled progression has been reported.
- **Azithromycin** 250–500 mg daily shows evidence of reducing the rate of recurrence of retinochoroiditis and its use in combination with pyrimethamine, folinic acid and prednisolone is a promising new regimen. Clarithromycin may be a good alternative to azithromycin.
- **Co-trimoxazole** (trimethoprim 160 mg/sulfamethoxazole 800 mg) twice daily in combination with prednisolone is a low-cost and better-tolerated option, but might not be quite as effective as classic therapy.
- **Clindamycin** 300 mg four times daily may be added to triple therapy (see above) or used instead of pyrimethamine. Pseudomembranous colitis is a potential adverse effect.
- **Atovaquone** theoretically attacks encysted bradyzoites, but does not seem to prevent recurrence *in vivo*; dosing is 750 mg two to four times daily.
- **Topical steroid and mydriatic** may be given for anterior uveitis.

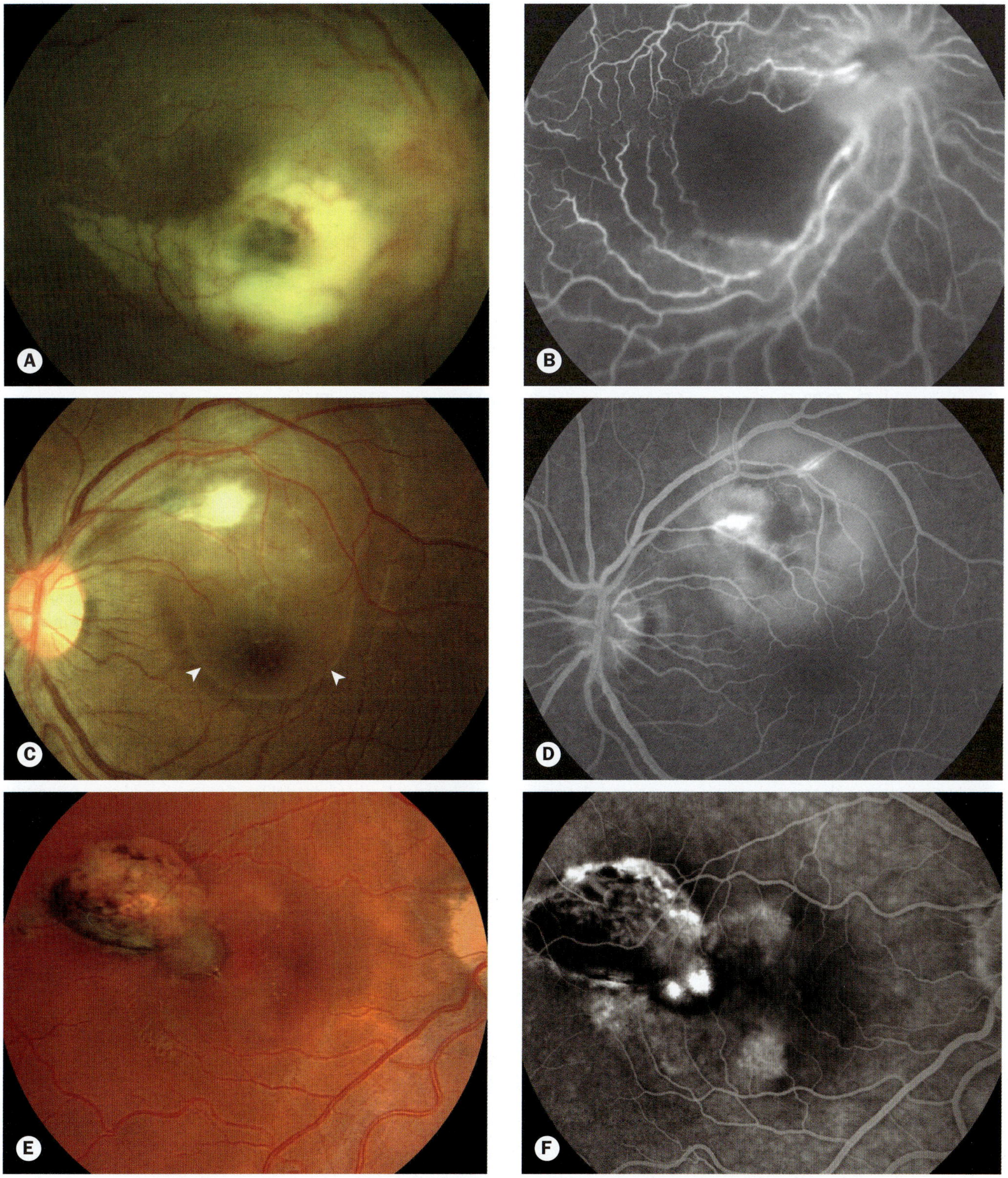

Fig. 12.32 Uncommon complications of *Toxoplasma* retinitis. **(A)** Periarteritis resulting in branch retinal artery occlusion; **(B)** FA showing extensive non-perfusion at the posterior pole; **(C)** serous macular detachment (arrow heads); **(D)** FA of **(C)** showing hyperfluorescence due to pooling of dye; **(E)** macular neovascularization adjacent to an old scar; **(F)** FA of **(E)** showing corresponding hyperfluorescence. *(Courtesy of C Pavesio – figs A–D; P Gili – figs E and F.)*

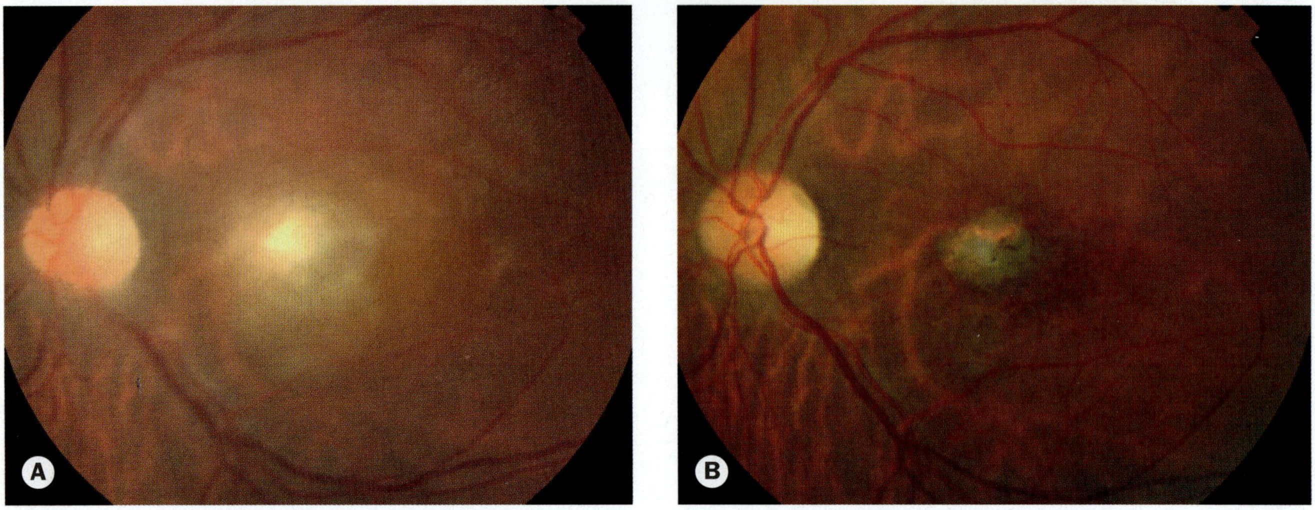

Fig. 12.33 Progression of *Toxoplasma* retinitis. **(A)** Moderate activity; **(B)** 3 months later, following antibiotic treatment. *(Courtesy of S Chen.)*

- **Antimicrobial maintenance therapy** is used in immunocompromised patients.
- **Pregnancy.** Treatment of recurrent ocular toxoplasmosis during pregnancy should be chosen carefully and only started if absolutely necessary, as several of the drugs discussed above have the potential to harm the fetus. Intravitreal therapy (see above) for reactivated disease, or systemic treatment with azithromycin, clindamycin and possibly prednisolone may be appropriate. Specific treatment to prevent transmission to the fetus is not generally given except in newly acquired infection, when urgent specialist management is appropriate. Spiramycin alone or in combination is commonly chosen.
- **Vitrectomy** may be performed in selected cases.
- **Prevention of recurrence.** Co-trimoxazole (160 mg trimethoprim combined with 800 mg sulfamethoxazole) taken three times daily for 12 months has been shown to reduce the recurrence rate from 22% to 3% for up to 3 years. After that period the likelihood of recurrence is as high as in patients who have never received prophylaxis.

Toxocariasis

Introduction

Toxocariasis is caused by infestation with a common intestinal ascarid (roundworm) of dogs, *Toxocara canis*. Puppies are more commonly infected than adult dogs and are also more likely to spread the organism. The feline variant – *Toxocara cati* – may also be causative. Human infestation is by ingestion of soil or food contaminated with ova shed in canine faeces. Young children are at particular risk from the soil of parks and playgrounds. Once ingested, ova develop into larvae, which penetrate the intestinal wall and travel to various organs such as the liver, lungs, skin, brain and eyes, with resultant inflammation.

Clinical features

- **Asymptomatic** infestation is common.
- **Visceral toxocariasis**, also known as visceral larva migrans, is systemic infection of variable severity that usually occurs in a child aged 2–7 years. Fever, abdominal pain, pneumonitis, lymphadenopathy, hepatomegaly and myocarditis are some of the possible features. Spontaneous recovery is usual. Death is very rare and usually occurs in individuals hypersensitive to parasitic antigens.
- **Covert toxocariasis** is associated with mild systemic symptoms.
- **Ocular toxocariasis** (ocular larva migrans) generally occurs independently of visceral larva migrans and is associated with a lower parasitic load. It is typically unilateral and in around two-thirds causes some degree of permanent visual impairment. In contrast to visceral toxocariasis, it tends to occur in older children and adults.
  - Chronic endophthalmitis (Fig. 12.34A) typically presents with leukocoria, strabismus, floaters or unilateral visual loss. Features may include anterior uveitis, vitritis, chorioretinitis, papillitis and a fundus granuloma (see below). A dense greyish-white exudate, similar to the snowbanking seen in PP, may involve the peripheral retina and pars plana. Complications leading to a poor visual outcome include tractional retinal or ciliary body detachment with hypotony leading to phthisis bulbi (Fig. 12.34B).
  - Posterior pole or peripheral granuloma without inflammation (Fig. 12.35A–C) classically occurs in an older child or adult with unilateral impaired vision or as an incidental finding. A one to two disc diameter-sized round yellow-white granuloma is present in the posterior fundus or periphery. Vitreoretinal traction may lead to complications due to macular distortion and/or retinal detachment.
  - Chorioretinal scar (Fig. 12.35D).
  - Diffuse unilateral subacute neuroretinitis (DUSN). See below.

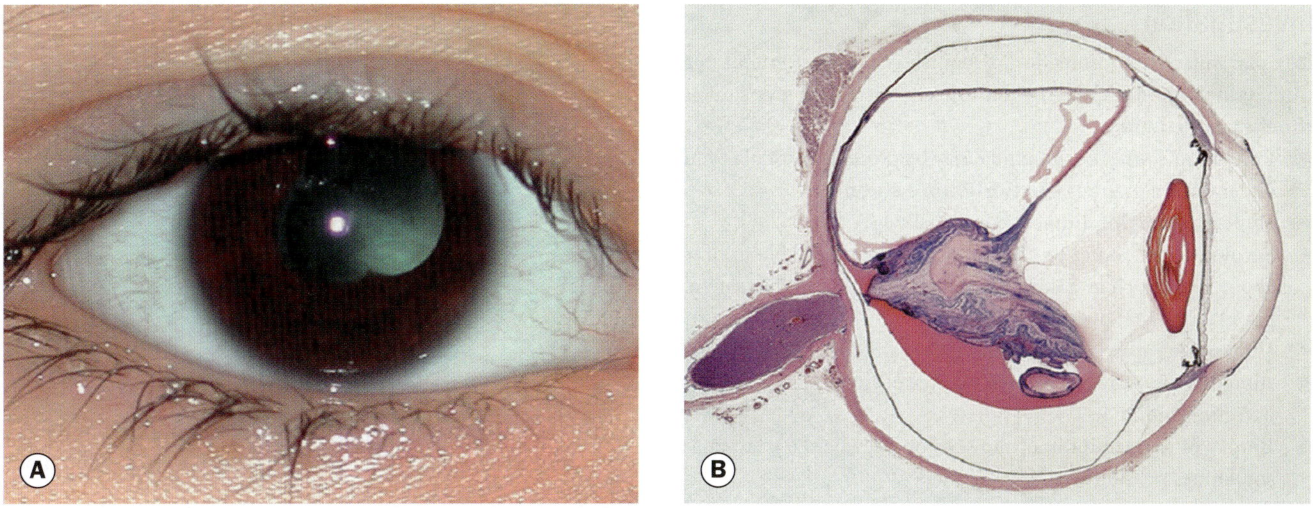

Fig. 12.34 Chronic *Toxocara* endophthalmitis. **(A)** Leukocoria; **(B)** a pathological specimen showing an inflammatory mass and total retinal detachment. *(J Harry and G Misson, from* Clinical Ophthalmic Pathology, *Butterworth-Heinemann 2001 – fig. B.)*

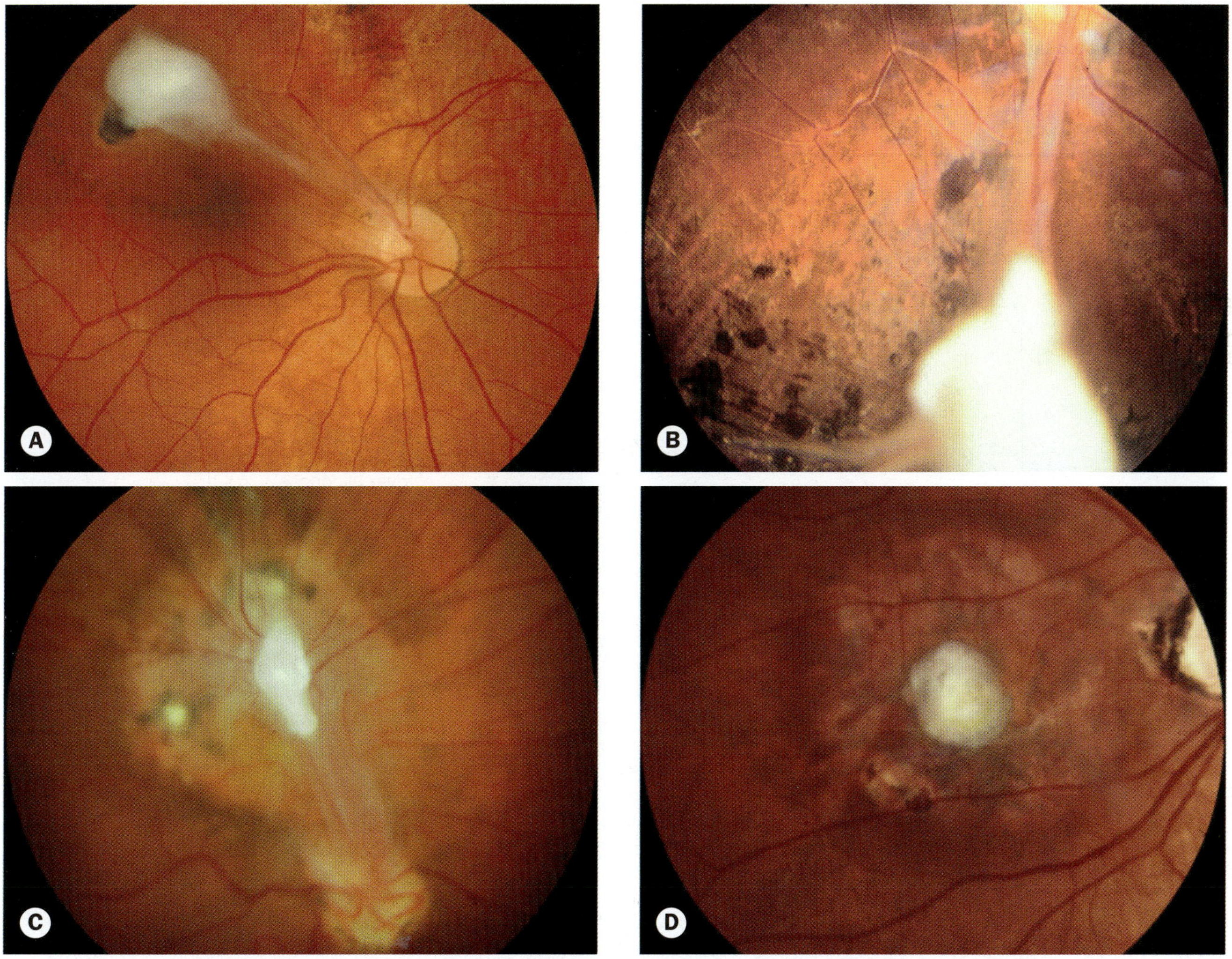

Fig. 12.35 *Toxocara* granuloma. **(A)** Granuloma with a vitreous band; **(B)** peripheral granuloma with a vitreous band extending to the disc; **(C)** mid-peripheral granuloma with underlying chorioretinal scarring; **(D)** chorioretinal scar at the macula with granuloma.

Investigation

It is particularly important to distinguish a *Toxocara* granuloma from retinoblastoma. Other helminthic organisms can give similar clinical manifestations.

- **Full blood count.** Eosinophilia may be present, particularly in visceral larva migrans and can become chronic.
- **Hypergammaglobulinaemia** especially IgE.
- **Serology.** Antibodies to *Toxocara canis* are detectable in only about 50% of ocular cases. Positivity is common in the general population (14% overall in the USA).
- **Ultrasonography** may be useful if the vitreous is hazy.
- **Aqueous or vitreous sampling** for eosinophilia, antibody detection and PCR.
- **Biopsy of a granuloma** of the skin or elsewhere for larvae is sometimes possible.

Ocular treatment

- **Prevention** by good hygiene practices and deworming of pets.
- **Steroids.** Topical, regional and systemic may be considered.
- **Anthelmintic agents** such as mebendazole and thiabendazole can be considered in ocular toxocariasis, remembering that worm death may promote inflammation.
- **Vitrectomy** for sight-threatening tractional sequelae.

Onchocerciasis

Introduction

Onchocerciasis, which affects the eyes and skin, is the second most common cause of infectious blindness in the world. It is endemic in areas of Africa and other regions and disease is particularly severe in savanna regions, where in some areas more than 50% of older adults are blind from the condition. Chronic onchocerciasis shortens lifespan by reducing resistance to other diseases. The parasitic helminth *Onchocerca volvulus* is causative. The vector is the *Simulium* blackfly, which breeds in fast-flowing water, hence the colloquial term 'river blindness'. Larvae are transmitted when the fly bites to obtain blood. They migrate to subcutaneous sites to form onchocercomas, where microfilariae are produced by adult worms (Fig. 12.36). Degenerating microfilariae excite an intense inflammatory reaction accounting for most of the clinical manifestations of the disease. The rickettsia *Wolbachia* lives symbiotically in adult worms and microfilaria and is important for microfilarial production. Diagnosis is by skin-snip biopsy, serology, tear or urine antigen detection (oncho-dipstick) and PCR of lesion fluid.

Clinical features

- **Systemic features** are principally dermatological and include pruritus, a maculopapular rash (onchodermatitis – Fig. 12.37A) involving the buttocks and extremities and areas of hypo- and hyperpigmentation on the shins ('leopard skin' – Fig. 12.37B). Scratching of itchy areas leads to lichenification. Onchocercomata are non-tender subcutaneous nodules (Fig. 12.37C) that enclose 2–3 adult worms. Severe lymphadenopathy can occur, with secondary lymphoedema. Eosinophilia is typical.
- **Live microfilariae** may be seen in the cornea, vitreous and suspended in the AC after the patient has postured face-down for a few minutes followed by immediate slit lamp examination.
- **Anterior uveitis** is an early feature. Pear-shaped pupillary dilatation may be seen and is due to PS.

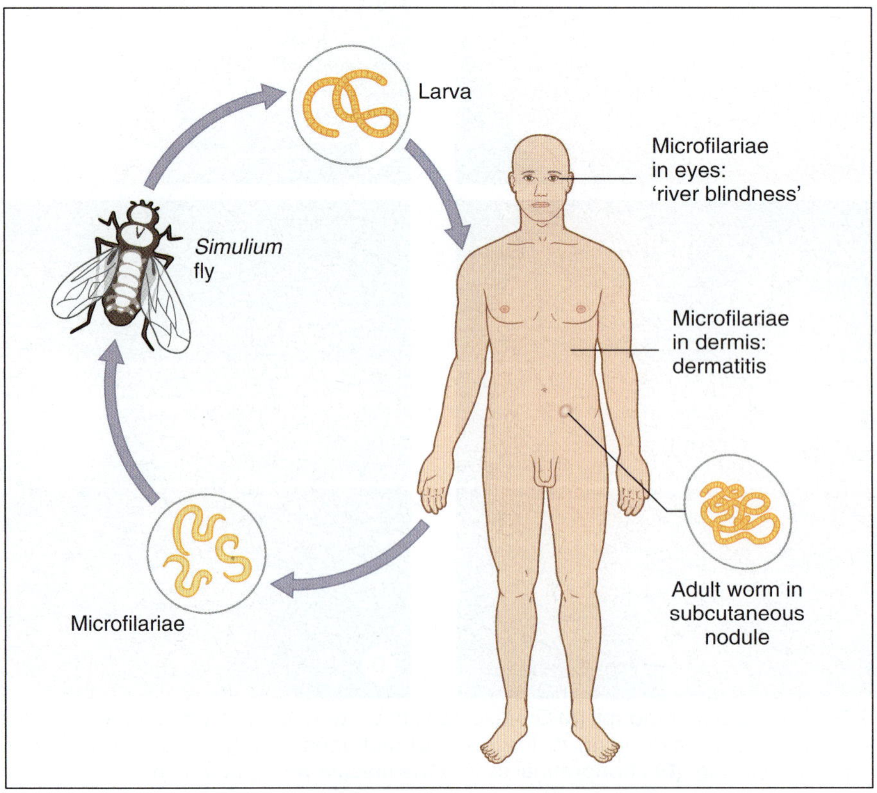

Fig. 12.36 Life cycle of *Onchocerca volvulus*.

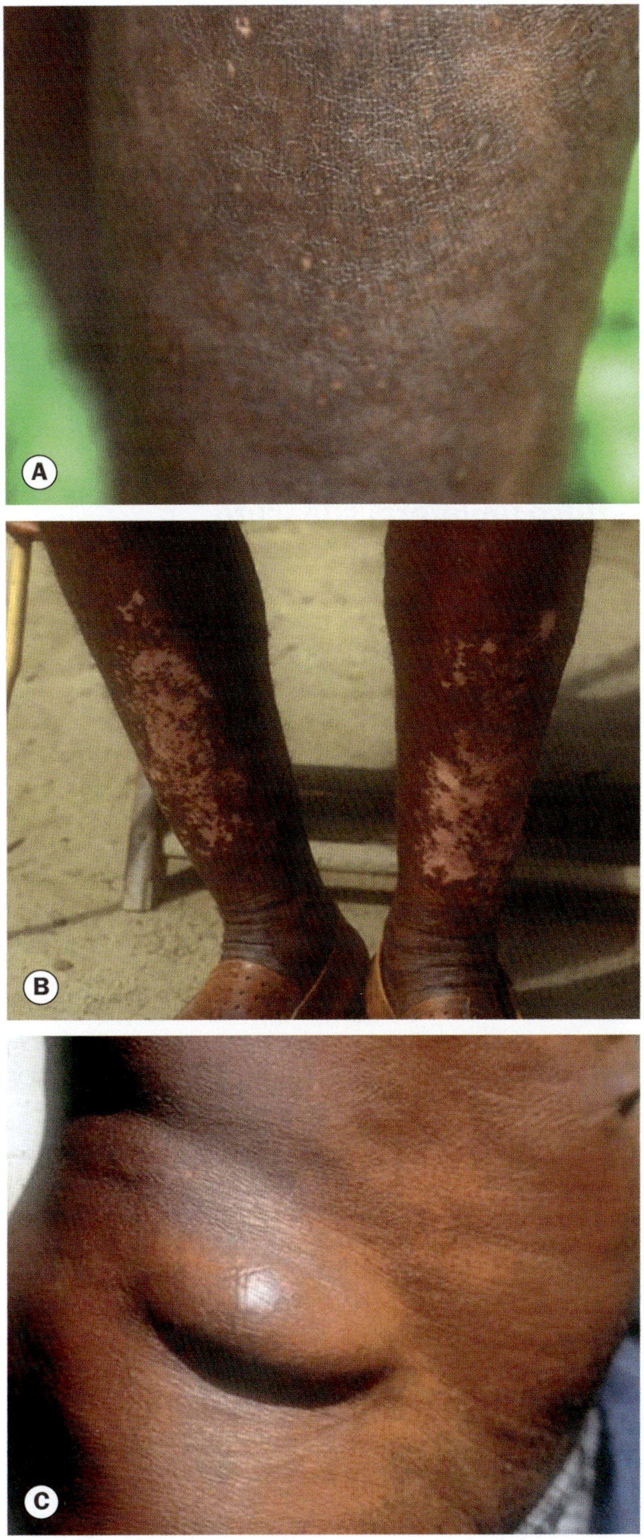

Fig. 12.37 Onchocerciasis systemic features. **(A)** Maculopapular rash; **(B)** 'leopard skin'; **(C)** subcutaneous nodule (onchocercoma). *(Courtesy of C Gilbert.)*

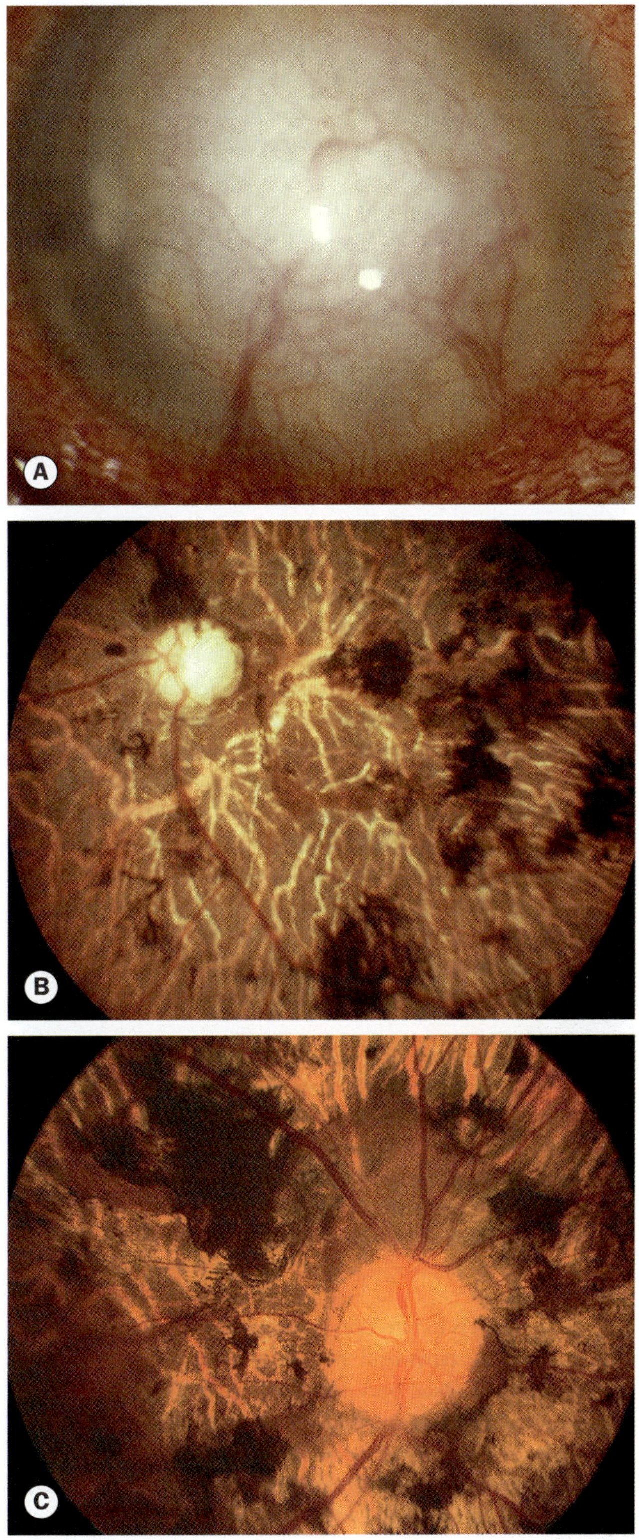

Fig. 12.38 Ocular onchocerciasis. **(A)** Corneal scarring; **(B)** intraretinal pigment clumping and RPE atrophy; **(C)** choroidal pigment clumping and chorioretinal atrophy.

- **Keratitis.** Punctate keratitis (snowflake opacities) affects a third of patients and consists of infiltrates surrounding dead microfilariae. Initial lesions are most commonly located at 3 and 9 o'clock in the anterior third of the stroma. Slowly progressing sclerosing keratitis may eventually involve the entire cornea (Fig. 12.38A).
- **Chorioretinitis** is usually bilateral and predominantly involves the temporal fundus, sparing the macula until late. Widespread choroidal sclerosis and atrophy can ensue (Fig. 12.38B and C). A perpetuating autoimmune response is hypothesized for progressive longer-term chorioretinopathy that may persist after control of infection.
- **Optic neuritis** may be acute.

Treatment

- **Ivermectin** (supplied in many countries by Merck at no charge) kills microfilariae (but not adult worms) and is given at least annually for many years. It has been effective in substantially reducing transmission rates and morbidity and no recent new cases have been reported in many communities. Ivermectin occasionally precipitates inflammation, so prophylactic prednisolone may be considered in patients with visible AC microfilariae. Ivermectin may cause toxic encephalopathy in patients with *Loa loa* infection.
- **Moxidectin** is a newer drug that may be superior to ivermectin.
- **Doxycycline** 100–200 mg per day for 6 weeks targets *Wolbachia*, indirectly preventing microfilarial embryogenesis and substantially reducing numbers for an extended period. It also has some effect on adult worms and may be a useful adjunct to ivermectin or moxidectin.
- **Suramin** is effective against adult worms. It is given intravenously.
- **Steroids.** Anterior uveitis is responsive.

TIP Ivermectin given annually is effective in reducing transmission rates and ocular morbidity in onchocerciases.

Cysticercosis

Introduction

Cysticercosis refers to infection by *Cysticercus cellulosae*, the larval form of the pork tapeworm *Taenia solium*. Ingesting cysts of *T. solium* in undercooked pork leads to intestinal tapeworm development (taeniasis). The infested human then sheds eggs that lead to larval infection (cysticercosis) when ingested by the same or another individual. Inflammation develops in response to antigens released by dead organisms.

Clinical features

- **Systemic disease** may involve the lungs, muscle and CNS (neurocysticercosis). MRI and CT imaging are effective at demonstrating cysts and plain X-rays may show calcified cysts. Serology and stool analysis are useful for diagnosis.
- **Ocular features** include cysts of the conjunctiva and rarely the AC may show a free-floating cyst (Fig. 12.39A). Larvae can enter the subretinal space (Fig. 12.39B) and may cause exudative retinal detachment (Fig. 12.39C). They can also pass into the vitreous where released toxins can incite an intense vision-threatening inflammatory reaction. A cyst may occasionally involve the orbit, eyelids or rectus muscle (Fig. 12.39D).

Treatment

Systemic steroids to control inflammation are combined with surgical removal of the larvae from the AC, vitreous and subretinal space. Anthelmintic agents such as albendazole may be appropriate in systemic disease, but should be used with caution under specialist guidance and often with steroid co-administration.

Diffuse unilateral subacute neuroretinitis (DUSN)

Introduction

DUSN is a clinical syndrome due to the presence of a single motile subretinal nematode such as *Toxocara canis*, *Baylisascaris procyonis* and *Ancylostoma caninum*. Misdiagnosis (e.g. multifocal choroiditis) is common as the worm is often small and may be overlooked.

Clinical features

- **Presentation** is with insidious monocular visual decrease. The disease is diagnosed clinically as special investigations are not helpful. Electroretinography (ERG) is subnormal, even in early disease.
- **Acute disease.** Crops of grey–white outer retinal lesions (Fig. 12.40),vitritis, papillitis and retinal vasculitis.
- **End-stage disease.** Optic atrophy, retinal vascular attenuation and diffuse RPE degeneration.

Treatment

Photocoagulation (200 μm, 0.2–0.5 s, 150–300 mW) is the treatment of choice when a worm can be visualized (<50%). If necessary, a slit beam or very light laser burns are first used to shepherd (sometimes lure) the photosensitive nematode away from the fovea. Systemic albendazole (400 mg for 30 days) or vitrectomy may be appropriate in some cases. Steroid cover may be prudent with all treatment modalities.

VIRAL UVEITIS

Uveitis in human immunodeficiency virus infection

Introduction

Human immunodeficiency virus infection/acquired immunodeficiency syndrome (HIV/AIDS) is transmitted by unprotected sexual intercourse, via contaminated blood or needles and vertically from mother to child transplacentally, during birth or breastfeeding. HIV depletes $CD4^+$ T cells, which are vital to the initiation of

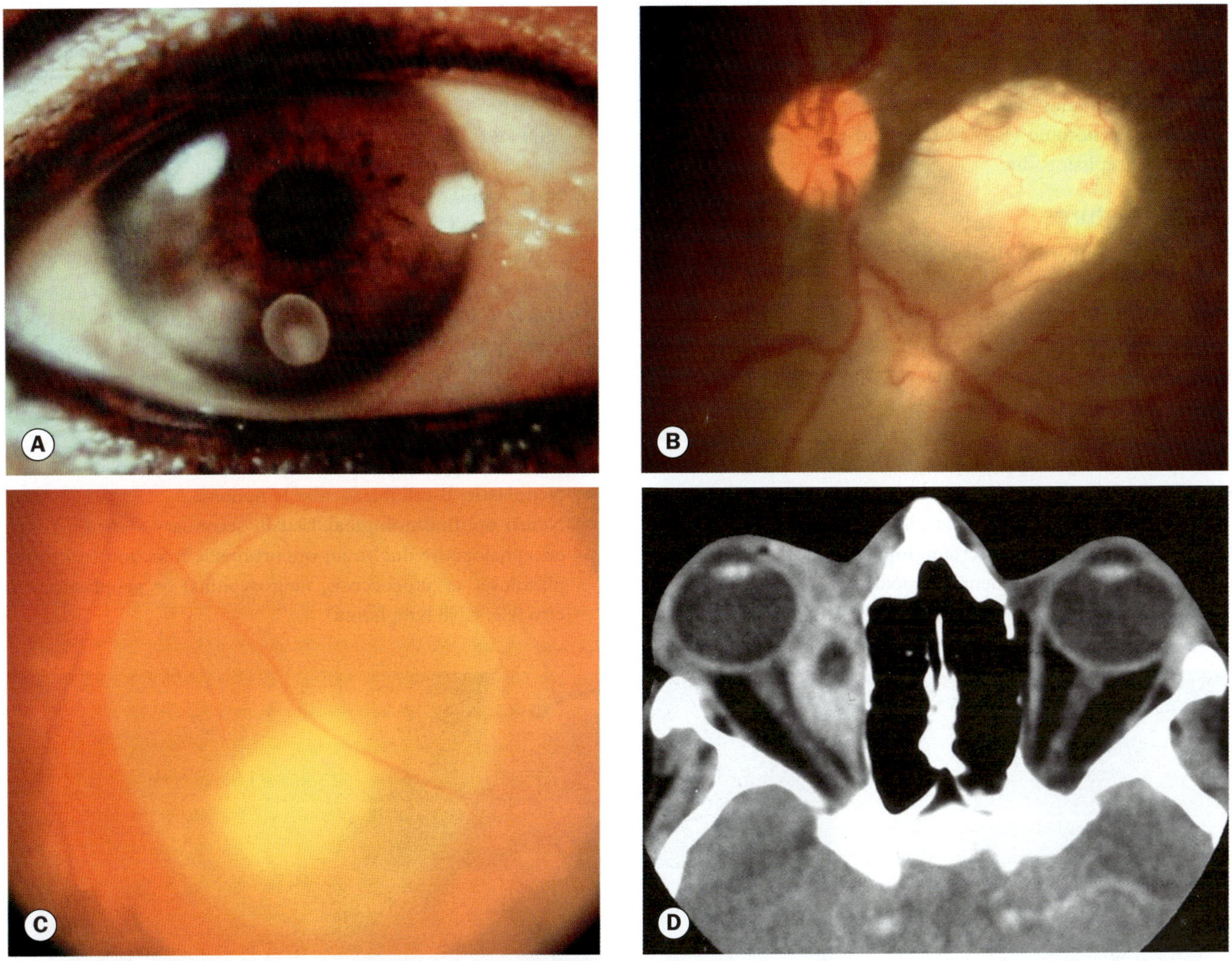

Fig. 12.39 Ocular cysticercosis. **(A)** Anterior chamber cyst; **(B)** subretinal cyst showing tract of the larva; **(C)** subretinal cyst with overlying exudative retinal detachment; **(D)** axial CT scan showing a cyst in the right medial rectus muscle. *(Courtesy of Dr RSR Naik – fig. A; A Pearson – fig. C.)*

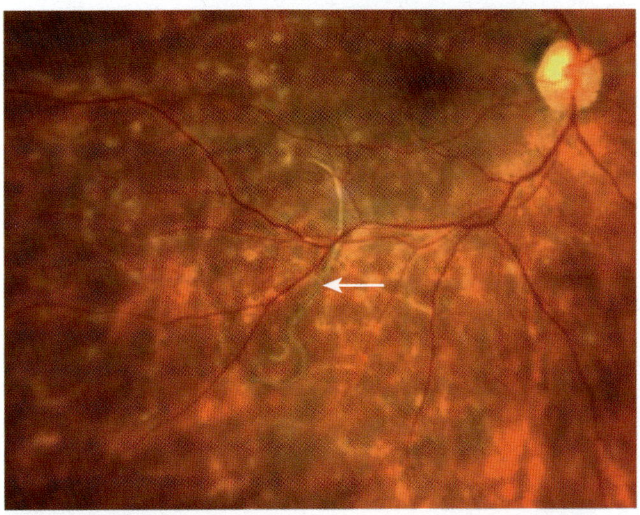

Fig. 12.40 Diffuse unilateral subacute neuroretinitis showing subretinal nematode (arrow) and multifocal grey–white spots. *(Courtesy of SR Rathinam.)*

the immune response to pathogens. Although there is currently no cure or vaccine, the progression of disease can be slowed radically by combination drug therapy: antiretroviral therapy (ART). ART is now recommended for all HIV-positive individuals irrespective of $CD4^+$ T cell count. Prophylaxis against opportunistic infections may also be instituted.

Systemic features

- **Stages of infection**: (a) a flu-like illness may occur 2–4 weeks after infection, sometimes including a rash; (b) clinical latency is a predominantly asymptomatic period of several (average 8) years, sometimes with minor clinical features such as persistent generalized lymphadenopathy; (c) AIDS develops in about half of HIV-positive individuals within 10 years and is defined as HIV infection with either a $CD4^+$ T count <200 cells/µl or the development of one or more AIDS-defining conditions.
- **AIDS-defining clinical conditions** include particular opportunistic infections such as respiratory or oesophageal

candidiasis, *Pneumocystis jirovecii* pneumonia (Fig. 12.41A), cryptosporidiosis and cytomegalovirus retinitis, specific tumours including Kaposi sarcoma (Fig. 12.41B) and certain lymphomas and other manifestations such as HIV wasting syndrome (Fig. 12.41C) and progressive multifocal leukoencephalopathy.

Ocular features

- **Eyelid.** Blepharitis, Kaposi sarcoma, multiple molluscum lesions and herpes zoster ophthalmicus.
- **Orbit.** Cellulitis (e.g. aspergillosis, contiguous sinus infection), B-cell lymphoma.
- **Conjunctiva.** Kaposi sarcoma, squamous cell carcinoma and microvasculopathy (up to 80%).
- **Cornea.** Keratoconjunctivitis sicca and an increased incidence of keratitis, e.g. herpes simplex and zoster and fungal.
- **Anterior uveitis** associated with ocular infections, or (commonly) with drug toxicity, e.g. rifabutin, cidofovir.
- **HIV-related retinal microangiopathy.** Retinal microangiopathy is the most frequent retinopathy in patients with AIDS, developing in up to 70% of patients. It is associated with a declining $CD4^+$ T cell count and higher plasma HIV-RNA levels and is a marker for increased cytomegalovirus (CMV) retinitis risk. Postulated causes include immune complex deposition, HIV infection of the retinal vascular endothelium and abnormalities of flow. It manifests with cotton-wool spots and/or retinal haemorrhages (Fig. 12.41D) and sometimes capillary abnormalities such as microaneurysms. In contrast to CMV retinitis, lesions are usually asymptomatic and almost invariably disappear spontaneously after several weeks.
- **Other viral retinitis**: cytomegalovirus retinitis (most common), progressive retinal necrosis, acute retinal necrosis.
- **Protozoal**: *Toxoplasma* retinochoroiditis, often atypical.
- **Fungal**: *Pneumocystis* choroiditis, *Histoplasma* chorioretinitis, cryptococcal choroiditis, candidiasis.
- **Bacterial**: syphilis, tuberculosis.
- **Neoplastic**: B-cell intraocular lymphoma.
- **Neuro-ophthalmological.** Usually secondary to meningitis or encephalopathy due to an opportunistic infection (e.g. toxoplasmosis, cryptococcosis, neurosyphilis) or neoplastic process (e.g. CNS lymphoma).

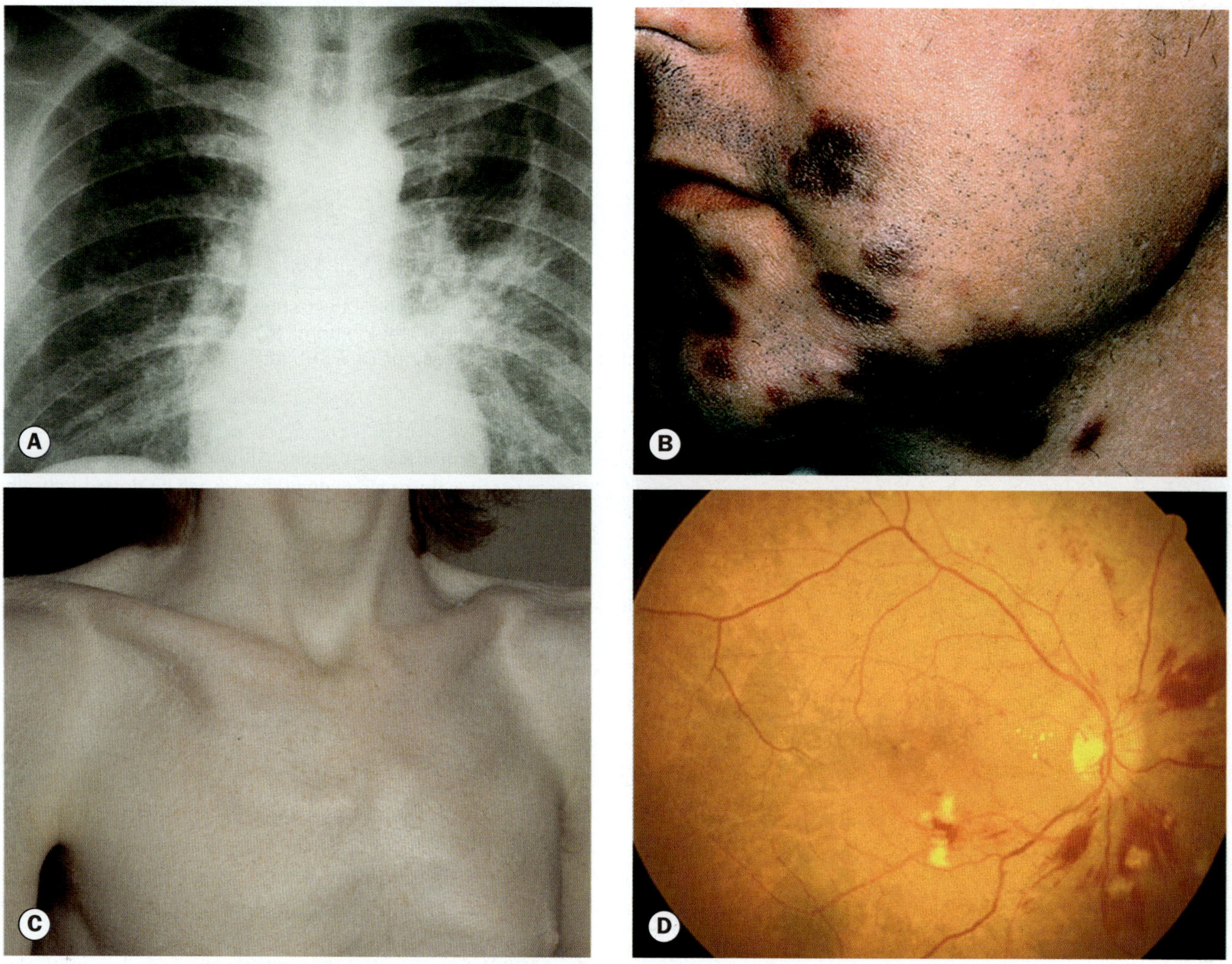

Fig. 12.41 Complications of AIDS. **(A)** X-ray showing *Pneumocystis* pneumonia; **(B)** Kaposi sarcoma; **(C)** HIV wasting syndrome; **(D)** HIV microangiopathy.

TIP Retinal microangiopathy is associated with a declining CD4 T-cell count and is a marker for increased risk of developing cytomegalovirus retinitis.

Cytomegalovirus retinitis

Introduction

Infection with cytomegalovirus (CMV), a herpesvirus, is very common in the general population, causing no or minimal constitutional symptoms in most healthy individuals. CMV retinitis is seen in patients immunocompromised from a variety of causes. It is a common opportunistic ocular infection in patients with AIDS, in whom it may represent reactivation of latent infection. Without treatment, severe visual loss is essentially inevitable. Since the advent of ART the incidence and severity have declined, though the prevalence remains high, partly due to increasing survival rates in AIDS patients in whom systemic steroid therapy may be a risk factor. There is a very strong association with a low $CD4^+$ count.

Systemic features

Severe involvement of a range of organs including the lungs, CNS and skin can occur in the immunocompromised.

Ocular features

- **Presentation** is with reduced vision from macular involvement or with floaters from vitritis. One eye is usually affected initially, progressing to both eyes in 50% of patients if untreated. Indolent retinitis (see below) frequently starts in the periphery without symptoms and progresses over weeks.
- **Anterior uveitis** can occur but is usually mild with little or no injection. It is considered separately later in this chapter.
- **Cataract** is a common later-stage finding.
- **Vitritis** is typically mild, except in immune recovery (see below).
- **Retinitis.** The characteristic appearance is of one or two areas of dense white retinal infiltration associated prominently with flame-shaped retinal haemorrhages ('pizza pie' or 'Margherita pizza'), beginning peripherally (centrally in 10%) and extending along the course of the vascular arcades (Fig. 12.42A). Peripheral areas tend to appear granular, with fewer rounder haemorrhages and little vasculitis. Indolent (more peripheral and less aggressive – Fig. 12.42B) and fulminant clinical patterns have been distinguished (Fig. 12.42C). The visual acuity can be significantly reduced if the macula is involved.
- **Optic neuritis** may result from direct spread or from primary involvement.
- **Retinal necrosis** is evident in areas where active inflammation has settled, leaving irregular pigmentation, atrophy and holes, frequently leading to retinal detachment (Fig. 12.42D), a major cause of visual morbidity (up to 50%).
- **Frosted branch angiitis (FBA)** describes marked vascular sheathing that occurs in about 6% (see Fig. 12.42D). This appearance is seen in other conditions (see Fig. 12.71) and the term is also used for a distinct idiopathic disorder (primary FBA).
- **Immune recovery uveitis (IRU).** This is a cause of limited visual outcome in CMV retinitis, thought to be due to a rejuvenated immune response against residual viral antigen following immune reconstitution with ART. Manifestations can be severe, progressing to phthisis in some cases.

Treatment

Close liaison with an infectious disease physician is critical. **ART** is the mainstay of management, restoring the patient's innate ability to suppress CMV activity. Discontinuation of antiviral treatment is considered when the $CD4^+$ count reaches >100–150 cells/µl.

- **Valganciclovir** is a pro-drug of ganciclovir that is taken orally and is as effective for both induction (900 mg twice daily for up to 3 weeks) and maintenance (900 mg daily). Neutropenia is a common side effect due to bone marrow suppression, but can be effectively treated with filgrastim (granulocyte colony-stimulating factor).
- **Intravitreal injection** of ganciclovir (2 mg/injection), foscarnet (1.2 mg), or cidofovir (20 µg) may occasionally be indicated for lesions close to the macula or optic nerve. The marketing authorization for ganciclovir implant has been withdrawn.
- **Vitrectomy** with endolaser demarcation and silicone oil tamponade is successful in around 75% of CMV-related retinal detachments.
- **Steroids** may be required for IRU, though intravitreal and systemic administration should be used with caution.
- **Prognosis.** This is poor, despite treatment, if the macula is involved (Fig. 12.43).
- **Screening** of patients with low CD4 counts: 3-monthly if < 50/µl, 6-monthly 50–100/µl, yearly if >100/µl.

Progressive retinal necrosis

Introduction

Progressive retinal necrosis (PRN, also known as progressive or posterior outer retinal necrosis, PORN) is a rare but devastating form of necrotizing retinitis which is usually caused by varicella zoster virus (VZV) and possibly other herpesviruses. It occurs predominantly in patients with AIDS, but may be associated with other immunocompromised states, particularly drug-induced. The prognosis is extremely poor, with no perception of light the outcome in more than half of affected eyes.

Ocular features

- **Presentation** is with rapidly progressive unilateral or bilateral visual loss.
- **Anterior uveitis and vitritis are minimal**, in contrast to CMV retinitis and acute retinal necrosis (ARN) (see below).
- **Retinitis.** Three stages are recognized:
  - **Early.** Multifocal homogeneous yellow–white deep retinal infiltrates (Fig. 12.44A). The macula may be involved at an early stage, often giving a cherry-red spot.

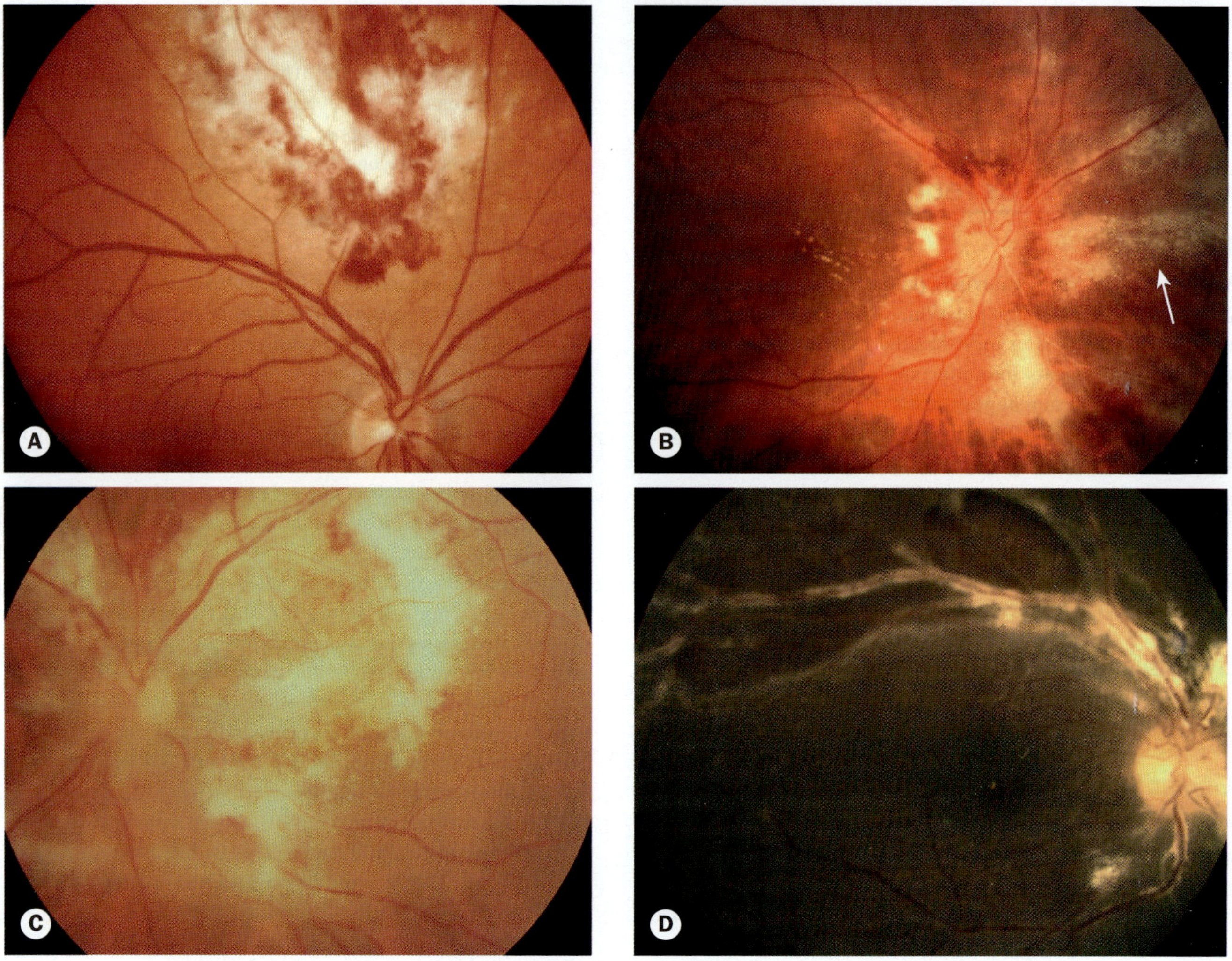

Fig. 12.42 Cytomegalovirus retinitis. **(A)** Early retinitis; **(B)** indolent retinitis with typical granular appearance (arrow) and retinal vasculitis; **(C)** advanced disease showing extensive macular exudation; **(D)** large posterior retinal tear with shallow localized detachment – there is vascular sheathing reminiscent of frosted branch angiitis. *(Courtesy of C Barry – fig. D.)*

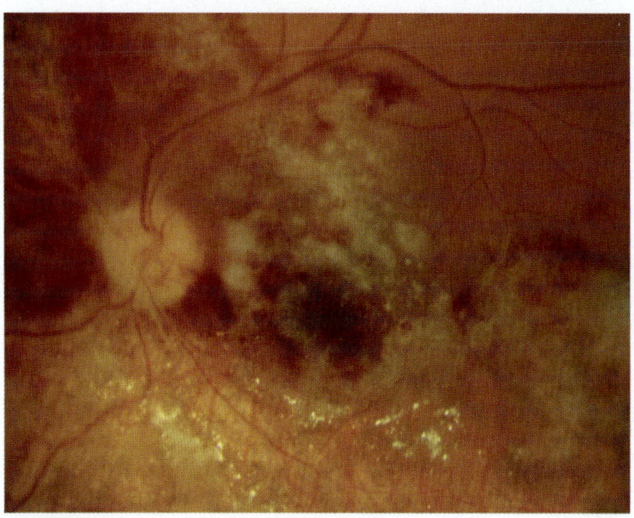

Fig. 12.43 Regressing CMV retinitis after treatment.

- **Established/middle.** The signs typically spread rapidly around the retina, with very extensive full-thickness necrosis (Fig. 12.44B). Signs of vasculitis are absent or mild and significant haemorrhage is uncommon. As inflammation clears, perivenular translucency is seen (Fig. 12.44C).
- **Late.** Retinal atrophy may follow as the arteriolar blood supply decreases (Fig. 12.44D). Rhegmatogenous retinal detachment (RRD) is common, as is optic atrophy.

Investigation

Vitreous and/or aqueous PCR assay for viral DNA; antibody assay is less effective.

Treatment

Immune rescue with ART together with aggressive antiviral therapy, e.g. intravitreal and intravenous ganciclovir and foscarnet. Vitreoretinal surgery for retinal detachment often yields poor results.

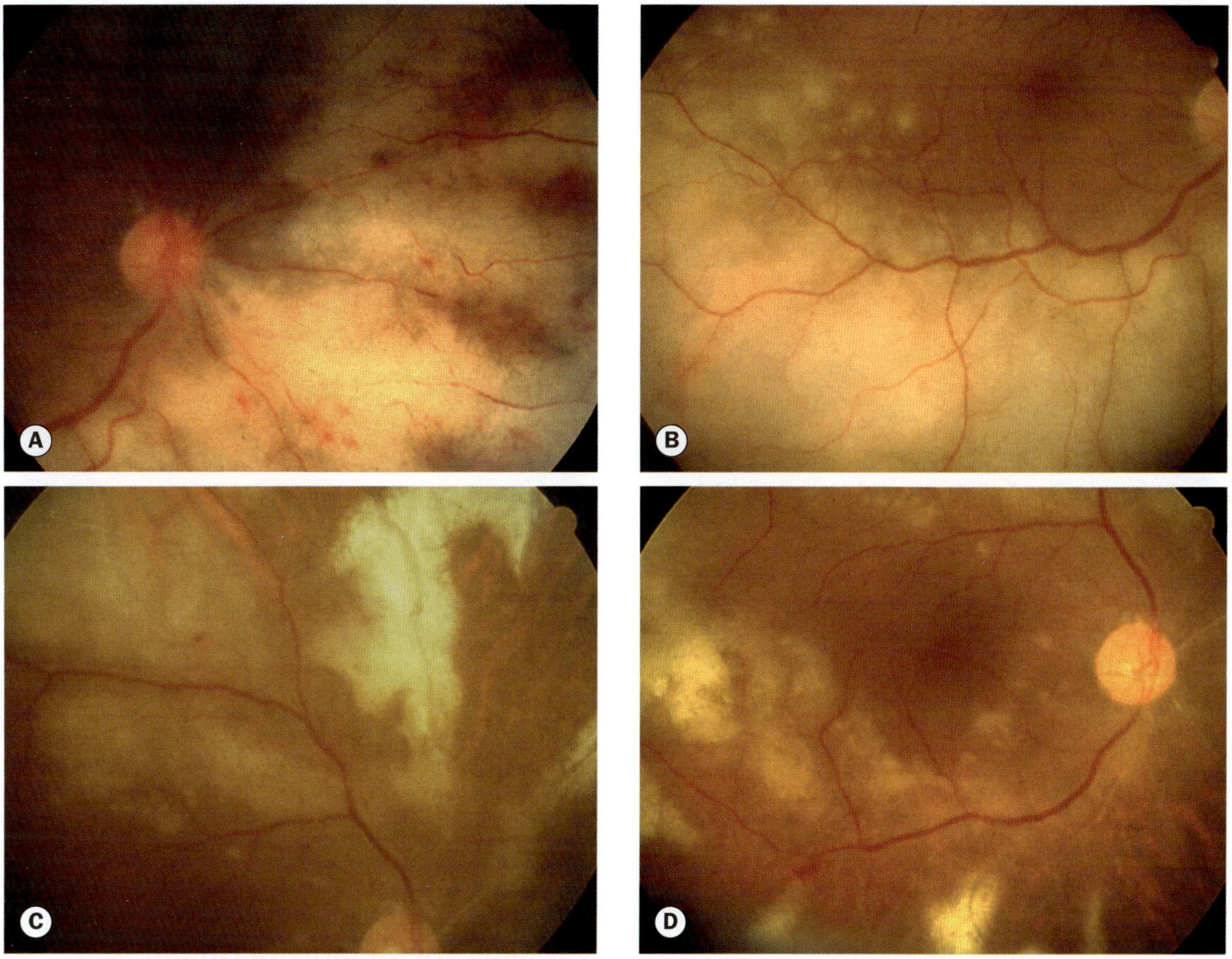

Fig. 12.44 Progressive retinal necrosis. **(A)** On presentation, showing multi-focal homogenous deep retinal infiltrates in the absence of vitritis; **(B)** pre-treatment showing deep yellow–white infiltrates with well-defined borders; **(C)** and **(D)** post-treatment showing regression of lesions, vascular attenuation and early retinal atrophy. *(Courtesy of C Herbort.)*

TIP Anterior uveitis and vitritis are minimal in a patient with progressive retinal necrosis, which is in contrast to CMV retinitis and acute retinal necrosis where significant inflammation occurs.

Acute retinal necrosis

Introduction

Acute retinal necrosis (ARN) is a rare but devastating necrotizing retinitis. It typically affects otherwise healthy individuals and tends to be caused by herpes simplex virus (HSV) in younger and VZV in older patients (other herpesviruses are also suspected). The prognosis is relatively poor, with more than half of patients eventually achieving only 6/60 as a result of retinal and optic nerve ischaemia or RRD.

- **Systemic features.** ARN has been reported following and occurring simultaneously with HSV encephalitis and herpetic skin infection.
- **Ocular features.** Presentation is initially unilateral with blurred vision and floaters. Pain is usually a feature. The American Uveitis Society criteria for diagnosis are as follows:
  - Prominent anterior uveitis and vitritis (panuveitis). Episcleritis and scleritis may occur.
  - One or more discrete foci of peripheral retinal necrosis. Deep yellow-white infiltrates with well-defined borders are seen (Fig. 12.45A). Retinal haemorrhages can occur, but are generally less prominent than in CMV retinitis. The acute lesions resolve after 6–12 weeks, leaving behind necrotic retina with hyperpigmented borders (Fig. 12.45B). Secondary RRD is a major cause of visual morbidity.
  - Circumferential spread of retinal involvement. Posterior pole involvement is late. Optic neuritis is sometimes a feature.
  - Occlusive retinal vasculitis including arteritis. Preretinal neovascularization can develop and may lead to vitreous haemorrhage.

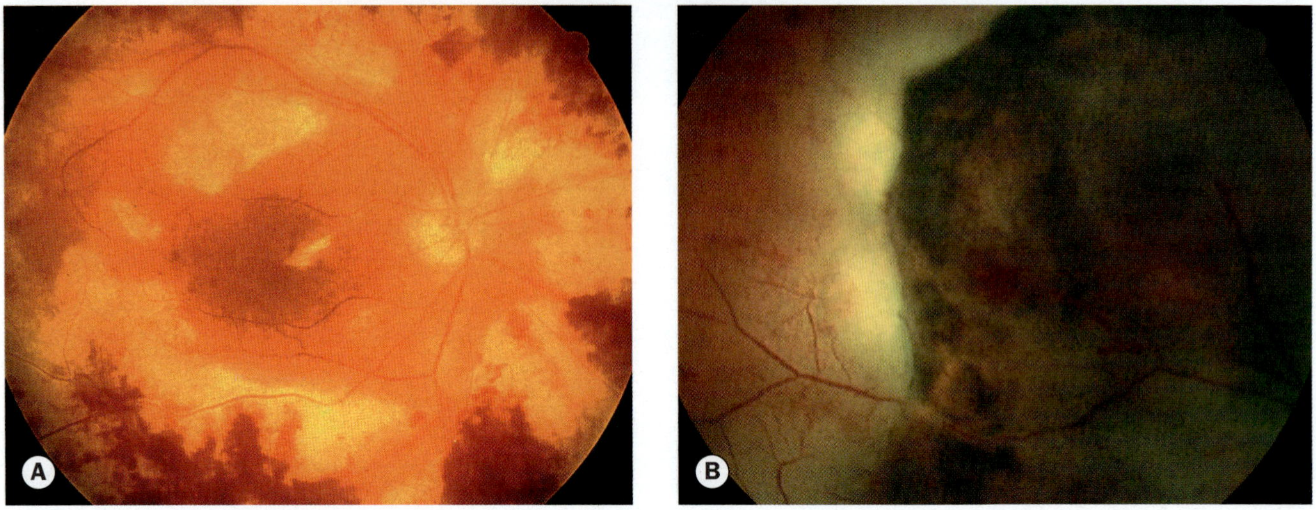

Fig. 12.45 Acute retinal necrosis. **(A)** Advanced disease reaching the posterior pole; **(B)** full-thickness retinal necrosis. *(Courtesy of C Barry – fig. B.)*

- Rapid progression of disease in the absence of treatment.

Investigation

Vitreous and/or aqueous PCR assay for viral DNA. Antibody assay is less effective.

Treatment

- **Aciclovir**: intravenously (15 mg/kg every 8 hours) for 10–14 days and then orally 800 mg five times daily for 6–12 weeks. This may hasten resolution of the acute retinal lesions and dramatically reduces the risk of second eye involvement. Long-term therapy is occasionally required.
- **Oral valaciclovir or famciclovir** may be substituted for oral aciclovir, with similar outcomes but better tolerability. Valaciclovir 2 g, orally, three times daily can be used as an induction dose, followed by a maintenance dose of 1 g, orally, three times daily.
- **Intravitreal ganciclovir or foscarnet** may improve the prognosis.
- **Systemic steroids** may be started 24 hours after initiation of antiviral therapy, especially in severe cases.
- **Laser retinopexy** around necrotic areas has been used in the past, but has no effect on the retinal detachment rate and should be avoided.
- **Vitrectomy** for RRD, commonly with silicone oil tamponade.

Herpes simplex anterior uveitis

Introduction

Anterior uveitis may occur with or without active corneal disease (see Ch. 7). Patchy and occasionally sectoral iris atrophy that includes the pigment epithelium (Fig. 12.46A) is common, as is elevated IOP. The pupil may be larger than its fellow. As in Fuchs uveitis syndrome (FUS), KPs may be fine, stellate and diffusely distributed across the cornea, but can also be large and grouped. There is often a past history of herpes simplex keratitis, cold sores and sometimes genital herpes. Recurrent episodes of herpetic iritis involve the same eye in almost all patients. Distinguishing herpetic from cytomegalovirus iridocyclitis (see below) can be difficult.

Treatment

Topical steroids (e.g. prednisolone acetate 1% four times daily) and a topical cycloplegic, in combination with an oral antiviral, e.g. aciclovir 400 mg five times a day. There is evidence that famciclovir or valaciclovir is better tolerated than aciclovir. Steroids may be delayed and used with caution if active epithelial disease is present, when a topical antiviral may be added. Raised IOP is treated as necessary.

Varicella zoster virus (VZV) anterior uveitis

Introduction

Anterior uveitis of variable severity occurs in around 50% of patients with herpes zoster ophthalmicus (HZO) and generally starts 1–3 weeks after the acute skin rash (occasionally in patients with HZO without dermatitis – zoster sine herpete). Zoster-associated iridocyclitis may be recurrent, when diagnosis is usually straightforward due to a past history of ipsilateral HZO. As with herpes simplex, signs may be of granulomatous inflammation. Sectoral iris atrophy is often present (Fig. 12.46B), corneal sensation may be reduced and IOP raised. PCR analysis of aqueous is indicated exceptionally. Anterior segment inflammation can occur in primary VZV infection (chickenpox), particularly in the immunocompromised; neuroretinitis is rare. Uveitis has been reported following VZV vaccination.

Treatment

Topical steroids and mydriatics, in addition to standard systemic antiviral treatment of shingles. Systemic steroids are required rarely (e.g. optic neuritis). All patients with HZO must be monitored by an ophthalmologist dependent on severity, e.g. up to weekly for at least 6 weeks to detect occult ocular inflammation and subsequently possibly long-term to detect late complications.

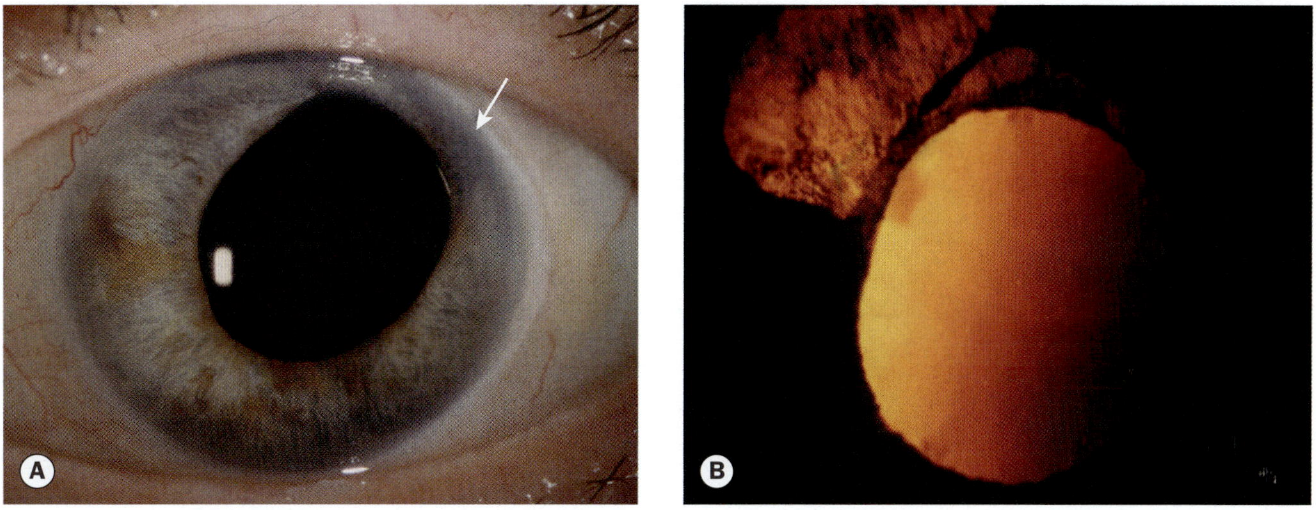

Fig. 12.46 **(A)** Iris atrophy (arrow) with corectopia in herpes simplex anterior uveitis; **(B)** sectoral iris atrophy in herpes zoster anterior uveitis.

Persistence or recurrence of anterior uveitis may respond to a week-long course of aciclovir 800 mg five times a day and long-term systemic antiviral prophylactic treatment may be considered for repeated recurrence. VZV vaccination offers protection against shingles. See also Chapter 7.

Cytomegalovirus anterior uveitis

Introduction

Cytomegalovirus (CMV) iridocyclitis in the immunocompetent is more common than previously realized, albeit still less prevalent than HSV- and VZV-related inflammation. It may be recurrent or chronic and unilateral or bilateral. Elevated IOP is very common. CMV has been reported as a cause of Posner–Schlossman syndrome (see Ch. 11). Little or no ciliary injection, limited flare, few cells, corneal endotheliitis, KP of a range of morphology and sectoral iris atrophy have been reported. PS are rare. A key diagnostic indicator, in some cases only, may be a failure to respond to aciclovir and/or steroids. PCR and antibody assay of an aqueous sample should be considered if there is clinical suspicion.

Treatment

Oral valganciclovir in proven infection, which sometimes requires long-term continuation. IOP elevation may be persistent.

Rubella

Rubella (German measles) is a common childhood infection and usually follows a benign and short-lived course. However, transplacental transmission of virus to the fetus from an infected mother can lead to congenital abnormalities of multiple organ systems, with severity generally worse the earlier in gestation infection occurs. Latent rubella virus may cause CAU relatively unresponsive to steroids and has been implicated in the causation of FUS. Reported ocular features of congenital rubella include cataract, anterior uveitis, 'salt and pepper' pigmentary retinopathy (Fig. 12.47A and B), glaucoma and microphthalmos.

Measles and subacute sclerosing panencephalitis

Congenital infection with the measles virus can cause spontaneous abortion or congenital systemic and ocular anomalies including cataract and retinopathy. Infection acquired in childhood typically features conjunctivitis and epithelial keratitis. Occasionally retinitis with macular and disc oedema can occur. Subacute sclerosing panencephalitis (SSPE) is a rare progressive degenerative disease of the CNS. The condition usually affects children and teenagers. The onset of symptoms is 6–15 years after infection with measles. The disease classically manifests initially with personality change and behavioral problems, followed some months later by involuntary choreoathetoid movements and myoclonus. Further neurological deterioration slowly occurs and eventually death follows. Papilloedema, nystagmus and optic neuritis can occur during the course of the disease. Posterior uveitis is common and may be the presenting feature. Ischaemic retinal vein occlusion secondary to vasculitis has been reported but is rare (Fig. 12.48A). The classical macular lesion appears white or grey–white, resolving to leave areas of scarring and irregular RPE atrophy (Fig. 12.48B).

Mumps

Iridocyclitis and interstitial keratitis are rare complications of mumps.

Vaccinia

Smallpox vaccination using the vaccinia virus has been resumed for some groups as a result of the perceived risk of bioterrorism. Though rare, a range of anterior segment manifestations has been described, both from autoinoculation in vaccines and in close contacts.

Zika

Zika virus is transmitted by an infected *Aedes* mosquito. The virus can be passed from a pregnant woman to her fetus, resulting in

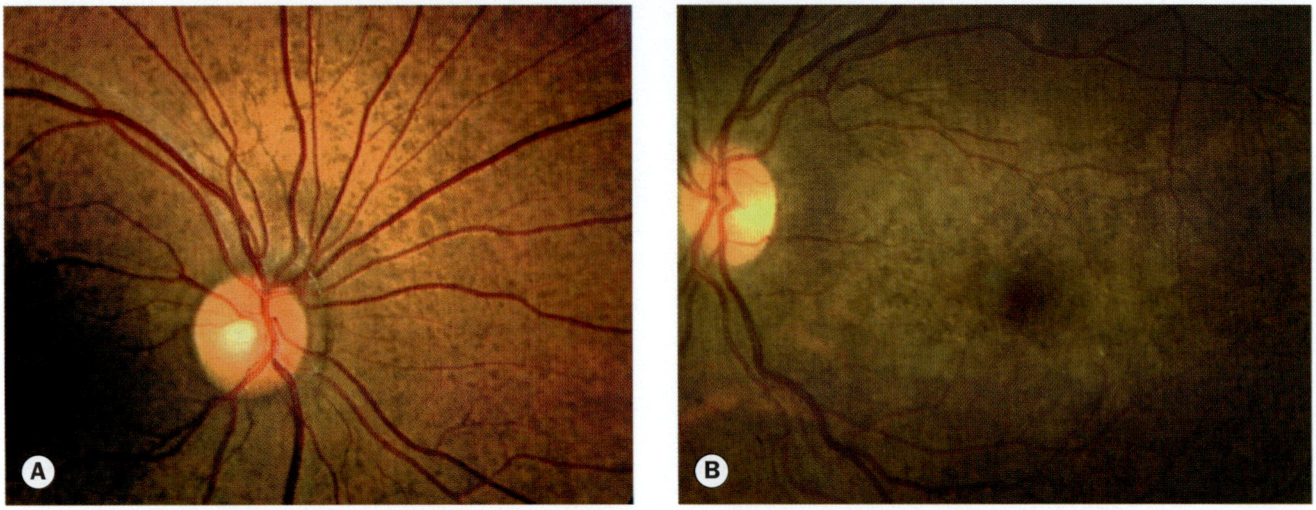

Fig. 12.47 Rubella retinopathy. **(A)** 'Salt and pepper' appearance; **(B)** predominantly manifesting in the macula.

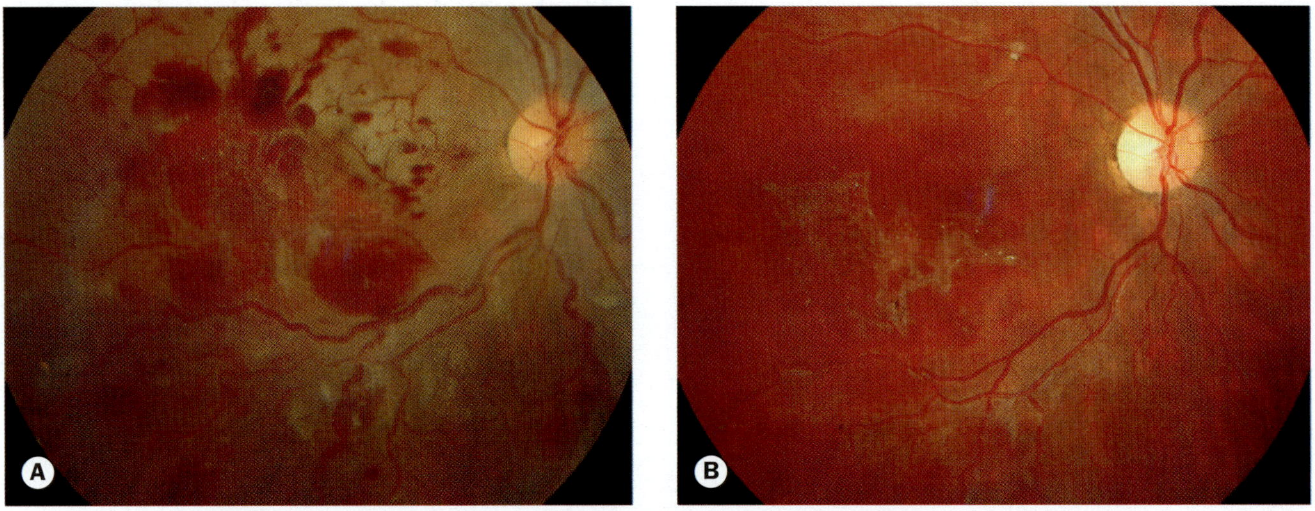

Fig. 12.48 Subacute sclerosing panencephalitis. **(A)** Retinal vein occlusion secondary to vasculitis in a 16-year-old girl; **(B)** 11 months later showing subtle optic atrophy, resorbing haemorrhages, macular scarring and irregular RPE atrophy. *(Courtesy of ADN Murray.)*

significant birth defects, including microcephaly. In congenital Zika, ocular effects include chorioretinal and macular atrophy, focal pigmentary changes in the macular region, optic nerve abnormality and glaucoma. In adults with an acute infection, conjunctivitis is the most common ocular manifestation, followed by uveitis. The virus may persist in the lacrimal gland and in other tissues of the eye, particularly in the retinal pigment epithelium.

Ebola

The Ebola virus, which is responsible for epidemics in West Africa, has the potential to cause clinical disease in sporadic outbreaks. In survivors, 'post-Ebola virus disease syndrome' (PEVDS) may result in ocular disease, arthritis, hearing loss, abdominal pain and neuropsychiatric disorders. Uveitis occurs in up to one-third of survivors and may result in acute or chronic visual loss. This can manifest as anterior, posterior or panuveitis, with most cases occurring within 2 months of discharge. Up to 15% subsequently develop a cataract. Optic nerve swelling has been reported to occur in 10% of survivors. The virus has been detected in the aqueous in the acute situation and can infect and persist in retinal pigment epithelial cells. Treatment with topical and oral corticosteroids is effective but needs to be started at the onset of symptoms to prevent long-term visual loss.

FUNGAL UVEITIS

Presumed ocular histoplasmosis syndrome (POHS)

Introduction

Histoplasma capsulatum infection occurs following inhalation of the yeast form of this dimorphic fungus and can lead to the systemic mycosis histoplasmosis – pulmonary involvement is the most common feature. It is common in AIDS. POHS is relatively common

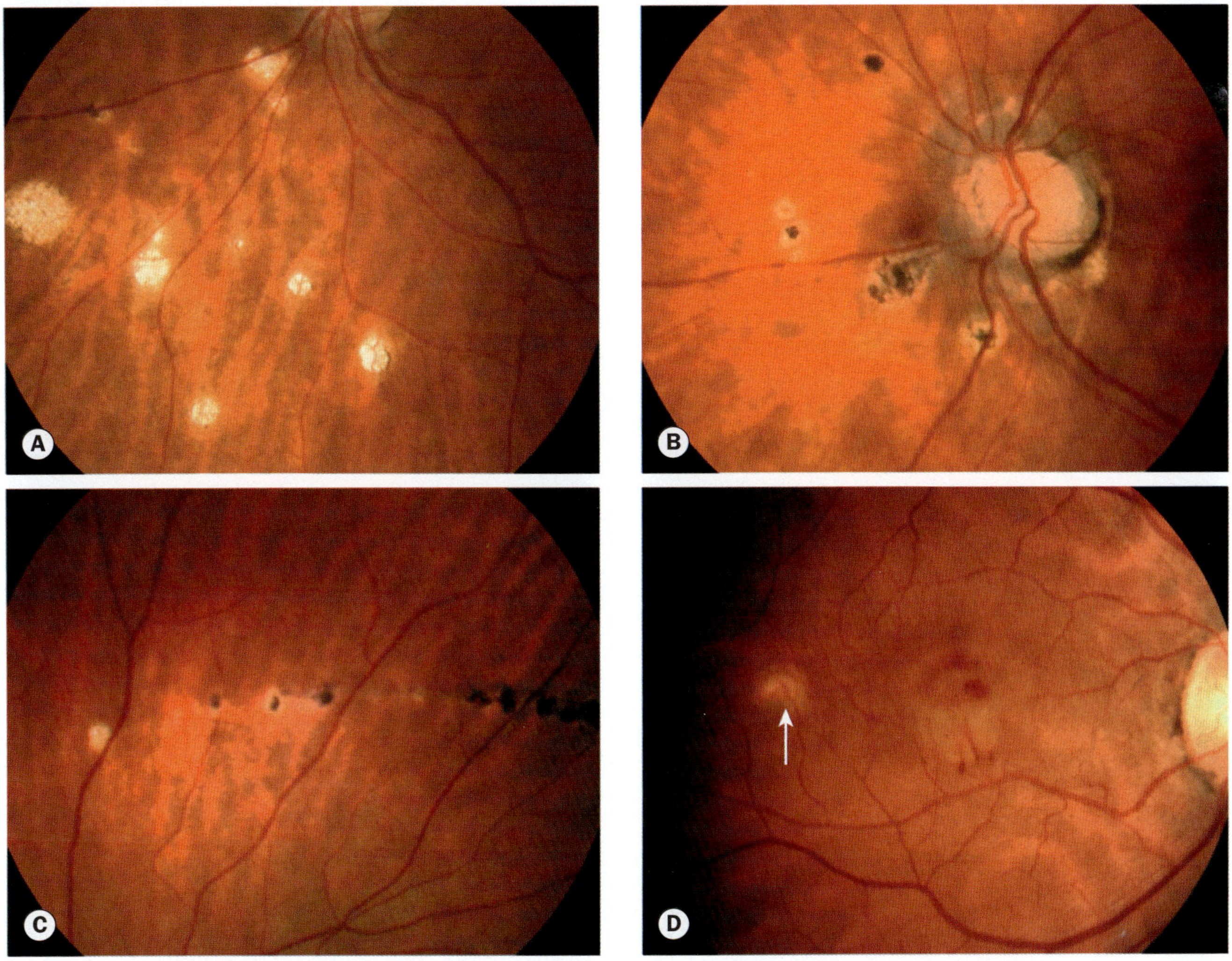

Fig. 12.49 Presumed ocular histoplasmosis syndrome. **(A)** Peripheral 'histo' spots; **(B)** circumferential peripapillary atrophy and 'histo' spots; **(C)** linear streaks; **(D)** macular neovascularization, showing a focal area of oedema and a few haemorrhages with a small 'histo' spot temporally (arrow).

in areas of endemic histoplasmosis (e.g. the Mississippi river valley in the USA). Causality has never been definitively confirmed, but over 90% react positively to histoplasmin testing. It is believed that eye disease represents an immune-mediated response to microbial antigen, rather than immediate damage due to active infection.

Ocular features

Sixty per cent have bilateral signs.

- **Presentation.** POHS is usually asymptomatic unless macular neovascularization supervenes. Signs may be discovered at a routine eye examination.
- **Classic triad**: (a) multiple white atrophic chorioretinal 'histo' spots about 200 μm in diameter (Fig. 12.49A); (b) peripapillary atrophy (Fig. 12.49B); (c) vitritis is absent. Linear mid-peripheral scars (Fig. 12.49C) also occur (5%).
- **Macular neovascularization** (MNV) is a late manifestation occurring in less than 5% of affected eyes. It is usually associated with a pre-existing macular histo spot. Associated subretinal fluid and haemorrhage lead to a fall in vision (Fig. 12.49D).
- **Acute chorioretinitis** is almost always asymptomatic and rarely identified, but discrete oval–round whitish lesions <400 μm in diameter that may develop into classic punched-out histo spots have been described.

Investigations

Skin testing is no longer undertaken.

- **HLA testing.** POHS is associated with HLA-B7 and DRw2.
- **Serological testing** is helpful if positive, but is usually negative in the absence of systemic mycosis.
- **FA and OCT** when MNV is suspected.

Treatment

Spontaneous regression of MNV may occasionally occur, but without treatment 60% of eyes with MNV have a final visual acuity of less than 6/60.

- Intravitreal anti-vascular endothelial growth factor (VEGF) injection for MNV.
- Amsler grid testing of the fellow eye at least weekly, particularly if a macular histo spot is present (25% risk of MNV).

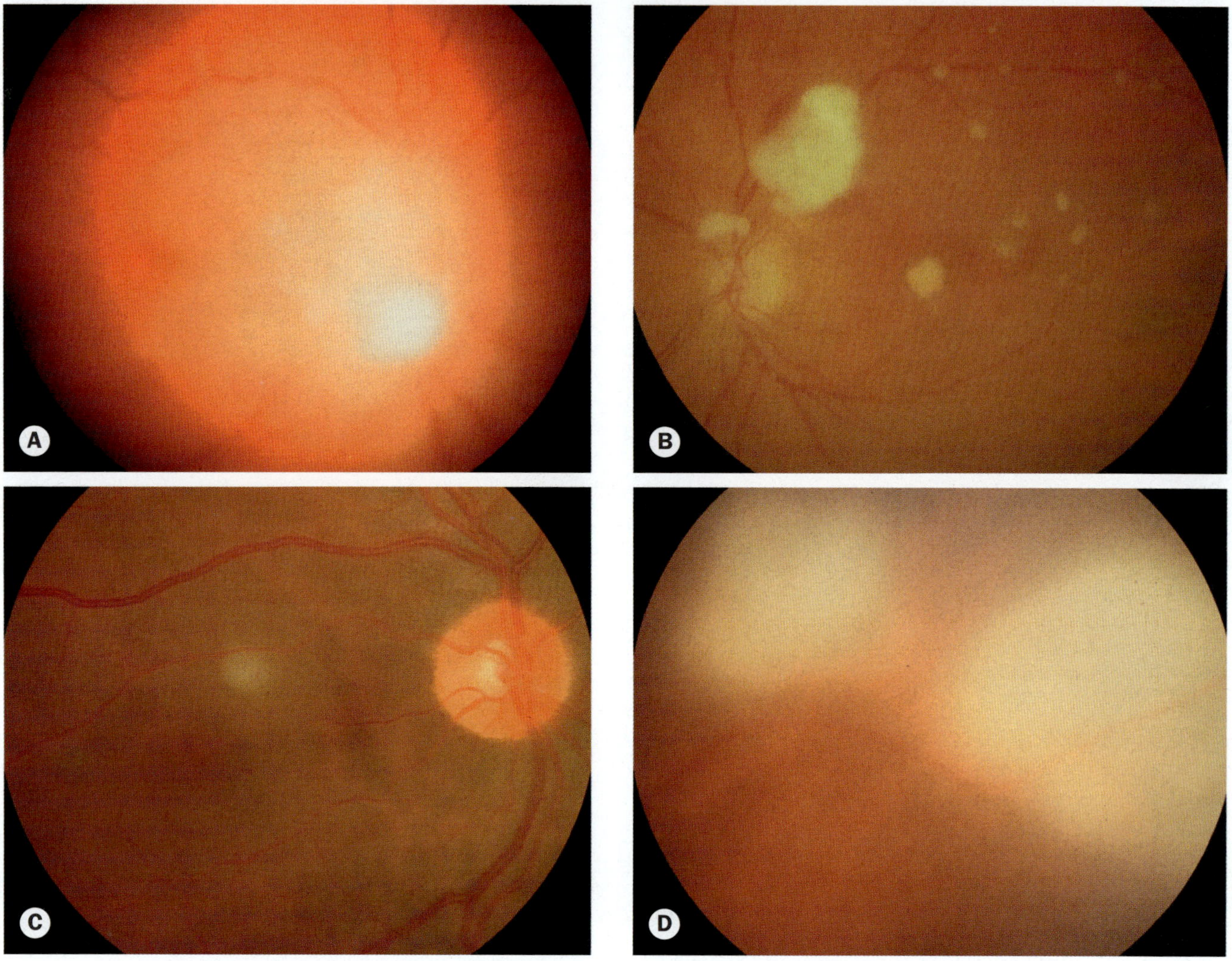

Fig. 12.50 *Candida* endophthalmitis. **(A)** Severe vitritis; **(B)** 'cotton ball' colonies; **(C)** focal chorioretinitis; **(D)** retinal necrosis.

Endogenous *Candida* endophthalmitis

Introduction

Candida (usually the commensal *C. albicans*) can be introduced into the eye from the external environment by trauma or surgery or can spread from fungal keratitis, but endogenous infection is an important alternative route. Risk factors for metastatic spread include intravenous drug abuse, a septic focus associated with an indwelling catheter, chronic lung disease such as cystic fibrosis, general debilitation and diabetes. It is relatively uncommon in AIDS.

TIP *Candida* endophthalmitis is often acquired from an endogenous source like an indwelling catheter or secondary to intravenous drug abuse.

Clinical features

- **Presentation.** Systemic candidiasis may already have been diagnosed. Up to a third of patients with untreated candidaemia will develop ocular involvement. Peripheral fundus lesions may cause little or no visual disturbance while central lesions or severe vitritis will manifest earlier. Progression is typically much slower than bacterial endophthalmitis. Bilateral involvement is common.
- **Anterior uveitis** is uncommon or mild in early disease but may become prominent later.
- **Vitritis.** May be marked (Fig. 12.50A), with fluffy 'cotton ball' (Fig. 12.50B) or 'string of pearls' colonies, sometimes progressing to abscess formation.
- **Chorioretinitis**: one or more small creamy white lesions with overlying vitritis (Fig. 12.50C). Retinal necrosis (Fig. 12.50D) may lead to retinal detachment, with severe proliferative vitreoretinopathy.

Investigation

- **Vitreous biopsy** (preferably using a vitreous cutter rather than a needle) to identify the organism (PCR and culture) and identify sensitivities.
- **Systemic investigation,** e.g. blood and urine cultures.

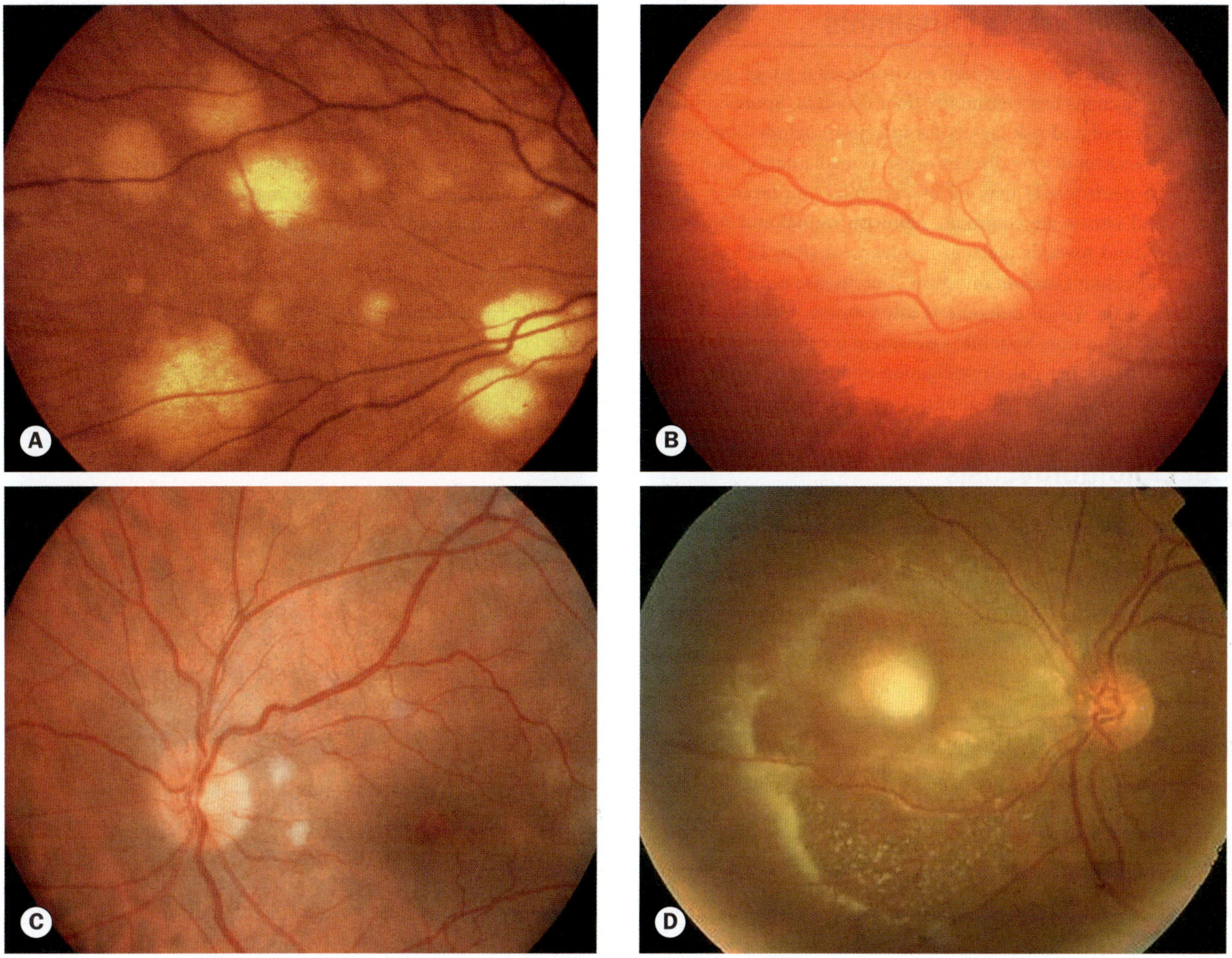

Fig. 12.51 Fungal infection with secondary uveitis. **(A)** Multifocal choroidal pneumocystosis lesions; **(B)** large coalescent pneumocystosis lesion; **(C)** multifocal cryptococcal choroiditis; **(D)** macular disease in *Aspergillus* infection. *(Courtesy of S Mitchell – fig. A; A Curi – figs C and D.)*

Treatment

- **Antifungal treatment.** The agent should be chosen with local microbiological specialist guidance. Infectious Diseases Society of America guidelines suggest intravenous amphotericin-B in combination with oral flucytosine, but resistance is a concern. Voriconazole orally or intravenously has a broad spectrum of antifungal action with low reported resistance and high ocular penetration. Adjunctive intravitreal treatment may be given (100 μg in 0.1 ml), with serial injections probably needed.
- **Pars plana vitrectomy** should be considered at an early stage, especially for severe or unresponsive disease. As well as providing a substantial culture specimen, it reduces fungal and antigen load, facilitates therapeutic agent penetration and clears the ocular media.

Pneumocystis choroiditis

The fungus *Pneumocystis jirovecii*, a pulmonary commensal, is a major cause of mortality in uncontrolled AIDS. Systemic antimicrobial prophylaxis has replaced pulmonary-only preventative treatment with inhaled pentamidine and along with immune reconstitution has dramatically reduced the incidence of *Pneumocystis* choroiditis. Multiple slowly progressing deep round yellow–orange lesions (Fig. 12.51A and B), commonly bilateral, are characteristic. There is minimal vitritis and visual loss is often negligible.

Cryptococcus choroiditis

Cryptococcus neoformans, a dimorphic yeast, enters the body through inhalation and can spread to the eye in the bloodstream or from the CNS via the optic nerve. As with pneumocystosis, cryptococcosis was formerly responsible for much morbidity, but clinically significant infection is now much less common since the advent of more effective therapy for AIDS. Ocular involvement may occur directly (e.g. multifocal choroiditis – Fig. 12.51C) with vasculitis and exudate or more commonly indirectly with papilloedema and ocular motility dysfunction.

Aspergillus endophthalmitis

Aspergillus species are common environmental fungi, but cause disease in humans less commonly than *Candida*. Spores undergo airborne spread and risk factors for infection include intravenous drug abuse, chronic lung disease, organ transplantation and blood disorders; neutropenia may be of particular importance. Iridocyclitis and vitritis are common. Yellowish retinal and subretinal infiltrates tend towards macular involvement (Fig. 12.51D) at an earlier stage than *Candida* infection. The disease progresses more rapidly and the visual outcome is often worse. Occlusive retinal vasculitis is common. Systemic assessment is critical; endocarditis presents a particular risk. Investigation and treatment are similar to that of *Candida* endophthalmitis.

Coccidioidomycosis

Coccidioides immitis acquired by inhalation usually causes a mild pulmonary infection, but wider systemic involvement can occur, and reinfection can lead to chronic lung disease. Ocular features include severe granulomatous anterior uveitis and multifocal choroiditis. Investigation and treatment are similar to that of *Candida* endophthalmitis.

BACTERIAL UVEITIS

Tuberculosis

Introduction

Tuberculosis (TB) is a chronic granulomatous infection usually caused in humans by *Mycobacterium tuberculosis*. TB is primarily a pulmonary disease but may spread by the bloodstream to other sites. Ocular involvement commonly occurs without clinically overt systemic disease. Immune deficiency is a risk factor, when atypical mycobacteria such as *M. avium* may cause disease.

Ocular features

- **Anterior uveitis** is common and is usually granulomatous. Iris nodules may be present and broad PS may form.
- **Vitritis** is very common and may be secondary to anterior, intermediate or posterior primary foci. Macular complications include cystoid oedema and epiretinal membrane formation.
- **Choroidal granuloma (tubercle)**: focal elevated dome-shaped lesions (Fig. 12.52A) that may be unilateral or bilateral and solitary or multiple (Fig. 12.52B). Extensive infiltration may occur in individuals with AIDS. A large abscess-like tubercle is termed a tuberculoma.
- **Choroiditis** independent of tubercles, typically multifocal and in a centrifugally spreading serpiginous pattern (serpiginoid), has increasingly been recognized (Fig. 12.53A and B). Choroiditis that tracks retinal vessels may have reasonable specificity for TB.
- **Retinal vasculitis** is preferentially venous. Retinal haemorrhages are common. Vascular occlusion with extensive ischaemia (Fig. 12.54A and B) and preretinal or disc neovascularization can occur. It is hypothesized that at least some cases of Eales disease (see Ch. 13) represent a hypersensitivity reaction to TB.
- **Other manifestations include** reddish-brown eyelid nodules (lupus vulgaris), conjunctivitis, phlyctenulosis, interstitial keratitis, scleritis, exudative retinal detachment and optic neuropathy including neuroretinitis.

Investigation

The diagnosis is often made clinically, considering evidence of previous TB exposure and other negative investigations. A systemic assessment by an appropriate specialist should be arranged.

- **A tuberculin skin test** may show a positive result within 48 hours.
- **T-SPOT.*TB*** is a blood test where the number of antimycobacterial effector T cells that produce interferon-gamma are counted. Because the test does not rely on the production of an antibody response, it can detect latent tuberculosis. The prevalence of tuberculosis in a given community influences the predictive value of the test: a sensitivity of 81% and a specificity of 86% has been reported.
- **Other investigations** include sputum testing with PCR and the interferon-gamma release assay (IGRA) blood test. This is approximately as sensitive as skin testing (80% in active disease) but has the advantage of being independent of previous BCG vaccination. HIV status must be determined. Chest X-ray, CT, positron emission tomography (PET)/CT are among other tests that may be considered.
- **Ocular.** Aqueous or vitreous sampling rarely yields demonstrable (smear – acid-fast bacilli on Ziehl–Neelsen staining – or culture – Lowenstein–Jensen medium) mycobacteria. PCR is highly specific but of variable sensitivity. OCT is useful for macular evaluation. Fluorescein angiography may be helpful in establishing whether choroiditis is active, as well as confirming preretinal neovascularization and demonstrating ischaemia. FAF allows activity staging, lesions becoming progressively hypoautofluorescent with healing.

Treatment

- **Prolonged multi-drug therapy** (often four initially) should be prescribed and monitored by a specialist with experience in systemic TB management. If ethambutol is used, monitoring for optic neuropathy should take place. Rifabutin can cause anterior uveitis. Non-adherence to treatment is common. Treatment with TB medication in patients with uveitis associated with latent TB halves the risk of uveitis recurrence and delays the onset of first recurrence.
- **Topical and systemic steroids** may be used concomitantly to reduce inflammation-induced damage, particularly in the early weeks of treatment, when they may retard paradoxical worsening of the fundus appearance.
- **Laser** may be applied to ischaemic retina to treat preretinal neovascularization.

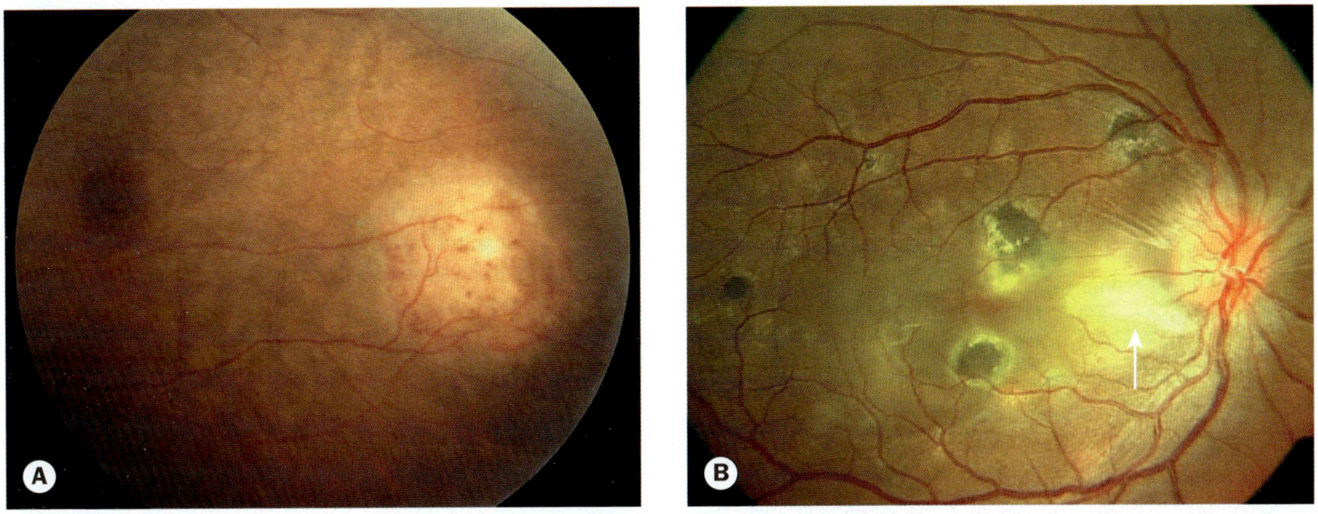

Fig. 12.52 Tuberculous choroiditis. **(A)** Choroidal granuloma; **(B)** active multifocal choroidal tuberculosis (arrow). *(Courtesy of SR Rathinam – fig. B.)*

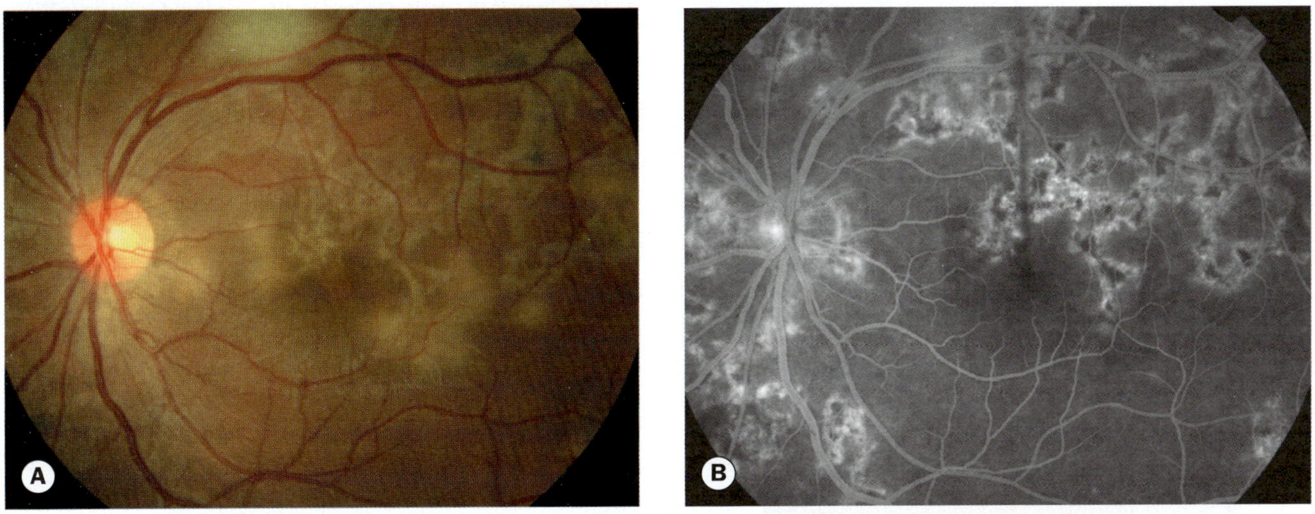

Fig. 12.53 Serpiginoid tuberculous choroiditis. **(A)** Clinical appearance – a granuloma is seen superiorly; **(B)** FA showing corresponding areas of hyper- and hypofluorescence. *(Courtesy of C Pavesio.)*

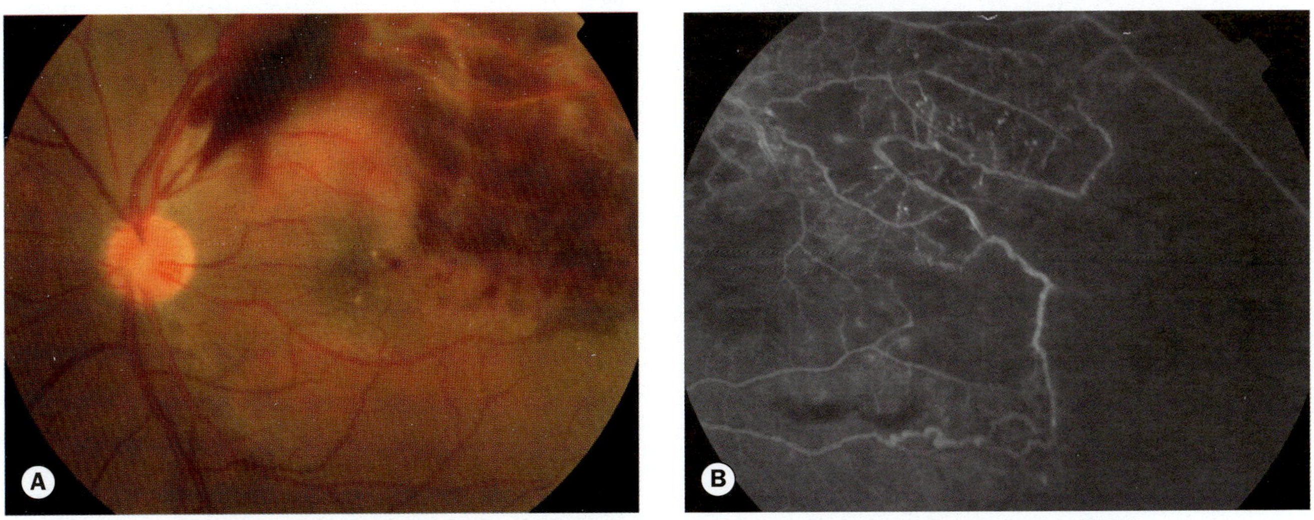

Fig. 12.54 Occlusive tuberculous periphlebitis. **(A)** Superior retinal branch occlusion; **(B)** FA showing extensive hypofluorescence due to capillary non-perfusion. *(Courtesy of C Pavesio.)*

Acquired syphilis

Introduction

Syphilis is caused by the spirochaete bacterium *Treponema pallidum*. In adults the disease is usually sexually acquired when organisms enter through a skin or mucous membrane abrasion. Transmission by kissing, blood transfusion or percutaneous injury is rare. Transplacental infection of the fetus can also occur, when the mother has become infected during or shortly before pregnancy (congenital syphilis – see Ch. 7).

Systemic features

The natural history of untreated syphilis is variable.

- **Primary syphilis** is characterized by a painless ulcer (chancre), commonly on the genitalia or anus.
- **Secondary syphilis** consists of a maculopapular rash (Fig. 12.55) and other systemic features.
- **Latent syphilis.**
- **Tertiary syphilis** occurs in about 40% of untreated cases and is characterized by cardiovascular manifestations such as aortitis, neurosyphilis and gummatous infiltration of bone and viscera.

Ocular features

- **Anterior uveitis** occurs in about 4% of patients with secondary syphilis. It may be granulomatous or non-granulomatous and is bilateral in 50%. Roseolae (Fig. 12.56A) are dilated iris capillaries that may develop into yellowish nodules. IOP may be elevated.

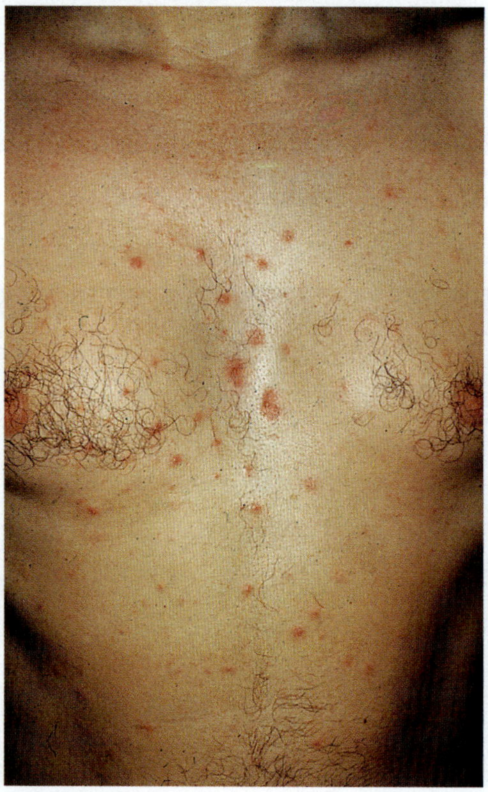

Fig. 12.55 Maculopapular rash in secondary disease in acquired syphilis.

- **Chorioretinitis** can be localized (Fig. 12.56B) but is often multifocal, bilateral and associated with vitritis and exudative retinal detachment can ensue.
- **Acute syphilitic posterior placoid chorioretinopathy (ASPPC)** is characterized by large pale-yellowish subretinal lesions in the posterior pole (Fig. 12.56C). It is thought to be a secondary infection of the choriocapillaris and occurs more commonly in the immunocompromised.
- **Retinitis** has a 'ground glass' appearance. Associated vasculitis may be occlusive and involve both arteries and veins. This heals leaving diffuse chorioretinal scars (Fig. 12.56D).
- **Optic neuritis and neuroretinitis.**
- **Other features** include conjunctivitis, episcleritis and scleritis, IU, glaucoma, cataract and miscellaneous neuro-ophthalmic features related to CNS involvement including Argyll Robertson pupils (see Ch. 19).

Investigation

- **Serology** is the mainstay and is discussed under Investigations earlier in this chapter.
- **Systemic assessment** by an appropriate specialist, including lumbar puncture to rule out neurosyphilis. HIV status should be established.
- **Aqueous and/or vitreous sampling** for PCR is sometimes indicated, such as when HIV positivity makes serology less reliable.

Treatment

This should be under the supervision of a specialist in infectious diseases, but usually consists of an extended course of parenteral penicillin. Alternatives may be required, for instance in penicillin allergy, but are less effective and parallel confirmatory allergen testing and desensitization may be considered. Topical and systemic steroids may be given in conjunction with antibiotics to ameliorate inflammatory damage. The Jarisch–Herxheimer reaction is a systemic response to treponemal antigens released on commencement of therapy and may include progression of ocular signs.

TIP Commencement of treatment for syphilis can cause an exacerbation of ocular symptoms and signs.

Lyme disease

Introduction

Lyme disease (borreliosis), like syphilis, is caused by a spirochaete. The disease is endemic in regions of North America, Europe and Asia, but can be difficult to diagnose. The responsible organism, *Borrelia burgdorferi*, is transmitted through tick bites, with deer being an important vector (Fig. 12.57A). An adult tick (Fig. 12.57B) can be distinguished from a head louse by the tick having eight legs – it is an arachnid – and the louse six (though larval ticks have only six). Several days after a bite an annular skin lesion, erythema chronicum migrans (Fig. 12.57C), forms at the

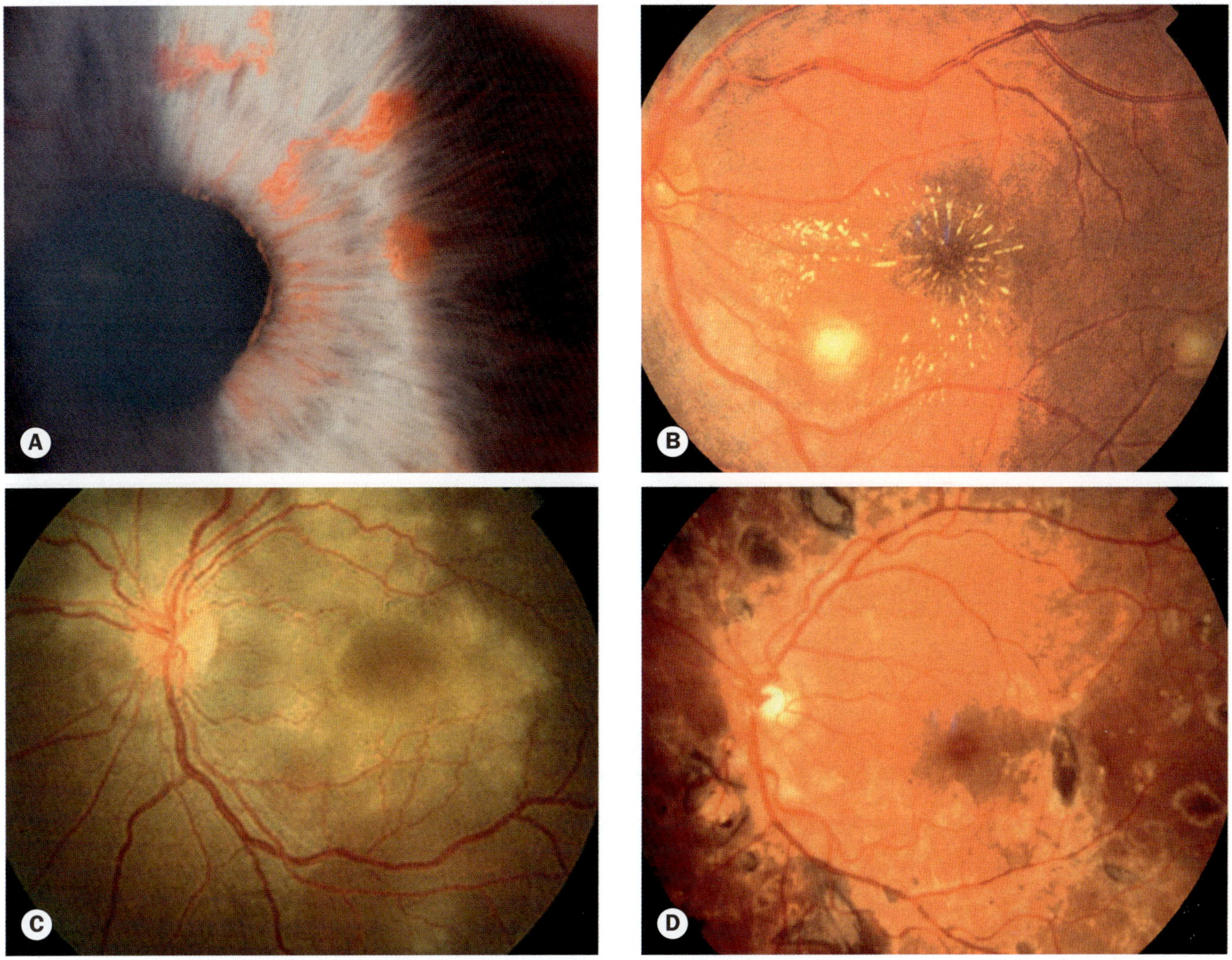

Fig. 12.56 Ocular syphilis. **(A)** Roseolae; **(B)** focal infiltration with macular star; **(C)** acute posterior placoid chorioretinitis; **(D)** old multifocal chorioretinitis.

site in 60–80%, often accompanied by constitutional symptoms (stage 1). Neurological (e.g. cranial nerve palsies, meningitis), cardiac (4–8% e.g. arrhythmia) and other manifestations may follow within a few weeks. Late (stage 3) complications include chronic arthritis of large joints, polyneuropathy and encephalopathy. Some patients develop chronic symptoms that may not respond to antibiotics.

Ocular features

These are varied and tend to occur in established stage 2 and stage 3 (late) disease.

- **Uveitis** is relatively uncommon but can be anterior (granulomatous or non-granulomatous), intermediate (the most common), or posterior including multifocal choroiditis, vasculitis and neuroretinitis.
- **Other manifestations** include early (stage 1) transient conjunctivitis, bilateral stromal keratitis, episcleritis (Fig. 12.57D), scleritis, orbital myositis, optic neuritis, papilloedema and ocular motor and facial nerve palsy (up to 25% of facial nerve palsy in endemic areas).

Investigations

Serology should be performed at least a month after infection, but false positives can occur. PCR of CSF or synovial fluid is performed in appropriate cases. Diagnosis relies on a combination of clinical features and positive serology. Co-infection with other tick-borne diseases is possible.

TIP Lyme disease can be difficult to diagnose in the early stages and many of the later symptoms are non-specific in nature. The diagnosis depends on a history of exposure to ticks and a combination of clinical features and positive serology.

Treatment

Treatment of early acute disease is highly effective and involves oral doxycycline (not children or in pregnancy), amoxicillin or erythromycin. Untreated, many patients with early or

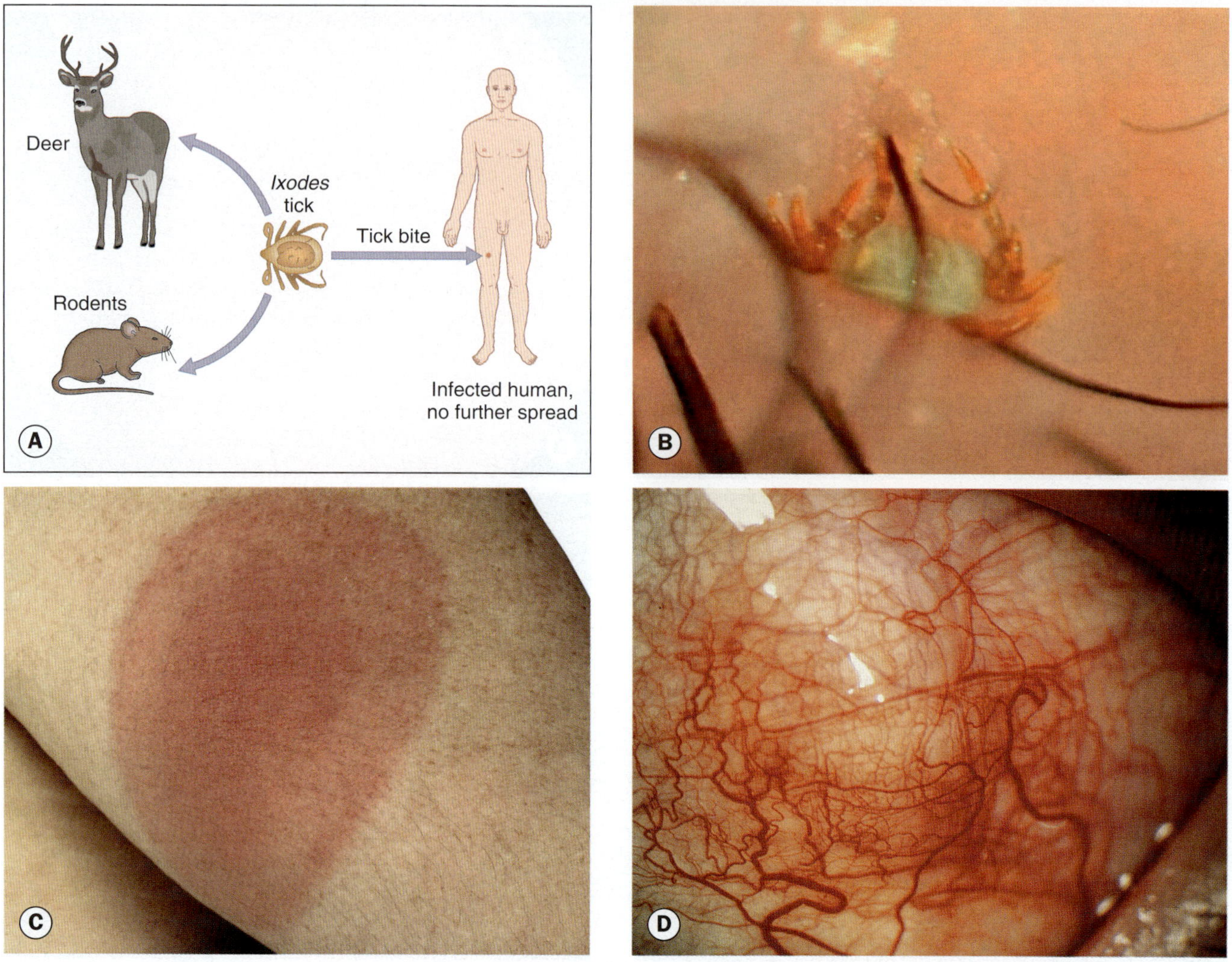

Fig. 12.57 Lyme disease. **(A)** Transmission; **(B)** tick attached to eyelid; **(C)** erythema chronicum migrans; **(D)** nodular episcleritis.

asymptomatic disease will experience no further problems. Patients with established disease, including ocular, may require extended intravenous penicillin or ceftriaxone. Keratitis and uveitis may need steroid treatment. Systemic steroids should not be given without concomitant antibiotics. Appropriate personal protection (clothing, insect repellent) should be adopted in endemic areas to reduce the risk of tick bite. Lyme disease vaccine is available, but does not offer complete or prolonged protection.

Brucellosis

Brucellosis is caused by the Gram-negative bacteria *Brucella melitensis* and *B. abortus*. It is usually transmitted from animals to man through milk products or uncooked meat. A variety of constitutional and ocular (20%) features are reported, the latter including chronic anterior and posterior uveitis, papilloedema and retinal haemorrhages. Investigation should include serology and blood culture. Treatment is with a combination of two antibiotics, e.g. streptomycin and doxycycline, with adjunctive steroids if required. Patients with known brucellosis should undergo ophthalmic examination.

Endogenous bacterial endophthalmitis

Introduction

This is an intraocular infection that originates from sources within the body. The incidence has increased in recent years. A wide range of organisms can be responsible – Gram-positives predominate in North America and Europe and Gram-negatives in East Asia. Risk factors include debilitating disease of many types as well as other factors such as intravenous drug abuse (where *Bacillus* species predominate). Spread can occur from any potential focus such as an indwelling catheter, tooth abscess, endocarditis (especially *Streptococcus*), urinary tract infection (especially *E. coli*) or septic joint. Patients are usually systemically unwell and mortality is relatively high – 5–10%. The two systemic diseases that confer an increase in mortality are pneumonia and renal/UTI infection, mainly because these infections are caused by virulent organisms. The visual prognosis is poorer than with postoperative endophthalmitis.

Ocular features

Diagnosis is frequently delayed. The main distinction is from endogenous fungal endophthalmitis.

- **Symptoms**: blurred vision, pain and redness.
- **Signs** are broadly similar to those of postoperative endophthalmitis (see Ch. 10), though retinal infiltrates may be an early feature, reflecting the route of infection.

Investigation

The search for a septic focus (blood and urine cultures, septic arthritis, endocarditis, lumbar puncture etc.) should be in collaboration with an appropriate physician. Aqueous and vitreous samples should be taken for microscopy and culture.

Treatment

- **Systemic infection** is treated with intravenous antibiotics according to clinical suspicion and local microbiological advice. Broad spectrum empirical treatment may be necessary.
- **Endophthalmitis** is treated with intravitreal and an oral fluoroquinolone. The place of systemic steroids is undefined. Pars plana vitrectomy may improve prognosis in some patients.

TIP Systemic antibiotics are key to the treatment of endogenous endophthalmitis, in contrast to postoperative endophthalmitis. The search for a septic focus should be made in collaboration with an appropriate physician.

Cat-scratch disease

Introduction

Cat-scratch disease (bartonellosis) is caused by *Bartonella henselae*, a Gram-negative rod. Infection is usually transmitted by the scratch (or bite) of an apparently healthy cat, though feline contact is not always described. One or more red papules at the site of inoculation are followed by fever and regional lymphadenopathy (Fig. 12.58A), though general symptoms are frequently absent. Severe systemic disease occasionally occurs. The visual prognosis is usually reasonable.

Ocular features

The eyes are affected in 5–10%. Neuroretinitis (see Ch. 19) is the most common manifestation and consists of disc oedema with macular exudate in a star conformation (Fig. 12.58B); focal retinochoroiditis, vasculitis and, rarely, an optic nerve head angiomatous lesion have been reported. Conjunctivitis with a 2–4 mm conjunctival granuloma and associated pre-auricular lymphadenopathy (Parinaud oculoglandular syndrome) may occasionally be seen. It is unusual for both eyes to be involved.

Investigation

Includes serology for *B. henselae.*

Treatment

Doxycycline 100 mg twice daily for 4–6 weeks should be used in immunocompetent adults. Oral erythromycin can be used in children. Other oral antibiotics, e.g. co-trimoxazole, azithromycin, rifampicin or ciprofloxacin are effective. Steroids have been used in some cases. Treatment is not usually given for mild systemic symptoms alone.

Leprosy

Introduction

Leprosy (Hansen disease) is a chronic granulomatous infection caused by *Mycobacterium leprae* and *M. lepromatosis.* The mode of spread remains uncertain, though nasal secretions have been implicated. Infection is thought to lead to a chronic immune response that leads to the peripheral neuropathy that is the primary pathogenetic mechanism. Genetic factors are

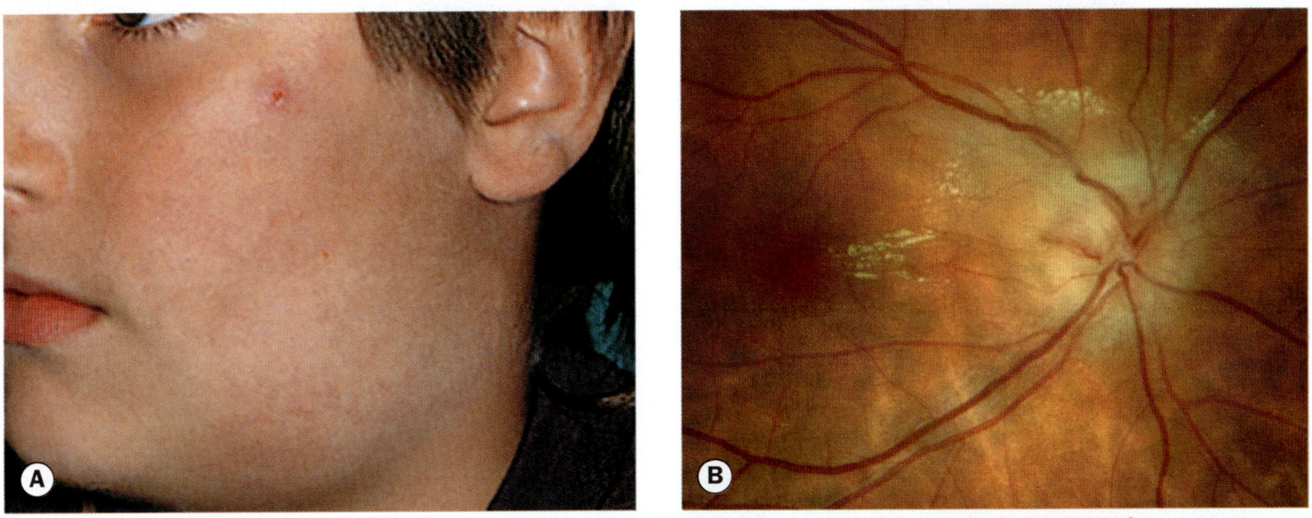

Fig. 12.58 Cat-scratch disease. **(A)** Ulcerated papule on the cheek caused by a cat scratch 2 weeks previously, with enlargement of submandibular lymph nodes; **(B)** neuroretinitis, manifesting with a partial macular star. *(Courtesy of BJ Zitelli and HW Davis, from* Atlas of Pediatric Physical Diagnosis, *Mosby 2002 – fig. A.)*

probably important – only 5% of the general population is thought to be vulnerable to leprosy on substantial contact with the organism.

Systemic features

- **Tuberculoid ('paucibacillary' in WHO classification).** One or more hypopigmented macules and anaesthetic skin patches.
- **Borderline (multibacillary).** The most common form. Similar to tuberculoid, but more numerous and extensive lesions.
- **Lepromatous (multibacillary).** Widespread cutaneous thickening with leonine facial appearance (Fig. 12.59A), peripheral plaques and nodules, upper respiratory tract involvement and peripheral nerve lesions facilitating trauma that may result in shortening and loss of digits.

Ocular features

Ocular signs are principally due to direct bacterial invasion.

- **Keratitis**: thickened, beaded corneal nerves, punctate subepithelial lesions, pannus and vascularization (Fig. 12.59B).
- **Anterior uveitis**: chronic and low-grade and is classically described as 'plasmoid' (prominent fibrin).
- **Miosis and iris atrophy** (Fig. 12.59C) result from impaired dilator pupillae innervation.
- **Iris pearls** (pathognomonic): usually under 0.5 mm in diameter (Fig. 12.59D).
- **Other features**: episcleritis and scleritis, retinal pearls, uveal effusion, cataract, glaucoma, decreased corneal sensation, facial nerve palsy, eyelid deformities and phthisis bulbi.

Investigation

Skin and occasionally ocular specimens show acid-fast bacilli. The lepromin test distinguishes between tuberculoid and lepromatous leprosy.

Treatment

- **Systemic.** Combination regimens of extended duration with antibiotics such as dapsone, rifampicin and clofazimine. BCG vaccination offers some protection.
- **Ocular.** Anterior uveitis is treated with steroids. Specific complications are addressed as indicated.

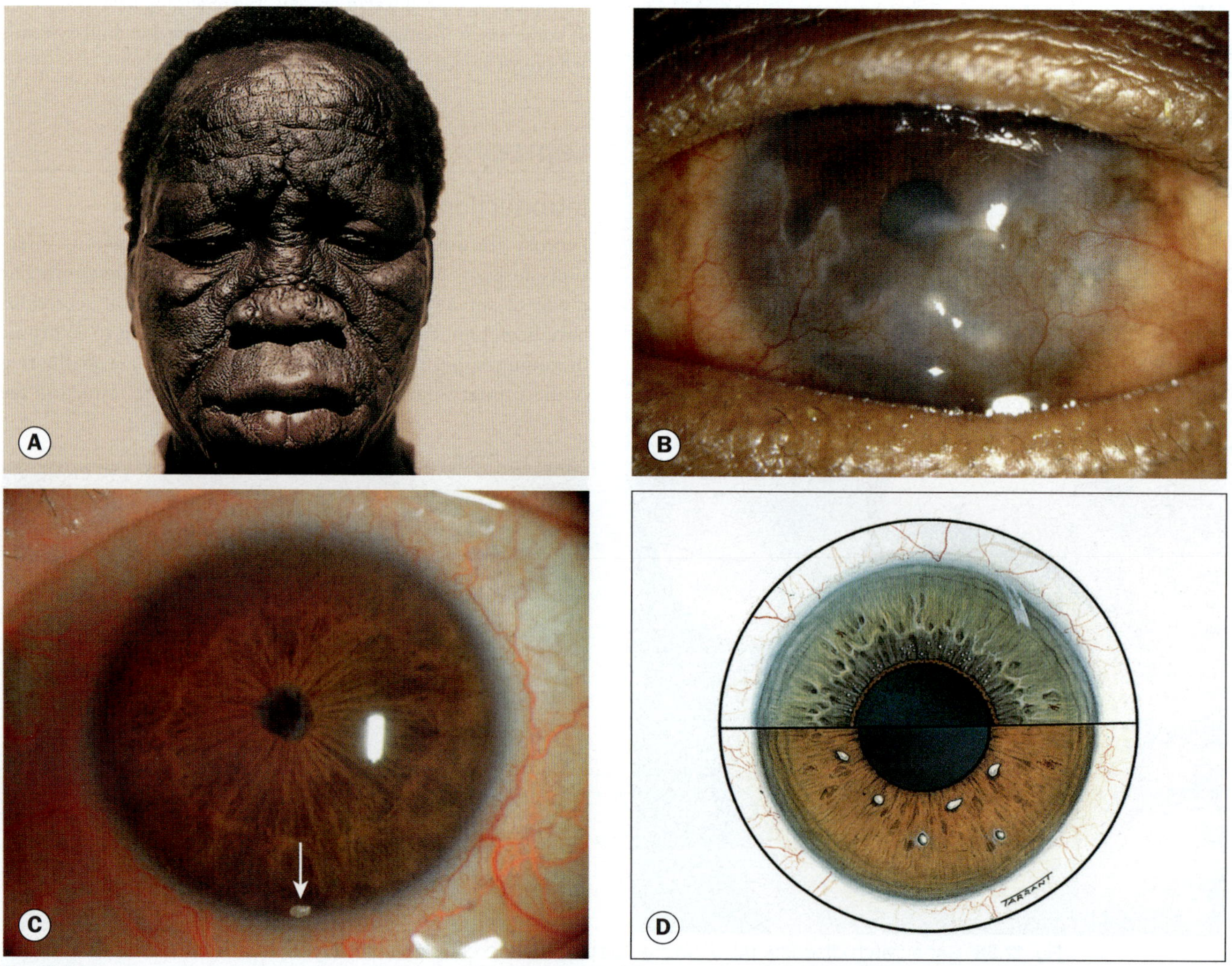

Fig. 12.59 Lepromatous leprosy. **(A)** Leonine facial appearance; **(B)** corneal involvement with pannus; **(C)** lepromatous chronic anterior uveitis with miosis and an anterior chamber pearl (arrow); **(D)** iris pearls. *(Courtesy of RT Emond, PD Welsby and HA Rowland, from* Colour Atlas of Infectious Diseases, *Mosby 2003 – fig. A; ADN Murray – fig. B.)*

MISCELLANEOUS IDIOPATHIC CHORIORETINOPATHIES

Introduction

The term 'white dot syndromes' has been used in the past to describe several different idiopathic inflammatory conditions of the posterior pole. These conditions tend to occur between the second to sixth decades of life, are more likely to affect women than men, usually have a self-limiting course and the visual prognosis depends on the condition. However, the term is considered by many uveitis specialists to be outdated because the white dots are a variable finding and the diseases are not driven by the same pathophysiological processes. Patients with other entities may present with similar clinical manifestations and it is critical to exclude alternative diagnoses, including infection and neoplasia. Recent advances in the field of ocular imaging have allowed better characterization of these conditions. Indocyanine green angiography enables two main disease categories to be recognized: (a) choriocapillaritis and (b) stromal choroiditis (Table 12.10).

Multiple evanescent white dot syndrome (MEWDS)

Introduction

MEWDS is an uncommon idiopathic disease of acute onset, typically occurring in young adult females, with 25–50% describing a preceding viral-like illness. Influenza vaccination has been reported to occasionally trigger the disease. The exact pathogenesis is not known, although immune-induced inflammation of the choriocapillaris has been suspected. The condition can be difficult to diagnose as the characteristic fundal white dots disappear fairly soon after the symptoms start (Fig. 12.60A). Multimodal imaging is key to making the diagnosis, as changes that are not clinically apparent are obvious on FAF, OCT and ICG angiography.

Table 12.10 ICG Angiographic Classification of Choroiditis

1A. Primary choriocapillaritis (trigger not known)
• Multiple evanescent white dot syndrome (MEWDS)
• Acute posterior multifocal placoid pigment epitheliopathy (APMPPE)
• Serpiginous choroidopathy
• Multifocal choroiditis (MFC)
• Punctate inner choroidopathy (PIC)
1B. Secondary choriocapillaritis (the pathogen triggers the immune response)
• Acute syphilitic posterior placoid chorioretinitis (ASPPC)
• TB-related serpiginous choroiditis
2A. Primary stromal choroiditis (stroma is target of inflammation)
• HLA-A29 birdshot retinochoroidopathy
• Vogt–Koyanagi–Harada disease (VKH)
• Sympathetic ophthalmia
2B. Secondary stromal choroiditis (secondary to systemic inflammation)
• Sarcoidosis
• Tubercular chorioretinitis
• Syphilitic chorioretinitis

Clinical features

- **Presentation.** Common: painless monocular blurring (6/9–6/60), subjective scotomas and photopsia. Less common: floaters, dyschromatopsia.
- **Subtle posterior vitritis** in 50%.
- **Posterior pole lesions.** Numerous small (100–300 μm), ill-defined, deep grey–white patches sparing the fovea, which has a characteristic orange granular appearance and a dulled reflex.
- **Optic disc oedema** is occasionally present.
- **Recovery** occurs over weeks, often leaving subtle residual signs. Recurrence occasionally (10%) occurs. If there is recurrence, idiopathic multifocal choroiditis (see below) should be suspected, as these two diseases can overlap.

Investigation

- **Visual fields.** The blind spot is commonly enlarged, with a temporal field defect.
- **FA** shows subtle early hyperfluorescence in the areas corresponding to white dots, with late staining (Fig. 12.60B). Vessel wall leakage and disc staining may be seen.
- **FAF** reveals hyperautofluorescent spots during active inflammation which correspond to the macular lesions (Fig. 12.60C). FAF has been used to demonstrate subclinical lesions in patients with only foveal granularity.
- **ICGA** shows hypofluorescent spots in the late angiographic phase (Fig. 12.60D) that are often more numerous than visible clinically or on FA. Some authorities suggest that this could be a sign of flow void at the level of the choriocapillaris, while others interpret this as outer retinal involvement leading to reduced late uptake of ICG by the RPE.
- **OCT** shows inner-segment/outer-segment junction (ellipsoid zone) disruption (Fig. 12.60E). It is sometimes associated with reflective focal lesions that cross the external limiting membrane.

Treatment

This is generally not required as the symptoms and signs start to improve spontaneously in most cases by 8–10 weeks (Fig. 12.60F).

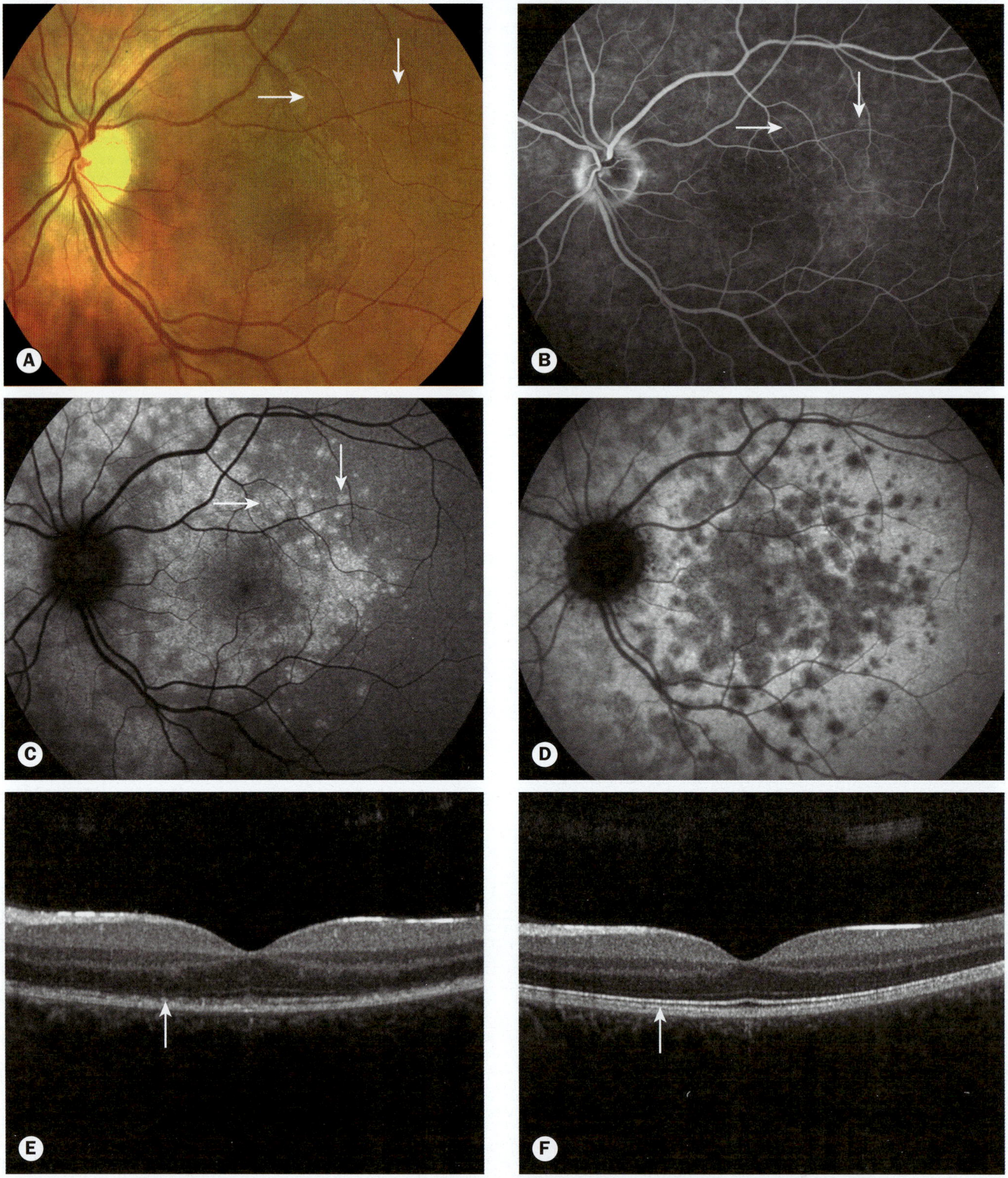

Fig. 12.60 Multiple evanescent white dot syndrome: images **A–E** taken on presentation shortly after the onset of symptoms. **(A)** Numerous lesions that are already fading (arrows); **(B)** venous phase FA showing punctate hyperfluorescence (arrows); **(C)** FAF showing numerous focal hyperautofluorescent spots (arrows); **(D)** ICGA showing hypofluorescent spots in the late angiographic phase that are often more numerous than visible clinically; **(E)** OCT of **(A)** showing disruption of the ellipsoid/interdigitation zones (arrow); **(F)** OCT 12 months later, showing a normal scan with restoration of the outer retinal layers (arrow).

Acute idiopathic blind spot enlargement syndrome (AIBSE)

AIBSE is a rare condition reported in young to middle-aged women and is likely to be a variant of MEWDS. Features include photopsia and decreased vision, with blind spot enlargement and mild disc swelling. Recovery to normal or near-normal without treatment is usual.

Acute posterior multifocal placoid pigment epitheliopathy (APMPPE)

Introduction

APMPPE is an uncommon bilateral idiopathic inflammatory disorder. It affects young to middle-aged adults of both genders equally. There is a viral prodrome in one-third and it is speculated to occur as a result of cell-mediated immunity to viral antigen. The exact pathogenesis is not known, but it has been suggested that inflammation at the level of the choriocapillaris results in hypoperfusion and ischaemia of the RPE and photoreceptors. Associated cerebral vasculitis can occur but is uncommon and can cause stroke. Erythema nodosum and other systemic manifestations of vasculitis have been reported. The clinical picture of APMPPE can be mimicked by other entities, such as sarcoidosis and tuberculosis.

Clinical features

- **Symptoms.** Subacute moderate visual impairment with central/paracentral scotomas and photopsia. If the macula is involved the visual acuity can deteriorate (ranging from 6/12 to 6/60). The fellow eye is affected within a few days or weeks. Headache and other neurological symptoms are common and can commence many months after ocular disease onset.
- **Anterior uveitis and vitritis** are usually very mild.
- **Fundus.** Multiple large deep yellow–white placoid lesions, initially at the posterior pole (Fig. 12.61A). Within weeks the majority fade, with residual RPE disturbance of varying severity. Subretinal macular fluid may be seen. Vasculitis and papillitis are rare.
- **Prognosis.** The visual symptoms and retinal appearance typically improve within weeks and the long-term prognosis for most patients is good. However, there appears to be a subgroup of patients whose symptoms may recur and who have a longer period of disease activity. In 25% visual recovery is limited to 6/15 or worse as a consequence of RPE and photoreceptor damage to the fovea. Factors that predict a poor prognosis include: (a) age older than 60 years, (b) unilaterality, (c) an interval before involvement of the second eye of at least 6 months, (d) disease recurrence, (e) leakage from choroidal veins.

Investigation

- **Alternative diagnoses** should be excluded.
- **HLA-B7** and **HLA-DR2** are associated in a substantial proportion of patients.
- **FA** of active lesions shows early dense hypofluorescence (blockage) (Fig. 12.61B) and late hyperfluorescent staining (Fig. 12.61C). Late hyperfluorescence may result from vascular leakage, which resolves in healed lesions.
- **FAF** shows scattered hypoautofluorescence surrounded by hyperautofluorescence corresponding to placoid lesions (Fig. 12.61D).
- **ICGA**: active placoid lesions manifest as early and late hypofluorescence secondary to poor choriocapillaris perfusion (Fig. 12.61E).
- **OCT** of the macula shows focal disruption of the outer retina (Fig. 12.61F).
- **OCT angiography (OCTA)** may show abnormal flow in the choriocapillaris.
- **CNS imaging** and lumbar puncture should be performed in patients with neurological symptoms to rule out retinal vasculitis.

Treatment

Treatment is not usually required, but steroids should be considered for patients with macular involvement. Steroids and possibly ciclosporin may be given for cerebral vasculitis. Patients should be instructed to seek medical advice urgently if neurological symptoms occur.

Serpiginous choroidopathy

Introduction

Serpiginous choroidopathy (choroiditis) is usually bilateral, though asymmetrical. Inflammation occurs in the outer retina and choriocapillaris. It typically occurs in middle age, affects men more frequently than women and is associated with HLA-B7. The disease is generally recurrent over years, with a relatively poor prognosis and almost 25% of affected eyes have a final visual acuity of less than 6/60. Tuberculosis (see Fig. 12.53) and syphilis (see Fig. 12.56D) can occasionally result in a similar clinical picture ('serpiginoid'), which can pose a diagnostic challenge, as the therapeutic approach to these diseases is significantly different.

Clinical features

- **Symptoms.** Initially unilateral blurring of central vision, scotoma or metamorphopsia.
- **Anterior uveitis and vitritis** are common but usually mild.
- **Fundus.** Active lesions (Fig. 12.62A) are grey–white and may remain active for several months before becoming scalloped and atrophic. The disease typically starts around the optic disc and extends gradually (Fig. 12.62B), though a variant starting at the central macula (5%) is recognized. Recurrence is usually contiguous with or adjacent to existing areas, eventually resulting in extensive chorioretinal atrophy (Fig. 12.62C).
- **Complications.** MNV (15–35%), subretinal fibrosis, preretinal neovascularization.

Investigation

- **Tuberculosis** should be excluded, especially in endemic areas. Test for syphilis.
- **FAF** shows the extent of the inflammation. Active lesions show a hyperautofluorescent halo on the edges of areas of

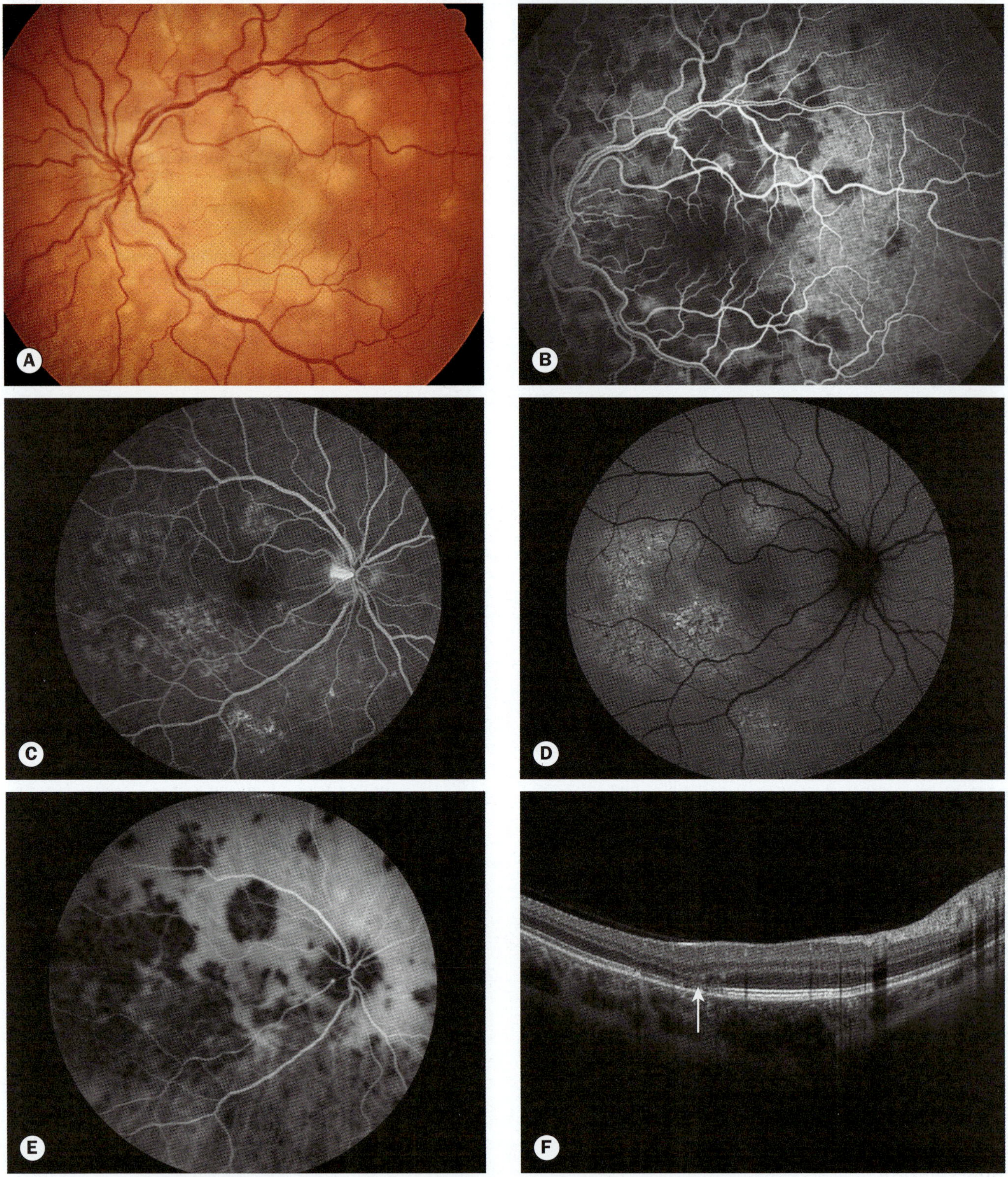

Fig. 12.61 Acute posterior multifocal placoid pigment epitheliopathy. **(A)** Retinal appearance; **(B)** FA early venous phase showing dense foci of hypofluorescence (blockage) corresponding to the placoid lesions; **(C)** FA venous phase on presentation of a different case showing multifocal areas of hyperfluorescence (leakage); **(D)** FAF of **(C)** showing scattered areas of hyperautofluorescence surrounding small hypoautofluorescent lesions; **(E)** ICGA of **(C)** at 8 minutes showing multifocal placoid areas of hypofluorescence secondary to poor perfusion of the choriocapillaris; **(F)** OCT of **(C)** showing localized disruption of the ellipsoid zone and thinning of the outer retinal and ellipsoid zones (arrow). *(Courtesy of C Barry – figs A and B.)*

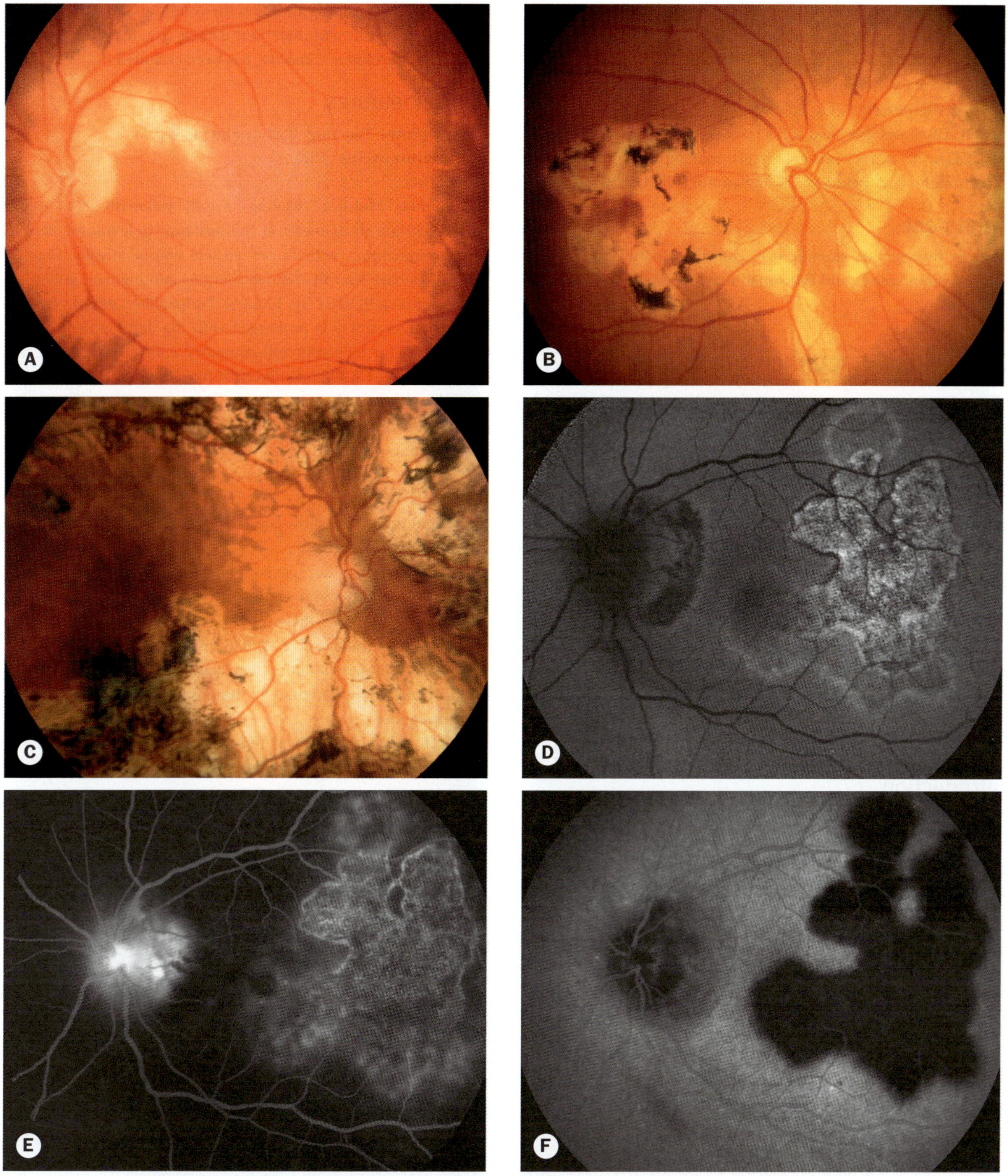

Fig. 12.62 Serpiginous choroidopathy. **(A)** Early active disease; **(B)** extension around the macula in typical snake-like fashion; **(C)** advanced scarring; **(D)** FAF of a different patient showing a border of hyperautofluorescence indicative of active inflammation; **(E)** FA of **(D)** showing late hyperfluorescence; **(F)** ICGA of **(D)** showing an area of late hypofluorescence. *(Courtesy of R Bates – fig. B.)*

hypoautofluorescence (Fig. 12.62D). Inactive lesions are dark and uniformly hypoautofluorescent. It is a useful technique to monitor disease progression.

- **FA** of active lesions shows early hypofluorescence and late hyperfluorescence (Fig. 12.62E).
- **OCTA** shows flow void at the level of the choriocapillaris.
- **ICGA** of active lesions reveals marked hypofluorescence throughout all phases of the angiogram (Fig. 12.62F)

Treatment

Oral or intravenous steroids may control activity. A variety of immunosuppressives and infliximab may be effective, alone or in combination.

Relentless placoid chorioretinitis (RPC)

This refers to a rare entity showing features of both APMPPE and serpiginous choroiditis and is also referred to as ampiginous choroiditis. In contrast to APMPPE which is limited to the posterior pole, RPC is characterized by the presence of hundreds of lesions, located anteriorly and posterior to the equator. The clinical course is often prolonged and relapsing.

Persistent placoid maculopathy (PPM)

This rare condition features lesions similar to those of the macular variant of serpiginous choroidopathy, but which generally behave in a more benign fashion unless complicated by MNV (common).

Idiopathic multifocal choroiditis (MFC)

Introduction

MFC is an uncommon, usually bilateral but asymmetrical, chronic/recurrent disease that typically affects young and middle-aged adult women. Many people present with flu-like symptoms before the onset of ocular disease. The severity and prognosis are very variable.

The aetiology is unknown and the condition is diagnosed clinically after systemic and infectious disease (e.g. tuberculosis, West Nile virus choroiditis, *Candida*) has been excluded.

Clinical features

- **Symptoms.** Blurring, floaters and photopsia.
- **Anterior uveitis** (50%).
- **Vitritis.**
- **Fundus.** Multiple discrete, ovoid, yellowish-grey lesions 50–350 μm in diameter at the posterior pole and/or periphery, sometimes with linear clusters and/or streaks. Inactive lesions have sharply defined margins and pigmented borders resembling POHS (Fig. 12.63A). Peripapillary atrophy may be seen. The course is prolonged with the development of new lesions and recurrent inflammatory episodes. MNV occurs in 25–35%, CMO and subretinal fibrosis resembling SFU (see below) can develop.
- **Optic disc** oedema and blind spot enlargement may be present.

Investigation

- **Visual fields** may show large defects not corresponding to the examination findings.
- **FA.** Early hypofluorescence and late hyperfluorescence. Old inactive lesions show window defects. If a neovascular membrane develops in the macular region, hyperfluorescence is seen due to leakage (Fig. 12.63B).
- **ICGA** shows hypofluorescent acute lesions which may not be clinically apparent. Old lesions remain hypofluorescent throughout.
- **OCT** shows elevation of the RPE with sub-RPE material of intermediate reflectivity and surrounding disruption of the outer retina.
- **OCTA** shows well-demarcated areas of reduced flow at the level of the choriocapillaris.
- **ERG** remains normal until there is advanced retinal atrophy.

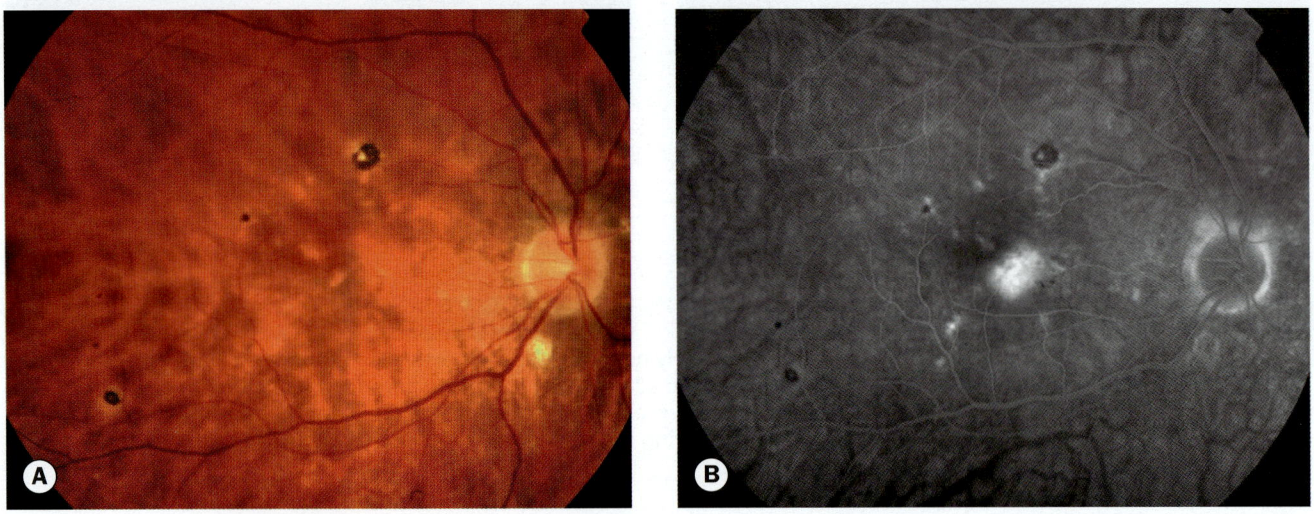

Fig. 12.63 Idiopathic multifocal choroiditis. **(A)** Inactive lesions; **(B)** late venous phase fluorescein angiogram showing hyperfluorescence at the fovea due to leakage from neovascularization in the macula.

Treatment

Systemic and local steroids. Steroid-resistant patients require immunosuppressive therapy (cyclosporine or tacrolimus, together with mycophenolate mofetil). MNV is treated with steroids and anti-VEGF agents.

Punctate inner choroidopathy (PIC)

Introduction

PIC typically affects young myopic women. Both eyes are involved in 80%, but the involvement is usually asymmetrical. It is likely to be a form of idiopathic multifocal choroiditis, but involvement predominantly involves the macula.

Clinical features

- **Symptoms.** Blurring, scotoma, floaters and photopsia.
- **Anterior uveitis and vitritis** are usually absent or very mild.
- **Fundus.** Several small yellow–white macular spots with fuzzy borders at the level of the inner choroid and retina (Fig. 12.64A), sometimes with an overlying serous sensory retinal detachment. These evolve into sharply demarcated atrophic scars with little pigmentation, similar to the histo spots of POHS.
- **Prognosis.** Central vision may be compromised by a lesion at the fovea or, more commonly, by MNV (up to 40% – Fig. 12.64B and C). Visual acuity improves to 6/7.5 in 50% of cases.

Investigation

- **Visual field** testing shows enlargement of the blind spot in about 40% of cases and central and paracentral scotomas.
- **FAF** shows hypoautofluorescent spots and areas of hyperautofluorescence (Fig. 12.64D)
- **FA** shows early hyperfluorescence and late staining of lesions and demonstrates MNV (Fig. 12.64E).
- **OCTA/OCT** shows submacular MNV (Fig. 12.64F) and acute hyper-reflective material with disruption of the outer retina in the acute stage.
- **ICG** shows multiple mid-phase hypofluorescent lesions in the posterior pole. Choroidal vessels may show localized points of hyperfluorescence situated close to the vessel walls, indicating vasculitis of smaller choroidal vessels and choriocapillaris.

Treatment

- No treatment is advised for most patients unless there is evidence of MNV.
- Anti-VEGF medication should be used for choroidal neovascular formation in the macular region.
- Steroids and systemic immunosuppressive therapy can be helpful in the management of recurrent CMV.

Progressive subretinal fibrosis and uveitis syndrome (SFU)

SFU, also known as diffuse subretinal fibrosis, is an extremely rare chronic condition. It typically affects myopic young women, causing gradual blurring of vision in one then both eyes. Anterior uveitis and vitritis accompanies subretinal mounds at the posterior pole and midperiphery (Fig. 12.65A) progressing to widespread subretinal fibrosis (Fig. 12.65B). Steroids may be effective early in the disease, but the prognosis is poor. Some experts view SFU as part of a spectrum with MFC/MCP and PIC.

Birdshot retinochoroidopathy

Introduction

Birdshot retinochoroidopathy (also known as birdshot uveitis) is an uncommon idiopathic inflammatory disease usually affecting middle-aged women. It is chronic, bilateral and manifests with severe retinitis and stromal choroiditis that are independent inflammatory events. Nearly all patients are HLA-A29 positive.

Clinical features

- **Symptoms.** Insidious impairment of central vision associated with floaters, nyctalopia, dyschromatopsia and photopsia.
- **Vitritis** is present in either or both eyes.
- **Fundus.** Multiple ill-defined ovoid cream-coloured choroidal patches, less than one disc diameter in size, in the posterior pole and midperiphery (Fig. 12.66A). The lesions often appear to radiate outward from the disc but usually spare the macula itself and are more concentrated in the inferotemporal area. Inactive lesions consist of well-delineated atrophic spots (Fig. 12.66B). CMO, epiretinal membrane and MNV may develop.
- **Visual field testing** (not visual acuity) is the appropriate functional test for monitoring disease evolution and response to treatment.
- **Prognosis.** About one-third of patients have an eventual best visual acuity of less than 6/60. However, results are starting to improve with aggressive and sustained immunomodulatory treatment. Choroiditis responds well to this treatment, but the retina less so.

Investigation

- **HLA-A29**: over 95% of patients are positive (versus 7% of the general population).
- **OCT** will confirm macular oedema.
- **Autofluorescence** will generally show more numerous hypoautofluorescent lesions than are seen on examination.
- **FA** shows extensive vascular leakage (Fig. 12.66C), with disc and vessel staining, and can show diffuse macular oedema. Strikingly, the fovea is often spared and true cystoid macular oedema is less common (15%).
- **ICGA**: lesions are more numerous. These are hypofluorescent (Fig. 12.66D), persist into the late phases and do not correspond to the retinal lesions.
- **OCTA** shows areas of flow void in the choroidal stroma, with initial sparing of the choriocapillaris. With progression of the disease the choriocapillaris can be affected.
- **ERG** is normal in early disease but with time shows rod and cone abnormalities.

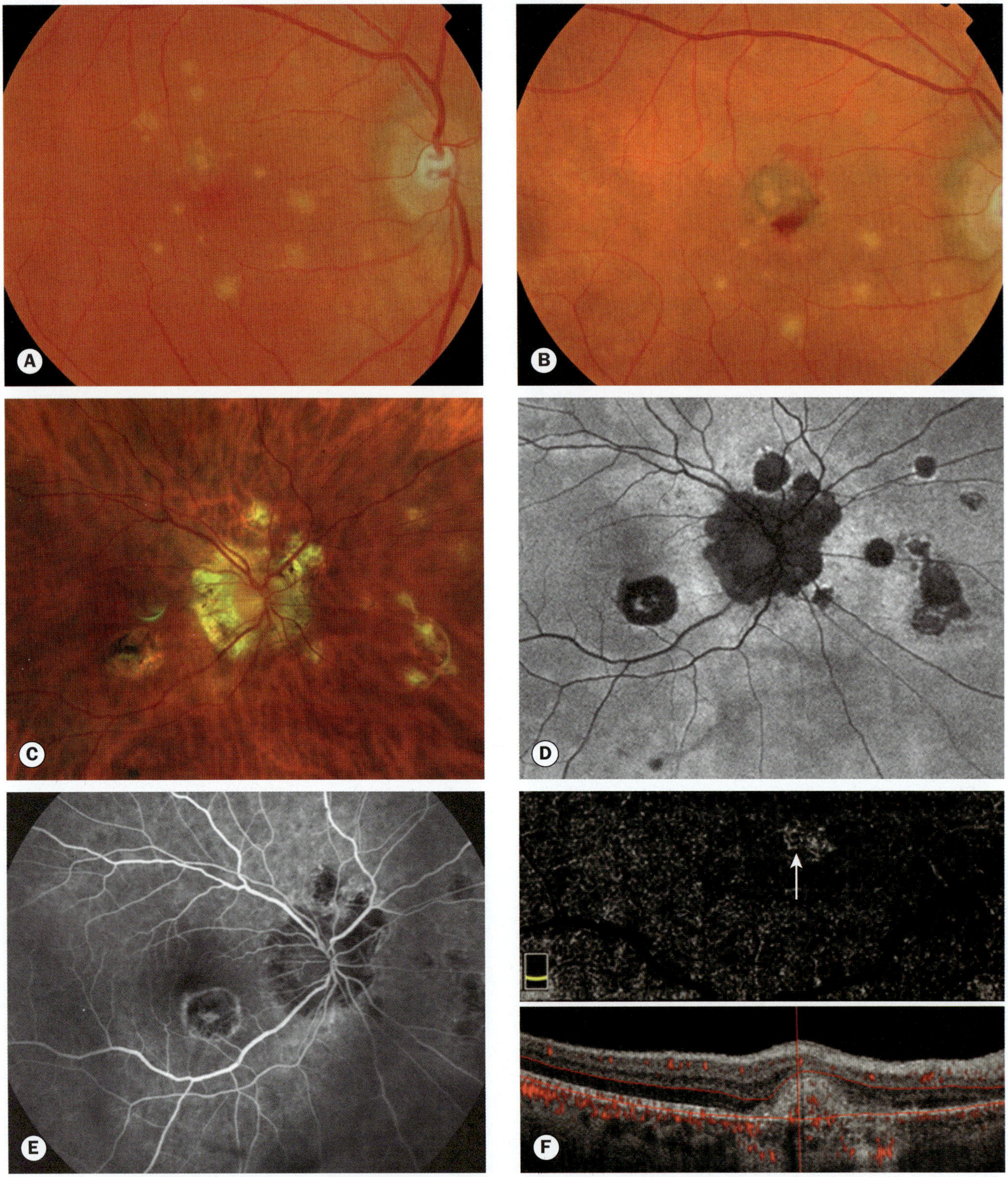

Fig. 12.64 Punctate inner choroidopathy. **(A)** Active lesions – there is a suspicion of neovascularization (MNV) immediately above the fovea; **(B)** the same eye 2 weeks later, showing active neovascularization; **(C)** colour image of a different patient with subretinal fibrosis due to MNV and scattered old PIC lesions; **(D)** FAF of **(C)** showing extensive areas of hyperautofluorescence and hypoautofluorescent scars; **(E)** early phase FA of **(C)** showing a discrete hyperfluorescent spot at the fovea due to MNV, with parapapillary hypofluorescence; **(F)** OCTA showing fibrotic submacular MNV (arrow) and corresponding OCT showing hyperreflective dome-shaped material with disruption of the outer retina. *(Courtesy of S Chen – figs A and B; A Ambresin – figs C–F.)*

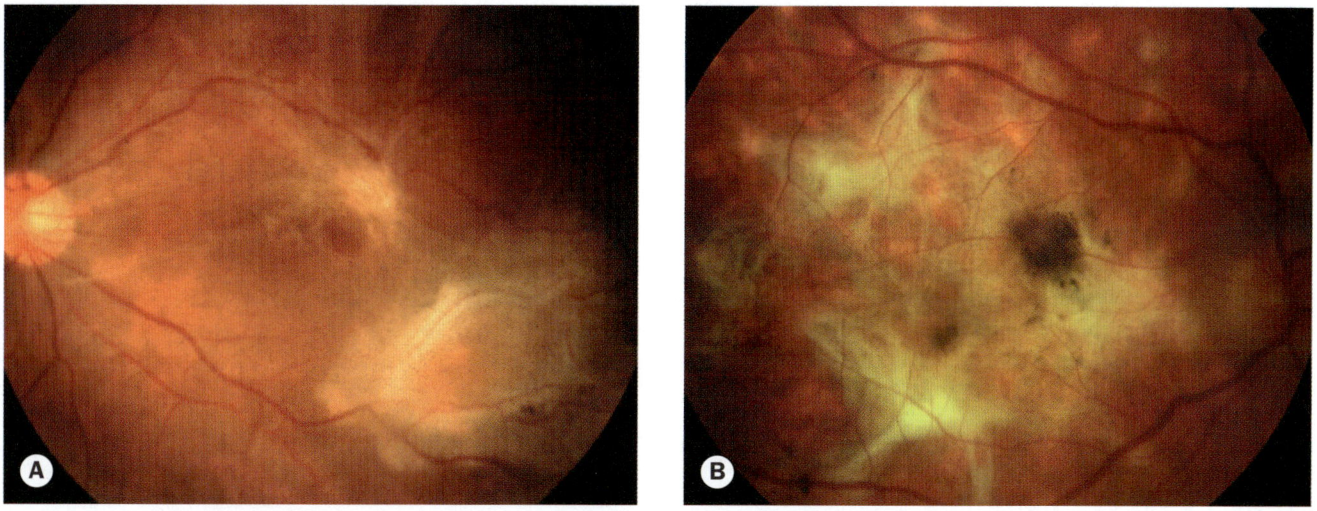

Fig. 12.65 Progressive subretinal fibrosis and uveitis syndrome. **(A)** Early and **(B)** advanced disease.

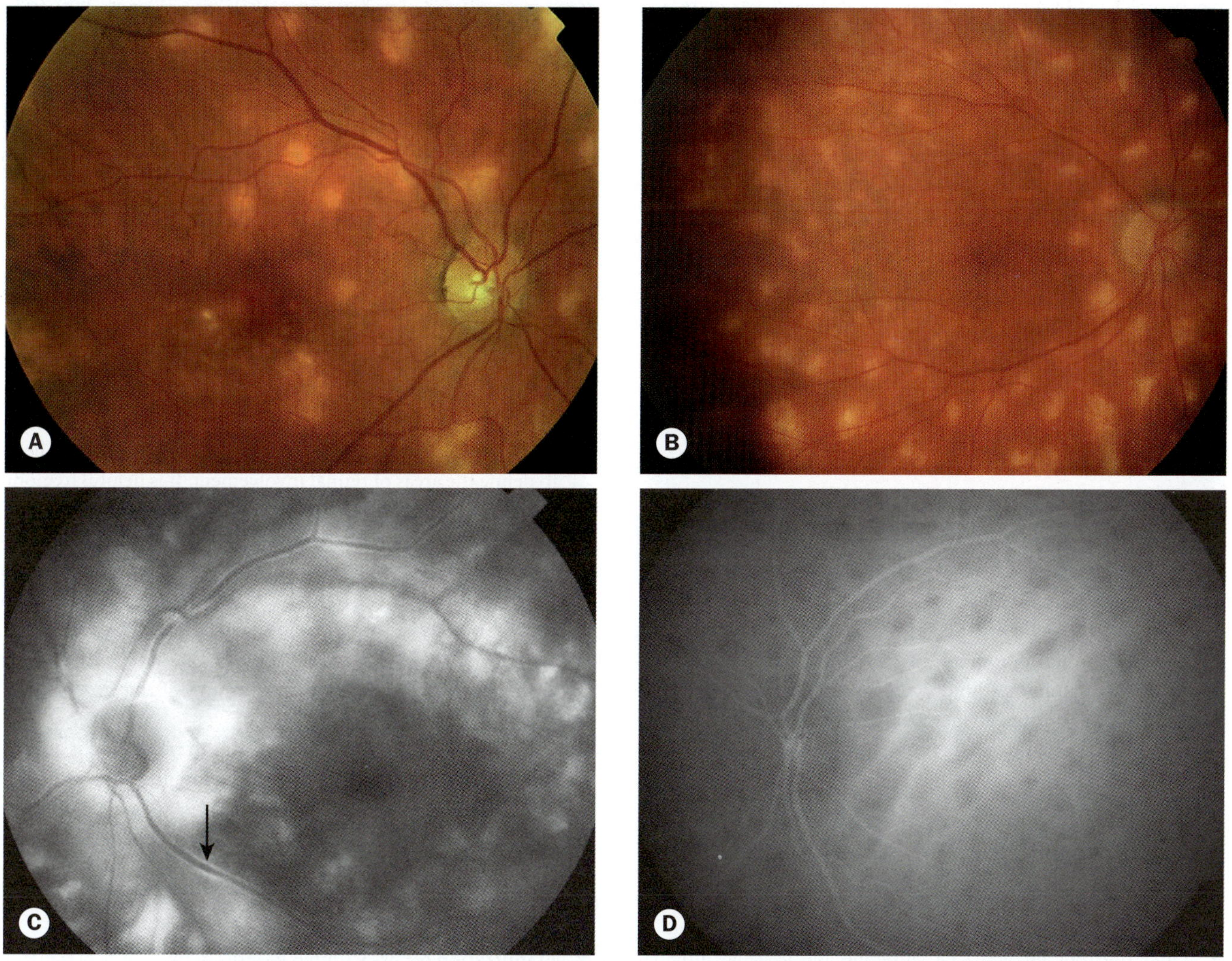

Fig. 12.66 Birdshot retinochoroidopathy. **(A)** Active stage; **(B)** inactive lesions; **(C)** late phase FA showing disc and vessel leakage, vessel wall staining (arrow); **(D)** early phase ICG showing numerous hypofluorescent lesions.

TIP HLA-A29 histocompatibility antigen is present in almost all patients with birdshot retinochoroidopathy when PCR methodology is used.

Treatment

- The first step is to use sub-Tenon triamcinolone acetonide (40 mg), particularly in patients with monocular disease.
- Up to 90% of patients need systemic treatment. Early referral to a uveitis specialist should be considered.
- Systemic steroids are used initially, but immunomodulatory treatment is often needed (cyclosporine or mycophenolate followed by infliximab).

OTHER INFLAMMATORY CONDITIONS OF THE POSTERIOR POLE

Acute macular neuroretinopathy (AMN)

AMN is a rare self-limited condition that typically affects healthy young adult women. The disease may affect one or both eyes and may be preceded by a flu-like illness. The incidence has increased since the start of the COVID-19 pandemic. Symptoms consist of decreased vision and paracentral scotomas. Red–brown wedge-shaped lesions are observed in a flower petal arrangement around the centre of the macula corresponding to the scotomas. FA is normal or shows faint hypofluorescence. Acute AMN is most easily identified by wedge-shaped parafoveal lesions on infra-red imaging (Fig. 12.67A). OCT shows a characteristic hyperreflectivity that starts in the outer plexiform layer (Fig. 12.67B). Over time the outer retinal layers become thinner and disruption occurs to the outer segments and RPE. Symptoms and signs fade slowly over months, but the scotoma often remains.

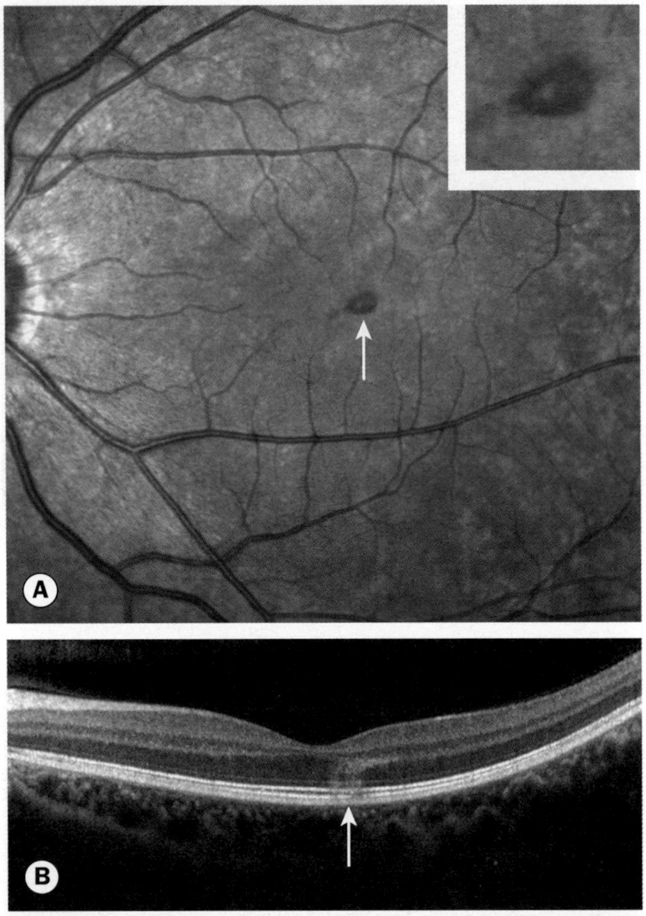

Fig. 12.67 Acute macular neuroretinopathy. **(A)** Infra-red image showing a parafoveal lesion (arrow); **(B)** OCT showing hyperreflectivity in the outer retinal layers (arrow). *(Courtesy of P Charbel Issa.)*

Acute zonal occult outer retinopathy (AZOOR)

Introduction

The acute zonal outer retinopathies (AZOR) are a group of rare conditions characterized by acute visual symptoms in one or both eyes of young or middle-aged women, some of whom have an antecedent viral-like illness. Acute zonal occult outer retinopathy (AZOOR) is the most common of the AZOR syndromes and is characterized by minimal fundoscopic signs early in the disease course. The other postulated members of the group have more evident findings. The pathogenesis is unknown.

Clinical features

- **Photopsia** and mild vitritis are frequent and subtle vasculitis is sometimes seen.
- **Visual field.** There is an acute onset of one or more zones of visual field loss. Field loss may progress and recovery is infrequent.
- **Later findings** include RPE clumping and vascular attenuation in the involved area and peripapillary region, although the fundus may remain normal.

Investigations

- **FAF** may demonstrate abnormalities (Fig. 12.68A) and helps to define the areas of retinal involvement. It is helpful to monitor for signs of progression.
- **OCT and FAF** show similar signs to MEWDS, but the choriocapillaris is preserved and demonstrates no evidence of hypofluorescence on ICGA. OCT shows loss of the outer retina in one or more zones (Fig. 12.68B). Chronically, atrophy of the RPE and thinning of the outer retinal layer is found, followed in time by thinning of the inner retinal layer.
- **ERG** is a less important investigation these days, but characteristically shows a-wave and b-wave amplitude reduction and delayed 30 Hz flicker (cones tend to be affected more than rods). Electro-oculography (EOG) shows absence or severe reduction of the light rise.

Prognosis

- **Stabilization** occurs within 6 months in up to 90% of patients. Final visual acuity is 6/12 in at least one eye in most cases. Recurrence is sometimes seen.

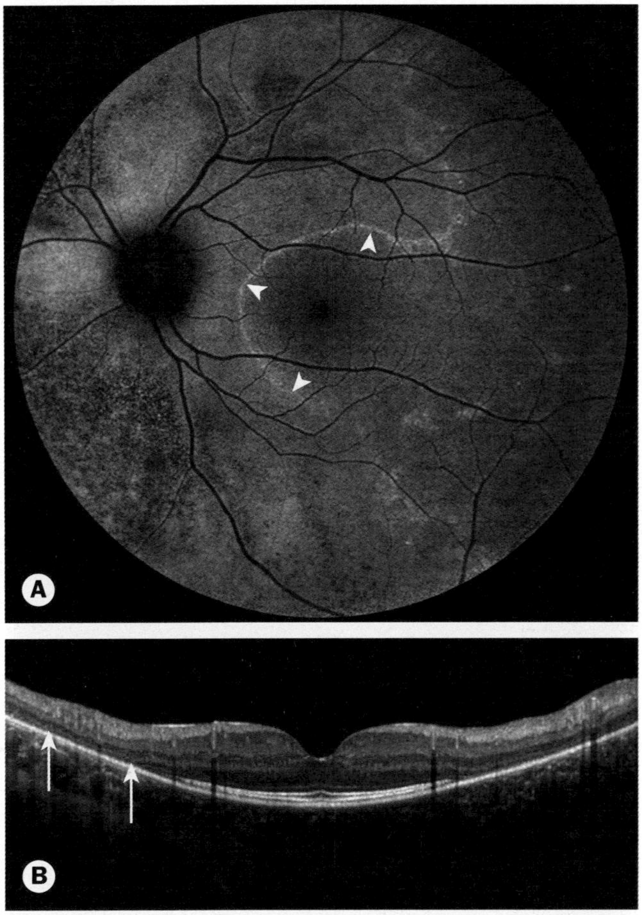

Fig. 12.68 AZOOR. **(A)** FAF showing speckled hypoautofluorescence nasal to the disc, indicating RPE/choroidal atrophy. Note the abrupt transition between abnormal and normal retina (arrow heads showing hyperautofluorescence); **(B)** OCT image of **(A)** showing abnormality of the ellipsoid and interdigitation zones (arrows). *(Courtesy of P Charbel Issa.)*

Treatment

- **There is no proven treatment**, although there are reports of favourable outcomes from systemic steroids.

Acute idiopathic maculopathy (AIM)

AIM is a rare, self-limited condition that is most frequently unilateral and may be preceded by a flu-like illness. Patients are young adults who describe sudden marked reduction in central vision. A viral prodrome is common and associated systemic infections have been noted. An irregularly yellow or grey exudative retinal detachment is seen at the macula (Fig. 12.69A and B) associated with small haemorrhages and papillitis. Within a few weeks the exudative changes resolve (Fig. 12.69C). An irregular bull's eye appearance may develop following resolution and can be associated with persistent visual loss. OCT shows hyper-reflectivity at the photoreceptor outer-segment layer and RPE thickening. FAF shows stippled hyperautofluorescence that becomes hypofluorescent. FA shows early irregular mild hyperfluorescence at the detachment, with subsequent intense staining (Fig. 12.69D). No treatment is needed.

Acute multifocal retinitis

Acute multifocal retinitis is a very rare self-limited condition that may be preceded by a flu-like illness, which is possibly an atypical presentation of cat-scratch disease. It causes sudden onset mild visual loss in young adults. Multiple areas of retinitis are seen posterior to the equator (Fig. 12.70) along with mild vitritis, disc oedema and sometimes a macular star. Recovery occurs over 2–4 months. Treatment as for cat-scratch disease may be considered.

Solitary idiopathic choroiditis (SIC)

SIC is a rare entity that presents with mild visual loss or is asymptomatic. A discrete post-equatorial dull-yellow choroidal elevation with ill-defined margins is seen; vitritis is present during active disease. Contiguous subretinal fluid and a macular star may be present. With healing the lesion develops a better-defined margin with resolution of subretinal fluid and exudation. Treatment of a vision-threatening lesion is with systemic steroids.

Frosted branch angiitis (FBA)

FBA describes a characteristic fundus picture, usually bilateral and may represent a specific entity (primary) or a common pathway in response to multiple stimuli. Secondary FBA may be associated with infectious retinitis, notably cytomegalovirus retinitis and other conditions such as lymphoma and leukaemia. Primary (idiopathic) FBA is rare and typically affects children and young adults, in whom presentation is with bilateral visual loss (6/30 to PL), floaters and/or photopsia. There may be a viral prodrome. Florid sheathing of retinal arterioles and venules is seen (Fig. 12.71). Anterior uveitis, vitritis and retinal oedema are common. Treatment is with systemic steroids, though some authorities believe the prognosis, which is usually good in the primary form, is unaffected.

Idiopathic retinal vasculitis, aneurysms and neuroretinitis syndrome (IRVAN)

Idiopathic retinal vasculitis, aneurysms and neuroretinitis syndrome is a rare entity that typically affects one or both eyes of healthy young women. Fundus signs consist of arteritis and multiple aneurysmal dilatations of arteriolar branches and on the optic nerve head, together with anterior uveitis and vitritis.

Disc oedema and a macular star (neuroretinitis) are common. Marked macular and circumpapillary exudative retinopathy can develop (Fig. 12.72A). The vascular changes are demonstrated very well on FA (Fig. 12.72B). Extensive peripheral capillary nonperfusion may lead to preretinal neovascularization and early panretinal photocoagulation should be considered. Intravitreal anti-VEGF treatment and steroids have been associated with good results in some patients and may be given in combination.

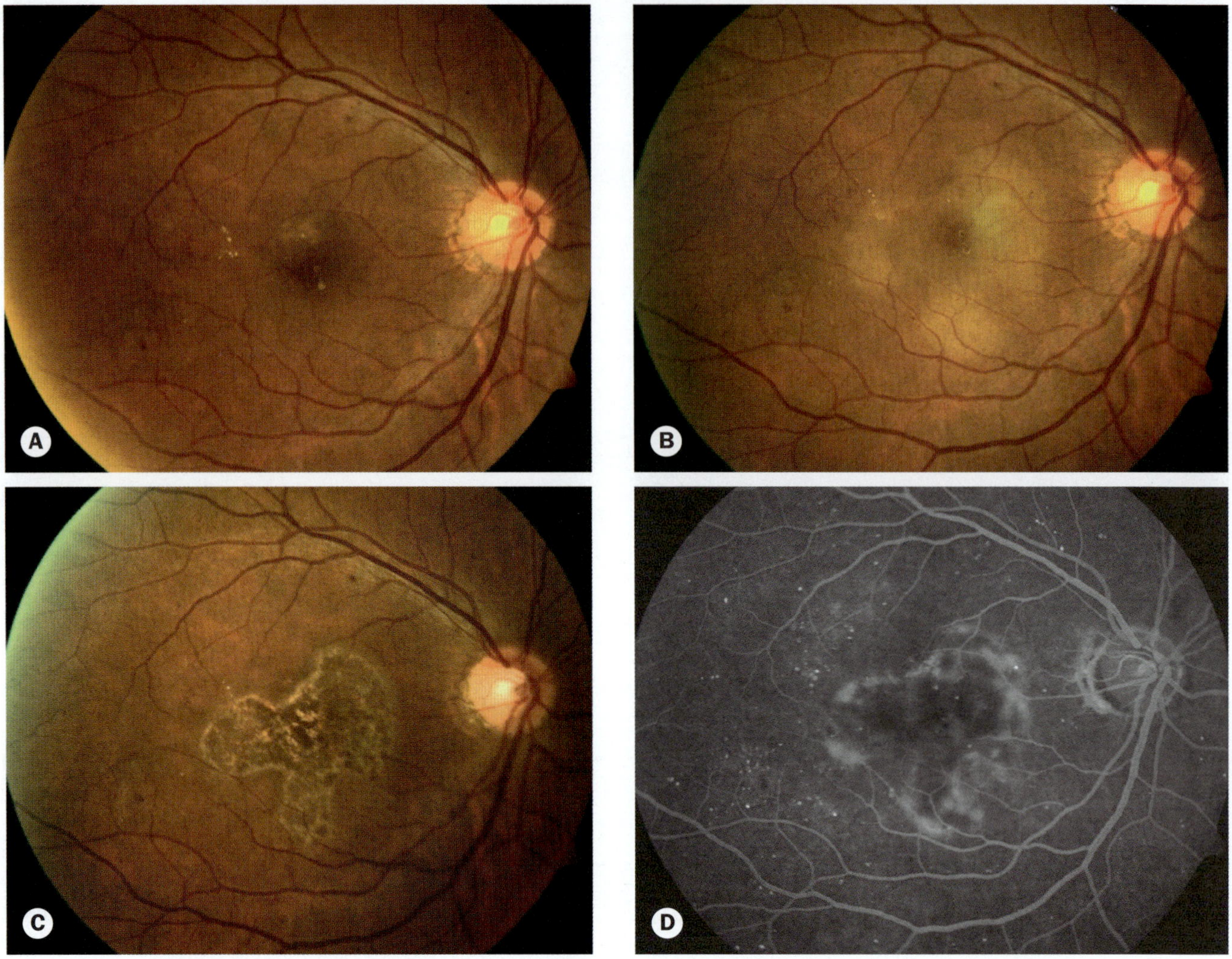

Fig. 12.69 Acute idiopathic maculopathy. **(A)** and **(B)** Development of macular sensory retinal detachment over the course of a month; **(C)** macular appearance after a further month; **(D)** FA showing hyperfluorescence of subretinal fluid. *(Courtesy of S Chen.)*

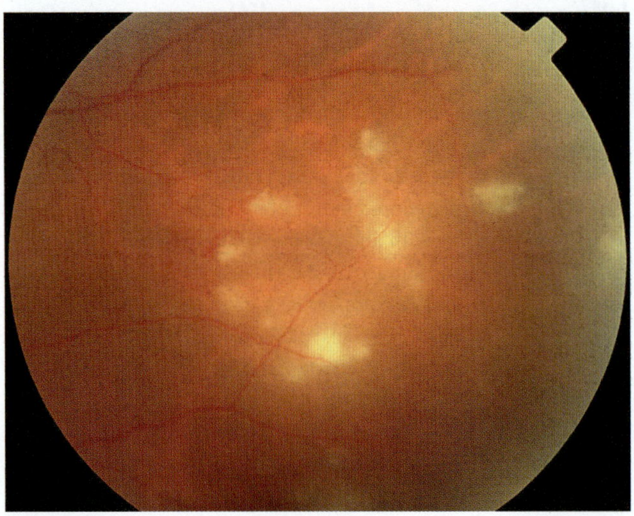

Fig. 12.70 Acute multifocal retinitis.

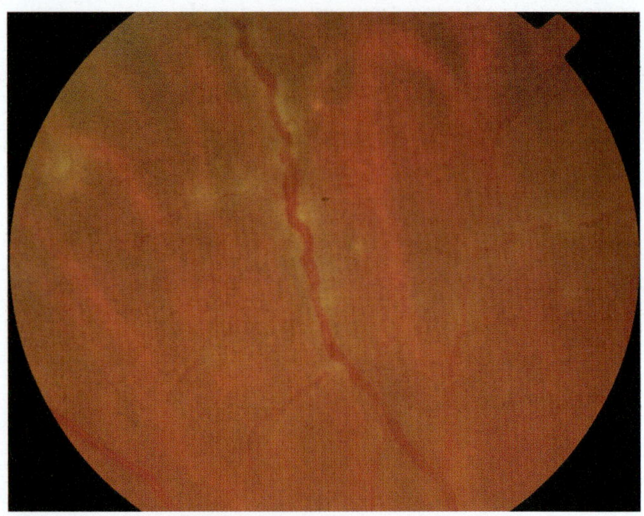

Fig. 12.71 Frosted branch angiitis in patient with lymphoma. *(Courtesy of T James.)*

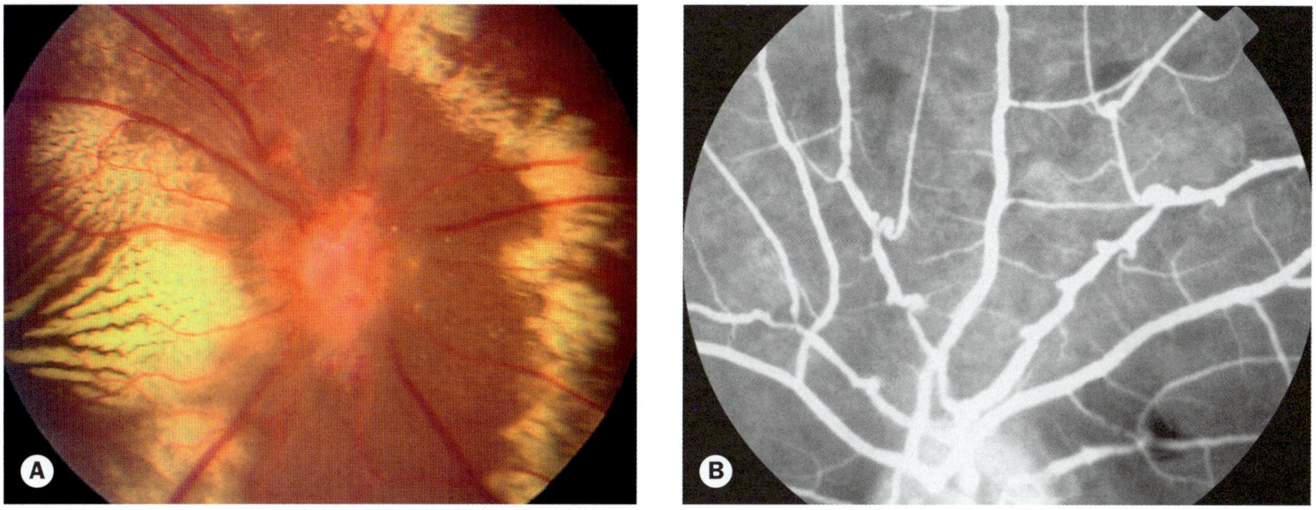

Fig. 12.72 Idiopathic retinal vasculitis, aneurysms and neuroretinitis syndrome. **(A)** Circinate pattern of hard exudates surrounding the disc. There is also venous irregularity and obscuration of the optic nerve head; **(B)** FA showing multiple aneurysms at arteriolar bifurcations and marked variation in arteriolar calibre. *(Courtesy of J Donald Gass, from* Stereoscopic Atlas of Macular Diseases, *Mosby 1997 – fig. A; RF Spaide, from* Diseases of the Retina and Vitreous, *WB Saunders 1999 – fig. B.)*

Chapter 13

Retinal Vascular Disease

RETINAL CIRCULATION

Arterial system

- **The central retinal artery**, an end artery, enters the optic nerve approximately 1 cm behind the globe. It is composed of three anatomical layers:
  - The intima, the innermost, is composed of a single layer of endothelium resting on a collagenous zone.
  - The internal elastic lamina separates the intima from the media.
  - The media consists mainly of smooth muscle.
  - The adventitia is the outermost and is composed of loose connective tissue.
- **Retinal arterioles** arise from the central retinal artery. Their walls contain smooth muscle, but in contrast to arteries the internal elastic lamina is discontinuous.

Capillaries

Retinal capillaries supply the inner two-thirds of the retina, with the outer third being supplied by the choriocapillaris. The inner capillary network (plexus) is located in the ganglion cell layer, with an outer plexus in the inner nuclear layer. Capillary-free zones are present around arterioles (Fig. 13.1A) and at the fovea (foveal avascular zone – FAZ). Retinal capillaries are devoid of smooth muscle and elastic tissue. Their walls consist of the following (Fig. 13.1B):

- **Endothelial cells** form a single layer on the basement membrane and are linked by tight junctions that form the inner blood–retinal barrier.
- **The basement membrane** lies beneath the endothelial cells with an outer basal lamina enclosing pericytes.
- **Pericytes** lie external to endothelial cells and have multiple pseudopodial processes that envelop the capillaries. Pericytes have contractile properties and are thought to participate in autoregulation of the microvascular circulation.

Venous system

Retinal venules and veins drain blood from the capillaries.

- **Small venules** are larger than capillaries but have a similar structure.
- **Larger venules** contain smooth muscle and merge to form veins.
- **Veins** contain a small amount of smooth muscle and elastic tissue in their walls and are relatively distensible. Their diameter gradually enlarges as they pass posteriorly towards the central retinal vein.

DIABETIC RETINOPATHY

Introduction

Diabetes is a major concern for healthcare systems throughout the world. The prevalence of diabetes is relentlessly increasing, particularly in working-age adults. Diabetic retinopathy is the commonest cause of new blindness in most industrialised countries, mainly because of a delay in obtaining medical treatment. However, with effective screening and by embracing and implementing the conclusions of the Early Treatment Diabetic Retinopathy Study (ETDRS) and the anti-VEGF clinical trials, the risk of severe visual loss can be reduced to less than 5%.

Ophthalmic complications of diabetes

- **Common**
  - Maculopathy: diabetic macular oedema and macular ischaemia.
  - Retinopathy: sequelae arising from retinal ischaemia (neovascularization of the optic disc and retina) and vitreous haemorrhage.
  - Unstable refraction.
- **Uncommon**
  - Recurrent styes.

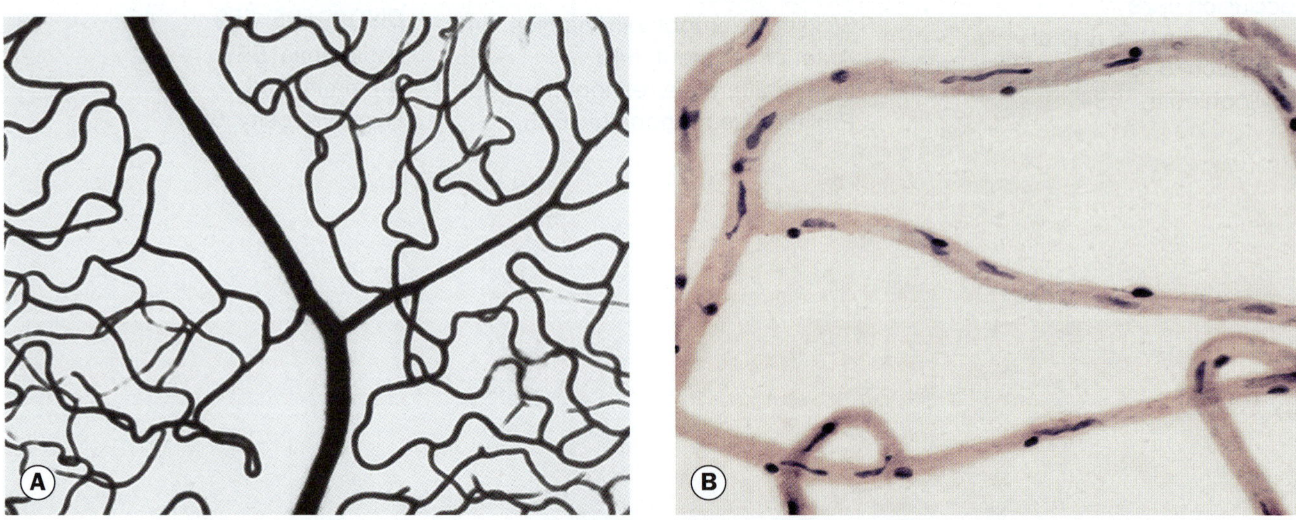

Fig. 13.1 Normal retinal capillary bed. **(A)** Periarteriolar capillary-free zone – flat preparation of Indian ink-injected retina; **(B)** endothelial cells with elongated nuclei and pericytes with rounded nuclei – trypsin digest preparation. *(Courtesy of J Harry and G Misson, from* Clinical Ophthalmic Pathology, *Butterworth-Heinemann 2001.)*

- Xanthelasma.
- Accelerated age-related cataract.
- Tractional retinal detachment.
- Neovascularization of the iris and angle.
- Neovascular glaucoma (NVG).
- Ocular motor nerve palsies.
- Reduced corneal sensitivity.

- **Rare.** Papillopathy, pupillary light–near dissociation, Wolfram syndrome (progressive optic atrophy and multiple neurological and systemic abnormalities), acute-onset cataract, rhino-orbital mucormycosis.

Prevalence

The reported prevalence of diabetic retinopathy (DR) in people with diabetes varies substantially among studies and even among contemporary populations in the same country, but is probably around 40%. People with diabetes are often unaware that they might have retinopathy. The prevalence of DR in type 2 diabetes is 67% 10 years after the diagnosis has been made and 10% will have proliferative disease. DR is more common in type 1 diabetes than in type 2 diabetes.

Risk factors

- **Duration of diabetes** is the most important predictor of diabetic retinopathy. DR rarely develops within 5 years of the onset of diabetes or before puberty. People with type 1 diabetes are at particular long-term risk. Duration is a stronger predictor for proliferative disease than for maculopathy.
- **Poor control of diabetes.** The Diabetes Control and Complication Trial (DCCT) shows that tight blood glucose control, particularly when instituted early, can prevent or delay the development or progression of DR (subsequently confirmed by the United Kingdom Prospective Diabetes Study). However, a sudden improvement in control may be associated with progression of retinopathy. The higher the glycated haemoglobin (HbA1c) the greater the risk of complications of diabetes such as PDR. In people with advanced retinopathy even the most rigorous control of blood glucose may not prevent progression.
- **Hypertension** is very common in those with type 2 diabetes and should be rigorously controlled (<140/80 mmHg). Tight control of blood pressure appears to be particularly beneficial in type 2 diabetics with maculopathy.
- **Nephropathy**, if severe, is associated with worsening of DR. Conversely, treatment of renal disease (e.g. renal transplantation) may be associated with improvement of retinopathy and a better response to photocoagulation.
- **Drugs.** Pioglitazone is associated with a significant risk of worsening of diabetic macular oedema.
- **Pregnancy** is sometimes associated with rapid progression of DR. Predicating factors include (a) greater pre-pregnancy severity of retinopathy, (b) poor pre-pregnancy control of diabetes, (c) control exerted too rapidly during the early stages of pregnancy and (d) pre-eclampsia. The risk of progression is related to the severity of DR in the first trimester. Approximately 5% with mild DR and a third of those with moderate DR will progress to PDR during the pregnancy. If substantial DR is present, frequency of review should reflect individual risk and can be up to 2-weekly. Diabetic macular oedema usually resolves spontaneously after pregnancy and might not need to be treated if it develops in late pregnancy.
- **Other risk factors** include hyperlipidaemia, cataract surgery and anaemia.

TIP The risk of severe visual loss can be significantly reduced by regular retinal screening and by embracing and implementing the conclusions of the various clinical trials in diabetes.

Pathogenesis

DR is predominantly a microangiopathy in which small blood vessels are particularly vulnerable to damage from high glucose levels. Direct hyperglycaemic effects on retinal cells are also likely to play a role.

Many angiogenic stimulators and inhibitors have been identified. Vascular endothelial growth factor (VEGF) appears to be of particular importance in the former category.

Classification

The classification used in the Early Treatment Diabetic Retinopathy Study (ETDRS – the modified Airlie House classification) is widely used internationally. An abbreviated version is set out in Table 13.1, in conjunction with management guidelines. The following descriptive categories are also in widespread use in clinical practice:

- **Background diabetic retinopathy (BDR)** is characterized by microaneurysms, dot and blot haemorrhages and exudates. These are generally the earliest signs of DR and persist as more advanced lesions appear.
- **Diabetic maculopathy** strictly refers to the presence of any retinopathy at the macula, but is commonly reserved for significant changes, particularly vision-threatening oedema and ischaemia.
- **Preproliferative diabetic retinopathy (PPDR)** manifests with cotton-wool spots, venous beading, intraretinal microvascular anomalies (IRMA) and moderate to severe retinal haemorrhages. PPDR indicates progressive retinal ischaemia, with a heightened risk of progression to retinal neovascularization.
- **Proliferative diabetic retinopathy (PDR)** is characterized by neovascularization on or within one disc diameter of the disc (NVD) and/or new vessels elsewhere (NVE) in the fundus.
- **High-risk PDR** is defined as any one of the following: (a) presence of vitreous haemorrhage or preretinal haemorrhage, (b) presence of any active neovascularization, (b) location of neovascularization on or within one disc diameter of the optic disc, (d) NVD >1/3-disc area or NVE >1/2-disc area.
- **Advanced diabetic eye disease** is characterized by tractional retinal detachment, significant persistent vitreous haemorrhage and neovascular glaucoma.

Table 13.1 Abbreviated Early Treatment Diabetic Retinopathy Study (ETDRS) Classification of Diabetic Retinopathy

Category/description	Management
Non-proliferative diabetic retinopathy (NPDR)	
No DR	Review in 12 months
Very mild NPDR Microaneurysms only	Review most patients in 12 months
Mild NPDR Any or all of: microaneurysms, retinal haemorrhages, exudates, cotton-wool spots, up to the level of moderate NPDR. No intraretinal microvascular anomalies (IRMA) or significant beading	Review range 6–12 months, depending on severity of signs, stability, systemic factors and patient's personal circumstances
Moderate NPDR • Severe retinal haemorrhages (more than ETDRS standard photograph 2A: about 20 medium–large per quadrant) in 1–3 quadrants or mild IRMA • Significant venous beading can be present in no more than 1 quadrant • Cotton-wool spots commonly present	Review in approximately 6 months Proliferative diabetic retinopathy (PDR) in up to 26%, high-risk PDR in up to 8% within a year
Severe NPDR The 4–2–1 rule; one or more of: • Severe haemorrhages in all 4 quadrants • Significant venous beading in 2 or more quadrants • Moderate IRMA in 1 or more quadrants	Review in 4 months PDR in up to 50%, high-risk PDR in up to 15% within a year
Very severe NPDR Two or more of the criteria for severe NPDR	Review in 2–3 months High-risk PDR in up to 45% within a year
Proliferative diabetic retinopathy (PDR)	
Mild–moderate PDR New vessels on the disc (NVD) or new vessels elsewhere (NVE), but extent insufficient to meet the high-risk criteria	Treatment considered according to severity of signs, stability, systemic factors and patient's personal circumstances such as reliability of attendance for review. If not treated, review in up to 2 months
High-risk PDR • NVD greater than ETDRS standard photograph 10A (about 1/3-disc area) • Any NVD with vitreous haemorrhage • NVE greater than 1/2-disc area with vitreous haemorrhage	Treatment advised – see text Should be performed immediately when possible and certainly same day if symptomatic presentation with good retinal view
Advanced diabetic eye disease See text for description	See text

Signs

Microaneurysms

Microaneurysms are localized outpouchings, mainly saccular, of the capillary wall that may form either by focal dilatation of the capillary wall where pericytes are absent, or by fusion of two arms of a capillary loop (Fig. 13.2A). Most develop in the inner capillary plexus (ganglion cell layer), frequently adjacent to areas of capillary non-perfusion (Fig. 13.2B). Loss of pericytes (Fig. 13.2C) may also lead to endothelial cell proliferation with the formation of 'cellular' microaneurysms (Fig. 13.2D). Microaneurysms may leak plasma constituents into the retina as a result of breakdown in the blood–retinal barrier, or may thrombose. They tend to be the earliest sign of DR.

- **Signs.** Tiny red dots, often initially temporal to the fovea (Fig. 13.3A). May be indistinguishable clinically from dot haemorrhages.
- **Fluorescein angiography (FA)** allows differentiation between dot haemorrhages and non-thrombosed microaneurysms. Early frames show tiny hyperfluorescent dots (Fig. 13.3B), typically more numerous than visible clinically. Late frames show diffuse hyperfluorescence due to leakage.
- **OCT** shows microaneurysms in the middle retinal layers. Normal vessels look similar to microaneurysms, but are usually seen in the inner retinal layers.

Retinal haemorrhages

- **Retinal nerve fibre layer haemorrhages** arise from the larger superficial precapillary arterioles (Fig. 13.4A) and assume their characteristic shape (Fig. 13.4B) because of the architecture of the retinal nerve fibre layer.
- **Intraretinal haemorrhages** arise from the venous end of capillaries and are located in the compact middle layers of the retina (see Fig. 13.4A) with a resultant red 'dot/blot' configuration (Fig. 13.4C).

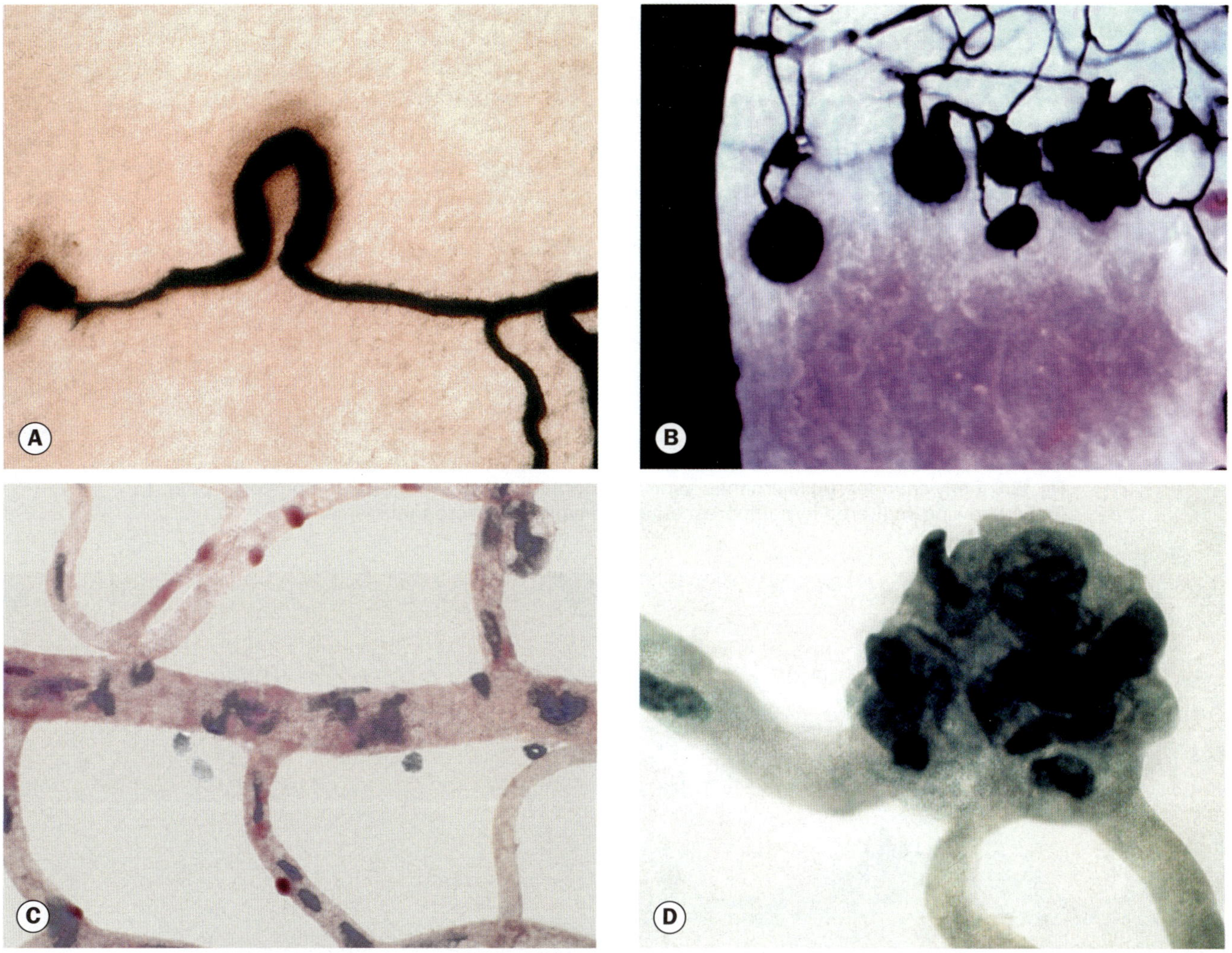

Fig. 13.2 Microaneurysms – histopathology. **(A)** Two arms of a capillary loop that may fuse to become a microaneurysm – flat preparation of Indian ink-injected retina; **(B)** an area of capillary non-perfusion and adjacent microaneurysms – flat preparation of Indian ink-injected retina; **(C)** eosinophilic (dark pink) degenerate pericytes – trypsin digest preparation; **(D)** microaneurysm with endothelial cell proliferation (cellular microaneurysm) – trypsin digest preparation. *(Courtesy of J Harry and G Misson, from* Clinical Ophthalmic Pathology, *Butterworth-Heinemann 2001.)*

- **Deeper dark round haemorrhages** (Fig. 13.4D) represent haemorrhagic retinal infarcts and are located within the middle retinal layers (see Fig. 13.4A). The extent of involvement is a significant marker of the likelihood of progression to PDR.

Exudates

Exudates are caused by chronic localised retinal oedema. They develop at the junction of normal and oedematous retina. They are composed of lipoprotein and lipid-filled macrophages located mainly within the outer plexiform layer (Fig. 13.5A). Hyperlipidaemia may increase the likelihood of exudate formation.

- **Signs**
  - Waxy yellow lesions (Fig. 13.5B) with relatively distinct margins arranged in clumps and/or rings at the posterior pole, often surrounding leaking microaneurysms.
  - With time, the number and size tend to increase (Fig. 13.5C) and the fovea may be involved.
  - When leakage ceases, exudates absorb spontaneously over a period of months, either into healthy surrounding capillaries or by phagocytosis.
  - Chronic leakage leads to enlargement and the deposition of crystalline cholesterol (Fig. 13.5D).
- **FA** will commonly show hypofluorescence only with large dense exudates. Although background choroidal fluorescence is masked, retinal capillary fluorescence is generally preserved overlying the lesions.

Diabetic macular oedema (DMO)

Diabetic maculopathy (macular oedema, exudates or ischaemia) is the most common cause of moderate visual impairment in diabetic patients, particularly type 2. Diffuse retinal

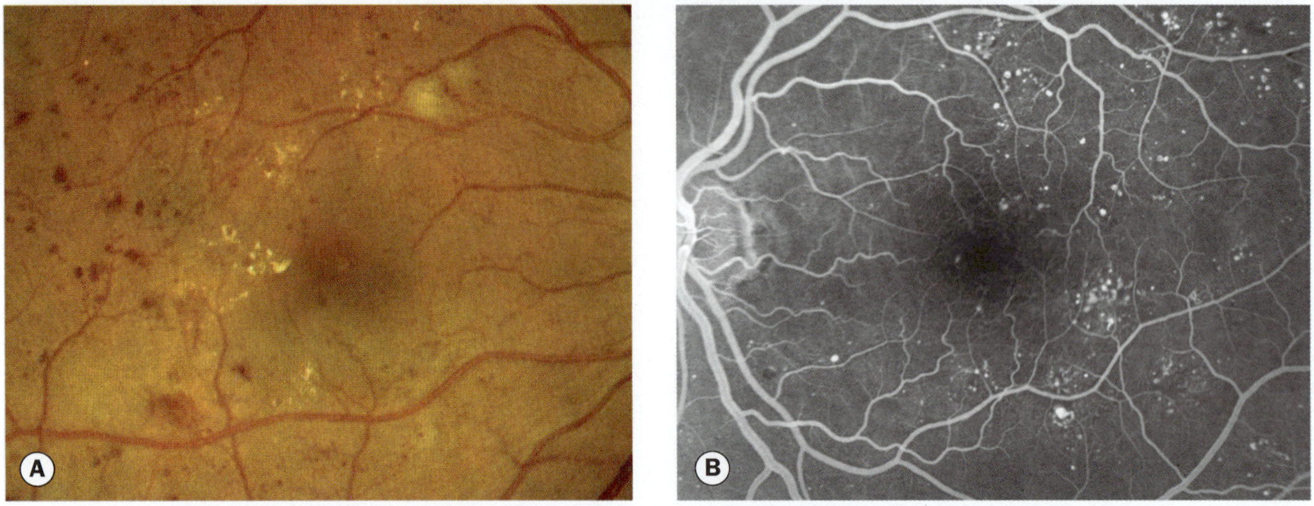

Fig. 13.3 Early changes. **(A)** Microaneurysms and dot/blot haemorrhages at the posterior pole; **(B)** FA showing scattered hyperfluorescent spots typical of microaneurysms.

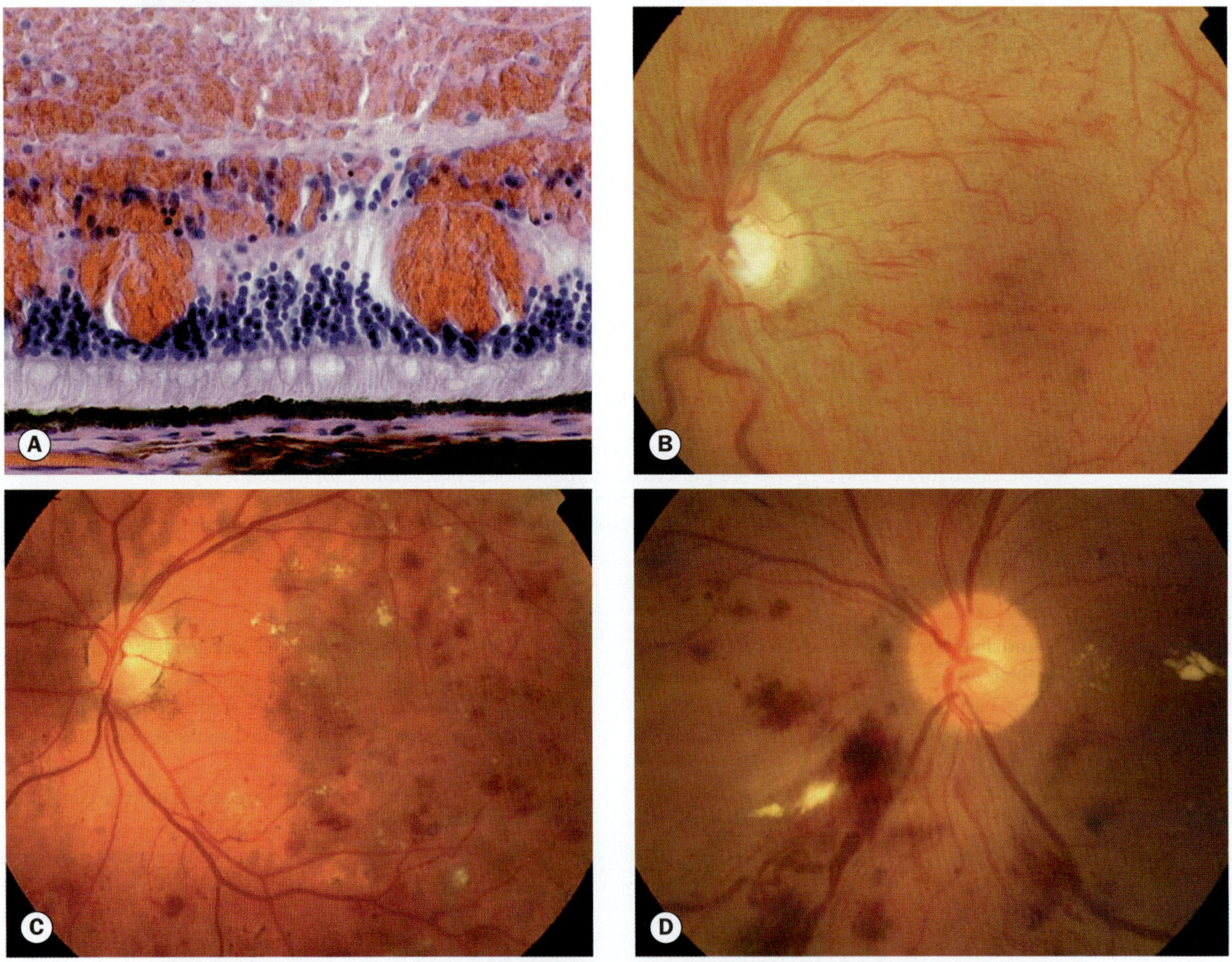

Fig. 13.4 Retinal haemorrhages. **(A)** Histology showing blood lying diffusely in the retinal nerve fibre and ganglion cell layers and as globules in the outer layers; **(B)** retinal nerve fibre layer (flame) haemorrhages; **(C)** dot and blot haemorrhages; **(D)** deep dark haemorrhages. *(Courtesy of J Harry and G Misson, from* Clinical Ophthalmic Pathology, *Butterworth-Heinemann 2001 – fig. A.)*

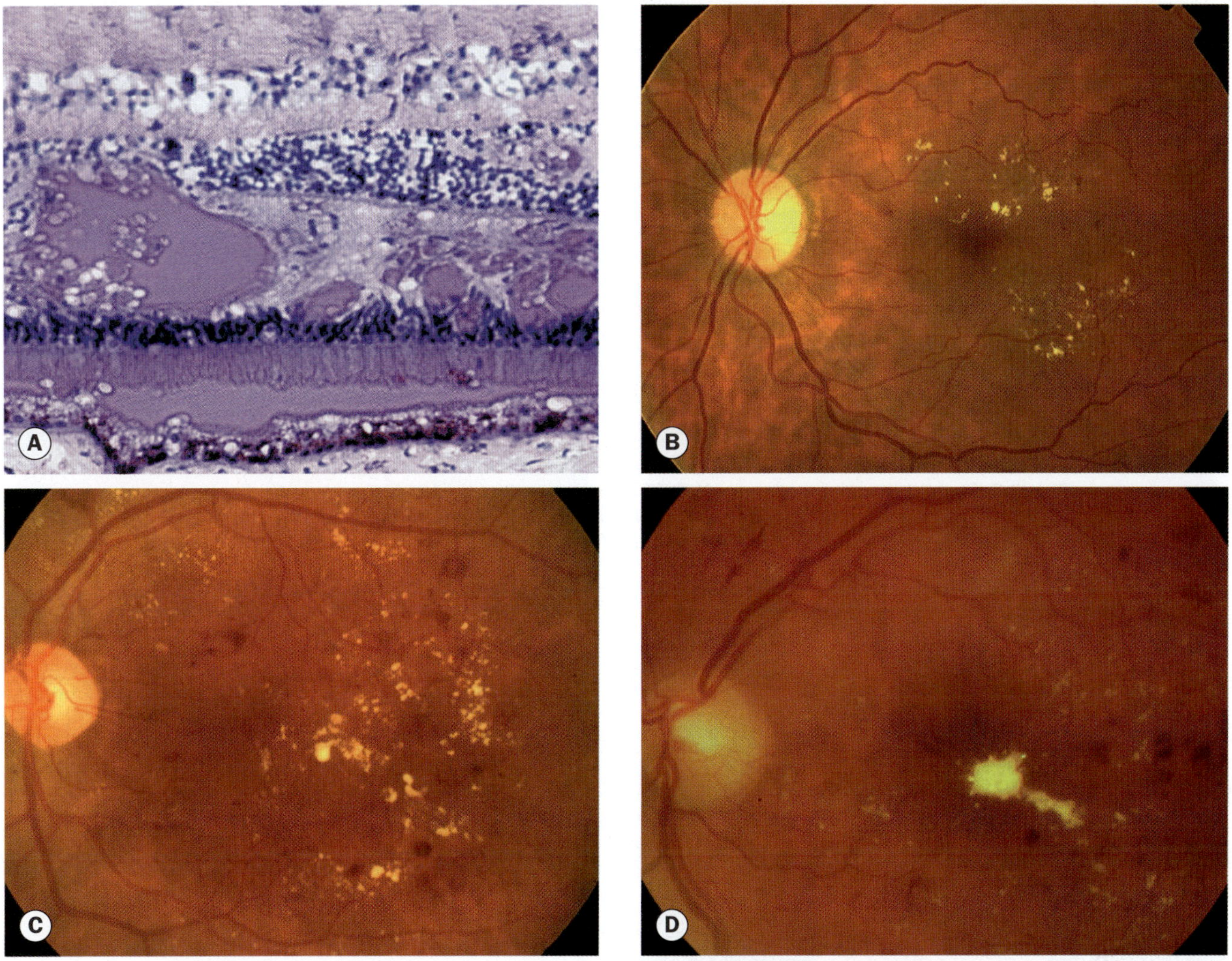

Fig. 13.5 Exudates. **(A)** Histology showing irregular eosinophilic deposits mainly in the outer plexiform layer; **(B)** small exudates and microaneurysms; **(C)** more extensive exudates forming a circinate pattern; **(D)** exudates involving the fovea, including central crystalline cholesterol deposition.

oedema is caused by extensive capillary leakage and localized oedema by focal leakage from microaneurysms and dilated capillary segments. The fluid is initially located between the outer plexiform and inner nuclear layers. Later it may also involve the inner plexiform and nerve fibre layers, until eventually the entire thickness of the retina becomes oedematous. This is readily detectable using OCT (Fig. 13.6A) and FA (Fig. 13.6B).

- **Clinically significant macular oedema (CSMO)** is defined in the ETDRS as:
  - Retinal thickening within 500 µm (or 1/3-disc diameter) of the centre of the macula (Fig. 13.7, upper left).
  - Hard exudates within 500 µm of the centre of the macula, with adjacent retinal thickening, which may lie more than 500 µm from the foveal centre (Fig. 13.7, upper right).
  - Retinal thickening 1-disc area or larger, any part of which is within one disc diameter of the centre of the macula (Fig. 13.7, lower centre).
- **Focal maculopathy**: well-circumscribed retinal thickening associated with complete or incomplete rings of exudates (Fig. 13.8A). FA shows late, focal hyperfluorescence due to leakage, usually with good macular perfusion (Fig. 13.8B).
- **Diffuse maculopathy**: diffuse retinal thickening, which may be associated with cystoid changes. There are typically also scattered microaneurysms and small haemorrhages. Landmarks may be obscured by oedema, which may render localization of the fovea impossible (Fig. 13.9A). FA shows mid- and late-phase diffuse hyperfluorescence (Fig. 13.9B).

Ischaemic maculopathy

- **Signs.** The retina often shows dot and blot haemorrhages and cotton wool spots, but the macula may look relatively normal despite reduced visual acuity (Fig. 13.10A).
- **FA** shows capillary non-perfusion at the fovea (an enlarged FAZ) and frequently other areas of capillary non-perfusion at the posterior pole and periphery (Fig. 13.10B and see OCTA appearance in Fig. 14.26D).

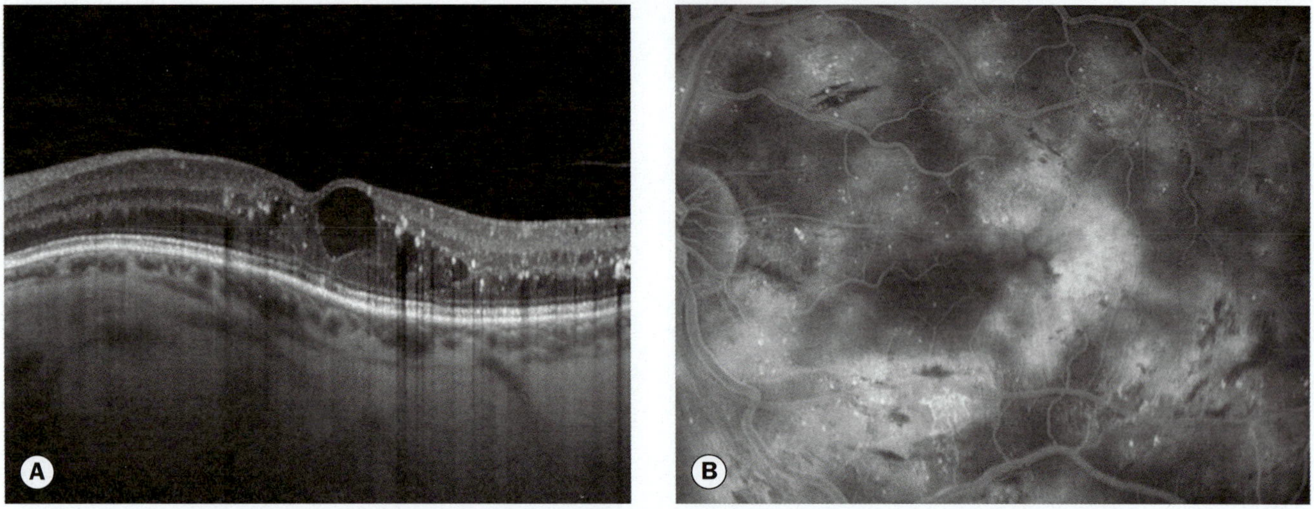

Fig. 13.6 Cystoid macular oedema. **(A)** OCT showing retinal thickening and cystoid spaces; **(B)** FA showing leaking microaneurysms and central diffuse hyperfluorescence with a flower petal configuration. *(Courtesy of A Ambresin – fig. A.)*

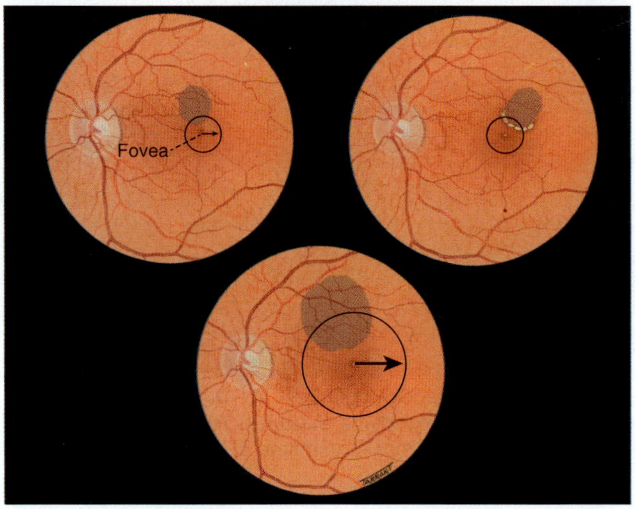

Fig. 13.7 Clinically significant macular oedema (see text).

Cotton-wool spots

Cotton-wool spots are composed of accumulations of neuronal debris within the nerve fibre layer. They result from ischaemic disruption of nerve axons, the swollen ends of which are known as cystoid bodies, seen on light microscopy as globular structures in the nerve fibre layer (Fig. 13.11A). As cotton-wool spots heal, debris is removed by autolysis and phagocytosis.

- **Signs.** Small fluffy whitish superficial lesions that obscure underlying blood vessels (Fig. 13.11B and C). They are clinically evident only in the post-equatorial retina, where the nerve fibre layer is of sufficient thickness to render them visible.
- **FA** shows focal hypofluorescence due to local ischaemia and blockage of background choroidal fluorescence.
- **OCT** shows cotton-wool spots in the retinal nerve fibre layer, which show a hyperreflective pattern in the acute stage. About 80% of the cotton-wool spots have hyporeflective cavities appearing as cysts.

Venous changes

Venous anomalies seen in retinal ischaemia consist of generalized dilatation and tortuosity, looping (Fig. 13.12A), beading (focal narrowing and dilatation) (Fig. 13.12B) and sausage-like segmentation (Fig. 13.12C). The extent of the retinal area exhibiting venous changes correlates well with the likelihood of developing proliferative disease.

Intraretinal microvascular abnormalities

Intraretinal microvascular abnormalities (IRMA) are arteriolar–venular shunts that run from retinal arterioles to venules, thus bypassing the capillary bed and are therefore often seen adjacent to areas of marked capillary hypoperfusion (Fig. 13.13A).

- **Signs.** Fine, irregular, red intraretinal lines that run from arterioles to venules, without crossing major blood vessels (Fig. 13.13B).
- **FA** shows focal hypofluorescence associated with adjacent areas of capillary closure ('dropout') but without leakage (unlike neovascularization, where profuse leakage of fluorescein occurs).
- **OCT.** Unlike new vessels, IRMA do not breach the ILM.

Arterial changes

Subtle retinal arteriolar dilatation may be an early marker of ischaemic dysfunction. When significant ischaemia is present signs include peripheral narrowing, 'silver wiring' and obliteration, similar to the late appearance following a branch retinal artery occlusion.

Proliferative retinopathy

Although preretinal new vessels may arise anywhere in the retina, they are most commonly seen at the posterior pole. Fibrous tissue, initially fine, gradually develops as vessels increase in size.

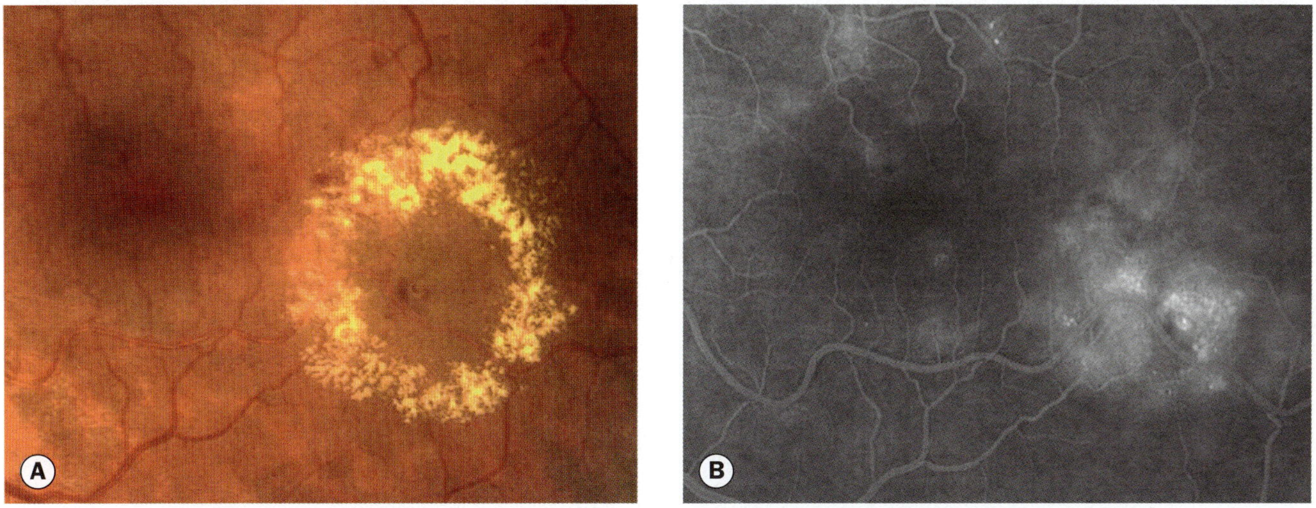

Fig. 13.8 Focal diabetic maculopathy. **(A)** A ring of hard exudates temporal to the macula; **(B)** FA late phase showing focal area of hyperfluorescence due to leakage corresponding to the centre of the exudate ring.

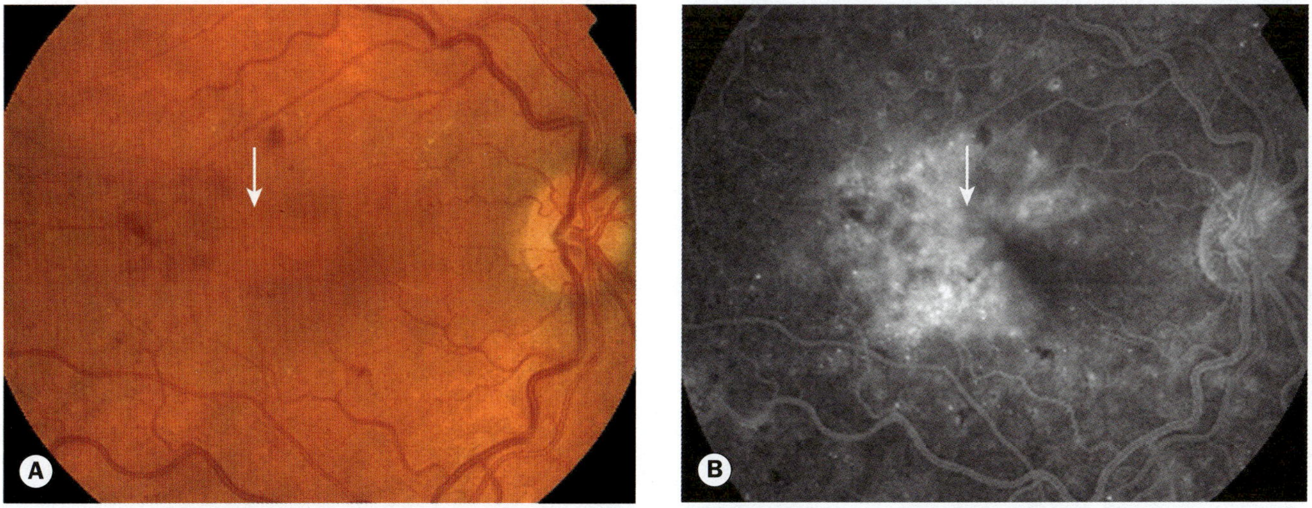

Fig. 13.9 Diffuse diabetic maculopathy. **(A)** Dot and blot haemorrhages – diffuse retinal thickening is present (arrow), which can be difficult to see clinically; **(B)** late phase FA showing extensive hyperfluorescence (arrow) at the posterior pole due to leakage in the same patient.

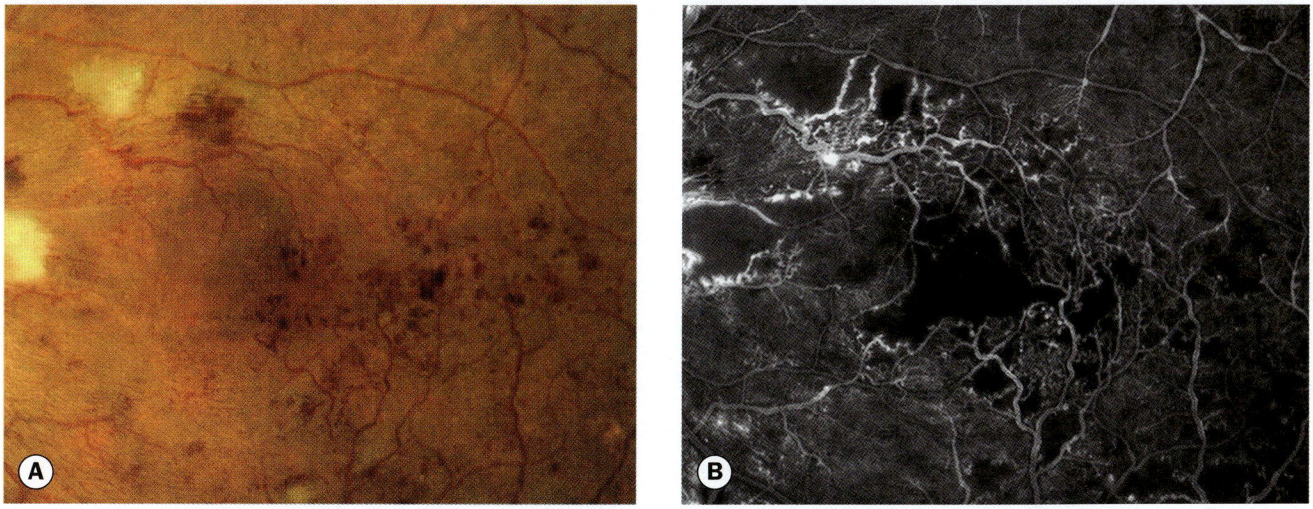

Fig. 13.10 Ischaemic diabetic maculopathy. **(A)** Dot and blot haemorrhages and cotton-wool spots; **(B)** FA venous phase showing hypofluorescence due to capillary non-perfusion at the macula and elsewhere.

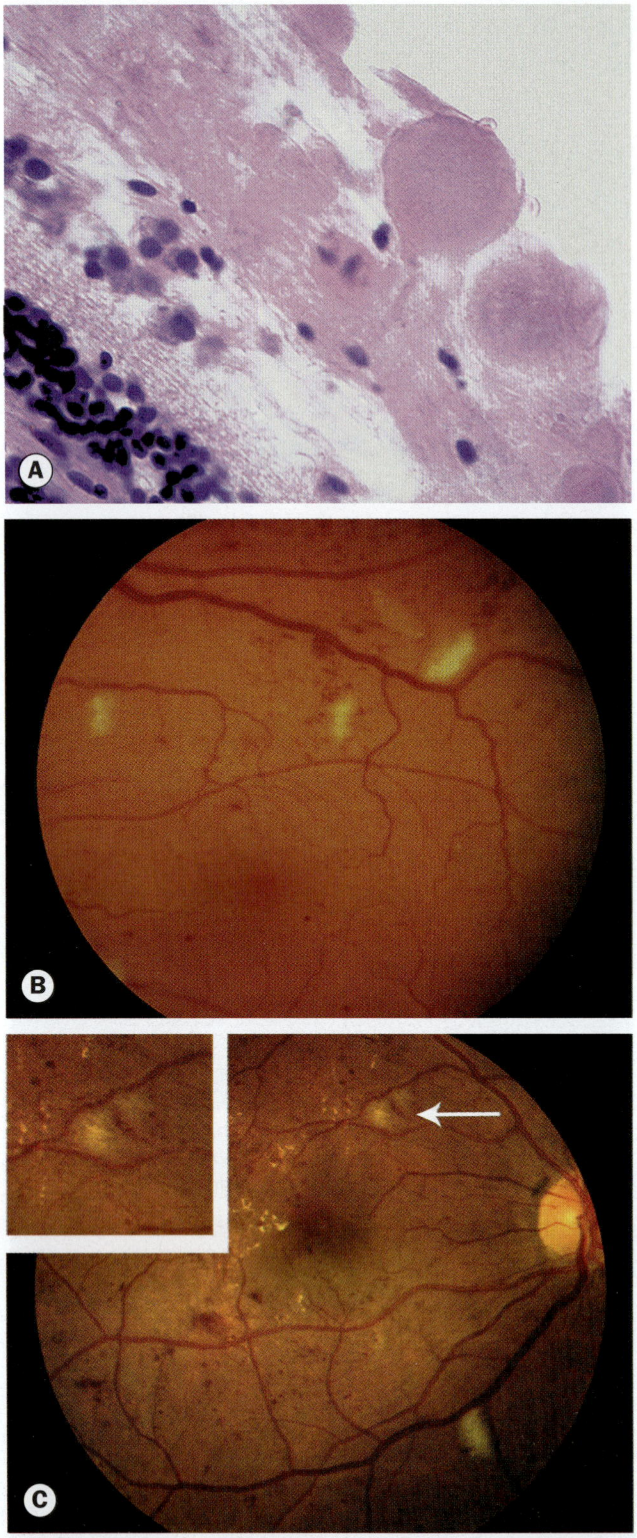

Fig. 13.11 Cotton-wool spots. **(A)** Histology showing cystoid bodies in the retinal nerve fibre layer; **(B)** clinical appearance; **(C)** pre-proliferative retinopathy showing IRMA (arrow).

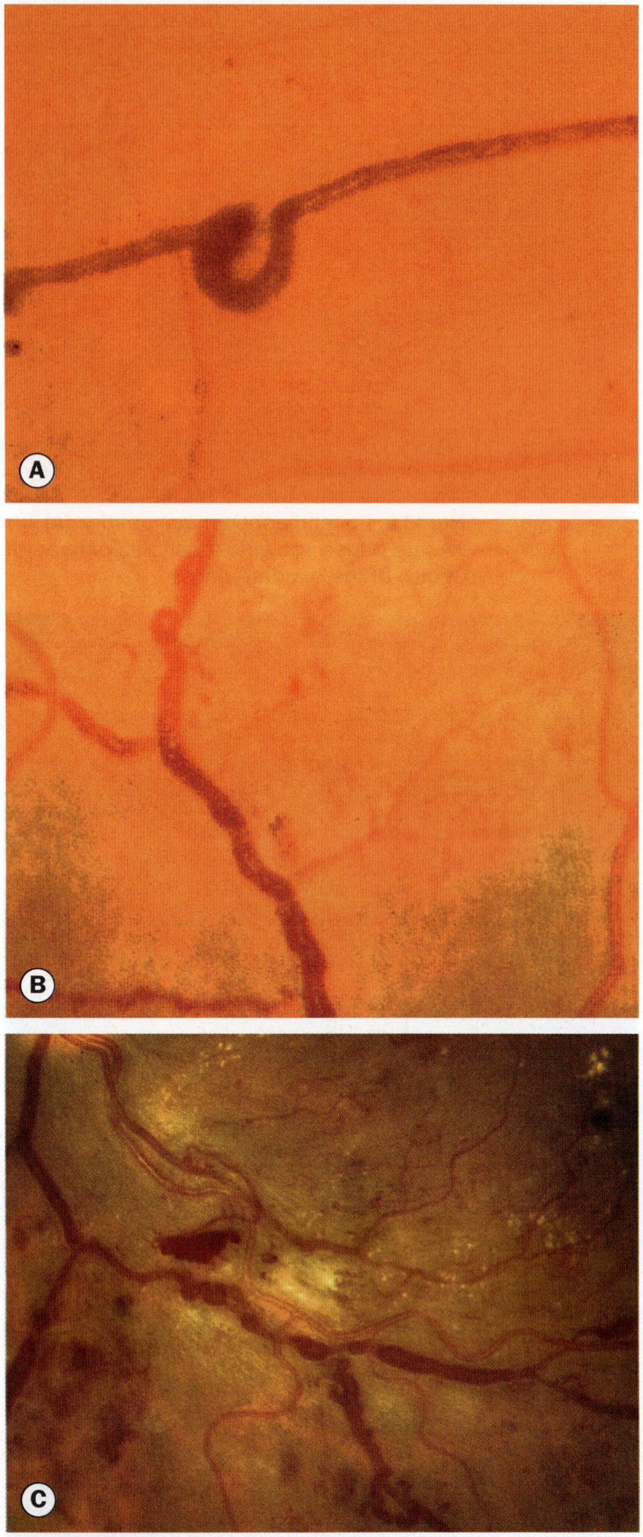

Fig. 13.12 Venous changes. **(A)** Looping; **(B)** beading; **(C)** severe segmentation.

TIP Anti-VEGF therapy and intravitreal steroids are the main therapeutic options used in the treatment of diabetic macular oedema.

TIP Improvement in best-corrected visual acuity after three injections of anti-VEGF medication is a strong predictor of long-term response in a patient with diabetic macular oedema.

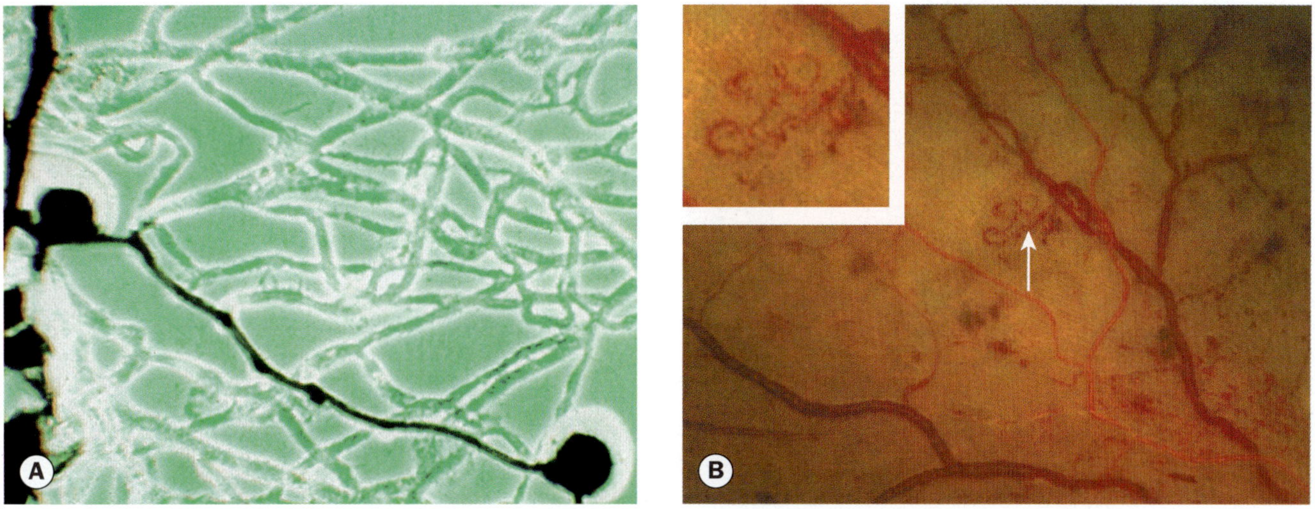

Fig. 13.13 Intraretinal microvascular abnormalities. **(A)** Histology showing arteriolar–venular shunt and a few microaneurysms within a poorly perfused capillary bed – flat preparation of Indian ink-injected retina; phase contrast microscopy; **(B)** clinical appearance (arrow).

- **New vessels at the disc** (NVD) describes neovascularization on or within one disc diameter of the optic nerve head (Fig. 13.14).
- **NVE** describes neovascularization further away from the disc (Fig. 13.15).
- **New vessels on the iris** (NVI – Fig. 13.16), also known as rubeosis iridis, carry a high likelihood of progression to neovascular glaucoma (see Ch. 11).
- **FA** (see Fig. 13.14C) highlights neovascularization during the early phases of the angiogram and shows irregular expanding hyperfluorescence during the later stages due to intense leakage of dye from neovascular tissue. FA can be used to confirm the presence of new vessels (NV) if the clinical diagnosis is in doubt and also delineates areas of ischaemic retina that might be selectively targeted for laser treatment.
- **OCT** of the retina is good at detecting new vessels (100%), but not regression (45%) or reactivation (10%). However, OCT angiography is useful for the objective monitoring of disease after treatment.

Treatment

General

- **Patient education** is critical, including the need to comply with review and treatment schedules in order to optimize visual outcomes. In type 2 diabetes this may involve counselling on weight reduction programs and emphasizing the benefits of regular exercise.
- **Diabetic control** should be optimized.
- **Other risk factors**, particularly systemic hypertension and hyperlipidaemia, should be controlled in conjunction with the patient's diabetologist.
- **Fenofibrate** 200 mg daily has been shown to reduce the progression of DR in type 2 diabetics and prescription should be considered. The decision is independent of whether the patient already takes a statin.
- **Smoking** has not been definitively shown to affect retinopathy, but patients should be advised to stop smoking in order to reduce the risk of macrovascular complications.
- **Other modifiable factors** such as anaemia and renal failure should be addressed as necessary.

TIP The key to the prevention of diabetic retinopathy is patient education and long-term control of blood sugar.

Ophthalmic treatment of diabetic macular oedema

Until recently laser photocoagulation was the mainstay of treatment for DMO, reducing the risk of moderate visual loss by 50% overall compared with observation. The availability of intravitreal anti-VEGF agents and strong evidence to support their efficacy has dramatically altered the approach to management in recent years. Many of the current guidelines for care have arisen from the conclusions of large prospective randomised controlled trials undertaken by the Diabetic Retinopathy Clinical Research Network (DRCR.net). It should be remembered that these studies provide average results in groups of patients and that individual responses may vary considerably, with some patients deriving little or no benefit from these interventions. Options should always be discussed fully with the patient. **In particular, patients with good vision (6/7.5 or better) who otherwise meet criteria for treatment might prefer to be monitored once the risks and benefits of various interventions are considered.** The need for meticulous follow-up and the cost of the proposed treatment may also be an issue for some patients and needs to be considered when discussing therapy.

- **Intravitreal anti-VEGF agents**
  - *DRCR.net Protocol I* concludes that intravitreal ranibizumab more effectively improves visual acuity than focal/grid laser treatment for centre-involved DMO. Laser treatment should be deferred for 6 months after commencement of anti-VEGF therapy. Good outcomes can be expected for at least 5 years, despite a sequential reduction in the number of anti-VEGF injections.
  - *DRCR.net Protocol T* concludes that there are no differences in visual acuity at 5 years irrespective of whether aflibercept, bevacizumab or ranibizumab is used in patients with

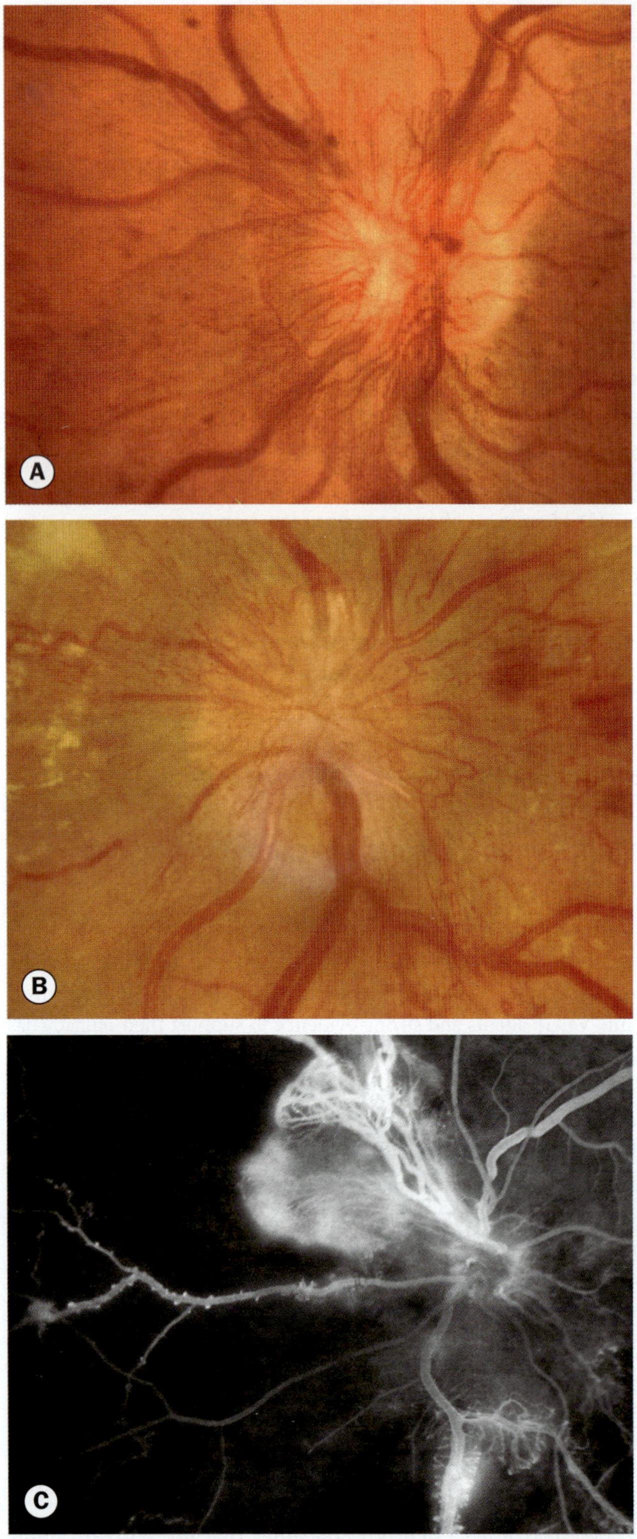

Fig. 13.14 New vessels at the disc (NVD). **(A)** Moderate; **(B)** severe with cotton-wool spots; **(C)** FA showing leaking disc vessels, with extensive peripheral capillary dropout and a small focus of leaking vessels elsewhere.

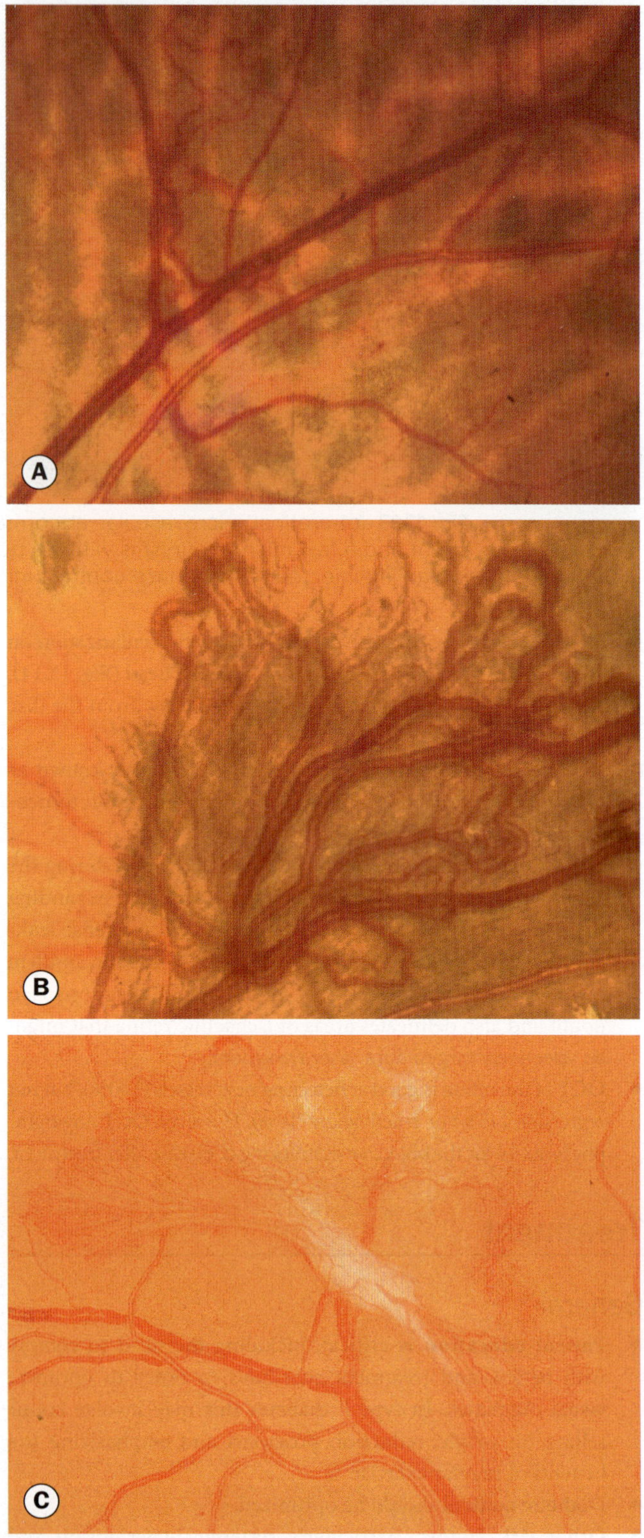

Fig. 13.15 New vessels elsewhere (NVE). **(A)** Mild; **(B)** severe; **(C)** associated with fibrosis.

TIP Intravitreal triamcinolone is a good therapeutic option in pregnant women with diabetic maculopathy, but this treatment can cause cataract and a rise in IOP.

TIP Panretinal photocoagulation continues to be the mainstay of proliferative diabetic retinopathy treatment in most healthcare systems.

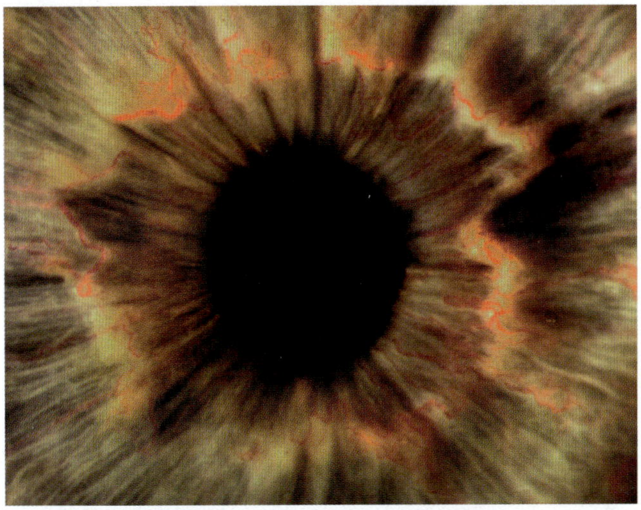

Fig. 13.16 New vessels on the iris (rubeosis iridis).

diabetic maculopathy and a visual acuity of better than 6/15. However, aflibercept is more likely to improve visual acuity than bevacizumab in those with vision of 6/15 or worse (Fig. 13.17).

  - Faricimab is the latest monoclonal antibody that is available for the treatment of diabetic maculopathy. It works by neutralising angiopoietin-2 and VEGF-A, leading to reduced vascular permeability and inflammation, inhibition of angiogenesis and improved vascular stability. It is as effective in improving vision as aflibercept and ranibizumab with a similar side-effect profile (YOSEMITE and RHINE studies). After four initial monthly injections of 6 mg faricimab a treat-and-extend approach can be adopted, leading up to a 16-week dosing regimen (depending on visual acuity and OCT findings).

- **Laser photocoagulation**
  - Although anti-VEGF therapy has replaced laser treatment for most cases, macular laser is a well-proven therapeutic option. It is significantly less effective than other options, but it has its place and could be considered in cases with off-centre retinal thickening when exudates threaten the fovea.
  - Focal laser. Frequency doubled YAG, diode or argon burns are applied to leaking microaneurysms 500–3000 µm from the foveola using a spot size 50–100 µm, duration 0.02–0.1 seconds with sufficient power to obtain a mild greyish reaction beneath the microaneurysm.
  - Modified grid laser (Fig. 13.18). A 'modified' grid includes focal treatment to foci of leakage, usually microaneurysms. The use of grid laser is no longer recommended.
- **Subthreshold macular laser therapy.** This modality uses a train of very short laser pulses (typically 100–300 microseconds) 'on', combined with a relatively longer interval 'off' (typically 1700–1900 microseconds), allowing energy dissipation. This minimises collateral damage to the retina and choroid whilst stimulating the retinal pigment epithelium. Subfoveal therapy is possible. There are positive reports of favourable results using this technology (Fig. 13.19), but there are no clinical trials showing superiority to conventional laser or anti-VEGF treatment.
- **Intravitreal triamcinolone and sustained-release steroid implants.** In pseudophakic eyes intravitreal triamcinolone steroid injection followed by prompt laser is comparable to ranibizumab with regard to visual improvement and reduced retinal thickening. This is a good therapeutic option in pregnancy or where there is a contraindication to anti-VEGF treatment (for example recent myocardial infarct). However, there is a significant risk of inducing an elevation of intraocular pressure (IOP) and this must be monitored regularly. In a phakic eye there is an increased risk of cataract. Sustained-release intravitreal steroid implants (e.g. Ozurdex and Iluvien) have demonstrated promising results.
- **Pars plana vitrectomy (PPV)** may be indicated when macular oedema is associated with tangential traction from a thickened and taut posterior hyaloid (see Ch. 14 – vitreomacular traction syndrome). It has also been suggested that some eyes without a taut posterior hyaloid may also benefit from vitrectomy. Clinically, a taut thickened posterior hyaloid is characterized by an increased glistening of the premacular vitreous face. FA typically shows diffuse leakage and prominent CMO, but OCT is usually the definitive assessment. There are several other indications for PPV in the management of diabetic eye disease (see later).
- **Specific recommendations**
  - CSMO not involving the centre of the macula (particularly where exudates threaten the fovea) may be treated with laser treatment in the form of continuous-wave focal or modified grid laser photocoagulation. If available, subthreshold macular laser treatment, intravitreal anti-VEGF therapy or an intravitreal steroid implant may be reasonable alternatives for this indication.
  - CSMO involving the centre of the macula, but with a visual acuity of better than 6/15 can be treated with aflibercept, bevacizumab, faricimab or ranibizumab. However, bevacizumab reduces OCT swelling less effectively and is more likely to result in persistent DMO than other agents. Alternatively, subthreshold laser can be considered. If laser is to be used, it is prudent to treat no closer than 500 µm from the perceived centre of the macula.
  - CSMO involving the centre of the macula, but with a visual acuity of 6/15 or worse and significant foveolar thickening should be considered for aflibercept or faricimab treatment with initial induction using monthly injections for 3–6 months. An 'as-needed' approach can subsequently be adopted. Focal/grid laser should be deferred for 6 months. An intravitreal dexamethasone implant (Ozurdex) is an alternative treatment that may be considered in patients with absolute or relative contraindications to anti-VEGF injections. In pseudophakic patients who have a transient but significant reduction in macular oedema switching to a fluocinolone acetonide implant (Iluvien) is a reasonable alternative, as it is longer acting and therefore will reduce the need for repeated dexamethasone injections.

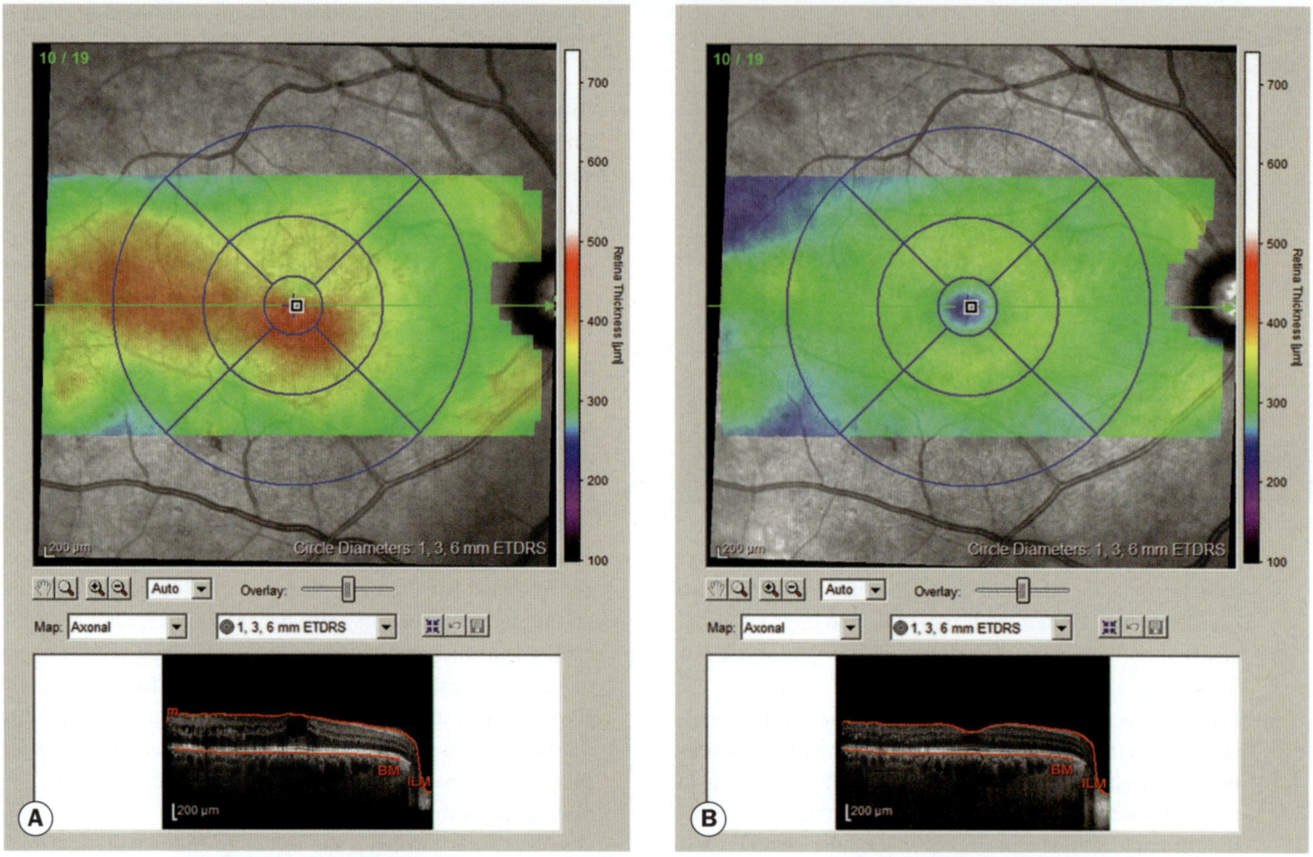

Fig. 13.17 Anti-VEGF treatment for clinically significant macular oedema. **(A)** Macula thickness map and OCT appearance prior to treatment showing diffuse thickening of the macular region; **(B)** 6 months after treatment showing resolution.

- In eyes with PDR and co-existing DMO, ranibizumab, faricimab or aflibercept treatment alone should be considered (rather than panretinal photocoagulation [PRP] and ranibizumab or PRP and aflibercept).
- In eyes with persistent DMO after 6 months of anti-VEGF monotherapy, consider adding laser or switching to an intravitreal dexamethasone implant if there are no contraindications. The simultaneous use of an intravitreal dexamethasone implant and ranibizumab injection appears to provide better visual acuity results than monotherapy with ranibizumab alone, in centre-involved diabetic maculopathy.
- Eyes with markedly reduced vision due to DMO often have associated macular ischaemia and therefore a poor prognosis. Optimal management for this group of patients has not been determined. Depending on circumstances, including the severity of macular oedema and the level of ischaemia, any of the interventions discussed above may be considered.
- In resistant cases, pars plana vitrectomy may be considered, particularly if vitreomacular traction or a marked epiretinal membrane is present.

Laser treatment for proliferative retinopathy

- **Scatter laser treatment** (panretinal photocoagulation – Fig. 13.20A) continues to be the mainstay of PDR treatment in most healthcare systems. The Diabetic Retinopathy Study (DRS) establishes the characteristics of high-risk proliferative disease and demonstrates the benefit of PRP. For instance, severe NVD without haemorrhage carries a 26% risk of visual loss at 2 years that is reduced to 9% with PRP. However, recent research *(Protocol S from DRCR.net)* shows that a course of injections of intravitreal ranibizumab is as effective as photocoagulation in patients at high risk of PDR at 5 years (see below). In addition, the CLARITY study provides 1-year data which show that intravitreal aflibercept injections are as effective as PRP in the treatment of PDR.
- **Informed consent**
  - Patients should be advised that PRP may cause visual field defects of sufficient severity to legally preclude driving a motor vehicle. However, most patients who start with good vision are able to maintain their binocular visual field to the standard legally required in most countries.
  - They should be made aware that there is a risk to central vision (because of developing or exacerbating macular oedema; a risk that can be reduced by fractionating the

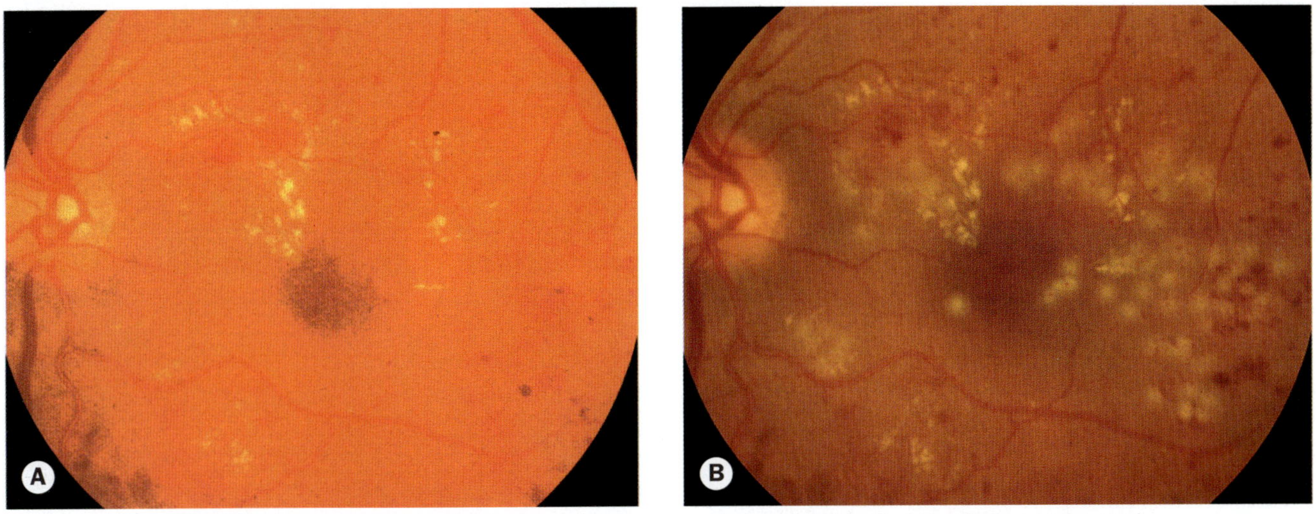

Fig. 13.18 Laser for clinically significant macular oedema. **(A)** Prior to modified macular grid laser treatment; **(B)** patient in **(A)** immediately following grid laser.

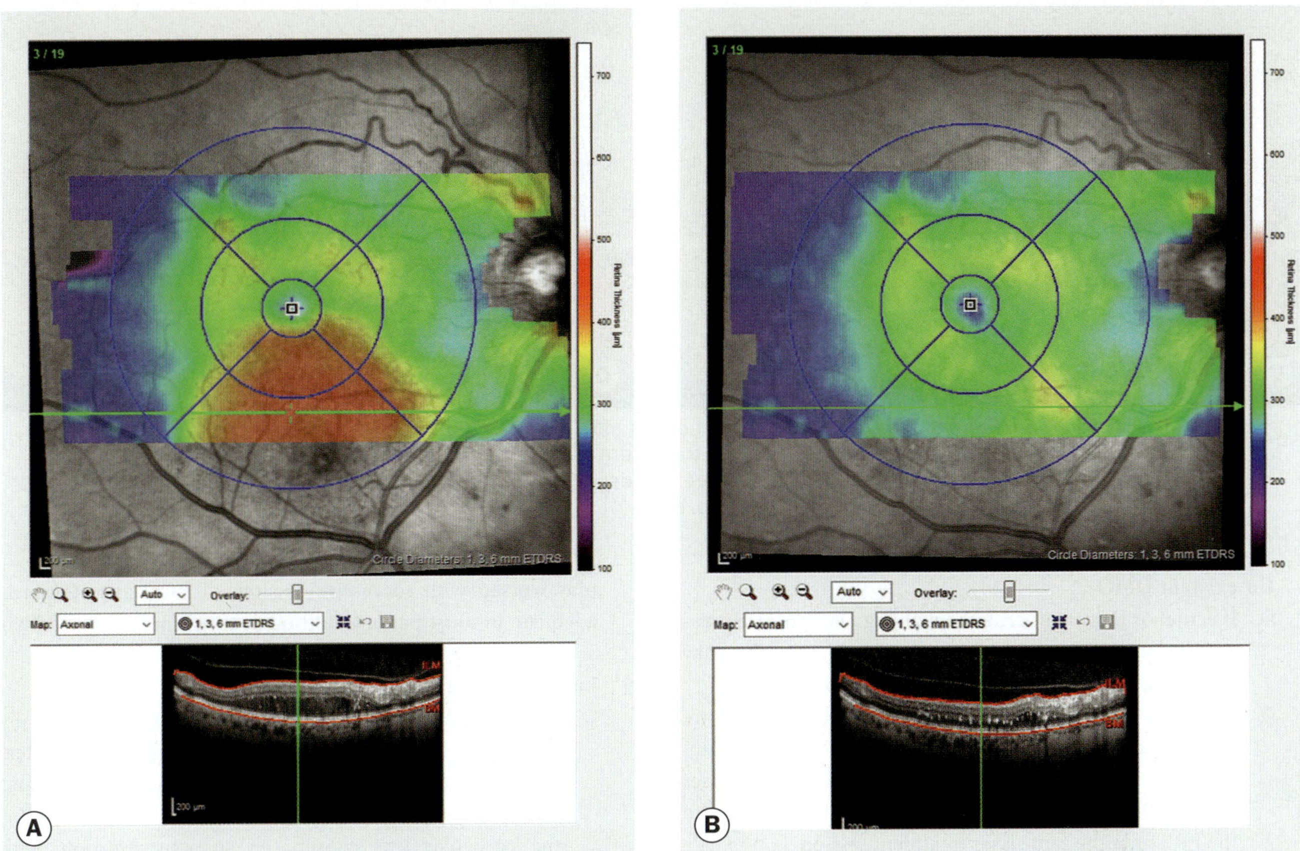

Fig. 13.19 Subthreshold (micropulse) diode laser for clinically significant macular oedema. **(A)** Macula thickness map and OCT appearance prior to treatment showing thickening of the macular region below the fovea; **(B)** 3 months after treatment showing no oedema.

treatment over 2–3 sessions) and that night and colour vision may be affected.

- The 5-year results of the *DRCR.net Protocol S* and CLARITY studies and the 2-year results from the YOSEMITE and RHINE studies should be discussed, as the patient may choose to be treated with an anti-VEGF agent instead of PRP. However, they should also be made aware of the risks associated with repeated injections and the relatively short-term nature of these studies.

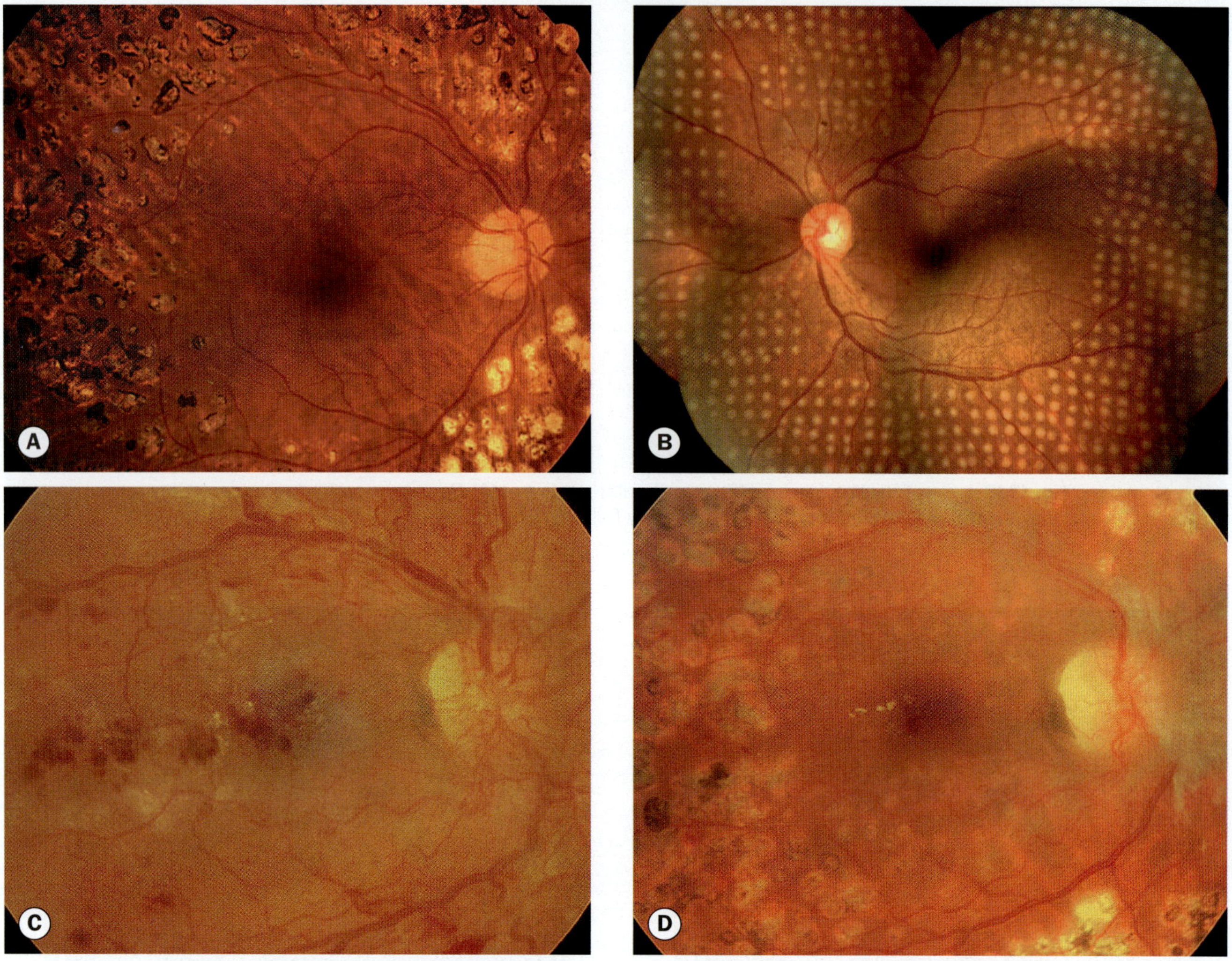

Fig. 13.20 **(A)** Retinal appearance several months after laser; **(B)** composite image of 'pattern scan' multispot array treatment; **(C)** before treatment of severe proliferative diabetic retinopathy; **(D)** 3 months later the new vessels have regressed – there is residual fibrosis at the disc. *(Courtesy of C Barry – fig. A; S Chen – fig. B.)*

- **Co-existent DMO**
  - If actual or imminent central-involving DMO is also present, an anti-VEGF agent should be considered. This may be used as monotherapy or as an adjunct to PRP.
  - Alternatively, in the case of CSMO not involving the centre of the macula and active PDR, laser treatment to the macula could be considered in addition to PRP. In such cases the macular laser treatment should be carried out prior to the PRP or at the same laser treatment session.
- **Lens.** A contact lens is used to provide a stable magnified fundus view. A panfundoscopic lens is generally preferred to a three-mirror lens. Some practitioners prefer to use a high-magnification/smaller-area contact lens (e.g. Mainster, Area Centralis) for the more posterior component of treatment. It is essential to constantly bear in mind that an inverted and laterally reversed image is seen.
- **Anaesthesia.** The amount of treatment it is possible to apply during one session may be limited by patient discomfort. This tends to be least at the posterior pole and greatest in the periphery and over the horizontal neurovascular bundles and may worsen with successive sessions. Topical anaesthesia is adequate in most patients, although sub-Tenon or peribulbar anaesthesia can be administered if necessary.
- **Laser parameters**
  - Spot size. A retinal burn diameter of 400 μm is usually desired for PRP. The diameter selected at the user interface to achieve this depends on the contact lens used and the operator must be aware of the correction factor for the particular lens chosen. As an approximation, with panfundoscopic-type lenses the actual retinal spot diameter is twice that selected on the laser user interface; 200 μm is typically selected for PRP, equating to a 400 μm actual retinal diameter once relative magnification is factored in. With the Mainster and Area Centralis, the retinal diameter equates closely to the interface selection, so 400 μm may be selected.
  - Duration depends on the type of laser: 0.05–0.1 s was conventionally used with the argon laser, but newer lasers allow much shorter pulses to be used and 0.01–0.05 s (10–50 ms) is the currently recommended range. Multispot strategies

available on some machines utilize a combination of short pulse duration (e.g. 20 ms), very short intervals and pre-programmed delivery arrays to facilitate the application of a large number of pulses in a short period (Fig. 13.20B). True subthreshold PRP is also under investigation and shows promising results. Shorter pulse duration seems to require a greater total number of burns for an adequate response and may be slower to achieve regression.

- Power should be sufficient to produce only a light intensity burn.
- Spacing. Burns should be separated by 1–1.5 burn widths.
- Extent of treated area. The initial treatment session should consist of 1500 burns in most cases, though more may be applied if there is a risk of imminent sight loss from vitreous haemorrhage. The more extensive the treatment at a single session, the greater the likelihood of complications. Reported figures vary, but 2500–3500 burns are likely to be required for regression of mild PDR, 4000 for moderate PDR and 7000 for severe PDR. The number of burns offers only approximate guidance, as the effective extent of treatment is dependent on numerous variables.
- Pattern of treatment. Treatment is generally restricted to the area outside the temporal macular vascular arcades. It is good practice to delineate a 'barrier' of laser burns temporal to the macula early in the procedure to help to reduce the risk of accidental macular damage. Many practitioners leave two disc diameters untreated at the nasal side of the disc, to preserve paracentral field. In very severe PDR it is advisable to treat the inferior fundus first, since any vitreous haemorrhage will gravitate inferiorly and obscure this area, precluding further treatment. Areas of vitreoretinal traction should be avoided.

- **Review** is dependent on PDR severity and the requirement for successive treatment applications. Initial treatment should be fractionated over 2–3 sessions. Once an adequate number of burns have been applied review can be set for 4–6 weeks.

TIP In a patient with proliferative diabetic retinopathy and macular oedema, first treat the oedema then undertake panretinal photocoagulation.

- **Indicators of regression** include blunting of vessel tips, shrinking and disappearance of NV, often leaving 'ghost' vessels or fibrosis (Fig. 13.20C and D), regression of IRMA, decreased venous changes, absorption of retinal haemorrhages, disc pallor. Contraction of regressing vessels or associated induction of vitreous separation can precipitate vitreous haemorrhage. Significant fibrous proliferation can lead to tractional retinal detachment (see below). Patients should remain under observation, as recurrence can occur with a requirement for additional PRP.

VEGF inhibition for proliferative retinopathy

PRCR.net Protocol S concludes that intravitreal ranibizumab treatment is as effective as PRP in patients at high risk of PDR for up to 5 years. The macular oedema rate is reduced and the visual field is slightly better maintained with anti-VEGF treatment. Irrespective of the therapeutic option, approximately half will experience a vitreous haemorrhage over that period. Anti-VEGF treatment should be avoided and PRP provided if follow-up is likely to be poor or if cost is an issue.

- Treatment of rubeosis iridis (see Ch. 11).
- Treatment of PDR prior to cataract surgery (see Ch. 10).

Targeted retinal photocoagulation (TRP)

Wide-field FA allows accurate delineation of peripheral capillary non-perfusion (Fig. 13.21). Selective treatment of these areas with scatter laser has been reported as effectively leading to regression of NV whilst minimizing potential complications.

Advanced diabetic eye disease

Advanced diabetic eye disease is a serious vision-threatening complication of DR that occurs in patients in whom treatment has been inadequate or unsuccessful. Occasionally, advanced disease is evident at presentation.

Clinical features

- **Haemorrhage** may be preretinal (retrohyaloid), intragel or both (Fig. 13.22A). Intragel haemorrhages usually take longer to clear than preretinal because the former is usually more substantial. In some eyes, altered blood becomes compacted on the posterior vitreous face to form an 'ochre membrane'. Ultrasonography is used in eyes with dense vitreous haemorrhage to detect the possibility of associated retinal detachment.
- **Tractional retinal detachment** (Fig. 13.22B and C) is caused by progressive contraction of fibrovascular membranes over areas of vitreoretinal attachment. Posterior vitreous detachment in eyes with PDR is often incomplete due to the strong adhesions between cortical vitreous and areas of fibrovascular proliferation. Haemorrhage often occurs at these sites due to stress exerted on NV.
- **Rubeosis iridis** (iris neovascularization – NVI) may occur in eyes with PDR and if severe may lead to neovascular glaucoma (see Ch. 11). NVI is particularly common in eyes with severe

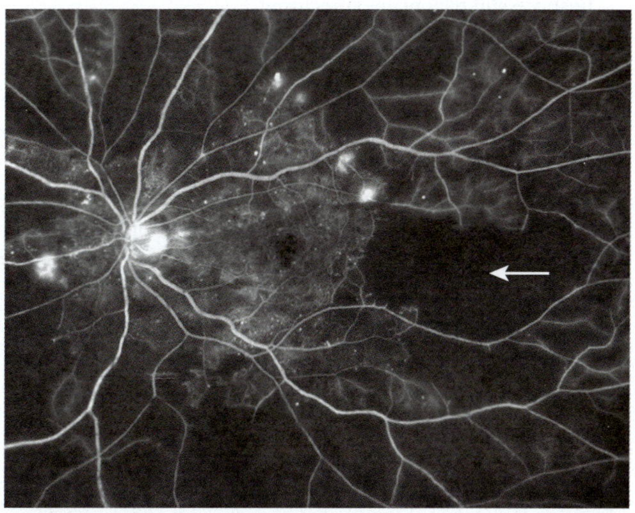

Fig. 13.21 Wide-field FA showing widespread areas of capillary non-perfusion – the arrow indicates a well-defined example. *(Courtesy of A Ambresin.)*

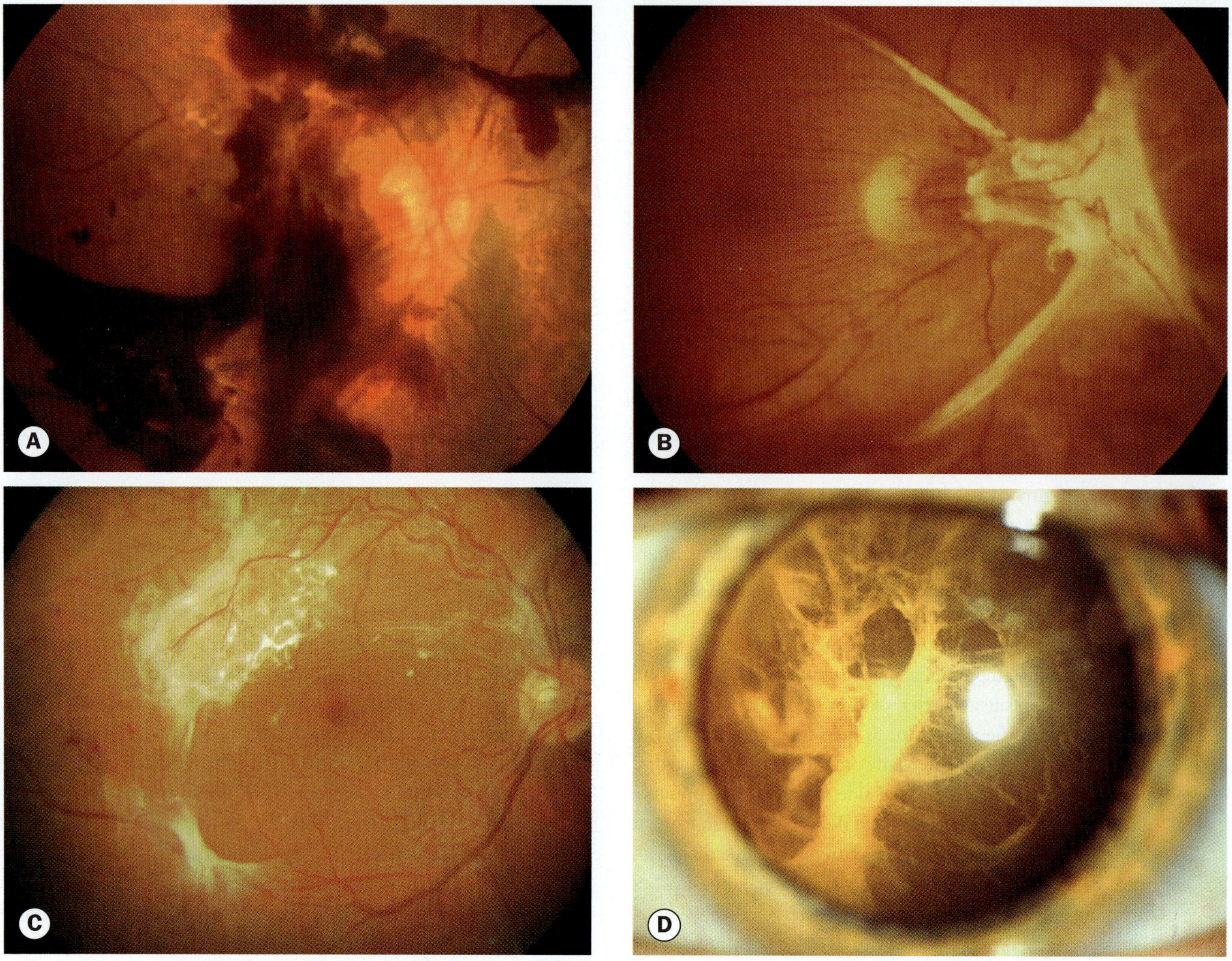

Fig. 13.22 Advanced diabetic eye disease. **(A)** Retrohyaloid and intragel haemorrhage; **(B)** preretinal traction; **(C)** tractional retinal detachment; **(D)** significant vitreous haemorrhage. *(Courtesy of S Chen – fig. A; C Barry – fig. D.)*

retinal ischaemia or persistent retinal detachment following unsuccessful pars plana vitrectomy.

Indications for pars plana vitrectomy

Vitrectomy in DR is typically combined with extensive endolaser PRP. Visual results depend on the specific indication for surgery and the severity of pre-existing disease.

- **Severe persistent vitreous haemorrhage** that precludes adequate PRP is the most common indication (Fig. 13.22D). In the absence of rubeosis iridis, vitrectomy has traditionally been considered within 3 months of the initial vitreous haemorrhage in type 1 diabetics and in most cases of bilateral haemorrhage. However, the outcome may be better with earlier surgery and the availability of intravitreal anti-VEGF therapy may further modify the approach.
- ***DRCR.net protocol AB*** concludes that eyes with vitreous haemorrhage that undergo initial vitrectomy with PRP recover vision faster than those treated initially with aflibercept. However, the vision is similar in the two groups 2 years later, which suggests that either option is a reasonable first-line treatment of vitreous haemorrhage from PDR.
- **Progressive tractional RD** threatening or involving the macula must be treated without delay. However, extramacular tractional detachments may be observed, since they often remain stationary for prolonged periods.
- **Combined tractional and rhegmatogenous RD** should be treated urgently.
- **Premacular retrohyaloid haemorrhage** (Fig. 13.23A), if dense and persistent should be considered for early vitrectomy because, if untreated, the internal limiting membrane or posterior hyaloid face may serve as a scaffold for subsequent fibrovascular proliferation and consequent tractional macular detachment or macular epiretinal membrane formation. Dispersion with Nd:YAG laser (hyaloidotomy) is often successful (Fig. 13.23B and C).
- **Anterior segment neovascularization and media opacities,** which prevent visualization of the posterior pole, should be considered for vitrectomy and intraoperative laser therapy.

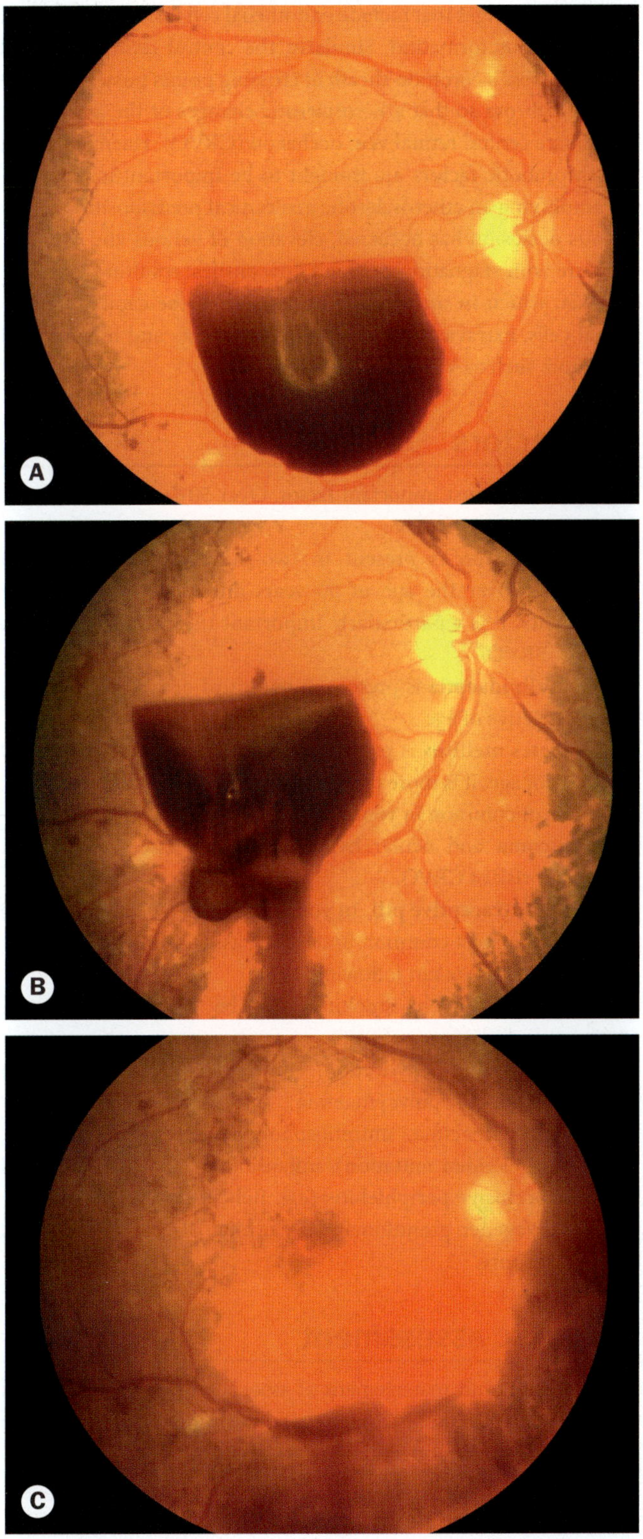

Fig. 13.23 Large premacular retrohyaloid haemorrhage. **(A)** Before; **(B)** and **(C)** after Nd:YAG laser hyaloidotomy. *(Courtesy of S Chen.)*

TIP Persistent vitreous haemorrhage or progressive tractional retinal detachment threatening the macula should be treated as soon as possible with a pars plana vitrectomy.

Diabetic papillopathy

Diabetic papillopathy (diabetic papillitis) has been speculated to be an uncommon variant of anterior ischaemic optic neuropathy, though is more commonly bilateral and tends to exhibit more diffuse disc swelling.

- **Pathogenesis.** The underlying pathogenesis is not known. The condition is more likely to occur in people with small optic discs and after a rapid decrease in the blood glucose level.
- **Clinical features.** It occurs mainly in younger people with diabetes and manifests with mild painless visual impairment that is unilateral in more than half of cases. Hyperaemic disc swelling is characteristic and disc telangiectasia is often present (Fig. 13.24A and B). Crowding of the fellow disc may be found.
- **Resolution** occurs over several months (Fig. 13.24C), often leaving mild disc pallor. Final visual acuity (VA) is 6/12 or better in 80%, subject to the effect of co-existing DR.
- **Differential diagnosis.** The telangiectasia should not be mistaken for neovascularization. Distinction from retinal vein occlusion (RVO)-type papillophlebitis (see below) rests on the presence of more extensive retinal haemorrhages and venous congestion in the latter, but may not be possible. Raised intracranial pressure should be excluded if there is bilateral disc swelling.
- **Treatment.** There is no validated treatment. Intravitreal anti-VEGF agents and steroids via various routes have been tried, with no significant benefit.

NON-DIABETIC RETINOPATHY

Up to 10% of individuals over the age of 40 without diabetes mellitus exhibit – usually very mild – retinopathic features such as microaneurysms, dot and blot haemorrhages and cotton-wool spots that would be consistent with a diagnosis of DR. Assuming that an alternative ocular cause such as RVO or idiopathic macular telangiectasia has been excluded, this 'non-diabetic' retinopathy tends to be associated with increased cerebrovascular and cardiovascular risk and may be particularly prevalent in patients with known or incipient hypertension. There is evidence suggesting that it may be a marker of preclinical diabetes in some patients; higher venular calibre may also denote this. Appropriate management is undefined, though evaluation and optimal management of systemic vascular risk factors may be prudent. The signs commonly disappear spontaneously and this is more likely in those with lower levels of cardiovascular risk.

RETINAL VENOUS OCCLUSIVE DISEASE

Introduction

Retinal vein thrombosis is strongly associated with age-related local and systemic factors. It is the second most common retinal vascular disease after DR. The condition affects 5 in 1000 people in the industrialised world. In branch retinal vein occlusion (BRVO) arteriosclerotic thickening of a branch retinal arteriole is associated with compression of a venule at an arteriovenous crossing point, exacerbated by sharing an adventitial sheath. This leads to

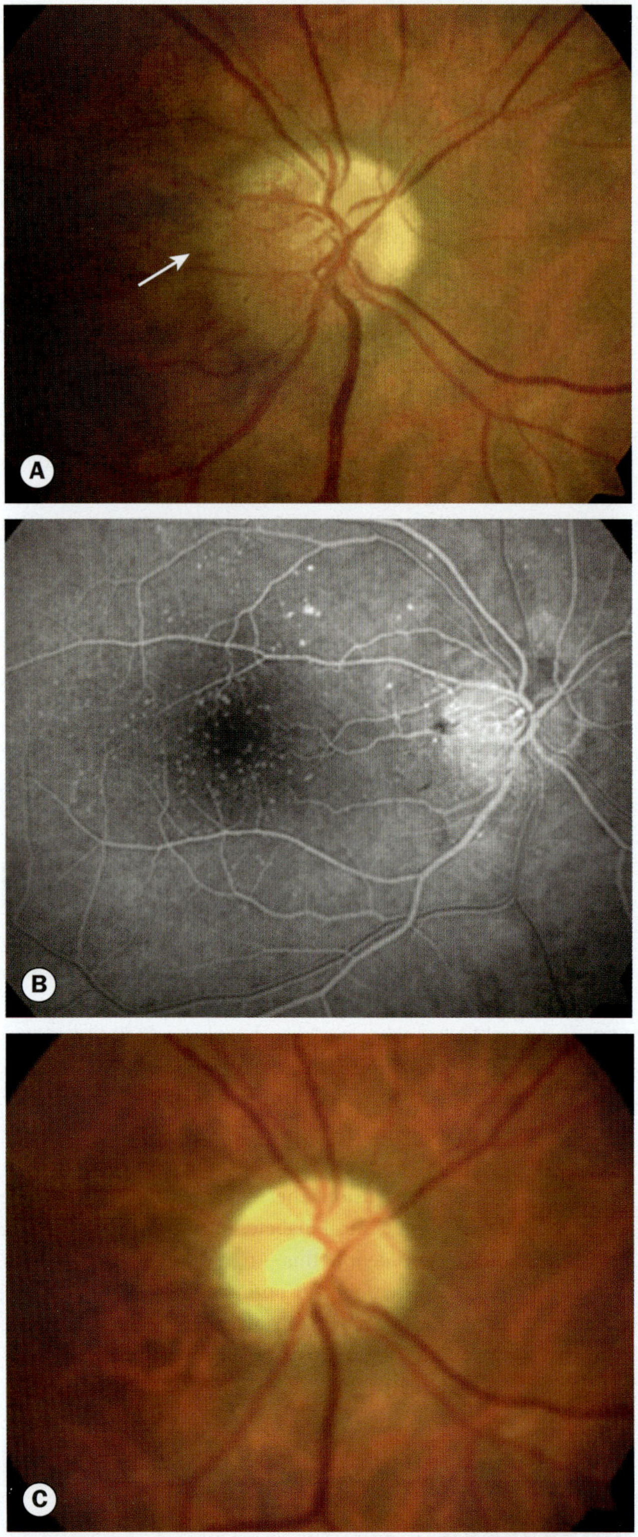

Fig. 13.24 Diabetic papillopathy. **(A)** Hyperaemic disc swelling and telangiectasia (arrow) with no visual symptoms; **(B)** fluorescein angiogram of optic disc shown in **(A)** showing telangiectasia and signs of early background retinopathy; **(C)** disc appearance 2 months later after spontaneous resolution.

secondary changes that include endothelial cell loss, turbulent flow and thrombus formation. Similarly, the central retinal vein and artery possess a common sheath at crossing points posterior to the lamina cribrosa so that atherosclerotic changes of the artery may precipitate central retinal vein occlusion (CRVO). Haematological pro-thrombotic factors are thought to be important in a minority, amplifying an atherosclerotic anatomical predisposition. Once venous occlusion has occurred, elevation of venous and capillary pressure with stagnation of blood flow ensues, resulting in retinal hypoxia, which in turn results in damage to the capillary endothelial cells, extravasation of blood constituents and liberation of mediators such as VEGF.

Risk factors

- **Age** is the most important factor. Over 50% of cases occur in patients older than 65.
- **Hypertension** is present in two-thirds or more of RVO patients over the age of 50 years and in 25% of younger patients. It is a particularly important risk factor in patients with BRVO.
- **Hyperlipidaemia** is present in one-third or more of patients, irrespective of age.
- **Diabetes mellitus** is present in up to 15% of patients over 50 years of age. It is more prevalent in Asian and African patients, but is uncommon in younger patients.
- **Glaucoma** and ocular hypertension are associated with a higher risk of CRVO.
- **Oral contraceptive pill.** In younger females the contraceptive pill is the most common underlying association and probably should not be taken following RVO.
- **Smoking.** Current smoking may be associated with an increased incidence of RVO.
- **Uncommon.** Dehydration, myeloproliferative disorders (e.g. myeloma, polycythaemia), thrombophilia (e.g. hyperhomocysteinaemia, antiphospholipid antibody syndrome, factor V Leiden mutation), inflammatory disease associated with occlusive periphlebitis (e.g. Behçet syndrome, sarcoidosis, Wegener granulomatosis), orbital disease and chronic renal failure.

Systemic assessment

The detection and management of associated systemic disease is aimed principally at reducing the risk of future vascular occlusive events, both ocular and systemic.

All patients

- **Blood pressure (BP).**
- **Erythrocyte sedimentation rate (ESR)** or **plasma viscosity (PV).**
- **Full blood count (FBC).**
- **Random blood glucose.** Further assessment for diabetes if indicated.
- **Random total and high-density lipoprotein (HDL) cholesterol.** Additional lipid testing may be considered.

- **Plasma protein electrophoresis.** To detect dysproteinaemias such as multiple myeloma.
- **Other tests.** Some authorities advocate routine investigation for systemic end-organ damage related to the cardiovascular risk factors commonly found in patients with RVO. This is intended to help the prevention of further non-ocular damage, as well as facilitating systemic management to reduce the risk of recurrent ocular venous occlusion.
  - Urea, electrolytes and creatinine to detect renal disease associated with hypertension. Chronic renal failure is also a rare cause of RVO.
  - Thyroid function testing. There is a higher prevalence of thyroid disease in RVO patients.
  - Electrocardiography (ECG). Left ventricular hypertrophy is associated with hypertension.

Selected patients according to clinical indication

These tests might be considered in (a) patients under the age of 50; (b) in bilateral RVO; (c) patients with previous thromboses or a family history of thrombosis; and (d) some patients in whom investigation for the common associations is negative. Evidence of a causative link for many of these is limited.

- **Chest X-ray.** Sarcoidosis, tuberculosis, left ventricular hypertrophy in hypertension.
- **C-reactive protein (CRP).** Sensitive indicator of inflammation.
- **Plasma homocysteine level.** To exclude hyperhomocysteinaemia, for which there is reasonable evidence of an increased RVO risk.
- **'Thrombophilia screen'.** By convention this refers to heritable thrombophilia. Tests might typically include thrombin time, prothrombin time and activated partial thromboplastin time, antithrombin functional assay, protein C, protein S, activated protein C resistance, factor V Leiden mutation, prothrombin G20210A mutation, lupus anticoagulant and in particular, anticardiolipin antibody (IgG and IgM).
- **Autoantibodies.** Rheumatoid factor, antinuclear antibody (ANA), anti-DNA antibody, antineutrophil cytoplasmic antibody (ANCA).
- **Serum angiotensin-converting enzyme (ACE).** Sarcoidosis.
- **Treponemal serology.** See Chapter 12.
- **Carotid duplex imaging** to exclude ocular ischaemic syndrome.

Branch retinal vein occlusion

Diagnosis

- **Symptoms and VA** depend on the anatomical location of the occlusion. If the macula is involved, a sudden painless onset of blurred vision and metamorphopsia is experienced. Peripheral occlusion may be asymptomatic.
- **Iris** neovascularization (NVI) and neovascular glaucoma (NVG) are much less common in BRVO than in CRVO (2–3% at 3 years).
- **Fundus**
  - Dilatation and tortuosity of the affected venous segment, with flame-shaped and dot/blot haemorrhages, principally in the retinal area drained by the thrombosed vein though an occasional haemorrhage may be identified elsewhere. Cotton-wool spots and retinal oedema may be present, but this is not inevitable.
  - The superotemporal quadrant is most commonly affected.
  - The site of occlusion may be identifiable as an arteriovenous crossing point (Fig. 13.25).
  - The acute features usually resolve within 6–12 months leaving venous sheathing and sclerosis and variable persistent/recurrent haemorrhage (Fig. 13.26). The severity of residual signs is highly variable.
  - Collateral vessels may form near areas of limited capillary perfusion after weeks to months. They usually connect a poorly functioning to a normally functioning segment of the venous circulation and typically appear as tortuous or looping channels. They may cross the horizontal raphe between the inferior and superior vascular arcades (Fig. 13.27A). The appearance of collaterals is associated with a better prognosis.
  - Chronic macular oedema is the most common cause of persistent poor VA after BRVO (Fig. 13.27B).
  - Retinal neovascularization occurs in about 8% of eyes by 3 years. The risk is much higher in eyes with more than about five disc areas of non-perfusion on FA (over one-third of eyes) (Fig. 13.27C and D). NVE are more common than NVD. NVE usually develop at the border of ischaemic retina drained by an occluded vein. They typically appear within 6–12 months, but may develop at any time.
  - Recurrent vitreous and preretinal haemorrhage and occasionally tractional retinal detachment can occur secondary to neovascularization.
- **FA** demonstrates peripheral and macular ischaemia (capillary non-perfusion, staining of vessel walls, vessel 'pruning' – small branches failing to fill), haemorrhage and oedema with collateral vessels commonly forming in established cases (Fig. 13.27D). Venous filling is delayed. In late or subtle cases, FA may be diagnostic.

TIP The commonest underlying cause of a branch retinal vein occlusion is systemic hypertension, which needs to be effectively treated to reduce the risk of late cardiovascular and cerebrovascular complications.

Management

- **Systemic arterial hypertension** and hyperlipidaemia, if present, should be treated. Further investigations are required in order to determine the underlying cause in patients younger than 50 years, in those with bilateral BRVO at presentation or in those with a history of recurrent BRVO.
- **Observation** without intervention is usually indicated if VA is 6/9 or better, or slightly worse but improving.
- **NVE or NVD** are generally regarded as an indication for sector photocoagulation, though some authorities withhold treatment unless vitreous haemorrhage occurs because early

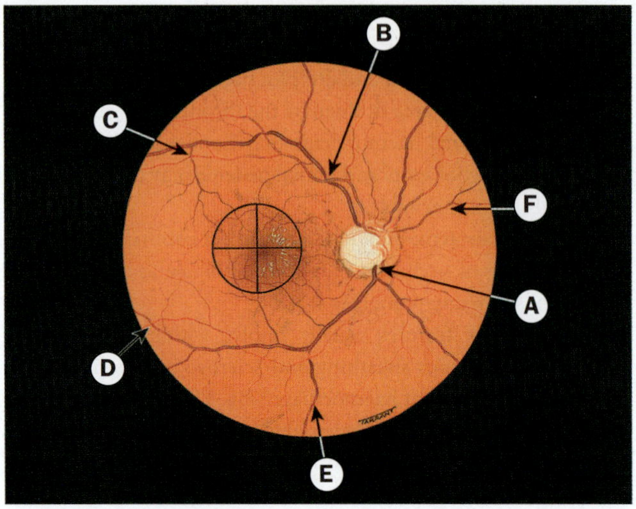

Fig. 13.25 Classification of retinal branch vein occlusion according to site of blockage. **(A)** Major at the disc; **(B)** major away from the disc; **(C)** minor macular; **(D–F)** peripheral not involving the macula.

intervention does not appear to affect the visual outcome. Burns of mild–moderate intensity, 400–500 µm actual diameter, 0.05 s duration and spaced one burn width apart are applied to the ischaemic area (Fig. 13.28A). FA can be used to confirm dubious NV if necessary and to demonstrate ischaemic areas that might be specifically targeted with laser (Fig. 13.28B). Laser may be combined with 4- to 6-weekly intravitreal anti-VEGF injection.

- **NVI** is an indication for urgent sector PRP. Secondary glaucoma is likely to be less aggressive than in CRVO. See Chapter 11 for the detailed management of NVG.
- **Intravitreal anti-VEGF agents** (Fig. 13.28C and D). These have been widely adopted for the treatment of macular oedema secondary to BRVO. All available agents are effective in these circumstances, but repeated injections are needed. The BRAVO study shows that ranibizumab is superior to traditional grid laser treatment at 12 months. This conclusion is confirmed by the VIBRANT study, which reveals that VA gains established after monthly injections of aflibercept can be

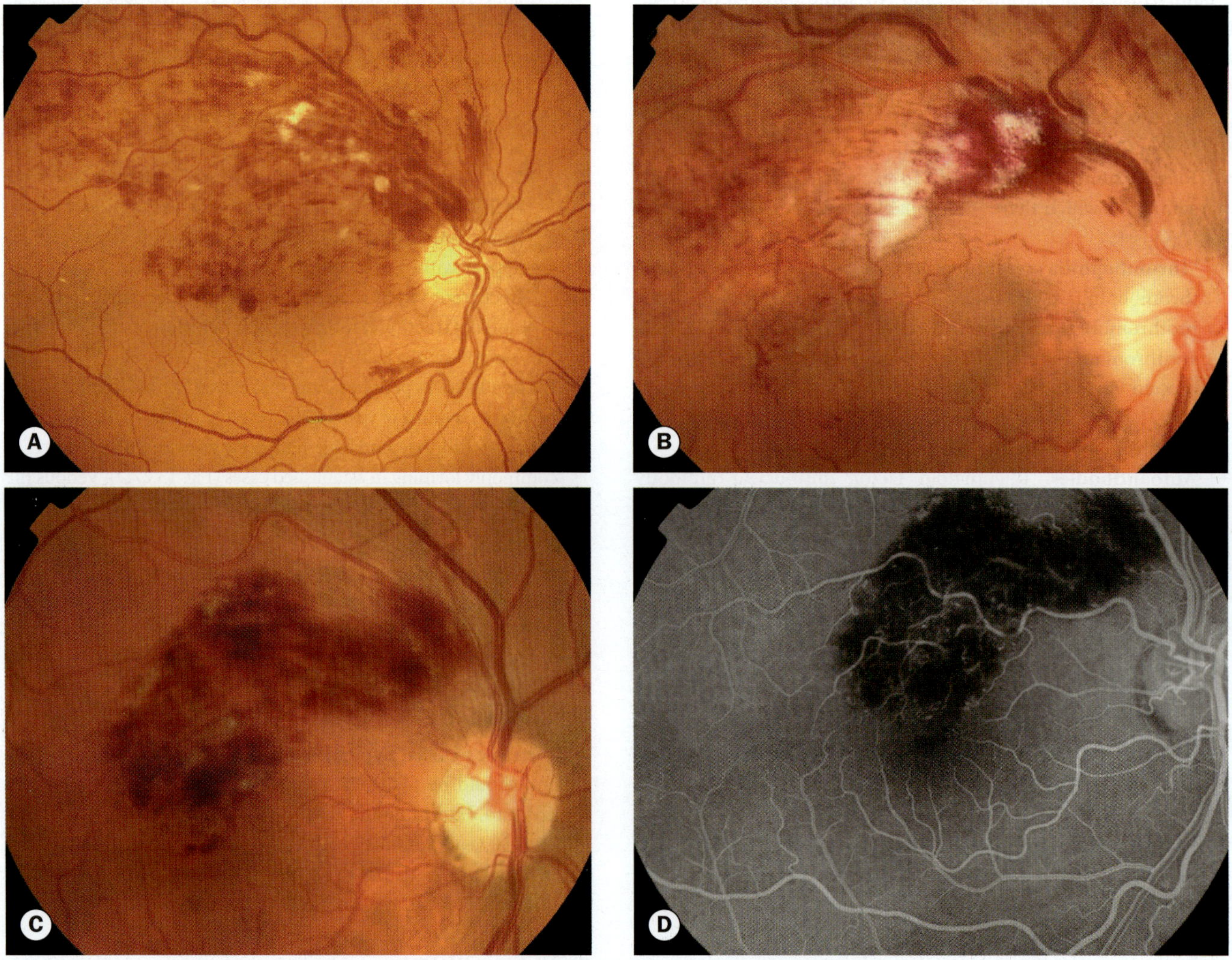

Fig. 13.26 Fresh BRVO. **(A)** Upper temporal branch vein occlusion with macular extension; **(B)** upper temporal venous engorgement and cotton-wool spots; **(C)** predominantly macular haemorrhage; **(D)** FA showing hypofluorescence. *(Courtesy C Barry – fig. A.)*

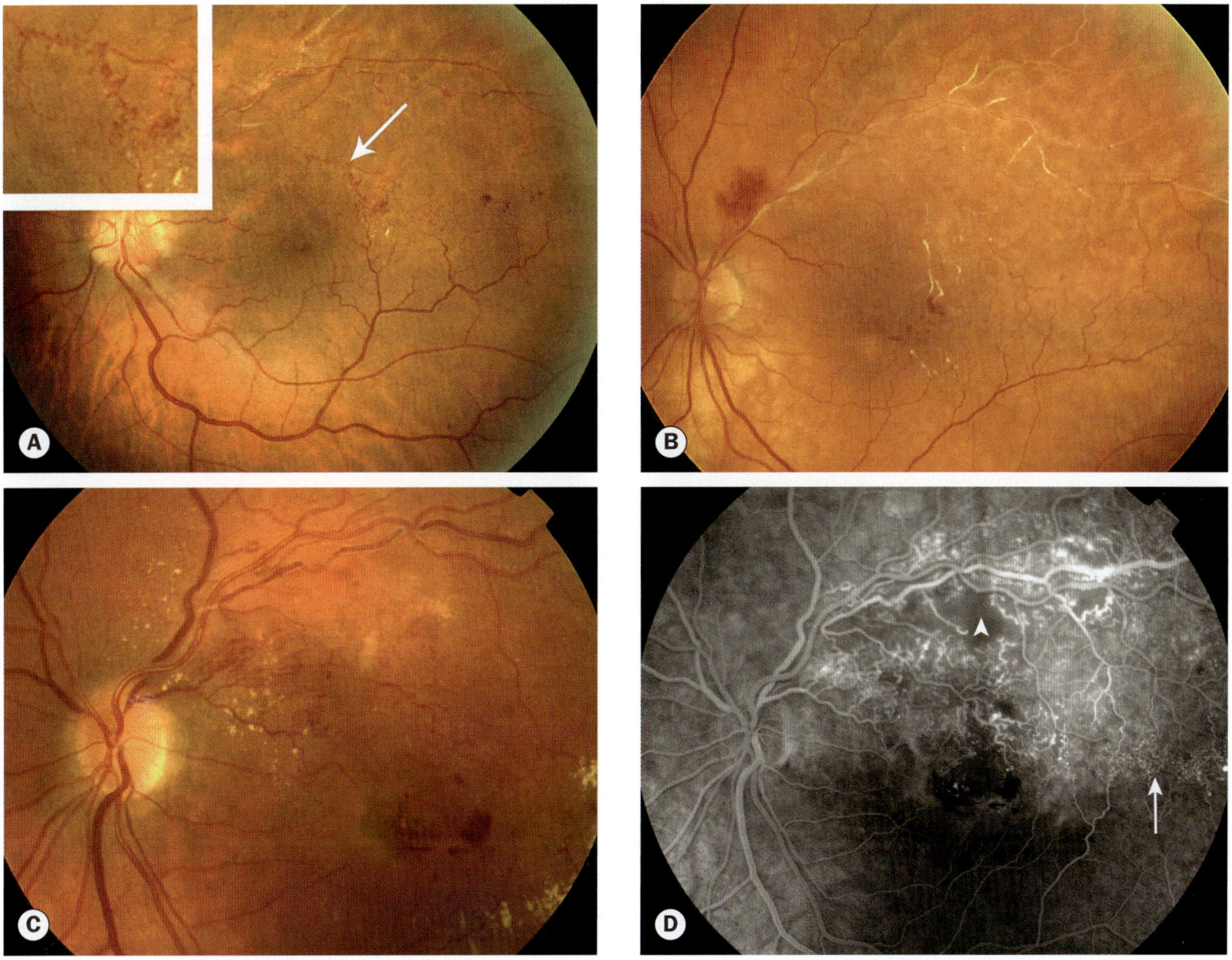

Fig. 13.27 Old BRVO. **(A)** Upper temporal branch vein occlusion with shunt vessels (arrow); **(B)** upper temporal occlusion with venous sclerosis and chronic macular oedema; **(C)** resorbing haemorrhages, exudates and collateral vessels; **(D)** FA of **(C)** showing areas of non-perfusion (arrowhead) and collateral vessels (arrow).

maintained with 'when required' treatment. Commence treatment as soon as the diagnosis is made. Combining intravitreal injections with laser may allow a reduction in the frequency of injections, but the optimal regimen has yet to be defined.

- **Intravitreal dexamethasone implant.** This confers visual improvement in BRVO substantially superior to observation alone. The treatment can be repeated after 4–6 months. Adverse effects include an increased glaucoma and cataract risk. As with anti-VEGF therapy, it may be used alone or in conjunction with laser.
- **Laser to the macula.** With the advent of intravitreal treatment, macular laser has become less popular and should be regarded as an adjunctive or combination modality. If VA remains 6/12 or worse after 3–6 months because of macular oedema that is associated with good central macular perfusion on FA, laser may be considered: 20–100 mild burns of diameter 50–100 μm and duration 0.01–0.05 s, concentrating on areas of leakage on FA. Pulses at the shorter end of the duration range seem to inflict less damage to the retina whilst exerting an approximately comparable therapeutic effect. Treatment should not encroach within 0.5 disc diameters of the foveal centre. Retinal haemorrhages and blood vessels – especially collaterals – should not be treated.
- **Subthreshold (micropulse) laser** appears to be as effective as conventional photocoagulation for macular oedema and inflicts considerably less retinal damage. The onset of action is slower.
- **Intravitreal triamcinolone** in a preservative-free preparation is as effective as laser in eyes with macular oedema but has a less sustained effect and a relatively high rate of cataract formation and IOP elevation.
- **Review** in cases that do not require early intervention should usually take place after 3 months and then at 3- to 6-monthly intervals for up to 2 years, principally to detect neovascularization.

TIP OCT allows rapid quantitative analysis of the macula and has become important in the assessment and subsequent management of retinal vein occlusion.

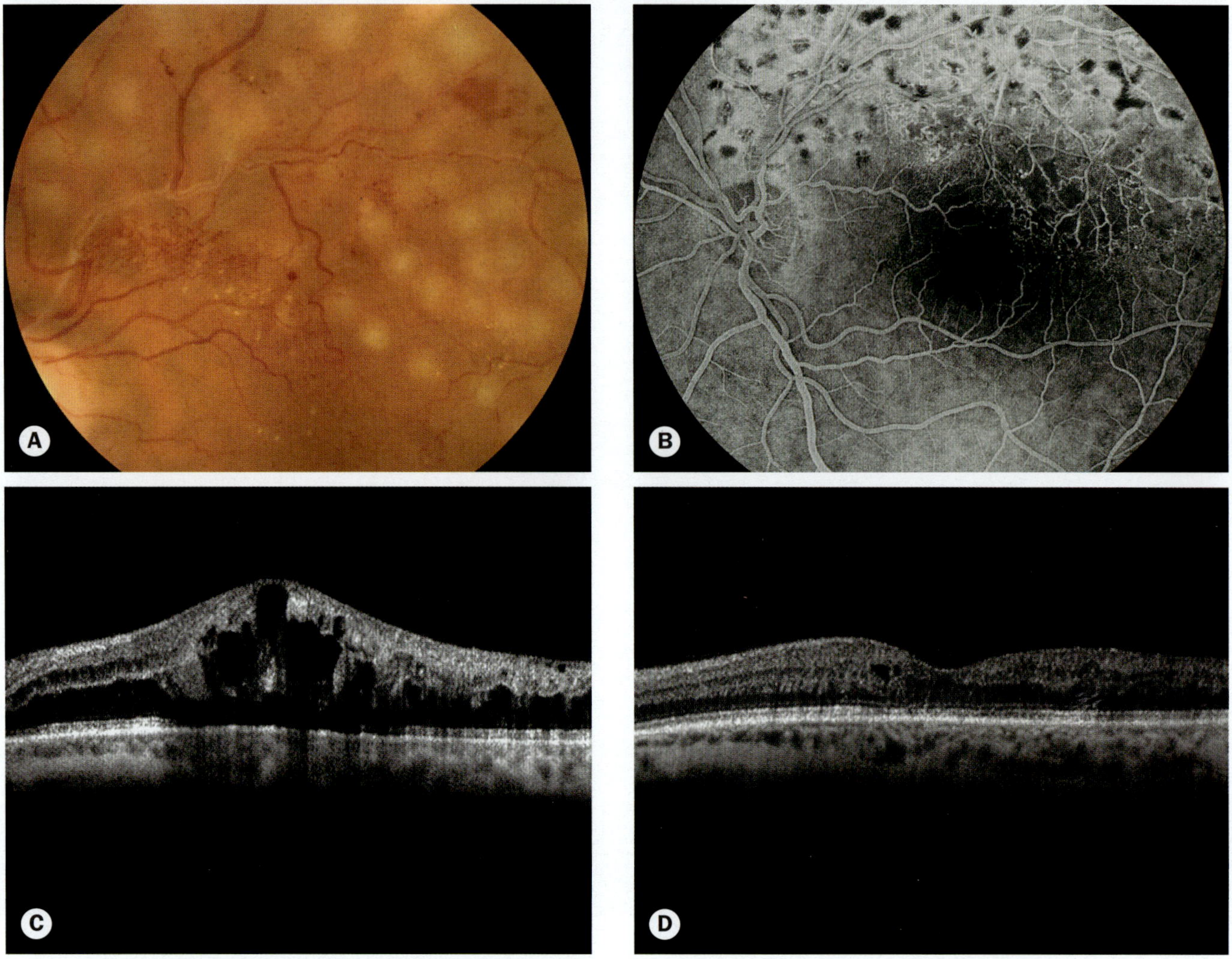

Fig. 13.28 Treatment of branch retinal vein occlusion. **(A)** Sector laser photocoagulation for neovascularization; **(B)** FA appearance after sector laser photocoagulation; **(C)** OCT of cystoid macular oedema before and **(D)** 4 weeks after bevacizumab intravitreal injection. *(Courtesy of C Barry – fig. A; S Chen – figs C and D.)*

Prognosis

- BRVO generally has a good visual prognosis, with 50–60% of patients maintaining a final VA of better than 6/15, even without treatment.
- Poor prognostic factors are chronic macular oedema, macular BRVO and new vessel formation leading to vitreous haemorrhage.
- About a quarter are left with a VA of 6/60 or worse.
- Developing BRVO in one eye slightly increases the risk of a similar event occurring in the fellow eye.

Hemiretinal vein occlusion

Hemiretinal vein occlusion is regarded as a variant of CRVO by some authorities and may be ischaemic or non-ischaemic. It is less common than either BRVO or CRVO and involves occlusion of the superior or inferior branch of the central retinal vein (CRV). A *hemispheric* occlusion blocks a major branch of the CRV at or near the optic disc. The less common *hemicentral* occlusion involves one trunk of a dual-trunked CRV that has persisted in the anterior part of the optic nerve head as a congenital variant.

Prognosis depends on the severity of retinal ischaemia, but management has been less well studied than BRVO and CRVO. Extensive retinal ischaemia implies a risk of neovascular glaucoma and should be managed in the same way as ischaemic CRVO (see below), otherwise management, particularly of macular oedema, may be as for BRVO.

Diagnosis

- **Symptoms.** A sudden onset altitudinal visual field defect (Fig. 13.29A).
- **VA** reduction varies depending on the site of the occlusion.
- **NVI** is more common than in BRVO but less than in CRVO.
- **Fundus** shows the features of BRVO, involving the superior (Fig. 13.29B) or inferior retinal hemisphere (Fig. 13.30A). NVD may be more common than in either CRVO or BRVO.
- **FA** shows masking by haemorrhages, hyperfluorescence due to leakage and variable capillary non-perfusion (Fig. 13.30B).

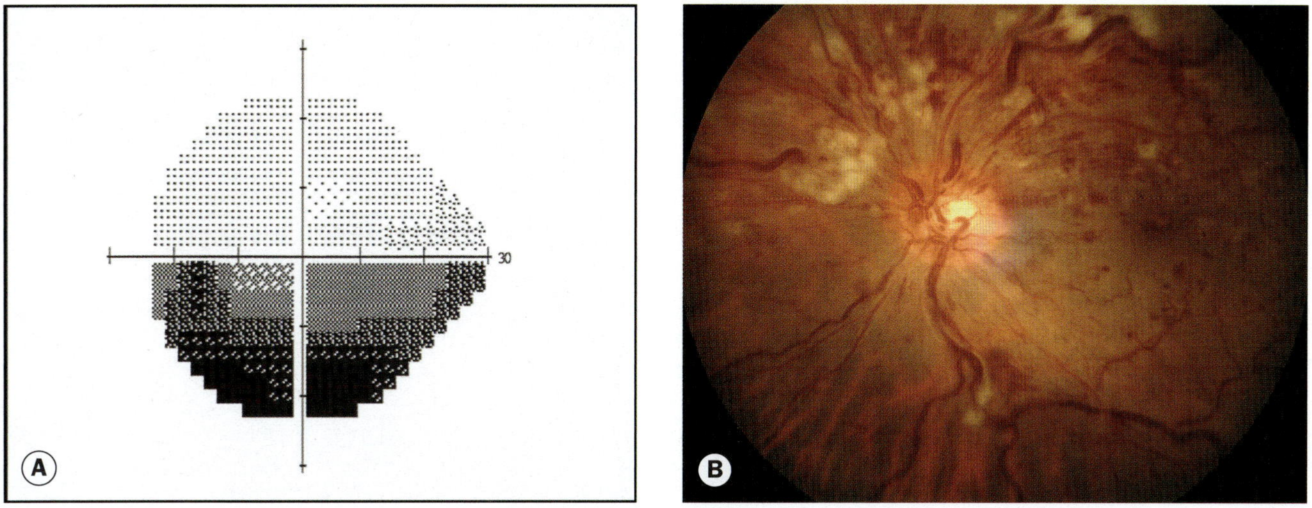

Fig. 13.29 Ischaemic hemiretinal vein occlusion. **(A)** Inferior altitudinal visual field defect; **(B)** superior ischaemic occlusion showing cotton-wool spots and haemorrhages.

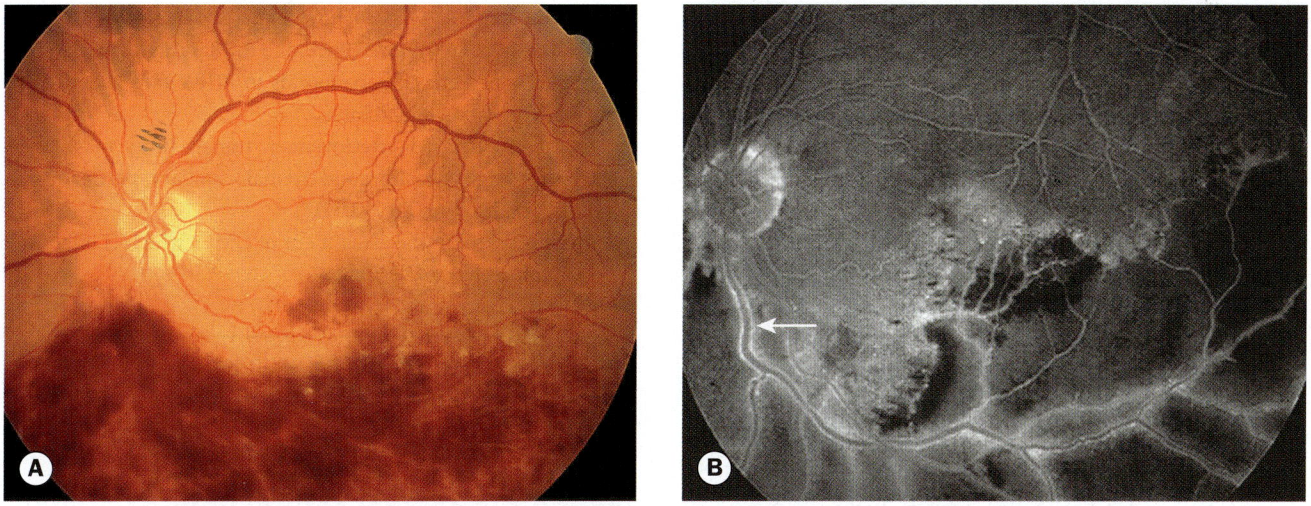

Fig. 13.30 **(A)** Inferior hemiretinal vein occlusion; **(B)** FA late phase showing extensive hypofluorescence due to capillary non-perfusion, with mild perivascular hyperfluorescence (arrow). *(Courtesy of C Barry.)*

Impending central retinal vein occlusion

Impending (partial) CRVO on average occurs in younger patients than those developing more severe occlusion. The prognosis is usually good, but a proportion will deteriorate to ischaemic CRVO. The distinction between 'impending' and mild non-ischaemic CRVO (see below) is not clear and may be artificial. Symptoms may be absent or consist of only minor or transient blurring that is characteristically worse on waking. On examination, there is mild retinal venous dilatation and tortuosity (Fig. 13.31A), with relatively few small, scattered dot and blot haemorrhages (Fig. 13.31B). There may be mild macular oedema. Fundus autofluorescence (FAF) may reveal a fern-like perivenular appearance (see below) and FA generally demonstrates an impaired retinal circulation. Treatment is empirical, with lack of an established evidence base. Correcting any predisposing systemic conditions, avoiding dehydration and lowering IOP to improve perfusion have been postulated. Antiplatelet agents, other anticoagulant measures and haemodilution are of no proven benefit, but may be considered in some cases.

Non-ischaemic central retinal vein occlusion

Diagnosis

Non-ischaemic CRVO, sometimes called 'venous stasis retinopathy' (also sometimes used to describe ocular ischaemic syndrome – see later) is more common than the ischaemic form. Around a third will progress to ischaemic CRVO, often within months.

- **Symptoms.** A sudden painless monocular fall in vision.

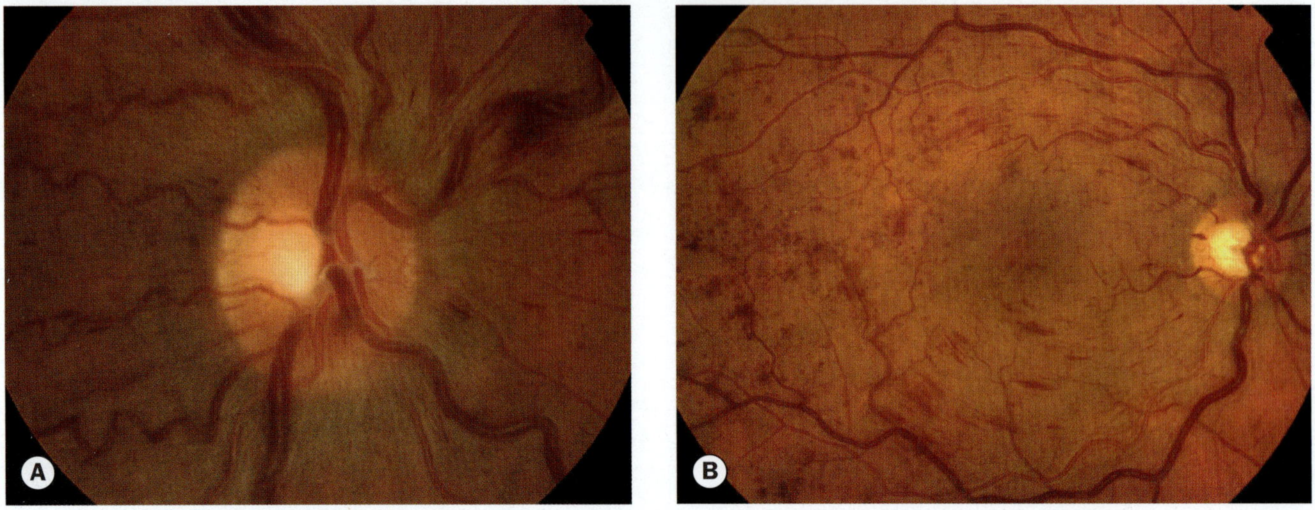

Fig. 13.31 Impending central retinal vein occlusion. **(A)** Retinal venous dilatation and tortuosity; **(B)** scattered dot and blot haemorrhages.

- **VA** is impaired to a variable degree dependent on severity. Eyes with initially good VA tend to have a good prognosis and vice versa. Initial VA in the middle range (6/30–6/60) is an unreliable predictor of outcome. VA worse than 6/60 commonly indicates that substantial ischaemia is present. In cases that do not become ischaemic, vision returns to normal or near normal in about 50%.
- **Relative afferent pupillary defect (RAPD).** Absent or mild.
- **Fundus.** Signs are present in all quadrants.
  - Tortuosity and dilatation of all branches of the central retinal vein, with dot, blot and flame haemorrhages to a mild–moderate extent (Fig. 13.32A and B). Cotton-wool spots, optic disc and macular oedema are common but generally mild.
  - Patchy (or perivenular) ischaemic retinal whitening (PIRW) in a perivenular pattern at the posterior pole is an early sign occurring in younger patients with non-ischaemic CRVO.
  - Most acute signs resolve over 6–12 months. Later findings are variable, depending on severity but may include persistent scattered retinal haemorrhages (Fig. 13.32C); venous tortuosity, sheathing and sclerosis; epiretinal gliosis; macular pigmentary and atrophic changes; peripheral and optic disc collateral vessels.
  - The main cause of poor vision is chronic macular oedema and secondary atrophy.
  - Disc collaterals are common following CRVO, appearing as a small vascular loop on the optic nerve head. They are also known as optociliary shunts or retinochoroidal collaterals and are thought to represent a compensatory circulation in response to impaired nerve perfusion. Their development is believed to be associated with a markedly decreased risk of neovascularization. They can form in a range of conditions besides CRVO, including chronic glaucoma and chronic optic nerve compression.
- **FAF** in acute RVO may show a characteristic fern-like perivenular hypoautofluorescence due to masking of background signal by oedema. It corresponds to PIRW (see above) but is more commonly identifiable.
- **FA** shows delayed arteriovenous transit time, masking by haemorrhage, usually good retinal capillary perfusion and some late leakage (Fig. 13.32D).
- **OCT** is useful in the assessment of CMO, which is often mild in a non-ischaemic lesion.

TIP A VA of <6/60 and a RAPD normally indicates significant retinal ischaemia and a poor visual prognosis in a patient with central retinal vein occlusion.

Ischaemic central retinal vein occlusion

Ischaemic CRVO is characterized by substantially decreased retinal perfusion with capillary closure and retinal hypoxia. Macular ischaemia and NVG are the major causes of visual morbidity.

Diagnosis

- **Symptoms.** Sudden and severe monocular painless visual impairment. Occasionally presentation may be with pain, redness and photophobia due to neovascular glaucoma, a prior reduction in vision having passed unnoticed or been ignored.
- **VA** is usually 'counting fingers' or worse. The visual prognosis is generally extremely poor due to macular ischaemia.
- **RAPD** is present.
- **NVI.** Rubeosis iridis (Fig. 13.33A) develops in about 50% of eyes, usually between 2 and 4 months ('hundred-day glaucoma') and there is a high risk of neovascular glaucoma. The pupillary margin should be examined at each review prior to pharmacological mydriasis.
- **Gonioscopy.** Angle neovascularization (Fig. 13.33B) may occur in the absence of neovascularization at the pupillary

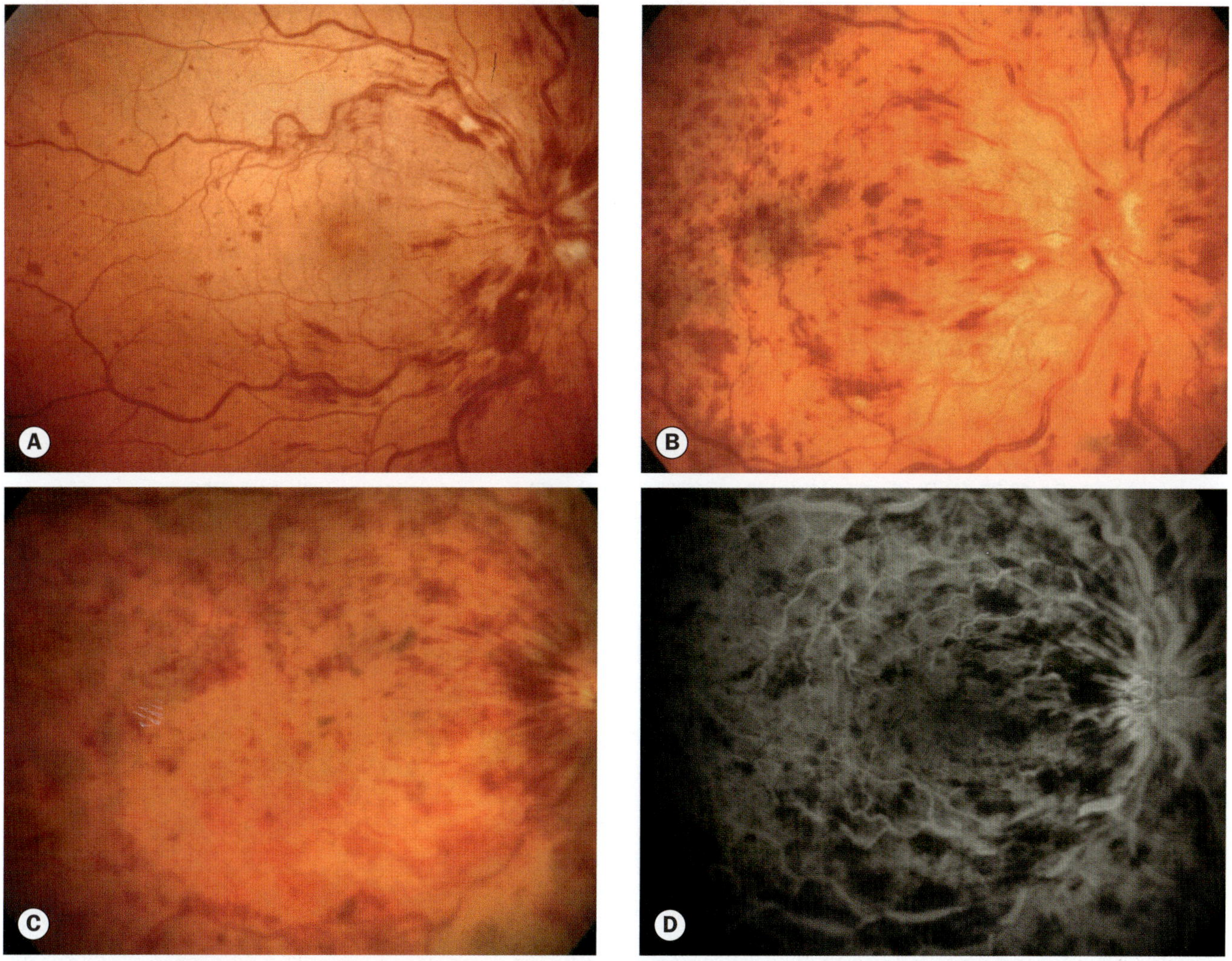

Fig. 13.32 Non-ischaemic central retinal vein occlusion (CRVO). **(A)** Acute – tortuosity and dilatation of all branches, with dot, blot and flame haemorrhages; **(B)** extensive flame-shaped haemorrhages; **(C)** resorbing haemorrhages; **(D)** FA of **(C)** late phase showing masking by blood and staining of vessel walls (arrow) but good capillary perfusion.

margin. Routine gonioscopy should therefore be performed prior to pupillary dilatation.

- **Fundus**
  - Severe tortuosity and engorgement of all branches of the central retinal vein. There are extensive deep blot and flame-shaped haemorrhages involving the peripheral and posterior retina and cotton-wool spots are typically prominent (Fig. 13.34A). There is usually optic disc swelling and hyperaemia (Fig. 13.34B).
  - Most acute signs resolve over 9–12 months. The macula may develop atrophic retinal and RPE changes, RPE hyperplasia, epiretinal membrane and chronic CMO. Rarely, subretinal fibrosis resembling that associated with exudative age-related macular degeneration may develop.
  - Retinal neovascularization occurs in about 5% of eyes – much less commonly than with BRVO, but severe vitreous haemorrhage can occur, obscuring vision and preventing retinal laser.
  - Optic disc collaterals (opticociliary shunts – see under non-ischaemic CRVO) are common and may protect the eye from anterior and posterior segment neovascularization. Their development probably indicates a dramatic reduction in the risk of this complication (Fig. 13.34C).
- **FA** shows a marked delay in arteriovenous transit time, masking by retinal haemorrhages, extensive areas of capillary non-perfusion and vessel wall staining and leakage (Fig. 13.34D). The presence of more than 10 disc areas of retinal capillary non-perfusion is associated with a substantially increased risk of neovascularization.
- **OCT** enables quantification of CMO.
- **Electroretinogram (ERG)** is depressed and the extent of this has sometimes been used to assess neovascular risk.

Treatment of the complications of CRVO

The management of non-ischaemic CRVO is generally much less aggressive than ischaemic CRVO, so it is important to distinguish the two as far as possible.

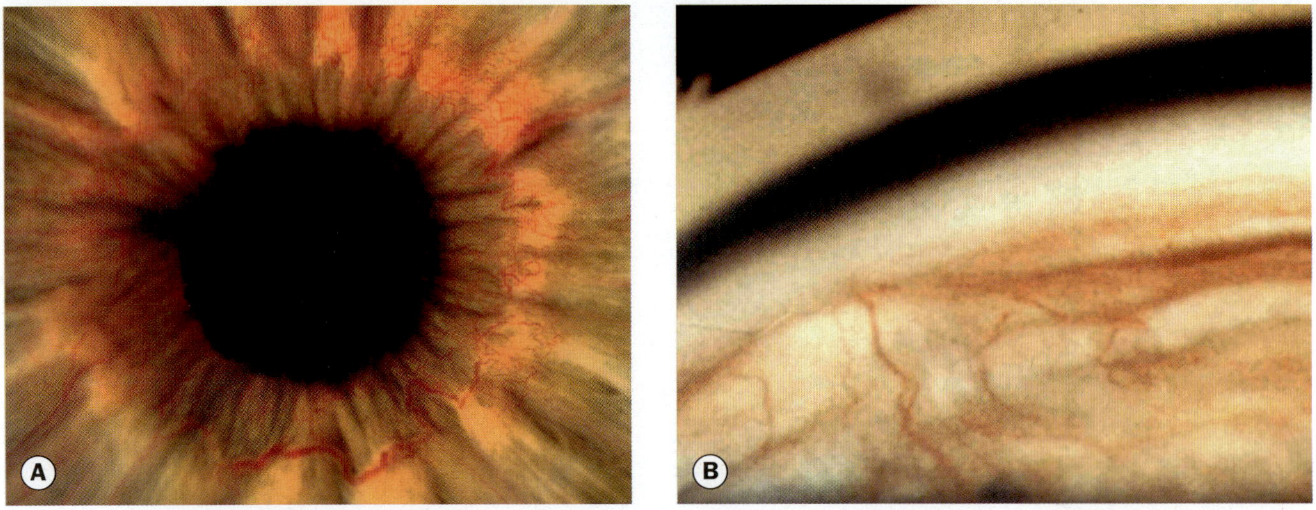

Fig. 13.33 **(A)** Rubeosis iridis at the pupillary border; **(B)** neovascularization with early PAS in a predominantly open angle.

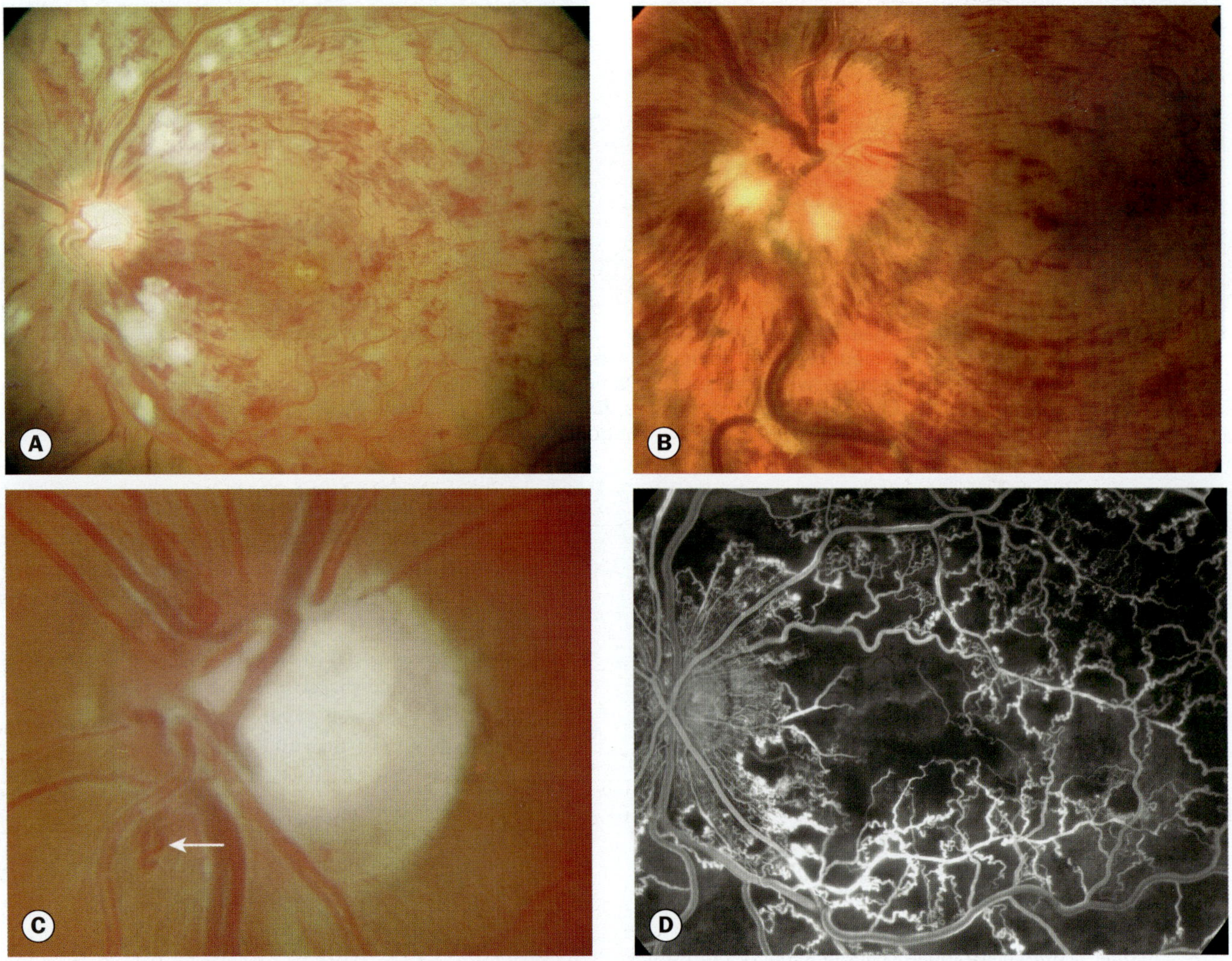

Fig. 13.34 Ischaemic central retinal vein occlusion. **(A)** Numerous cotton-wool spots, flame and deep blot haemorrhages in the acute stage; **(B)** venous distension with cotton-wool spots at the disc; **(C)** shunt vessels (arrow); **(D)** FA showing extensive hypofluorescence due to capillary non-perfusion.

- **Systemic assessment** as described above is essential, followed by appropriate systemic management (discussed below).
- **Treatment of macular oedema.** Treatment is generally indicated for VA worse than 6/9 and/or with significant central macular thickening (e.g. >250 μm) on OCT, but is unlikely to be of benefit if VA is 6/120 or worse. Intravitreal anti-VEGF agents or dexamethasone implant are the current standard of care.
  - Intravitreal anti-VEGF agents. The CRUISE study concludes that monthly injections of ranibizumab for 6 months is more likely to improve VA than placebo. The COPERNICUS study provides similar results using intravitreal aflibercept even when an 'as-needed' protocol is adopted. Bevacizumab is also effective in these circumstances and is therefore commonly used in clinical practice.
  - Intravitreal dexamethasone implant. The GENEVA trial of a sustained-release biodegradable dexamethasone (700 μg) intravitreal implant (Ozurdex) shows that substantial visual and anatomical (Fig. 13.35A and B) improvement can be expected over the first 2 months following a single implantation and although this declines to baseline by 6 months, the treatment can then be repeated. As with triamcinolone, there is a slightly higher rate of IOP elevation and cataract. Administration within 90 days of CMO onset is likely to be associated with an improved outcome. Treatment can be repeated after 4–6 months. The COMRADE study concludes that eyes treated with ranibizumab have significantly better VA than those receiving intravitreal dexamethasone (0.7 mg) at 6 months.
  - Intravitreal triamcinolone (Fig. 13.35C). The SCORE study shows an improvement of three or more lines of vision at 1 year in over 25% of patients (versus 7% of controls) treated with an average of two injections of 1 mg triamcinolone, using a preservative-free preparation developed for intraocular use. There is a slightly higher rate of IOP elevation and cataract than with observation. Risk factors for a rise of IOP of >10 mmHg include: higher dose (4 mg vs 1 mg), younger age and higher baseline IOP.
  - Laser photocoagulation. Although macular oedema is anatomically improved, laser is not beneficial for visual outcome, except in some younger patients.
  - Investigational treatments include chorioretinal anastomosis, vitrectomy with radial optic neurotomy and local recombinant tissue plasminogen activator (rtPA) CRV infusion.
- **Treatment of neovascularization**
  - There is no benefit in performing PRP **before** the development of iris and angle neovascularization.
  - Frequent follow-up is key and PRP should be performed without delay in eyes that develop NVI or angle neovascularization. This initially involves placing 1500–2000 burns of 0.05–0.1 s duration, spaced one burn width apart, with sufficient energy to produce a moderate reaction, avoiding areas of haemorrhage (Fig. 13.35D). Treatment may be fractionated and further photocoagulation is commonly required.
  - Adjunctive intravitreal anti-VEGF injections are commonly administered every 6 weeks until the eye stabilizes, leading to more rapid resolution of NV than that found in patients undergoing PRP alone. This also has the advantage of reducing macular oedema.
  - Patients may still develop neovascular glaucoma, but the risk is reduced. The onset of NVG may be delayed by up to 18 months, so these patients need to be followed at 3-monthly intervals for at least 2–3 years.
  - The management of NVG is discussed in Chapter 11.
  - Vitreous haemorrhage may respond to intravitreal anti-VEGF, but definitive treatment is with vitrectomy and endolaser.
- **Review**
  - Ischaemic CRVO. Where possible, patients with ischaemic CRVO should be seen monthly for 6 months. Subsequent monitoring should usually be for 2–3 years to detect significant ischaemia, macular oedema and NVI. Once a disc collateral has developed, the risk of neovascularization reduces.
  - Non-ischaemic CRVO. In an obviously non-ischaemic occlusion, initial follow-up should take place after 3 months. Structured arrangements for review of test results should be in place. The patient should be instructed to make contact if the vision deteriorates as this may indicate the development of significant ischaemia. Pain or redness, which may indicate neovascular glaucoma and occasionally inflammation without rubeosis, should also be reported. Subsequent review is dependent on the clinical picture and response to treatment, with discharge from follow-up usually taking place at 18–24 months.

Prognosis

The main cause for poor vision after a CRVO is chronic macular oedema. The prognosis for ischaemic CRVO is extremely poor due to macular ischaemia and neovascular glaucoma.

- **The prognosis** is usually determined by the initial visual acuity:
  - 6/18 or better: the VA is likely to remain so.
  - 6/24–6/60: the clinical course is variable and the final VA is difficult to predict.
  - Worse than 6/60: improvement is unlikely.

Systemic management in retinal vein occlusion

- **Control of systemic risk factors.** Although there is no conclusive evidence that vascular mortality is higher in RVO patients, cardiovascular risk factors are commonly identified after a retinal vein occlusion and should be dealt with. As well as conferring systemic benefit this may also reduce the risk of recurrent RVO. Smoking should be actively discouraged.
- **Antiplatelet therapy.** The role of aspirin or alternative antiplatelet agents in reducing the risk of further retinal venous occlusion is unclear. This medication is not usually prescribed unless there is a clear systemic indication.
- **Hormone replacement therapy (HRT).** The risk of HRT remains undefined. Most authorities would avoid continuing or commencing oestrogen-containing HRT following RVO. Appropriate expert advice should be obtained. The presence of

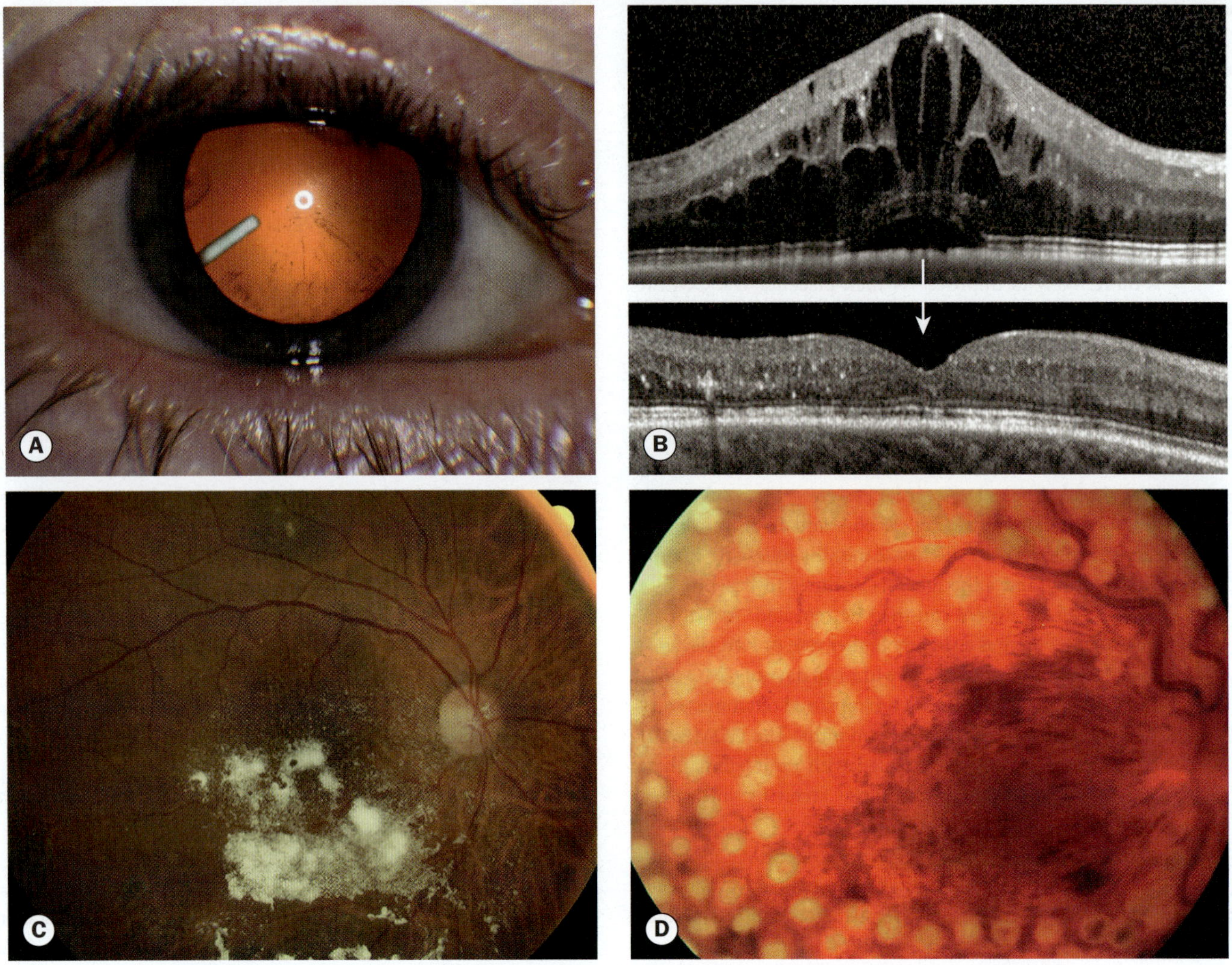

Fig. 13.35 Treatment of central retinal vein occlusion complications. **(A)** Ozurdex (dexamethasone 0.7mg) implant in the vitreous cavity; **(B)** OCT showing significant macular oedema before and 6 months after intravitreal Ozurdex implant, showing resorption of oedema; **(C)** triamcinolone after intravitreal administration; **(D)** panretinal photocoagulation. *(Courtesy of S Chen – fig C.)*

other thrombophilia risk factors is associated with a substantially increased risk of systemic venous thrombosis in conjunction with HRT.

- **Oral contraceptive pill.** This should probably be discontinued following RVO.
- **Others.** A range of systemic treatment modalities (e.g. isovolaemic haemodilution, plasmapheresis, recombinant tissue plasminogen infusion) has been employed to try to improve visual outcomes in RVO, but clear evidence for benefit is lacking. Dehydration should be avoided.

Papillophlebitis

Papillophlebitis is an uncommon, poorly defined condition that typically affects individuals under the age of 50 years who may have a higher prevalence of hypertension and diabetes. Some or all cases may simply be a variant of CRVO occurring in younger people, though optic disc swelling or inflammation of the central retinal vein have been speculated as the initiating event in at least some instances. There is likely to be some diagnostic overlap with diabetic papillopathy. Papillophlebitis typically causes only mild to moderate reduction of vision with no RAPD and has a generally good prognosis. Disc oedema is the dominant finding and retinal haemorrhages and other signs such as cotton-wool spots are predominantly peripapillary and confined to the posterior pole (Fig. 13.36). CMO may be present and posterior or anterior segment neovascularization have been reported occasionally in concert with capillary non-perfusion on FA. It may be bilateral, when raised intracranial pressure must be ruled out. Investigation should probably be as for CRVO in a young individual. Distinction from diabetic papillopathy may be difficult. Treatment with intravitreal anti-VEGF or steroid has been reported.

RETINAL ARTERIAL OCCLUSIVE DISEASE

Aetiology

The outer retina is supplied by the ciliary arteries via the choriocapillaris and the inner retina by the central retinal artery (CRA).

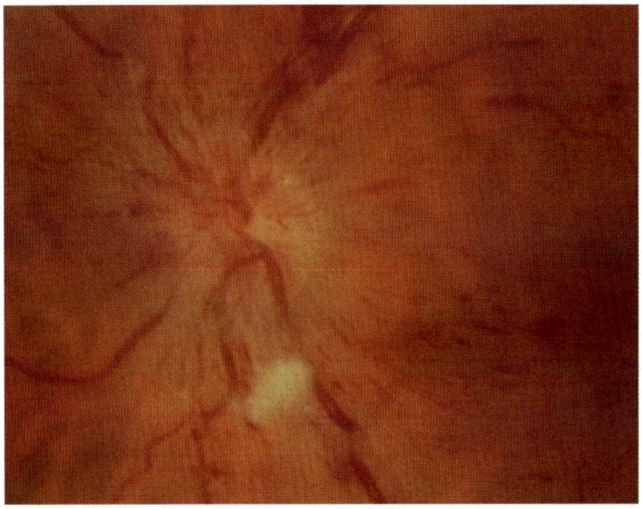

Fig. 13.36 Papillophlebitis.

The ophthalmic artery gives rise to both the CRA – its first branch – and the ciliary arteries (see Fig. 19.5A). The latter also supply the anterior segment via the rectus muscles.

- **Atherosclerosis-related embolism and thrombosis** are thought to be responsible for the majority of cases of retinal artery occlusion, but the proportion of cases due to each of these is unknown. The origin of emboli is most commonly an atheromatous carotid plaque and since the ophthalmic artery is the first branch of the internal carotid artery, embolic material has an easy route to the eye. Emboli can be refractile yellow–white cholesterol (Hollenhorst) plaques (Fig. 13.37A), greyish elongated fibrin-platelet aggregates (Fig. 13.37B and C), non-scintillating white calcific particles (Fig. 13.37D) and, rarely, vegetations from bacterial endocarditis, cardiac myxomatous material and fat. Other cardiac causes include arrhythmia and mitral valve prolapse.
- **Inflammation** in or around the vessel wall (e.g. giant cell arteritis – GCA, systemic lupus erythematosus, granulomatosis with polyangiitis, polyarteritis nodosa), vasospasm (e.g. migraine) and systemic hypotension contribute in a minority.
- **Thrombophilic disorders** that may be associated with retinal artery occlusion (one-third of young patients) include hyperhomocysteinaemia, antiphospholipid antibody syndrome, inherited defects of various natural anticoagulants and sickle cell haemoglobinopathy.
- **Susac syndrome**, a rare immune-mediated vasculo-occlusive disease of young people, consists of the triad of branch retinal artery occlusion, encephalopathy and sensorineural hearing loss. Women predominate and both eyes are usually affected. Retinal microaneurysms are found in 70% of affected individuals. Arteriolar wall hyperfluorescence remote from the BRAO on FA is typical of the condition. Treatment of Susac syndrome involves immunosuppressive and immunomodulatory medication.

Systemic assessment

Following diagnosis and initial evaluation by an ophthalmologist many elements of the assessment may be carried out by a specialist stroke team. **Urgent specialist vascular evaluation is essential following a retinal arterial event**, including amaurosis fugax. The risk of a stroke is relatively high in the first few days after a transient ischaemic attack (TIA) and occurs in 25% at 3 years. The detection of atrial fibrillation is of particular importance as admission for anticoagulation may be indicated.

TIP Urgent specialist cardiovascular evaluation is essential in a patient with a retinal artery occlusion in order to reduce the risk of a stroke or a similar event occurring in the fellow eye.

All patients

Many or most patients will already be aware of vascular risk factors and/or disease.

- **Smoking** should be enquired about.
- **Symptoms of GCA** (1–2% of central retinal artery occlusion – CRAO) such as headache, jaw claudication, scalp tenderness, limb girdle pain, weight loss and existing polymyalgia rheumatica (see Ch. 19). GCA is extremely unlikely under 55–60 years. It constitutes an ophthalmic emergency.
- **Pulse** should be palpated to detect arrhythmia, particularly atrial fibrillation.
- **Blood pressure,** checking for systemic hypertension.
- **Cardiac auscultation** for a murmur.
- **Carotid auscultation** is of limited value as the absence of a bruit does not exclude significant stenosis.
- **ECG** to detect arrhythmia and other cardiac disease.
- **ESR** or **PV** and **CRP** to identify possible GCA.
- **Other blood tests** include FBC (platelets may be raised in GCA), glucose, lipids and urea and electrolytes, the latter to exclude derangement including dehydration.
- **Carotid duplex scanning** is a non-invasive screening test involving a combination of high-resolution real-time ultrasonography with Doppler flow analysis. If significant stenosis is present, surgical management may be considered.

Selected patients

The following additional tests can be considered on a targeted basis in some patients, particularly if younger and with no known cardiovascular risk factors, or if there is an atypical clinical picture (Fig. 13.38A and B).

- **Further carotid imaging** (see Ch. 19).
- **Cranial magnetic resonance imaging (MRI) or computed tomography (CT)** may be indicated to rule out intracranial or orbital pathology.
- **Echocardiography.** Usually performed in young patients or if there is a specific indication such as a history of rheumatic fever, known cardiac valvular disease, or intravenous drug use.
- **Chest X-ray.** Sarcoidosis, tuberculosis, left ventricular hypertrophy in hypertension.
- **24-hour ECG** to exclude intermittent arrhythmia.
- **Additional blood tests**
  - Fasting plasma homocysteine level to exclude hyperhomocysteinaemia.

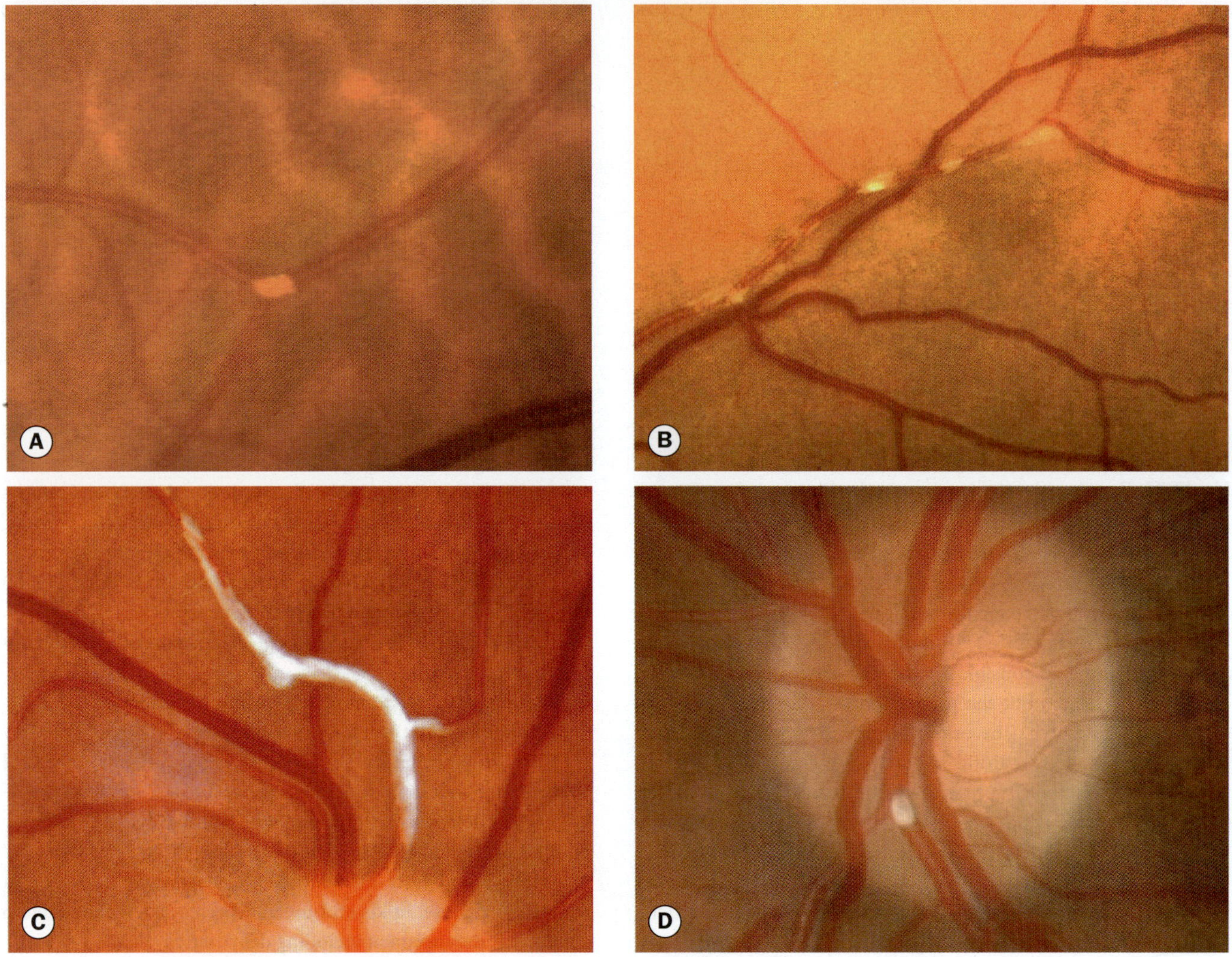

Fig. 13.37 Retinal emboli. **(A)** Hollenhorst plaque; **(B)** fibrin-platelet emboli; **(C)** large fibrin-platelet embolus extending from the disc; **(D)** calcific embolus at the disc. *(Courtesy of S Chen – fig. B; C Barry – fig. D.)*

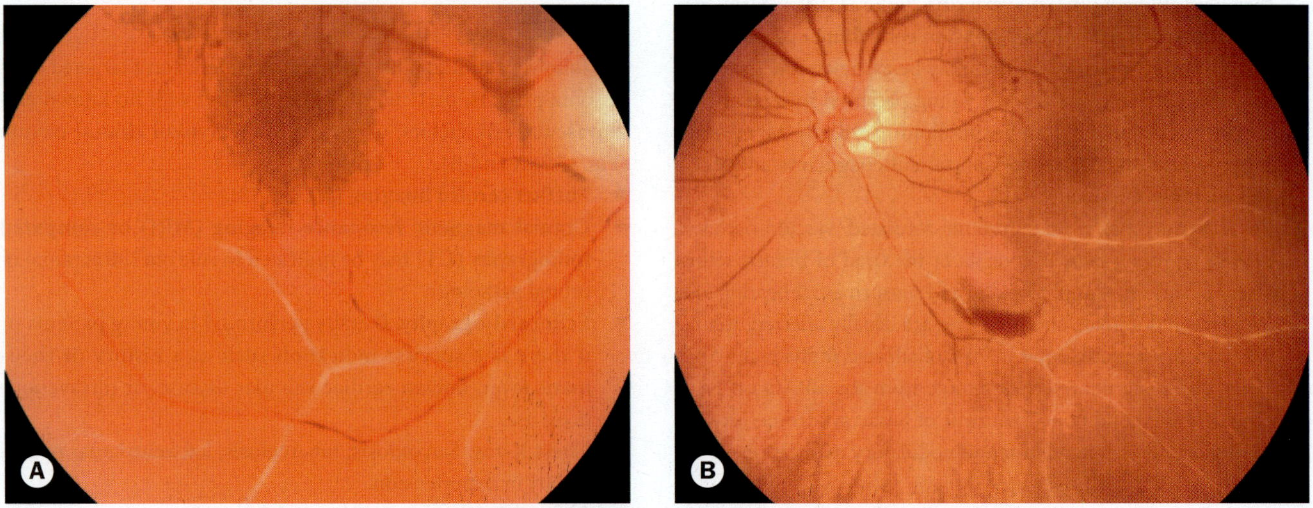

Fig. 13.38 **(A)** and **(B)** Multiple bilateral branch retinal artery occlusions in polyarteritis nodosa.

- 'Thrombophilia screen'. By convention refers to heritable thrombophilias, which have predominantly been implicated in venous rather than arterial thromboses.
- Plasma protein electrophoresis to detect dysproteinaemias such as multiple myeloma.
- Thyroid function tests, especially if atrial fibrillation is present. It may be associated with dyslipidaemia.
- Autoantibodies. Rheumatoid factor, anticardiolipin antibody, antinuclear antibody, anti-double stranded DNA antibodies, principally looking for vasculitis in younger patients.
- Syphilis serology.
- Blood cultures.

Amaurosis fugax

Amaurosis fugax is characterized by transient painless monocular loss of vision, often described as a curtain coming down over the eye. The Amaurosis Fugax Study Group divides the causes into five categories (embolic, hemodynamic, ocular, neurologic and idiopathic), but in clinical practice it is typically used to refer to transient visual loss of embolic origin. It is common for patients to be unaware of whether transient unilateral visual loss affects one eye or the ipsilateral hemifield of both (the latter indicating cerebral rather than more anterior ischaemia). Embolic visual loss, which may be complete, usually lasts a few minutes. Recovery is generally in the same pattern as the loss, although usually more gradual. Frequency of attacks may vary from several times a day to once every few months. The attacks may sometimes be accompanied by an ipsilateral cerebral TIA, with contralateral neurological features. Investigation and systemic management of embolic-pattern amaurosis fugax is the same as that of retinal arterial occlusion and should be undertaken urgently because of the high risk of stroke.

Branch retinal artery occlusion

- **Symptoms.** Sudden and profound painless altitudinal or sectoral visual field loss. Branch retinal artery occlusion (BRAO) can sometimes go unnoticed, particularly if central vision is spared.
- **VA** is variable. In patients where central vision is severely compromised, the prognosis is commonly poor unless the obstruction is relieved within a few hours (see below).
- **RAPD** is often present.
- **Fundus** signs may be subtle.
  - Attenuation of arteries and veins with sludging and segmentation of the blood column ('cattle trucking'/'box-car' appearance).
  - Cloudy white oedematous (ground glass) retina corresponding to the area of ischaemia (Fig. 13.39A and C).
  - One or more occluding emboli may be seen, especially at bifurcation points (see Fig. 13.39A).
  - The affected artery is likely to remain attenuated. Occasionally, recanalization may leave absent ophthalmoscopic signs.
- **Visual field testing** confirms the defect, which rarely recovers.
- **FA** shows delay in arterial filling and hypofluorescence of the involved segment due to blockage of background fluorescence by retinal swelling (Fig. 13.39B and D).
- **Review** in 3 months is warranted to review the appearance of the fundus, the visual fields, provide advice on prognosis and confirm that systemic management has been carried out appropriately.

Central retinal artery occlusion

- **Symptoms.** Sudden profound loss of vision, painless except in GCA.
- **VA** is severely reduced except if a cilioretinal artery supplying a critical macular area preserves central vision (see below). Absence of light perception usually indicates either GCA or ophthalmic artery occlusion. The prognosis is poor in all cases unless recovery occurs in the first few hours.
- **RAPD** is profound, sometimes total (amaurotic pupil).
- **Fundus** shows similar changes to BRAO but involving all retinal quadrants.
  - The orange reflex from the intact choroid stands out at the thin foveola, in contrast to the surrounding pale retina, giving rise to a 'cherry-red spot' appearance (Fig. 13.40A and B).
  - The peripapillary retina may appear especially swollen and opaque.
  - An occasional small haemorrhage is not unusual.
  - Emboli are visible in 20%, when Nd:YAG embolysis may be considered (see below).
  - In eyes with a cilioretinal artery part of the macula will remain of normal colour (Fig. 13.40C).
  - Retinal signs can sometimes be subtle. Retinal oedema may take several hours to develop.
  - Over a few days to weeks the retinal cloudiness and 'cherry-red spot' gradually disappear although the arteries remain attenuated. Later signs include optic atrophy, vessel sheathing and patchy inner retinal atrophy and RPE changes.
  - Around 2% of eyes with CRAO develop retinal or disc neovascularization.
  - Rubeosis iridis may occur in up to about 1 in 5 eyes, typically earlier than in CRVO (4–5 weeks compared with 3 months, though sometimes later) and along with very poor vision may indicate ophthalmic artery occlusion.
- **OCT** may show a highly reflective embolic plaque within the superficial optic nerve head.
- **FA** shows a variable delay in arterial filling and masking of background choroidal fluorescence by retinal oedema. A patent cilioretinal artery will fill during the early phase (Fig. 13.40D).
- **Electroretinography** may be helpful to establish the diagnosis if in doubt, particularly to distinguish from optic nerve disease, typically when signs are subtle. A diminished b-wave is present.
- **Ophthalmic review.** The patient should be seen by an ophthalmologist after 3–4 weeks and a minimum of

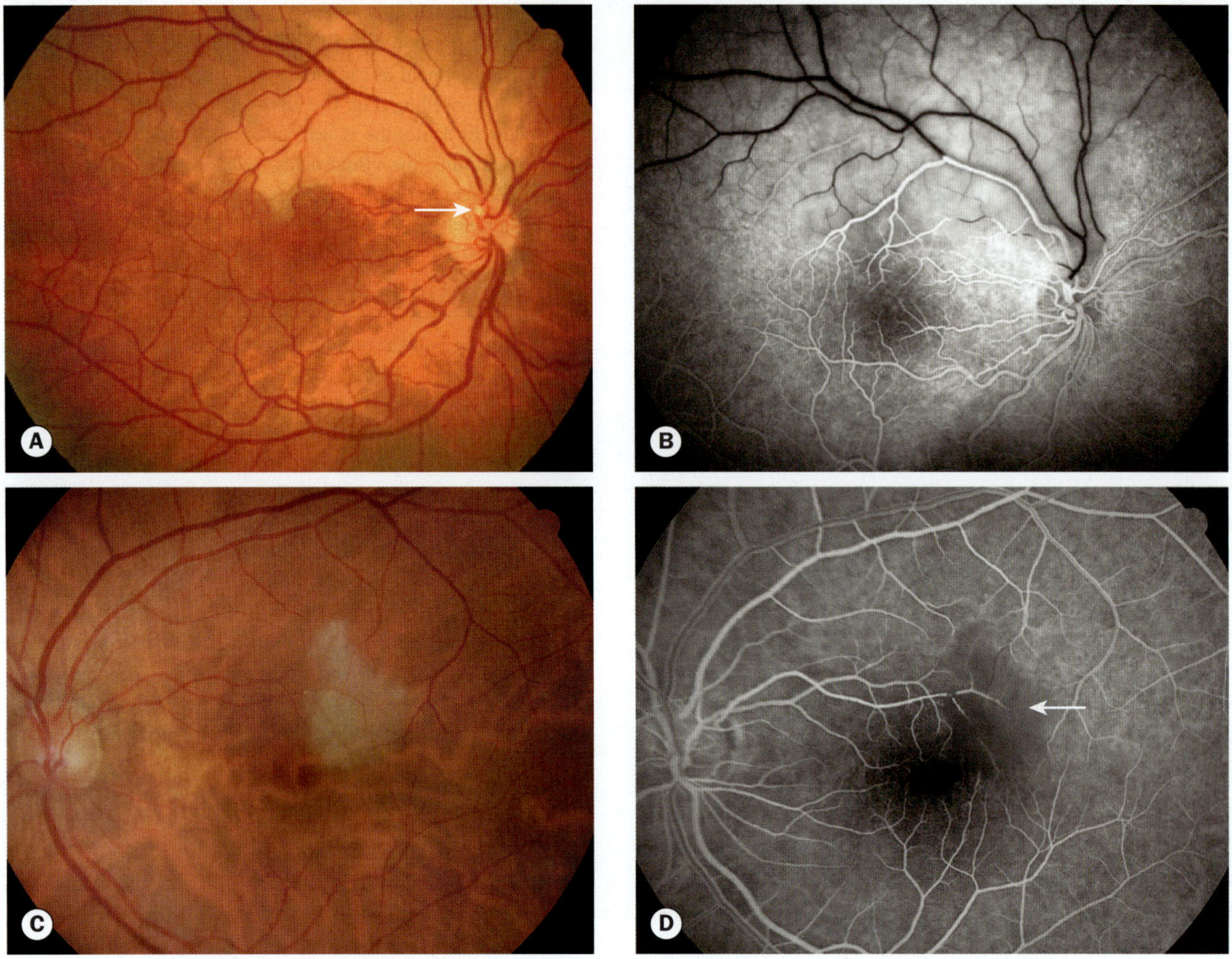

Fig. 13.39 Embolic branch retinal artery occlusions. **(A)** Superior branch retinal artery occlusion due to an embolus at the disc (arrow); **(B)** FA of **(A)** showing lack of arterial filling of the involved artery and hypofluorescence of the involved segment due to blockage of background fluorescence by retinal swelling; **(C)** small macular branch artery occlusion; **(D)** FA of **(C)** showing hypofluorescence (arrow). *(Courtesy of C Barry – figs A and B; S Chen – figs C and D.)*

twice subsequently at monthly intervals in order to detect incipient neovascularization, particularly of the anterior segment. In this event, PRP should be performed as for ischaemic CRVO and intravitreal injection of VEGF inhibitor might be considered. Appropriate systemic management is critical.

Cilioretinal artery occlusion

A cilioretinal artery is present in about one-third of eyes, providing the central macula with a second arterial supply derived from the posterior ciliary circulation. Its main importance is that when present it may facilitate preservation of central vision following central retinal artery occlusion, provided the fovea is supplied.

- **Isolated.** This is rare (Fig. 13.41A and B). It may occur in young patients with an associated systemic vasculitis.
- **Combined with CRVO.** This (Fig. 13.41C) is not uncommon, but occlusion is transient and the prognosis is better than in isolated cilioretinal artery occlusion.
- **Combined with anterior ischaemic optic neuropathy** (Fig. 13.41D), typically affects patients with GCA and carries a very poor prognosis.

Treatment of acute retinal artery occlusion

Retinal artery occlusion is an emergency because it causes irreversible visual loss unless the retinal circulation can be re-established before the development of retinal infarction. Theoretically, timely dislodgement of thrombus or emboli may ameliorate subsequent visual loss. In primate studies, partial recovery is possible if the ischaemia is reversed within 4 hours. The time when irreversible retinal damage occurs with no visual recovery is not known in humans, but has been postulated to

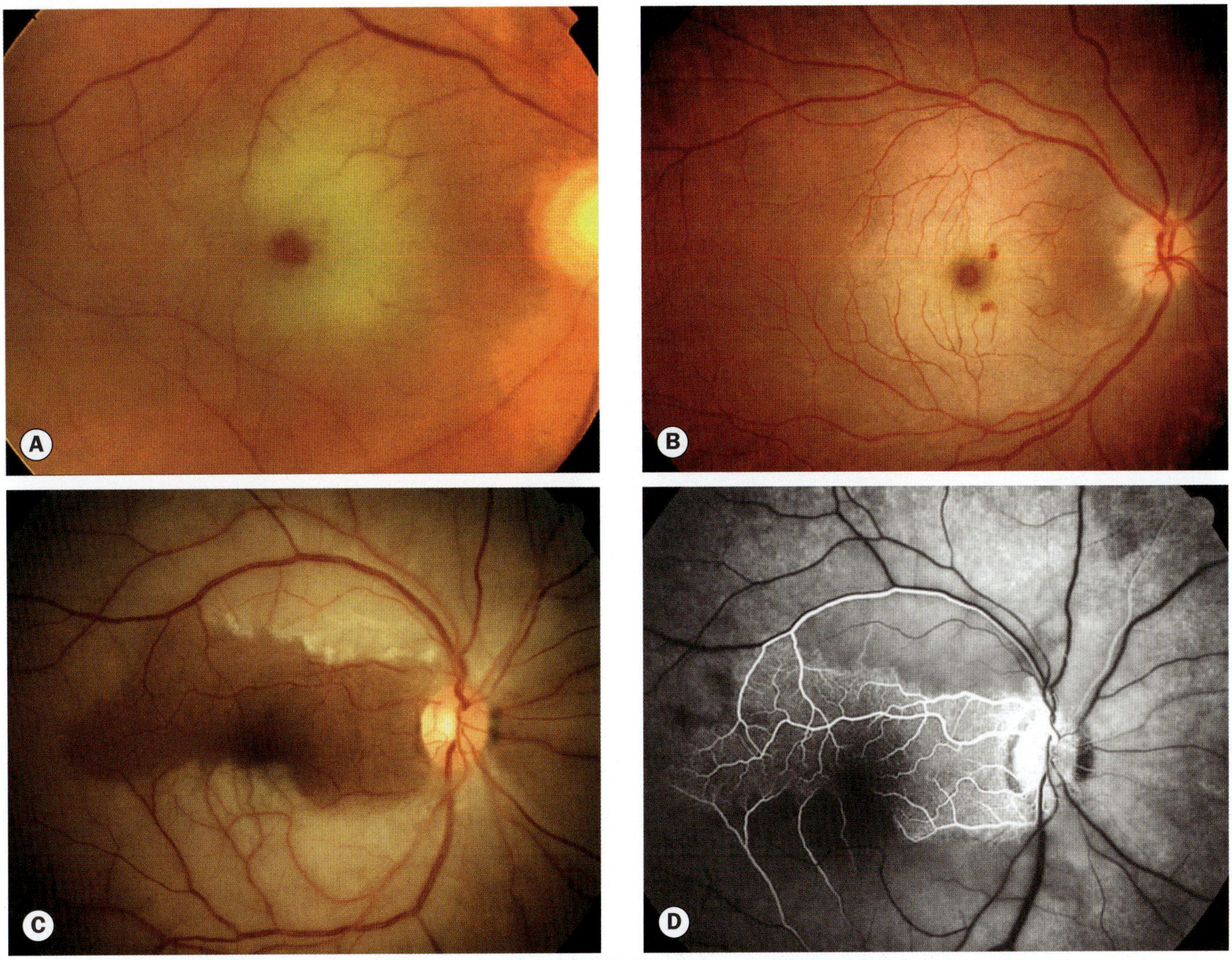

Fig. 13.40 Central retinal artery occlusion (CRAO). **(A)** Acute CRAO with a 'cherry-red spot' at the macula; **(B)** recent CRAO with 'cherry-red spot' and small area of normal retina adjacent to the disc; **(C)** CRAO with a patent cilioretinal artery; **(D)** FA showing blockage of background fluorescence by retinal oedema but normal perfusion of a sector of retina in the eye in **(C).**

be about 6 hours in studies determining the effect of tissue plasminogen activator on thrombolysis. Unfortunately, treatment is usually not effective. In two-thirds the final VA is worse than 6/120 and only one-fifth are left with a VA of 6/12 or better. The various therapeutic options should be discussed before use, including the lack of evidence for clear benefit and the associated risks. The following can be tried in patients with an occlusion of less than 6 hours' duration at presentation though evidence of benefit is limited:

- **Ocular massage** using a three-mirror contact lens (allows direct artery visualization). The aim is to mechanically collapse the arterial lumen and cause prompt changes in arterial flow, improving perfusion and potentially dislodging an embolus or thrombus. One described method consists of positive pressure for 10–15 seconds followed by release, continued for 3–5 minutes. Self-massage through closed eyelids can be continued by the patient.
- **Anterior chamber paracentesis** using a 27-gauge needle to withdraw 0.1–0.2 ml of aqueous has been advocated by some authorities. Povidone-iodine 5% and topical antibiotic are instilled a few minutes prior to the procedure, with a short course of antibiotic afterwards. It may be prudent for ocular massage to be avoided following paracentesis.
- **Topical apraclonidine 1%**, timolol 0.5% and intravenous acetazolamide 500 mg to achieve a more sustained lowering of intraocular pressure.
- **'Rebreathing'** into a paper bag in order to elevate blood carbon dioxide and respiratory acidosis has been advocated, as this may promote vasodilatation. Similarly, breathing a high oxygen (95%) and carbon dioxide (5%) mixture, 'carbogen', has been advocated for a possible dual effect of retarding ischaemia and vasodilatation.

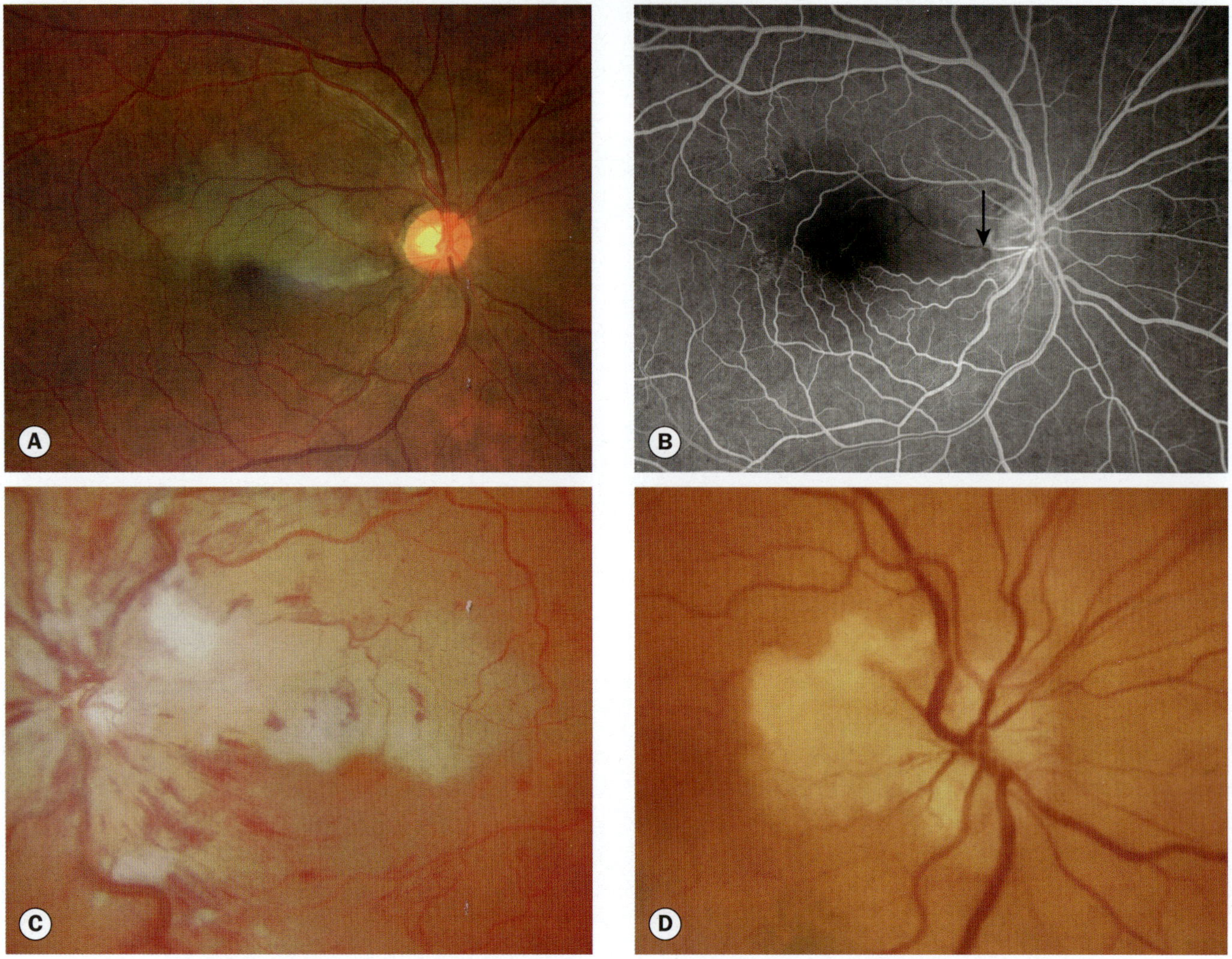

Fig. 13.41 Cilioretinal artery occlusion. **(A)** Secondary to embolus; **(B)** FA of **(A)** showing the occluded vessel (arrow) and hypofluorescence in the affected area due to reduced filling and masking by retinal oedema; **(C)** combined with central retinal vein occlusion; **(D)** combined with anterior ischaemic optic neuropathy. *(Courtesy of C Mishra – figs A and B.)*

- **Transluminal Nd:YAG** laser embolysis/embolectomy has been advocated for BRAO or CRAO where an occluding embolus is visible. Although experience with this technique is limited, surprisingly good final visual results have been reported. A variable number of shots of 0.5–1 mJ or higher (to a maximum of 2.4 mJ) are applied directly to the embolus using a fundus contact lens. Embolectomy has been said to occur if the embolus is ejected into the vitreous via a hole in the arteriole. The main complication is subretinal and vitreous haemorrhage in approximately half, which may be curtailed with pressure on the globe.
- **Thrombolysis.** Extrapolating from successful treatment of stroke and myocardial infarction, various strategies have been used to deliver thrombolytic agents to the ophthalmic artery, including local arterial (internal carotid and ophthalmic) and intravenous infusion. On the basis of observational data and in the absence of other effective treatment, patients with acute CRAO who are seen within 4.5 hours of onset of visual loss could be considered for treatment with intravenous tissue plasminogen activator (tPA). The commonest regimen used is intravenous (IV) alteplase (0.9mg/kg, with 10% given over 1 minute and the remainder over 59 minutes). Patients undergoing this treatment should be fully informed of the benefits and risks of treatment. A large multicentre trial of local intraocular thrombolysis with recombinant tissue plasminogen activator (rtPA) showed no benefit over conservative treatment that included isovolaemic haemodilution. This finding may reflect the rapidity of retinal dysfunction that occurs secondary to ischaemia and perhaps the resistance to dissolution of embolic, versus thrombotic obstruction.

TIP To reduce the risk of stroke and ischaemic heart disease, the systemic factors responsible for a central retinal artery occlusion need to be determined and treated.

Systemic management following retinal arterial occlusion

- **The risk of stroke is relatively high** in the first few days following retinal artery occlusion or amaurosis fugax. Urgent referral to a specialist stroke clinic is imperative. Of those with a CRAO who are sent for urgent systemic evaluation, 30% will have severe carotid disease, coincidental stroke or extreme hypertension and 20% will have simultaneous myocardial infarction or critical heart disease. Almost 95% will subsequently need a change in their systemic medication and 25% will require urgent surgical intervention.
- **General risk factors** as discussed above should be addressed and smoking should be discontinued. Urgent referral to an appropriate physician is mandatory for significant cardiac arrhythmia.
- **Antiplatelet therapy** is commenced provided there are no contraindications. An immediate loading dose of 600 mg may be given. Alternative/additional agents include dipyridamole and clopidogrel. If fibrinolysis (see above) is being considered, this should be discussed with a physician prior to starting antiplatelet treatment.
- **Oral anticoagulation** (e.g. warfarin) may be prescribed for some patients, particularly those with atrial fibrillation.
- **Carotid endarterectomy** may be indicated in patients with symptomatic stenosis greater than 70%.

Asymptomatic retinal embolus

It is not uncommon to identify a retinal embolus on routine examination of an asymptomatic older patient. This indicates a substantially increased risk of stroke and ischaemic heart disease and management should consist of evaluation and treatment of risk factors discussed above. A higher threshold for carotid surgery is appropriate.

OCULAR ISCHAEMIC SYNDROME

Introduction

Ocular ischaemic syndrome (OIS) results from chronic ocular hypoperfusion secondary to severe (more than 90%) ipsilateral atherosclerotic carotid stenosis. It typically affects older patients and may be associated with diabetes, hypertension, cardio- and cerebrovascular disease. The male:female ratio is about 2:1. Five-year mortality is around 40%, most frequently from cardiac disease. OIS, along with non-ischaemic CRVO, is sometimes termed 'venous stasis retinopathy' but it may be prudent to avoid this term.

Diagnosis

OIS is unilateral in 80%. The signs are variable and may be subtle such that the condition is missed or misdiagnosed.

- **Symptoms.** Gradual loss of vision over weeks or months, although occasionally loss may be sudden or intermittent (amaurosis fugax). Ocular and periocular pain may also be present (40%). Patients may notice unusually persistent after-images, or worsening of vision with sudden exposure to bright light ('bright light amaurosis fugax'), with slow adaptation. The prognosis for vision is often very poor, though patients with better acuity at presentation are more likely to retain this. About 25% will deteriorate to light perception by the end of 1 year.
- **Anterior segment**
  - Diffuse episcleral injection and corneal oedema.
  - Aqueous flare with few cells (ischaemic pseudo-iritis).
  - Iris atrophy with a mid-dilated, poorly reacting pupil.
  - Rubeosis iridis is common, developing in up to 90% and often progresses to neovascular glaucoma. The IOP may remain low due to poor ocular perfusion.
  - Cataract in advanced cases.
- **Fundus**
  - Venous dilatation, arteriolar narrowing, deep round and flame haemorrhages and occasionally disc oedema (Fig. 13.42A) and cotton-wool spots.
  - Proliferative retinopathy with NVD and occasionally NVE.
  - Spontaneous arterial pulsation, most pronounced near the optic disc, is present in most cases or may be easily induced by exerting gentle pressure on the globe (digital ophthalmodynamometry).
  - Macular oedema can occur.
  - In diabetic patients the retinopathy may be more severe ipsilateral to carotid stenosis.
- **FA.** Delayed choroidal filling and prolonged arteriovenous transit is the major feature. Non-perfusion, vessel wall staining and retinal oedema may also be evident (Fig. 13.42B–D).
- **Carotid imaging** may involve duplex ultrasonography, digital subtraction angiography, MR or CT angiography.

Management

- **Anterior segment inflammation** is treated with topical steroid and a mydriatic as appropriate.
- **Neovascular glaucoma** is managed medically or surgically (see Ch. 11).
- **Proliferative retinopathy** can be treated with PRP although the outcome is considerably less certain than in proliferative diabetic retinopathy. Intravitreal anti-VEGF agents may be beneficial.
- **Macular oedema** may respond to intravitreal steroid or anti-VEGF agents, or to carotid surgery.
- **Carotid surgery.** Endarterectomy or stenting may be performed to reduce the risk of stroke. It may be beneficial for proliferative retinopathy and neovascular glaucoma and may help to stabilize vision. Endarterectomy cannot be performed where there is total obstruction, and in this situation extracranial–intracranial arterial bypass surgery is sometimes carried out. It should be noted that an increase in ocular perfusion following surgery can sometimes be associated with a rise in IOP.

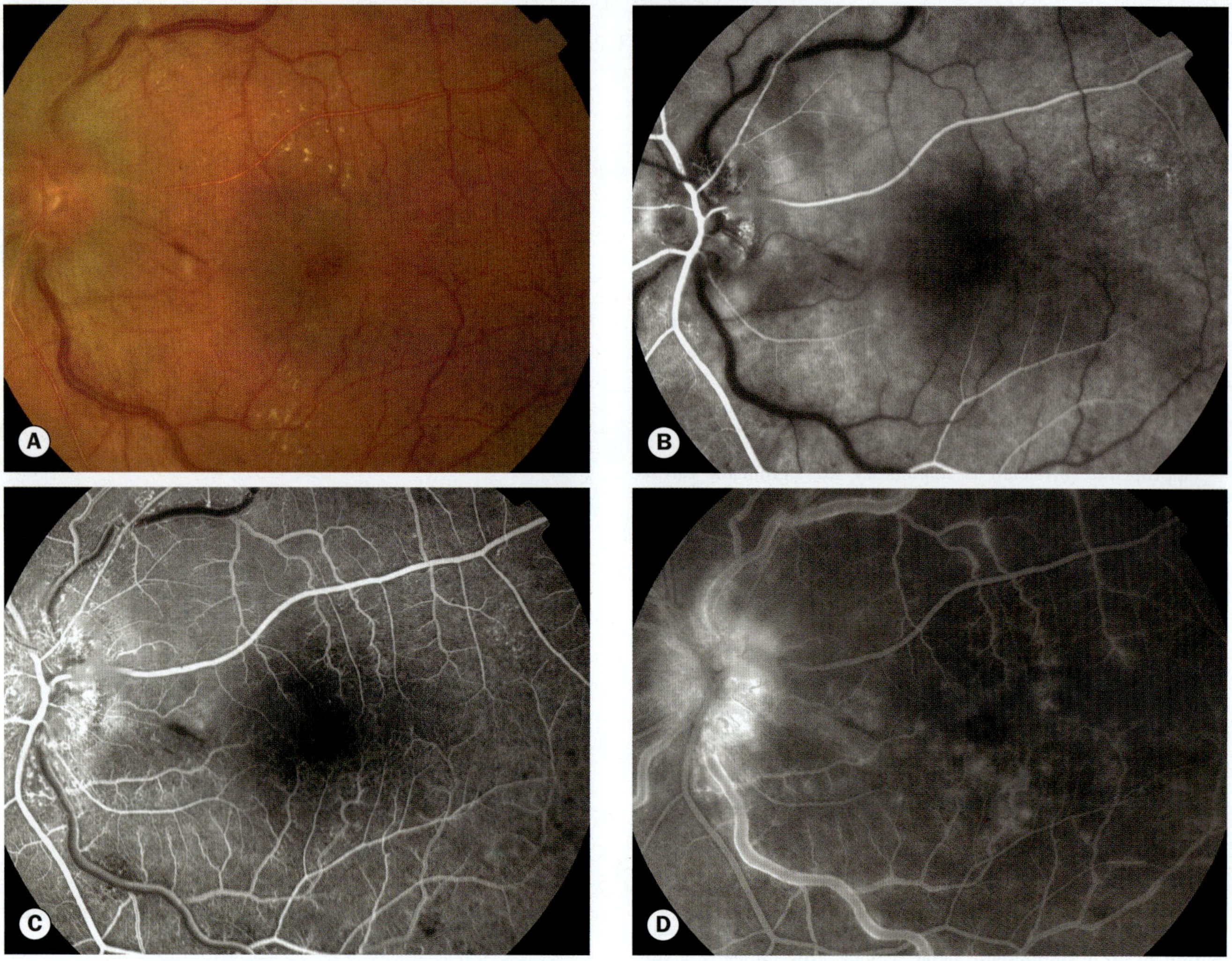

Fig. 13.42 Ocular ischaemic syndrome showing AV filling delay. **(A)** Venous dilatation, arteriolar narrowing, a few scattered flame haemorrhages and hard exudates, and disc oedema; **(B)** early FA (20s) and **(C)** FA early phase (35s) showing delayed choroidal filling and prolonged arteriovenous transit; **(D)** FA late phase (5min) showing disc and perivascular hyperfluorescence, with spotty hyperfluorescence at the posterior pole due to leakage.

Surgery tends to be of greater benefit when performed before the onset of severe ocular ischaemia.

- **Investigation and management of cardiovascular risk factors** in conjunction with the appropriate medical specialists is essential. OIS is occasionally the only manifestation of marked systemic vascular disease. Full investigation should be carried out, broadly similar to that for retinal arterial occlusion.

HYPERTENSIVE EYE DISEASE

Retinopathy

Systemic arterial hypertension is common. In addition to heart, kidneys and brain, the eye is often affected by hypertension. Ocular effects can be observed in the retina, choroid and optic nerve. The primary response of the retinal arterioles to systemic hypertension is vasoconstriction, which is less marked in older individuals because of involutional sclerosis conferring increased rigidity. Arteriolosclerosis refers to hardening and loss of elasticity of small vessel walls, manifested most obviously by arteriovenous (AV) nipping (nicking) at crossing points. The presence of this sign makes it probable that hypertension has been present for many years, even if the BP is currently controlled. Mild AV changes may be seen in the absence of hypertension. In sustained hypertension the inner blood–retinal barrier is disrupted, increased vascular permeability leading to flame-shaped retinal haemorrhages and oedema.

- **Grade 1.** Mild generalized retinal arteriolar narrowing (Fig. 13.43A).
- **Grade 2.** Focal arteriolar narrowing (Fig. 13.43B) and arteriovenous nipping (Fig. 13.43C). A 'copper wiring' opacified appearance of arteriolar walls may be seen (Fig. 13.43D).
- **Grade 3.** Grade 2 plus retinal haemorrhages (dot, blot, flame), exudates (chronic retinal oedema may result in the deposition of hard exudates around the fovea as a 'macular star' – Fig. 13.43E) and cotton-wool spots.
- **Grade 4.** Severe grade 3 plus optic disc swelling, which is a marker of 'malignant' hypertension (Fig. 13.43F).

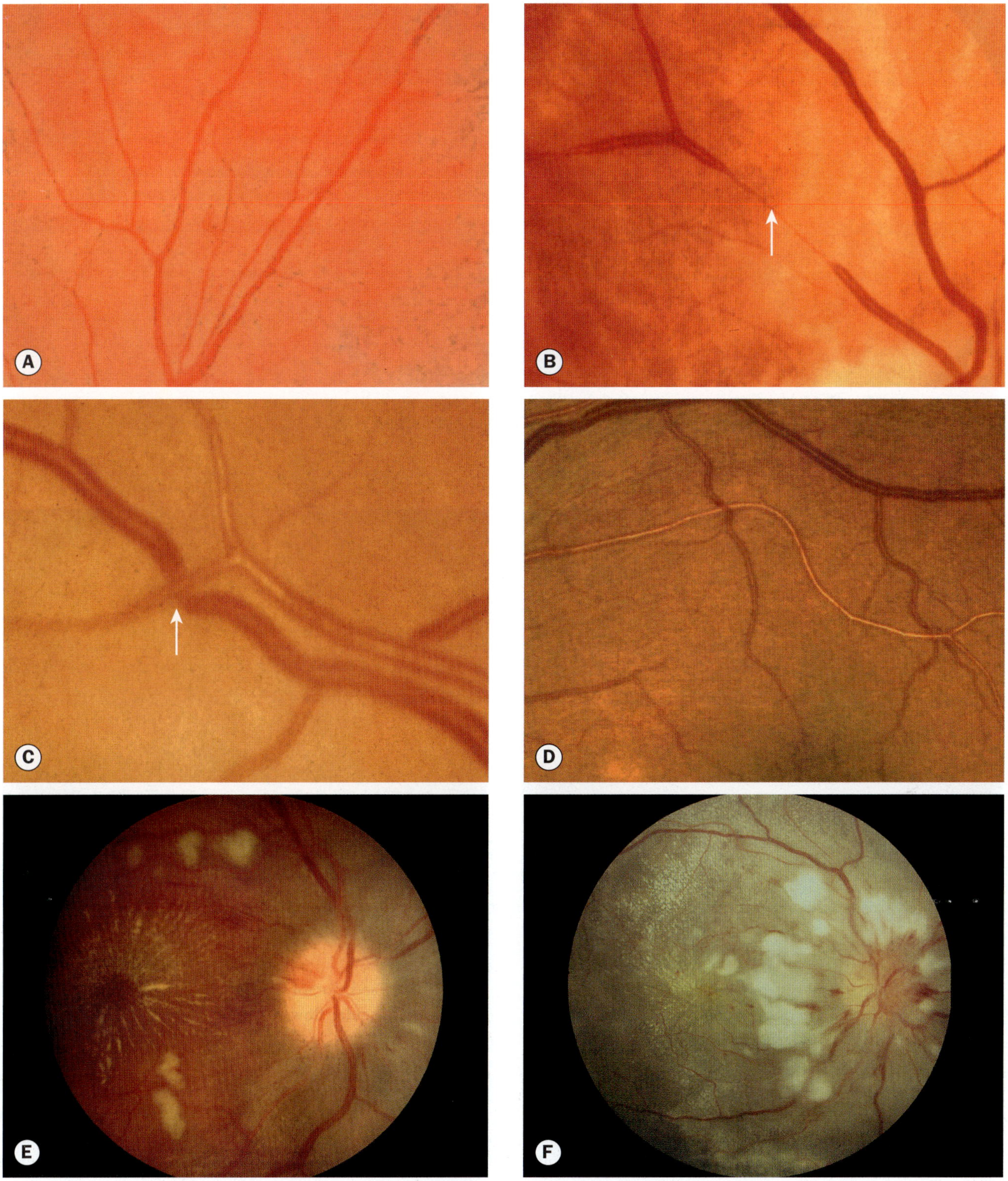

Fig. 13.43 Hypertensive retinopathy. **(A)** Generalized arteriolar attenuation; **(B)** focal arteriolar attenuation (arrow); **(C)** arteriovenous nipping (arrow); **(D)** 'copper wiring'; **(E)** grade 3 retinopathy with macular star; **(F)** grade 4 hypertensive retinopathy showing extensive cotton-wool spots and slight disc swelling.

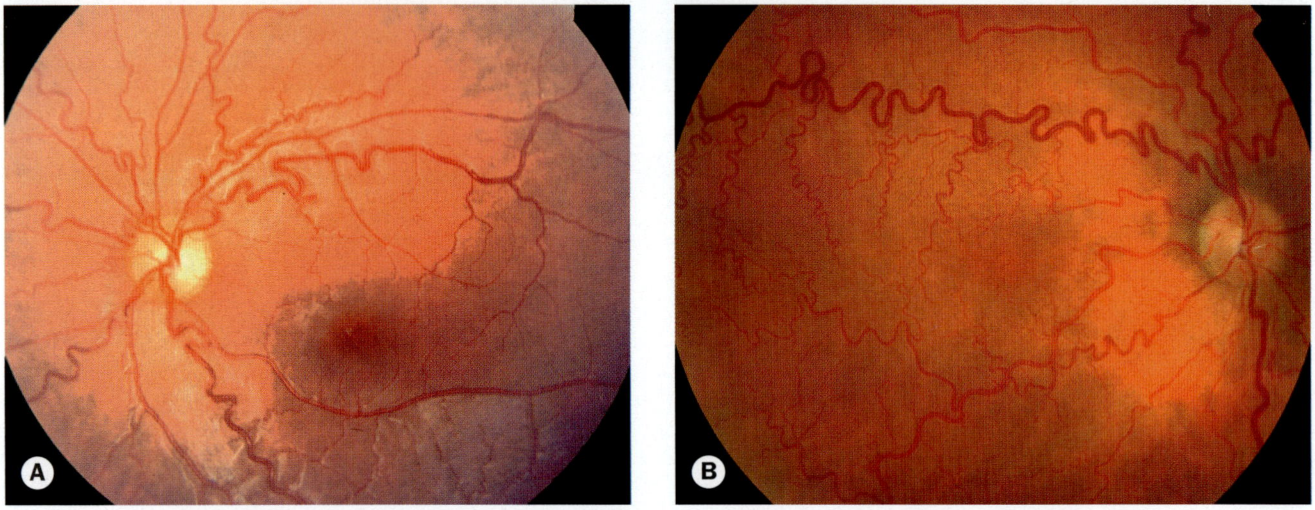

Fig. 13.44 Vascular tortuosity. **(A)** Selective venous tortuosity – the arterioles are unaffected; **(B)** mixed arteriolar and venular tortuosity. *(Courtesy of S Chen – fig. B.)*

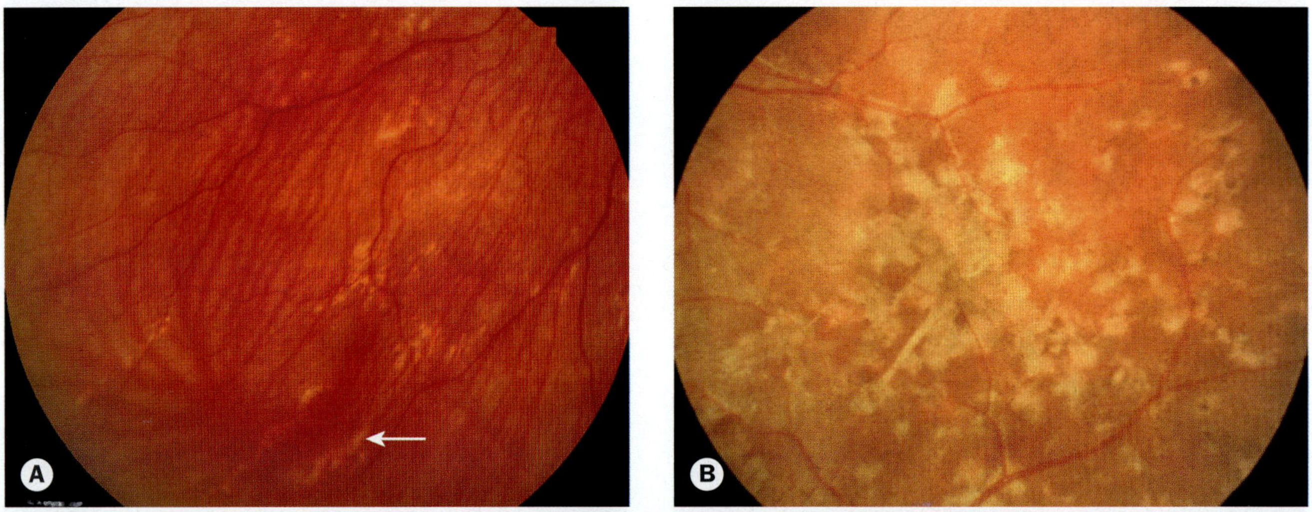

Fig. 13.45 Hypertensive choroidopathy. **(A)** Siegrist lines (arrow); **(B)** Elschnig spots.

- **Markers of preclinical systemic disease.**
  - Reduced retinal arteriolar calibre (see Fig. 13.43A) is an early pre-hypertensive sign and if identified should prompt BP monitoring.
  - Wider venular calibre is relatively specific for impaired glucose metabolism.
  - Low arteriolar calibre and high venular calibre are both thought to be markers of preclinical cardiovascular disease.
  - Increased venular tortuosity (Fig. 13.44A) can be associated with chronic hypertension and pre-hypertension, though evidence on arteriolar tortuosity is conflicting – straightening of arterioles has been reported in some studies. Numerous other causes of retinal vascular tortuosity (Fig. 13.44B) have been described, notably conditions associated with high and low vascular flow.

Choroidopathy

Hypertensive choroidopathy is rare but may occur as the result of an acute hypertensive crisis (accelerated hypertension) in young adults.

- **Siegrist streaks** are flecks arranged linearly along choroidal vessels and are indicative of fibrinoid necrosis associated with malignant hypertension (Fig. 13.45A).
- **Elschnig spots** are focal choroidal infarcts seen as small black spots surrounded by yellow haloes (Fig. 13.45B).
- **Exudative retinal detachment**, sometimes bilateral, may occur in acute severe hypertension such as that associated with toxaemia of pregnancy.

PARACENTRAL ACUTE MIDDLE MACULOPATHY (PAMM)

PAMM is an uncommon condition of the macula which occurs mainly in individuals aged 60–75 years, presumably as a complication of retinal microvasculopathy or systemic vascular disease. In younger individuals no cause may be found. The patient notices a sudden positive scotoma close to fixation in one eye and has no other visual or ocular symptoms. Fundus examination reveals subtle whitish parafoveal lesions within the retina. When an OCT scan is undertaken in the acute phase a placoid, hyperreflective band is seen at the level of the inner nuclear layer, with a normal outer retina (Fig. 13.46). Partial resolution is the most common outcome, although full resolution may occasionally occur. The main differential is acute macular neuroretinopathy, which can be excluded with an OCT (see Ch. 12). There is no treatment. Systemic diseases like arterial hypertension and diabetes need to be excluded.

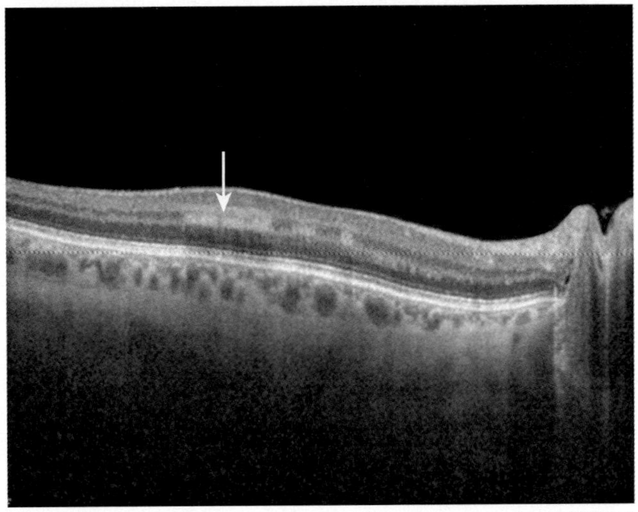

Fig. 13.46 Paracentral acute middle maculopathy (PAMM) in a 74-year old severely hypertensive woman. OCT in the acute phase shows a placoid, hyperreflective band at the level of the INL (arrow), sparing the outer retina. *(Courtesy of G Kontos.)*

SICKLE-CELL RETINOPATHY

Sickling haemoglobinopathies

Sickling haemoglobinopathies are caused by one or more abnormal haemoglobins that induce red blood cells to adopt an anomalous shape (Fig. 13.47) under conditions of physiological stress such as hypoxia and acidosis, with resultant vascular occlusion. Mutant haemoglobin variants S and C can be found in combination with the normal adult haemoglobin A or, less commonly, with other mutant haemoglobin variants. Retinopathy can occur in sickle-cell disease (homozygous for mutant haemoglobin S, i.e. SS), sickle-cell C disease (SC – the most likely to develop severe retinopathy) and sickle-cell thalassaemia disease. It is rare in patients with sickle-cell trait (SA – found in 10% of African-Americans), unless there is other co-existing systemic disease such as diabetes or an inflammatory disorder. Carbonic anhydrase inhibitors (CAI) should be avoided in these disorders as they can precipitate sickling and vascular occlusion.

Anterior segment

- **Conjunctiva.** Dark red corkscrew- or comma-shaped vessels that are typically transient.
- **Iris.** Patches of ischaemic atrophy, often extending from the pupillary edge to the collarette and occasionally rubeosis.
- **Hyphaema** may be spontaneous or follow minor trauma. Careful IOP control (avoiding CAI) is critical to reduce the risk of RVO in the presence of a hyphaema.

Non-proliferative retinopathy

- **Venous changes.** Tortuosity (see Fig. 13.44) is very common and is thought to be due to peripheral arteriovenous shunting.
- **Optic disc 'sign of sickling'.** Dark red blots on the disc surface due to small vessel occlusion.
- **'Salmon patches'.** Orange–red mid-peripheral superficial intraretinal haemorrhages (Fig. 13.48A) that may break through to become preretinal or subretinal. The initiating event is thought to be a vascular occlusion. Salmon patches resolve to leave schisis cavities containing refractile deposits, 'black sunbursts' (see below) when the RPE is sufficiently stimulated, or a combination lesion.
- **Black sunbursts.** Patches of peripheral RPE hyperplasia and chorioretinal atrophy (see Fig. 13.48A) that evolve from some salmon patches. The extent and morphology of pigmentation is variable, but an outer pale band is generally present.
- **Arteriolar changes.** Occlusions can involve branch, central or macular vessels (Fig. 13.48B) and if seen acutely may benefit from measures such as 100% oxygen and exchange transfusion. 'Silver wiring' of arterioles in the peripheral retina signifies previously occluded vessels. Corkscrewing of peripheral vessels may also be seen.
- **Macular (retinal) depression sign.** An oval depression in the temporal macular retina due to retinal thinning following arteriolar occlusion, with irregularity of the light reflex. Vascular anomalies such as microaneurysms and epiretinal membranes may occur.
- **Peripheral areas of whitening or darkening.**
- **Angioid streaks** (see Ch. 14) occur in up to 6%.

Proliferative retinopathy

Diagnosis

The development of proliferative retinopathy is usually insidious, with no symptoms unless vitreous haemorrhage or retinal detachment occurs.

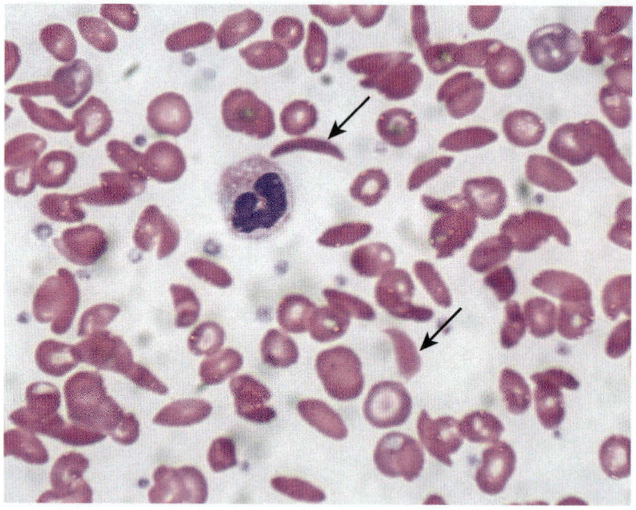

Fig. 13.47 Several sickle cells (arrows) in a peripheral smear of a patient with homozygous (HbSS) sickle-cell anaemia.

- **Stage 1.** Peripheral arteriolar occlusion.
- **Stage 2.** Peripheral arteriovenous anastomosis (Fig. 13.49A) proximal to non-perfused areas.
- **Stage 3.** 'Sea fan' neovascularization (Fig. 13.49B) develops at the edge of perfused retina, usually with a single supplying arteriole and a single draining venule. Disc neovascularization may rarely occur.
- **Stage 4.** Vitreous haemorrhage from the NV.
- **Stage 5.** Rhegmatogenous retinal detachment caused by a retinal break associated with extensive fibrovascular proliferation (Fig. 13.49C). Tractional detachment may also occur (Fig. 13.49D).
- FA in stage 3 shows filling of sea fans and peripheral capillary non-perfusion (Fig. 13.49E) followed by leakage from the NV (Fig. 13.49F). Wide-field imaging is especially suited to evaluation of this condition.

TIP Avoid the use of carbonic anhydrase inhibitors in patients with sickel-cell anaemia as these drugs can cause sickling and vascular occlusion.

Treatment

- **Observation** if vitreous haemorrhage has not occurred, particularly in middle-aged and older patients. Many neovascular complexes involute spontaneously as a result of auto-infarction or fibrotic strangulation, subsequently appearing as greyish fibrovascular lesions.
- **Laser or cryotherapy** ablation of peripheral non-perfused retina is probably the optimal approach, though ablation of neovascularization may also be used. Ablation of feeder vessels is now rarely performed due to a high incidence of subsequent macular neovascularization.
- **Vitreoretinal surgery** may be required for tractional retinal detachment and/or persistent vitreous haemorrhage. Caution is required as anterior segment ischaemia, potentially severe, is very common following scleral explant application.

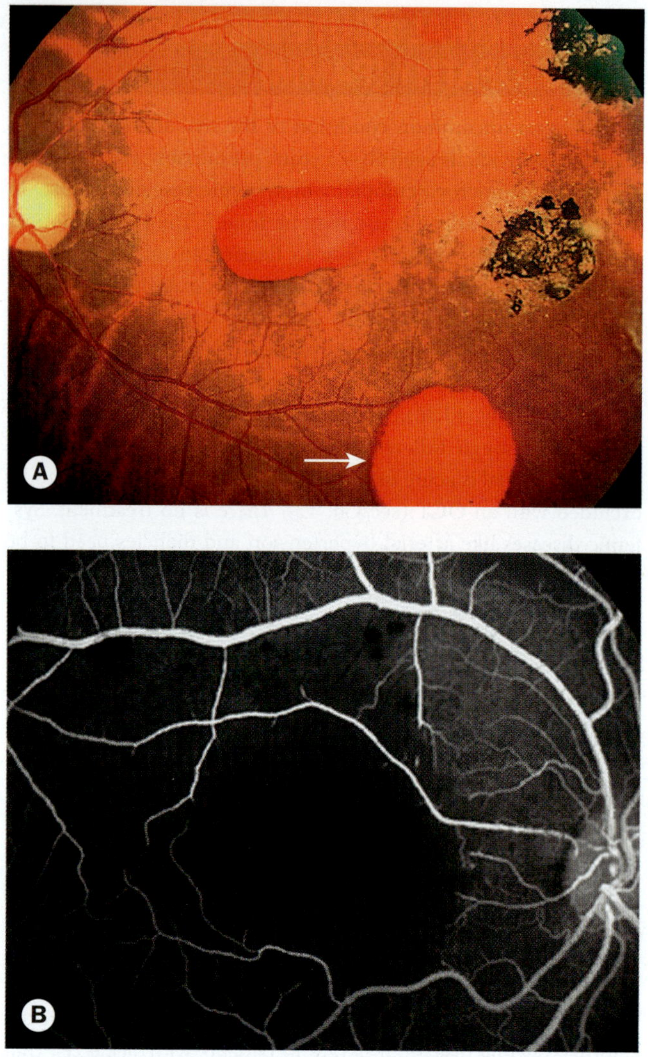

Fig. 13.48 Non-proliferative sickle cell retinopathy. **(A)** RPE hyperplasia ('black sunburst') and preretinal haemorrhages ('salmon patch') (arrow); **(B)** FA showing macular ischaemia.

THALASSAEMIA RETINOPATHY

Thalassaemia is a common genetic disorder in which a mutation gives rise to abnormal haemoglobin with a consequent failure of normal red blood cell maturation. Ocular involvement occurs in patients with thalassaemia major and thalassaemia intermedia. Changes are caused by the disease itself as well as treatment with blood transfusions and iron chelating agents such as desferrioxamine. A major mechanism is tissue deposition of iron (siderosis) from the lysing of abnormal red cells. The ocular features predominantly affect the posterior segment and are non-proliferative, though vitreous haemorrhage has been reported. Visual dysfunction is rarely severe. Manifestations include cataract, a smooth featureless iris, vascular tortuosity, angioid streaks, optic neuropathy and pigmentary retinal mottling, including pattern dystrophy-like macular changes. The fundus appearance may resemble that of pseudoxanthoma elasticum.

Chapter 14

Acquired Macular Disorders

INTRODUCTION

The macula (Fig. 14.1A) is a round area at the posterior pole, lying inside the temporal vascular arcades. It measures between 5 and 6 mm in diameter and subserves the central 15–20° of the visual field. Histologically, it shows more than one layer of ganglion cells, in contrast to the single ganglion cell layer of the peripheral retina. The inner layers of the macula contain the yellow xanthophyll carotenoid pigments lutein and zeaxanthin in far higher concentration than the peripheral retina (hence the full name 'macula lutea' – yellow plaque).

- **The fovea** is a depression in the retinal surface at the centre of the macula (Fig. 14.1B–D), with a diameter of 1.5 mm – about the same as the optic disc.
- **The foveola** forms the central floor of the fovea and has a diameter of 0.35 mm (see Fig. 14.1B). It is the thinnest part of the retina and is devoid of ganglion cells, consisting only of a high density of cone photoreceptors and their nuclei (Fig. 14.2), together with Müller cells.
- **The umbo** is a depression in the very centre of the foveola (see Fig. 14.1B) which corresponds to the foveolar light reflex (see Fig. 14.1A), loss of which may be an early sign of damage.
- **The foveal avascular zone** (FAZ – see Fig. 14.1B), a central area containing no blood vessels but surrounded by a continuous network of capillaries, is located within the fovea but extends beyond the foveola. The exact diameter varies with age and in disease and its limits can be determined with accuracy only by fluorescein angiography (average 0.6 mm).

Retinal pigment epithelium

- **Structure**
  - The retinal pigment epithelium (RPE) is composed of a single layer of cells that are hexagonal in cross-section. The cells consist of an outer non-pigmented basal element containing the nucleus and an inner pigmented apical section containing abundant melanosomes.
  - The cell base is in contact with Bruch membrane and at the cell apices multiple thread-like villous processes extend between the outer segments of the photoreceptors.

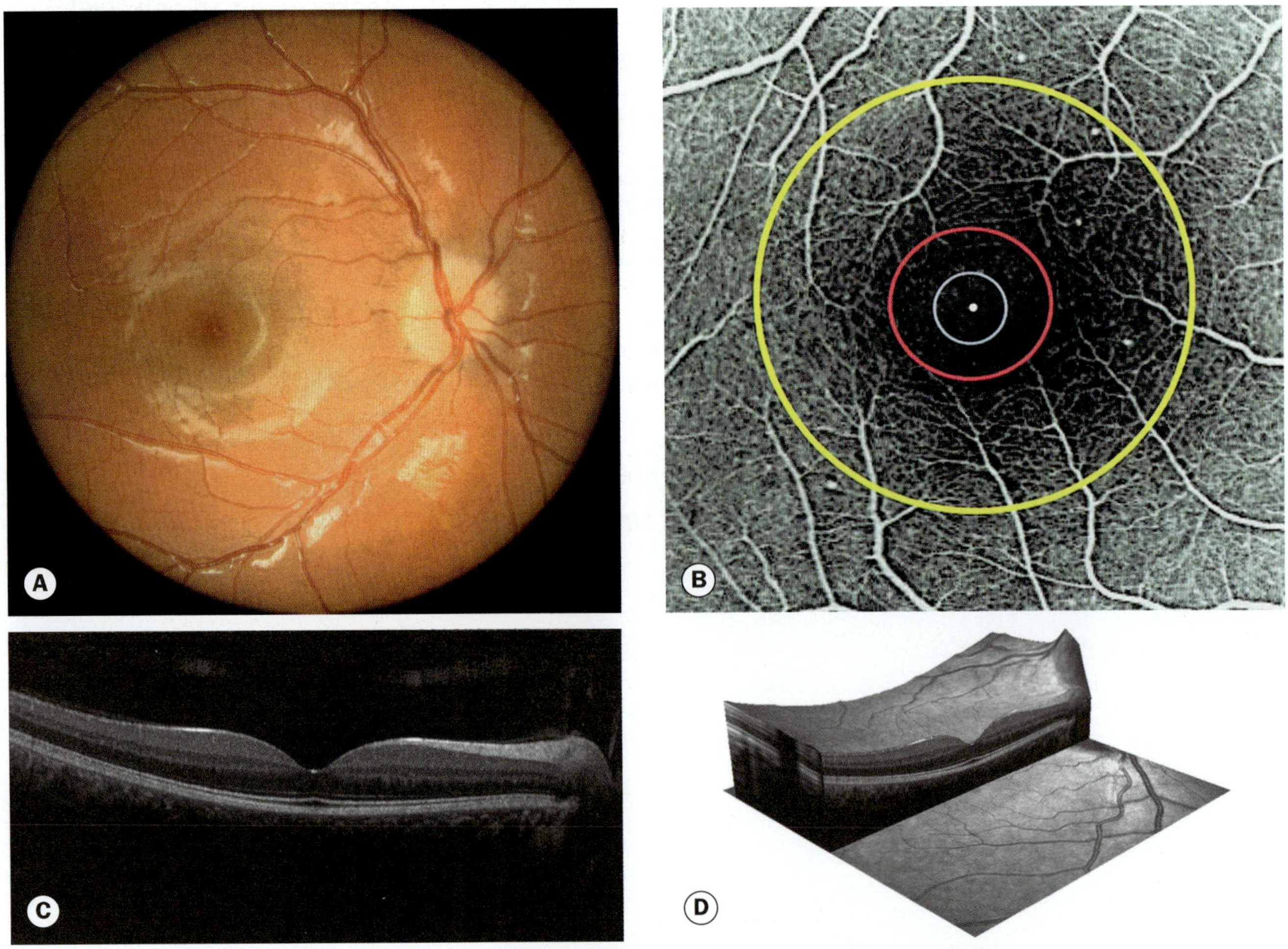

Fig. 14.1 Anatomical landmarks. **(A)** Normal foveola (almost punctate central reflex) and macula light reflexes (band-like reflex encircling the fovea); **(B)** fluorescein angiogram – fovea (yellow circle), approximate extent of the foveal avascular zone (red circle), foveola (lilac circle), umbo (central white spot); **(C)** OCT showing the foveal depression; **(D)** three-dimensional OCT.

- At the posterior pole, particularly at the fovea, RPE cells are taller and thinner, more regular in shape and contain more numerous and larger melanosomes than in the periphery.

- **Function**
  - RPE cells and intervening tight junctional complexes (zonula occludentes) constitute the outer blood–retinal barrier, preventing extracellular fluid leaking into the subretinal space from the choriocapillaris and actively pumping ions and water out of the subretinal space.
  - Its integrity and that of Bruch membrane is important for continued adhesion between the two, thought to be due to a combination of osmotic and hydrostatic forces, possibly with the aid of hemidesmosomal attachments.
  - Facilitation of photoreceptor turnover by the phagocytosis and lysosomal degradation of outer segments following shedding.
  - Preservation of an optimal retinal milieu. Maintenance of the outer blood–retinal barrier is a key factor, as are the inward transport of metabolites (mainly small molecules such as amino acids and glucose) and the outward transport of metabolic waste products.
  - Storage, metabolism and transport of vitamin A in the visual cycle.
  - The dense RPE pigment serves to absorb stray light.

Bruch membrane

- **Structure.** Bruch membrane separates the RPE from the choriocapillaris and on electron microscopy consists of five distinct elements:
  - The basal lamina of the RPE.
  - An inner collagenous layer.
  - A thicker band of elastic fibres.
  - An outer collagenous layer.
  - The basal lamina of the inner layer of the choriocapillaris.
- **Function.** The RPE utilizes Bruch membrane as a route for the transport of metabolic waste products out of the retinal environment. Changes in its structure are thought to be important in the pathogenesis of many macular disorders – for example, intact Bruch membrane may be important in the suppression of macular neovascularization (MNV).

CLINICAL EVALUATION OF MACULAR DISEASE

Symptoms

- **Blurred vision** and difficulty with close work is an early symptom. Onset can be rapid in some conditions, such as MNV.
- **A positive scotoma**, in which patients complain of something obstructing central vision, is a symptom of more severe disease. This is in contrast to optic neuropathy, which typically causes a missing area in the visual field (negative scotoma).
- **Metamorphopsia** (distortion of perceived images) is a common symptom that does not occur in optic neuropathy.
- **Micropsia** (decrease in image size) is caused by spreading apart of foveal cones and is uncommon.
- **Macropsia** (increase in image size) is due to crowding together of foveal cones and is uncommon.
- **Colour** discrimination may be disturbed, but is generally less evident than in even relatively mild optic neuropathy.
- **Difficulties related to dark adaptation**, such as poor vision in dim light and persistence of after-images, may occur.

TIP Metamorphopsia is a common early symptom of macular disease and can be evaluated with an Amsler grid.

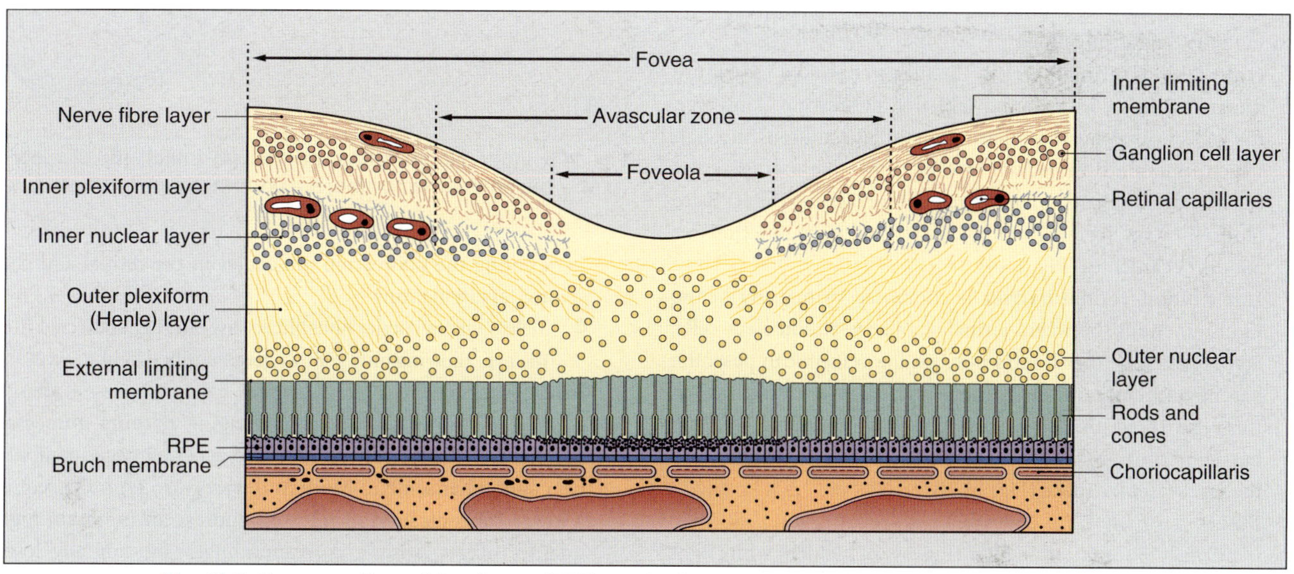

Fig. 14.2 Cross-section of the fovea. (RPE = retinal pigment epithelium.)

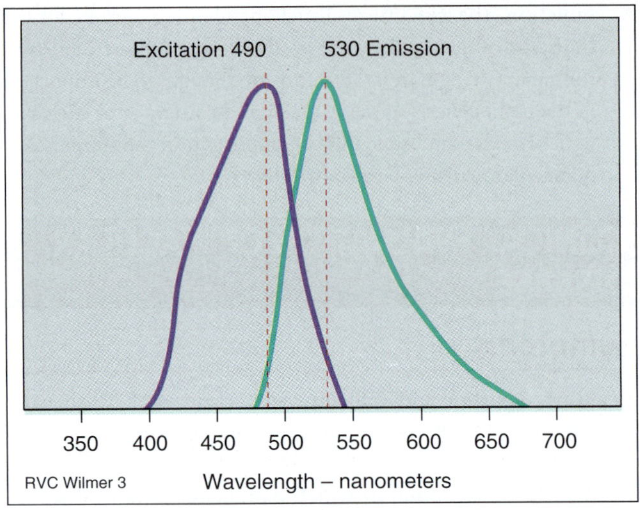

Fig. 14.3 Excitation and emission of fluorescein.

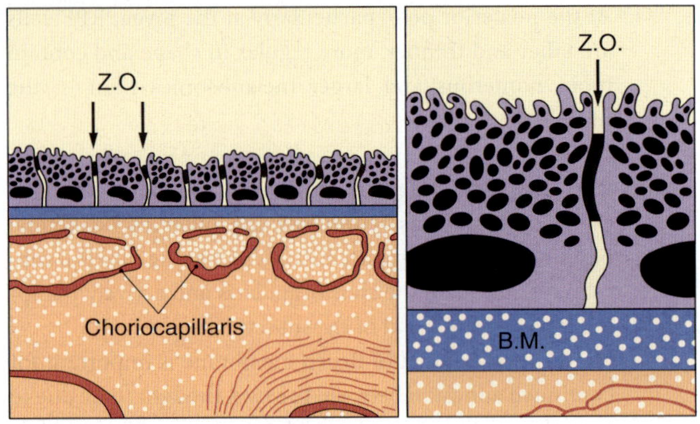

Fig. 14.4 The outer blood–retinal barrier. (B.M. = Bruch membrane; Z.O.= zonula occludentes.)

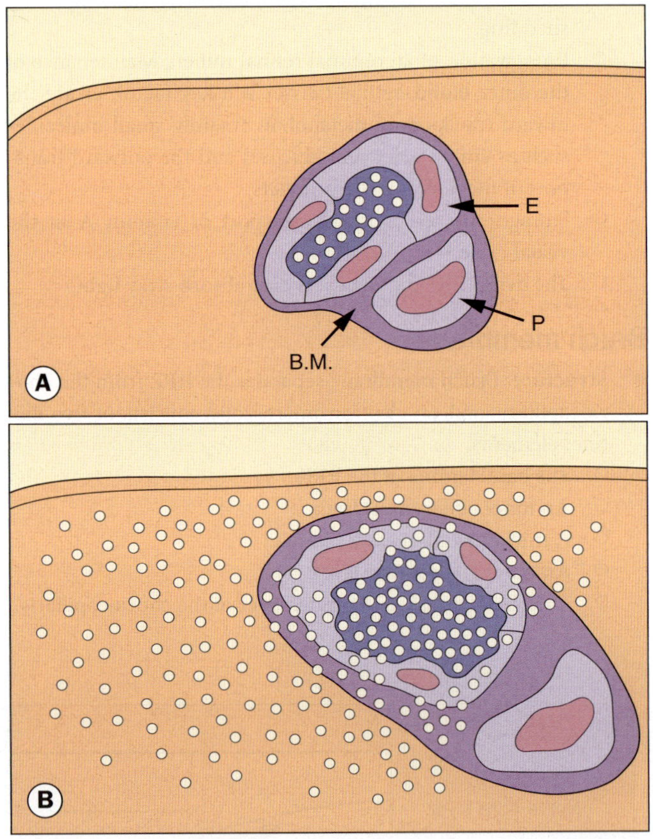

Fig. 14.5 Inner blood–retinal barrier. **(A)** Intact; **(B)** disrupted. (B.M. = basement membrane; E = endothelial cell; P = pericyte.)

INVESTIGATION OF MACULAR DISEASE

Fundus fluorescein angiography

Introduction

Fluorescein angiography (FA) should be performed only if the findings are likely to influence management.

- **Fluorescence** is the property of certain molecules to emit light of a longer wavelength when stimulated by light of a shorter wavelength. The excitation peak for fluorescein is about 490 nm (in the blue part of the spectrum) – the wavelength of maximal absorption of light energy by fluorescein. Stimulated molecules will emit yellow–green light of about 530 nm (Fig. 14.3).
- **Fluorescein** (sodium fluorescein) is an orange water-soluble dye that, when injected intravenously, remains largely intravascular (>70% bound to serum proteins). It is excreted in the urine over 24–36 hours.
- **FA** involves photographic surveillance of the passage of fluorescein through the retinal and choroidal circulations following intravenous injection.
- **Outer blood–retinal barrier.** The major choroidal vessels are impermeable to both bound and free fluorescein. However, the walls of the choriocapillaris contain fenestrations through which unbound molecules escape into the extravascular space, crossing Bruch membrane but on reaching the RPE are blocked by intercellular complexes termed tight junctions or zonula occludentes (Fig. 14.4).
- **Inner blood–retinal barrier** is composed principally of the tight junctions between retinal capillary endothelial cells, across which neither bound nor free fluorescein can pass; the basement membrane and pericytes play only a minor role in this regard (Fig. 14.5A). Disruption of the inner blood–retinal barrier permits leakage of both bound and free fluorescein into the extravascular space (Fig. 14.5B).
- **Filters**
  - Cobalt blue excitation filter (Fig. 14.6). Incident white light from the camera is filtered so that blue light enters the eye, exciting the fluorescein molecules in the retinal and choroidal circulations.
  - Yellow–green barrier filter blocks any blue light reflected from the eye, allowing only yellow–green emitted light to pass.
- **Image capture** in modern digital cameras uses a charge-coupled device (CCD). Digital imaging permits immediate picture availability, easy storage and access, image manipulation and enhancement. Modern devices also typically require a lower concentration of injected fluorescein to obtain high-quality images, with a correspondingly substantially lower incidence of adverse effects.

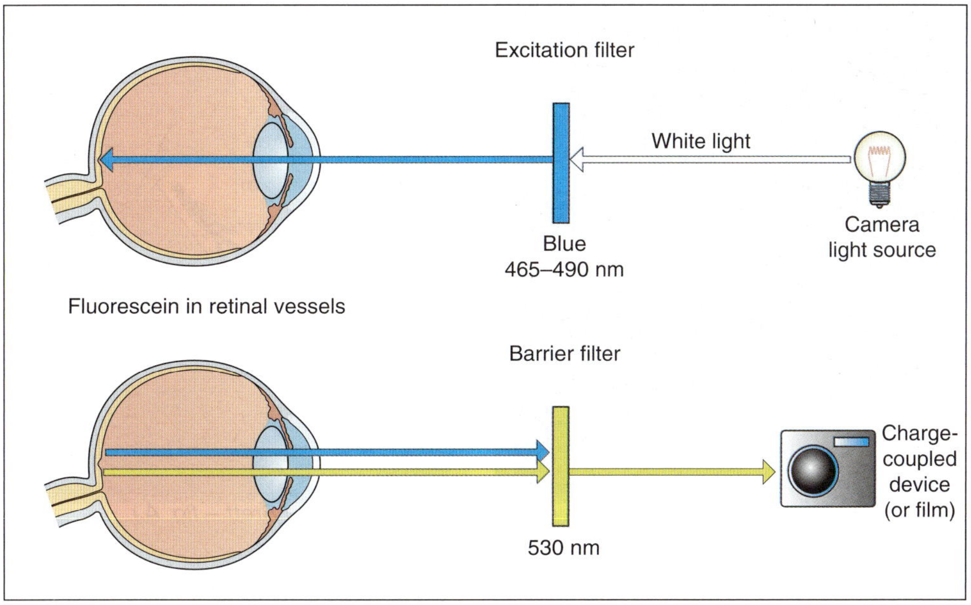

Fig. 14.6 Principles of fluorescein angiography.

- **Contraindications**
  - Fluorescein allergy is an absolute contraindication and a history of a severe reaction to any allergen is a strong relative contraindication. Preventative anti-allergy pre-treatment may be helpful in some cases.
  - Other relative contraindications include renal failure (a lower fluorescein dose is used), pregnancy, moderate–severe asthma and significant cardiac disease.
  - Allergy to iodine-containing media or seafood is not a contraindication to FA or to indocyanine green angiography (ICGA).

Technique

Facilities must be in place to address possible adverse events. This includes adequate staffing, a resuscitation trolley that includes drugs for the treatment of anaphylaxis, a couch (or reclining chair) and a receiver in case of vomiting. Significant nausea and vomiting are less common using the lower fluorescein concentrations required by modern digital cameras.

- Adequate pharmacological mydriasis is important to obtain high-quality images. Media opacity such as cataract may reduce picture quality.
- The procedure is explained and formal consent taken. It is important to mention common and serious adverse effects (Table 14.1), particularly the invariable skin and urine staining.
- The patient should be seated comfortably in front of the fundus camera and colour photographs, red-free (green incident light, to enhance red detail) and autofluorescence images taken as indicated.
- An intravenous cannula is inserted; a standard cannula is often preferred rather than a less secure 'butterfly' winged infusion set. After cannulation, the line should be flushed with normal saline to check patency and exclude extravasation.
- Fluorescein, usually 5 ml of a 10% solution, is drawn up into a syringe and injected over the course of 5–10 seconds, taking care not to rupture the cannulated vein (Fig. 14.7A and B).
- Oral administration at a dose of 30 mg/kg is an alternative if venous access cannot be obtained or is refused. A 5 ml vial of 10% (100 mg/ml) sodium fluorescein contains 500 mg and pictures should be taken over 20–60 minutes following ingestion.
- Images are taken at 1–2 second intervals initially to capture the critical early transit phases, beginning 5–10 seconds after injection, tapering frequency through subsequent phases.
- With monocular pathology, control pictures of the opposite eye should be taken, usually after the initial transit phase has been photographed in the index eye.
- If appropriate, images may be captured as late as 10–20 minutes.
- Stereo images may be helpful to demonstrate elevation and are usually taken by manually repositioning the camera sideways or by using a special device (a stereo separator) to adjust the image. These are actually pseudo-stereo images as true stereo requires simultaneous image capture from different angles.

Table 14.1 Adverse Events in Fluorescein Angiography
Discoloration of skin and urine (invariable)
Extravasation of injected dye, giving a painful local reaction (treat with cold compress)
Nausea, vomiting (now rare with lower concentrations of fluorescein)
Itching, rash
Sneezing, wheezing
Vasovagal episode or syncope (usually due to anxiety but sometimes to ischaemic heart disease)
Anaphylactic and anaphylactoid reactions (1:2000 angiograms)
Myocardial infarction (extremely rare)
Death (1:220000 in the largest study)

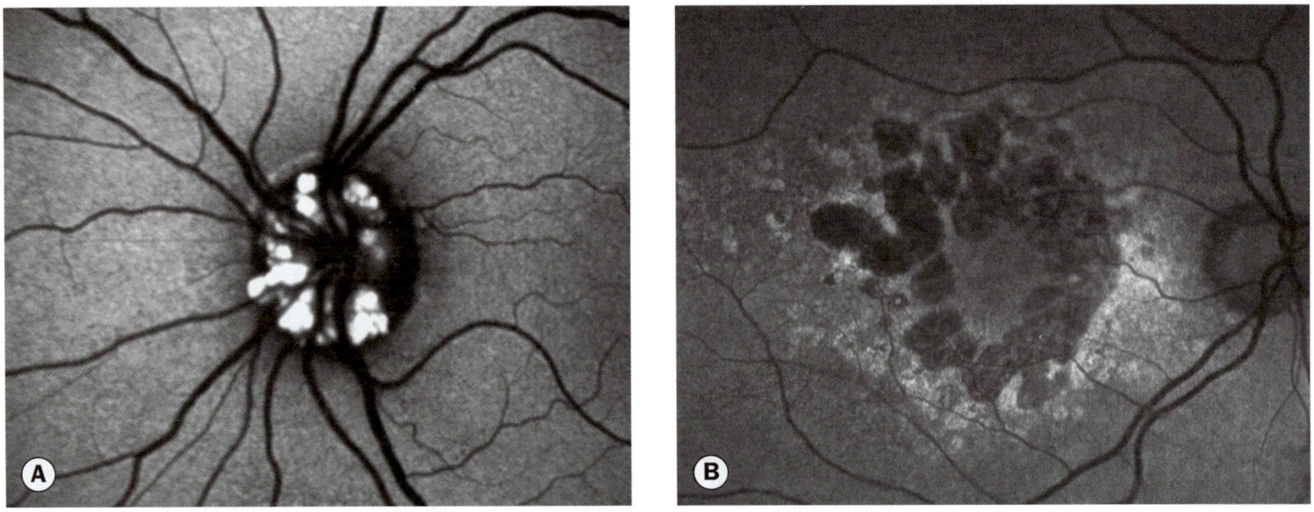

Fig. 14.11 FAF image. **(A)** Optic disc drusen; **(B)** hyperautofluorescence surrounding geographic atrophy.

digital cameras have enhanced autofluorescence detection capability, though imaging is most effective with scanning laser ophthalmoscopy. Autofluorescent lesions classically include optic nerve head drusen (Fig. 14.11A) and astrocytic hamartoma, but with increased availability of high-sensitivity imaging, patterns associated with a wide range of posterior segment pathology have been characterized, e.g. areas surrounding geographic atrophy, which show an accumulation of lipofuscin in the RPE cells (lipofuscin is chemically a complex mixture of lipid, oxidized proteins and trace metals which results from the oxidation of membrane lipids and proteins by free radicals) (Fig. 14.11B).

- **Pseudofluorescence** (false fluorescence) refers to non-fluorescent reflected light visible prior to fluorescein injection. This passes through the filters due to the overlap of wavelengths passing through the excitation then the barrier filters. It is more evident when filters are wearing out.
- **Increased fluorescence** may be caused by (a) enhanced visualization of normal fluorescein density, or (b) an increase in fluorescein content of tissues.
- **A window defect** is caused by atrophy or absence of the RPE as in atrophic age-related macular degeneration (Fig. 14.12A), a full-thickness macular hole, RPE tears and some drusen. This results in unmasking of normal background choroidal fluorescence, characterized by very early hyperfluorescence that increases in intensity and then fades without changing size or shape (Fig. 14.12B and C).
- **Pooling** in an anatomical space occurs due to breakdown of the outer blood–retinal barrier (RPE tight junctions):
  - In the subretinal space, e.g. central serous chorioretinopathy (Fig. 14.13A). This is characterized by early hyperfluorescence, which, as the responsible leak tends to be only small (Fig. 14.13B), slowly increases in intensity and area (Fig. 14.13C), the maximum extent remaining relatively well defined.
  - In the sub-RPE space, as in pigment epithelial detachment (Fig. 14.14A). This is characterized by early hyperfluorescence (Fig. 14.14B) that increases in intensity but not in size (Fig. 14.14C).
- **Leakage** of dye is characterized by fairly early hyperfluorescence, increasing with time in both area and intensity. It occurs as a result of breakdown of the inner blood–retinal barrier due to:
  - Dysfunction or loss of existing vascular endothelial tight junctions as in background diabetic retinopathy (DR), retinal vein occlusion (RVO), cystoid macular oedema (Fig. 14.15A) and disc swelling (Fig. 14.15B).
  - Primary absence of vascular endothelial tight junctions as in MNV, proliferative diabetic retinopathy (Fig. 14.15C), tumours and some vascular anomalies such as Coats disease.
- **Staining** is a late phenomenon consisting of the prolonged retention of dye in entities such as drusen, fibrous tissue, exposed sclera and the normal optic disc and is seen in the later phases of the angiogram, particularly after the dye has left the choroidal and retinal circulations.

Causes of hypofluorescence

Reduction or absence of fluorescence may be due to: (a) optical obstruction (masking or blockage) of normal fluorescein density (Fig. 14.16) or (b) inadequate perfusion of tissue (filling defect).

- **Masking of retinal fluorescence.** Preretinal lesions such as blood will block all fluorescence (Fig. 14.17A–C).
- **Masking of background choroidal fluorescence** allows persistence of fluorescence from superficial retinal vessels:
  - Deeper retinal lesions, e.g. intraretinal haemorrhages, dense exudates.
  - Subretinal or sub-RPE lesions, e.g. blood (Fig. 14.18A–C).
  - Increased density of the RPE, e.g. congenital hypertrophy (Fig. 14.19A and B).
  - Choroidal lesions, e.g. naevus (Fig. 14.19C).
- **Filling defects** may result from:
  - Vascular occlusion, which may involve the retinal arteries, veins or capillaries (capillary drop-out – Fig. 14.20A), or

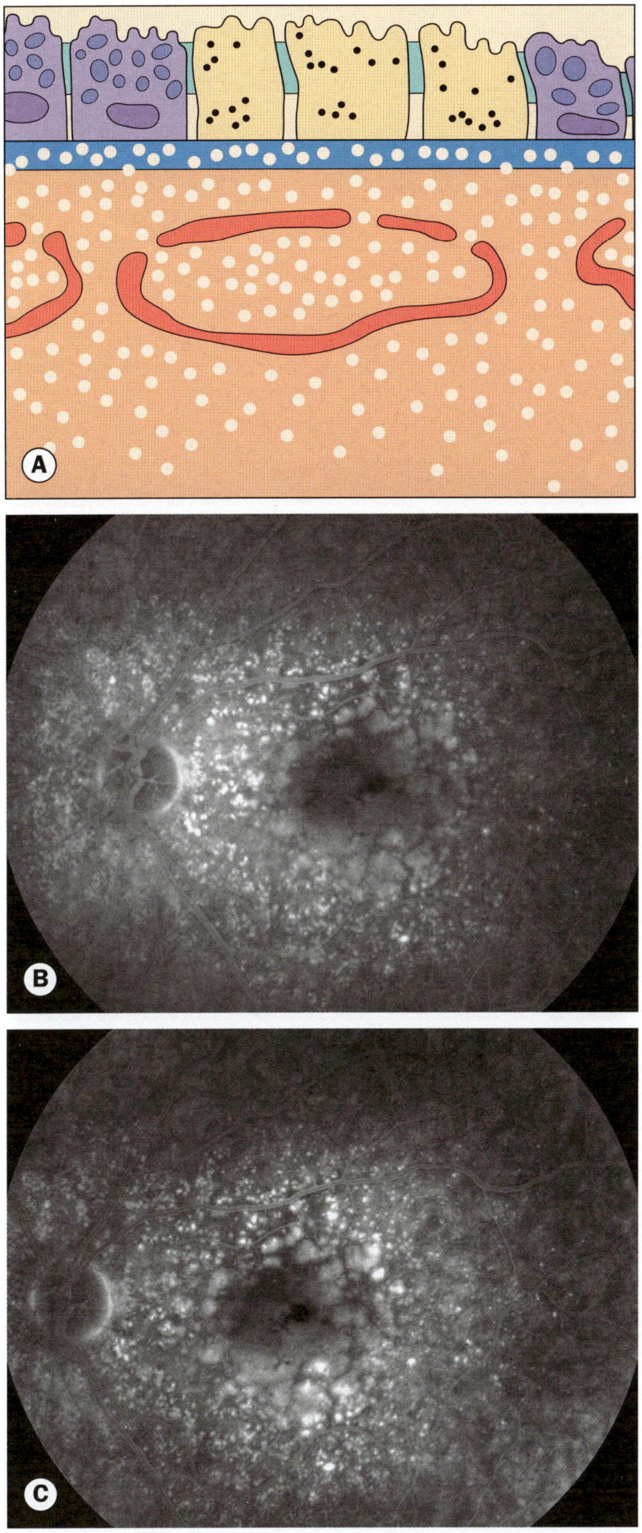

Fig. 14.12 Hyperfluorescence caused by window defects associated with dry age-related macular degeneration. (A) Diagrammatic representation; (B) fluorescein angiographic appearance at 2.5 minutes; (C) at 5.5 minutes.

the choroidal circulation. FA is sometimes used to demonstrate optic nerve head filling defects as in anterior ischaemic optic neuropathy.

- Loss of the vascular bed as in myopic degeneration and choroideremia (Fig. 14.20B).

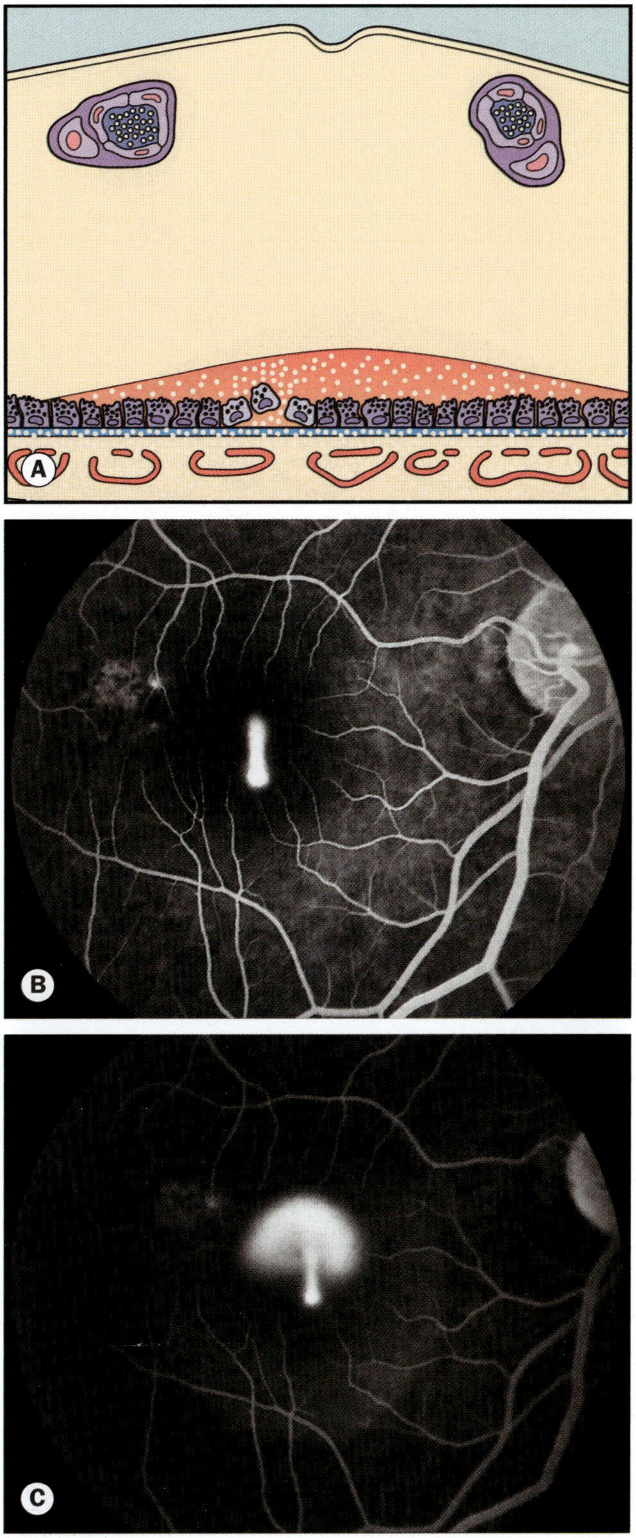

Fig. 14.13 Hyperfluorescence caused by pooling of dye in the subretinal space in central serous chorioretinopathy. (A) Diagrammatic representation; (B) and (C) fluorescein angiographic appearance.

Systematic approach to fluorescein angiogram analysis

A fluorescein angiogram should be interpreted methodically to optimize diagnostic accuracy.

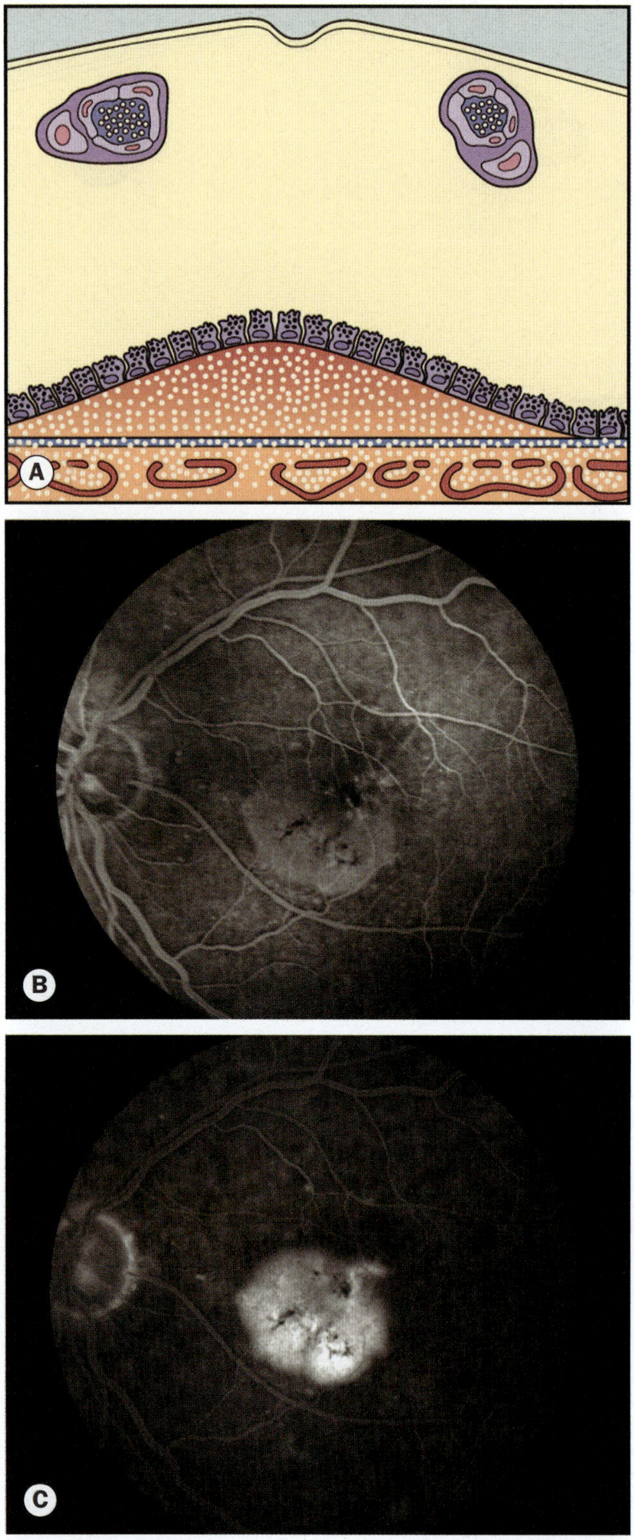

Fig. 14.14 Hyperfluorescence caused by pooling of dye in the subretinal pigment epithelium (RPE) space in RPE detachment. **(A)** Diagrammatic representation; **(B)** and **(C)** fluorescein angiographic appearance.

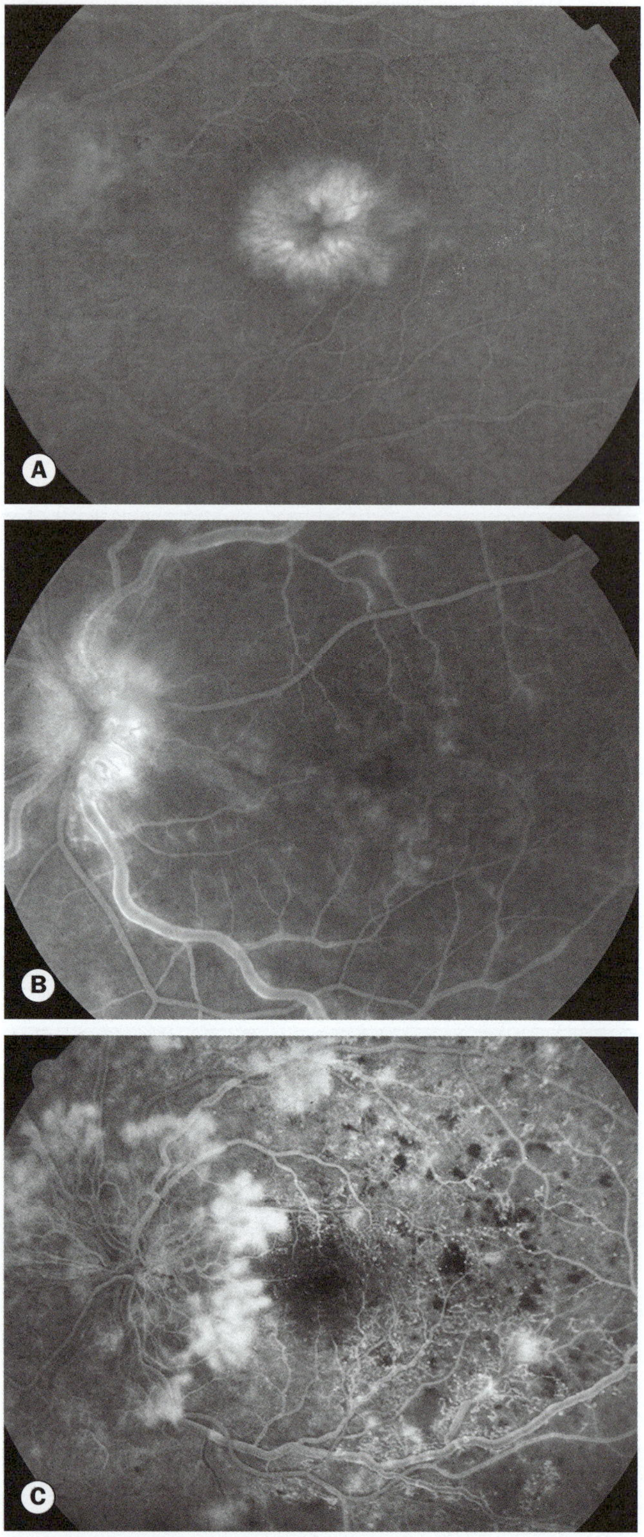

Fig. 14.15 Causes of hyperfluorescence due to leakage. **(A)** Cystoid macular oedema; **(B)** disc swelling; **(C)** proliferative diabetic retinopathy showing leakage from extensive vessels around the disc.

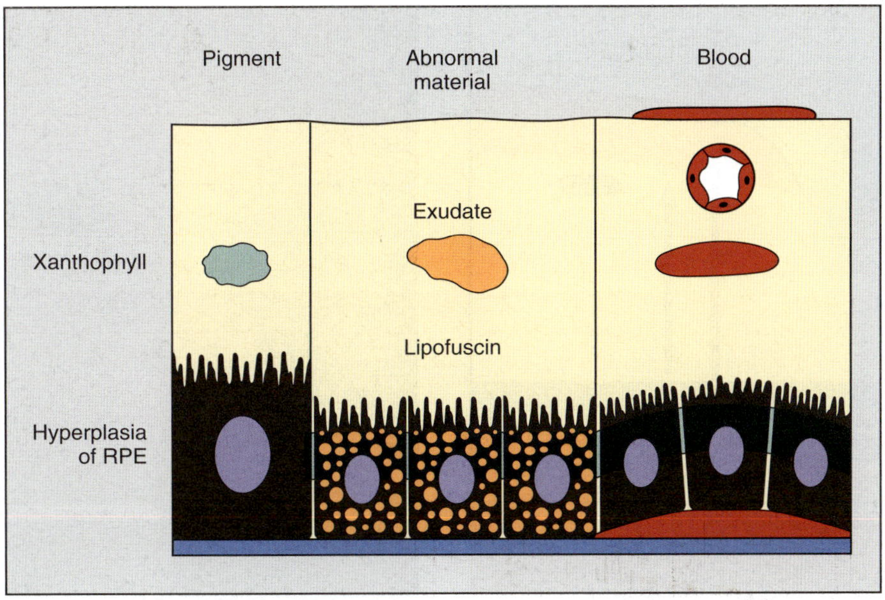

Fig. 14.16 Causes of hypofluorescence.

- Clinical findings, including the patient's age and gender, should be noted before assessing the images.
- Note whether images of right, left or both eyes have been taken.
- Comment on any colour and red-free images and on any pre-injection demonstration of pseudo- or autofluorescence.
- Looking at the post-injection images, indicate whether the overall timing of filling, especially arm-to-eye transit time, is normal.
- Briefly scan through the sequence of images in time order for each eye in turn, initially concentrating on the eye with the greatest number of shots as this is likely to be the one about which there is greater concern. On the first review, look for any characteristic major diagnostic, especially pathognomonic features; for example, a lacy filling pattern or a 'smokestack' (see later).
- Go through the run for each eye in greater detail, noting the evolution of any major features found on the first scan and then providing a description of any other findings using the methodical consideration of the causes of hyper- and hypofluorescence set out above.

Indocyanine green angiography

Introduction

- **Advantages over FA.** Whilst FA is an excellent method of studying the retinal circulation, it is of limited use in delineating the choroidal vasculature, due principally to masking by the RPE. In contrast, the near-infrared light utilized in indocyanine green angiography (ICGA) penetrates ocular pigments such as melanin and xanthophyll, as well as exudate and thin layers of subretinal blood, making this technique eminently suitable. An additional factor is that about 98% of ICG molecules bind to serum protein (mainly albumin); considerably higher than the binding of fluorescein. As choriocapillaris fenestrations are impermeable to larger protein molecules, most ICG is retained within choroidal vessels. Infrared light is also scattered less than visible light, making ICGA superior to FA in eyes with media opacity. ICG stains the RPE in the late stages of the angiogram.
- **Image capture.** ICG fluorescence is only 1/25th that of fluorescein so modern digital ICGA uses high-sensitivity videoangiographic image capture by means of an appropriately adapted camera. Both the excitation (805 nm) and emission (835 nm) filters are set at infrared wavelengths (Fig. 14.21). Alternatively, scanning laser ophthalmoscopy (SLO) systems provide high contrast images, with less scattering of light and fast image acquisition rates facilitating high-quality ICG video.
- **The technique** is similar to that of FA, but with an increased emphasis on the acquisition of later images (up to about 45 minutes) than with FA. A dose of 25–50 mg in 1–2 ml water for injection is used.
- **Phases of ICGA**: (a) early – up to 60 seconds post-injection, (b) early mid-phase – 1–3 minutes (Fig. 14.22A), (c) late mid-phase – 3–15 minutes, (Fig. 14.22B) and (d) late phase – 15–45 minutes.

Adverse effects

ICGA is generally better tolerated than FA.

- Nausea, vomiting and urticaria are uncommon, but anaphylaxis probably occurs with approximately equal incidence to FA.
- Serious reactions are exceptionally rare.
- ICGA is relatively contraindicated in liver disease (excretion is hepatic) and as with FA in patients with a history of a severe reaction to any allergen, moderate or severe asthma and significant cardiac disease. Its safety in pregnancy has not been established.

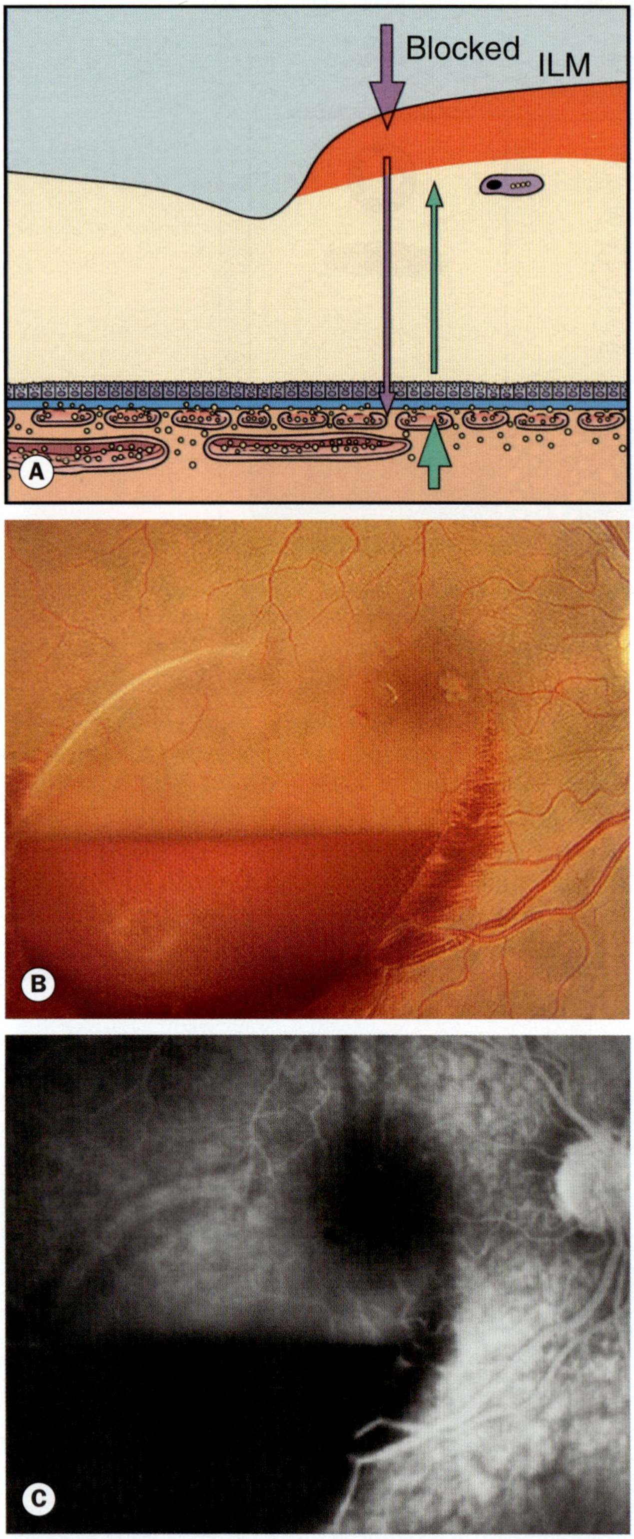

Fig. 14.17 Hypofluorescence – masking of all signal, including from retinal vessels, by preretinal haemorrhage. (ILM = internal limiting membrane.) **(A)** Diagrammatic representation; **(B)** clinical appearance; **(C)** fluorescein angiographic appearance.

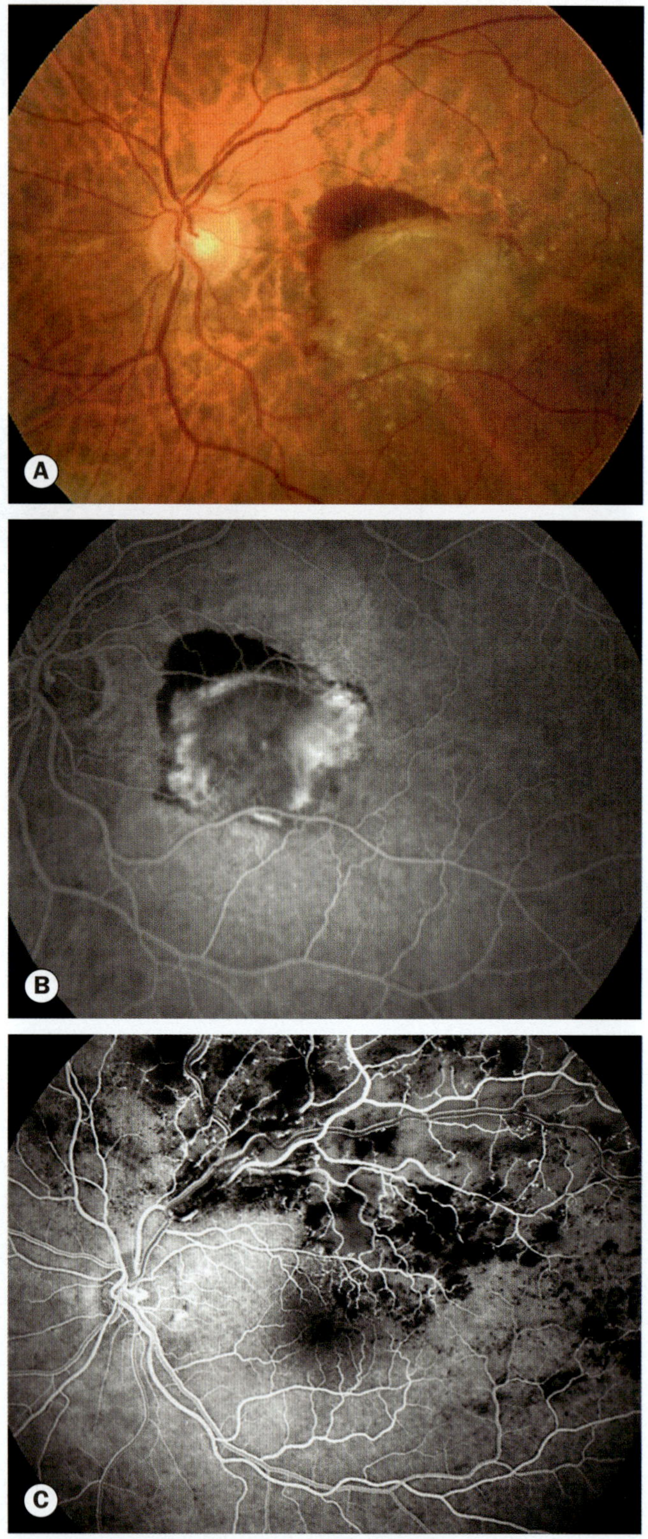

Fig. 14.18 Hypofluorescence – blockage by sub- and intraretinal haemorrhage, showing persistence of signal from retinal vessels. **(A)** Clinical appearance in a patient with age-related macular degeneration; **(B)** fluorescein angiographic appearance of **(A)**; **(C)** upper temporal branch vein occlusion.

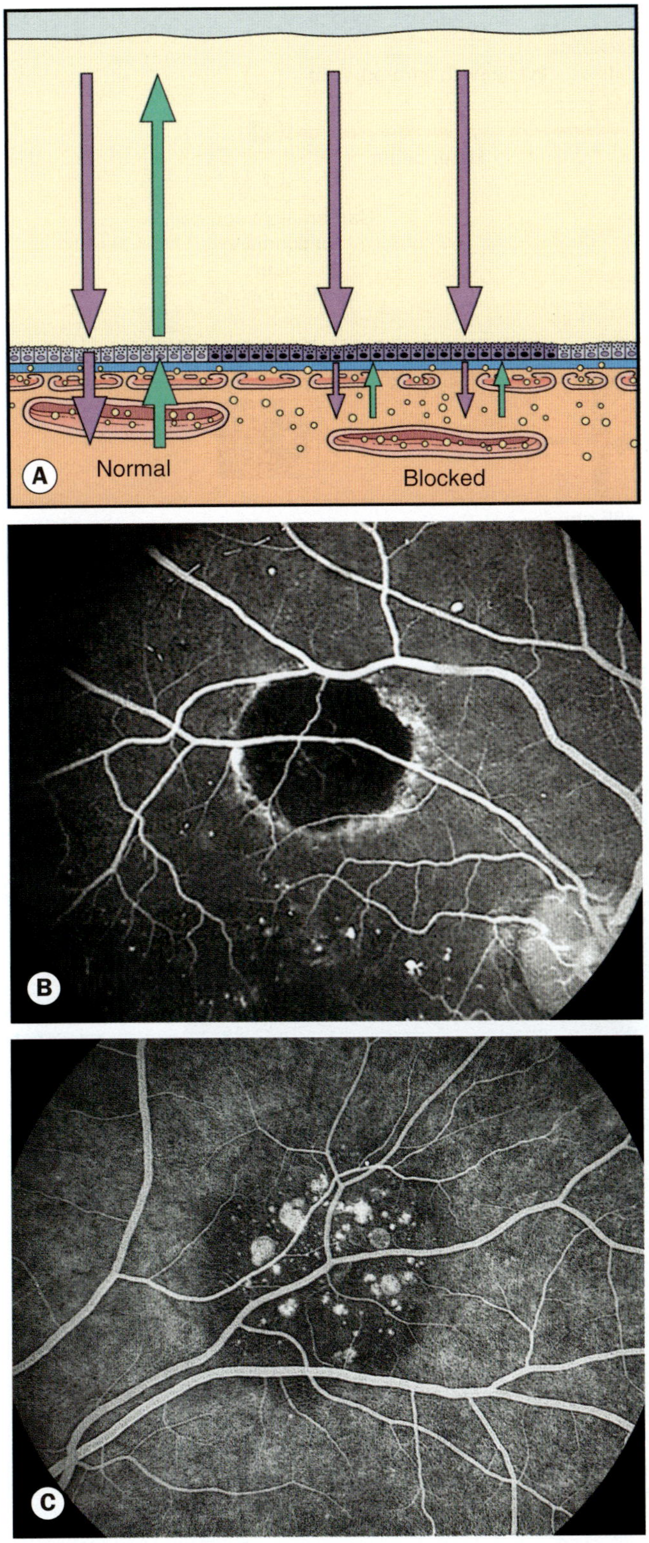

Fig. 14.19 Hypofluorescence caused by blockage of background fluorescence. **(A)** Diagrammatic representation; **(B)** fluorescein angiographic appearance of congenital hypertrophy of the retinal pigment epithelium; **(C)** choroidal naevus (with staining of drusen).

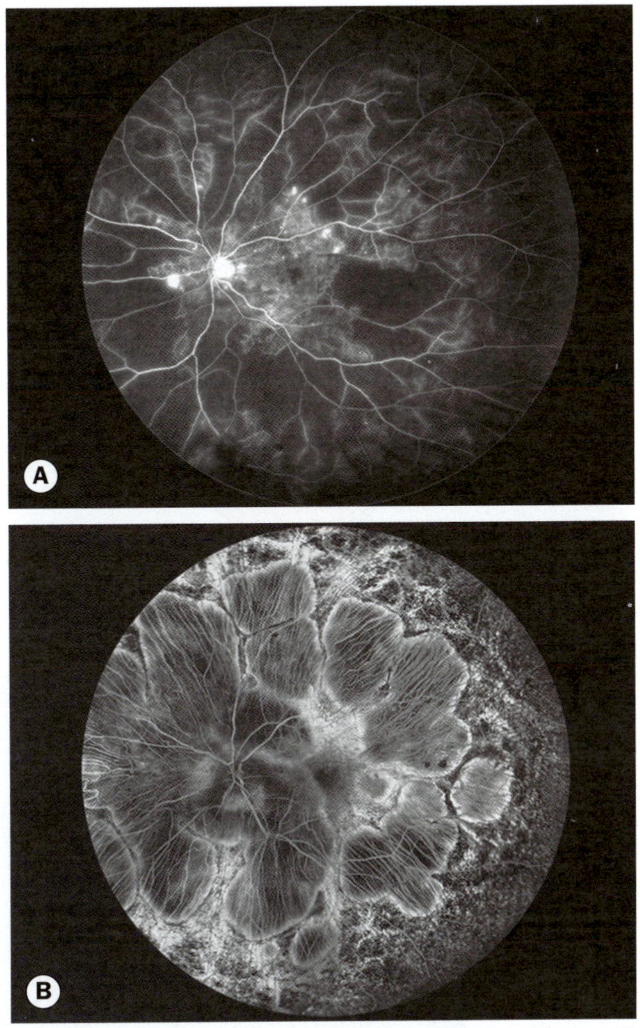

Fig. 14.20 Hypofluorescence caused by filling defects. **(A)** Capillary drop-out in diabetic retinopathy; **(B)** choroideremia.

Diagnosis

Examples of pathological images are shown under the discussion of individual conditions where relevant.

- **Hyperfluorescence**
  - A window defect similar to those seen with FA.
  - Leakage from retinal or choroidal vessels (Fig. 14.23), the optic nerve head or the RPE; gives rise to tissue staining or to pooling.
  - Abnormal retinal or choroidal vessels with an anomalous morphology (see Fig. 14.23) and/or exhibiting greater fluorescence than normal.
- **Hypofluorescence**
  - Blockage (masking) of fluorescence. Pigment and blood are self-evident causes, but fibrosis, infiltrate, exudate and serous fluid also block fluorescence. A particular phenomenon to note is that in contrast to its FA appearance, a pigment epithelial detachment appears predominantly hypofluorescent on ICGA.

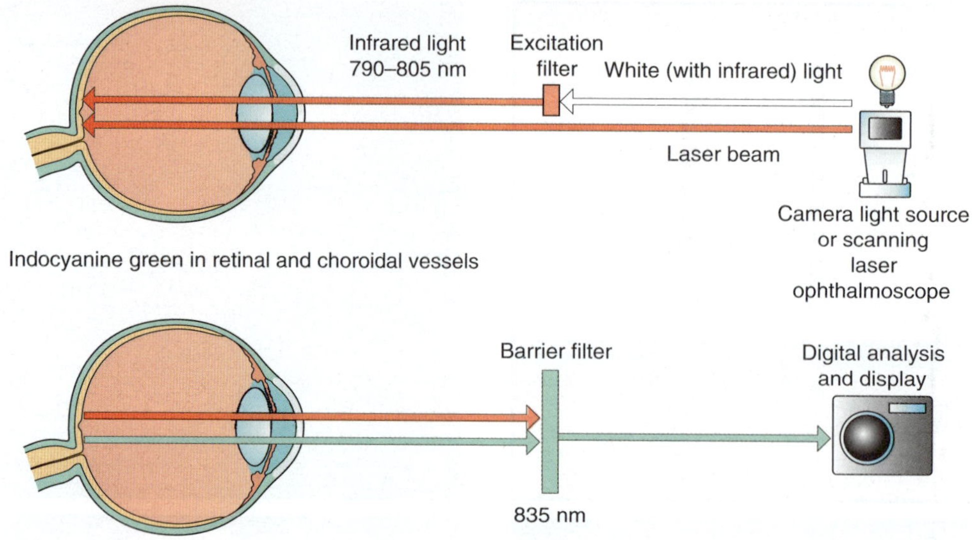

Fig. 14.21 Principles of indocyanine green angiography.

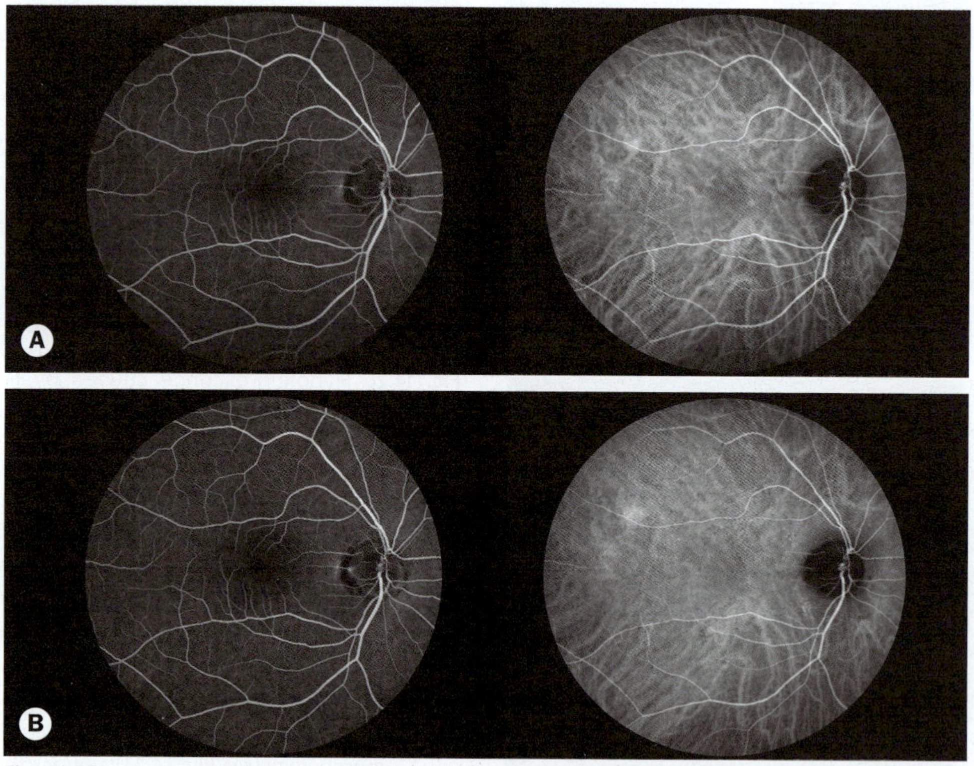

Fig. 14.22 Normal fluorescein angiogram, left, with normal indocyanine green angiogram, right. **(A)** Early mid-phase (1–3 minutes) showing greater prominence of choroidal veins as well as retinal vessels; **(B)** late mid-phase (3–15 minutes) showing fading of choroidal vessels but retinal vessels are still visible; diffuse tissue staining is also present.

- Filling defect due to obstruction or loss of choroidal or retinal circulation. Choriocapillaris non-perfusion manifests as dark geographic areas of hypofluorescence, whereas choroidal stromal foci impair diffusion of the ICG molecule and manifests as regular round evenly distributed dark dots in the early phase.

Indications

- **Polypoidal choroidal vasculopathy (PCV)**: ICGA is far superior to FA for the imaging of PCV (see Fig. 14.23).
- **Exudative age-related macular degeneration (AMD).** Conventional FA remains the primary method of assessment, but ICGA can be a useful adjunct, particularly if PCV is suspected.

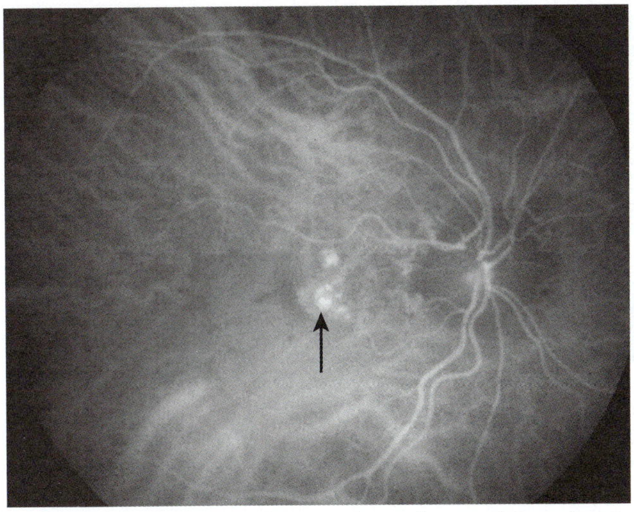

Fig. 14.23 ICGA image showing hyperfluorescence due to polyps (arrow) and leakage in polypoidal choroidal vasculopathy.

- **Retinal angiomatous proliferation (Type 3 MNV).** ICGA is diagnostic in most cases, showing a hot spot in mid and or late frames.
- **Chronic central serous chorioretinopathy (CSR)** in which it is often difficult to interpret areas of leakage on FA. However, ICGA shows choroidal leakage and the presence of dilated choroidal vessels. Previously unidentified lesions elsewhere in the fundus are also frequently visible using ICGA.
- **Posterior uveitis.** ICGA can provide useful information beyond that available from FA in relation to diagnosis and the extent of disease involvement (see Ch. 15).
- **Choroidal tumours** may be imaged effectively, but ICGA is inferior to clinical assessment for diagnosis.
- **Breaks in Bruch membrane** such as lacquer cracks and angioid streaks are more effectively defined on ICGA than on FA.
- If **FA is contraindicated.**

Optical coherence tomography

Introduction

Optical coherence tomography (OCT) is a non-invasive, non-contact imaging system providing high-resolution cross-sectional images of the posterior segment. OCT is analogous to B-scan ultrasonography but uses near-infrared light interferometry rather than sound waves, with images created by the analysis of interference between reflected reference waves and those reflected by tissue. Most instruments in current use employ spectral/Fourier domain technology, in which the mechanical movement required for image acquisition in older 'time domain' machines has been eliminated and the information for each point on the A-scan is collected simultaneously, speeding data collection and improving resolution. Promising newer modalities include swept-source (SS) OCT that can acquire images at a much higher rate and with extremely high retinal element resolution and better imaging depth. So-called 'adaptive optics' allows correction of higher-order optical aberrations to improve resolution. Wide-field, intraoperative, functional and Doppler (blood flow measurement) OCT applications may all have clinical utility in the future.

The diagnosis and monitoring of macular pathology has been revolutionized by the advent of OCT imaging, e.g. AMD, diabetic maculopathy, macular hole, epiretinal membrane and vitreomacular traction, CSR and retinal venous occlusion.

This technology allows a distinction to be made between retinal detachment and retinoschisis.

TIP OCT imaging is key to the diagnosis, monitoring and treatment of macular disease.

Normal appearance

Fine retinal structures such as the external limiting membrane and ganglion cell layer can be defined (Fig. 14.24). Detailed quantitative information on retinal thickness can be displayed numerically (Fig. 14.25). Three-dimensional images can be constructed and different retinal layers studied in relief. False-colour topographical maps are rarely used these days.

OCT angiography

OCT angiography (OCTA) is a non-invasive diagnostic technique that allows the blood flow in the retina and choroid to be visualized without the need for an injection of contrast medium. The disadvantage of this technology is that the classic abnormalities of traditional angiography (leakage, staining, pooling) are not shown. The images are based on the detection of red blood cell movement within the microvasculature of the back of the eye, using a series of OCT B-scans. These scans are performed vertically in the same retinal position. Differences between the scans generate detectable changing contrast as the red cells move through the vessels. A two-dimensional horizontal map is then created of the microcirculation, within the various layers of the retina and choroid. Importantly, it is the flow that is visualized rather than the vessel walls and flow that is too slow or too fast may not be detected by the technology.

Applications

- **Macular neovascular membrane**:
  - Visualization of flow in the outer retina.
  - Abnormal vasculature in areas featuring blood vessels (e.g. choroid) (Fig. 14.26A and B).
- **Non-exudative neovascular membrane.** In dry AMD to diagnose a non-exudative neovascular membrane.
- **Choroidal vessels.** Visualization of abnormal choroidal vessels, particularly after treatment.
- **Diabetic retinopathy**:
  - Diagnosis of preretinal neovascularization and to differentiate intraretinal microvascular abnormalities (IRMA) from new vessels.
  - Detection of microvascular changes without clinical retinopathy.

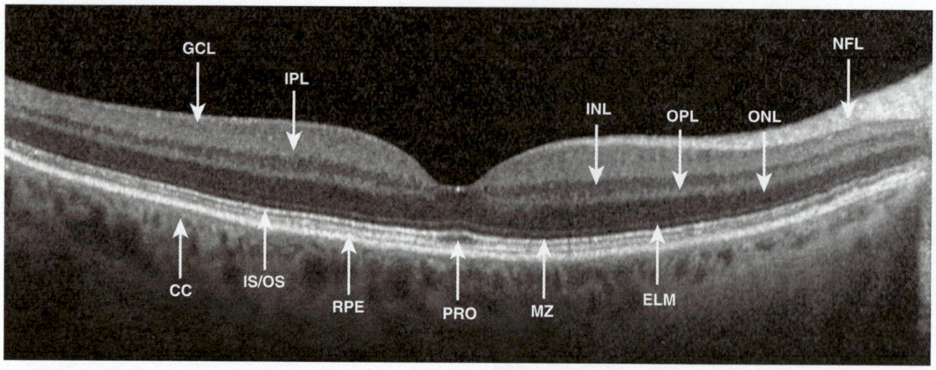

Fig. 14.24 High resolution image of a normal retina provided by spectral-domain OCT. (CC = choriocapillaris; ELM = external limiting membrane; GCL = ganglion cell layer; INL = inner nuclear layer; IPL = inner plexiform layer; IS/OS = photoreceptor inner-segment/outer-segment junction (also called ellipsoid zone); MZ = myoid zone; NFL = nerve fibre layer; ONL = outer nuclear layer; OPL = outer plexiform layer; PRO = photoreceptor outer segments; RPE = retinal pigment epithelium.)

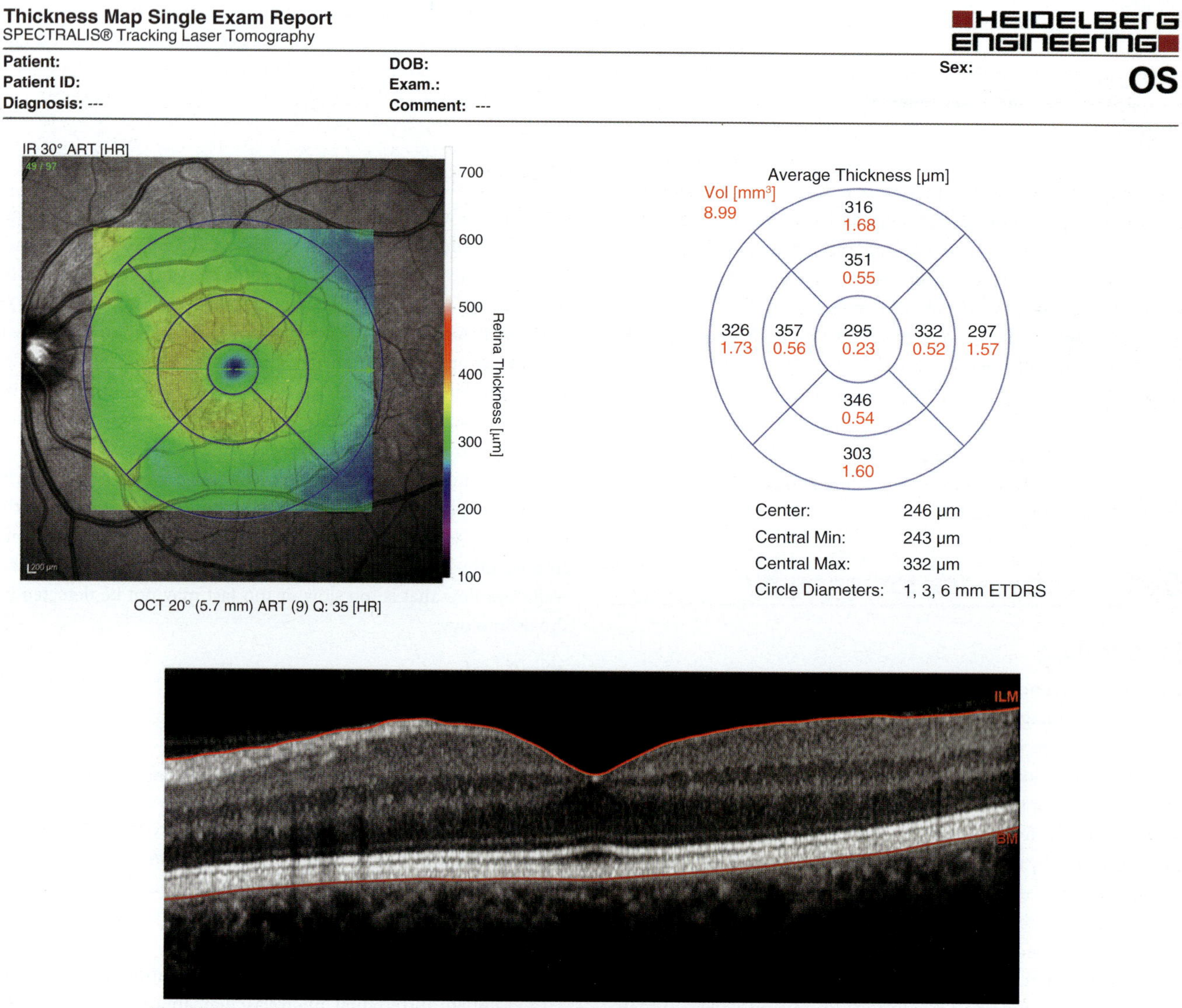

Fig. 14.25 OCT printout showing retinal thickness measurement.

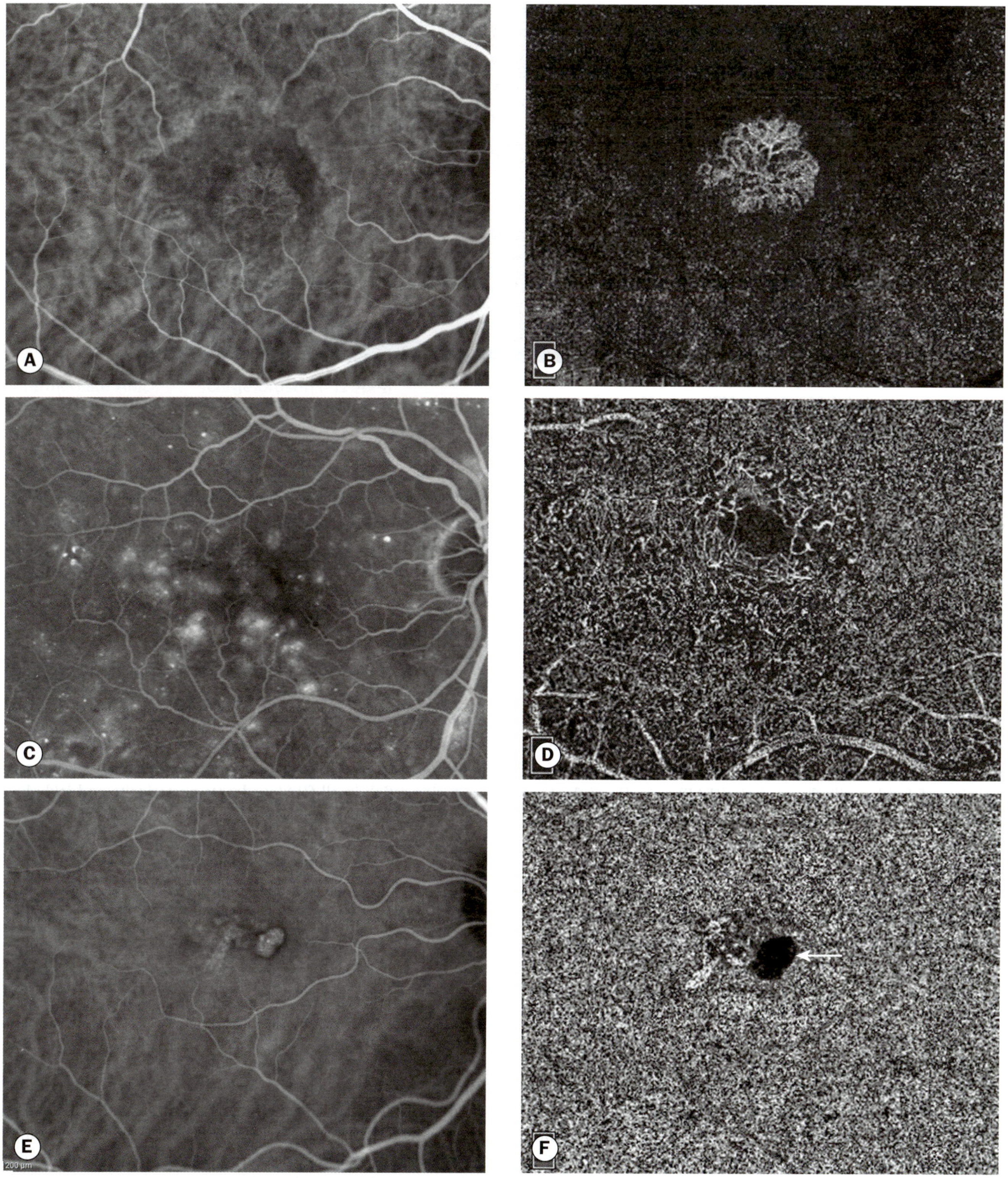

Fig. 14.26 OCT angiography. **(A)** FA showing macular neovascular membrane; **(B)** OCT angiogram of **(A)**; **(C)** FA at 2 minutes in diabetic macular oedema; **(D)** OCT angiogram of deep capillary plexus showing loss of the perifoveal network; **(E)** FA late phase showing polypoidal choroidal vasculopathy; **(F)** OCT angiogram; the black area is a polyp (arrow) and does not show blood flow because of turbulence within the polyp. *(Courtesy of A Ambresin.)*

consist of small (25–75 µm) yellowish nodules (Fig. 14.29B) that tend to cluster and increase in number with time and can progress to serous PED. FA characteristically gives a 'stars in the sky' appearance (Fig. 14.29C). The condition has been linked to a variant of the *CFH* gene.

- **Type 2 membranoproliferative glomerulonephritis** is a chronic renal disease that occurs in older children and adults. A minority of patients develop bilateral diffuse drusen-like lesions. The *CFH* gene has again been implicated.

Antioxidant supplementation

Introduction

There is substantial evidence, notably from the Age-Related Eye Disease Study (AREDS, now known as AREDS1) and the follow-up AREDS2, that taking high-dose antioxidant vitamins and minerals on a regular basis can decrease the risk of the development of advanced AMD in individuals with certain dry AMD features. The recommendation was made in AREDS1 that individuals aged over 55 should undergo examination for the following high-risk characteristics and if one or more are present should consider antioxidant supplementation:

- Extensive intermediate- (≥63–125 µm) drusen.
- One or more large (≥125 µm) drusen.
- GA in one or both eyes.
- Late AMD in one eye (greatest benefit in AREDS1).

In AREDS1 the reduction in risk of progression to advanced AMD at 10 years was in the order of 25–30% for those with the more advanced of these signs at baseline who took supplements. However, supplements did not discernibly reduce progression in those with early or no AMD at baseline.

AREDS2

The regimen used in AREDS1 consisted of vitamin C, vitamin E, the beta-carotene form of vitamin A and 80 mg daily of zinc (with copper to prevent zinc-induced anaemia). However, high zinc doses are potentially associated with genitourinary tract problems and there are data suggesting that 25 mg of zinc may be the maximal level that is absorbed. Beta-carotene increases the incidence of lung cancer in current and former smokers. AREDS2 looked at adjusting the beta-carotene and zinc components and also whether additional or alternative supplements could enhance outcomes. AREDS2 found:

- The carotenoids lutein and zeaxanthin are a safe alternative to beta-carotene and are probably superior (possible 18% reduction in risk of advanced AMD above that conferred by the AREDS1 regimen).
- Lutein and zeaxanthin supplementation added to the original AREDS1 regimen was only associated with a statistically significantly reduced (26%) risk of AMD in patients in whom the dietary intake of these was not already high (self-described and blood testing). There was evidence that competition for absorption between different carotenoids may have prevented the demonstration of superiority in other patients. This group also showed a one-third reduction in the likelihood of cataract surgery.
- Adding omega-3 fatty acids to the regimen did not seem to enhance outcomes.
- Lowering the zinc dose did not lead to a statistically significant prognostic worsening and is likely to be associated with a lower incidence of side-effects such as gastrointestinal and urinary problems.
- Recommended daily supplementation based on AREDS2:
  - Vitamin E (400 IU).
  - Vitamin C (500 mg).
  - Lutein (10 mg).
  - Zeaxanthin (2 mg).
  - Zinc (25–80 mg; the lower dose may be equally effective).
  - Copper (2 mg; this may not be required with the lower zinc dose).

Other considerations

- A green leafy vegetable intake confers a lower risk of AMD and for individuals with a strong family history of AMD and those with early AMD who do not meet the AREDS criteria, this may be a prudent lifestyle choice.
- Cessation of smoking should be advised.
- Protective measures against exposure to excessive sunlight should be considered.
- Some authorities consider that evidence still supports the regular consumption of oily fish.

TIP In a patient with dry AMD and high-risk characteristics, the risk of developing severe AMD can be reduced with regular anti-oxidant dietary supplementation.

Non-exudative (dry, non-neovascular) AMD

Introduction

This is a common condition, with geographic atrophy threatening central visual loss in up to 5 million people worldwide. Loss of photoreceptors and RPE cells in the macula results in retinal atrophy, with the late stages referred to as geographic atrophy (GA). Although the process of atrophy is slow, GA can eventually result in significant loss of visual acuity. GA also remains an inevitable long-term progressive outcome for many patients with wet AMD. Lesion size is the main measure of disease progression and FAF is the commonest imaging method that is used in clinical trials to report lesion growth. Activation of complement factors C3 and C5 plays an important role in the pathogenesis of dry AMD. Current research is aimed at manipulating the complement system by inhibiting the effects of these factors in the macular region.

Diagnosis

- **Symptoms** consist of gradual impairment of vision over months or years. Both eyes are usually affected, but often asymmetrically. Vision may fluctuate and is often better in bright light.
- **Signs** in approximately chronological order:
  - Numerous intermediate–large soft drusen, which may become confluent.
  - Focal hyper- and/or hypopigmentation of the RPE (Fig. 14.30A and B).

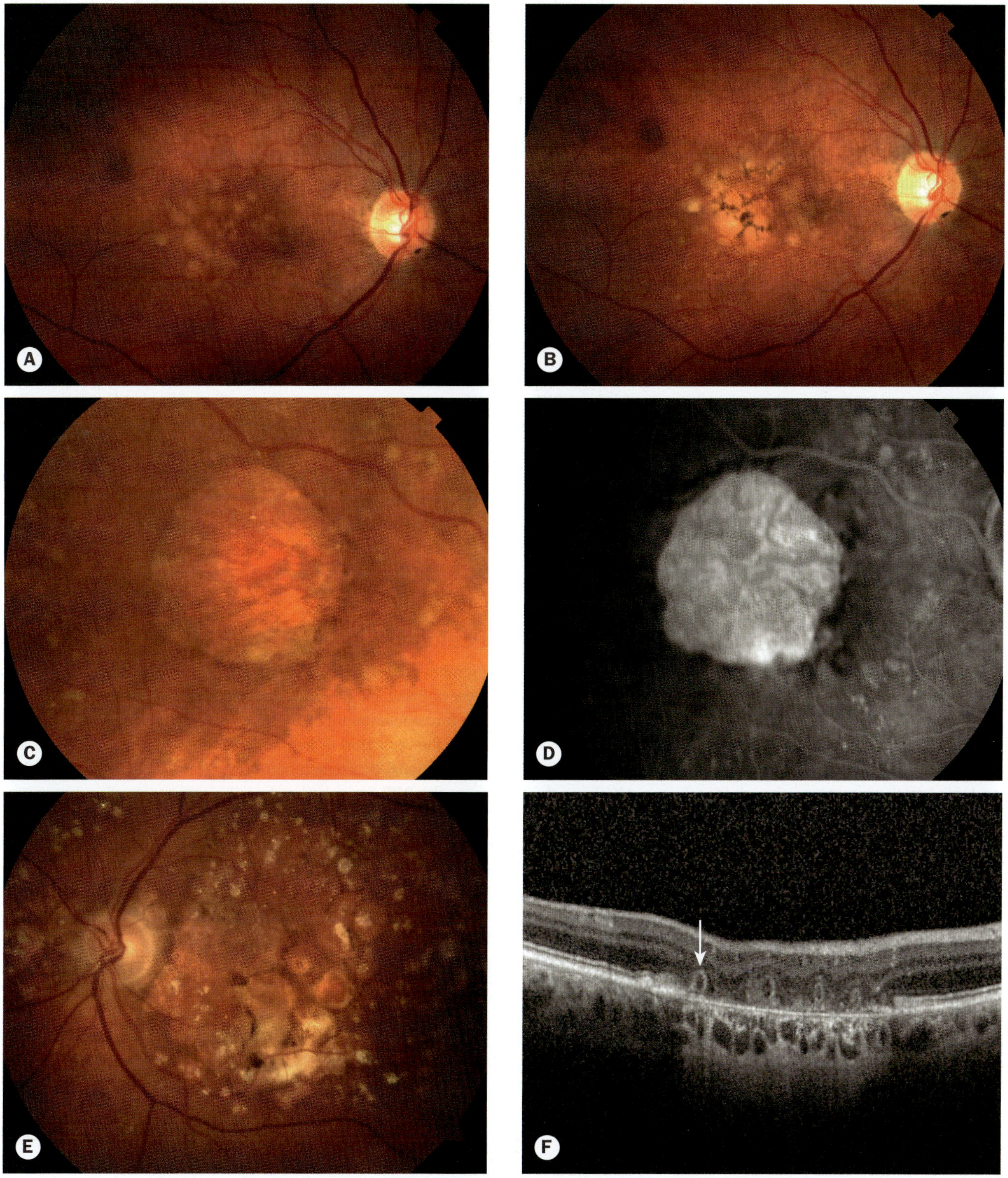

Fig. 14.30 Age-related macular degeneration without neovascularization. **(A)** Drusen and mild pigmentary changes; **(B)** same eye as **(A)** 4 years later with moderate retinal atrophy and pigmentary abnormalities; **(C)** geographic atrophy; **(D)** late FA of eye in **(C)**; **(E)** substantial geographic atrophy and pigmentary abnormalities; **(F)** OCT showing outer retinal tubulations (arrow). *(Courtesy of S Chen – figs A, B, E.)*

- Sharply circumscribed areas of RPE atrophy associated with variable loss of the retina and choriocapillaris (Fig. 14.30C and D).
- Enlargement of atrophic areas, within which larger choroidal vessels may become visible and pre-existing drusen disappear (GA – Fig. 14.30E). Visual acuity may be severely impaired if the fovea is involved. Rarely, MNV may develop in an area of GA.
- Drusenoid RPE detachment (see below).

- **OCT**
  - Drusen – see above.
  - Loss of RPE and morphological alterations of the overlying retina of increasing severity are seen in GA, including increased hyper-reflectivity initially in the outer retinal layers and eventual photoreceptor loss.
  - Outer retinal tubulations may be seen. These are thought to consist of degenerating photoreceptors aggregated into tubular structures that appear as roundish hyporeflective spaces (Fig. 14.30F), often around the margin of GA.
  - Outer retinal corrugations. This recently described phenomenon is an undulating hyper-reflective layer on OCT thought to correspond to the histological finding of basal *laminar* deposit, a layer that accumulates between the RPE and the RPE basement membrane (the inner layer of Bruch membrane) in AMD. Basal *linear* deposit is a distinct finding consisting of membranous debris laid down between the RPE basement membrane and the inner collagenous layer of Bruch membrane that may progress focally to form drusen.
- **Microperimetry** is an accurate method of testing central vision (see Fig. 1.26).
- **FAF** allows visualization of areas of atrophy and shows areas of hyperautofluorescence in the junctional zone at higher risk of progression to geographic atrophy (see Fig. 14.11B).
- **FA** of atrophic areas shows a window defect due to unmasking of background choroidal fluorescence (see Fig. 14.12), if the underlying choriocapillaris is still intact. Exposed sclera may exhibit late staining.

Management

- **Prophylaxis**
  - Antioxidant supplementation if indicated.
  - Risk factors should be addressed, e.g. smoking, ocular sun protection, cardiovascular, dietary.
- **An Amsler grid** should be provided for home use, with advice to self-test on a regular basis and to seek professional advice urgently in the event of any change in vision.
- **Provision of low vision aids** and visually impaired certification for individuals with significant visual loss, as this may facilitate access to social and financial support.
- **Potential new therapies**
  - Thirteen different complement inhibitors have been studied in clinical trials of dry AMD. However, many have been ineffective despite the theoretical promise. Factors like the timing of intervention, dosing schedule and selective permeability of these drugs may be responsible for the less than expected performance. Intravitreal avacincaptad pegol (C5 inhibitor) or pegcetacoplan (C3 inhibitor) result in a reduction in geographic atrophy growth in the short term.
  - Visual cycle modulation by reducing the rate of vitamin A processing using emixustat has not proved helpful in slowing the growth of atrophy.
  - Photocoagulation of drusen leads to a substantial reduction in their extent, but does not reduce the risk of progression to AMD.
  - Saffron (20 mg/day): short-term results suggest an improvement in retinal function.
- **Experimental surgery**
  - Patients should be fully informed of the risks associated with the surgery and the slender likelihood of long-term central visual improvement.
  - Miniature intraocular telescope implantation may provide benefit in selected cases.
  - RPE cells (derived from stem cells) implanted behind the macula have resulted in improved vision in some patients.
  - Macular translocation surgery has a high complication rate and has not been successful in improving vision.
  - Visual prostheses of various types are under investigation.

Retinal pigment epithelial detachment

Pathogenesis

Pigment epithelial detachment (PED) from the inner collagenous layer of Bruch membrane is caused by disruption of the physiological forces maintaining adhesion. The basic mechanism is thought to be the reduction of hydraulic conductivity of a thickened and dysfunctional Bruch membrane, thus impeding movement of fluid from the RPE towards the choroid. Immune-mediated processes may also be important.

Four types are recognised: serous, fibrovascular, drusenoid and haemorrhagic (discussed below).

TIP The diagnosis of pigment epithelial detachment relies on careful examination and OCT imaging of the macula.

Serous PED

- **Symptoms.** Patients can be asymptomatic, but usually present with blurred central vision (sometimes induced hypermetropia) and metamorphopsia in one eye.
- **Signs**
  - An orange dome-shaped elevation with sharply delineated edges, often with a pale margin of subretinal fluid (Fig. 14.31A). Multiple lesions may occur.
  - An associated pigment band may indicate chronicity.
  - Associated blood, lipid exudation, chorioretinal folds or irregular subretinal fluid may indicate underlying MNV.
  - If no drusen are seen, PCV (see below) should be suspected.
- **FA**: a well-demarcated oval area of hyperfluorescent pooling (Fig. 14.31B) that increases in intensity but not in area with time. An indentation (notch) may signify MNV.

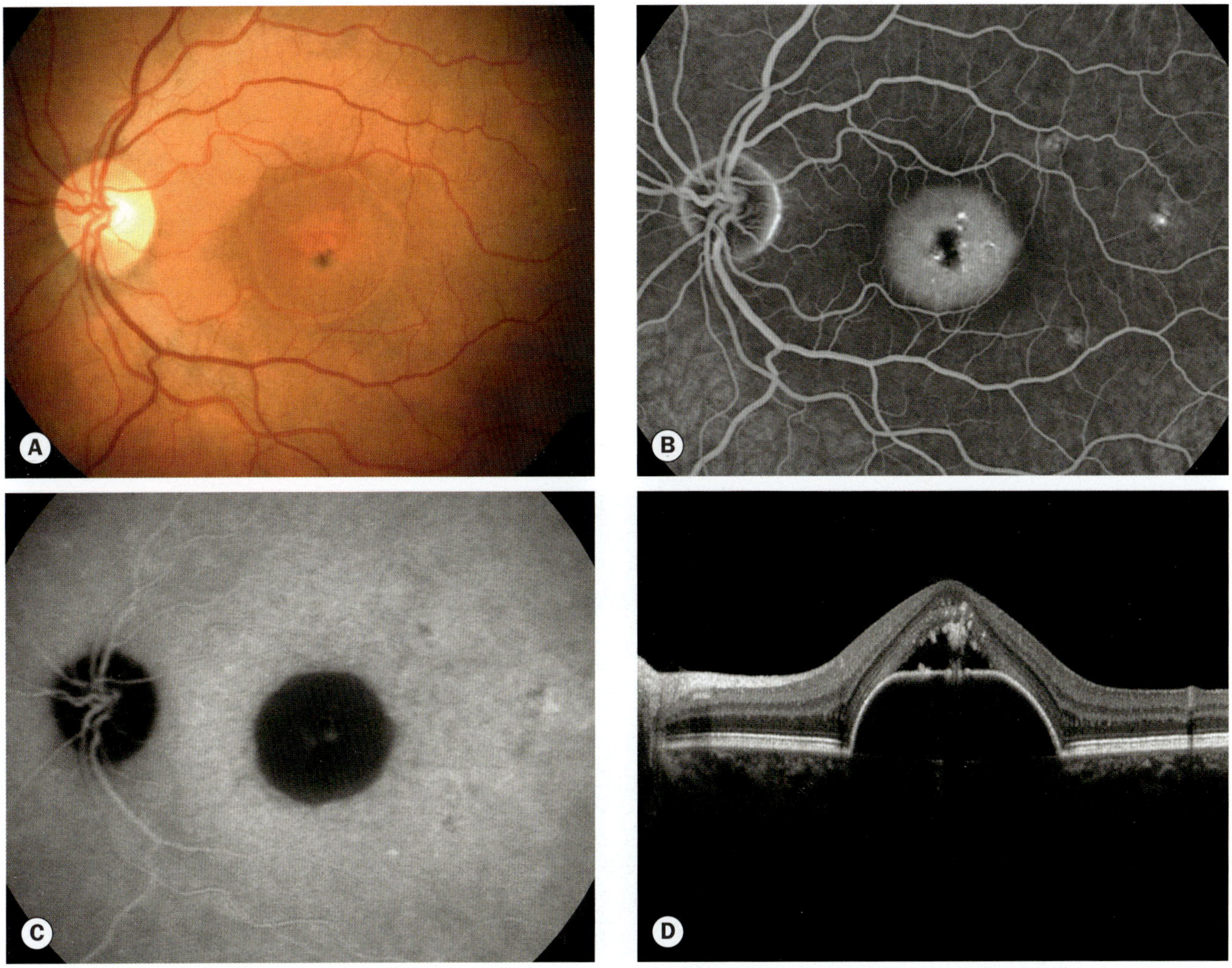

Fig. 14.31 Detachment of the retinal pigment epithelium (RPE). **(A)** Clinical appearance; **(B)** FA at 10 minutes showing hyperfluorescence; **(C)** ICGA at 10 minutes showing hypofluorescence; **(D)** OCT showing separation of the RPE from Bruch membrane. Subretinal hypo/hyper-reflective material is present under the sensory retina.

- **ICGA**: an oval hypofluorescent area with a surrounding hyperfluorescent ring (Fig. 14.31C). Occult MNV (focal hot spot or diffuse plaque) is detected in over 90%.
- **OCT** shows separation of the RPE from Bruch membrane by an optically empty area (Fig. 14.31D). MNV may be indicated by a notch between the main elevation and a second small mound.
- **Natural course**
  - Persistence with increasing atrophy and gradually worsening vision.
  - Patients aged over 60 have a worse prognosis (6/60 or less), but speed of deterioration varies.
  - Resolution leaving GA with visual loss (spontaneous resolution with relative preservation of vision is more common in younger patients).
  - RPE tear formation (see below) or haemorrhage from MNV can occur, with sudden visual loss.
  - Up to a third of eyes develop clinical MNV within 2 years, but the proportion is much higher angiographically.
- **Management**
  - Observation may be appropriate in clinically stable patients without readily detectable MNV, especially those younger than 60.
  - Intravitreal injection of anti-vascular endothelial growth factor (VEGF) agents may stabilize or improve vision and should be considered, particularly when there is associated MNV. However, there is a 5–20% risk of RPE tear.
  - Combining photodynamic therapy (PDT) with intravitreal anti-VEGF or intravitreal triamcinolone injection (IVTA) can also be effective, though the RPE tear risk persists.

Fibrovascular PED

By definition (Macular Photocoagulation Study classification), fibrovascular PED represents a form of 'occult' MNV (Type 1, see below).

- **Signs.** The PED is much more irregular in outline and elevation than serous PED.

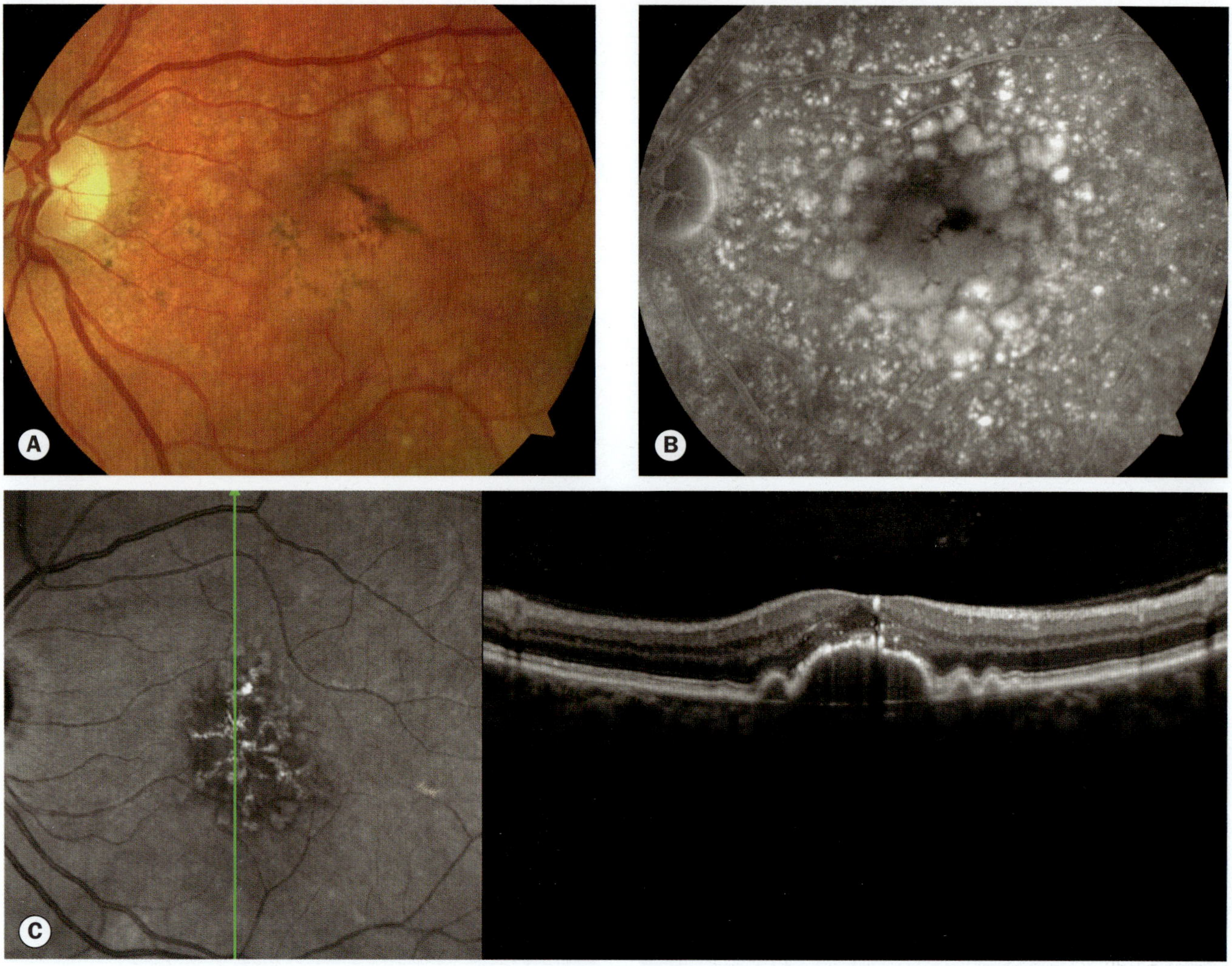

Fig. 14.32 Drusenoid detachment of the retinal pigment epithelium. **(A)** Clinical appearance; **(B)** FA late phase showing moderate hyperfluorescence due to staining; **(C)** OCT appearance showing confluent soft drusen and a drusenoid RPE detachment. *(Courtesy of P Charbel Issa – fig. C.)*

- **OCT.** Less uniform than a serous PED. Both fluid and fibrous proliferation are shown, the latter as irregular scattered reflections.
- **FA** shows markedly irregular granular (stippled) hyperfluorescence, with uneven filling of the PED, leakage and late staining.
- **ICGA** demonstrates MNV more effectively.
- **Management** is essentially as for serous PED with MNV.

Drusenoid PED

Drusenoid PED develops from confluent large soft drusen and is often bilateral.

- **Signs.** Shallow elevated pale areas with irregular scalloped edges (Fig. 14.32A).
- **FA.** Early diffuse hypofluorescence with patchy relatively faint early hyperfluorescence, progressing to moderate irregular late staining (Fig. 14.32B).
- **ICGA.** Hypofluorescence predominates.
- **OCT** shows homogeneous hyper-reflectivity within the PED, in contrast to optically empty serous PED. There is usually no subretinal fluid (Fig. 14.32C).
- **Natural course.** The outlook is usually better than other forms of PED, with only gradual visual loss, though probably around 75% still progress to develop GA and 25% MNV by 10 years from diagnosis. Long-term stability is common: at 3 years, only about one-third will have GA or MNV.
- **Management.** Observation in most cases, with no evidence to support the efficacy of any intervention.

Haemorrhagic PED

Virtually every haemorrhagic PED has underlying MNV or polypoidal choroidal vasculopathy (PCV): the latter should always be considered if no drusen are present.

- **Symptoms.** Sudden impairment of central vision.
- **Signs**
  - Elevated dark red dome-shaped lesion with a well-defined outline (Fig. 14.33A and B).

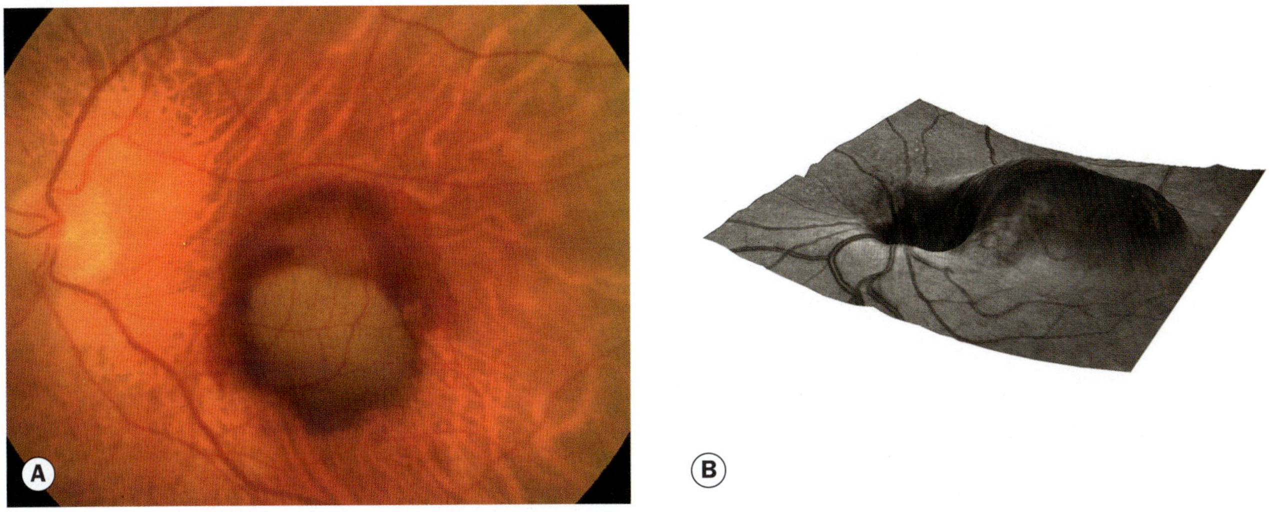

Fig. 14.33 Haemorrhagic detachment of the retinal pigment epithelium (RPE). (A) Subretinal blood is present in the lighter red areas and sub-RPE blood in the darker red areas; (B) three-dimensional OCT scan (detachment in the presence of glaucomatous cupping).

  - Blood may break through into the subretinal space, assuming a more diffuse outline and a lighter red colour.
- **FA.** Dense masking of background fluorescence, but overlying vessels are visible.
- **Management** of large haemorrhagic lesions is described below under 'Haemorrhagic AMD', but the prognosis for central vision is generally poor. MNV associated with a small haemorrhagic PED can be managed conventionally. Management of PCV is discussed separately.

TIP Patients with a large pigment epithelial detachment should be warned that there is a risk of inducing a pigment epithelial tear with anti-VEGF injection.

Retinal pigment epithelial tear

Tears may occur spontaneously, following laser (including PDT), or after intravitreal injection.

- An RPE tear occurs at the junction of attached and detached RPE. Two opposing forces play a role: traction from MNV contraction and adhesive forces from the attached RPE. The tear appears on the opposite side of the neovascular membrane and the contracted RPE monolayer comes to rest on the side of the MNV.
- **Risk factors**
  - Older patients.
  - Long duration.
  - Large PED with a small ratio of MNV size to PED.
  - Wrinkles in the RPE on SD-OCT imaging.
- **Symptoms.** Sudden fall in vision with foveal involvement.
- **Signs.** A crescent-shaped pale area of RPE dehiscence is seen, next to a darker area corresponding to the retracted and folded flap (Fig. 14.34A).
- **FA** late phase shows hypofluorescence over the flap due to the thickened folded RPE, with adjacent hyperfluorescence, initially over the exposed choriocapillaris where the RPE is absent and later due to scleral staining. The two areas are often separated by a sharply defined border (Fig. 14.34B).
- **OCT.** Loss of the normal dome shape of the RPE layer in the PED, with hyper-reflectivity of the folded RPE (Fig. 14.34C and D).
- **The prognosis** for vision in patients with subfoveal tears is poor. Good visual acuity (VA) is usually maintained if the fovea is spared.

Macular neovascularization (MNV)

Introduction

Macular neovascularization (MNV) consists of a blood vessel complex that extends through Bruch membrane from the choriocapillaris into the sub-RPE (type 1) or subretinal (type 2) space. The neovascularization may also start in the outer retina (type 3), hence the new term 'macular neovascularization' (MNV) rather than 'choroidal neovascularization' (CNV). The aim of the new nomenclature is to improve accuracy of communication. MNV occurs in many different disorders, usually when Bruch membrane and/or RPE function has been compromised by a degenerative, inflammatory, traumatic or neoplastic process. AMD is the most common causative association, followed by myopic degeneration. The present discussion relates to MNV arising *de novo* as the primary lesion in neovascular AMD, but MNV may also develop secondary to retinal angiomatous proliferation and polypoidal choroidal vasculopathy (RAP and PCV – see below), both of which are considered to be variants of neovascular AMD. The prognosis of untreated MNV is poor, with 'counting fingers' vision a common outcome. An understanding of the pathogenesis has improved over recent years. The promotion and inhibition of blood vessel growth by cytokines is important, particularly vascular endothelial growth factor (VEGF), which binds to endothelial cell receptors, promoting proliferation and vascular leakage. The inhibitory mediators pigment epithelium-derived factor (PEDF) and complement factor H (CFH) are also

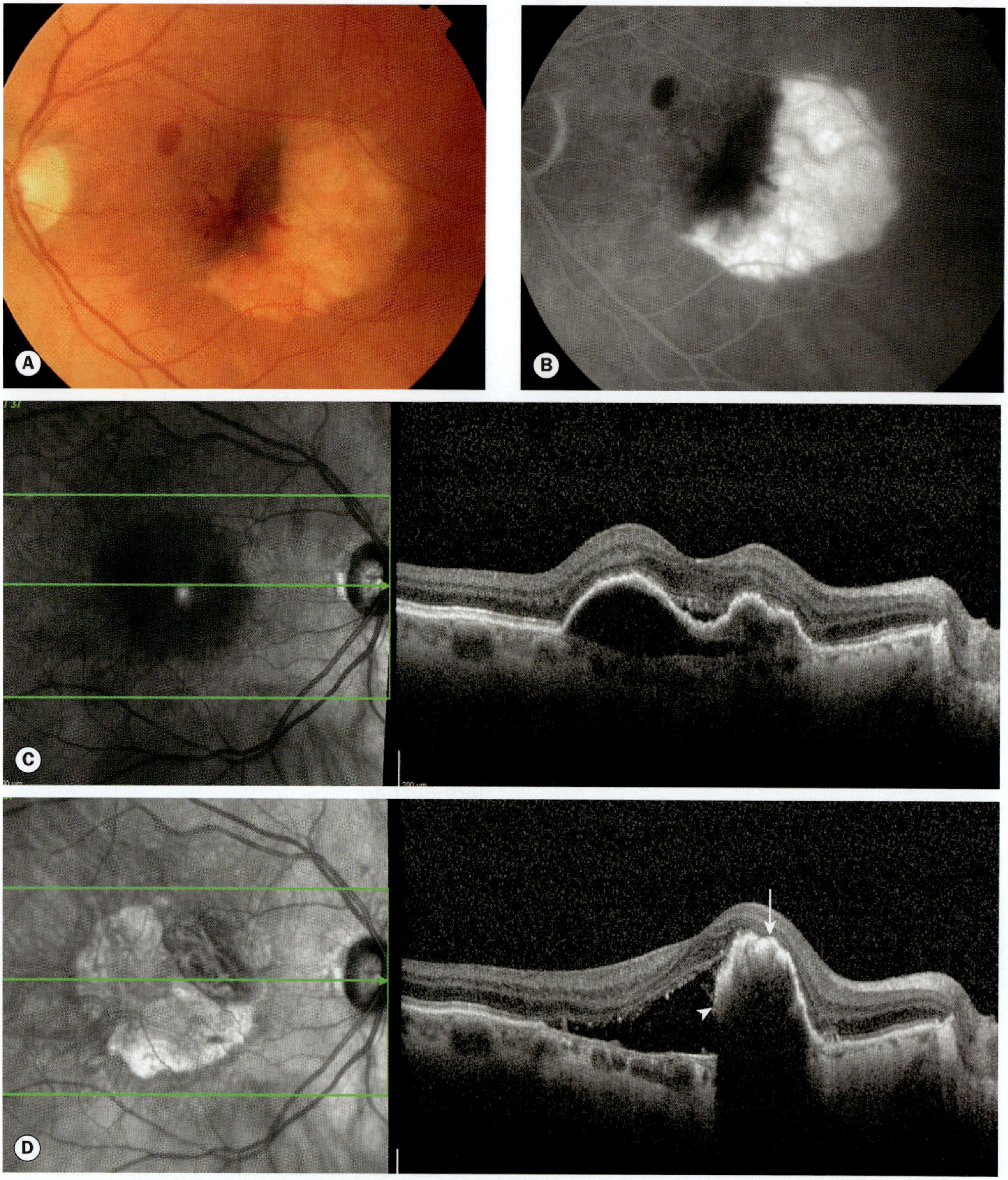

Fig. 14.34 Retinal pigment epithelium (RPE) tear. **(A)** Clinical appearance of pigment epithelial tear; **(B)** FA late phase showing relative hypofluorescence of the folded flap with adjacent hyperfluorescence where the RPE is missing; **(C)** OCT showing multilobed PED with subretinal fluid prior to tear; **(D)** OCT after tear (arrowhead) showing corrugation of the elevated RPE (arrow). *(Courtesy of A Ambresin – figs C and D.)*

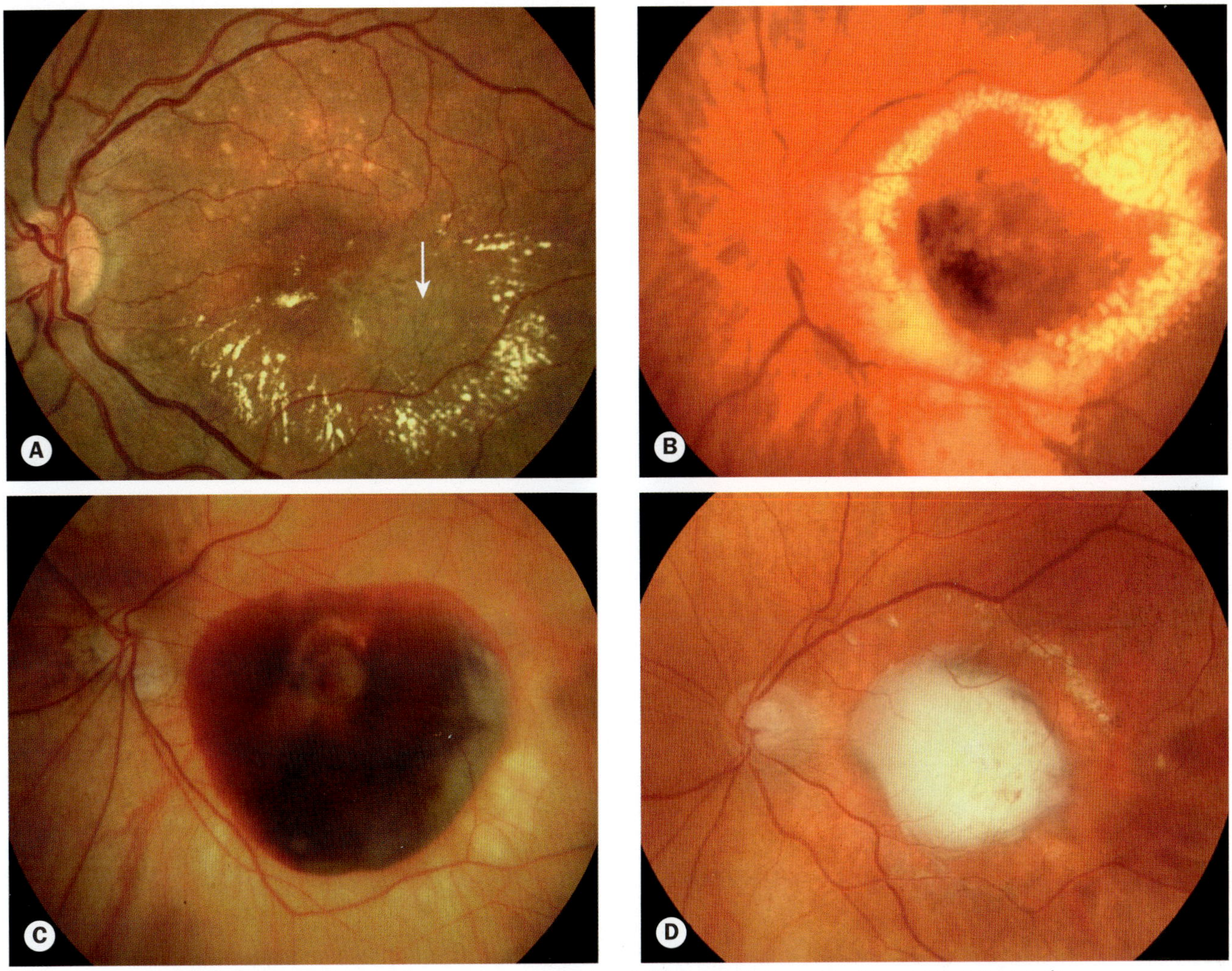

Fig. 14.35 Signs in macular neovascularization (MNV). **(A)** MNV visible as a grey–green submacular area (arrow) with surrounding exudation; **(B)** extensive lipid deposition; **(C)** haemorrhage – intra- and subretinal; **(D)** 'disciform' scarring.

thought to play key roles. Supplementary endothelial progenitor cells are thought to be recruited from systemic reservoirs, enhancing growth of the new vessel complex.

Clinical features

- **Symptoms.** Acute or subacute painless blurring of vision, usually with metamorphopsia. Haemorrhage may give a positive scotoma.
- **Signs**
  - The MNV itself may be identifiable as a grey–green or pinkish-yellow lesion (Fig. 14.35A).
  - Associated medium–large drusen are a typical finding in the same or fellow eye.
  - Localized subretinal fluid, sometimes with cystoid macular oedema (CMO).
  - Intra- and subretinal lipid deposition, sometimes extensive (Fig. 14.35B).
  - Haemorrhage (Fig. 14.35C) is common, e.g. subretinal, preretinal/retrohyaloid, vitreous.
  - There may be an associated serous, fibrovascular drusenoid or haemorrhagic PED.
  - Retinal and subretinal cicatrization ('disciform' scar) in an evolved or treated lesion (Fig. 14.35D).

Fluorescein angiography

FA was previously used to diagnose MNV and to plan and monitor the response to laser photocoagulation or PDT.

- **Current indications include:**
  - Diagnosis of MNV prior to committing to anti-VEGF treatment. FA should usually be performed urgently on the basis of clinical suspicion.
  - As an adjunct to diagnosis of an alternative form of neovascular AMD such as PCV and RAP.
  - Exceptionally, localization for extrafoveal photocoagulation, or guidance for PDT.
- **Terminology** used to describe MNV on FA is derived from the Macular Photocoagulation Study:
  - **Occult** (70%). New term: **Type 1 MNV.** The limits of the neovascular membrane cannot be fully defined on FA (Fig. 14.36A–D). Variants are fibrovascular PED (see above) and 'late leakage of an undetermined source' (LLUS). Type 1

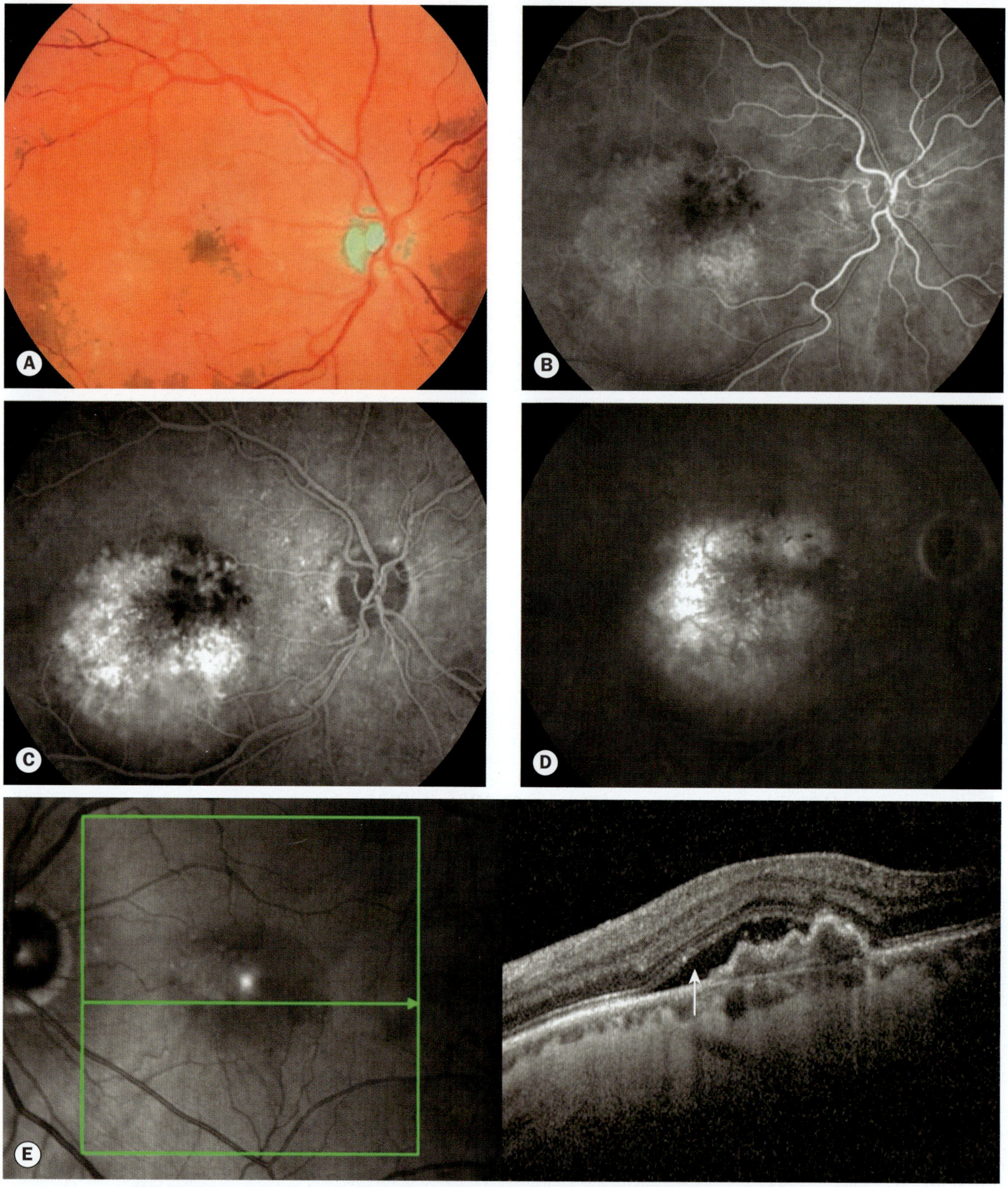

Fig. 14.36 Type 1 macular neovascularization (occult). **(A)** Specks of blood at the fovea; **(B–D)** FA showing diffuse hyperfluorescence but the limits of the membrane cannot be defined; **(E)** OCT showing a PED with thickening of the overlying RPE and variable internal reflectivity associated with adjacent subretinal fluid (arrow). *(Courtesy of A Ambresin – fig. E.)*

MNV is commonly associated with AMD but can also occur secondary to other conditions such as trauma and pseudoxanthoma elasticum. It is present above Bruch membrane, but below the RPE (Fig. 14.36E).

- ○ **Classic** (20%). New term: **Type 2 MNV.** Neovascular membrane fills with dye in a well-defined 'lacy' pattern during early transit subsequently leaking into the subretinal space over 1–2 minutes, with late staining of fibrous tissue (Fig. 14.37A–D). Most MNV is subfoveal; extrafoveal being defined as ≥200 µm from the centre of the foveal avascular zone on FA. It is present below the neurosensory retina, but above the RPE (Fig. 14.37E). Predominantly or minimally classic MNV is present when the classic element is greater or less than 50% of the total lesion respectively.
- ○ **Retinal angiomatous proliferation** (10%). New term: **Type 3 MNV.** Neovascularisation originates from the retinal circulation (typically the deep capillary plexus) and grows towards the outer retina. Stippled hyperfluorescence is seen over an area of elevated RPE that expands to coalesce in the later stages of the angiogram (see Fig. 14.39C and D).

Indocyanine green angiography

ICGA demonstrates MNV as a focal hyperfluorescent 'hot spot' (Fig. 14.38) or 'plaque'. Benefits adjunctive to FA include:

- Increased sensitivity in the detection of MNV, for example if low-density haemorrhage, fluid or pigment preclude adequate FA visualization.
- The distinction of MNV from other conditions that may have a similar presentation, particularly PCV, RAP and CSR.
- The delineation of occult MNV may still have utility for combined modality treatment and for patients who refuse intravitreal therapy.

Optical coherence tomography

Optical coherence tomography (OCT) is critical in the diagnosis and quantitative monitoring of the response to MNV treatment. Typically, MNV is shown as a thickening and fragmentation of the RPE and choriocapillaris. Subretinal and sub-RPE fluid, blood and scarring are demonstrated. Outer retinal tubulations (see Fig. 14.30F) may be present, often in a branching pseudodendritic conformation. On OCT the classification is based on the location of the pathology.

- **Type 1 MNV**: neovascularization is above Bruch membrane, but below the retinal pigment epithelium and manifests as a pigment epithelial detachment that is often multilobulated in appearance. OCT shows an elevation of the RPE by material with heterogenous reflectivity and vascular elements may be seen (see Fig. 14.36E).
- **Type 2 MNV**: neovascularization is below the neurosensory retina, but above the retinal pigment epithelium. It may be associated with subretinal hyperreflective material and separation of the neurosensory retina from the RPE. Subretinal fluid, haemorrhage or intraretinal fluid may be present (see Fig. 14.37E).
- **Type 3 MNV**: OCT findings similar to type 1, with irregular PEDs, subretinal fluid and intraretinal cysts. In some patients dilated vascular elements are seen at the outer border of the lesion (see Fig. 14.39E).

Type 3 MNV (retinal angiomatous proliferation)

Introduction

The major component of the neovascular complex is initially located within the retina. The process may originate in the deep retinal capillary plexus or within the choroid; in the latter case with the early formation of a retinal-choroidal anastomosis (RCA). The disease is frequently bilateral and symmetrical and is probably underdiagnosed. It may constitute 10–20% of neovascular AMD in White people.

Diagnosis

- **Presentation** is similar to that of MNV, but PED and exudate are more frequent. Haemorrhages are also more common and tend to be superficial and multiple.
- **Stage 1**: Intraretinal neovascularization (IRN). Dilated telangiectatic retinal vessels and small angiomatous lesions, typically accompanied by intra-, sub- and preretinal haemorrhage, oedema and exudate (Fig. 14.39A).
- **Stage 2**: Subretinal neovascularization (SRN) extends into the subretinal space associated with increasing oedema and exudate. A serous PED may be present.
- **Stage 3**: MNV. Perfusion is principally via the choroid, with RCA formation. MNV is clearly evident clinically or angiographically; a disciform scar will often form.
- **ICGA** is diagnostic in most cases, showing a hot spot in mid and/or late frames (Fig. 14.39B) and frequently a perfusing retinal arteriole and draining venule ('hairpin loop' when linked).
- **FA** is usually similar to occult or minimally classic MNV (Fig. 14.39C and D), but may show focal intraretinal hyperfluorescence.
- **OCT** is commonly associated with marked intra- and subretinal fluid (Fig. 14.39E). Neovascularization can be seen as a hyper-reflective area leading to a PED. Other features depend on the stage.

Treatment

Type 3 MNV is extremely sensitive to anti-VEGF treatment, especially in the early stages. Favourable outcomes in combination with PDT have been reported. Limited success has been reported for other modalities, including PDT alone and photocoagulation of feeder vessels, though the latter may be used in resistant cases.

Haemorrhagic AMD

- **The visual prognosis** for most eyes with extensive subretinal or sub-RPE haemorrhage is poor.
- **Clinical trials** assessing surgical drainage of extensive subretinal or sub-RPE haemorrhage with MNV excision have

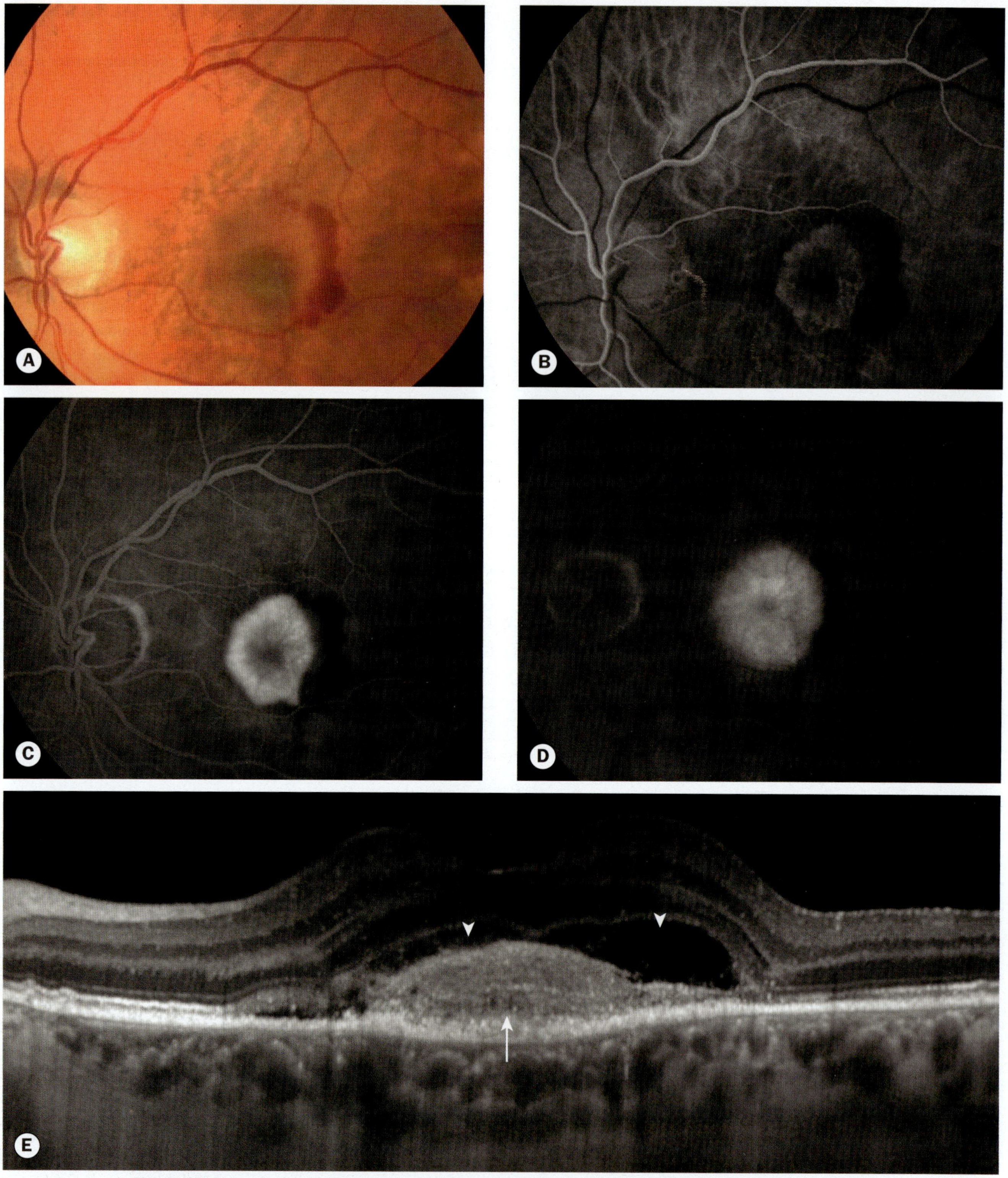

Fig. 14.37 Type 2 subfoveal macular neovascularization (classic). **(A)** Colour image showing grey–green area and small haemorrhage; **(B)** early FA showing 'lacy' hyperfluorescent pattern and an area of hypofluorescence secondary to the haemorrhage; **(C)** late venous phase – more intense hyperfluorescence with leakage and staining; **(D)** persistent staining at 10 minutes; **(E)** OCT showing subretinal fluid (arrowheads) and subretinal hyper-reflective material (arrow) above the RPE. *(Courtesy of A Ambresin – fig. E.)*

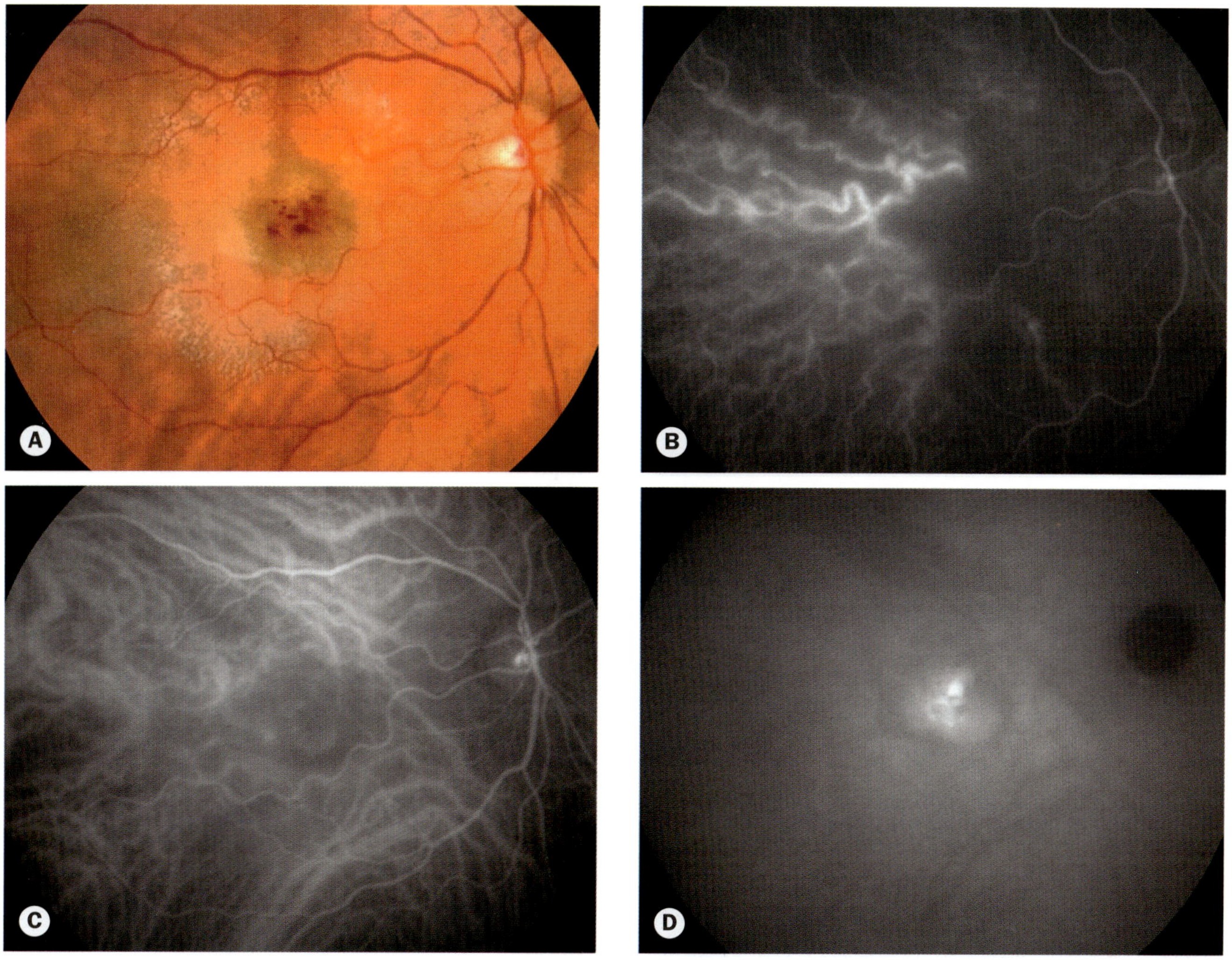

Fig. 14.38 ICGA of macular neovascularization (MNV). **(A)** Blood and fluid at the macula surrounded by hard exudates; **(B–D)** showing a small area of increasing hyperfluorescence ('hot spot') from underlying MNV.

not shown any significant improvement in prognosis and an increased rate of rhegmatogenous retinal detachment. However, better results have been reported using intravitreal anti-VEGF injection and liquefaction of blood by intravitreal (or subretinal, requiring vitrectomy) recombinant tissue plasminogen activator (rtPA). In addition, pneumatic displacement may be appropriate for large or thick haemorrhage.

- **Anticoagulant treatment.** If the patient takes a coumarin anticoagulant, liaison with the prescribing physician is worthwhile to assess if this could be stopped as there is an association with massive macular haemorrhage. Antiplatelet drugs do not usually require discontinuation, though aspirin may be associated with a greater risk of MNV than other agents.
- **Alternative pathology** (e.g. PCV, macroaneurysm) that may be associated with extensive haemorrhage should always be considered.

Treatment with anti-VEGF agents

- **Principles.** Inhibitors of VEGF block its interaction with receptors on the endothelial cell surface and so retard or reverse vessel growth. They have become the predominant means of treatment for MNV, dramatically improving the visual prognosis. Genetic factors are associated with a variability in response so that visual outcomes can differ from patient to patient. Intravitreal injection is the standard method of administration. Notable (but rare) risks include retinal detachment, damage to the lens, RPE tears and endophthalmitis. Sustained elevation of intraocular pressure (IOP) and sterile uveitis may occasionally occur. Systemically, there may be a slightly increased incidence of stroke. All available anti-VEGF agents seem to have potential for benefit in a range of vascular eye diseases. As a general principle, the better the visual acuity at the onset of treatment the better the visual acuity at follow-up. There is some evidence that younger age at treatment onset may confer a worse outcome. Treatment should be initiated within 2–3 weeks of symptom onset.
- **Landmark studies.** The following large, randomized, double-masked, sham-controlled trials provide the evidential basis for anti-VEGF-treatment in individuals with neovascular age-related macular degeneration.

slightly greater severity than less intensive administration. There is a suggestion that systemic adverse events may, counterintuitively, be less common with regular monthly injections than discontinuous schedules.
  - Three initial monthly injections followed by monthly review with re-injection when deterioration occurs as assessed by VA (e.g. loss of five letters or more) and OCT (e.g. retinal thickness increase of 100 μm or more).
  - 'Treat and extend' entails administering three initial injections at monthly intervals and then gradually increasing the period between injections until deterioration is evident. If possible, a tailored interval is determined for each patient.
  - Minor intraocular inflammation may occur after the injection. The endophthalmitis rate is about 1%.
- **Bevacizumab (Avastin).** In contrast to ranibizumab, bevacizumab is a complete antibody originally developed to target blood vessel growth in metastatic cancer deposits. Its use for AMD and other indications is 'off label'. It is very much cheaper than ranibizumab and aflibercept. Clinical trial results suggest that it is approximately comparable to ranibizumab in efficacy and safety, though some studies have suggested that the risk of serious systemic adverse events is marginally higher with bevacizumab than ranibizumab. Treatment strategies in AMD are similar to those used for ranibizumab. The dose of bevacizumab is usually 1.25 mg/0.05 ml.
- **Brolucizumab (Beavu).** The drug is significantly smaller than other anti-VEGF agents and has high binding affinity. It lasts longer in the eye and thus permits less frequent dosing. The HAWK and HARRIER studies show non-inferiority to aflibercept with an improved dosing interval. Approximately half of the patients on this agent can be maintained on a 3-monthly injection schedule at 1 year.
- **Faricimab (Vabysmo).** This is a new bispecific antibody that inhibits angiopoietin-2 and VEGF-A. The TENAYA and LUCERNE trials show non-inferiority to aflibercept at 2 years, with dosing determined by visual acuity and central subfield macular thickness measured with OCT. The drug is generally well tolerated, but a small number develop intraocular inflammation. Almost 80% of patients can be managed on a 12-week dosing schedule and 60% on a 16-week schedule. It may have a significant impact on care by reducing the frequency of injections.
- **Pegaptanib (Macugen).** Pegaptanib sodium was the first anti-VEGF agent approved by regulatory authorities for ocular treatment. The results are similar to outcomes with PDT and its use is now extremely limited.
- **Biosimilars.** These are medicines that are highly similar to other biological medicines that are already in use, with no clinical differences in terms of safety and effectiveness. Two ranibizumab biosimilars have received regulatory approval for use: Byooviz and Ongavia/Ranivisio. At least 11 biosimilars to ranibizumab, aflibercept and bevacizumab are in late-stage development.
- **Technique of intravitreal injection.** Various protocols are in use. A typical approach is set out in Table 14.3 and applies to anti-VEGF injection – there are slight differences for intravitreal steroid administration.
- Patients can return to normal activity after 24 hours, but should be warned to seek advice urgently should they experience any deterioration in their vision or symptoms of inflammation.

TIP In patients with AMD secondary to MNV, the better the visual acuity at the onset of anti-VEGF treatment the better the final visual acuity.

Treatment with photodynamic therapy (PDT)

Verteporfin is a light-activated compound preferentially taken up by dividing cells including neovascular tissue. It is infused intravenously and then activated by diode laser to cause thrombosis. The main indication is subfoveal predominantly classic MNV with visual acuity of 6/60 or better. Severe adverse effects are rare. PDT should not be used in patients with porphyria. With the advent of anti-VEGF treatment, PDT is now rarely used for MNV, but combination therapy (see below) and refusal of intravitreal treatment remain indications. Reduced-intensity regimens have been used with good effect in CSR.

Combination and other experimental therapies

Although anti-VEGF therapy has revolutionized the management of MNV, further investigation is attempting to achieve outcomes that are even better, particularly a reduction in the frequency of intravitreal injections. To date, regimens that include the combination of PDT with anti-VEGF treatment have not been shown to be superior to anti-VEGF treatment alone, but investigation is ongoing, including parallel inhibition of anti-VEGF agents with inhibition of other cytokines and with low-intensity macular radiotherapy. Other avenues of potential therapeutic advantage are sustained-release anti-VEGF systems and gene therapy utilizing adenoviral vectors to facilitate the production of cytokines within the eye.

Laser

Thermal argon or diode laser ablation of MNV is now rarely used, though may still be suitable for the treatment of small classic extrafoveal membranes well away from the macular centre and possibly some cases of PCV and RAP.

PACHYCHOROID DISEASE SPECTRUM

This term refers to a group of macular disorders that share the common features of a thick choroid, dilated and hyperpermeable choroidal vessels, attenuation of the choriocapillaris and retinal pigment epithelial dysfunction. These changes may lead to serous retinal detachment. Normal subfoveal choroidal thickness is approximately 300 μm and the median choroidal thickness is about 260 μm (depending on the technique of measuring), but varies considerably with age, gender and race. If a neovascular membrane is present it tends to be a slow-growing type 1 MNV producing flat, irregular RPE detachments. These disorders can be investigated using OCT and ICG angiography. The following variants are recognized:

Table 14.3 Technique of Intravitreal Injection

- The procedure and its risks should be explained to the patient and appropriate consent obtained.
- The environment should be appropriate, e.g. a dedicated 'clean room' with adequate illumination.
- The indication and the eye to be treated should be checked and the eye marked.
- It should be confirmed that anterior and posterior segment examination (including IOP) has been carried out recently to exclude contraindications.
- Confirmation should be obtained that a syringe of the drug to be injected is available.
- Bilateral injections are optimally administered at separate sessions to minimize risk, but if necessary different instruments and drug batches should be used.
- A surgical mask should be worn.
- Topical anaesthetic and mydriatic agents are instilled.
- Povidone-iodine 5% (chlorhexidine if allergic to iodine) is applied to the ocular surface and at least 3 minutes allowed prior to injection.
- Subconjunctival lidocaine 1% or 2% may be used to supplement the topical agent. Some practitioners prefer lidocaine gel, though concerns have been expressed regarding the possibility of microorganism retention within this.
- Hands are washed using a standard surgical procedure and sterile gloves donned.
- The periocular skin, eyelids and lashes are cleaned with 5–10% povidone-iodine.
- As for other forms of intraocular surgery, a sterile periocular drape may be advisable.
- The sterile pouch containing a pre-prepared syringe is opened, or a sterile syringe is used to draw up the appropriate volume of drug from a vial of ready-prepared drug. A needle (typically 30-gauge, 0.5 inch) on the syringe is primed to expel any air.
- A sterile speculum is placed in the eye.
- The patient is instructed to look away from the injection site – this is most commonly inferotemporal because of ease of access, though any quadrant can be used; the 3 and 9 o'clock positions are avoided because of the risk of neurovascular damage.
- A gauge is used to identify an injection site 3.5–4.0 mm posterior to the limbus (pars plana).
- Forceps can be used to stabilize the eye and, if wished, to apply anterior traction to the conjunctiva so that the conjunctival hole does not overlie the scleral track.
- The needle is advanced perpendicularly through the sclera towards the centre of the eyeball and the required volume of drug (usually 0.05 ml) is injected into the vitreous cavity. Some practitioners try to 'step' the needle track.
- The needle is removed and discarded.
- It has become usual practice not to use post-injection antibiotics as there is a suggestion that serial use may increase the rate of infection by promoting bacterial resistance.
- Elevated IOP can occlude the central retinal artery and it is important routinely to ensure this remains perfused after the procedure by checking the patient's vision (subjectively is adequate), directly visualizing the artery, or optimally by checking the IOP (particularly in glaucoma patients). If occlusion occurs, urgent paracentesis should be carried out; simply lying down may restore blood flow.
- A clear plastic eye shield may be used until the local anaesthetic has worn off and during sleep for the first night or two, but practice varies.

- **Polypoidal choroidal vasculopathy** (see below).
- **Central serous chorioretinopathy** (see below).
- **Pachychoroid neovasculopathy.** This is possibly an early stage of polypoidal choroidal vasculopathy and features macular neovascularization above focal areas of pachychoroid. The condition is treated with anti-VEGF injections combined with full-dose PDT.
- **Pachychoroid pigment epitheliopathy (PPE).** This condition manifests with alteration of the retinal pigment epithelium, usually without neurosensory detachment, although this may occasionally occur. Patients present with normal visual acuity and large choroidal vessels beneath elevations of RPE and sub-RPE drusen-like deposits.
- **Peripapillary pachychoroid syndrome.** This rare condition tends to affect elderly males. It is characterised by peripapillary choroidal thickening associated with intraretinal fluid and/or subretinal fluid on the nasal side of the fovea and occasionally optic disc oedema. The condition is similar to chronic central serous retinopathy. Macular neovascularization is not present. Photodynamic therapy with verteporfin may be considered, but is not always needed.

Polypoidal choroidal vasculopathy

Introduction

Polypoidal choroidal vasculopathy (PCV, also called: pachychoroid aneurysmal type 1 choroidal neovascularization) is characterized by a branching vascular network of inner choroidal vessels with multiple terminal aneurysmal protuberances that appear to be the source of bleeding and exudation. It is more common in patients of African and East Asian ethnic origin than in White patients and is more common in women than men (5:1). The disease is often bilateral but tends to be asymmetrical. Risk factors include cigarette smoking, increased body mass index and increased levels of inflammatory biomarkers (e.g. C-reactive protein). Overall, it is relatively common and the presence of prominent haemorrhage should lead to the consideration of PCV, particularly if there is an absence of drusen and the patient is relatively young and Asian or African.

Diagnosis

- **Presentation** is usually in late middle age with the sudden onset of unilateral visual impairment.

- **Signs**
  - Terminal swellings are frequently visible as reddish-orange nodules beneath the RPE in the peripapillary or macular area (Fig. 14.41A) and less commonly the periphery.
  - Multiple recurrent serosanguineous retinal and RPE detachments.
  - Deterioration can be slow with intermittent bleeding and leakage, resulting in macular damage and visual loss. Up to 50% may have a favourable outlook, with eventual spontaneous resolution of exudation and haemorrhage.
- **FA** shows an intense localized area of hyperfluorescence (Fig. 14.41B).
- **ICGA** is the key investigation in PCV.
  - Hyperfluorescent nodules and a network of large choroidal vessels with surrounding hypofluorescence appear in the early phase. The polyp-like swellings rapidly begin to leak (Fig. 14.41C–F).
  - The previously darker surrounding region becomes hyperfluorescent by the late phase.
  - A cluster of grape-like lesions may carry a higher risk of severe visual loss.
- **OCTA** shows the polyps (see Fig. 14.26F).
- **OCT**
  - Multiple large pigment epithelial detachments, particularly the 'double-hump' sign and the 'inverted V', associated with pachychoroid (Fig. 14.41G).
  - Round-oval polyps may be attached to the posterior surface of the PED.
  - A branching vascular network may be seen underlying a flat PED adjacent to the polyp.
  - Choroidal thickening may be demonstrated.

Treatment

The favourable prognosis without treatment in a significant proportion of cases should be borne in mind and asymptomatic polyps may be observed.

- **Combination treatment.** The results of combination therapy of ranibizumab plus verteporfin PDT are superior to ranibizumab monotherapy in respect of best-corrected visual acuity and complete polyp regression. Fewer injections are required (EVEREST-II trial).
- **Anti-VEGF agents** are less effective than when they are used in typical MNV, but may suppress leakage and bleeding.
- **PDT** alone may lead to regression of polyps and result in an extended treatment effect. Early PDT provides a better outcome compared to delayed PDT. Consider PDT as a rescue therapy in an eye with PCV that is refractory to a course of anti-VEGF monotherapy.
- **Laser photocoagulation** of feeder vessels or polyps may be effective in selected cases, specifically if the changes are juxta-foveal.

TIP In a patient with AMD who has not responded to anti-VEGF treatment after 3 months, undertake ICGA to check for polypoidal choroidal vasculopathy.

Central serous chorioretinopathy

Overview

Central serous chorioretinopathy (CSR) is an idiopathic disorder characterized by a localized serous detachment of the sensory retina at the macula secondary to leakage from the choriocapillaris through one or more hyperpermeable RPE sites (see Fig. 14.13). CSR has been classified as one of the 'pachychoroid' spectrum disorders; in eyes with unilateral CSR almost two-thirds of fellow eyes have signs of pachychoroid pigment epitheliopathy. CSR typically affects one eye of a young or middle-aged White man. The male to female ratio is 3:1; females with CSR tend to be older. It presents in two forms: acute (self-resolving within 3–6 months) and chronic. A SNP involving the complement factor H gene on chromosome 1 predisposes to the chronic form of CSR in White individuals. The use of steroids in any form (including endogenous Cushing syndrome) is significantly linked to this condition. Numerous other risk factors and associations have been reported (including *Helicobacter pylori* infection, renal dialysis, systemic hypertension, psychological stress, pregnancy and sleep apnoea syndrome).

Clinical features

- **Symptoms.** Unilateral blurring, metamorphopsia, micropsia and mild dyschromatopsia.
- **Signs**
  - VA is typically 6/9–6/18, but may improve with a low-strength convex lens (correction of acquired hypermetropia from retinal elevation).
  - Round or oval detachment of the sensory retina at the macula (Fig. 14.42A and see Fig. 14.13).
  - The subretinal fluid may be clear (particularly in early lesions) or turbid. Precipitates may be present on the posterior retinal surface.
  - One or more depigmented RPE foci (often small PEDs) of variable size may be visible within the neurosensory detachment. Small patches of RPE atrophy (Fig. 14.42B) and hyperplasia elsewhere in the posterior pole may indicate the site of previous lesions and are typically seen easily on FAF imaging (Fig. 14.42C).
  - Chronic lesions may be associated with substantial underlying atrophic change. Fluid can sometimes track downwards in a gravity-dependent fashion (gravitational tract), best shown on FAF imaging (Fig. 14.42D) and can occasionally progress to bullous CSR (see below).
  - The optic disc should be examined to exclude a congenital pit as the cause of a neurosensory detachment (see Ch. 19).
- **Course**
  - Spontaneous resolution within 3–6 months, with return to near-normal or normal vision in around 80%. Recurrence is seen in up to 50%.
  - Some patients (about 15%) follow a chronic course lasting more than 12 months. Prolonged detachment is associated with gradual photoreceptor and RPE degeneration and permanently reduced vision. Multiple recurrent attacks may also give a similar clinical picture.

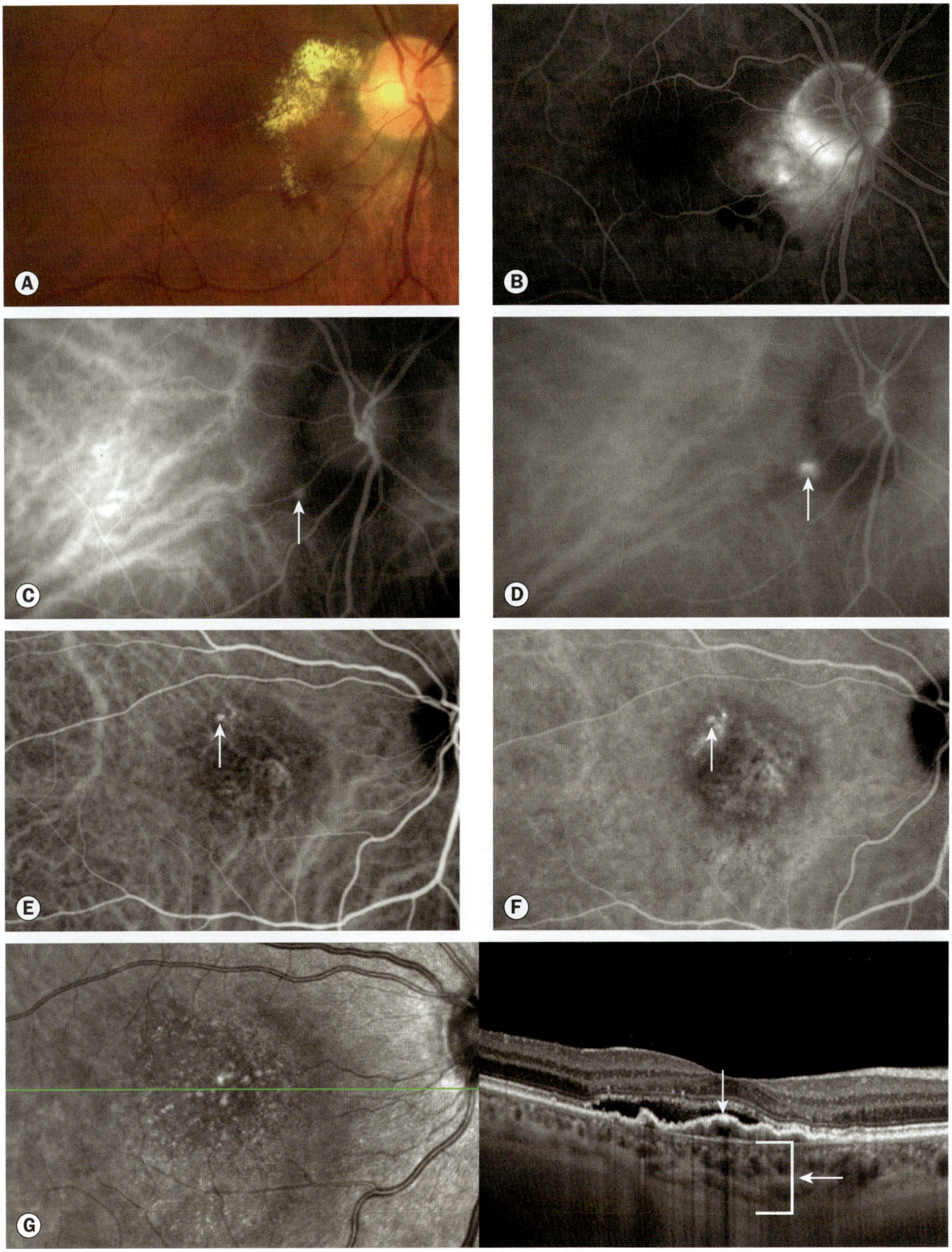

Fig. 14.41 Polypoidal choroidal vasculopathy. **(A)** Reddish-orange nodular terminal swellings with surrounding leakage in the parapapillary region; **(B)** FA appearance of **(A)** in late venous phase showing intense localized area of hyperfluorescence; **(C)** early ICGA of **(A)** showing polyp (arrow); **(D)** late ICGA appearance; **(E)** ICGA of a different patient showing a polyp at 2 minutes (arrow); **(F)** ICGA at 10 minutes showing several polyp-like swellings with leakage (arrow); **(G)** OCT of **(E)** showing multiple vascularized PEDs (arrow), subretinal fluid and pachychoroid (box). *(Courtesy of A Ambresin – figs E–G.)*

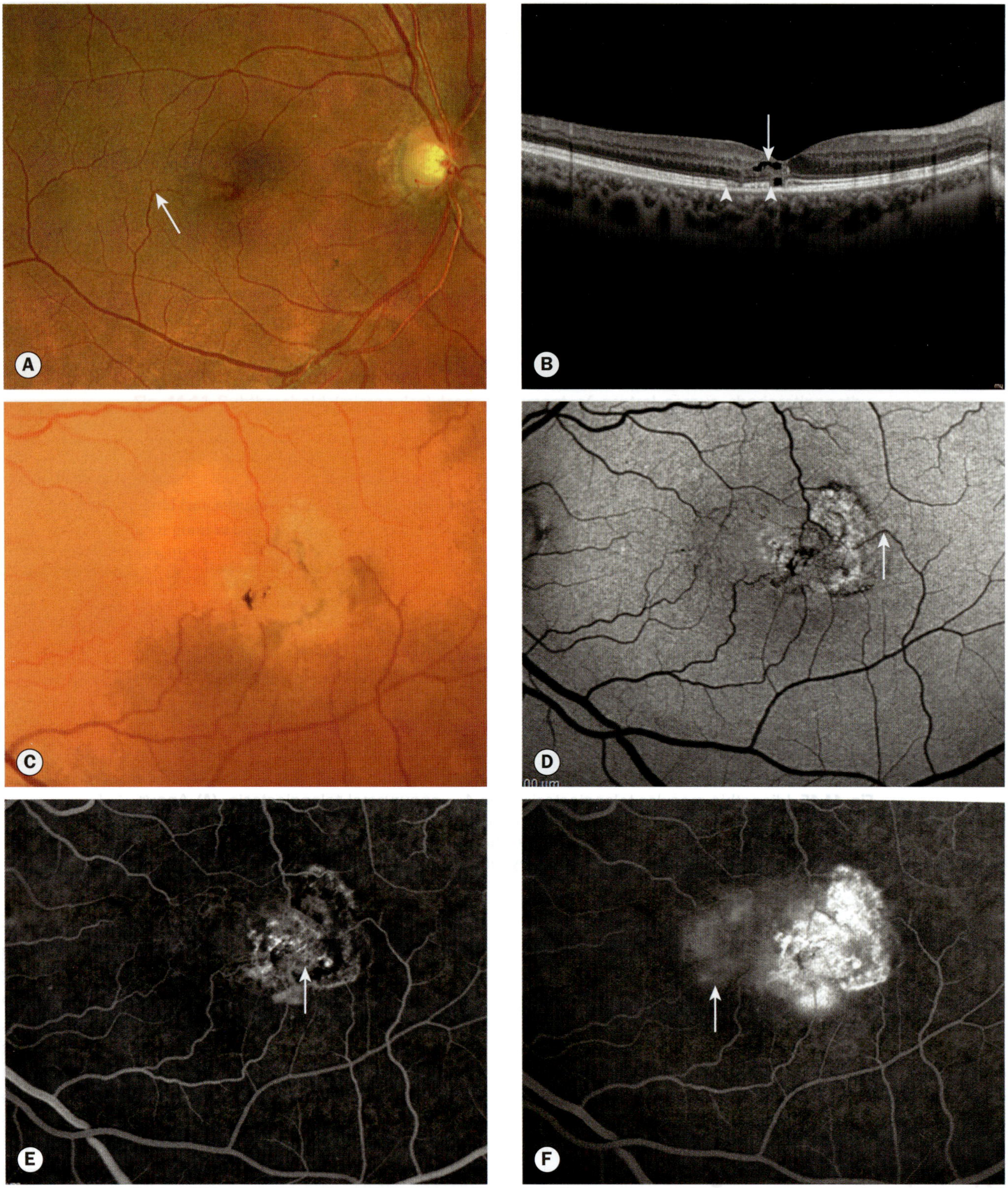

Fig. 14.46 MacTel. **(A)** Early disease showing subtle changes temporal to the fovea and a venule that turns into the deep retina (arrow); **(B)** OCT of **(A)** showing localized loss of the outer nuclear layer and ellipsoid zone (arrowheads), with cavitation (arrow); **(C)** advanced disease with changes mainly temporal to the fovea and confined to the MacTel zone; **(D)** FAF of patient in **(C)** showing a dilated venule that suddenly turns at right-angles into the deep retina (arrow) and macular hyperautofluorescence; **(E)** early phase FA of patient in **(C)** showing a neovascular membrane (arrow); **(F)** FA showing late leakage (arrow). *(Courtesy of P Charbel Issa.)*

  - Greyish loss of parafoveal retinal transparency extending up to one disc diameter from the foveola, initially temporal to and later surrounding the fovea (Fig. 14.46C).
  - Fine superficial crystalline retinal deposits are common.
  - Mildly ectatic capillaries can be seen in the later stages. These telangiectatic vessels are present in the inner and outer retina and are best seen in a fluorescein angiogram.
  - The vascular alterations may be demonstrated more readily by red-free photography. Blunted, slightly dilated venules are often associated with ectatic capillaries and in later disease stages, with pigment hyperplasia. These venules seem to turn at right angles into the deeper retina and are often associated with pigment clumps at the tips. The abnormal vessels can proliferate to subretinal neovascularization distinct from MNV, but similar to retinal angiomatous proliferation and indicate the proliferative stage of the condition.
  - Intraretinal cavities may simulate a lamellar hole (see Fig. 14.46B).
  - Small RPE plaques develop in many patients, usually associated with the right-angled venules.
  - Aneurysms are uncommon, but have been reported. Vascular leakage is mild; exudation with cystoid macular oedema is not a feature of this disease.
- **OCT** is a key aid to the diagnosis. The formation of hyporeflective inner retinal cavities of variable size, morphologically distinct from those seen in CMO, are a characteristic finding (see Fig. 14.46B). An inner lamellar cyst that enlarges with progressive disease is commonly seen underlying the fovea. Thinning and disruption of the photoreceptor layers is also common, but is a late sign. Pigment clumps are shown as intraretinal hyper-reflective plaques with posterior shadowing. There is usually no overall macular thickening, because outer retinal thinning is counteracted by inner retinal thickening. Hyper-reflective inner retinal dots corresponding to telangiectatic vessels may be present.
- **FAF** changes occur early in the disease course and may precede clinically detectable signs. Heightened foveal autofluorescence is a common early finding, which gradually increases in extent (Fig. 14.46D).
- **FA** in early disease shows bilateral perifoveal telangiectasia with early leakage from the abnormal vessels progressing to diffuse leakage, though without CMO. The cystoid spaces identifiable on OCT do not show hyperfluorescence on FA. FA is also used to confirm MNV (Fig. 14.46E and F).
- **Macular pigment optical density** (MPOD) imaging shows a possibly pathognomonic pattern of oval reduction in density corresponding to the late distribution of hyperfluorescence on FA. MPOD is preserved from 6° outwards.
- **Prognosis.** Visual acuity generally does not deteriorate to less than 6/60, with an average acuity of 6/12. The development of subretinal neovascularization is most often preceded by enlargement of pigment clumps. Spread of the pigment increases the risk of developing poor vision and proliferative disease, particularly in females. MNV in MacTel tends to carry a better prognosis than in AMD.
- **Treatment.** Intravitreal anti-VEGF agents can decrease leakage on FA in the non-proliferative stage but are not helpful visually and may even have negative long-term effects. They are only useful in the proliferative stage, especially for MNV. Preliminary studies of an intravitreal implant (Renexus) which secretes ciliary neurotrophic factor, have shown slowing of retinal degeneration.

Type 3: occlusive telangiectasia

This extremely rare condition presents in late middle age and carries a poor visual prognosis. The manifestations relate to capillary occlusion rather than telangiectasia (progressive occlusion of parafoveal capillaries with marked aneurysmal dilatation of terminal capillaries). It is distinct from type 1 and type 2 macular telangiectasia.

CYSTOID MACULAR OEDEMA

Introduction

Cystoid macular oedema (CMO) results from the accumulation of fluid in the outer plexiform and inner nuclear layers of the retina with the formation of tiny cyst-like cavities (Fig. 14.47A). Fluid may initially accumulate intracellularly in Müller cells, with subsequent rupture. Coalescence of smaller cavities may occur over time with subsequent progression to a foveal lamellar hole with irreversible impairment of central vision. CMO is a non-specific manifestation of any type of macular oedema. Causes include:

- **Ocular surgery and laser**, e.g. phacoemulsification, panretinal photocoagulation and miscellaneous other procedures.
- **Retinal vascular disease**, e.g. diabetic retinopathy, retinal vein occlusion.
- **Inflammation**, e.g. intermediate uveitis, severe or chronic uveitis of any kind.
- **Drug-induced**, e.g. topical prostaglandin derivatives.
- **Retinal dystrophies**, e.g. retinitis pigmentosa.
- **Conditions involving vitreomacular traction**, e.g. epiretinal membrane.
- **MNV.**
- **Fundus tumours**, e.g. retinal capillary haemangioma.
- **Systemic disease**, e.g. chronic renal failure.

Diagnosis

- **Symptoms** may include blurring, distortion and micropsia.
- **Signs**
  - Loss of the foveal depression, thickening of the retina and multiple cystoid areas in the sensory retina (Fig. 14.47B), best seen with red-free light using a fundus contact lens.
  - Optic disc swelling is sometimes present.
  - A lamellar hole may be visible.
  - Features of associated disease.
- **Amsler chart** demonstrates central blurring and distortion.
- **FA.** A petaloid pattern is seen due to dye accumulation in microcystic spaces in the outer plexiform layer (Fig. 14.47C).
- **OCT** shows retinal thickening with cystic hyporeflective spaces and loss of the foveal depression (Fig. 14.47D). A lamellar hole may be demonstrated in advanced cases.

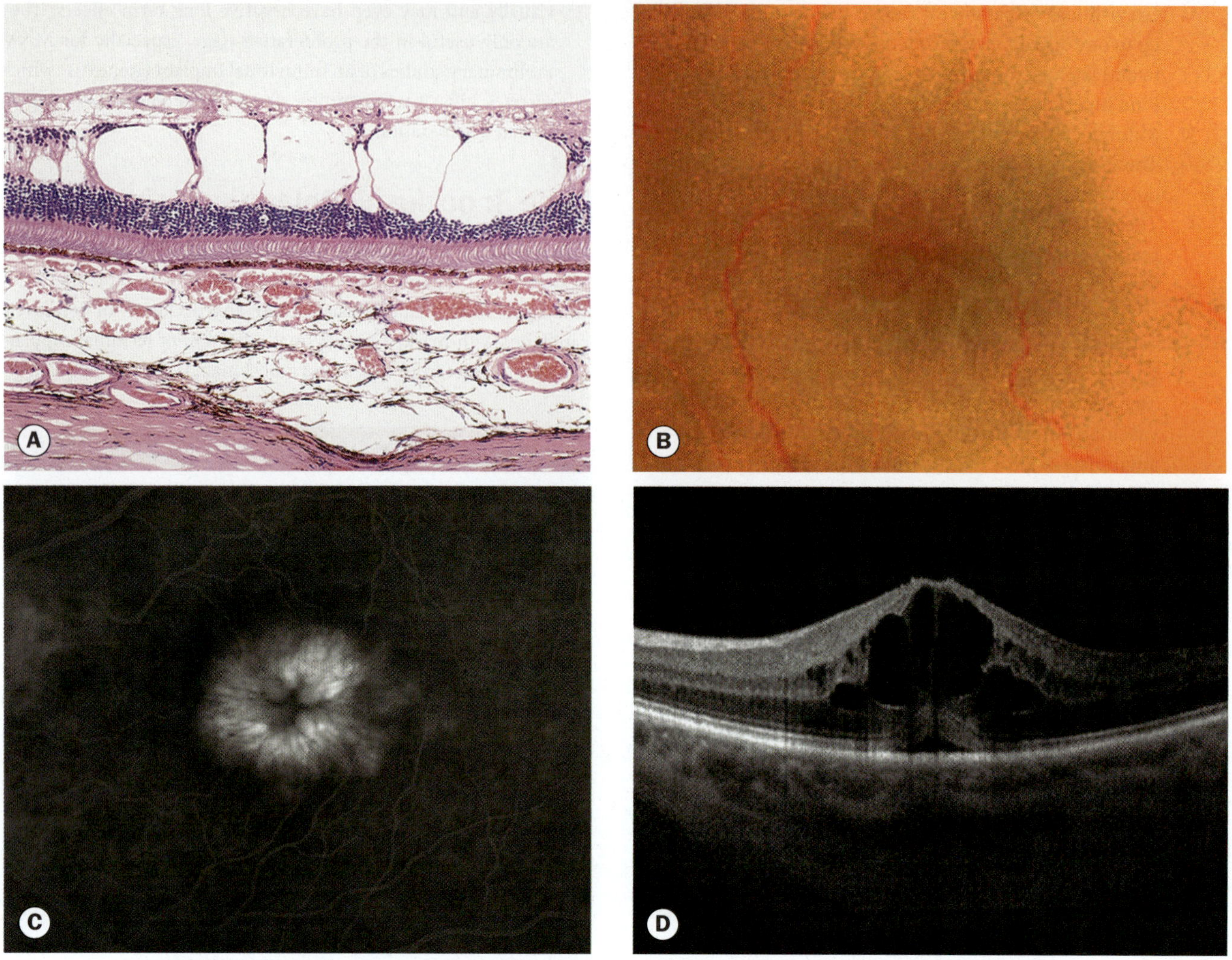

Fig. 14.47 Cystoid macular oedema. **(A)** Histology showing cystic spaces in the outer plexiform and inner nuclear layer; **(B)** clinical appearance of severe oedema; **(C)** FA late phase showing a 'flower petal' pattern of hyperfluorescence; **(D)** OCT showing hyporeflective spaces within the retina, macular thickening and loss of the foveal depression. *(Courtesy of J Harry and G Misson, from* Clinical Ophthalmic Pathology, *Butterworth-Heinemann 2001 – fig. A; Donald M Gass, from* Stereoscopic Atlas of Macular Diseases, *Mosby 1997 – fig. B.)*

MICROCYSTIC MACULAR OEDEMA

Microcystic changes of the inner nuclear layer distinct from classic CMO can occur in eyes with optic neuritis and some other forms of optic neuropathy. It is believed to be caused by retrograde degeneration of the inner retinal layers that manifests with impaired fluid resorption.

VITREOMACULAR INTERFACE DISORDERS

Epiretinal membrane

Introduction

An epiretinal membrane (ERM) is a transparent, avascular, fibrocellular structure that develops on or above the surface of the retina. Proliferation of the cellular component and contraction of the membrane leads to visual symptoms, primarily due to retinal wrinkling, obstruction and localized elevation with or without pseudocyst formation and CMO.

- **Idiopathic**
  - No apparent cause, as a relatively common ageing process. The prevalence of early ERM (cellophane) is approximately 6.5% and advanced ERM (preretinal macular fibrosis), approximately 2.5%.
  - Residual vitreous tissue remains on the retinal surface following cortical separation in around 50% of eyes, with subsequent proliferation. The predominant cellular constituent is glial cells, probably derived from the indigenous posterior hyaloid membrane (PHM) cell population (laminocytes). ERM development can occur at any stage of posterior vitreous detachment (PVD). It is now believed that the process of PVD from initiation to completion often extends over the course of years.
  - About 10% are bilateral.
  - Tend to be milder than secondary ERMs.

- **Secondary**
  - Occur following retinal detachment surgery (most frequent cause of secondary ERM), retinal break, panretinal photocoagulation, retinal cryotherapy, retinal vascular disease, inflammation and trauma.
  - Binocularity is dependent on whether both eyes are affected by the causative factors.
  - Cell type more varied, with prominent pigment cells – thought to be derived from the RPE.

Diagnosis

- **Symptoms.** Blurring and metamorphopsia. Mild cases are often asymptomatic.
- **Signs**
  - VA is highly variable, depending on severity.
  - An irregular translucent sheen (cellophane maculopathy) is present in early ERM, often best detected using green (red-free) light (Fig. 14.48A).
  - As the membrane thickens and contracts it becomes more obvious (macular pucker) and typically causes mild distortion of blood vessels (Fig. 14.48B).
  - Advanced ERM may give severe distortion of blood vessels, marked retinal wrinkling and striae and may obscure underlying structures (Fig. 14.48C).
  - Associated findings may include macular pseudohole (Fig. 14.48D), CMO, retinal telangiectasia and small haemorrhages.
- **Amsler grid** testing typically shows distortion.
- **OCT** shows a highly reflective surface layer associated with retinal thickening (Fig. 14.48E). Disruption of the inner-segment/outer-segment junction may be associated with a worse visual outcome following surgery. OCT is also useful to exclude significant vitreomacular traction (see later).
- **FA has been superseded by OCT** for routine assessment of ERM, but if undertaken it highlights vascular tortuosity and demonstrates leakage. It is sometimes indicated to investigate the cause of an ERM, such as a prior retinal vein occlusion.

Treatment

- **Observation** if the membrane is mild and non-progressive. Spontaneous resolution of visual symptoms sometimes occurs, typically due to complete separation of the ERM from the retina. CMO or tractional detachment may require fairly prompt surgery to minimize secondary degenerative change.
- **Surgical removal** of the membrane via vitrectomy usually improves or eliminates distortion (the main benefit), with an improvement in visual acuity of at least two lines in around 75% or more; in about a quarter VA is unchanged and around 2% get worse. The surgical complications are principally those occurring after vitrectomy (see Ch. 16). Removal of the internal limiting membrane (ILM) in concert with ERM peeling may be beneficial, but remains controversial. Visual improvement commonly does not occur for several months postoperatively. Recurrence is rare.

Full-thickness macular hole

Introduction

Full-thickness macular hole (FTMH) is a relatively common cause of central visual loss, with a prevalence of approximately 3:1000. The onset is most common in females aged 60–70. Careful examination of the fellow eye is important as macular holes are bilateral on presentation in about 30%. The role of vitreomacular traction (VMT) in the aetiology of macular hole has increasingly been defined over recent years and is considered at greater length as a separate topic later in this chapter. A new OCT-based classification has been published by the International Vitreomacular Traction Study (IVTS) Group and replaces the older Gass classification of macular hole, which was based on careful clinical examination and divided macular holes into four stages. Other causes of full-thickness macular hole include high myopia (which can lead to macular retinal detachment) and blunt ocular trauma. Lesions that may sometimes have a similar appearance include macular pseudohole and lamellar hole (see 'Vitreoretinal traction' below). The clinical appearance of a macular hole is typical, but the differential diagnosis includes cystoid macular oedema, subfoveal drusen, CSR and adult vitelliform macular dystrophy.

Symptoms

Presentation of a full-thickness dehiscence may be with impairment of central vision in one eye, or as a relatively asymptomatic deterioration, first noticed when the fellow eye is occluded or at a routine sight test. Symptoms are absent or mild prior to the development of a full-thickness lesion. Metamorphopsia may be present.

Signs and OCT features

- **Vitreomacular adhesion – VMA**: no distortion of the foveal contour. This term was proposed to denote the OCT finding of oblique foveal vitreoretinal traction before the appearance of clinical changes.
- **Vitreomacular traction – VMT**: distortion of foveal contour in the absence of a hole. Clinically stage 1a: 'Impending' macular hole. Appears as flattening of the foveal depression with an underlying yellow spot. Pathologically, the inner retinal layers detach from the underlying photoreceptor layer, often with the formation of a cyst-like schisis cavity. With loss of structural support, the photoreceptor layer commonly undergoes centrifugal displacement. Clinically stage 1b: occult macular hole, indicates foveal detachment and is characterised by a yellowish ring (Fig. 14.49A).
- **Small or medium FTMH with VMT**: small is less than 250 µm or medium is 250–400 µm measured at its narrowest point with OCT. Clinically stage 2: small full-thickness hole measuring less than 400 µm in diameter. The defect may be central, slightly eccentric or crescent-shaped (Fig. 14.49B). A dehiscence is present in the inner retina with persistent vitreofoveolar adhesion. The posterior hyaloid remains attached to the fovea. Nearly all will progress to the next stage, with further visual decline.

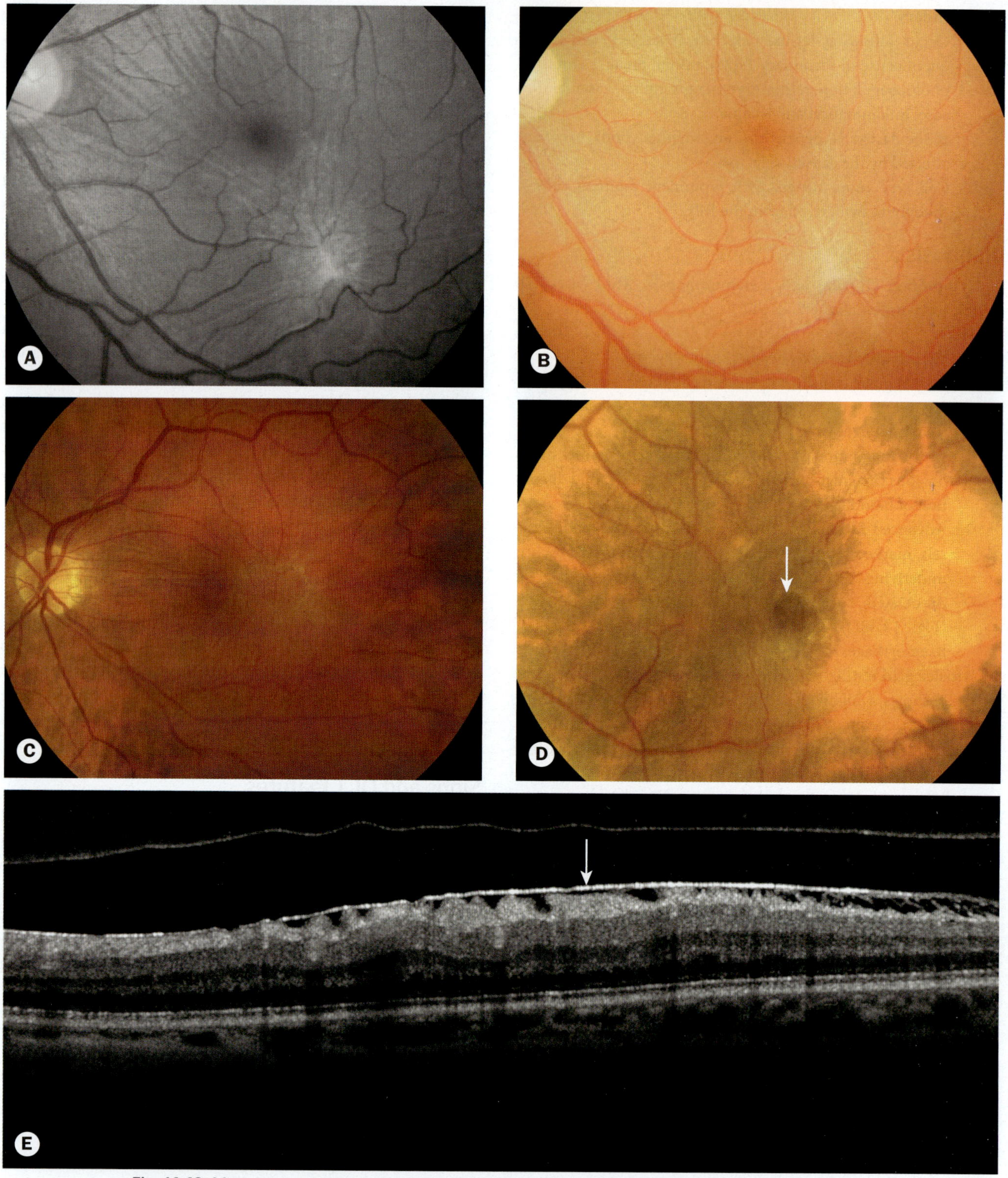

Fig. 14.48 Macular epiretinal membrane. **(A)** Translucent membrane seen with red-free light; **(B)** colour image of the patient in **(A)**; **(C)** advanced membrane; **(D)** macular pseudohole (arrow); **(E)** OCT showing a highly reflective thin membrane anterior to the macula (arrow), with corrugations of the retinal surface and a PVD.

- **Large FTMH with VMT**: greater than 400 μm in diameter. Clinically stage 3: large full-thickness macular hole measuring more than 400 μm associated with a red base in which yellow–white dots may be seen (Fig. 14.49C). A surrounding grey cuff of subretinal fluid is usually present (Fig. 14.49D) and an overlying retinal operculum (sometimes called a pseudo-operculum) may be visible. Visual acuity is commonly reduced to 6/60, but is occasionally better, particularly with eccentric fixation. An operculum (see Fig. 14.50C) consists primarily of glial tissue and condensed vitreous cortex, though 40% contain

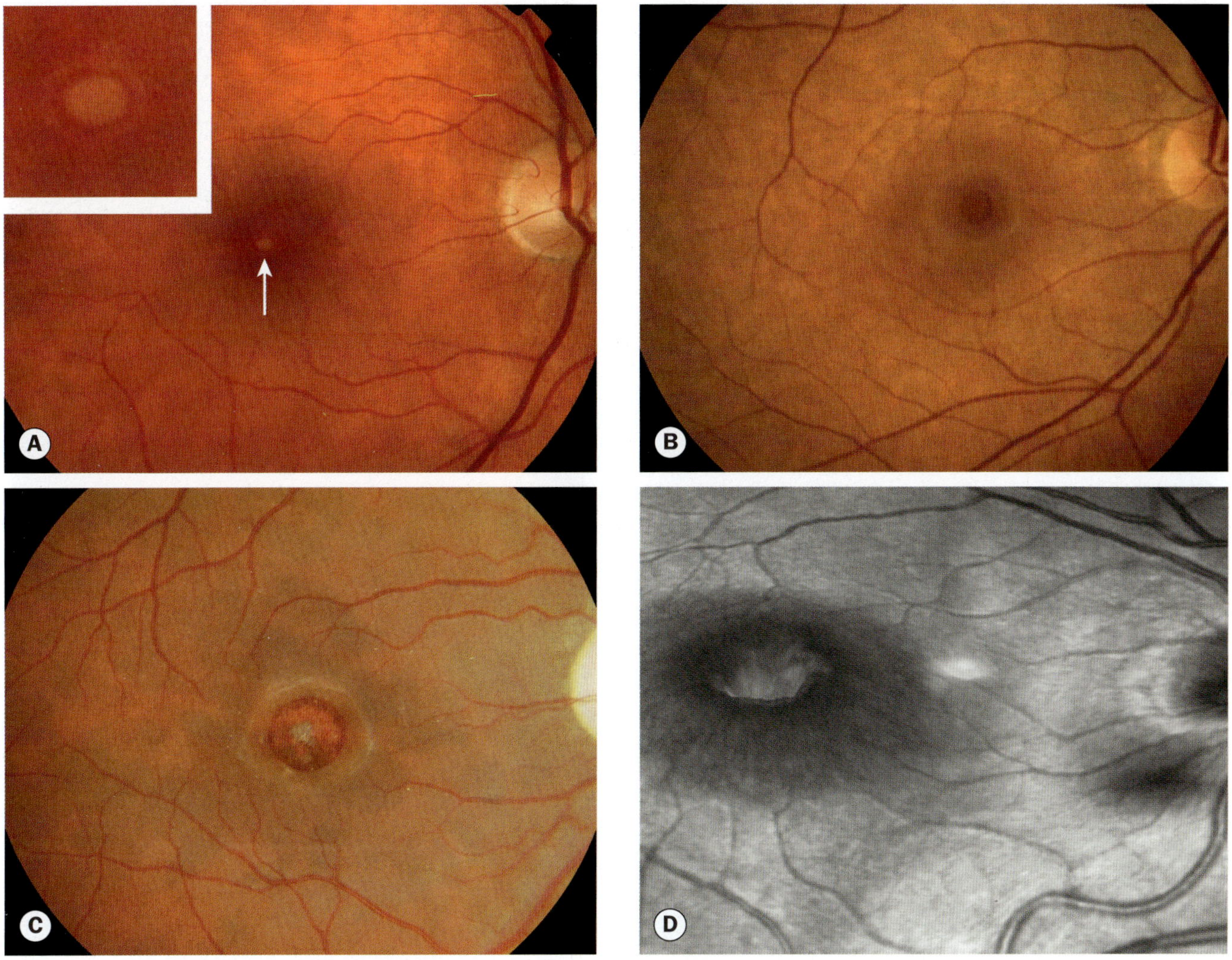

Fig. 14.49 Macular hole. **(A)** Occult – stage 1b (arrow); **(B)** small full-thickness – stage 2; **(C)** full-thickness – stage 3; **(D)** three-dimensional OCT of stage 4 hole (with surrounding subretinal fluid).

photoreceptor elements. By definition, there is persistent parafoveal attachment of the vitreous cortex.

- **Small, medium or large FTMH without VMT.** Clinically stage 4: full-thickness macular hole with complete posterior vitreous detachment, suggested (but not confirmed) by the presence of a Weiss ring. A significant proportion of idiopathic macular holes have an associated ERM.
- **Spontaneously resolved macular hole.** Macular holes may heal spontaneously, often resuming a near-normal or even normal clinical and OCT appearance. A tiny outer retinal – often inner-segment/outer-segment junction – or other subfoveolar defect may persist after spontaneous or surgical closure. Solar retinopathy commonly gives a similar appearance, as does scarring from several other conditions where the foveal centre is a focus of damage.
- **Macular microhole** refers to a small (<150 µm) full-thickness foveal retinal defect and is synonymous with a small full-thickness macular hole (stage 2 above). Symptoms are often minimal and may consist of mild central blurring, metamorphopsia (distortion) or disturbed reading vision. Visual acuity is typically impaired less than with a larger FTMH and the abnormality may not be noticed immediately. The full-thickness defect typically heals within a few weeks and by the time of initial examination only a well-demarcated red spot rather than a visibly full-thickness defect may be present. At this stage OCT may show only a small defect in the inner-segment/outer-segment layer (see Fig. 14.50D).

Investigations

- **Amsler grid** testing will usually show non-specific central distortion rather than a scotoma.
- **The Watzke–Allen test** is performed by projecting a narrow slit beam over the centre of the hole vertically and horizontally, preferably using a fundus contact lens. A patient with a macular hole will report that the beam is thinned or broken. Patients with other pathology usually see a distorted beam of uniform thickness.
- **OCT** is extremely useful in diagnosis and staging (Fig. 14.50A–D) and can show the dynamic nature of the pathology.

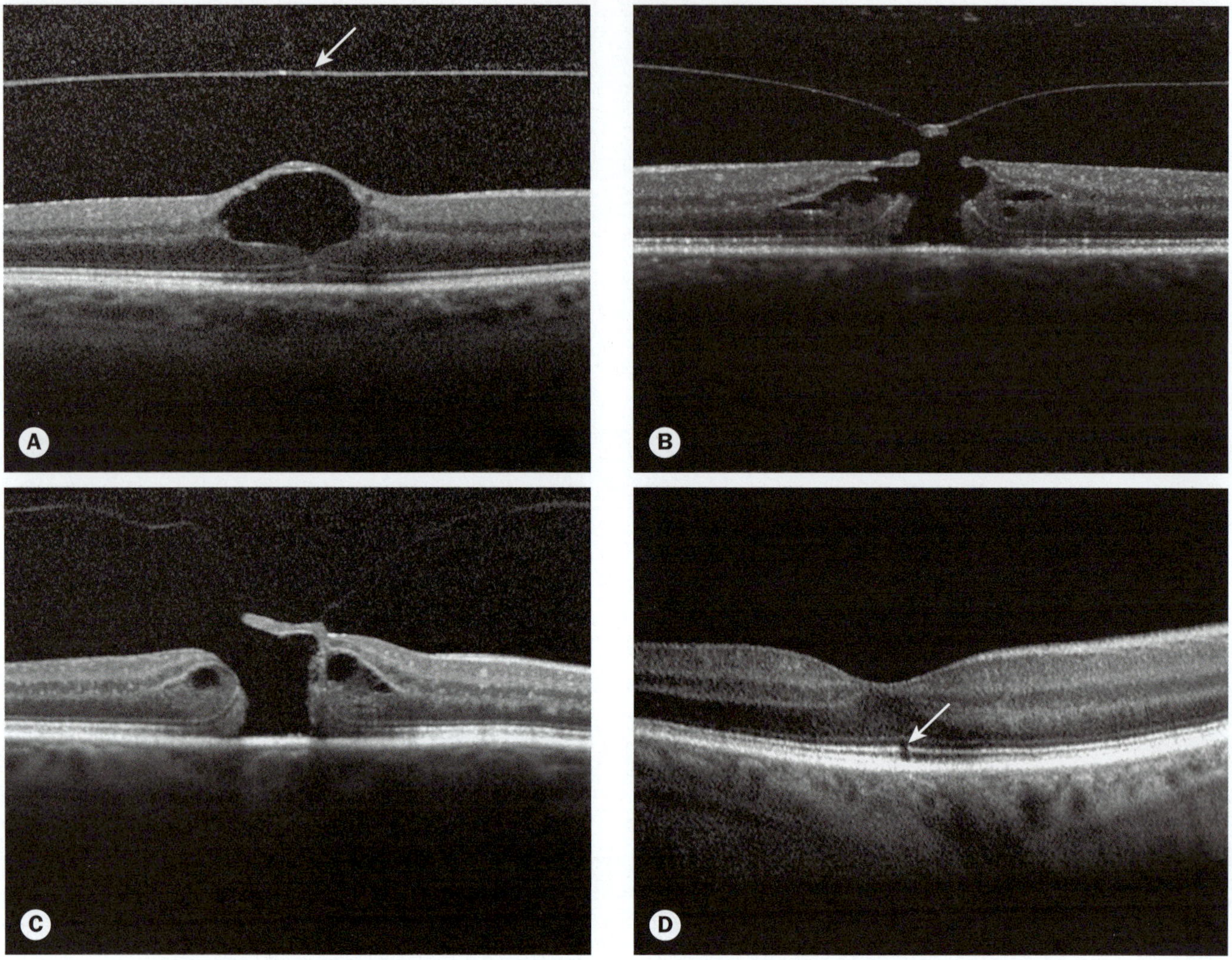

Fig. 14.50 OCT of macular hole. **(A)** The posterior hyaloid is detached from the macular surface (arrow) leaving a lamellar hole. Note the intact layer of inner retina; **(B)** FTMH with separation between inner and outer retina and a small foveal operculum which is attached to the posterior hyaloid face; **(C)** FTMH with intraretinal cystic spaces and overlying operculum (sometimes called a pseudo-operculum); **(D)** resolved macular microhole showing tiny focal inner/outer-segment junction deficit (arrow).

- **FAF** shows a markedly hyperfluorescent foveolar spot in stages 3 and 4 and punctate fluorescence in stage 2.
- **FA** in a full-thickness hole shows an early well-defined window defect. In light of the effectiveness of OCT in this condition there is no need to undertake fluorescein angiography.

TIP OCT is key to the confirmation of the diagnosis of macular hole and for staging purposes.

Treatment

- **The clinical stage and duration** are the most important variables that influence the management and prognosis.
- **Observation.** About 50% of stage 1 holes resolve following spontaneous vitreo-foveolar separation, so these are managed conservatively. About 10% of full-thickness holes also close spontaneously, sometimes with marked visual improvement. Spontaneous resolution is more common with smaller FTMH. Treatment is not needed for spontaneously healed holes, though vitrectomy with ERM peeling is sometimes indicated. Patients whose other eye is healthy should be warned that the risk of the fellow eye becoming involved within 5 years is around 10%. The risk is less if there is already a PVD present.
- **Pharmacological vitreolysis** with ocriplasmin may be suitable for small early-stage holes. It is discussed under 'Vitreomacular traction' below.
- **Intravitreal gas or air.** Preliminary studies suggest that closure may follow an injection of a small bolus of gas into the vitreous.
- **Surgery** may be considered in stage 2 or greater holes and for some lamellar holes. Symptom duration before surgery is strongly and consistently associated with poorer anatomical and visual outcome after surgery. Better results are usually achieved in patients with smaller holes present for under 6 months.

- Operative treatment consists of vitrectomy, together with (a) peeling of the ILM facilitated by vital dye staining, (b) relief of vitreomacular traction by either induction of a total PVD if not already present or removal of the perifoveal vitreous and (c) gas tamponade. The reattachment rate is improved by postoperative face-down positioning (8 hours daily for 5 days). An extensive period of postoperative positioning is not required with modern techniques.
- The hole is closed in most cases and visual improvement occurs over the course of months in 80–90% of eyes, with a final visual acuity of 6/12 or better in approximately 65%. Worsening of visual acuity occurs in up to 10% of eyes. Mild residual abnormality on OCT such as a defect in the inner-segment/outer-segment junction or other disturbance adjacent to the RPE is common and may also provide a diagnostic indicator of a spontaneously healed macular hole or microhole.
- Complications are the same as those occurring after vitrectomy (see Ch. 16).

Vitreomacular traction

Introduction

Physiological PVD (see Ch. 16) usually proceeds gradually over an extended period to encompass complete separation from the macula and optic nerve head: complete PVD. If adhesion of the gel persists at the central macula, an anomalous PVD is present and can precede a range of macular conditions.

- **Vitreomacular adhesion (VMA)** refers to residual attachment of the vitreous within a 3 mm radius of the central macula in the presence of perifoveal vitreous separation. In most cases it constitutes a stage in a dynamic process of PVD so may not incur pathological sequelae. There is no distortion of the foveal contour or any secondary retinal changes. Focal VMA involves an area of attachment of ≤1500 μm diameter, broad VMA >1500 μm.
- **Vitreomacular traction (VMT)** is defined as the presence of retinal changes on OCT with evident perifoveal (within 3 mm) PVD. Distortion of the foveal surface contour and/or other structural retinal changes may be present. Focal (Fig. 14.51A) and broad types are defined as for VMA. Concurrent VMT is associated with other macular disease, e.g. AMD, RVO, DR. Isolated VMT is not associated with other macular disease.
- **Full-thickness macular hole (FTMH).** A foveal lesion featuring interruption of all retinal layers from the internal limiting membrane to the RPE (see above) (Fig. 14.51B). Other considerations include the status of the vitreous (with or without VMT) and the presence of an identifiable cause such as trauma.
- **Lamellar macular hole.** This is a partial-thickness defect of the inner retina at the fovea but maintenance of an intact photoreceptor layer (see Fig. 14.51A). Its pathogenesis is incompletely defined, but may develop from anomalous PVD, sometimes following a foveal pseudocyst, or represent abortive FTMH formation in some patients. Classically, lamellar hole was described as a sequel to CMO.
- **Macular pseudohole.** This lesion mimics the clinical appearance of a FTMH, but is caused by distortion of the perifoveal retina into heaped edges by ERM, without any loss of retinal tissue and near-normal foveal thickness; there is a central defect in the membrane. VMT may be present (see Fig. 14.48D).
- **Epiretinal membrane (ERM).** ERM is independent of the IVTS classification, but most eyes with broad vitreomacular traction have an associated ERM. Vitreous remnants on the retinal surface following PVD provide a mechanism for the development of idiopathic ERM.

Diagnosis

- **Symptoms** in VMT include decreased vision, metamorphopsia, photopsia and micropsia, but are usually milder in lamellar holes and pseudoholes and absent in VMA.
- **Signs** in VMT may include retinal surface thickening, wrinkling and distortion, foveal pseudocyst, CMO, macular schisis

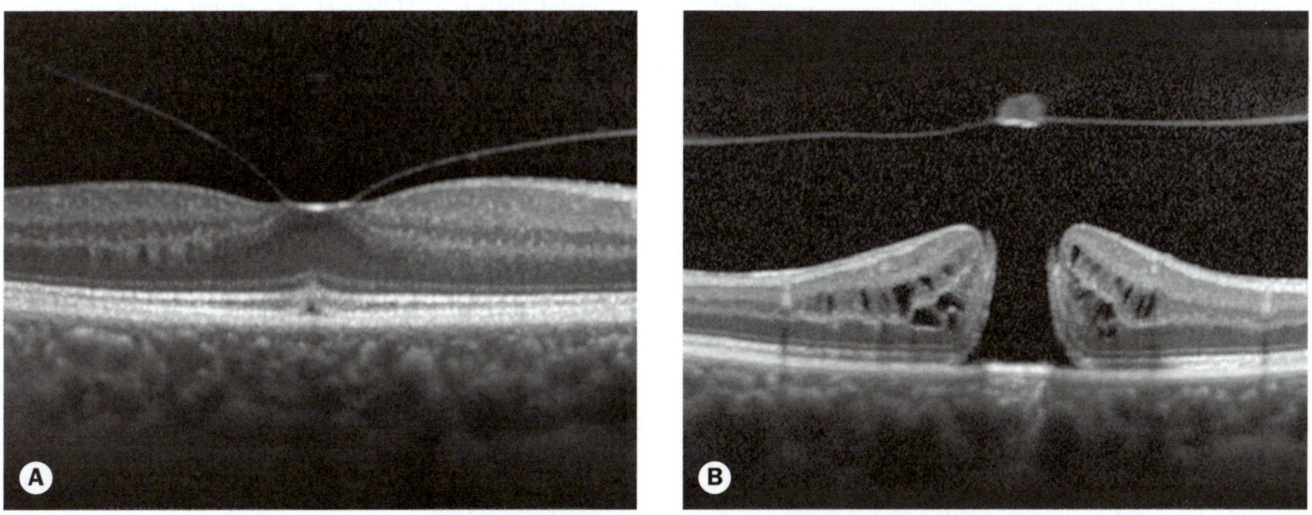

Fig. 14.51 Vitreomacular traction (VMT). **(A)** OCT showing VMT; **(B)** OCT of full-thickness macular hole without VMT, showing interruption of all retinal layers, macular oedema and a small operculum.

or detachment and capillary leakage. The limit of the attached gel may be visible as a whitish band or reflex. Visible changes may be subtle. Both lamellar holes and pseudoholes can appear as a discrete reddish oval or round foveal spot.
- **OCT** is the key investigation.

Treatment

Treatment of FTMH and ERM is considered under separate topics above.

- **Observation.** Spontaneous separation occurs in a proportion of patients with VMT and is more likely in milder cases. Observation is appropriate in patients with VMA and in many cases of VMT.
- **Pharmacological vitreolysis.** Intravitreal injection of ocriplasmin, a recombinant form of human plasmin, releases VMT in over 25% of eyes and may close macular holes where VMT is present (40% versus 10% with placebo). Results are generally inferior to vitrectomy. Smaller areas of VMT and smaller macular holes have better outcomes. The presence of ERM is a poorer prognostic indicator for ocriplasmin treatment. Diffuse retinal dysfunction of uncertain mechanism, including substantially decreased acuity, has been reported as a rare side effect.
- **Pars plana vitrectomy** with peeling of the adherent area and any associated ERM usually gives good results in VMT. The benefit of vitrectomy for lamellar and pseudoholes is less clear-cut, but is probably greater if significant ERM is present.

DEGENERATIVE MYOPIA

Introduction

Myopia is the result of complex hereditary and environmental factors. There is strong evidence for a causative association with long-term intensive near visual activity, particularly reading and using personal computers. A refractive error of more than −6 dioptres constitutes a common definition of high myopia, in which axial length is usually greater than 26 mm. It affects over 2% of adult Western European or American populations and may be as high as 10% in East Asians. Pathological or degenerative myopia is characterized by progressive anteroposterior elongation of the scleral envelope associated with a range of secondary ocular changes, principally thought to relate to mechanical stretching of the involved tissues. It is a significant cause of legal blindness, with maculopathy the most common cause of visual loss.

Low-dose atropine (0.01%) instilled at bed-time can significantly slow the progression of myopia in children. Although there is no consensus, a reasonable approach is to offer this treatment to children between the ages of 5 and 15 years whose myopia is increasing at more than 1 dioptre per year.

These children should also be encouraged to spend more time outdoors in sunshine.

In children aged 7–11 years with less than 5 dioptres of myopia, a high-add (+2.50 D) centre-distance soft multifocal contact lens can be considered. The BLINK trial concludes that this slows the rate of myopia progression and that the response is dose-dependent

Table 14.4 lists systemic associations of high myopia.

Table 14.4 Systemic Associations of High Myopia
Down syndrome
Stickler syndrome
Marfan syndrome
Prematurity
Noonan syndrome
Ehlers–Danlos syndrome
Pierre–Robin syndrome

Diagnosis

- **A pale tessellated** (tigroid) appearance is due to diffuse attenuation of the RPE with visibility of large choroidal vessels (Fig. 14.52A).
- **Focal chorioretinal atrophy** is characterized by patchy visibility of choroidal vessels and often sclera (Fig. 14.52B).
- **Anomalous optic nerve head.** This may appear unusually small, large or anomalous with a 'tilted' conformation (Fig. 14.52C). Peripapillary chorioretinal atrophy is very common, most commonly as a temporal crescent of thinned or absent RPE.
- **Acquired optic disc pit** formation is not uncommon and is thought to be due to expansion of the peripapillary region as the eye enlarges over time.
- **Lattice degeneration** (see Ch. 16).
- **Lacquer cracks** are ruptures in the RPE–Bruch membrane–choriocapillaris complex characterized by fine irregular yellow lines criss-crossing at the posterior pole (Fig. 14.52D) in around 5% of highly myopic eyes and can be complicated by MNV.
- **Subretinal 'coin' haemorrhages** (Fig. 14.52E) may develop from lacquer cracks in the absence of MNV.
- **Fuchs spot** (Fig. 14.52F) is a raised, circular, pigmented lesion at the macula developing after a subretinal haemorrhage has absorbed.
- **Staphyloma** is a peripapillary or macular ectasia of the posterior sclera (Fig. 14.53A and B) due to focal thinning and expansion present in about a third of eyes with pathological myopia. Associations include macular hole formation and 'dome-shaped macula' (see below).
- **(Peripapillary) intrachoroidal cavitation**, formerly described as peripapillary detachment of pathological myopia (PDPM), may occur adjacent to the nerve, commonly inferiorly (Fig. 14.53C). Clinically, it may be evident as a small yellowish-orange peripapillary area typically inferior to the disc. It can usually be identified on OCT (Fig. 14.53D). Visual field defects are common and frequently mimic glaucoma.
- **Rhegmatogenous retinal detachment (RD)** is much more common in high myopia, the pathogenesis including increased frequency of PVD, lattice degeneration, asymptomatic atrophic holes, myopic macular holes (see below) and occasionally giant retinal tears.
- **MNV**
  - 10% of highly myopic eyes develop MNV.

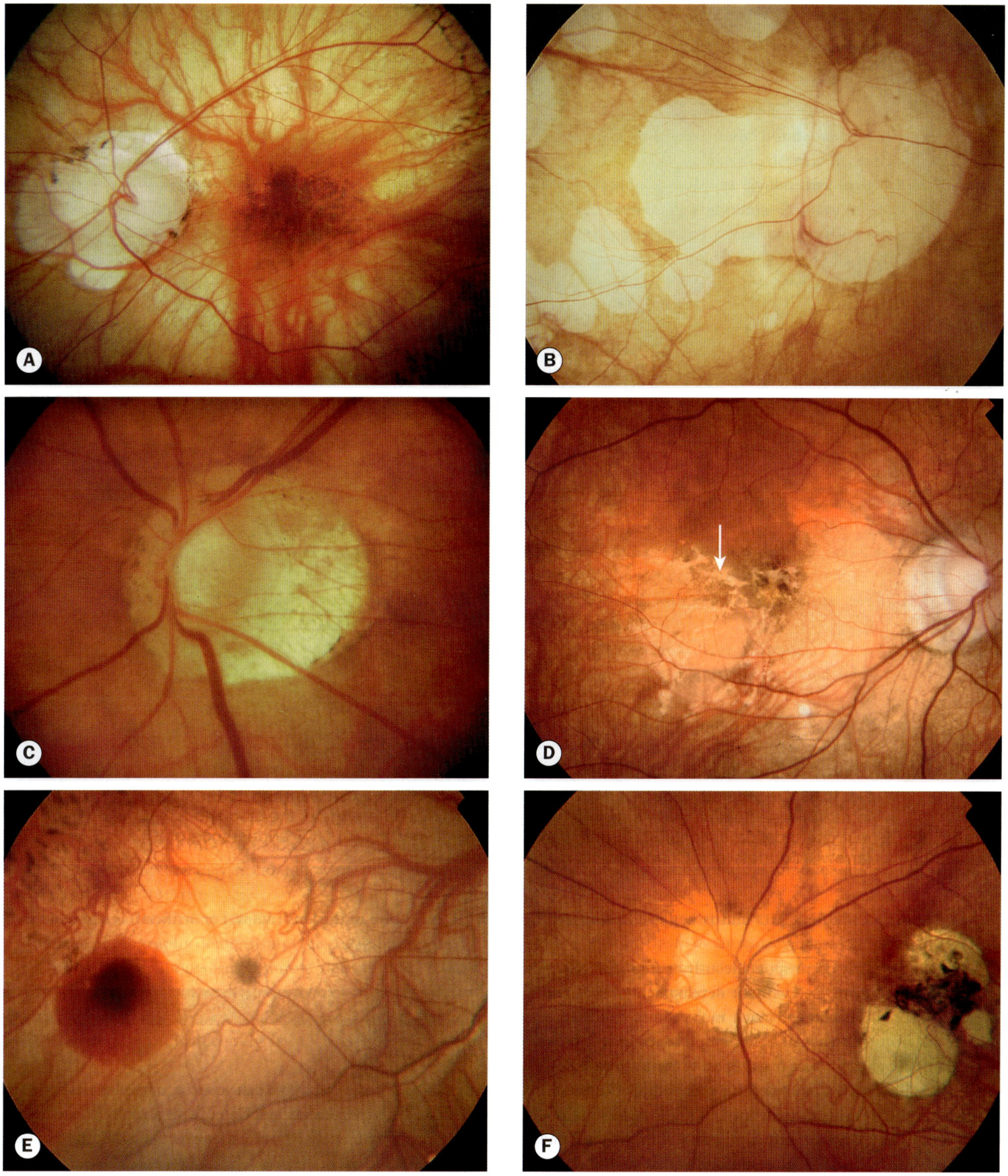

Fig. 14.52 High myopia. **(A)** Tessellated fundus; **(B)** focal chorioretinal atrophy and tilted disc; **(C)** tilted disc with parapapillary atrophy; **(D)** lacquer cracks (arrow); **(E)** 'coin' haemorrhage; **(F)** Fuchs spot.

- The prognosis is better in younger patients with myopia-related MNV than in AMD.
- Anti-VEGF therapy is generally the treatment of choice. The injection frequency may be less than that needed for AMD, but RD risk is higher.

- **Macular retinoschisis** (foveoschisis) and macular retinal detachment without macular hole formation may occur in highly myopic eyes with posterior staphyloma, probably as a result of vitreous traction. Some cases are associated with intrachoroidal cavitation (see above). Retinoschisis may be

INTRODUCTION

General

The inherited retinal degenerations ('retinal dystrophies') are a group of disorders that commonly exert their major effect on the retinal pigment epithelium (RPE)–photoreceptor complex and the choriocapillaris to cause a range of visual impairment. The most common example is retinitis pigmentosa. Hereditary retinal diseases are now the leading cause of blindness certification in the working-age population (age 16–64 years) in the UK. Some inherited retinal degenerations manifest in early childhood while others do not present until later in life. Isolated dystrophies have features confined to the eye, whilst syndromic dystrophies are part of a wider disease process that also affects tissues elsewhere in the body. In a patient with an inherited retinal degeneration, genetic sequencing should be undertaken to determine the exact causative gene, as mutations in a number of genes can cause the same clinical phenotype (genetic heterogeneity) and different phenotypes can be caused by the same gene (phenotypical heterogeneity). Mutations in more than 250 genes have been linked to inherited retinal degenerations and a table of genes associated with these conditions can be found online (https://sph.uth.edu/retnet/). Identification of the causative gene allows the identification of patients who might benefit from novel therapies, although this may only be possible within a clinical trial setting.

TIP Mutations in different genes (genetic heterogeneity) can cause the same clinical phenotype in an individual with an inherited retinal degeneration.

Anatomy

There are two types of retinal photoreceptor:

- **The rods** are the most numerous (120 million) and are of the densest concentration outside the macular region. They are most sensitive in dim illumination and are responsible for night, motion sense and peripheral vision. If rod dysfunction occurs earlier or is more severe than cone dysfunction, it will result initially in poor night vision (nyctalopia). Rod and cone loss results in loss of visual field.
- **The cones** are far fewer in number (6 million) and are concentrated at the fovea. There are three types of cones: **L** (long; the commonest) responding to red wavelengths of light; **M** (medium) responding to yellow-green wavelengths; and **S** (short, only about 2% of the total) responding to blue wavelengths. They are most sensitive in bright light and mediate day vision, colour vision, central and fine vision. Cone dysfunction therefore results in poor central vision, impairment of colour vision (dyschromatopsia) and occasionally problems with day vision (hemeralopia).
- **Photoreceptor structure.** Each photoreceptor consists of an outer segment which is the light-sensitive portion of the cell and an inner segment which is the manufacturing portion of the cell, containing mitochondria and endoplasmic reticulum (Fig. 15.1). These segments are joined by the cilium. In each rod outer segment there are about 1000 separate discs, while in the cones the discs are joined to a boundary membrane with an aperture that allows the discs to be in contact with the extracellular space and therefore with each other. Photopigments exist as transmembrane proteins within the discs. New discs are formed in the region of the cilium and older discs are shed from the tips of the outer segments and undergo phagocytosis by the retinal pigment epithelium (RPE). For rods the discs are shed in packets at the onset of morning light. The process is slower for cones and occurs at night.

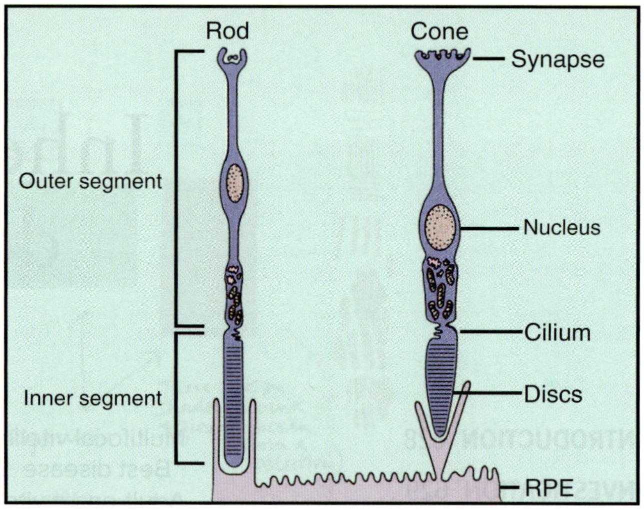

Fig. 15.1 Photoreceptor structure. (RPE = Retinal pigment epithelium.)

Inheritance

All inherited retinal degenerations are caused by genetic variants, most of which are inherited and a few of which occur *de novo*. A new mutation (allelic variant) can occur in an individual and can subsequently be passed to future generations.

- **Autosomal dominant** (AD) conditions often exhibit variable expressivity and tend to have a later onset and milder course than recessive disorders.
- **Recessive** conditions may be autosomal (AR) or X-linked. They generally have an earlier onset and a more severe course than AD conditions. In some cases, female carriers of X-linked conditions show characteristic fundus findings.
- **X-linked dominant** conditions are very rare and are usually lethal in boys (e.g. Aicardi syndrome).
- **Mitochondrial** DNA is inherited solely via the maternal line. Inherited retinal degenerations associated with mitochondrial DNA variants often occur as part of a wider systemic disease. Heteroplasmy describes the presence of more than one type of mitochondrial DNA within a cell. Because cells contain thousands of mitochondria, a low level of heteroplasmy is common in normal individuals. The presence and severity of an inherited retinal degeneration depends on the proportion of faulty mitochondria. The manifestations of mitochondrial-inherited ocular disease usually do not appear before adulthood, as many cell divisions are required for a cell to accumulate enough mutant mitochondria to cause symptoms.

- **Digenic** conditions are due to the combined effect of mutations in two different genes.

TIP Mutations in the same gene can cause different phenotypes (phenotypical heterogeneity) in an individual with an inherited retinal degeneration.

Classification

As well as division by inheritance pattern, dystrophies can be considered as generalized, in which the clinical effects involve the entire fundus (rod-cone or cone-rod, depending on which photoreceptor type is predominantly dysfunctional), or central (local, macula) in which only the macula is affected. They can also be classified according to the element that is the focus of the pathological process (e.g. photoreceptors, RPE or choroid) and by whether they are stationary (non-progressive) or progressive.

INVESTIGATION

After taking a careful history (especially a detailed family history) and undertaking a clinical examination, the main investigations that are usually needed to make a diagnosis of inherited retinal degeneration are OCT and fundus autofluorescence (FAF). Supplementary investigations include electrophysiological and genetic testing.

Electroretinography

Introduction

The electroretinogram (ERG) measures retinal electrical activity. When stimulated by light of adequate intensity, ionic flow – principally sodium and potassium – is induced in or out of cells such that a potential is generated. This retinal electrical activity can be recorded with an electrode placed at or near the cornea and a reference electrode placed on the forehead. The potential between the two electrodes is then amplified and displayed (Fig. 15.2). The normal ERG is predominantly biphasic (Fig. 15.3A):

- **The a-wave** is an initial fast corneal-negative deflection generated by the photoreceptors.
- **The b-wave** is a subsequent slower positive large-amplitude deflection. Although it is generated from Müller and bipolar cells, it is directly dependent on functional photoreceptors and its magnitude makes it a convenient measure of photoreceptor integrity. Its amplitude is measured from the a-wave trough to the b-wave peak. The b-wave is enhanced with dark adaptation and increased light stimulus.
- **Reduced ratio.** As a general principle, a reduced ratio between a- and b-waves indicates inner retinal dysfunction.
- **The c-wave** is a third (negative) deflection generated by the RPE and photoreceptors.
- **Latency** is the interval to the commencement of the a-wave after the stimulus is applied.
- **Implicit time** is the interval from the stimulus to the b-wave peak.

Electroretinography may be used for the diagnosis of a range of different retinal disorders on the basis of characteristic patterns of change, as well as monitoring of disease progress in dystrophies and other conditions such as some forms of uveitis (e.g. birdshot retinochoroiditis) and drug toxicity (e.g. hydroxychloroquine).

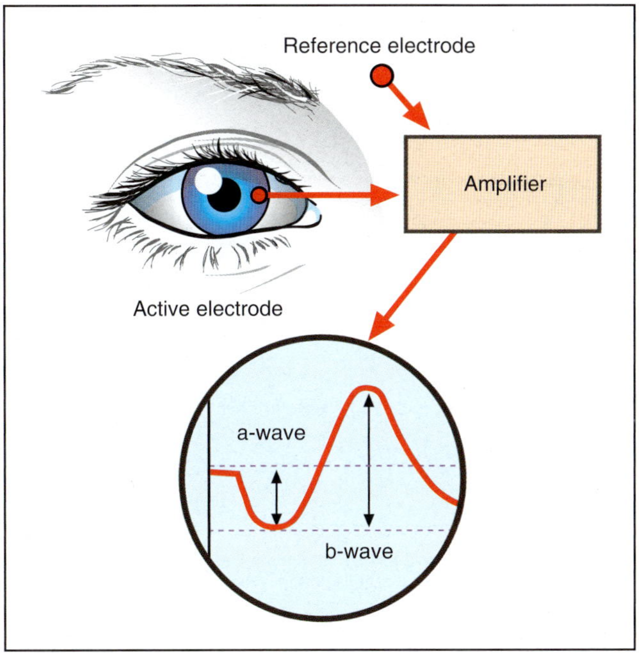

Fig. 15.2 Principles of electroretinography.

TIP High-quality retinal imaging techniques and specific genetic testing in a patient with an inherited retinal degeneration is more commonly used than electroretinography.

Full-field ERG

Guidelines for the preparation of a patient who requires an ERG and the minimum set of responses that need to be obtained have been published by the International Society for Clinical Electrophysiology of Vision (ISCEV-2022 update). A standard full-field ERG (Fig. 15.3B) consists of six recordings and is taken during diffuse stimulation of the entire retinal area. It is used to assess generalized retinal disorders, but may not detect localized pathology. The first three recordings are elicited after a minimum of 20 minutes of dark adaptation (scotopic) and the last three after 10 minutes of adaptation to moderately bright diffuse illumination (photopic). Several responses are usually averaged to improve the signal-to-noise ratio. It may be difficult to dark-adapt children for 30 minutes and therefore dim light (mesopic) conditions can be utilized to evoke predominantly rod-mediated responses to low-intensity white or blue light stimuli.

- **Scotopic ERG**
  - Rod responses are elicited with a very dim flash of 0.01 cd•s/m^2, resulting in a small b-wave and a barely visible a-wave.
  - Combined rod and cone responses are elicited with a very bright white flash, resulting in a prominent a-wave and b-wave.
  - Oscillatory potentials are elicited by using a bright flash and changing the recording parameters. The oscillatory

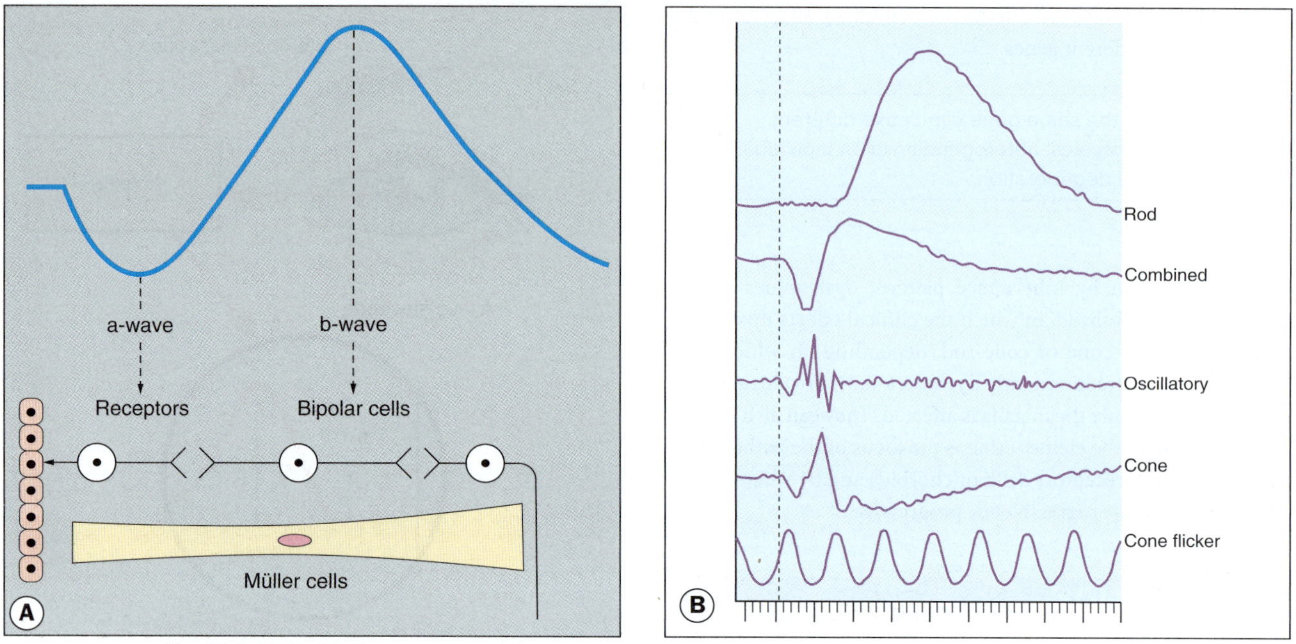

Fig. 15.3 ERG. **(A)** Components and origins of the electroretinogram; **(B)** normal electroretinographic recordings (dark-adapted responses at 3 and 10 minutes are incorporated in the combined tracing).

wavelets occur on the ascending limb of the b-wave and are generated by cells in the inner retina.

- **Photopic ERG**
  - Cone responses are elicited with a single bright flash, resulting in an a- and a b-wave with subsequent small oscillations.
  - Cone flicker is used to isolate cones by using a flickering light stimulus at a frequency of 30 Hz to which rods cannot respond. It provides a measure of the amplitude and implicit time of the cone b-wave. Cone responses can be elicited in normal eyes up to 50 Hz, after which point individual responses are no longer recordable ('critical flicker fusion').

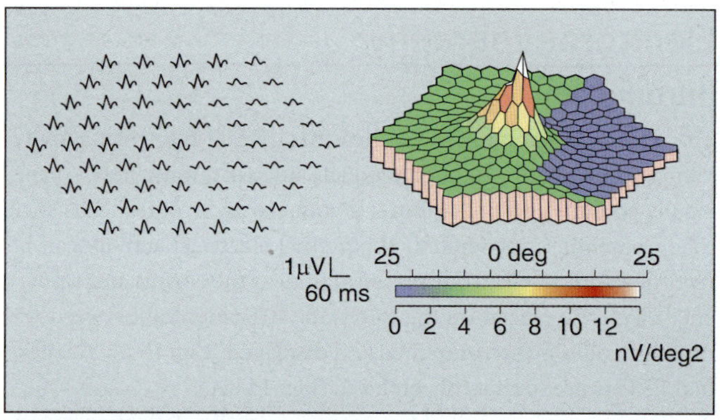

Fig. 15.4 Multifocal electroretinogram.

Multifocal ERG

Multifocal ERG is a method of producing topographical maps of retinal function (Fig. 15.4). The stimulus is scaled for variation in photoreceptor density across the retina. At the fovea, where the density of receptors is high, a lesser stimulus is employed than in the periphery where receptor density is lower. As with conventional ERG, many types of measurements can be made. Both the amplitude and timing of the troughs and peaks can be measured and reported, and the information can be summarized in the form of a three-dimensional plot which resembles the hill of vision.

Focal ERG

Focal (foveal) ERG can be used to assess macular disease, but is rarely utilized.

Pattern ERG

A similar stimulus to that used in visual evoked potentials (see Ch. 19), pattern reversal, is used to target ganglion cell function, typically in order to detect subtle optic neuropathy and early glaucoma (see Fig. 11.25A and B).

Electro-oculography

The electro-oculogram (EOG) measures the standing potential between the electrically positive cornea and the electrically negative back of the eye (Fig. 15.5). It reflects the activity of the RPE and the photoreceptors. The ISCEV (www.iscev.org) has determined standards for clinical EOG. In general, diffuse or widespread disease of the RPE is needed to significantly affect the response. The EOG is always abnormal if there is widespread photoreceptor dysfunction. As there is much variation in EOG amplitude in normal subjects, the result is calculated by dividing the maximal height of the potential in the light ('light peak') by the minimal height of the potential in the dark ('dark trough'). This is expressed as a ratio (Arden ratio) with a normal value that is typically more than 1.7.

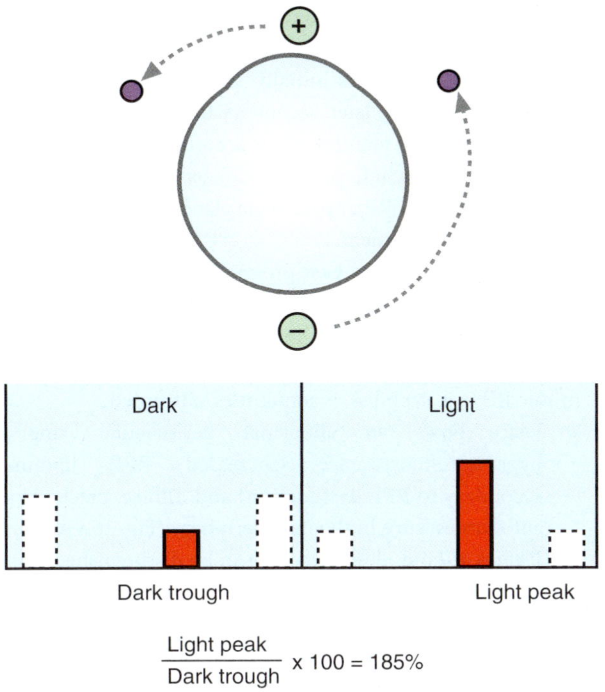

Fig. 15.5 Principles of electro-oculography.

Dark adaptometry

Dark adaptation (DA) is the phenomenon by which the visual system adapts to decreased illumination and evaluation of this is particularly useful in the investigation of nyctalopia. The retina is exposed to an intense light for a time sufficient to bleach 25% or more of the rhodopsin in the retina. Following this, normal rods are insensitive to light and cones respond only to very bright stimuli. Subsequent recovery of light sensitivity can be monitored by placing the subject in the dark and periodically presenting spots of light of varying intensity in the visual field and asking the subject if they are perceived. The threshold at which the subject just perceives a light is recorded, the flashes repeated at regular intervals and the increased sensitivity of the eye to light plotted: the dark adaptation curve (Fig. 15.6).

- **The cone branch** of the curve represents the initial 5–10 minutes of darkness during which cone sensitivity rapidly improves. The rod photoreceptors are also recovering, but more slowly during this time.
- **The 'rod-cone' break** normally occurs after 7–10 minutes when cones achieve their maximum sensitivity and the rods become perceptibly more sensitive than cones.
- **The rod branch** of the curve is slower and represents the continuation of improvement of rod sensitivity. After 15–30 minutes, the fully dark-adapted rods allow the subject to perceive a spot of light over 100 times dimmer than would be possible with cones alone. If the flashes are focused onto the foveola (where rods are absent), only a rapid segment corresponding to cone adaptation is recorded.

Genetic testing

This should be undertaken in association with a geneticist who has access to a laboratory that can undertake the necessary tests.

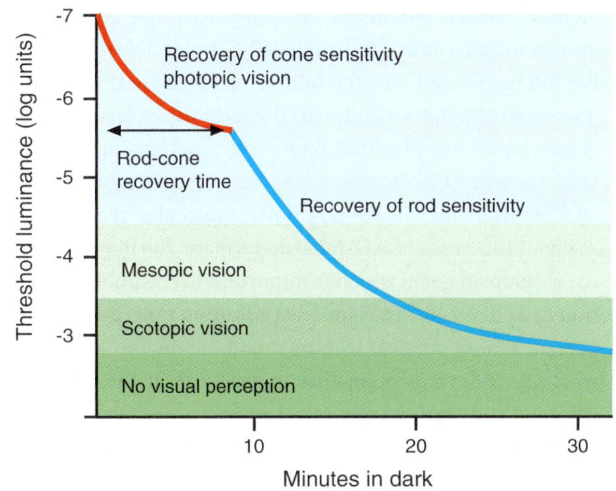

Fig. 15.6 Dark adaptation curve.

- **Single gene testing** is used in patients with a family history of a known genetic mutation, in order to confirm the molecular diagnosis.
- **Sequencing** using targeted panels of all known inherited retinal degeneration genes has been developed and yields high diagnostic rates. Once a genetic defect is identified, Sanger single gene sequencing can be undertaken to confirm the mutation.

TIP A monogenetic retinal degeneration can develop at any age and although the genetic abnormality can often be determined using modern techniques, a substantial number of patients with an inherited retinal degeneration remain without a genetic diagnosis.

GENERALIZED PHOTORECEPTOR DYSTROPHIES

Retinitis pigmentosa

Introduction

- **Definition.** Retinitis pigmentosa (RP), or pigmented retinal degeneration, denotes a clinically and genetically diverse group of inherited diffuse retinal degenerative diseases initially predominantly affecting the rod photoreceptors, with subsequent less marked degeneration of cones and retinal pigment epithelium.
- **Prevalence.** It is the most common hereditary retinal degeneration, with a prevalence of 1:3000 to 1:5000. The age of onset, rate of progression, eventual visual loss and associated ocular features are frequently related to the mode of inheritance. However, the severity of disease at a given age can vary in different patients with the same gene defect.
- **Inheritance.** RP may occur as a sporadic disorder or can be inherited in an AD, AR or X-linked pattern. Sporadic cases are also AD, AR or X-linked, but they have no other known affected family members. The reasons for this include: (a) incomplete penetrance, (b) AR inheritance in small families, (c) non-paternity, (d) death before onset of the disease.

- **Genetic defect.** Mutations in more than 100 gene loci are known to cause non-syndromic RP. Genetic defects that cause RP can be divided into the following: (a) those that affect the phototransduction cascade, (b) the retinoid cycle, (c) photoreceptor structure, (d) other biological functions of the photoreceptor and RPE. Despite advances in genetics, about half of affected individuals have no known molecular genetic abnormality. Most cases of AD-inherited RP are due to mutations of the rhodopsin gene, which is important in the phototransduction cascade. X-linked is the least common inheritance pattern and in 90% of cases is due to mutations in the *RPGR* gene, which encodes a protein that is localized in the connecting cilium of rod photoreceptors.
- **Syndromic RP.** In 20–30% of cases, RP, often atypical (see below), is associated with a systemic disorder. These conditions are usually of AR or mitochondrial inheritance.
- **Leber congenital amaurosis.** Around 5% of RP belongs to the very early-onset severe type grouped together as Leber congenital amaurosis (see separate topic).

Diagnosis

The classic triad of findings comprises bone-spicule retinal pigmentation, arteriolar attenuation and 'waxy' disc pallor. There is often significant symmetry in the retinal appearance of the two eyes. There may be a family history of RP and a pedigree should be prepared.

- **Symptoms**
  - Nyctalopia and dark adaptation difficulties are frequently presenting symptoms, but peripheral visual problems may be noticed.
  - Reduced central vision tends to be a later feature, but can be involved earlier if a cataract develops.
  - Photopsia is not uncommon.
- **Signs**
  - Visual acuity may be normal. Contrast sensitivity may be affected at an earlier stage than visual acuity.
  - Bilateral mid-peripheral intraretinal perivascular 'bone-spicule' pigmentary changes and RPE atrophy associated with arteriolar narrowing (Fig. 15.7A and B).
  - There is a gradual increase in density of the pigment with anterior and posterior spread and a tessellated fundus appearance develops due to unmasking of large choroidal vessels (Fig. 15.7C).
  - Peripheral pigmentation may become severe, with marked arteriolar narrowing and disc pallor (Fig. 15.7D).
  - The macula may show atrophy, epiretinal membrane (ERM) formation and cystoid macular oedema (CMO).
  - Myopia is common.
  - Optic disc drusen occur more frequently in patients with RP.
- **Female carriers** of the X-linked form may have normal fundi or show a golden-metallic ('tapetal') reflex at the macula (Fig. 15.8A) and/or small peripheral patches of bone-spicule pigmentation. The most striking feature of the carrier state is centrifugal hyperautofluorescent lines on FAF imaging (Fig. 15.8B).
- **RP *sine pigmento*** is characterized by an absence or paucity of pigment accumulation and is not a separate form of the disease. Every patient with RP is initially '*sine pigmento*', as the bone spicules only develop later, secondary to photoreceptor degeneration. Functional manifestations are similar to typical RP.
- **Complications** include posterior subcapsular cataract (common in all forms of RP), open-angle glaucoma (3%) and posterior vitreous detachment.
- **Prognosis.** AD has the best prognosis. X-linked is the most severe form with reduction of central vision to 6/60 or less by the fifth decade of life. AR is intermediate in severity.
- **Investigation.** Investigation for infectious conditions that mimic RP (e.g. syphilis), is sometimes warranted.
  - FAF shows an abnormal perimacular ring of hyper-autofluorescence (increased RPE lipofuscin secondary to RPE dysfunction) and diffuse, patchy hypo-autofluorescence in the mid-periphery (Fig. 15.9A). Using FAF as a stand-alone test, RP can be distinguished from a normal fundus in 95% of cases.
  - OCT contributes to the analysis of macular involvement in RP and has prognostic value. Macular oedema can be detected in about 15% and macular atrophy in about 40% of patients with RP.
  - Perimetry initially demonstrates small mid-peripheral scotomas that gradually coalesce and may deteriorate to leave a tiny island of residual central vision (Fig. 15.9B) that may subsequently be extinguished. Microperimetry is useful for central visual assessment.
  - Full-field ERG is a sensitive diagnostic test, but is rarely needed. In early disease it shows reduced scotopic rod and combined responses (Fig. 15.10). Photopic responses reduce with progression and eventually the ERG becomes extinguished.
  - Dark adaptation is prolonged and measuring this using the Dark Adaptation Test may be useful in equivocal early cases.
  - Genetic analysis may identify the particular mutation responsible in an individual patient and facilitate genetic counselling, including the risk of transmission to offspring.

TIP Identifying the precise mutation responsible for an inherited retinal degeneration aids genetic counselling and can facilitate enrolment in a clinical trial.

Management

- **Treatment.** No specific treatment is commercially available, but gene therapy is showing promise in early trials. Luxturna is an approved and commercially available gene therapy for patients with *RPE 65* mutations.
- **Annual follow-up** is recommended in order to detect treatable vision-threatening complications, provide support and maintain contact in case of therapeutic innovation.
- **Cataract surgery** is often beneficial.
- **Low-vision aid** provision, rehabilitation and social service access when appropriate.
- **Smoking** should be avoided.

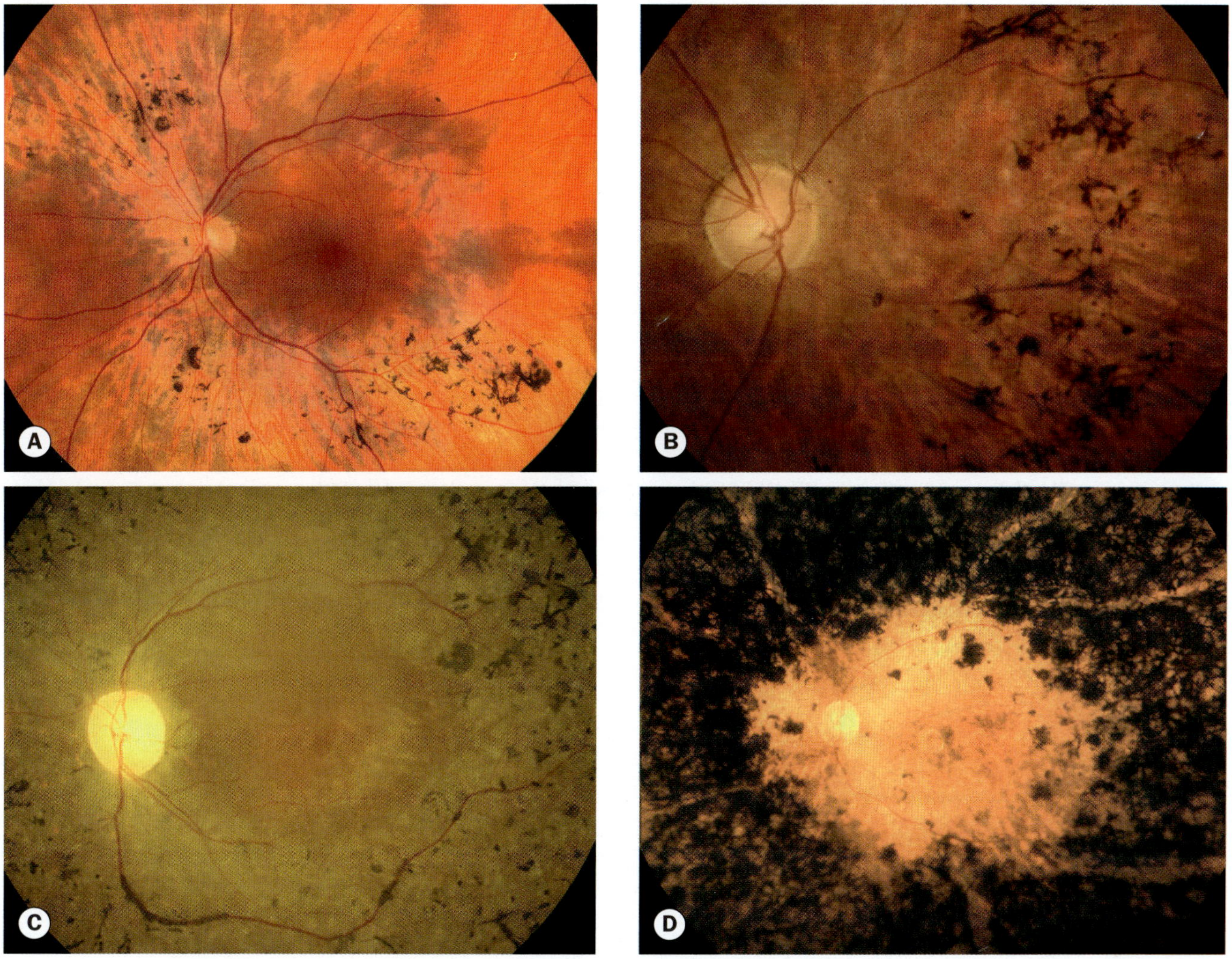

Fig. 15.7 Progression of retinitis pigmentosa. **(A)** Early changes; **(B)** moderate changes; **(C)** advanced changes showing a waxy disc and vessel attenuation; **(D)** wide-field image in end-stage disease. *(Courtesy of P Saine – fig. A.)*

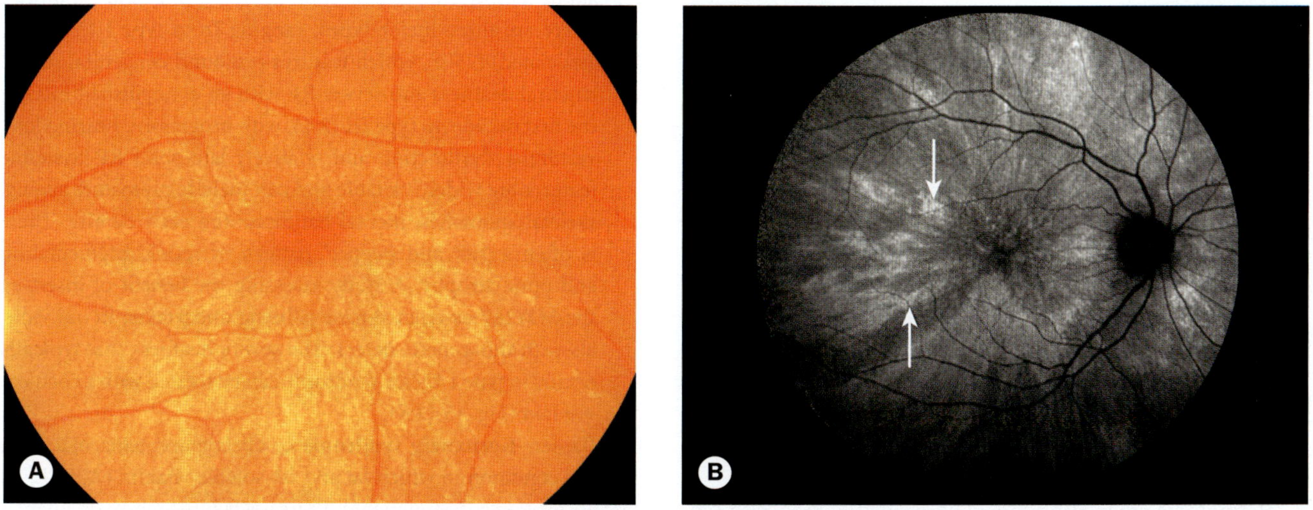

Fig. 15.8 Findings in carriers of X-linked retinitis pigmentosa. **(A)** 'Tapetal' reflex at the macula; **(B)** FAF showing characteristic radial hyperautofluorescent streaks (arrows). *(Courtesy of P Charbel Issa – fig. B.)*

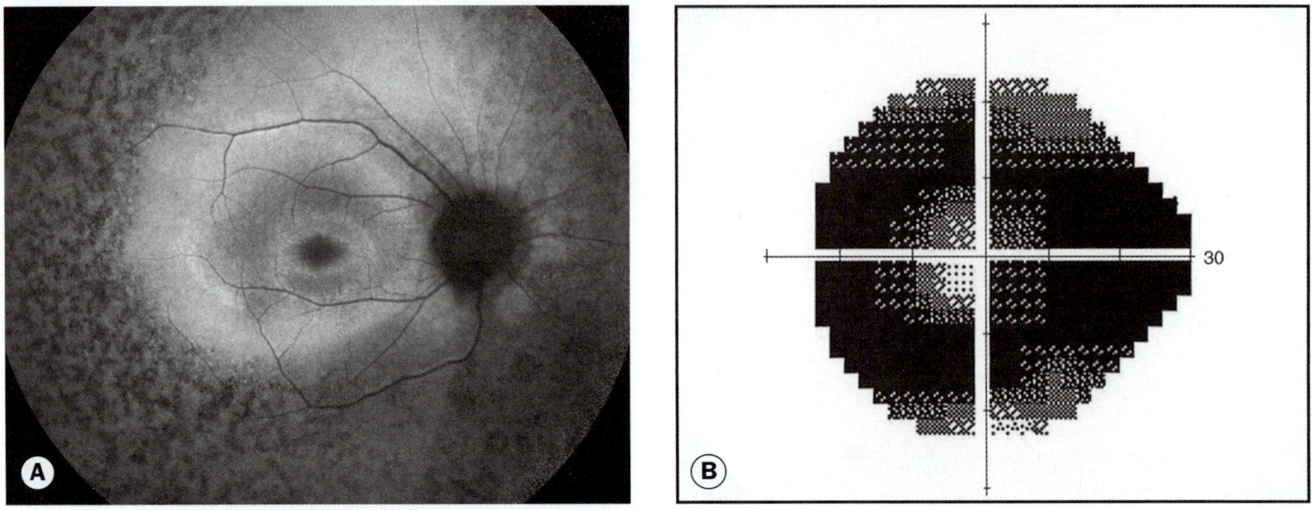

Fig. 15.9 Investigations in RP. **(A)** FAF showing two posterior pole hyperautofluorescent rings and mottled hypoautofluorescence in the mid-periphery; **(B)** perimetry: visual field constriction in advanced retinitis pigmentosa.

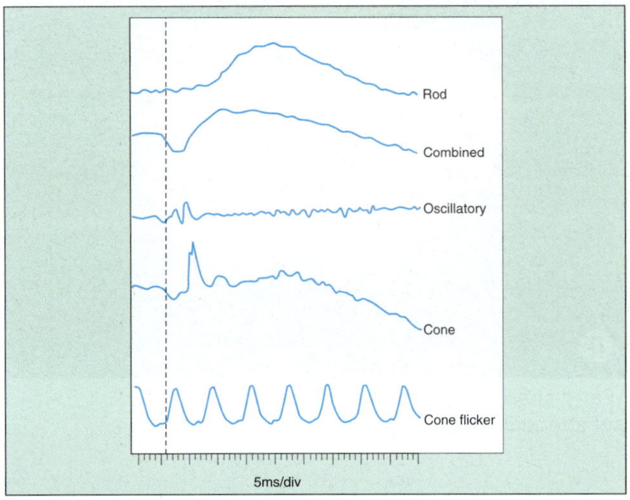

Fig. 15.10 ERG in early retinitis pigmentosa showing reduced scotopic rod and combined responses.

- **Light exposure.** Some forms of RP may be modified by reducing light exposure and therefore blocking short-wavelength light below approximately 550 nm might be beneficial. Indoor amber spectacles blocking to 511–527 nm may improve contrast sensitivity and reduce glare.
- **CMO** in RP may respond to oral acetazolamide and sometimes topical carbonic anhydrase inhibitors.
- **Dietary supplementation.** The use of high-doses of vitamin A has been explored, but there is no consensus on its potential beneficial effect, which might be gene-dependent. Caution is advisable in light of potential adverse effects. Several other supplements and drugs (e.g. lutein, zeaxanthin, calcium-channel blockers) have shown potential benefits, but their efficacy and safety in RP have not been fully ascertained.
- **Retinotoxic medication** should be avoided or used with caution. Examples include isotretinoin and other retinoids, phenothiazines, hydroxychloroquine, tamoxifen and vigabatrin.

TIP Therapeutic options that can be helpful in selected cases of retinitis pigmentosa include phacoemulsification with IOL implantation and medical treatment for macular oedema.

Atypical retinitis pigmentosa

Introduction

The term 'atypical RP' has conventionally been used to group together heterogeneous disorders clinically having features in common with typical pigmentary retinal degeneration. The precise conditions included within this category vary between authors.

Atypical RP associated with a systemic disorder (syndromic RP)

- **Usher syndrome** (AR, genetically heterogeneous) accounts for about 5% of all cases of profound deafness in children and about half of all cases of combined deafness and blindness. There are three major types, ranging from type I (*MYOA7*-associated) (75%), which features profound congenital sensorineural deafness and severe RP with an extinguished ERG in the first decade, to type III (2%), with progressive hearing loss, vestibular dysfunction and relatively late-onset RP. Systemic features are widely variable and can include premature ageing, skeletal anomalies, mental handicap and early demise. There is often a 'salt and pepper' pattern of retinal pigmentation and optic atrophy. A study assessing the benefit of inserting the *MYOA7*-associated gene is being undertaken in individuals with this genetic defect. The severe deafness that typically occurs in type 1 Usher syndrome can be treated with a cochlear implant (Fig. 15.11A).
- **Bassen–Kornzweig syndrome** or abetalipoproteinaemia (AR) is a condition in which fat and fat-soluble vitamin (A, D, E, K) absorption is dysfunctional. There is a failure to thrive in infancy, with the development of severe spinocerebellar ataxia. A blood film shows 'thorny' red cells (acanthocytosis – Fig. 15.11B).

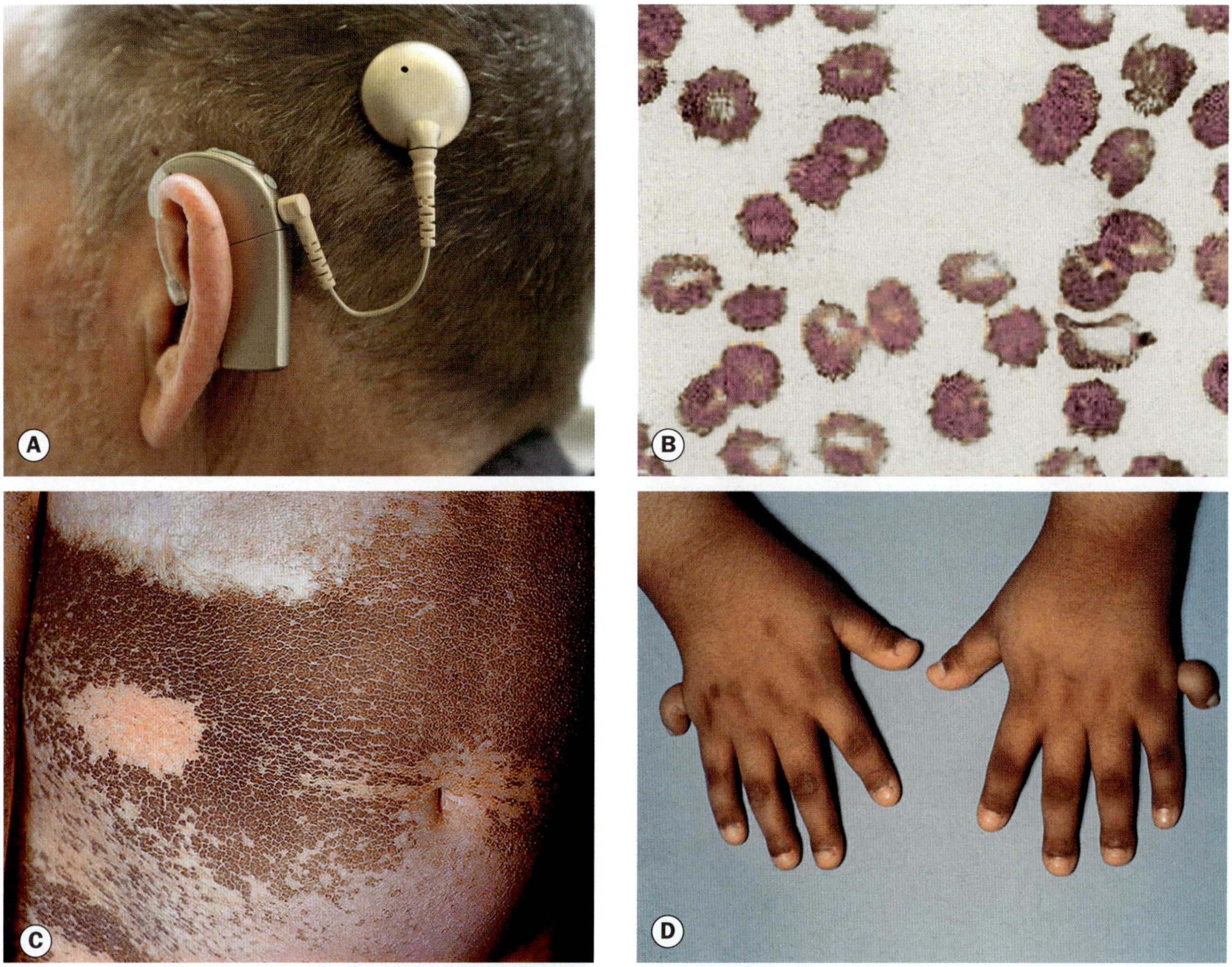

Fig. 15.11 Selected systemic associations of retinitis pigmentosa. **(A)** Cochlear implant to treat deafness in type 1 Usher syndrome; **(B)** acanthocytosis in Bassen–Kornzweig syndrome; **(C)** ichthyosis in adult Refsum disease; **(D)** polydactyly in Bardet–Biedl syndrome.

The fundus exhibits scattered white dots followed by RP-like changes developing towards the end of the first decade. Other features include ptosis, ophthalmoplegia, strabismus and nystagmus. Vitamin supplementation and a low-fat diet should be implemented.

- **Refsum disease** (AR) is rare and consists of genetically and clinically distinct infantile and adult forms. Phytanic acid accumulates throughout the body, with substantial and varied skin (Fig. 15.11C), neurological and visceral features. Retinal changes may be similar to RP or take on a salt and pepper appearance and there may be other ocular features such as cataract and optic atrophy. A low phytanic acid diet can retard progression.
- **Bardet–Biedl syndrome** (most cases AR; genetically heterogenous) is rare and occurs as a consequence of mutations in the genes responsible for proteins involved in non-motor cilia function. It can encompass a range of systemic abnormalities including polydactyly (Fig. 15.11D), dysfunction of the kidneys and mental handicap. Visual symptoms include nyctalopia, visual field constriction and later, loss of visual acuity. There is typically a bull's-eye maculopathy due to cone-rod dystrophy and less frequently RP. Almost 80% have severe changes by the age of 20 years.

Sector retinitis pigmentosa

Sector (sectoral) RP (AD) is characterized by involvement of inferior quadrants only (Fig. 15.12). Progression is slow and many cases are apparently stationary. Unilateral RP can also occur.

Kearns–Sayre syndrome

Kearns-Sayre syndrome is rare and is most commonly due to single deletions in mitochondrial DNA. The retinal disease is **not an atypical form** of RP. Patients typically present within the first two decades of life with chronic progressive external ophthalmoplegia, bilateral ptosis (see Fig. 19.101A) and subsequently develop a salt and pepper retinal appearance, most striking at the macula (see Fig. 19.101B). Cardiac abnormalities and other systemic problems may occur.

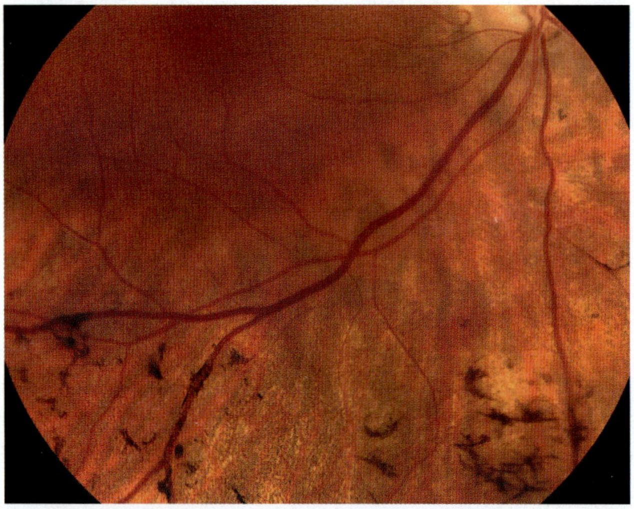

Fig. 15.12 Sectoral retinitis pigmentosa.

Leber congenital amaurosis

Leber congenital amaurosis (AR, genetically heterogeneous) is a severe inherited retinal degeneration affecting rods and cones. It usually has a recessive inheritance pattern and is genetically heterogenous. Variants in three of the at least 28 different genes known to be responsible for this disease are inherited in an AD manner. Mutation in the *RPE65* gene is one of the major causes. Some cases are association with mental handicap, deafness, epilepsy, central nervous system and renal anomalies, skeletal malformations and endocrine dysfunction.

- **Presentation** is with blindness at birth or early infancy, associated with roving eye movements or nystagmus and photoaversion.
- **Signs** are variable but may include:
  - Absent or diminished pupillary light reflexes.
  - The fundi may be normal in early life apart from mild arteriolar narrowing.
  - Initially mild peripheral pigmentary retinopathy (Fig. 15.13A), salt and pepper changes and, less frequently, yellow flecks.

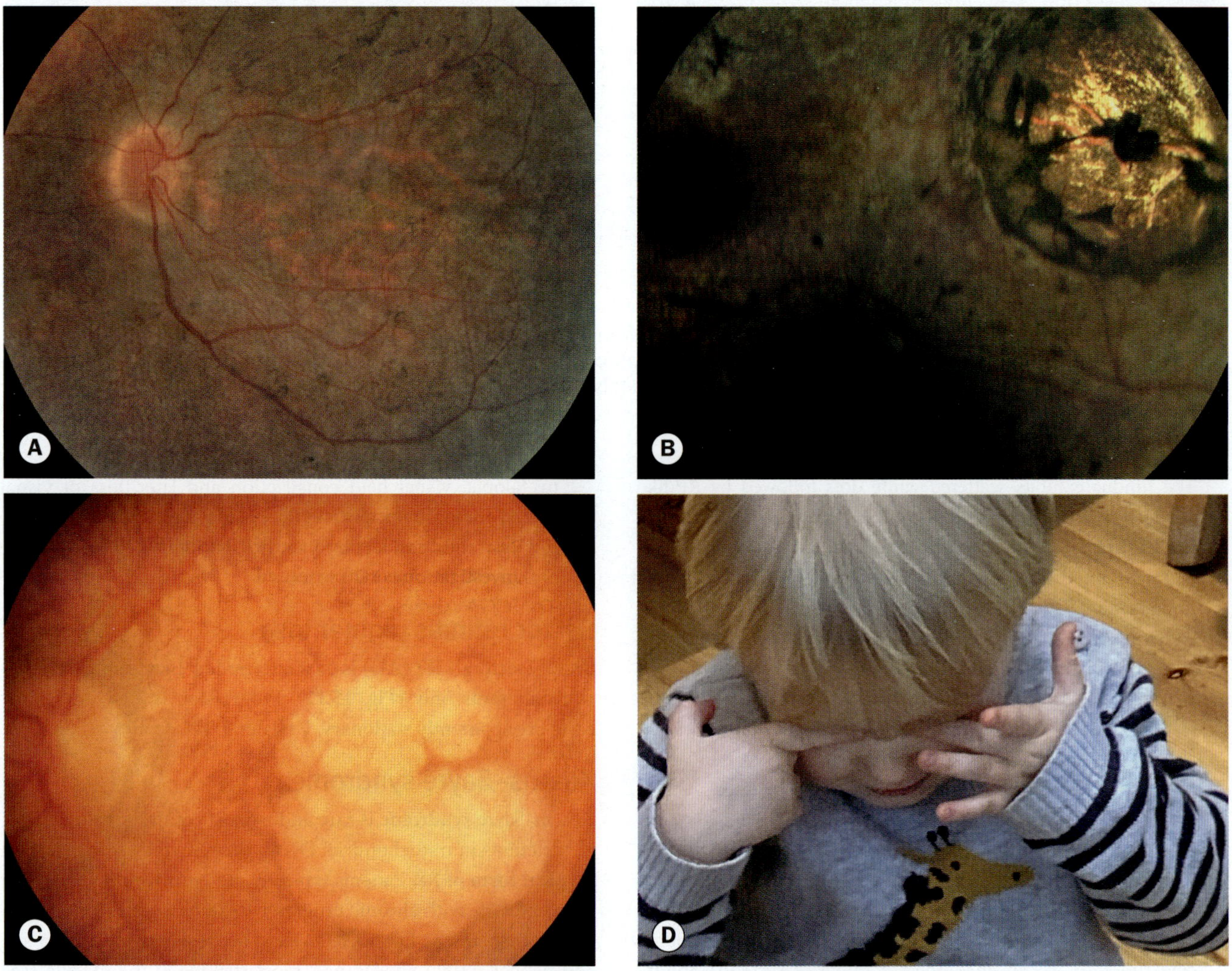

Fig. 15.13 Leber congenital amaurosis. **(A)** Mild pigmentary retinopathy; **(B)** macular pigmentation and optic disc drusen; **(C)** macular atrophy; **(D)** oculodigital syndrome. *(Courtesy of A Moore – figs A and B.)*

  - In some sub-forms, severe macular pigmentation (Fig. 15.13B) or macular atrophy may occur (Fig. 15.13C).
  - Pigmentary retinopathy, optic atrophy and severe arteriolar narrowing in later childhood.
  - Oculodigital syndrome: constant rubbing of the eyes may cause orbital fat atrophy with enophthalmos (Fig. 15.13D) and subsequent keratoconus or keratoglobus.
  - Other associations include strabismus, hypermetropia or myopia and cataract.
  - FAF shows hypoautofluorescence in children with *RPE 65* gene mutation.
- **Treatment**
  - Low visual aids, advice on schooling, rehabilitation and access to social services.
  - A single subretinal injection of adeno-associated virus (AAV)-mediated *RPE65* gene therapy (Luxturna) has shown remarkable results in some cases of LCA. Postoperative ocular inflammation, which occurs in about 50% of cases, responds to immunosuppressive treatment. Some other genetic causes are currently subject to clinical trials.

Pigmented paravenous chorioretinal atrophy

Pigmented paravenous chorioretinal atrophy (predominantly AD) is usually asymptomatic and non-progressive. The ERG is normal. Paravenous bone-spicule pigmentation (Fig. 15.14) is seen, together with sharply outlined zones of chorioretinal atrophy that follow the course of the major retinal veins. Changes may also encircle the optic disc. The optic disc and vascular calibre are usually normal.

CRB-1 associated retinal dystrophy

CRB-1 encodes a transmembrane protein with the main role of maintaining the zonula adherens junctions between photoreceptors, Müller cells and the external limiting membrane and is key to the preservation of an organized photoreceptor layer. Variants of this gene (AR inheritance) are associated with a wide and complex range of phenotypes, the commonest of which is Leber congenital amaurosis in infants (10% of all cases), retinitis pigmentosa in teens and cone-rod dystrophies at any age. Distinctive features include the presence of nummular pigmented deposits and small yellow or white dots (Fig. 15.15A). FAF shows circumferential hyperautofluorescence in the macular region and alongside retinal arterioles. (Fig. 15.15B). OCT reveals preserved para-arteriolar RPE and abnormally laminated, thickened retina (Fig. 15.15C). There is no treatment, but *CRB-1* gene therapy may offer help in the future.

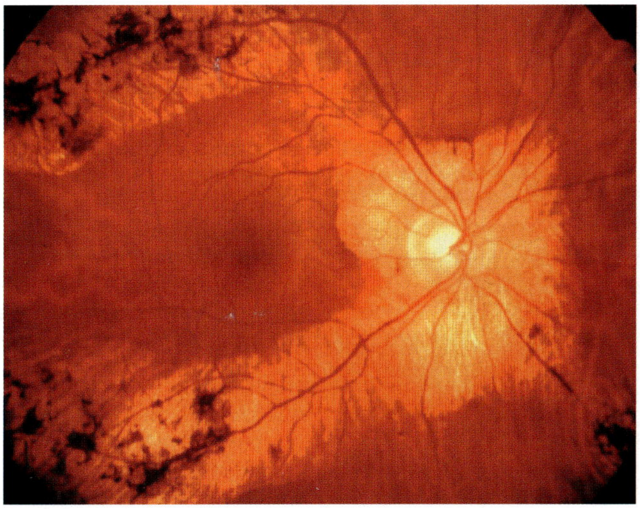

Fig. 15.14 Pigmented paravenous retinochoroidal atrophy. *(Courtesy of C Barry.)*

Cone and cone-rod dystrophy

Introduction

Progressive cone and cone-rod dystrophies are a clinically and genetically heterogenous group of inherited retinal diseases characterized by cone photoreceptor degeneration, which may be followed by rod photoreceptor loss. The majority are AR, with some AD and X-linked inheritance and mutations in at least 30 genes have been implicated. As with other retinal dystrophies, the age of onset, severity and rate of progression can vary substantially. Affected individuals typically present with progressive loss of central vision, disturbance of colour vision and photophobia. The prognosis is usually poor, with an eventual visual acuity of 6/60 or worse.

Diagnosis

- **Symptoms.** Gradual bilateral impairment of central and colour vision, which may be accompanied by photophobia.
- **Signs.** The features may evolve through the stages below.
  - The macula may be virtually normal or show non-specific central pigmentary changes or atrophy.
  - Golden sheen may be seen in X-linked disease (Fig. 15.16A).
  - A bull's-eye maculopathy is classically described, but is not universal. Other causes of a bull's-eye appearance are given in Table 15.1.
  - Progressive RPE atrophy at the macula with eventual atrophy (Fig. 15.16B).
- **Investigation**
  - Colour vision: severe deuteron–tritan defect out of proportion to visual acuity in some patients.
  - OCT shows loss of the outer retinal layers in the macula and foveal region (Fig. 15.17A). In advanced disease there is complete atrophy of the macula.
  - FAF is often the key diagnostic test, showing various annular patterns concentric with the fovea (Fig. 15.17B).
  - FA is never needed these days. However, if undertaken it typically shows a round hyperfluorescent window defect with a hypofluorescent centre, resulting in a bull's-eye appearance (Fig. 15.17C).
  - ERG: cone responses are subnormal, but rod responses are preserved until late (Fig. 15.17D).
  - Genetic testing.

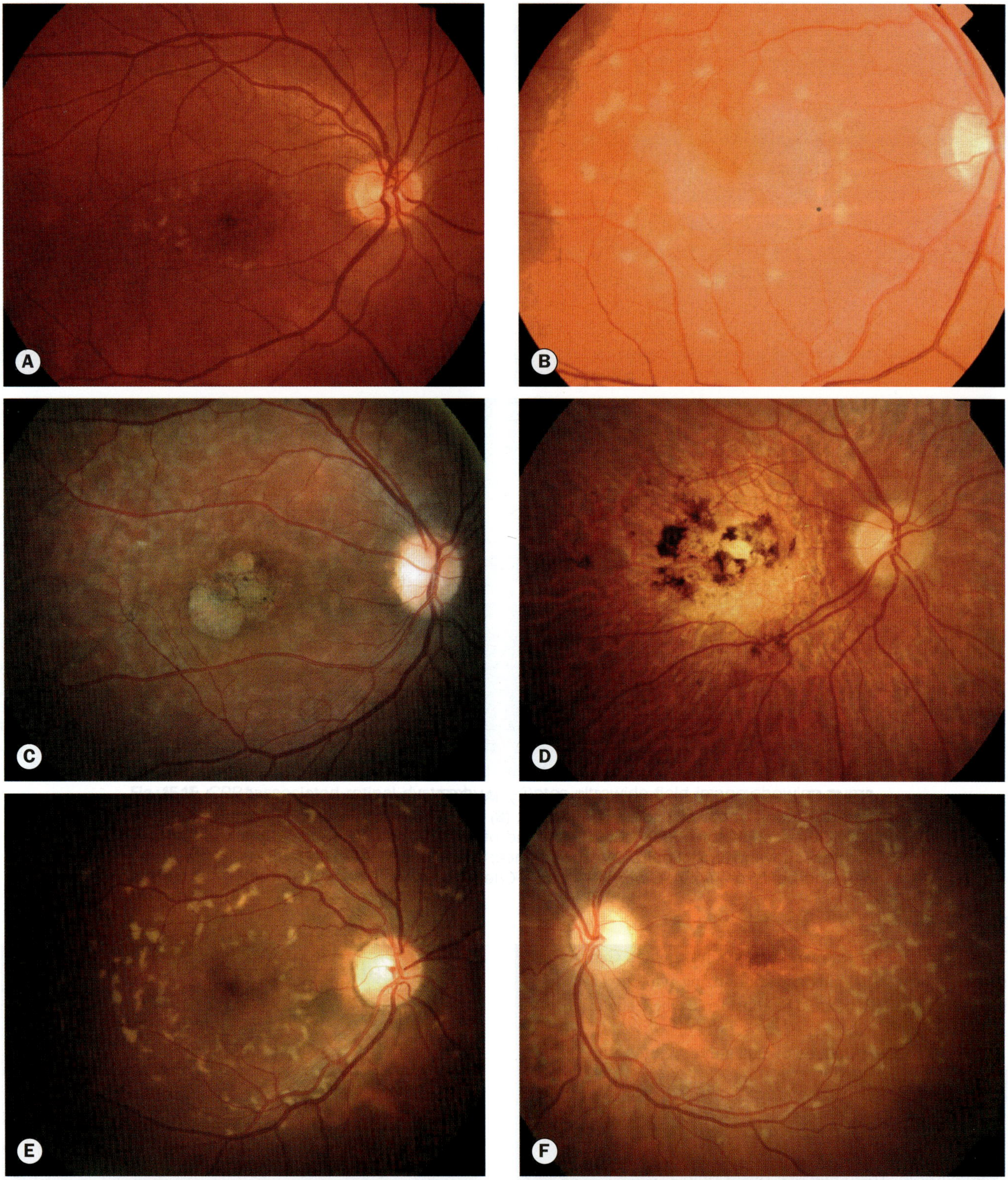

Fig. 15.18 Stargardt disease/fundus flavimaculatus. **(A)** Non-specific macular mottling; **(B)** 'snail slime' maculopathy surrounded by flecks; **(C)** quasi bull's-eye maculopathy surrounded by flecks – note the 'beaten-bronze' paramacular appearance; **(D)** geographic atrophy; **(E)** posterior pole flecks; **(F)** posterior pole flecks extending to the mid-periphery.

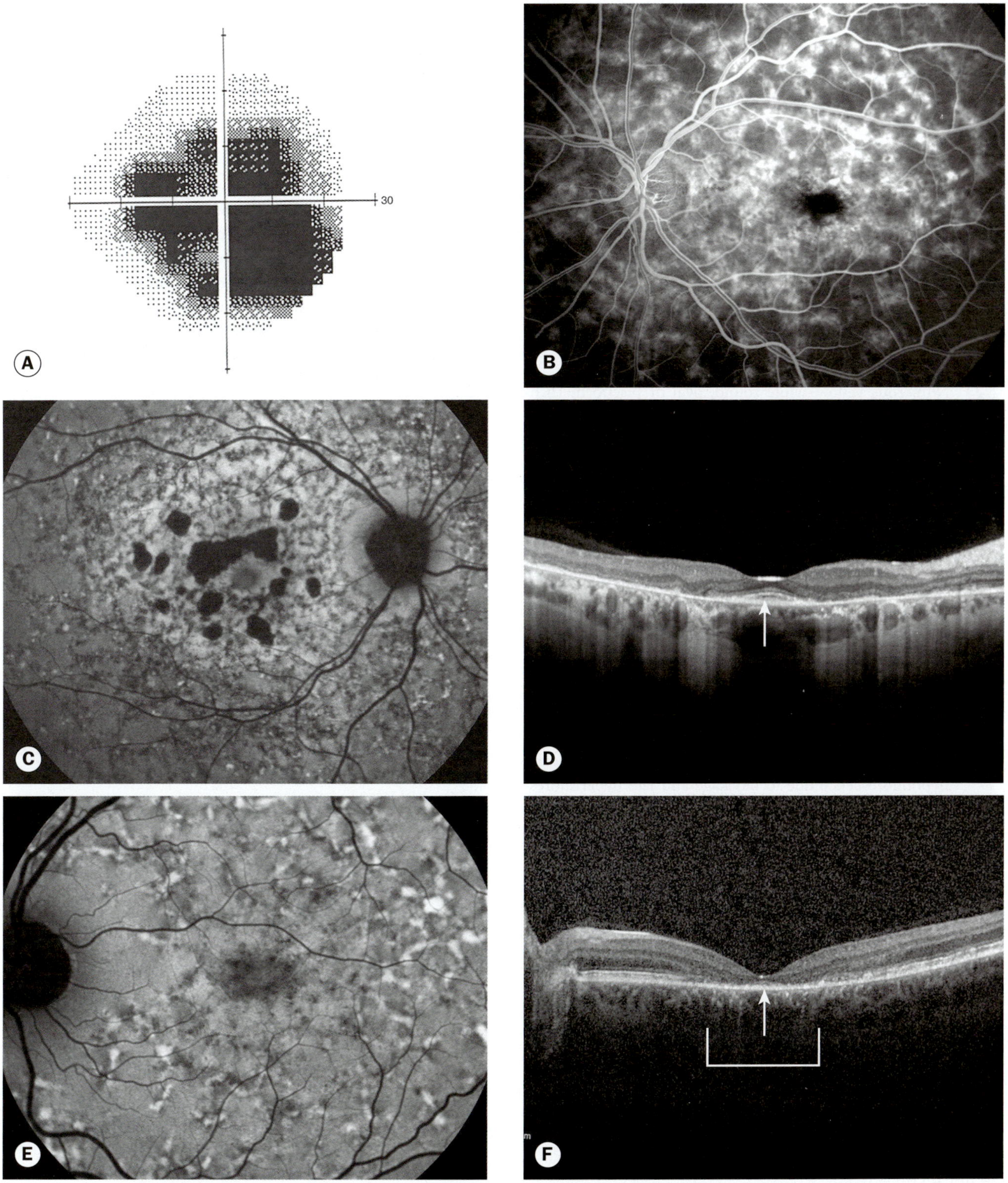

Fig. 15.19 Imaging in Stargardt disease/fundus flavimaculatus. **(A)** Central visual field loss; **(B)** FA showing hyperfluorescent flecks; **(C)** FAF in early onset disease showing macular hypoautofluorescent and surrounding hyperautofluorescent flecks. The black areas in the macula represent RPE atrophy; **(D)** OCT of **(C)** showing RPE and outer retinal atrophy with relative sparing of the fovea (arrow). Increased backscatter from the choroid indicates atrophic changes of the RPE; **(E)** FAF showing hyperfluorescent flecks in late disease; **(F)** OCT of **(E)** showing significant outer retinal thinning notably in the foveola (arrow). Adjacent ellipsoid zone shows altered reflectivity. *(Courtesy of S Chen – fig. C; P Charbel Issa – figs D, E and F.)*

Diagnosis

- **Symptoms.** Gradual impairment of central vision occurs that may be out of proportion to examination findings and manifests with difficulty when reading. A quarter of childhood-onset STGDT1 do not have any retinal lesions at presentation and malingering may be suspected, but OCT imaging soon clarifies this misconception.
- **Signs**
  - The macula may initially be normal or show non-specific mottling and fine flecks (Fig. 15.18A), progressing to an oval 'snail slime' (Fig. 15.18B) or 'beaten-bronze' appearance (Fig. 15.18C) and subsequently to atrophy (Fig. 15.18D) that may tend to a bull's-eye configuration. Rarely, a small number of patients may develop macular neovascularization (MNV).
  - Numerous yellow–white round, oval or pisciform (fish-shaped) lesions at the level of the RPE. These may be confined to the posterior pole (Fig. 15.18E) or extend to the mid-periphery (Fig. 15.18F).
  - New lesions develop as older ones become ill-defined and atrophic.
  - The structure and function of the parapapillary retina is spared, but can be involved in late-stage severe disease.
- **Investigation**
  - Visual fields show central loss (Fig. 15.19A) and microperimetry can accurately document progression.
  - FA: This has been superseded by OCT and FAF and is not usually needed. The classic feature is a 'dark choroid' due to masking of background choroidal fluorescence by lipofuscin accumulation in the RPE. The macula shows mixed hyper- and hypofluorescence. Fresh flecks show early hypofluorescence due to blockage and late hyperfluorescence due to staining and old flecks show RPE window defects (Fig. 15.19B).
  - Indocyanine green angiography (ICGA) shows hypofluorescent spots, often more numerous than seen clinically.
  - FAF is key to the diagnosis in early cases and shows a characteristic appearance with hyperautofluorescent flecks (Fig. 15.19C and E) and macular hypoautofluorescence.
  - OCT demonstrates outer retinal atrophy (Fig. 15.19D and F).
  - ERG: photopic is normal to subnormal, scotopic may be normal.
  - EOG is commonly subnormal, especially in advanced cases.

TIP Stargardt disease is the most commonly inherited macular dystrophy and is usually associated with mutations in the *ABCA4* gene.

Treatment

- **General measures** should be considered as for RP. Protection from excessive high-energy light exposure may be particularly important.
- **Avoid vitamin A** supplementation as it may accelerate lipofuscin accumulation.
- **Clinical trials** have been initiated assessing the effect of: (a) gene therapy using a lentiviral vector for *ABCA4*, (b) stem cell therapy, (c) pharmatherapy to reduce lipofuscin accumulation, (d) metformin taken by mouth.

Bietti crystalline corneoretinal dystrophy

Bietti dystrophy (AR, *CYP4V2* gene) is characterized by deposition of crystals in the retina and the superficial peripheral cornea. It is a rare condition, but is more prevalent in Chinese and Japanese people than in other ethnic groups. The *CYP4V2* enzyme is involved in fatty acid oxidation, but the specific function is not understood and it is not known how this leads to the specific signs found in this condition. The rate of progression is variable. There is no treatment.

- **Presentation.** Young adults with slowly progressive visual loss constitute the typical case.
- **Signs**
  - Superficial peripheral corneal crystals.
  - Numerous fine yellow–white crystals scattered throughout the posterior fundus (Fig. 15.20A and B) are followed by localized atrophy of the RPE and choriocapillaris at the macula.
  - Diffuse atrophy of the choriocapillaris subsequently develops, with a decrease in size and number of the crystals.
  - There is gradual confluence and expansion of the atrophic areas into the periphery, leading to diffuse chorioretinal atrophy in end-stage disease.
- **Investigation**
  - OCT demonstrates the crystalline deposits and macular changes (Fig. 15.20C).
  - ERG is subnormal.
  - FA in moderate disease shows characteristic large hypofluorescent patches corresponding to choriocapillaris loss, with intact overlying retinal vessels (Fig. 15.20D). The patches become confluent over time.

Familial benign fleck retina

Familial benign fleck retina (benign flecked retina syndrome) is a very rare AR disorder. Individuals with the condition are asymptomatic, so the condition is usually discovered by chance. Numerous diffusely distributed yellow–white polymorphous lesions spare the fovea and extend to the far periphery (Fig. 15.21). The flecks show autofluorescence and are probably composed of lipofuscin. The ERG is normal and the prognosis is excellent.

Alport syndrome

Alport syndrome (predominantly X-linked) is caused by mutations in several different genes, all of which encode particular forms of type IV collagen, a major basement membrane component. It is characterized by chronic renal failure and is often associated with high-tone sensorineural hearing loss by the age of 20. There are scattered yellowish punctate flecks in the perimacular area, which

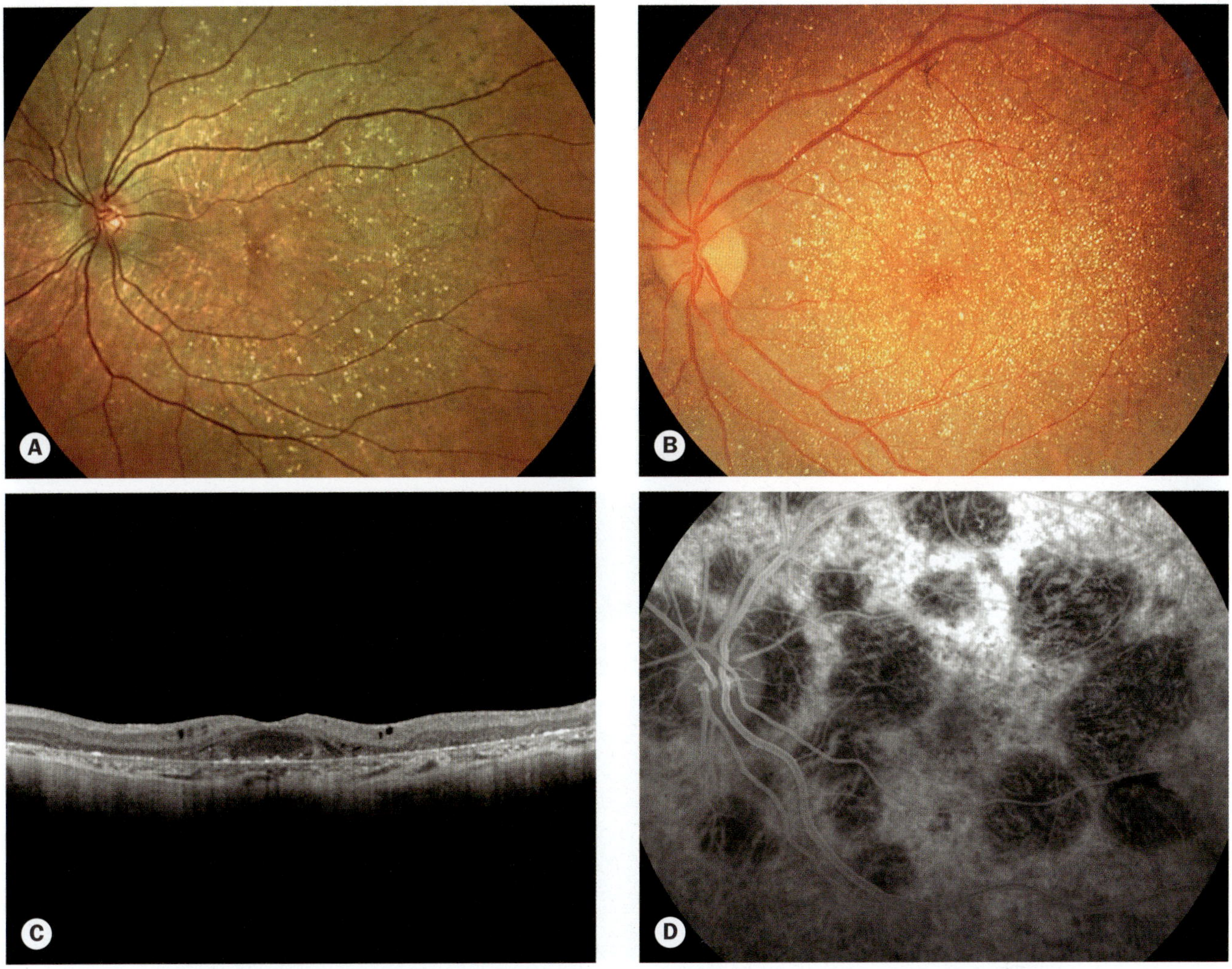

Fig. 15.20 Bietti corneoretinal crystalline dystrophy. **(A)** Wide-field image showing crystalline deposits; **(B)** crystals mainly in the macular region; **(C)** OCT of A showing crystalline deposits in the inner retina, diffuse outer retinal atrophy and choroidal thinning – there is relative foveal sparing; **(D)** FA showing characteristic hypofluorescent patches secondary to RPE atrophy. *(Courtesy of C Barry – figs A and C.)*

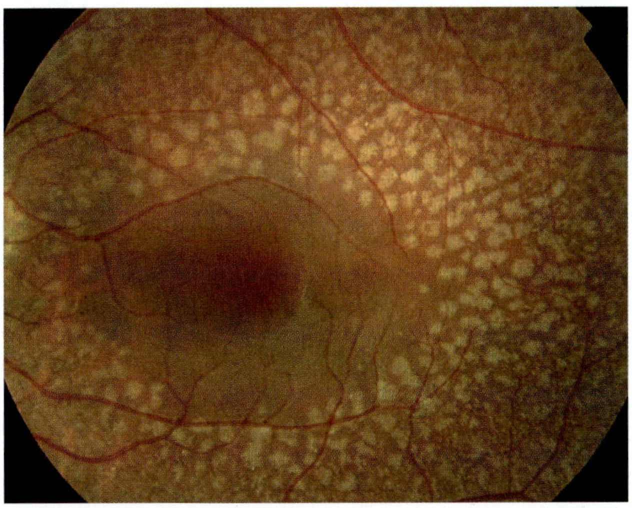

Fig. 15.21 Familial benign fleck retina.

are often subtle (Fig. 15.22A), and larger peripheral flecks, some of which may become confluent, but rarely threaten vision (Fig. 15.22B). OCT is helpful to demonstrate the retinal changes and typically shows temporal macular thinning (Fig. 15.22C). The ERG is normal and the prognosis for vision is excellent. Anterior lenticonus occurs in about 20% and posterior polymorphous corneal dystrophy may occasionally be seen.

Congenital stationary night blindness

Introduction

Congenital stationary night blindness (CSNB) refers to a group of disorders characterized by nyctalopia from birth, but non-progressive retinal dysfunction. The fundus appearance may be normal or abnormal. A number of genetic mutations have been reported that result in abnormal phototransduction and post-phototransduction transmission.

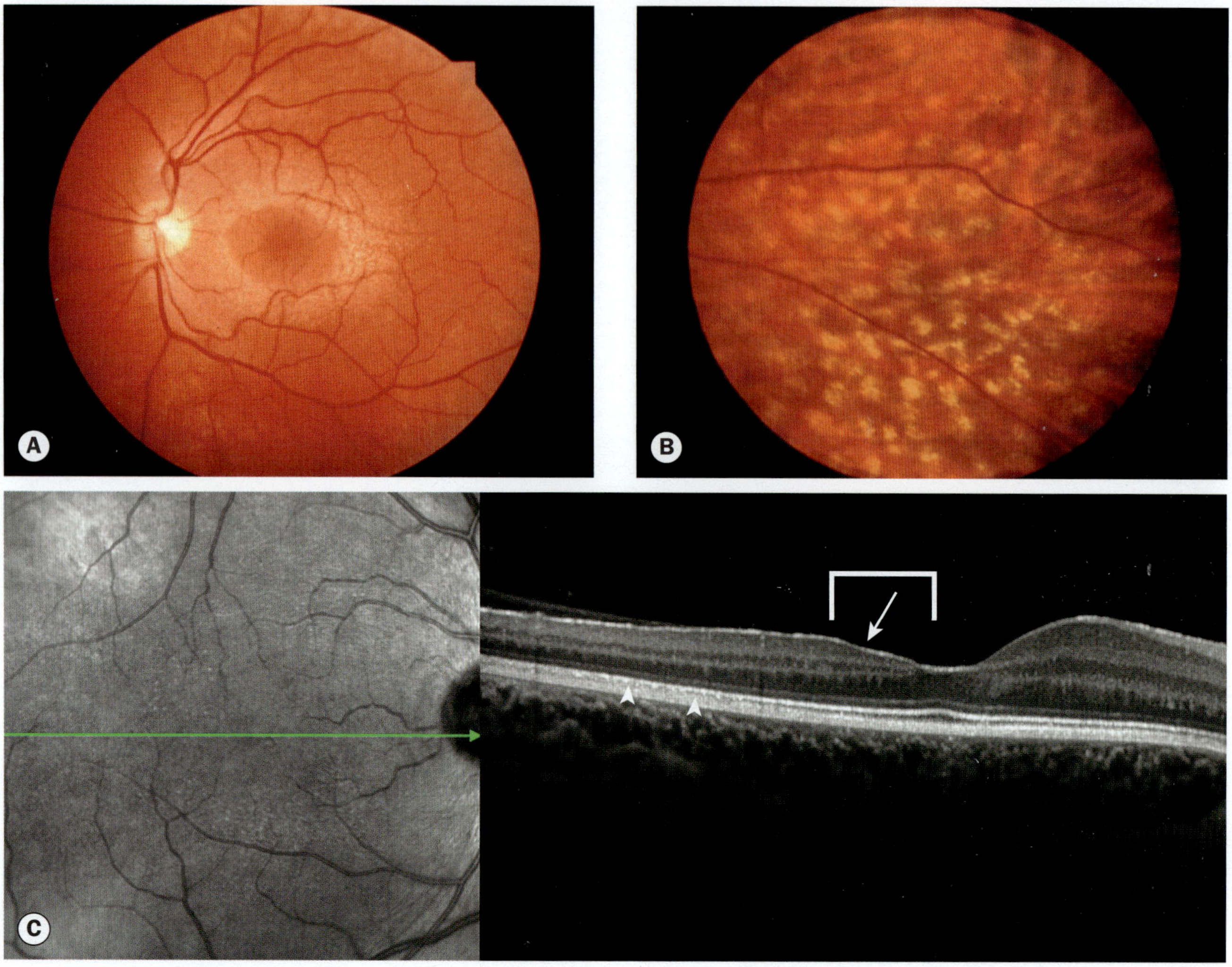

Fig. 15.22 Alport syndrome. **(A)** Subtle perimacular flecks; **(B)** peripheral flecks; **(C)** infrared image showing retinal flecks and corresponding OCT showing temporal macular thinning (arrow) and outer retinal disruption (arrowheads). *(Courtesy of P Herrmann.)*

With a normal fundus appearance

CSNB with a normal fundus appearance is sometimes classified into type 1 (complete) and type 2 (incomplete) forms that are generally due to mutations in different genes. The former is characterized by a complete absence of rod pathway function and essentially normal cone function clinically and on ERG, the latter by impairment of both rod and cone function. Mutations in numerous genes have been implicated, with X-linked, AD and AR inheritance patterns. The AD form is usually associated with normal visual acuity, but many AR and X-linked patients have poor vision with nystagmus and often significant myopia.

With an abnormal fundus appearance

- **Oguchi disease** (AR). The fundus has an unusual golden-yellow colour in the light-adapted state (Fig. 15.23A), which becomes normal after prolonged dark adaptation (Mizuo or Mizuo–Nakamura phenomenon – Fig. 15.23B). Rod function is absent after 30 minutes of dark adaptation but recovers to a near-normal level after a long period of dark adaptation.
- **Fundus albipunctatus** is an AR or AD condition that may be the same entity as retinitis punctata albescens. The fundus shows a multitude of subtle, tiny yellow–white spots at the posterior pole (Fig. 15.24A), sparing the fovea – sometimes the macula – and extending to the periphery. In contrast to retinitis punctata albescens, the retinal blood vessels, optic disc, peripheral fields and visual acuity are believed to remain normal, though the natural history is not yet absolutely defined. FA shows mottled hyperfluorescence, indicating depigmentation of the RPE. The ERG is variably abnormal; both cones and rods may be affected.
- **Retinitis punctata albescens** (AR or AD) is rare and is characterized by scattered whitish-yellow spots, most numerous at the equator, usually sparing the macula and associated with arteriolar attenuation (Fig. 15.24B). This form of flecked retina may be a variant of fundus albipunctatus, as mutations in *RLBP1* (retinaldehyde-binding protein-1) have been identified in both conditions. However, those identified as having retinitis punctata albescence tend to have a more serious and

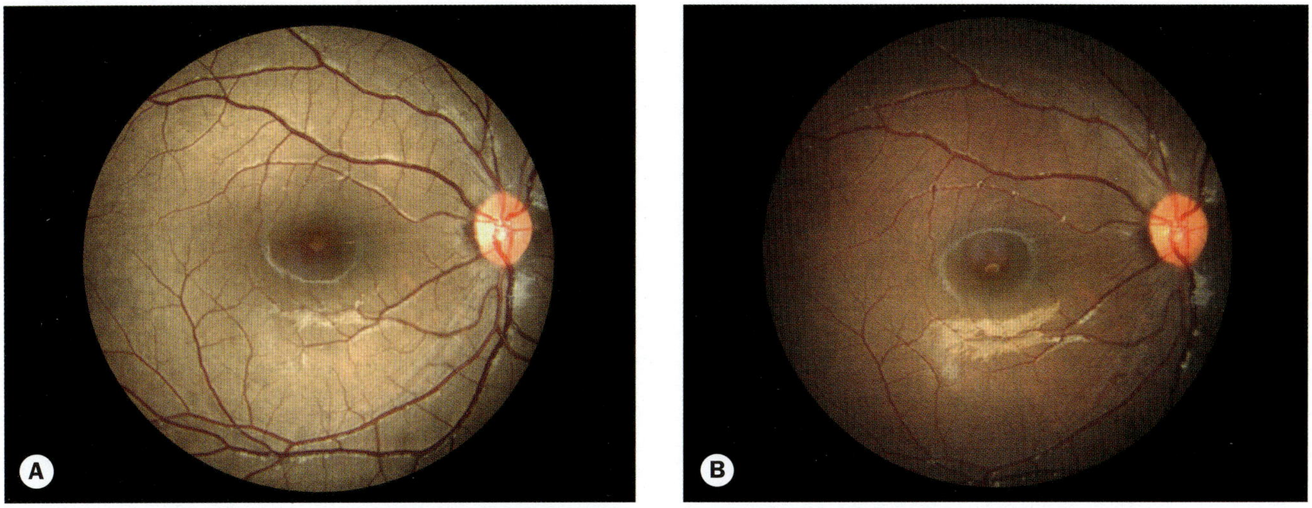

Fig. 15.23 Mizuo phenomenon in Oguchi disease. **(A)** In the light-adapted state; **(B)** in the dark-adapted state. *(Courtesy of C Mishra.)*

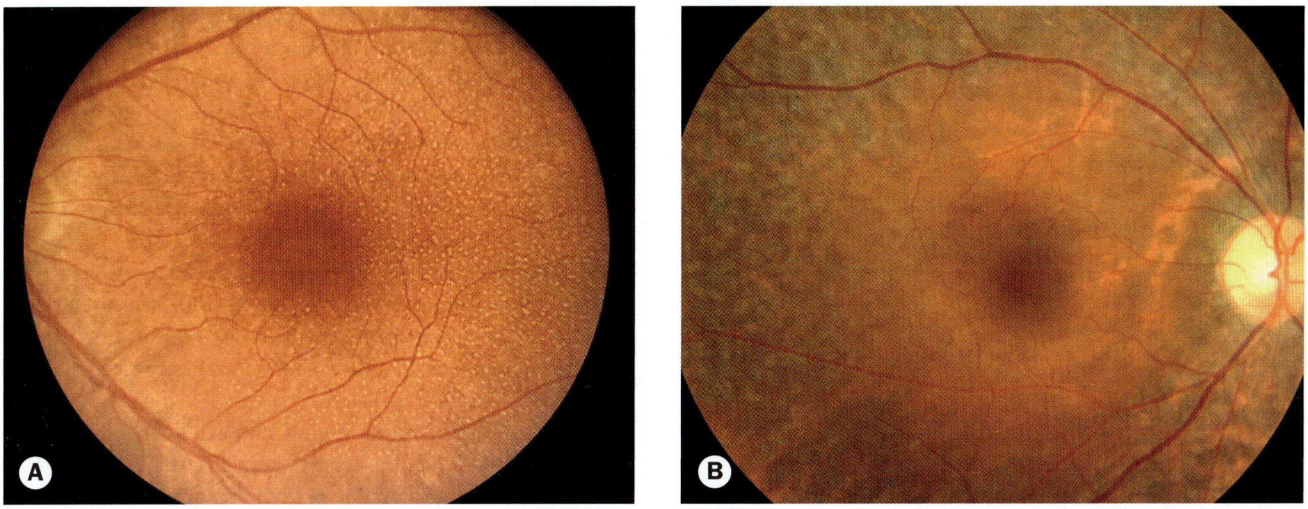

Fig. 15.24 Clinical appearance. **(A)** Fundus albipunctatus; **(B)** retinitis punctata albescens. *(Courtesy of C Barry.)*

progressive disease, while those with fundus albipunctatus tend to have a stable disease with night blindness being the major symptom. The relationship between these two conditions will become more transparent once the natural history has been elucidated.

Congenital achromatopsia

This is a group of congenital disorders in which colours cannot be perceived and visual acuity is reduced, particularly in brightly illuminated environments (hemeralopia). Mutations affecting the cone-specific cyclic nucleotide gated (CNG) channel beta (B3) and alpha (A3) subunits are responsible for about 50% and 25% of complete achromatopsia, respectively. Animal models of the disease have shown successful restoration of cone-mediated vision following gene therapy for the *CNGA3* and *CNGB3* mutations.

Rod monochromatism (complete achromatopsia)

In rod monochromatism (AR) visual acuity is poor, typically 6/60. There is congenital nystagmus and photophobia. Colour vision is totally absent, all colours appearing as shades of grey. The macula usually appears normal, but may be hypoplastic. The photopic (cone) ERG is abnormal and the scotopic may also be subnormal.

Blue cone monochromatism (incomplete achromatopsia)

Blue cone monochromatism (X-linked) features only slightly subnormal acuity at 6/6–6/9, but colour vision is completely absent. Nystagmus and photophobia are not typical features. There is a normal macula. The ERG is normal except for the absence of cone responses to red and white light.

MACULAR DYSTROPHIES

Best vitelliform macular dystrophy

Introduction

Best vitelliform macular dystrophy (early- or juvenile-onset vitelliform macular dystrophy) is the second most common macular dystrophy, after Stargardt disease. It is due to allelic variation in the bestrophin (*BEST1)* gene on chromosome 11q13. Bestrophin is found on the plasma membrane of the RPE and functions as a transmembrane ion channel. Inheritance is usually AD with variable penetrance and expressivity. Although there is significant variability even in the same family, the prognosis is usually reasonably good until middle age, after which visual acuity declines in one or both eyes due to macular atrophy, scarring or MNV.

Diagnosis

- **Signs.** There is gradual evolution through the following stages:
  - **Pre-vitelliform** is characterized by a subnormal EOG in an asymptomatic infant or child with a normal fundus.
  - **Vitelliform** develops in infancy or early childhood and does not usually impair vision. A round, sharply delineated ('sunny side up egg yolk') macular lesion between 0.5 and 2 disc diameters in size develops within the RPE (Fig. 15.25A). The size of the lesions and stage of development in the two eyes may be asymmetrical and sometimes only one eye is involved initially. Occasionally the condition may be extramacular and multiple.
  - **Pseudohypopyon** may occur when part of the lesion regresses (Fig. 15.25B), often at puberty.
  - **Vitelliruptive.** The lesion breaks up and visual acuity drops (Fig. 15.25C).
  - **Atrophic** in which all pigment has disappeared leaving an atrophic area of RPE.
- **Investigation**
  - FAF: the yellowish material is intensely hyperautofluorescent. In the later atrophic stages hypoautofluorescent areas supervene.
  - FA shows corresponding hypofluorescence due to masking (Fig. 15.25D).
  - OCT shows material beneath, above and within the RPE (Fig. 15.25E).
  - EOG is severely subnormal during all stages (Arden index less than 1.5) and is also abnormal in carriers with clinically normal fundi.

Multifocal vitelliform lesions without Best disease

Rarely, multifocal vitelliform lesions (Fig. 15.26), identical to those in Best dystrophy but distributed around the macular vascular arcades and optic disc, may become manifest in adult life and give rise to diagnostic problems. However, in these patients the EOG is normal and the family history is negative. Occasionally genetically confirmed Best dystrophy with an abnormal EOG may present with multifocal lesions. The relationship between multifocal vitelliform lesions, juvenile vitelliform (Best) dystrophy and adult-onset vitelliform macular dystrophy is incompletely defined, though some cases of each are associated with mutations in the same genes.

Adult-onset vitelliform macular dystrophy (foveomacular vitelliform dystrophy)

When symmetrical yellow deposits that resemble Best disease develop in the macula of older individuals (usually over 40 years), the term 'adult-onset vitelliform macular (foveomacular) dystrophy' is used. In contrast to juvenile Best disease, the foveal lesions are often smaller. The lesions gradually increase and then decrease in size over many years, leaving an area of atrophic outer retina and RPE. This process is accompanied by a loss of visual acuity. There is genetic heterogeneity including mutations in the *PRPH2*, *IMPG2* or the *BEST1* gene. Vitelliform macular lesions may also be observed in a wide range of other conditions including acute idiopathic exudative polymorphous vitelliform maculopathy and acute laser damage. This appearance may occur secondary to basal laminar drusen, reticular pseudodrusen and chronic vitreomacular traction. Adult-onset vitelliform macular dystrophy may also be grouped in the phenotypical spectrum of pattern dystrophy (see next). There is no treatment for the condition.

- **Symptoms.** Often the condition is discovered by chance, but may present in late middle or old age with decreased central vision. The vision is often reduced by one or more lines at presentation and mild deterioration occurs subsequently. The prognosis varies from case to case.
- **Signs.** A round or oval slightly elevated yellowish subfoveal deposit (Fig. 15.27A), generally smaller than the lesions of Best disease, is seen in one or both eyes. There may be central pigmentation and numerous associated drusen are present in some cases. The material may persist, absorb, or break up and disperse at a late stage, leaving atrophy of very variable severity. Choroidal neovascularization sometimes supervenes.
- **Investigation**
  - Fluorescein angiography is almost never needed, but can occasionally be useful to show absence of MNV. In adult-onset vitelliform macular dystrophy FA typically shows central hypofluorescence surrounded by a small irregular hyperfluorescent ring. In the late phases the entire lesion shows hyperfluorescence (Fig. 15.27B).
  - FAF imaging shows intense hyperautofluorescence corresponding to the deposited material, which is typically much more obvious than on clinical examination (Fig. 15.27C). When atrophy supervenes, there is hypoautofluorescence.
  - OCT shows hyper-reflective material between the RPE and outer retina, similar to Best disease (Fig. 15.27D and see Fig. 15.25E).
  - ERG and EOG are usually normal, indicating localized retinal pathology.

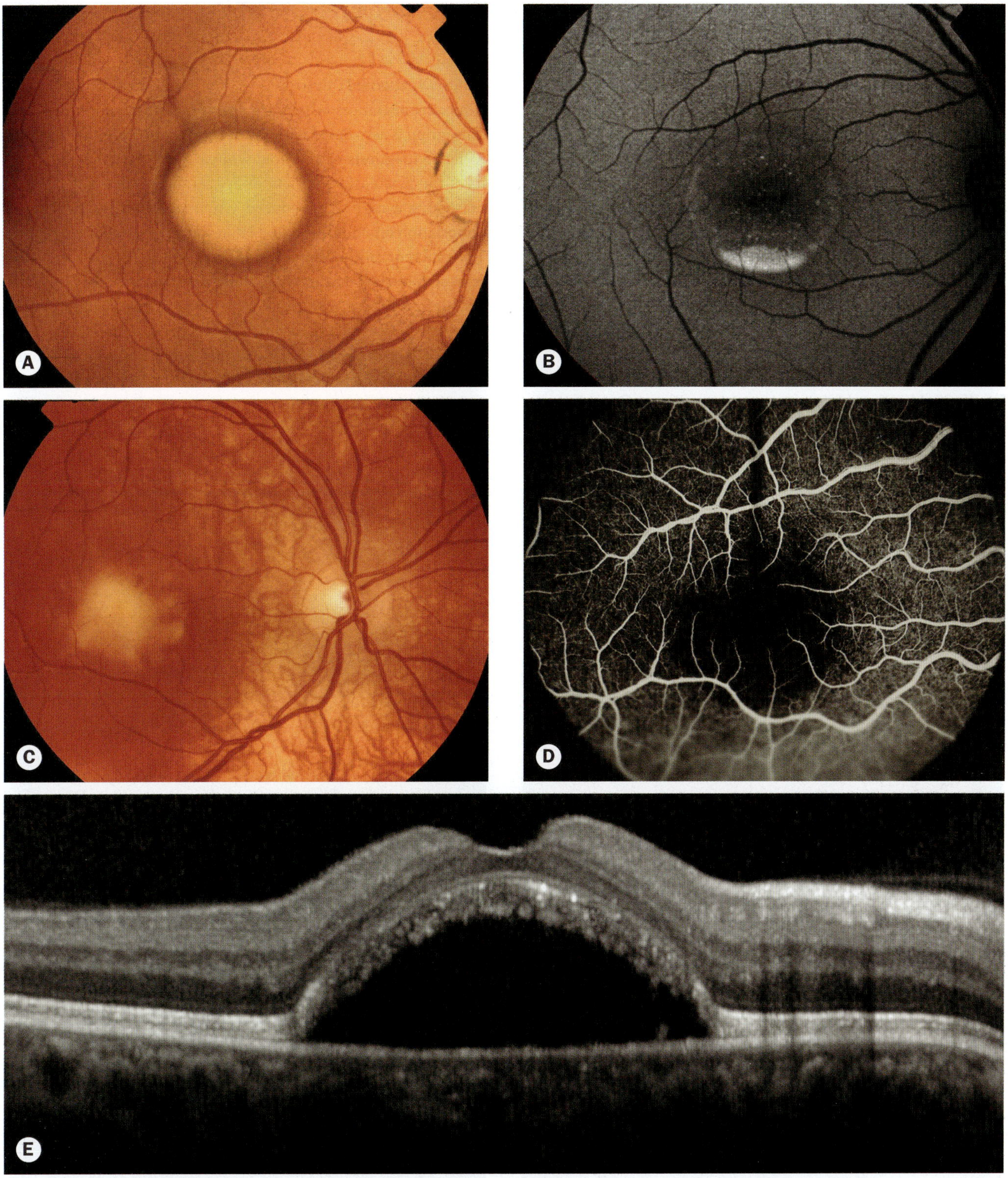

Fig. 15.25 Best dystrophy. **(A)** Vitelliform stage; **(B)** FAF image of pseudohypopyon; **(C)** vitelliruptive stage; **(D)** FA showing central hypofluorescence; **(E)** OCT image of eye in **(B)** in the vitelliform stage, showing subretinal hyporeflective component. *(Courtesy of P Charbel Issa – figs B and E.)*

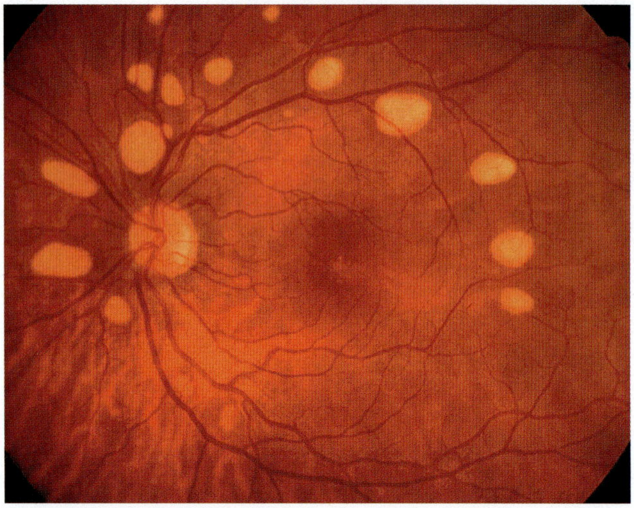

Fig. 15.26 Multifocal vitelliform lesions without Best disease. *(Courtesy of C Barry.)*

Pattern dystrophy of the retinal pigment epithelium

Pattern (patterned) dystrophy of the RPE encompasses several clinical appearances which are autosomal dominantly inherited. This group is associated with the accumulation of lipofuscin in the RPE and manifests with yellow, whitish, grey or pigmented deposits at the macula in a variety of appearances. The most common presenting symptom is reduced visual acuity or mild metamorphopsia in early adulthood or later, but many are asymptomatic. The different clinical appearances are believed in many cases to represent variable expression of a mutation in *PRPH2*, which encodes peripherin-2, a protein involved in compaction of outer segment discs of photoreceptors. Other genes and conditions can give rise to a similar appearance and notably, a pattern dystrophy-like appearance can occur in response to a range of pathogenic stimuli. Pattern dystrophies may be associated with systemic diseases, e.g. pseudoxanthoma elasticum, myotonic dystrophy and

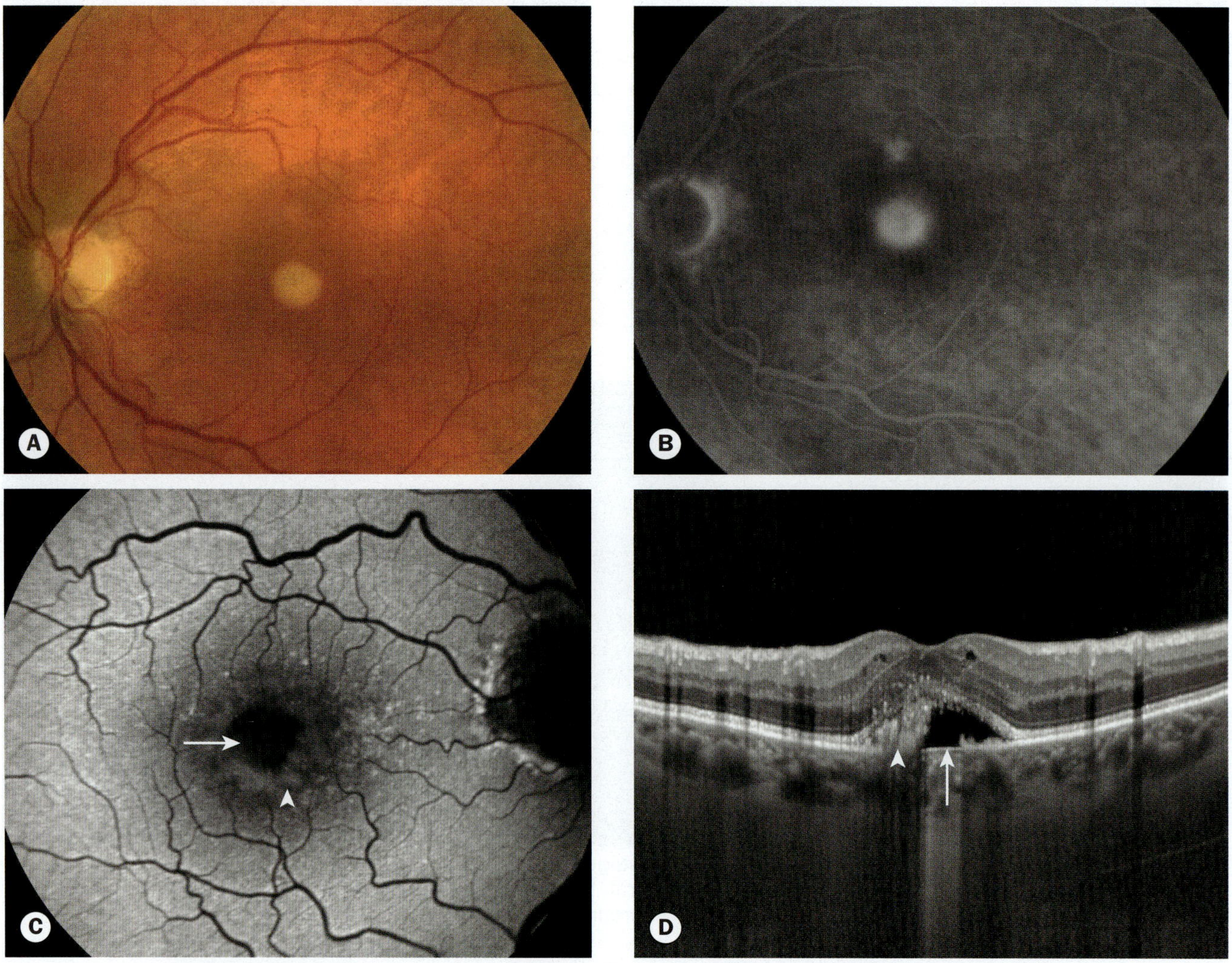

Fig. 15.27 **(A)** Adult-onset macular vitelliform dystrophy (monogenic); **(B)** FA showing corresponding hyperfluorescence; **(C)** FAF of a different patient showing hyperautofluorescence vitelliform lesion in the inferior macula (arrowhead) and RPE atrophy (arrow); **(D)** vertical OCT scan showing subretinal material (arrowhead) and an adjacent small central area with increased choroidal backscatter, indicating RPE atrophy (arrow).

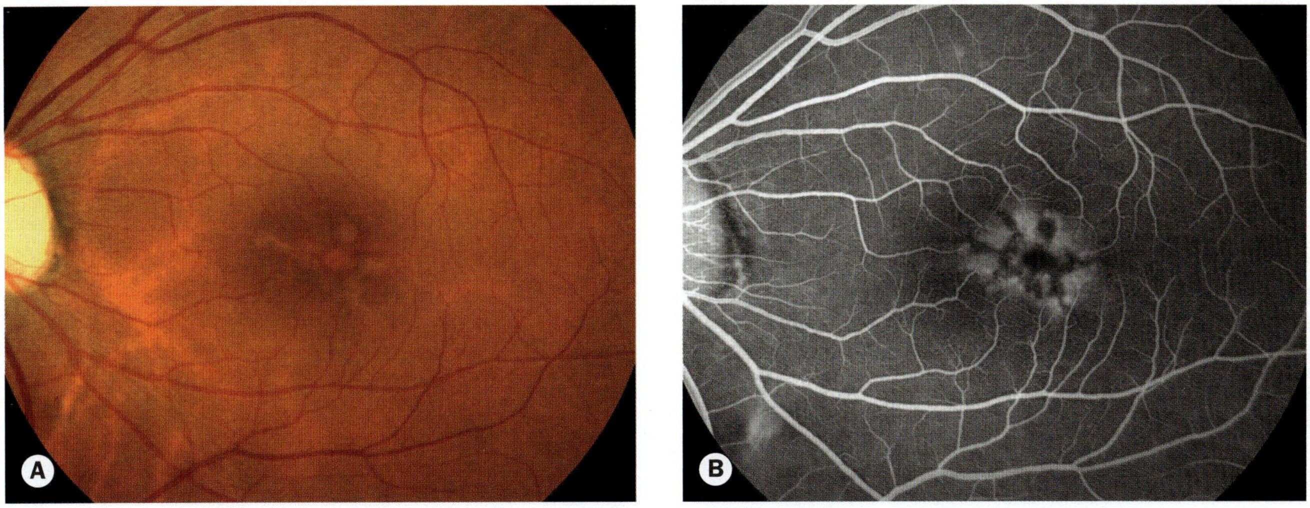

Fig. 15.28 Butterfly-shaped pattern dystrophy of the RPE. **(A)** Spokes of yellowish material and pigment radiating from the foveola; **(B)** FA of the eye in **(A)** showing central and spoke-like radiating hypofluorescence with surrounding hyperfluorescence.

MIDD. These dystrophies usually progress at a very slow rate and the prognosis is generally good. There is no treatment. Based on the pigment distribution the pattern dystrophies have been classified into **five prominent patterns**. Importantly, one pattern may change into another in the same patient.

- **Butterfly-shaped pigment dystrophy:** foveal yellow and melanin pigmentation, commonly in a spoke-like or butterfly wing-like conformation (Fig. 15.28A). FA shows central and radiating hypofluorescence with surrounding hyperfluorescence (Fig. 15.28B).
- **Reticular dystrophy (Sjögren):** a network of pigmented lines at the posterior pole. This includes **macroreticular** (spider-shaped) where pigment granules are initially seen at the fovea, followed by reticular pigmentation that spreads to the periphery.
- **Multifocal pattern dystrophy simulating fundus flavimaculatus:** multiple, widely scattered, irregular yellow lesions which may be similar to those seen in fundus flavimaculatus.
- **Adult-onset foveomacular vitelliform dystrophy** – see above.
- **Fundus pulverulentus** is extremely rare. Macular pigment mottling develops.

North Carolina macular dystrophy

North Carolina macular dystrophy is a rare non-progressive condition. It was first described in families living in the mountains of North Carolina and subsequently in many unrelated families in other parts of the world. Inheritance is AD with complete penetrance, but highly variable expressivity. A third are asymptomatic, a third have mild central visual loss and a third have moderate central visual loss. A few develop MNV with severe central visual loss. Most affected individuals have a mutation of the *MCDR1* locus of chromosome 6q, which results in dysregulation of the *PRDM13* gene. Patients show a characteristic retinal phenotype and distribution of drusen that differs from the drusen found in patients with AMD. Despite the variability of macular phenotype, multimodal retinal imaging reveals consistent findings.

- **Grade 1** is characterized by yellow–white, drusen-like peripheral (Fig. 15.29A) and macular deposits that develop during the first decade but may remain asymptomatic throughout life.
- **Grade 2** is characterized by deep, confluent macular deposits (Fig. 15.29B). The long-term visual prognosis is guarded because some patients develop neovascular maculopathy and subretinal scarring.
- **Grade 3** is characterized by atrophic macular lesions associated with variable impairment of visual acuity.
- **FAF** shows characteristic peripheral hyperautofluorescent streaks (Fig. 15.29C). The atrophic macula shows hyperautofluorescence in the early stages (Fig. 15.29D), followed by late hypoautofluorescence.
- **OCT** shows mild irregularity in the outer retina (Fig. 15.29E and F).

Familial dominant drusen

Familial dominant drusen (Doyne honeycomb choroiditis, malattia leventinese) is thought to represent an early-onset variant of age-related macular degeneration. Inheritance is AD with variable expressivity. A mutation in the gene *EFEMP1* (chromosome 2p16) is responsible, which results in increased lipid accumulation in drusen. Significant differences in severity and progression can occur in the two eyes of the same patient and between patients in the same family. Typically, asymptomatic yellow–white, elongated, radially orientated drusen centred on the macula develop in the second decade (Fig. 15.30A). The drusen may involve the disc margin nasal to the disc. With age the lesions become increasingly dense and acquire a honeycomb pattern (Fig. 15.30B). Initially the visual symptoms are insidious and nyctalopia is not usually experienced. Central visual loss with acuity less than 6/60 may occur in the seventh and eighth decades due to RPE degeneration, macular atrophy or occasionally MNV. Investigations include OCT and FAF. The ERG is normal, but the EOG is subnormal in those with advanced disease.

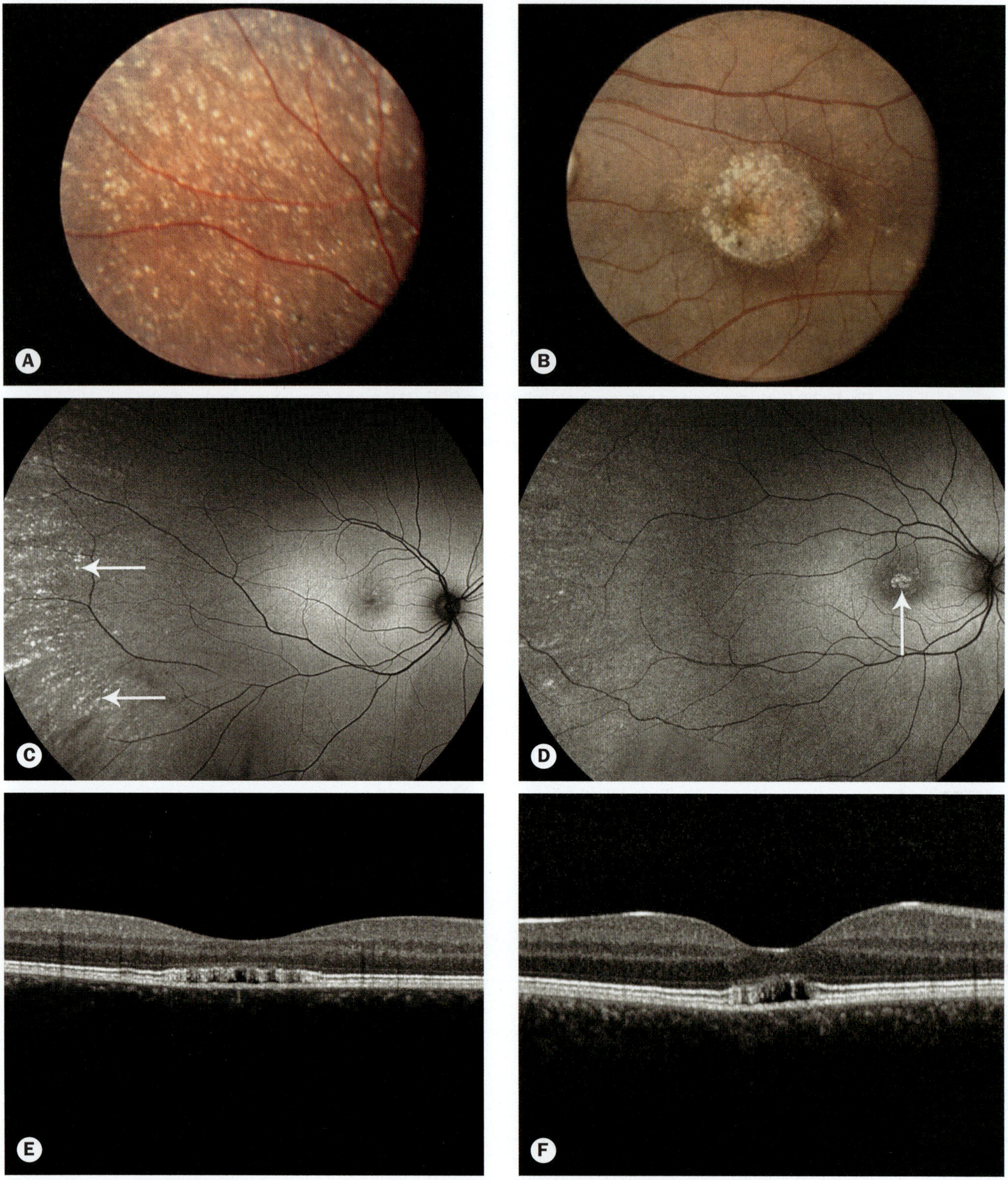

Fig. 15.29 North Carolina macular dystrophy. **(A)** Peripheral flecks; **(B)** confluent macular flecks; **(C)** FAF of an asymptomatic individual, showing peripheral hyperautofluorescent flecks (arrows); **(D)** FAF of her symptomatic daughter showing hyperautofluorescence in the macular region (arrow); **(E)** OCT of **(D)** in the intermediate stage showing localized outer retinal disruption; **(F)** OCT 2 years later showing progressive outer retinal disruption. *(Courtesy of P Charbel Issa.)*

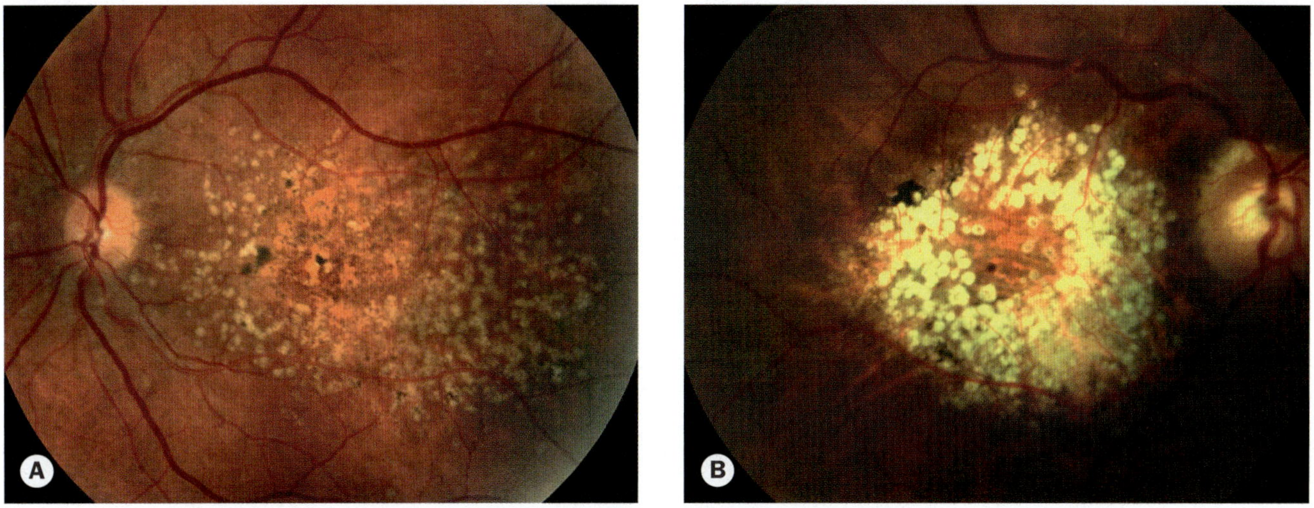

Fig. 15.30 Familial dominant drusen. **(A)** Typical earlier radially orientated lesions extending nasal to the disc; **(B)** high-density drusen with RPE degeneration. *(Courtesy of S Chen.)*

Sorsby fundus dystrophy

Sorsby fundus dystrophy (SFD) is a rare disorder that results in bilateral visual loss, typically in late middle age. Inheritance is AD with full penetrance but variable expressivity; allelic variation in the gene *TIMP3* (chromosome 22q) is responsible. The predominant pathological feature is confluent amorphous deposits found between the basement membrane of the RPE and the inner layer of Bruch membrane. Early presentation may be in the third decade with nyctalopia, when confluent yellow–white drusen-like deposits may be seen in the macula, along the arcades and nasal to the disc (Fig. 15.31A), or in the fifth decade with sudden visual loss due to exudative maculopathy secondary to MNV and subretinal scarring (Fig. 15.31B). When early-onset drusen are associated with MNV in young adulthood this diagnosis should be considered. Peripheral chorioretinal atrophy may occur by the seventh decade and result in loss of ambulatory vision. OCT shows reticular pseudodrusen. The ERG is initially normal but may be subnormal in later disease. Prolonged rod-mediated dark adaptation is a sensitive test in early disease. Patients with MNV may respond to anti-VEGF treatment.

Concentric annular macular dystrophy

The prognosis is good in the majority of cases of (benign) concentric annular macular dystrophy, an AD disorder, although a minority develop progressive loss of acuity and nyctalopia. Presentation is in adult life with mild impairment of central vision. A paracentral ring scotoma is present on visual field testing.

Central areolar choroidal dystrophy

Central areolar choroidal dystrophy, also termed central choroidal sclerosis, is a genetically heterogeneous but typically AD condition presenting in the third or fourth decades with gradual impairment of central vision. Non-specific foveal granularity progresses to well-circumscribed RPE atrophy and loss of the choriocapillaris (Fig. 15.32A) and subsequently slowly expanding geographic atrophy with prominence of large choroidal vessels (Fig. 15.32B). There is no treatment and the prognosis is for central vision is poor.

Dominant cystoid macular oedema

Bilateral CMO (AD) commonly presents in adolescence with gradual impairment of central vision. Treatment is ineffective and macular atrophy inevitably ensues.

Sjögren–Larsson syndrome

Sjögren–Larsson syndrome (AR) is a neurocutaneous disorder which occurs secondary to defective enzyme activity (fatty aldehyde dehydrogenase; *ALDH3A2* encoded on chromosome 17p with 11 distinct mutations). It is characterized by congenital ichthyosis, neurological problems and mild to moderate intellectual disability. Presentation is with photophobia and poor vision, and glistening yellow–white crystalline deposits develop at the macula (Fig. 15.33), appearing during the first 2 years of life. Pigmentary retinopathy (50%), cataract and colobomatous microphthalmos may also occur.

Maternally inherited diabetes and deafness

Maternally inherited diabetes and deafness (MIDD) constitutes around 1% of all cases of diabetes, with inheritance via mitochondrial DNA. Most patients develop progressive dystrophic macular changes (Fig. 15.34A), but vision is not usually affected. The abnormal fundal appearance can be difficult to see clinically, but FAF (Fig. 15.34B) and OCT (Fig. 15.34C) show typical abnormalities.

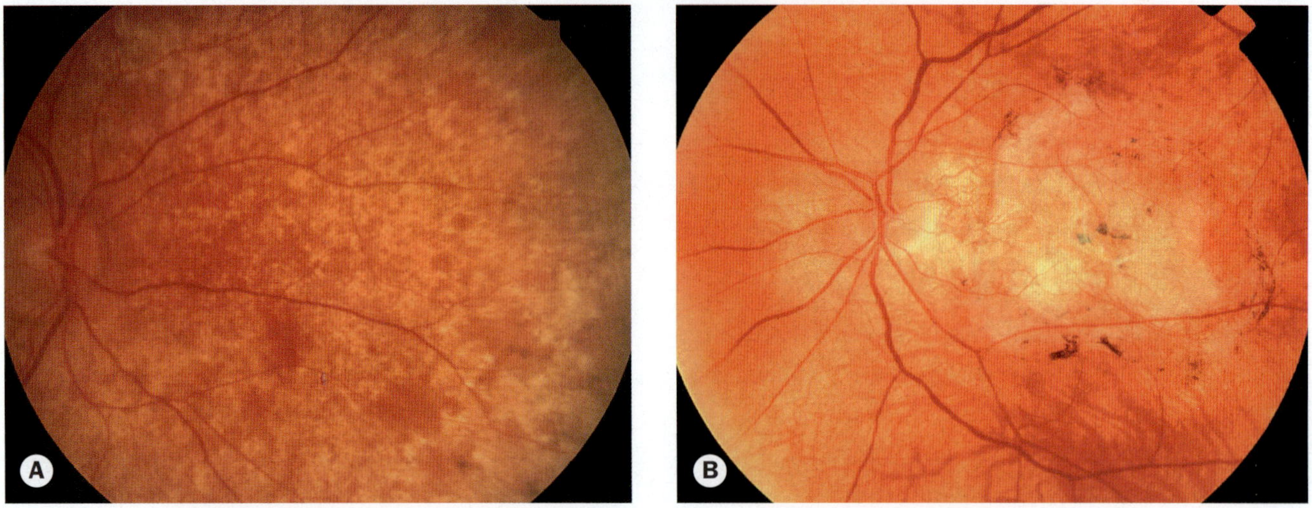

Fig. 15.31 Sorsby fundus dystrophy. **(A)** Confluent flecks nasal to the disc; **(B)** scarring in end-stage disease.

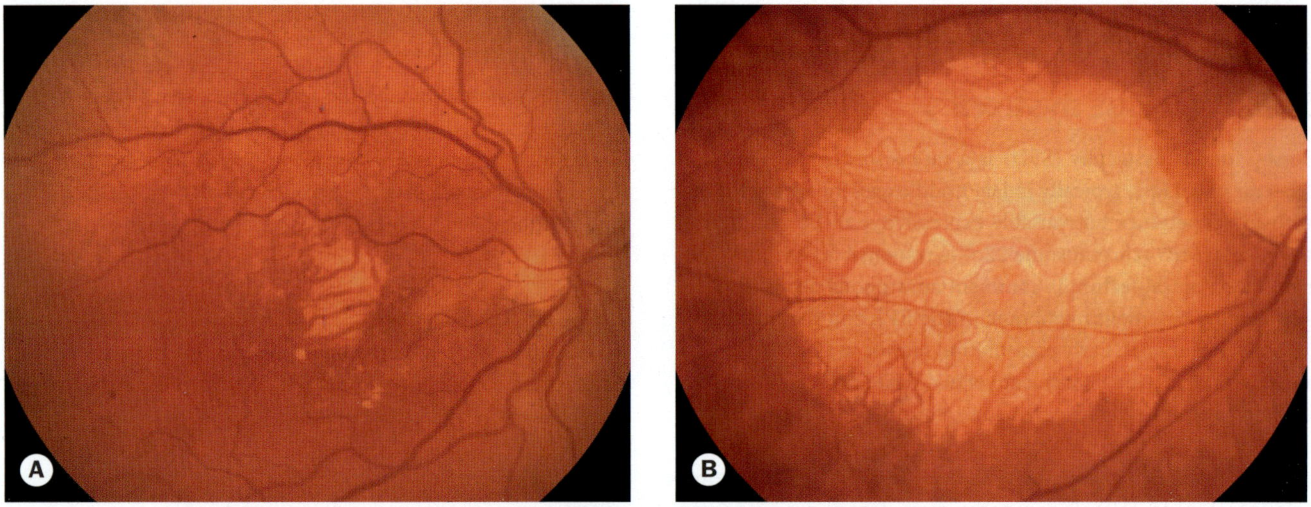

Fig. 15.32 Central areolar choroidal dystrophy. **(A)** Early; **(B)** end-stage.

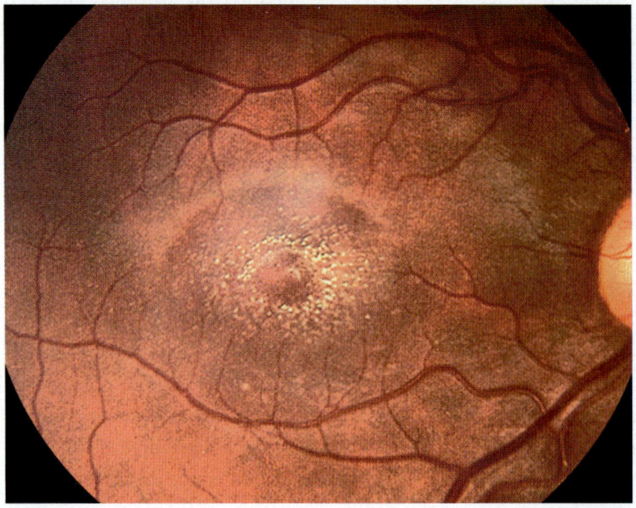

Fig. 15.33 Macular crystals in Sjögren–Larsson syndrome. *(Courtesy of D Taylor and C S Hoyt, from* Pediatric Ophthalmology and Strabismus, *Elsevier Saunders 2005.)*

GENERALIZED CHOROIDAL DYSTROPHIES

Choroideremia

Choroideremia is a progressive diffuse degeneration of the choroid, RPE and photoreceptors. Inheritance is X-linked, so that males are predominantly affected. However, it is important to identify female carriers, as 50% of their sons will develop choroideremia and 50% of their daughters will be carriers. The prognosis is very poor. Although most patients retain some vision until the sixth decade, severe visual loss occurs thereafter. The gene responsible is *CHM*; a contiguous extended gene deletion can lead to deafness and mental handicap.

- **Symptoms.** Nyctalopia, often beginning in adolescence, is followed by reduced peripheral vision and some years later, by loss of central vision. Clinically problematic disease occurs almost exclusively in males, but females may rarely also develop severe disease due to skewed inactivation of the X-chromosome.

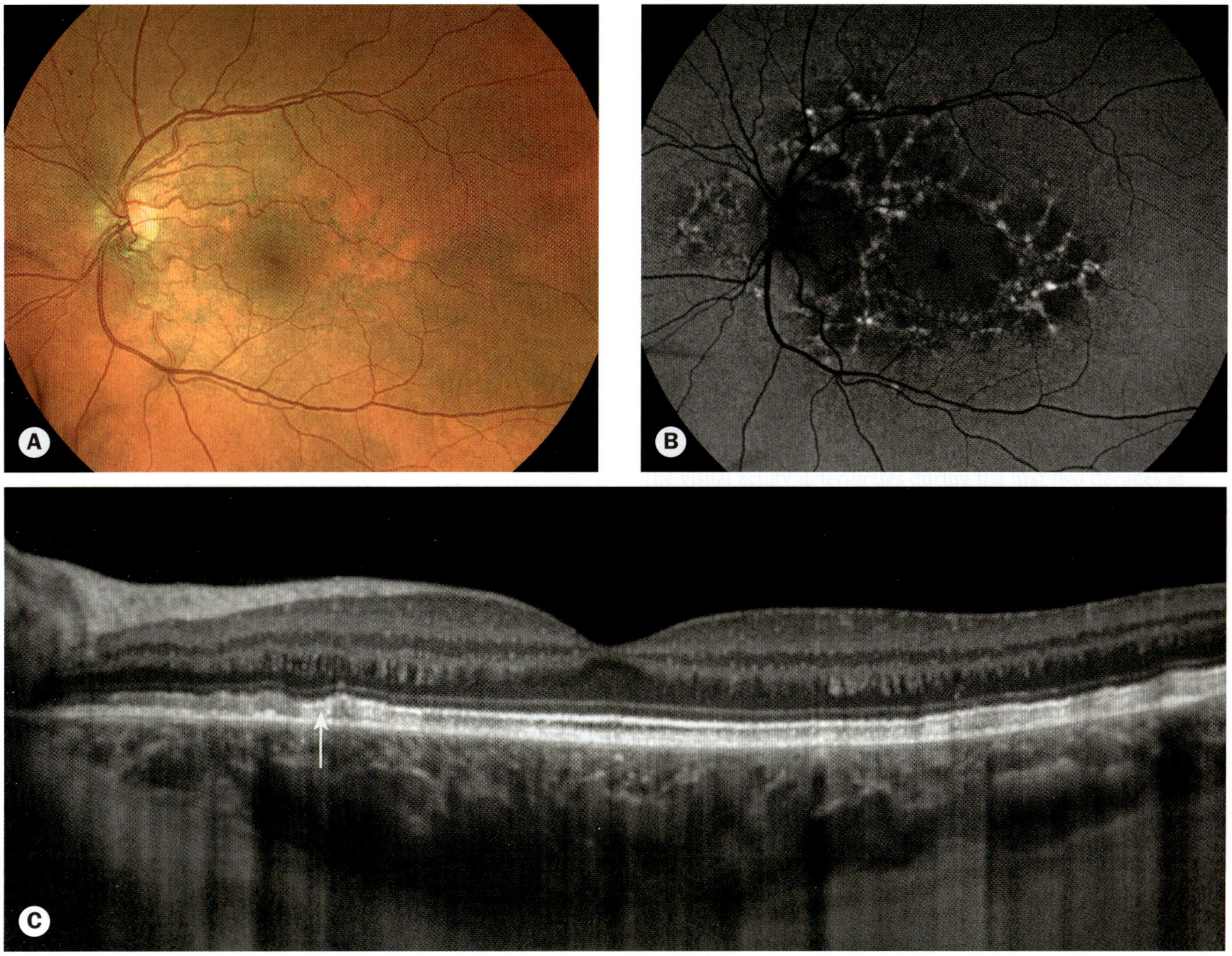

Fig. 15.34 Macular changes in maternally inherited diabetes and deafness. **(A)** Subtle atrophic changes are present in the macular region; **(B)** FAF of **(A)** showing macular hypoautofluorescence, surrounded by a reticular pattern of hyperautofluorescence; **(C)** OCT of **(A)** showing mild eccentric changes at the interface between RPE and photoreceptor outer segments (arrow), with subtle elevation of the ellipsoid zone and loss of the hyper-reflective line of the interdigitation zone.

- **Signs**
  - Female carriers show mild, patchy peripheral RPE atrophy and mottling (Fig. 15.35A). The visual acuity, fields and ERG are usually normal.
  - Males initially exhibit mid-peripheral RPE abnormalities that may, on cursory examination, resemble RP. Over time, chorioretinal atrophy spreads peripherally and centrally (Fig. 15.35B). The end-stage appearance consists of isolated choroidal vessels coursing over bare sclera. In contrast to primary retinal dystrophies, the fovea is spared until late.
- **Investigation**
  - FAF shows foveal sparing with a characteristic speckled pattern of autofluorescence (Fig. 15.35C).
  - ERG: scotopic is non-recordable; photopic is severely subnormal.
  - FA shows filling of the retinal and large choroidal vessels but not of the choriocapillaris. The intact fovea is hypofluorescent and is surrounded by hyperfluorescence due to an extensive window defect (Fig. 15.35D). This investigation is rarely needed.
  - ICGA shows chorioretinal loss with preserved larger choroidal vessels (Fig. 15.35E).
- **Treatment.** Clinical trials of specific gene therapy for choroideremia are ongoing.

Gyrate atrophy

Gyrate atrophy (AR) is caused by a mutation in the *OAT* gene (chromosome 10q) encoding the main ornithine degradation enzyme, ornithine aminotransferase. Deficiency of the enzyme leads to elevated ornithine levels in the plasma, urine, cerebrospinal fluid and aqueous humour. The visual prognosis is generally poor, with legal blindness occurring around the age of 50.

- **Symptoms.** Myopia and nyctalopia in adolescence, with a subsequent gradual worsening of vision.

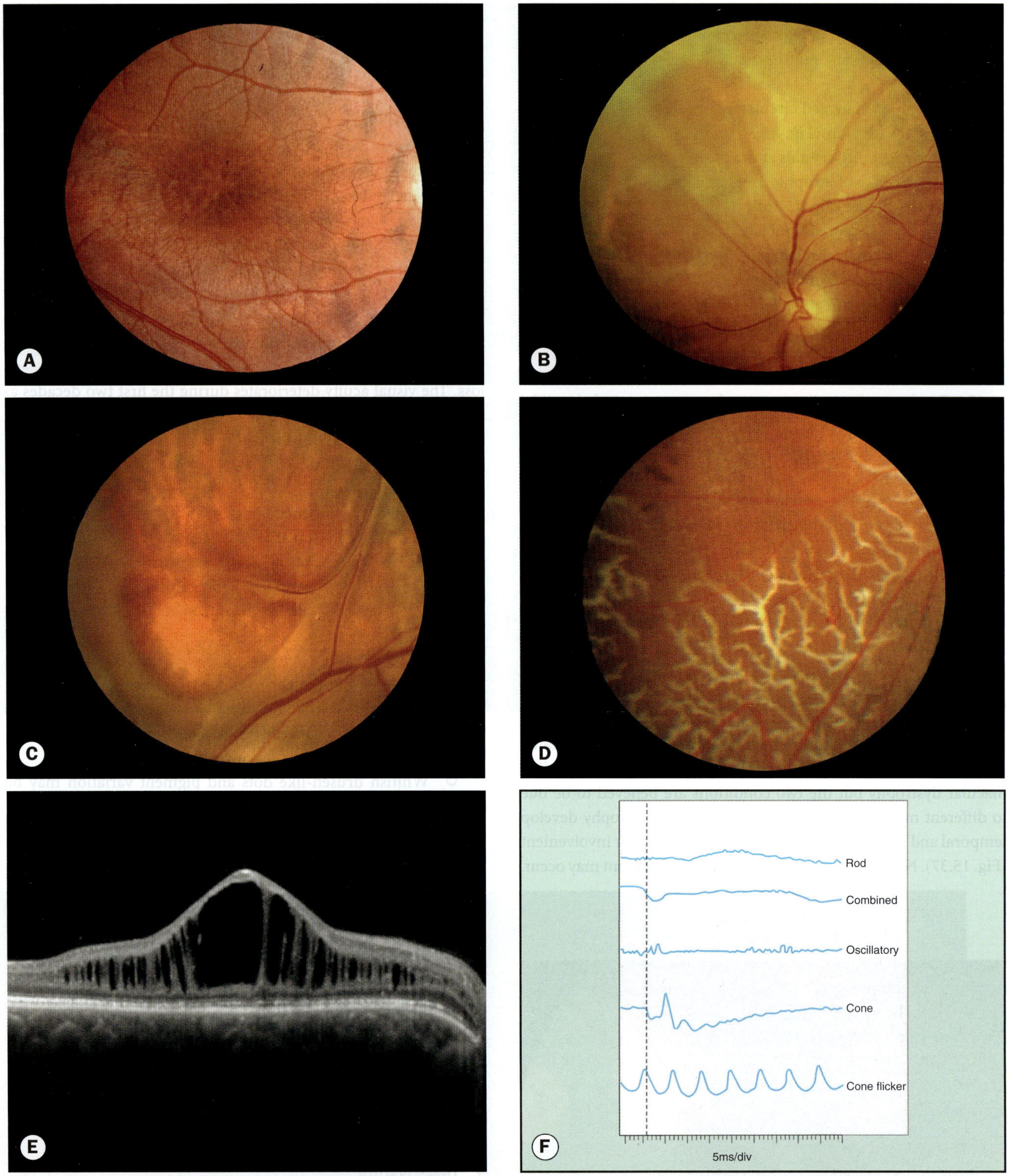

Fig. 15.38 Juvenile retinoschisis. **(A)** 'Bicycle wheel'-like maculopathy; **(B)** large, typically oval, inner leaf defects; **(C)** 'vitreous veils'; **(D)** peripheral dendritic lesions; **(E)** OCT showing macular schisis; **(F)** ERG showing selective decrease in b-wave amplitude in the combined response (electronegative). *(Courtesy of C Barry – fig. C; P Charbel Issa – fig. E.)*

- ERG is normal in eyes with isolated maculopathy. Eyes with peripheral schisis show a characteristic selective decrease in amplitude of the b-wave as compared with the a-wave on scotopic and photopic testing (Fig. 15.38F).
- FA is almost never needed, but if undertaken it may show mild window defects in the macula and no leakage, in contrast to CMO.
- Genetic testing for mutations in the *RS1* gene.

Treatment

- **Topical or oral carbonic anhydrase inhibitors** (e.g. dorzolamide eye drops three times daily) may reduce foveal schisis and improve visual acuity in some patients.
- **Vitrectomy** may be required for vitreous haemorrhage or retinal detachment repair, but is technically challenging.
- **Gene therapy** is under investigation, with the aim of restoring normal function of the protein abnormality underlying retinoschisis.

Stickler syndrome

Introduction

Stickler syndrome (hereditary arthro-ophthalmopathy) is a genetically heterogeneous disorder of collagen connective tissue. The condition affects approximately 1 in 7500 to 9000 people. At least eight clinically and genetically distinct sub-groups of Stickler syndrome are now recognized and it is possible to identify the underlying genetic mutation in 95% of cases. Inheritance is AD (STL1–STL3) or AR (STL4-STL8) with complete penetrance but variable expressivity. Stickler syndrome is the most common inherited cause of retinal detachment in children. Importantly, there is a high risk of childhood blindness secondary to bilateral retinal detachment in the three dominantly inherited sub-groups. Stickler syndrome should be considered in any infant with cleft palate, deafness or joint hypermobility in association with myopia. In general, the prognosis has been poor, but is improving with elevated standards of care.

- **Stickler syndrome type I (STL1 – membranous vitreous type)** is the most common form and is the result of mutations in the *COL2A1* gene, which encodes type 2 procollagen. The classic ocular and systemic features are present as originally described by Stickler, though there is also a predominantly ocular (non-syndromic) form of STL1.
- **STL2 (beaded vitreous type)** is caused by mutations in the *COL11A1* gene. Patients have congenital non-progressive high myopia, sensorineural deafness and other features of Stickler syndrome type 1.
- **STL3 (non-ocular type)** is due to mutations in the *COL11A2* gene. Affected individuals have the typical systemic features, but no ocular manifestations.
- **STL4-STL8 (AR types)** are extremely rare.
- **Systemic features** include mid-facial hypoplasia, joint hypermobility (Fig. 15.39A), Pierre-Robin-type features (micrognathia, cleft palate – Fig. 15.39B and glossoptosis – backward displacement of the tongue), bifid uvula (Fig. 15.39C), mild spondyloepiphyseal dysplasia and early-onset osteoarthritis. Deafness may be sensorineural or caused by recurrent otitis media.
- **Kniest dysplasia** is usually caused by a defect in the type II collagen gene *COL2A1*, which is also involved in Stickler syndrome type 1. Inheritance can be AD, but most cases represent a *de novo* mutation. High myopia, vitreous degeneration, retinal detachment and ectopia lentis can occur. Systemic features may include short stature, a round face and arthropathy.

Diagnosis

The three characteristic ocular features are high myopia, vitreoretinal degeneration with an associated extremely high rate of retinal detachment and cataract.

- **Signs**
  - In STL1 patients exhibit an optically empty vitreous, a retrolenticular membrane and circumferential equatorial membranes that extend a short way into the vitreous cavity (Fig. 15.39D and E).
  - In STL2 patients the vitreous has a fibrillary and beaded appearance.
  - Radial lattice-like degeneration associated with RPE hyperplasia, vascular sheathing and sclerosis.
  - Retinal detachment develops in approximately 50% in the first decade of life, often as a result of multiple or giant tears that may involve both eyes (Fig. 15.39F). This should not be confused with retinal dialysis.
  - Presenile cataract characterized by frequently non-progressive peripheral cortical wedge-shaped, fleck or lamellar opacities is common.
  - Ectopia lentis can occur, but is uncommon.
  - Glaucoma (5–10%) is associated with congenital angle anomaly.

Treatment

- Prophylactic 360° retinal laser or cryotherapy reduces the incidence of retinal detachment. Regular screening with prophylactic treatment of retinal breaks is essential. Long-term review of all patients is mandatory.
- Retinal detachment repair is challenging and vitrectomy is generally indicated. Proliferative vitreoretinopathy is a particularly common complication and re-detachment may occur.
- Cataract in Stickler is often visually inconsequential, particularly when early. If surgery is required, a careful preoperative retinal evaluation with treatment of breaks should be performed. Vitreous loss and postoperative retinal detachment are relatively common.
- Glaucoma treatment may be required. If early-onset and presumably related to angle anomaly, management is generally as for congenital glaucoma (see Ch. 11).

TIP Prophylactic treatment is key to preserving vision in the high-risk sub-groups of Stickler syndrome, as this reduces the risk of visual loss secondary to retinal detachment.

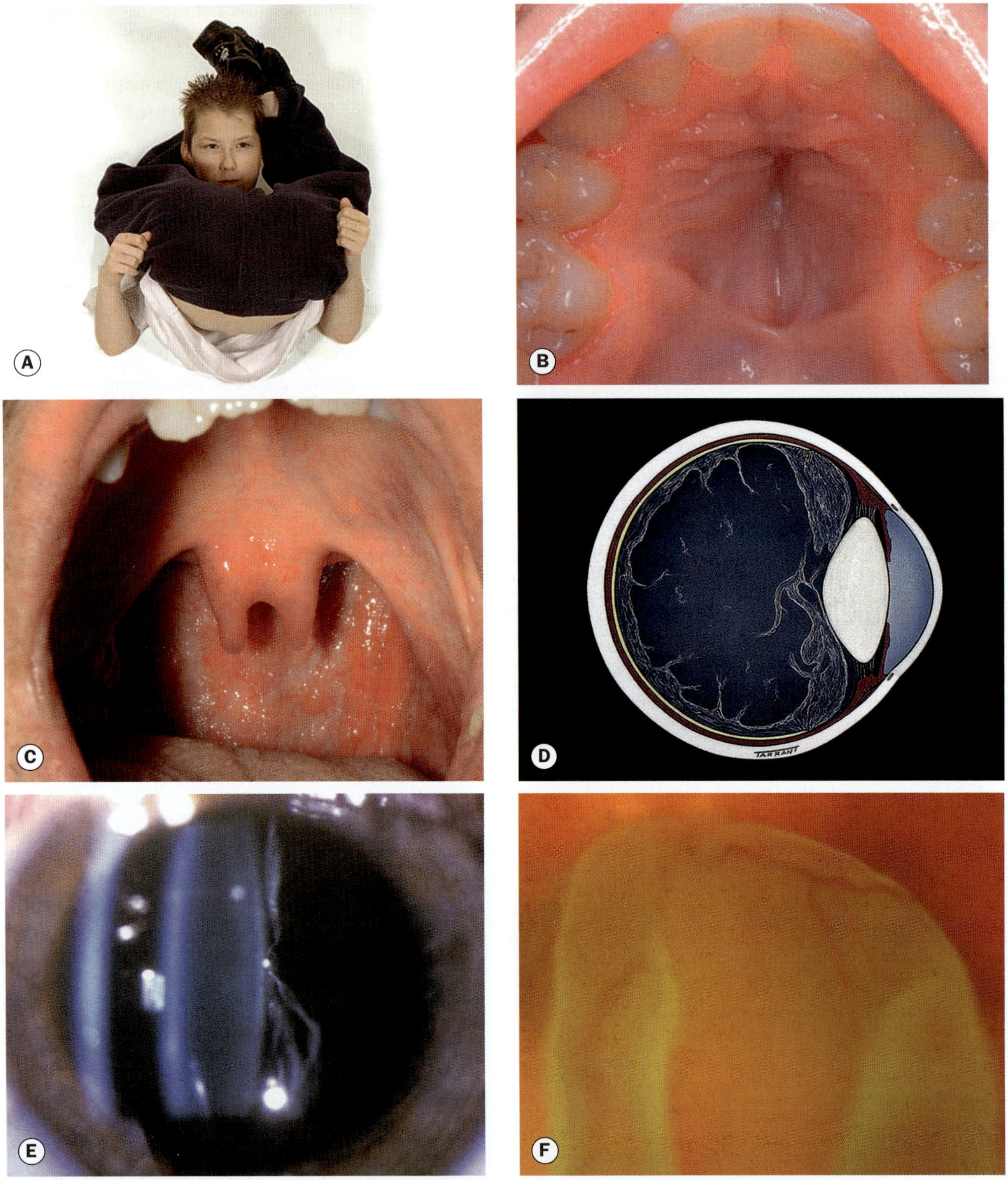

Fig. 15.39 Stickler syndrome. **(A)** Hypermobility of joints; **(B)** cleft and high-arched palate; **(C)** bifid uvula; **(D)** vitreous appearance; **(E)** slit lamp appearance in type 1; **(F)** 360° giant retinal tear with detachment *(Courtesy of M Snead – figs A, E and F; Ken K Nischal – fig. B.)*

Wagner syndrome

Wagner syndrome (VCAN-related vitreoretinopathy) is a rare condition having some features in common with Stickler syndrome, but no association with systemic abnormalities. Erosive vitreoretinopathy is now known to be the same disorder. Inheritance is AD and mutations in the gene *VCAN* can be responsible. Severity is variable, with up to 50% developing retinal detachment, often before the age of 15.

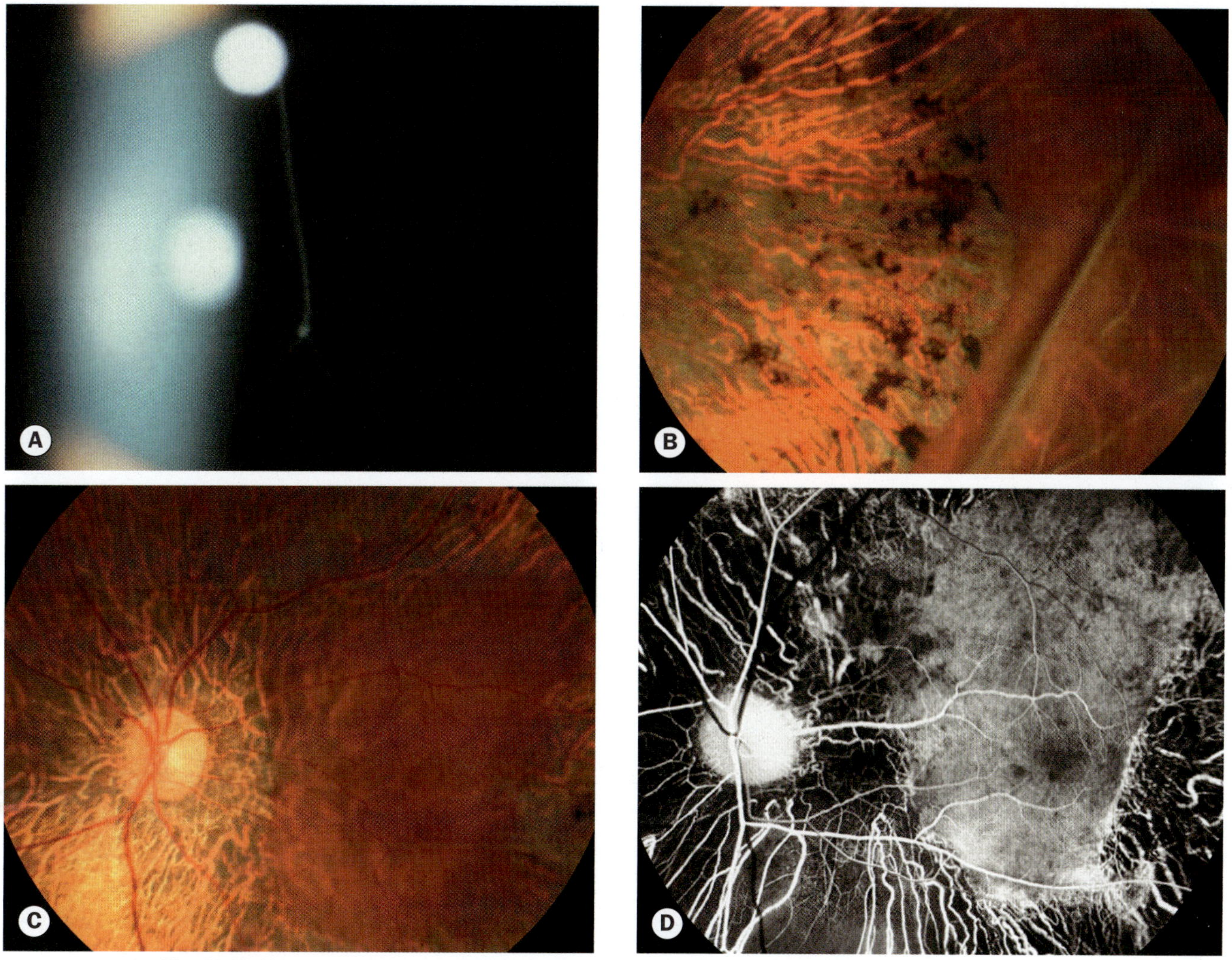

Fig. 15.40 Wagner syndrome. **(A)** Vitreous appearance; **(B)** peripheral chorioretinal atrophy and preretinal membranes; **(C)** progressive chorioretinal atrophy; **(D)** FA showing gross loss of the choriocapillaris. *(Courtesy of E Messmer.)*

- **Signs**
  - Patients tend to have low to moderate myopia.
  - The key abnormal finding is an optically empty vitreous cavity (Fig. 15.40A) lacking structural elements and it is thought this leads to reduced 'scaffolding' support for the retina.
  - The peripheral retinal vasculature is deficient.
  - Greyish-white avascular strands and membranes extend into the vitreous cavity and there may be a circumferential ridge-like condensation of the gel at or anterior to the retinal periphery (Fig. 15.40B).
  - Peripheral retinal changes including progressive chorioretinal atrophy (Fig. 15.40C) occur and nyctalopia is commonly troublesome. The visual fields gradually constrict.
  - Cataract is common in younger adults and glaucoma can develop.
- **Investigation.** FA shows non-perfusion due to choriocapillaris loss (Fig. 15.40D). The ERG may initially be normal, but later shows a reduction of scotopic b-wave amplitudes and diffuse cone-rod loss.
- **Treatment.** Retinal breaks and detachment are treated as they occur, but extensive prophylaxis is avoided.

Familial exudative vitreoretinopathy

Familial exudative vitreoretinopathy is a rare, slowly progressive condition characterized by failure of vascularization of the temporal retinal periphery, similar to that seen in retinopathy of prematurity. The avascular peripheral retina leads to hypoxia and stimulates neovascularization which can lead to vitreoretinal traction, subretinal exudation and haemorrhages, tractional retinal detachment and foveal displacement. Inheritance is most commonly AD and rarely X-linked or AR, with high penetrance and variable expressivity. To date, mutations in 10 genes have been implicated which affect normal retinal angiogenesis. The clinical appearance is often asymmetrical and can vary significantly even among affected members of the same family. Presentation is in childhood. The prognosis is frequently poor, especially with early aggressive onset.

- **Signs**
  - High myopia may be present.
  - Stage 1: peripheral avascularity. There is abrupt termination of retinal vessels at the temporal equator. Vitreous degeneration and peripheral vitreoretinal

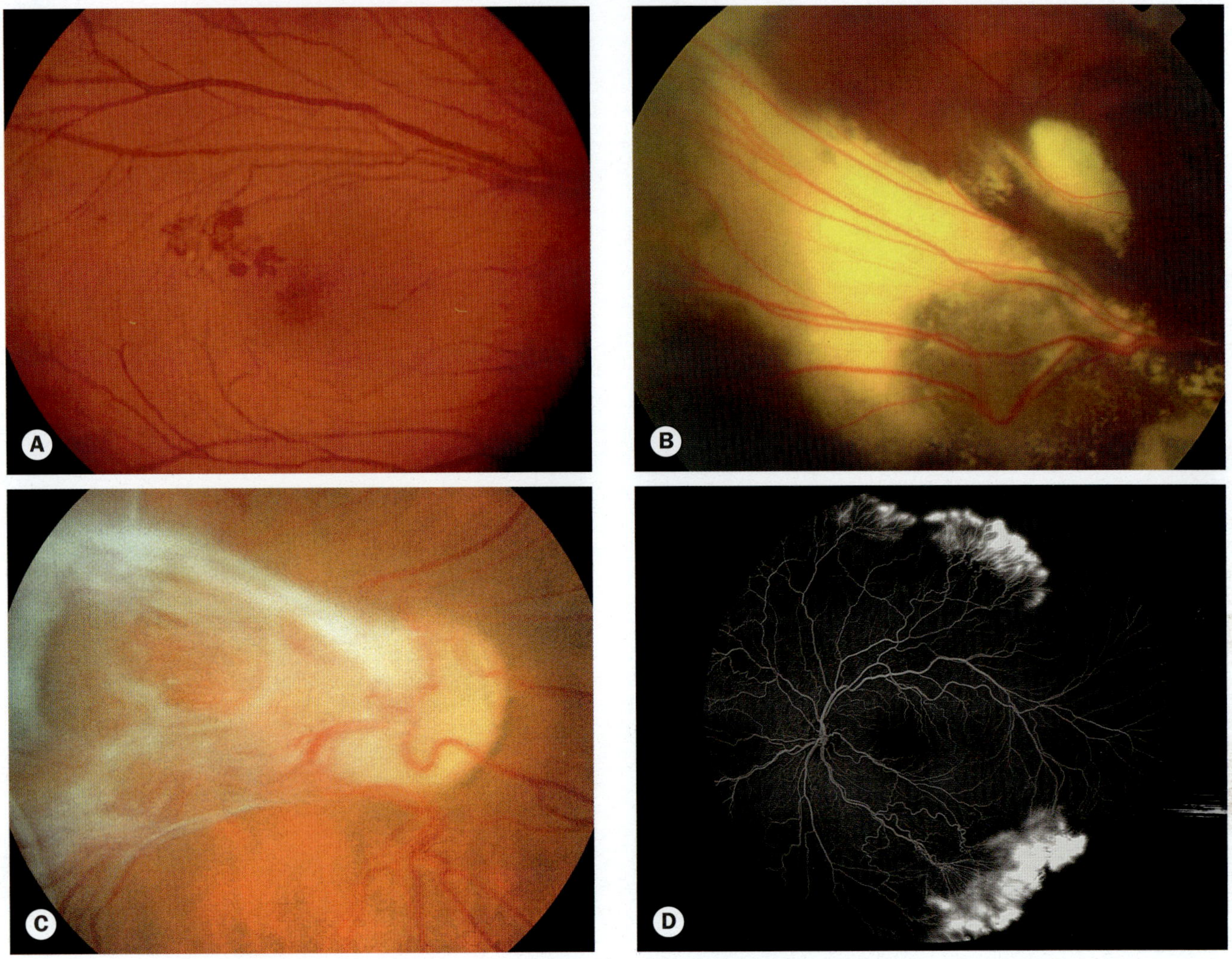

Fig. 15.41 Familial exudative vitreoretinopathy. **(A)** Straightening of the macular vessels and peripheral telangiectasia; **(B)** subretinal exudation; **(C)** 'dragging' of the disc and macula, with underlying macular tractional detachment; **(D)** wide-field FA showing vascular straightening and abrupt termination with leaking capillaries in familial exudative vitreoretinopathy. *(Courtesy of C Hoyng – fig. B.)*

attachments are associated with areas of 'white without pressure'. Vascular straightening may be present (Fig. 15.41A).

- Stage 2: peripheral vascular tortuosity and telangiectasia progresses to preretinal fibrovascular proliferation with or without subretinal exudation (Fig. 15.41B).
- Stage 3: tractional and/or rhegmatogenous macular-sparing retinal detachment, with or without exudation.
- Stages 4 and 5 are macula-involving (Fig. 15.41C) and total retinal detachment, respectively.
- Vitreous haemorrhage, cataract and neovascular glaucoma can occur.

- **Investigation.** Wide-field FA is invaluable (Fig. 15.41D) in confirming the diagnosis, ensuring accurate targeting and completeness of ablation of avascular retina and identifying asymptomatic cases with subtle features.
- **Treatment**
  - Management depends on the clinical stage of the disease.
  - Laser ablation of avascular retina is recommended, usually once neovascularization has occurred.
  - Vitrectomy for retinal detachment is challenging but often successful.
  - Intravitreal anti-VEGF treatment can be useful as a temporizing measure.
  - Lifelong monitoring is required. Although the disease has a progressive course during childhood it tends to become latent after the second decade. However, late progression with sight-threatening complications can occur at any age after varying periods of quiescence.
  - Relatives should be screened.

Enhanced S-cone syndrome and Goldmann–Favre syndrome

This is a rare inherited progressive retinal degeneration which has a highly variable phenotype. The human retina has three cone

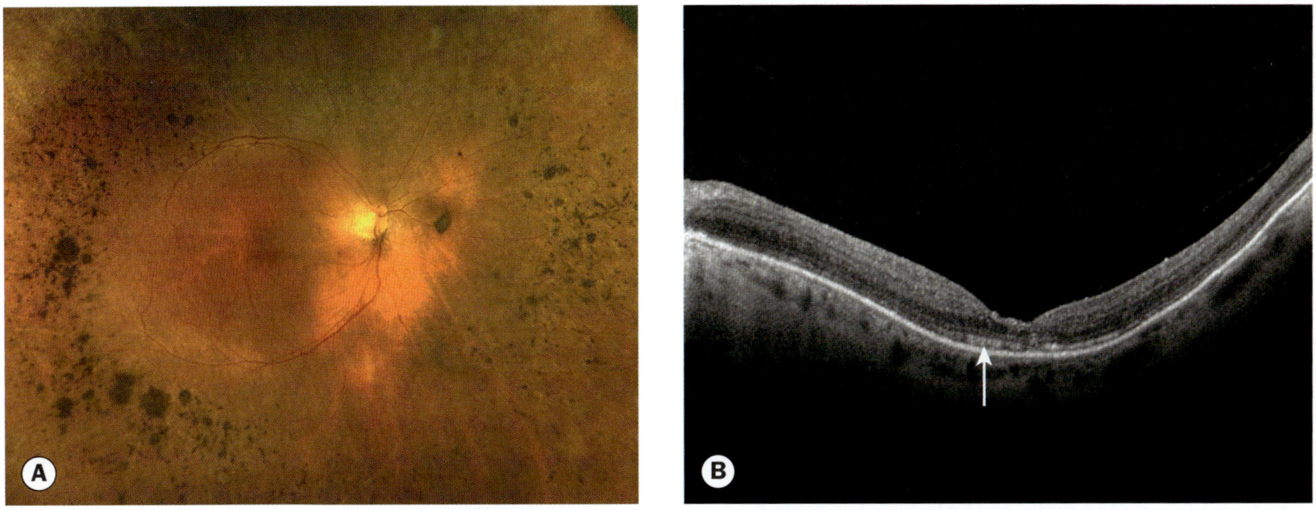

Fig. 15.42 Enhanced S-cone and Goldmann–Favre syndrome. **(A)** Optos image showing characteristic nummular pigmentation around the vascular arcades; **(B)** OCT showing disrupted foveal lamination with a thickened subfoveal ellipsoid zone (arrow). *(Courtesy of S de Silva.)*

photoreceptor types: short-wave sensitivity (S), middle-wave sensitivity (M) and long-wave sensitivity (L). Most inherited retinal dystrophies exhibit progressive attenuation of rods and all classes of cones. However, enhanced S-cone syndrome is characterized by hyperfunction of S-cones and severe impairment of M- and L-cones, with non-recordable rod function. Goldmann–Favre syndrome, which is caused by mutations in the same gene, represents a severe variant.

- **Inheritance** is AR with variable expressivity. The gene implicated is *NR2E3*, which encodes for a ligand-dependent transcription factor.
- **Presentation** is with nyctalopia in childhood and sometimes hemeralopia (reduced vision in bright light). Colour vision is decreased, but the tritan axis is preserved. Pigmentary changes along the vascular arcades or mid-periphery may be associated in more advanced cases with round pigment clumps (Fig. 15.42A). Macular changes may include cystoid maculopathy (without fluorescein leakage) and schisis. Vitreous degeneration and peripheral retinoschisis can occur.
- **OCT** shows disrupted foveal lamination with a thickened subfoveal ellipsoid zone (Fig. 15.42B).
- **ERG** shows no rod response and the scotopic maximum response and photopic ERG waveforms are similar.
- **Prognosis** is subject to considerable clinical variability; while some patients maintain good visual acuity and show little progression, some patients develop extensive retinal degeneration and visual loss. About 30% have a visual acuity of 6/36 or worse by late middle age.
- **There is no treatment** other than supportive measures.

Snowflake vitreoretinal degeneration

This rare AD condition (gene *KCNJ13*) has some similarities to Wagner syndrome. Retinal detachment is less common and the prognosis is usually very good.

- **Signs** (Fig. 15.43)

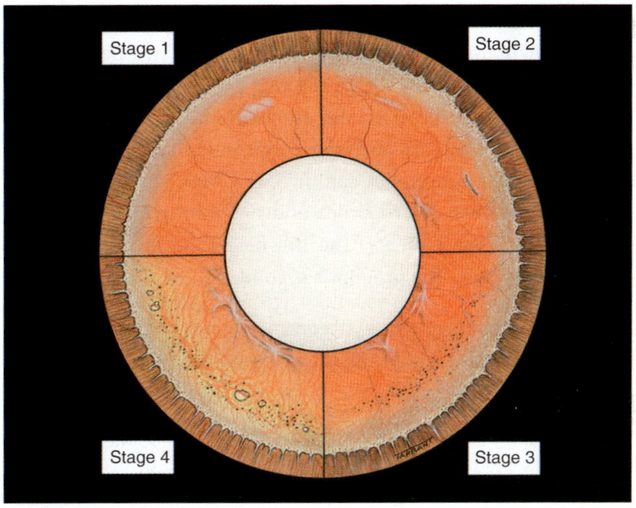

Fig. 15.43 Snowflake degeneration.

  - Stage 1 shows extensive areas of 'white without pressure' in patients typically under the age of 15 years.
  - Stage 2 shows snowflake-like yellow–white crystalline deposits in areas of 'white with pressure' in patients aged between 15 and 25.
  - Stage 3 manifests with vascular sheathing and pigmentation posterior to the area of snowflake degeneration in patients aged between 25 and 50.
  - Stage 4 is characterized by increased pigmentation, gross vascular attenuation, areas of chorioretinal atrophy and less prominent snowflakes in patients over the age of 60. The macula remains normal.
  - Other possible features include mild myopia, vitreous fibrillary degeneration and liquefaction, a waxy optic nerve head, corneal guttae, retinal detachment and early-onset cataract.
- **Investigation.** The ERG shows a low scotopic b-wave amplitude.

Autosomal dominant neovascular inflammatory vitreoretinopathy

A rare but interesting inherited (gene *CAPN5*) disorder, autosomal dominant neovascular inflammatory vitreoretinopathy features panuveitis, often of onset in early adulthood. The initial symptom is typically floaters due to vitritis, with the development of peripheral vascular closure with peripheral and then disc neovascularization, fundus pigmentation, epiretinal and subretinal fibrocellular membranes. Complications include vitreous haemorrhage, tractional retinal detachment, CMO, cataract and neovascular glaucoma. The ERG shows selective loss of b-wave amplitude. The prognosis can be poor. Peripheral retinal photocoagulation and vitreous surgery may be required.

Autosomal dominant vitreoretinochoroidopathy

Autosomal dominant vitreoretinochoroidopathy can be caused by *BEST1* mutations. Presentation is in adult life if symptomatic, but frequently discovery is by chance. Vitreous cells and fibrillary degeneration develop, with a non-progressive or very slowly progressive encircling band of pigmentary disturbance between the ora serrata and equator, with a discrete posterior border. Within the band there can be arteriolar attenuation, neovascularization, punctate white opacities and later chorioretinal atrophy. Complications are uncommon, but can include CMO, vitreous haemorrhage and cataract. Microcornea and nanophthalmos have been described in some patients. The full-field ERG is subnormal in older patients only. The prognosis is good.

ALBINISM

Introduction

Albinism is a genetically determined, heterogeneous group of disorders of melanin synthesis in which either the eyes alone (ocular albinism) or the eyes, skin and hair (oculocutaneous albinism) may be affected. The latter may be either tyrosinase-positive or tyrosinase-negative. The different mutations are thought to act through a common pathway involving reduced melanin synthesis in the eye during development. Molecular genetics allows 7 subtypes of non-syndromic oculocutaneous albinism (OCA) to be determined (OCA 1–7). Patients with oculocutaneous albinism have an increased risk of cutaneous basal cell and squamous cell carcinoma.

TIP Patients with oculocutaneous albinism are at increased risk of cutaneous basal cell and squamous cell carcinoma and should take precautions to avoid exposure to sunlight.

Tyrosinase-negative oculocutaneous albinism (OCA type 1)

Individuals who have tyrosinase-negative (complete) albinism are incapable of synthesizing any melanin and have white hair and very pale skin (Fig. 15.44A) throughout life with a lack of melanin pigment in all ocular structures. The condition is caused by mutations in *TYR* gene (chromosome 11q14), responsible for the enzyme tyrosinase, usually with AR inheritance.

- **Signs**
  - VA is usually <6/60 due to foveal hypoplasia.
  - Nystagmus is typically pendular and horizontal. It usually increases in bright illumination and tends to lessen in severity with age.
  - The iris is diaphanous and translucent (Fig. 15.44B), giving rise to a 'pink-eyed' appearance (Fig. 15.44C).
  - The fundus lacks pigment and shows conspicuously large choroidal vessels. There is also foveal hypoplasia with absence of the foveal pit and poorly formed perimacular vascular arcades (Fig. 15.44D).
  - The optic chiasm has fewer uncrossed nerve fibres than normal – the majority of fibres from each eye cross to the contralateral hemisphere. This can be demonstrated with visual evoked potentials.
  - Other features include high refractive errors of various types, a positive angle kappa, squint and absent stereopsis.

Tyrosinase-positive oculocutaneous albinism (OCA type 2)

Individuals who have tyrosinase-positive (incomplete) albinism synthesize variable amounts of melanin. Their hair may be white, yellow or red and darkens with age. Skin is pale at birth but usually darkens by 2 years of age (Fig. 15.45A). Inheritance is usually AR. The condition is caused by hundreds of different mutations in the *OCA2* gene (chromosome 15q12), which plays a role in tyrosine transport in melanosomes. This is the commonest form of albinism in Africa and accounts for a third of cases worldwide.

- **Ocular signs**
  - VA is usually impaired due to foveal hypoplasia.
  - Iris may be blue or dark brown with variable translucency.
  - Fundus shows variable hypopigmentation (Fig. 15.45B).

Oculocutaneous albinism OCA (types 3–7)

OCT type 3 is seen especially in Black Africans. The other subtypes are rare and have been reported in single families.

Systemic associations

- **Chediak–Higashi syndrome**: a rare AR disorder arising from a mutation of a lysosomal regulator protein. This leads to failure of phagolysosome formation and recurrent pyogenic infections (especially *Staphylococcus*).
- **Hermansky–Pudlak syndrome**: an extremely rare AR lysosomal storage disease with platelet dysfunction (easy bruising and excessive bleeding). In some cases, pulmonary fibrosis and granulomatous colitis with bleeding may occur.
- **Waardenburg syndrome**: an AD condition with a range of systemic presentations including a white forelock, poliosis, synophrys ('monobrow'), deafness and sometimes limb and

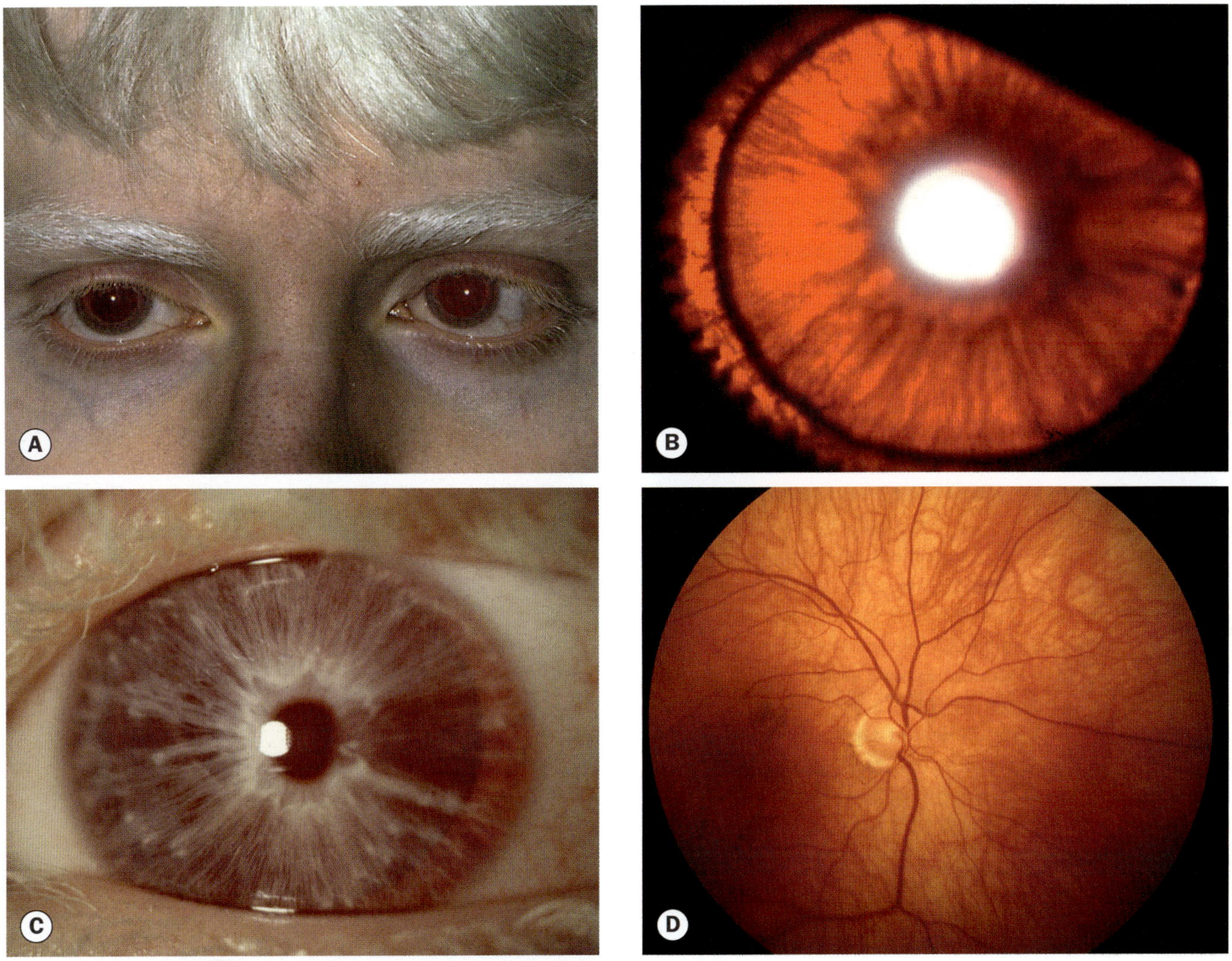

Fig. 15.44 Signs in tyrosinase-negative oculocutaneous albinism. **(A)** White hair and pale skin; **(B)** marked iris translucency; **(C)** 'pink eyed' appearance; **(D)** severe fundus hypopigmentation and foveal aplasia.

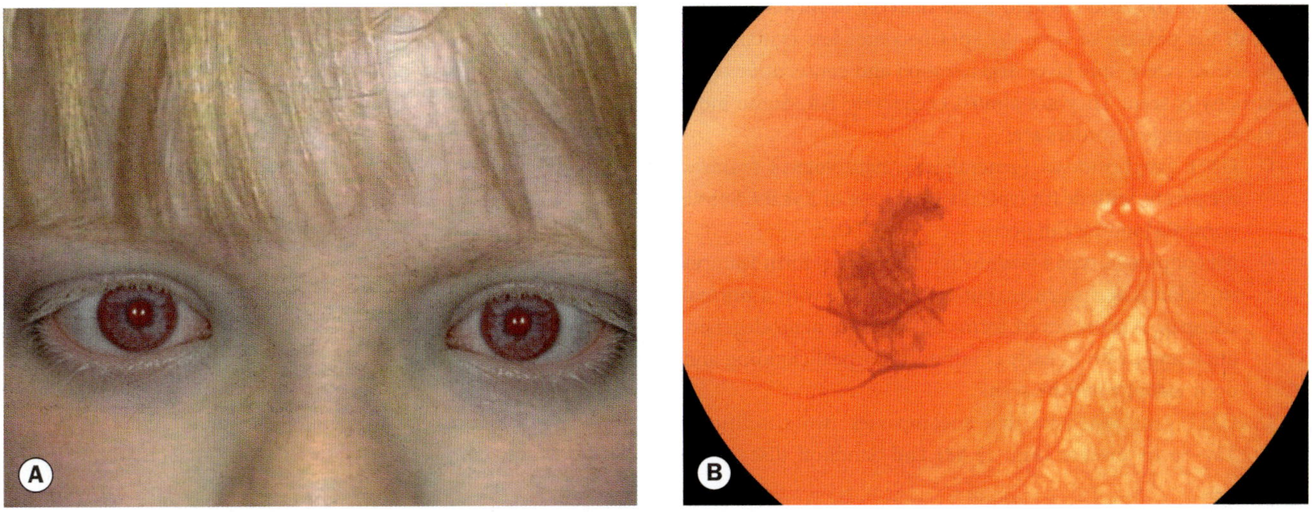

Fig. 15.45 Tyrosinase-positive oculocutaneous albinism. **(A)** Fair hair and normal skin colour; **(B)** mild fundus hypopigmentation.

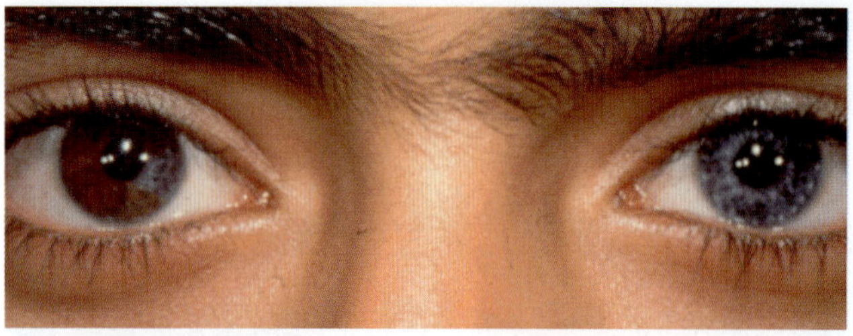

Fig. 15.46 Waardenburg syndrome with iris heterochromia (segmental in the right eye) and synophrys.

neurological anomalies. Ocular features include lateral displacement of the medial canthi, hypochromic irides with segmental or total heterochromia (Fig. 15.46) and choroidal depigmentation.

Ocular albinism (OA)

In this variant, involvement is predominantly ocular, with normal skin and hair, although occasionally hypopigmented skin macules may be seen. Two types are recognized: OA1 (Nettleship Falls syndrome) and OA2 (Forsius–Eriksson syndrome). Inheritance is always X-linked. Female carriers are asymptomatic, but may show partial iris translucency, macular stippling and mid-peripheral scattered areas of depigmentation and granularity (Fig. 15.47). Affected males have hypopigmented irides and fundi.

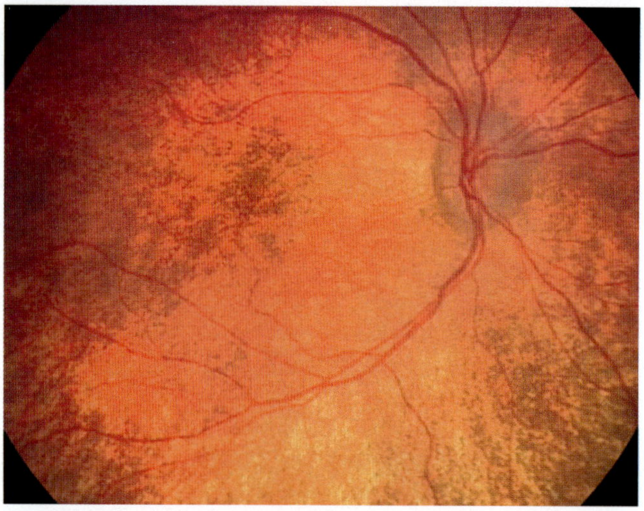

Fig. 15.47 Carrier of X-linked ocular albinism. *(Courtesy of M Pennesi.)*

CHERRY-RED SPOT AT THE MACULA

A cherry-red spot at the macula is a clinical sign seen in the context of thickening and loss of transparency of the retina at the posterior pole. The fovea is the thinnest part of the retina, allowing persistent transmission of the underlying vascular choroidal hue when the surrounding retina becomes relatively opaque. Causes include:

- **Metabolic storage diseases.** A group of rare inherited metabolic diseases, often enzyme deficiencies, leads to the pathological accumulation of lipid-based material in various tissues. With the passage of time the spot becomes less evident due to retinal nerve fibre layer degeneration and consecutive optic atrophy is seen. They are almost exclusively AR. Some individual storage disorders are:
    - GM1 gangliosidosis (generalized): neurological features are severe, with death typically by the age of 2 years. Subtle corneal clouding can occur.
    - Mucolipidosis type I (sialidosis): a late-onset form features myoclonus and seizures, but is compatible with a normal life span. A more severe form causes severe neurodegeneration and death in early childhood. Corneal clouding and optic atrophy may be seen.
    - GM2 gangliosidosis: this encompasses two conditions, Tay–Sachs disease (Fig. 15.48) and Sandhoff disease. In both, there is progressive neurological deterioration, with early blindness and death.
    - Niemann–Pick disease: of the three main types (A–C), only the first two feature a cherry-red spot. Abnormal ocular motility occurs in type C (chronic neuropathic).
    - Farber disease: systemically, aphonia, dermatitis, lymphadenopathy, psychomotor retardation, renal and cardiopulmonary disease may develop. Ocular features additional to cherry-red spot development include pinguecula-like conjunctival lesions and nodular corneal opacity.
- **Central retinal and cilioretinal artery occlusion** (see Ch. 13). Retinal clouding results from oedema; the appearance is an acute sign only.
- **Retinotoxicity** due to specific agents including quinine, dapsone, gentamicin, carbon monoxide and methanol.
- **Commotio retinae** (see Ch. 22); oedema due to blunt trauma.

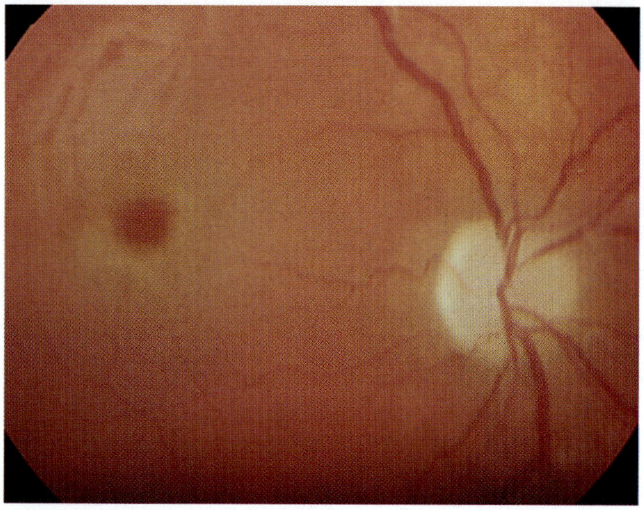

Fig. 15.48 Cherry-red spot at the macula in a baby with Tay–Sachs disease.

Chapter 16

Retinal Detachment

INTRODUCTION

Anatomy of the peripheral retina

Pars plana

The ciliary body starts 1 mm from the limbus and extends posteriorly for about 6 mm. The anterior 2 mm consist of the pars plicata, the remaining 4 mm, the flattened pars plana. In order not to endanger either the lens or retina, the optimal location for a pars plana surgical incision or intravitreal injection is 4 mm and 3.5 mm posterior to the limbus in phakic and pseudophakic eyes, respectively. An incision through the mid-pars plana will usually be located anterior to the vitreous base (see below).

Ora serrata

The ora serrata (Fig. 16.1) is the junction between the retina and ciliary body. In retinal detachment (RD), fusion of the sensory retina with the retinal pigment epithelium (RPE) and choroid limits forward extension of subretinal fluid (SRF) at the ora. However, there is no equivalent adhesion between the choroid and sclera and choroidal detachments may progress anteriorly to involve the ciliary body (ciliochoroidal detachment).

- **Dentate processes** are tapering extensions of retina onto the pars plana. They are more marked nasally than temporally and display marked variation in contour.
- **Oral bays** are scalloped edges of pars plana epithelium between dentate processes.
- **Meridional folds** (Fig. 16.2) are small radial folds of thickened retinal tissue in line with dentate processes, most commonly in the superonasal quadrant. A fold may occasionally exhibit a small retinal hole at its apex. A meridional complex is a configuration in which a dentate process, usually with an associated meridional fold, is aligned with a ciliary process.
- **Enclosed oral bays** (see Fig. 16.2) are small islands of pars plana surrounded by retina as a result of the meeting of two adjacent dentate processes. They should not be mistaken for retinal holes.

Vitreous base

The vitreous base (Fig. 16.3) is a 3–4 mm wide zone straddling the ora serrata, throughout which the cortical vitreous is strongly attached. Following posterior vitreous detachment (PVD), the posterior hyaloid face remains attached at the vitreous base. Pre-existing retinal holes within the attached vitreous base do not lead to RD. Blunt trauma may cause an avulsion of the vitreous base, with tearing of the non-pigmented epithelium of the pars plana along the base's anterior border and of the retina along the base's posterior border.

Innocuous peripheral retinal degenerations (Fig. 16.4A)

Peripheral retinal degenerations and other lesions carrying the potential to lead to RD are described separately.

- **Microcystoid (peripheral cystoid) degeneration** consists of tiny vesicles with indistinct boundaries on a greyish-white background, making the retina appear thickened and less transparent. The degeneration starts adjacent to the ora serrata and extends circumferentially and posteriorly with a smooth undulating posterior border. Microcystoid degeneration is

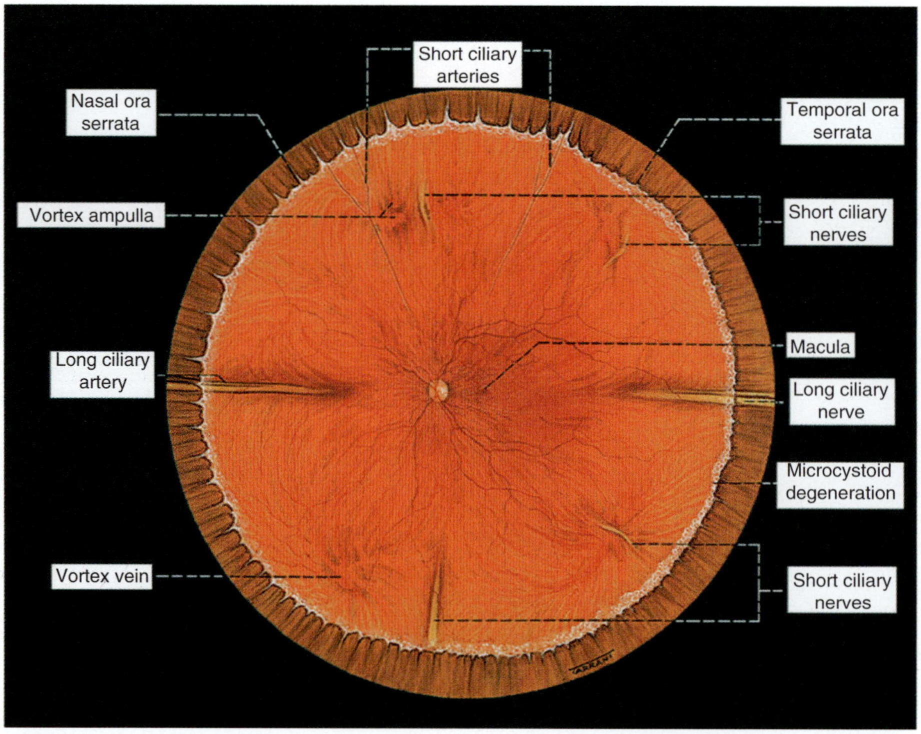

Fig. 16.1 The ora serrata and normal anatomical landmarks.

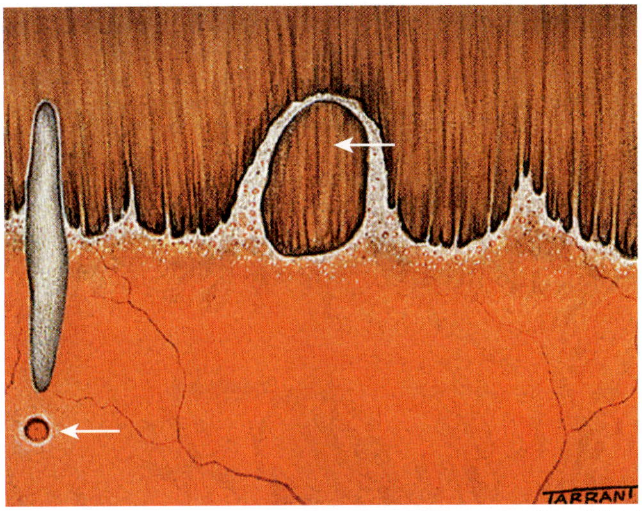

Fig. 16.2 Normal variants of the ora serrata: meridional fold with a small retinal hole at its base (arrow); enclosed oral bay (arrow).

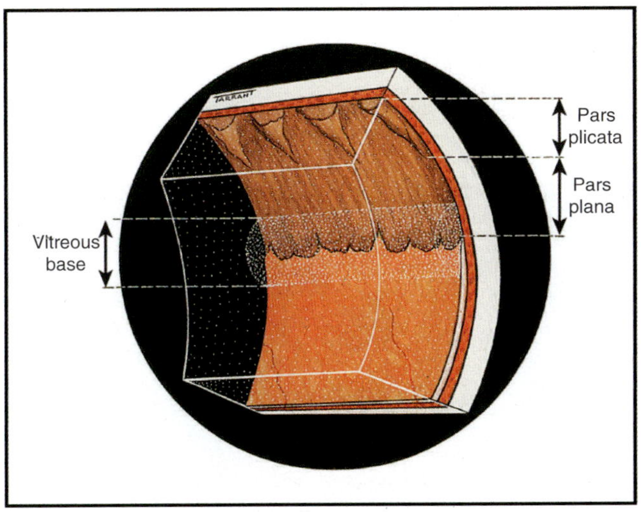

Fig. 16.3 The vitreous base.

present in most adult eyes, increasing in extent with age. It is not causally related to RD, though it may give rise to typical degenerative retinoschisis.
- **Paving stone degeneration** is characterized by discrete yellow–white patches of focal chorioretinal atrophy that may have pigmented margins (Fig. 16.4B and C). It is typically found between the equator and the ora and is more common in the inferior fundus. It is present to some extent in at least 25% of normal eyes.
- **Reticular (honeycomb) degeneration** is an age-related change consisting of a fine network of perivascular pigmentation that sometimes extends posterior to the equator (Fig. 16.4D).
- **Peripheral drusen.** Clustered or scattered small pale discrete lesions (Fig. 16.4E) that may have hyperpigmented borders. They are similar to drusen at the posterior pole and usually occur in the eyes of older individuals.
- **Pars plana cyst.** Clear-walled cysts, usually small, are derived from non-pigmented ciliary epithelium. They are present in 5–10% of eyes and are more common temporally. They do not predispose to RD.

Sites of vitreous adhesion

Physiological

The peripheral cortical vitreous is loosely attached to the internal limiting membrane (ILM) of the sensory retina. Sites of stronger adhesion in the normal eye include:
- Vitreous base (very strong).
- Optic disc margins (fairly strong).
- Perifoveal (fairly weak).
- Peripheral blood vessels (usually weak).

Pathological

Abnormal adhesions may lead to retinal tear formation following PVD, or to vitreomacular interface disease. Most are discussed in detail later in this chapter.
- Lattice degeneration.
- Retinal pigment clumps.
- Cystic retinal tufts.
- Vitreous base anomalies, such as extensions and posterior islands.
- 'White with pressure' and 'white without pressure'.
- Zonular traction tufts.
- Vitreomacular traction (see Ch. 14).
- Preretinal new vessels, e.g. proliferative diabetic retinopathy.

Definitions

- **Retinal detachment (RD).** RD refers to separation of the neurosensory retina (NSR) from the RPE. This results in the accumulation of subretinal fluid (SRF) in the potential space between the NSR and RPE.
- **Rhegmatogenous** (Greek *rhegma* – break) **RD** requires a full-thickness defect in the sensory retina, which permits fluid derived from synchytic (liquefied) vitreous to gain access to the subretinal space. Rhegmatogenous retinal detachment (RRD), as opposed to the presence merely of a cuff of SRF surrounding a retinal break, is said to be present when fluid extends further than one optic disc diameter from the edge of the break.
- **Tractional RD.** The NSR is pulled away from the RPE by contracting vitreoretinal membranes in the absence of a retinal break.
- **Exudative** (serous, secondary) **RD.** SRF is derived from the vessels of the NSR and/or choroid.
- **Combined tractional–rhegmatogenous RD** results when a retinal break is caused by traction from an adjacent area of fibrovascular proliferation.
- **Subclinical RD** is generally used to refer to an asymptomatic break surrounded by a relatively small amount of SRF, by definition extending further than one disc diameter away from the edge of the break but less than two disc diameters posterior to the equator. It does not usually give rise to a subjective visual field defect. The term is sometimes also used to describe an asymptomatic RD of any extent.

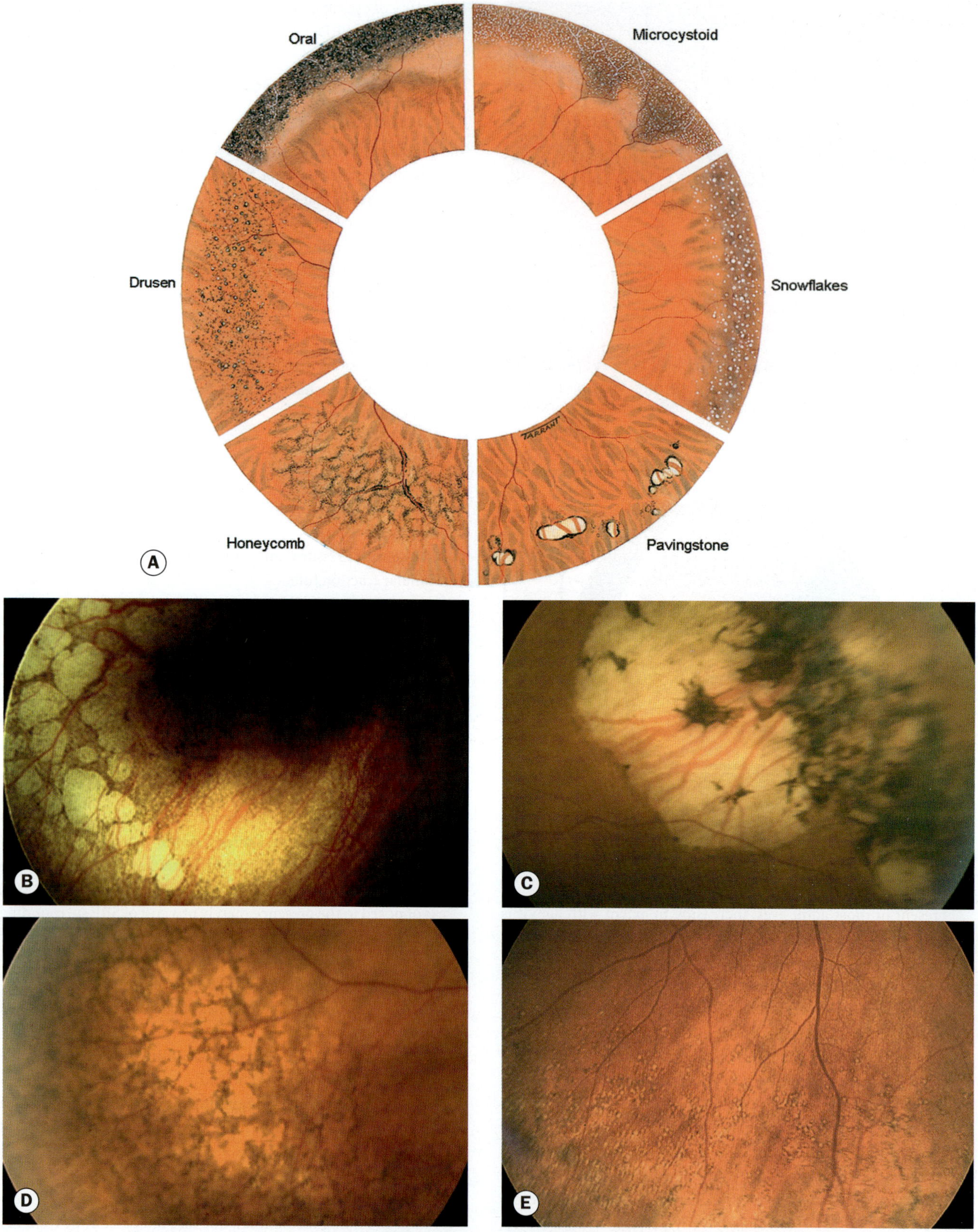

Fig. 16.4 Innocuous peripheral retinal degenerations. **(A)** Composite diagram; **(B)** and **(C)** paving stone; **(D)** honeycomb (reticular); **(E)** peripheral drusen.

Ultrasonography

Introduction

Ultrasonography (US) utilizes high frequency sound waves that produce echoes as they strike the interface between acoustically distinct structures. B-scan (two-dimensional) US is a key tool in the diagnosis of RD in eyes with opaque media, particularly severe vitreous haemorrhage.

Technique

- The examiner holds the US probe with the dominant hand (Fig. 16.5A).
- Methylcellulose or an ophthalmic gel is placed on the tip of the probe to act as a coupling agent.
- A cross-sectional view of the eye (Fig. 16.5B) is obtained and the image can be viewed on a monitor.
- The B-scan probe incorporates a marker for orientation that correlates with a point on the display screen, usually to the left.
- Vertical scanning is performed with the marker on the probe orientated superiorly (Fig. 16.6A).
- Horizontal scanning is performed with the marker orientated towards the nose (Fig. 16.6B).
- The eye is then examined with the patient looking straight ahead, up, down, left and right. For each position a vertical and horizontal scan can be performed.
- The examiner then moves the probe in the opposite direction to the movement of the eye. For example, when examining the right eye, the patient looks to the left and probe is moved to the patient's right, the nasal fundus anterior to the equator is scanned and vice versa. Dynamic scanning is performed by asking the patient to move the eye, whilst the probe position is maintained.

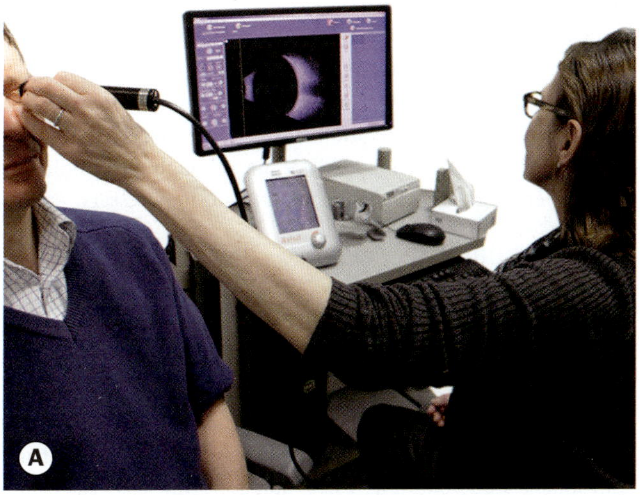

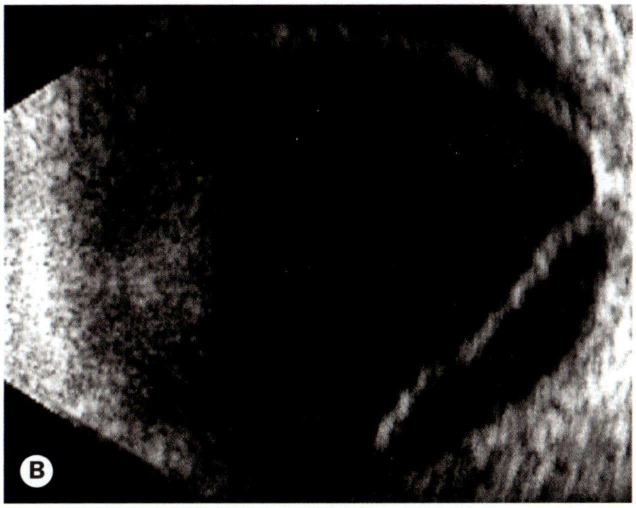

Fig. 16.5 (A) Technique of ultrasonography; **(B)** B-scan ultrasonogram showing retinal detachment. *(Courtesy of P Terry.)*

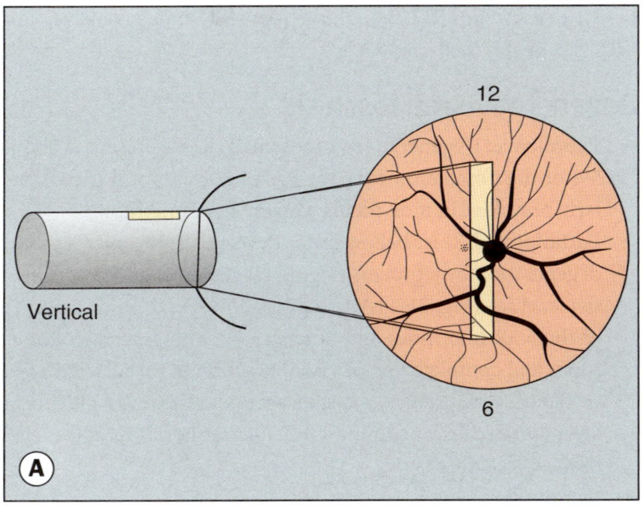

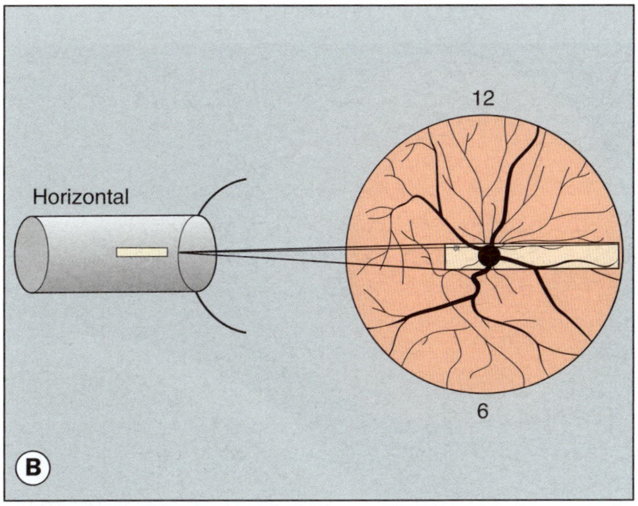

Fig. 16.6 Technique of ultrasound scanning of the globe. **(A)** Vertical scanning with the marker pointing towards the brow; **(B)** horizontal scanning with the marker pointing towards the nose.

- Gain adjusts the amplification of the echo signal, similar to volume control of a radio. Higher gain increases the sensitivity of the instrument in displaying weak echoes such as vitreous opacities. Lower gain only allows display of strong echoes such as the retina and sclera, though improves resolution because it narrows the beam.

PERIPHERAL LESIONS PREDISPOSING TO RETINAL DETACHMENT

Patients with any predisposing lesion, or indeed any high-risk features for RD, should be educated about the nature of symptoms of PVD and RD and the need to seek review urgently if these occur.

Lattice degeneration

- **Prevalence.** Lattice degeneration is present in about 8% of the population. It probably develops early in life, with a peak incidence during the second and third decades. It is found more commonly in moderate myopes. The lifetime risk of a RD in an individual with lattice degeneration is approximately 1%. However, lattice degeneration is present in about 40% of eyes with RD. In these patients, detachment of the retina is caused by premature PVD and tractional tears.
- **Pathology.** There is discontinuity of the ILM with variable atrophy of the underlying NSR. The vitreous overlying an area of lattice is synchytic but the vitreous attachments around the margins are exaggerated (Fig. 16.7).
- **Signs.** Lattice is most commonly bilateral, temporal and superior.
  - Spindle-shaped areas of retinal thinning, commonly located between the equator and the posterior border of the vitreous base.
  - Sclerosed vessels forming an arborizing network of white lines is characteristic (Fig. 16.8A).
  - Some lesions may be associated with 'snowflakes', remnants of degenerate Müller cells (Fig. 16.8B).
  - Associated hyperplasia of the RPE is common (Fig. 16.8C).
  - Small holes are common (Fig. 16.8D).

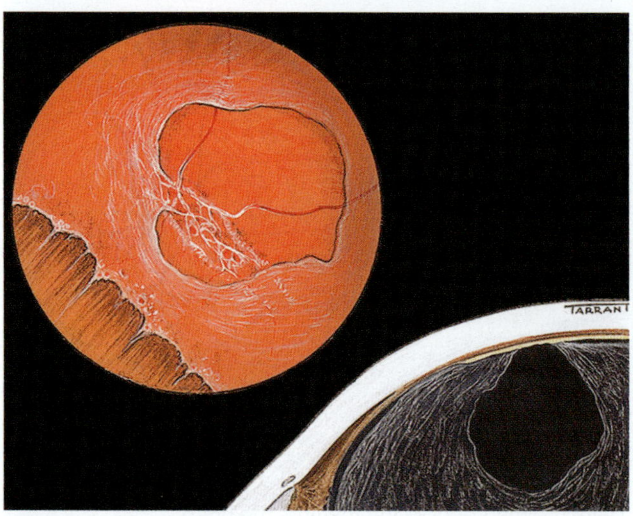

Fig. 16.7 Vitreous changes associated with lattice degeneration.

- **Complications** do not occur in most eyes with lattice degeneration.
  - Tears may develop consequent to a PVD, when lattice is sometimes visible on the flap of the tear.
  - Atrophic holes may rarely (2%) lead to RD. The risk is higher in young myopes. In these patients the RD may not be preceded by acute symptoms of PVD (see below) and SRF usually spreads slowly so that diagnosis may be delayed.
- **Management.** In an asymptomatic patient with lattice degeneration the areas of lattice do not need to be treated prophylactically, even if retinal holes are seen. However, the patient should be advised of the symptoms of RD and written information should be provided. An associated asymptomatic U-tear should be managed as discussed later in the chapter.

TIP Prophylactic treatment of lattice and snailtrack degeneration is not required, as the lifetime risk of retinal detachment secondary to these conditions is low.

Snailtrack degeneration

Snailtrack degeneration is characterized by sharply demarcated bands of tightly packed 'snowflakes' that give the peripheral retina a white frost-like appearance (Fig. 16.9). It is viewed by some as a precursor to lattice degeneration. Marked vitreous traction is seldom present so that U-tears rarely occur, although round holes are relatively common. Prophylactic treatment is unnecessary.

Cystic retinal tuft

A cystic retinal tuft (CRT), also known as a granular patch or retinal rosette, is a congenital abnormality consisting of a small, round or oval, discrete elevated whitish lesion, typically in the equatorial or peripheral retina, more commonly temporally. It may be associated with pigmentation at its base. It is comprised principally of glial tissue. Strong vitreoretinal adhesion is commonly present and both small round holes (Fig. 16.10) and horseshoe tears can occur. It is an under-recognized lesion, though this may change with the adoption of wide-field imaging. CRT are present in up to 5% of the population (bilateral in 20%) and may be the causative lesion in 5–10% of eyes with RD, though the risk of RD in a given eye with CRT is probably well under 1%.

Degenerative retinoschisis

- **Prevalence.** Degenerative retinoschisis (RS) is present in about 5% of the population over the age of 20 years and is particularly prevalent in individuals who are hypermetropic.
- **Pathology.** RS is believed to develop from microcystoid degeneration by a process of gradual coalescence of degenerative cavities (Fig. 16.11A), resulting in separation or splitting of the NSR into inner and outer layers, with severing of neurones and complete loss of visual function in the affected area. In typical retinoschisis the split occurs in the outer plexiform layer and in the less common reticular retinoschisis at the level of the nerve fibre layer.
- **Symptoms**
  - Photopsia and floaters are absent because there is no vitreoretinal traction.

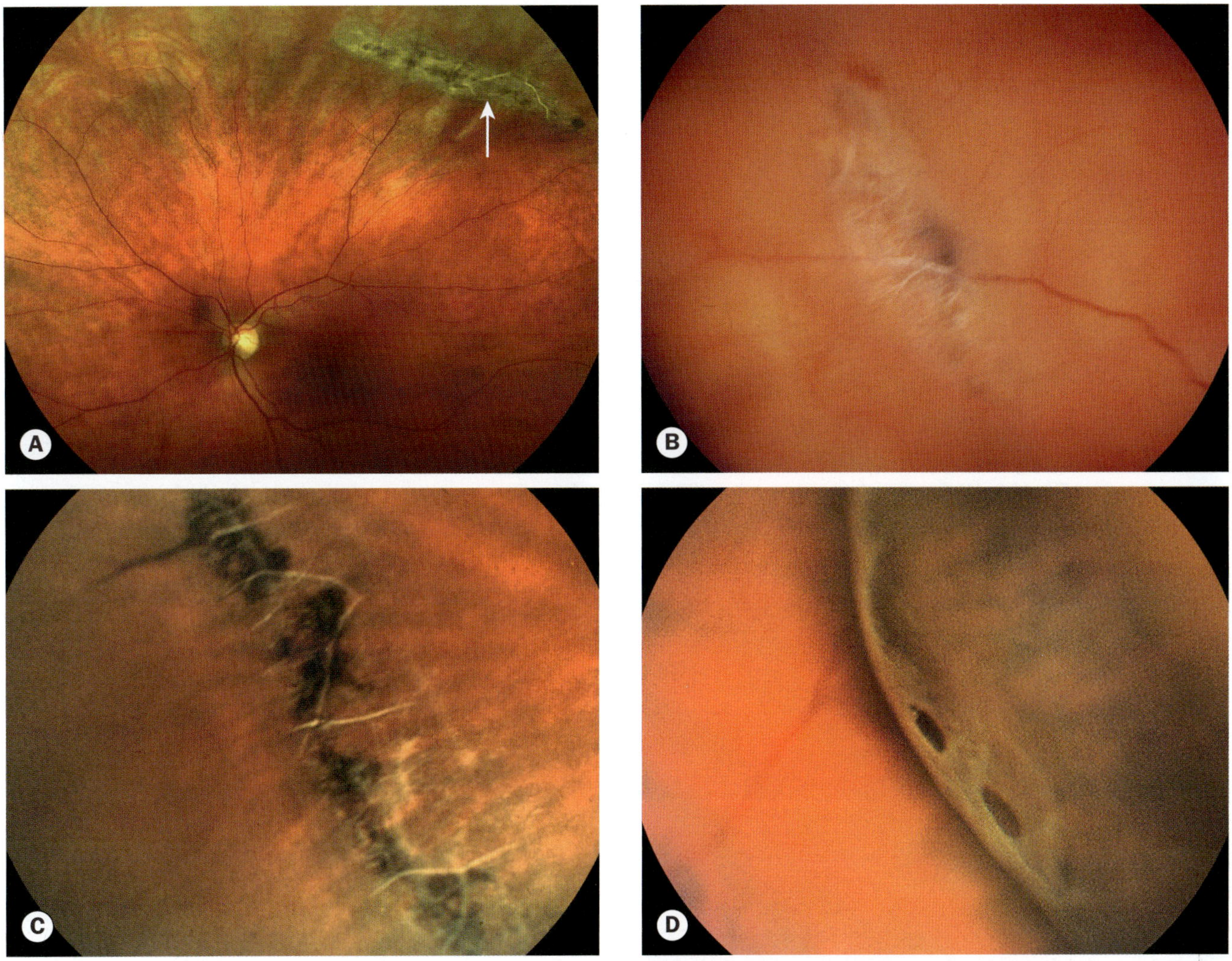

Fig. 16.8 Clinical features of lattice degeneration. **(A)** Small island of lattice with an arborizing network of white lines (arrow) using wide-field photography; **(B)** lattice associated with 'snowflakes'; **(C)** lattice associated with pigmentary changes; **(D)** small holes within lattice seen on scleral indentation. *(Courtesy of NE Byer, from* The Peripheral Retina in Profile, A Stereoscopic Atlas*, Criterion Press, Torrance, CA, 1982 – figs B and D.)*

- It is rare for the patient to notice a visual field defect, even with spread posterior to the equator.
- Occasionally symptoms result from vitreous haemorrhage or a progressive RD.

- **Signs.** RS is bilateral in up to 80%. Distinction between the typical and reticular types is difficult clinically, though the inner layer is thinner and tends to be more elevated in the latter. Differentiation is based principally on behaviour, with complications much more common in the reticular form.
  - Early retinoschisis usually involves the extreme inferotemporal periphery of both fundi, appearing as an exaggeration of microcystoid degeneration with a smooth immobile dome-shaped elevation of the retina (Fig. 16.11B). This can be shown with optical coherence tomography (OCT) (Fig. 16.11C) and is easily distinguished from a rhegmatogenous RD (Fig. 16.11D).
  - The elevation is convex, smooth, thin and relatively immobile, unlike the opaque and corrugated appearance of a rhegmatogenous RD (Fig. 16.12A).
  - The thin inner leaf of the schisis cavity may be mistaken, on cursory examination, for an atrophic longstanding rhegmatogenous RD but demarcation lines and secondary cysts in the inner leaf are absent.
  - The lesion may progress circumferentially until it has involved the entire periphery. The typical form usually remains anterior to the equator. The reticular type is more likely to spread posteriorly.
  - The presence of a pigmented demarcation line is likely to indicate the presence of associated RD.
  - The surface of the inner layer may show 'snowflakes', whitish remnants of Müller cell footplates, as well as sclerosis of blood vessels and the schisis cavity may be bridged by grey–white tissue strands.
  - Breaks may be present in one or both layers. Inner layer breaks are small and round (Fig. 16.12B), whilst the less common outer layer breaks are usually larger, with rolled edges (Fig. 16.12C) and located behind the equator.

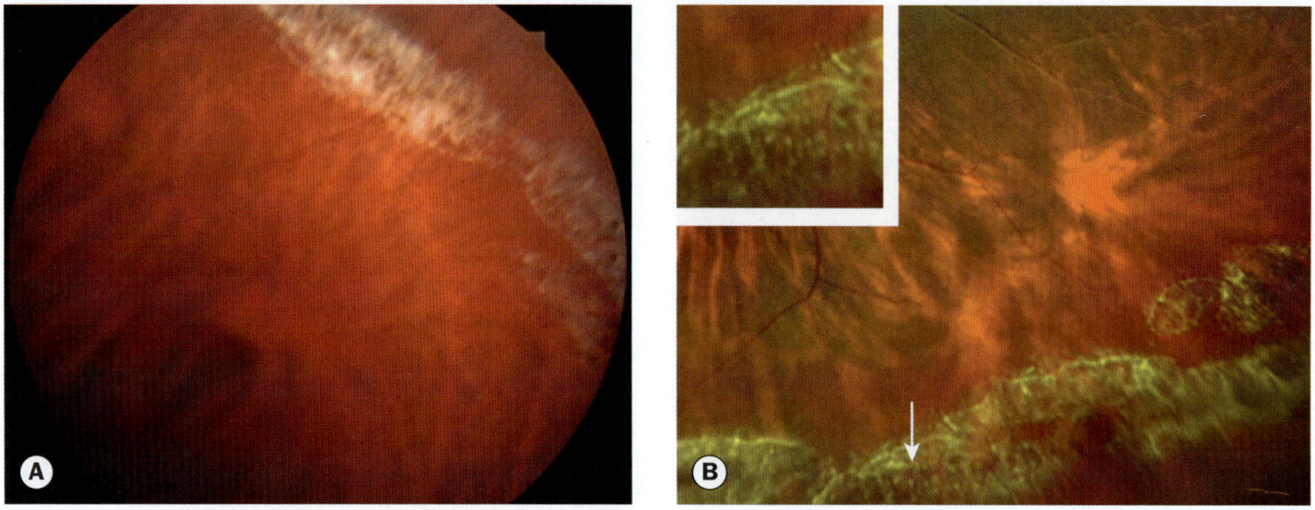

Fig. 16.9 (A) Snailtrack degeneration; **(B)** islands of snailtrack degeneration, some of which contain holes (arrow).

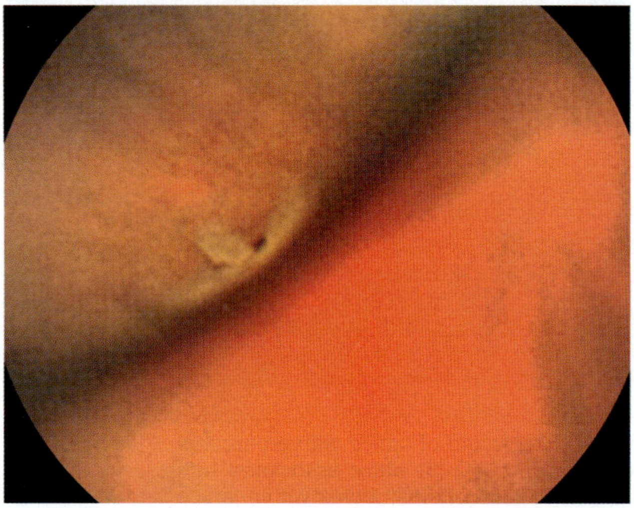

Fig. 16.10 Cystic retinal tuft with small round hole. *(Courtesy of NE Byer, from* The Peripheral Retina in Profile, A Stereoscopic Atlas, *Criterion Press, Torrance, CA 1982.)*

- Microaneurysms and small telangiectatic vessels are common, particularly in the reticular type.
- If a visual field defect is detectable, it is absolute, rather than relative as in RD.

- **Complications** are uncommon and are thought to be much more likely in the reticular form.
  - RD is rare; even in an eye with breaks in both layers the incidence is only around 1%. The detachment is almost always asymptomatic, infrequently progressive and rarely requires surgery.
  - Posterior extension of RS to involve the fovea is very rare but can occur. Progression is generally slow.
  - Vitreous haemorrhage is rare.
- **Management.** Though RD is rare, discussion of the symptoms is prudent in all patients, especially those with double layer breaks.
  - A small peripheral RS discovered on incidental examination, especially if breaks are not present in both layers, does not require routine review.
  - A large RS should be observed periodically, particularly if breaks are present in both layers or it extends posterior to the equator. Photography and visual field testing are useful, with OCT imaging when posterior extension is present. OCT is also useful for distinguishing between RS and RD (see Fig. 16.11C and D).
  - Retinopexy or surgical repair may be indicated for relentless progression towards the fovea, when complication by RD should be excluded.
  - Recurrent vitreous haemorrhage may necessitate vitrectomy.
  - Progressive symptomatic RD should be addressed promptly. More than one procedure may be necessary. Scleral buckling may be adequate for smaller RD with small outer layer breaks, but vitrectomy is generally indicated for more complex RD.

Zonular traction tuft

This refers to a common (15%) phenomenon caused by an aberrant zonular fibre extending posteriorly to be attached to the retina near the ora serrata, and exerts traction on the retina at its base. It is typically located nasally. The risk of retinal tear formation is around 2% and periodic long-term review is generally recommended.

White with pressure and white without pressure

- **'White with pressure' (WWP)** refers to retinal areas in which a translucent white–grey appearance can be induced by scleral indentation (Fig. 16.13A). Each area has a fixed configuration that does not change when indentation is moved to an adjacent area. It may also be observed along the posterior border of islands of lattice degeneration, snailtrack degeneration and the outer layer of acquired retinoschisis. It is frequently seen in normal eyes and may be associated with abnormally strong attachment of the vitreous gel, though may not indicate a higher risk of retinal break formation.

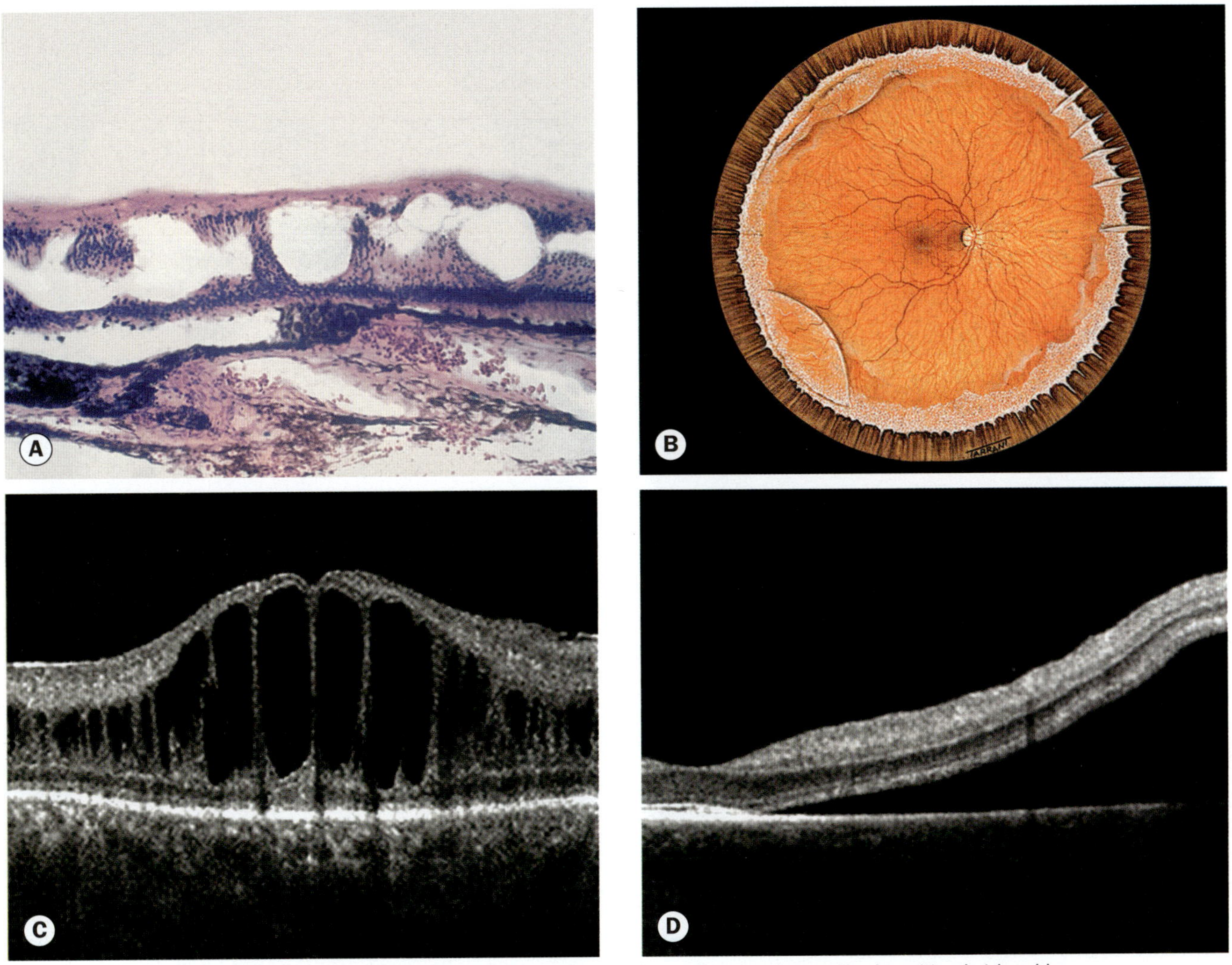

Fig. 16.11 Development of retinoschisis. **(A)** Histology showing intraretinal cavities bridged by Müller cells; **(B)** circumferential microcystoid degeneration with progression to retinoschisis supero- and inferotemporally; **(C)** OCT showing separation principally in the outer plexiform layer; **(D)** OCT of rhegmatogenous retinal detachment in comparison. *(Courtesy of J Harry and G Misson, from* Clinical Ophthalmic Pathology, *Butterworth-Heinemann 2001 – fig. A.)*

- **'White without pressure' (WWOP)** has the same appearance as WWP but is present without scleral indentation (Fig. 16.13B). WWOP corresponds to an area of fairly strong adhesion of condensed vitreous (Fig. 16.13C). On cursory examination a normal area of retina surrounded by WWOP may be mistaken for a flat retinal hole. However, retinal breaks, including giant tears, occasionally develop along the posterior border of WWOP (see Fig. 16.13B). For this reason, if WWOP is found in the fellow eye of a patient with a spontaneous giant retinal tear, prophylactic therapy should be considered. Regular review should be considered for treated and untreated eyes, though evidence for the benefit of this is limited.

Myopic choroidal atrophy

Diffuse choroidal/chorioretinal atrophy in myopia is characterized by diffuse or circumscribed (Fig. 16.14) choroidal depigmentation, commonly associated with thinning of the overlying retina and occurs typically in the posterior pole and equatorial area of highly myopic eyes. Retinal holes developing in the atrophic retina may occasionally lead to RD. Because of lack of contrast, small holes may be very difficult to visualize.

POSTERIOR VITREOUS DETACHMENT

Introduction

PVD refers to separation of the cortical vitreous, along with the delineating posterior hyaloid membrane (PHM), from the neurosensory retina posterior to the vitreous base. PVD occurs due to vitreous gel liquefaction with age (synchysis) to form fluid-filled cavities (Fig. 16.15A) and subsequently condensation (syneresis), with access to the preretinal space allowed by a dehiscence in the cortical gel and/or PHM. The prevalence of PVD increases with age; while less than 10% of individuals under 50 years have a PVD, this rises to two-thirds of those over 70 years. It is usually a spontaneous event, but it can be induced by events such as cataract surgery, trauma, uveitis and panretinal photocoagulation. Perifoveal

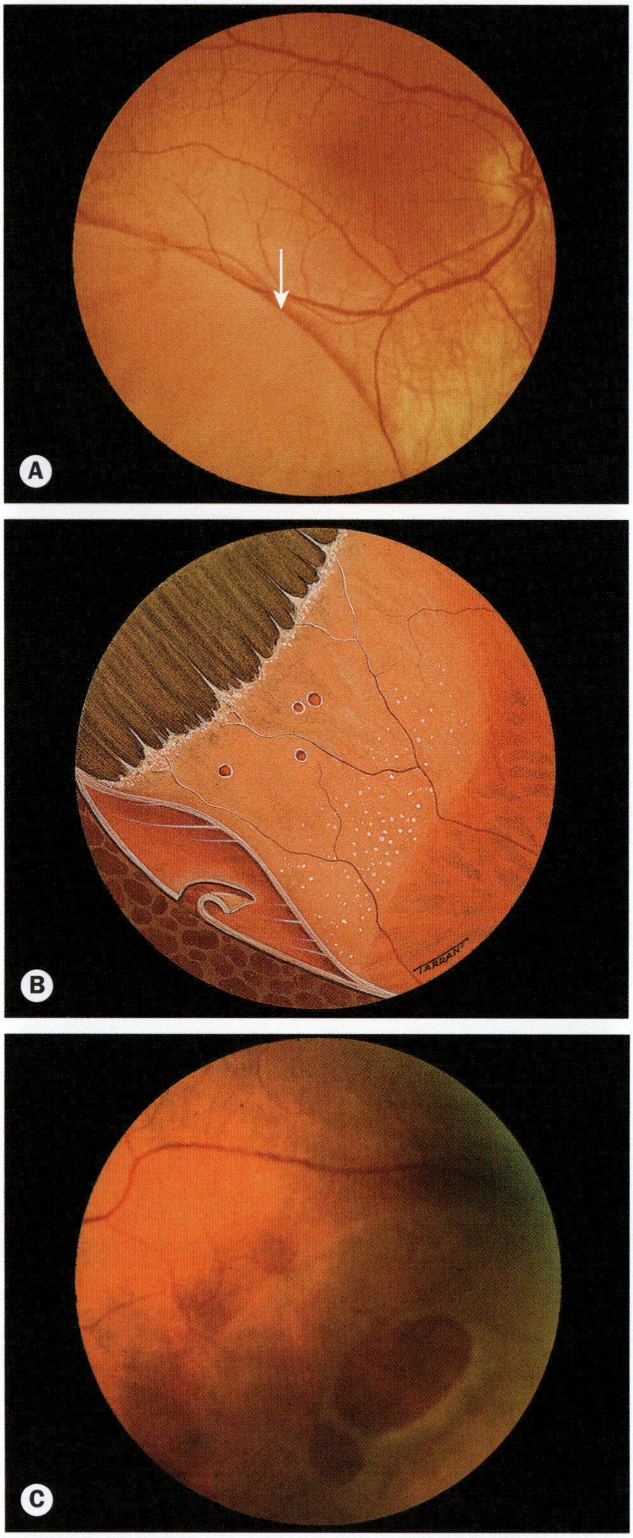

Fig. 16.12 Retinoschisis. **(A)** Early changes (arrow); **(B)** inner and outer layer breaks; **(C)** large outer layer break.

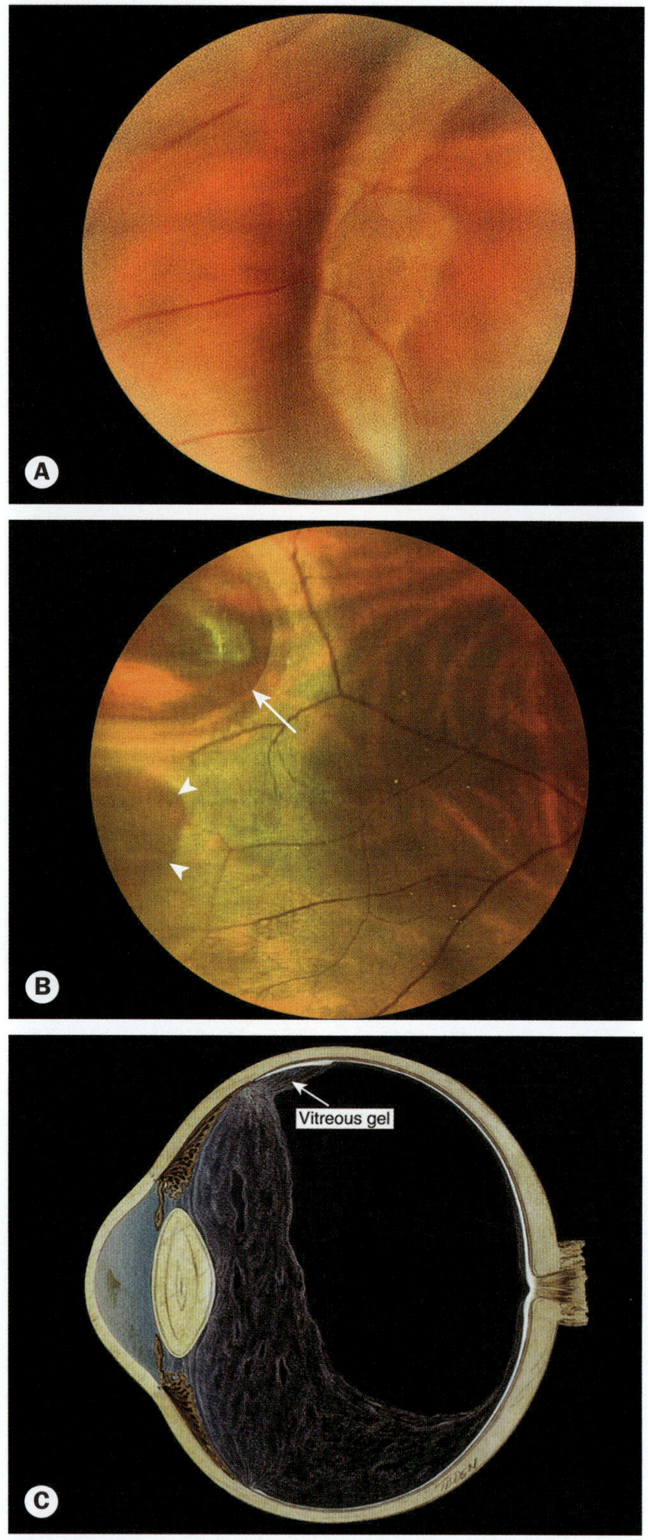

Fig. 16.13 **(A)** White with pressure; **(B)** white without pressure showing retinal tear (arrow) and adjacent pseudo-break (arrowheads); **(C)** strong attachment of condensed vitreous gel to an area of 'white without pressure'. *(Courtesy of NE Byer, from* The Peripheral Retina in Profile, A Stereoscopic Atlas, *Criterion Press, Torrance, CA 1982 – fig. A; S Chen – fig. B; CL Schepens, ME Hartnett and T Hirose, from* Schepens' Retinal Detachment and Allied Diseases, *Butterworth-Heinemann 2000 – fig. C.)*

TIP Degenerative retinoschisis has a convex, smooth, thin and relatively immobile appearance and should be distinguished from a rhegmatogenous retinal detachment, which is slightly opaque and has a corrugated appearance.

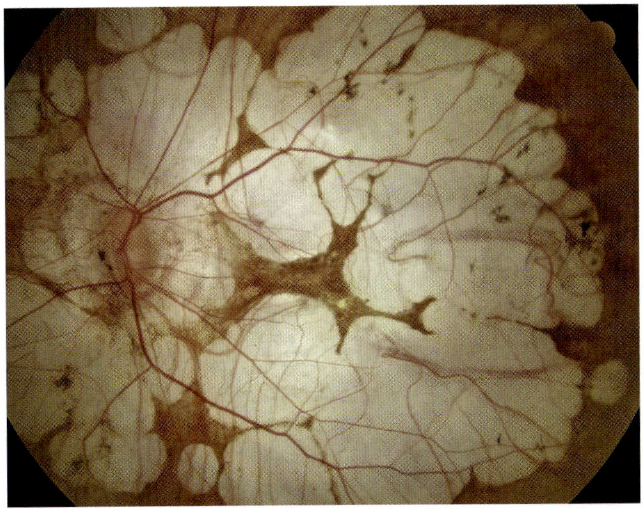

Fig. 16.14 Myopic choroidal atrophy. *(Courtesy of S Chen.)*

hyaloid detachment is followed by foveal separation, then detachment from the posterior retina as far as the equator, attachment initially being retained at the optic disc. Subsequently complete detachment of the cortical vitreous as far anteriorly as the vitreous base takes place (Fig. 16.15B). This process can occur in stages over many months. With the exception of the vitreous base, physiological attachments to the retina and other structures are disengaged in the course of a normal PVD. Overall, about 10% of all patients with an acute symptomatic PVD will have a retinal tear. However, if a vitreous haemorrhage is present, this rises to about 60%.

Clinical features

- **Symptoms** are usually, though not invariably, present.
  - Flashing lights (photopsia) in PVD is often described as a lightning-like arc induced by eye or head movement and is more noticeable in dim illumination. It is almost always seen in the temporal periphery. The mechanism is uncertain, but may relate to traction on the optic disc and possibly at sites of vitreoretinal adhesion, including actual or potential retinal tears.
  - Floaters (myodesopsia) are mobile vitreous opacities most evident against a bright pale background. They are often described as spots, cobwebs or flies (muscae volitantes) and are commonly present in individuals without a PVD, especially myopes. A Weiss ring (Fig. 16.15C and D) is the detached former attachment to the margin of the optic disc and may be seen by the patient as a circle or other large solitary lesion. Its presence does not necessarily indicate total PVD, nor does its absence confirm the absence of PVD since it may be destroyed during the process of separation. Floaters can also be due to vitreous blood.
  - Blurred vision. A diffuse haze may be due to dispersed haemorrhage within the vitreous gel, with a variable accompanying reduction in visual acuity (VA). Bleeding can arise from a torn retinal blood vessel or from the site of a retinal break. Blurring can also be caused by a visually significant PHM or floaters in the visual axis, which may also cause impairment (usually slight) of acuity.
- **Signs**
  - The detached PHM can often be seen clinically on slit lamp examination as a crumpled translucent membrane in the mid-vitreous cavity behind which the cavity is optically clear (Fig. 16.16A).
  - Haemorrhage may be indicated by the presence of red blood cells in the anterior vitreous or as (usually small) focal intragel collections, or preretinally, when it sometimes forms a crescent shape bordering the limit of PHM detachment. Its presence should prompt a careful search for a retinal break (40–90%), particularly with larger amounts – in such cases breaks tend to be posterior.
  - Pigment granules in the anterior vitreous on slit lamp examination (the Shafer sign or 'tobacco dust' – see Fig. 16.21) are larger, darker and less reflective than red blood cells. Their presence raises the possibility of a retinal break (up to 95% sensitivity), with loss of continuity allowing communication between the RPE and vitreous cavity.
  - Vitreous cells, if numerous, may signify the presence of a break.
  - Retinal breaks (see below).
- **Investigation.** B-scan ultrasound (Fig. 16.16B) can demonstrate the extent of PVD. OCT can show separation of the posterior vitreous face and retina (Fig. 16.16C).

TIP A retinal break is usually present in a patient with a PVD who has pigment granules ('tobacco dust') in the vitreous on slit lamp examination.

Management

Patients with substantial acute symptoms of a PVD should be examined as soon as possible, usually within 24–48 hours, with greater urgency in the presence of risk factors including myopia, a past or family history of RD, high-risk syndromes such as Stickler, pseudophakia and symptoms such as a visual field defect, reduced vision or very prominent floaters. Enquiry should be made about the presence of any condition predisposing to non-PVD vitreous haemorrhage, usually diabetes mellitus. If there is only a single small floater and no photopsia, evidence suggests that the risk of retinal break in the symptomatic eye is insignificantly higher than that of the asymptomatic fellow eye, so that urgent assessment may not necessarily be required.

- **Examination.** The anterior vitreous should be assessed for the presence of blood and pigment. Careful retinal examination including visualization of the ora serrata for 360° should be performed and should generally include binocular indirect ophthalmoscopy or contact lens scleral indentation. The asymptomatic fellow eye should always be examined. If 10 or more vitreous cells are present in a 1 mm slit lamp field the incidence of a retinal break in a fellow asymptomatic eye has been reported as over 30%.
- **Subsequent management.** Recommendations for review vary and the following is a general guide.
  - If there are no suspicious findings (e.g. vitreous blood) on examination and no pre-existing risk factors as discussed

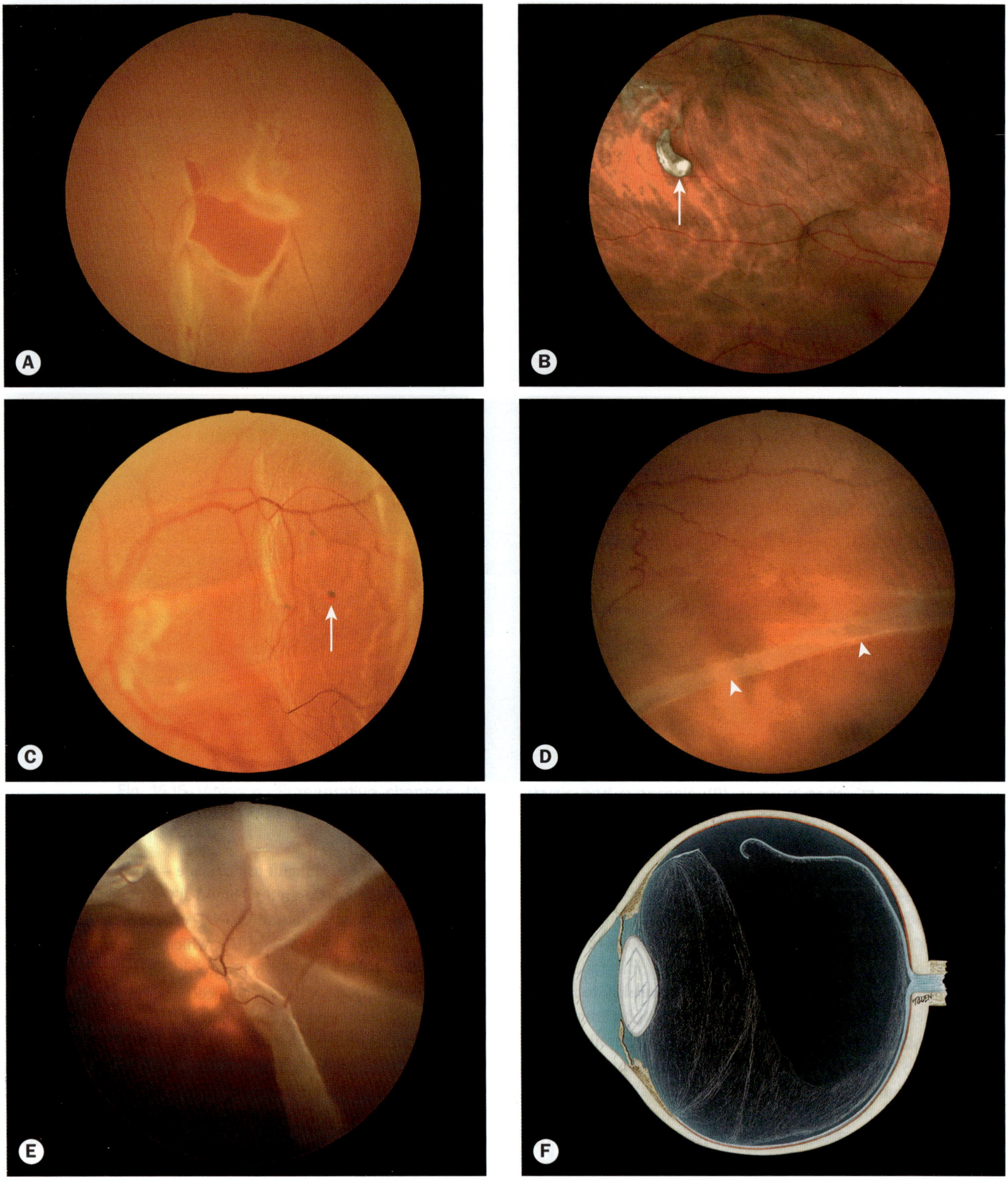

Fig. 16.17 Retinal tears. **(A)** Large U-tear; **(B)** operculated tear (arrow); **(C)** atrophic hole (arrow) with subretinal fluid; **(D)** retinal dialysis (arrowheads); **(E)** giant retinal tear; **(F)** vitreous attached to the anterior edge of a giant tear. *(Courtesy of C Barry – figs D and E; CL Schepens, ME Hartnett and T Hirose, from* Schepens' Retinal Detachment and Allied Diseases, *Butterworth-Heinemann 2000 – fig. F.)*

attached to the anterior margin of the break. It is most frequently located in the immediate post-oral retina or, less commonly, at the equator.

Management

The management of many categories of break remains imperfectly defined and approaches differ between retinal subspecialists. There has been a trend in recent years towards less aggressive prophylactic treatment of asymptomatic and operculated breaks, with substitution by observation and patient education. Patients should always be instructed about the symptoms of vitreous detachment and RD, optimally supplemented by written information, and should seek review urgently in the event of new visual symptoms. The risk associated with prophylaxis is small, but includes new break formation and epiretinal membrane formation. Severe complications are rare.

- **Risk factors for progression to detachment**
  - Miscellaneous factors include a history of RD in the fellow eye, prior cataract surgery (particularly if vitreous loss occurred), myopia, a family history of RD and systemic conditions such as Marfan, Stickler and Ehlers–Danlos syndromes. Evidence suggests that prophylactic treatment should be considered for asymptomatic breaks, including round operculated and atrophic holes prior to cataract surgery, laser capsulotomy and intravitreal injection, particularly when other risk factors are present.
  - Symptomatic breaks associated with an acute PVD are at higher risk than asymptomatic breaks detected on routine examination.
  - Size. Larger breaks carry a higher risk of progression.
  - Persistent vitreoretinal traction. An operculated tear, in which the focus of vitreous traction has detached from the break, is safer than a break, typically a U-tear, in which traction persists. Round holes are rarely associated with ongoing vitreoretinal traction. Apparent demonstration of a complete PVD clinically or on ultrasonography, with no residual attachment in the region of the break, is a favourable feature, though cannot be relied upon.
  - Shape. U-tears are at higher risk than round holes.
  - Location. Superior breaks are at higher risk of progression to RD, probably due to the protective effect of gravity upon inferior breaks. With superotemporal tears, the macula is threatened early in the event of RD. Equatorial breaks are more likely to progress than oral breaks, as the latter are usually located within the vitreous base.
  - Pigmentation around a retinal break indicates chronicity and a degree of stability.
  - Aphakia, now rare, confers a higher risk.
- **Acutely symptomatic U-tears.** Up to 90% of these lead to RD. Treatment (see below) reduces the risk to 5% so urgent intervention is needed.
- **Operculated tears,** particularly in a person who is asymptomatic, are believed to be at low risk of progression to RD and can safely be observed in most cases. A recommended review schedule (symptomatic or asymptomatic) is an initial interval of 2–4 weeks, then 1–3 months, then 6–12 months, then annually. The presence of an intact bridging vessel overlying the break may indicate ongoing vitreoretinal traction – which may also cause vitreous haemorrhage – and treatment should be considered.
- **Asymptomatic U-tears.** The risk of progression to RD is low at 5%, which is a similar rate to that in treated symptomatic U-tears and observation as for operculated tears is generally safe in the absence of factors indicating higher risk.
- **Traumatic retinal breaks**, including acute dialyses, should always be treated.
- **An asymptomatic dialysis** can sometimes be followed without treatment. However, most cases are treated surgically if an associated RD is present.
- **Asymptomatic subclinical RD.** Progression is not invariable in RD discovered incidentally, with about 10% becoming symptomatic over 2–3 years and a decision regarding intervention should be made on a case-by-case basis. For example, many practitioners would prefer to treat rather than observe a large superotemporal RD that extends posterior to the equator, but may observe a small inferior longstanding RD. With any option, fully informed patient consent and regular review is vital. Surgery is generally indicated if progression occurs.
- **Asymptomatic flat round holes** do not require prophylactic treatment, but some guidelines recommend review every 1–2 years.

TIP A patient with a symptomatic retinal break associated with an acute PVD is at risk of RD and needs rapid treatment.

Treatment techniques

Retinal breaks without RD can be treated with laser (via a slit lamp or binocular indirect ophthalmoscopy [BIO]) or cryotherapy. In most cases laser is the optimal technique as it is more precise, causing less collateral retinal damage, with a lower risk of epiretinal membrane formation. Adequate treatment of the base of a very peripheral lesion may only be possible with BIO or cryotherapy due to the requirement for indentation to visualize the area. Cryotherapy may be preferred for multiple contiguous tears or extensive lesions and in eyes with hazy media or small pupils.

- **Laser retinopexy.** Using slit lamp delivery under topical anaesthesia (occasionally regional or even general anaesthesia is required), typical settings are a duration of 0.1 second, a spot size of 200–300 µm with a three-mirror contact lens or 100–200 µm with a wide-field lens and a starting power of 200 mW. The power should be adjusted as appropriate to obtain moderate blanching. With head-mounted BIO delivery, the spot size is estimated and adjusted by adjusting the condensing lens (usually 20 D) position. The lesion is surrounded with two to three rows of confluent burns (Fig. 16.18). With both forms of laser, care should be taken to identify appropriate landmarks frequently to avoid inadvertent macular damage.

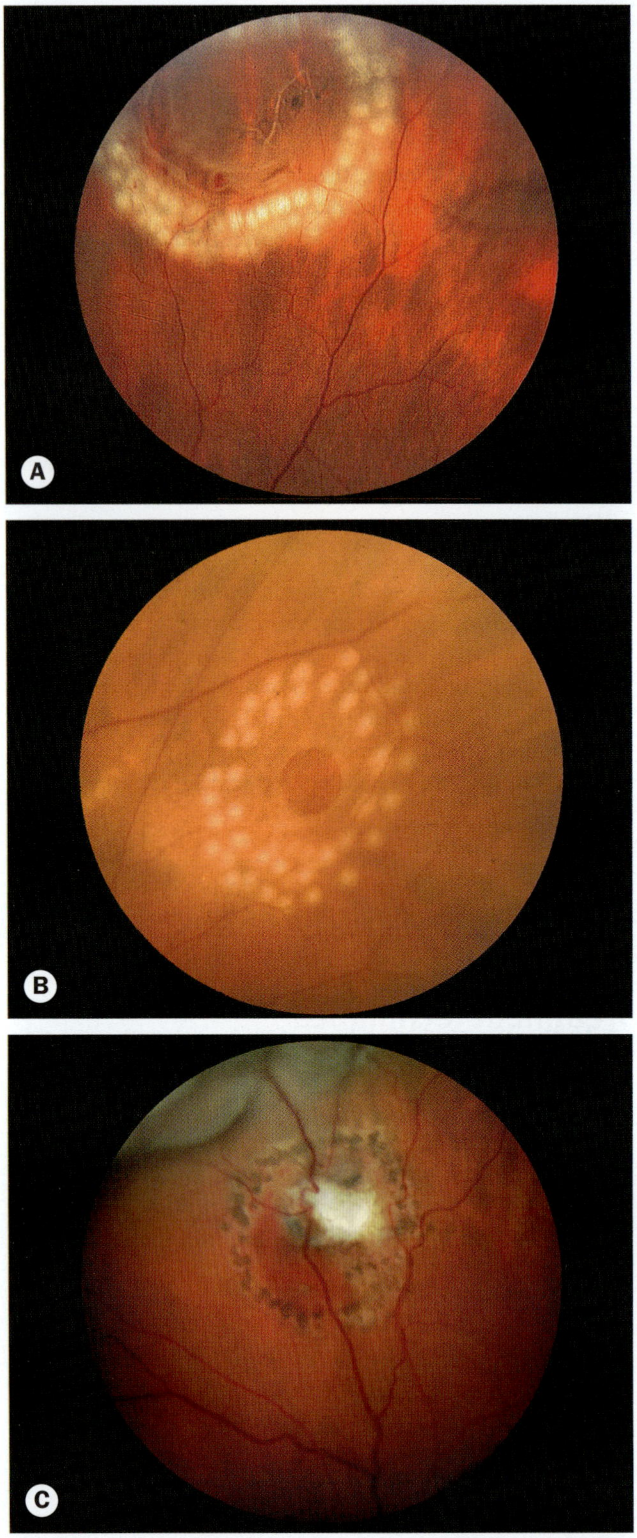

Fig. 16.18 Laser retinopexy after treatment. **(A)** U-tear; **(B)** retinal hole; **(C)** recent penetrating injury.

- **Cryoretinopexy.** Subconjunctival or regional anaesthesia is commonly required. For lesions behind the equator, a small conjunctival incision may be necessary for access. A lid speculum is used. The cryotherapy probe tip must be exposed beyond its rubber sleeve. The instrument should initially be purged (e.g. 10 seconds at −25 °C, repeating after 1 minute). The treatment temperature is set (typically −85 °C). It is useful to check the effectiveness of the instrument by activating it in sterile water for 10 seconds, when a 5-mm ice ball should form. Under BIO visualization, the lesion is indented and the foot pedal depressed until visible whitening of the retina is seen. It is critical not to remove the tip from the treated area until thawing occurs (2–3 seconds). Care should be taken to maintain orientation of the probe whilst the tip is not visible and not to mistake indentation by the shaft of the probe for that of the tip. The lesion is surrounded by a single row of applications, in most cases achieved by one or two applications to a tear. The eye is usually padded afterwards and oral analgesia is commonly prescribed.

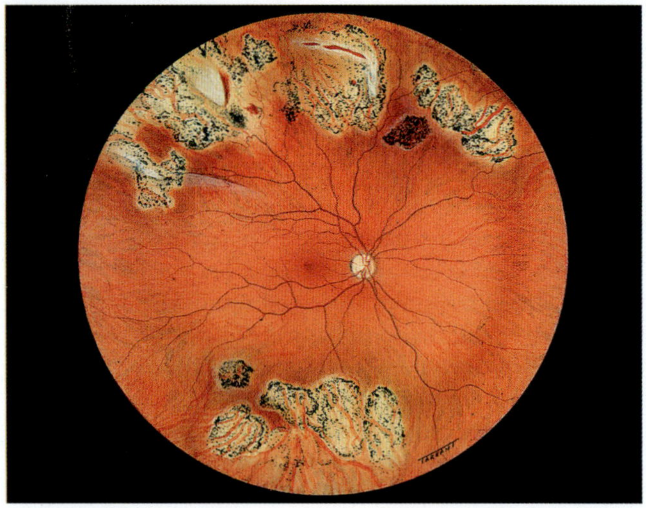

Fig. 16.19 Pigmentation and chorioretinal atrophy following prophylactic cryotherapy to several retinal breaks.

- **After treatment** the patient should avoid strenuous physical exertion for about a week until an adequate adhesion has formed (Fig. 16.19). Review should usually take place after 1–2 weeks.

RHEGMATOGENOUS RETINAL DETACHMENT

Introduction

Pathogenesis

Rhegmatogenous RD affects about 1 in 10 000 of the population each year, with both eyes eventually affected in about 10%. In most cases it is characterized by the presence of a retinal break in concert with vitreoretinal traction that allows accumulation of liquefied vitreous under the neurosensory retina, separating it from the RPE. Even though a retinal break is present, a RD will almost never occur if the vitreous is not at least partially liquefied and traction is absent. Over 40% of RDs occur in myopic eyes and the higher the refractive error the greater the risk. Vitreous degeneration and PVD and predisposing lesions such as lattice and snailtrack degeneration are more common in myopia. Highly myopic eyes are also at risk from RD due to small round holes in chorioretinal atrophy and from macular holes. Vitreous loss during cataract surgery and laser capsulotomy also carries a greater risk of RD in highly myopic eyes.

Identification of retinal breaks

- **Distribution of breaks** in eyes with RD is approximately as follows: 60% superotemporal quadrant, 15% superonasal, 15% inferotemporal and 10% inferonasal. The upper temporal region should therefore be examined in detail if a break cannot be detected initially. It should also be remembered that about 50% of eyes with RD have more than one break, often within 90° of each other.
- **Configuration of SRF.** SRF spread is governed by (a) gravity, by (b) anatomical limits (ora serrata and optic nerve) and by (c) the location of the primary retinal break. If the primary break is located superiorly, the SRF first spreads inferiorly on the same side of the fundus as the break and then superiorly on the opposite side, so that the likely location of the primary retinal break can be predicted.
- **Modified Lincoff's rules:**
  - A shallow inferior RD in which the SRF is slightly higher on the temporal side points to a primary break located inferiorly on that side (Fig. 16.20A).
  - A primary break located at 6 o'clock will cause an inferior RD with equal fluid levels (Fig. 16.20B).
  - In a bullous inferior RD, the primary break usually lies above the horizontal meridian (Fig. 16.20C).
  - If the primary break is located in the upper nasal quadrant the SRF will revolve around the optic disc and then rise on the temporal side until it is level with the primary break (Fig. 16.20D).
  - A subtotal RD with a superior wedge of attached retina points to a primary break located in the periphery nearest its highest border (Fig. 16.20E).
  - When the SRF crosses the vertical midline above, the primary break is near to 12 o'clock, the lower edge of the RD corresponding to the side of the break (Fig. 16.20F).

Symptoms

The classic premonitory symptoms reported in about 60% of patients with spontaneous rhegmatogenous RD are flashing lights and floaters associated with acute PVD. After a variable period of time a curtain-like relative peripheral visual field defect may ensue and can progress to involve central vision. In some patients this may not be present on waking in the morning, due to spontaneous absorption of SRF while inactive overnight, only to reappear later in the day. A lower field defect is usually appreciated more quickly by the patient than an upper defect. The quadrant of the visual field in which the field defect first appears is useful in predicting the location of the primary retinal break, which will be in the opposite quadrant. The location of photopsia is of no value in predicting the site of the primary break. Loss of central vision may be due to involvement of the fovea by SRF or, infrequently, obstruction of the visual axis by a large bullous RD.

Signs

General

- **Relative afferent pupillary defect** (Marcus Gunn pupil) is present in an eye with an extensive RD.
- **Intraocular pressure (IOP)** is often lower by about 5 mmHg compared with the normal eye. If the intraocular pressure is extremely low, an associated choroidal detachment may be present. It may be raised, characteristically in Schwartz–Matsuo syndrome, in which RRD is associated with an apparent mild anterior uveitis, often due to a dialysis secondary to previous blunt trauma in a young man. The aqueous cells are believed in most cases to be displaced photoreceptor outer segments that compromise trabecular outflow. Both the aqueous 'cells' and the elevated IOP typically resolve following repair of the RD.

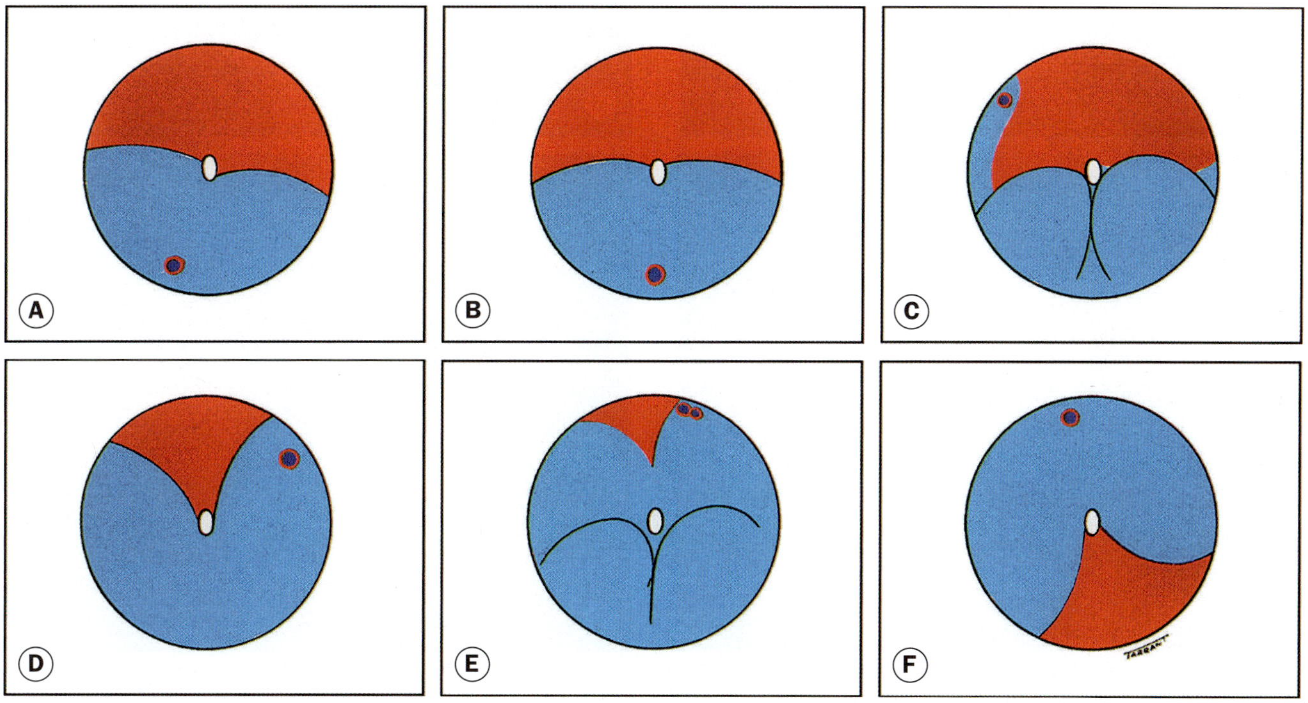

Fig. 16.20 Distribution of subretinal fluid in relation to the location of the primary retinal break (see text).

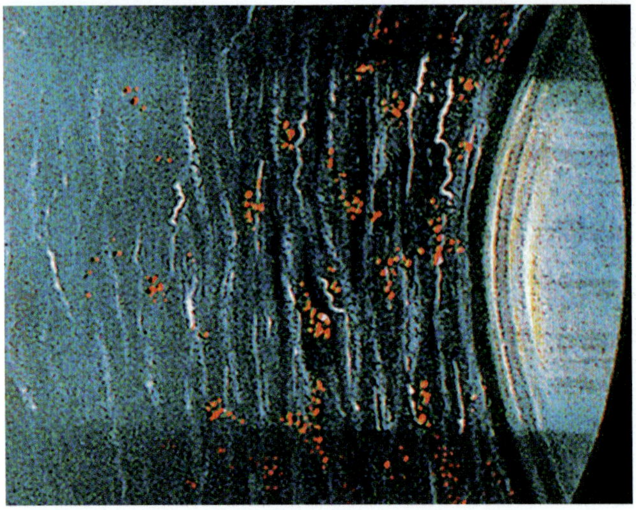

Fig. 16.21 'Tobacco dust' in the anterior vitreous.

- **Iritis** is common but usually mild and should be differentiated from Schwartz–Matsuo syndrome (above). Occasionally it may be severe enough to cause posterior synechiae and the underlying RD may be overlooked.
- **'Tobacco dust'** consisting of pigment cells is commonly seen in the anterior vitreous (Fig. 16.21). Substantial vitreous blood or inflammatory cells are also highly specific.
- **Retinal breaks** (see Fig. 16.17) appear as discontinuities in the retinal surface. They are usually red because of the colour contrast between the sensory retina and underlying choroid. However, in eyes with hypopigmented choroid (e.g. high myopia), the colour contrast is decreased and small breaks may be overlooked.
- **Retinal signs** depend on the duration of RD and the presence or absence of proliferative vitreoretinopathy (PVR) as described below.

Fresh retinal detachment

- **The RD** has a convex configuration and a slightly opaque and corrugated appearance as a result of retinal oedema (Fig. 16.22A–C). There is loss of the underlying choroidal

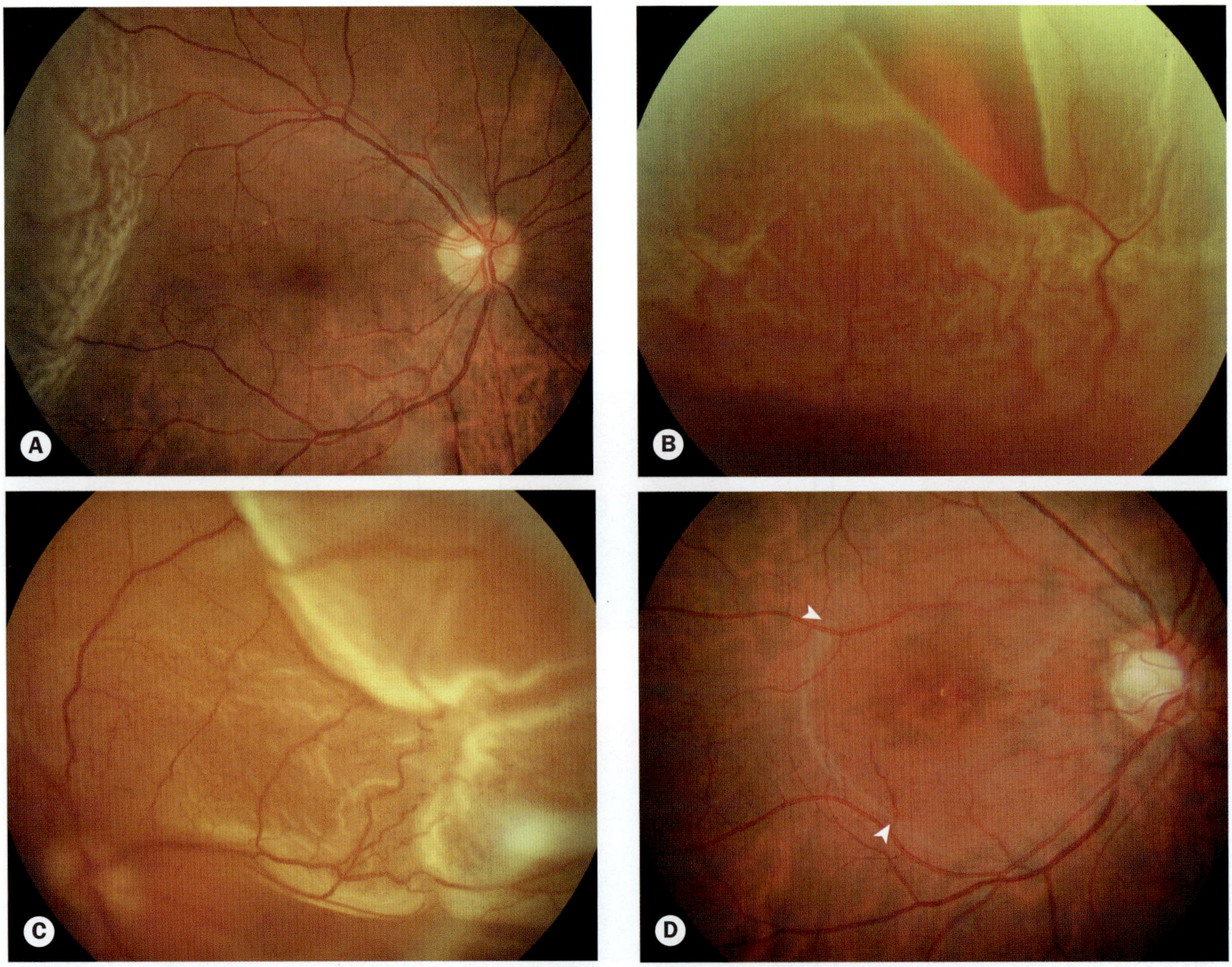

Fig. 16.22 Fresh retinal detachment. **(A)** Temporal detachment with macula on; **(B)** superior bullous detachment with large tear; **(C)** typical corrugated appearance of detached retina with macula off; **(D)** macular hole surrounded by shallow subretinal fluid (arrowheads) confined to the posterior pole. *(Courtesy of S Chen – fig. A.)*

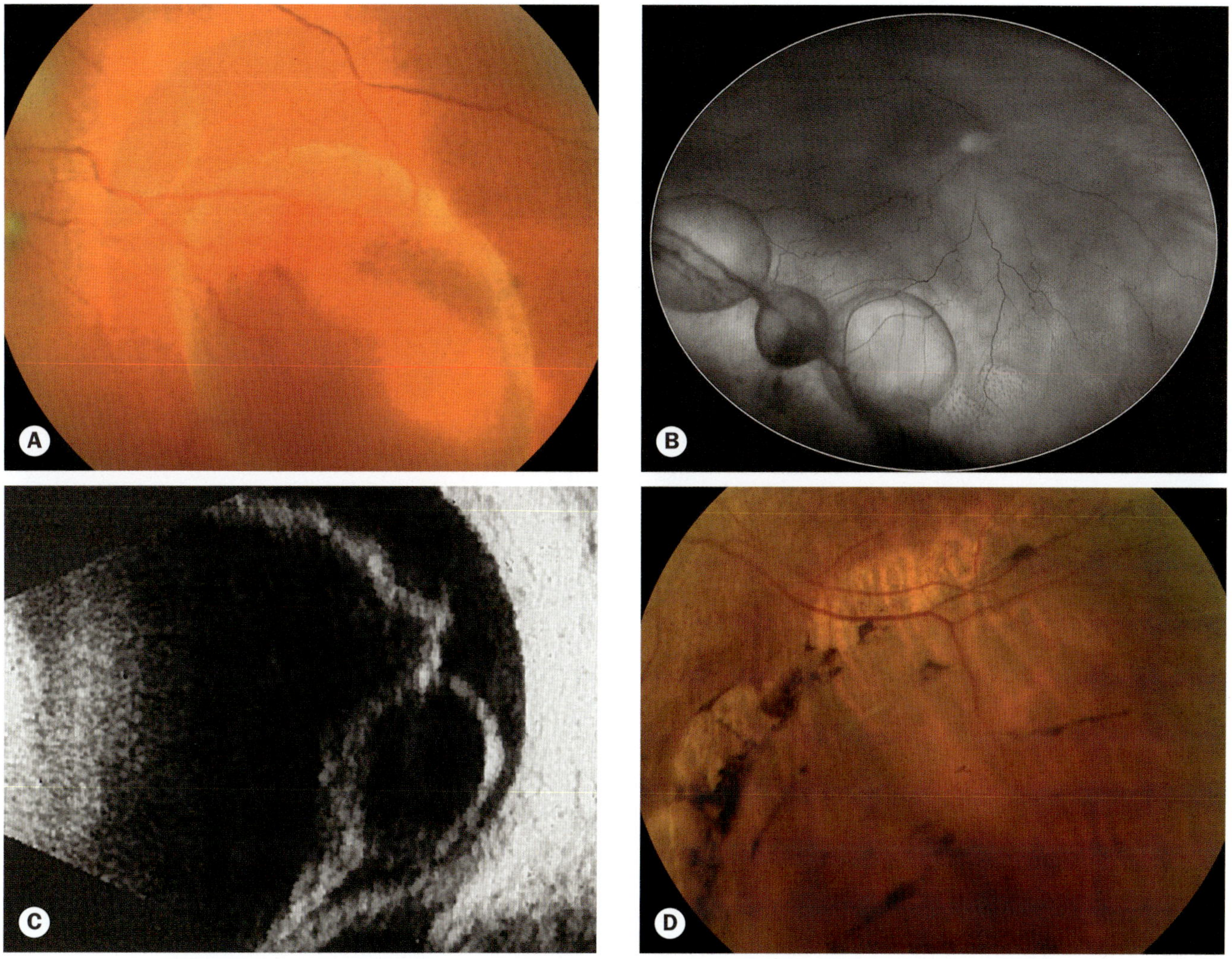

Fig. 16.23 Longstanding retinal detachment. **(A)** Retinal cysts; **(B)** multiple cysts in chronic total detachment (red-free wide-field image); **(C)** B-scan ultrasonogram demonstrating cyst; **(D)** demarcation line surrounding localized inferior subretinal fluid. *(Courtesy of C Barry – fig. B; RF Spaide, from* Diseases of the Retina and Vitreous, *WB Saunders 1999 – fig. C.)*

pattern and retinal blood vessels appear darker than in flat retina.

- **SRF** extends up to the ora serrata, except in the rare cases caused by a macular hole in which fluid is initially confined to the posterior pole (Fig. 16.22D).
- **Macular pseudohole.** Because of the thinness of the foveal retina, the impression of a macular hole may be given if the posterior pole is detached. This should not be mistaken for a true macular hole, which may give rise to RD in highly myopic eyes or following blunt trauma.
- **B-scan ultrasonography** shows good mobility of the retina and vitreous.

Longstanding retinal detachment

- **Retinal thinning** secondary to atrophy is a characteristic finding and should not lead to a misdiagnosis of retinoschisis.
- **Intraretinal cysts** (Fig. 16.23A–C) may develop if the RD has been present for about 1 year. These tend to disappear after retinal reattachment.
- **Subretinal demarcation lines** ('high water' or 'tide' marks) caused by proliferation of RPE cells at the junction of flat and detached retina (Fig. 16.23D) are common, taking about 3 months to develop. Pigmentation tends to decrease over time. Although representing sites of increased adhesion, they do not invariably limit the spread of SRF.

Proliferative vitreoretinopathy

Proliferative vitreoretinopathy (PVR) is caused by epiretinal and subretinal membrane formation, contraction of which leads to tangential retinal traction and fixed retinal fold formation (Fig. 16.24). Usually, PVR occurs following surgery for rhegmatogenous RD or penetrating injury, though it may also occur in eyes

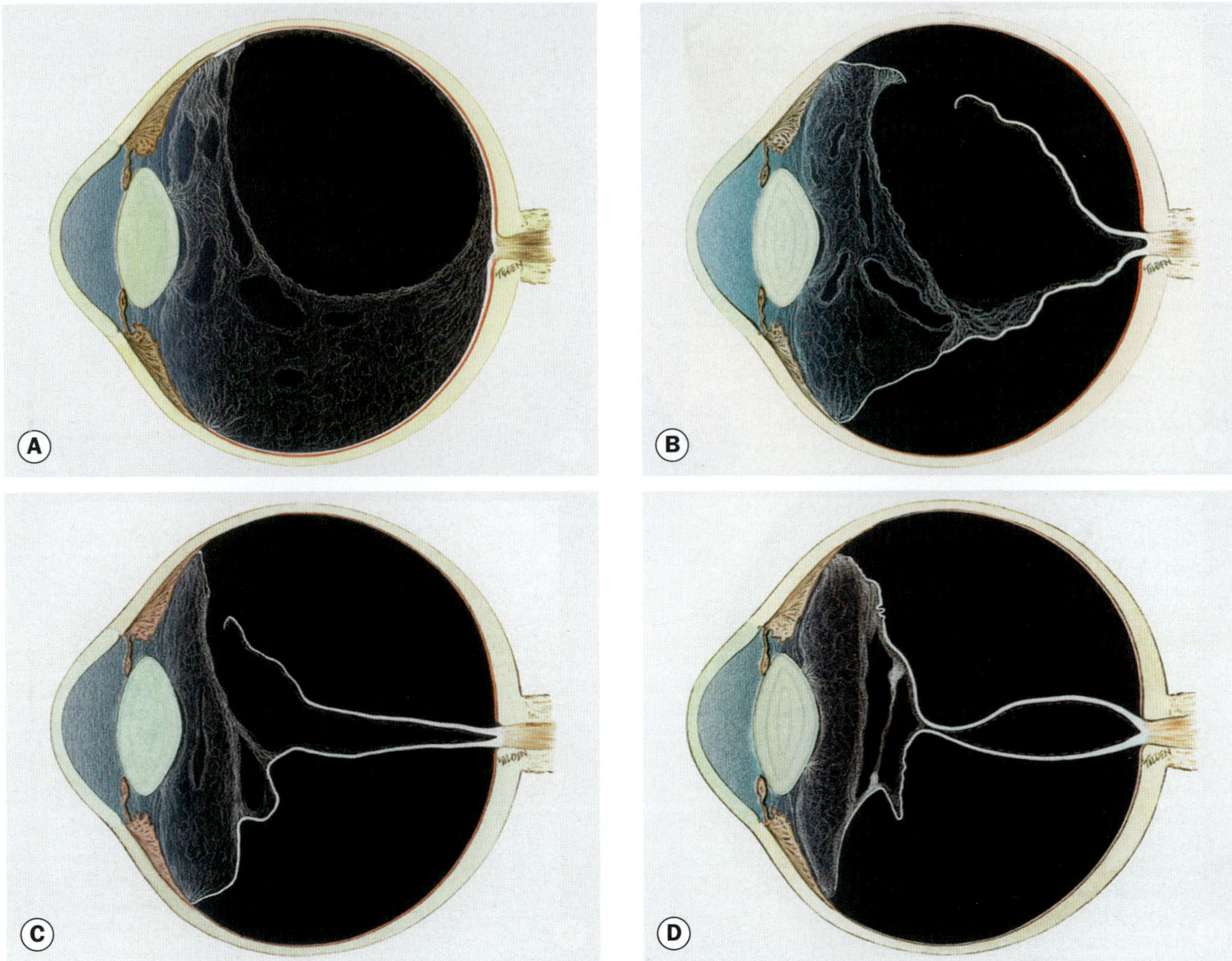

Fig. 16.24 Development of proliferative vitreoretinopathy (PVR). **(A)** Extensive vitreous syneresis; **(B)** total retinal detachment without PVR; shrunken vitreous is condensed and attached to the equator of the retina; **(C)** early PVR with anteriorly retracted vitreous gel and equatorial circumferential retinal folds; **(D)** advanced PVR with a funnel-like retinal detachment bridged by dense vitreous membranes. *(Courtesy of CL Schepens, ME Hartnett and T Hirose, from* Schepens' Retinal Detachment and Allied Diseases, *Butterworth-Heinemann 2000.)*

with rhegmatogenous RD that have not had previous retinal surgery. The main features are retinal folds and rigidity so that retinal mobility induced by eye movements or scleral indentation is decreased. Progression from one stage to the next is not inevitable.

- **Grade A** (minimal) PVR is characterized by diffuse vitreous haze and tobacco dust. There may also be pigmented clumps on the inferior surface of the retina. Although these findings occur in many eyes with RD, they are particularly severe in eyes with early PVR.
- **Grade B** (moderate) PVR is characterized by wrinkling of the inner retinal surface (Fig. 16.25A), decreased mobility of vitreous gel, rolled edges of retinal breaks, tortuosity of blood vessels and retinal stiffness (Fig. 16.25B). The epiretinal membranes responsible for these findings typically cannot be identified clinically.
- **Grade C** (marked) PVR is characterized by rigid full-thickness retinal folds (often star-shaped) with heavy vitreous condensation and strands (Fig. 16.25C and D). It can be either anterior (A) or posterior (P), the approximate dividing line being the equator of the globe. The severity of proliferation in each area is expressed by the number of clock hours of retina involved although proliferations need not be contiguous.
- **Advanced disease** shows gross reduction of retinal mobility with retinal shortening and a characteristic funnel-like triangular conformation (see Fig. 16.24D).
- **Management.** PVR is usually managed by undertaking a pars plana vitrectomy, with removal of the membranes. Peeling the internal limiting membrane (ILM) at the time of surgery in patients with advanced PVR improves the success rate of surgery. It is sometimes necessary to perform a relaxing retinotomy to relieve traction. Perfluorocarbon liquid is used to stabilize the retina, which is then replaced with long-acting gas or silicone oil (see later in this chapter).

Differential diagnosis

The tractional and exudative forms of RD are described later in the chapter.

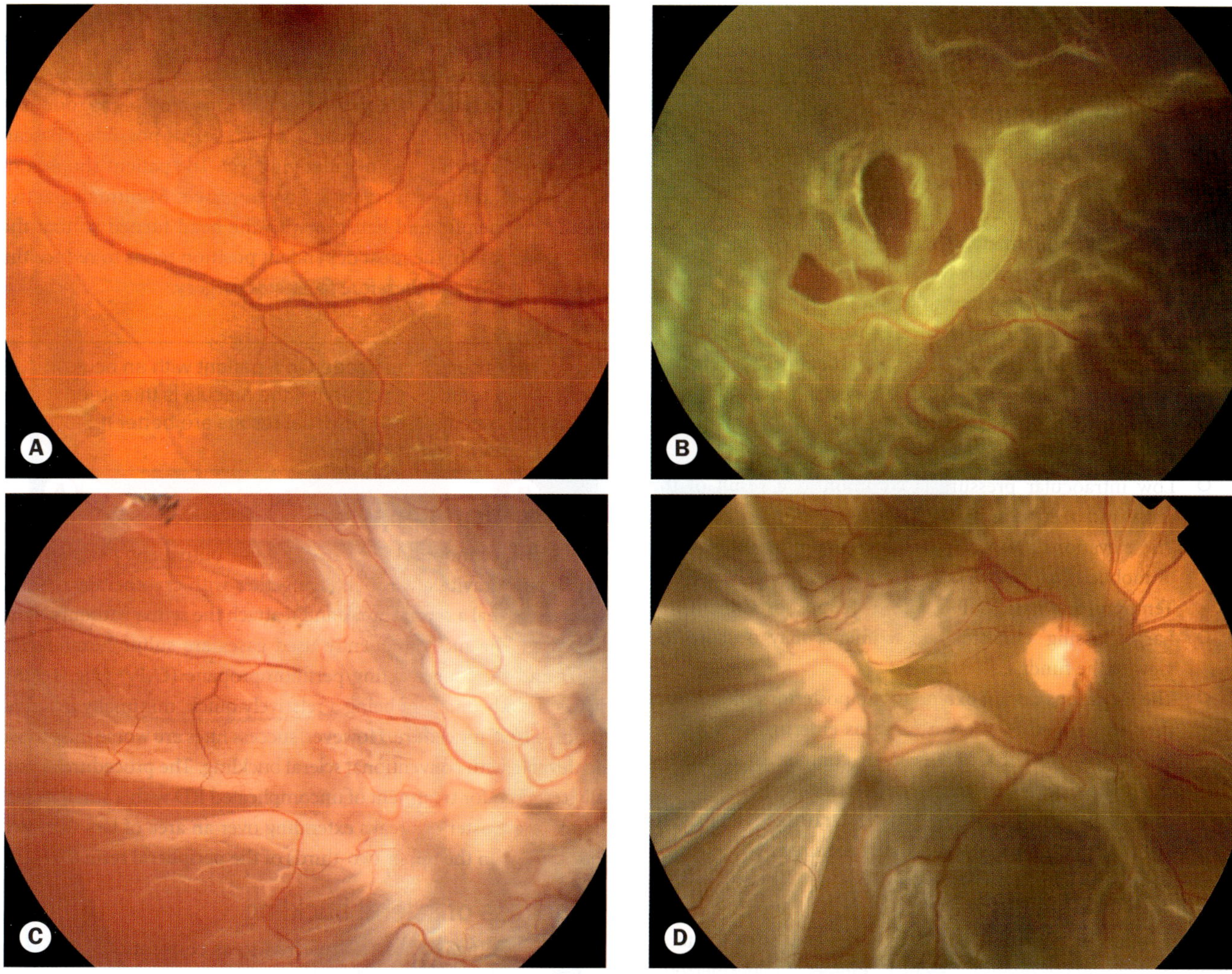

Fig. 16.25 Proliferative vitreoretinopathy (PVR). **(A)** Early retinal wrinkling in minimal grade B; **(B)** marked grade B with rolled retinal break edges; **(C)** grade C with upper temporal tear; **(D)** grade C with prominent star fold.

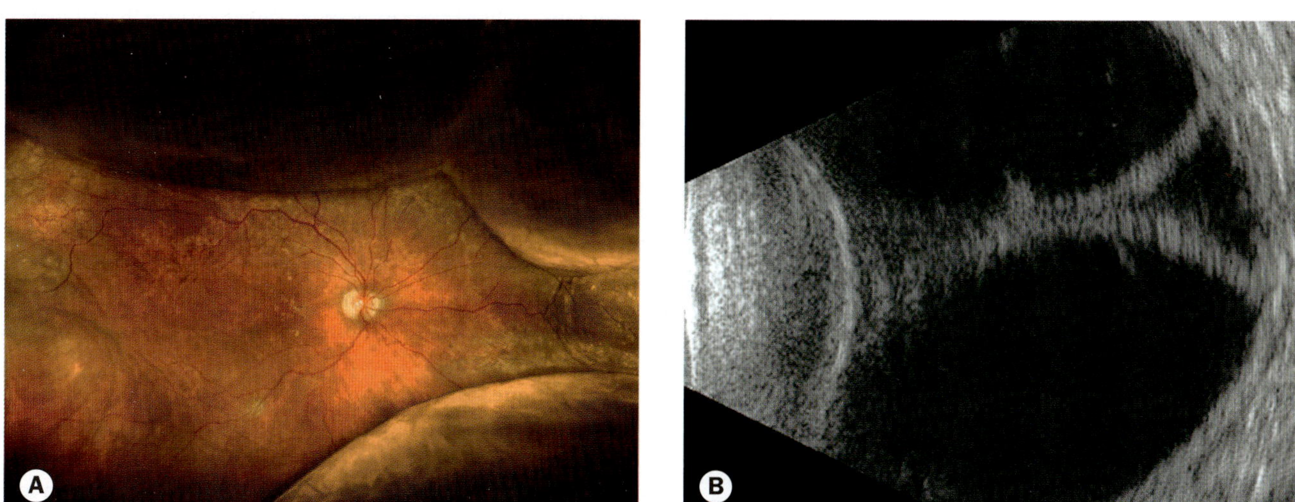

Fig. 16.26 Choroidal effusion. **(A)** Secondary to hypotony; **(B)** B-scan showing limitation of posterior fluid spread by the vortex veins. *(Courtesy of S Chen – fig. A; R Bates – fig. B.)*

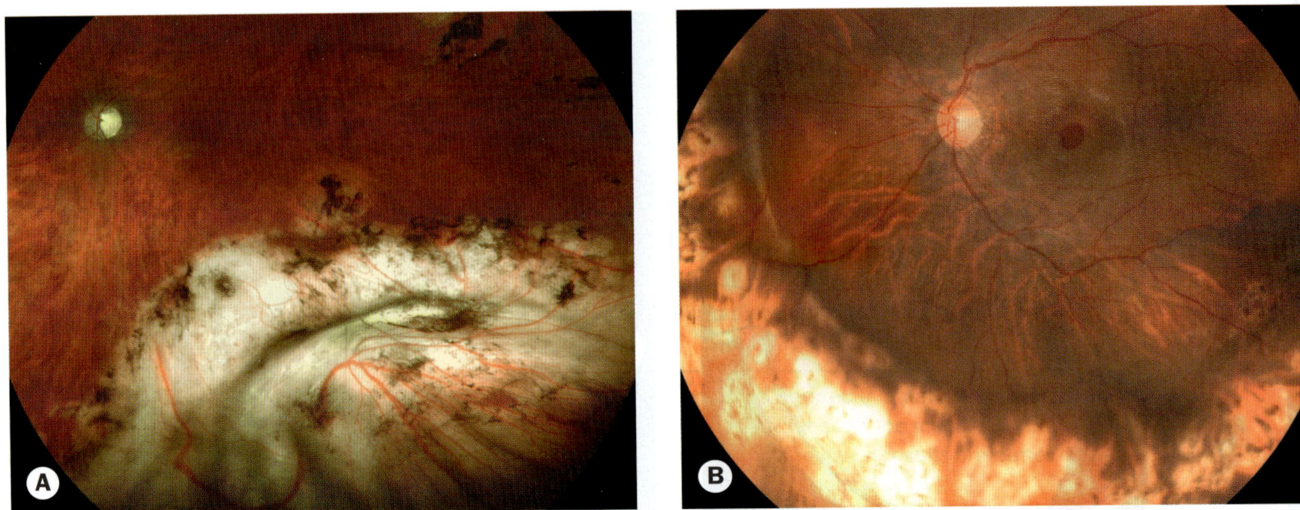

Fig. 16.29 Scleral buckling (wide-field view). **(A)** Buckle induced by radial explant; **(B)** buckle induced by circumferential explant (full-thickness macular hole present). *(Courtesy of S Chen – fig. A; B Sim – fig. B.)*

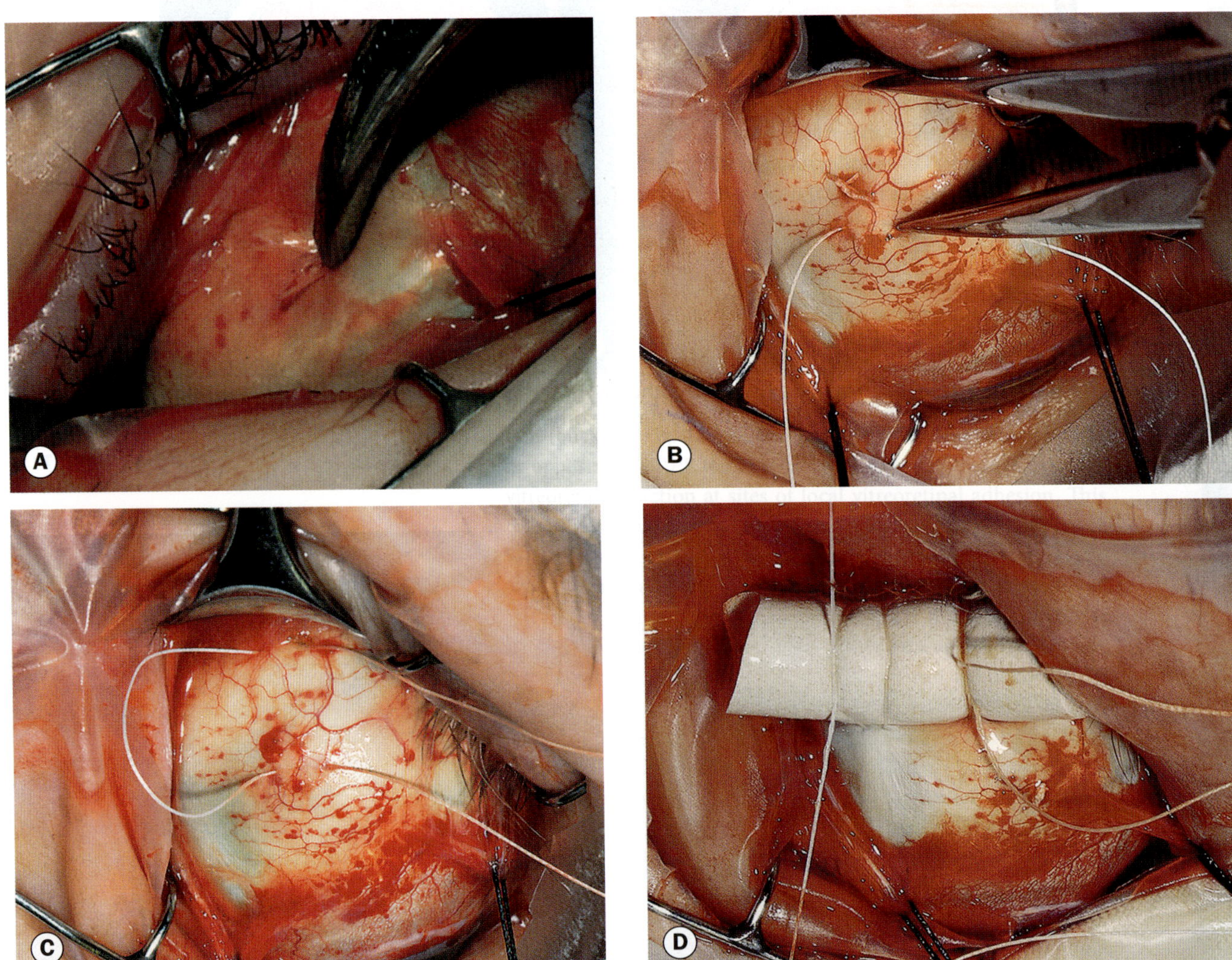

Fig. 16.30 Technique of scleral buckling. **(A)** Marking the retinal break; **(B)** suture inserted and caliper used to measure the position of the second suture; **(C)** mattress suture in place; **(D)** suture is tied over the sponge.

Drainage of subretinal fluid

Drainage of SRF via the sclera (e.g. the D-ACE: Drainage-Air-Cryotherapy-Explant) surgical technique (Fig. 16.31A) is advocated by many practitioners, citing more rapid retinal reattachment in the presence of deep or longstanding viscous SRF. Others prefer to avoid external drainage because of the potential complications associated with the technique, such as retinal perforation or incarceration in the drainage site (Fig. 16.31B) and choroidal haemorrhage (Fig. 16.31C and D) and would rather perform a pars plana vitrectomy as a primary option.

Complications of scleral buckling

- **Diplopia** due to the mechanical effect of the buckle is common. Early spontaneous resolution is typical, though intervention is sometimes necessary.
- **Cystoid macular oedema** occurs in up to 25%, but usually responds to treatment. Other macular complications include epiretinal membrane (around 15%), persistent subfoveal fluid and foveal structural disruption, usually in macula-off detachments.
- **Anterior segment ischaemia** due to vascular compromise. This is a particular risk with an encircling band and with predisposing systemic conditions such as sickle haemoglobinopathies.
- **Buckle extrusion, intrusion or infection** (Fig. 16.32). Removal is usually required, with intensive antibiotic therapy if needed.
- **Elevated IOP.** An early IOP spike usually resolves rapidly, but occasionally can persist. Angle closure can occur.
- **Choroidal detachment** usually resolves spontaneously, presumably as scleral oedema settles and allows improved vortex vein function.
- **Surgical failure**
  - Missed breaks. A thorough search should always be made for the presence of multiple breaks, particularly if the configuration of the RD does not correspond to the position of the primary break.

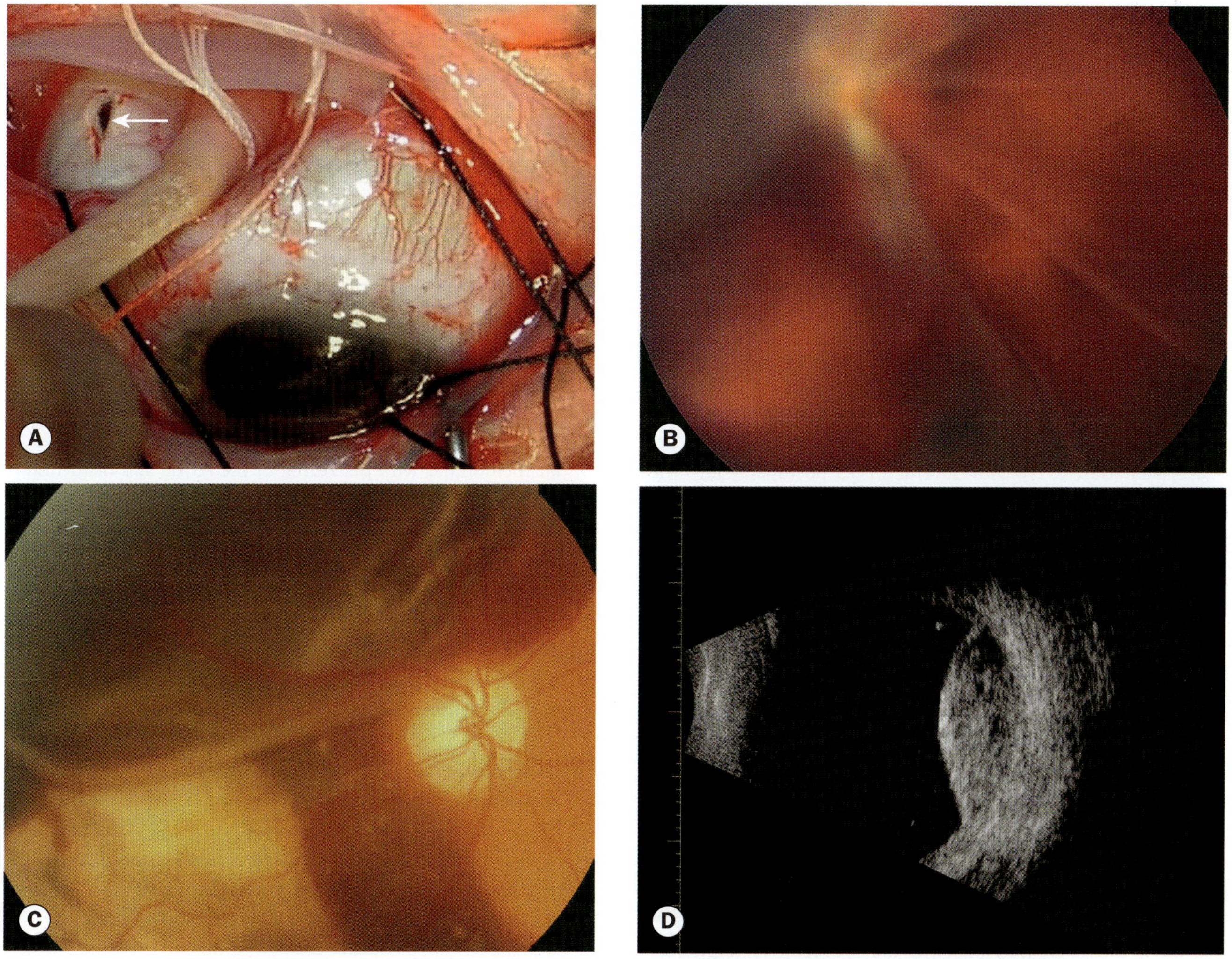

Fig. 16.31 Drainage of subretinal fluid during scleral buckling. **(A)** A circumferential explant is visible but has not yet been tightened into place. Fluid drainage can be encouraged by applying gentle pressure adjacent to the sclerostomy (arrow); **(B)** retinal incarceration into the drainage site; **(C)** subretinal haemorrhage; **(D)** ultrasound appearance showing subretinal haemorrhage. *(Courtesy of S Chen – figs A and B; P Terry – fig. D.)*

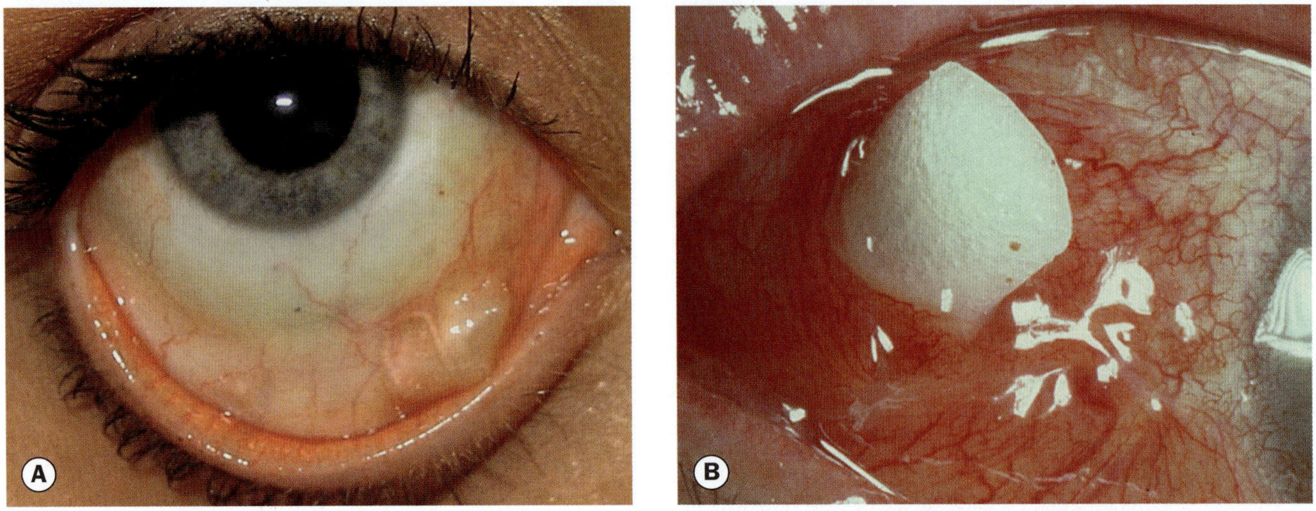

Fig. 16.32 Complications of scleral buckling. **(A)** Buckle extrusion; **(B)** plomb extrusion. *(Courtesy of S Chen – fig. A.)*

- ○ Buckle failure may occur due to inadequate size, incorrect positioning (Fig. 16.33A–D), or inadequate height. The explant may have to be replaced or repositioned to address the first two, but drainage of SRF or intravitreal gas injection may suffice for the latter, though pars plana vitrectomy (PPV) may be preferred as a more definitive measure. 'Fish-mouthing' (Fig. 16.33E and F) describes the phenomenon of a tear, typically a large superior equatorial U-tear in a bullous RD, to open widely following scleral buckling, requiring further operative treatment.
- ○ Proliferative vitreoretinopathy is the most common cause of late failure. The tractional forces associated with PVR can occasionally open old breaks and create new ones. Presentation is typically several weeks postoperatively with re-detachment.
- ○ Reopening of a retinal break in the absence of PVR can occur as a result of inadequate cryotherapy or scleral buckling, or sometimes when buckle height decreases either with time or following late surgical removal.

TIP The three commonest causes of failed retinal detachment surgery are: proliferative vitreoretinopathy, failure to close all breaks and the development of new breaks.

Pars plana vitrectomy

PPV is discussed later in this chapter.

TRACTIONAL RETINAL DETACHMENT

The main causes of tractional RD are proliferative retinopathy secondary to diabetes, retinopathy of prematurity and penetrating posterior segment trauma (see Ch. 22).

Pathogenesis of diabetic tractional retinal detachment

Tractional RD is caused by progressive contraction of fibrovascular membranes over large areas of vitreoretinal adhesion. In contrast to acute PVD in eyes with rhegmatogenous RD, PVD in diabetic eyes is gradual and frequently incomplete. It is thought to be caused by leakage of plasma constituents into the vitreous gel from a fibrovascular network adherent to the posterior vitreous surface. Owing to the strong adhesions of the cortical vitreous to areas of fibrovascular proliferation, PVD is usually incomplete. In the rare event of a subsequent complete PVD, the new blood vessels are avulsed and RD does not develop. Vitreoretinal traction can be any of the following:

- **Tangential**, caused by the contraction of epiretinal fibrovascular membranes with puckering of the retina and distortion of blood vessels.
- **Anteroposterior**, due to the contraction of fibrovascular membranes extending from the posterior retina, usually in association with the major arcades, to the vitreous base anteriorly and/or bridging (trampoline).
- **The result of contraction** of fibrovascular membranes stretching from one part of the retina to another or between vascular arcades, tending to pull the two involved points together.

Diagnosis

- **Symptoms.** Photopsia and floaters are usually absent because vitreoretinal traction develops insidiously and is not associated with acute PVD. A visual field defect usually progresses slowly and may be stable for months or even years.
- **Signs** (Fig. 16.34A)
  - ○ The RD has a concave configuration and breaks are absent.
  - ○ Retinal mobility is severely reduced and shifting fluid is absent.

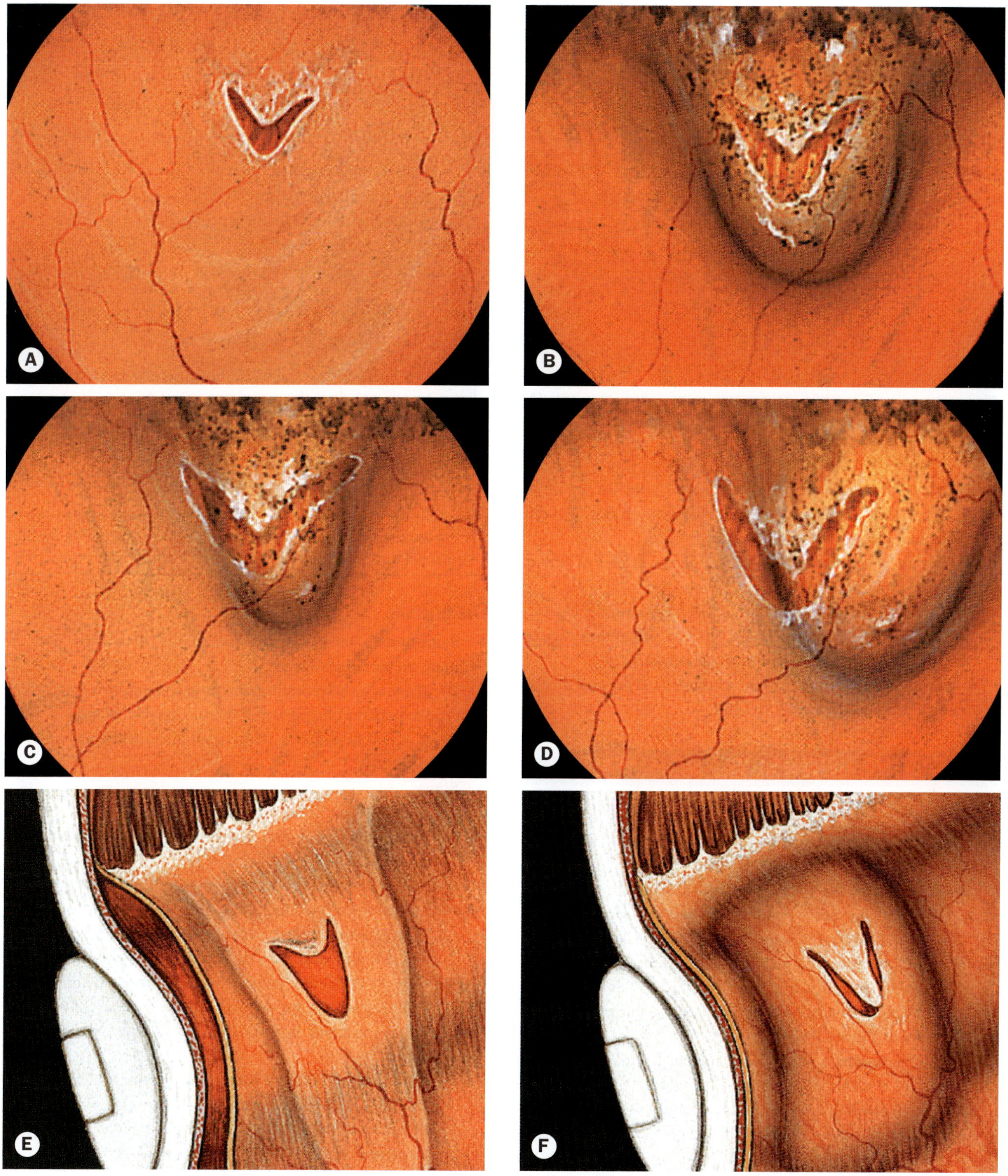

Fig. 16.33 Treatment of a fresh upper temporal retinal detachment and causes of failure. **(A)** Prior to surgery; **(B)** successful outcome; **(C)** tear is still open because the plomb is undersized; **(D)** tear is still open because the plomb is incorrectly positioned; **(E)** 'fish-mouthing' of a U-tear that is communicating with a radial fold; **(F)** flat retina following insertion of a radial buckle.

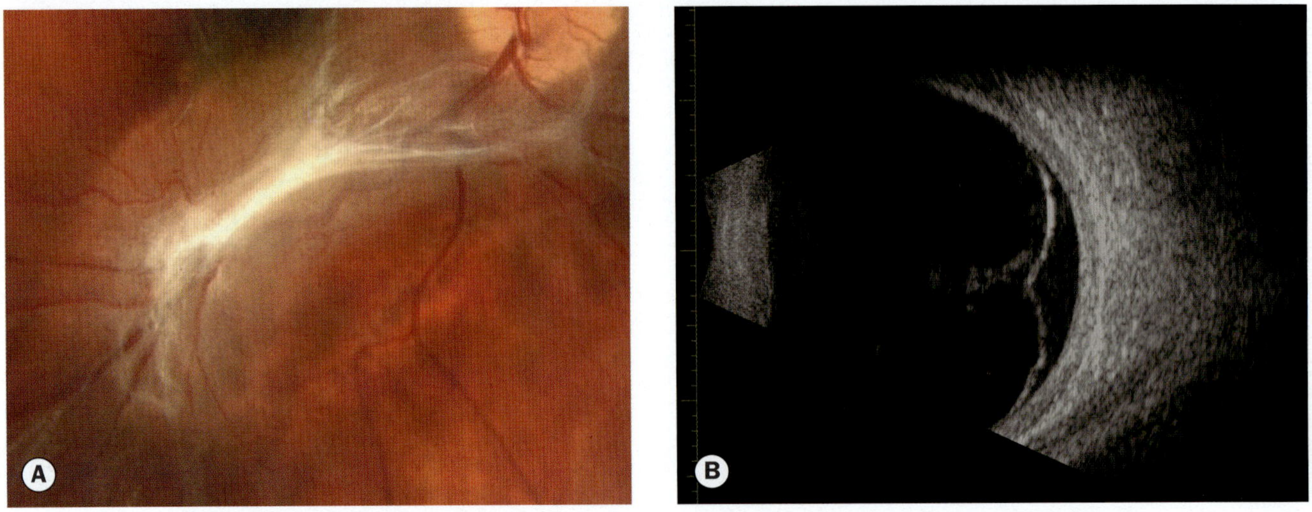

Fig. 16.34 Tractional retinal detachment. **(A)** Localized tractional detachment secondary to preretinal fibrosis; **(B)** B-scan. *(Courtesy of P Terry – fig. B.)*

  - The SRF is shallower than in a rhegmatogenous RD and seldom extends to the ora serrata.
  - The highest elevation of the retina occurs at sites of vitreoretinal traction.
  - If a break occurs in a tractional RD, it assumes the characteristics of a rhegmatogenous RD and progresses rapidly (combined tractional–rhegmatogenous RD).
- **B-scan ultrasonography** shows incomplete PVD and a relatively immobile retina (Fig. 16.34B).

EXUDATIVE RETINAL DETACHMENT

Pathogenesis

Exudative RD is characterized by the accumulation of SRF in the absence of retinal breaks or traction. It may occur in a variety of vascular, inflammatory and neoplastic diseases involving the retina, RPE and choroid in which fluid leaks outside the vessels and accumulates under the retina. As long as the RPE is able to compensate by pumping the leaking fluid into the choroidal circulation, RD does not occur. However, when the mechanism is overwhelmed or functions less than normally, fluid accumulates in the subretinal space. Causes include:

- **Choroidal tumours** such as melanoma, haemangioma and metastases. An intraocular tumour should be considered the cause of an exudative RD until proved otherwise.
- **Inflammation** such as Harada disease and posterior scleritis.
- **Bullous central serous chorioretinopathy** is a rare cause.
- **Iatrogenic** causes include RD surgery and panretinal photocoagulation.
- **Choroidal neovascularization**, which may leak and give rise to extensive subretinal accumulation of fluid at the posterior pole.
- **Hypertensive choroidopathy**, as may occur in toxaemia of pregnancy, is a very rare cause.
- **Idiopathic**, such as uveal effusion syndrome (see above).

TIP An exudative retinal detachment (which is often caused by a choroidal tumour) is characterized by 'shifting' subretinal fluid.

Diagnosis

- **Symptoms.** Depending on the cause, both eyes may be involved simultaneously.
  - There is no vitreoretinal traction, so photopsia is absent.
  - Floaters may be present if there is associated vitritis.
  - A visual field defect may develop suddenly and progress rapidly.
- **Signs**
  - The RD has a convex configuration, as with a rhegmatogenous RD, but its surface is smooth and not corrugated.
  - The detached retina is very mobile and exhibits the phenomenon of 'shifting fluid' in which SRF detaches the area of retina under which it accumulates (Fig. 16.35A and B). For example, in the upright position the SRF collects under the inferior retina, but on assuming the supine position for several minutes, the inferior retina flattens and SRF shifts posteriorly, detaching the superior retina.
  - The cause of the RD, such as a choroidal tumour (Fig. 16.36A), may be apparent when the fundus is examined or on B-scan ultrasonography, or the patient may have an associated systemic disease responsible for the RD (e.g. Harada disease, toxaemia of pregnancy).
  - 'Leopard spots' consisting of scattered areas of subretinal pigment clumping may be seen after the detachment has flattened (Fig. 16.36B).

Treatment

Treatment depends on the cause. Some cases resolve spontaneously, whilst others are treated with systemic corticosteroids

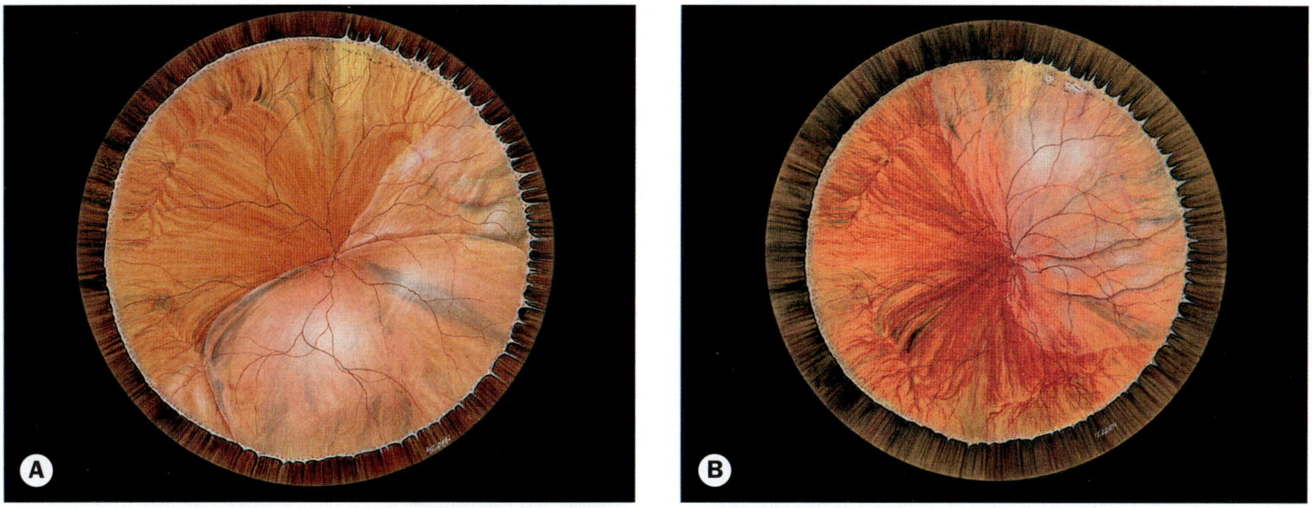

Fig. 16.35 Exudative retinal detachment with shifting fluid. **(A)** Inferior collection of subretinal fluid with the patient sitting; **(B)** the subretinal fluid shifts upwards when the patient assumes the supine position. *(Courtesy of CL Schepens, E Hartnett and T Hirose, from* Schepens' Retinal Detachment and Allied Diseases, *Butterworth-Heinemann 2000.)*

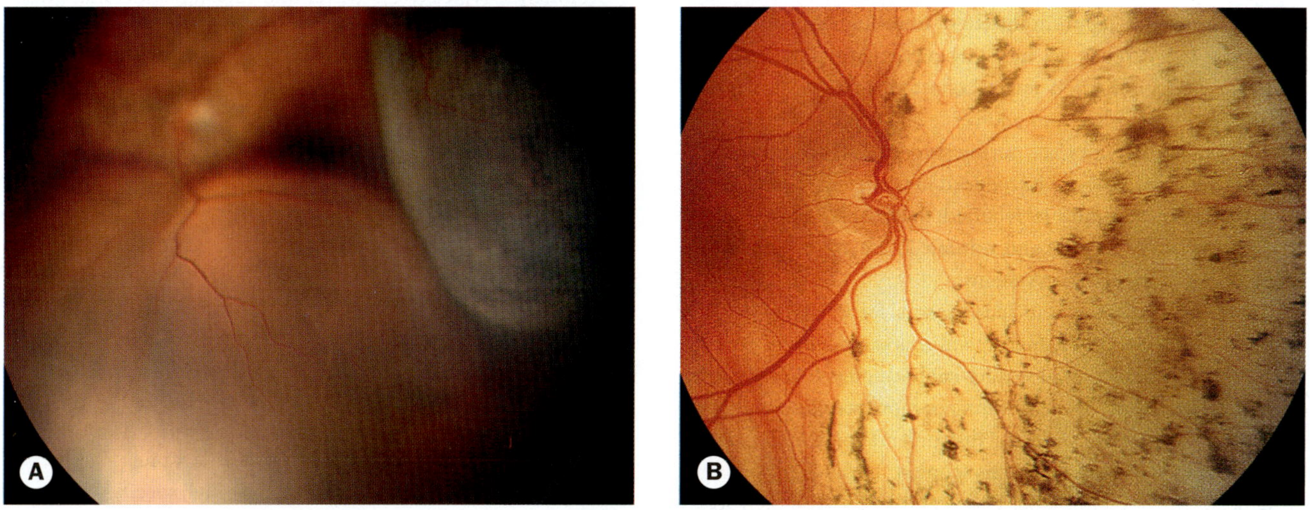

Fig. 16.36 Exudative retinal detachment. **(A)** Caused by a choroidal melanoma; **(B)** 'leopard spot' pigmentation following resolution of exudative retinal detachment. *(Courtesy of B Damato – fig. A.)*

(Harada disease and posterior scleritis). In some eyes with bullous central serous chorioretinopathy, the leak in the RPE can be sealed by laser photocoagulation.

PARS PLANA VITRECTOMY

Introduction

Instrumentation

The diameter of the shaft of vitrectomy instrumentation has conventionally been 0.9 mm (20-gauge), but smaller 23-gauge, 25-gauge and even 27-gauge sutureless systems (transconjunctival microincision vitrectomy – MIVS) are increasingly becoming the standard of care, offering shorter operating time, less trauma and scarring, and faster rehabilitation. Early concerns about an increased risk of postoperative endophthalmitis do not seem to have been borne out and operative success rates are comparable to larger-gauge instrumentation.

- **Intraocular illumination** is supplied by a fibreoptic probe (light pipe – see Fig. 16.37A). Initially, reduced illumination was a problem with the narrow calibre MIVS systems, because of the limitations of halogen bulbs. Brighter sources consisting of xenon and potentially less phototoxic mercury vapour sources have been introduced that match or exceed the levels of 20-gauge systems. These minimize retinal phototoxicity by filtering out higher-energy ultraviolet and blue light. Some systems offer adjustable lighting characteristics to increase the contrast of particular structures. Wide-angle lighting and self-retaining 'chandelier' sources are available – the latter offer the advantages of freeing both of the surgeon's hands to carry out true bimanual surgery (which can be particularly useful in challenging cases) and of reducing phototoxicity (by increasing the working distance of the light probe from the retina). Extremely small-gauge dual chandelier probes are available to eliminate shadowing from the working field.

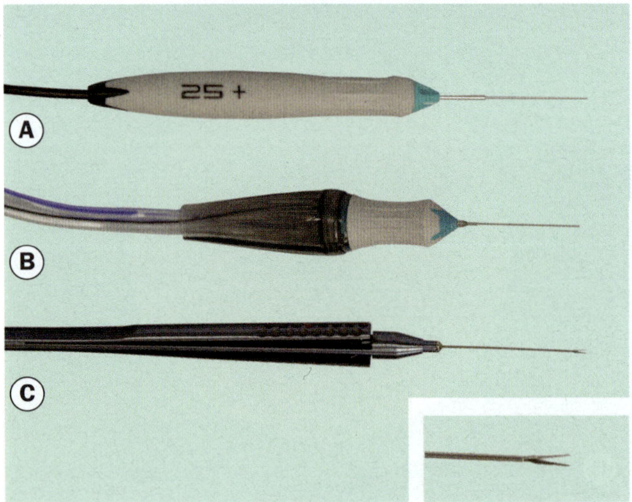

Fig. 16.37 **(A)** Illumination pipe; **(B)** cutter; **(C)** micro-forceps.

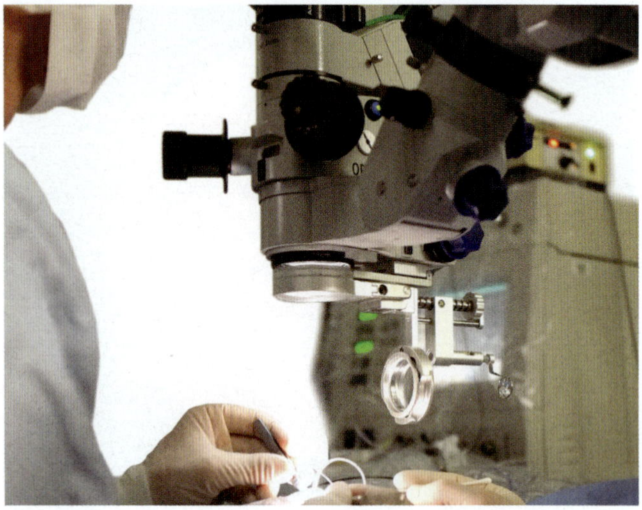

Fig. 16.38 Viewing system for pars plana vitrectomy.

- **Vitreous cutter** (Fig. 16.37B) has an inner guillotine blade that oscillates at very high speed (from 1500 up to 5000–7500 cuts per minute [cpm] in the latest 'ultra-high speed' cutters), cutting the vitreous gel into tiny pieces and simultaneously removing it by suction into a collecting cassette. Faster cutting speeds translate into a lower level of traction exerted on the vitreoretinal interface during surgery. Safer more efficient fluidic control has been introduced in tandem.
- **An infusion cannula** is required in order to maintain the vitreous cavity pressure and volume. These are generally self-retaining in small-gauge systems.
- **Accessory instruments** include scissors, forceps (Fig. 16.37C), flute needle and endodiathermy and endolaser delivery systems. With the introduction of smaller-calibre cutters that are able to manipulate fibrovascular membranes more precisely and safely, the requirement for additional instrumentation may decrease.
- **Wide-angle viewing systems** consist of an indirect lens beneath the operating microscope and an incorporated series of prisms to reinvert the image (Fig. 16.38). The field of view extends almost to the ora serrata. Higher magnification smaller field lenses are available for macular surgery.

Tamponading agents

These achieve intraoperative retinal flattening in combination with internal drainage of SRF and are commonly used postoperatively for internal tamponade of retinal breaks.

- **Expanding gases.** Although air can be used, an expanding gas is usually preferred in order to achieve prolonged tamponade. Postoperative positioning of the patient is used to maximize the effective vector and maintain surface tension around the break.
  - Sulfur hexafluoride (SF_6) doubles its volume if used at a 100% concentration and lasts 10–14 days.
  - Perfluoroethane (C_2F_6) triples its volume at 100% and lasts 30–35 days.
  - Perfluoropropane (C_3F_8) quadruples its volume at 100% and lasts 55–65 days.
- **Gas concentration.** Because the eye is usually left almost entirely gas-filled at the end of the procedure, most are used at only an isovolumetric (non-expansile) concentration (e.g. 20–30% for SF_6 and 12–16% for C_3F_8). Low-pressure environments, typically air travel and nitrous oxide anaesthesia, must be avoided until gas absorption is complete, as these will increase the intraocular gas pressure.

TIP If gas has been used at the time of RD repair, air travel should be avoided because the gas bubble can expand with a change in atmospheric pressure and cause an acute rise in IOP.

- **Silicone oils** have low specific gravity – they are lighter than water and thus buoyant. They are commonly used for both intraoperative retinal manipulation and prolonged postoperative intraocular tamponade and are particularly helpful in the management of proliferative vitreoretinopathy. 1000 cs silicone is easier to inject and to remove whilst 5000 cs is more viscous but may be less prone to emulsification.
- **Heavy liquids** (perfluorocarbons) have high specific gravity and thus settle inferiorly in the vitreous cavity (Fig. 16.39). Perfluoro-n-octane is most commonly used as it allows good visibility and low viscosity. It acts as an intraoperative mechanical device and can be used to flatten the posterior retina, open retinal folds and improve visualization of additional membranes. Although primarily developed for RD surgery, other indications include haemostasis (by localizing bleeding), expression of liquefied blood from behind the retina and anterior floating of dislocated lens fragments or intraocular lens (IOL). Cases of retinal toxicity and inflammation have been reported.

Indications

Although many simple rhegmatogenous RD can be treated successfully by scleral buckling techniques, PPV has greatly improved the prognosis for more complex detachments. As techniques have improved and surgeons' familiarity and confidence has grown, the threshold for vitrectomy surgery has fallen. Many vitreoretinal surgeons now feel that morbidity and success rates are better with vitrectomy than with scleral buckling for all pseudophakic and aphakic RD and for those that would otherwise require external drainage of

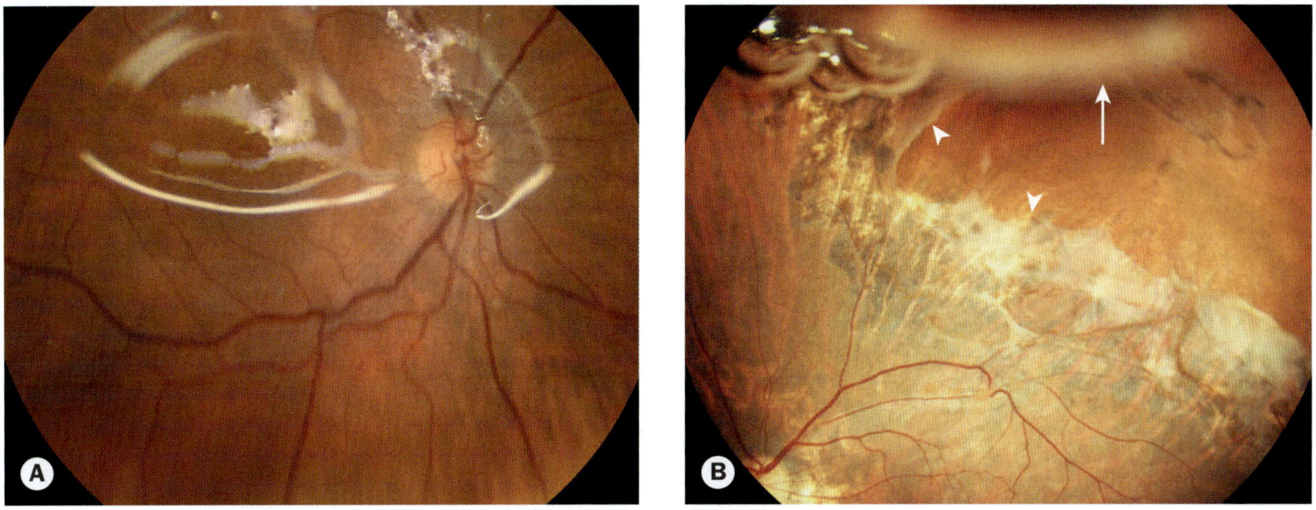

Fig. 16.39 **(A)** Perfluorocarbon visible at the posterior pole (see light reflex); **(B)** giant tear (arrowheads) unrolled with heavy liquid (arrow). *(Courtesy of C Barry – fig. B.)*

SRF. A recent survey of vitreoretinal trends in the USA reveals that more than 80% of primary RD surgery is undertaken using a PPV approach. The guidelines below are therefore not absolute.

Rhegmatogenous retinal detachment

- **When retinal breaks cannot be visualized** as a result of haemorrhage, vitreous debris, posterior capsular opacity, IOL edge effects. Vitrectomy is crucial to provide an adequate retinal view. Scleral buckling carries a high risk of failure if any breaks are missed.
- **When retinal breaks are unlikely to be closed by scleral buckling**, such as giant tears, large posterior breaks and in the presence of PVR (Fig. 16.40A–C).

Tractional retinal detachment

- **Indications in diabetic RD**
  - Tractional RD threatening or involving the macula (Fig. 16.40D). Vitrectomy is always combined with anti-VEGF agents and/or internal panretinal photocoagulation to prevent postoperative neovascularization that may cause vitreous haemorrhage or rubeosis iridis. Extramacular tractional RD may be observed without surgery because, in many cases, it remains stationary for a long time provided proliferative retinopathy has been controlled.
  - Combined tractional–rhegmatogenous RD should be treated urgently, even if the macula is not involved, because SRF is likely to spread quickly.
- **Indications in penetrating trauma**
  - Prevention of tractional RD. Unlike diabetic retinopathy where epiretinal membrane proliferation occurs mostly on the posterior retina, fibrocellular proliferation after penetrating trauma tends to develop on the pre-equatorial retina and/or the ciliary body. Treatment is usually aimed at visual rehabilitation and minimizing the tractional process.
  - Late tractional RD, which may be associated with an intraocular foreign body or retinal incarceration, occasionally develops months after otherwise successful surgery.

Technique

Goals of surgery

- **To separate the posterior hyaloid** from the retinal surface.
- **To remove the epiretinal tissue** in order to release the central and/or peripheral retinal traction.
- **To close retinal breaks** if present.

Basic vitrectomy

- **An infusion cannula** is inserted (3.5 mm behind the limbus in pseudophakic or aphakic eyes and 4 mm in phakic eyes) at the level of the inferior border of the lateral rectus muscle. Limbal peritomy (conjunctival dissection) is required for conventional large-gauge systems, but is unnecessary in small-gauge systems.
- **Further sclerotomies** are made at the 10 and 2 o'clock positions, through which the vitreous cutter and fibreoptic probe are introduced (Fig. 16.41). These sclerotomies are self-sealing with modern small-gauge systems, though wound leak occasionally occurs (Fig. 16.42).
- **Excision.** The central vitreous gel and posterior hyaloid face are excised.
- **Two types of epithelial membrane** are encountered:
  - Non-vascular membranes found in PVR and macular pucker.
  - Fibrovascular membranes found in patients with proliferative diabetic retinopathy.
- **The surgical techniques** employed involve delamination, segmentation and *en-bloc* dissection.
- **Intraoperative tissue staining** can be helpful. In particular trypan blue can be used to stain an epiretinal membrane and triamcinolone to stain vitreous.
- **The above basic steps** apply to all vitrectomy surgery. Subsequent steps depend on the specific indication.
- **Sutures.** Transconjunctival small-gauge systems do not require postoperative suturing.

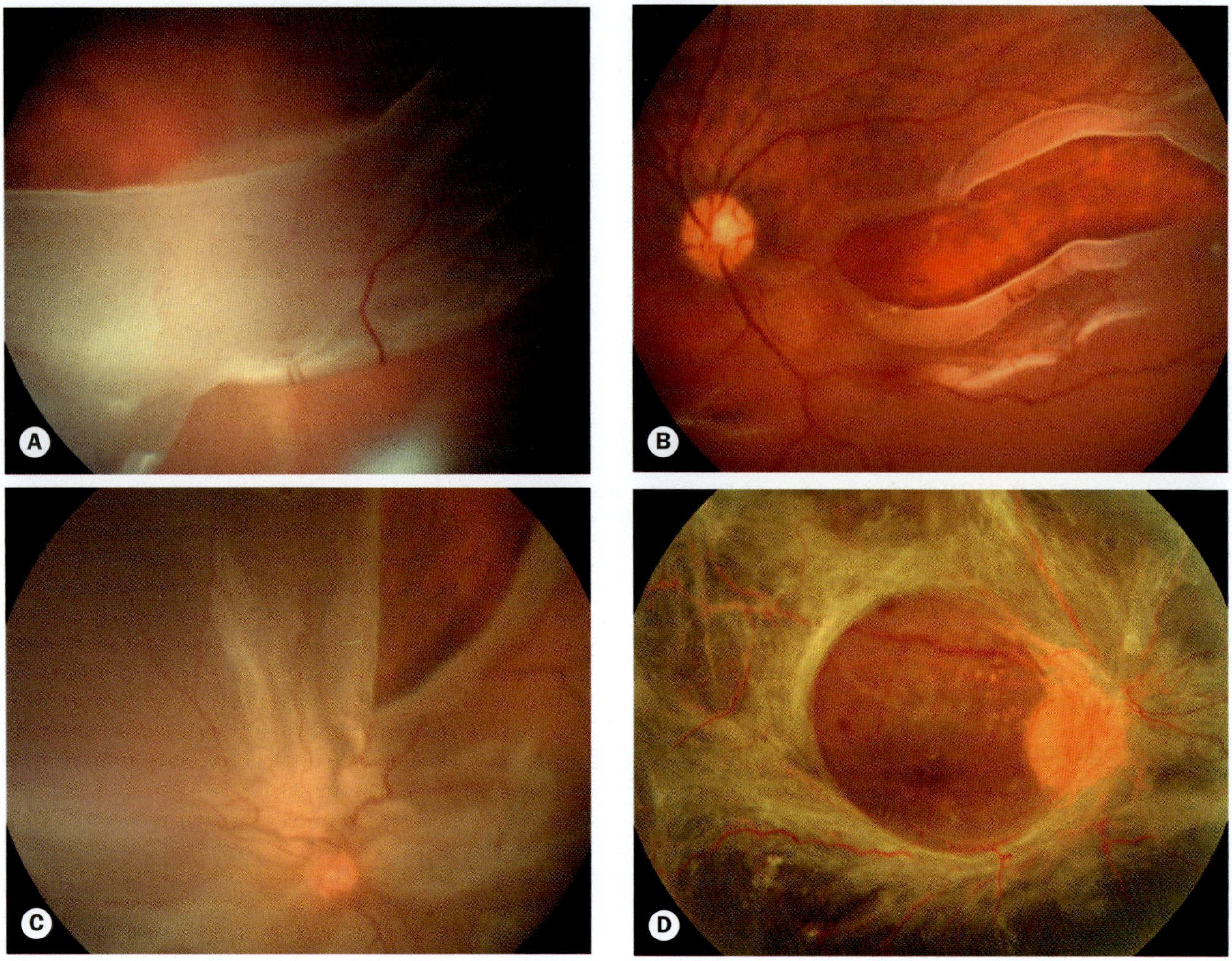

Fig. 16.40 Some indications for pars plana vitrectomy. **(A)** Giant retinal tear; **(B)** large posterior tear; **(C)** proliferative vitreoretinopathy in the presence of a large tear; **(D)** tractional retinal detachment. *(Courtesy of C Barry – fig. B; S Chen – fig. D.)*

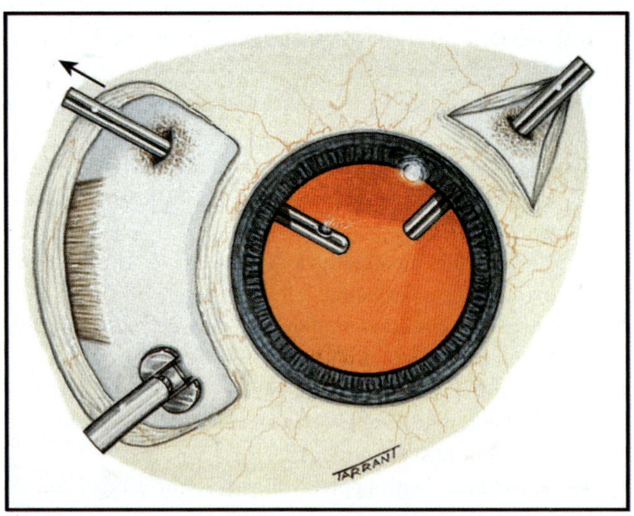

Fig. 16.41 Infusion cannula, light pipe and cutter in position (right eye).

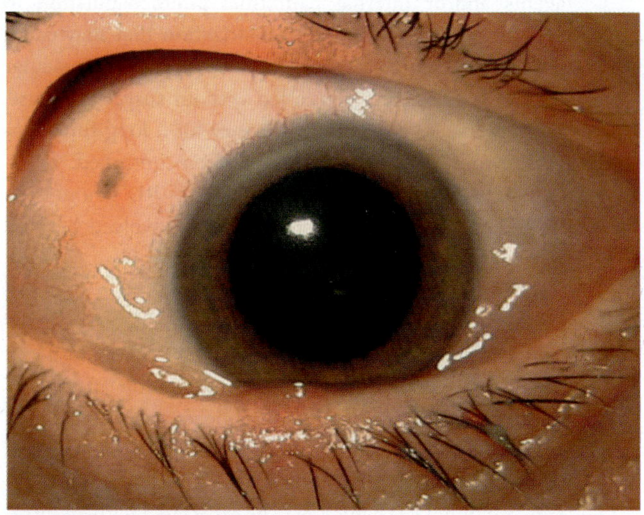

Fig. 16.42 Wound leak following sutureless vitrectomy. *(Courtesy of S Chen.)*

Proliferative vitreoretinopathy

The aims of surgery in PVR are to release both transvitreal traction by vitrectomy and tangential (surface) traction by membrane dissection in order to restore retinal mobility and allow closure of retinal breaks.

Localized fixed retinal folds may be freed by the removal of the central plaque of epiretinal membrane. This can usually be achieved by engaging the tip of vertically cutting scissors or a pick-type instrument in the edge of a valley between two adjacent folds (Fig. 16.43). The membrane is either surgically dissected or simply peeled from the surface of the retina. Small-gauge cutters may be used in some cases to engage membranes directly and forceps can facilitate this. A relieving retinotomy should be considered if the mobility of the retina is believed to be insufficient for sustained reattachment.

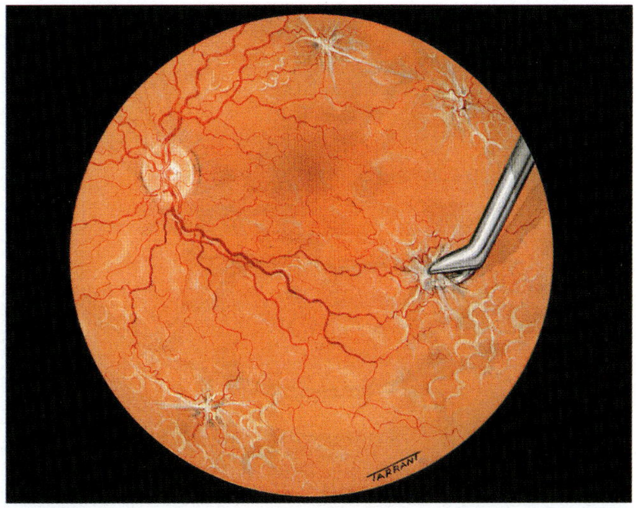

Fig. 16.43 Dissection of retinal folds in proliferative vitreoretinopathy.

Tractional retinal detachment

The goal of vitrectomy in tractional RDs is to release anteroposterior and/or circumferential vitreoretinal traction. Because the membranes are vascularized and the retina often friable, they cannot be simply peeled from the surface of the retina as this would result in haemorrhage and tearing of the retina. The three methods of removing fibrovascular membranes in diabetic tractional RDs are the following:

- **Delamination** involves the horizontal cutting of individual vascular pegs connecting a membrane to the surface of the retina (Fig. 16.44A). This allows the complete removal of fibrovascular tissue from the retinal surface (Fig. 16.44B).
- **Segmentation** involves the vertical cutting of epiretinal membranes into small segments (Fig. 16.44C and D). It is used to release circumferential vitreoretinal traction when delamination is difficult or impossible.
- ***En-bloc* dissection.** The key step is to separate posterior hyaloid from the retina. An incision is made in the epiretinal membrane using an illuminated pick. The membrane is then peeled away using an end-gripping membrane forceps (Fig. 16.45).

Complications

The rate of complications has decreased significantly in recent years because of technological advances and specialized training in the field. Complications can nevertheless occur intraoperatively and postoperatively.

Intraoperative complications

- **Posterior retinal breaks.**
- **Peripheral retinal breaks.**
- **Rarely, choroidal haemorrhage.**

Postoperative complications

- **Retinal breaks** and rhegmatogenous RD.
- **Retinal fold** (Fig. 16.46). This is less likely to occur by placing the patient face down immediately after surgery.
- **Inflammation**, particularly in patients with diabetes.
- **Raised intraocular pressure.**
  - Overexpansion of intraocular gas, usually when the concentration or volume of expansile gas is inadvertently too great. Medical measures alone may be sufficient in some cases, but if a substantial elevation of IOP occurs excess gas can be removed at the slit lamp via the pars plana by using a 30-gauge needle on a 1 ml syringe.

TIP Excessive concentrations of intraocular gas can result in a significant rise in IOP. Excess gas can be removed at the slit lamp by inserting a 30-gauge needle into the vitreous cavity via the pars plana.

  - Silicone oil-associated glaucoma. Early glaucoma may be caused by direct pupillary block by silicone oil (Fig. 16.47A). This occurs particularly in an aphakic eye with an intact iris diaphragm. In aphakic eyes this can be prevented by performing an inferior (Ando) iridectomy at the time of surgery to allow free passage of aqueous to the anterior chamber. Intraocular gas can also cause pupillary block. Late glaucoma is caused by emulsified silicone in the anterior chamber (Fig. 16.47B) causing trabecular obstruction and scarring. The risk may be reduced by early oil removal, though glaucoma can still occur. A long tube seton may be required (Fig. 16.47C).
  - Other mechanisms include ghost cell, inflammatory and steroid-induced glaucoma (see Ch. 11). Angle closure can also result from ciliochoroidal effusion with anterior rotation of the lens–iris diaphragm, which may respond to cycloplegia and steroids.
- **Cataract**
  - Gas-induced. A large or long-lasting intravitreal gas bubble typically gives rise to feathering of the posterior subcapsular lens, but this is usually transient.
  - Silicone-induced. Almost all phakic eyes with silicone oil eventually develop cataract (Fig. 16.47D).
  - Delayed. Following vitrectomy, substantial nuclear sclerosis commonly develops, especially if the patient is over 50 years of age.
- **Band keratopathy** is not uncommon with extended silicone oil tamponade.

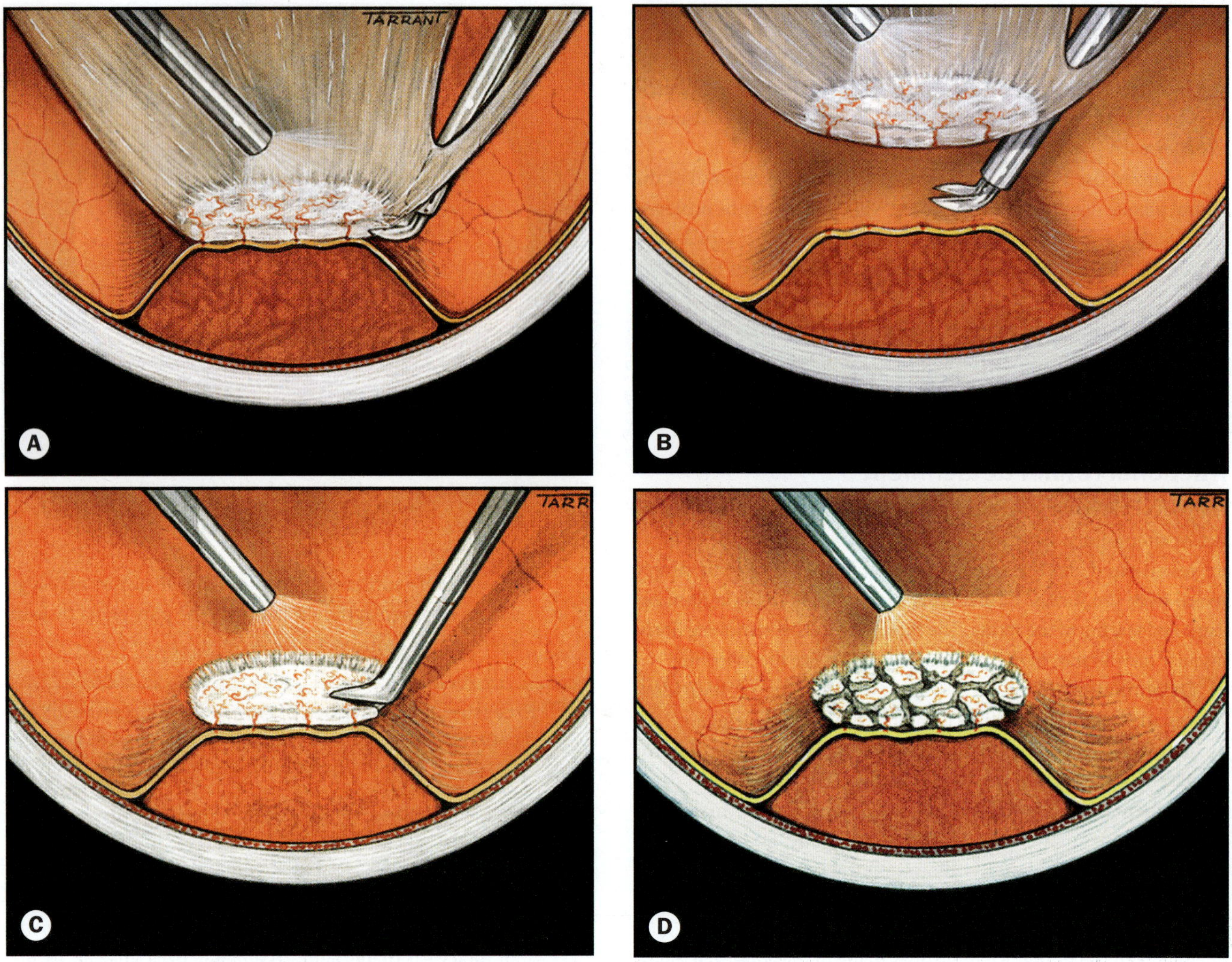

Fig. 16.44 **(A)** Delamination with horizontally cutting scissors; **(B)** completed; **(C)** segmentation with vertically cutting scissors; **(D)** completed.

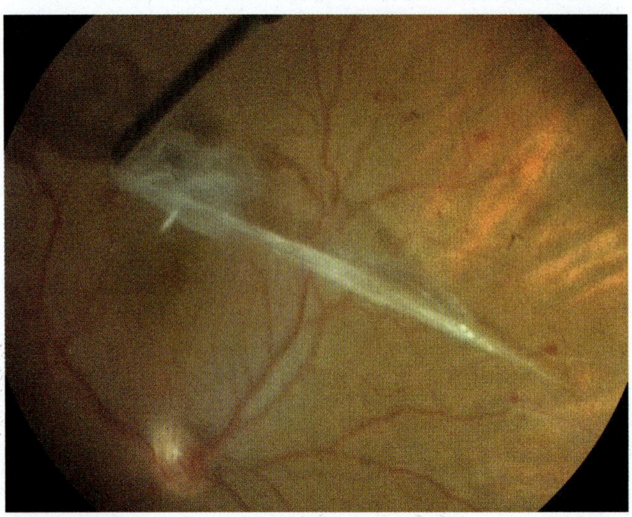

Fig. 16.45 *En-bloc* dissection of epiretinal membrane. *(Courtesy of V Tanner.)*

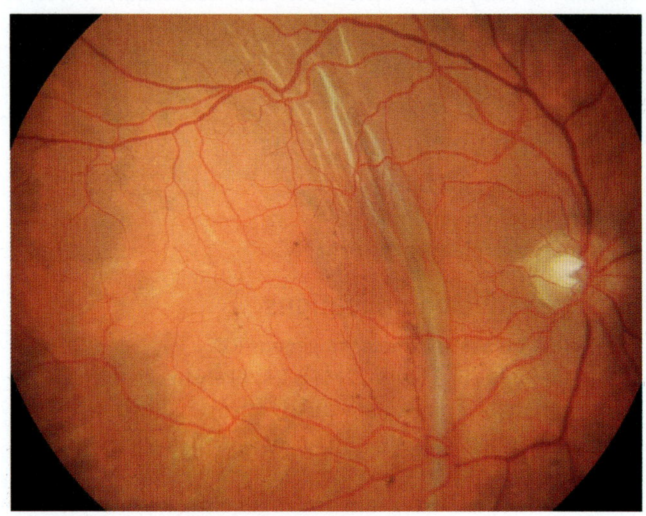

Fig. 16.46 Postoperative retinal fold.

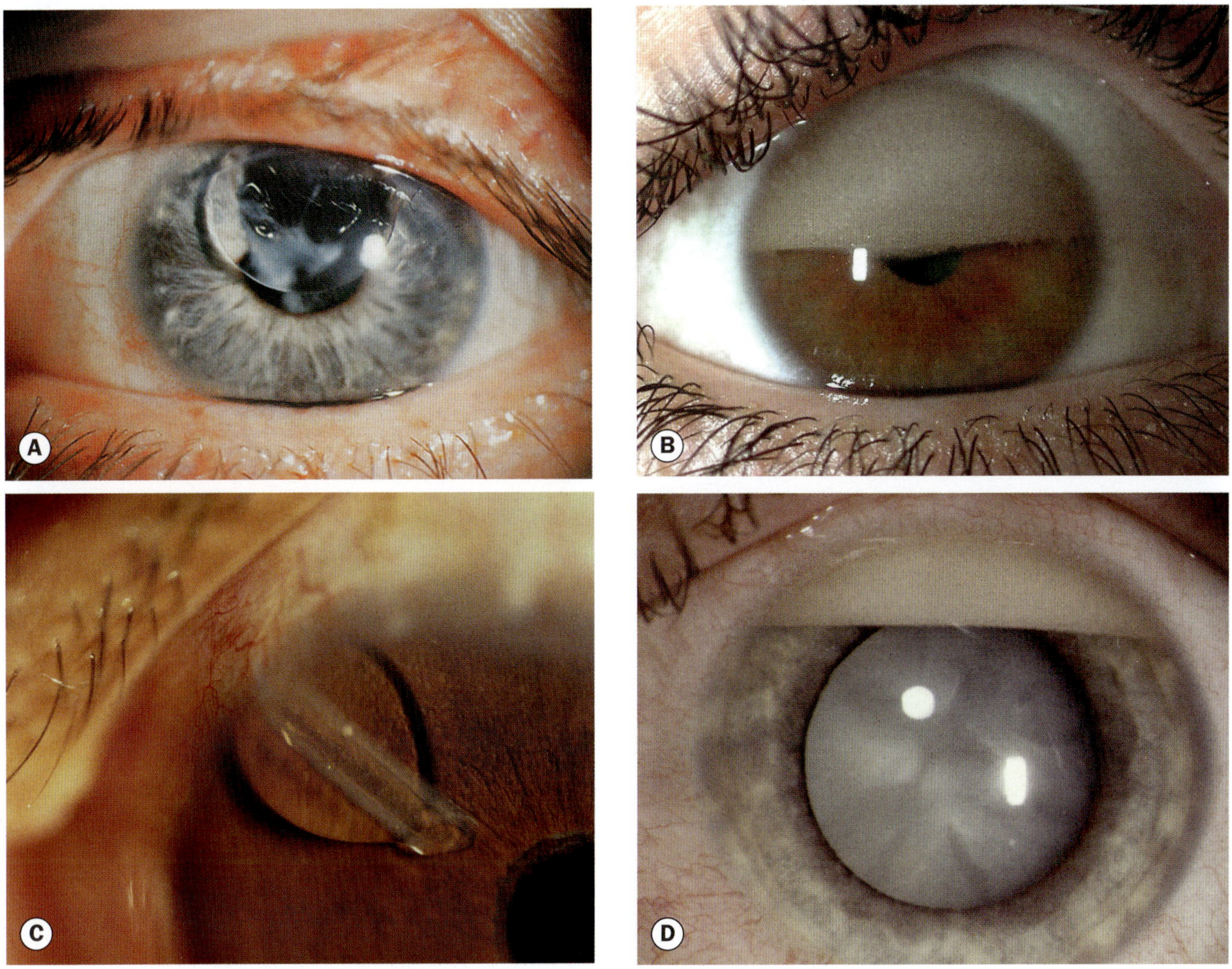

Fig. 16.47 Some complications of silicone oil injection. **(A)** Pupillary block glaucoma caused by oil in the anterior chamber; **(B)** late glaucoma due to emulsified oil in the anterior chamber; an inverted pseudo-hypopyon (hyperoleon) is seen; **(C)** Baerveldt tube inserted for secondary glaucoma with small silicone bubble beneath the tube; **(D)** cataract with a hyperoleon.

Chapter 17

Vitreous Opacities

Introduction

The vitreous is a transparent extracellular gel consisting of collagen, soluble proteins, hyaluronic acid and water. The total vitreous volume is approximately 4.0 ml. The few cells normally present in the gel are located predominantly in the cortex and include hyalocytes, astrocytes and glial cells. The vitreous provides structural support to the globe while allowing a clear and optically uniform path to the retina. Once liquefied or surgically removed it does not re-form. Vitreous opacities can be caused by a variety of pathological processes primarily involving other ocular sites. Apart from vitreous haemorrhage, the conditions discussed below are those in which the vitreous gel is the primary site of pathology.

Muscae volitantes

Muscae volitantes (Latin for 'hovering flies'), commonly referred to as 'floaters', is an ubiquitous entoptic phenomenon of fly-, cobweb- or thread-like condensations that are best seen against a pale background. It is thought to predominantly represent tiny embryological remnants in the vitreous gel. A sudden exacerbation can occur due to vitreous haemorrhage or, more commonly, a change in the conformation of the gel, such as a posterior vitreous detachment (see Fig. 16.15).

Vitreous haemorrhage

Vitreous haemorrhage is a common condition with many causes (Table 17.1). Symptoms vary according to severity. Mild haemorrhage (Fig. 17.1A) causes sudden onset floaters and diffuse blurring of vision, but may not affect visual acuity, whilst a dense bleed may result in severe visual loss (Fig. 17.1B). B-scan ultrasonography in non-clotted vitreous haemorrhage generally shows a uniform appearance and once cellular aggregates develop, small particulate echoes become visible (Fig. 17.1C). Ultrasonography is critical in the evaluation of an eye with dense vitreous haemorrhage to exclude an underlying retinal tear or detachment (Fig. 17.1D). Treatment is dictated by severity and cause, but an increasingly low threshold is being adopted for early vitrectomy (see Ch. 16) in cases of dense haemorrhage.

TIP Undertake ultrasound investigation in an eye with a dense vitreous haemorrhage to exclude a retinal detachment or choroidal melanoma.

Table 17.1 Causes of Vitreous Haemorrhage

- Acute posterior vitreous detachment associated either with a retinal tear or avulsion of a peripheral vessel
- Proliferative retinopathy
  - Diabetic
  - Retinal vein occlusion
  - Sickle cell disease
  - Eales disease
  - Vasculitis
- Miscellaneous retinal disorders
  - Macroaneurysm
  - Telangiectasia
  - Capillary haemangioma
- Trauma
- Systemic
  - Bleeding disorders
  - Terson syndrome

Terson syndrome

Terson syndrome refers to the combination of intraocular and subarachnoid haemorrhage secondary to aneurysmal rupture, most commonly arising from the anterior communicating artery. However, intraocular haemorrhage may also occur with subdural haematoma and acute elevation of intracranial pressure from other causes. The haemorrhage is frequently bilateral and is typically intraretinal and/or preretinal (Fig. 17.2), although occasionally subhyaloid blood may break into the vitreous. It is probable that intraocular bleeding is due to retinal venous stasis secondary to increase in cavernous sinus pressure. Vitreous haemorrhage usually resolves spontaneously within a few months and the long-term visual prognosis is good in most. Early vitrectomy may be considered in some cases.

Asteroid hyalosis

Asteroid hyalosis is a common degenerative process in which calcium pyrophosphate particles collect within the vitreous gel. It is seen clinically as numerous tiny round yellow–white opacities of varying size and density (Fig. 17.3A and B). These move with the vitreous during eye movements but do not sediment inferiorly when the eye is immobile. Only one eye is affected in 75% of patients. It rarely causes visual problems and the majority of patients are asymptomatic. An association with diabetes has been suggested, but is unproven. The prevalence of asteroid hyalosis increases with age and affects 3% of those aged 75–86 years. It is more common in men than in women. Optical coherence tomography (OCT) (Fig. 17.3C) and ultrasonography (Fig. 17.3D) show high reflectivity foci.

TIP Because asteroid hyalosis rarely causes visual symptoms, dual pathology should be considered if the visual acuity is reduced.

Synchysis scintillans

Synchysis (synchisis) scintillans occurs as a consequence of chronic vitreous haemorrhage, often in a blind eye. The condition is usually discovered when frank haemorrhage is no longer present. The crystals are composed of cholesterol and are derived from plasma cells or degraded products of erythrocytes and lie either freely or engulfed within foreign body giant cells.

Numerous flat golden-brown refractile particles are seen (Fig. 17.4A), which tend to sediment inferiorly when the eye is immobile. Occasionally the anterior chamber may also be involved (Fig. 17.4B).

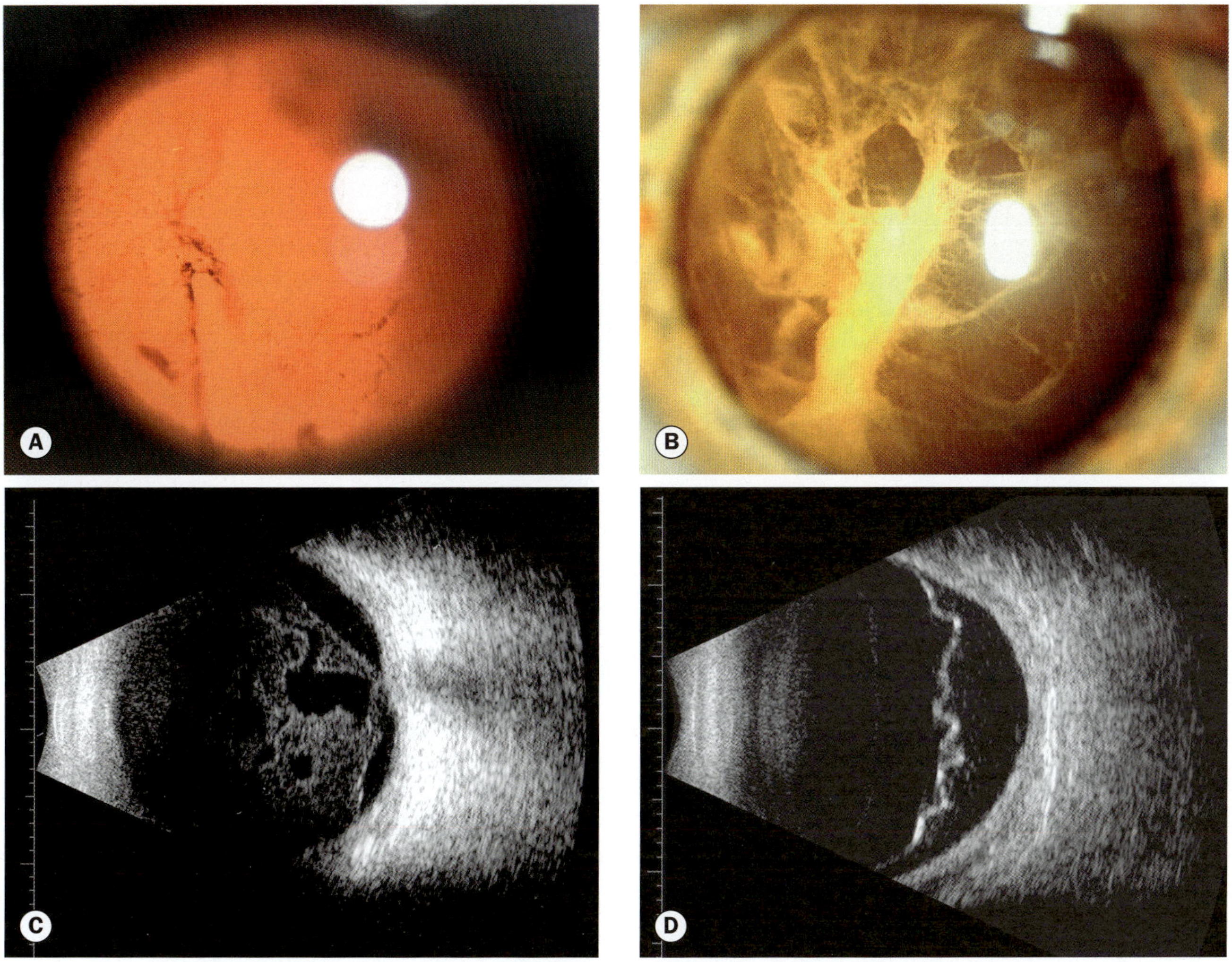

Fig. 17.1 (A) Mild vitreous haemorrhage seen against the red reflex; **(B)** resorbing vitreous haemorrhage; **(C)** B-scan image showing vitreous haemorrhage and flat retina; **(D)** B-scan image showing retinal detachment. *(Courtesy of C Barry – fig. B; P Terry – figs C and D.)*

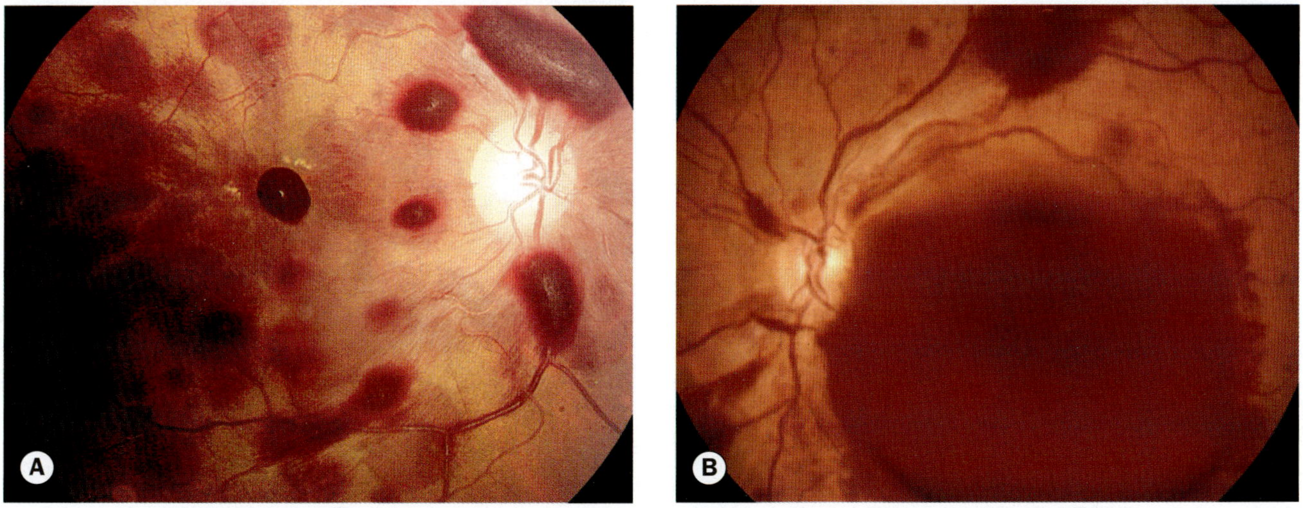

Fig. 17.2 Terson syndrome. **(A)** Acute intra- and preretinal haemorrhages in a 48-year-old man with subarachnoid haemorrhage; **(B)** macular involvement. *(Courtesy of A Agarwal, from* Gass' Atlas of Macular Diseases*, Elsevier 2012 – fig. A.)*

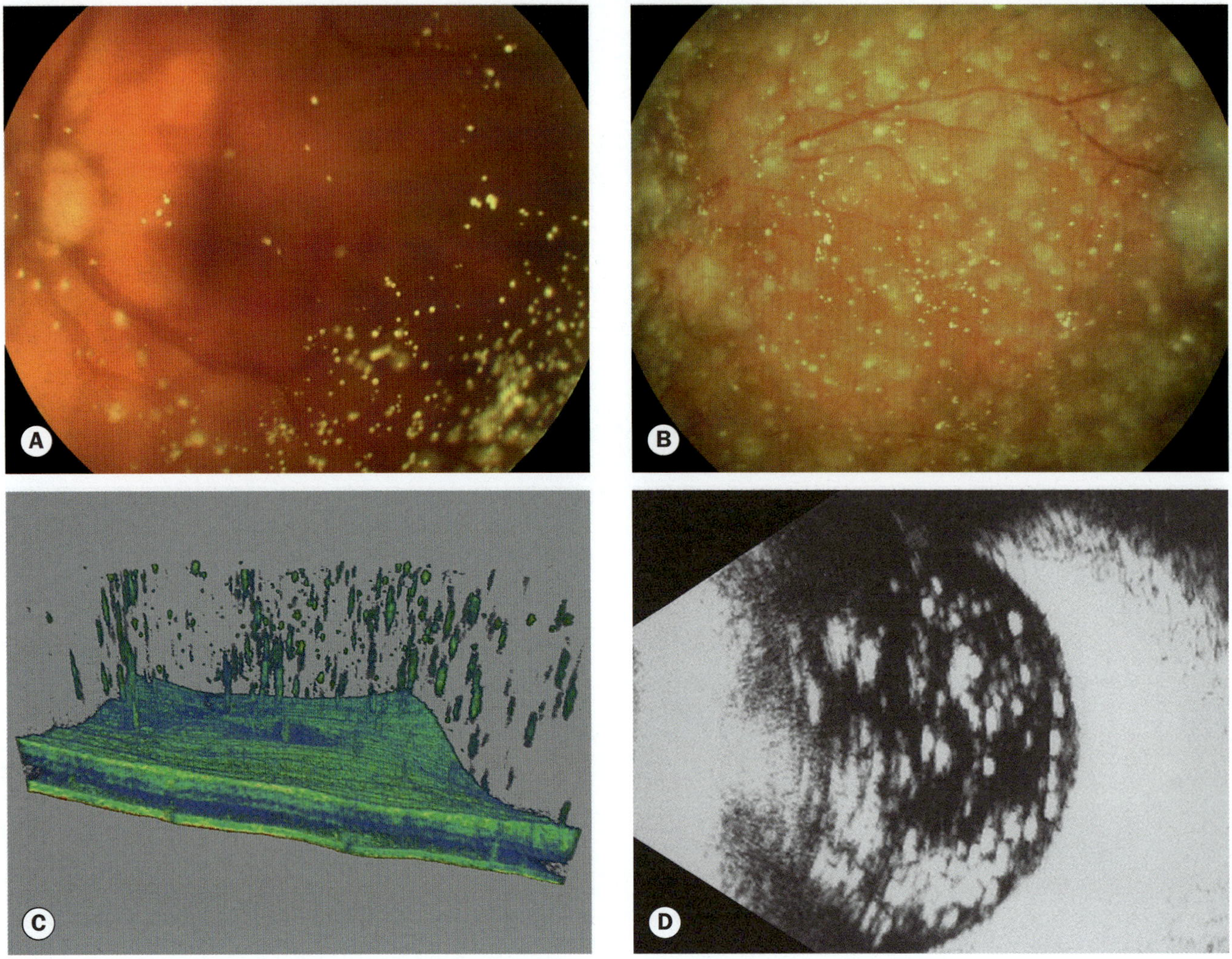

Fig. 17.3 Asteroid hyalosis. **(A)** Mild; **(B)** severe; **(C)** 3-dimensional OCT reconstruction; **(D)** B-scan ultrasonogram. *(Courtesy of S Chen – fig. C.)*

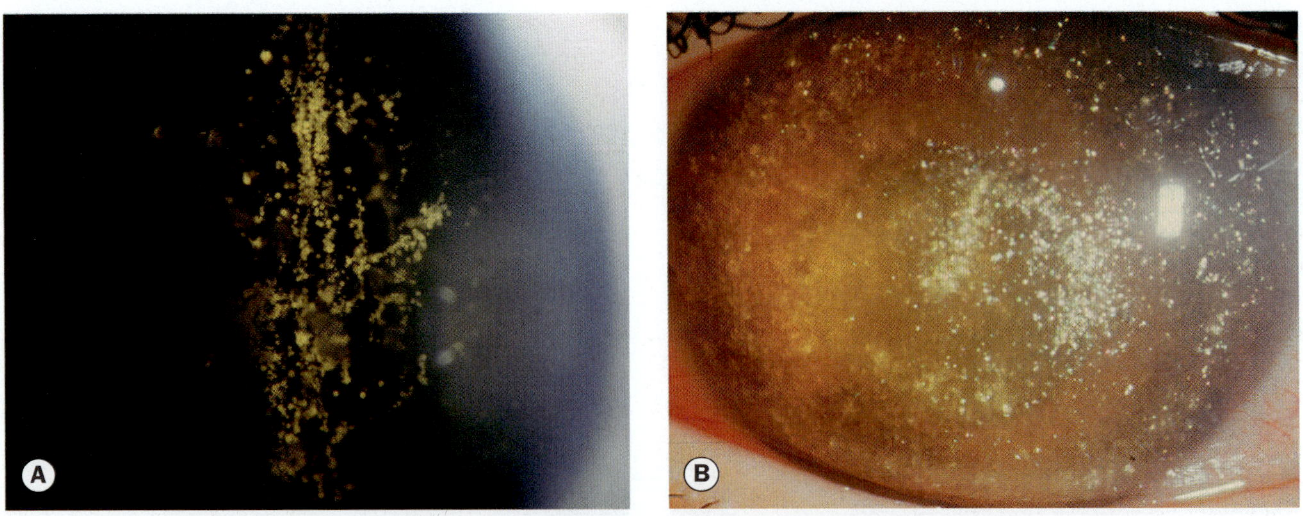

Fig. 17.4 Synchysis scintillans. **(A)** Golden-brown particles in the vitreous; **(B)** in the anterior chamber of a degenerate eye. *(Courtesy of P Gili – fig. B.)*

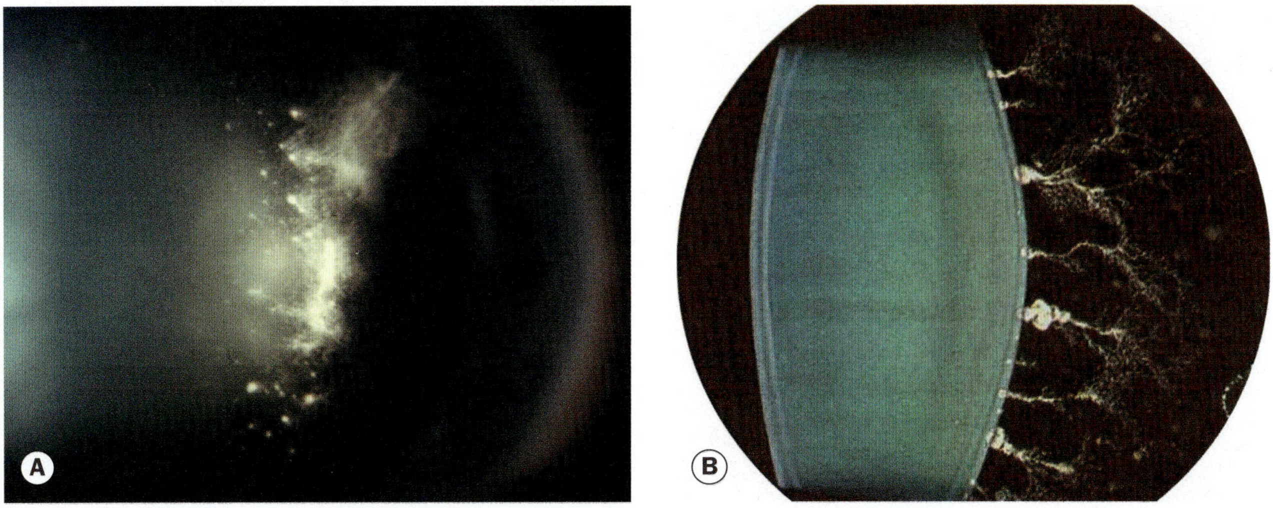

Fig. 17.5 Amyloidosis. **(A)** Vitreous deposits involving the anterior gel, showing a characteristic 'glass wool' appearance; **(B)** opacities attached to the posterior lens by thick footplates.

Amyloidosis

Amyloidosis is a localized or systemic condition in which there is extracellular deposition of fibrillary protein. Vitreous involvement typically occurs in familial amyloidosis, also characterized by polyneuropathy, prominent corneal nerves and pupillary light-near dissociation. Vitreous opacities may be unilateral or bilateral and are initially perivascular. Later they involve the anterior gel and take on a characteristic sheet-like ('glass wool') appearance (Fig. 17.5A). The opacities may become attached to the posterior lens by thick footplates (Fig. 17.5B). Dense opacification resulting in significant visual impairment may require vitrectomy.

Vitreous cyst

Vitreous cysts can be congenital or acquired, acquired cysts being caused by a range of pathology such as trauma and inflammation. Congenital cysts are pigmented or non-pigmented, the former usually arising from the ciliary body pigment epithelium, the latter from remnants of the primary hyaloid vascular system. They are generally fixed – non-pigmented cysts are typically attached to the optic disc – but can be found floating freely in the posterior (occasionally anterior) segment (Fig. 17.6). Treatment is seldom required, but laser cystotomy or vitrectomy can be performed for troublesome symptoms.

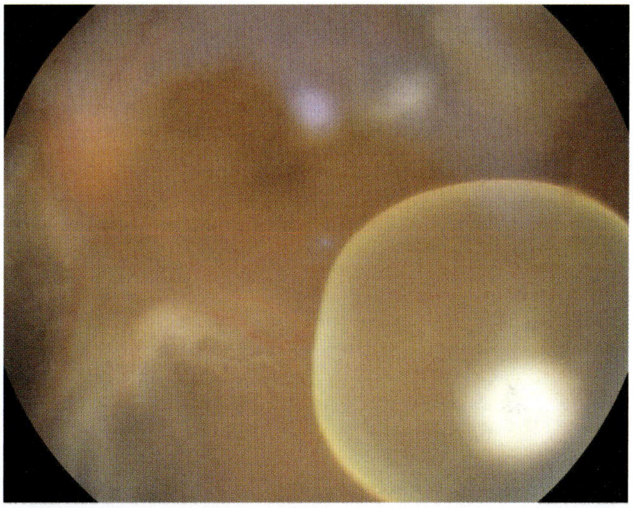

Fig. 17.6 Vitreous cyst.

Persistent fetal vasculature

In addition to non-pigmented vitreous cysts, remnants of the hyaloid vessels can form a Bergmeister papilla, seen as a tuft at the optic disc (Fig. 17.7), a Mittendorf dot on the posterior lens surface and the more marked manifestations for which the term persistent fetal vasculature is generally reserved, previously

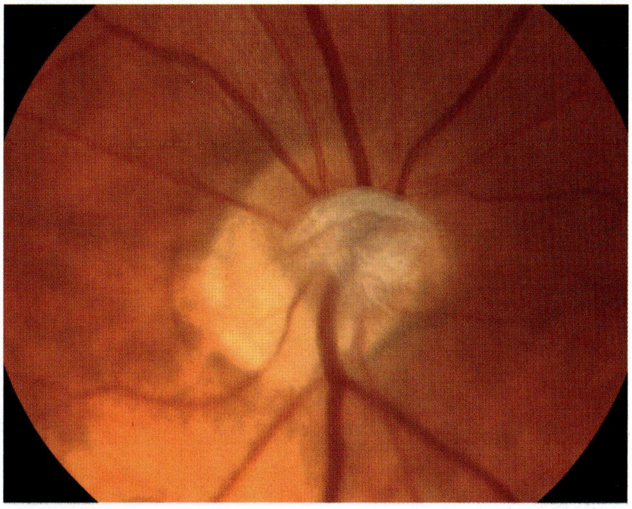

Fig. 17.7 Bergmeister papilla.

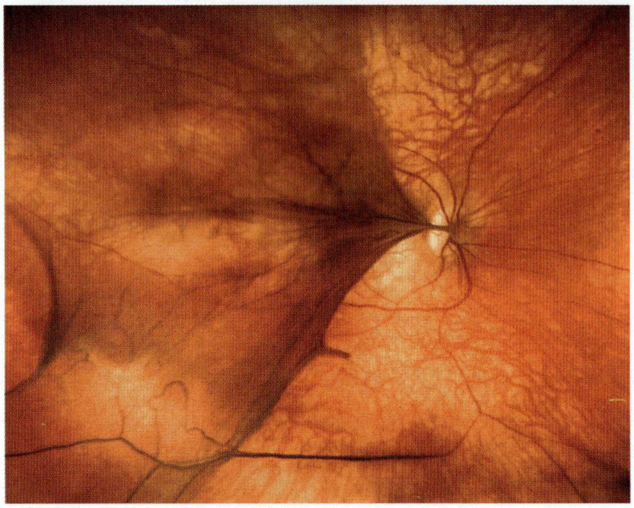

Fig. 17.8 Congenital vitreous veil.

termed persistent hyperplastic primary vitreous (see Ch. 20). A congenital vitreous veil is a translucent, curtain-like structure found in normal vitreous, which may be vascularized (Fig. 17.8). It is extremely rare and is of unknown aetiology. Treatment is not needed.

Chapter

Strabismus 18

INTRODUCTION

Definitions

- **The visual axis** passes from the fovea, through the nodal point of the eye, to the point of fixation. In normal binocular single vision (BSV) the visual axes of the two eyes intersect at the point of fixation, the images being aligned by the fusion reflex and combined by binocular responsive cells in the visual cortex to give BSV.
- **Orthophoria** implies perfect ocular alignment in the absence of any stimulus for fusion; this is uncommon.
- **Heterophoria** ('phoria') implies a tendency of the eyes to deviate when fusion is blocked (latent squint).
  - Slight phoria is present in most normal individuals and is overcome by the fusion reflex. The phoria can be either a small inward imbalance (esophoria) or an outward imbalance (exophoria).
  - When fusion is insufficient to control the imbalance, the phoria is described as decompensating and is often associated with symptoms of binocular discomfort (asthenopia) or double vision (diplopia).
- **Heterotropia** ('tropia') implies a manifest deviation in which the visual axes do not intersect at the point of fixation.
  - The images from the two eyes are misaligned so that either double vision is present or, more commonly in children, the image from the deviating eye is suppressed at cortical level.
  - A childhood squint may occur because of failure of the normal development of binocular fusion mechanisms or as a result of oculomotor imbalance secondary to a difference in refraction between the two eyes (anisometropia).
  - Failure of fusion, for example secondary to poor vision in one eye, may cause heterotropia in adulthood, or a squint may develop because of weakness or mechanical restriction of the extraocular muscles, or damage to their nerve supply.
  - Horizontal deviation of the eyes (latent or manifest) is the most common form of strabismus.
  - Upward displacement of one eye relative to the other is termed a *hypertropia* and a latent upward imbalance a *hyperphoria.*
  - Downward displacement is termed a *hypotropia* and a latent imbalance a *hypophoria.*
- **The anatomical axis** is a line passing from the posterior pole through the centre of the cornea. Because the fovea is usually slightly temporal to the anatomical centre of the posterior pole of the eye, the visual axis does not usually correspond to the anatomical axis of the eye.
- **Angle kappa** is the angle, usually about 5°, subtended by the visual and anatomical axes (Fig. 18.1).
  - The angle is positive (normal) when the fovea is temporal to the centre of the posterior pole resulting in a nasal displacement of the corneal reflex and negative when the converse applies.
  - A large angle kappa may give the appearance of a squint when none is present (pseudo-squint) and is seen most commonly as a pseudoexotropia following displacement of the macula in retinopathy of prematurity, where the angle may significantly exceed +5° (Fig. 18.1B–D).

Anatomy of the extraocular muscles

Principles

The lateral and medial orbital walls are at an angle of 45° with each other. The orbital axis therefore forms an angle of 22.5° with both lateral and medial walls, though for the sake of simplicity this angle is usually regarded as being 23° (Fig. 18.2A). When the eye is looking straight ahead at a fixed point on the horizon with the head erect (primary position of gaze), the visual axis forms an angle of 23° with the orbital axis (Fig. 18.2B). The actions of the extraocular muscles depend on the position of the globe at the time of muscle contraction (Fig. 18.2C and D).

- **The primary action** of a muscle is its major effect when the eye is in the primary position.
- **Subsidiary actions** are the additional effects, which depend on the position of the eye.
- **The Listing plane** is an imaginary coronal plane passing through the centre of rotation of the globe. The globe rotates on the axes of Fick, which intersect in the Listing plane (Fig. 18.3).
  - The globe rotates left and right on the vertical Z axis.
  - The globe moves up and down on the horizontal X axis.
  - Torsional movements (wheel rotations) occur on the Y (sagittal) axis which traverses the globe from front to back (similar to the anatomical axis of the eye).
  - Intorsion occurs when the superior limbus rotates nasally and extorsion on temporal rotation.
- **The anatomy** of the muscles is illustrated in Fig. 18.4A and B.

Horizontal recti

When the eye is in the primary position, the horizontal recti are purely horizontal movers on the vertical Z axis and have only primary actions.

- **Medial rectus** originates at the annulus of Zinn at the orbital apex and inserts 5.5 mm behind the nasal limbus. Its sole action in the primary position is adduction.
- **Lateral rectus** originates at the annulus of Zinn and inserts 6.9 mm behind the temporal limbus. Its sole action in the primary position is abduction.

Vertical recti

The vertical recti run in line with the orbital axis and are inserted in front of the equator. They therefore form an angle of 23° with the visual axis (see Fig. 18.2C).

- **Superior rectus** originates from the upper part of the annulus of Zinn and inserts 7.7 mm behind the superior limbus.
  - The primary action is elevation (Fig. 18.5A); secondary actions are adduction and intorsion.

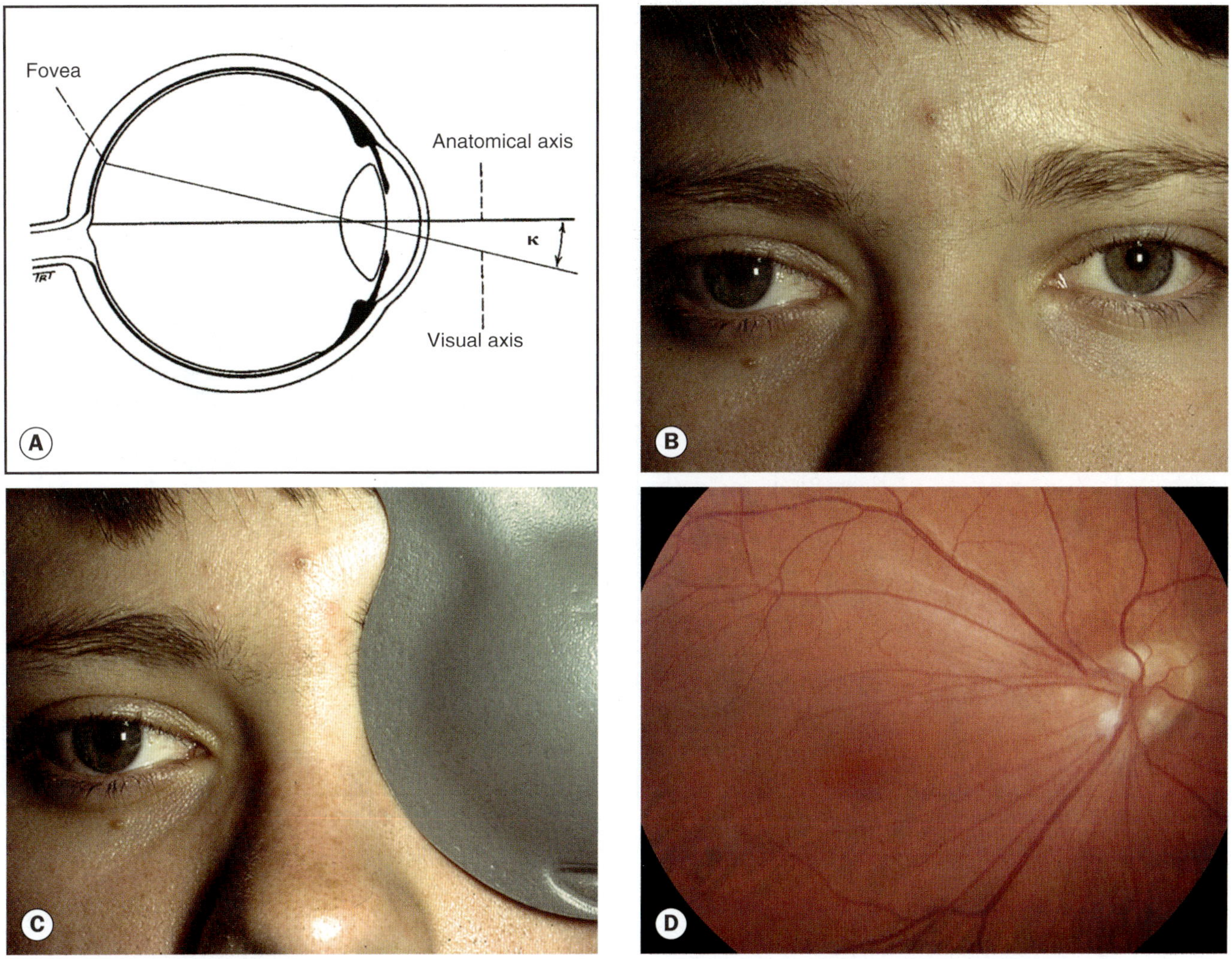

Fig. 18.1 Angle kappa. **(A)** The angle subtended by the visual and anatomical axis; **(B)** large positive angle kappa manifesting as a pseudo-exotropia; **(C)** no movement of the affected eye on occlusion of the opposite eye; **(D)** displacement of the fovea secondary to ROP in the same patient. *(Courtesy of ADN Murray.)*

- When the globe is abducted 23°, the visual and orbital axes coincide. In this position it has no subsidiary actions and can act only as an elevator (Fig. 18.5B). This is therefore the optimal position of the globe for testing the function of the superior rectus muscle.
- If the globe were adducted 67°, the angle between the visual and orbital axes would be 90°. In this position the superior rectus could act only to intort the eye (Fig. 18.5C).

- **Inferior rectus** originates at the lower part of the annulus of Zinn and inserts 6.5 mm behind the inferior limbus.
  - The primary action is depression; secondary actions are adduction and extorsion.
  - When the globe is abducted 23°, the inferior rectus acts purely as a depressor. As for superior rectus, this is the optimal position of the globe for testing the function of the inferior rectus muscle.
  - If the globe were adducted 67°, the inferior rectus could act to extort the eye.

Spiral of Tillaux

The spiral of Tillaux (Fig. 18.6) is an imaginary line joining the insertions of the four recti and is an important anatomical landmark when performing surgery. The insertions are located progressively further away from the limbus in a spiral pattern. The medial rectus insertion is closest (5.5 mm), followed by the inferior rectus (6.5 mm), lateral rectus (6.9 mm) and superior rectus (7.7 mm).

Oblique muscles

The obliques are inserted behind the equator and form an angle of 51° with the visual axis (see Fig. 18.2D).

- **Superior oblique** originates superomedial to the optic foramen. It passes forwards through the trochlea at the angle between the superior and medial walls and is then reflected

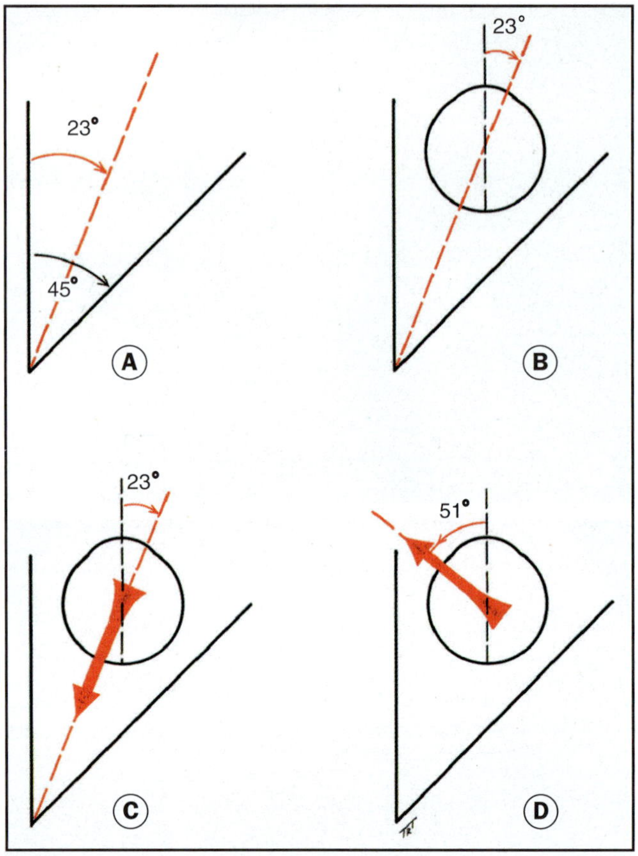

Fig. 18.2 Anatomy of the extraocular muscles (see text).

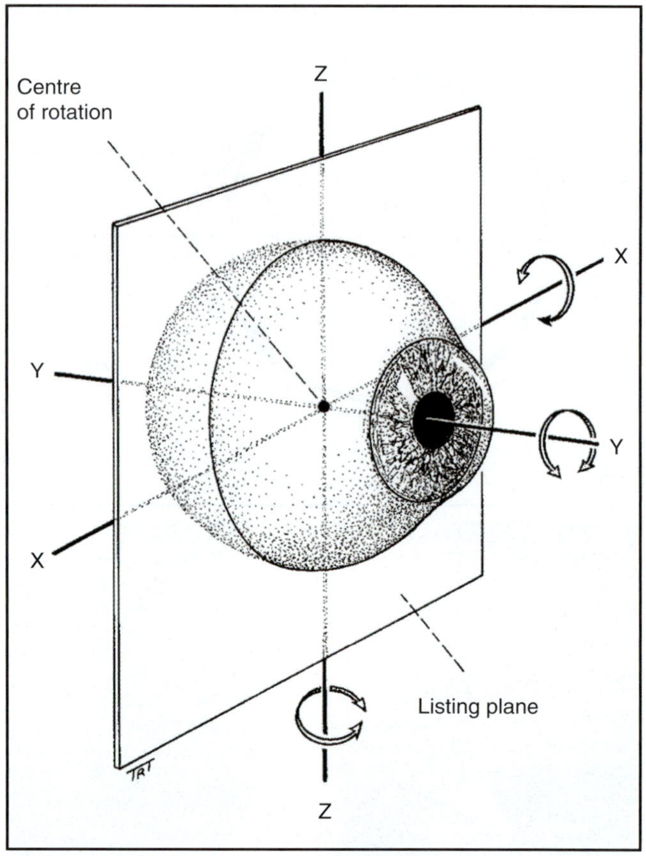

Fig. 18.3 The Listing plane and axes of Fick.

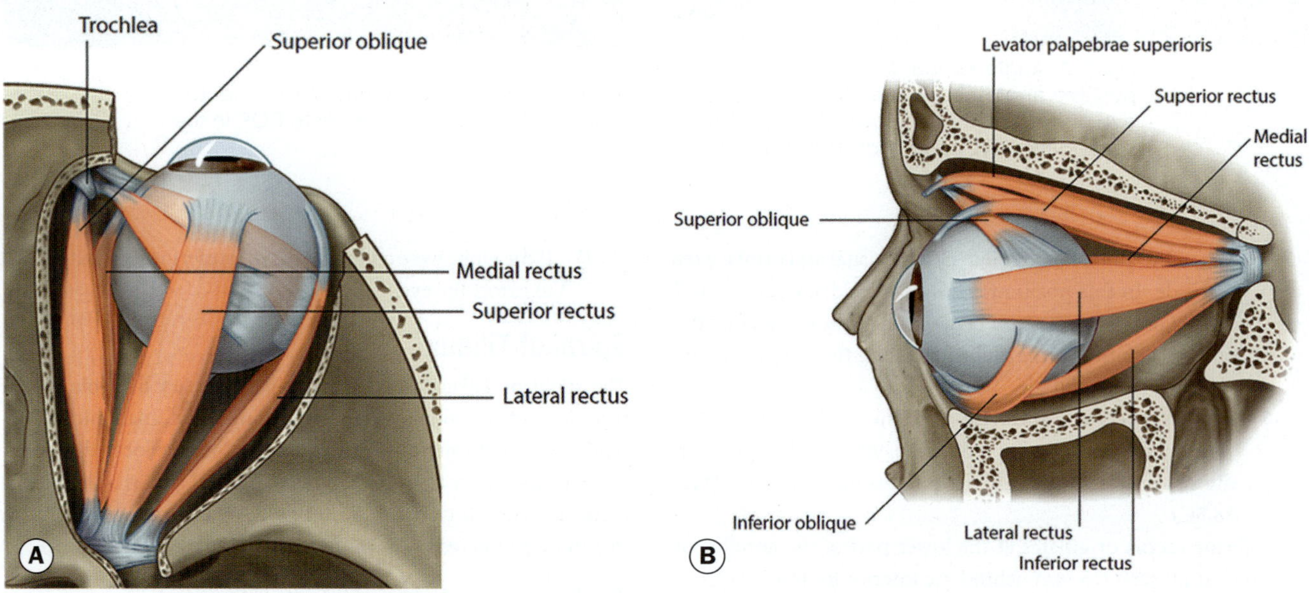

Fig. 18.4 Anatomy of the muscles of the eyeball. **(A)** Superior view; **(B)** lateral view.

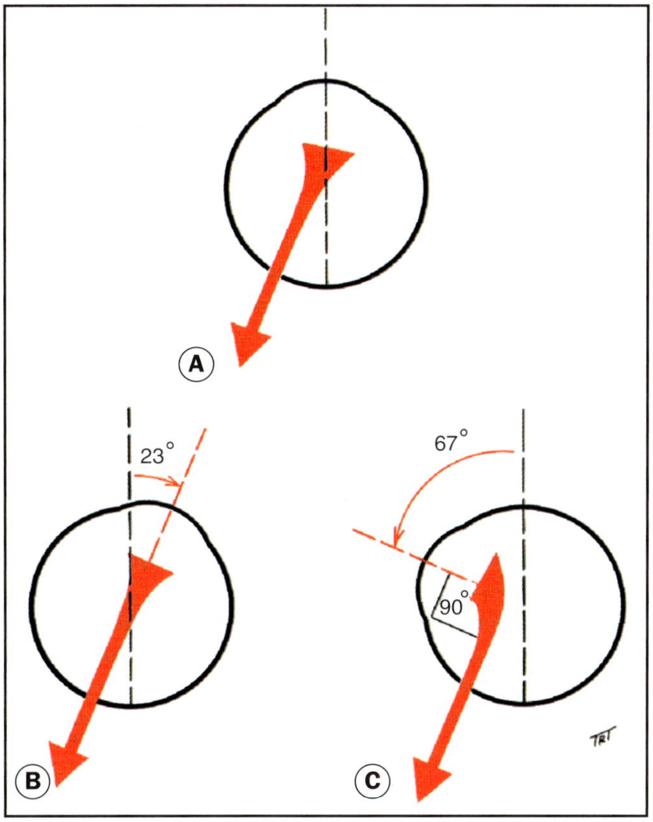

Fig. 18.5 Actions of the right superior rectus muscle (see text).

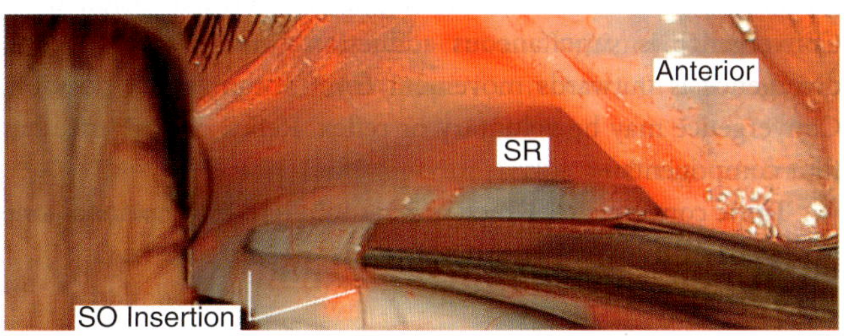

Fig. 18.7 Insertion of the superior oblique (SO) tendon; SR = superior rectus as viewed from the temporal aspect.

backwards and laterally to insert in the posterior upper temporal quadrant of the globe (Fig. 18.7).

- The primary action is intorsion (Fig. 18.8A); secondary actions are depression and abduction.
- The anterior fibres of the superior oblique tendon are primarily responsible for intorsion and the posterior fibres for depression, allowing separate surgical manipulation of these two actions (see below).
- When the globe is adducted 51°, the visual axis coincides with the line of pull of the muscle. In this position it can act only as a depressor (Fig. 18.8B). This is, therefore, the best position of the globe for testing the action of the superior oblique muscle. Thus, although the superior oblique has an abducting action in primary position, the main effect of superior oblique weakness is seen as failure of depression in adduction.

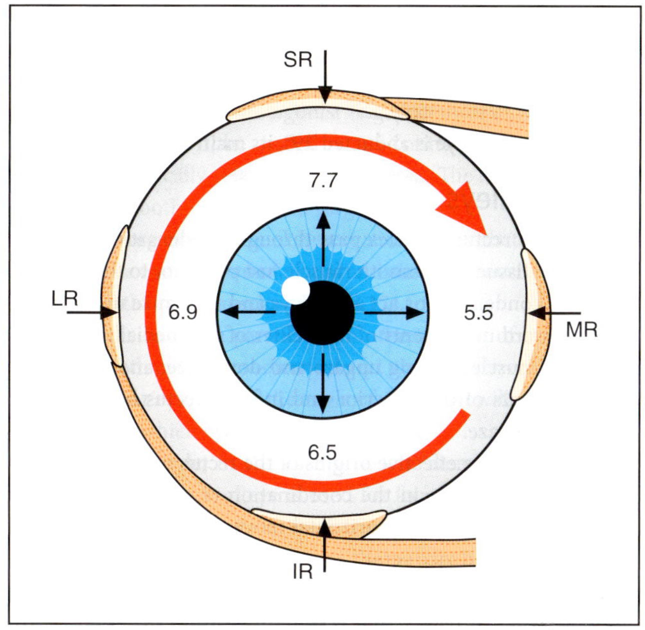

Fig. 18.6 Spiral of Tillaux. IR = inferior rectus; LR = lateral rectus; MR = medial rectus; SR = superior rectus.

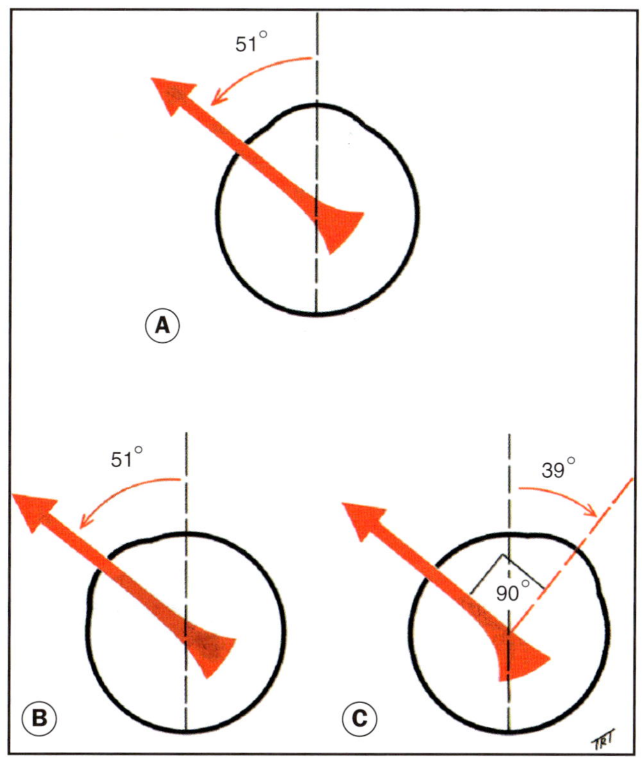

Fig. 18.8 Actions of the right superior oblique muscle (see text).

- When the eye is abducted 39°, the visual axis and the superior oblique make an angle of 90° with each other. In this position the superior oblique can cause only intorsion (Fig. 18.8C).

- **Inferior oblique** originates from a small depression just behind the orbital rim lateral to the lacrimal sac. It passes backwards and laterally to insert in the posterior lower temporal quadrant of the globe close to the macula.

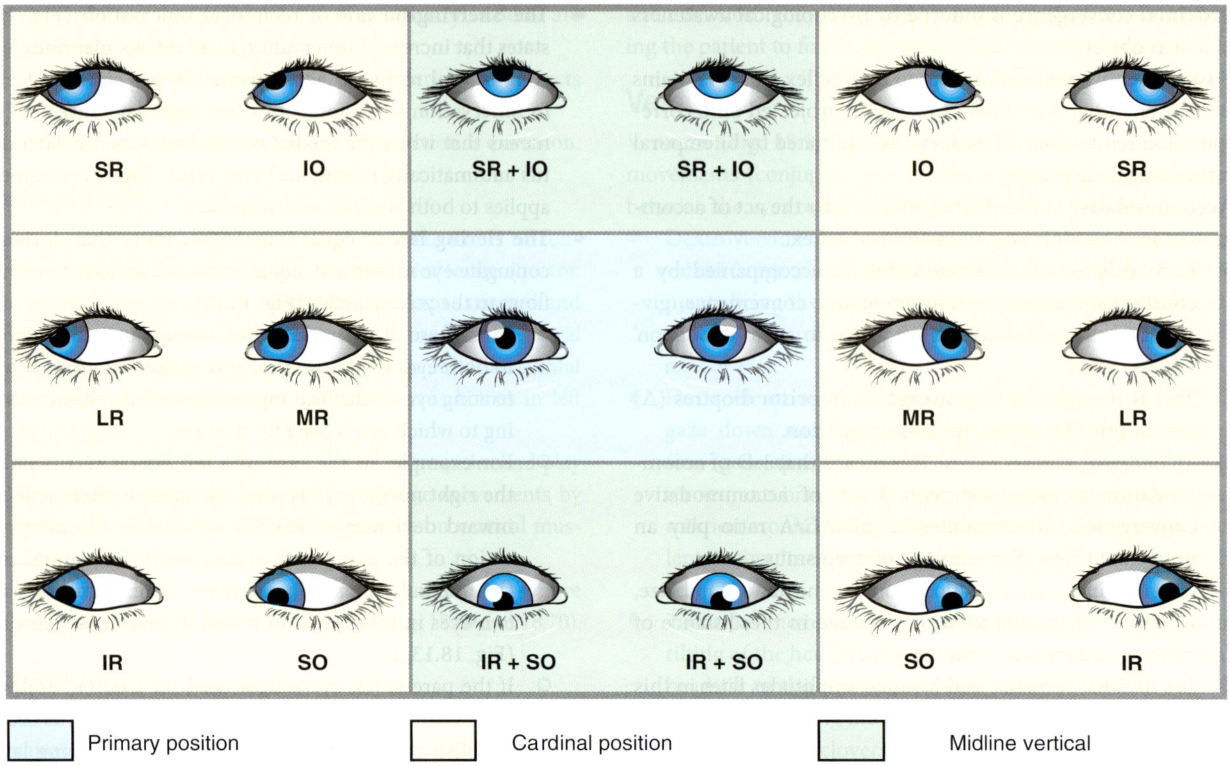

Fig. 18.10 Diagnostic positions of gaze. IO = inferior oblique; IR = inferior rectus; LR = lateral rectus; MR = medial rectus; SO = superior oblique; SR = superior rectus.

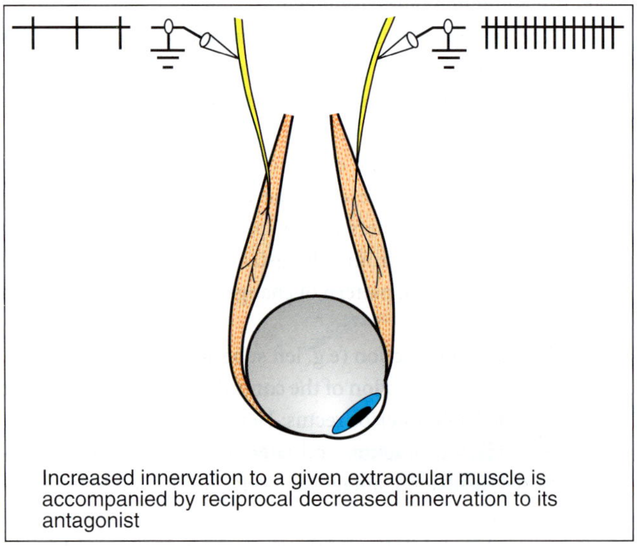

Fig. 18.11 Sherrington law of reciprocal innervation.

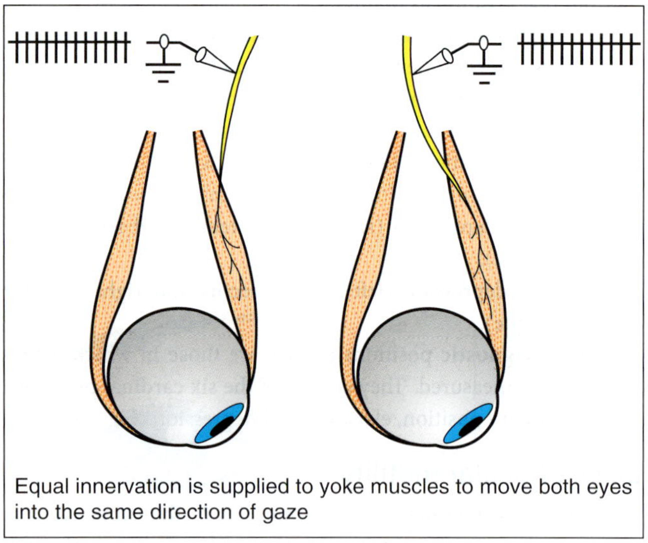

Fig. 18.12 Hering law of equal innervation of yoke muscles.

- Normal routing of visual pathways with overlapping visual fields.
- Binocularly driven neurones in the visual cortex.
- Normal retinal (retinocortical) correspondence (NRC) resulting in 'cyclopean' viewing.
- Accurate neuromuscular development and coordination, so that the visual axes are directed at, and maintain fixation on, the object of regard.
- Approximately equal image clarity and size for both eyes.
- BSV is based on NRC, which requires first an understanding of uniocular visual direction and projection.

- **Visual direction** is the projection of a given retinal element in a specific direction in subjective space.
  - The principal visual direction is the direction in external space interpreted as the line of sight. This is normally the visual direction of the fovea and is associated with a sense of direct viewing.

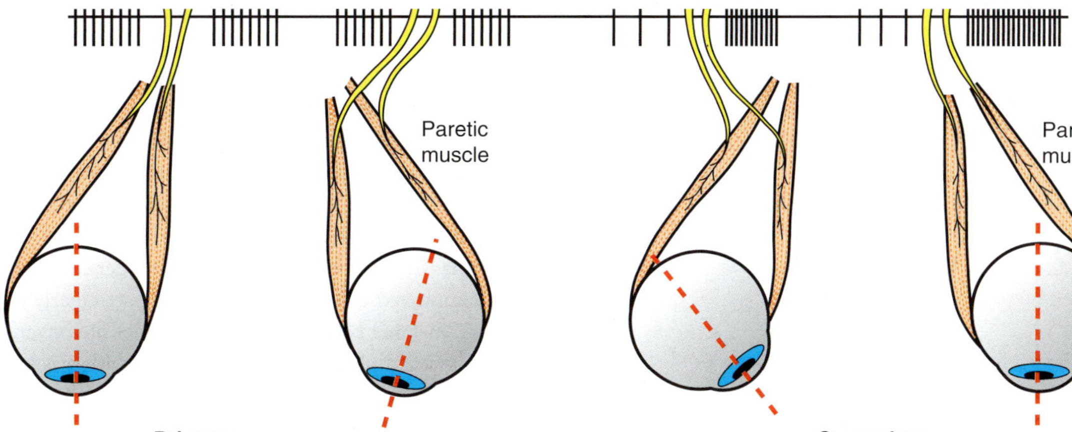

Fig. 18.13 Primary and secondary deviations in paretic strabismus.

- Secondary visual directions are the projecting directions of extrafoveal points with respect to the principal direction of the fovea, associated with indirect (eccentric) viewing.

- **Projection** is the subjective interpretation of the position of an object in space on the basis of stimulated retinal elements.
  - If a red object stimulates the right fovea (F) and a black object that lies in the nasal field stimulates a temporal retinal element (T), the red object will be interpreted by the brain as having originated from the straight-ahead position and the black object will be interpreted as having originated in the nasal field (Fig. 18.14A). Similarly, nasal retinal elements project into the temporal field, upper retinal elements into the lower field and vice versa.
  - With both eyes open, the red fixation object is now stimulating both foveae, which are corresponding retinal points. The black object is now not only stimulating the temporal retinal elements in the right eye but also the nasal elements of the left eye. The right eye therefore projects the object into its nasal field and the left eye projects the object into its temporal field.
  - Because both of these retinal elements are corresponding points, they will both project the object into the same position in space (the left side) and there will be no double vision.
- **Retinomotor values**
  - The image of an object in the peripheral visual field falls on an extrafoveal element. To establish fixation on this object a saccadic version of accurate amplitude is required.
  - Each extrafoveal retinal element therefore has a retinomotor value proportional to its distance from the fovea, which guides the amplitude of saccadic movements required to 'look at it'.
  - Retinomotor value, zero at the fovea, increases progressively towards the retinal periphery.
- **Corresponding points** are areas on each retina that share the same subjective visual direction (for example, the foveae share the primary visual direction).
  - Points on the nasal retina of one eye have corresponding points on the temporal retina of the other eye and vice versa. For example, an object producing images on the right nasal retina and the left temporal retina will be projected into the right side of visual space. This is the basis of normal retinal correspondence.
  - This retinotopic organization is reflected back along the visual pathways, each eye maintaining separate images until the visual pathways converge onto binocularly responsive neurones in the primary visual cortex.
- **The horopter** is an imaginary plane in external space, relative to both the observer's eyes for a given fixation target, all points on which stimulate corresponding retinal elements and are therefore seen singly and in the same plane (Fig. 18.14B). This plane passes through the intersection of the visual axes and therefore includes the point of fixation in BSV.
- **The Panum fusional space** (or volume) is a zone in front of and behind the horopter in which objects stimulate slightly non-corresponding retinal points (retinal disparity).
  - Objects within the limits of the fusional space are seen singly and the disparity information is used to produce a perception of binocular depth (stereopsis). Objects in front of and behind the Panum space appear double.
  - This is the basis of physiological diplopia. The Panum space is shallow at fixation (6 seconds of arc) and deeper towards the periphery (30–40 seconds of arc at 15° from the fovea).
  - The retinal areas stimulated by images falling within the Panum fusional space are termed Panum fusional areas.
  - Therefore, objects on the horopter are seen singly and in one plane. Objects in Panum fusional areas are seen singly and stereoscopically. Objects outside Panum fusional areas appear double.
  - Physiological diplopia is usually accompanied by physiological suppression.
- **BSV** is characterized by the ability to fuse the images from the two eyes and to perceive binocular depth:

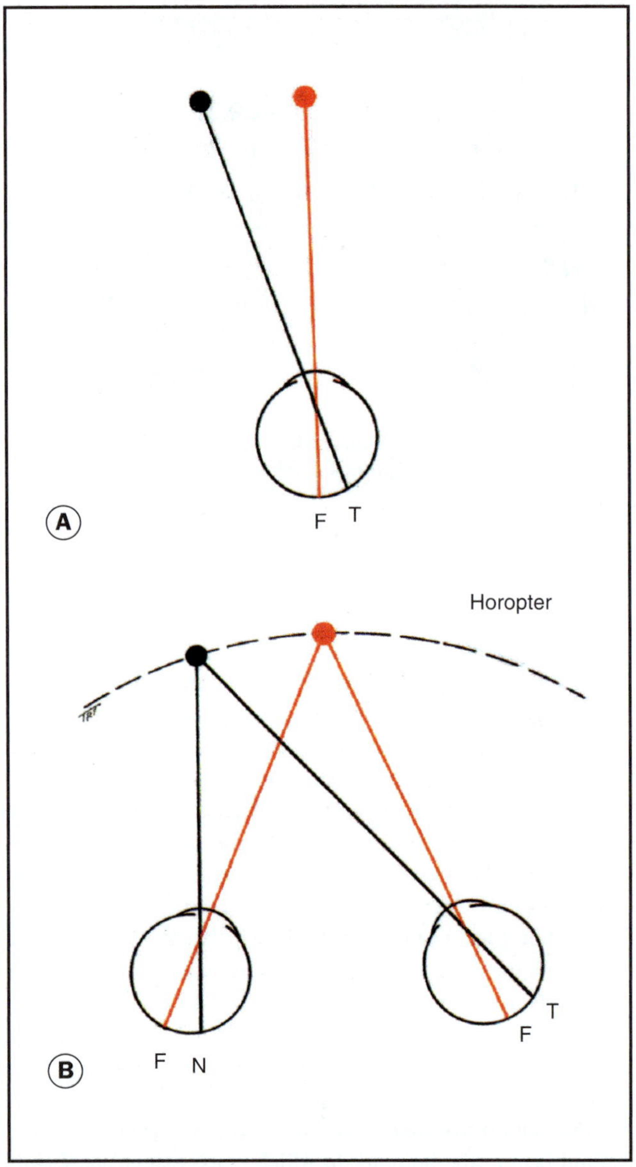

Fig. 18.14 Principles of projection. F = fovea; N = nasal retinal element; T = temporal retinal element. **(A)** When a red object stimulates the right fovea and a black object, which lies in the nasal field, stimulates the temporal retina, the red object will be interpreted by the brain as having originated from the straight-ahead position and the black object will be interpreted as having originated in the nasal field; **(B)** the horopter is an imaginary plane in external space. All points on the horopter stimulate corresponding retinal elements and are therefore seen singly and in the same plane.

- Sensory fusion involves the integration by the visual areas of the cerebral cortex of two similar images, one from each eye, into one image. It may be central, which integrates the image falling on the foveae, or peripheral, which integrates parts of the image falling outside the foveae. It is possible to maintain fusion with a central visual deficit in one eye, but peripheral fusion is essential to BSV and may be affected in patients with advanced field changes in glaucoma and pituitary lesions.
- Motor fusion involves the maintenance of motor alignment of the eyes to sustain bifoveal fixation. It is driven by retinal image disparity, which stimulates fusional vergences.

- **Fusional vergence** involves disjugate eye movements to overcome retinal image disparity. Fusional convergence helps to control an exophoria whereas fusional divergence helps to control an esophoria. The fusional vergence mechanism may be decreased by fatigue or illness, converting a phoria to a tropia. The amplitude of fusional vergence mechanisms can be improved by orthoptic exercises, particularly in the case of near fusional convergence for the relief of convergence insufficiency. Amplitudes can be measured with prisms or a synoptophore. Normal values are:
  - Convergence: about 15–20 Δ for distance and 25 Δ for near.
  - Divergence: about 6–10 Δ for distance and 12–14 Δ for near.
  - Vertical: 2–3 Δ.
  - Cyclovergence: about 8°.
- **Stereopsis** is the perception of depth. It arises when objects behind and in front of the point of fixation (but within Panum fusional space) stimulate horizontally disparate retinal elements simultaneously. The fusion of these disparate images results in a single visual impression perceived in depth. A solid object is seen stereoscopically (in three dimensions) because each eye sees a slightly different aspect of the object.
- **Sensory perceptions.** At the onset of a squint two sensory perceptions arise based on the normal projection of the retinal areas stimulated; confusion and pathological diplopia may result. These require simultaneous visual perception, that is, the ability to perceive images from both eyes simultaneously. Young children readily suppress diplopia but it is persistent and usually troublesome with strabismus in older children and adults, when it arises after the sensitive period for binocularity (see below).
  - Confusion is the simultaneous appreciation of two superimposed but dissimilar images caused by stimulation of corresponding retinal points (usually the foveae) by images of different objects (Fig. 18.15).
  - Pathological diplopia is the simultaneous appreciation of two images of the same object in different positions and results from images of the same object falling on non-corresponding retinal points. In esotropia the diplopia is homonymous (uncrossed – Fig. 18.16A), in exotropia the diplopia is heteronymous (crossed – Fig. 18.16B).

Sensory adaptations to strabismus

The ocular sensory system in children has the ability to adapt to anomalous states (confusion and diplopia) by two mechanisms: suppression and abnormal retinal correspondence (ARC). These occur because of the plasticity of the developing visual system in children under the age of 6–8 years. Occasional adults who develop sudden-onset strabismus are able to ignore the second image after a time and therefore do not complain of diplopia.

- **Suppression** involves active inhibition by the visual cortex of the image from one eye when both eyes are open. Stimuli for suppression include diplopia, confusion and a blurred image

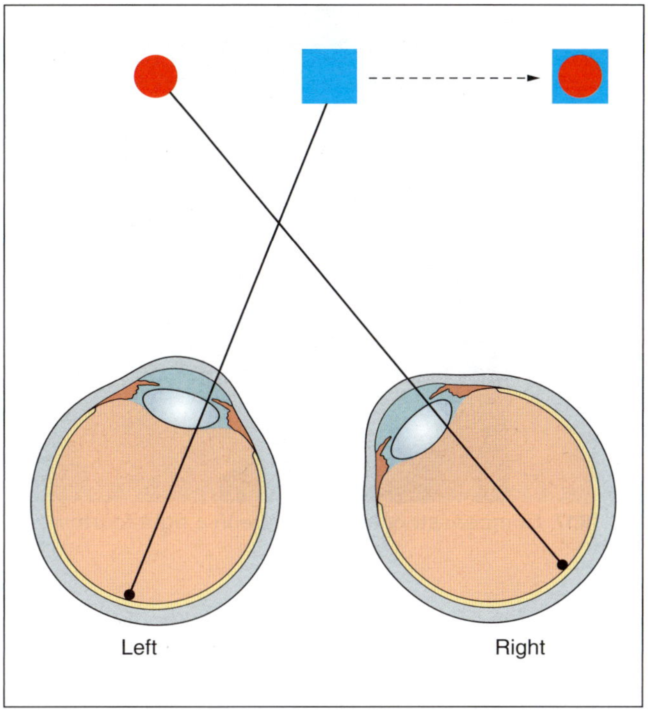

Fig. 18.15 Confusion.

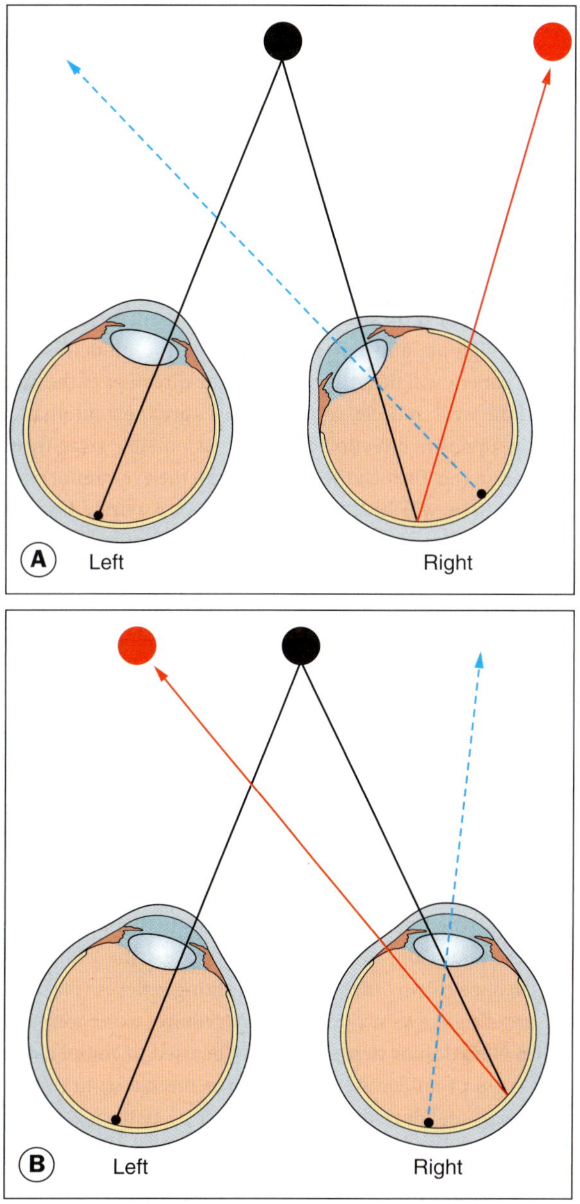

Fig. 18.16 Diplopia. **(A)** Homonymous (uncrossed) diplopia in right esotropia with normal retinal correspondence; **(B)** heteronymous (crossed) diplopia in right exotropia with normal retinal correspondence.

from one eye resulting from astigmatism/anisometropia. Clinically, suppression may be:

- Central or peripheral. In central suppression the image from the fovea of the deviating eye is inhibited to avoid confusion. Diplopia, on the other hand, is eradicated by the process of peripheral suppression, in which the image from the peripheral retina of the deviating eye is inhibited.
- Monocular or alternating. Suppression is monocular when the image from the dominant eye always predominates over the image from the deviating (or more ametropic) eye, so that the image from the latter is constantly suppressed. This type of suppression leads to amblyopia. When suppression alternates (switches from one eye to the other), amblyopia is less likely to develop.
- Facultative or obligatory. Facultative suppression occurs only when the eyes are misaligned. Obligatory suppression is present at all times, irrespective of whether the eyes are deviated or straight. Examples of facultative suppression include intermittent exotropia and Duane syndrome.

- **Abnormal (anomalous) retinal correspondence (ARC)** is a condition in which non-corresponding retinal elements acquire a common subjective visual direction, i.e. fusion occurs in the presence of a small-angle manifest squint; the fovea of the fixating eye is paired with a non-foveal element of the deviated eye. Binocular responses in ARC are never as good as in normal bifoveal BSV. It represents a positive sensory adaptation to strabismus (as opposed to negative adaptation by suppression), which allows some anomalous binocular vision in the presence of a heterotropia. It is most frequently encountered in small-angle esotropia (microtropia), but is less common in accommodative esotropia because of the variability of the angle of deviation and in large-angle deviations because the separation of the images is too great.
- **Microtropia** is discussed further later in this chapter (see Fig. 18.28)
- **Consequences of strabismus**
  - The fovea of the squinting eye is suppressed to avoid confusion.
  - Diplopia will occur, since corresponding retinal elements receive different images.
  - To avoid diplopia, the patient will develop either peripheral suppression of the squinting eye or ARC.
  - If constant unilateral suppression occurs this will subsequently lead to strabismic amblyopia.

Motor adaptation to strabismus

Motor adaptation involves the adoption of a compensatory head posture (CHP) and occurs primarily in children with congenitally abnormal eye movements who use the CHP to maintain BSV. In these children loss of a CHP may indicate loss of binocular function and the need for surgical intervention. These patients may present in adult life with symptoms of decompensation, often unaware of their CHP. Acquired paretic strabismus in adults may be consciously controlled by a CHP provided the deviation is neither too large nor too variable with gaze (incomitance). The CHP eliminates diplopia and helps to centralize the binocular visual field. The patient will turn the head into the direction of the field of action of the weak muscle, so that the eyes are then automatically turned the opposite direction and as far as possible away from its field of action (i.e. the head will turn where the eye cannot).

- **A face turn** will be adopted to control a purely horizontal deviation. For example, if the left lateral rectus is paralysed, diplopia will occur in left gaze. The face will be turned to the left, which deviates the eyes to the right, away from the field of action of the weak muscle and area of diplopia. A face turn may also be adopted in a paresis of a vertically acting muscle to avoid the side where the vertical deviation is greatest (e.g. in a right superior oblique weakness the face is turned to the left).
- **A head tilt** is adopted to compensate for torsional and/or vertical diplopia. In a right superior oblique weakness, the right eye is relatively elevated and the head is tilted to the left (Fig. 18.17), towards the hypotropic eye. This reduces the vertical separation of the diplopic images and permits fusion to be regained. If there is a significant torsional component preventing fusion, tilting the head in the same left direction will reduce this by invoking the righting reflexes (placing the extorted right eye in a position that requires extorsion).
- **Chin elevation or depression** may be used to compensate for weakness of an elevator or depressor muscle or to minimize the horizontal deviation when an 'A' or 'V' pattern is present.

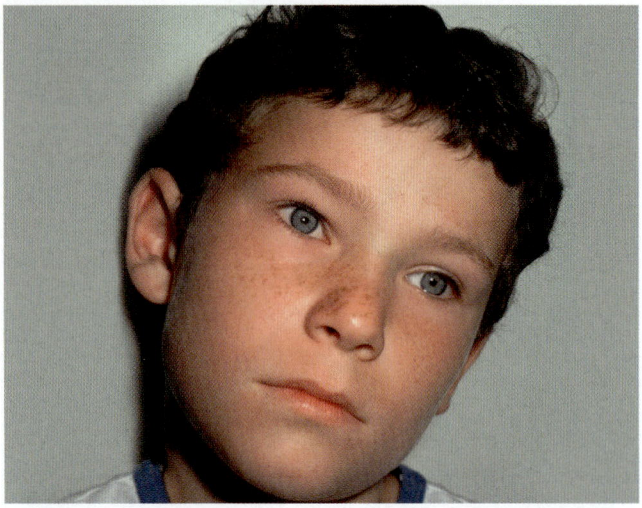

Fig. 18.17 Compensatory head posture in a right fourth nerve palsy.

AMBLYOPIA

Classification

Amblyopia is the unilateral, or rarely bilateral, decrease in best-corrected visual acuity (VA) caused by form vision deprivation and/or abnormal binocular interaction, for which there is no identifiable pathology of the eye or visual pathway.

- **Strabismic** amblyopia results from abnormal binocular interaction where there is continued monocular suppression of the deviating eye.
- **Anisometropic** amblyopia is caused by a difference in refractive error between the eyes and may result from a difference of as little as 1 dioptre. The more ametropic eye receives a blurred image, in a mild form of visual deprivation. It is frequently associated with microstrabismus and may co-exist with strabismic amblyopia.
- **Stimulus deprivation** amblyopia results from vision deprivation. It may be unilateral or bilateral and is typically caused by opacities in the media (e.g. cataract) or ptosis that covers the pupil.
- **Bilateral ametropic** amblyopia results from high symmetrical refractive errors, usually hypermetropia.
- **Meridional** amblyopia results from image blur in one meridian. It can be unilateral or bilateral and is caused by uncorrected astigmatism (usually >1 D) persisting beyond the period of emmetropization in early childhood.

Diagnosis

In the absence of an organic lesion, a difference in best-corrected VA of two Snellen lines or more (or >1 log unit) is indicative of amblyopia. VA in amblyopia is usually better when reading single letters than letters in a row. This 'crowding' phenomenon occurs to a certain extent in normal individuals but is more marked in amblyopes and must be taken into account when testing preverbal children.

Treatment

It is essential to examine the fundi to diagnose any visible organic disease prior to commencing treatment for amblyopia. Organic disease and amblyopia may co-exist and a trial of patching may still be indicated in the presence of organic disease. If acuity does not respond to treatment, investigations such as electrophysiology or imaging should be reconsidered. The sensitive period during which acuity of an amblyopic eye can be improved is usually up to 7–8 years in strabismic amblyopia and may be longer (into the teens) for anisometropic amblyopia where good binocular function is present.

- **Occlusion** of the normal eye, to encourage use of the amblyopic eye, is the most effective treatment. The regimen, full-time or part-time, depends on the age of the patient and the density of amblyopia.
  - The younger the patient, the more rapid the likely improvement but the greater the risk of inducing amblyopia in the normal eye. It is therefore very important to monitor VA regularly in both eyes during treatment.

- The better the VA at the start of occlusion, the shorter the duration required, although there is wide variation between patients.
- If there has been no improvement after 6 months of effective occlusion, further treatment is unlikely to be fruitful.
- Poor compliance is the single greatest barrier to improvement and must be monitored. Amblyopia treatment benefits from time spent at the outset on communication of the rationale and the difficulties involved.

- **Penalization**, in which vision in the normal eye is blurred with atropine, is an alternative method. It may work best in the treatment of mild–moderate amblyopia (6/24 or better), especially when due to anisometropic hypermetropia. Patch occlusion is likely to produce a quicker response than atropine, which has conventionally been reserved for use when compliance with patch occlusion is poor. Penalization offers the particular advantage of being difficult to thwart even if the child objects. It also creates less of a psychosocial problem than patching, especially in the school-going child. Weekend instillation may be adequate.

TIP Organic disease needs to be excluded before commencing treatment for amblyopia.

CLINICAL EVALUATION

History

- **Age of onset**
  - The earlier the onset, the more likely the need for surgical correction.
  - The later the onset, the greater the likelihood of an accommodative component (mostly arising between 18 and 36 months).
  - The longer the duration of squint in early childhood the greater the risk of amblyopia, unless fixation is freely alternating. Inspection of previous photographs may be useful for the documentation of strabismus or CHP.
- **Symptoms** may indicate decompensation of a pre-existent heterophoria or more significantly a recently acquired (usually paretic) condition. In the former, the patient usually complains of discomfort, blurring and possibly diplopia of indeterminate onset and duration in comparison to the acquired condition with the sudden onset of diplopia.
  - The type of diplopia (horizontal, cyclovertical) should be established, together with the direction of gaze in which it predominates and whether any BSV is retained.
  - In adults it is very important to determine exactly what problems the squint is causing as a basis for decisions about treatment.
  - It is not unusual for patients to present with spurious symptoms that mask embarrassment over a psychosocially noticeable squint.
- **Variability** is significant because intermittent strabismus indicates some degree of binocularity. An equally alternating deviation suggests symmetrical VA in both eyes.
- **General health** or developmental problems may be significant (e.g. children with cerebral palsy have an increased incidence of strabismus). In older patients, poor health and stress may cause decompensation and in acquired paresis patients may report associations or causal factors (trauma, neurological disease, diabetes etc.).
- **Birth history**, including period of gestation, birth weight and any problems *in utero*, with delivery or in the neonatal period.
- **Family history** is important because strabismus is frequently familial, although no definitive inheritance pattern is recognized. It is also important to know what therapy was necessary in other family members.
- **Previous ocular history** including refractive prescription and compliance with spectacles or occlusion, previous surgery or prisms is important to future treatment options and prognosis.

TIP In children, the later the onset of esotropia, the greater the likelihood of an accommodative component to the deviation.

Visual acuity

Testing in preverbal children

The evaluation can be separated into the qualitative assessment of visual behaviour and the quantitative assessment of VA using preferential looking tests. Assessment of visual behaviour is achieved as follows:

- **Fixation and following** may be assessed using bright attention-grabbing targets (a face is often best). This method indicates whether the infant is visually alert and is of particular value in a child suspected of being blind.
- **Comparison** between the behaviour of the two eyes may reveal a unilateral preference. Occlusion of one eye, if strongly objected to by the child, indicates poorer acuity in the other eye. However, it is possible to have good visual attention with each eye but unequal VA and all risk factors for amblyopia must be considered in the interpretation of results.
- **Fixation behaviour** can be used to establish unilateral preference if a manifest squint is present.
  - Fixation is promoted in the squinting eye by occluding the dominant eye while the child fixates a target of interest (preferably incorporating a light).
  - Fixation is then graded as *central* or *non-central* and *steady* or *unsteady* (the corneal reflection can be observed).
  - The other eye is then uncovered and the ability to *maintain* fixation is observed.
  - If fixation immediately returns to the uncovered eye, then VA is probably impaired.
  - If fixation is maintained through a blink, then VA is probably good.

  - If the patient alternates fixation, then the two eyes probably have equal vision.
- **The 10 Δ test** is similar and can be used regardless of whether a manifest squint is present. It involves the promotion of diplopia using a 10 Δ vertical prism. Alternation between the diplopic targets suggests equal VA.
- **Rotation test** is a gross qualitative test of the ability of an infant to fixate with both eyes open. The test is performed as follows:
  - The examiner holds the child facing him or her and rotates briskly through 360°.
  - If vision is normal, the eyes will deviate in the direction of rotation under the influence of the vestibulo-ocular response. The eyes flick back to the primary position to produce a rotational nystagmus.
  - When rotation stops, nystagmus is briefly observed in the opposite direction for 1–2 seconds and should then cease due to suppression of post-rotary nystagmus by fixation.
  - If vision is severely impaired, the post-rotation nystagmus does not stop as quickly when rotation ceases because the vestibulo-ocular response is not blocked by visual feedback.
- **Preferential looking** tests can be used from early infancy and are based on the fact that infants prefer to look at a pattern rather than a homogeneous stimulus. The infant is exposed to a stimulus and the examiner observes the eyes for fixation movements, without themselves knowing the stimulus position.
  - Tests in common use include the Teller and Keeler acuity cards, which consist of black stripes (gratings) of varying widths and Cardiff acuity cards (Fig. 18.18), which consist of familiar pictures with variable outline width.
  - Low-frequency (coarse) gratings or pictures with a wider outline are seen more easily than high-frequency gratings or thin outline pictures and an assessment of resolution (not recognition) VA is made accordingly.
  - Since grating acuity often exceeds Snellen acuity in amblyopia, Teller cards may overestimate VA. These methods may not be reliable if a proper forced-choice staircase protocol is not followed during testing and neither method has high sensitivity to the presence of amblyopia. The results must be considered in combination with risk factors for amblyopia.
- **Pattern visual evoked potentials** (VEP) give a representation of spatial acuity but are more commonly used in the diagnosis of optic neuropathy.

Testing in verbal children

The tests described below should be performed at 3–4 metres from the target, as it is easier to obtain compliance than at 6 metres, with little or no clinical detriment. It is important to note that amblyopia can only be accurately diagnosed using a crowded test requiring target recognition and that logMAR tests (logarithm of the minimal angle of resolution – see Ch. 1) provide the best measure against which improvement with amblyopia therapy can be assessed. These are readily available in formats suited to normal children from 2 years onwards.

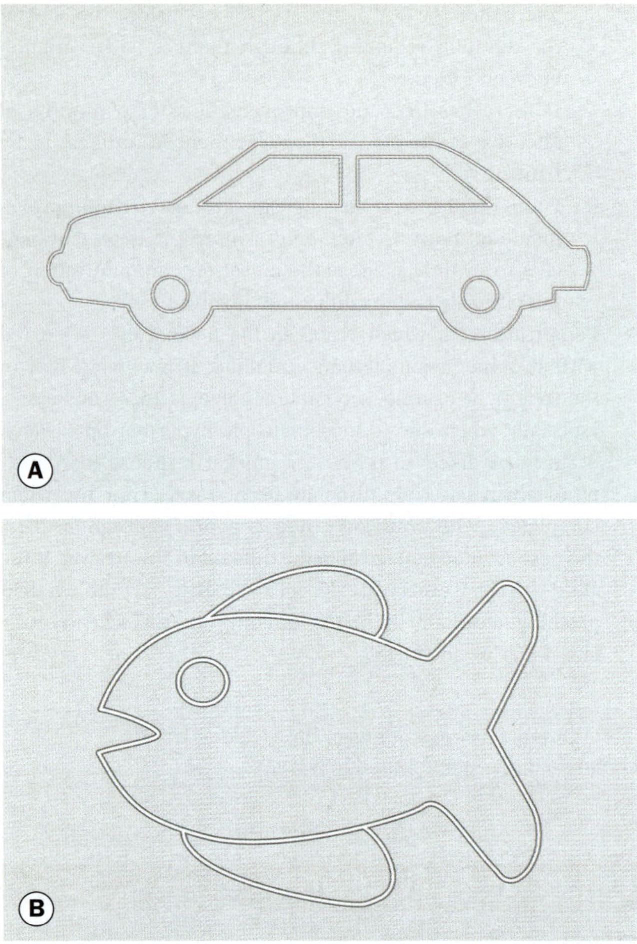

Fig. 18.18 Cardiff acuity cards, shown at a distance of 100 cm. **(A)** Car with thin outline (6/7.5); **(B)** fish with thick outline (6/15).

- **At age 2 years** most children will have sufficient language skills to undertake a picture naming test such as the crowded Kay pictures (Fig. 18.19A).
- **At age 3 years** most children will be able to undertake the matching of letter optotypes as in the Keeler logMAR (Fig. 18.19B), Sonksen or Otago crowded tests. If a crowded letter test proves too difficult it is preferable to perform the crowded Kay pictures than to use single optotype letters.
- **Older children** may continue with the crowded letter tests, naming or matching them. LogMAR tests are in common usage and are preferable to Snellen for all children at risk of amblyopia.

Tests for stereopsis

Stereopsis is measured in seconds of arc (1° = 60 minutes of arc; 1 minute = 60 seconds); the lower the value the better the stereoacuity. It is useful to remember that normal spatial resolution (VA) is 1 minute and normal stereoacuity is 60 seconds (also 1 minute, but conventionally expressed in seconds). Various tests, using differing principles, are employed to assess the stereoacuity. Random dot tests (e.g. TNO, Frisby) provide the most definitive evidence of high-grade BSV. Where this is weak and/or based on ARC (see above), contour-based tests (e.g. Titmus) may provide more reliable information.

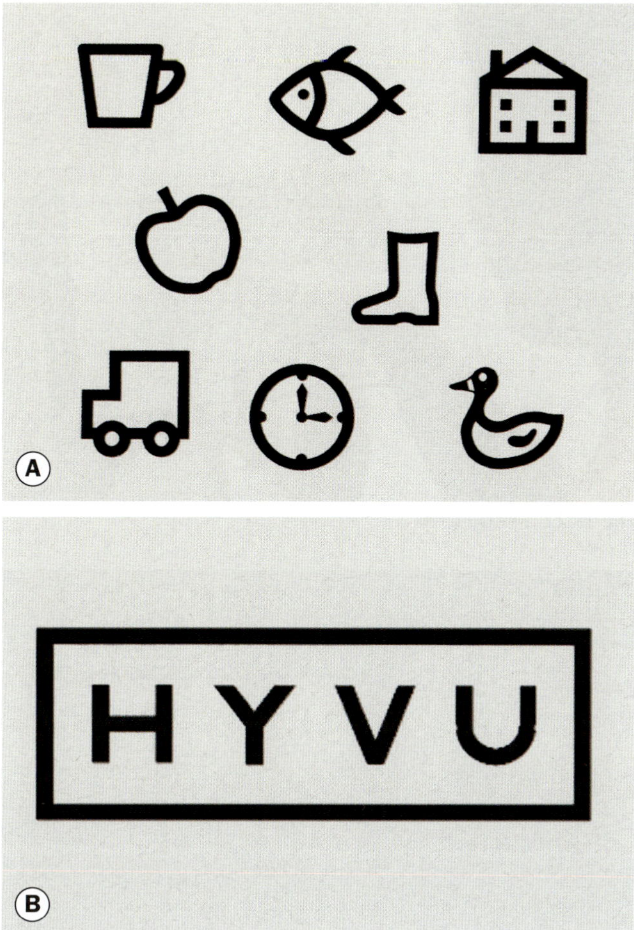

Fig. 18.19 **(A)** Kay pictures; **(B)** Keeler logMAR crowded test.

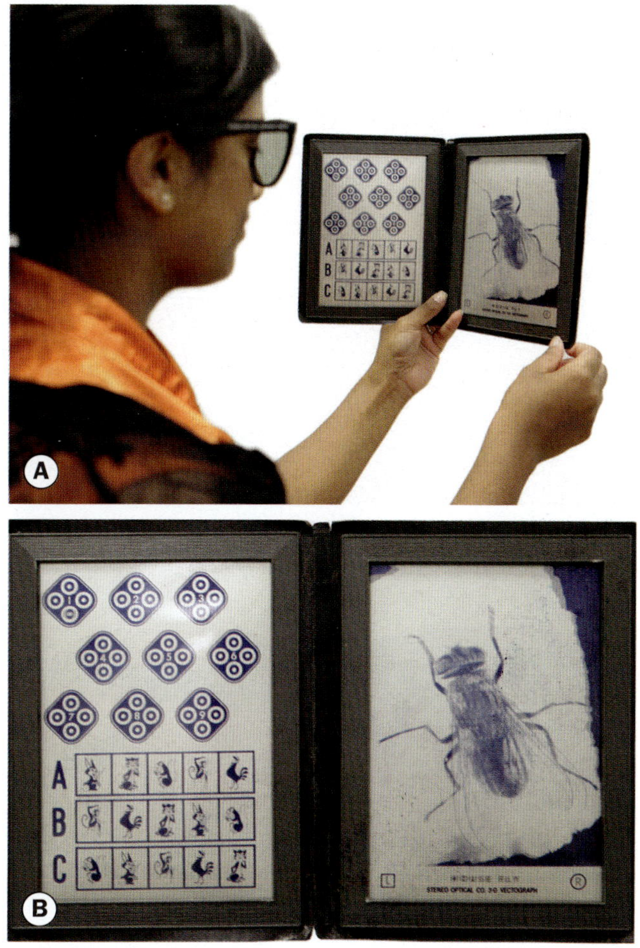

Fig. 18.20 Titmus test.

Titmus

The Titmus test consists of a three-dimensional polarized vectograph comprising two plates in the form of a booklet viewed through polarized spectacles. The spectacles should be worn before the plates are viewed. On the right is a large fly and on the left is a series of nine squares (within each of which there are four circles) and animals (Fig. 18.20). The test should be performed at a distance of 40 cm.

- **The fly** is a test of gross stereopsis (3000 seconds) and is especially useful for young children. It should appear to stand out from the page and the child is encouraged to pick up the tip of one of its wings between finger and thumb.
- **The animal** component consists of three rows of stylized animals (400–100 seconds), one of which will appear forward of the plane of reference.
- **The circles** comprise a graded series measuring 800–40 seconds; one of a set of four circles should appear to stand out from the plate surface.
- If the child has less than 800 seconds of stereopsis and prefers fixing with the right eye (left suppression), the bottom circle of first square of four circles is displaced to the left (and vice versa if fixing with the left eye).

TNO

The TNO random dot test consists of seven plates of randomly distributed paired red and green dots viewed with red–green spectacles and measures from 480 down to 15 seconds of arc at 40 cm. Within each plate the dots of one colour forming the target shape (squares, crosses etc. – Fig. 18.21) are displaced horizontally in relation to paired dots of the other colour so that they have a different retinal disparity to those outside the target. Control shapes are visible without the spectacles.

Frisby

The Frisby stereotest consists of three transparent plastic plates of varying thickness. On the surface of each plate are printed four squares of small randomly distributed shapes (Fig. 18.22). One of the squares contains a 'hidden' circle, in which the random shapes are printed on the reverse of the plate. The test does not require special spectacles because disparity (600–15 seconds) is created by the thickness of the plate; the working distance must be measured.

Lang

The Lang stereotest does not require special spectacles. The targets (a star, moon, car and elephant) are seen alternately by each eye

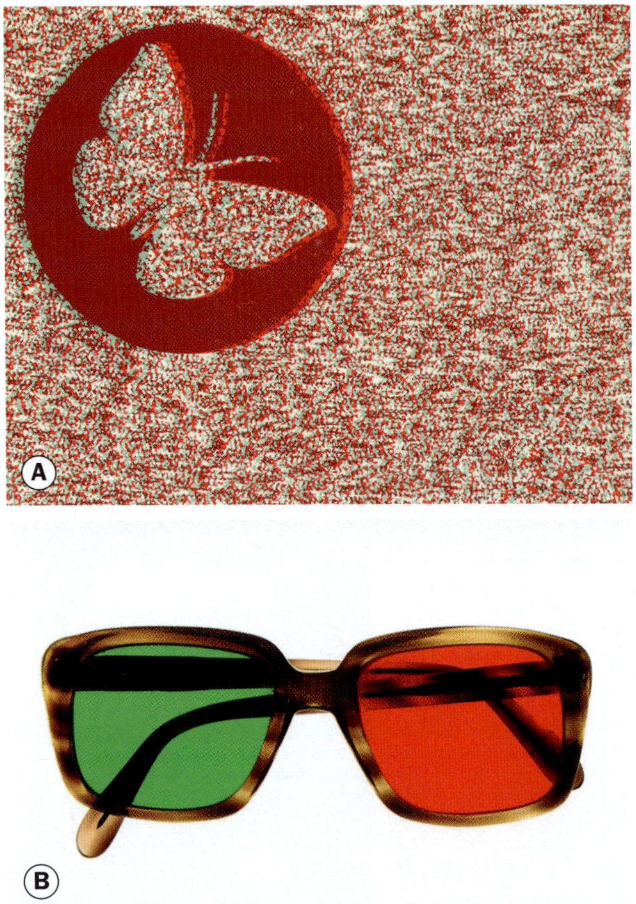

Fig. 18.21 TNO test. Shapes are only visible to an individual with stereopsis. **(A)** Test target, **(B)** red–green spectacles.

through the built-in cylindrical lens elements. The star is monocularly visible but provides a stereoscopic effect to observers with binocular vision. The star helps to attract and maintain the interest of small children. Displacement of the dots creates disparity (1200–200 seconds) and the patient is asked to name or point to a simple shape, such as a star, on the card (Fig. 18.23).

Tests for binocular fusion in infants without manifest squint

Base-out prism

This is a simple method for detecting fusion in children. The test is performed by placing a 20 Δ base-out prism in front of one eye (the right eye in Fig. 18.24). This displaces the retinal image temporally with resultant diplopia.

- There will be a shift of the right eye to the left to resume fixation (right adduction) with a corresponding shift of the left eye to the left (left abduction) in accordance with the Hering law (Fig. 18.24B).
- The left eye will then make a corrective re-fixational saccade to the right (left re-adduction) (Fig. 18.24C).
- On removal of the prism both eyes move to the right (Fig. 18.24D).

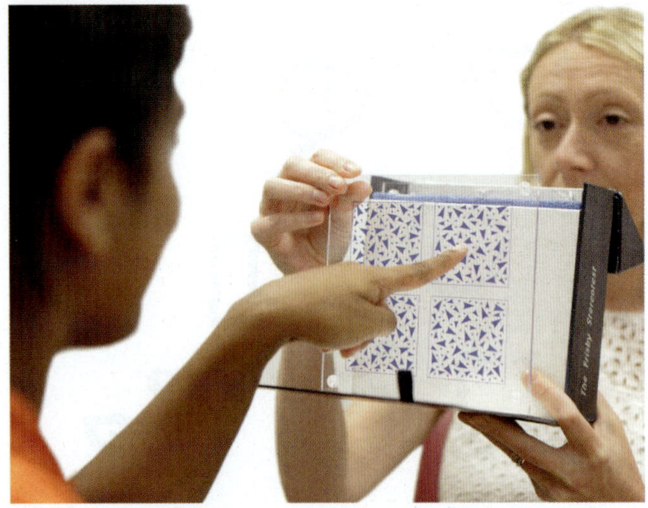

Fig. 18.22 Frisby test.

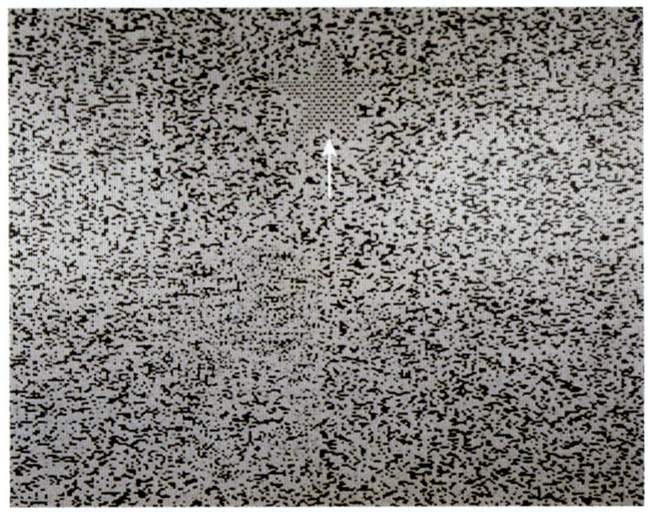

Fig. 18.23 Lang test (arrow shows the star).

- The left eye then makes an outward fusional movement (Fig. 18.24E).
- Most children with good BSV should be able to overcome a 20 Δprism from the age of 6 months. If not, weaker prisms (16 Δ or 12 Δ) may be tried, but the response is then more difficult to identify.

Binocular convergence

Simple convergence to an interesting target can be demonstrated from 3 to 4 months. Both eyes should follow the approaching target symmetrically 'to the nose'. Over-convergence in the infant may indicate an incipient esotropia. Divergence may be due either to a tendency to a divergent deviation or simply lack of interest.

Tests for sensory anomalies

Worth four-dot test

This is a dissociation test that can be used with both distance and near fixation and differentiates between BSV, ARC and suppression.

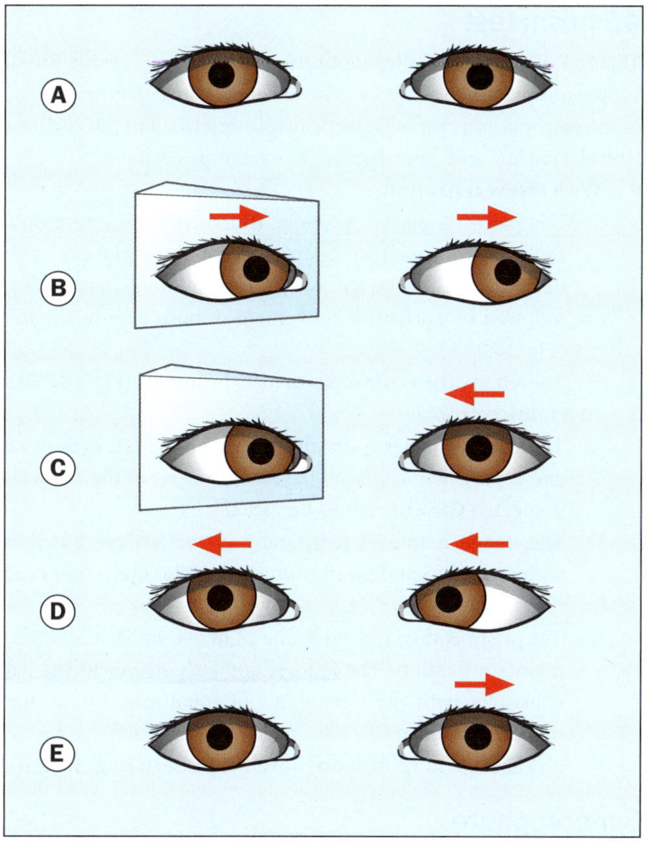

Fig. 18.24 Base-out prism test (see text).

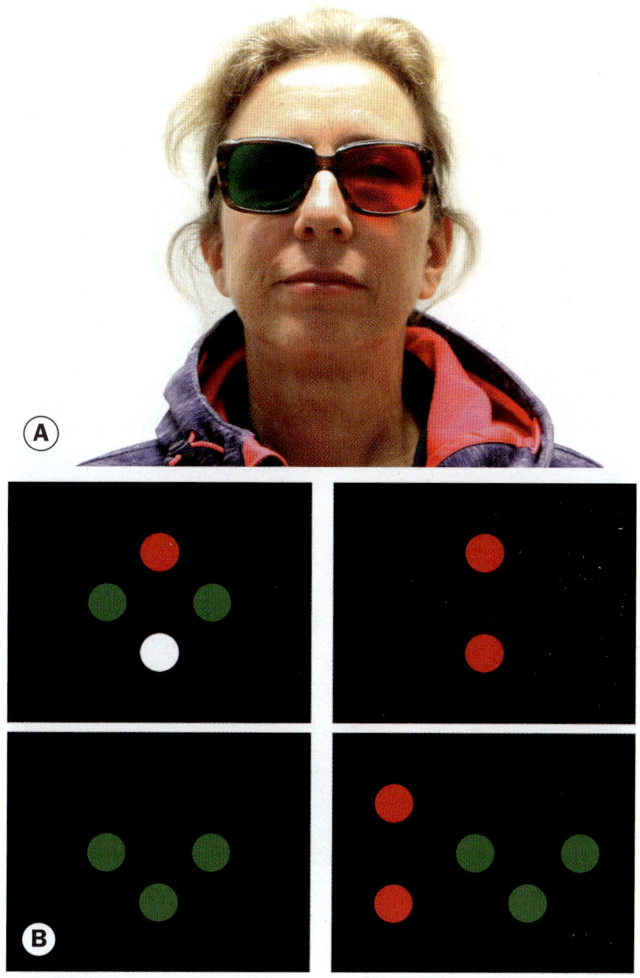

Fig. 18.25 Worth four-dot test. **(A)** Red–green glasses; **(B)** possible results (see text).

Results can only be interpreted if the presence or absence of a manifest squint is known at time of testing.

- **Procedure**
  - The patient wears a green lens in front of the right eye, which filters out all colours except green and a red lens in front of the left eye which will filter out all colours except red (Fig. 18.25A).
  - The patient then views a box with four lights: one red, two green and one white.
- **Results** (Fig. 18.25B)
  - If BSV is present, all four lights are seen.
  - If all four lights are seen in the presence of a manifest deviation, harmonious ARC (see 'Synoptophore' below) is present.
  - If two red lights are seen, right suppression is present.
  - If three green lights are seen, left suppression is present.
  - If two red and three green lights are seen, diplopia is present.
  - If the green and red lights alternate, alternating suppression is present.

Bagolini striated glasses

This is a test for detecting BSV, ARC or suppression. Each lens has fine striations that convert a point source of light into a line, as with the Maddox rod (see below).

- **Procedure.** The two lenses are placed at 45° and 135° in front of each eye and the patient fixates on a focal light source (Fig. 18.26A). Each eye perceives an oblique line of light, perpendicular to that perceived by the fellow eye (Fig. 18.26B). Dissimilar images are thus presented to each eye under binocular viewing conditions.
- **Results** (Fig. 18.26C) cannot be interpreted unless it is known whether strabismus is present.
  - If the two streaks intersect at their centres in the form of an oblique cross (an 'X'), the patient has BSV if the eyes are straight, or harmonious ARC in the presence of manifest strabismus.
  - If the two lines are seen but they do not form a cross, diplopia is present.
  - If only one streak is seen, there is no simultaneous perception and suppression is present.
  - In theory, if a small gap is seen in one of the streaks, a central suppression scotoma (as found in microtropia) is present. In practice this is often difficult to demonstrate and the patient describes a cross. The scotoma can be confirmed with the 4 Δ prism test (see below).

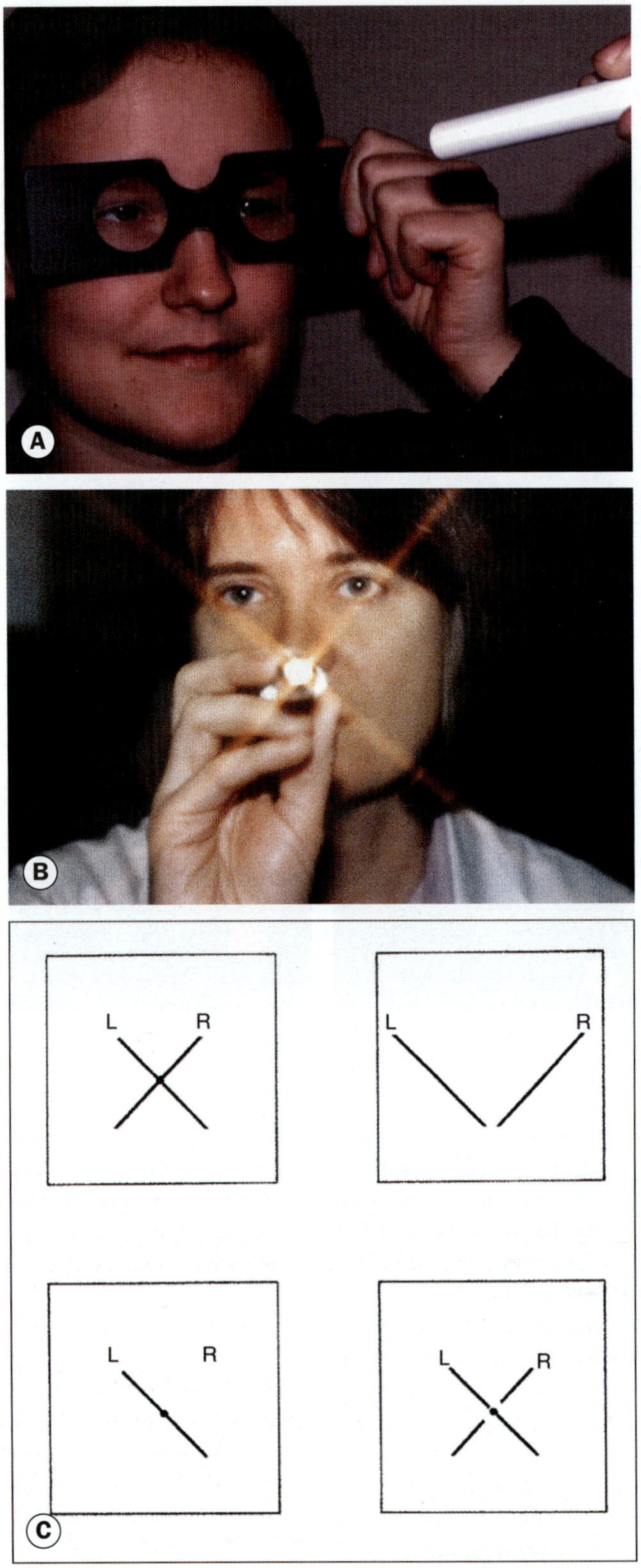

Fig. 18.26 Bagolini test. **(A)** Striated glasses; **(B)** appearance of a point of light through Bagolini lenses; **(C)** possible results.

TIP The 4Δ prism base-out test is useful to distinguish bifoveal fixation from foveal suppression (central suppression scotoma), which occurs during binocular viewing in patients with monofixation syndrome.

4Δ prism test

This test distinguishes bifoveal fixation (normal BSV) from foveal suppression (also known as a central suppression scotoma – CSS) in microtropia and employs the principle described in the 20 Δ test (the Hering law and convergence) to overcome diplopia.

- **With bifoveal fixation**
  - The prism is placed base-out (microtropia is commonly esotropic not exotropic) in front of the right eye with deviation of the image away from the fovea temporally, followed by corrective movement of both eyes to the left (Fig. 18.27A).
  - The left eye then converges to fuse the images (Fig. 18.27B).
- **In left microtropia**
  - The patient fixates a distance target with both eyes open and a 4 Δ prism is placed base-out in front of the eye with suspected CSS (the left in Fig. 18.28).
  - The image is moved temporally in the left eye but falls within the CSS and no movement of either eye is observed (Fig. 18.28A).
  - The prism is then moved to the right eye which adducts to maintain fixation. The left eye similarly moves to the left consistent with the Hering law of equal innervation, but the second image falls within the CSS of the left eye and so no subsequent re-fixation movement is seen (Fig. 18.28B).

Synoptophore

The synoptophore compensates for the angle of squint and allows stimuli to be presented to both eyes simultaneously (Fig. 18.29A). It can thus be used to investigate the potential for binocular function in the presence of a manifest squint and is of particular value in assessing young children (from age 3 years), who generally find the test process enjoyable. It can also detect suppression and ARC.

- The instrument consists of two cylindrical tubes with a mirrored right-angled bend and a +6.50 D lens in each eyepiece (Fig. 18.29B, top). This optically sets the testing distance as equivalent to about 6 metres.
- Pictures are inserted in a slide carrier situated at the outer end of each tube. The two tubes are supported on columns that enable the pictures to be moved in relation to each other and any adjustments are indicated on a scale.
- The synoptophore can measure horizontal, vertical and torsional misalignments simultaneously and is valuable in determining surgical approach by assessing the different contributions in the cardinal positions of gaze.

Grades of binocular vision

Binocular vision can be graded on the synoptophore as below (Fig. 18.29B, bottom).

- **First grade** (simultaneous perception – SP) is tested by introducing two dissimilar but not mutually antagonistic pictures, such as a bird and a cage.
  - The subject is then asked to put the bird into the cage by moving the arm of the synoptophore.
  - If the two pictures cannot be seen simultaneously, then suppression is present.

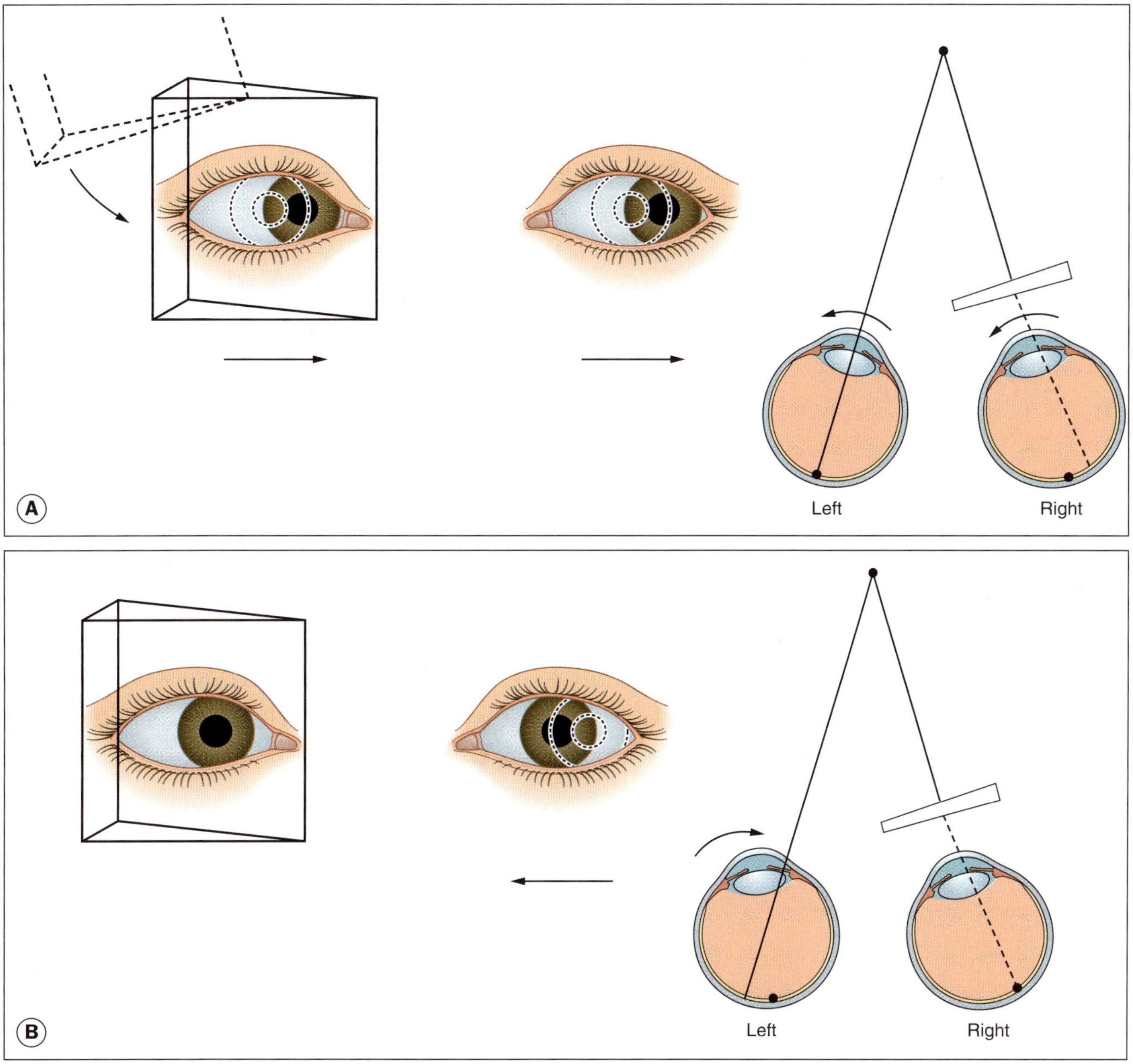

Fig. 18.27 4Δ prism test in bifoveal fixation. **(A)** Shift of both eyes away from the prism base; **(B)** fusional re-fixation movement of the left eye.

- Some retinal 'rivalry' will occur although one picture is smaller than the other, so that while the small one is seen foveally, the larger one is seen parafoveally (and is thus placed in front of the deviating eye).
- Larger macular and paramacular slides are used if foveal slides cannot be superimposed.

- **Second grade** (fusion). If simultaneous perception slides can be superimposed then the test proceeds to the second grade, which is the ability of the two eyes to produce a composite picture (sensory fusion) from two similar pictures, each of which is incomplete in one small different detail.
  - The classic example is two rabbits, one lacking a tail and the other lacking a bunch of flowers. If fusion is present, one rabbit complete with tail and flowers will be seen.
  - The range of fusion (motor fusion) is then tested by moving the arms of the synoptophore so that the eyes have to converge and diverge in order to maintain fusion.
  - The presence of simple fusion without any range is of little value in everyday life.
- **Third grade** (stereopsis) is the ability to obtain an impression of depth by the superimposition of two pictures of the same object which have been taken from slightly different angles. The classic example is a bucket, which should be appreciated in three dimensions.

Detection of abnormal retinal correspondence

ARC is detected on the synoptophore as follows:

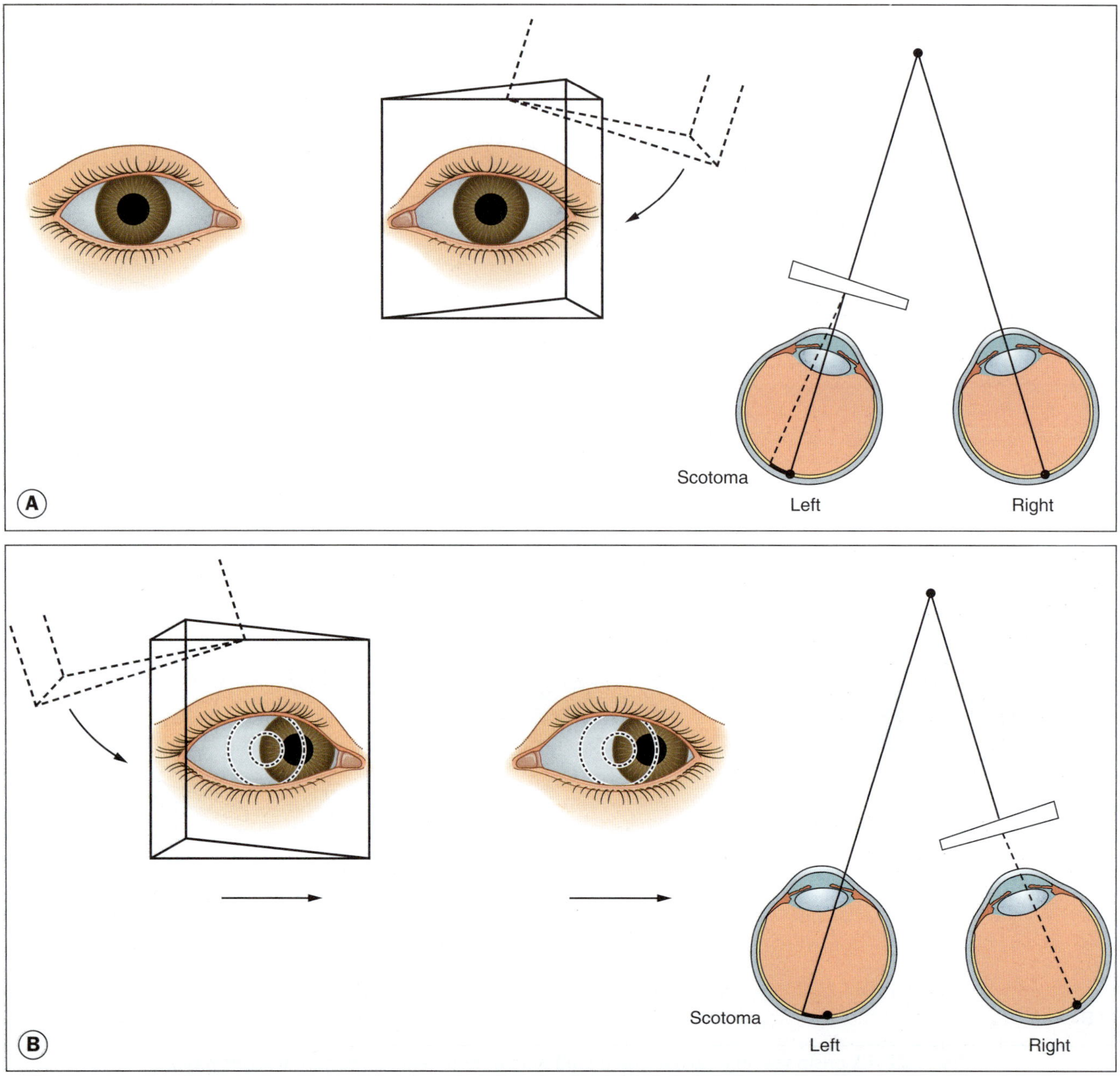

Fig. 18.28 4Δ prism test in left microtropia with a central suppression scotoma. **(A)** No movement of either eye; **(B)** both eyes move to the left but there is absence of re-fixation.

- The subjective angle of deviation is that at which the SP slides are superimposed. The examiner determines the objective angle of the deviation by presenting each fovea alternately with a target by extinguishing one or other light and moving the slide in front of the deviating eye until no movement of the eyes is seen.
- If the subjective and objective angles coincide then retinal correspondence is normal.
- If the objective and subjective angles are different, ARC is present. The difference in degrees between the subjective and objective angles is the angle of anomaly. ARC is said to be harmonious when the objective angle equals the angle of anomaly and inharmonious when it exceeds the angle of anomaly. It is only in harmonious ARC that binocular responses can be demonstrated. The inharmonious form may represent a lesser adaptation or an artefact of testing.

Measurement of deviation

Hirschberg test

The Hirschberg test gives a rough objective estimate of the angle of a manifest strabismus and is especially useful in young or uncooperative patients or when fixation in the deviating eye is poor. It is also useful in excluding pseudostrabismus. A pen torch is shone into the eyes from arm's length and the patient asked to

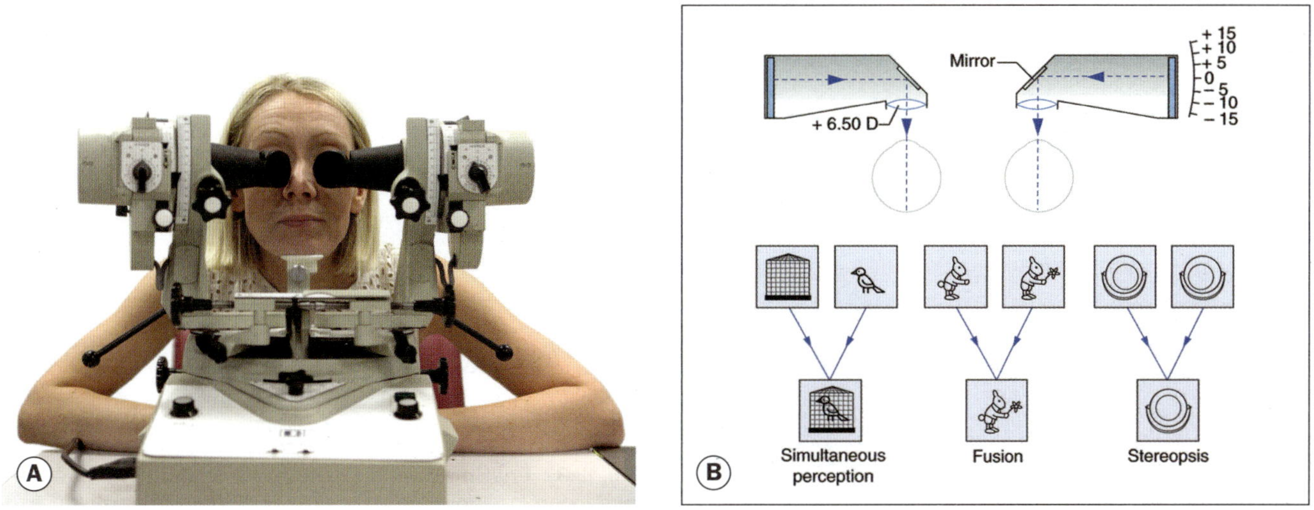

Fig. 18.29 (A) Synoptophore; **(B)** optical principles and grading of binocular vision.

fixate the light. The corneal reflection of the light will be (more or less) centred in the pupil of the fixating eye, but will be decentred in a squinting eye, in the direction opposite to that of the deviation (Fig. 18.30). The distance of the corneal light reflection from the centre of the pupil is noted; each millimetre of deviation is approximately equal to 7° (1° ≈ 2 prism dioptres). For example, if the reflex is situated at the temporal border of the pupil (assuming a pupillary diameter of 4 mm), the angle is about 15°; if it is at the limbus, the angle is about 45°. As the pupil size varies, the estimated angle varies.

Krimsky and prism reflection tests

Corneal reflex assessment can be combined with prisms to give a more accurate approximation of the angle in a manifest deviation.

- **The Krimsky test** involves placement of prisms in front of the fixating eye until the corneal light reflections are symmetrical (Fig. 18.31A and B). This test reduces the problem of parallax and is more commonly used than the prism reflection test.
- **The prism reflection test** involves the placement of prisms in front of the deviating eye until the corneal light reflections are symmetrical.

Cover–uncover test

The cover–uncover test consists of two parts:

- **The cover test** detects heterotropia. It is helpful to begin the near test using a light to observe the corneal reflections and to assess fixation in the deviating eye. It should then be repeated for near using an accommodative target and for distance as follows:
  - The patient fixates on a straight-ahead target.
  - If a right deviation is suspected, the examiner covers the fixing left eye and notes any movement of the right eye to take up fixation.
  - No movement indicates orthotropia (Fig. 18.32A) or left exotropia (Fig. 18.32B).
  - Adduction of the right eye to take up fixation indicates right exotropia and abduction, right esotropia (Fig. 18.32C).
  - Downward movement indicates right hypertropia and upward movement right hypotropia.
  - The test is repeated on the opposite eye.
- **The uncover test** detects heterophoria. It should be performed both for near (using an accommodative target) and for distance as follows:

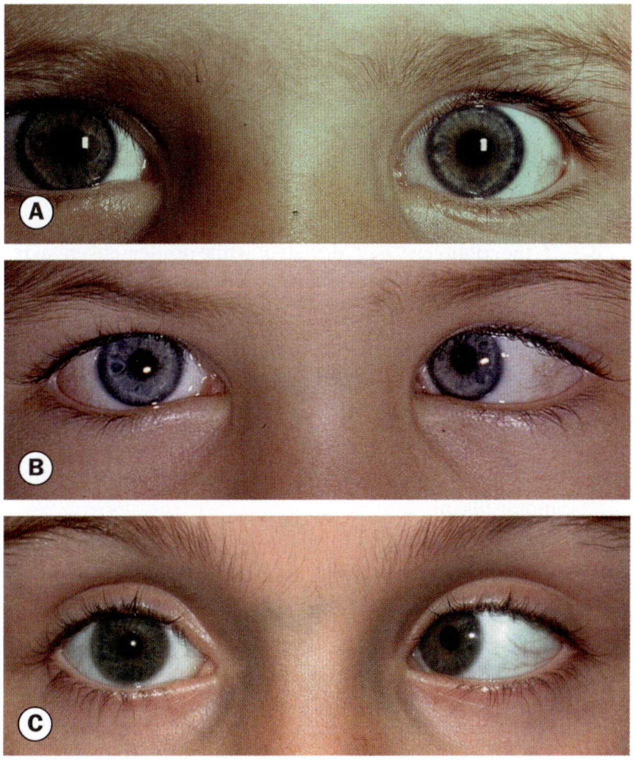

Fig. 18.30 Hirschberg test of a convergent squint. **(A)** The right corneal reflex is near the inner border of the pupil indicating an angle of about 10°; **(B)** the left corneal reflex is near the temporal border of the pupil indicating an angle of 15–20°; **(C)** the left corneal reflex is near the limbus indicating an angle of close to 40°. *(Courtesy of ADN Murray.)*

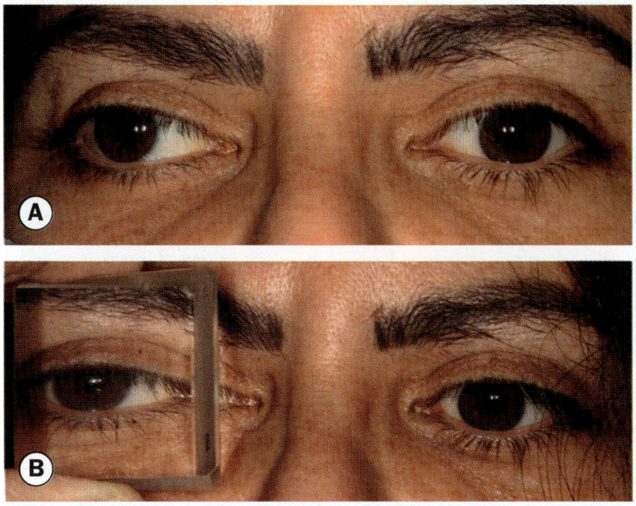

Fig. 18.31 Krimsky test. **(A)** Right exotropia; **(B)** large base-in prism placed in front of the right eye, showing alignment of the corneal light reflexes. *(Courtesy of M Parulekar.)*

- The patient fixates a straight-ahead distant target.
- The examiner covers the right eye and, after 2–3 seconds, removes the cover.
- No movement indicates orthophoria (Fig. 18.33A). A keen observer will frequently detect a very slight latent deviation in most normal individuals, as few individuals are truly orthophoric, particularly on near fixation.
- If the right eye had deviated while under cover, a re-fixation movement (recovery to BSV) is observed on being uncovered.
- Adduction (nasal recovery) of the right eye indicates exophoria (Fig. 18.33B) and abduction esophoria (Fig. 18.33C).
- Upward or downward movement indicates a vertical phoria.
- After the cover is removed, the examiner notes the speed and smoothness of recovery as evidence of the strength of motor fusion.
- The test is repeated for the opposite eye.
- Most examiners perform the cover test and the uncover test sequentially, hence the term cover–uncover test.

TIP When undertaking cover testing, the patient must fixate on an accommodative target rather than on a light source.

Alternate cover test

The alternate cover test induces dissociation to reveal the total deviation when fusion is disrupted. It should be performed only after the cover–uncover test.

- The right eye is covered for several seconds.
- The occluder is quickly shifted to the opposite eye for 2 seconds, then back and forth several times. After the cover is removed, the examiner notes the speed and smoothness of recovery as the eyes return to their pre-dissociated state.
- A patient with a well-compensated heterophoria will have straight eyes before and after the test has been performed whereas a patient with poor control may decompensate to a manifest deviation.

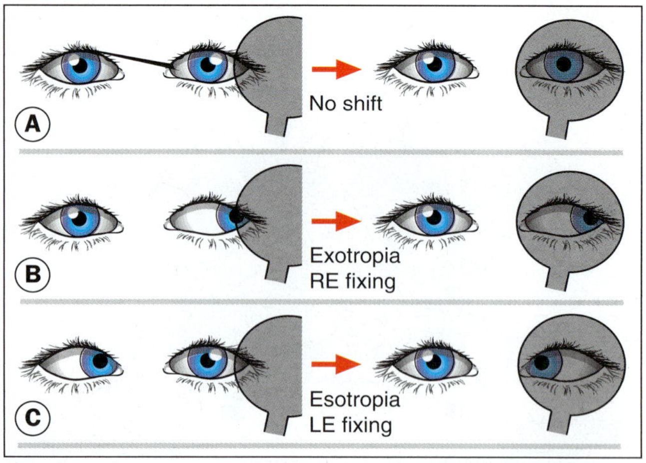

Fig. 18.32 Possible results of the cover test. **(A)** With the right eye fixing, no movement indicates orthotropia or **(B)** left exotropia; **(C)** with the left eye fixing, abduction of the right eye indicates esotropia.

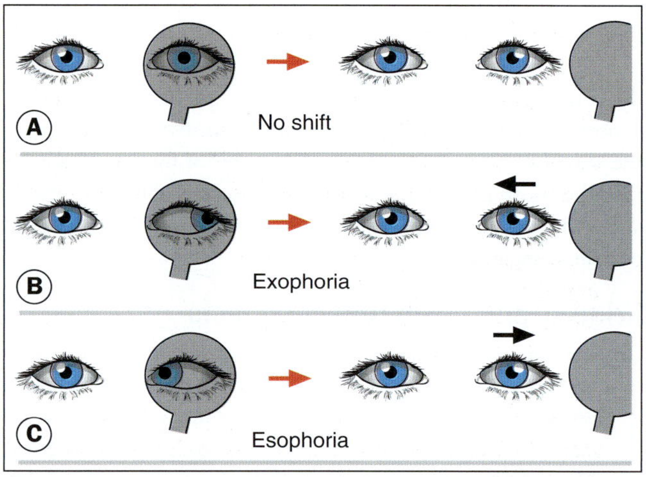

Fig. 18.33 Possible results of the uncover test. **(A)** No movement indicates orthophoria; **(B)** adduction indicates exophoria; **(C)** abduction indicates esophoria.

Prism cover test

The prism cover test measures the angle of deviation and includes the alternate cover test with prisms. It is performed with the patient fixing on a distant target in the primary position and in the eight diagnostic positions of gaze. It is repeated in the primary position with near fixation and in patients with intermittent exotropia, with fixation in the far distance. It is performed as follows:

- The alternate cover test is first performed to establish the direction and approximate extent of deviation.
- Prisms of increasing strength are placed in front of one eye with the base opposite the direction of the deviation (i.e. the apex of the prism is pointed in the direction of the deviation). For example, in a convergent strabismus the prism is held base-out and in a right hypertropia, base-down before the right eye.

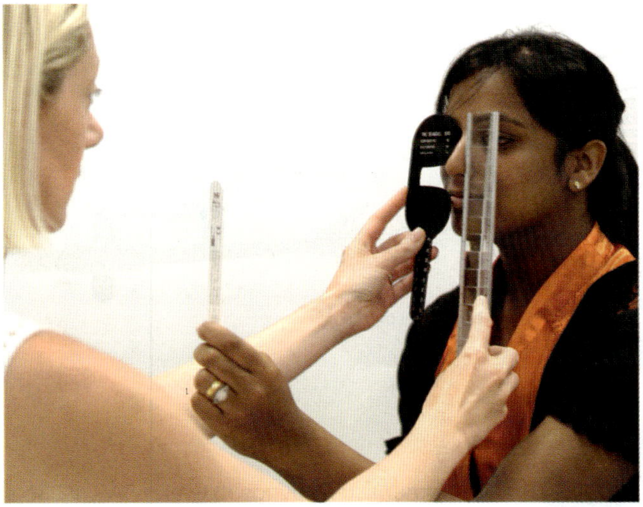

Fig. 18.34 Prism cover test.

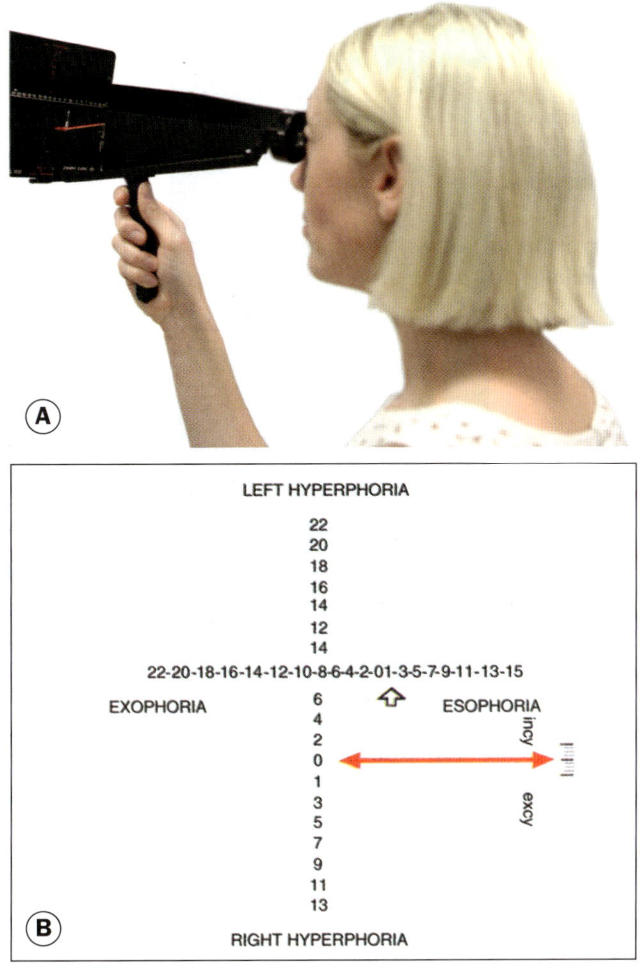

Fig. 18.35 Patient's view using the Maddox wing.

- The alternate cover test is performed continuously as stronger prisms are introduced, typically using a prism bar consisting of a column of prisms of progressive strength (Fig. 18.34). The amplitude of the re-fixation movement should gradually decrease as the strength of prism approaches the extent of deviation.
- The end-point is approached when no movement is seen. To ensure the maximum angle is found, the prism strength can be increased further until a movement is observed in the opposite direction (the point of reversal) and then reduced again to find the neutral value; the angle of deviation is then taken from the strength of the prism.

Maddox wing

The Maddox wing dissociates the eyes for near fixation (1/3 m) and measures heterophoria. The instrument is constructed in such a way that the right eye sees only a white vertical arrow and a red horizontal arrow, whereas the left eye sees only horizontal and vertical rows of numbers (Fig. 18.35).

- Horizontal deviation is measured by asking the patient to which number the white arrow points.
- Vertical deviation is measured by asking the patient which number intersects with the red arrow.
- The amount of cyclophoria is determined by asking the patient to move the red arrow so that it is parallel with the horizontal row of numbers.

Maddox rod

The Maddox rod consists of a series of fused cylindrical red or white glass rods that convert the appearance of a white spot of light into a red or white streak. The optical properties of the rods cause the streak of light to be at an angle of 90° with the long axis of the rods. When the glass rods are held horizontally, the streak will be vertical and vice versa.

- The rod is placed in front of the right eye (Fig. 18.36A). This dissociates the two eyes: the red streak seen by the right eye cannot be fused with the unaltered white spot of light seen by the left eye (Fig. 18.36B).
- The amount of dissociation (Fig. 18.36C) is measured by the superimposition of the two images using prisms. The base of the prism is placed in the position opposite to the direction of the deviation.
- Both vertical and horizontal deviations can be measured in this way but the test cannot differentiate a phoria from a tropia.
- The double Maddox rod test is used to determine cyclodeviations. Traditionally, a red Maddox is placed before the right eye and a white Maddox before the left. A Maddox rod is placed in front of each eye in a trial frame or phoropter with the lines arranged vertically so that the patient sees horizontal line images. The patient or examiner rotates the axes of the rods until the lines are perceived to be parallel. To facilitate the patient's recognition of the two lines, it is often helpful to dissociate the lines by placing a small prism base-up or base-down in front of one eye. The degree of deviation and the direction (incyclo- or excyclo-) can be determined by the angle of rotation that causes the line images to appear horizontal and parallel.

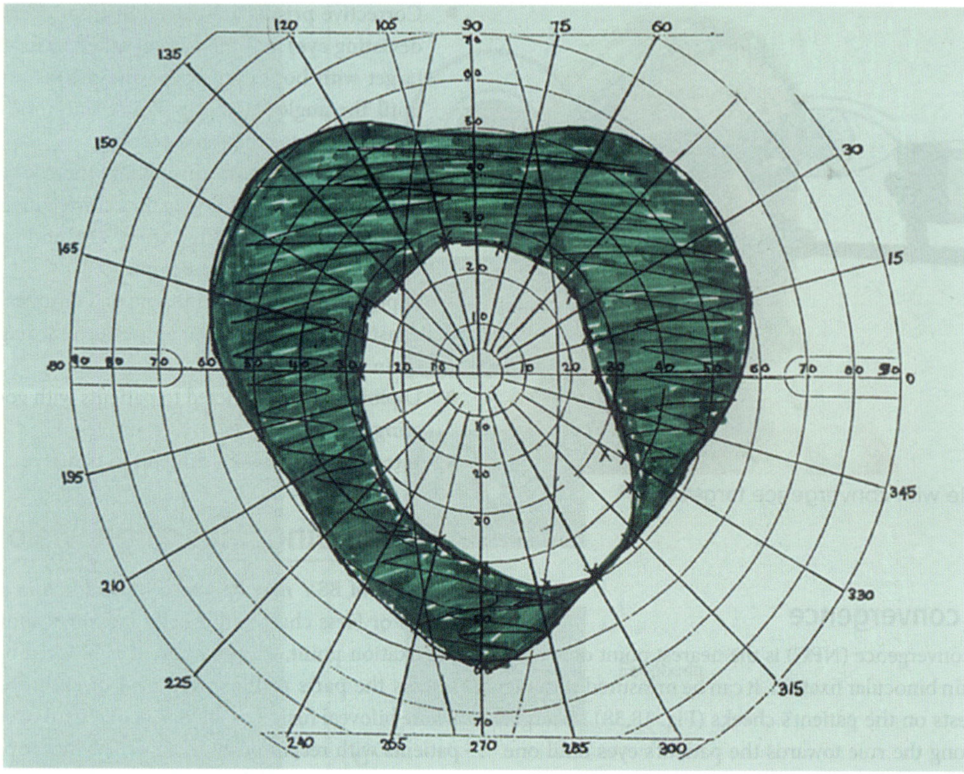

Fig. 18.39 Field of binocular single vision (clear area between the green colour) using a Goldmann perimeter. *(Courtesy of ADN Murray.)*

reversed and the procedure repeated. Software is available that facilitates the plotting of a Hess chart using a standard desktop computer screen.

Lees screen

This apparatus (Fig. 18.40) consists of two opalescent glass screens at right-angles to each other, bisected by a two-sided plane mirror that dissociates the eyes; each of the eyes can see only one of the two screens. Each screen has a tangent pattern (two-dimensional projection of a spherical surface) that is revealed only when the screen is illuminated. The patient is positioned facing the non-illuminated screen with his or her chin stabilized on a rest. Using a pointer, the examiner indicates a target point on the illuminated tangent pattern and the patient positions a pointer on the non-illuminated screen, at a position perceived to be superimposed on the dot indicated by the examiner. The non-illuminated screen is briefly illuminated by the examiner using a footswitch to facilitate recording of the dot indicated by the patient. When the procedure has been completed for one eye, the patient is rotated through 90° to face the previously illuminated screen and the procedure repeated.

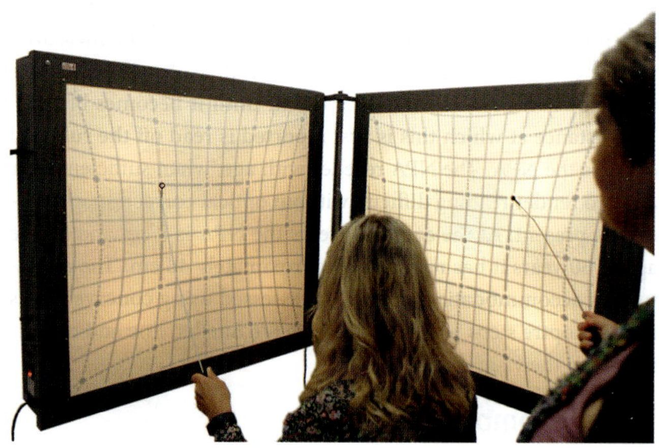

Fig. 18.40 Lees screen.

Interpretation

Fig. 18.41 shows a typical Hess chart appearance in right lateral rectus paresis of recent onset.

- The smaller chart indicates the eye with the paretic muscle (right eye).
- The larger chart indicates the eye with the overacting yoke muscle (left eye).
- The smaller chart will show its greatest restriction in the main direction of action of the paretic muscle (right lateral rectus).
- The larger chart will show its greatest expansion in the main direction of action of the yoke muscle (left medial rectus).
- The degree of disparity between the plotted point and the template in any position of gaze gives an estimate of the angle of deviation (each square = 5°).

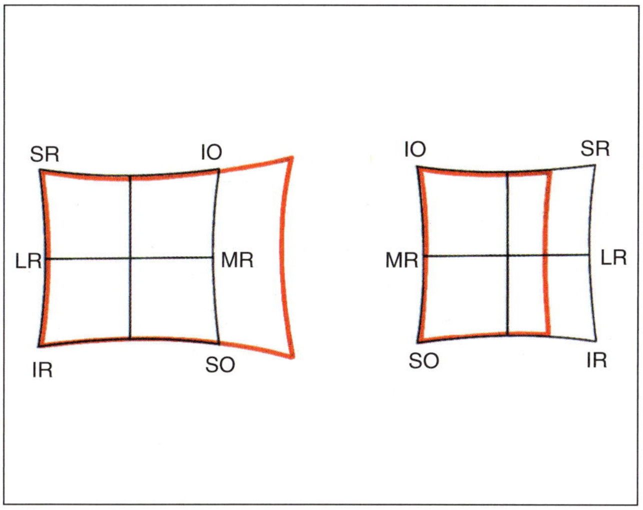

Fig. 18.41 Hess chart of a recent right lateral rectus palsy. IO = inferior oblique; IR = inferior rectus; LR = lateral rectus; MR = medial rectus; SO = superior oblique; SR = superior rectus.

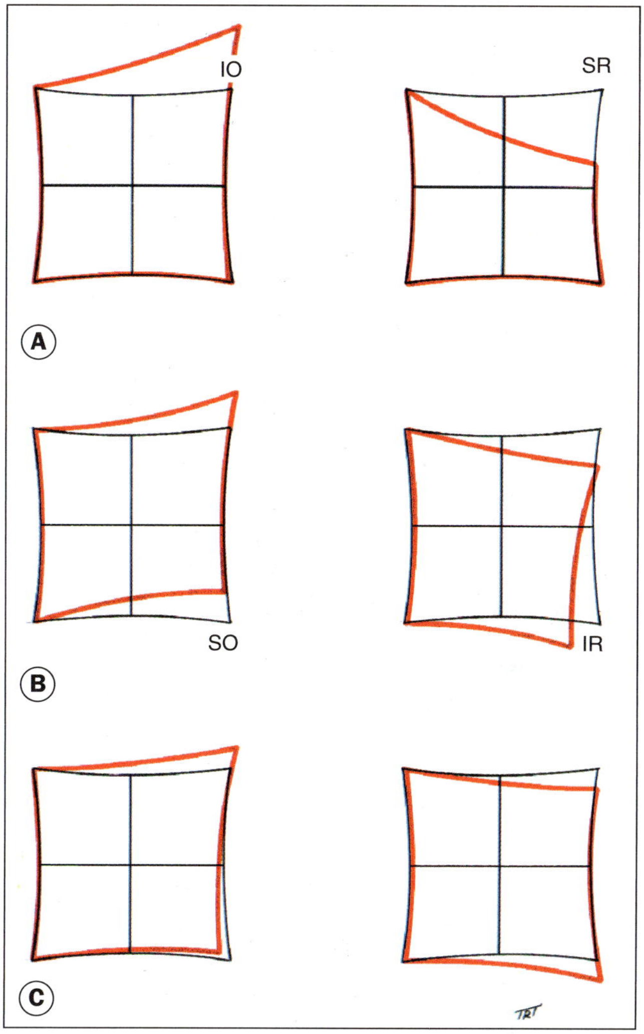

Fig. 18.42 Hess chart showing changes with time of a right superior rectus palsy. IO = inferior oblique; SR = superior rectus; SO = superior oblique. **(A)** Underaction of the affected superior rectus and overaction of the yoke muscle (left inferior oblique); **(B)** secondary overaction of the ipsilateral antagonist (right inferior rectus) results in a weakness of the yoke muscle (left superior oblique); **(C)** with further passage of time, concomitance occurs and it can be difficult to determine which was the primary paretic muscle.

Changes with time

Progressive changes in the Hess chart with time are characteristic and useful both as a prognostic indicator and to guide management.

- In right superior rectus palsy, the Hess chart will show underaction of the affected muscle with an overaction of its yoke muscle, the left inferior oblique (Fig. 18.42A). Because of the great incomitance of the two charts, the diagnosis is straightforward. If the paretic muscle recovers its function, both charts will revert to normal.
- Secondary contracture of the ipsilateral antagonist (right inferior rectus) will manifest as an overaction which will lead to a secondary (inhibitional) palsy of the antagonist of the yoke muscle (left superior oblique), which will show up on the chart as an underaction (Fig. 18.42B). This could lead to the incorrect impression that the left superior oblique is the primarily paretic muscle.
- With further passage of time, the two charts become progressively more concomitant, such that it may be impossible to determine the initiating muscle weakness (Fig. 18.42C).

Examples

The clinical features of extraocular muscle palsies are discussed in detail in Chapter 19.

- **Left third nerve palsy** (Fig. 18.43)
  - The area enclosed on the left chart is much smaller than that on the right.
  - Left exotropia – note that the fixation spots in the inner charts of both eyes are deviated laterally. The deviation is greater on the right chart (when the left eye is fixating), indicating that secondary deviation exceeds the primary, typical of a paretic squint.
  - Left chart shows underaction of all muscles except the lateral rectus.
  - Right chart shows overaction of all muscles except the medial rectus and inferior rectus, the 'yokes' of the spared muscles.
  - The primary angle of deviation (fixing right eye – FR) in the primary position is −20° and R/L 10°.
  - The secondary angle (fixing left eye – FL) is −28° and R/L 12°.
  - In inferior rectus palsy, the function of the superior oblique muscle can only be assessed by observing intorsion on attempted depression. This is best performed by observing a conjunctival landmark using the slit lamp.
- **Recently acquired right fourth nerve palsy** (Fig. 18.44)
  - Right chart is smaller than the left.
  - Right chart shows underaction of the superior oblique and overaction of the inferior oblique.
  - Left chart shows overaction of the inferior rectus and underaction (inhibitional palsy) of the superior rectus.

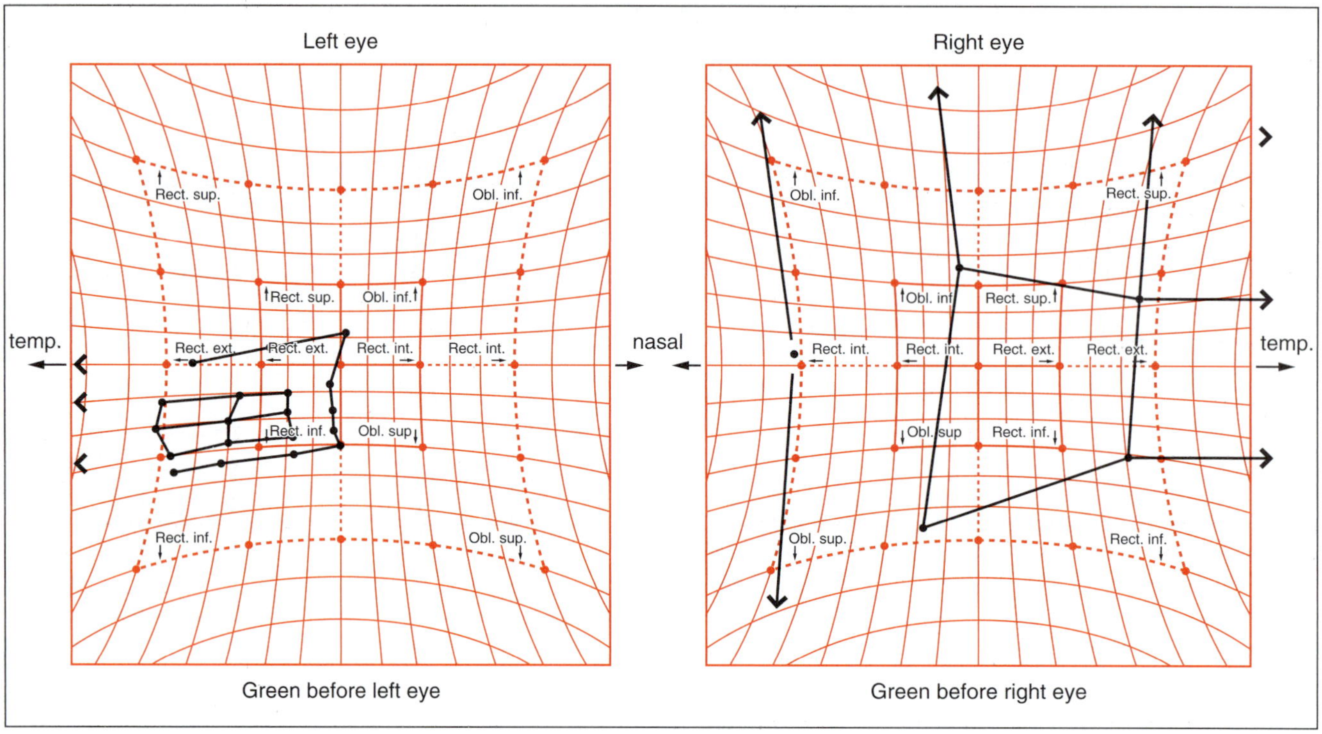

Fig. 18.43 Hess chart of a left third nerve palsy (see text).

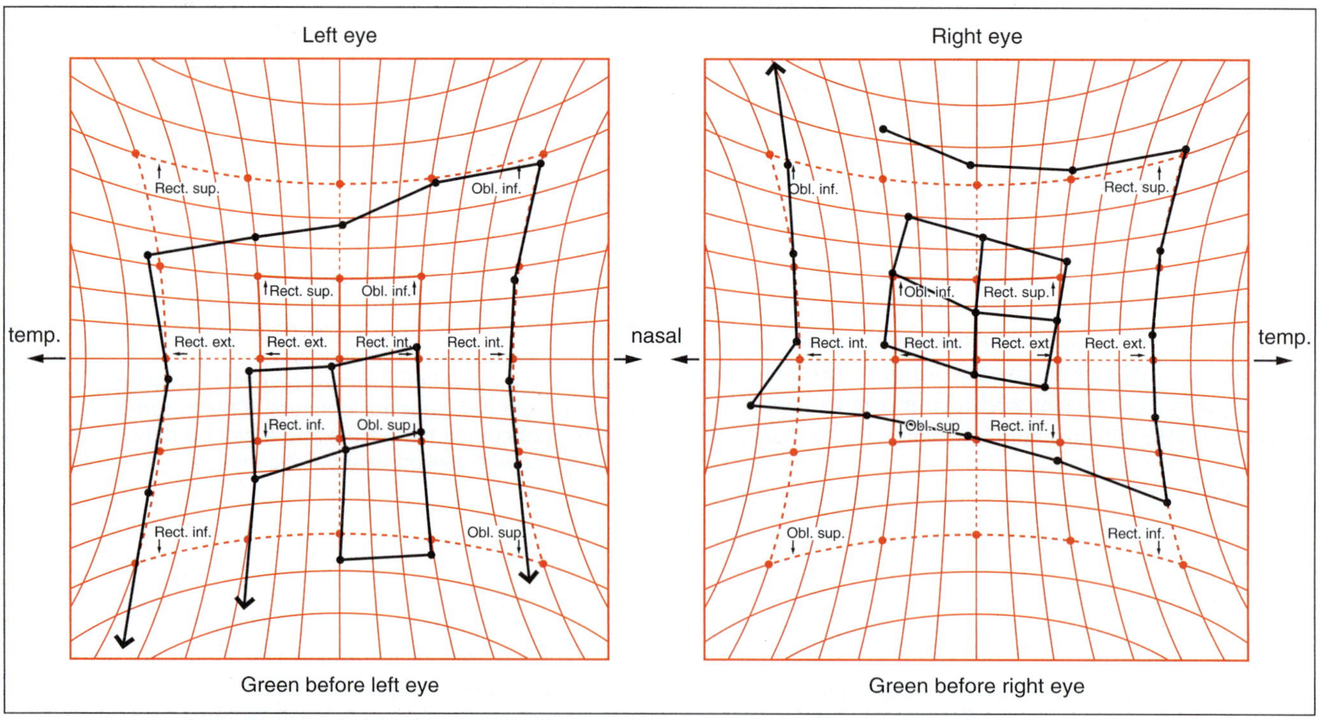

Fig. 18.44 Hess chart of a recently acquired right fourth nerve palsy (see text).

   - The primary deviation (FL) is R/L 8°, while the secondary deviation (FR) is R/L 17°.
- **Congenital right fourth nerve palsy** (Fig. 18.45)
   - No difference in overall chart size.
   - Primary and secondary deviation R/L 4°.
   - Right hypertropia – note that the fixation spot of the right inner chart is deviated upwards and the left is deviated downwards.
   - Hypertropia increases on laevoversion and reduces on dextroversion.

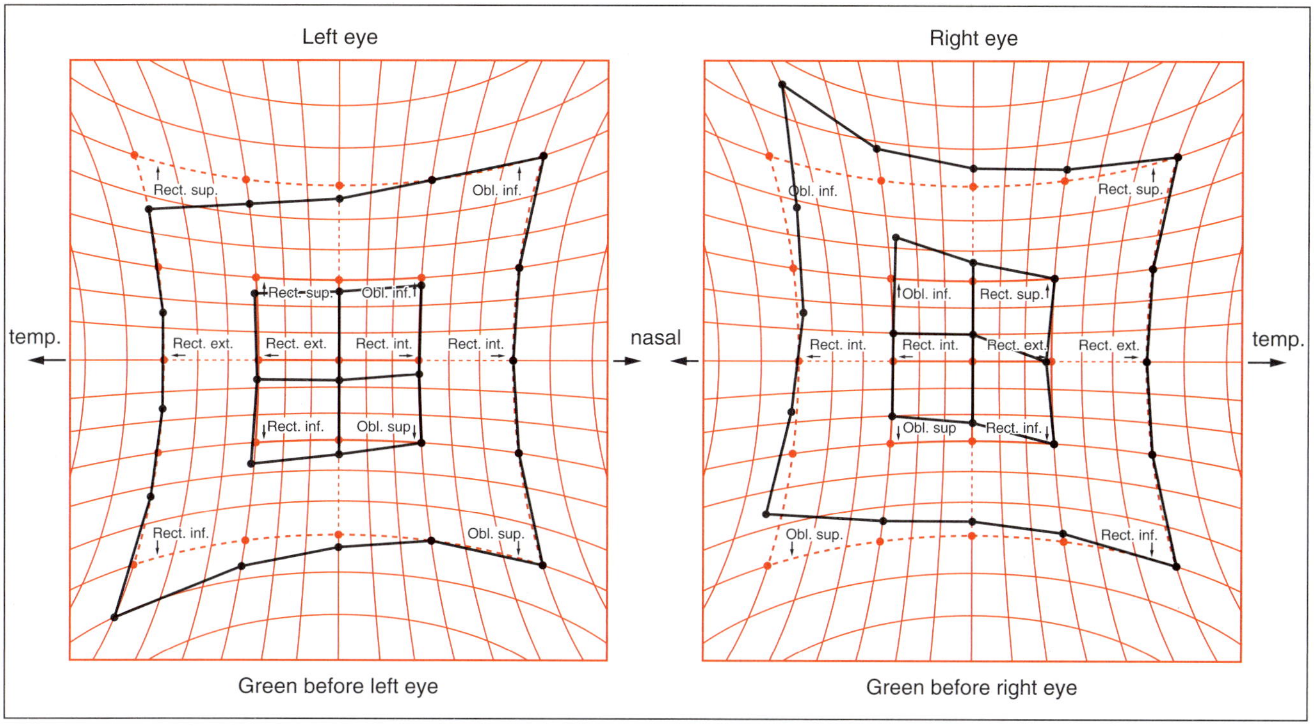

Fig. 18.45 Hess chart of a congenital right fourth nerve palsy (see text).

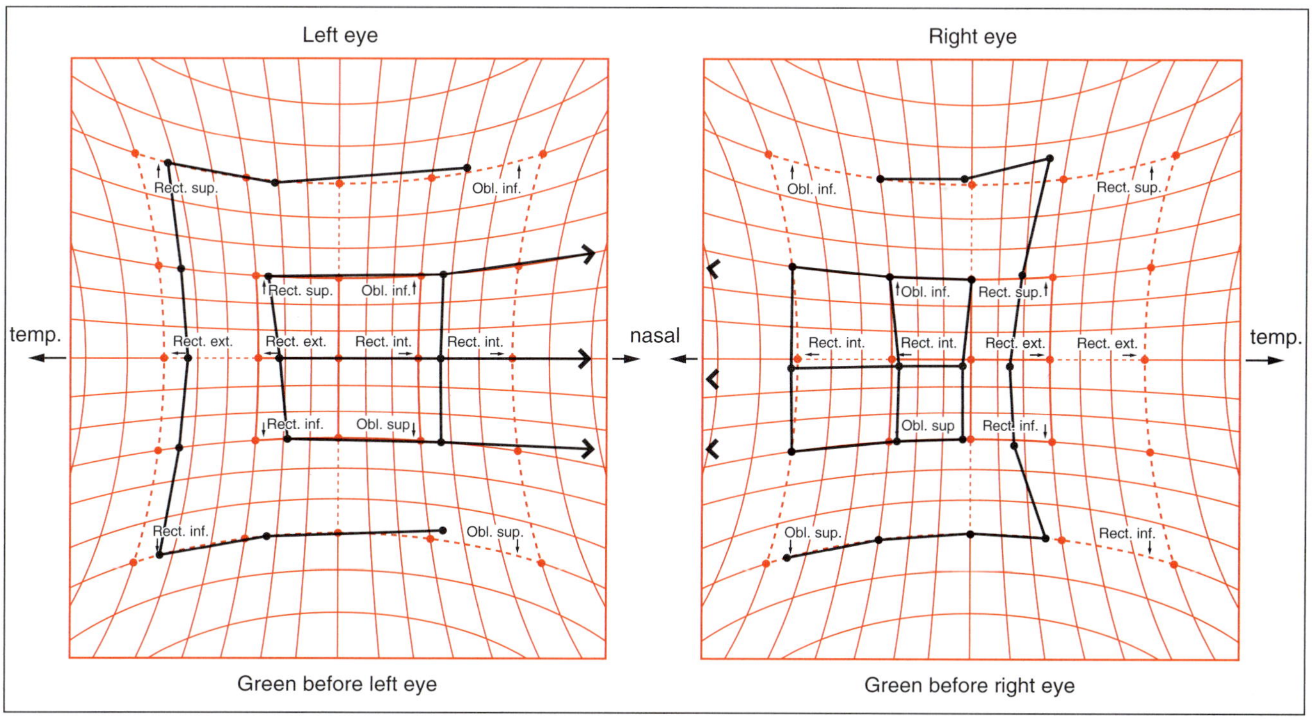

Fig. 18.46 Hess chart of a right sixth nerve palsy (see text).

- Right chart shows underaction of the superior oblique and overaction of the inferior oblique.
- Left chart shows overaction of the inferior rectus and underaction (inhibitional palsy) of the superior rectus.

- **Right sixth nerve palsy** (Fig. 18.46)
  - Right chart is smaller than the left.
  - Right esotropia – note that the fixation spot of the right inner chart is deviated nasally.
  - Right chart shows marked underaction of the lateral rectus and slight overaction of the medial rectus.
  - Left chart shows marked overaction of the medial rectus.

- The primary angle FL is +15° and the secondary angle FR +20°.
- Inhibitional palsy of the left lateral rectus has not yet developed.

Refraction and fundoscopy

Dilated fundoscopy is mandatory in the context of strabismus, principally to exclude any underlying ocular pathology such as macular scarring, optic disc hypoplasia or retinoblastoma as the cause of the deviation. More commonly, strabismus is secondary to refractive error; hypermetropia (hyperopia), astigmatism, anisometropia and myopia may all be associated.

Cycloplegia

The most common refractive error to cause strabismus is hypermetropia. Accurate measurements of hypermetropia necessitate effective paralysis of the ciliary muscle (cycloplegia), in order to neutralize the masking effect of accommodation. In a young child the risk of penalization amblyopia should be avoided by always inducing cycloplegia in both eyes at one sitting, particularly if atropine is used.

- **Cyclopentolate** (0.5% under 6 months and 1% subsequently). One drop, repeated after 5 minutes, usually results in maximal cycloplegia within 30 minutes, with recovery of accommodation within 2–3 hours and resolution of mydriasis within 24 hours. The adequacy of cycloplegia can be determined by comparing retinoscopy readings with the patient fixating for distance and then for near (dynamic retinoscopy). Topical anaesthesia with a well-tolerated agent such as proxymetacaine prior to instillation of cyclopentolate is useful in preventing ocular irritation and reflex tearing, thus affording better retention of the cyclopentolate in the conjunctival sac and effective cycloplegia.
- **Atropine** (0.5% under the age of 12 months and 1% subsequently) has a somewhat stronger cycloplegic effect than cyclopentolate. In most cases this is clinically insignificant, but may be helpful in instances such as high hypermetropia or heavily pigmented irides. As the onset of cycloplegia is slower, a parent or carer may be supplied with topical atropine for instillation at home twice daily over 1–3 days prior to attendance (but not on the day of examination) as either eye drops or ointment. Drops are easier to instil, but there may be less risk of overdose with ointment. The atropine should be discontinued if there are signs of systemic toxicity, such as flushing, fever or restlessness and immediate medical attention sought. The visual effects may last for up to 2 weeks.

Change of refraction with age in childhood

Because refraction changes with age, it is important to check this in patients with strabismus at least every year and more frequently in younger children and if acuity is reduced. At birth most babies are hypermetropic. After the age of 2 years there may be an increase in hypermetropia and a decrease in astigmatism. Hypermetropia may continue to increase until the age of about 6 years, levelling off between the ages of 6 and 8 and subsequently decreasing.

When to prescribe

Most children are mildly hypermetropic (1–3 D). There is some evidence that fully correcting hypermetropia in a normal child may reduce physiological emmetropization.

- **Hypermetropia.** In general, up to 4 D of hypermetropia should not be corrected in a child without a squint unless they are experiencing problems with near vision. With hypermetropia greater than this a two-thirds correction is usually given. However, in the presence of esotropia, the full cycloplegic correction should be prescribed, even under the age of 2 years.
- **Astigmatism.** A cylinder of 1.50 D or more should probably be prescribed, especially in anisometropia after the age of 18 months.
- **Myopia.** The necessity for correction depends on the age of the child. Under the age of 2 years, −5.00 D or more of myopia should be corrected; between the ages of 2 and 4 the amount is −3.00 D. Older children should have correction of even low myopia to allow clear distance vision. Under-correction and bifocals may retard progression and are under investigation.
- **Anisometropia.** After the age of 3 the full difference in refraction between the eyes should be prescribed if it is more than 1 D, with full hypermetropic correction in squint.

TIP In the presence of esotropia, the full cycloplegic hypermetropic correction should be prescribed, even in children under the age of 2 years.

PSEUDOSTRABISMUS

Pseudostrabismus is the clinical impression of ocular deviation when no squint is present.

- **Epicanthic folds** may simulate an esotropia (Fig. 18.47A).
- **Abnormal interpupillary distance**, if short may simulate an esotropia and if wide an exotropia (Fig. 18.47B).
- **Angle kappa** is the angle between the visual and anatomical (pupillary) axes (see Fig. 18.1).
  - Normally, the fovea is situated temporal to the anatomical centre of the posterior pole. The eyes are therefore slightly abducted to achieve bifoveal fixation and a light shone onto the cornea will therefore cause a reflex just nasal to the centre of the cornea in both eyes (Fig. 18.48A). This is termed a positive angle kappa.
  - A large positive angle kappa (e.g. temporally displaced macula) may give a pseudoexotropia (Fig. 18.48B and see Fig. 18.1B).
  - A negative angle kappa occurs when the fovea is situated nasal to the posterior pole (e.g. high myopia). In this situation, the corneal reflex is situated temporally to the centre of the cornea and it may simulate an esotropia (Fig. 18.48C).

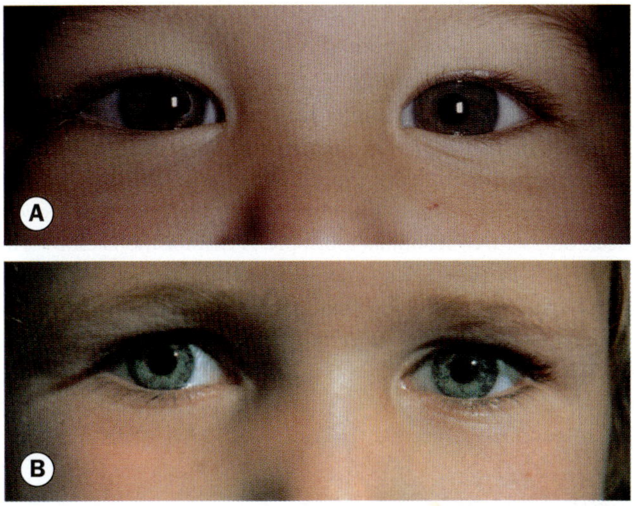

Fig. 18.47 Pseudostrabismus. **(A)** Prominent epicanthic folds simulating esotropia; **(B)** wide interpupillary distance simulating exotropia.

HETEROPHORIA

Heterophoria may present clinically with associated visual symptoms when the fusional amplitudes are insufficient to maintain alignment, particularly at times of stress or poor health.

- **Signs.** Both esophoria and exophoria can be classified by the distance at which the angle is greater: respectively, convergence excess or weakness, divergence weakness or excess and mixed.
- **Treatment**
  - Orthoptic treatment is of most value in convergence weakness exophoria.
  - Any significant refractive error should be appropriately corrected.
  - Symptom relief may otherwise be obtained using temporary stick-on Fresnel prisms and may be subsequently incorporated into spectacles (maximum usually 10–12 Δ, split between the two eyes).
  - Surgery may occasionally be required for larger deviations.

VERGENCE ABNORMALITIES

Convergence insufficiency

Convergence insufficiency (CI) typically affects individuals with high near visual demand, such as students.

- **Signs.** Remote NPC independent of any heterophoria and poor fusional convergence amplitudes.
- **Treatment** involves orthoptic exercises aimed at normalizing the near point and maximizing fusional amplitudes. With good compliance, symptoms should be eliminated within a few weeks but if persistent can be treated with base-in prisms.
- **Accommodative insufficiency** (AI) is occasionally also present. It may be idiopathic (primary) or post-viral and typically affects school-age children. The minimum reading correction to give clear vision is prescribed but is often difficult to discard.

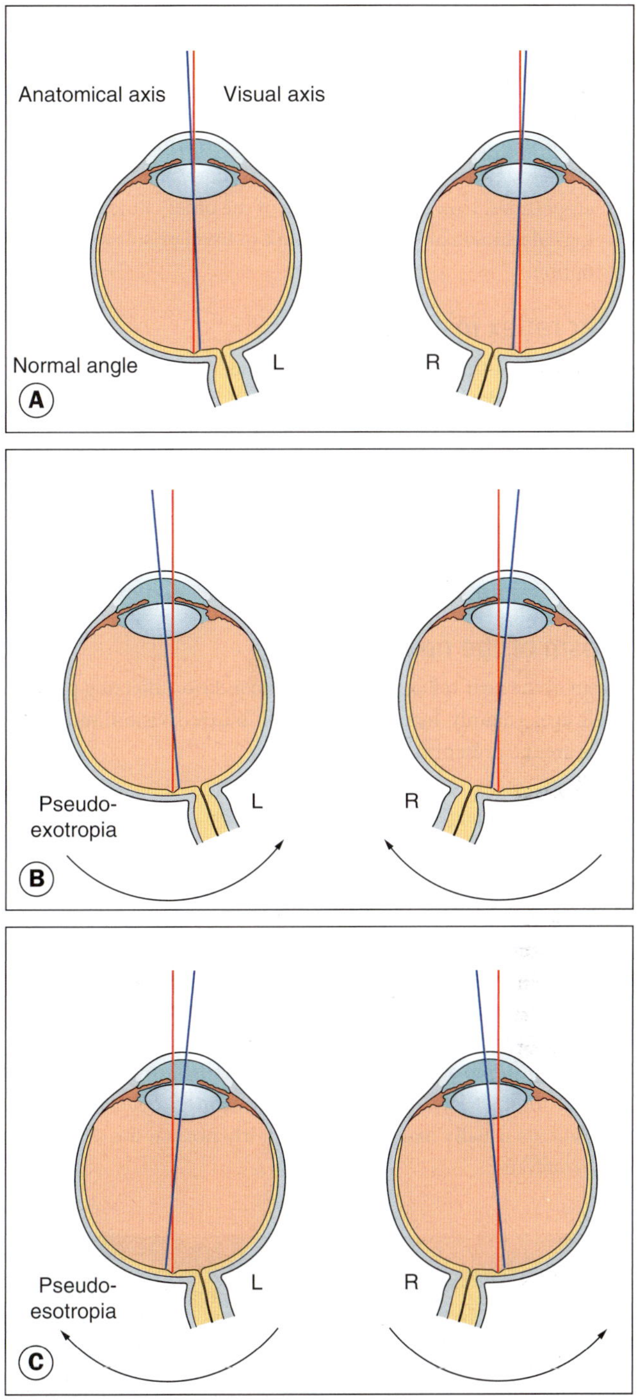

Fig. 18.48 Angle kappa. **(A)** Normal; **(B)** positive, simulating an exotropia; **(C)** negative, simulating an esotropia.

Divergence insufficiency and divergence paralysis

- **Divergence insufficiency** is recognized these days as being part of a common condition called 'sagging eye syndrome – SES,' which occurs in elderly adults (see later in this chapter). If symmetrical, age-related distance esotropia (ARDE) results and if asymmetrical, unilateral hypotropia with excyclotropia results ('cyclovertical strabismus').

- **Divergence paralysis** is a rare condition typically associated with underlying neurological disease such as intracranial space-occupying lesions, cerebrovascular accidents and head trauma. Presentation may be at any age and it may be difficult to distinguish from sixth nerve palsy. It is primarily a concomitant esodeviation with reduced or absent divergence fusional amplitudes. However, it has none of the other clinical or radiological features of SES. It is difficult to treat; prisms are the best option.

Near reflex insufficiency

- **Paresis** of the near reflex presents as dual convergence and accommodation insufficiency. Mydriasis may be seen on attempted near fixation. Treatment involves reading glasses, base-in prisms and possibly botulinum toxin (orthoptic exercises have no effect). It is difficult to eradicate.
- **Complete paralysis** in which no convergence or accommodation can be initiated may be of functional origin, due to midbrain disease or after head trauma; recovery is possible.

Spasm of the near reflex

Spasm of the near reflex is a functional condition affecting patients of all ages (mainly females). Diplopia, blurred vision and headaches are the presenting symptoms.

- **Signs**
  - Esotropia, pseudomyopia and miosis.
  - Spasm may be triggered when testing ocular movements (Fig. 18.49A).
  - Observation of miosis is the key to the diagnosis (Fig. 18.49B).
  - Refraction with and without cycloplegia confirms the pseudomyopia, which must not be corrected optically.
- **Treatment** involves reassurance and advising the patient to discontinue any activity that triggers the response. If persistent, atropine and a full reading correction are prescribed but it is difficult later to abandon treatment without recurrence. Patients usually manage to live a fairly normal life despite the symptoms.

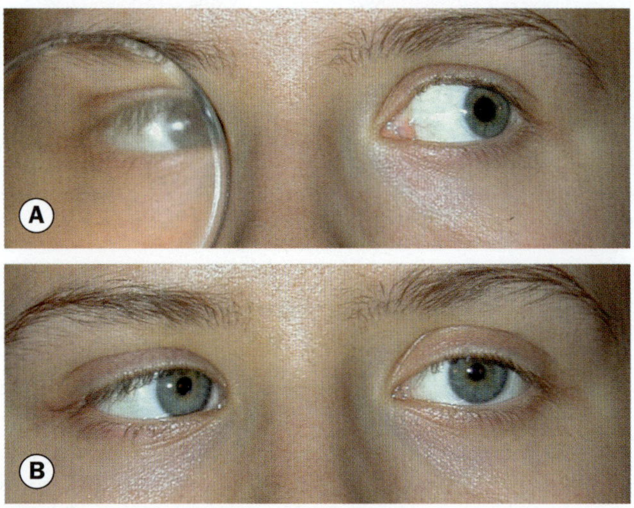

Fig. 18.49 (A) Spasm of the near reflex precipitated on testing ocular movements; **(B)** right esotropia and miosis.

ESOTROPIA

Esotropia (manifest convergent squint) may be concomitant or incomitant. In a concomitant esotropia the variability of the angle of deviation is within 5 Δ in different horizontal gaze positions. In an incomitant deviation the angle differs in various positions of gaze as a result of abnormal innervation or restriction. This section deals only with concomitant esotropia. A classification is shown in Table 18.1. However, all squints are different and not all fit neatly into a classification. For example, a microtropia may occur with a number of the other categories. It is more important to understand the part played by binocular function, refractive error and accommodation in the pathophysiology of each individual squint and to tailor treatment accordingly.

Early-onset esotropia

Up to the age of 4 months, infrequent episodes of convergence are normal but thereafter ocular misalignment is abnormal. Early-onset (essential infantile) esotropia is an idiopathic esotropia developing within the first 6 months of life in an otherwise normal infant with no significant refractive error and no limitation of ocular movements.

Signs

- The angle is usually fairly large (>30 Δ) and stable.
- Fixation in most infants is alternating in the primary position (Fig. 18.50).
- There is cross-fixating in side gaze, so that the child uses the left eye in right gaze (Fig. 18.51A) and the right eye on left gaze (Fig. 18.51B). Such cross-fixation may give a false impression of bilateral abduction deficits, as in bilateral sixth nerve palsy.
- Abduction can usually be demonstrated, either by the doll's head manoeuvre or by rotating the child.

Table 18.1 Classification of Esotropia

Accommodative

• Refractive
  • Fully accommodative
  • Partially accommodative
• Non-refractive
  • With convergence excess
  • With accommodation weakness
  • Mixed

Non-accommodative
• Early onset (essential infantile) • Microtropia • Basic • Convergence excess • Convergence spasm • Divergence insufficiency • Divergence paralysis • Sensory • Consecutive • Acute onset • Cyclic

- Should these fail, uniocular patching for a few hours will often unmask the ability of the other eye to abduct.
- Nystagmus is usually horizontal.
- Latent nystagmus (LN) is seen only when one eye is covered and the fast phase beats towards the side of the fixing eye. This means that the direction of the fast phase reverses according to which eye is covered.
- Manifest latent nystagmus (MLN) is the same except that nystagmus is present with both eyes open, but the amplitude increases when one is covered.
- The refractive error is usually normal for the age of the child (about +1 to +2 D).
- Asymmetry of optokinetic nystagmus is present.
- Inferior oblique overaction may be present initially or develop later.
- Dissociated vertical deviation (DVD) develops in 80% by the age of 3 years.

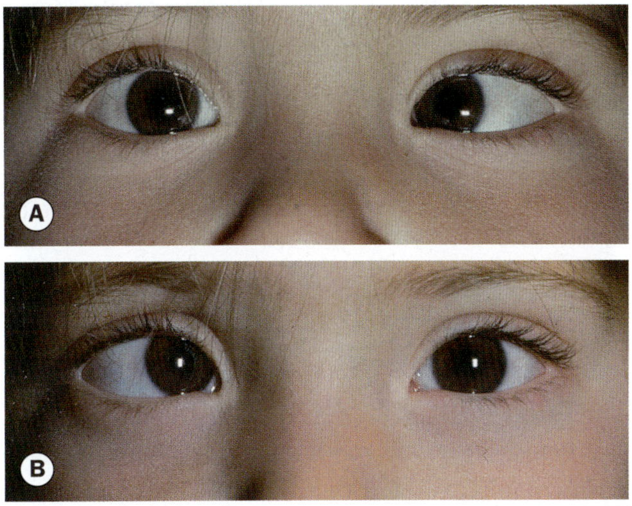

Fig. 18.50 Alternating fixation in early-onset esotropia. **(A)** Fixating with right eye; **(B)** fixating with left eye. *(Courtesy of ADN Murray.)*

- **Differential diagnosis** includes bilateral congenital sixth nerve palsy, secondary (sensory) esotropia due to organic eye disease, nystagmus blockage syndrome in which convergence dampens a horizontal nystagmus and mechanical limitations of eye movement such as Duane and Möbius syndromes and strabismus fixus.

Initial treatment

- **Timing of surgery.** After an initial period of variability, the angle of esotropia becomes constant at about 4–5 months of age. Once any amblyopia and significant refractive error have been appropriately corrected, the eyes should be surgically aligned within 4 months of the date of onset of constant esotropia. Evidence is accumulating that surgical alignment within that time frame may achieve a superior sensory outcome and improved binocular function.
- **The initial procedure** can be either recession of both medial rectus muscles or unilateral medial rectus muscle recession with lateral rectus muscle resection. Angles larger than 50 Δ will require recession of both medical rectus muscles as well as resection of one lateral rectus muscle.
- **Angles larger than 65 Δ** may require recession of both medial rectus muscles as well as resection of both lateral rectus muscles.
- **Large recessions.** Recessions of medial rectus muscles of more than 6.5 mm have been abandoned as they lead to late over-corrections.
- **Significant inferior oblique overaction** should be dealt with surgically.
- **An acceptable goal** is alignment of the eyes to within 8 Δ, associated with peripheral fusion and central suppression (Fig. 18.52). This small-angle residual strabismus is often stable, even though bifoveal fusion is not achieved.

Subsequent treatment

- **Under-correction** may require further recession of the medial recti, resection of one or both lateral recti or surgery to the other eye, depending on the initial procedure.

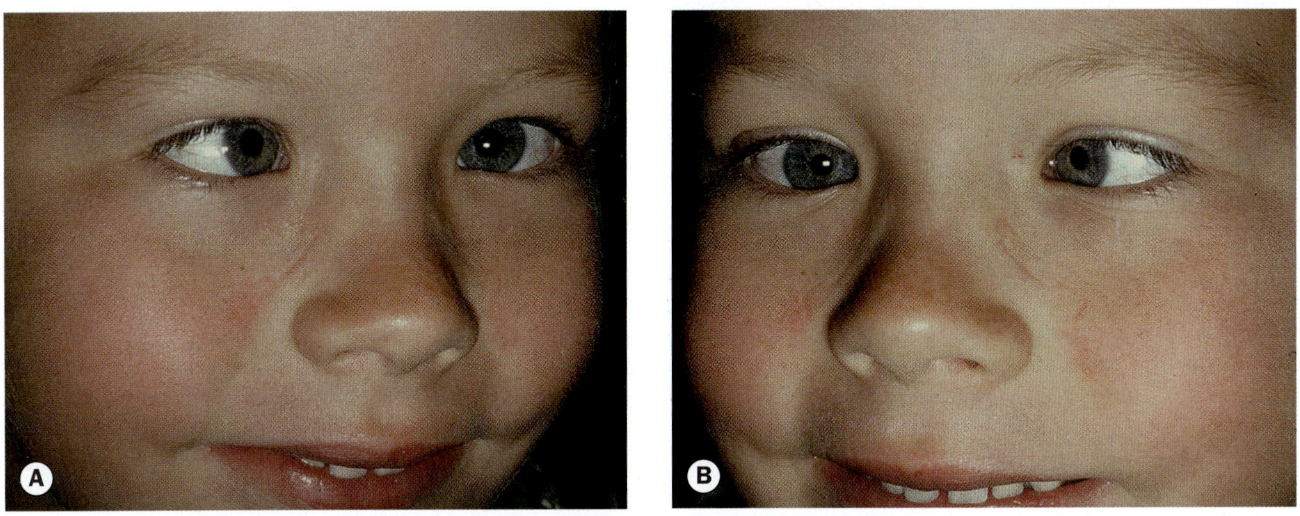

Fig. 18.51 Cross-fixation in early-onset esotropia. **(A)** Left fixation on right gaze; **(B)** right fixation on left gaze. *(Courtesy of ADN Murray.)*

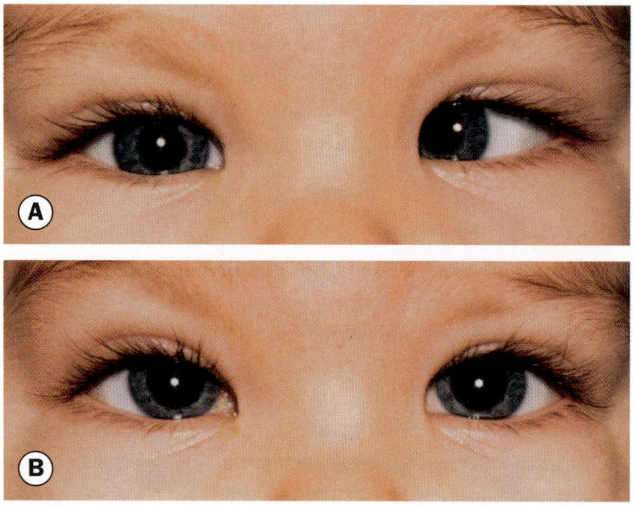

Fig. 18.52 Early-onset esotropia. **(A)** Before surgery; **(B)** after surgery.

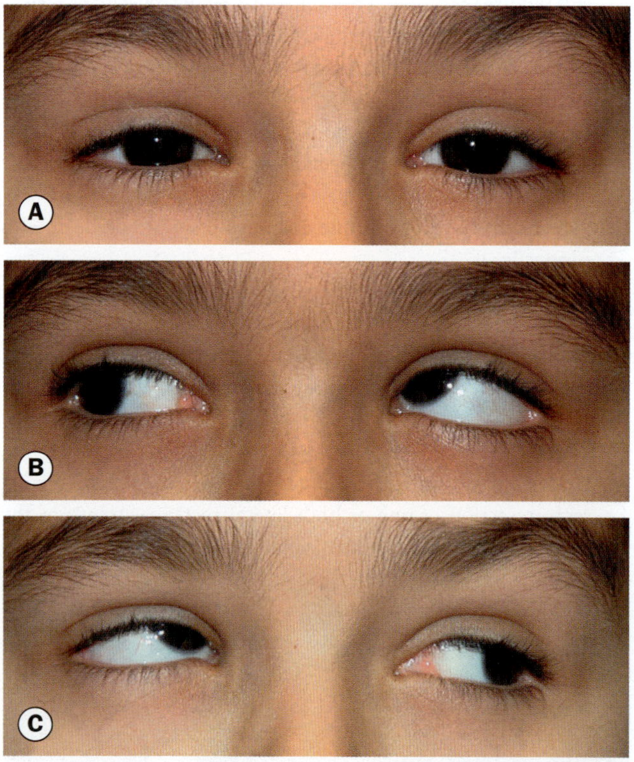

Fig. 18.53 Bilateral inferior oblique overaction. **(A)** Straight eyes in the primary position; **(B)** left inferior oblique overaction on right gaze; **(C)** right inferior oblique overaction on left gaze.

- **Inferior oblique overaction** may develop subsequently, most commonly at age 2 years (Fig. 18.53). The parents should therefore be warned that further surgery may be necessary despite an initially good result. Initially unilateral, it frequently becomes bilateral within 6 months. Inferior oblique weakening procedures include disinsertion, recession and myectomy.
- **DVD** (Fig. 18.54) is characterized by up-drift with excyclorotation (extorsion) of the eye when under cover, or spontaneously during periods of visual inattention. When the cover is removed the affected eye will move down without a corresponding down-drift of the other eye. It is usually bilateral. Surgical treatment may be indicated for psychosocial reasons. Options include superior rectus recession with or without posterior fixation sutures, resection or tuck of the inferior rectus muscle and inferior oblique anterior transposition.
- **Amblyopia** subsequently develops in about 50% of cases as unilateral fixation preference commonly develops postoperatively.
- **An accommodative element** should be suspected if the eyes are initially straight or almost straight after surgery and then start to become convergent. Regular refraction is therefore important.

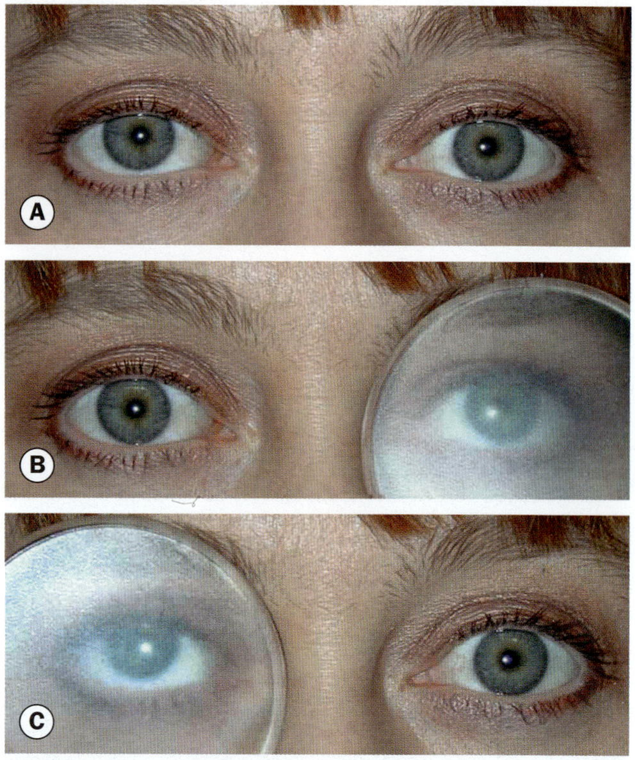

Fig. 18.54 Dissociated vertical deviation. **(A)** Straight eyes in the primary position; **(B)** up-drift of left eye under cover; **(C)** up-drift of right eye under cover.

TIP Inferior oblique overaction needs to be distinguished from dissociated vertical deviation.

Accommodative esotropia

Near vision involves both accommodation and convergence. Accommodation is the process by which the eye focuses on a near target, by altering the curvature of the crystalline lens. Simultaneously, the eyes converge, in order to fixate bifoveally on the target. Both accommodation and convergence are quantitatively related to the proximity of the target and have a fairly constant relationship to each other (AC/A ratio) as described previously. Abnormalities of the AC/A ratio are an important cause of certain types of esotropia.

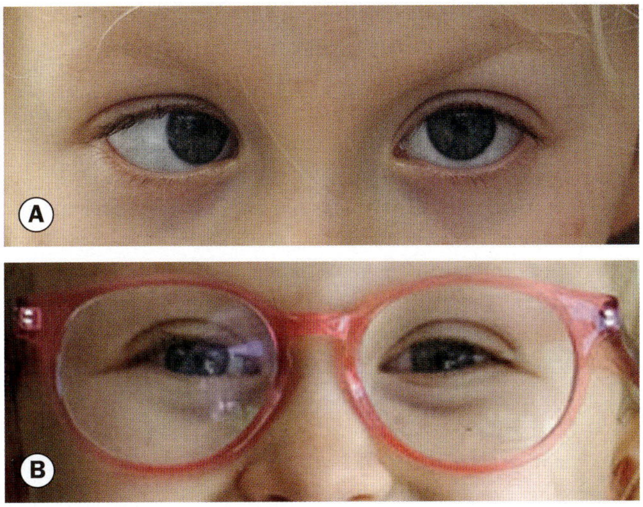

Fig. 18.55 Fully accommodative esotropia. **(A)** Right esotropia without glasses; **(B)** straight eyes for near and distance with glasses.

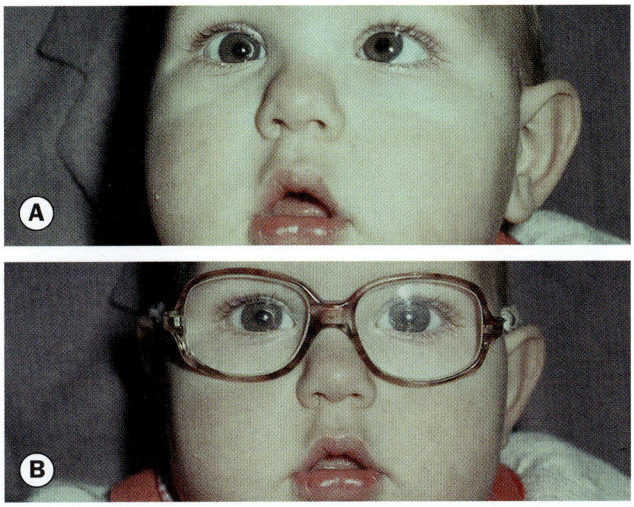

Fig. 18.56 Fully accommodative esotropia in a baby. **(A)** Esotropia without glasses; **(B)** straight eyes for near and distances with glasses. *(Courtesy of ADN Murray.)*

Refractive accommodative esotropia

In this type of accommodative esotropia, the AC/A ratio is normal and esotropia is a physiological response to excessive hypermetropia, usually between +2.00 and +7.00 D. The considerable degree of accommodation required to focus clearly on even a distant target is accompanied by a proportionate amount of convergence, which is beyond the patient's fusional divergence amplitude. It cannot therefore be controlled and a manifest convergent squint results. The magnitude of the deviation varies little (usually <10 Δ) between distance and near. The deviation typically presents at the age of 18 months to 3 years (range 6 months to 7 years).

- **Fully accommodative esotropia** is characterized by hypermetropia with esotropia when the refractive error is uncorrected (Fig. 18.55A). The deviation is eliminated and BSV is present at all distances following optical correction of hypermetropia (Fig. 18.55B). This may occasionally be seen in a baby (Fig. 18.56), which illustrates the point that irrespective of age all children with esotropia should undergo cycloplegic refraction.
- **Partially accommodative esotropia** is reduced but not eliminated by full correction of hypermetropia (Fig. 18.57). Amblyopia is frequent as well as bilateral congenital superior oblique weakness. Most cases show suppression of the squinting eye although ARC may occur, but of lower grade than in microtropia.

Non-refractive accommodative esotropia

In this type of accommodative esotropia the AC/A ratio is high so that a unit increase of accommodation is accompanied by a disproportionately large increase in convergence. This occurs independently of refractive error, although hypermetropia frequently coexists. Subtypes are set out below.

- **Convergence excess**
    - High AC/A ratio due to increased accommodative convergence (accommodation is normal, convergence is increased).
    - Normal near point of accommodation.

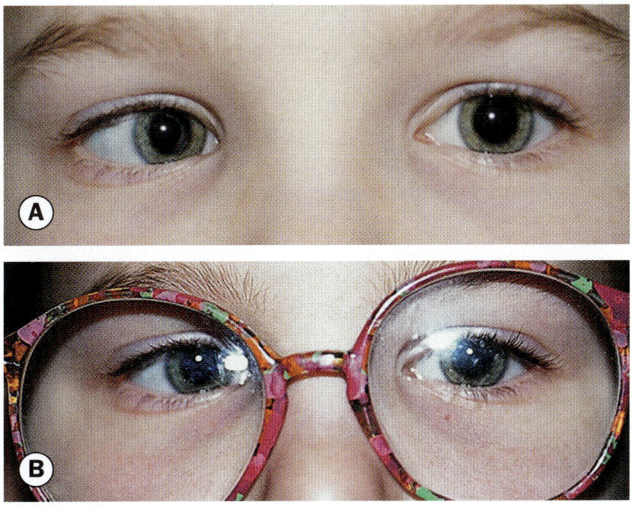

Fig. 18.57 Partially accommodative esotropia. **(A)** Right esotropia without glasses; **(B)** angle is reduced but not eliminated with glasses.

    - Straight eyes with BSV for distance (Fig. 18.58A).
    - Esotropia for near, usually with suppression (Fig. 18.58B).
    - Straight eyes through bifocals (Fig. 18.58C).
- **Hypoaccommodative convergence excess**
    - High AC/A ratio due to decreased accommodation (accommodation is weak, necessitating increased effort, which produces over-convergence).
    - Remote near point of accommodation.
    - Straight eyes with BSV for distance.
    - Esotropia for near, usually with suppression.

Treatment

- **Correction of refractive error** is the initial treatment.
    - In children under the age of 6 years, the full cycloplegic hypermetropic refraction revealed on retinoscopy should be prescribed, with a deduction only for the working

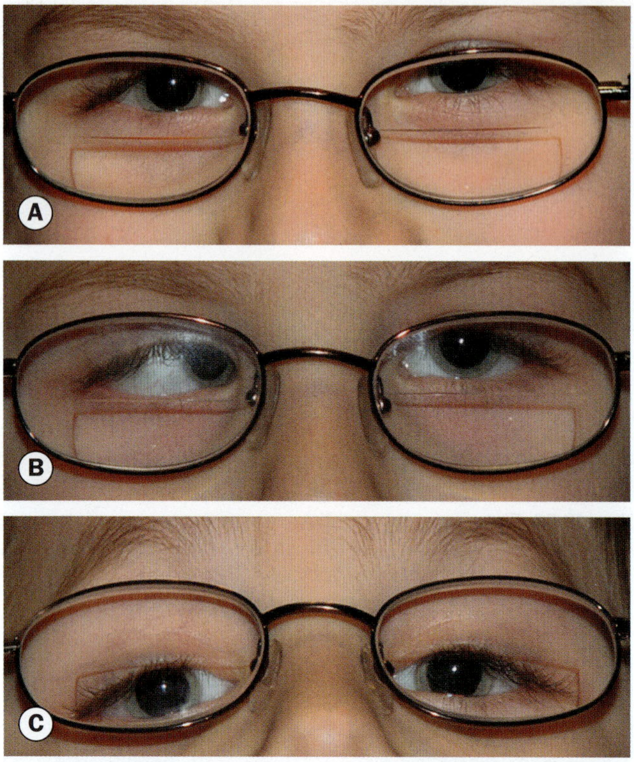

Fig. 18.58 Convergence excess esotropia. **(A)** Eyes straight for distance; **(B)** right esotropia for near; **(C)** eyes straight when looking through bifocals.

distance. In the child with fully accommodative refractive esotropia this will control the deviation for both near and distance.

  - After the age of 8 years, refraction should be performed without cycloplegia and the maximal amount of 'plus' that can be tolerated (manifest hypermetropia) prescribed.
  - For convergence excess esotropia bifocals may be prescribed to relieve accommodation (and thereby accommodative convergence), thus allowing the child to maintain bifoveal fixation and ocular alignment at near (see Fig. 18.58C). The minimum 'add' required to achieve this is prescribed.
  - The most satisfactory form of bifocals is the executive type in which the intersection crosses the lower border of the pupil. The strength of the lower segment should be gradually reduced and eliminated by the early teenage years.
  - Bifocals are also used in hypoaccommodative esotropia where the AC/A ratio is not overly excessive and there is a reasonable chance of discarding bifocal correction with time.
  - At higher levels surgery is the better long-term option. The ultimate prognosis for complete withdrawal of spectacles is related to the magnitude of the AC/A ratio and to the degree of hypermetropia and associated astigmatism. Spectacles may be needed only for close work.
- **Surgery** is aimed at restoring or improving BSV, or at improving the appearance of the squint and so the child's social functioning. It should be considered only if spectacles do not fully correct the deviation and after every attempt has been made to treat amblyopia.
  - Bilateral medial rectus recessions are performed in patients in whom the deviation for near is greater than that for distance.
  - If there is no significant difference between distance and near measurements and equal vision in both eyes, some perform unilateral medial rectus recession combined with lateral rectus resection, whereas others prefer bilateral medial rectus recessions.
  - In patients with residual amblyopia, surgery is usually performed on the amblyopic eye.
  - In partially accommodative esotropia, surgery to improve appearance is best delayed until requested by the child. This avoids early consecutive exotropia. It should aim to correct only the residual squint present with glasses.
  - The usual first procedure for convergence excess esotropia is recession of both medial rectus muscles. This relies on fusion to prevent a distance exotropia; a few patients become divergent after surgery and need a further procedure.
  - Medial rectus posterior fixation sutures (Faden operation) or fixation of the medial rectus to its surrounding pulley ('pulley fixation') can also be used either as a first procedure, or in the case of under-correction, following bimedial recessions.

Microtropia

Microtropia is a small angle (<10 Δ) squint. Binocular cooperation in microtropia is more substantial than in most manifest deviations and it may be considered more a description of binocular status than a specific diagnosis. This condition is also known as monofixation syndrome. It may be primary or secondary, the latter representing the sequela to strabismus surgery or other treatment (e.g. optical, such as fully accommodative esotropia controlled with glasses to a microtropia rather than true bifoveal BSV) for a larger deviation and occasionally to other pathology.

- Symptoms are rare unless there is an associated decompensating heterophoria.
- The small manifest angle of deviation may not be readily detectable on cover testing.
- There is a prominent association with anisometropia, commonly hypermetropia or hypermetropic astigmatism, with amblyopia (typically mild) of the more ametropic eye.
- There is normal motor fusion as demonstrated by fusional amplitudes.
- Anomalous retinal correspondence (ARC) is present, with associated abnormal BSV. The fovea of the fixating eye acquires an anomalous common visual direction with an extrafoveal location in the deviating eye. Under binocular conditions extrafoveal fixation occurs in the deviating eye with a central foveal suppression scotoma and peripheral fusion. However, when the preferred eye is covered, fixation in the deviating eye

then returns to the fovea and the eye is aligned. Stereopsis is usually present, but reduced.
- The 4 Δ prism test, discussed earlier in the chapter, is useful in assessment.

Treatment

Treatment involves correction of refractive error and occlusion for amblyopia as indicated. There is evidence that aggressive treatment sometimes leads to normalization. Most patients remain stable and symptom-free.

Other esotropias

Near esotropia (non-accommodative convergence excess)

- **Presentation** is usually in older children and young adults.
- **Signs**
  - No significant refractive error.
  - Orthophoria or small esophoria with BSV for distance.
  - Esotropia for near but normal or low AC/A ratio.
  - Normal near point of accommodation.
- **Treatment** involves bilateral medial rectus recessions.

Distance esotropia

- **Presentation** is in healthy young adults, who are often myopic.
- **Signs**
  - Intermittent or constant esotropia for distance.
  - Minimal or no deviation for near.
  - Normal bilateral abduction.
  - Fusional divergence amplitudes may be reduced.
  - Absence of neurological disease.
- **Treatment** is with prisms until spontaneous resolution or surgery in persistent cases.

Acute (late-onset) esotropia

- **Presentation** is at around 5–6 years of age.
- **Signs**
  - Sudden onset of diplopia and esotropia.
  - Normal ocular motility without significant refractive error.
  - Underlying sixth nerve palsy must be excluded.
- **Management**
  - Because the onset of comitant esotropia in an older child may indicate an underlying neurological disorder, it is important to check the pupil reflexes and exclude optic disc changes, nystagmus and a sixth nerve palsy. Neuroradiological examination may be needed.
- **Treatment** is aimed at re-establishing BSV to prevent suppression using prisms, botulinum toxin or surgery.

Secondary (sensory) esotropia

Secondary esotropia is caused by a unilateral reduction in VA that interferes with or abolishes fusion. Causes can include cataract, optic atrophy or hypoplasia, macular scarring or retinoblastoma (Fig. 18.59A and B). Fundus examination under mydriasis is therefore essential in all children with strabismus.

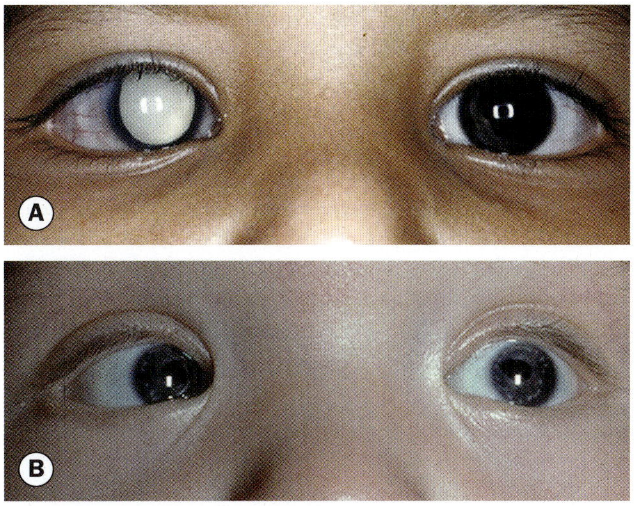

Fig. 18.59 Sensory esotropia. **(A)** Secondary to a retinoblastoma in the right eye; **(B)** secondary to microphthalmos and aphakia in Down syndrome. *(Courtesy of ADN Murray – fig. B.)*

Consecutive esotropia

Consecutive esotropia follows surgical over-correction of an exo-deviation. If it occurs following surgery for an intermittent exotropia in a child it should not be allowed to persist for more than 6 weeks without further intervention.

Sagging eye syndrome

- **Introduction.** This is one of the commonest causes of acquired strabismus in elderly non-myopic individuals and occurs in association with blepharoptosis and deepening of the superior sulcus. The condition arises as a consequence of age-related degeneration of the ligaments which interconnect the extraocular muscles. This results in bilateral inferior sagging of the lateral rectus pulley, causing esotropia and/or cyclovertical malalignment.
- **Symptoms.** Initially the individual notices intermittent binocular diplopia in the distance, which becomes permanent over a period of several months. The distance deviation is rarely more than 10 Δ.
- **Signs**
  - Distance esotropia, with no near esotropia.
  - Full horizontal ductions and clinically normal horizontal saccadic eye velocities.
  - Limited supraduction of both eyes.
  - Blepharoptosis.
  - Deep superior sulcus.
  - If downward displacement of the lateral rectus pulley is asymmetrical, unilateral hypotropia with excyclotropia results (see: Cyclovertical strabismus).
- **Treatment.** Most patients can be treated conservatively by using a prism incorporated in distance spectacles, as they do not have diplopia when undertaking near tasks. If surgery is needed, resection or plication of the lateral rectus or recession of the medial rectus can be considered.

High myopia esotropia ('heavy eye syndrome')

- **Introduction.** This is a cause of acquired esotropia in adults secondary to high myopia (average: −18 D; range −12 D to −21 D and axial length 27–35 mm). The condition occurs as a consequence of shifting of the lateral rectus and superior rectus muscles secondary to an elongated posterior portion of a highly myopic eyeball. Imaging consistently demonstrates inferior shift of the lateral rectus and nasal shift of the inferior and superior recti causing the eye to shift supero-temporally from the pulley array, converting the lateral rectus from abductor to infraductor.

- **Symptoms.** Patients present with diplopia associated with limitation of abduction and elevation.
- **Treatment.** Surgery involves loop myopexy, uniting adjacent borders of the lateral rectus and superior rectus with non-absorbable sutures. This condition responds poorly to lateral rectus tightening or medial rectus recession alone.

Cyclic esotropia

Cyclic esotropia is a very rare condition characterized by alternating manifest esotropia with suppression and BSV, each typically lasting 24 hours. The condition may persist for months or years and the patient may eventually develop a constant esotropia requiring surgery.

EXOTROPIA

Constant (early-onset) exotropia

- **Presentation** is often at birth.
- **Signs**
  - Normal refraction.
  - Large and constant angle.
  - DVD may be present.
- **Neurological anomalies** are frequently present, in contrast with infantile esotropia.
- **Treatment** is mainly surgical and consists of lateral rectus recession and medial rectus resection.
- **Differential diagnosis** is secondary exotropia, which may conceal serious ocular pathology.

Intermittent exotropia

Diagnosis

- **Presentation** is often at around 2 years with exophoria, which breaks down to exotropia under conditions of visual inattention, bright light (resulting in reflex closure of the affected eye), fatigue or ill health.
- **Signs.** The eyes are straight with BSV at times (Fig. 18.60A) and manifest with suppression at other times (Fig. 18.60B). Control of the squint varies with the distance of fixation and other factors such as concentration.

TIP Children with intermittent exotropia tend to close an eye when exposed to bright light.

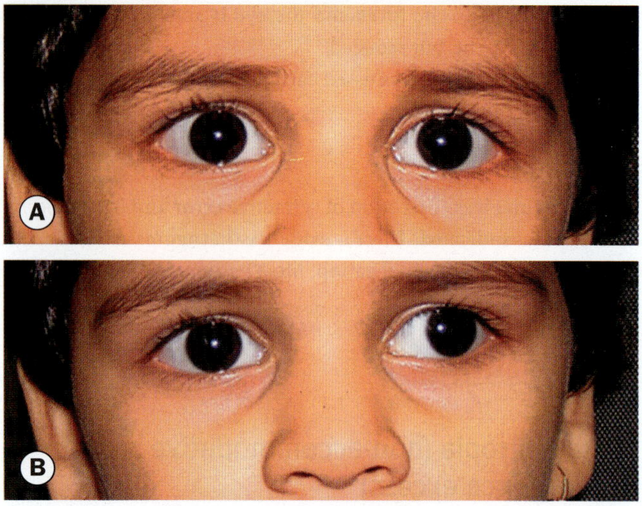

Fig. 18.60 Intermittent exotropia. **(A)** Eyes straight most of the time; **(B)** left exotropia under conditions of visual inattention or fatigue. *(Courtesy of M Parulekar.)*

Classification

- **Distance excess** exotropia, in which the angle of deviation is greater for distance than near and increases further beyond 6 metres. Simulated and true forms are recognized.
  - Simulated (formerly pseudo-divergence excess) is associated with a high AC/A ratio or with 'tenacious proximal fusion' (TPF – tonic fusional convergence that relaxes after occlusion). The distance angle initially seems to be larger than the near angle, but the deviation for near and distance is similar when the near angle is remeasured with the patient looking through +3.00 D lenses (high AC/A controlling exodeviation) or after 30–60 minutes of uniocular occlusion to relax TPF, the latter with a normal AC/A ratio).
  - True. The angle for near remains significantly less than that for distance with the above tests.
- **Basic** exotropia, in which control of the squint and the angle of deviation are the same for distance and near fixation.
- **Convergence insufficiency** exotropia, in which the deviation is greater for near fixation. It tends to occur in older children and adults and may be associated with acquired myopia or presbyopia.

Treatment

- **Spectacle correction** in myopic patients may, in some cases, control the deviation by stimulating accommodation and with it, convergence. In some cases, over-minus prescription may be useful.
- **Part-time occlusion** of the non-deviating eye may improve control in some patients and orthoptic exercises may be helpful for near exotropia.
- **Surgery.** Patients with effective and stable control of their intermittent exotropia are often just observed. Surgery is indicated if control is poor or is progressively deteriorating. Unilateral lateral rectus recession and medial rectus resection

are generally preferred except in true distance exotropia when bilateral lateral rectus recessions are more usual. Similar results are achieved with either approach. The exodeviation is rarely completely eliminated by surgery.

Sensory exotropia

Secondary (sensory) exotropia is the result of monocular or binocular visual impairment by acquired lesions, such as cataract, corneal scarring (Fig. 18.61A and B) or other media opacity. Treatment consists of correction of the visual deficit, if possible, followed by surgery if appropriate. A minority of patients develop intractable diplopia due to loss of fusion, even when good VA is restored to both eyes and the eyes are realigned.

Consecutive exotropia

Consecutive exotropia develops spontaneously in an amblyopic eye, or more frequently following surgical correction of an esodeviation. Postoperative divergence occurring hours to months after initial alignment is usually due to muscle slippage (see Fig. 18.75). If it occurs years later, it is usually due to a stretched scar. Most cases present in adult life with psychosocial concerns and can be greatly helped by surgery. Careful evaluation of the risk of postoperative diplopia is required, although serious problems are uncommon. About 75% of patients are still well aligned 10 years after surgery, although re-divergence may occur.

Congenital cranial dysinnervation disorders

Congenital cranial dysinnervation disorders (CCDD) or congenital innervation dysgenesis syndromes constitute a group of disorders originally believed to be the result of congenital muscular fibrosis, but now known to be the result of brainstem or cranial nerve developmental disturbance, in most cases having an identifiable genetic basis. Systemic associations are recognized for several.

Duane retraction syndrome

In Duane retraction syndrome (DRS) there is failure of innervation of the lateral rectus by a hypoplastic sixth nerve nucleus, with anomalous innervation of the lateral rectus by fibres from the third nerve. The condition is often bilateral. Up to half of patients have associated systemic defects such as deafness, external ear abnormalities, speech disorder and skeletal abnormalities. Associated mutations in several genes have been found. Approximately 10% of cases are familial.

Clinical features

- **A face turn** is typical and confers BSV with the face in the turned position, thus avoiding amblyopia.
- **Complete or partial restriction of abduction.**
- **Restricted adduction**, usually partial.

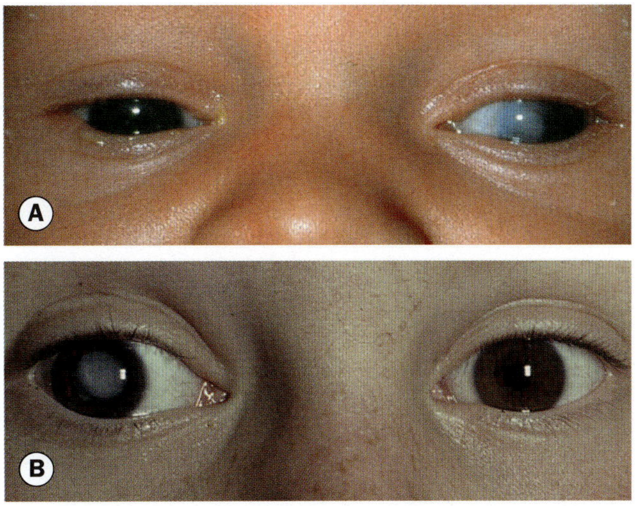

Fig. 18.61 Sensory exotropia. (A) Secondary to corneal opacity; (B) secondary to a dense cataract.

- **Retraction of the globe on adduction** as a result of co-contraction of the medial and lateral recti with resultant narrowing of the palpebral fissure.
- **An up-shoot or down-shoot in adduction** may be present. In some cases this is produced by a tight lateral rectus muscle slipping over or under the globe to produce an anomalous vertical movement.
- **Deficiency of convergence** in which the affected eye remains fixed in the primary position while the unaffected eye is converging.

TIP A face turn, which is commonly found in Duane retraction syndrome, confers binocular single vision with the face in the turned position.

Classification (Huber)

- **Type I**, the most common, is characterized by (Fig. 18.62):
  - Limited or absent abduction.
  - Normal or mildly limited adduction.
  - In the primary position, straight or slight esotropia.
- **Type II**, the least common, is characterized by (Fig. 18.63):
  - Limited adduction.
  - Normal or mildly limited abduction.
  - In primary position, straight or slight exotropia.
- **Type III** is characterized by:
  - Limited adduction and abduction.
  - In the primary position, straight or slight esotropia.
  - In some cases, phenotypic variants have been allied to differing genotypes.

Treatment

The majority of patients with Duane syndrome do not need any surgical intervention.

- Most young children maintain BSV by using a CHP to compensate for their lateral rectus weakness and surgery is needed

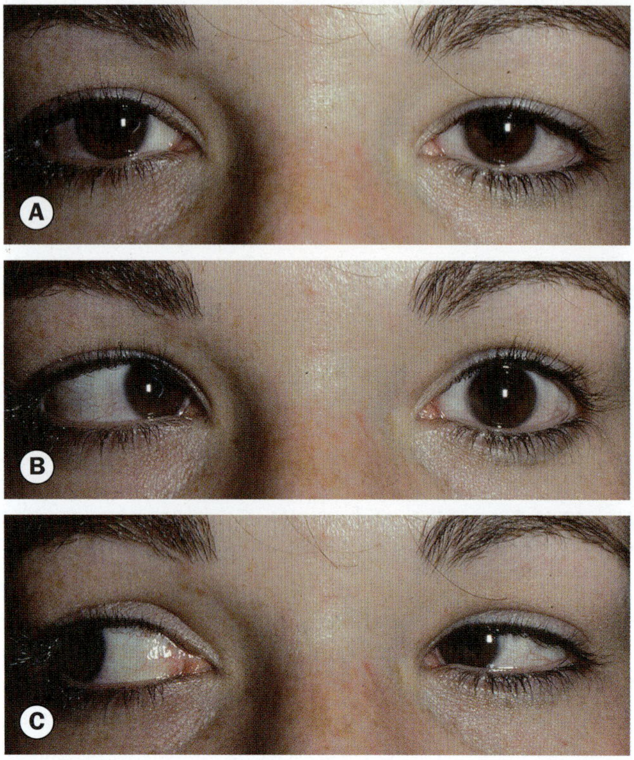

Fig. 18.62 Duane syndrome – Huber type I ('eso'). **(A)** Straight eyes in the primary position; **(B)** extremely limited left abduction; **(C)** narrowing of the left palpebral fissure on adduction. *(Courtesy of ADN Murray.)*

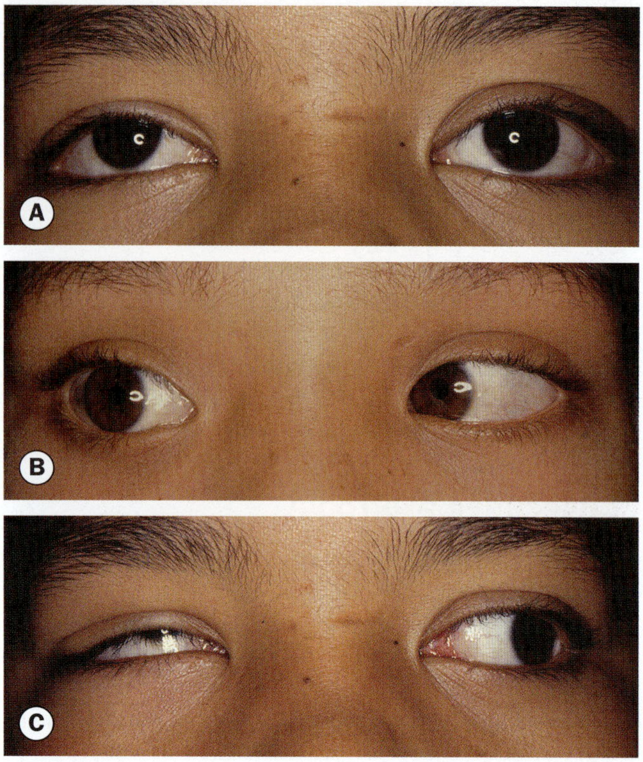

Fig. 18.63 Duane syndrome type II ('exo'). **(A)** Slight exotropia in the primary position; **(B)** limitation of right abduction with widening of the right palpebral fissure; **(C)** grossly limited right adduction with narrowing of the palpebral fissure. *(Courtesy of ADN Murray.)*

only if there is evidence of loss of binocular function. This may be indicated by failure to continue to use a CHP.

- In adults or children over the age of about 8 years surgery can reduce a head posture that is psychosocially unacceptable or causing neck discomfort. Surgery may also be necessary for cosmetically unacceptable up-shoots, down-shoots or severe globe retraction.
- Amblyopia, when present, is usually the result of anisometropia rather than strabismus.
- Depending on the clinical features, unilateral or bilateral medial rectus and/or lateral rectus recession are the procedures of choice. In order to improve abduction, transposition of the superior and inferior rectus muscles (or just the superior rectus muscle) to the lateral rectus muscle may be required.
- The lateral rectus of the involved side should not be resected, as this increases retraction.

Möbius syndrome

Möbius syndrome is a rare, usually sporadic, condition, the basic components of which are congenital non-progressive bilateral sixth and seventh cranial nerve palsies that are believed to relate to a developmental abnormality of the brainstem.

- **Systemic features**
  - Bilateral facial palsy, which is usually asymmetrical and often incomplete, giving rise to an expressionless facial appearance and problems with eyelid closure (Fig. 18.64A).
  - The fifth, eighth, tenth and twelfth (Fig. 18.64B) cranial nerves may also be affected.
  - Limb anomalies and mild mental handicap may be present.
- **Ocular features**
  - Bilateral sixth nerve palsy.
  - Horizontal gaze palsy (50%).
  - Occasionally, third and fourth nerve palsy and ptosis.

Congenital fibrosis of the extraocular muscles

Congenital fibrosis of the extraocular muscles (CFEOM) is a rare non-progressive, usually autosomal dominant, disorder characterized by bilateral ptosis and restrictive external ophthalmoplegia. Numerous forms have been identified, of which CFEOM1 is the most common and there is considerable genetic heterogeneity. CFEOM1 is caused by mutations in the *KIF21A* gene, which produces a protein used for intracellular transport that plays a key role in some aspects of cranial nerve development and pathologically there is a hypoplastic superior division of the oculomotor nerve. Typically, vertical movements are severely restricted with inability to elevate the eyes above the horizontal plane.

In the primary position each eye is fixed below the horizontal by about 10°, with a corresponding compensatory chin elevation. The degree of residual horizontal movement varies markedly. Ptosis is common (Fig. 18.65).

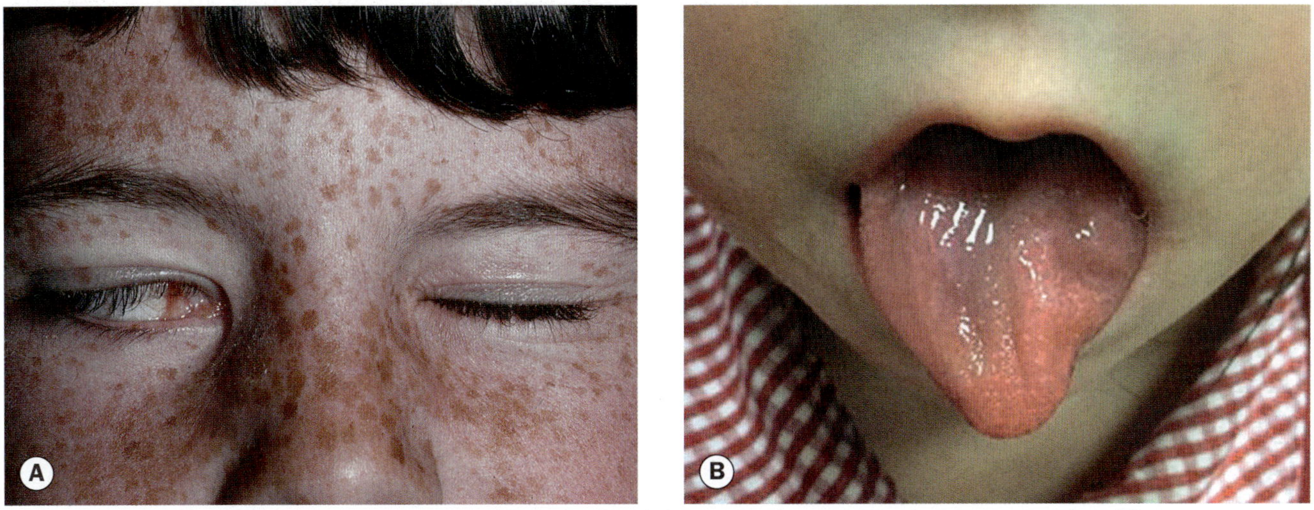

Fig. 18.64 Möbius syndrome. **(A)** Defective lid closure due to right facial nerve palsy; **(B)** atrophic tongue with fasciculations due to hypoglossal nerve palsy in a different child. *(Courtesy of D Hildebrand – fig. B.)*

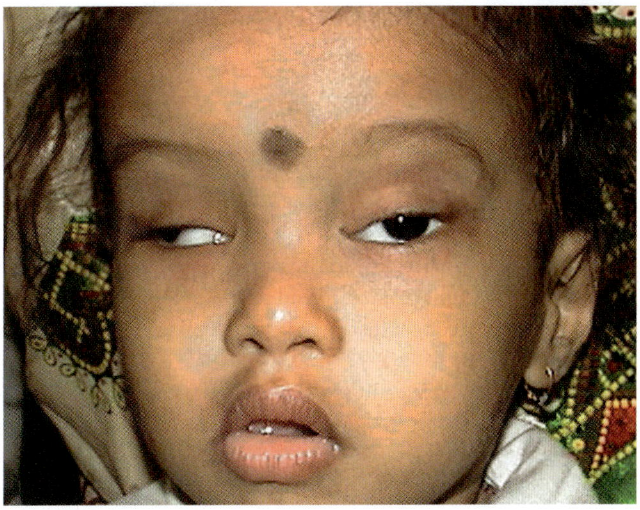

Fig. 18.65 Congenital fibrosis of the extraocular muscles – bilateral ptosis and divergent strabismus. *(Courtesy of M Parulekar.)*

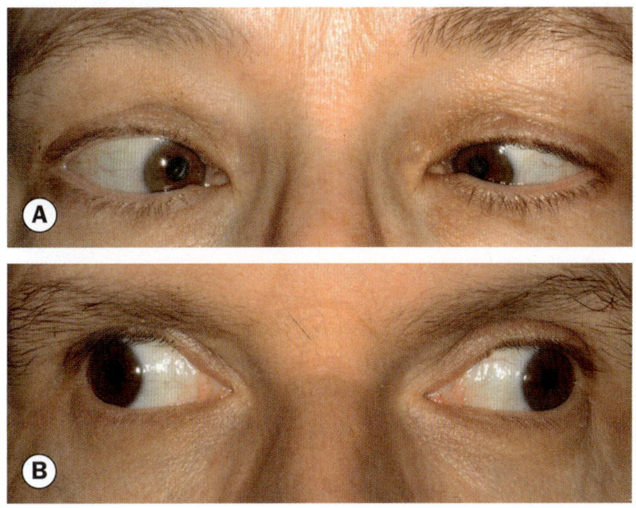

Fig. 18.66 Strabismus fixus. **(A)** Convergent; **(B)** divergent.

Strabismus fixus

Strabismus fixus is a rare condition in which both eyes are fixed by fibrous tightening of the medial recti (convergent strabismus fixus – Fig. 18.66A), or the lateral recti (divergent strabismus fixus – Fig. 18.66B). Congenital and acquired forms have been described.

Other CCDD syndromes with ophthalmic features

Marcus Gunn jaw-winking syndrome (see Ch. 2) is now believed to be a CCDD, as are horizontal gaze palsy and progressive scoliosis, many cases of congenital ptosis, congenital fourth cranial nerve palsy and congenital facial nerve palsy.

MONOCULAR ELEVATION DEFICIENCY

Monocular elevation deficiency (MED), formerly double elevator palsy, is a rare sporadic condition that in at least some cases may be categorized as a CCDD. It is thought to manifest primarily with a tight or contracted inferior rectus muscle or a hypoplastic or ineffective superior rectus muscle. There is a profound inability to elevate one eye across the horizontal plane, from abduction to adduction (Fig. 18.67), with orthophoria in the primary position in about one-third of cases. Chin elevation may be present. A base-up prism can be helpful.

BROWN SYNDROME

Brown syndrome is a condition involving mechanical restriction, typically of the superior oblique tendon. It is usually congenital but occasionally acquired. Recent evidence strongly suggests that at least some congenital cases should be categorized as a CCDD.

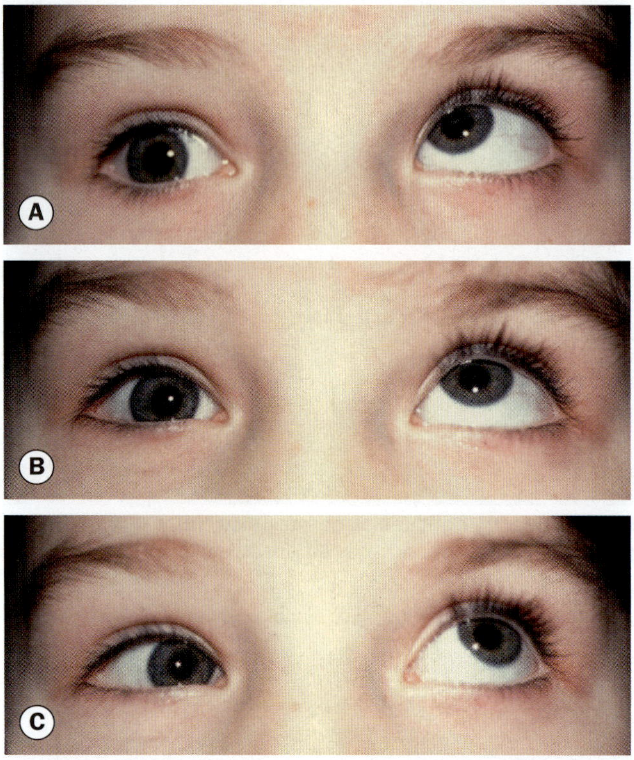

Fig. 18.67 Right monocular elevation deficiency. **(A)** Defective elevation in abduction; **(B)** in upgaze; and **(C)** in adduction.

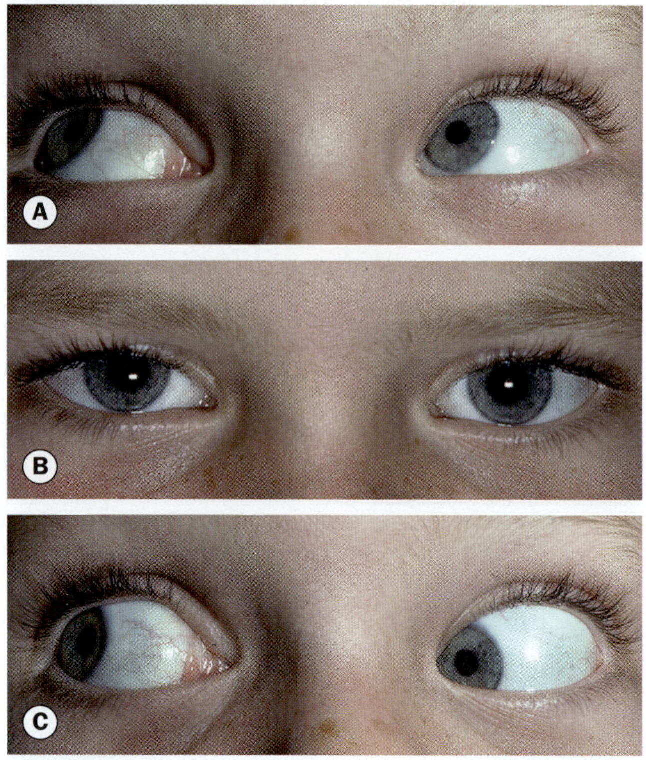

Fig. 18.68 Left Brown syndrome. **(A)** Limited left elevation in adduction; **(B)** straight in the primary position; **(C)** down-shoot in adduction. *(Courtesy of ADN Murray.)*

Classification

- **Congenital**
  - Idiopathic.
  - 'Congenital click syndrome', where there is impaired movement of the superior oblique tendon through the trochlea.
- **Acquired**
- Trauma to the trochlea or superior oblique tendon.
- Inflammation of the tendon, which may be caused by rheumatoid arthritis, pansinusitis or scleritis.

Types

All have limited elevation in adduction (Fig. 18.68A).

- **Mild**
  - No hypotropia in primary position.
  - No down-shoot in adduction.
- **Moderate**
  - No hypotropia in the primary position (Fig. 18.68B).
  - Down-shoot in adduction (Fig. 18.68C).
- **Severe**
  - Hypotropia in the primary position.
  - Down-shoot in adduction.
  - Chin-up head posture.
  - Face-turn away from the affected eye.

Treatment

- **Congenital** cases do not usually require treatment as long as binocular function is maintained with an acceptable head posture. Spontaneous improvement is often seen towards the end of the first decade. Indications for treatment include significant primary position hypotropia, deteriorating control and/or an unacceptable head posture. The recommended procedure for congenital cases is lengthening of the superior oblique tendon.
- **Acquired;** treatable aetiology should be addressed specifically. Depending on the cause, acquired cases may benefit from steroids, either orally or by injection near the trochlea.

TIP Congenital Brown syndrome does not usually require treatment as long as binocular function is maintained with an acceptable head posture.

ALPHABET PATTERNS

'V' or 'A' patterns occur when the relative contributions of the superior rectus and inferior oblique to elevation, or of the inferior rectus and superior oblique to depression, are abnormal, resulting in derangement of the balance of their horizontal vectors in up- and downgaze. They can also be caused by anomalies in the position of the rectus muscle pulleys. Assessment is by measuring horizontal deviations in the primary position, upgaze and downgaze. They can occur in both concomitant and incomitant deviations.

'V' pattern

A 'V' pattern (Fig. 18.69) is said to be significant when the difference between upgaze and downgaze is ≥15 Δ.

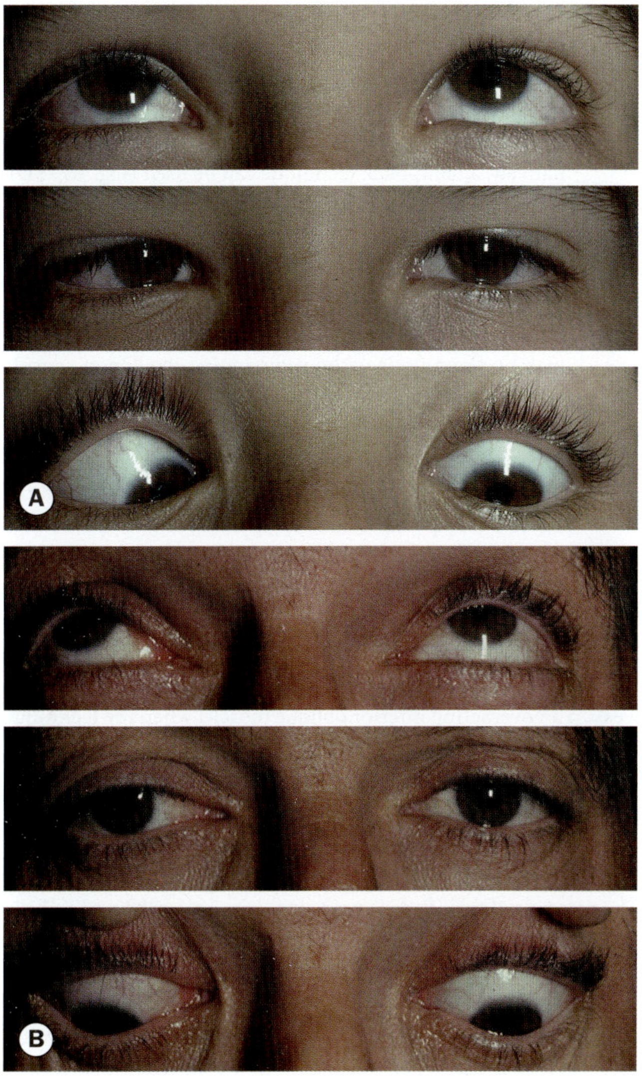

Fig. 18.69 'V' pattern. **(A)** Esotropia; **(B)** exotropia.

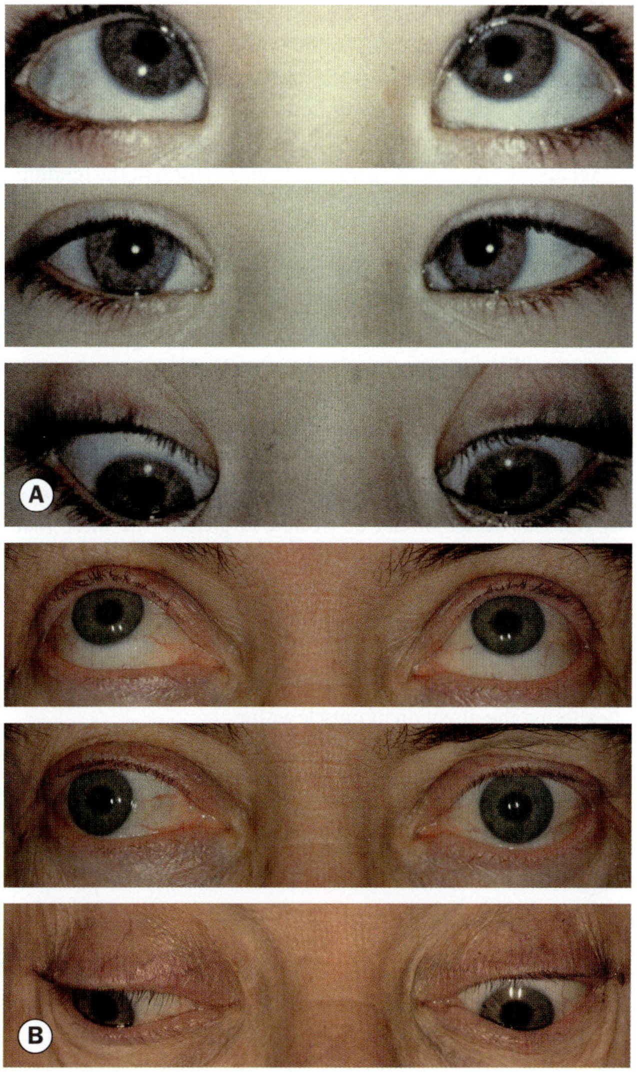

Fig. 18.70 'A' pattern. **(A)** Esotropia; **(B)** exotropia.

Causes

- Inferior oblique overaction associated with fourth nerve palsy.
- Superior oblique underaction with subsequent inferior oblique overaction, seen in infantile esotropia as well as other childhood esotropias. The eyes are often straight in upgaze with a marked esodeviation in downgaze.
- Superior rectus underaction.
- Brown syndrome.
- Craniofacial anomalies featuring shallow orbits and downslanting palpebral fissures.

Treatment

Treatment is by inferior oblique weakening or superior oblique strengthening when oblique dysfunction is present. Without oblique muscle dysfunction, treatment is as follows:

- **'V' pattern esotropia** (Fig. 18.69A) can be treated by bilateral medial rectus recessions and downward transposition of the tendons.
- **'V' pattern exotropia** (Fig. 18.69B) can be treated by bilateral lateral rectus recessions and upward transposition of the tendons.

'A' pattern

An 'A' pattern (Fig. 18.70) is considered significant if the difference between upgaze and downgaze is ≥10 Δ. A particular complaint may be difficulty with reading if the patient is binocular.

Causes

- Primary superior oblique overaction is usually associated with exodeviation in the primary position of gaze.
- Inferior oblique underaction/palsy with subsequent superior oblique overaction.
- Inferior rectus underaction.

Treatment

Patients with oblique dysfunction are treated by superior oblique posterior tenotomy, which will correct 20 Δ of 'A' pattern. Total tenotomy will correct up to 50 Δ of 'A' pattern. Treatment of cases without oblique muscle dysfunction is as follows:

- **'A' pattern esotropia** (Fig. 18.70A) is treated by bilateral medial rectus recessions and upward transposition of the tendons.
- **'A' pattern exotropia** (Fig. 18.70B) is treated by bilateral lateral rectus recessions and downward transposition of the tendons.

SURGERY

The most common aims of surgery on the extraocular muscles are to correct misalignment to improve appearance and, if possible, to restore BSV. Surgery can also be used to reduce an abnormal head posture and to expand or centralize a field of BSV. However, the first step in the management of childhood strabismus involves correction of any significant refractive error and/or treatment of amblyopia. Once maximal visual potential is reached in both eyes, any residual deviation can be treated surgically. The three main types of procedure are:

- **Strengthening**, to enhance the pull of a muscle.
- **Weakening** to decrease the effective strength of action of a muscle.
- **Vector adjustment** procedures that have the primary aim of altering the direction of muscle action.

> **TIP** Before surgical realignment is undertaken any significant refractive error and/or underlying amblyopia must be corrected.

Strengthening procedures

- **Resection** shortens a muscle to enhance its effective pull. It is suitable only for a rectus muscle and involves the following steps:
  - The muscle is exposed and two absorbable sutures inserted at a measured distance behind its insertion (Fig. 18.71A–E).
  - The muscle anterior to the sutures is excised (Fig. 18.71F–H) and the cut end reattached to the original insertion.
- **Plication (tucking)** has a similar effect to resection, but has the advantage that it is less traumatic, does not sacrifice the anterior ciliary vessels and can be easily reversed if needed. It can be used to enhance the action of the rectus muscles and is today frequently preferred to a resection. It can also be used to tighten a lax superior oblique muscle in congenital fourth nerve palsy (Fig. 18.72).
- **Advancement** of the muscle nearer to the limbus can be used to enhance the action of a previously recessed rectus muscle.

Weakening procedures

Recession

Recession slackens a muscle by moving it away from its insertion.

- **Rectus muscle recession**
  - The muscle is exposed and two absorbable sutures are tied through the outer quarters of the tendon (Fig. 18.73A and B).
  - The tendon is disinserted from the sclera and the amount of recession is measured and marked on the sclera with calipers (Fig. 18.73C).
  - The detached end of the muscle is sutured to the sclera at the measured distance behind its original insertion. Alternatively, a hang-back technique can be used (Fig. 18.73D).
- **Inferior oblique recession**
  - The muscle belly is exposed through an inferotemporal fornix incision.
  - A squint hook is passed behind the posterior border of the muscle, which must be clearly visualized. Care is taken to pick up the muscle without disrupting the Tenon capsule and fat posterior to it.
  - An absorbable suture is passed through the anterior border of the muscle at its insertion and tied.
  - The muscle is disinserted, and the cut end sutured to the sclera 3 mm posterior and temporal to the temporal edge of the inferior rectus insertion.

Disinsertion

Disinsertion (or myectomy) involves detaching a muscle from its insertion without reattachment. It is most commonly used to weaken an overacting inferior oblique muscle, when the technique is the same as for a recession except that the muscle is not sutured. Very occasionally, disinsertion is performed on a severely contracted rectus muscle.

Posterior fixation suture

The principle of this (Faden) procedure is to suture the muscle belly to the sclera posteriorly so as to decrease the pull of the muscle in its field of action without affecting the eye in the primary position. The Faden procedure may be used on the medial rectus to reduce convergence in a convergence excess esotropia and on the superior rectus to treat DVD. When treating DVD, the superior rectus muscle may also be recessed. The belly of the muscle is then anchored to the sclera with a non-absorbable suture about 12 mm behind its insertion. Alternatively, instead of a posterior fixation suture the muscle belly can be sutured posteriorly to its pulley ('pulley fixation'), which has the same effect and avoids placement of the suture into the sclera.

Transposition

Transposition refers to the relocation of one or more extraocular muscles to substitute for the action of an absent or severely deficient muscle. The most common indication is severe lateral rectus weakness due to acquired sixth cranial nerve palsy (see Fig. 19.79). Other applications include CCDD (e.g. Duane syndrome), alphabet patterns and monocular elevation deficit. A variety of techniques involving recti and oblique muscles have been described.

Adjustable sutures

Indications

The results of strabismus surgery can be improved by the use of adjustable suture techniques on the rectus muscles. While

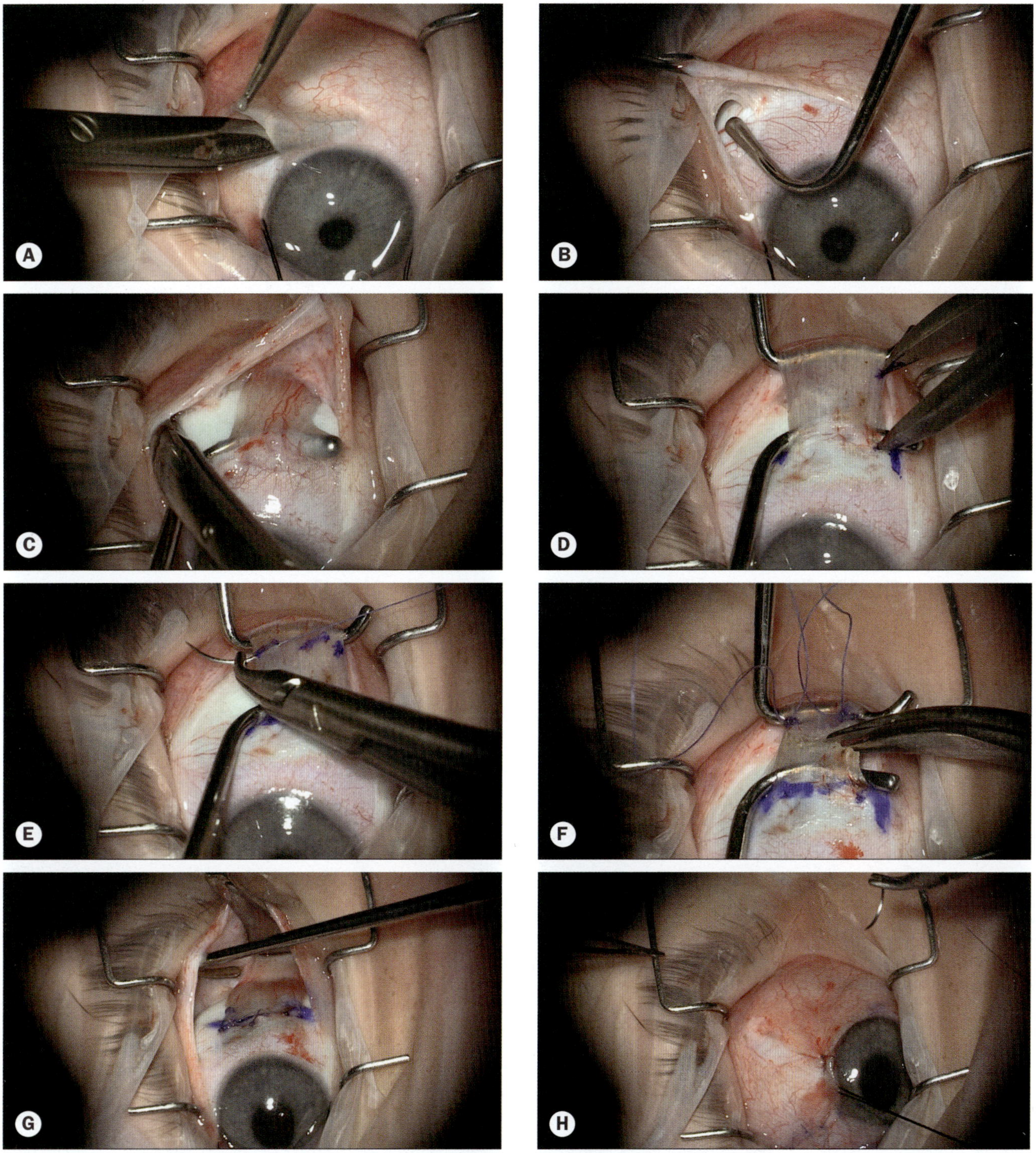

Fig. 18.71 Resection of a horizontal rectus muscle. **(A)** Conjunctival incision with traction sutures to expose the operation site; **(B)** insertion of squint hook; **(C)** isolation of the muscle; **(D)** calipers set to the desired amount of resection; **(E)** muscle marked and initial 6-0 vicryl suture inserted; **(F)** muscle crushed, cauterized and then cut anterior to the sutures; **(G)** sutured muscle in position; **(H)** conjunctival closure. *(Courtesy of D Hildebrand.)*

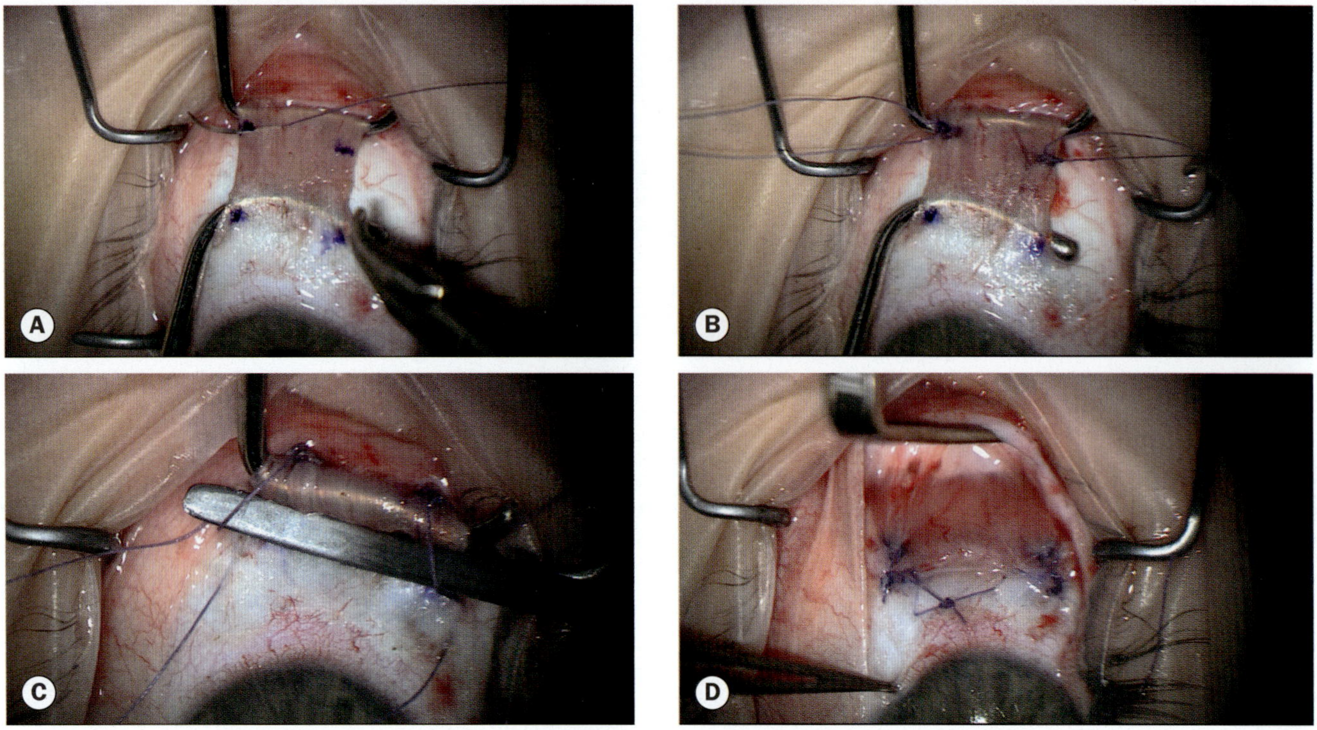

Fig. 18.72 Plication of medial rectus. **(A)** Muscle isolated and marked; **(B)** sutures inserted; **(C)** muscle folded over a fine repositor; **(D)** sutures in position. *(Courtesy of D Hildebrand.)*

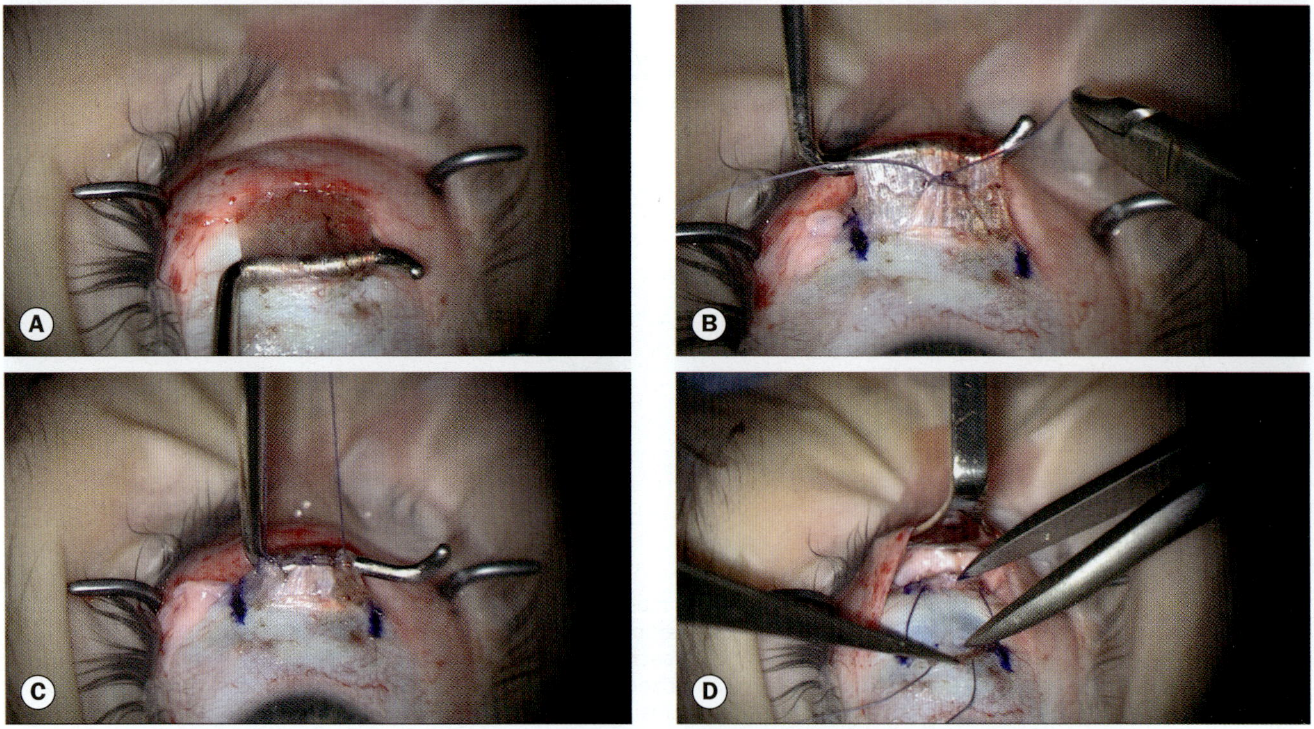

Fig. 18.73 Recession of a horizontal rectus muscle. **(A)** The muscle is exposed then hooked and stretched with a Chavasse squint hook; **(B)** a single double-armed suture is placed with a central knot; and **(C)** locked at the upper and lower borders; **(D)** the tendon is disinserted from the sclera and the amount of recession is measured and marked on the sclera with calipers. The detached end of the muscle is sutured to the sclera at the measured distance behind its original insertion. Alternatively, a hang back technique can be used. *(Courtesy of D Hildebrand.)*

many ophthalmologists use this technique in all adults, adjustable sutures are particularly indicated when a precise outcome is essential and when the results with more conventional procedures are likely to be unpredictable. Examples include: (a) restrictive strabismus (thyroid myopathy, blow-out fracture of the floor of the orbit), (b) previous trauma or surgery, (c) slipped or lost muscles, (d) incomitant deviations (Duane syndrome, Möbius syndrome, myasthenia gravis or paralytic strabismus), (e) combined horizontal, vertical and torsional strabismus. The surgery can be done on any patient who can cooperate. Some older children will tolerate postoperative adjustment under topical anaesthesia. If not, an option is to keep the child nil by mouth in the recovery room and re-anaesthetize the child if necessary to undertake the adjustment.

Operative procedure

- The muscle is exposed, sutures inserted and the tendon disinserted from the sclera as for a rectus muscle recession.
- The two ends of the suture are passed, side by side, through the stump of the insertion.
- A second suture is knotted and tied tightly around the muscle suture anterior to its emergence from the stump: noose knot (Fig. 18.74A).
- One end of the suture is cut short and the two ends tied together to form a loop (Fig. 18.74B).
- The conjunctiva is left open.

Postoperative adjustment

This is performed under topical anaesthesia, usually a few hours after surgery when the patient is fully awake.

- The accuracy of alignment is assessed.
- If ocular alignment is satisfactory, the muscle suture is tied off and its long ends cut short.
- If more recession is required, the noose knot is pulled anteriorly along the muscle suture, thereby providing additional slack to the recessed muscle and enabling it to move posteriorly when the patient is asked to look towards the field of action of the recessed muscle (Fig. 18.74C).
- If less recession is required, the muscle suture is pulled anteriorly and the knot tightened against the muscle stump (Fig. 18.74D).

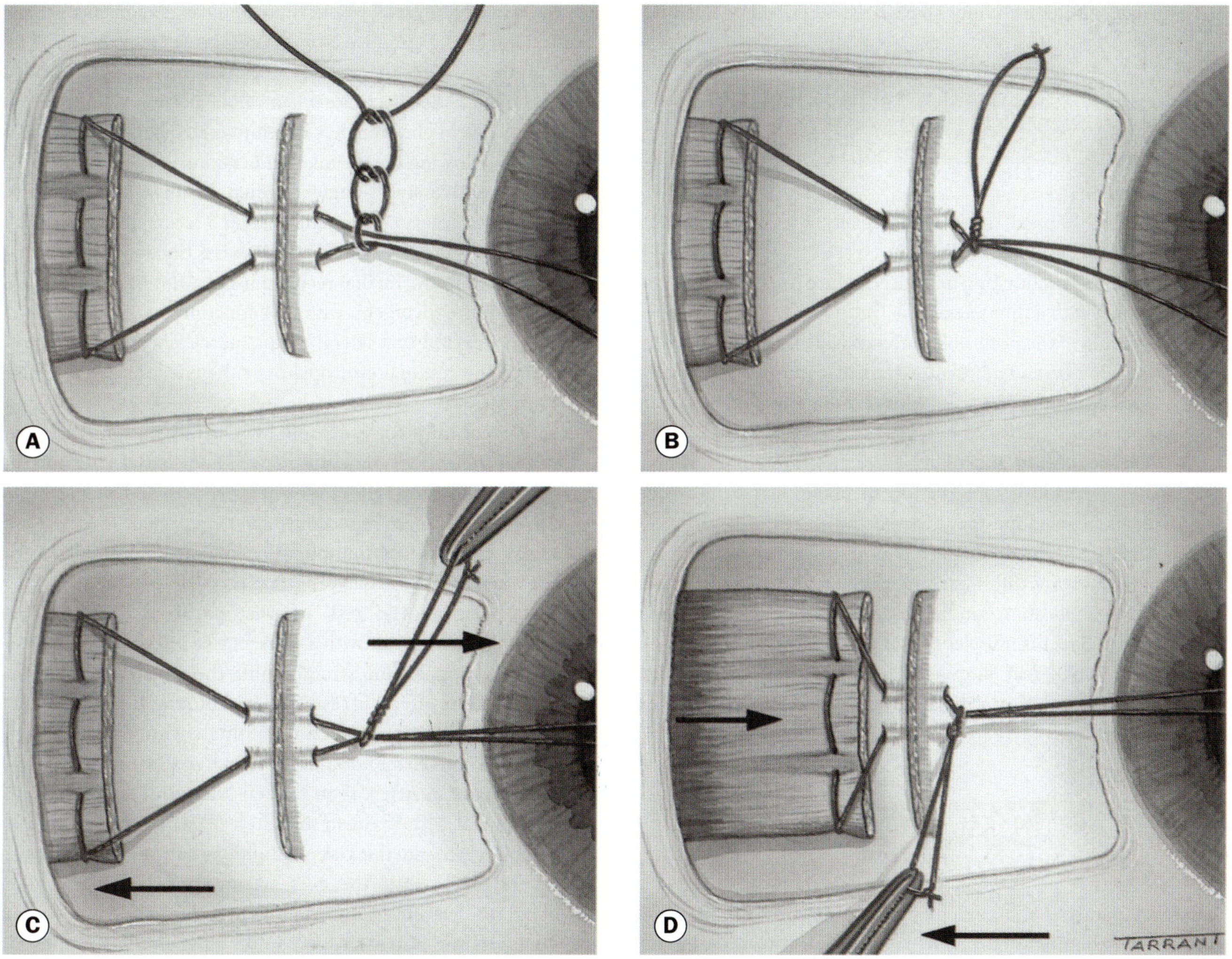

Fig. 18.74 Adjustable sutures (see text).

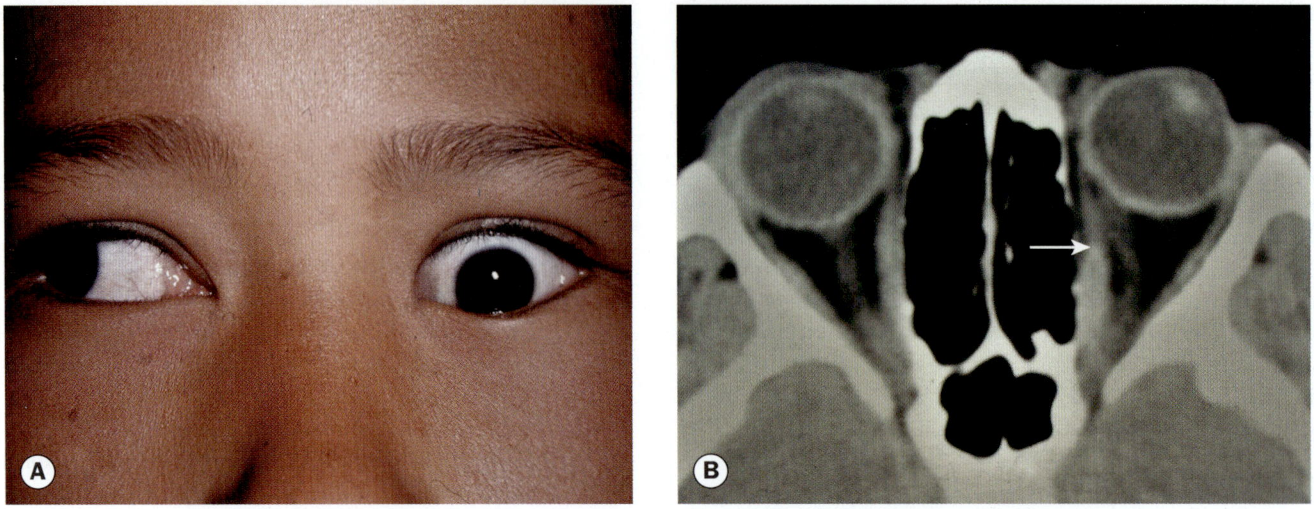

Fig. 18.75 Slipped left medial rectus muscle after surgery. **(A)** Clinical appearance on gaze to the right showing a large-angle exotropia with reduced adduction of the left eye; **(B)** axial CT scan showing the retracted muscle within the muscle sheath (arrow). *(Courtesy of ADN Murray.)*

- Once alignment is satisfactory, the main knot is secured, the sliding loop removed and the conjunctiva closed.
- A variety of other techniques have been described.

COMPLICATIONS OF STRABISMUS SURGERY

- **Operative**
  - Lost or 'slipped' muscle (especially the medial rectus muscle) (Fig. 18.75).
  - Globe perforation by a misplaced suture (especially in high myopia with a thin sclera).
  - Opening of the posterior Tenon capsule leading to fibrosis involving fat and adjacent extraocular muscles (especially when operating on the inferior oblique muscle).
- **Postoperative**
  - Over-correction and under-correction are common and after a period of observation to obtain stable measurements, reoperation may be needed.
  - Anterior segment ischaemia is more likely to occur in older patients with systemic vascular disease, but is rare. This complication can be avoided by not removing more than two rectus muscles of one eye at one time.
  - A stretched scar may occur years after initial surgery and can result in a malalignment that requires further surgery.

BOTULINUM TOXIN CHEMODENERVATION

Temporary paralysis of an extraocular muscle can be induced by an injection of botulinum toxin (BT) under topical anaesthesia and electromyographic (EMG) control. The effect takes several days to develop, is usually maximal at 1–2 weeks following injection and has generally worn off by 3 months. An extraocular muscle lengthens while it is paralyzed by botulinum and its antagonist contracts. These changes may produce long-term improvements in the alignment of the eyes. Results are best when there is fusion to stabilize the alignment. Side effects are uncommon, although about 16% of adults and 25% of children may develop some degree of temporary ptosis. The following are the main indications:

- **Postoperative small-angle residual strabismus** (2–8 weeks following surgery). For example, after a recession for esotropia that has resulted in a small under-correction, an injection can be given into the medial rectus muscle. After the injection the eye becomes divergent, with no adduction for 3 months. During this period that lateral rectus muscle shortens enough to reduce the residual esotropia once the effect of the toxin has worn off.
- **To correct infantile esotropia** by injecting both medial recti, so that the eyes become divergent. The lateral rectus muscles shorten and the angle of esotropia reduces and may even be corrected. If not, the procedure can be repeated.
- **Active thyroid ophthalmopathy**, inflamed or prephthisical eye when surgery is inappropriate.
- **To determine the risk of postoperative diplopia.** For example, in an adult with a consecutive left divergent squint and left suppression, straightening the eyes may make suppression less effective resulting in diplopia. If postoperative diplopia testing by correcting the angle with prisms is negative, then the risk of double vision after surgery is very low. If testing is positive, then the left lateral rectus muscle can be injected with toxin so that the eyes will either straighten or converge and the risk of diplopia can be assessed over several days while the eyes are straight. If diplopia does occur, the patient is able to judge whether it is troublesome.
- **To assess the potential for BSV** in a patient with a constant manifest squint by straightening the eyes temporarily. The

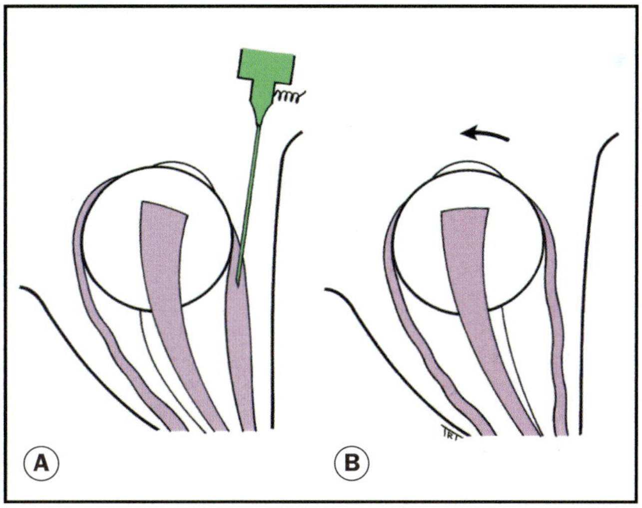

Fig. 18.76 Principles of botulinum toxin chemodenervation in left sixth nerve palsy (see text).

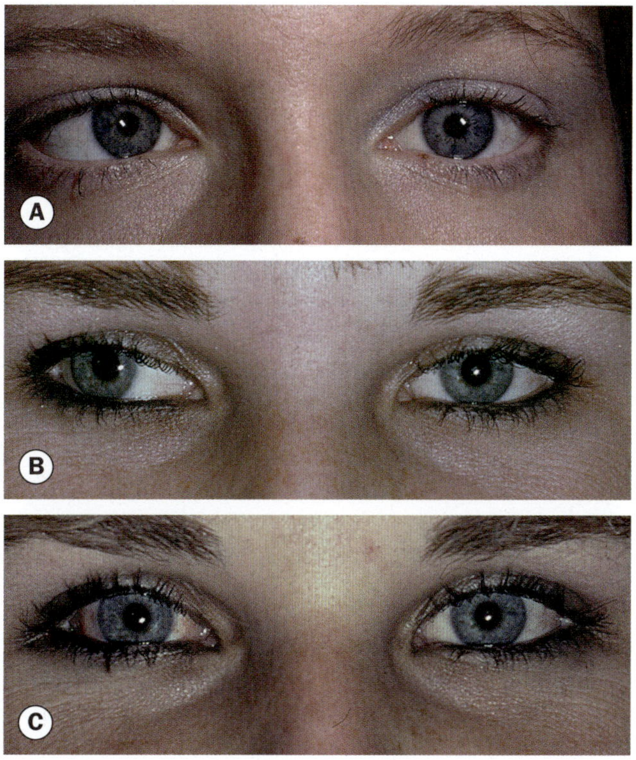

Fig. 18.77 Chronic right sixth nerve palsy with diplopia treated with botulinum injection. **(A)** Esotropia secondary to right abduction weakness; **(B)** after the injection into the right medial rectus muscle, showing marked exotropia; **(C)** three months later ocular alignment achieved after medial rectus recession and vertical rectus muscle transposition surgery. *(Courtesy of ADN Murray.)*

deviation can then be corrected surgically if appropriate. A small proportion of patients maintain BSV long-term after the effects of the toxin have worn off.

- **In lateral rectus palsy** botulinum toxin can be injected into the ipsilateral medial rectus to give symptomatic relief during recovery and to see whether there is any lateral rectus action when there is medial rectus contracture (Fig. 18.76A). The temporary paralysis of the muscle causes relaxation so that the horizontal forces on the globe are more balanced, thus allowing assessment of lateral rectus function (Fig. 18.76B). Medial rectus recession or muscle transposition surgery may subsequently be required to achieve ocular alignment (Fig. 18.77A–C). A similar approach can be used for fourth nerve palsy, with injection into the ipsilateral inferior oblique or contralateral inferior rectus.
- **Patients with a psychosocially unacceptable deviation** who have undergone multiple squint operations can be treated by repeated BT injections, which may reduce in frequency with time.

Chapter

19 Neuro-ophthalmology

NEUROIMAGING

Computed tomography

Physics

Computed tomography (CT) uses X-ray beams to obtain tissue density values from which detailed cross-sectional images are formed by a computer. Tissue density is represented by a grey scale, white being maximum density (e.g. bone) and black being minimum density (e.g. air). Advanced CT scanners are able to acquire thinner slices leading to improved spatial resolution, together with faster examination times, without a proportionate increase in radiation dose. Images are acquired in an axial form and can be viewed in any plane using computer reconstruction. This multiplanar information can be an advantage over magnetic resonance (MR) with regard to anatomical detail. CT is widely available, easy to perform, relatively inexpensive and quick, but unlike MR exposes the patient to ionizing radiation.

Contrast enhancement

Iodinated contrast material improves sensitivity and specificity but is contraindicated in patients allergic to iodine and in those with renal failure. Contrast is not indicated in acute haemorrhage, bony injury or localization of foreign bodies because it may mask visualization of these high-density structures.

Indications

- **Orbital trauma**, for the detection of bony lesions such as fractures (blood, herniation of extraocular muscles into the maxillary sinus (Fig. 19.1A) and surgical emphysema).
- **Evaluation of the extraocular muscles** in thyroid eye disease (Fig. 19.1B). CT and MRI (see below) have complementary advantages in the assessment of orbital disease.
- **Bony involvement of orbital tumours** is better assessed using CT than MR (Fig. 19.1C).
- **Orbital cellulitis** for assessment of intraorbital extension and subperiosteal abscess formation.

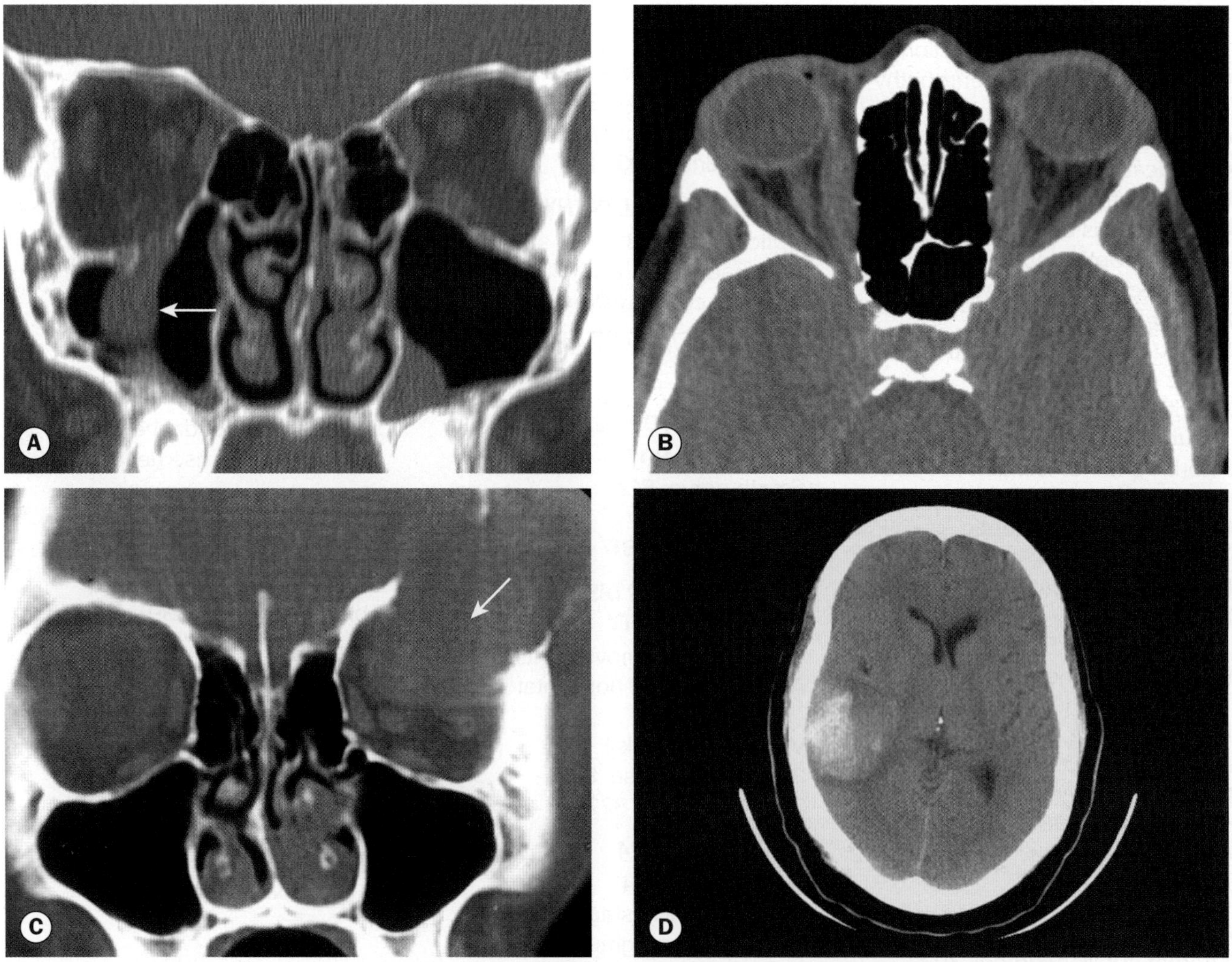

Fig. 19.1 CT scans. **(A)** Coronal image of a blow-out fracture, showing a defect in the right orbital floor and soft tissue prolapse (arrow) into the maxillary sinus; **(B)** axial image showing bilateral enlargement of extraocular muscles; **(C)** coronal image showing loss of the left superior bony orbit (arrow) secondary to a tumour; **(D)** axial image showing an acute parenchymal haematoma in the right temporal lobe. *(Courtesy of N Sibtain – fig. D.)*

- **Detection of intraorbital calcification** as in meningioma and retinoblastoma.
- **Detection of acute cerebral** (Fig. 19.1D) or **subarachnoid haemorrhage**, which is harder to visualize on MR within the first few hours of onset.
- **When MR is contraindicated** (e.g. ferrous foreign body).

Magnetic resonance imaging

Physics

Magnetic resonance imaging (MRI) depends on the rearrangement of positively charged hydrogen nuclei (protons) when a tissue is exposed to a short electromagnetic pulse. When the pulse subsides, the nuclei return to their normal position, re-radiating some of the absorbed energy. Sensitive receivers pick up this electromagnetic echo. Unlike CT, it does not subject the patient to ionizing radiation. The signals are analyzed and displayed as a cross-sectional image that may be axial, coronal or sagittal.

Basic sequences

Weighting refers to two methods of measuring the relaxation times of the excited protons after the magnetic field has been switched off. Various body tissues have different relaxation times so that a given tissue may be T1- or T2-weighted (i.e. best visualized on that particular type of image). In practice, both types of scans are usually performed. It is easy to tell the difference between CT and MR images because bone appears white on CT but is not clearly demonstrated on MR.

- **T1-weighted** images are generally optimal for viewing normal anatomy. Hypointense (dark) structures include vitreous (Fig. 19.2A) and cerebrospinal fluid (CSF) (Fig. 19.2B). Hyperintense (bright) structures include fat, blood, contrast agents and melanin.

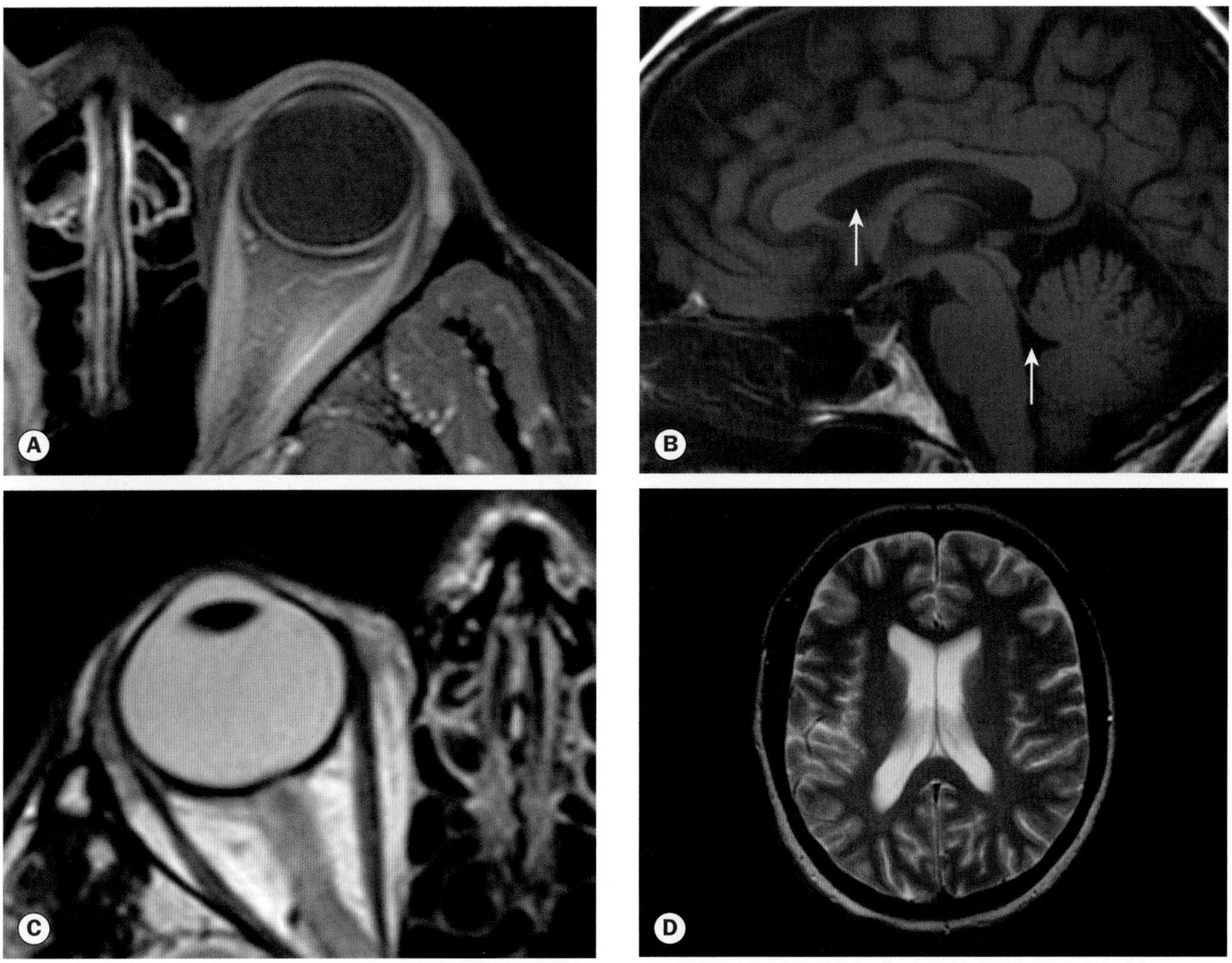

Fig. 19.2 MR scans. **(A)** T1-weighted axial image through the globe in which vitreous is hypointense (dark) and orbital fat is hyperintense (bright); **(B)** T1-weighted midline sagittal image through the brain in which the CSF is hypointense in the lateral and fourth ventricles (arrows); **(C)** T2-weighted axial image through the globe in which vitreous and orbital fat are hyperintense; **(D)** T2-weighted axial image through the brain in which the CSF in the lateral ventricles is hyperintense

- **T2-weighted** images, in which water is shown as hyperintense, are useful for viewing pathological changes because oedematous tissue (e.g. inflammation) will display a brighter signal than normal surrounding tissue. Vitreous (Fig. 19.2C) and CSF (Fig. 19.2D) are hyperintense as they have high water content. Blood vessels appear black on T2 imaging unless they are occluded.

Image enhancement

- **Gadolinium contrast** acquires magnetic moment when placed in an electromagnetic field. Administered intravenously, it remains intravascular unless there is a breakdown of the blood–brain barrier. It is only visualized on T1-weighted images and enhancing lesions such as tumours and areas of inflammation will appear bright. Ideally MR is performed both before (Fig. 19.3A) and after (Fig. 19.3B) administration of gadolinium for most clinical indications. Special head or surface coils can also be used to improve spatial definition of the image. Adverse effects with gadolinium are uncommon and usually relatively innocuous.
- **Fat-suppression techniques** are useful for imaging the orbit because the bright signal of orbital fat on conventional T1-weighted imaging frequently obscures other orbital contents. Fat suppression eliminates this bright signal and better delineates normal structures (optic nerve and extraocular muscles) as well as tumours, inflammatory lesions and vascular malformations. The two types of fat-suppression sequence used for orbital imaging are:
    - T1 fat saturation used with gadolinium allows areas suspicious using other techniques to be enhanced, e.g. suppressing orbital fat signal to visualize optic nerve sheath or perineural lesions (Fig. 19.3C).
    - STIR (short T1 inversion recovery) is the optimal sequence for detecting intrinsic lesions of the intraorbital optic nerve (e.g. glioma- Fig. 19.3D; optic neuritis – Fig. 19.3E). STIR images have very low signal from fat but still have high signal from water.
- **FLAIR** (fluid-attenuated inversion recovery) sequences suppress the bright CSF on T2-weighted images to allow better visualization of adjacent pathological tissue such as periventricular plaques of demyelination (Fig. 19.3F).
- **DWI/ADC** (diffusion-weighted imaging and apparent diffusion coefficient). DWI measures aberrance in expected Brownian motion of free water, and is useful in acute ischaemic stroke to identify abnormalities at a very early stage – within minutes – and in distinguishing ischaemic damage reversible with treatment from irreversible damage such that intervention (e.g. with a thrombolytic agent) is unlikely to be of benefit.
- **FIESTA and CISS** (fast imaging employing steady-state acquisition and constructive interference in steady-state) are newer high-resolution sequences. In neuro-ophthalmology, a particular application may be the investigation of cranial nerve palsy.

Limitations

- Bone appears black and is not directly imaged.
- Recent haemorrhage is not detected, so MRI is inappropriate in patients with suspected acute intracranial bleeding.
- It cannot be used in patients with magnetic foreign objects (e.g. cardiac pacemakers, intraocular foreign bodies and ferromagnetic aneurysm clips).
- Substantial patient cooperation is required, including remaining motionless. It is poorly tolerated by claustrophobic patients as it involves lying in an enclosed space for many minutes.

Neuro-ophthalmic indications

MRI is the technique of choice for lesions of the intracranial visual pathways.

- **The optic nerve** is best visualized on coronal STIR images in conjunction with coronal and axial T1 fat saturation post-gadolinium images. Axial T1 images are useful for displaying normal anatomy. MRI can detect lesions of the intraorbital part of the optic nerve (e.g. neuritis, glioma) as well as intracranial extension of optic nerve tumours.
- **Optic nerve sheath lesions** (e.g. meningioma) are of similar signal intensity to the nerve on T1- and T2-weighted images but enhance avidly with gadolinium.
- **Sellar masses** (e.g. pituitary tumours) are best visualized by T1-weighted contrast-enhanced studies. Coronal images optimally demonstrate the contents of the sella turcica as well as the suprasellar and parasellar regions and are usually supplemented by sagittal images.
- **Cavernous sinus pathology** is best demonstrated on coronal images; contrast may be required.
- **Intracranial lesions of the visual pathways** (e.g. inflammatory, demyelinating, neoplastic and vascular). MRI allows further characterization of these lesions as well as better anatomical localization.

Angiography

Magnetic resonance angiography

Magnetic resonance angiography (MRA) is a non-invasive method of imaging the intra- and extracranial carotid and vertebrobasilar circulations (Fig. 19.4A) to demonstrate abnormalities such as stenosis, dissection, occlusion, arteriovenous malformations and aneurysms. The motion sensitivity of MR is utilized to visualize blood flow within vessels and does not require contrast. However, because of the reliance on active flow, thrombosed aneurysms may be missed and turbulent flow may lead to difficulties in interpretation. The technique has limited facility in the detection of very small aneurysms. MRA adds about 10 minutes to the standard MRI acquisition time.

Magnetic resonance venography

Over recent years, increasing attention has been paid to intracranial venous system pathology, particularly dural sinus occlusion and stenosis. Historically, the venous phase of conventional digital subtraction angiography (DSA) has been used for intracranial venous assessment and still offers high sensitivity and specificity. However, both CT and MRI can be used to similar purpose and are relatively non-invasive and low-risk compared to DSA. Technological advances have conferred greatly improved accuracy. Whilst

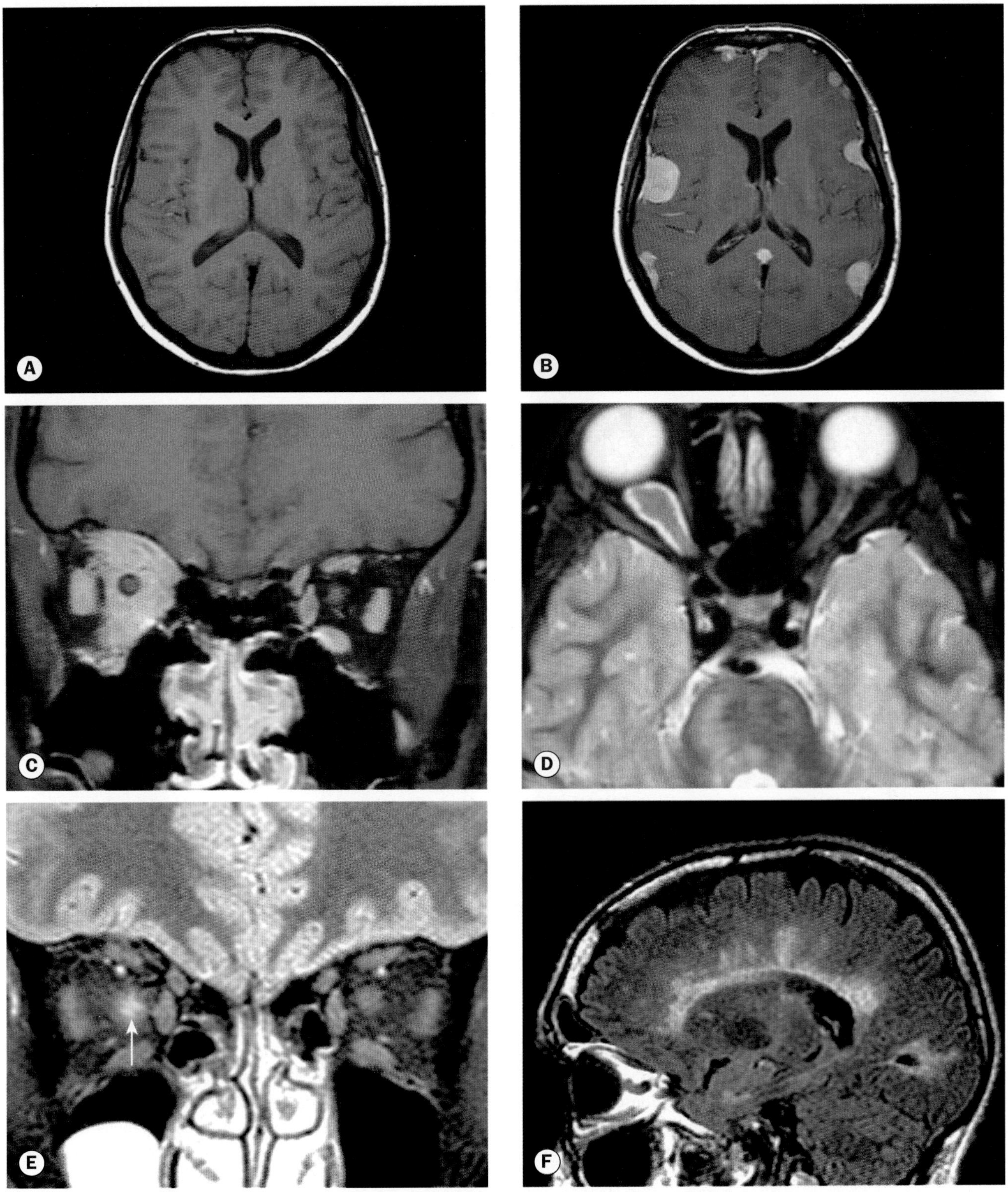

Fig. 19.3 Enhancement techniques. **(A)** Pre-contrast axial T1-weighted MR image of the brain in a patient with neurofibromatosis type 2 and multiple meningiomas; **(B)** gadolinium enhancement of the tumours; **(C)** coronal fat-saturated gadolinium enhanced T1-weighted image of a patient with lymphoma of the right orbit. Note the avid contrast enhancement of the extra-ocular muscles and the tumour which surrounds the optic nerve sheath; **(D)** axial STIR image showing a right optic nerve glioma in a patient with neurofibromatosis type 1. The STIR sequence is useful as it increases the contrast between the 'bright' pathological process and 'dark' surrounding fat; **(E)** coronal STIR image of right retrobulbar neuritis showing a bright signal (arrow), within a swollen optic nerve; **(F)** sagittal FLAIR image showing multiple periventricular plaques of demyelination. *(Courtesy of N Sibtain – fig. F.)*

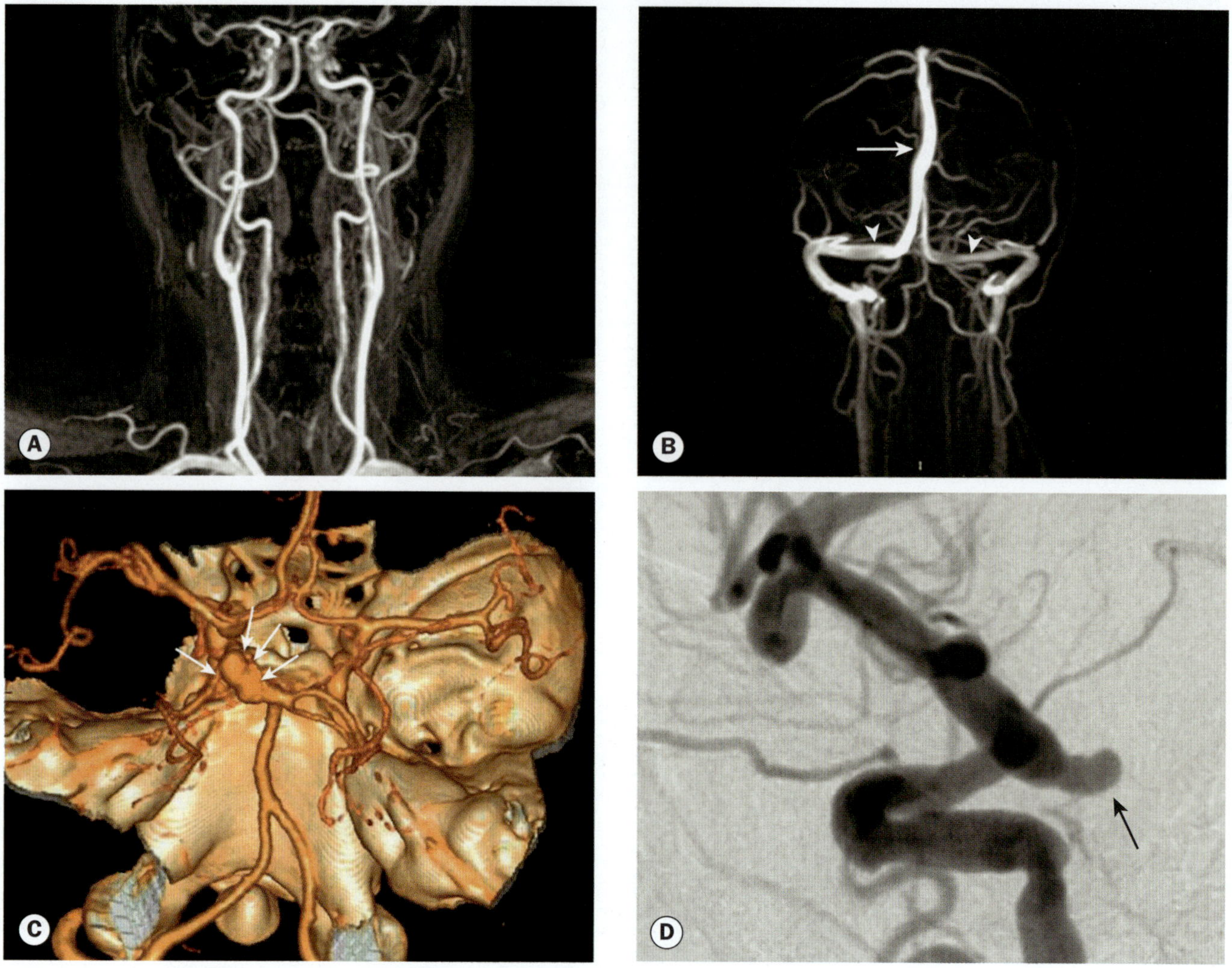

Fig. 19.4 Cerebral angiography. **(A)** Normal MRA of the external carotid and vertebral circulation; **(B)** maximum intensity phase-contrast MR venogram in a normal subject. The superior sagittal sinus (arrow) divides to form the sigmoid sinuses (arrowheads); **(C)** CT angiogram showing a left posterior communicating aneurysm (arrows); **(D)** conventional catheter angiogram with subtraction showing an aneurysm arising from the internal carotid artery at its junction with the posterior communicating artery (arrow). *(Courtesy of N Sibtain – fig. C.)*

CTV (see below) is generally faster and offers high spatial resolution, it entails a significant radiation dose and always requires contrast for image acquisition. Magnetic resonance venography (MRV) can be used with contrast or using non-contrast enhanced techniques, among other indications making it suitable for patients to whom contrast cannot be given. Substantial advances in MRV pulse sequences now allow excellent visualization of the venous system (Fig. 19.4B) and increasing reliance on MRV seems to be evident. However, local resource availability, experience and expertise are critical in determining the choice of technique.

Computed tomographic angiography

Computed tomographic angiography (CTA) has been emerging as the method of choice in the investigation of intracranial aneurysms (Fig. 19.4C). It enables acquisition of extremely thin slice images of the brain following intravenous contrast. Images of the vessels can be reconstructed in three dimensions and viewed from any direction, aiding the approach to treatment. The investigation is safe and quick and does not carry the 1% risk of stroke associated with conventional catheter angiography.

Computed tomographic venography

Computed tomographic venography (CTV) is a rapid high-resolution technique in which patient motion artefact is of lesser importance than with MRV. CTV is believed to be at least as sensitive as MRV in the diagnosis of cerebral venous thrombosis. Both techniques may provide complementary findings in difficult diagnostic situations. However, contrast is always required, and a significant radiation dose is delivered. Visualization of skull base structures is limited by bony artefact relative to MRV. The technique is similar to that of CTA.

Conventional catheter angiography

Conventional intra-arterial catheter angiography is usually performed under local anaesthetic. A catheter is passed via the femoral artery into the internal carotid and vertebral arteries in the neck

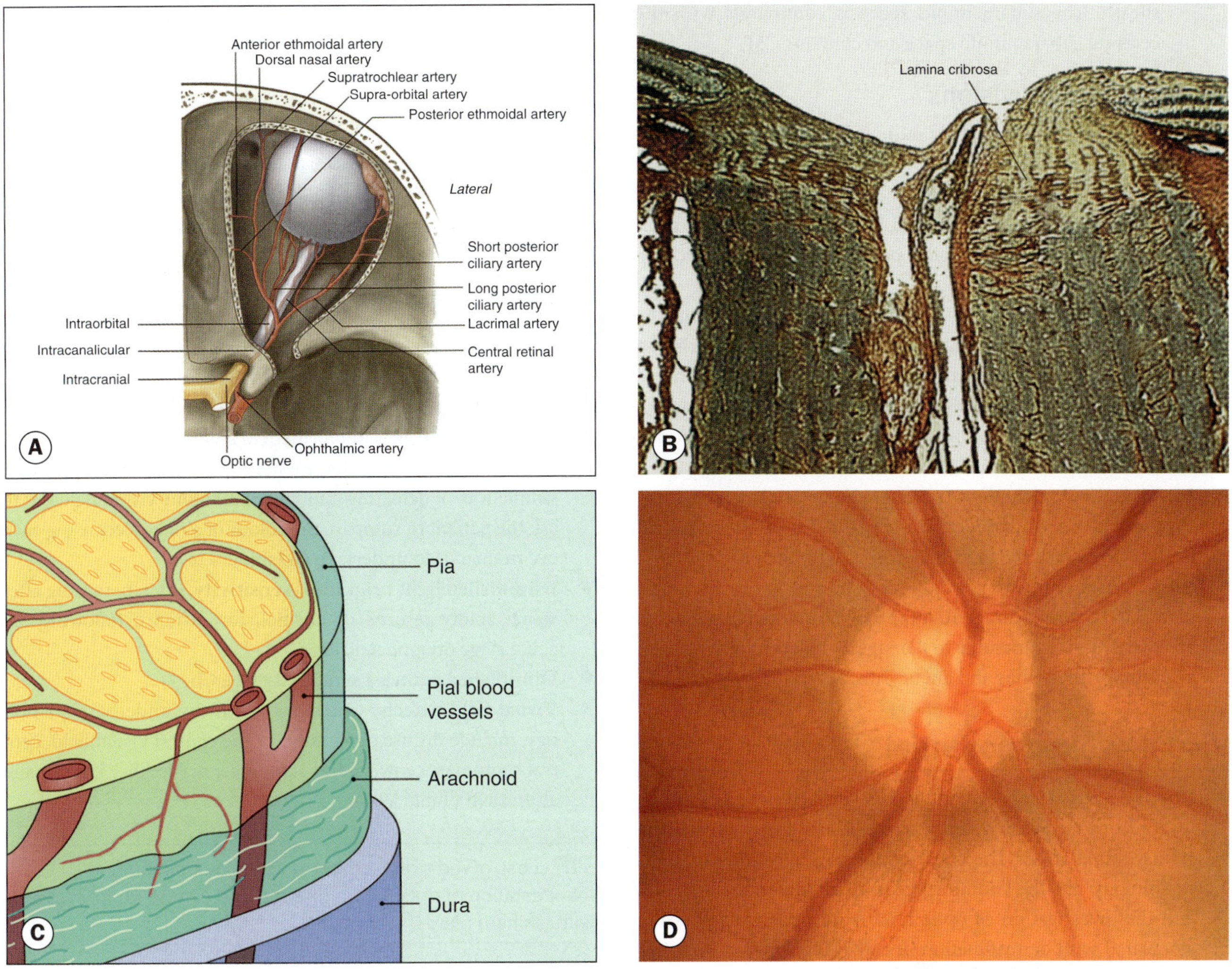

Fig. 19.5 Anatomy of the optic nerve. **(A)** Subdivisions of the nerve and retrobulbar circulation; **(B)** longitudinal section showing lamina cribrosa; **(C)** surrounding sheaths and pial blood vessels; **(D)** appearance of the normal optic disc

under fluoroscopic guidance. Following contrast injection, images are acquired in rapid succession. Digital subtraction results in images of the contrast-filled vessels with the exclusion of background structures such as bone (Fig. 19.4D). Until recently, this technique was the first-line investigation in the diagnosis of intracranial aneurysms but may now be reserved for cases where CTA is equivocal or negative.

OPTIC NERVE

Anatomy

Circulation (Fig. 19.5A)

- **The ophthalmic artery** arises from the internal carotid artery and runs inferior to the optic nerve in the optic canal.
- **The central retinal artery** is the continuation of the ophthalmic artery after it passes into the optic nerve 8–12 mm behind the globe. This supplies blood to the inner retina.
- **Long posterior ciliary arteries.** The blood supply to the optic nerve head arises from the circle of Zinn–Haller, which receives blood from 4–5 long posterior ciliary arteries, choroidal vessels and the pial arterial network.

General structure (Fig. 19.5B)

- **Afferent fibres.** The optic nerve carries approximately 1.2 million afferent nerve fibres, each of which originates in a retinal ganglion cell. Most of these fibres synapse in the lateral geniculate body, although some reach other centres, notably the pretectal nuclei in the midbrain. Nearly one-third of the fibres subserve the central 5° of the visual field. Within the optic nerve itself the nerve fibres are divided into about 600 bundles by fibrous septae derived from the pia mater.
- **Surrounding layers** (Fig. 19.5C)
  - The innermost layer is the delicate and vascular pia mater.
  - The outer sheath comprises the arachnoid mater and the tougher dura mater, which is continuous with the sclera; optic nerve fenestration involves incision of this outer

sheath. The subarachnoid space is continuous with the cerebral subarachnoid space and contains CSF.

Anatomical subdivisions

The optic nerve is approximately 50 mm long from globe to chiasm. It can be subdivided into four segments (see Fig. 19.5A):

- **Intraocular** segment (optic nerve head) is the shortest, being 1 mm deep and approximately 1.5 mm in vertical diameter. The ophthalmoscopically visible portion is called the optic disc (Fig. 19.5D).
- **Intraorbital** segment is 25–30 mm long and extends from the globe to the optic foramen at the orbital apex. Its diameter is 3–4 mm because of the addition of the myelin sheaths to the nerve fibres. At the orbital apex the nerve is surrounded by the tough fibrous annulus of Zinn, from which originate the four rectus muscles.
- **Intracanalicular** segment traverses the optic canal and measures about 6 mm. Unlike the intraorbital portion, it is fixed to the canal, since the dura mater fuses with the periosteum.
- **Intracranial** segment joins the chiasm and varies in length from 5 to 16 mm (average 10 mm). Long intracranial segments are particularly vulnerable to damage by adjacent lesions such as pituitary adenomas and aneurysms.

Visual evoked potential

- **Principle** (Fig. 19.6). Visual (visually) evoked potential (VEP) tests record electrical activity of the visual cortex created by retinal stimulation. The most common indications in ophthalmology are the monitoring of visual function in babies and the investigation of optic neuropathy, particularly when associated with demyelination. It can also be used to monitor macular pathway function and to investigate functional (non-physiological) visual loss.
- **Technique.** The stimulus is either a flash of light (flash VEP) or a black-and-white checkerboard pattern on a screen that periodically reverses polarity (pattern VEP). Several tests are performed and the average potential is calculated.
- **Interpretation.** Latency (delay) and amplitude are assessed. In optic neuropathy both parameters are affected, with prolongation of latency and a decrease in amplitude. Threshold VEP (by using different-sized check stimuli) can detect early or subclinical dysfunction as smaller check size responses may become abnormal earlier than responses to larger stimuli.

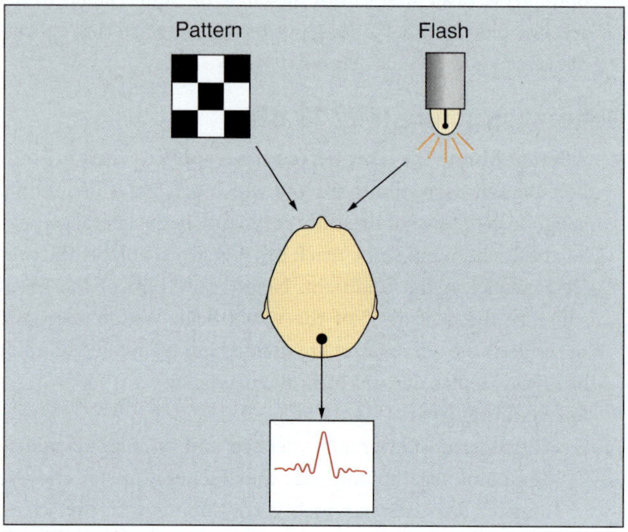

Fig. 19.6 Principles of the visual evoked potential test.

Signs of optic nerve dysfunction

- **Reduced visual acuity** for distance and near is common, but is non-specific. Acuity may be preserved in some conditions.
- **Relative afferent pupillary defect** (see below).
- **Dyschromatopsia** is impairment of colour vision, which in the context of optic nerve disease mainly affects red and green. A simple way of detecting a monocular colour vision defect is to ask the patient to compare the colour of a red object using each eye in turn or to undertake an Ishihara test.
- **Diminished light brightness sensitivity**, often persisting after visual acuity returns to normal, for instance following the acute stage of optic neuritis.
- **Diminished contrast sensitivity** (see Ch. 1).
- **Visual field defects**, which vary with the underlying pathology, include diffuse depression of the central visual field, central scotomas, centrocaecal scotomas, nerve fibre bundle and altitudinal (Table 19.1).

TIP Loss of red-green colour vision is a common manifestation of optic nerve disease and can be rapidly tested with Ishihara plates.

Classification of optic neuropathy by cause

- **Inflammatory.** Optic neuritis, including demyelinating, parainfectious, infectious and non-infectious and neuroretinitis.
- **Glaucomatous.** See Chapter 11.

Table 19.1 Focal Visual Field Defects in Optic Neuropathies

1. Central scotoma
   - Demyelination
   - Toxic and nutritional
   - Leber hereditary optic neuropathy
   - Compression
2. Enlarged blind spot
   - Papilloedema
   - Congenital anomalies
3. Respecting horizontal meridian
   - Anterior ischaemic optic neuropathy
   - Glaucoma
   - Disc drusen
4. Upper temporal defects not respecting vertical meridian
   - Tilted discs

- **Ischaemic.** Anterior non-arteritic, anterior arteritic, posterior ischaemic and diabetic papillopathy.
- **Hereditary.** Leber hereditary optic neuropathy, other hereditary optic neuropathies.
- **Nutritional and toxic.** See also Chapter 21.
- **Papilloedema.** Secondary to raised intracranial pressure.
- **Traumatic.** See Chapter 22.
- **Compressive.** Including secondary to an orbital lesion.
- **Infiltrative.** Inflammatory conditions (e.g. sarcoidosis), tumours and infective agents.

Optic atrophy

Introduction

Optic atrophy refers to the late-stage changes that take place in the optic nerve resulting from axonal degeneration in the pathway between the retina and the lateral geniculate body, manifesting with disturbance in visual function and in the appearance of the optic nerve head.

Primary optic atrophy

Primary optic atrophy occurs without antecedent swelling of the optic nerve head. It may be caused by lesions affecting the visual pathways at any point from the retrolaminar portion of the optic nerve to the lateral geniculate body. Lesions anterior to the optic chiasm result in unilateral optic atrophy, whereas those involving the chiasm and optic tract will cause bilateral changes.

- **Signs**
  - Flat white disc with clearly delineated margins (Fig. 19.7A).
  - Reduction in the number of small blood vessels on the disc surface.
  - Attenuation of peripapillary blood vessels and thinning of the retinal nerve fibre layer (RNFL).
  - The atrophy may be diffuse or sectoral depending on the cause and level of the lesion. Temporal pallor of the optic

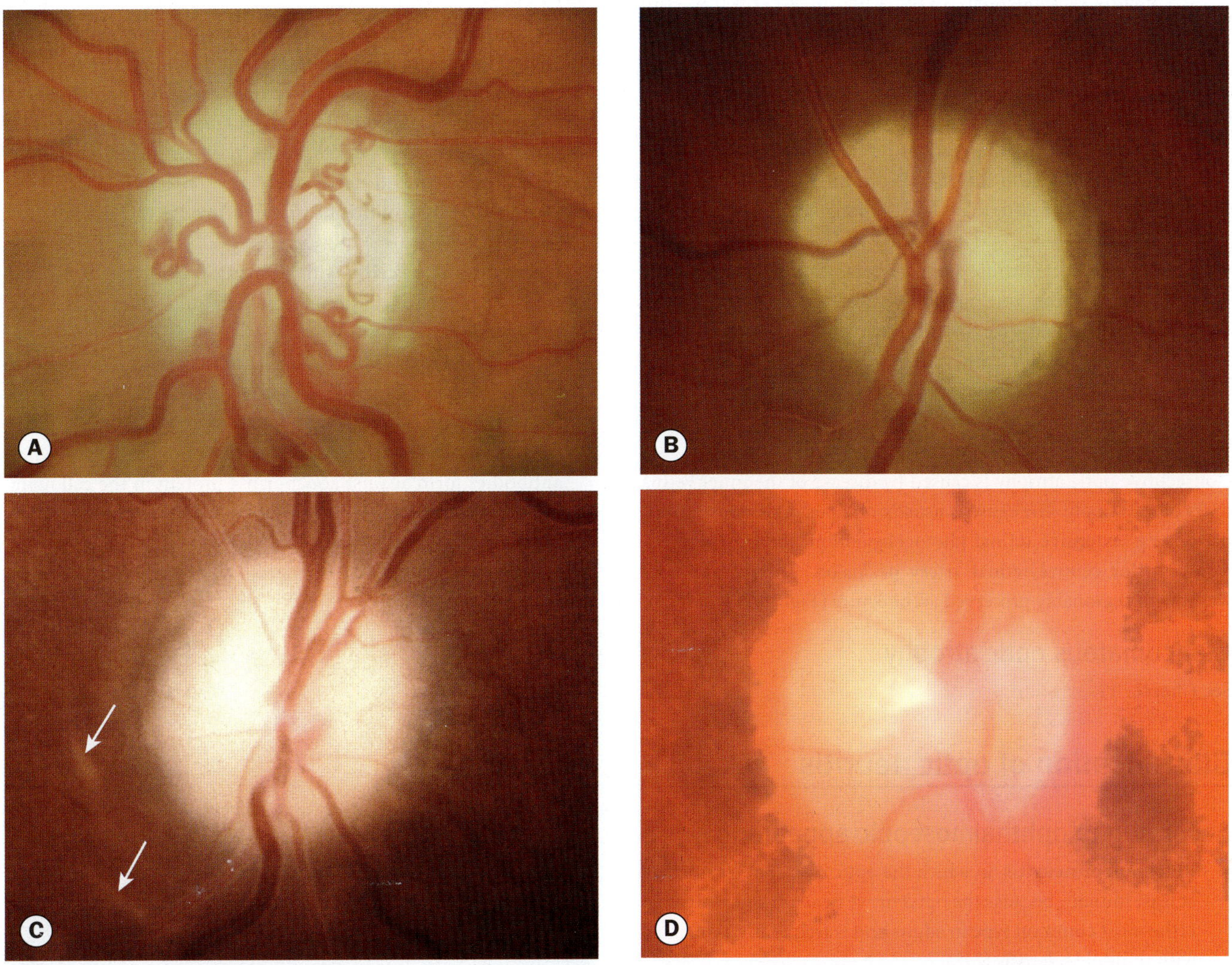

Fig. 19.7 Optic atrophy. **(A)** Primary due to compression, showing a flat white disc and shunt vessels; **(B)** primary due to nutritional neuropathy – note predominantly temporal pallor; **(C)** secondary due to chronic papilloedema – note Paton lines (arrows); **(D)** consecutive due to vasculitis.

nerve head may indicate atrophy of fibres of the papillomacular bundle and is classically seen following demyelinating optic neuritis. Band atrophy is a similar phenomenon caused by involvement of the fibres entering the optic disc nasally and temporally. It occurs in lesions of the optic chiasm or tract and gives nasal as well as temporal pallor.

- **Important causes**
  - Optic neuritis.
  - Compression by tumours and aneurysms.
  - Hereditary optic neuropathies.
  - Toxic and nutritional optic neuropathy, which may give temporal pallor, particularly in early/milder cases when the papillomacular fibres are preferentially affected (Fig. 19.7B).
  - Trauma.

Secondary optic atrophy

Secondary optic atrophy is preceded by longstanding swelling of the optic nerve head.

- **Signs** vary according to the cause and its course.
  - Slightly or moderately raised white or greyish disc with poorly delineated margins due to gliosis (Fig. 19.7C).
  - Obscuration of the lamina cribrosa.
  - Reduction in the number of small blood vessels on the disc surface.
  - Peripapillary circumferential retinochoroidal folds, especially temporal to the disc (Paton lines – see Fig. 19.7C), sheathing of arterioles and venous tortuosity may be present.
- **Causes** include chronic papilloedema, anterior ischaemic optic neuropathy and papillitis. Intraocular inflammatory causes of marked disc swelling are sometimes considered to cause secondary rather than consecutive atrophy (see below).

Consecutive optic atrophy

Consecutive optic atrophy is caused by disease of the inner retina or its blood supply. The cause is usually obvious on fundus examination, e.g. extensive retinal photocoagulation, retinitis pigmentosa or prior central retinal artery occlusion. The disc appears waxy, with reasonably preserved architecture (Fig. 19.7D).

Glaucomatous optic atrophy

See Chapter 11.

Classification of optic neuritis

According to ophthalmoscopic appearance

- **Retrobulbar neuritis**, in which the optic disc appears normal, at least initially, because the optic nerve head is not involved. It is the most common type in adults and is frequently associated with multiple sclerosis (MS).
- **Papillitis** is characterized by hyperaemia and oedema of the optic disc, which may be associated with peripapillary flame-shaped haemorrhages (Fig. 19.8). Cells may be seen in the posterior vitreous. Papillitis is the most common type of optic neuritis in children, but can also affect adults.
- **Neuroretinitis** is characterized by papillitis in association with inflammation of the RNFL and a macular star figure (see below). It is the least common type and is only rarely a manifestation of demyelination.

According to aetiology

- **Demyelinating.** This is by far the most common cause.
- **Parainfectious**, following a viral infection or immunization.
- **Infectious.** This may be sinus-related, or associated with conditions such as cat-scratch disease, syphilis, Lyme disease, cryptococcal meningitis and herpes zoster.
- **Non-infectious** causes include sarcoidosis and systemic autoimmune diseases such as systemic lupus erythematosus, polyarteritis nodosa and other vasculitides.

Demyelinating optic neuritis

Overview

Demyelination is a pathological process in which normally myelinated nerve fibres lose their insulating myelin layer. The myelin is phagocytosed by microglia and macrophages, subsequent to which astrocytes lay down fibrous tissue in plaques. Demyelinating disease disrupts nervous conduction within the white matter tracts of the brain, brainstem and spinal cord.

Demyelinating conditions that may involve the visual system include the following:

- **Isolated optic neuritis** with no clinical evidence of generalized demyelination, although in a high proportion of cases this subsequently develops.
- **Multiple sclerosis** (MS), by far the most common demyelinating disease (see below).
- **Neuromyelitis optica spectrum disorder** (NMOSD), previously called Devic disease, is a rare autoimmune disease where antibodies form against aquaporin 4 protein in the cell membranes of astrocytes.

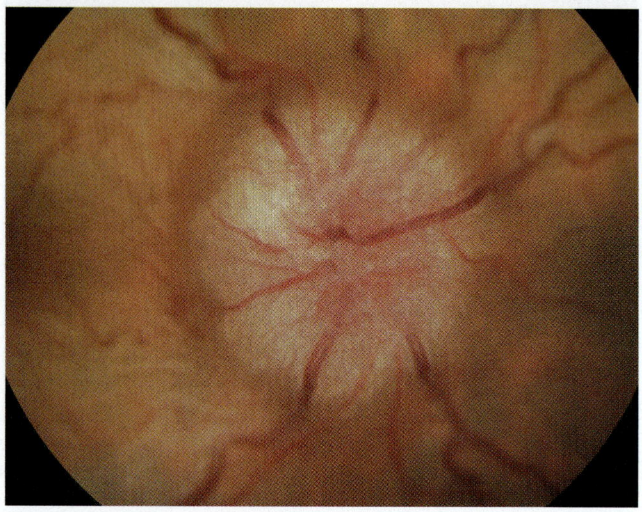

Fig. 19.8 Papillitis.

- It may occur at any age, but typically affects middle-aged women.
- The condition is characterized by bilateral optic neuritis and within a few weeks, long-segment transverse myelitis (demyelination of the spinal cord) (see Fig. 19.9D). Most patients experience repeated attacks, separated by periods of remission.
- The NMO-IgG blood test, which is highly specific, is positive in 70% of patients and is an important marker of the condition.
- Acute treatment involves the use of high-dose intravenous steroids followed by oral steroids. If steroids are ineffective, plasmapheresis may be used. Immunosuppressive drugs are used for long-term therapy. Eculizumab, inebilizumab and satralizumab have recently been approved for use in adults with NMOSD who are anti-aquaporin antibody positive.

- **MOG antibody disorder** (MOGAD) is a recently identified rare auto-immune disease that results in inflammation of the optic nerve and spinal cord. Antibodies form against myelin oligodendrocyte glycoprotein (MOG). Bilateral simultaneous optic neuropathy is a common presenting feature.
- **Schilder disease**, a very rare relentlessly progressive generalized disease with an onset prior to the age of 10 years and death within 1–2 years. Bilateral optic neuritis without subsequent improvement may occur.

Multiple sclerosis

MS is an idiopathic demyelinating disease involving central nervous system white matter. Infection with Epstein–Barr virus (EBV) significantly increases the chances of developing multiple sclerosis. However, EBV in itself is not sufficient to trigger MS and other unknown factors play a role. It is more common in women than men.

- **Presentation** is typically in the third–fourth decades, generally with relapsing/remitting demyelination that may switch later to an unremitting pattern and less commonly with progressive disease from the outset.

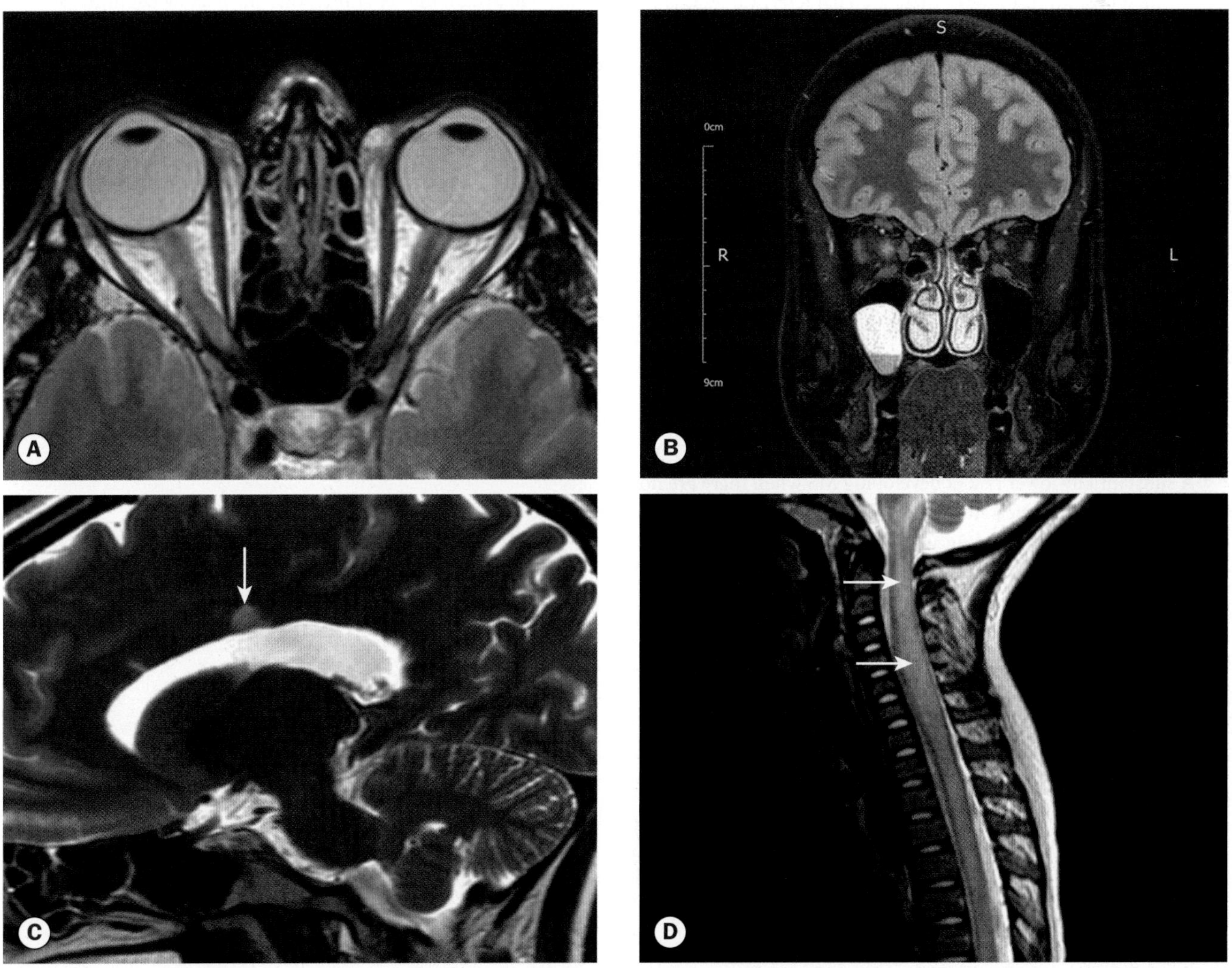

Fig. 19.9 Demyelination. **(A)** Axial T2-weighted image of right optic neuritis in a patient with multiple sclerosis; **(B)** coronal STIR image of **(A)**; **(C)** T2-weighted STIR image showing typical hyperintense demyelinating plaques in the supratentorial white matter (arrow), particularly in the corpus callosum; **(D)** MRI showing transverse myelitis in NMOSD (Devic disease) (arrows).

- **Systemic features** may include:
  - Spinal cord, e.g. weakness, stiffness, sphincter disturbance, sensory loss.
  - Brainstem, e.g. diplopia, nystagmus, dysarthria, dysphagia.
  - Cerebral, e.g. hemiparesis, hemianopia, dysphasia.
  - Psychological, e.g. intellectual decline, depression, euphoria.
  - Transient features, e.g. the Lhermitte sign (electrical sensation on neck flexion) and the Uhthoff phenomenon (sudden worsening of vision or other symptoms on exercise or increase in body temperature).
- **Ophthalmic features**
  - Common: optic neuritis (usually retrobulbar), internuclear ophthalmoplegia, nystagmus.
  - Uncommon: skew deviation, ocular motor nerve palsies, hemianopia.
  - Rare: intermediate uveitis and retinal periphlebitis.
- **Investigations**
  - Lumbar puncture shows oligoclonal bands on protein electrophoresis of cerebrospinal fluid in 90–95%.
  - MRI shows changes in the optic nerve appearance on STIR imaging. Almost always there are characteristic lesions in the white matter of the brain (plaques) (Fig. 19.9A–C).
  - VEPs are abnormal (conduction delay and a reduction in amplitude) in up to 100% of patients with clinically definite MS.

Association between optic neuritis and multiple sclerosis

- The overall 15-year risk of developing MS following an acute episode of optic neuritis is about 50%. With no lesions on MRI the risk is 25%, but the risk is over 70% in patients with one or more lesions on MRI. The presence of MRI lesions is therefore a very strong predictive factor.
- MS is not considered a hereditary disease, but the probability of developing the disease is higher in closely related relatives. There is an association between MS and HLA DR15 and DQ6.
- A substantially lower risk of developing MS when there are no MRI lesions is conferred by the following factors, providing critical support in deciding whether to commence immunomodulatory MS-prophylactic treatment following an optic neuritis episode:
  - Male gender.
  - Absence of a viral syndrome preceding the optic neuritis.
  - Negative test for Epstein–Barr virus.
  - Optic disc swelling, disc/peripapillary haemorrhages or macular exudates.
  - Vision reduced to no light perception.
  - Absence of periocular pain.
- Optic neuritis is the presenting feature of MS in up to 30%.
- Optic neuritis occurs at some point in 50% of patients with established MS.

TIP In optic neuritis secondary to multiple sclerosis the vision usually improves without treatment over a period of several months.

Clinical features of demyelinating optic neuritis

- **Symptoms**
  - Subacute monocular visual impairment.
  - Usual age range 20–50 years (mean around 30).
  - Some patients experience tiny white or coloured flashes or sparkles (phosphenes).
  - Discomfort or pain in or around the eye is present in over 90% and typically exacerbated by ocular movement. It may precede or accompany the visual loss and usually lasts a few days.
  - Frontal headache and tenderness of the globe may also be present.
- **Signs**
  - Visual acuity (VA) is usually 6/18–6/60, but may rarely be worse.
  - Other signs of optic nerve dysfunction (see above), particularly impaired colour vision and a relative afferent pupillary defect.
  - The optic disc is normal in two-thirds of cases (retrobulbar neuritis); the remaining one-third show papillitis (see Fig. 19.8).
  - Temporal disc pallor may be seen in the fellow eye (see Fig. 19.7B for similar appearance), indicative of previous optic neuritis.
- **Visual field defects** (Fig. 19.10)
  - Diffuse depression of sensitivity in the entire central 30° is the most common.
  - Altitudinal/arcuate defects and focal central/centrocaecal scotomas are also frequent.
  - Focal defects are frequently accompanied by an element of superimposed generalized depression.
- **Course.** Vision worsens over several days to 3 weeks and then begins to improve. Most recover within 4 weeks. Initial recovery is fairly rapid and then slower over 6–12 months.

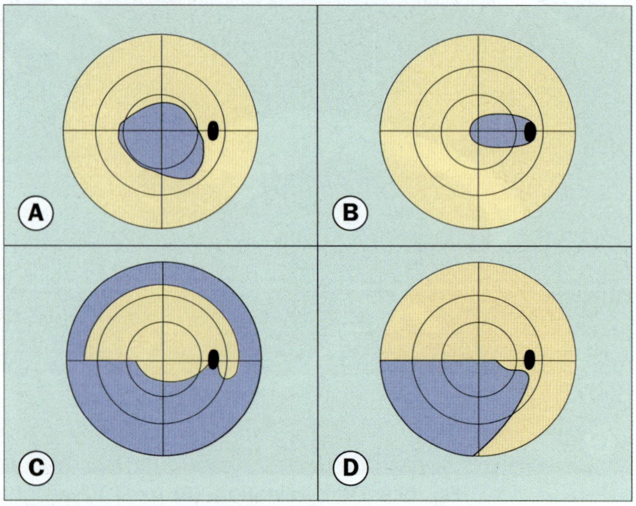

Fig. 19.10 Visual field defects in optic neuritis. **(A)** Central scotoma; **(B)** centrocaecal scotoma; **(C)** nerve fibre bundle; **(D)** altitudinal.

Prognosis

More than 90% of patients recover VA to 6/9 or better. Subtle parameters of visual function, such as colour vision, may remain abnormal. A mild relative afferent pupillary defect may persist. Temporal optic disc pallor or more marked optic atrophy may ensue. About 10% develop chronic optic neuritis with slowly progressive or stepwise visual loss.

Management following demyelinating optic neuritis

Nearly 80–85% of patients with MS experience a relapsing course. If left untreated most will develop neurological disability over time. Disease modifying therapies early in the course of active relapsing MS can prevent relapses and reduce neurological disability. Some of these medications are associated with potentially serious side effects and careful monitoring is required, preferably in a specialist clinic.

Indications for steroid treatment in optic neuritis

- **Starting treatment.** Optic nerve axon preservation and final visual acuity may be improved by starting intravenous steroid therapy within 48 hours of the onset of symptoms.
- **Speed of recovery.** When the VA is worse than 6/12 within the first week of onset, treatment may speed up recovery by 2–3 weeks and delay the onset of clinical MS over the short term. This may be relevant in the patients with poor vision in the fellow eye, but the limited benefit must be balanced against the risks of high-dose steroids.
- **Steroid regimen.** Intravenous methylprednisolone sodium succinate 1 g daily (250 mg six-hourly) for 3 days, followed by oral prednisolone (1 mg/kg daily) for 11 days, subsequently tapered over 3 days.
- **Oral prednisolone** may increase the risk of recurrence of optic neuritis if used without prior intravenous steroid.

Disease modifying therapies for MS

- **Interferon beta** (IFNß) is used in the early stages, but can cause transient flu-like symptoms. Four interferon drugs are currently approved to treat MS and vary in their administration routes and frequency of injection: subcutaneous IFNß-1a and -1b, intramuscular IFNß-1a and long-acting subcutaneous peginterferon beta-1a (given every 2 weeks). The long-term safety profile and efficacy makes IFNß an important first-line therapeutic option.
- **Glatiramer acetate** (subcutaneous injection) is used to reduce the frequency of relapses of MS and possibly decreases disability progression. An injection site reaction occurs in about one-third. The method of action is not known, but it may possibly act as a decoy, diverting the autoimmune response against myelin.
- **Monoclonal antibody** treatment is showing promise in the treatment of MS, but use of these agents has been associated with systemic side effects, notably opportunistic infections and abnormal liver function. The following medication can be considered in difficult cases: natalizumab, ocrelizumab and alemtuzumab.
- **Natalizumab** is used for highly active relapsing–remitting MS in patients who have not responded favourably to treatment with interferon beta or glatiramer acetate and reduces relapses by about two-thirds, slowing disability by half.
- **Ocrelizumab** is helpful for highly active disease and primary progressive disease, but may rarely cause progressive multifocal leukoencephalopathy (which can be fatal).
- **Alemtuzumab** may be the most cost-effective of these medications because of the favourable dosing strategy.

Approach to treatment of MS

- **A multidisciplinary approach** is important in these patients.
- **First attack** suggestive of MS: intravenous corticosteroids, interferon beta or glatiramer acetate.
- **Relapsing MS:** (a) inactive disease: regular clinical monitoring; (b) active and highly active disease: disease modifying therapy (alemtuzumab, cladribine, fingolimod, natalizumab, ocrelizumab, mitoxantrone).
- **Progressive MS**: ocrelizumab.

Parainfectious optic neuritis

Optic neuritis may be associated with viral infections such as measles, mumps, chickenpox, rubella, whooping cough and glandular fever and may also occur following immunization. Children are affected much more frequently than adults. Presentation is usually 1–3 weeks after a viral infection, with acute severe visual loss generally involving both eyes. Bilateral papillitis is the rule. Occasionally there may be a neuroretinitis or the discs may be normal. The prognosis for spontaneous visual recovery is very good and treatment is not required in the majority of patients. However, when visual loss is severe and bilateral or involves an only seeing eye, intravenous steroids should be considered, with antiviral cover where appropriate.

Infectious optic neuritis

- **Sinus-related** optic neuritis is uncommon and is sometimes characterized by recurrent attacks of unilateral visual loss associated with severe headache and spheno-ethmoidal sinusitis. Possible mechanisms include direct spread of infection, occlusive vasculitis and mucocoele. Treatment is with systemic antibiotics and, if appropriate, surgical drainage.
- **Cat-scratch fever** (benign lymphoreticulosis) is usually caused by *Bartonella henselae* inoculated by a cat scratch or bite (see below and also Ch. 12). Numerous ophthalmological features have been described, notably neuroretinitis.
- **Syphilis** may cause acute papillitis or neuroretinitis during the primary or secondary stages (see Ch. 12).
- **Lyme disease** (borreliosis) is a spirochaetal infection caused by *Borrelia burgdorferi* transmitted by a tick bite (see Ch. 12). It may cause neuroretinitis and occasionally acute retrobulbar neuritis, which may be associated with other neurological manifestations and can mimic MS.

- **Cryptococcal meningitis** in patients with acquired immunodeficiency syndrome (AIDS) may be associated with acute optic neuritis, which may be bilateral (see Ch. 12).
- **Varicella zoster virus** may cause papillitis by spread from contiguous retinitis (i.e. acute retinal necrosis, progressive retinal necrosis – see Ch. 12) or associated with herpes zoster ophthalmicus. Primary optic neuritis is uncommon but may occur in immunocompromised patients, some of whom may subsequently develop viral retinitis.

TIP Bilateral severe visual loss secondary to optic neuritis may occur in children 1–3 weeks after a viral infection, but the prognosis for visual recovery is good.

Non-infectious optic neuritis

Sarcoidosis

Optic neuritis affects 1–5% of patients with neurosarcoidosis. It may occasionally be the presenting feature of sarcoidosis, but usually develops during the course of established systemic disease. The optic nerve head may exhibit a lumpy appearance suggestive of granulomatous infiltration and there may be associated vitritis (Fig. 19.11). The response to steroid therapy is often rapid, though vision may decline if treatment is tapered or stopped prematurely and some patients require long-term low-dose therapy. Methotrexate may also be used as an adjunct to steroids or as monotherapy in steroid-intolerant patients.

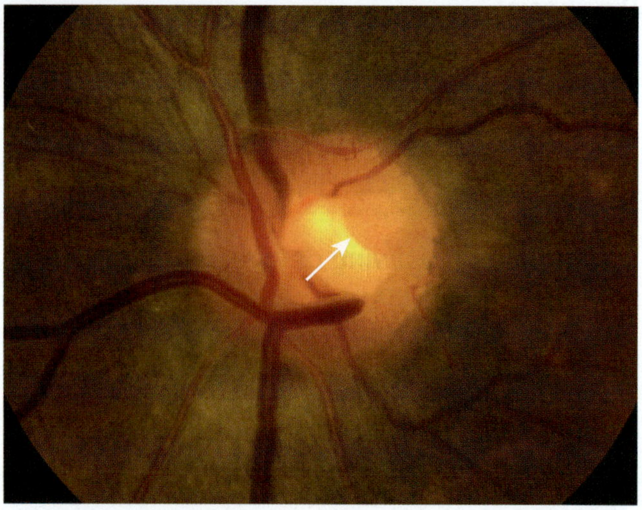

Fig. 19.11 Sarcoid granuloma of the optic nerve head (arrow).

Autoimmune

Autoimmune optic nerve involvement may take the form of retrobulbar neuritis or anterior ischaemic optic neuropathy (see below). Some patients may also experience slowly progressive visual loss suggestive of compression. Treatment is with systemic steroids and other immunosuppressants.

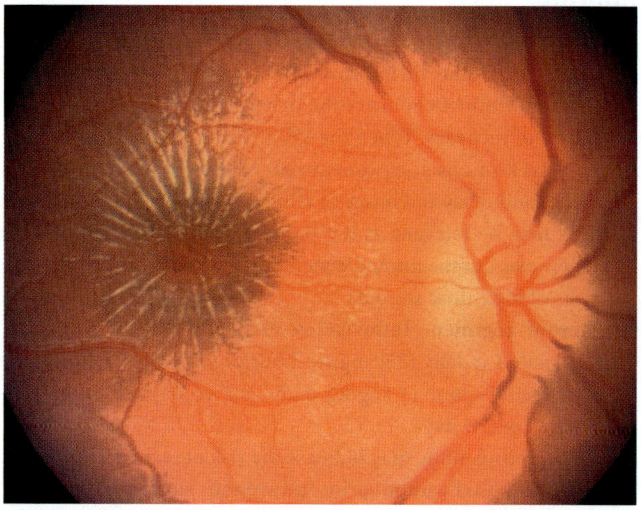

Fig. 19.12 Neuroretinitis showing disc swelling and a macular star.

Neuroretinitis

Introduction

Neuroretinitis refers to the combination of optic neuritis and signs of retinal, usually macular, inflammation. Cat-scratch fever is responsible for 60% of cases. About 25% of cases are idiopathic (Leber idiopathic stellate neuroretinitis). Other notable causes include syphilis, Lyme disease, mumps and leptospirosis.

Diagnosis

- **Symptoms.** Painless unilateral visual impairment, usually gradually worsening over about a week.
- **Signs**
  - VA is impaired to a variable degree.
  - Signs of optic nerve dysfunction are usually mild or absent, as visual loss is largely due to macular involvement.
  - Papillitis associated with peripapillary and macular oedema.
  - A macular star (Fig. 19.12) typically appears as disc swelling settles. The macular star resolves with a return to normal or near-normal VA over 6–12 months.
  - Venous engorgement and splinter haemorrhages may be present in severe cases.
  - Fellow eye involvement occasionally develops.
- **Optical coherence tomography (OCT)** demonstrates sub- and intraretinal fluid to a variable extent.
- **Fluorescein angiography (FA)** shows diffuse leakage from superficial disc vessels.
- **Blood tests** may include serology for *Bartonella* and other causes according to clinical suspicion (see also Ch. 12).

Treatment

This is specific to the cause and often consists of antibiotics. Recurrent idiopathic cases may require treatment with steroids and/or other immunosuppressants.

Non-arteritic anterior ischaemic optic neuropathy

Introduction

Non-arteritic anterior ischaemic optic neuropathy (NAION) is caused by occlusion of the short posterior ciliary arteries resulting in partial or total infarction of the optic nerve head. Predispositions include structural crowding of the optic nerve head so that the physiological cup is either very small or absent, hypertension (very common), diabetes mellitus, hyperlipidaemia, collagen vascular disease, antiphospholipid antibody syndrome, hyperhomocysteinaemia, sudden hypotensive events, cataract surgery and sleep apnoea syndrome. This condition may occasionally follow air travel or exposure to high altitude. Patients are usually over the age of 50, but are typically younger than those who develop arteritic ION (see below).

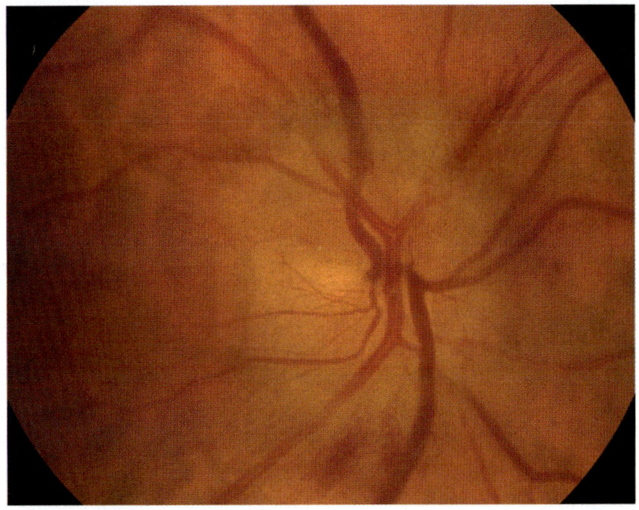

Fig. 19.13 Non-arteritic anterior ischaemic optic neuropathy showing optic disc swelling.

Diagnosis

- **Symptoms**
  - Sudden painless monocular visual loss, which is frequently discovered on awakening, suggesting that nocturnal hypotension may play a role.
- **Signs**
  - VA is normal or only slightly reduced in about 30%. The remainder have moderate to severe impairment.
  - Visual field defects are typically inferior altitudinal but central, paracentral, quadrantic and arcuate defects may also be seen.
  - Dyschromatopsia is usually proportional to the level of visual impairment, in contrast to optic neuritis in which colour vision may be severely impaired when VA is reasonably good.
  - Diffuse or sectoral hyperaemic disc swelling, often associated with a few peripapillary splinter haemorrhages (Fig. 19.13).
  - Disc swelling gradually resolves and pallor ensues 3–6 weeks after onset.
- **Investigation** should include assessment of the blood pressure and determination of the fasting lipid profile and blood glucose. It is also very important to exclude occult giant cell arteritis (see below). Atypical features may prompt special investigations, such as neuroimaging.
- **Prognosis.** Improvement in vision is common although recurrence occurs in about 6%. About 50% of eyes achieve 6/9 or better, though 25% will only reach 6/60 or worse.
- **Fellow eye.** Involvement of the fellow eye occurs in about 10% of patients after 2 years and 15% after 5 years.

Treatment

- There is no definitive treatment.
- Optic nerve fenestration has not been shown to be of benefit.
- Some authorities advocate short-term systemic steroid treatment.
- Any underlying systemic predispositions should be treated.
- Although aspirin is effective in reducing systemic vascular events and is frequently prescribed in patients with NAION, it does not appear to reduce the risk of involvement of the fellow eye.

Arteritic anterior ischaemic optic neuropathy

Arteritic anterior ischaemic optic neuropathy (AAION) is caused by giant cell arteritis (GCA). About 50% of patients with GCA have polymyalgia rheumatica (PMR) at diagnosis, while around 20% of PMR patients will develop GCA. PMR is characterized by pain and stiffness in proximal muscle groups, typically the shoulders and biceps, that is worse on waking. Symptoms can be severe but generally respond dramatically to a low–medium dose (initially 15–20 mg daily) of oral prednisolone. The causative relationship between GCA and PMR remains uncertain.

Diagnosis of giant cell arteritis

GCA is a granulomatous necrotizing arteritis (Fig. 19.14A) with a predilection for large and medium-size arteries, particularly the major aortic branches and the superficial temporal (STA), ophthalmic, posterior ciliary and proximal vertebral arteries. The severity and extent of involvement are associated with the quantity of elastic tissue in the media and adventitia and intracranial arteries are usually spared as they possess little elastic tissue. Smoking, low body mass index and early menopause may be independent risk factors. Patients are usually elderly (average 70 years) and the condition is extremely rare under the age of 50. Women are affected four times more commonly than men. The diagnosis of both GCA and PMR is mainly made on the basis of clinical findings. The American College of Rheumatology criteria may be helpful in diagnostic decision-making (Table 19.2). The classification was updated in 2022, to incorporate recent developments (like the halo sign on temporal artery ultrasound).

- **Symptoms**
  - Scalp tenderness, first noticed when combing the hair, is common.

Table 19.2 American College of Rheumatology 1990 Classification Criteria for Giant Cell Arteritis

- Age at disease onset 50 years or older
- New headache
- Temporal artery tenderness to palpation or decreased pulsation
- Erythrocyte sedimentation rate of 50 mm/h or greater
- Abnormal artery biopsy: biopsy specimen showing vasculitis characterized by a predominance of mononuclear cell infiltration or granulomatous inflammation, usually with multinucleated giant cells

For purposes of classification, a patient shall be said to have giant cell (temporal) arteritis if at least three of these five criteria are present.

- Headache, which may be localized to the frontal, occipital or temporal areas or be more generalized.
- Jaw claudication (cramp-like pain on chewing), caused by ischaemia of the masseter muscles, is virtually pathognomonic.
- Non-specific symptoms such as weight loss, fever, night sweats, malaise and depression are common.
- Double vision may occur.
- AAION (see below).

- **Other features**
  - Superficial temporal arteritis is characterized by thickened, tender, inflamed and nodular arteries (Fig. 19.14B), though the signs may be subtle.
  - Pulsation is initially present, but later ceases, a sign strongly suggestive of GCA, since a non-pulsatile superficial temporal artery is highly unusual in a normal individual.
  - Ocular motor palsies, including a pupil-involving third nerve palsy, can manifest.
  - Scalp gangrene may occur in very severe cases.
  - Rare complications include dissecting aneurysms, aortic incompetence, myocardial infarction, renal failure and brainstem stroke.
- **Investigations**
  - Erythrocyte sedimentation rate (ESR) is often very high, with a level of >60 mm/hr, although in approximately 20% of patients it is normal, even low–normal.
  - C-reactive protein (CRP) is raised.
  - Full blood count: elevated platelets and normocytic normochromic anaemia are commonly present. Platelet level is a stronger predictor for GCA than ESR or CRP.
  - Liver function tests are abnormal in one-third.
  - Autoantibodies are normal.
  - Temporal artery biopsy (TAB) should be performed if GCA is suspected. Steroid treatment (see below) should never be withheld pending biopsy, which should ideally be performed within 3 days of commencing steroids. Systemic steroid administration of duration greater than 7–10 days may suppress histological evidence of active arteritis although this is not invariable. In patients with ocular involvement, it is advisable to take the biopsy from the ipsilateral side. The ideal location is the temple because it lessens the risk of major nerve damage. At least 2.5 cm of artery should be collected and serial sections examined because of the phenomenon of 'skip' lesions in which inflamed segments of arterial wall are interspersed with histologically normal areas. On meta-analysis the estimated sensitivity of TAB has been reported to be 77%. A negative TAB should not prevent ongoing treatment in the presence of a convincing clinical picture of GCA as approximately 20% have normal histology. A contralateral biopsy may be positive in 5% following a negative initial biopsy.
  - Colour Doppler and duplex ultrasonography shows a hypoechoic halo around the superficial temporal artery lumen in around 75% due to oedema in the artery wall (Fig. 19.14C). There is good evidence that ultrasound provides a valid non-invasive alternative to TAB. However, a hypoechoic halo is not pathognomonic of GCA, as atherosclerosis and other inflammatory arterial conditions can cause a false positive halo. Doppler imaging is a useful aid to locating the artery for biopsy when it cannot be palpated.
  - Extracranial large vessel imaging. Aortic imaging with ultrasonography, MRA or positron emission tomography (PET) scanning may be used to exclude aortic aneurysm or dissection due to aortitis. Serial long-term imaging is increasingly being advocated to exclude these potentially life-threatening complications, the risk of which has now been demonstrated to be substantially increased in and following GCA.
  - Shoulder joint (axillary) imaging. Recent work suggests that particular inflammatory features in the shoulder joints and axilla on MRI and ultrasonography may be useful diagnostically in PMR.

Treatment of giant cell arteritis without AAION

Treatment in the absence of visual symptoms is with oral prednisolone. An initial dose of 1 mg/kg daily is typical, the subsequent duration of treatment being governed by the response of symptoms and the level of the ESR or CRP. Symptoms may recur without a corresponding rise in ESR or CRP and vice versa. Most patients need treatment for 1–2 years, although some may require indefinite maintenance therapy. Rapid tapering should generally not occur, with added caution when the dose is reduced to below about 10 mg a day. CRP may play an important role in monitoring disease activity, as the level seems to fall more rapidly than the ESR in response to treatment.

Arteritic anterior ischaemic optic neuropathy

Arteritic anterior ischaemic optic neuropathy (AAION) affects 30–50% of untreated patients with GCA, of whom one-third develop involvement of the fellow eye, usually within a week of the first. Posterior ischaemic optic neuropathy is much less common.

- **Symptoms**
  - Sudden, profound unilateral visual loss not uncommonly preceded by transient visual obscurations (amaurosis fugax) and sometimes by double vision.

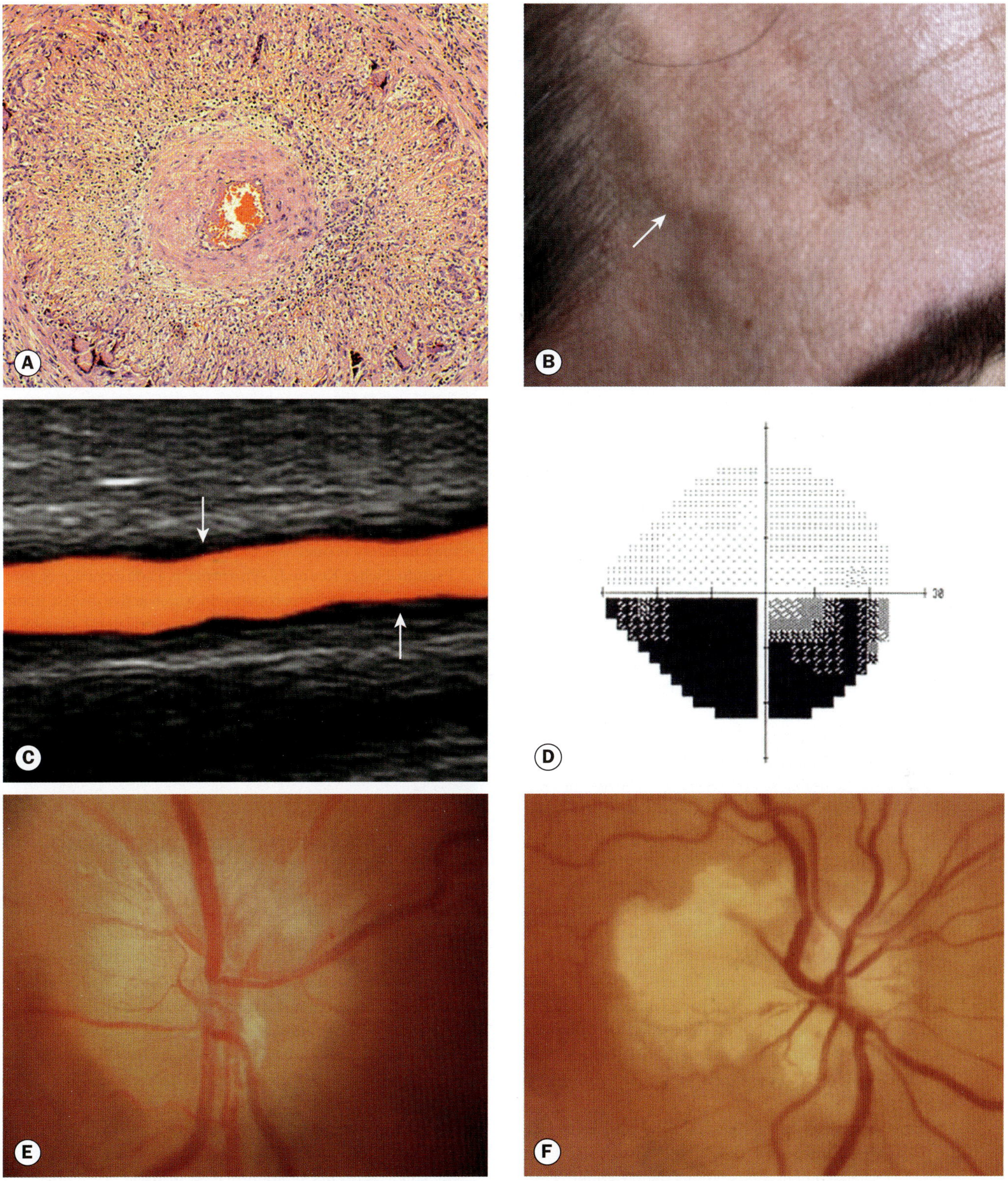

Fig. 19.14 Giant cell arteritis. **(A)** Histology showing transmural granulomatous inflammation, disruption of the internal elastic lamina, proliferation of the intima and gross narrowing of the lumen; **(B)** the superficial temporal artery is often pulseless, nodular and thickened; **(C)** ultrasound showing a hypoechoic halo around the superficial temporal artery lumen (arrows); **(D)** lower altitudinal visual field defect in arteritic ischaemic optic neuropathy; **(E)** pale swelling of the upper half of the optic disc of the patient in **(D)**; **(F)** ischaemic optic neuropathy and cilioretinal artery occlusion. *(Courtesy of J Harry and G Misson, from* Clinical Ophthalmic Pathology*, Butterworth-Heinemann 2002 – fig. A.)*

  - Periocular pain is common.
  - Other GCA symptoms are common. Most cases of AAION occur within a few weeks of the onset of GCA, although at presentation about 20% do not have systemic symptoms.
  - Simultaneous bilateral involvement is rare but rapid involvement of the second eye, with resultant total blindness, should always be regarded as a substantial risk.
- **Signs**
  - Severe visual loss is the rule. However, the upper or lower circulation can be affected leading to an altitudinal visual field defect (Fig. 19.14D).
  - A strikingly pale 'chalky white' oedematous disc (Fig. 19.14E) is particularly suggestive of GCA.
  - Over 1–2 months, the swelling gradually resolves and severe optic atrophy ensues.
- **Prognosis** is very poor. Visual loss is usually permanent, although, very rarely, prompt administration of systemic steroids may be associated with partial recovery.

TIP Immediate systemic steroid treatment should be prescribed for a patient with ischaemic optic neuropathy secondary to temporal arteritis, to reduce the risk of visual loss in the fellow eye.

- **Treatment** is aimed at preventing blindness of the fellow eye, as visual loss in the index eye is unlikely to improve even with immediate treatment. The second eye may still become involved in 25% despite early steroid administration. The regimen is as follows:
  - Intravenous methylprednisolone, 500 mg to 1 g/day for 3 days followed by oral prednisolone 1–2 mg/kg daily. After 3 more days the oral dose is reduced to 50–60 mg (not less than 0.75 mg/kg) for 4 weeks or until symptom resolution and ESR/CRP normalization. A typical subsequent regimen consists of reducing the daily dose by 10 mg/day every 2 weeks until 20 mg/day is reached, with tapering afterwards titrated against ESR/CRP and symptoms, e.g. a 2.5 mg reduction every 2–4 weeks to 10 mg then a 1 mg reduction every 1–2 months.
  - Enteric-coated prednisolone may be appropriate, particularly in patients with a history of peptic ulceration.
  - Steroid treatment should be accompanied by bone and gastrointestinal protection, e.g. a weekly bisphosphonate, calcium/vitamin D supplementation and a proton pump inhibitor.
  - Monitoring should be performed by a physician with appropriate training and should look particularly for steroid-related complications. A full blood count, ESR/CRP, urea and electrolytes, random glucose and blood pressure should be checked at each visit. Every 1–2 years, a chest X-ray or more sophisticated imaging should be performed to exclude an aortic aneurysm and bone mineral density should be assessed.
  - Antiplatelet therapy, e.g. aspirin 600 mg stat then 100 mg/day should be commenced as this has been shown to reduce the risk of visual loss and stroke.
  - Any significant symptomatic relapse should be treated with an aggressive increase in steroid dose; intravenous methylprednisolone should be given if visual disturbance occurs.
  - Immunosuppressives such as methotrexate may be used as adjuncts in steroid-resistant cases or as steroid-sparing agents when extended treatment is required, though with caution as their benefit is considerably less proven than that of steroids.
  - Tocilizumab (a humanized monoclonal antibody against interleukin-6 receptor) may be helpful for relapsing or refractory GCA, especially when used in association with steroid tapering.

Other manifestations

- **Cilioretinal artery occlusion** may occasionally be combined with AAION (Fig. 19.14F).
- **Central retinal artery occlusion** is often combined with occlusion of a posterior ciliary artery – with resultant choroidal hypoperfusion – as the two can arise from the ophthalmic artery by a common trunk.
- **Ocular ischaemic syndrome** due to involvement of the ophthalmic artery is rare.
- **'Pseudo-Foster Kennedy syndrome'** is a consequence of anterior ischaemic optic neuropathy, in which active disease in one eye (Fig. 19.15A) is associated with contralateral atrophy in the other eye secondary to a previous episode (Fig. 19.15B). It should be distinguished from true Foster Kennedy syndrome, which is uncommon and is classically caused by a frontal space-occupying lesion, characterized by ipsilateral compressive optic atrophy and contralateral papilloedema secondary to raised intracranial pressure.

Posterior ischaemic optic neuropathy

Posterior ischaemic optic neuropathy (PION) is much less common than the anterior variety. It is caused by ischaemia of the retrolaminar portion of the optic nerve supplied by the surrounding pial capillary plexus, which in turn is supplied by pial branches of the ophthalmic artery. Only a small number of capillaries actually penetrate the nerve and extend to its central portion among the pial septae. The diagnosis of PION should be made only after other causes of retrobulbar optic neuropathy have been excluded, such as compression or inflammation. Initially, the optic disc appears normal, but pallor develops over weeks.

- **Operative** (perioperative) PION develops following a variety of surgical procedures, most notably involving the heart and the spine. It occurs in about 0.02% of these procedures. The major risk factors appear to be anaemia and intraoperative hypovolaemic hypotension. Bilateral involvement is common and the visual prognosis is poor. Prompt blood transfusion and treatment of facial/orbital swelling may be of benefit.
- **Arteritic** PION is associated with GCA and carries a poor visual prognosis.
- **Non-arteritic** PION is associated with the same systemic risk factors as NAION, but is not associated with a crowded optic

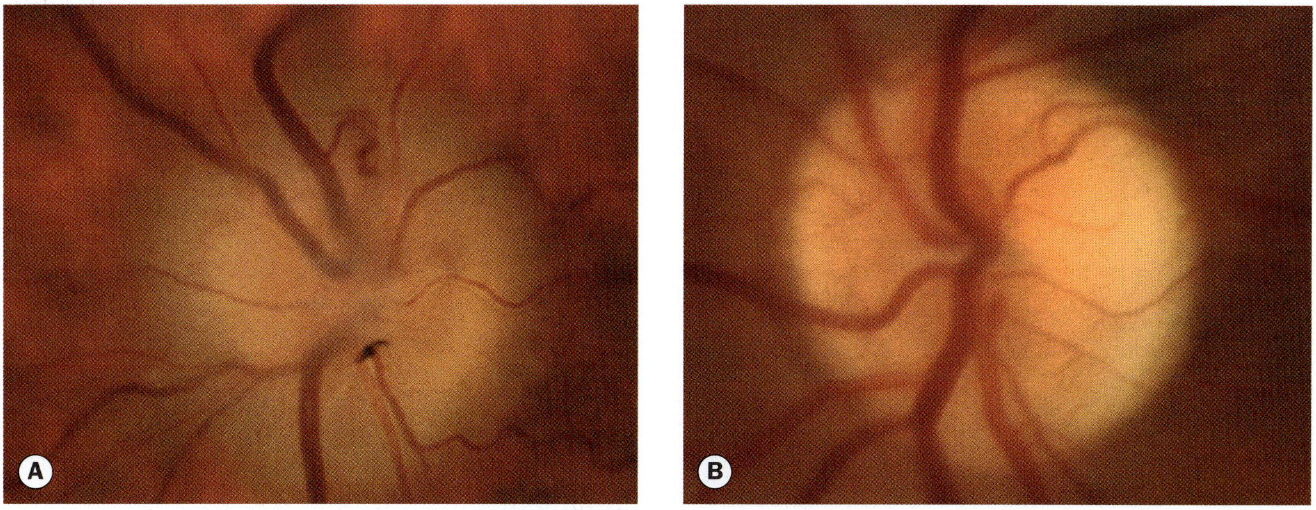

Fig. 19.15 'Pseudo-Foster Kennedy syndrome'. (A) Swollen disc in the acute phase; (B) opposite eye showing subtle optic atrophy.

disc. The visual prognosis is similar to NAION. Some practitioners prescribe a short course of high-dose systemic steroid in early cases.

Diabetic papillopathy

The cause of diabetic papillopathy is unknown, but it possibly represents a mild form of non-arteritic ischaemic optic neuropathy. Younger patients (under 50 years) are more likely to be affected and usually present with slight visual symptoms. The optic disc shows either hyperaemic oedema or marked telangiectasia of the inner surface microvasculature, which can be mistaken for neovascularization (see Fig. 13.24). Diabetic retinopathy is usually present, with macular oedema in 25% and retinal neovascularization in about 10%. It should be differentiated from NAION, which has a poor prognosis. There is no treatment, but the disc oedema slowly resolves over a period of 2–10 months resulting in a final visual acuity of 6/12 or better in 80% of cases, subject to the effect of co-existing diabetic retinopathy.

- **The criteria for diagnosis** include:
  - The presence of diabetes (type 1 in 70%, type 2 in 30%).
  - Optic disc oedema (unilateral in about 60%).
  - Mild optic nerve dysfunction.
  - Absence of ocular inflammation or raised intracranial pressure.

Leber hereditary optic neuropathy

Introduction

Leber hereditary optic neuropathy (LHON) is a rare ganglion cell degeneration that typically affects the papillomacular bundle. The condition is caused by maternally inherited mitochondrial DNA point mutations, most frequently (50–90%) at nucleotide position 11778 (G to A) in the *MT-ND4* gene; primarily affecting respiratory chain complex genes. It is the commonest inherited mitochondrial disorder. The condition typically affects males between the ages of 15 and 35 years, although in atypical cases the condition may affect females and present at any age between 10 and 60 years. The diagnosis of LHON should therefore be considered in any patient with bilateral optic neuropathy, irrespective of age.

Diagnosis

- **Symptoms.** Typically, acute or subacute severe painless unilateral (50%) loss of central vision occurs. In initially unilateral cases, the fellow eye becomes similarly affected within weeks or months.
- **Signs** during the acute stage are often subtle and easily overlooked and in some patients the disc may be entirely normal.
  - Colour vision is likely to be subnormal.
  - There is often a relative afferent pupillary defect.
  - In typical cases there is disc hyperaemia with obscuration of the disc margins (Fig. 19.16A).
  - Dilated capillaries on the disc surface, which may extend onto adjacent retina (telangiectatic microangiopathy – Fig. 19.16B).
  - Swelling of the peripapillary nerve fibre layer (pseudo-oedema).
  - Dilatation and tortuosity of posterior pole vasculature.
  - Subsequently, the vessels and pseudo-oedema regress and severe optic atrophy supervenes (Fig. 19.16C), with nerve fibre layer dropout most pronounced in the papillomacular bundle.
  - Telangiectatic microangiopathy may be present in asymptomatic female relatives.
  - Surprisingly, the pupillary light reactions may remain fairly brisk.
- **LHON plus** refers to rare variants with additional manifestations such as neuromuscular dysfunction.
- **Prognosis** is poor, although some visual recovery may occur in a minority of cases even years later. Most patients suffer permanent bilateral visual loss with a final VA of 6/60 or less. The prognosis is better if the age of onset is less than 20 years and especially if the age of onset is less than

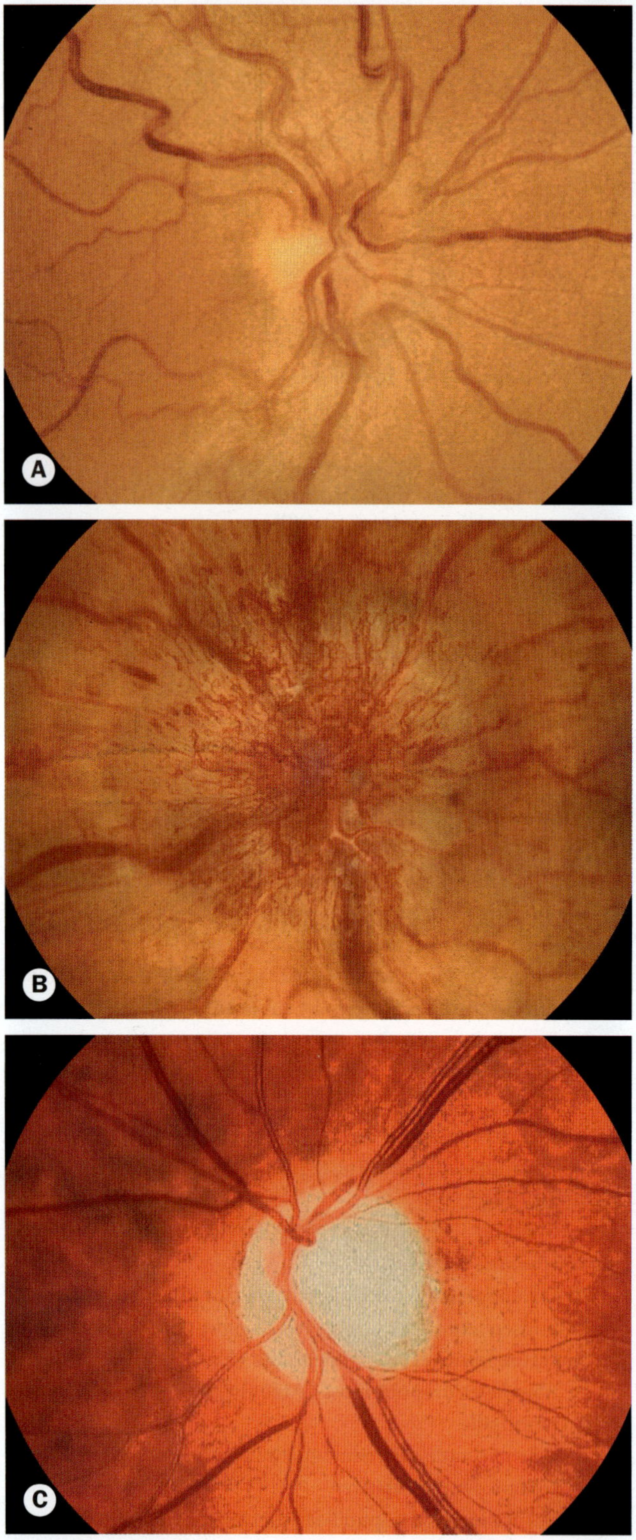

Fig. 19.16 Leber hereditary optic neuropathy. **(A)** Acute stage showing hyperaemic disc swelling with blurring of margins; **(B)** marked telangiectatic microangiopathy; **(C)** late – atrophic appearance.

TIP Undertake genetic testing for Leber hereditary optic neuropathy in any patient who presents with bilateral optic neuropathy of unknown cause.

10 years. The 11778 mutation carries the worst prognosis and the 14484 mutation has the best chance of spontaneous visual recovery.

- **Investigations**
  - OCT. Patients show peripapillary retinal thinning. Unaffected carriers frequently show variable thickening of the temporal RNFL, perhaps due to compensatory mitochondrial accumulation.
  - Visual field defects usually consist of central or centrocaecal scotomas, with preserved peripheral vision.
  - FA shows no leakage from the disc or microangiopathic vessels.
  - Genetic testing to look for the three common causative mutations.

Treatment

- Apart from symptomatic measures such as low vision aids, treatment is generally ineffective.
- Mitochondrial 'cocktails' have been tried, which include various vitamins, co-factors (CoQ_{10}), creatine and alpha-lipoic acid, with anecdotal success. Subspecialist prescription of one or more of these may be worthwhile, particularly in early disease or prior to second eye involvement.
- Counterintuitively, the cyanocobalamin (but not the hydroxocobalamin) form of vitamin B_{12} has been reported to worsen outcomes.
- Smoking and excessive alcohol consumption should be discouraged.
- Idebenone (900 mg/day) appears to be neuroprotective in this condition and may have a role to play in some patients.
- Intravitreal gene therapy is showing promising results; an adeno-associated virus vector expressing normal *ND4* complementary DNA is used in patients with the 11778 mutation.

Miscellaneous hereditary optic neuropathies (atrophies)

This heterogeneous group of rare disorders are characterized primarily by bilateral optic atrophy. There is no effective treatment, though the measures described above for LHON may be tried.

Dominant optic atrophy (Kjer type optic atrophy, optic atrophy type 1)

- **Inheritance** is autosomal dominant (AD). This is the most common hereditary optic neuropathy, with an incidence of around 1:50 000. It is frequently due to a mutation in the *OPA1* gene on chromosome 3, which causes mitochondrial dysfunction, but other genes can be responsible and X-linked and autosomal recessive (AR) forms have been reported. There is usually high penetrance but variable expressivity in the dominant forms.
- **Presentation** is typically, though not always, in childhood with insidious visual loss. There is usually a family history, but the course may be variable even within the same family.
- **Optic atrophy** may be subtle and temporal (Fig. 19.17A and B) or diffuse (Fig. 19.17C and D). There may be enlargement of the cup.

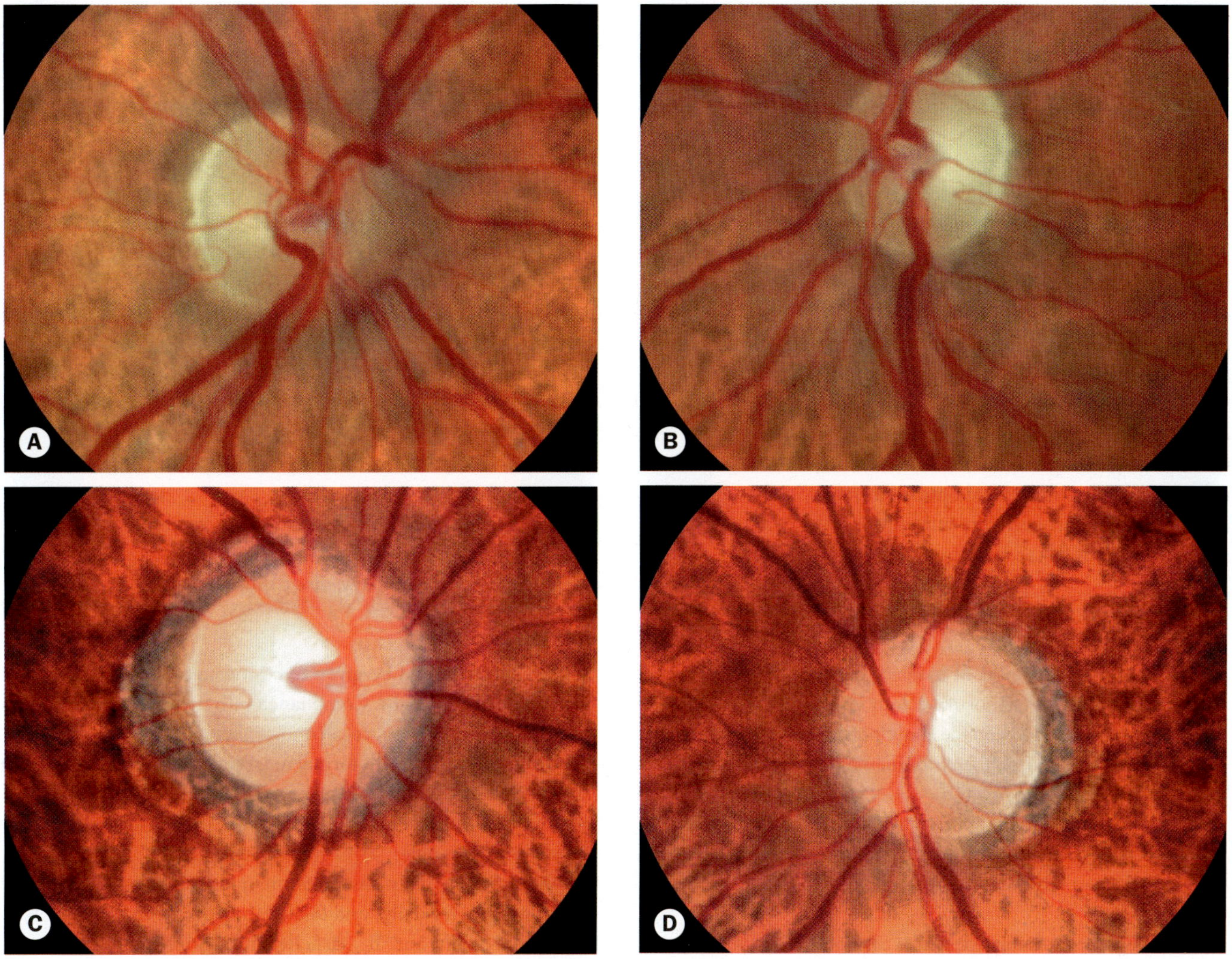

Fig. 19.17 Hereditary optic atrophy. **(A** and **B)** Bilateral temporal disc pallor; **(C** and **D)** bilateral diffuse pallor.

- **Prognosis** is variable (final VA 6/12–6/60) with considerable differences within and between families. Very slow progression over decades is typical.
- **Systemic abnormalities.** Twenty per cent develop sensorineural hearing loss. Other features are less common.

Behr syndrome

- **Inheritance** is AR; heterozygotes may have mild features.
- **Presentation** is in early childhood with reduced vision.
- **Optic atrophy** is diffuse.
- **Prognosis** is variable, with moderate to severe visual loss and nystagmus.
- **Systemic abnormalities** include spastic gait, ataxia and mental handicap.

Wolfram syndrome

Wolfram syndrome is also referred to as DIDMOAD (diabetes insipidus, diabetes mellitus, optic atrophy and deafness).

- **Inheritance.** Three genetic forms are recognized, caused by a variety of mutations in *WFS1*, which gives Wolfram syndrome 1, *CISD2* – Wolfram syndrome 2 – and probably a form caused by a mitochondrial DNA mutation, with inheritance being AR, AD or via the maternal mitochondrial line.
- **Presentation** is usually between the ages of 5 and 21 years. Diabetes mellitus is typically the first manifestation, followed by visual problems.
- **Optic atrophy** is diffuse and severe and may be associated with disc cupping.
- **Prognosis** is typically poor (final VA is <6/60).
- **Systemic abnormalities** (apart from DIDMOAD) are highly variable, presumably in part due to genetic heterogeneity and may include anosmia, ataxia, seizures, mental handicap, short stature, endocrine abnormalities and elevated CSF protein. Life expectancy is usually substantially reduced.

Nutritional optic neuropathy

Introduction

Nutritional optic neuropathy (tobacco-alcohol amblyopia) is an uncommon but underdiagnosed acquired optic neuropathy.

The mechanism is thought to be deficient mitochondrial function, similar to that of the heritable optic neuropathies, and like these the papillomacular bundle is preferentially affected. In Western developed countries the condition typically affects individuals with high alcohol and tobacco consumption. Most patients have neglected their diet and the features are most likely to be due principally to deficiency in the B-complex vitamins, particularly cyanocobalamin (B_{12}) and thiamine (B_1), but also riboflavin (B_2), niacin (B_3) and pyridoxine (B_6). Copper, folic acid and protein deficiency may also be important and direct toxic effects of alcohol and tobacco may also be significant. A strict vegan diet can also be causative, as can dietary deficiency in elderly patients. A similar clinical picture may be seen due to toxicity from medication or environmental (e.g. occupational) toxins. In under-resourced geographic regions, nutritional aetiological factors due to inadequate dietary intake predominate and nutritional optic neuropathy can be epidemic. Pernicious anaemia sufferers may develop the condition due to reduced vitamin B_{12} absorption.

Diagnosis

- **Symptoms**
  - The insidious onset of painless bilateral central blurring associated with abnormal colour vision.
  - Enquiry should be made about potentially causative medication (see Ch. 21), environmental toxin exposure and a vegan diet.
  - A family history of optic neuropathy should be excluded.
  - Peripheral neurological symptoms (sensory loss, gait disturbance) raise the suspicion of a peripheral neuropathy.
- **Signs**
  - VA is very variably affected.
  - The discs at presentation are normal in most cases, but some patients show subtle pallor, often temporal, splinter-shaped haemorrhages on or around the disc, or minimal oedema.
  - The pupil reactions are often normal, but may respond weakly in more severe cases.
  - Other ocular and systemic features of nutritional deficiency should be sought (and investigations carried out accordingly), e.g. Korsakoff syndrome, Wernicke disease and pernicious anaemia. Xerophthalmia and beriberi should be considered in developing nations.
- **Colour vision testing.** A reduction in colour vision is disproportionate to the reduction in acuity. Red desaturation is likely to be present. Ishihara chart testing is a simple, moderately quantitative test that is widely available.
- **Visual field defects** are bilateral, relatively symmetrical, centrocaecal scotomas. The margins of the defects are difficult to define with a white target but are more substantive with a red target.
- **OCT** may show peripapillary RNFL thickening and will help to exclude macular pathology.
- **Fundus autofluorescence (FAF)** is useful to exclude macula changes secondary to a cone or cone-rod dystrophy, that may present with colour deficiency and a central scotoma.
- **Prognosis** is good in early cases provided patients comply with treatment although visual recovery may be slow. Colour perception returns more slowly than measured acuity. In advanced cases there is likely to be a substantial permanent deficit, but it is highly unusual for complete loss of useful vision to occur, with preservation of peripheral field usual even in quite severe cases.
- **Blood tests.** B_{12} (cobalamin) and folate (serum and red cell) and possibly other vitamin levels such as B_1 (thiamine) and B_2, a full blood count and film (macrocytic anaemia) and serum protein levels. Screening for specific toxins or for LHON (see above) mutations may be indicated. A high serum methylmalonate and/or homocysteine level may be an indicator of potentially functional B_{12} deficiency, even in the presence of a low–normal B_{12}.
- **VEP.** The P100 amplitude is markedly reduced but with normal or near-normal latency.
- **MRI** is commonly considered to rule out intracranial pathology, particularly when an atypical clinical picture is present (e.g. marked asymmetry, disc pallor but good vision).

Treatment

Consideration should be given to co-management with a general physician or neurologist. Compliance with treatment and review is commonly poor in tobacco-alcohol amblyopia.

- **Dietary revision** with formal nutritional advice, incorporating increased fruit and leafy green vegetable intake.
- **Abstention from alcohol and tobacco** is a priority, but is not always achievable.
- **Vitamins.** A daily multivitamin preparation, plus thiamine (100 mg twice daily) and folate (1 mg daily). In someone who is both folate and B_{12} deficient it is prudent to correct the B_{12} deficiency first to avoid precipitating subacute combined degeneration of the cord.
- **Intramuscular hydroxocobalamin** (vitamin B_{12}) injections. The use of injected B_{12} has become less popular in recent years, as evidence shows that even in malabsorption states oral treatment may be effective. Hydroxocobalamin injections improve vision in tobacco-alcohol amblyopia, perhaps by reversing cyanide toxicity and should be considered in severe or unresponsive cases. Regimens range from 1 mg weekly for 8 weeks to monthly for several months. Injections every 3 months are typically continued for life.
- **Exposure to the identified agent** should be discontinued immediately in cases due to medication or environmental toxicity.

Papilloedema

Introduction

Papilloedema is swelling of the optic nerve head secondary to raised intracranial pressure (ICP). 'Disc swelling' and 'disc oedema' are non-specific terms that include papilloedema but also a disc swollen from other causes. All patients with papilloedema should be suspected of harbouring an intracranial mass. Not all patients

Table 19.3 Causes of Optic Disc Elevation

- Papilloedema
- Accelerated hypertension
- Anterior optic neuropathy
  - Ischaemic
  - Inflammatory
  - Infiltrative
  - Compressive including orbital disease
- Pseudopapilloedema
  - Disc drusen
  - Tilted optic disc
  - Peripapillary myelinated nerve fibres
  - Crowded disc in hypermetropia
- Mitochondrial optic neuropathies
  - Leber hereditary optic neuropathy
  - Methanol poisoning
- Intraocular disease
  - Central retinal vein occlusion
  - Uveitis
  - Posterior scleritis
  - Hypotony

with raised ICP will develop disc swelling. Causes of a swollen optic disc are given in Table 19.3.

TIP All patients with papilloedema should undergo urgent neuroradiological investigation to exclude intracranial pathology.

Cerebrospinal fluid

- **Circulation** (Fig. 19.18A)
  - Cerebrospinal fluid (CSF) is formed by the choroid plexus in the ventricles of the brain.
  - It leaves the lateral ventricles to enter the third ventricle through the foramina of Munro.
  - From the third ventricle, it flows through the Sylvian aqueduct to the fourth ventricle.
  - From the fourth ventricle, the CSF passes through the foramina of Luschka and Magendie to enter the subarachnoid space, flowing around the spinal cord and bathing the cerebral hemispheres.
  - Absorption is into the cerebral venous system through the arachnoid villi.
- **Normal CSF pressure** on lumbar puncture (not upright) is 10–18 cmH_2O in adults.
- **Causes of raised ICP** (Fig. 19.18B)
  - Idiopathic intracranial hypertension.
  - Obstruction of the ventricular system by congenital or acquired lesions.
  - Space-occupying intracranial lesions, including haemorrhage.
  - Impairment of CSF absorption due to meningitis, subarachnoid haemorrhage or trauma.
  - Cerebral venous sinus thrombosis (Fig. 19.19).
  - Cerebral oedema from blunt head trauma.
  - Severe systemic hypertension.

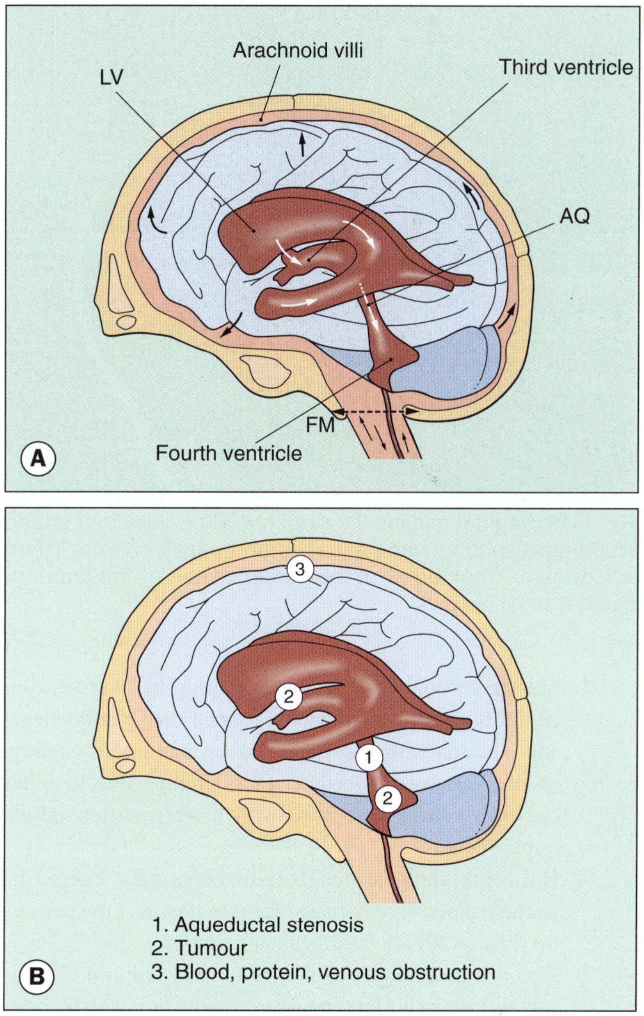

Fig. 19.18 (A) Circulation of cerebrospinal fluid; **(B)** causes of raised intracranial pressure – see text. AQ = aqueduct of Sylvius; FM = foramen magnum; LV = lateral ventricle.

  - Hypersecretion of CSF by a choroid plexus tumour (very rare).

Diagnosis of raised ICP

- **Headaches**, which characteristically occur early in the morning and may wake the patient from sleep, although less commonly they can occur at any time of day. The pain may be generalized or localized and may intensify with head movement, bending or coughing. They tend to get progressively worse over time. Very rarely, headache may be absent.
- **Nausea**, often episodic and with associated projectile vomiting may occur as an isolated feature or may precede the onset of headaches.
- **Deterioration of consciousness** as severity increases, initially with drowsiness and somnolence. A dramatic deterioration in the level of consciousness may be indicative of brainstem distortion and requires immediate attention.
- **Visual symptoms** are commonly absent in mild or early raised ICP.

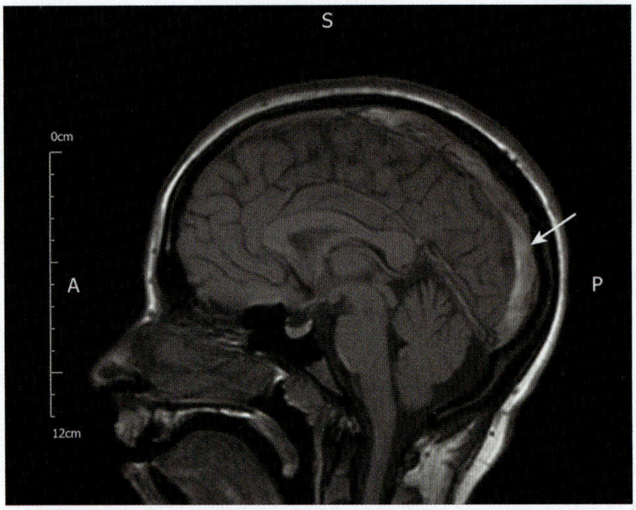

Fig. 19.19 Sagittal midline T1-weighted MR image in a young woman presenting with headache and papilloedema. There is extensive thrombosis of the posterior half of the superior sagittal sinus (arrow).

- Transient visual obscurations lasting up to 30 seconds in one or both eyes are frequent in established papilloedema and are sometimes precipitated by bending, coughing or the Valsalva manoeuvre. Disc swelling due to other causes is usually associated with more persistent visual impairment.
- Horizontal diplopia due to sixth nerve palsy caused by stretching of one or both abducens nerves over the petrous tip (Fig. 19.20) is a false localizing sign.
- Vision is generally normal or minimally reduced. Significant reduction is a late feature in conjunction with secondary optic atrophy.

- **Neurological examination should be performed.**
- **Investigations**
  - B-scan ultrasonography can be used to aid in distinguishing between papilloedema and other causes of a swollen or apparently swollen optic disc with 80–90% sensitivity and specificity by measuring the external diameter of the optic nerve sheath (ONSD), which is substantially distended (5.0–5.7 mm or greater at 3.0 mm behind the globe – Fig. 19.21A). The nerve must be scanned axially for the measurement to be accurate and there is a degree of operator dependence. In contrast to spontaneous venous pulsation (SVP – see below), ONSD does not normalize with short-term ICP fluctuation. The 'crescent sign' (Fig. 19.21B) refers to an echolucent area in the anterior intraorbital nerve thought to represent increased separation of the nerve and its sheath. Lateral gaze ('thirty-degree test') commonly leads to a 10% reduction in diameter on A-scan measurement in the presence of excess fluid (Fig. 19.21C and D), but not if normal or if increased ONSD is due to infiltration. Fluid-related ONSD can also be caused by other pathology, such as inflammation and trauma.
  - MRI to exclude a space-occupying lesion and/or enlarged ventricles. MRI can also be used to measure ONSD (average normal diameter approximately 5.5 mm ± 1 mm on MRI).

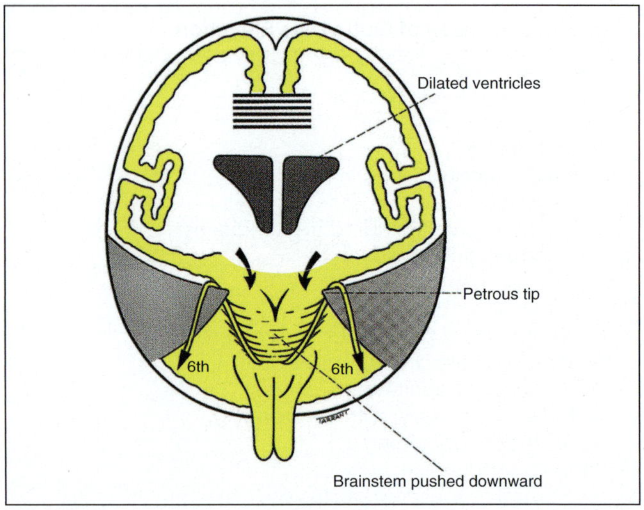

Fig. 19.20 Mechanism of sixth nerve palsy due to raised intracranial pressure.

  - In certain cases, vascular imaging such as venography may be performed, to rule out cerebral venous sinus thrombosis.
  - Lumbar puncture (LP) must not be carried out until imaging has excluded a space-occupying lesion that might cause downwards herniation of the intracranial contents towards the LP-induced low-pressure area. Clotting abnormality, including therapeutic anticoagulation, is also a contraindication unless reversed prior to the LP.

Stages of papilloedema

Papilloedema is nearly always bilateral, but may be asymmetrical.

- **Early** (Fig. 19.22A)
  - Mild disc hyperaemia with preservation of the optic cup.
  - Indistinct peripapillary retinal nerve striations and disc margins.
  - SVP is absent in about 20% of normal individuals and may be difficult to identify even when present. An identifiable venous pulsation in at least one eye means that the ICP is normal at that point in time, bearing in mind that diurnal fluctuation can occur.
- **Established** (acute – Fig. 19.22B)
  - Normal or reduced VA.
  - Severe disc hyperaemia, moderate elevation with indistinct margins and absence of the physiological cup.
  - Venous engorgement, peripapillary flame haemorrhages and frequently cotton-wool spots.
  - As the swelling increases, the optic nerve head appears enlarged.
  - Circumferential retinal folds (Paton lines) may develop, especially temporally (see Fig. 19.7C).
  - Macular fan: in younger patients small vesicles may form in the superficial retina, converging on the fovea in a fan shape with the apex at the fovea. This is not to be confused with a macular star, composed of exudates.
  - Enlarged blind spot.

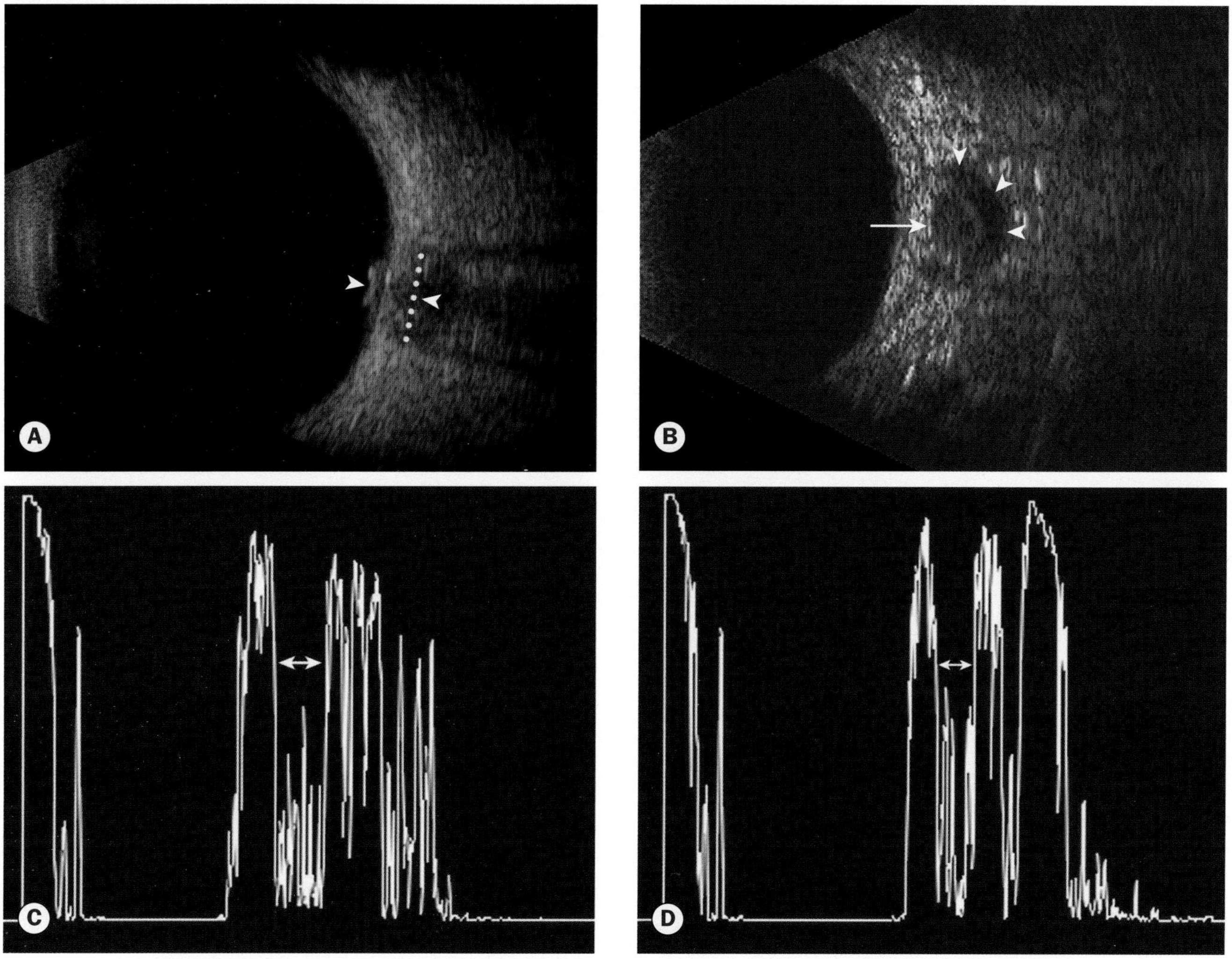

Fig. 19.21 Ultrasonography in papilloedema. **(A)** Optic nerve sheath diameter of 7.1 mm (stippled line), 3 mm posterior to the globe (arrowheads) ; **(B)** transverse B-scan showing crescent sign (arrowheads); optic nerve sheath diameter is measured 3 mm behind the globe (arrow); **(C)** A-scan in primary position with retrobulbar nerve diameter of 4.8 mm; **(D)** in lateral gaze diameter reduces to 3.5 mm – positive 30° test. *(Courtesy of L Lystad, B Hayden, A Singh, from* Ultrasound Clinics *2008;3:257–66 – figs B–D.)*

- **Chronic** (Fig. 19.22C)
  - VA is variable and the visual fields begin to constrict.
  - Disc elevation without cotton-wool spots and haemorrhages.
  - Optociliary shunts (see Ch. 13) and drusen-like crystalline deposits (corpora amylacea) may be present on the disc surface.
- **Atrophic** (secondary optic atrophy – Fig. 19.22D)
  - VA is severely impaired.
  - The optic discs are grey–white, slightly elevated, with few crossing blood vessels and indistinct margins.

Idiopathic intracranial hypertension

Introduction

Idiopathic intracranial hypertension, previously known as benign intracranial hypertension or pseudotumour cerebri, is characterized by elevated ICP that by definition has no identifiable cause. Obese young adult women are the most commonly affected group. Various medications including the contraceptive pill have been implicated (strictly 'secondary intracranial hypertension' if a cause is identified), as well as a range of conditions such as systemic lupus erythematosus, Lyme disease and sleep apnoea syndrome.

Diagnosis

- **Symptoms and signs** are similar to those of papilloedema, with headache in over 90%. Pulsatile tinnitus may be experienced, and cranial nerve palsies and occasionally other symptoms may occur. The long-term visual prognosis is usually good, but up to a quarter will have a degree of permanent impairment.
- **Investigation** is as for papilloedema: ONSD is increased and MRI may show slit-like ventricles and flattening of the pituitary gland ('empty sella' sign). MRV is usually carried out to exclude cerebral venous sinus thrombosis or

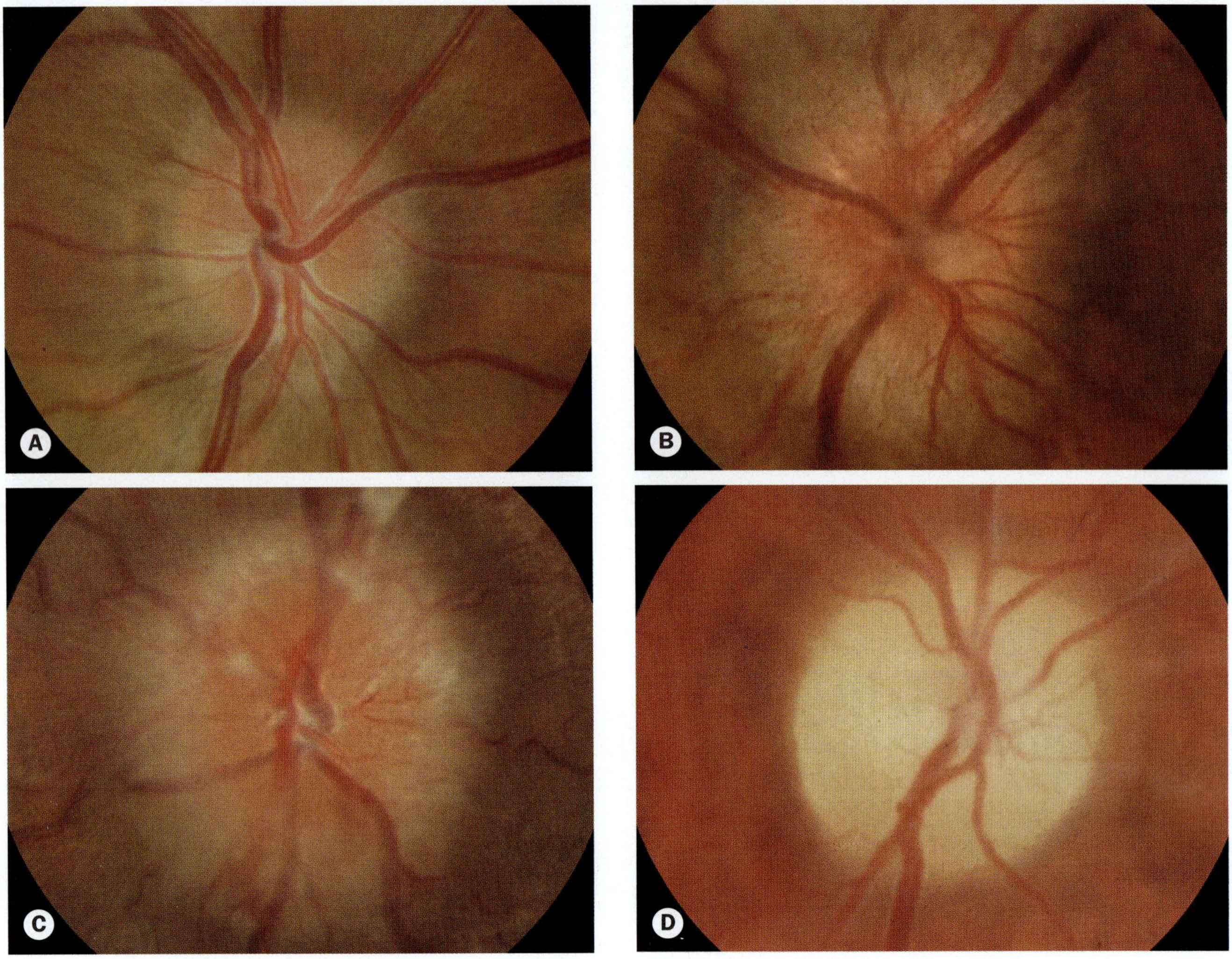

Fig. 19.22 Papilloedema. **(A)** Early; **(B)** acute established; **(C)** chronic; **(D)** atrophic.

stenosis. Additional investigation for an occult cause should be considered, especially in patients who do not fit the usual profile.

Treatment

- **Weight loss**, including via bariatric surgery, can be effective and formal dietary intervention is strongly recommended.
- **Medical.** Acetazolamide is the drug of first choice, although furosemide can also be considered. The use of steroids is controversial, but a short course is sometimes used in severe papilloedema. Intravenous mannitol is usually reserved for acute exacerbations.
- **Lumbar puncture.** This may be used for acute exacerbations, but usually has a short-lived effect.
- **Surgical.** In unresponsive cases optic nerve fenestration can be helpful. Other options include lumboperitoneal shunting and transverse dural sinus stenting, but these options have a high complication rate.
- **The ophthalmologist's role** is usually confined to diagnosis and the monitoring of visual function with VA, colour vision and fields, and optic nerve appearance/photography.

Congenital optic disc anomalies

Tilted disc

A tilted optic disc is a common anomaly, usually bilateral, describing an apparently oblique entry of the optic nerve into the globe. It is strongly associated with myopia and astigmatism. Tilting is defined as being present when the ratio of the longest diameter of the disc to the shortest (ovality index) is greater than 1.3 (Fig. 19.23A), but this will not include many subjectively apparently tilted discs. A major implication of tilting is difficulty in excluding superimposed glaucomatous damage, as the temporal, particularly the inferotemporal, neuroretinal rim is frequently very thin.

- **Signs.** Small, oval or D-shaped disc: the axis is most frequently directed inferonasally, but may be horizontal or nearly vertical.
  - The disc margin is indistinct where retinal nerve fibres are elevated.
  - Peripapillary chorioretinal thinning may be marked and situs inversus may be present. The temporal vessels deviate nasally before turning temporally (see Fig. 19.23A).

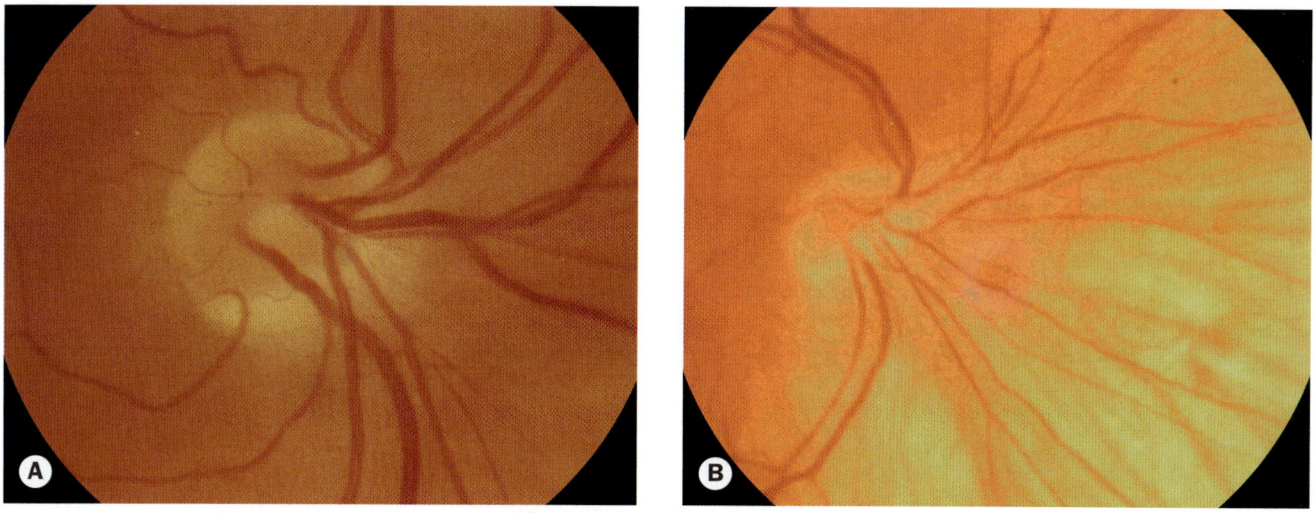

Fig. 19.23 Anatomical variants. **(A)** Tilted disc; **(B)** markedly tilted and torsional disc with situs inversus and associated inferonasal chorioretinal thinning.

- **Perimetry** may show superotemporal defects that do not respect the vertical midline.
- **OCT** may demonstrate sectoral peripapillary RNFL thinning, but the macular ganglion cell complex analysis is often – but not always – normal and thus may provide a more useful parameter for the exclusion of co-existent glaucomatous damage.
- **Complications** (rare) include choroidal neovascularization and sensory macular detachment.

Torsional disc

A torsional (torsioned) disc is said to be present when its long axis is inclined at more than 15° from the vertical meridian, a line at 90° to a horizontal line connecting the foveola to the centre of the optic disc (Fig. 19.23B). It is often present in association with tilting and is also associated with myopia.

Optic disc pit

- **Signs**
  - VA is normal in the absence of complications.
  - The disc is often larger than normal and contains a greyish round or oval pit of variable size, usually temporal (Fig. 19.24A–C) but occasionally central or elsewhere. Pits are bilateral in 10–15%.
  - Visual field defects are common and may mimic glaucoma. A central defect may indicate a macular detachment.
- **Serous macular detachment** develops in about half of eyes with non-central disc pits (median age 30 years). The source of the fluid is unclear.
  - A schisis-like retinal separation that extends from the pit is followed by serous detachment of the outer retinal layers (Fig. 19.24D). It is important to examine the optic disc carefully in all patients with central serous chorioretinopathy.
  - FA does not usually show hyperfluorescence of the detachment, which is demonstrated well on FAF and OCT.
- **Management.** Long-term follow-up is unnecessary. However, patients with this condition should be warned to return if their acuity changes or if they develop metamorphopsia. Options when macular detachment develops include:
  - Observation for spontaneous resolution, which occurs in up to 25%, but may worsen the eventual outcome.
  - Laser may be considered if vision is deteriorating. Light burns are applied along the temporal aspect of the disc. The success rate is 25–35%.
  - Vitrectomy with air–fluid exchange and postoperative prone positioning may be considered if laser is unsuccessful.

Optic disc drusen

Disc drusen are deposits, usually calcified, within the substance of the optic nerve head that are present in up to 2% of the population, often bilaterally (75%). They are usually sporadic but, in some cases, have AD inheritance. They are thought to consist of focal collections of axonal metabolic products.

- **Symptoms** are usually absent, but some patients may experience episodic blurring, possibly due to transient ischaemia related to a crowding effect.
- **Buried drusen.** Particularly in childhood, drusen may be obscured beneath the disc surface (Fig. 19.25A and B) and is a common cause of pseudopapilloedema. A lumpy disc appearance, an absent cup and anomalous vascular patterns including proximal branching, an increased number of major vessels and tortuosity suggest drusen, as well as a lack of papilloedematous features such as hyperaemia and vessel obscuration. Visibility of drusen typically increases in the early teens.
- **Exposed drusen.** Drusen at or close to the disc surface appear as whitish pearl-like lesions of a range of sizes (Fig. 19.25C and D). They tend to enlarge slowly over many years.
- **Retinal nerve fibre layer thinning** is common.
- **Visual field defects** of a range of configurations are present in up to 75% and are often progressive, though a substantial impact on sight is rare. No definitive treatment is recognized, though reducing IOP and other speculative measures may be tried in selected cases.

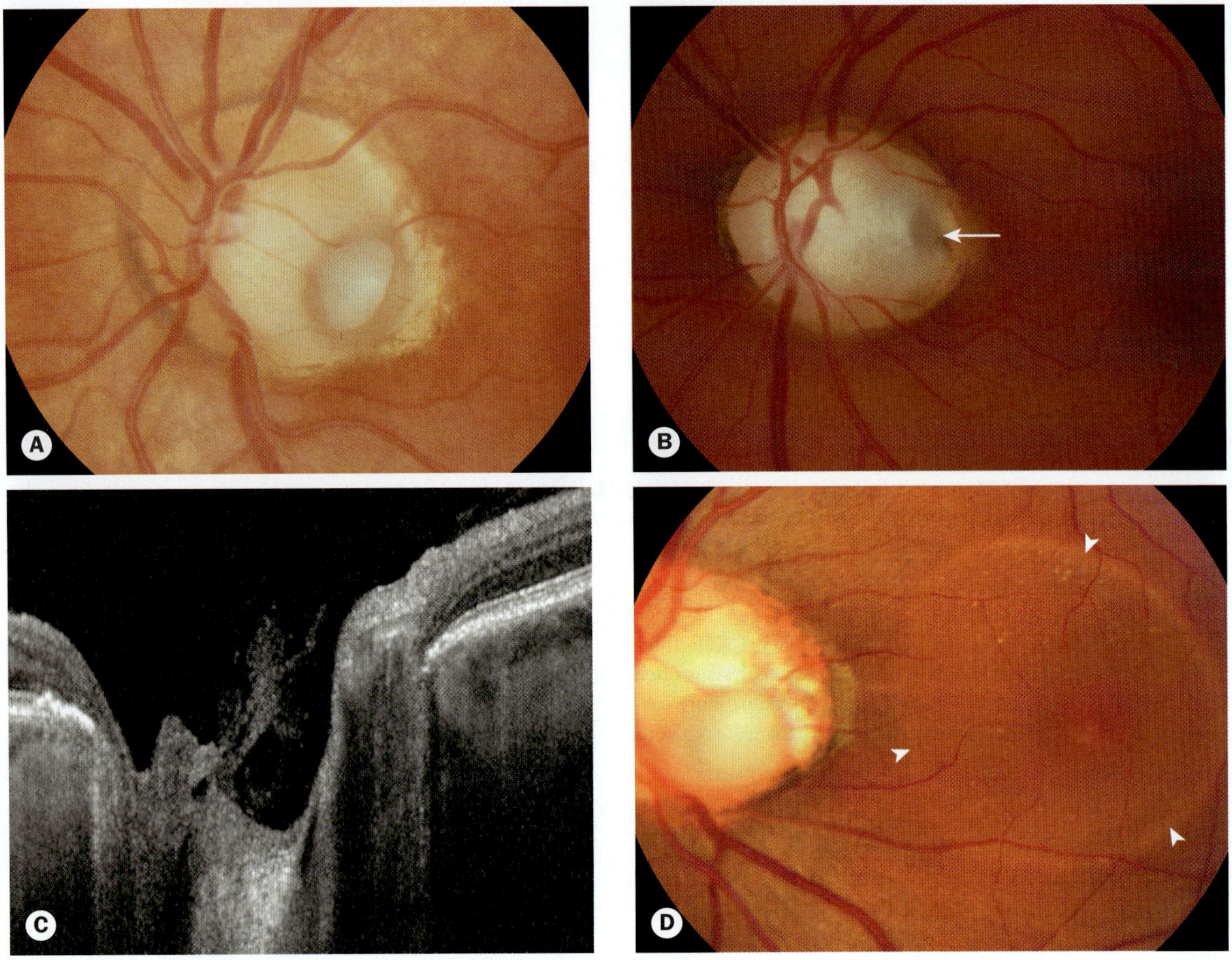

Fig. 19.24 Optic disc pit. (A) Inferotemporal; (B) temporal (arrow); (C) OCT of the optic disc; (D) macular detachment (arrowheads).

- **Associations** include retinitis pigmentosa and angioid streaks. Disc drusen are present in 90% of patients with Alagille syndrome.
- **Complications** (rare) include juxtapapillary choroidal neovascularization, vitreous haemorrhage and vascular occlusions, particularly anterior ischaemic optic neuropathy.
- **Imaging**
  - FAF usually demonstrates drusen extremely well (see Fig. 19.25B and D). Green-light FAF is the most sensitive of all en-face imaging techniques to detect optic disc drusen.
  - Ultrasonography (US) shows calcified drusen as highly reflective foci. US optic nerve features distinguishing raised ICP are discussed above.
  - OCT. Diffuse or focal RNFL thinning; OCT can be used for monitoring (Fig. 19.25E).
  - CT shows calcification but involves a substantial radiation dose and so is not indicated solely to confirm drusen (Fig. 19.25F).

TIP Buried optic disc drusen in children can mimic papilloedema.

Optic disc coloboma

The embryonic fissure of the developing eye is located inferiorly and slightly nasally and extends from the optic nerve to the margin of the pupil. A coloboma is a defect in one or more ocular structures due to the fissure's incomplete closure. The defect may be unilateral or bilateral and usually occurs sporadically in otherwise normal individuals (Fig. 19.26), though numerous systemic associations have been described, e.g. chromosomal abnormalities, CHARGE syndrome, Goldenhar syndrome and central nervous system abnormalities. An AD variety is caused by a mutation in the gene *PAX6*.

- **Signs**
  - VA is often decreased; amblyopia and refractive error may be present.
  - A disc pit is sometimes associated (Fig. 19.27A). Pit-like excavations are sometimes seen with a disc coloboma.
  - A disc coloboma may be associated with, or even continuous with, a large chorioretinal coloboma (Fig. 19.27B).
  - A focal, glistening white, bowl-shaped excavation, decentred inferiorly so that the inferior neuroretinal rim is thin or absent and normal disc tissue is confined

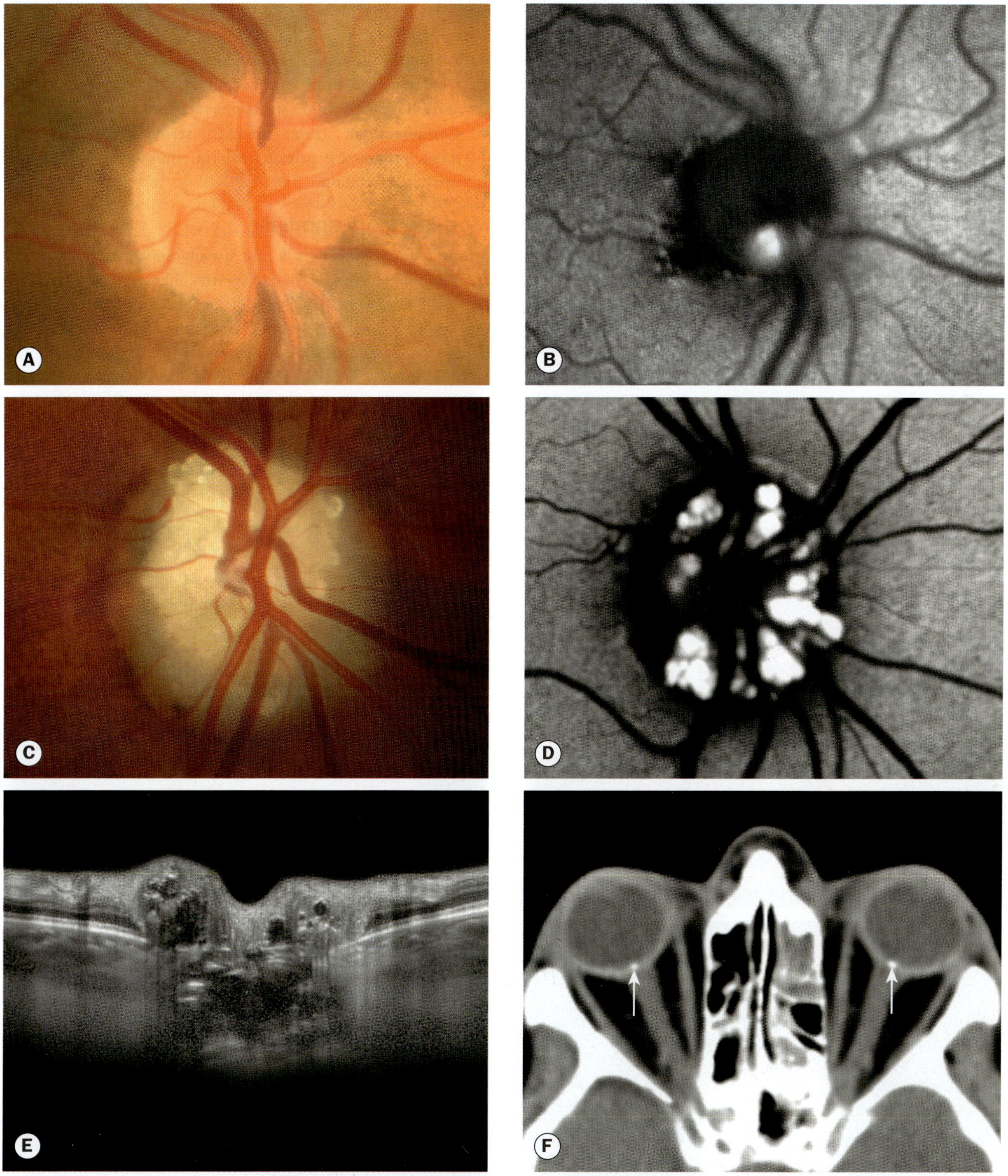

Fig. 19.25 Optic disc drusen. **(A)** Buried disc drusen; **(B)** fundus autofluorescence image of eye in **(A)**; **(C)** exposed disc drusen; **(D)** fundus autofluorescence; **(E)** OCT scan of the optic disc; **(F)** axial CT image of the orbits at the level of the optic nerves demonstrating focal calcification of the optic nerve heads (arrows).

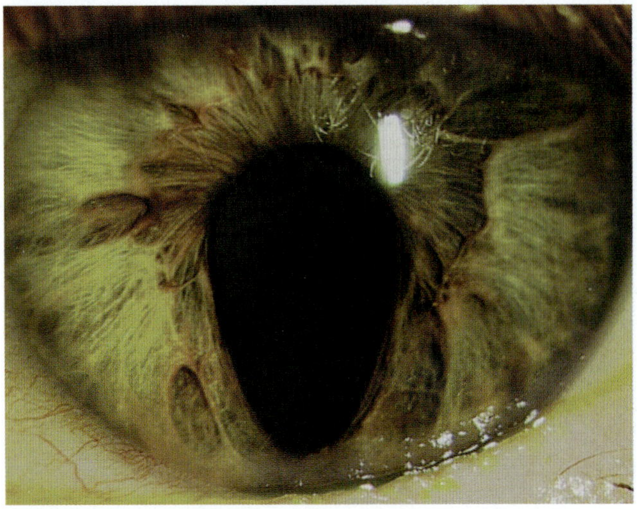

Fig. 19.26 Iris coloboma.

to a superior wedge of variable size depending on severity (Fig. 19.27C and D).

- **Perimetry** shows a superior defect.
- **Ocular associations** include microphthalmos, microcornea and coloboma of other structures such as the iris or lens.
- **Complications** (rare) include serous retinal detachment, progressive neuroretinal rim thinning and choroidal neovascularization.

Morning glory anomaly

Morning glory anomaly is a rare, usually unilateral and sporadic condition that has a spectrum of severity. Bilateral cases, which are rarer still, may be hereditary. As in coloboma, a *PAX6* gene mutation can be responsible. Systemic associations are uncommon, but the most important is frontonasal dysplasia, characterized by midfacial anomalies, a basal encephalocele and other midline brain malformations, including pituitary insufficiency (Fig. 19.28A).

- **Signs**
  - VA may be normal or impaired to a variable extent.

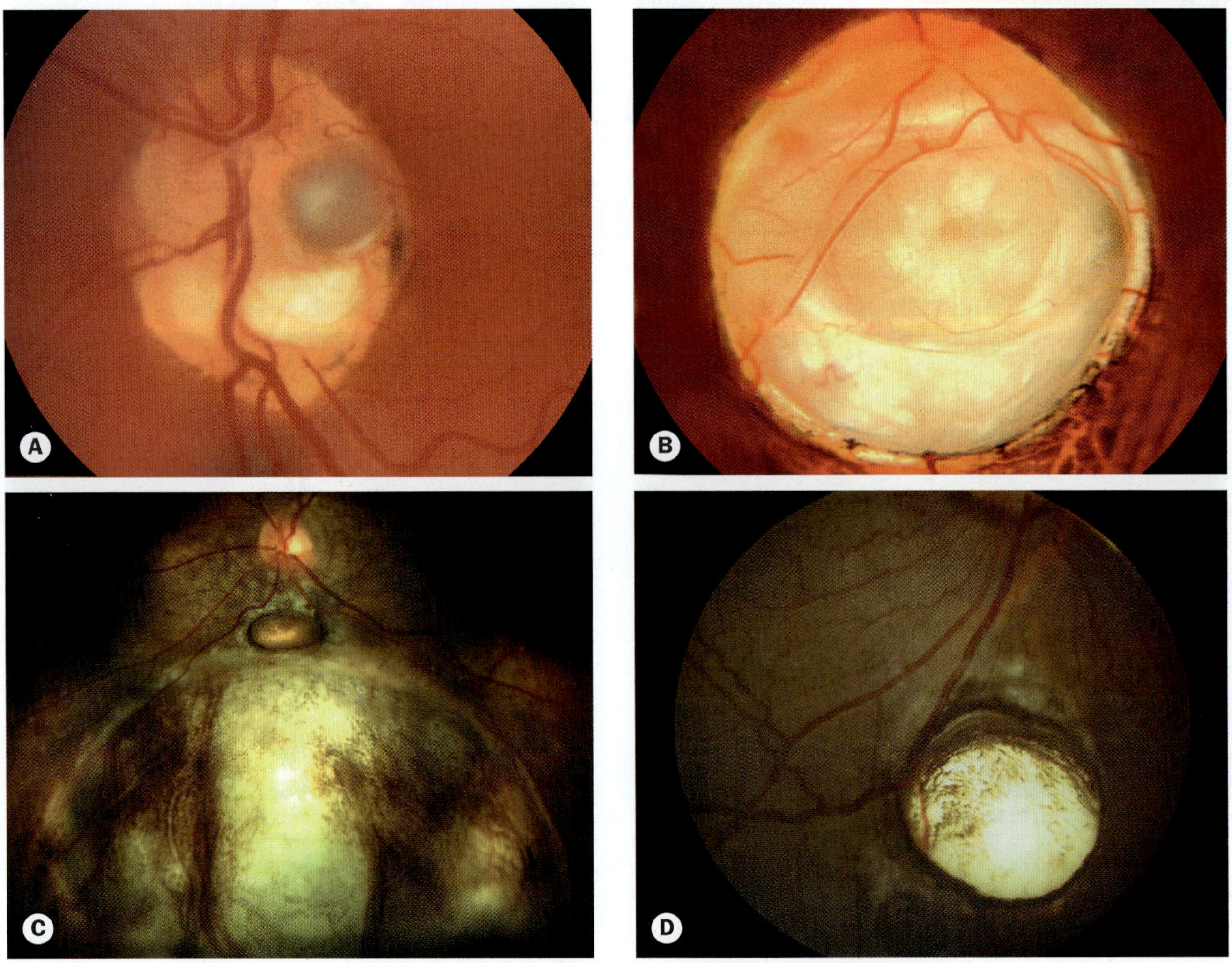

Fig. 19.27 Optic disc coloboma. **(A)** Coloboma with associated disc pit; **(B)** large disc coloboma; **(C)** montage of large chorioretinal coloboma; **(D)** isolated chorioretinal coloboma. *(Courtesy of P Gili – fig. B.)*

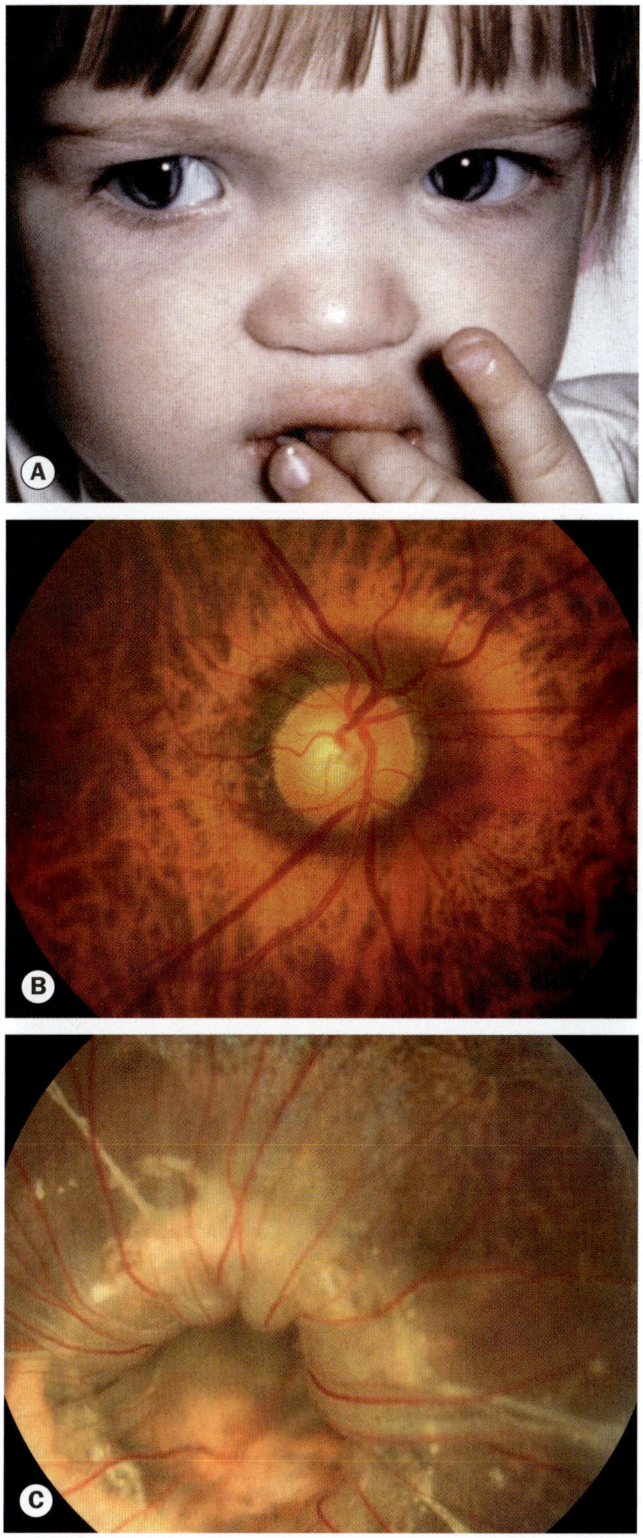

Fig. 19.28 (A) Hypertelorism and flat nasal bridge – note bilateral iris coloboma; **(B)** mild morning glory optic disc anomaly showing an annulus of chorioretinal pigmentary change surrounding the optic disc; **(C)** morning glory optic disc anomaly showing an enlarged, funnel-shaped excavation of the optic disc.

- A large disc with a funnel-shaped excavation surrounded by a ring-shaped chorioretinal disturbance (Fig. 19.28B and C).
- A white tuft of glial tissue overlies the central portion and represents persistent hyaloid vascular remnants.
- The blood vessels emerge from the rim of the excavation in a radial pattern like the spokes of a wheel. They are increased in number and it may be difficult to distinguish arteries from veins.

- **Complications** include serous retinal detachment (30%) and choroidal neovascularization.

Optic nerve hypoplasia

The hypoplastic optic nerve, unilateral or bilateral, carries a diminished number of nerve fibres. Its frequency seems to be increasing, though it remains relatively rare. Young maternal age, primiparity and maternal exposure to various agents have been linked. It may occur as an isolated anomaly in an otherwise normal eye, but systemic associations are common (see below).

- **Symptoms**
  - Severe bilateral cases present with blindness in early infancy with roving eye movements or nystagmus.
  - Unilateral or less severe bilateral cases usually present with squint.
  - Mild cases are easily overlooked.
- **Signs**
  - VA ranges from normal to severely impaired.
  - A relative afferent pupillary defect may be present. Both pupils may have sluggish light responses in bilateral cases.
  - Mild hypoplasia consists simply of a smaller than normal disc. A foveola disc-centre distance of three or more times the disc diameter strongly suggests hypoplasia.
  - Further along the hypoplastic spectrum, a small grey disc is seen, with central cupping-like deficiency of neural tissue and disc vessels emerging in a radial configuration. The vessels are sometimes tortuous.
  - The double-ring sign is characteristic and consists of a white ring of visible sclera surrounding a pigmented band thought to consist of migrated pigment epithelium (Fig. 19.29A). A thin outer pigmented line may also be seen.
- **Ocular associations** include astigmatism, amblyopia, field defects, foveal hypoplasia, aniridia and microphthalmos.
- **Systemic associations.** Optic disc hypoplasia is associated with a wide variety of developmental midline brain defects; pituitary and hypothalamic deficits are common. Historically, the most frequent association has been considered to be 'septo-optic dysplasia' (de Morsier syndrome) – bilateral optic nerve hypoplasia, absent septum pellucidum, corpus callosum agenesis (Fig. 19.29B–D) and hypopituitarism – but it is now believed that this complex does not exist as a specific entity.
- **Investigation.** All affected children should be screened for systemic associations, especially hormonal deficiencies and developmental delay.

Myelinated nerve fibres

Occasionally myelination of ganglion cell axons extends beyond the cribriform plate and is visible on retinal examination in about

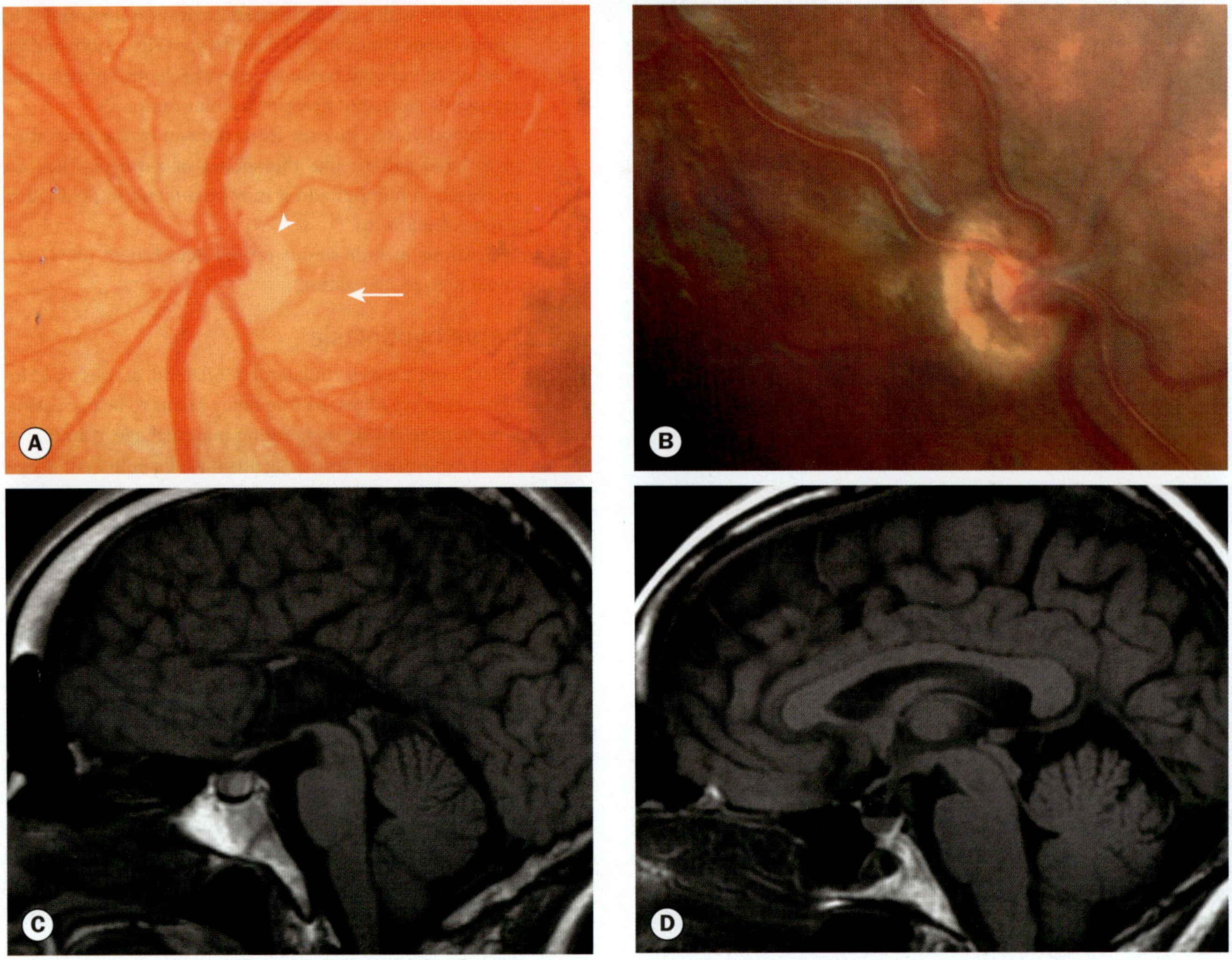

Fig. 19.29 (A) Moderately hypoplastic disc showing the double-ring sign. The arrowhead shows the edge of the disc and the arrow shows the edge of visible sclera; **(B)** markedly hypoplastic disc; **(C)** midline sagittal T1-weighted MR image demonstrating agenesis of the corpus callosum while **(D)** demonstrates a normal corpus callosum. *(Courtesy of D Hildebrand – fig. A; A Moore – fig. B.)*

1% of the population: myelinated or medullated nerve fibres (MNF). The condition is usually congenital and stable but both progression and an acquired form have been reported. MNF is occasionally familial. Systemic associations are very rare.

- **Signs**
  - VA is likely to be reduced if the central macula is involved. Perimetry may show an absolute scotoma corresponding to the involved area of retina.
  - One or more whitish striated patches with feathery borders. The location and size are variable (Fig. 19.30A–D) and two-thirds are not contiguous with the optic disc (Fig. 19.30B).
  - Retinal vessels in the involved area are obscured.
  - Between 5% and 10% of cases are bilateral.
  - The appearance can be mimicked by neoplastic infiltration and other conditions.
- **Ocular associations** include myopia, anisometropia, strabismus and amblyopia.
- **Imaging.** FAF shows hypoautofluorescence and there is masking of background fluorescence on FA. The RNFL is hyperreflective on OCT.
- **Treatment** consists of addressing refractive error, amblyopia and squint if present.

Aicardi syndrome

Aicardi syndrome consists of a range of central nervous system and other malformations in association with multiple bilateral depigmented chorioretinal lacunae clustered around a hypoplastic, colobomatous or pigmented optic disc (Fig. 19.31). Other ocular features can include cataract and coloboma. Inheritance is X-linked dominant; the condition is lethal *in utero* for males. Death usually occurs within the first few years of life in affected girls.

Bergmeister papilla

This relatively common anomaly consists of remnants of the hyaloid vessels (Fig. 19.32); see also Chapter 17.

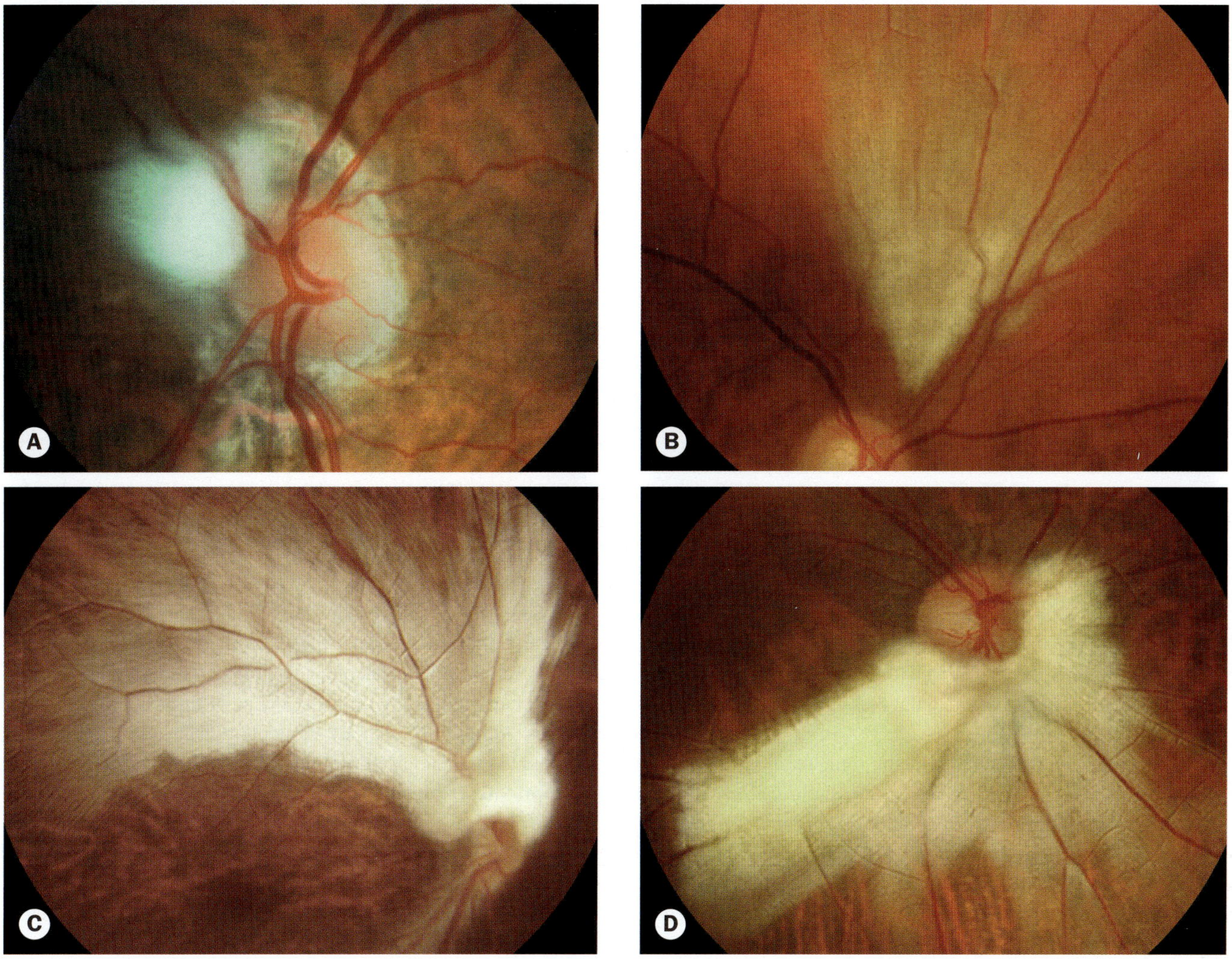

Fig. 19.30 Myelinated nerve fibres. **(A)** Mild juxtapapillary; **(B)** fan-shaped; **(C)** extensive superior to the disc; **(D)** extensive inferior to the disc.

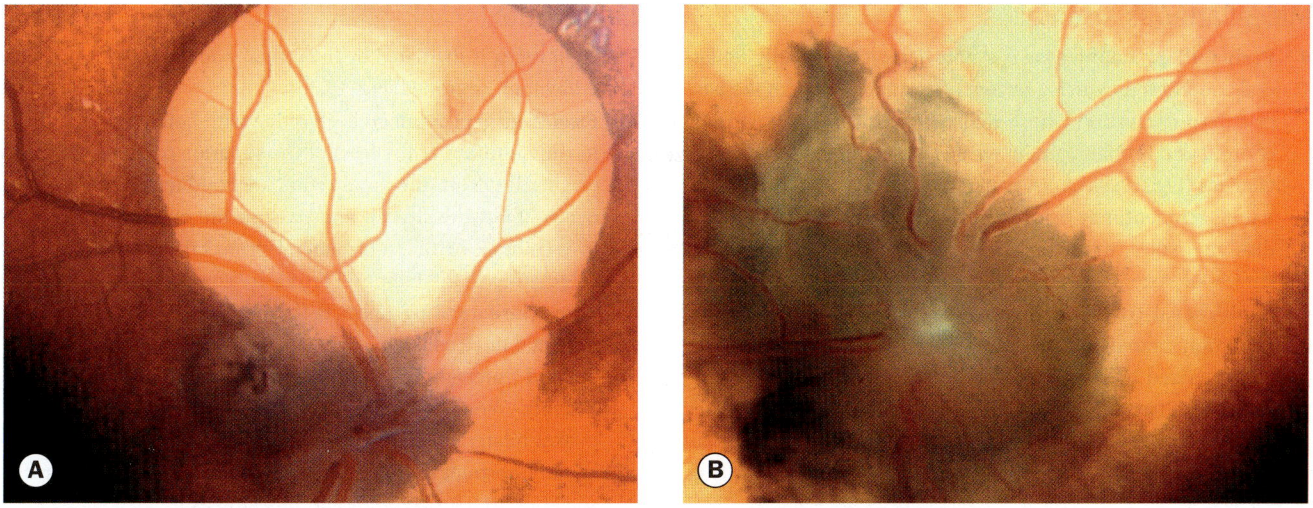

Fig. 19.31 The ocular fundus in Aicardi syndrome. **(A)** Right eye; **(B)** left eye.

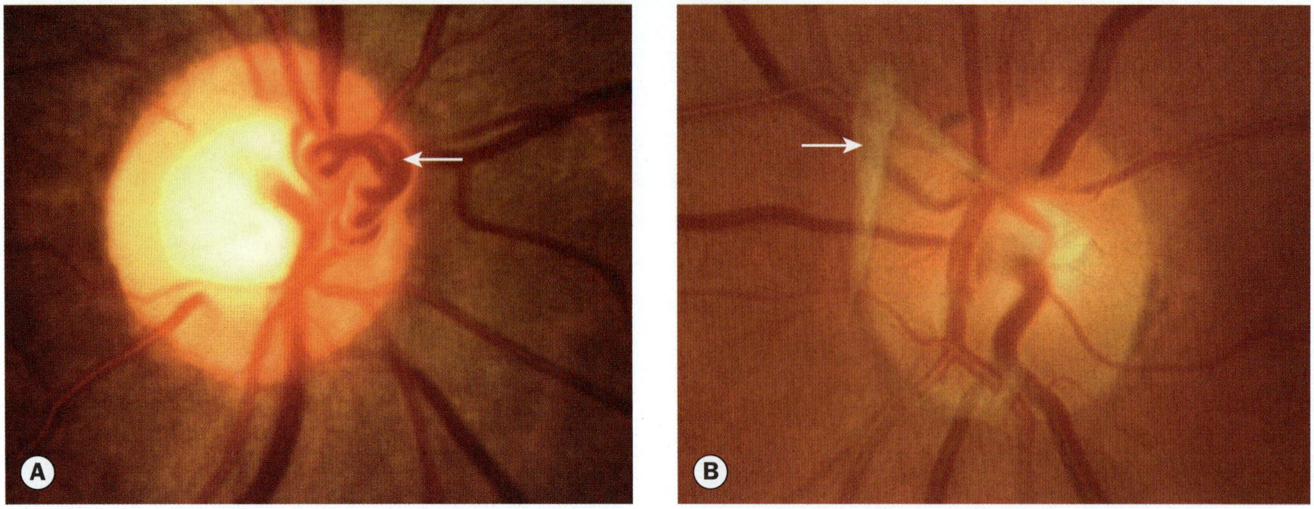

Fig. 19.32 Bergmeister papilla. **(A)** Prepapillary loop (arrow); **(B)** remnant of hyaloid vessel (arrow).

Acquired vascular abnormalities

- **Disc collaterals** are veno-venular shunts that develop within the existing vascular network to bypass an area of closure and are most frequently associated with retinal vein occlusion. The collaterals appear as distended flat vessels that start and end on the disc (Fig. 19.33A).
- **Optociliary shunts** are usually unilateral anastomoses between the retinal and choroidal circulations, consisting of enlarged pre-existing peripapillary capillaries. The vessels appear as large tortuous channels that disappear at the disc margin (Fig. 19.33B). The most common association is an optic nerve sheath meningioma. Other causes are discussed in Chapter 4.
- **Disc new vessels** manifest as fine, lace-like vessels that may extend onto adjacent retina. The vessels may be flat or elevated above the disc and may be associated with gliosis (Fig. 19.33C). Causes are discussed in Chapter 14.

Miscellaneous anomalies

- **Peripapillary staphyloma** is a non-hereditary, usually unilateral condition in which a relatively normal disc sits at the base of a deep excavation whose walls, as well as the surrounding choroid and retinal pigment epithelium (RPE), show atrophic changes (Fig. 19.34A). VA is markedly reduced and local retinal detachment may be present. Unlike other excavated optic disc anomalies, it is rarely associated with other congenital defects or systemic diseases.
- **Papillorenal (renal-coloboma) syndrome** is an AD genetic condition caused in most cases by a mutation in *PAX2* and characterized by renal and optic disc dysplasia. The discs do not exhibit true hypoplasia, but a failure of angiogenesis. They are normal in size with central excavation and replacement of the central retinal vasculature by cilioretinal vessels (Fig. 19.34B).
- **Optic disc dysplasia** is a descriptive term for a markedly deformed disc that does not conform to any recognizable category (Fig. 19.34C).
- **Megalopapilla** is a typically bilateral condition in which both the horizontal and vertical disc diameters are 2.1 mm or more, or the disc area is greater than 2.5 mm^2. Although the cup-to-disc ratio is greater than normal, the cup should retain its normal configuration with no evidence of focal neuroretinal rim loss. Although OCT may show peripapillary RNFL thinning, macular ganglion cell complex imaging is typically normal.
- **Optic nerve aplasia** is an extremely rare condition in which the optic disc is absent or rudimentary and retinal vessels are absent or few in number and abnormal. There may be retinal pigmentary disturbance, especially at the site where the optic disc might have been. Other ocular and systemic developmental defects may be present.

PUPILS

Anatomy

Light reflex

The light reflex is mediated by the retinal photoreceptors and subserved by four neurones (Fig. 19.35).

- **First** (sensory) connects each retina with both pretectal nuclei in the midbrain at the level of the superior colliculi. Impulses originating from the nasal retina are conducted by fibres that decussate in the chiasm and pass up the opposite optic tract to terminate in the contralateral pretectal nucleus. Impulses originating in the temporal retina are conducted by uncrossed fibres (ipsilateral optic tract) that terminate in the ipsilateral pretectal nucleus.
- **Second** (internuncial) connects each pretectal nucleus to both Edinger–Westphal nuclei. Thus, a uniocular light stimulus evokes bilateral and symmetrical pupillary constriction. Damage to internuncial neurones is responsible for light–near dissociation in neurosyphilis and pinealomas.
- **Third** (preganglionic motor) connects the Edinger–Westphal nucleus to the ciliary ganglion. The parasympathetic fibres pass through the oculomotor nerve, enter its inferior division

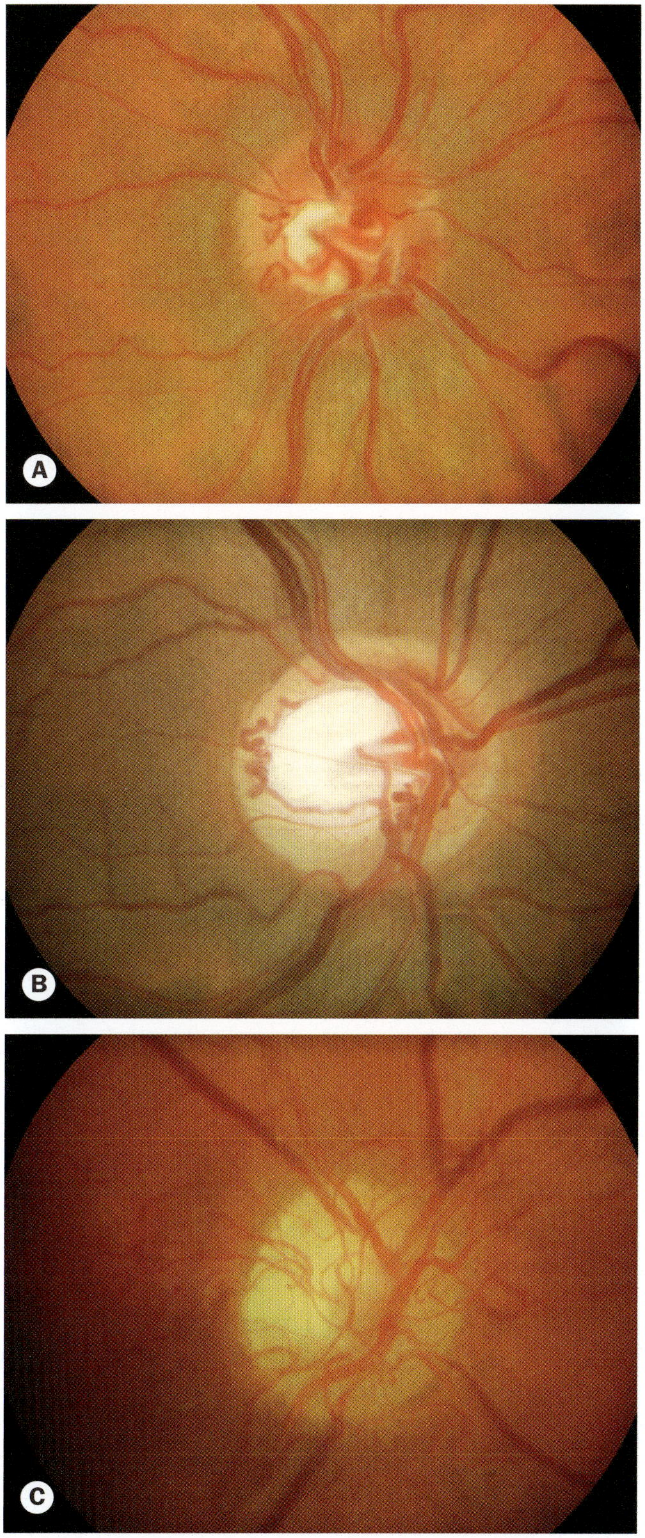

Fig. 19.33 Acquired vascular abnormalities. **(A)** Disc collaterals; **(B)** optociliary shunts (note disc pallor); **(C)** disc new vessels.

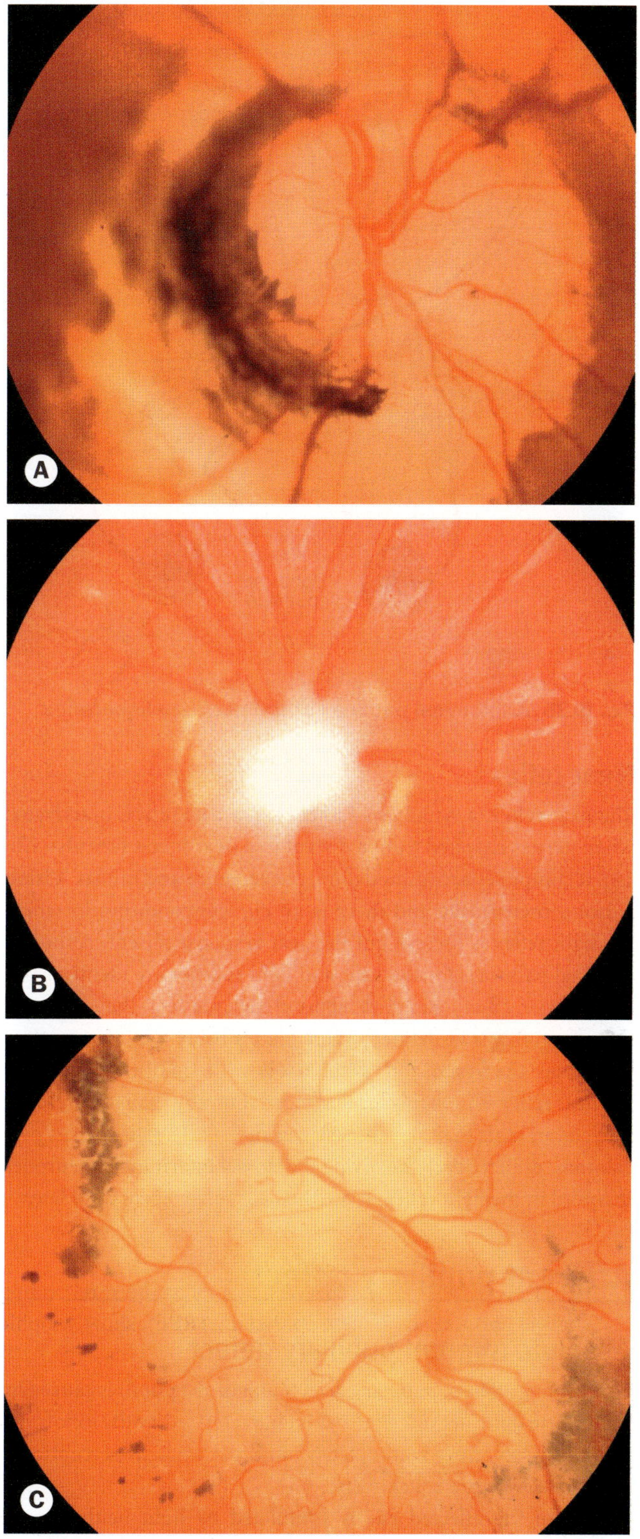

Fig. 19.34 Miscellaneous congenital disc anomalies. **(A)** Peripapillary staphyloma; **(B)** papillorenal syndrome; **(C)** optic disc dysplasia. *(Courtesy of D Taylor and CS Hoyt, from* Pediatric Ophthalmology and Strabismus, *Elsevier 2005 – fig. B.)*

and reach the ciliary ganglion via the nerve to the inferior oblique muscle.

- **Fourth** (postganglionic motor) leaves the ciliary ganglion and passes in the short ciliary nerves to innervate the sphincter pupillae. The ciliary ganglion is located within the muscle cone, just behind the globe. It should be noted that, although the ciliary ganglion serves as a conduit for other nerve fibres, only the parasympathetic fibres synapse there.

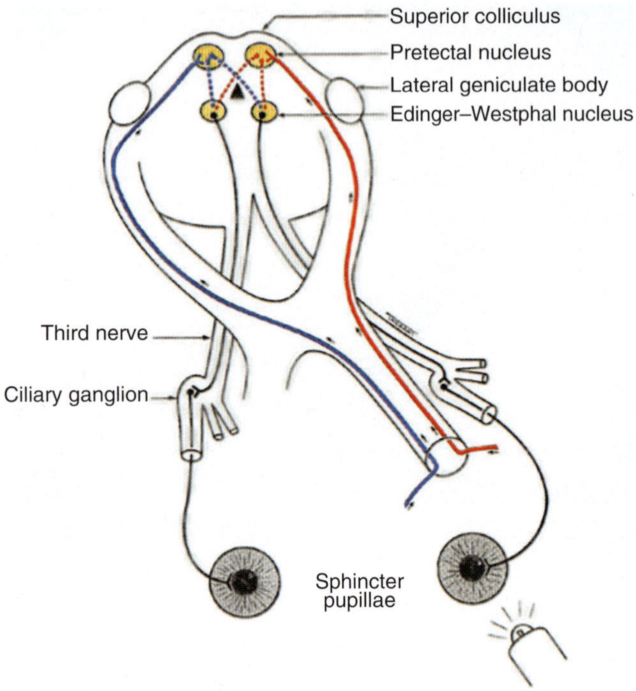

Fig. 19.35 Anatomical pathway of the pupillary light reflex.

Near reflex

The near reflex, a synkinesis rather than a true reflex, is activated when gaze is changed from a distant to a near target (see also Ch. 18). It comprises accommodation, convergence and miosis. Vision is not a prerequisite and there is no clinical condition in which the light reflex is present but the near response absent. Although the final pathways for the near and light reflexes are identical (i.e. third nerve, ciliary ganglion, short ciliary nerves), the centre for the near reflex is ill-defined. There are probably two supranuclear influences: the frontal and occipital lobes. The midbrain centre for the near reflex is probably located more ventrally than the pretectal nucleus and this may explain why compressive lesions such as pinealomas, preferentially involving the dorsal internuncial neurones involved in the light reflex, spare the near reflex fibres until later.

Afferent pupillary defect

Absolute afferent pupillary defect

An absolute afferent pupillary defect (amaurotic pupil) is caused by a complete optic nerve lesion and is characterized by the following:

- The involved eye is completely blind (i.e. no light perception).
- Both pupils are equal in size.
- When the affected eye is stimulated by light neither pupil reacts.
- When the normal eye is stimulated both pupils react normally.
- The near reflex is normal in both eyes.

Relative afferent pupillary defect

A relative pupillary defect (Marcus Gunn pupil) is caused by an incomplete optic nerve lesion or severe retinal disease, but never by a dense cataract. The clinical features are those of an amaurotic pupil but subtler. Thus, the pupils respond weakly to stimulation of the diseased eye and briskly to that of the normal eye. The difference between the pupillary reactions of the two eyes is highlighted by the 'swinging flashlight test' in which a light source is alternatively switched from one eye to the other and back, thus stimulating each eye in rapid succession. A left relative pupillary defect is characterized by the following:

- When the normal eye is stimulated, both pupils constrict (Fig. 19.36A).
- When the light is swung to the diseased eye, the stimulus delivered to the constriction mechanism is reduced and both pupils dilate instead of constricting (Fig. 19.36B).
- When the normal eye is again stimulated, both pupils constrict once more (Fig. 19.36C).
- When the diseased eye is stimulated, both pupils dilate (Fig. 19.36D).

It should be remembered that in afferent (sensory) lesions, the pupils are equal in size. Anisocoria (asymmetrical pupil diameter) implies disease of the efferent (motor) nerve or the iris itself.

TIP In afferent (sensory) lesions of the visual pathway the pupils are equal in size. Anisocoria (inequality of the pupillary size) indicates an abnormality of the efferent (motor) pathway.

Horner syndrome (oculosympathetic palsy)

Anatomy

The sympathetic supply involves three neurones (Fig. 19.37):

- **First** (central) starts in the posterior hypothalamus and descends, uncrossed, down the brainstem to terminate in the ciliospinal centre of Budge, in the intermediolateral horn of the spinal cord, located between C8 and T2.
- **Second** (preganglionic) passes from the ciliospinal centre to the superior cervical ganglion in the neck. During its long course, it is closely related to the apical pleura where it may be damaged by bronchogenic carcinoma (Pancoast tumour) or during surgery on the neck.
- **Third** (postganglionic) ascends along the internal carotid artery to enter the cavernous sinus where it joins the ophthalmic division of the trigeminal nerve. The sympathetic fibres reach the ciliary body and the dilator pupillae muscle via the nasociliary nerve and the long ciliary nerves.

Causes

The causes of Horner syndrome are shown in Table 19.4. Most commonly, isolated (without additional neurological features) postganglionic Horner syndrome is microvascular in aetiology, but this cannot be assumed.

Presentation

The majority of cases are unilateral. Causes of bilateral involvement include cervical spine injuries and autonomic diabetic neuropathy.

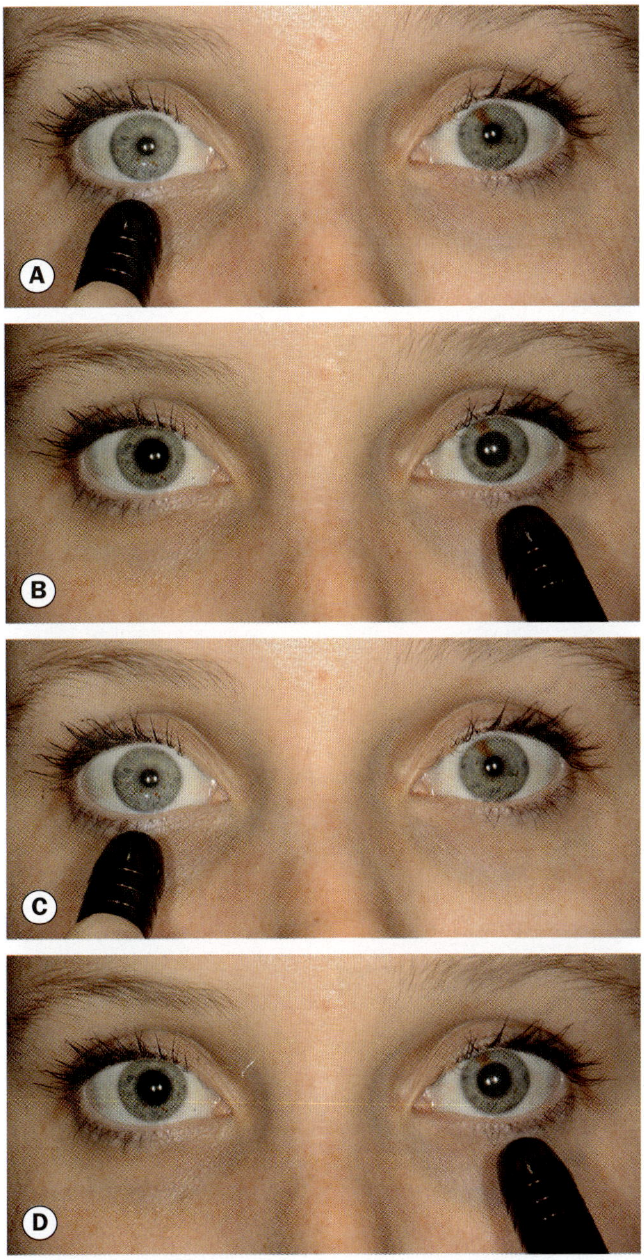

Fig. 19.36 'Swinging flashlight test' in a left afferent pupillary defect. **(A)** When the normal right eye is stimulated both pupils constrict; **(B)** when the light is swung to the diseased left eye, both pupils dilate; **(C)** when the normal eye is again stimulated, both pupils constrict once more; **(D)** when the diseased eye is stimulated, both pupils dilate.

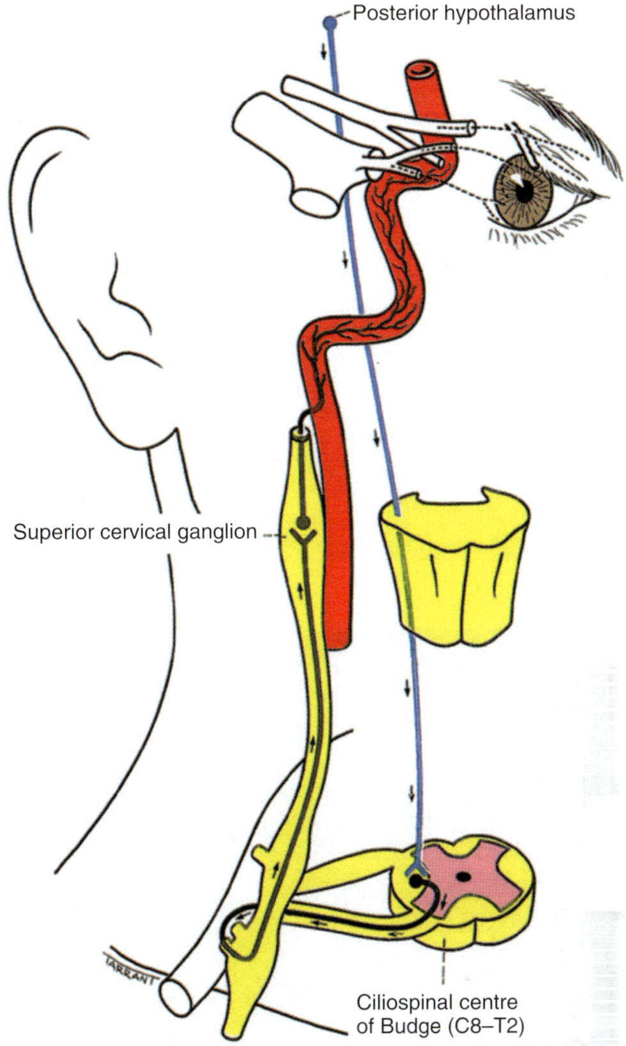

Fig. 19.37 Anatomical pathway of the sympathetic nerve supply.

Painful Horner syndrome, especially of acute onset, should raise the possibility of carotid dissection (Fig. 19.38).

- Mild ptosis (usually 1–2 mm) as a result of weakness of Müller muscle and miosis due to the unopposed action of the sphincter pupillae with resultant anisocoria (Fig. 19.39A and B).
- A key examination finding is that anisocoria is accentuated in dim light, since in contrast to a normal fellow pupil the Horner pupil will dilate only very slowly. The dark-induced anisocoria diminishes with time spent in the dark environment.
- Pupillary constriction to light and near stimuli is normal.
- Hypochromic heterochromia (irides of different colour, the Horner being lighter) may be seen if congenital or longstanding (Fig. 19.39C).
- Slight elevation of the inferior eyelid (inferior ptosis) as a result of weakness of the inferior tarsal muscle.
- Reduced ipsilateral sweating, but because the sudomotor fibres supplying the skin of the face run along the external carotid artery this occurs only if the lesion is below the superior cervical ganglion. Patients may mistakenly interpret the normal side to be sweating excessively.
- The cranial nerves and peripheral nervous system (e.g. T1 – grip strength), as well as the neck and regional lymph nodes should be examined, if necessary by a neurologist.

Pharmacological tests

Apraclonidine or cocaine is used to confirm the diagnosis, the latter now less commonly (see below). Hydroxyamphetamine and adrenaline may be used to differentiate a preganglionic (abnormal first- or second-order neurone) from a postganglionic lesion (abnormal third-order neurone), though as the distinction may

Table 19.4 Causes of Horner Syndrome

- Central (first-order neurone)
  - Brainstem disease – commonly stroke (e.g. lateral medullary infarction), but also tumour, demyelination
  - Syringomyelia
  - Lateral medullary (Wallenberg) syndrome
  - Cervical spinal cord lesion
  - Diabetic autonomic neuropathy
- Preganglionic (second-order neurone)
  - Pancoast tumour
  - Carotid and aortic aneurysm and dissection
  - Thoracic spinal cord lesion
  - Miscellaneous neck lesions (thyroid tumour, enlarged lymph nodes, trauma, postsurgical)
- Postganglionic (third-order neurone)
  - Internal carotid artery dissection
  - Nasopharyngeal tumour
  - Cavernous sinus mass
  - Otitis media
- Cluster headache (migrainous neuralgia)

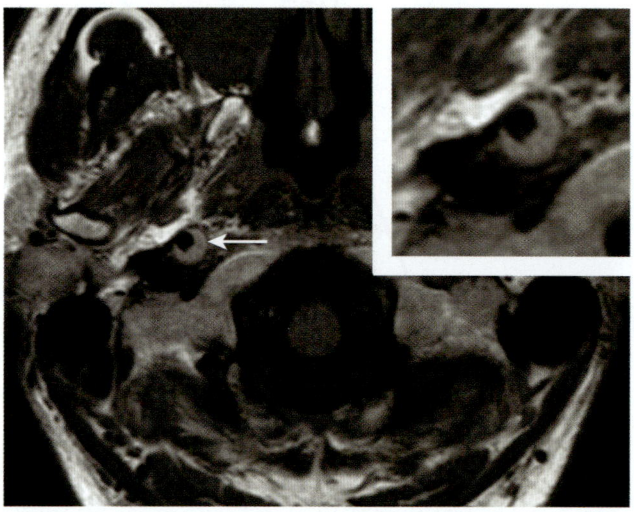

Fig. 19.38 Axial T1-weighted MR image just below the level of the skull base in a patient presenting with right-sided Horner syndrome. There is dissection of the right internal carotid artery. The true lumen is of reduced calibre and appears black, while the crescent-shaped false lumen appears bright due to stagnant methaemoglobin (arrow).

not alter investigation – carotid lesions may cause either pre- or postganglionic disease, for instance – some authorities limit pharmacological testing to confirmation of the presence of Horner syndrome.

- **Apraclonidine 0.5% or 1.0%.** One drop is instilled into both eyes to confirm or refute the presence of Horner syndrome. The pupils should be checked at 30 minutes and, if negative, rechecked at 45 minutes (Fig. 19.40). Apraclonidine should not be used in infants, as it can cross the blood–brain barrier. There is a latent period of approximately 7 days before the test becomes positive. It can have an extended duration of action, so subsequent pharmacological tests should not be performed for 3–5 days.
  - Result: A Horner pupil will dilate but a normal pupil will not be affected. The ptosis commonly also improves.

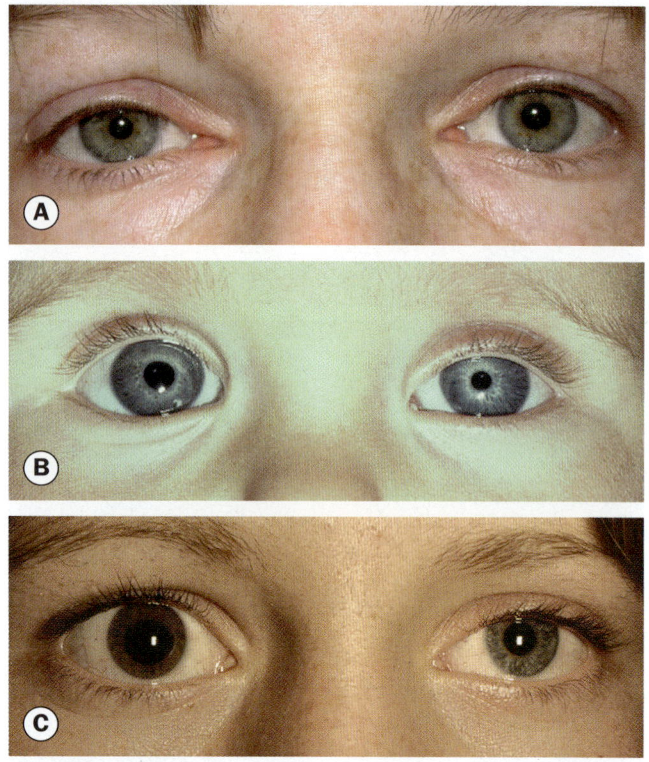

Fig. 19.39 Horner syndrome. **(A)** Right Horner syndrome; **(B)** congenital left Horner syndrome; **(C)** heterochromia iridis associated with a left congenital Horner syndrome in a young adult. *(Courtesy of ADN Murray – figs B and C.)*

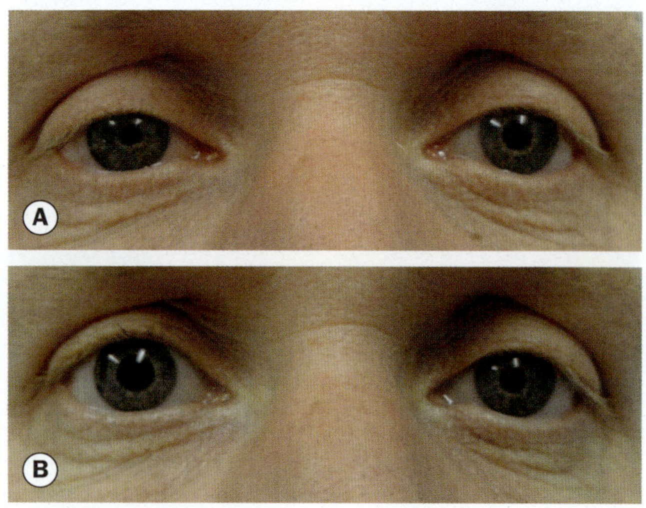

Fig. 19.40 Apraclonidine test in acquired Horner syndrome due to a traumatic right internal carotid artery dissection. **(A)** Before apraclonidine 1% showing right ptosis and miosis; **(B)** 45 minutes after instillation showing reversal of signs. *(Courtesy of D Hildebrand.)*

TIP An acute presentation of Horner syndrome should be regarded as an emergency and urgent radiological investigations should be undertaken to exclude treatable conditions.

Sensitivity is around 90% (it will detect most cases) and specificity close to 100% (it will very rarely falsely identify abnormality that is not actually present).

   - Explanation: Alpha-1 receptors are upregulated in the denervated dilator pupillae.
- **Cocaine 4%** is instilled into both eyes. As cocaine is less readily available than apraclonidine, this test is not commonly performed and may be reserved for acute lesions or those in which apraclonidine testing is equivocal but clinical suspicion is high.
   - Result: The normal pupil will dilate but the Horner pupil will not. Anisocoria of as little as 0.8 mm in a dimly lit room is significant.
   - Explanation: Cocaine blocks the re-uptake of noradrenaline secreted at the postganglionic nerve ending, which accumulates and causes dilatation of a normal pupil. In Horner syndrome, there is no noradrenaline being secreted, so cocaine has no effect.
- **Phenylephrine 1%** is more readily available than hydroxyamphetamine (see next) and adrenaline and is comparable in effect. As a result, it has replaced these drugs when testing to distinguish between pre- and postganglionic lesions. It is typically prepared by dilution of commonly available 2.5% or 10% solution.
   - Result: In an established (10 days) postganglionic lesion, the Horner pupil will dilate and ptosis may be temporarily relieved. A central or preganglionic Horner pupil and a normal pupil will not dilate or will dilate minimally.
   - Explanation: In postganglionic Horner syndrome the dilator pupillae muscle develops denervation hypersensitivity to adrenergic neurotransmitters due to its dysfunctional local motor nerve.
- **Hydroxyamphetamine 1%.** Two drops are instilled into each eye. It is slightly more sensitive than phenylephrine testing.
   - Result: A normal or preganglionic Horner pupil will dilate, but a postganglionic Horner will not.
   - Explanation: Hydroxyamphetamine potentiates the release of noradrenaline from functioning postganglionic nerve endings. In a lesion of the third-order neurone (postganglionic) there is no release of noradrenaline from the dysfunctional nerve.
- **Adrenaline 0.1%** has an action similar to that of phenylephrine.

Investigation

Specialist neurological or neuro-ophthalmological assessment should be sought for a confirmed Horner syndrome. An acute presentation should be regarded as an emergency. In contrast, if the features have been present for more than a year and there are no other localizing signs then the likely diagnostic yield from further investigation is very low. The mainstay of investigation is imaging. CT or MR angiography examining the region from the aortic arch to the circle of Willis will facilitate exclusion of neck (including carotid), apical lung, thyroid and skull base lesions. MR may be utilized if greater soft tissue definition is required, such as to exclude a brainstem stroke. Plain X-rays and carotid ultrasound imaging have limited utility.

Treatment

Any identified cause should be addressed as appropriate. The ptosis of Horner syndrome is mild but surgery can be considered at the patient's discretion. Apraclonidine may be helpful as a temporizing measure.

Adie pupil

Introduction

An Adie pupil (tonic pupil, Adie syndrome) is caused by denervation of the postganglionic parasympathetic supply to the sphincter pupillae and the ciliary muscle and may follow a viral illness. It is occasionally inherited in an AD pattern. Sites of dysfunction are presumed to be the ciliary ganglion and in Holmes–Adie syndrome, the dorsal root ganglion involved in reflex pathways. It typically affects young women and presents in one eye in 80%, though involvement of the second eye typically develops within months or years.

Diagnosis

- **Symptoms.** Patients may notice anisocoria, or may have blurring for near due to impaired accommodation.
- **Signs**
   - Large, regular (irregularity sometimes reported) pupil (Fig. 19.41A).
   - The direct light reflex is absent or sluggish (Fig. 19.41B).
   - On slit lamp examination, vermiform movements of the pupillary border are typically seen.
   - Constriction is also absent or sluggish in response to light stimulation of the fellow eye (consensual light reflex – Fig. 19.41C).
   - The pupil responds slowly to near, following which redilatation is also slow.
   - Accommodation may manifest similar tonicity, with slowed and impaired focusing for near and prolonged refocusing in the distance.
   - In longstanding cases the pupil may become small ('little old Adie').
- **Associations** include diminished lower limb deep tendon reflexes (Holmes–Adie syndrome – Fig. 19.41D) and other features of autonomic nerve dysfunction such as excessive sweating (Ross syndrome), orthostatic hypotension and occasionally bowel obstruction or urinary retention. Typical Adie-type pupils are often present in generalized dysautonomia, with a wide range of causes.
- **Pharmacological testing.** Instillation of 0.1–0.125% pilocarpine into both eyes leads to constriction of the abnormal pupil due to denervation hypersensitivity, with the normal pupil unaffected. Some diabetic patients may also show this response and very occasionally both pupils constrict in normal individuals.

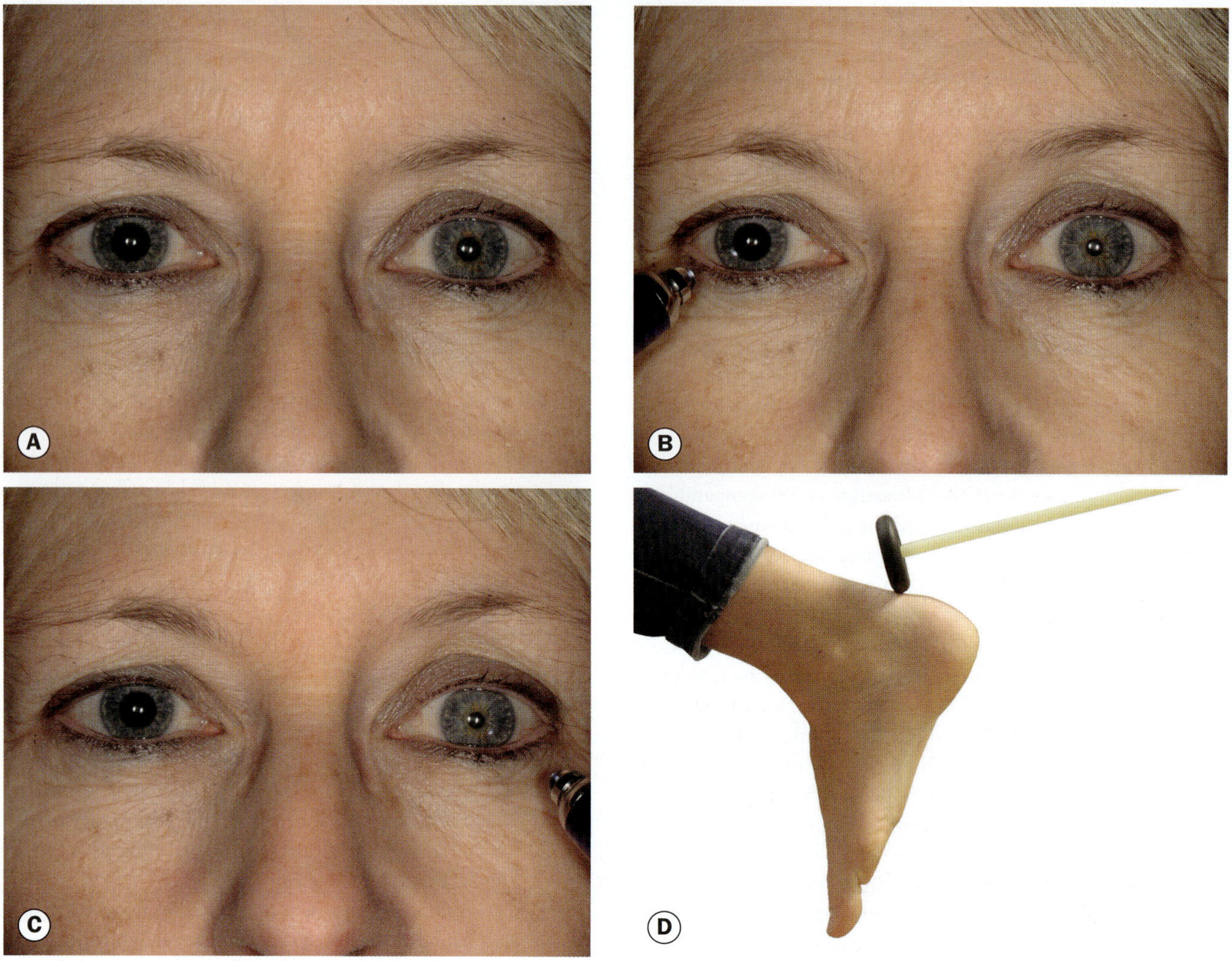

Fig. 19.41 Right Adie pupil. **(A)** Large right pupil; **(B)** absent direct light reflex; **(C)** consensual light reflex is similar; **(D)** diminished deep tendon reflex.

- **Syphilis serology** (see Ch. 12) should usually be checked in patients with bilateral tonic pupils.

Treatment

Treatment is not usually required, but reading glasses may be used to address near vision difficulties and sunglasses or low-concentration pilocarpine drops can be used for cosmetic reasons and to reduce photophobia. Thoracic sympathectomy can be considered for excessive sweating.

Miscellaneous pupillary abnormalities

- **Physiological anisocoria** (Fig. 19.42). Anisocoria of around 1 mm is present in about 20% of the normal population. The asymmetry persists to the same proportion under differing levels of illumination. Exceptionally, apraclonidine or cocaine testing may be needed to exclude Horner syndrome.
- **Pharmacological mydriasis** (Fig. 19.43). Dilatation of one or both pupils due to instillation of a mydriatic agent can be inadvertent (e.g. use of eye drops prescribed for someone else, rubbing the eye after touching a car sickness scopolamine skin patch) or deliberate for the purpose of malingering. The pupil does not constrict in bright light or on accommodation and there is no response to any concentration of pilocarpine. There are no other neurological features.
- **Argyll Robertson pupils** (Fig. 19.44) are caused by neurosyphilis and have been attributed to a dorsal midbrain lesion that interrupts the pupillary light reflex pathway but spares the more ventral pupillary near reflex pathway – light–near dissociation results. In dim light both pupils are small and may be irregular. In bright light neither pupil constricts, but on accommodation (near target) both constrict. The pupils do not dilate well in the dark, but cocaine induces mydriasis unless marked iris atrophy is present. After instillation of pilocarpine 0.1% into both eyes, neither pupil constricts, distinguishing Argyll Robertson pupils from bilateral longstanding tonic pupils. Other causes of light–near dissociation are shown in Table 19.5.
- **Tectal (dorsal midbrain) pupils** (Fig. 19.45). This phenomenon is a component of dorsal midbrain syndrome (see later). The pupils are dilated in both dim and bright light. There is light–near dissociation. Pilocarpine 0.1% has no effect.

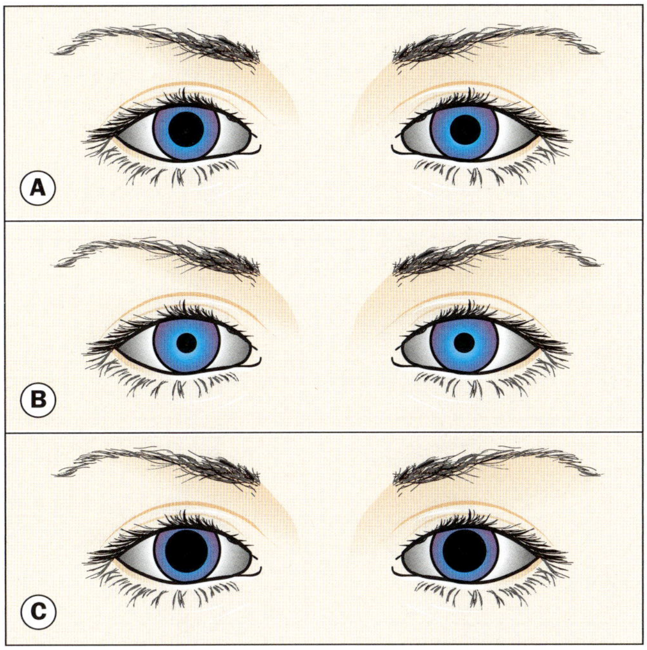

Fig. 19.42 Right physiological anisocoria. **(A)** In dim light the right pupil is slightly larger than the left; **(B)** in bright light both pupils constrict normally, but the right pupil is still fractionally larger than the left; **(C)** both pupils dilate with instillation of cocaine 4%. *(Courtesy of JJ Kanski, from* Signs in Ophthalmology: Causes and Differential Diagnosis, *Mosby 2010.)*

- **Benign episodic unilateral mydriasis (BEUM).** This idiopathic condition (Fig. 19.46) occurs most commonly in otherwise healthy young women and may represent a migrainous phenomenon or a range of heterogeneous aetiologies. Mydriasis tends to last for minutes or hours before resolving completely. There may be mild associated blurring and headache. The need for further investigation should be assessed on an individual basis. There is no – or limited – response to light or accommodation. Pilocarpine 0.1% induces no change, but pilocarpine 1% to both eyes gives bilateral miosis.

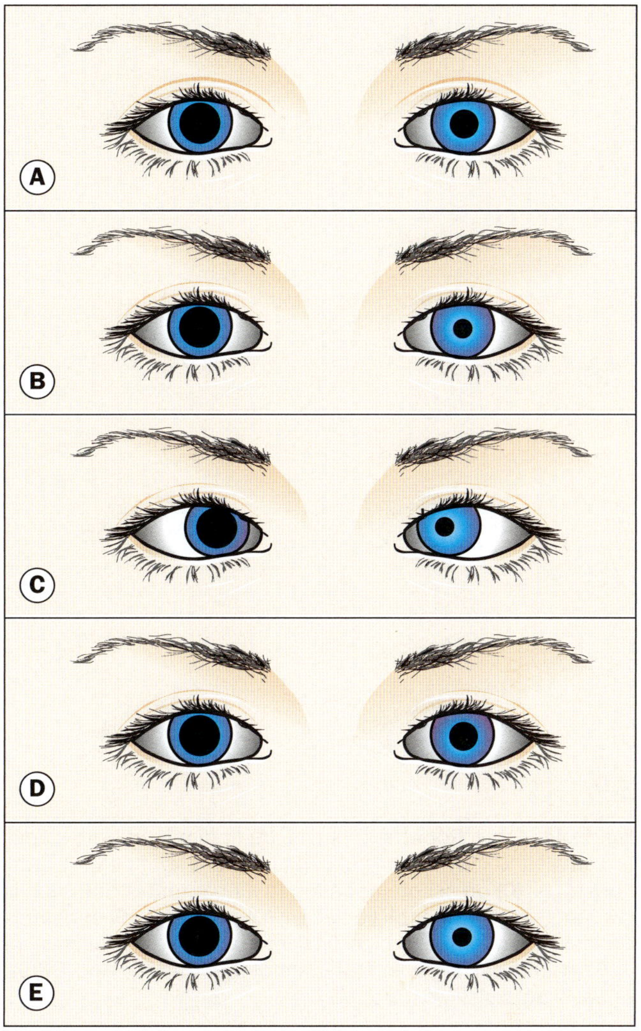

Fig. 19.43 Right pharmacological mydriasis. **(A)** Right mydriasis in dim illumination; **(B)** in bright light the right pupil does not constrict; **(C)** on accommodation the right pupil does not constrict; **(D)** neither pupil constricts after instillation of pilocarpine 0.1% into both eyes; **(E)** after instillation of 1% pilocarpine into both eyes the left pupil constricts but the right does not. *(Courtesy of JJ Kanski, from* Signs in Ophthalmology: Causes and Differential Diagnosis, *Mosby 2010.)*

CHIASM

Anatomy

Pituitary gland

The sella turcica (Turkish saddle) is a deep saddle-shaped depression in the superior surface of the body of the sphenoid bone in which the pituitary gland lies (Fig. 19.47). The roof of the sella is formed by a fold of dura mater, the diaphragma sellae, which stretches from the anterior to the posterior clinoids. The optic nerves and chiasm lie above the diaphragma sellae. Posteriorly, the chiasm is continuous with the optic tracts and forms the anterior wall of the third ventricle. A visual field defect in a patient with a pituitary tumour therefore generally indicates suprasellar extension. Tumours less than 10 mm in diameter (microadenomas) tend to remain confined to the sella, whereas those larger than 10 mm (macroadenomas) often extend outside the sella. Causes of chiasmal disease are listed in Table 19.6.

TIP A visual field defect in a patient with a pituitary tumour usually indicates suprasellar extension.

Parachiasmal vascular structures

- **Venous.** The cavernous sinuses lie lateral to the sella so that horizontally extending pituitary tumours affect the cavernous sinus and may damage the intracavernous parts of the third, fourth and sixth cranial nerves. Conversely, aneurysms arising from the intracavernous part of the internal carotid artery may erode into the sella and mimic pituitary tumours.

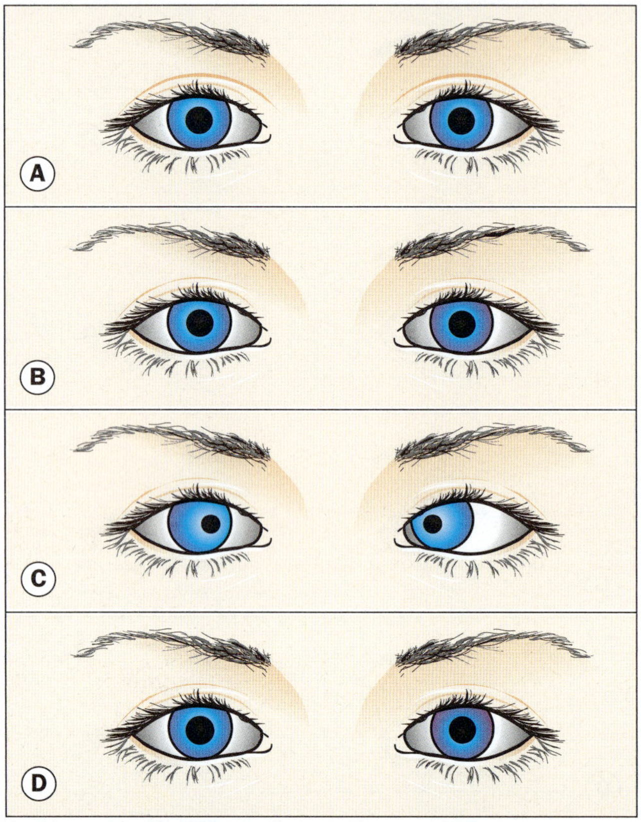

Fig. 19.44 Argyll Robertson pupils. **(A)** In dim light both pupils are small and may be irregular; **(B)** in bright light neither pupil constricts; **(C)** on accommodation to a near target both pupils constrict – light–near dissociation; **(D)** neither pupil constricts on instillation of pilocarpine 0.1% into both eyes. *(Courtesy of JJ Kanski, from* Signs in Ophthalmology: Causes and Differential Diagnosis, *Mosby 2010.)*

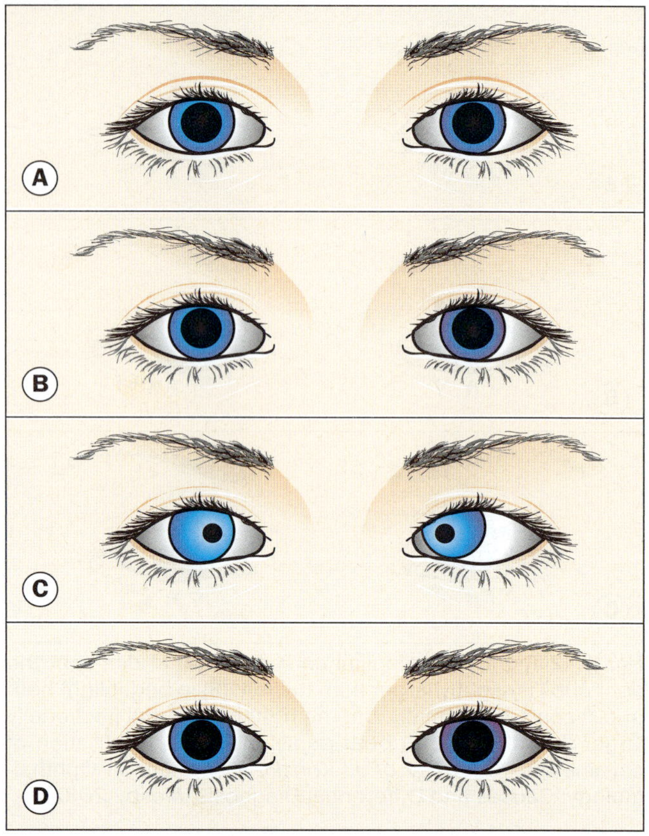

Fig. 19.45 Tectal (dorsal midbrain) pupils. **(A)** In dim light there is bilateral mydriasis, which may be asymmetrical; **(B)** in bright light neither pupil constricts; **(C)** on accommodation both pupils constrict normally – light–near dissociation; **(D)** neither pupil constricts on instillation of pilocarpine 0.1% into both eyes. *(Courtesy of JJ Kanski, from* Signs in Ophthalmology: Causes and Differential Diagnosis, *Mosby 2010.)*

Table 19.5 Causes of Light–Near Dissociation

- **Unilateral**
  - Afferent conduction defect
  - Adie pupil
  - Herpes zoster ophthalmicus
  - Aberrant regeneration of the third cranial nerve
- **Bilateral**
  - Neurosyphilis
  - Type 1 diabetes mellitus
  - Myotonic dystrophy
  - Parinaud (dorsal midbrain) syndrome
  - Familial amyloidosis
  - Encephalitis
  - Chronic alcoholism

- **Arterial** (Fig. 19.48). The internal carotid arteries curve posteriorly and upwards from the cavernous sinus and lie immediately below the optic nerves, following which they ascend vertically along the lateral aspect of the chiasm. The precommunicating portion of the anterior cerebral artery is closely related to the superior surface of the chiasm and optic nerves, so an aneurysm in this region can compress either, or both, the optic nerve or chiasm.

Physiology

Pituitary hormones

The lobules of the anterior part of the pituitary gland are composed of six cell types. Five of these secrete hormones and the sixth (follicular cell) has no secretory function. Pituitary adenomas of mixed-cell type are common; any of the six cell types may proliferate to produce an adenoma. The current classification of pituitary tumours is discussed further below.

- **The anterior pituitary lobe** is under the control of various inhibiting and promoting factors synthesized in the hypothalamus, passing to the pituitary through the hypothalamus–hypophyseal portal system:
  - Human growth hormone (HGH or GH) or somatotropin.
  - Follicle-stimulating hormone (FSH).
  - Luteinizing hormone (LH).
  - Prolactin (PRL).
  - Thyroid-stimulating hormone (TSH).
  - Adrenocorticotrophic hormone (ACTH), which regulates blood cortisol levels.
  - Beta-endorphin.

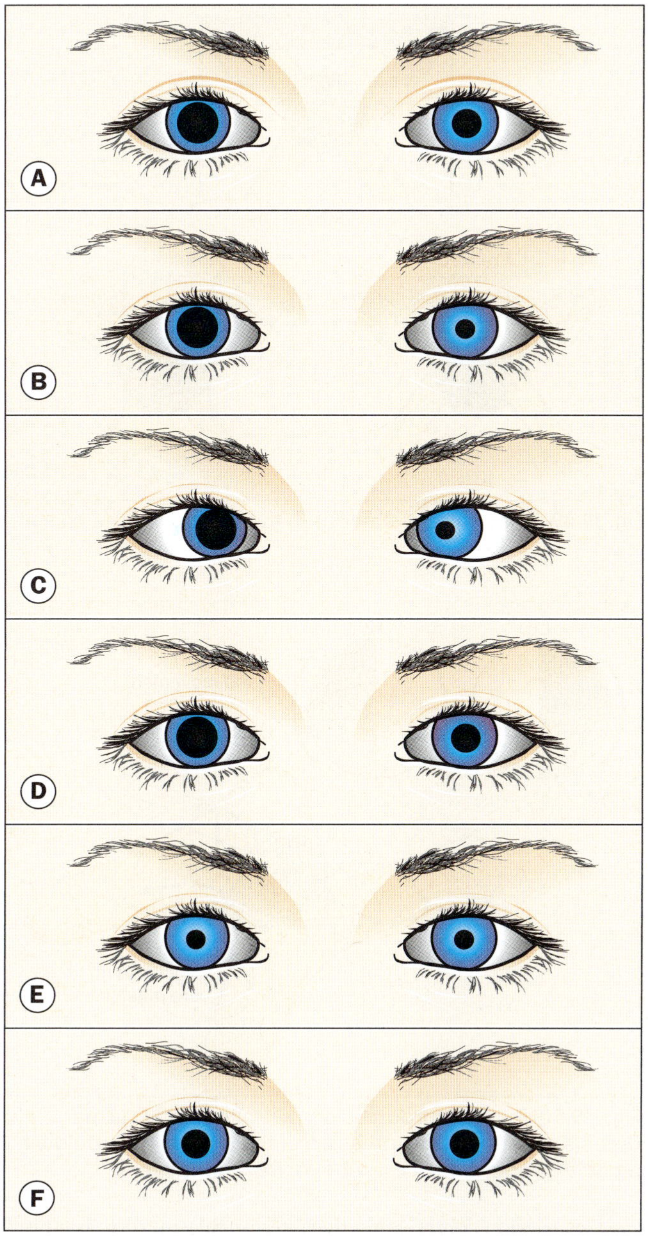

Fig. 19.46 Right benign episodic unilateral mydriasis (BEUM). **(A)** In dim light the right pupil is larger than the left; **(B)** in bright light the right pupil does not constrict; **(C)** on accommodation the right pupil does not constrict; **(D)** instillation of pilocarpine 0.1% to both eyes fails to constrict either pupil; **(E)** instillation of pilocarpine 1% to both eyes induces bilateral miosis; **(F)** after 24 hours both pupils are equal. *(Courtesy of JJ Kanski, from* Signs in Ophthalmology: Causes and Differential Diagnosis*, Mosby 2010.)*

- **The intermediate lobe** secretes melanocyte-stimulating hormone (MSH).
- **The posterior pituitary** releases antidiuretic hormone (ADH) and oxytocin.

Pituitary adenomas

Tumour classification is based on the type of hormone secreted. About 25% of primary pituitary tumours do not secrete any hormones and may be asymptomatic, cause hypopituitarism and/or ophthalmic features. An older classification system divided pituitary tumours into acidophilic, basophilic and chromophobic types based on their histological staining characteristics, but is now not commonly used.

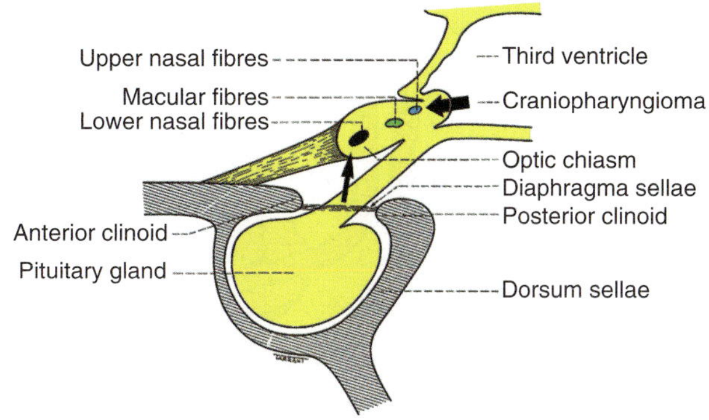

Fig. 19.47 Anatomy of the chiasm in relation to the pituitary gland.

Table 19.6 Causes of Chiasmal Disease

- **Tumours**
  - Pituitary adenomas
  - Craniopharyngioma
  - Meningioma
  - Glioma
  - Chordoma
  - Dysgerminoma
  - Nasopharyngeal tumours
  - Metastases
- **Non-neoplastic masses**
  - Aneurysm
  - Rathke pouch cysts
  - Fibrous dysplasia
  - Sphenoidal sinus mucocoele
  - Arachnoid cysts
- **Miscellaneous**
  - Demyelination
  - Inflammation, e.g. sarcoidosis
  - Trauma
  - Radiation-induced necrosis
  - Toxicity, e.g. ethambutol
  - Vasculitis

Ophthalmic features of large adenomas

Patients with a large pituitary lesion may first present with vague visual symptoms. A low threshold should be adopted for visual field assessment in patients with unexplained unilateral central visual impairment and chronic headache.

TIP A visual field test should be undertaken as the initial step in a patient with unexplained unilateral central visual impairment, in order to exclude compressive optic neuropathy.

- **Symptoms**
  - Headache may be prominent due to local effects but does not have the usual features associated with raised ICP, and diagnostic delay is therefore common.

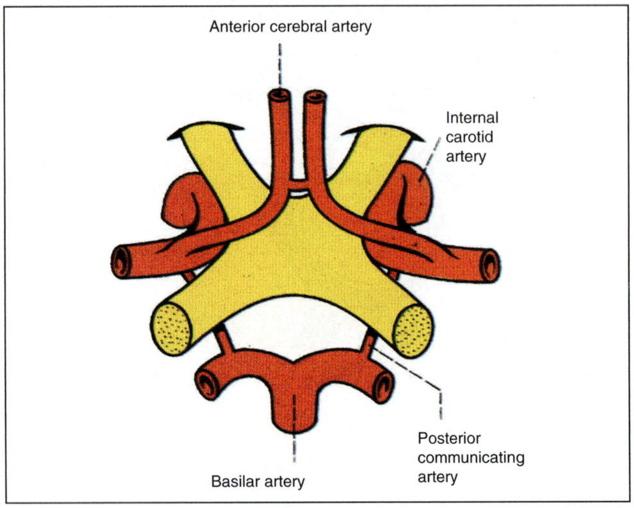

Fig. 19.48 Relationship between the chiasm and adjacent arterial structures.

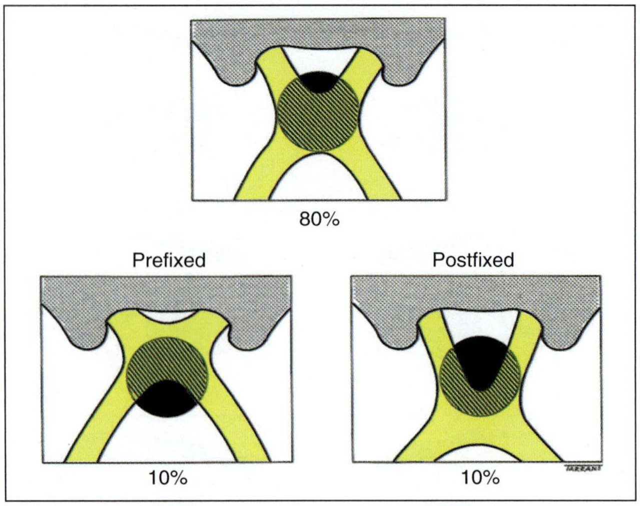

Fig. 19.49 Anatomical variations in the position of the chiasm.

- Visual symptoms may be vague, usually have a gradual onset and may not be noticed by the patient until well established.
- **Colour desaturation** across the vertical midline of the uniocular visual field is an early sign of chiasmal compression.
  - The patient is asked to compare the colour and intensity of a red pin or pen top as it is moved from the nasal to the temporal visual field in each eye.
  - Another technique is to simultaneously present red targets in precisely symmetrical parts of the temporal and nasal visual fields and to ask if the colours appear the same.
- **Optic atrophy** is present in approximately 50% of cases with field defects. When optic atrophy is present the prognosis for visual recovery after treatment is guarded. When nerve fibre loss is confined to fibres originating in the nasal retina (i.e. nasal to the fovea) only the nasal and temporal aspects of the disc will be involved, resulting in a band or 'bow tie'-shaped atrophy.
- **Papilloedema** is rare.
  - Visual field defects depend on the location and direction of enlargement of a compressive lesion, as well as the anatomical relationship between the pituitary and chiasm (Fig. 19.49 and see below). Patients may not present until central vision is affected from pressure on macular fibres.
  - Lower nasal optic nerve fibres traverse the chiasm inferiorly and anteriorly, hence the upper temporal quadrants of both visual fields are affected first by most expanding pituitary lesions, giving a bitemporal superior quadrantanopia progressing to the classic chiasmal visual field lesion, a bitemporal hemianopia (Fig. 19.50). Field loss is commonly asymmetrical between the two eyes (Fig. 19.51).
  - Upper nasal fibres traverse the chiasm high and posteriorly and therefore are involved first by a lesion such as a craniopharyngioma that arises above the chiasm (Fig. 19.52). If the lower temporal quadrants of the visual field are affected more profoundly than the upper, a pituitary adenoma is unlikely.

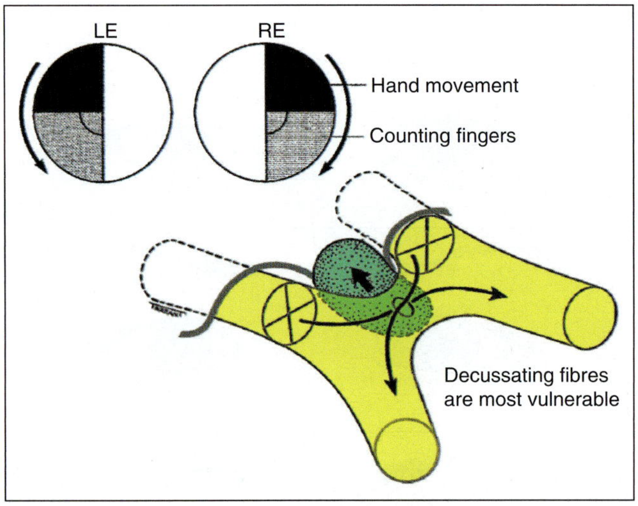

Fig. 19.50 Typical progression of bitemporal visual field defects caused by compression of the chiasm from below by a pituitary adenoma. LE= left eye; RE = right eye.

  - A lesion compressing the anterior chiasm, such as a pituitary adenoma in conjunction with a postfixed chiasm, may give rise to a 'junctional scotoma' – the syndrome of a central or paracentral defect on the side of optic nerve involvement together with a contralateral superotemporal defect (see Fig. 19.57). The precise mechanism is disputed, but is commonly attributed to simultaneous involvement of the fibres of one of the optic nerves together with contralateral inferonasal fibres looping forward into the nerve in the putative knee of Wilbrand.
  - Macular fibres decussate throughout the chiasm, but are concentrated posteriorly. A lesion that preferentially compresses the posterior chiasm, such as a pituitary adenoma in conjunction with a prefixed chiasm, may therefore cause bitemporal hemianopic changes predominantly affecting the central and paracentral fields. Predominant involvement of the optic tracts by a posterior lesion can give a homonymous hemianopia.

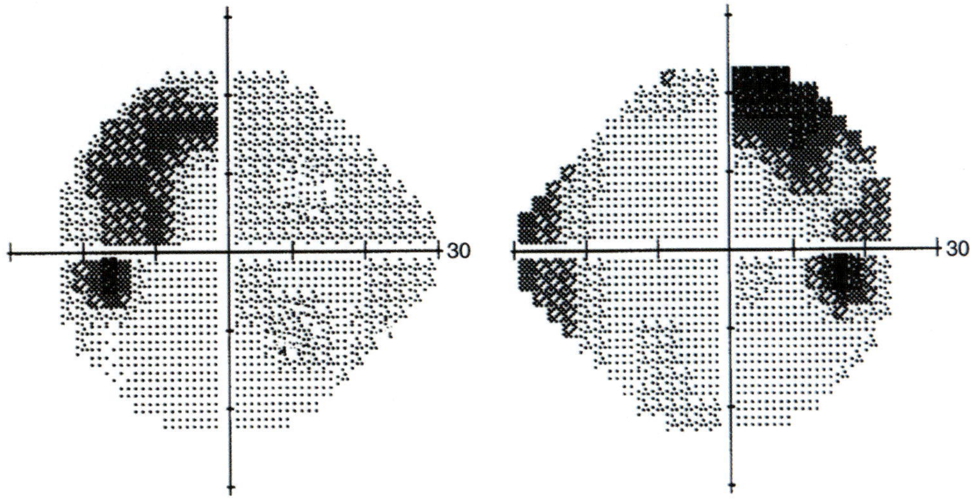

Fig. 19.51 Typically asymmetrical bitemporal hemianopia.

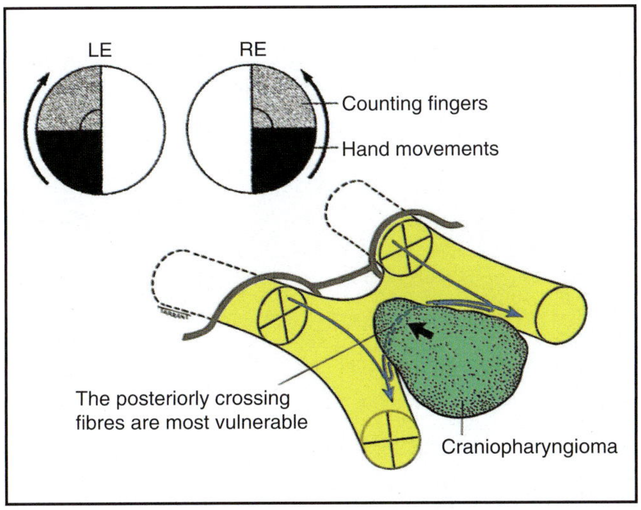

Fig. 19.52 Progression of bitemporal visual field defects caused by compression of the chiasm from above by a craniopharyngioma. LE = left eye; RE = right eye.

- Extensive loss of the temporal visual field in both eyes can disrupt sensory fusion, decompensating a phoria and causing problems with near vision. 'Postfixation blindness' refers to the presence of a non-seeing area distal to the fixation point due to the overlap of two blind hemifields (Fig. 19.53). Despite similar terminology, it is not linked to a postfixed chiasm. Patients may complain of difficulty with fine close-up tasks such as threading a needle and cutting fingernails and near VA measured binocularly may be worse than when measured with each eye individually. Double vision may result from slippage of the two fields with fusional failure ('hemifield slide') or less often from cranial nerve palsy (see next).
- Differential diagnosis of bitemporal defects includes dermatochalasis, tilted discs, optic nerve colobomas, nasal retinoschisis, nasal retinitis pigmentosa and functional ('non-physiological') visual loss.

- **Extraocular muscle paresis** due to disruption of the cranial nerves traversing the cavernous sinus.
- **See-saw nystagmus** (see later) is a rare feature.

Investigation

- **MRI** with gadolinium contrast (Fig. 19.54) utilizing multiple planes and thin sections demonstrates the relationship between a mass lesion and the chiasm and is usually the preferred imaging modality. Adenomas are typically hypointense on T1 and hyperintense on T2 images.
- **CT** will demonstrate enlargement or erosion of the sella.
- **Endocrinological evaluation** is complex, particularly as combined hormonal over- and under-secretion may be present and is usually undertaken by an endocrinologist.

Prolactin-secreting (lactotrophic) adenoma

Lactotrophic adenoma or prolactinoma (formerly known as chromophobe adenoma, though lesions can be weakly acidophilic) is the most common pituitary adenoma. Patients are typically young to middle-aged adults. In women excessive prolactin secretion leads to the infertility–amenorrhoea–galactorrhoea syndrome and in men may cause hypogonadism, impotence, sterility, decreased libido and occasionally gynaecomastia and galactorrhoea. Up to 95% remain as microadenomas, though those that do not may present initially with visual features.

Corticotrophic adenoma

A corticotrophic adenoma (a variant of basophil adenoma) secretes ACTH and causes Cushing disease (Cushing *syndrome* refers to the clinical picture of increased blood cortisol from any cause), which may include central obesity and moon face, cutaneous striae, pigmentation and other features such as hypertension.

Somatotrophic adenoma

Somatotrophic (acidophil) tumours secrete excessive GH, causing acromegaly in adults (once bone elongation has been completed) and gigantism in children. Presentation is in middle age with

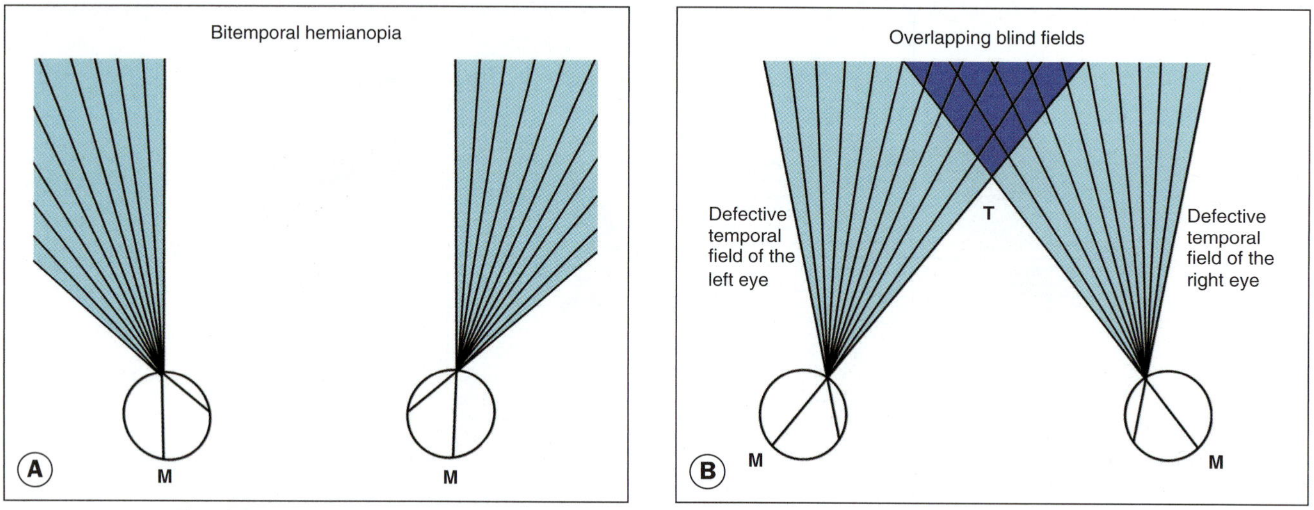

Fig. 19.53 Mechanism of postfixation blindness. M = macula; T = target. **(A)** Bitemporal hemianopia (light blue area); **(B)** when fixating on a target the area behind fixation is not visible (dark blue hatched area).

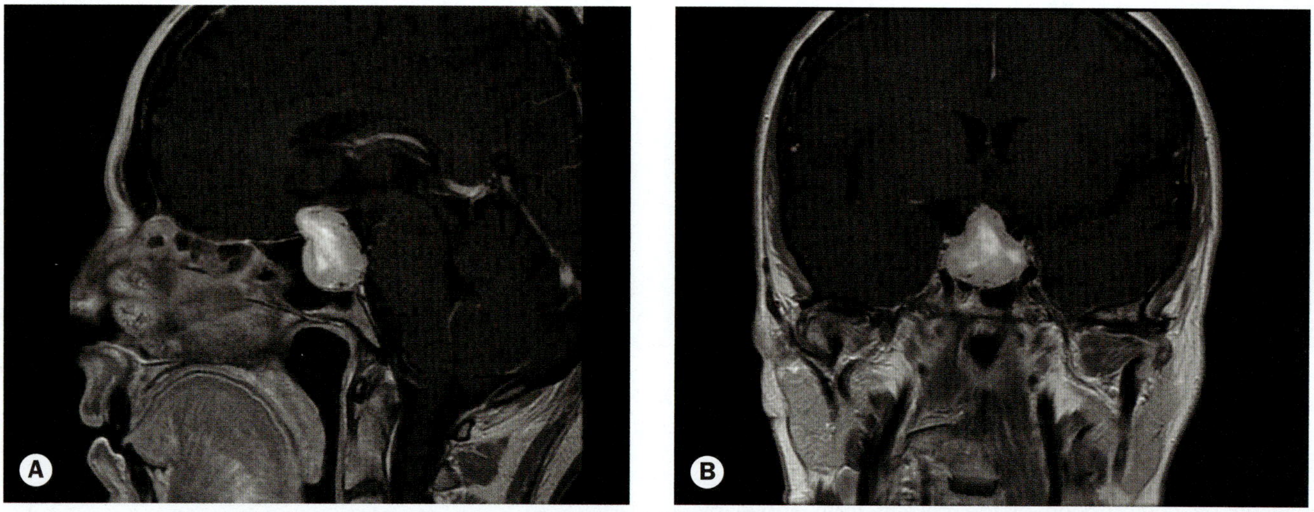

Fig. 19.54 T1-weighted gadolinium-enhanced MR of a pituitary adenoma expanding the pituitary fossa and compressing the optic chiasm. **(A)** Sagittal and **(B)** coronal images.

features including enlargement of the head, hands, feet and tongue, coarseness of features with prominent supraorbital ridges and nasolabial folds (Fig. 19.55), enlargement of the jaw with dental malocclusion and hirsutism in females. There are many complications, including diabetes mellitus, hypertension, cardiomyopathy and carpal tunnel syndrome.

Treatment of pituitary adenomas

- **Observation** may be appropriate for incidentally discovered and clinically silent tumours.
- **Medical therapy** is usually the initial step and consists of the reduction in tumour size and secretion using agents such as dopamine agonists (e.g. cabergoline and the older bromocriptine) and somatostatin analogues such as octreotide, with supplementary hormonal correction as appropriate.
- **Surgery** consists of tumour debulking rather than complete excision and is usually carried out endoscopically via a trans-sphenoidal approach through a gum incision behind the upper lip. Indications include the failure or intolerance of medical management and sometimes decompression for acute visual loss (see below). Visual field improvement is fastest in the earliest weeks and months following surgery.
- **Radiotherapy** is rarely employed due to the risk of complications. Newer techniques include intensity-modulated radiation therapy and stereotactic radiosurgery.
- **Monitoring.** Long-term ophthalmological review is required, with serial assessment of visual function.

Pituitary apoplexy

Pituitary apoplexy (PA) is caused by acute haemorrhage into or infarction of the pituitary gland and is usually associated with a previously undiagnosed adenoma. Sheehan syndrome is infarction of the pituitary usually associated with childbirth and is

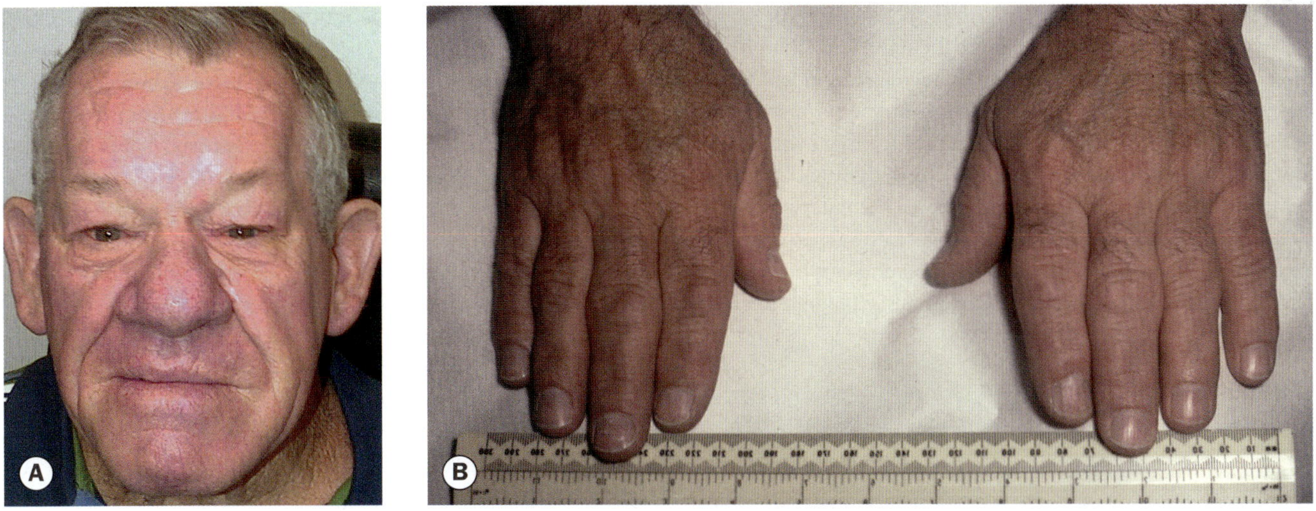

Fig. 19.55 Acromegaly. **(A)** Facial features; **(B)** hands.

generally regarded as a form of PA. PA typically manifests with the sudden onset of a severe headache, nausea and vomiting, sometimes with meningism and occasionally reduced consciousness or stroke. There is often reduced VA and/or a bitemporal hemianopia depending on the anatomical effects of the lesion. Double vision due to compromise of the adjacent ocular motor nerves is common. Acute hormonal insufficiency can lead to life-threatening complications such as an Addisonian crisis. Investigations include MR, urgent visual field testing and hormonal assessment. Acute medical management, including hormone administration and surgical decompression, may be necessary.

Craniopharyngioma

Craniopharyngioma is a slow-growing tumour arising from vestigial remnants of the Rathke pouch along the pituitary stalk. Affected children frequently present with dwarfism, delayed sexual development and obesity due to interference with hypothalamic function. Adults usually present with visual impairment.

Visual field defects are complex and may be due to involvement of the optic nerves, chiasm or tracts.

The initial defect frequently involves both inferotemporal fields because the tumour compresses the chiasm from above and behind, damaging the upper nasal fibres (see Fig. 19.52). MRI shows a solid tumour that appears isointense on T1 images (Fig. 19.56). Cystic components appear hyperintense on T1 images. Treatment is mainly surgical, but recurrences are common.

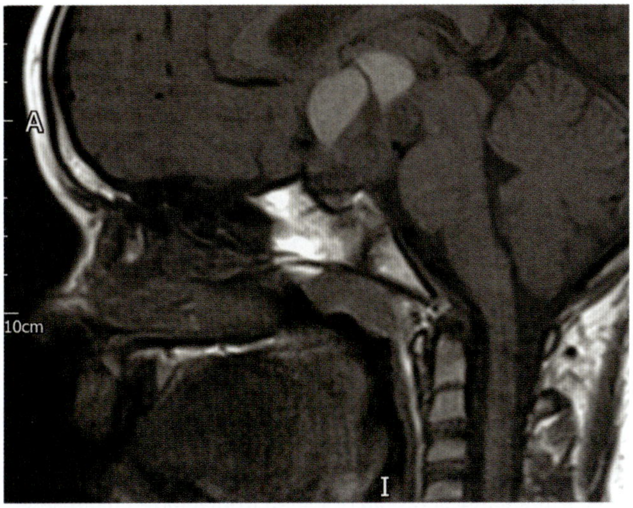

Fig. 19.56 Sagittal T1-weighted MR image of the pituitary and supra-sellar region of a patient with a large craniopharyngioma. The optic chiasm is compressed to the extent that it cannot be clearly distinguished on the surface of the tumour.

Meningioma

Intracranial meningiomas typically affect middle-aged women. Visual field defects and clinical signs depend on the location of the tumour (Fig. 19.57).

- **Tuberculum sellae** meningiomas often produce a junctional scotoma (see above and Fig. 19.57) due to their location.
- **Sphenoidal ridge** tumours compress the optic nerve early if the tumour is located medially and late if the lateral aspect of the sphenoid bone and middle cranial fossa are involved (Fig. 19.58A). A classic finding in the latter is fullness in the temporal fossa due to hyperostosis (Fig. 19.58B).
- **Olfactory groove** meningioma may cause loss of the sense of smell, as well as optic nerve compression.
- **Treatment** usually consists of surgery, but radiotherapy is sometimes required. Observation alone may be adequate.

RETROCHIASMAL PATHWAYS

Optic tracts

Overview

Retrochiasmal pathology results in partial or total binocular visual field defects involving contralateral visual space. This hemianopia (hemianopsia) involving the same side of the field in both eyes is homonymous, in contradistinction to the bitemporal hemianopia seen in chiasmal compression, which produces heteronymous loss, with opposite sides of the visual field affected in each eye.

Congruity

A homonymous hemianopia may be incomplete or complete. In the context of incomplete hemianopia, congruity refers to how closely the extent and pattern of field loss in one eye matches that of the other. Almost identical field defects in either eye are therefore highly congruous, while mismatching right and left visual field defects are incongruous. Hemianopia secondary to pathology in the anterior retrochiasmal visual pathways is characteristically incongruous, while that due to pathology further back (e.g. the posterior optic radiations) manifests a higher degree of congruity.

Clinical features

- **Homonymous hemianopia**

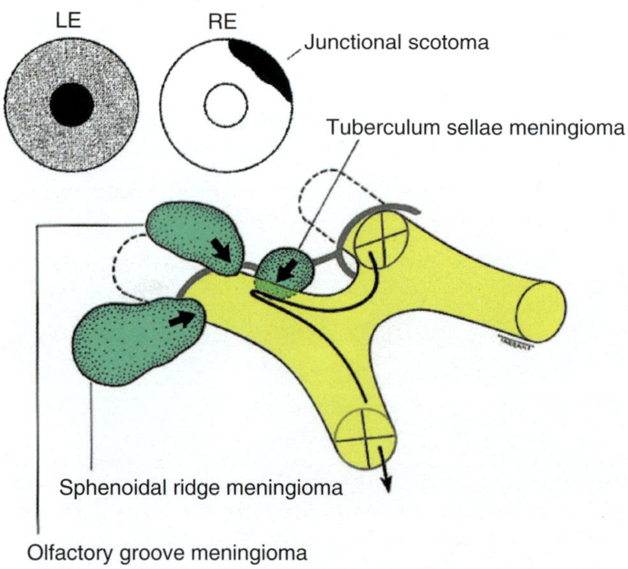

Fig. 19.57 Examples of optic nerve compression by meningioma; a junctional scotoma resulting from a tuberculum sellae lesion is also shown.

  - The optic tracts arise at the posterior aspect of the chiasm, diverge and extend posteriorly around the cerebral peduncles, to terminate in the lateral geniculate bodies.
  - Each optic tract contains crossed fibres from the contralateral nasal hemiretina and uncrossed fibres from the ipsilateral temporal hemiretina.
  - Nerve fibres originating from corresponding retinal elements are, however, not closely aligned.
  - Homonymous hemianopia caused by optic tract lesions is therefore characteristically incongruous.
  - Lesions of the lateral geniculate body also produce asymmetrical hemianopic defects.
  - The causes of optic tract disease are similar to those affecting the chiasm but the tract is particularly vulnerable when the chiasm is prefixed (see above).
- **Wernicke hemianopic pupil**
  - The optic tracts contain both visual and pupillomotor fibres. The visual fibres terminate in the lateral geniculate body but the pupillary fibres leave the optic tract anterior to the lateral geniculate body, projecting through the brachium of the superior colliculus to terminate in the pretectal nuclei.
  - An optic tract lesion may therefore give rise to an afferent pupillary conduction defect.
  - Characteristically, the pupillary light reflex will be normal when the unaffected hemiretina is stimulated and absent when the involved hemiretina is stimulated (i.e. light is shone from the hemianopic side).
  - In practice, this Wernicke hemianopic pupillary reaction is difficult to elicit because of scatter of light within the eye – a fine beam should be used.
- **Optic atrophy** may occur when the optic tracts are damaged because their fibres are the axons of the retinal ganglion cells. The ipsilateral disc manifests atrophy of the superior and inferior aspects of the neuroretinal rim (fibres from the temporal

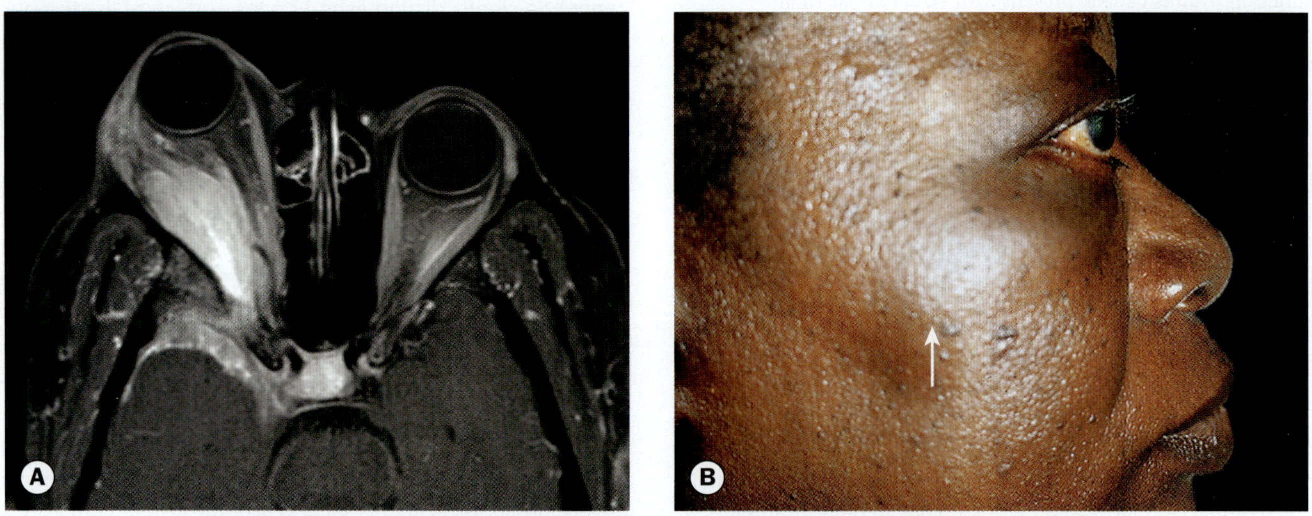

Fig. 19.58 Sphenoidal ridge meningioma. **(A)** Axial fat saturated T1-weighted, gadolinium-enhanced image in a patient with a right-sided sphenoid wing meningioma. The tumour involves the lateral aspect of the orbit and the right middle cranial fossa; **(B)** reactive hyperostosis (arrow).

retina), while the contralateral disc manifests a 'bow tie' pattern (nasal and nasal macular fibres).

- **Contralateral pyramidal signs** may occur when an optic tract lesion also damages the ipsilateral cerebral peduncle.

Optic radiations

Anatomy

The optic radiations extend from the lateral geniculate body to the striate cortex, which is located on the medial aspect of the occipital lobe, above and below the calcarine fissure (Fig. 19.59). As the radiations pass posteriorly, fibres from corresponding retinal elements lie progressively closer together. For this reason, incomplete hemianopia caused by posterior radiation lesions are more congruous than those involving the anterior radiations. Because these fibres are third-order neurones that originate in the lateral geniculate body, lesions of the optic radiations do not produce optic atrophy. The optic radiations and visual cortex have a dual blood supply from the middle and posterior cerebral arteries.

Temporal radiations

- **Visual field defect** consists of a contralateral superior homonymous quadrantanopia ('pie in the sky'), because the inferior fibres of the optic radiations, which subserve the upper visual fields, first sweep antero-inferiorly (Meyer loop) into the temporal lobe around the anterior tip of the temporal horn of the lateral ventricle (see 'a' in Fig. 19.59).
- **Associated features** are likely to include contralateral hemisensory disturbance and hemiparesis, because the temporal radiations pass very close to the sensory and motor fibres of the internal capsule before passing posteriorly and re-joining the superior fibres. Other features of temporal lobe disease include paroxysmal olfactory and gustatory hallucinations (uncinate fits), formed visual hallucinations and seizures, with receptive dysphasia if the dominant hemisphere is involved.

Anterior parietal radiations

- **Visual field defect** consists of a contralateral inferior homonymous quadrantanopia ('pie on the floor') because the superior fibres of the radiations, which subserve the inferior visual fields, proceed directly posteriorly through the parietal lobe to the occipital cortex. However, a lesion involving only the anterior parietal part of the radiations is rare. Hemianopia resulting from a parietal lobe lesion tends to be relatively congruous (see 'b' in Fig. 19.59).
- **Associated features** of dominant parietal lobe disease include acalculia, agraphia, left–right disorientation and finger agnosia. Non-dominant lobe lesions may cause dressing and constitutional apraxia and spatial neglect.

Main radiations

Deep in the parietal lobe, the optic radiations lie just external to the trigone and the occipital horn of the lateral ventricle. Lesions in this area usually cause a complete homonymous hemianopia (see 'c' in Fig. 19.59).

- **Optokinetic nystagmus** (OKN), elicited with a rotating striped optokinetic drum, may be useful in localizing the cause of an isolated homonymous hemianopia.
  - Physiological OKN involves smooth pursuit of a target, followed momentarily by a saccade in the opposite direction to fixate on the next target.
  - If a homonymous hemianopia is due to a lesion in the parietal lobe, the smooth pursuit pathways towards the side of the lesion are likely to be affected, making this component of OKN defective. OKN will therefore be asymmetrical: erratic when the drum is rotated towards the side of the lesion, but regular when the drum is rotated away from the side of the lesion.
  - If the lesion is in the occipital lobe, the smooth pursuit pathways are intact and OKN will be symmetrical – this is the Cogan dictum, which also states that the parietal lobe lesion is more likely to be a tumour and the occipital lesion an infarction.

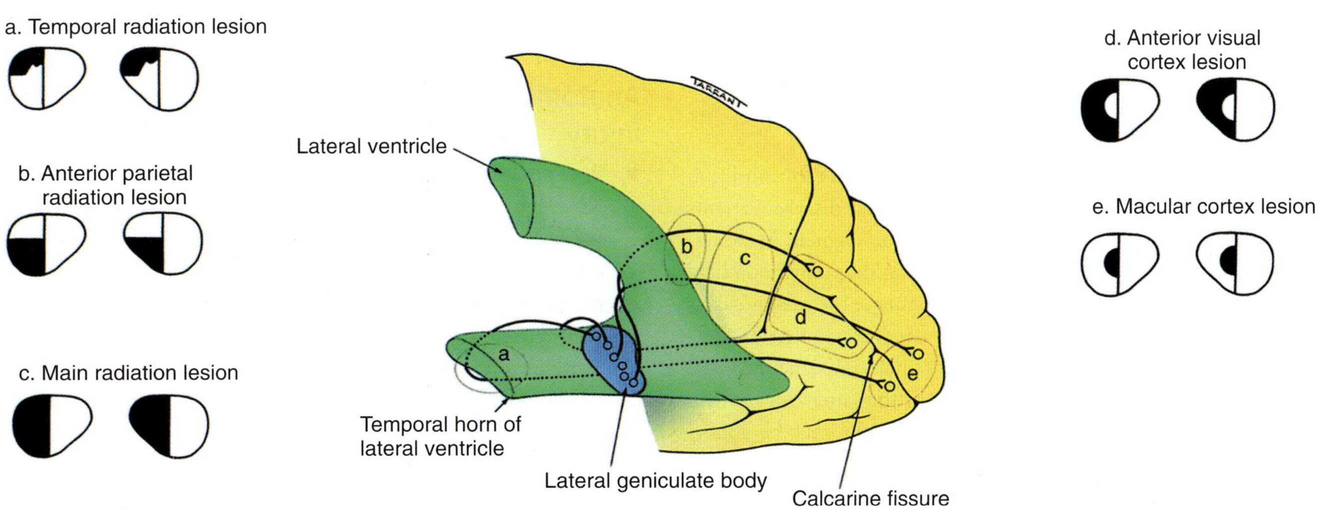

Fig. 19.59 Visual field defects caused by lesions of the optic radiations and visual cortex.

Occipital cortex

Clinical features

- **Visual field defects**
    - In the striate cortex the peripheral visual fields are represented anteriorly. This part of the occipital lobe is supplied by a branch of the posterior cerebral artery.
    - Central macular vision is represented posteriorly just lateral to the tip of the calcarine cortex, an area supplied mainly by a branch of the middle cerebral artery. Occlusion of the posterior cerebral artery will therefore tend to produce a macular-sparing congruous homonymous hemianopia (see 'd' in Fig. 19.59).
    - Damage to the tip of the occipital cortex, as might occur from a head injury, tends to give rise to congruous, homonymous, macular defects (see 'e' in Fig. 19.59), although macular sparing may sometimes occur with vascular lesions of the occipital lobe.
    - The front of the calcarine cortex subserves the temporal extremity of the visual field of the contralateral eye, the area of visual space that extends beyond the field of binocular single vision and is perceived monocularly. A lesion in this area may therefore give rise to a monocular temporal field defect in the contralateral eye, known as a temporal crescent.
- **Associated features** of visual cortex disease (cortical blindness) include formed visual hallucinations, denial of blindness (Anton syndrome) and the Riddoch phenomenon (only moving visual targets perceived).

Causes

- **Stroke** in the territory of the posterior cerebral artery is responsible for over 90% of homonymous hemianopia with no other neurological deficit.
- **Other causes** include trauma, tumours and rarely migraine. A range of uncommon inflammatory (including autoimmune and infective), degenerative and toxic disorders can also be causative, but will usually manifest with more widespread neurological features. Imaging and lumbar puncture are typically key to diagnosis. Mimicking by retinal disease such as acute zonal occult outer retinopathy (AZOOR) may occur.

Benson syndrome

Benson syndrome (posterior cortical atrophy) is a rare condition often referred to as a visual variant of Alzheimer disease. Patients may have normal VA, anterior and posterior segment examination, but commonly abnormal colour vision, homonymous field defects, visual agnosia, alexia and acalculia. The diagnosis is commonly missed. Other degenerative conditions often exhibiting early occipital cortical involvement include Alzheimer and Creutzfeldt–Jakob disease; presentation in the latter can be with acute visual symptoms only. Electroretinography may be abnormal. In immunocompromised states, including drug-induced, progressive multifocal leukoencephalopathy can present with isolated occipital features.

Balint syndrome

Balint syndrome refers to the combination of simultanagnosia (inability to discern the overall impression of an image whilst distinguishing individual components), optic ataxia (defective visually-directed reaching) and ocular apraxia (impairment of voluntary saccades). It is typically due to parieto-occipital disease, with a range of causes reported.

Posterior reversible encephalopathy syndrome

Posterior reversible encephalopathy syndrome (PRES) or reversible posterior leukoencephalopathy syndrome refers to a clinical presentation thought to result from vascular endothelial dysfunction seen in patients with malignant hypertension or eclampsia, treatment with some drugs (e.g. tacrolimus, ciclosporin) and rarely other associations such as autoimmune disease. Cortical visual deficits can occasionally be the presenting feature, others including headache and seizures.

CEREBRAL VISUAL IMPAIRMENT (CVI)

Introduction

'Cerebral visual impairment' is the term used to describe visual disability which cannot be attributed to a disorder of the eyes and anterior visual pathways. It is a consequence of abnormality in the parts of the brain that process visual information. CVI is the commonest cause of visual disability in children living in industrialised countries and affects up to 3% of mainstream school children. It can be a difficult diagnosis to make in subtle cases where the visual acuity is normal, particularly as brain imaging may reveal no significant abnormality. CVI can limit social interaction, mobility and learning.

Causes

- **Children:** especially premature birth and its cerebral complications (hypoxia and ischaemia), neonatal hypoglycemia, head injury, infections (meningitis and encephalitis), hydrocephalus, developmental brain defects.
- **Adults:** head injury, stroke, dementia.

Anatomical basis and outcomes of visual brain injury

- **The posterior parietal lobes** are connected to the occipital lobes by the superior longitudinal fasciculus. This functional pathway is called the 'dorsal stream', which creates a subconscious real-time dynamic three-dimensional reproduction of our surroundings. This is mapped to body position and allows accurate visually guided movement and visual search. Balint syndrome (when severe) and dorsal stream dysfunction (when less profound) results from bilateral posterior parietal pathology.
- **Bilateral middle temporal lobe** pathology slightly anterior to the occipital lobes causes difficulty in seeing moving targets (dyskinetopsia).

- **Infarction of both occipital lobes** that spares the middle temporal lobes can conversely result in either an ability to see moving objects but not static targets, or result in the Riddoch phenomenon, which occurs when a person who is otherwise blind can perceive moving objects. Retained ability to recognize emotion conveyed by facial expression despite cortical blindness is called 'effective blindsight'.

Symptoms

- **Difficulty with visual complexity**: difficulty in seeing an object when other stimuli are present (e.g. sounds) or where there is a visually complex environment.
- **Visual field preference.** The child prefers to look at objects in a particular visual field.
- **Absence of visually guided reach**: impairment of a child's ability to look at an object while reaching for it.
- **Visual latency.** The visual responses are slow and often delayed.
- **Preference** for familiar objects and rich, highly saturated colours like red and yellow.
- **Staring.** These children may have a need to look at rapidly moving objects (e.g. fixating on a rapidly moving fan) and non-purposeful gaze (e.g. tendency to stare at a light source).
- **Atypical visual reflexes.** For example, delayed or absent protective blink response.

Management

- **Key issues.** Early intervention, educational support and visual rehabilitation are central to helping these individuals develop and learn.
- **Identify the specific visual difficulty.** Take a structured history from the patient/child and a family member.
- **Provide an explanation** for the origin of the symptoms.
- **Devise strategies to compensate** for the impairment, preferably by using a trained multi-disciplinary team.

OCULAR MOTOR NERVES

Third nerve

Nuclear complex

The nuclear complex of the third (oculomotor) nerve is situated in the midbrain at the level of the superior colliculus, ventral to the Sylvian aqueduct (Fig. 19.60). It is composed of the following paired and unpaired sub nuclei:

- **Levator subnucleus** is an unpaired caudal midline structure that innervates both levator muscles. Lesions confined to this area will therefore give rise to bilateral ptosis.
- **Superior rectus subnuclei** are paired: each innervates the respective contralateral superior rectus. A nuclear third nerve palsy will therefore spare the ipsilateral and affect the contralateral, superior rectus.
- **Medial rectus, inferior rectus** and **inferior oblique subnuclei** are paired and innervate their corresponding ipsilateral muscles. Lesions confined to the nuclear complex are relatively uncommon. The most frequent causes are vascular disease, primary tumours and metastases. Involvement of the paired medial rectus subnuclei cause a wall-eyed bilateral internuclear ophthalmoplegia (WEBINO), characterized by exotropia with defective convergence and adduction. Lesions involving the entire nucleus are often associated with involvement of the adjacent and caudal fourth nerve nucleus.

Fasciculus

The fasciculus consists of efferent fibres that pass from the third nerve nucleus through the red nucleus and the medial aspect of the cerebral peduncle (see Fig. 19.60). They then emerge from the midbrain and pass into the interpeduncular space. The causes of nuclear and fascicular lesions are similar, except that demyelination may affect the fasciculus.

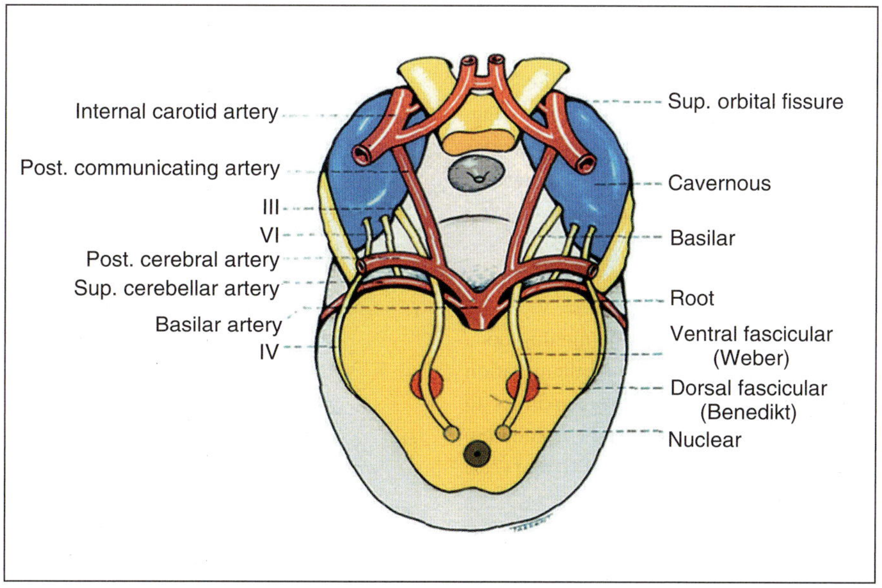

Fig. 19.60 Dorsal view of the course of the third (oculomotor) nerve. Post. = posterior; Sup. = superior.

- **Benedikt** syndrome involves the fasciculus as it passes through the red nucleus and is characterized by ipsilateral third nerve palsy and contralateral extrapyramidal signs such as hemi tremor.
- **Weber** syndrome involves the fasciculus as it passes through the cerebral peduncle and is characterized by ipsilateral third nerve palsy and a contralateral hemiparesis.
- **Nothnagel** syndrome involves the fasciculus and the superior cerebellar peduncle and is characterized by ipsilateral third nerve palsy and cerebellar ataxia.
- **Claude** syndrome is a combination of Benedikt and Nothnagel syndromes.

Basilar

The basilar part starts as a series of 'rootlets' that leave the midbrain on the medial aspect of the cerebral peduncle, before coalescing to form the main trunk. The nerve then passes between the posterior cerebral and superior cerebellar arteries, running lateral to and parallel with the posterior communicating artery (Fig. 19.61). As the nerve traverses the base of the skull along its subarachnoid course unaccompanied by any other cranial nerve, an isolated third nerve palsy is commonly basilar. The following are important causes:

- **Aneurysm** of the posterior communicating artery at its junction with the internal carotid artery (Fig. 19.62), typically presents acutely as a pupil-involving painful third nerve palsy. In a recent population-based study, compression from an aneurysm only accounted for 6% of acute third nerve palsies. Approximately two-thirds had pupillary involvement.
- **Head trauma**, resulting in extradural or subdural haematoma, may cause a tentorial pressure cone with downward herniation of the temporal lobe. This compresses the third nerve as it passes over the tentorial edge (Fig. 19.63), initially causing irritative miosis followed by mydriasis and complete third nerve palsy.

Intracavernous

The third nerve then enters the cavernous sinus by piercing the dura just lateral to the posterior clinoid process. Within the sinus, the third nerve runs in the lateral wall above the fourth nerve (Fig. 19.64). In the anterior part of the cavernous sinus, the nerve divides into superior and inferior branches that enter the orbit through the superior orbital fissure within the annulus of Zinn. The following are potential causes of intracavernous third nerve palsy:

- **Diabetes.**
- **Pituitary apoplexy** (see above).
- **Miscellaneous pathology** such as aneurysm, meningioma, carotid-cavernous fistula and granulomatous inflammation (Tolosa–Hunt syndrome). Because of its close proximity to other cranial nerves, intracavernous third nerve lesions are likely to be associated with involvement of the fourth and sixth nerves and the first division of the fifth nerve.

Intraorbital

- **Superior** division innervates the levator and superior rectus muscles.

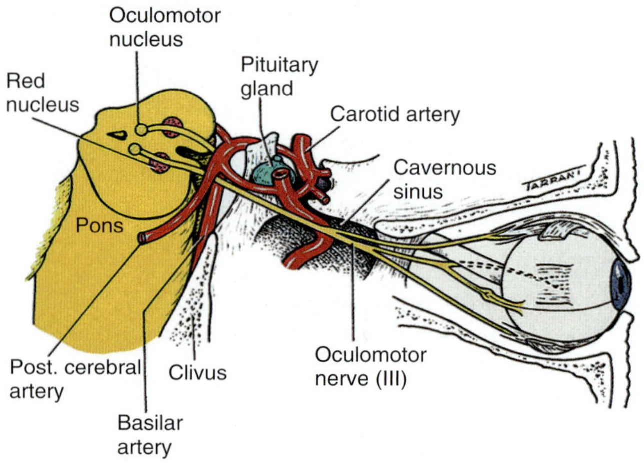

Fig. 19.61 Lateral view of the course of the third (oculomotor) nerve. Post. = posterior.

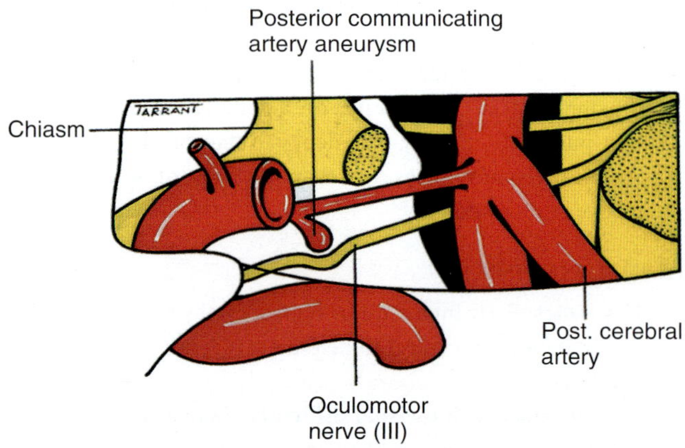

Fig. 19.62 Compression of the third (oculomotor) nerve by a posterior communicating aneurysm. Post. = posterior.

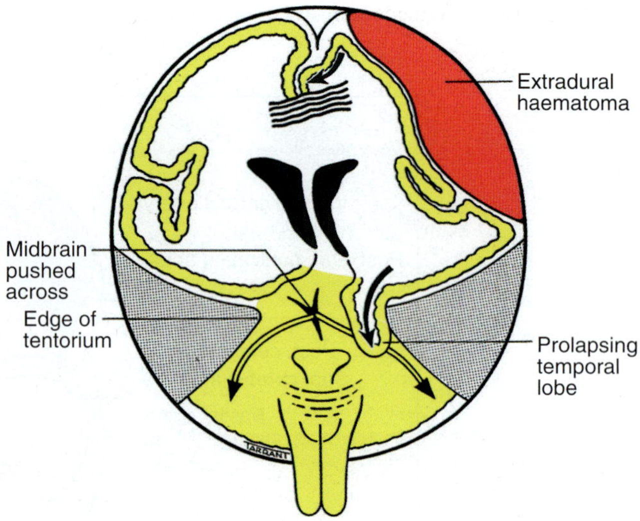

Fig. 19.63 Mechanism of third nerve palsy by extradural haematoma.

- **Inferior** division innervates the medial rectus, the inferior rectus and the inferior oblique muscles. The branch to the inferior oblique also contains preganglionic parasympathetic fibres from the Edinger–Westphal subnucleus, which

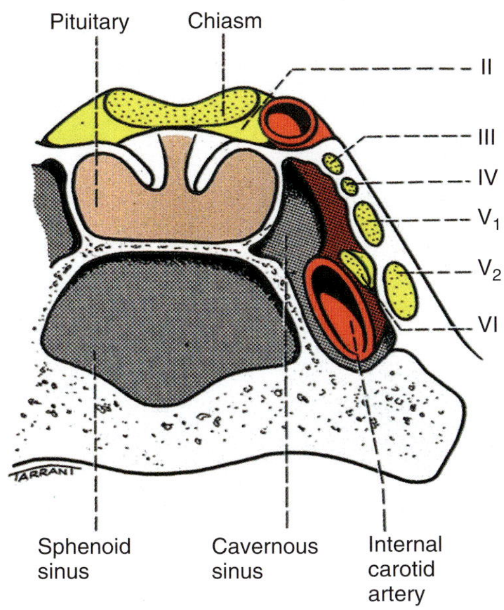

Fig. 19.64 Location of the cranial nerves in the cavernous sinus viewed from behind.

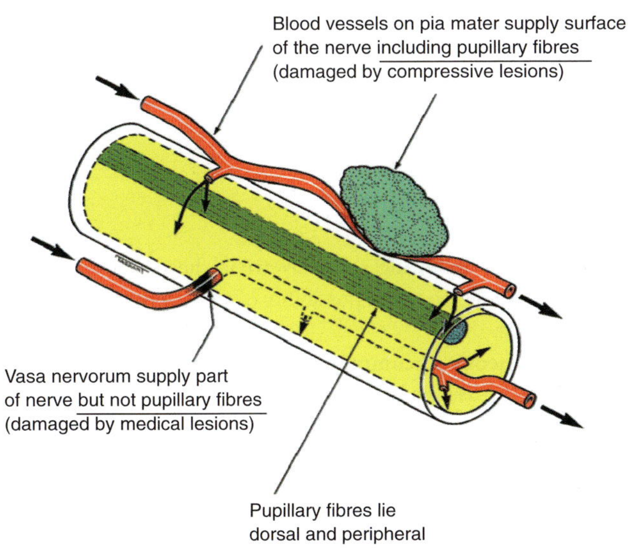

Fig. 19.65 Location of pupillomotor fibres within the trunk of the third nerve.

innervate the sphincter pupillae and the ciliary muscle. Lesions of the inferior division are characterized by limited adduction and depression, together with a dilated pupil. Both superior and inferior division palsies are commonly traumatic or vascular.

Pupillomotor fibres

Between the brainstem and the cavernous sinus, the pupillomotor parasympathetic fibres are located superficially in the superomedial part of the third nerve (Fig. 19.65). They derive their blood supply from the pial blood vessels, whereas the main interior trunk of the nerve is supplied by the vasa nervorum. Involvement or sparing of the pupil is important, as it frequently differentiates a 'surgical' from a 'medical' lesion:

- **'Surgical' lesions** such as aneurysms, trauma and uncal herniation characteristically involve the pupil by compressing the pial blood vessels and the superficially located pupillary fibres.
- **'Medical' lesions** such as occur in hypertension and diabetes usually spare the pupil (Fig. 19.66). This is because the microangiopathy associated with medical lesions involves the vasa nervorum, causing ischaemia of the main trunk of the nerve, leaving the superficial pupillary fibres intact.
- **These principles are not infallible** as pupillary involvement may be seen in some microangiopathic palsies, while pupillary sparing does not invariably exclude aneurysm or other compressive lesion. Pupillary involvement may develop a few days after the onset of diplopia as an aneurysm expands. Exceptionally, pupillary involvement may be the only sign of third nerve palsy (basal meningitis, uncal herniation). Like other features of third nerve palsy, pupillary involvement may be complete or partial, so mild pupillary signs may be clinically significant.

TIP Medical conditions (hypertension, diabetes) tend to cause a pupil-sparing third nerve palsy, but this principle is not infallible.

Signs

Partial involvement will give milder degrees of ophthalmoplegia. The other cranial nerves and peripheral nervous system should always be examined.

- **Profound ptosis** due to weakness of the levator muscle (Fig. 19.67A).
- **Abduction and depression in the primary position** ('down and out' – Fig. 19.67B) due to unopposed action of the lateral rectus and superior oblique muscles. The intact superior oblique muscle also causes intorsion of the eye at rest, which increases on attempted downgaze.
- **Limited adduction** due to medial rectus weakness (Fig. 19.66C and Fig. 19.67C).
- **Normal abduction** as the lateral rectus is intact (Fig. 19.66D).
- **Limited elevation** due to weakness of the superior rectus and inferior oblique (Fig. 19.66E and Fig. 19.67D).
- **Limited depression** due to weakness of the inferior rectus (Fig. 19.66F).
- **Dilated pupil and defective accommodation** due to parasympathetic palsy (Fig. 19.67).

Aberrant regeneration

Aberrant regeneration may follow acute traumatic and compressive, but not vascular, third nerve palsies. This is because the endoneural nerve sheaths, which may be breached in traumatic and compressive lesions, remain intact with vascular lesions. Bizarre defects in ocular motility, such as elevation of the upper eyelid on attempted adduction or depression (the pseudo-Graefe or pseudo-von Graefe phenomenon), are caused by misdirected regenerating axons that re-innervate the incorrect extraocular muscle (Fig. 19.68). The pupil may also be involved.

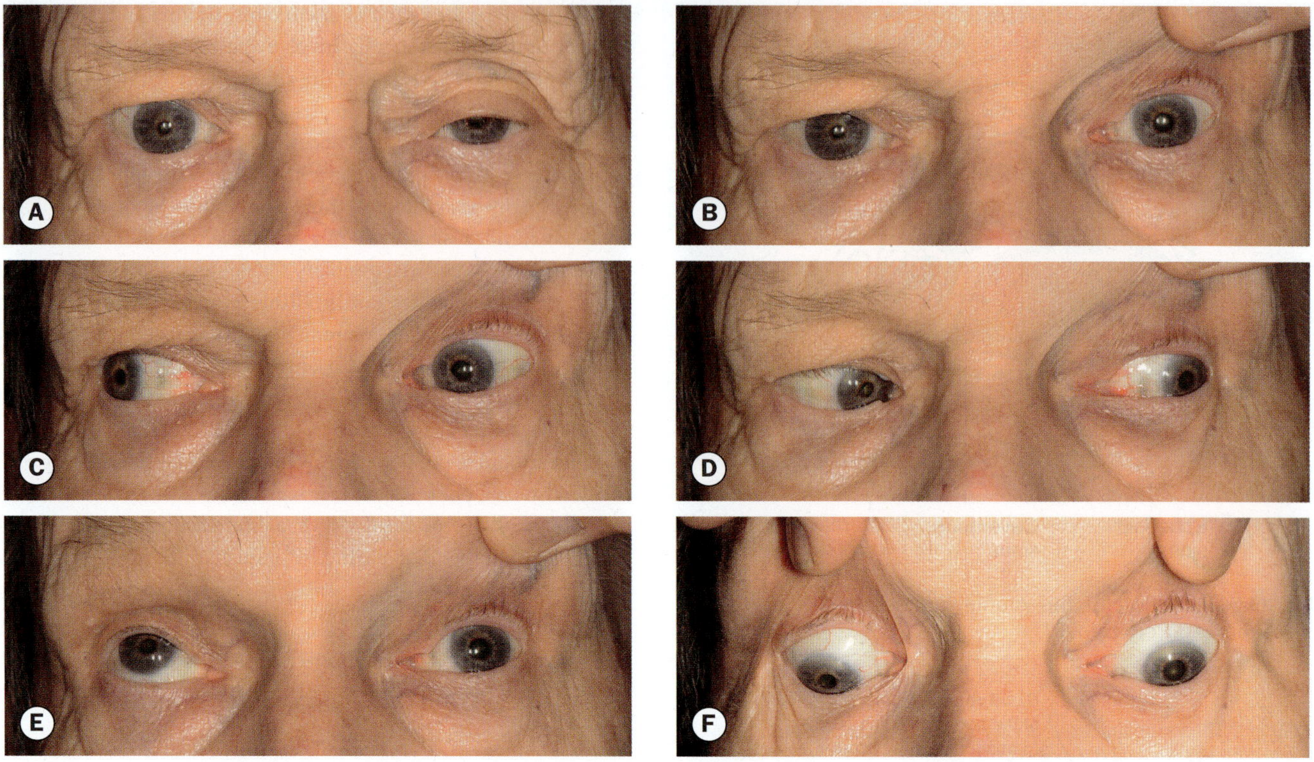

Fig. 19.66 Left third nerve palsy with pupil sparing. **(A)** Slight left ptosis; **(B)** subtle left exotropia in the primary position; **(C)** limitation of adduction; **(D)** normal abduction; **(E)** limitation of elevation; **(F)** slight limitation of depression.

Causes of isolated third nerve palsy

Clinical evaluation and imaging facilitate identification of a cause in most cases.

- **Microvascular** disease associated with systemic risk factors such as hypertension and diabetes are the most common cause of third nerve palsy, accounting for about 40% of cases. Marked periorbital pain is often associated, which is therefore not helpful in distinguishing an aneurysmal cause. In diabetes-related paresis, motility disturbance is typically profound, but there is usually (80%) relative or complete pupil sparing and when pupillary involvement does occur some degree of reaction to light is almost always preserved. As a general rule, where there is a complete third nerve palsy and a normally responsive pupil the cause is significantly more likely to be microvascular than secondary to an aneurysm.
- **Aneurysm** of the posterior communicating artery at its junction with the internal carotid is a very important cause of isolated third nerve palsy with involvement of the pupil. Pain is often, though not invariably, present and the extent of pupillary involvement characteristically exceeds the severity of motility dysfunction. An aneurysm of the internal carotid within the cavernous sinus tends to also involve other cranial nerves (see above).
- **Trauma**, both direct and secondary to subdural haematoma with uncal herniation. However, the development of third nerve palsy following relatively trivial head trauma should alert the clinician to the possibility of an underlying aneurysm or tumour.
- **Miscellaneous uncommon causes** include tumour, inflammatory disease such as syphilis, Lyme disease and sarcoidosis, GCA and vasculitis associated with collagen vascular disorders.
- **Episodic.** Brief episodes of third nerve dysfunction with spontaneous recovery may be idiopathic or occur with migraine, compression, ischaemia and alterations in intracranial pressure. Myasthenia gravis may mimic intermittent pupil-sparing third nerve paresis.

Investigation

- **Vascular risk factor** assessment similar to that for retinal arterial disease (see Ch. 13). Supplementary investigation may be required if a rarer aetiology such as infection (e.g. syphilis, Lyme disease) or vasculitis (including GCA) is suspected. In some cases, a lumbar puncture may be needed.
- **CT angiography** should be performed with great urgency if the clinical features are suspicious of an expanding aneurysm, especially if there is marked pupillary involvement with milder motility dysfunction and only partial ptosis.
- **MRI brain and orbits with venography**, including specific exclusion of a brainstem stroke or tumour, cavernous sinus or orbital apex lesion.
- **Conventional cerebral angiography** is occasionally indicated.

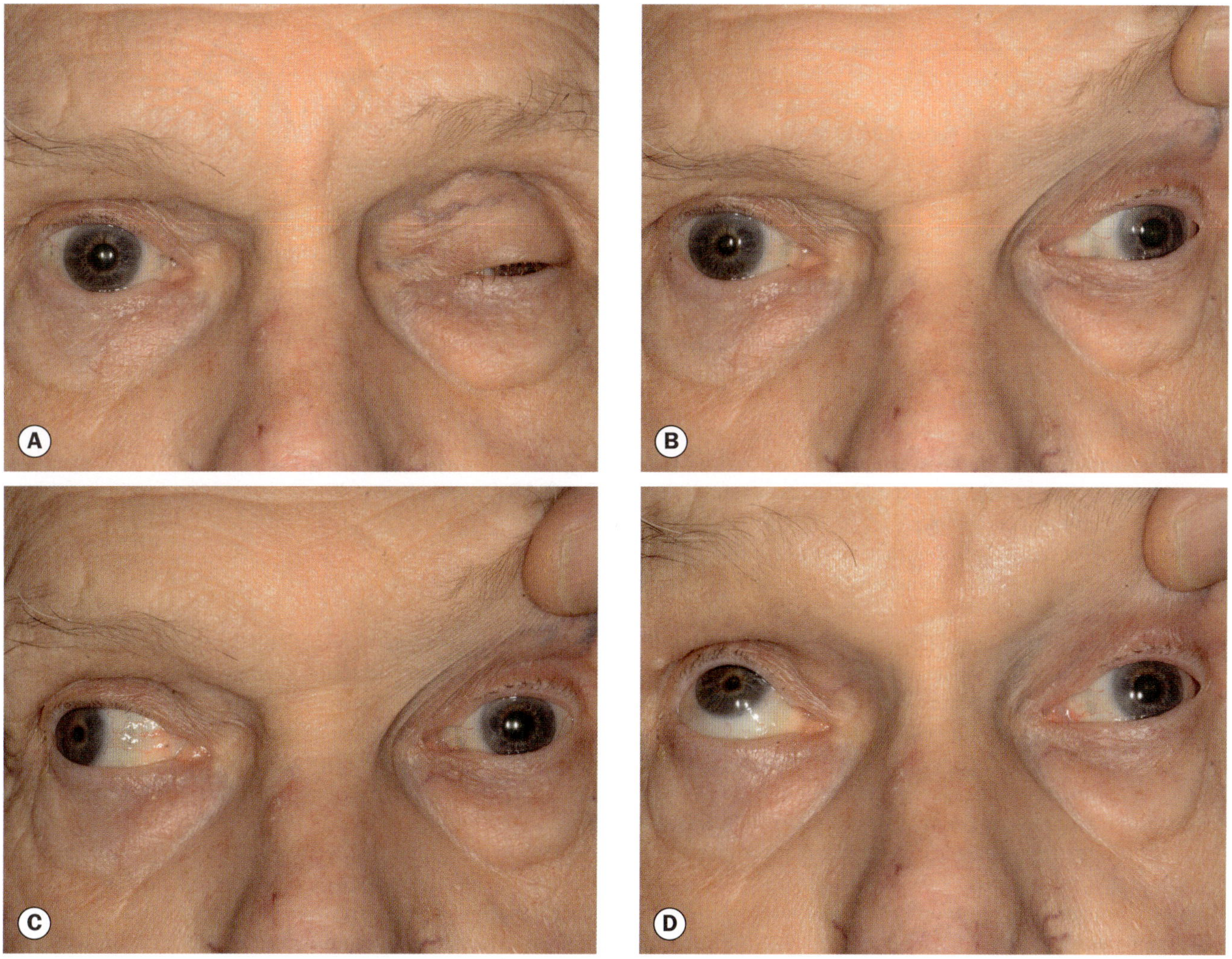

Fig. 19.67 Left third nerve palsy with pupil involvement. **(A)** Profound ptosis with the eye deviated down and out; **(B)** left exotropia in the primary position; **(C)** limited adduction; **(D)** limited elevation.

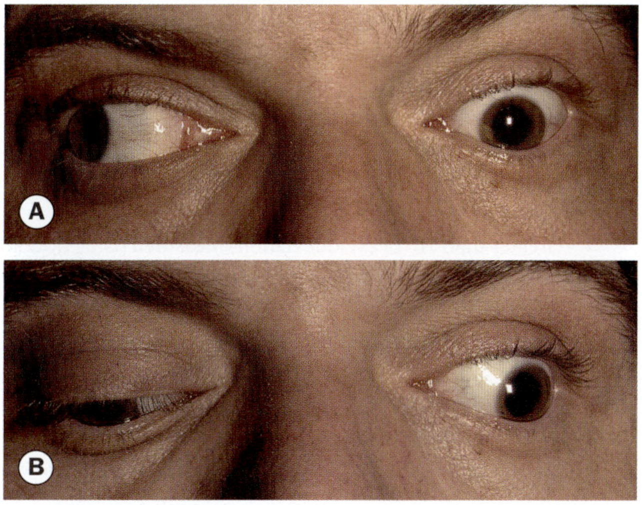

Fig. 19.68 Left third nerve palsy with aberrant regeneration. **(A)** Lid elevation with reduced adduction on attempted right gaze; **(B)** lid elevation with depression of the eye (pseudo von Graefe sign). *(Courtesy of ADN Murray.)*

TIP Urgent CT angiography is needed in a patient who presents with an acute third nerve palsy that involves the pupil, to exclude an expanding intracranial aneurysm.

Treatment

- **Observation** is usually appropriate in presumed microvascular cases; the majority will resolve over weeks or months. Temporary (e.g. Fresnel stick-on) prisms may be useful if the angle of deviation is small, but uniocular occlusion may be necessary to avoid diplopia if the ptosis component is partial or recovering. Botulinum toxin injection into the uninvolved lateral rectus muscle is sometimes used to prevent its contracture when recovery time is prolonged.
- **Surgical** treatment of the ocular motility element and ptosis should be contemplated only after spontaneous improvement has ceased, usually not earlier than 6–12 months from onset. Numerous innovative surgical techniques have been described.

Fourth nerve

Anatomy

The fourth (trochlear) cranial nerve (Fig. 19.69) supplies only the superior oblique muscle.

- **Key features**
  - It is a very long and slender nerve, increasing its vulnerability.
  - It is the only cranial nerve to emerge from the dorsal aspect of the brain.
  - It is the only decussated (crossed) cranial nerve besides the optic nerve, innervating the superior oblique muscle contralateral to its nucleus.
  - It has the fewest axons of any of the cranial nerves.
- **The nucleus** is located at the level of the inferior colliculi ventral to the Sylvian aqueduct. It is caudal to and continuous with the third nerve nuclear complex.
- **The fasciculus** consists of axons that curve posteriorly around the aqueduct and decussate completely in the anterior medullary velum.
- **The trunk** leaves the brainstem on the dorsal surface, just caudal to the inferior colliculus. It then curves laterally around the brainstem, runs forwards beneath the free edge of the tentorium and, like the third nerve, passes between the posterior cerebral artery and the superior cerebellar artery. It then pierces the dura and enters the cavernous sinus.
- **The intracavernous** part runs in the lateral wall of the sinus, inferior to the third nerve and above the first division of the fifth. In the anterior part of the cavernous sinus, it rises and passes through the superior orbital fissure above and lateral to the annulus of Zinn.
- **The intraorbital** part innervates the superior oblique muscle.

Causes of isolated fourth nerve palsy

- **Idiopathic** lesions are common and many of these are thought to be congenital although symptoms may not develop until decompensation occurs in adult life due to reduced fusional ability. In contrast to acquired lesions patients are not usually aware of the torsional aspect, but may develop vertical double vision that is often appreciated as of sudden or subacute onset. Examination of old photographs for the presence of a compensatory head posture may be helpful, as is the presence of an increased vertical prism fusional range. Occasionally cataract surgery can be associated with decompensation.
- **Trauma** frequently causes bilateral fourth nerve palsy. The long and slender nerves are particularly vulnerable as they decussate in the anterior medullary velum, through impact with the tentorial edge. Care must be taken not to mistake a bilateral palsy for a unilateral lesion, particularly when corrective surgery is contemplated.
- **Microvascular** lesions are relatively common, this aetiology often being presumed when appropriate systemic risk factors are present in the absence of features of congenital onset.
- **Aneurysms and tumours** are extremely rare.

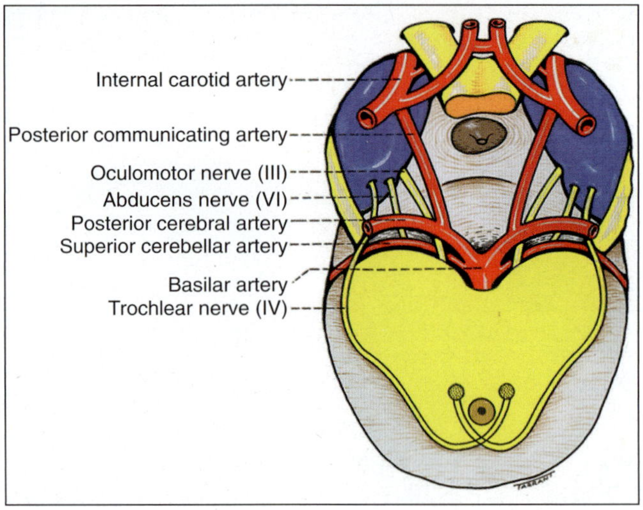

Fig. 19.69 Dorsal view of the course of the fourth (trochlear) nerve

Signs

The acute onset of vertical diplopia in the absence of ptosis, combined with a characteristic head posture, strongly suggests fourth nerve disease. The main actions of the superior oblique are intorsion (incyclotorsion) and depression in adduction. Peripheral lesions cause ipsilateral and nuclear lesions contralateral superior oblique weakness. Left paresis is characterized by:

- **Left hypertropia** ('left over right') in the primary position (Fig. 19.70A), increasing on right gaze (Fig. 19.70B).
- **Limitation of left depression,** most marked in adduction.
- **Left extorsion**, greatest in abduction.
- **Normal abduction** of the left eye.
- **Normal elevation** of the left eye.
- **A compensatory head posture** (Fig. 19.70C) avoids diplopia: vertical, torsional and worse on downgaze. To compensate for weakness of intorsion there is contralateral head tilt to the right. To alleviate the weakened depression of the eye the chin is slightly depressed. As this is most marked in adduction, the face may also be turned slightly to the right.
- **Bilateral involvement** should always be excluded, particularly following head trauma (Fig. 19.71A).
  - Right hypertropia in left gaze and left hypertropia in right gaze, though orthophoria may be present.
  - Greater than 10° of cyclodeviation (measured using double Maddox rods or by synoptophore – see Ch. 18).
  - 'V' pattern esotropia is often present (Fig. 19.71B–D). Absence of the secondary abduction function provided by the superior oblique muscles in downgaze allows the increased tone in the inferior rectus muscles to produce an esodeviation.
  - Bilaterally positive Bielschowsky head tilt test (see below).

TIP Trauma is the commonest cause of bilateral fourth nerve palsy.

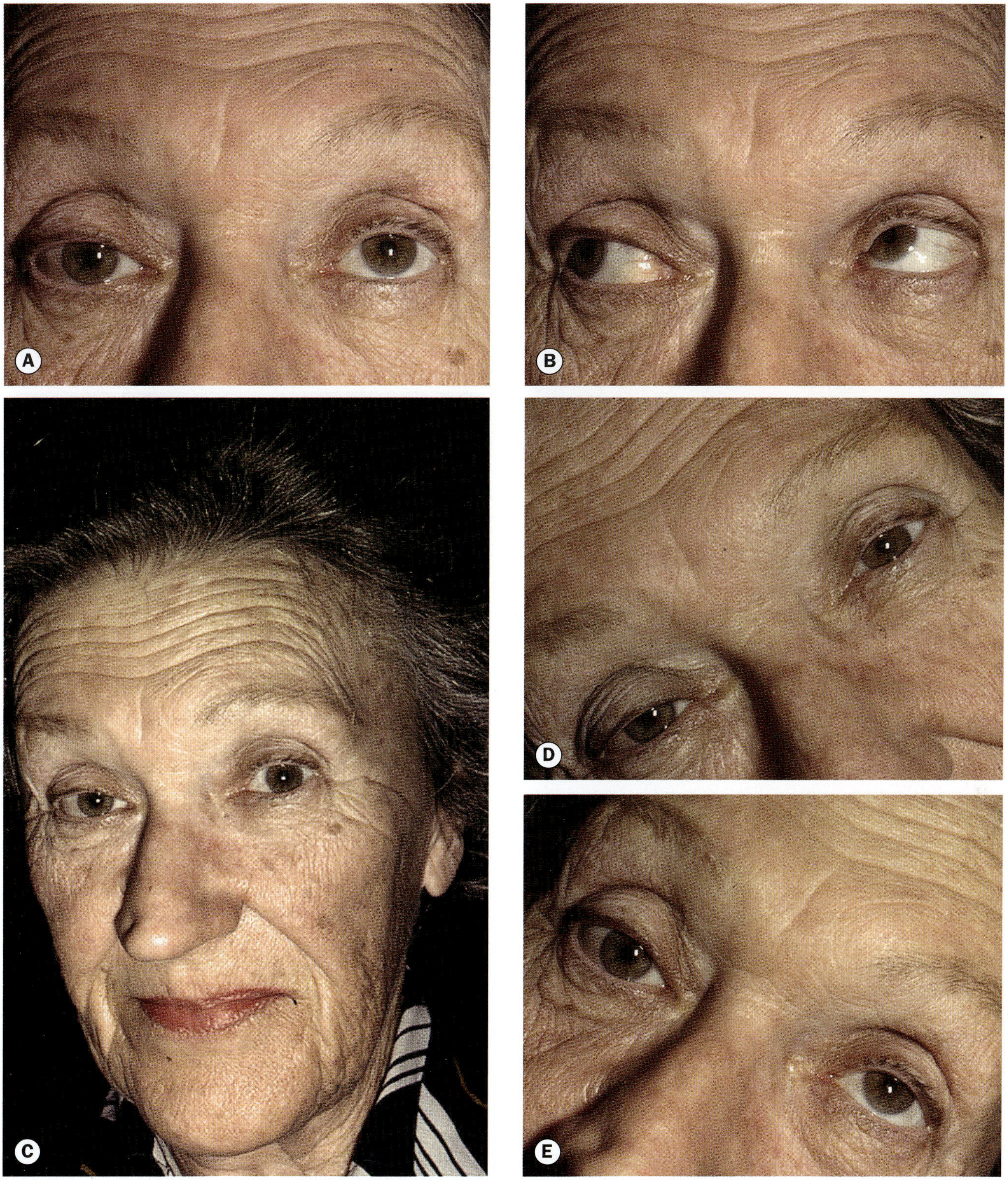

Fig. 19.70 Left fourth nerve palsy. **(A)** Left hypertropia (left over right) in the primary position; **(B)** increase in left hypertropia on right gaze due to left inferior oblique overaction; **(C)** compensatory head posture; head tilt to right, face turn to the right and chin depressed; **(D)** no hypertropia on right head tilt; **(E)** marked hypertropia on left head tilt: positive Bielschowsky test. *(Courtesy of ADN Murray.)*

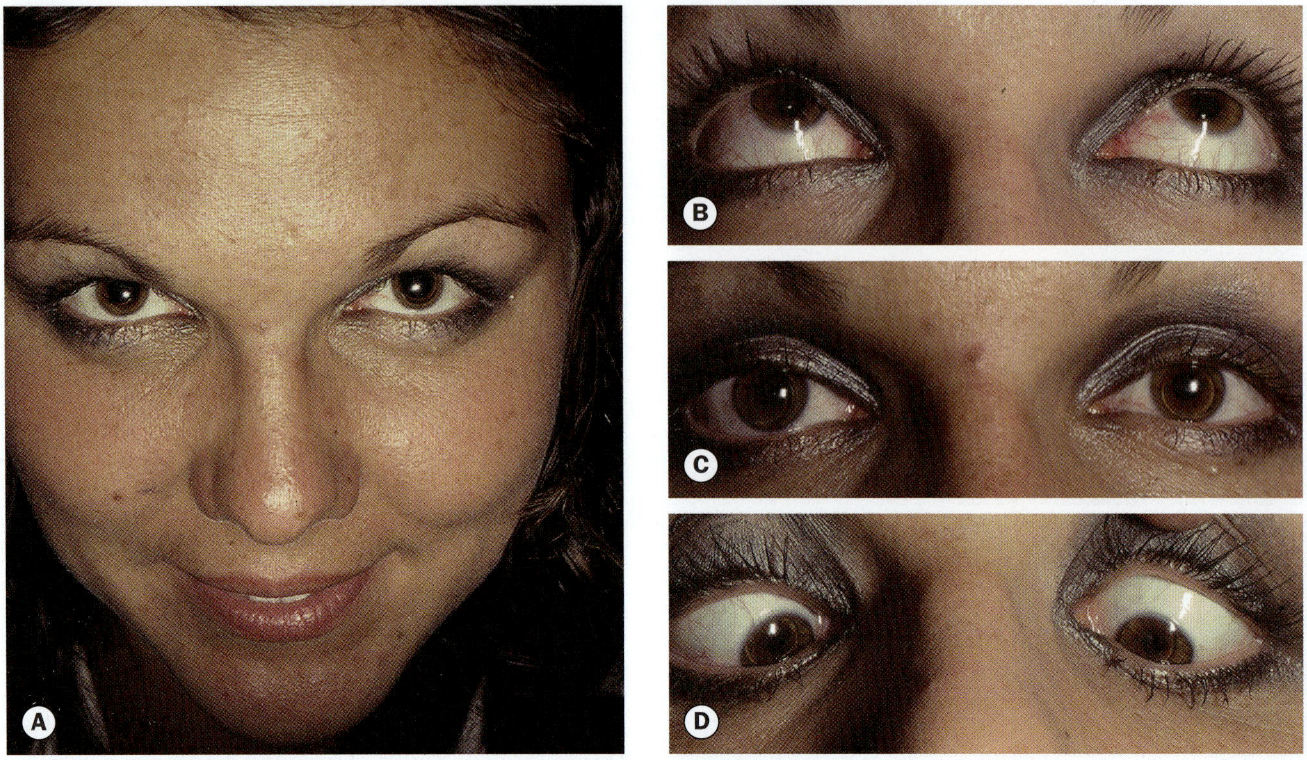

Fig. 19.71 Bilateral fourth nerve palsy. **(A)** Compensatory head posture with chin tilted down to prevent diplopia in the primary position; **(B)** upgaze; **(C)** looking straight ahead; **(D)** 'V' pattern in downgaze. *(Courtesy of ADN Murray.)*

Parks three-step test

This clinical test allows isolation of a single weak muscle in patients with vertical diplopia of acute onset. It is inaccurate in some circumstances, including patients who have undergone previous extraocular muscle surgery.

- **Step one.** In the primary position, the hypertropic eye is identified, narrowing the affected muscle to one of the depressors of the hypertropic eye (superior oblique or inferior rectus) or one of the elevators of the hypotropic eye (superior rectus or inferior oblique). In a fourth nerve palsy, the involved eye is higher (see Fig. 19.70A).
- **Step two.** The eyes are examined in right and left gaze to determine where the hypertropia is greater, thus assigning the weakness to the two of the four previously identified muscles having the greatest vertical action in that position. In superior oblique weakness (see Fig. 19.70B) the deviation is **w**orse **o**n **o**pposite **g**aze – **WOOG.**
- **Step three**
  - The Bielschowsky head tilt test (BHTT) is performed with the patient fixating on a target directly ahead, optimally at 3 metres (see Fig. 19.70D and E).
  - The head is tilted to each side in turn in order to assess the muscles responsible for cyclotorsion, with observation to determine the position in which the hypertropia is worse. On tilt to one side, the superior oblique and superior rectus (note that both are superior) muscles of the eye of that same side correctively intort and the inferior rectus and inferior oblique (note both are inferior) of the contralateral eye correctively extort. From the two muscles previously isolated, one can be eliminated.
  - In fourth nerve palsy the deviation is **b**etter **o**n **o**pposite **t**ilt – **BOOT** (see Fig. 19.70D). In practice, as the three-step test is almost always employed to confirm a fourth nerve palsy, the BHTT alone is often sufficient for a working diagnosis.

Investigation

Vascular investigation is sometimes indicated. Neuroimaging is not required routinely for an isolated non-progressive fourth nerve palsy, but should be considered if improvement does not occur.

Treatment

Congenital decompensated and presumed microvascular palsies commonly resolve spontaneously. Strabismus surgery is not infrequently required for traumatic and childhood cases, in the former for troublesome diplopia and the latter for a substantial compensatory head posture. The approach depends on the pattern and severity of weakness.

- **A small hypertropia** under 15 prism dioptres (Δ) can usually be treated either by inferior oblique weakening or by superior oblique tucking, though surgery to other muscles might be required in some circumstances.
- **A moderate–large deviation** may be treated by ipsilateral inferior oblique weakening combined with, or followed by, ipsilateral superior rectus weakening and/or contralateral inferior rectus weakening if required; defective elevation is a potential complication.

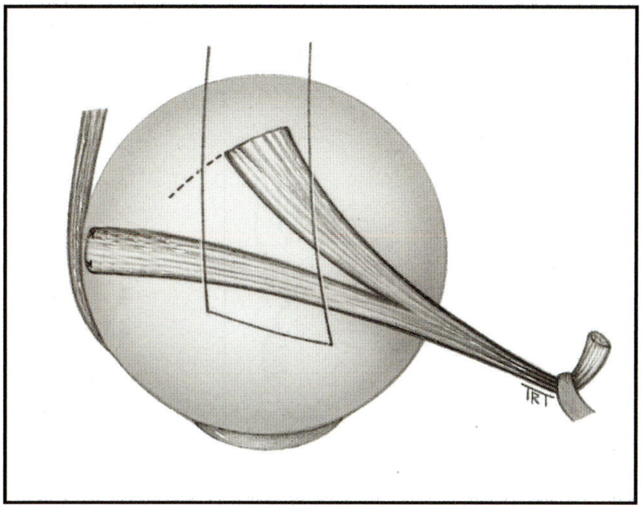

Fig. 19.72 Harada–Ito procedure for superior oblique palsy.

- **Excyclotorsion** may need to be addressed, particularly in bilateral cases. The Harada–Ito procedure involves splitting and anterolateral transposition of the lateral half of the superior oblique tendon (Fig. 19.72).
- **V-pattern esotropia** secondary to bilateral fourth nerve palsy can be treated by symmetrical recession of both **inferior rectus** muscles: e.g. 1.6 mm reduces a 'V' pattern by 18 Δ and 2.8 mm reduces a 'V' pattern by 34 Δ.

Sixth nerve

Brainstem

The nucleus of the sixth (abducens or abducent) nerve lies at the mid-level of the pons, ventral to the floor of the fourth ventricle (Fig. 19.73). The fibres (fasciculus) leave the brainstem ventrally at the pontomedullary junction.

- **Nuclear lesion.** A nuclear sixth nerve lesion also causes a failure of horizontal gaze towards the side of the damage due to involvement of the adjacent horizontal gaze centre (paramedian pontine reticular formation). Facial (seventh) nerve fibres wrap around the sixth nerve nucleus, so ipsilateral lower motor neurone (LMN) facial nerve palsy is also common. Isolated sixth nerve palsy is never nuclear in origin.
- **Foville (inferior medial pontine) syndrome** is most frequently caused by vascular disease or tumours involving the dorsal pons. It is characterized by ipsilateral involvement of the fifth to eighth cranial nerves, central sympathetic fibres (Horner syndrome) and horizontal gaze palsy.
- **Millard–Gubler (ventral pontine) syndrome** involves the fasciculus as it passes through the pyramidal tract and is most frequently caused by vascular disease, tumours or demyelination. As well as ipsilateral sixth nerve palsy, there is contralateral hemiplegia and often an ipsilateral LMN facial nerve palsy.
- **Raymond syndrome** involves the pyramidal tract and sixth nerve. In addition to an ipsilateral sixth nerve palsy there is contralateral hemiplegia.

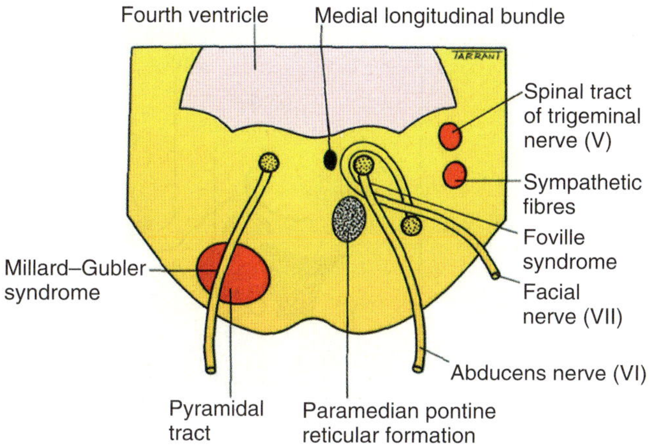

Fig. 19.73 The pons at the level of the sixth (abducens) nerve nucleus.

Basilar

The basilar part of the nerve enters the prepontine basilar cistern, passes upwards close to the base of the skull and is crossed by the anterior inferior cerebellar artery (Fig. 19.74). It pierces the dura below the posterior clinoid and angles forwards over the tip of the petrous bone, passing through or around the inferior petrosal sinus, through the Dorello canal (underneath the petroclinoid ligament), to enter the cavernous sinus.

- **A vestibular schwannoma** (also called an acoustic neuroma, although this is a misnomer as the tumour arises from the Schwann cells of the nerve, rather than the actual neurones) may damage the sixth nerve at the pontomedullary junction (Fig. 19.75). The first symptom is hearing loss and the first sign diminished corneal sensitivity. Hearing and corneal sensation should be checked in all patients with sixth nerve palsy.
- **Nasopharyngeal tumours** may invade the skull and its foramina and damage the nerve during its basilar course.
- **Raised intracranial pressure** may cause a downward displacement of the brainstem. This may stretch one or both sixth nerves over the petrous tip, when paresis is a false localizing sign.
- **Basal skull fracture** may cause unilateral or bilateral palsy.
- **Gradenigo syndrome**, most frequently caused by mastoiditis or acute petrositis, may result in damage of the sixth nerve at the petrous tip. The latter is frequently accompanied by facial weakness and pain and hearing difficulties.

TIP Hearing and corneal sensation should be tested in patients with a sixth nerve palsy, to exclude a vestibular schwannoma ('acoustic neuroma').

Intracavernous and intraorbital

- **The intracavernous** section runs below the third and fourth and the first division of the fifth nerves. The sixth nerve is the most medially situated and runs through the middle of the sinus in close relation to the internal carotid artery. Occasionally, intracavernous sixth nerve palsy is accompanied by a postganglionic Horner syndrome (Parkinson syndrome) due

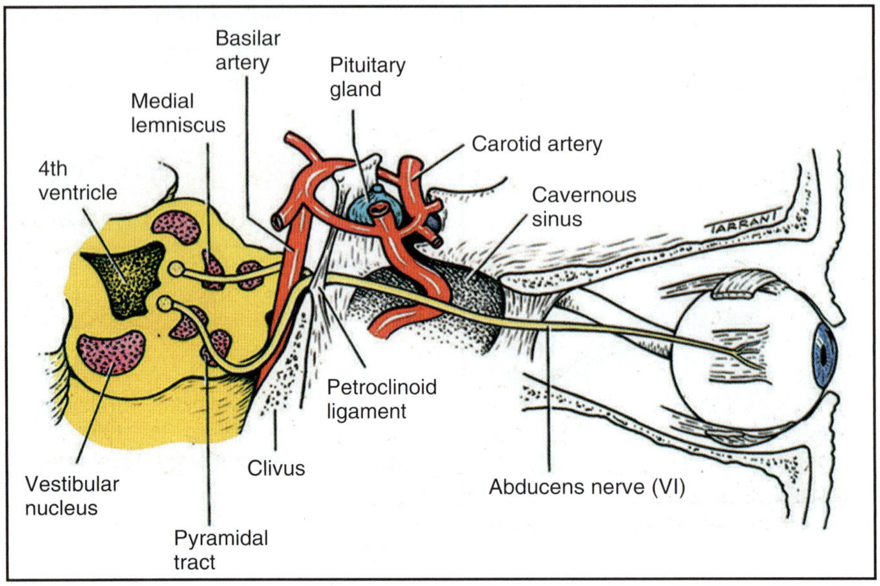

Fig. 19.74 Lateral view of the course of the sixth nerve.

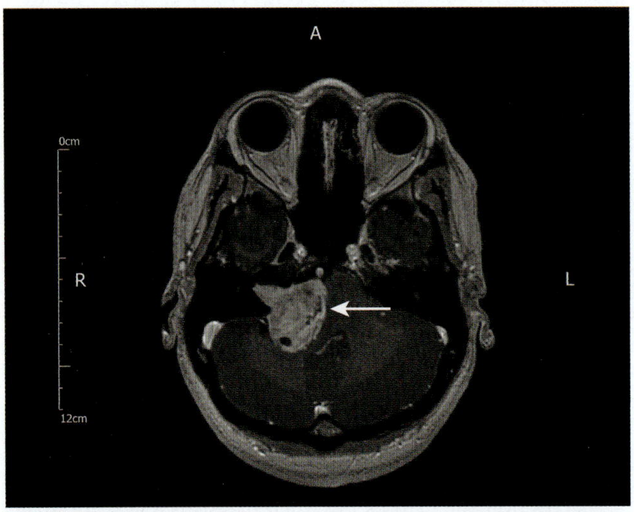

Fig. 19.75 Axial gadolinium-enhanced T1-weighted MR image through the posterior fossa showing the typical 'ice-cream cone' configuration of a large right-sided vestibular schwannoma (arrow).

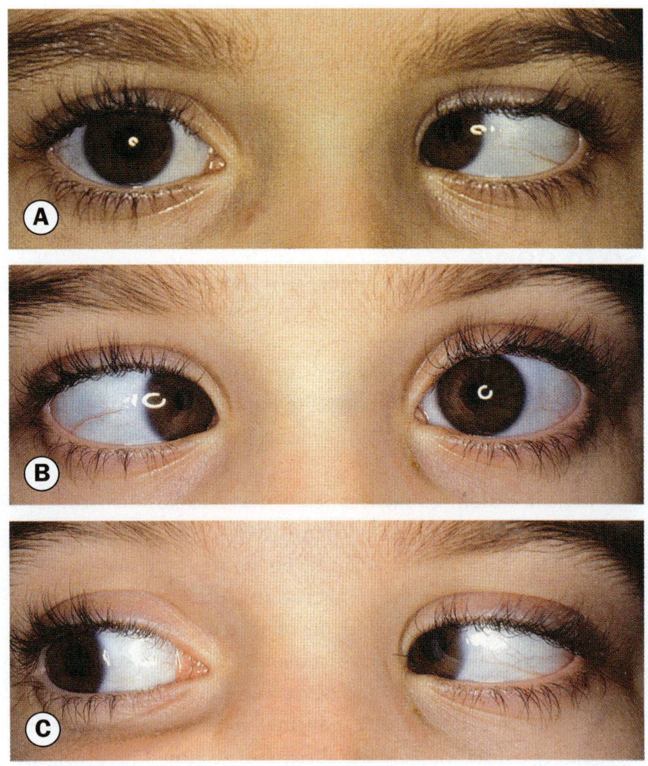

Fig. 19.76 Acute left sixth nerve palsy in a child. **(A)** Left esotropia in the primary position; **(B)** marked limitation of left abduction; **(C)** normal left adduction. *(Courtesy of ADN Murray.)*

to damage to the paracarotid sympathetic plexus. The causes of intracavernous sixth nerve and third nerve lesions (see above) are similar.

- **The intraorbital** part enters the orbit through the superior orbital fissure within the annulus of Zinn to innervate the lateral rectus.

Diagnosis

- **Symptoms.** Double vision is characteristically worse for a distant target and less or absent for near fixation. A careful review of systems should be conducted, including enquiry about other neurological symptoms, GCA, trauma and symptoms of ear disease.
- **Esotropia** in the primary position due to relatively unopposed action of the medial rectus (Figs 19.76A and 19.77A). The deviation (and symptomatic description) is characteristically worse for distance than near fixation.
- **Limitation of abduction** on the side of the lesion (Figs 19.76B and 19.77B).
- **Normal adduction** of the affected eye (Fig. 19.76C).

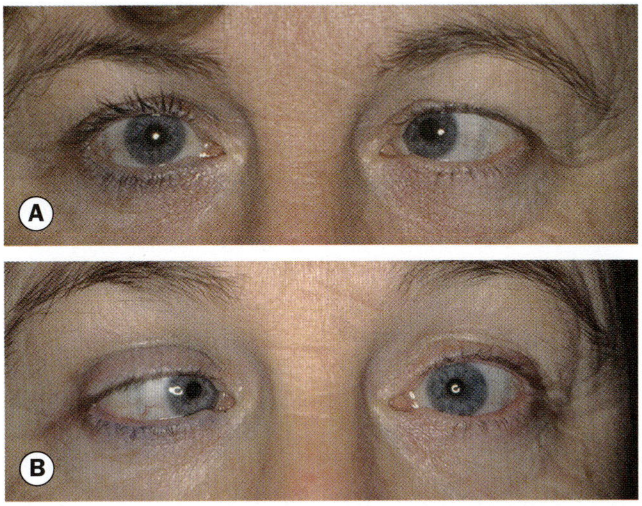

Fig. 19.77 Left sixth nerve palsy in an adult. **(A)** Left esotropia in the primary position; **(B)** limitation of left abduction.

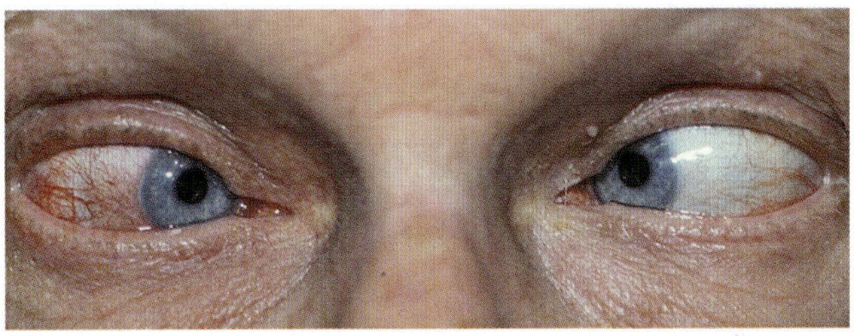

Fig. 19.78 Acute bilateral sixth nerve palsy. *(Courtesy of C Barry.)*

- **Bilateral acute sixth nerve palsy** (Fig. 19.78) is considerably less common than unilateral. The causes are similar, but it is important to exclude elevated intracranial pressure.
- **A compensatory face turn** is towards the side of the paralysed muscle in unilateral palsy.
- **Neurological examination.** The other cranial nerves and the peripheral nervous system should be examined, if necessary, by an appropriate specialist. In a child or any patient with relevant symptoms, an otorhinolaryngological review may be sought.

Investigation

Idiopathic and presumed microvascular lesions are common (up to 60%) in older patients, but a wide range of causes has been reported and a low threshold should be adopted for neuroimaging and other investigations even with isolated paresis. Also, as with third nerve palsy, improved imaging has led to increasingly common identification of a cause in lesions that might previously have been categorized as idiopathic. In contrast to fourth nerve palsy, a decompensated congenital aetiology is thought to be rare. The presence of bilateral paresis, additional relevant clinical findings or presentation in children and younger adults should prompt thorough investigation.

TIP Children or young adults presenting with bilateral sixth nerve palsy should undergo urgent neuroradiological investigation to find the cause.

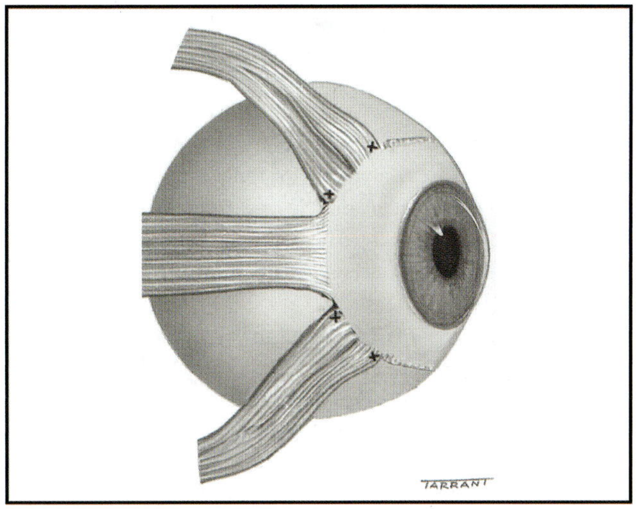

Fig. 19.79 Transposition of the superior and inferior rectus muscles in lateral rectus palsy.

Treatment

- **Observation** with monocular occlusion or prismatic (e.g. temporary Fresnel stick-on) correction of diplopia is appropriate in idiopathic and presumed microvascular lesions. Up to 90% will recover spontaneously, usually over weeks to several months. Young children should be treated with alternate patching to prevent amblyopia.
- **Botulinum toxin** injection into the ipsilateral medial rectus may be used to prevent contracture, assess residual function and sometimes to facilitate prismatic correction with a large deviation (see Fig. 18.76), but is rarely curative.
- **Surgery** should be considered only when adequate time has been allowed for maximal spontaneous improvement, typically at least 6–12 months from onset.
  - Partial palsy (paresis) is treated by adjustable medial rectus recession and lateral rectus resection in the affected eye, aiming for a small exophoria in the primary position to maximize the field of binocular single vision.
  - Complete palsy is treated by transposition of the superior and inferior recti to positions above and below the affected lateral rectus muscle (Fig. 19.79) coupled with weakening of the ipsilateral medial rectus (sometimes with injection of botulinum toxin – 'toxin transposition') (see Fig. 18.76). Three rectus muscles should not be detached from the globe at the same procedure because of the risk of anterior segment ischaemia.
- **Permanent prism.** Troublesome but mild residual deviation may be treated with a prism incorporated into spectacles as an alternative to surgery.

Seventh nerve

The seventh (facial) cranial nerve innervates the facial muscles, stimulates secretomotor activity in the lacrimal gland, submandibular and sublingual salivary glands, is involved in the sensation of taste from the anterior two-thirds of the tongue and controls the amplitude of sound from the inner ear.

Key features

- **Facial muscles.** The facial nerve provides motor innervation of muscles that are responsible for facial expression.
- **Innervation.** The facial muscles are innervated centrally by the cerebral cortex and peripherally by the ipsilateral seventh nerve. Central innervation is bilateral for the upper face and unilateral for the lower face.
- **Palsy.** Supranuclear lesions result in palsy of the lower face on the opposite side and peripheral lesions result in palsy of the upper and lower face on the same side.
- **Dry eye syndrome.** Loss of parasympathetic fibres causes reduced tear production and loss of taste from the anterior part of the tongue.
- **Hearing.** Loss of stapedius function causes hyperacusis.

Anatomy (Fig. 19.80)

- The facial nerve arises from the pons and consists of a large motor root and a smaller sensory root.
- The two roots cross the posterior cranial fossa and pass out of the cranial cavity through the internal acoustic meatus, next to the vestibulocochlear (VIII) nerve.
- After entering the facial canal in the petrous temporal bone, the two roots fuse and form the facial nerve, which soon enlarges as the geniculate ganglion.
- At the geniculate ganglion the facial nerve gives off the greater petrosal nerve, which carries preganglionic parasympathetic fibres to the lacrimal gland and mucous glands of the nasal cavity.
- The facial nerve continues along the bony canal giving off the nerve to the stapedius muscle (sound regulation) and chorda tympani (taste and parasympathetic fibres destined for the submandibular ganglion), before leaving the cranium through the stylomastoid foramen.
- The nerve then divides into the terminal branches at the posterior edge of the parotid gland, which then innervate the facial muscles.
- The **corneal reflex**, which is tested by stimulating the cornea with a thin strand of cotton-wool, results in the reflex closure of both eyelids. The afferent limb of this reflex is transmitted by the trigeminal nerve and the efferent limb by the facial nerve.

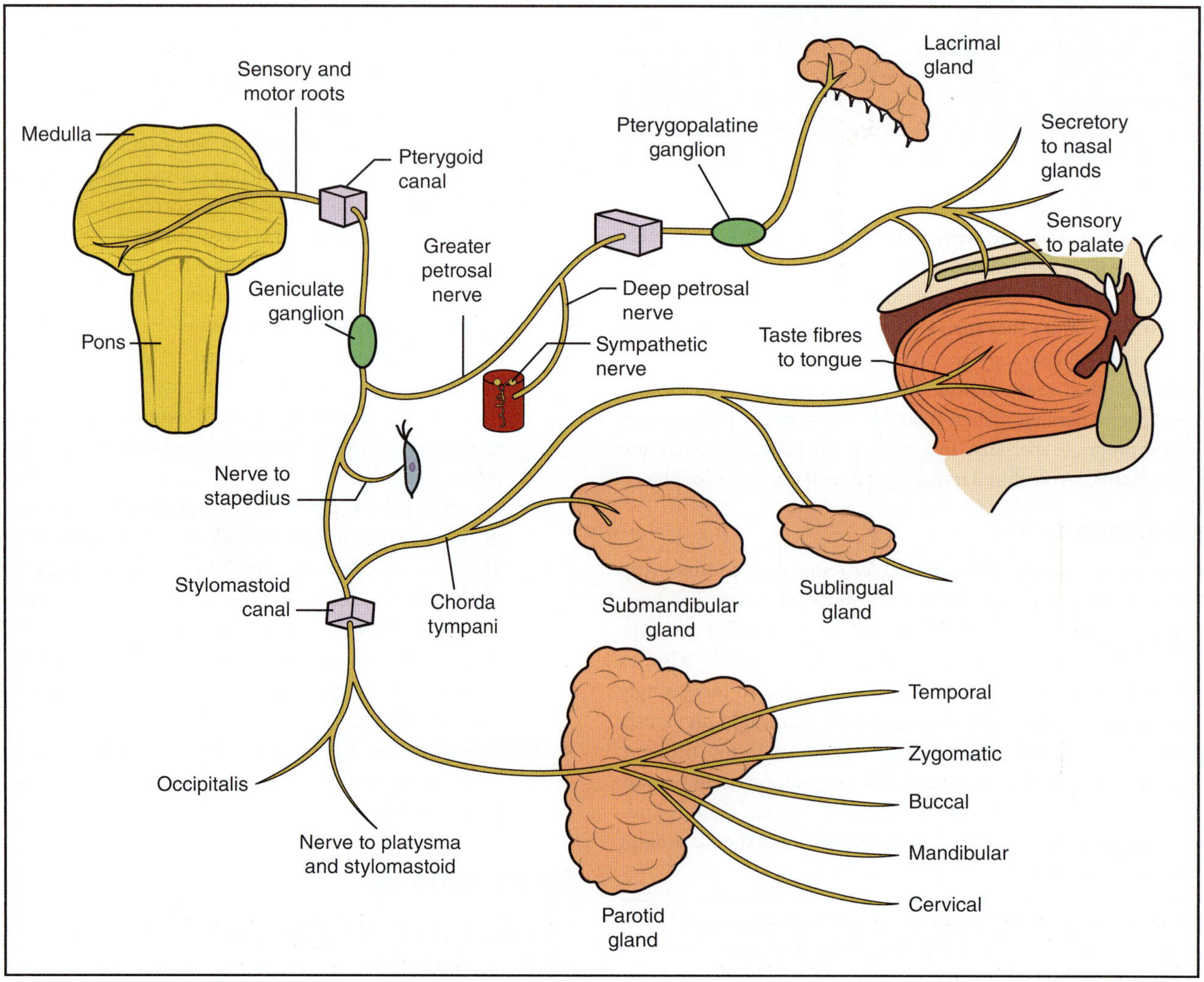

Fig. 19.80 Anatomy of the seventh nerve.

Physical signs

- **A supranuclear lesion** results in paralysis of the contralateral middle and lower parts of the face (Fig. 19.81A).
- **A nuclear lesion** results in complete paralysis of the facial muscles on the ipsilateral side.
- **Based on the anatomy**, the precise location of the lesion is possible:
  - Pons: ipsilateral facial paralysis, sixth nerve palsy, contralateral hemiplegia, paralysis of conjugate gaze to the side of the lesion (PPRF).
  - Cerebro-pontine angle: ipsilateral facial palsy, decreased secretion of tears and saliva, hyperacusis and loss of taste to the anterior 2/3 of the tongue.
  - Eighth (vestibulocochlear) nerve: additional findings include deafness and tinnitus.
  - Parotid gland: ipsilateral facial palsy manifesting with a feeling of numbness, associated with an expressionless face.
  - Ramsay Hunt syndrome results from reactivation of herpes zoster in the geniculate ganglion and manifests with: ipsilateral facial palsy, ear pain and vesicles on the face and in the ear.

Causes

- **Bell palsy** is an idiopathic form of facial nerve palsy and is responsible for 60–70% of cases (Fig. 19.81B). The symptoms develop rapidly over several hours. The patient often recovers within days to several weeks. The extent of nerve damage determines the outcome. Residual symptoms may include facial muscle weakness (Fig. 19.81C), a watery eye and synkinesis ('crocodile' tears).
- **Trauma** (10%) (see Fig. 19.81A). Check for periorbital or mastoid bruising and blood in the ear canal; can be iatrogenic.
- **Viral infection** (5%): herpes simplex (most common), cytomegalovirus, Epstein–Barr, mumps, rubella.
- **Lyme disease** (often bilateral).
- **Neoplastic** (2%): parotid malignancy, vestibular schwannoma.
- **Diabetes.**
- **Sarcoidosis** (often bilateral).

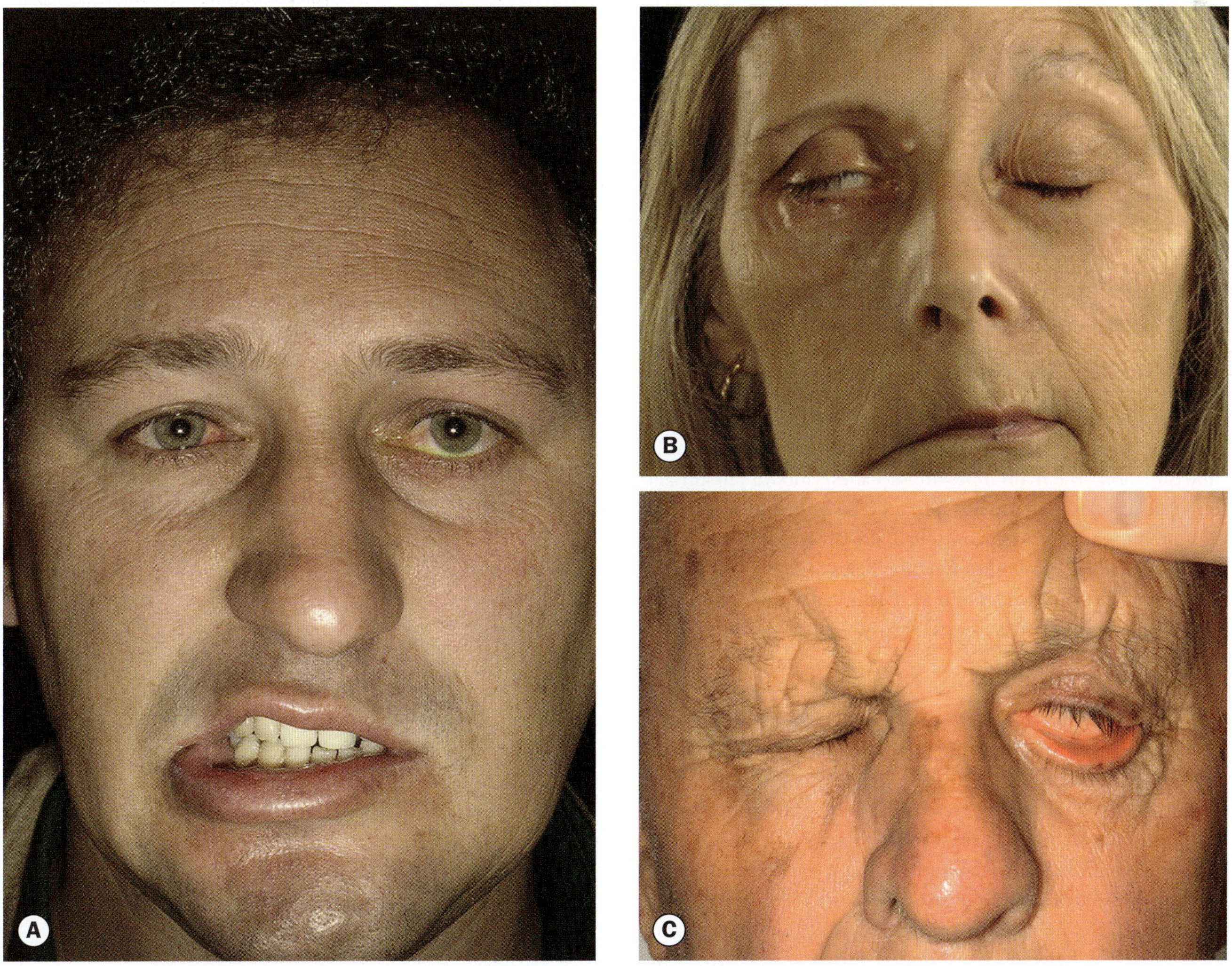

Fig. 19.81 Seventh nerve palsy. **(A)** Left upper motor neurone palsy secondary to cerebral trauma; **(B)** right lower motor neurone palsy (Bell palsy); **(C)** chronic left seventh nerve palsy showing severe paralytic ectropion and poor frontalis function. *(Courtesy of ADN Murray – fig. A; J Norris – figs B and C.)*

- **'Stroke mimics'**, e.g. hemiparesis and facial drooping caused by hypoglycaemia in elderly individuals, migraine, or sepsis are transient causes of focal neurological signs.

Management

- **Corneal protection**, especially if the fifth nerve is also affected.
- **Corticosteroids.** In Bell palsy systemic corticosteroids are helpful if started within 48–72 hours of onset: use prednisolone 60–80 mg daily for one week, then taper over one week.
- **Antiviral treatment** (acyclovir or valaciclovir) added to systemic corticosteroids in idiopathic facial nerve palsy is beneficial. Although the rate of recovery is not affected, the number of people left with long-term effects (excessive tearing or an abnormal facial movement) is reduced.
- **MRI scan of the brain** should be undertaken if the palsy is slow in onset or if there are any other neurological findings.
- **If bilateral**, undertake a chest X-ray and serum angiotensin-converting enzyme (SACE) test to exclude sarcoidosis.
- **Surgery.** Surgical decompression of the facial nerve in Bell palsy is not beneficial. In patients with long-term paralysis reconstructive surgery can offer some improvement but cannot fully restore natural movement or facial expressions.

TIP If the onset of a facial nerve palsy is slow or if there are other neurological signs, investigate with an MRI scan to exclude intra-cranial pathology.

SUPRANUCLEAR DISORDERS OF OCULAR MOTILITY

Conjugate eye movements

Conjugate eye movements (versions) are binocular movements in which the eyes move synchronously and symmetrically in the same direction. The main types are saccades, smooth pursuit and non-optical reflex movements. Saccadic and pursuit movements are supranuclear in origin, controlled at both cerebral and brainstem levels. Non-optical reflex function helps to stabilize the visual field with respect to head position. Disturbance of supranuclear eye movement function causes gaze palsy.

Saccades

- **Function.** Rapid voluntary or reflex alignment of the fovea with a target image, including transferral of fixation from one target to another.
- **Pathway.** There are separate horizontal and vertical pathways. Many cortical areas and the superior colliculi are involved in saccade generation, but classically initiation occurs in the premotor cortex frontal eye fields, from where impulses for horizontal movement pass to the contralateral paramedian pontine reticular formation (PPRF) – the horizontal gaze centre (Fig. 19.82). Each frontal lobe initiates contralateral saccades. Vertical pathways are less well mapped (see below).
- **Saccadic palsy.** This usually happens after damage or hyperactivity in the frontal eye field and results in a saccadic palsy to the contralateral side. If bilateral, there is a spasm of fixation and a need to use head trust to refixate. Hyperactivity (frontal adversive seizures) causes a deviation of the eyes to the contralateral side.

Smooth pursuit

- **Function.** To maintain fixation on a target with slow smooth movements once it has been located by the saccadic system. The stimulus is image movement near the fovea.
- **Pathway.** This is complex, involving several cortex regions as well as the PPRF, the superior colliculi, cerebellum and other structures. The pathways are ipsilateral, the cortex on one side controlling pursuit to the same side.
- **Pursuit palsy.** This usually happens following damage or hyperactivity in the parieto-occipital lobe. The damaging lesion causes a unilateral pursuit palsy to the ipsilateral direction. Hyperactivity causes a deviation of the eyes to the ipsilateral side usually associated with visual hallucinations.

Non-optical reflexes

- **Function.** The maintenance of eye position without conscious input following a change of head or body position. Other, visually directed (i.e. optical) mechanisms are also concerned with visual field stability. Both may be active in the doll's eye (oculocephalic) reflex, where the head of an unconscious patient is rotated causing the eyes to move in the opposite direction to preserve the image position on the retina
- **Pathway.** Movements are mediated mainly via the vestibular system. Signals originate in the inner ear labyrinths and in proprioceptors that provide information concerning head and neck movements. For horizontal movements, afferent fibres synapse in the vestibular nuclei and pass to the horizontal gaze centre.

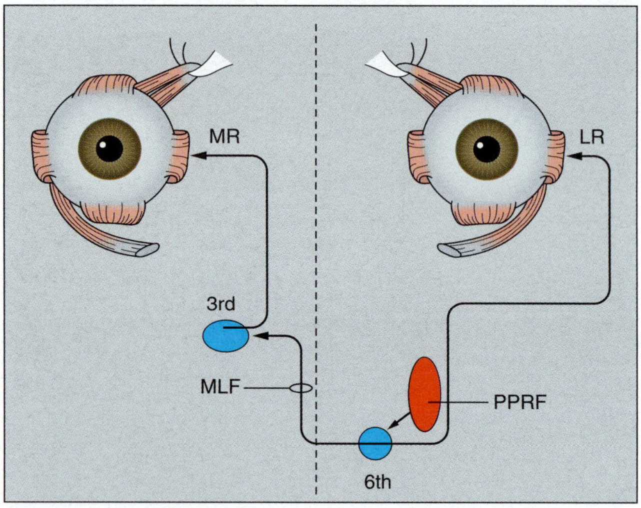

Fig 19.82 Anatomical pathways for horizontal eye movements. LR = lateral rectus; MLF = medial longitudinal fasciculus; MR = medial rectus; PPRF = paramedian pontine reticular formation.

Abnormalities of horizontal gaze

Anatomy

After initiation horizontal eye movements are generated in the horizontal gaze centre (PPRF – see Fig. 19.82) and mediated via a common pathway. From here, impulses travel directly to the ipsilateral sixth nerve nucleus and indirectly via internuclear neurones that cross the midline at the level of the pons and pass up the contralateral medial longitudinal fasciculus (MLF), to motor neurones in the medial rectus subnucleus of the contralateral third nerve complex. Stimulation of the horizontal gaze centre on one side therefore causes a conjugate movement of the eyes to the same side.

Horizontal gaze palsy

A lesion of the horizontal gaze centre in the PPRF gives ipsilateral horizontal gaze palsy, with an inability to look in the direction of the lesion.

Internuclear ophthalmoplegia

A lesion in the MLF is responsible for the clinical syndrome of internuclear ophthalmoplegia (INO). Causes include demyelination, stroke and tumours. Strabismus surgery can be performed for persistent diplopia.

- **Unilateral INO** (Fig. 19.83). Double vision is not typically a complaint.
  - Straight eyes in the primary position.
  - Defective adduction of the eye on the side of the lesion and nystagmus of the contralateral eye on abduction; note that the side of the lesion is named for the side of the adduction deficit.
  - Gaze to the side of the lesion is normal.
  - Convergence is intact if the lesion is anterior and discrete but impaired if the lesion is posterior or extensive.
- **Bilateral INO** (Fig. 19.84)
  - Limitation of left adduction and ataxic nystagmus of the right eye on right gaze.
  - Limitation of right adduction and ataxic nystagmus of the left eye on left gaze.
  - Convergence may be intact or impaired.
  - A rostral midbrain lesion may give an associated convergence deficit with resultant bilateral exotropia and abducting nystagmus: 'wall-eyed bilateral INO' – WEBINO.
- **One-and-a-half syndrome.** PPRF and MLF lesions combined on the same side give rise to the 'one-and-a-half syndrome' characterized by a combination of ipsilateral gaze palsy and INO. The only residual movement is abduction of the contralateral eye, which exhibits abduction nystagmus.

Vertical gaze palsy

Anatomy

Vertical eye movement initiation in the frontal lobes is simultaneously bilateral, with impulses mediated via the vertical gaze centre in the midbrain (rostral interstitial nucleus of the MLF). From the

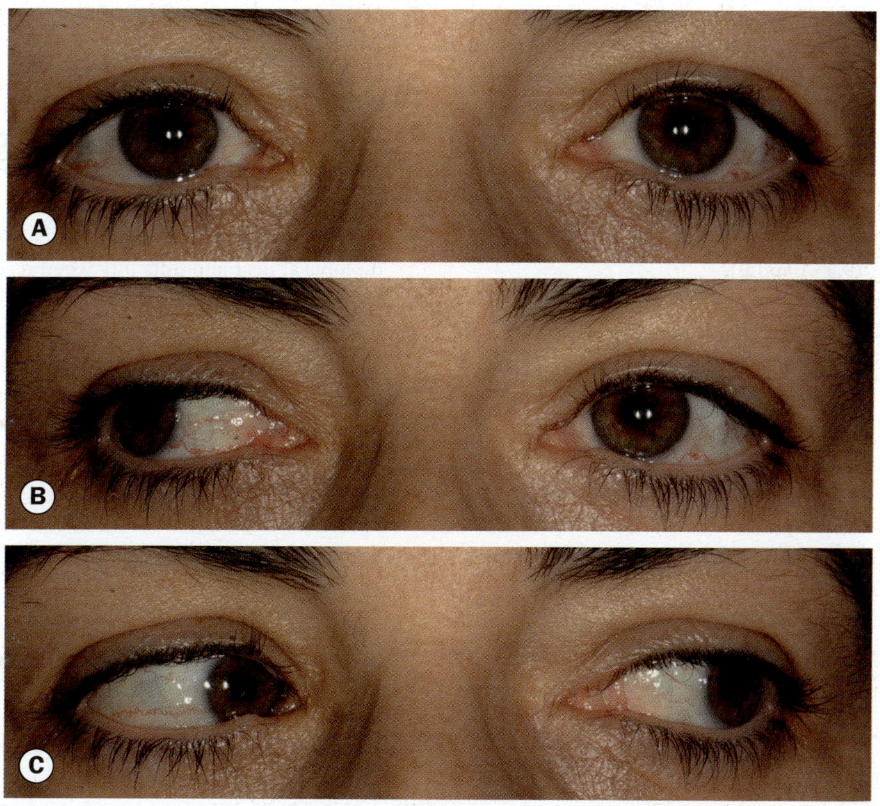

Fig. 19.83 Left internuclear ophthalmoplegia. **(A)** Straight in the primary position; **(B)** limitation of left adduction on right gaze; **(C)** normal left abduction on left gaze.

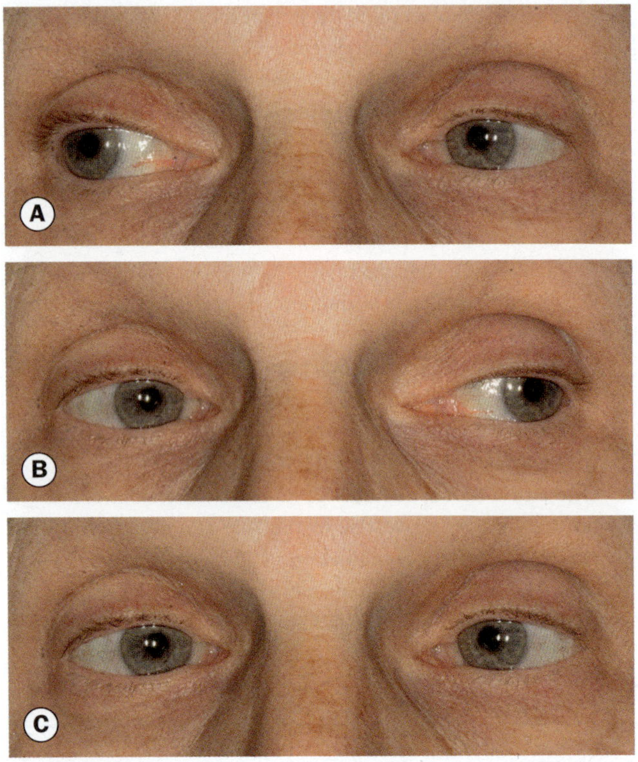

Fig. 19.84 Bilateral internuclear ophthalmoplegia. **(A)** Limitation of left adduction on right gaze; **(B)** less severe limitation of right adduction on left gaze; **(C)** convergence is intact.

vertical gaze centre, impulses pass to the subnuclei of the eye muscles controlling vertical gaze in both eyes. Cells subserving upward and downward eye movements are intermingled in the vertical gaze centre, although selective paralysis of upgaze and downgaze may occur in spite of this.

Parinaud (dorsal midbrain) syndrome

- **Signs**
  - Straight eyes in the primary position.
  - Supranuclear upgaze and downgaze palsy on saccadic movement (Fig. 19.85A and B).
  - Defective convergence.
  - Normal downgaze using doll's head manoeuvre (Fig. 19.85C).
  - Large pupils with light–near dissociation (see Fig. 19.45).
  - Lid retraction (Collier sign) (Fig. 19.85D).
  - Convergence–retraction nystagmus (Fig. 19.85E and F).
- **Causes**
  - Children: aqueduct stenosis, meningitis and pinealoma/pinealoblastoma (Fig. 19.86).
  - Young adults: demyelination, trauma and arteriovenous malformations.
  - The elderly: midbrain vascular accidents, mass lesions involving the periaqueductal grey matter and posterior fossa aneurysms.

Progressive supranuclear palsy

Progressive supranuclear palsy (Steele–Richardson–Olszewski syndrome) is a severe degenerative disease presenting in old age. Clinical features include:

- Supranuclear gaze palsy, initially primarily of downgaze and subsequently upgaze.
- Horizontal movements subsequently become impaired, with eventual global gaze palsy.
- Paralysis of convergence.
- Pseudobulbar palsy.
- Extrapyramidal rigidity, gait ataxia and dementia.

Parkinson disease

This is a chronic, progressive, neurodegenerative disorder of the CNS secondary to pathology in the basal ganglia and dopaminergic pathways. The cause is not known, but inherited and environmental factors (especially previous head injury and exposure to pesticides) play a role. There is no cure, but the symptoms can be controlled with levodopa (L-DOPA), MAO-B inhibitors or dopamine agonists. Clinical examination requires sensitivity to both the physical disability and mental state of the individual.

Clinical symptoms and signs

- **Early signs** include: tremor (usually of asymmetrical onset), rigidity, slowness of movement (bradykinesia) and altered sense of smell.
- **Postural instability**, sleep disturbance (REM sleep behaviour disorder) and neuropsychiatric problems may occur in time.
- **Dementia** is a late manifestation in up to 80% of affected individuals and is influenced by age and duration of disease.
- **MRI** shows absence of the swallow tail pattern in the substantia nigra (Fig. 19.87).

Ocular features

- **Visual abnormalities** like impaired colour vision and reduced contrast sensitivity are amongst the most frequent non-motor symptoms in the early stages.
- **Convergence insufficiency**, leading to binocular horizontal diplopia at near and difficulty when reading.
- **Jerkiness** and limitation of vertical eye movements.
- **Eye movement abnormalities.** Saccadic and smooth pursuit abnormality, including slow reaction time of horizontal gaze and hypometria ('under-reaching of task').
- **Decreased blink frequency**, associated with the characteristic 'stare' and resulting in ocular surface dryness (see Fig. 2.67D).
- **Apraxia of eyelid closure** and blepharospasm. Visual and auditory hallucinations of a complex nature may occur in the late stages in up to 40% of patients.

Skew deviation

- **Clinical signs.** Skew deviation is an uncommon acquired ocular misalignment, in which the eyes are deviated vertically and often exhibit cyclotorsional disturbance. Three categories have been described, corresponding to differing motility patterns and lesion sites. Both eyes can be deviated upwards, or one can be hypertropic and one hypotropic.

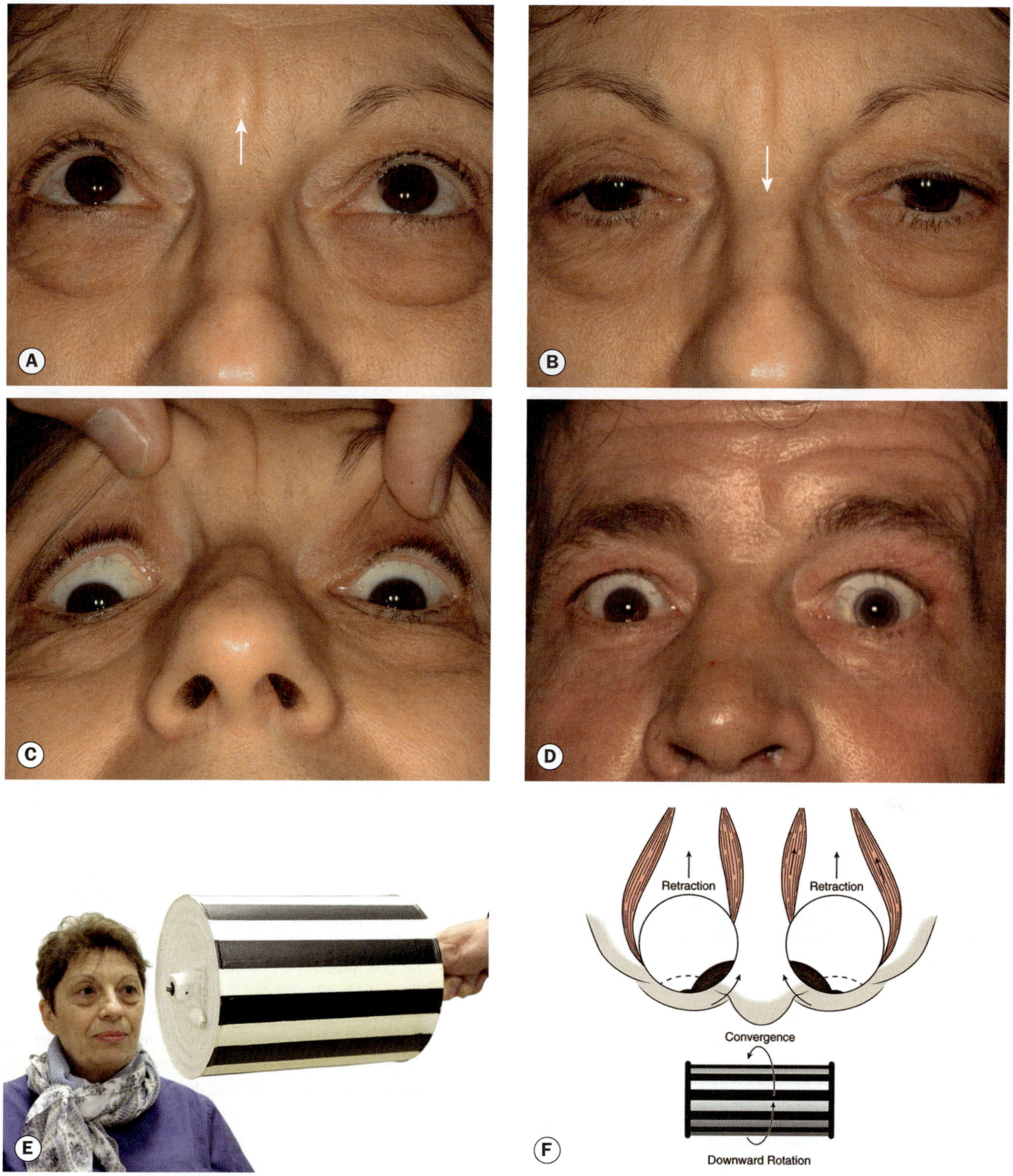

Fig. 19.85 Parinaud syndrome. **(A)** Defective upgaze; **(B)** defective downgaze on saccadic movement; **(C)** normal downward movement using doll's head manoeuvre; **(D)** Collier sign; **(E)** use of the OKN drum; **(F)** diagram showing the mechanism of convergence–retraction nystagmus – convergence occurs because the medial rectus muscle is stronger than the lateral rectus muscle.

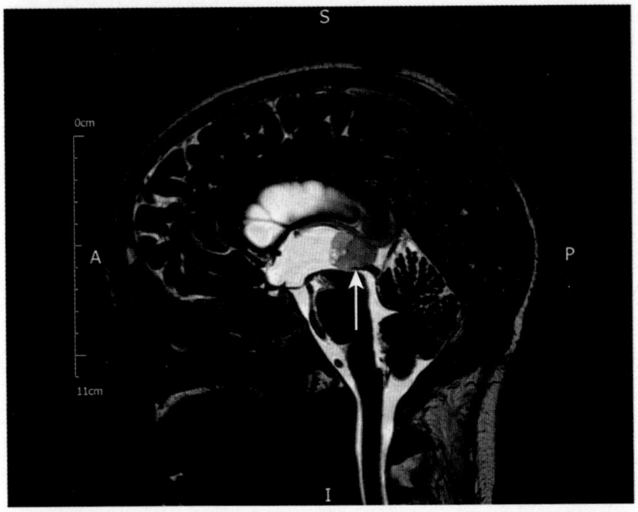

Fig. 19.86 High-resolution midline sagittal T2-weighted MR image in a patient with a pinealoblastoma (arrow) obstructing the aqueduct of Sylvius causing a dilated third ventricle.

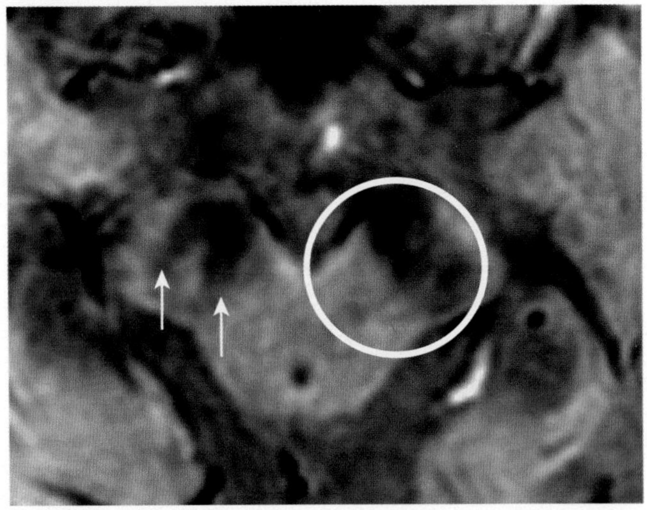

Fig. 19.87 Axial MRI image of early Parkinson disease showing unilateral loss of the swallow tail sign in the substantia nigra (circled). The arrows show the normal substantia nigra on the opposite side.

- **Cause.** The most frequent cause is an abnormality of the prenuclear vestibular input secondary to a brainstem or cerebellar stroke, which results in dysfunction of a primordial field stabilization mechanism.
- **Differential diagnosis.** Fourth nerve palsy and myasthenia gravis can occasionally present in a similar fashion.
- **The upright-supine test** is helpful to confirm the diagnosis of skew deviation: the patient fixates on an object 1/3 meter away and the alignment is measured with the patient in an upright position and then in a supine position. A positive test is defined as a more than 50% decrease in vertical alignment in the supine position, when compared to the upright position.
- **The prognosis** depends on the cause.
- **Treatment.** Prismatic correction in spectacles, botulinum injections and, in persistent cases, vertical muscle surgery can be considered.

NYSTAGMUS

Introduction

Physiological principles

Nystagmus is an involuntary oscillation of the eyes that can be a physiological (e.g. following the rotation of an optokinetic drum) or pathological phenomenon. In pathological nystagmus, each cycle of movement is usually initiated by an involuntary, defoveating drift of the eye away from the target, followed by a refixating saccadic movement.

- **Plane** may be horizontal, vertical, or torsional.
- **Amplitude** refers to the extent of excursion: fine or coarse.
- **Frequency** describes how rapidly the eyes oscillate: high, moderate or low.

Classification

A schematic such as that shown in Fig. 19.88 can be used for documentation.

- **Jerk** nystagmus is saccadic with a slow defoveating 'drift' movement and a fast corrective refoveating saccadic movement. The direction of nystagmus is described in terms of the direction of the fast component: right, left, up, down or rotatory.
- **Pendular** nystagmus is non-saccadic in that both foveating and defoveating movements are slow (i.e. the velocity of nystagmus is equal in both directions).
- **Mixed** nystagmus consists of pendular nystagmus in the primary position and jerk nystagmus on lateral gaze.

Physiological nystagmus

- **End-point** nystagmus is a fine jerk nystagmus of moderate frequency seen in extremes of gaze. The fast phase is in the direction of gaze (Fig. 19.89).
- **Optokinetic nystagmus (OKN)** is a jerk nystagmus induced by moving repetitive targets (e.g. OKN drum) across the visual field.
  - The slow phase is a pursuit movement in which the eyes follow the target. The fast phase is a saccadic movement in the opposite direction as the eyes fixate on the next target.
  - If the OKN tape or drum is moved from right to left, the left parieto-occipito-temporal region controls the slow (pursuit) phase to the left and the left frontal lobe controls the rapid (saccadic) phase to the right.
  - OKN nystagmus is useful for detecting functional (nonphysiological) blindness and for testing VA in the very young. It can be helpful in the assessment of an isolated homonymous hemianopia.

Vestibular nystagmus

- **Physiological** vestibular nystagmus is a jerk nystagmus caused by altered input from the vestibular nuclei to the horizontal gaze centres. The slow phase is initiated by the vestibular nuclei

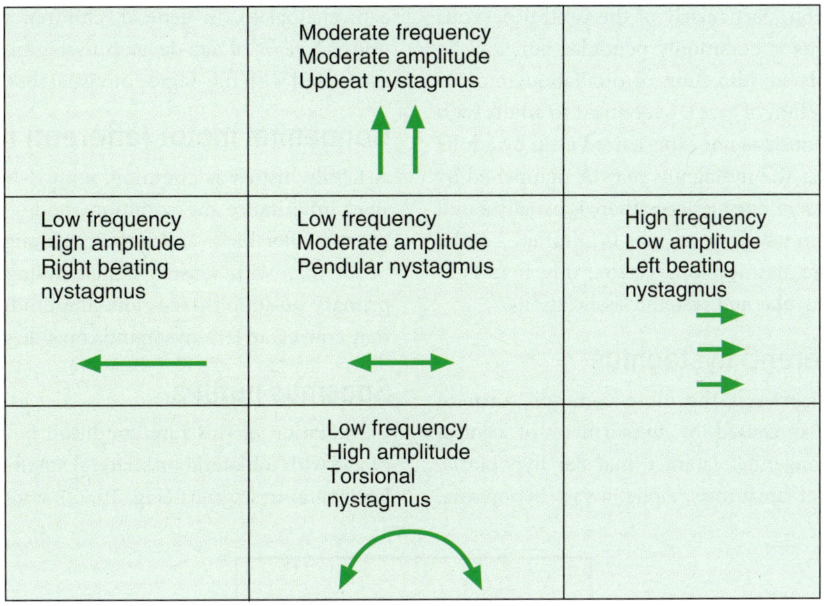

Fig. 19.88 Schematic for documenting nystagmus. *(Courtesy of JJ Kanski,* Signs in Ophthalmology: Causes and Differential Diagnosis, *Mosby 2010.)*

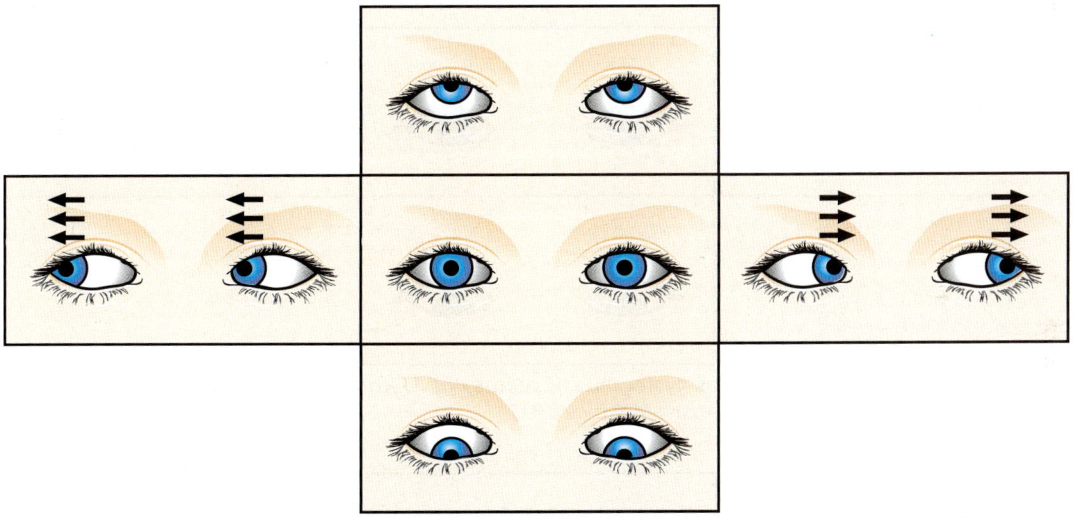

Fig. 19.89 Physiological nystagmus – end-point. *(Courtesy of JJ Kanski,* Signs in Ophthalmology: Causes and Differential Diagnosis, *Mosby 2010.)*

and the fast phase by the brainstem and frontomesencephalic pathway. Vestibular nystagmus may be elicited by caloric stimulation as follows:

- When cold water is poured into the right ear the patient will develop left jerk nystagmus (i.e. fast phase to the left).
- When warm water is poured into the right ear the patient will develop right jerk nystagmus (i.e. fast phase to the right). A useful mnemonic is 'COWS' (cold-opposite, warm-same) indicating the direction of the nystagmus.
- When cold water is poured into both ears simultaneously, a jerk nystagmus with the fast phase upwards develops. Warm water in both ears elicits nystagmus with the fast phase downwards (cold 'slows things down').
- An abnormal test indicates the presence of peripheral vestibular disease.

- **Pathological** peripheral vestibular nystagmus (Fig. 19.90) is caused by disease affecting the ear such as labyrinthitis, Ménière disease and middle or inner ear infections. It tends to be solely horizontal, vertical or torsional, increases in intensity with gaze in the direction of the fast phase and is dampened by fixation. It is typically of fine amplitude.

Infantile (congenital) nystagmus

Introduction

Early-onset (usually the first few months of life rather than truly congenital) nystagmus can occur secondary to poor vision or to a motor deficit with the nystagmus itself causing poor vision, though the distinction is not always clear. It can be associated with a serious systemic condition, particularly of the central nervous system. Infantile nystagmus is commonly pendular but may be jerk, horizontal and uniplanar (direction of oscillation remains constant regardless of direction of gaze). In contrast to adults with acquired nystagmus, oscillopsia is not experienced even by adults with congenital nystagmus. The nystagmus may be dampened by convergence and is not present during sleep. There is usually a null point – a position of gaze in which nystagmus is minimal – and a compensatory head posture may develop to favour this. Investigation should seek to detect ocular and systemic associations.

Sensory deficit (afferent) nystagmus

Sensory deprivation nystagmus is the more common form of infantile nystagmus and is caused by impairment of central vision in early life (e.g. congenital cataract, macular hypoplasia, albinism, Leber congenital amaurosis, optic nerve hypoplasia, achromatopsia). In general, children with bilateral poor vision under 2 years of age develop nystagmus, the severity of which is associated with the degree of visual loss.

Congenital motor (efferent) nystagmus

A family history is common, with X-linked (dominant or recessive) inheritance the common mode. Presentation is about 2–3 months after birth and persists throughout life. VA is generally better than with sensory deficit nystagmus, at 6/12–6/36. In the primary position there is low-amplitude pendular nystagmus that may convert to jerk nystagmus on side gaze (Fig. 19.91).

Spasmus nutans

Presentation of this rare condition is between 3 and 18 months of age with unilateral or bilateral small-amplitude high-frequency horizontal nystagmus (Fig. 19.92) associated with head nodding.

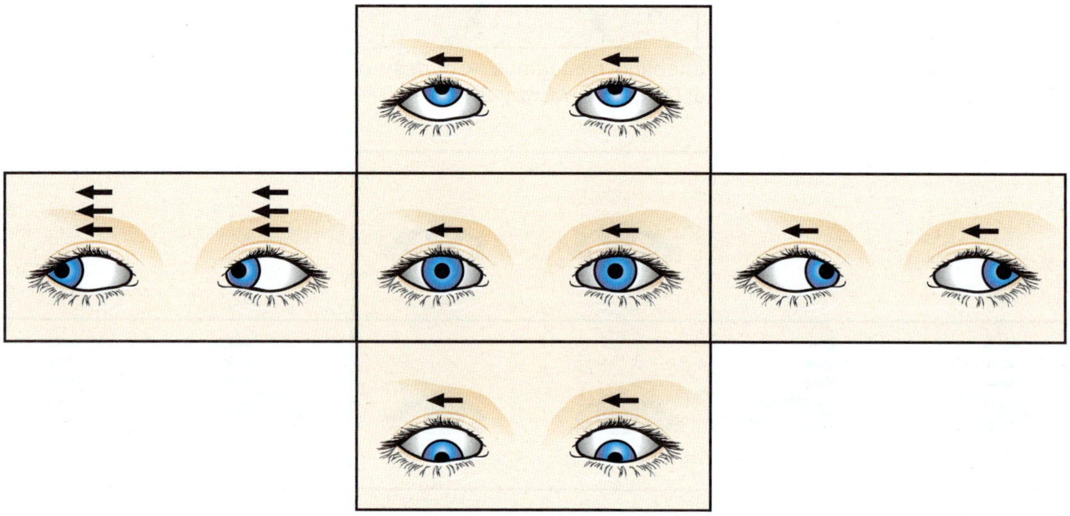

Fig. 19.90 Peripheral vestibular nystagmus. *(Courtesy of JJ Kanski,* Signs in Ophthalmology: Causes and Differential Diagnosis, *Mosby 2010.)*

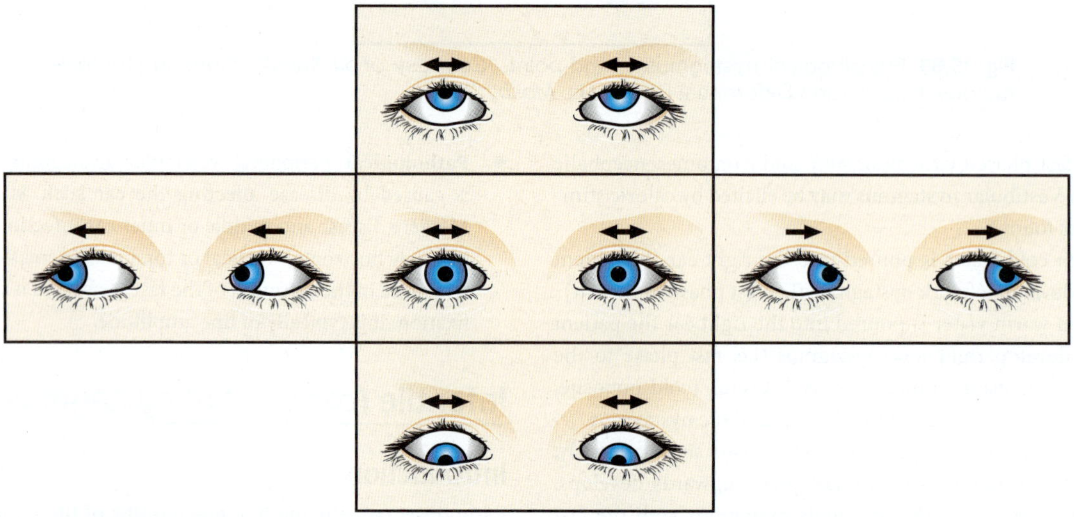

Fig. 19.91 Congenital motor (efferent) nystagmus, in this case pendular in the primary position and on vertical gaze, but converting to a gaze-evoked jerk nystagmus on left and right gaze. *(Courtesy of JJ Kanski,* Signs in Ophthalmology: Causes and Differential Diagnosis, *Mosby 2010.)*

It is frequently asymmetrical, with increased amplitude in abduction. Vertical and torsional components may be present. An idiopathic form spontaneously resolves by age 3 years, but glioma of the anterior visual pathway, empty sella syndrome and porencephalic cyst can also be causative.

Others

Other forms of nystagmus such as periodic alternating (see below) can be infantile in presentation.

Acquired nystagmus

Latent nystagmus

Latent nystagmus is associated with infantile esotropia and dissociated vertical deviation (see Ch. 18). With both eyes open there is no nystagmus, but horizontal nystagmus becomes apparent on covering one eye; the fast phase is in the direction of the uncovered fixating eye. Occasionally an element of latency may be superimposed on a manifest nystagmus so that when one eye is covered the amplitude of nystagmus increases (manifest-latent nystagmus).

Periodic alternating nystagmus

Periodic alternating nystagmus (PAN) is a conjugate horizontal jerk nystagmus that periodically reverses direction. During the active phase, the amplitude and frequency of nystagmus first progressively increase then decrease. This is followed by an interlude lasting 4–20 s during which time the eyes are steady and may show low-intensity, often pendular movements. A similar sequence in the opposite direction occurs thereafter, the whole cycle lasting between 1 and 3 minutes. PAN can be congenital or due to cerebellar disease, ataxia telangiectasia and drugs such as phenytoin.

Convergence–retraction nystagmus

Convergence–retraction nystagmus is a jerk nystagmus due to the co-contraction of extraocular muscles, often the medial recti. It can be induced by rotating an OKN drum downwards; the upward refixation saccade brings the two eyes towards each other in a convergence movement. There is classically associated retraction of the globe into the orbit. It is a component of Parinaud dorsal midbrain syndrome (see Fig. 19.85). Causes include lesions of the pretectal area such as pinealoma and vascular accidents.

Downbeat nystagmus

This is a vertical nystagmus with the fast phase beating downwards (Fig. 19.93), more easily elicited in lateral gaze and downgaze. It can be caused by lesions at the foramen magnum such as Arnold–Chiari malformation and syringobulbia, drugs such as lithium and phenytoin and a range of other conditions such as Wernicke encephalopathy, demyelination and hydrocephalus.

Upbeat nystagmus

Upbeat nystagmus is a vertical nystagmus with the fast phase beating upwards in all positions (Fig. 19.94); causes include posterior fossa lesions, drugs and Wernicke encephalopathy.

See-saw nystagmus

A pendular nystagmus, in which one eye elevates and intorts while the other depresses and extorts. It can be due to parasellar tumours (often with bitemporal hemianopia), syringobulbia and brainstem stroke.

Ataxic nystagmus

Ataxic nystagmus is a horizontal jerk nystagmus that occurs in the abducting eye of a patient with an INO (see above).

Bruns nystagmus

This consists of a coarse cerebellar horizontal jerk nystagmus in one eye and fine high-frequency vestibular nystagmus in the other and can be caused by cerebellopontine angle tumours such as vestibular schwannoma.

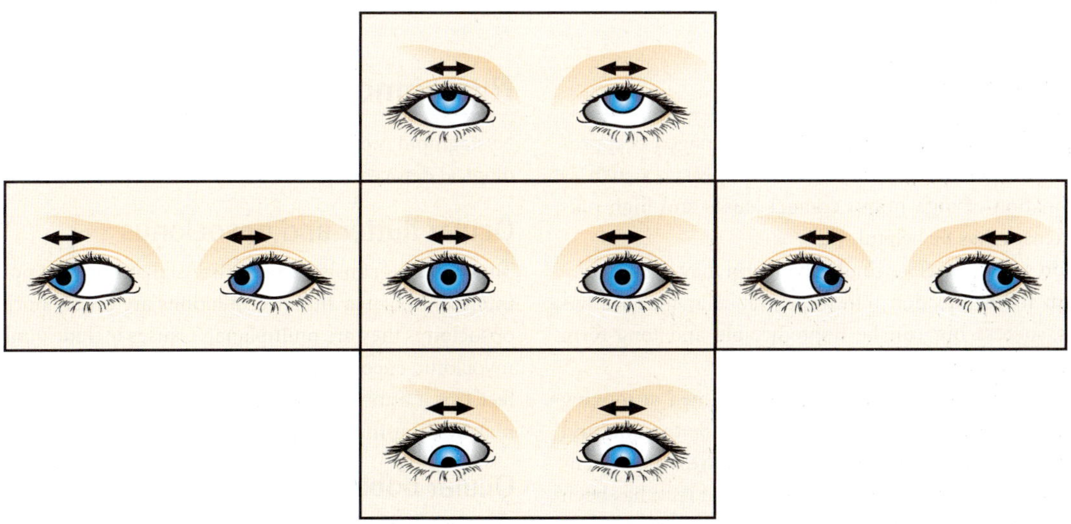

Fig. 19.92 Spasmus nutans – the nystagmus in this patient is pendular, uniplanar and of equal amplitude in all directions of gaze. *(Courtesy of JJ Kanski,* Signs in Ophthalmology: Causes and Differential Diagnosis, *Mosby 2010.)*

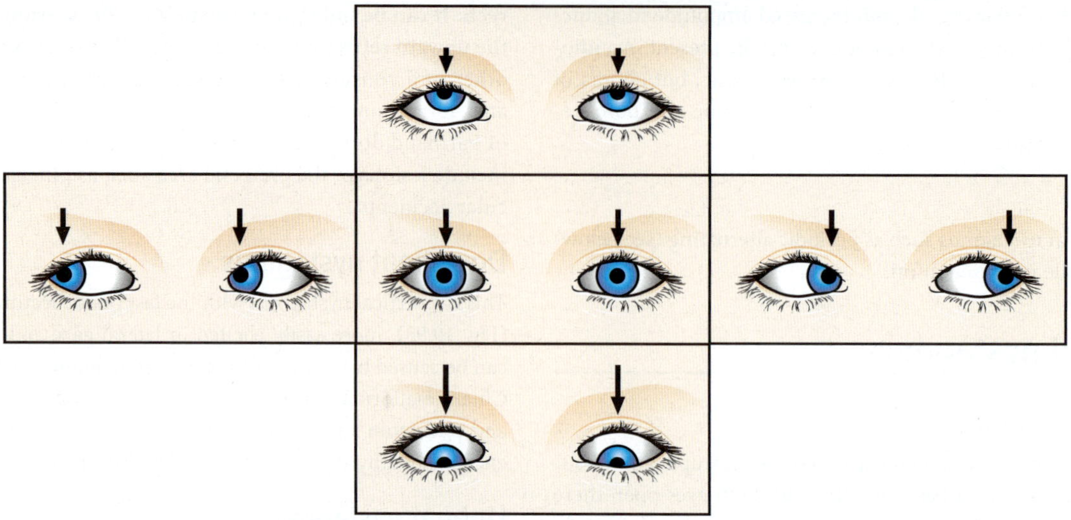

Fig. 19.93 Downbeat nystagmus (see text). *(Courtesy of JJ Kanski,* Signs in Ophthalmology: Causes and Differential Diagnosis, *Mosby 2010.)*

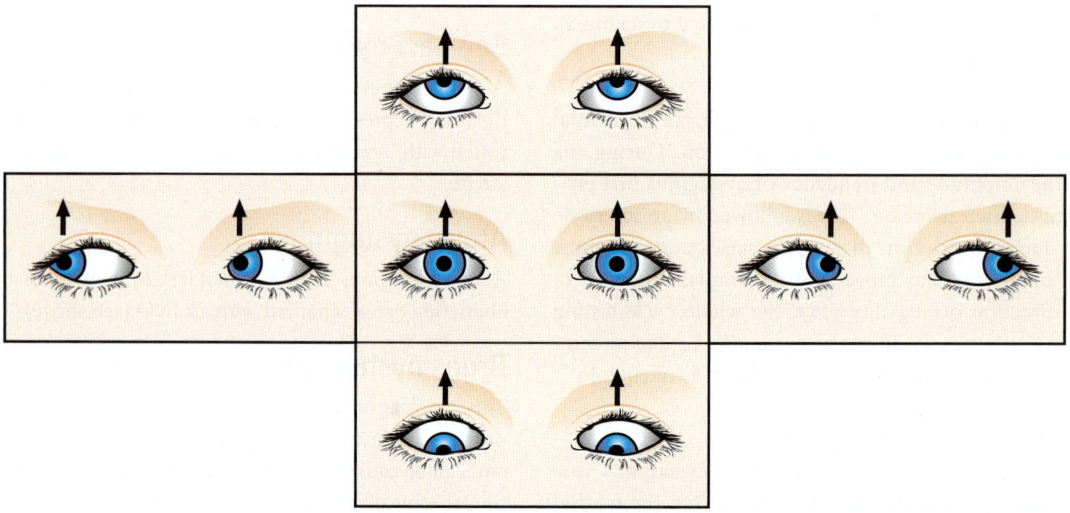

Fig. 19.94 Upbeat nystagmus. *(Courtesy of JJ Kanski,* Signs in Ophthalmology: Causes and Differential Diagnosis, *Mosby 2010.)*

Treatment of nystagmus

- **Amblyopia and refractive error** should be managed as appropriate. Contact lenses and other refractive measures such as the combination of high minus contact lenses and high plus spectacle lenses may be helpful.
- **Medication** such as baclofen and gabapentin may be helpful.
- **Botulinum toxin** injection into the extraocular muscles has had some success but can be unpredictable and long-term treatment is required.
- **Surgery** for nystagmus with a null point is aimed at moving muscles in order to mimic muscle tension while the eyes and face are straight and may be performed to address a compensatory head posture. Recession of all horizontal recti has been successful in reducing the amplitude of nystagmus in some patients without a significant null point.

Nystagmoid movements

Nystagmoid movements resemble nystagmus, but the initial pathological defoveating movement is a saccadic intrusion.

Ocular flutter and opsoclonus

These entities consist of saccadic oscillations with no intersaccadic interval; in ocular flutter oscillations are purely horizontal and in opsoclonus they are multiplanar. Causes include viral encephalitis, myoclonic encephalopathy in infants ('dancing eyes and dancing feet'), as a transient idiopathic occurrence in healthy neonates, or may be drug-induced.

Ocular bobbing

Ocular bobbing manifests with rapid downward conjugate eye movements with a subsequent slow drift up to the primary position. Causes include pontine lesions (usually haemorrhage), cerebellar lesions compressing the pons and metabolic encephalopathy.

Superior oblique myokymia

Superior oblique myokymia is a rare condition characterized by intermittent episodes of oscillopsia and diplopia in one eye (usually the right eye). The cause is not known, but the condition may follow ocular or head injury and rarely brainstem tumours. Some cases occur secondary to compression of the fourth nerve root by the adjacent superior cerebellar artery, resulting in ephaptic impulse transmission. There is no definitive treatment, but oral or topical beta-blockers can be helpful. In persistent cases, superior oblique muscle weakening procedures may be tried. It should be distinguished from **orbicularis oculi muscle myokymia (tic)** which is common, innocuous and usually settles spontaneously.

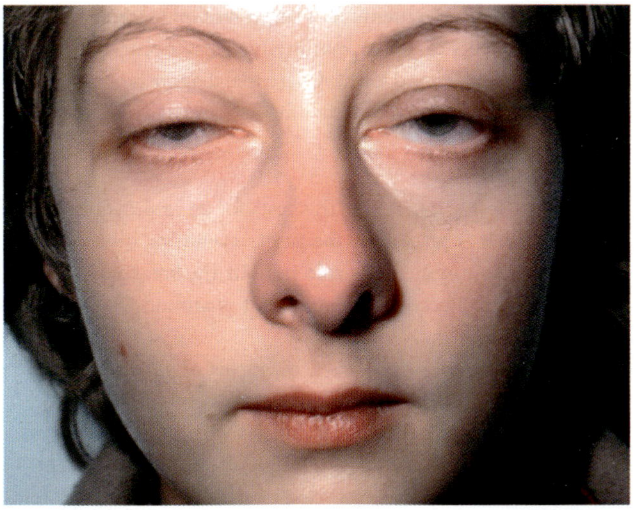

Fig. 19.95 Myopathic facial appearance in myasthenia gravis.

OCULAR MYOPATHIES

Myasthenia gravis

Introduction

Myasthenia gravis (MG) is an autoimmune disease in which antibodies mediate damage and destruction of acetylcholine receptors in striated muscle. The resultant impairment of neuromuscular conduction causes weakness and fatigability of skeletal musculature, but not of cardiac and involuntary muscles. The disease affects females twice as commonly as males. MG may be ocular, bulbar (affecting the cranial nerves arising from the lower brainstem) or generalized. Congenital and juvenile forms are rare. A similar clinical picture is found in the Lambert–Eaton myasthenic syndrome mediated by antibodies against pre-synaptic voltage-gated calcium channels. This is a paraneoplastic phenomenon associated with a lung tumour in 60%. Patients positive for anti-MuSK (muscle-specific kinase) antibody may have a distinct form of MG. A range of drugs can exacerbate MG and should be avoided if possible; those with ophthalmic relevance include many antibiotics and beta-blockers.

Systemic myasthenia

- **Symptoms** are typically of onset in the third decade and may include painless fatigue, often brought on by exercise, commonly in conjunction with ptosis and diplopia. Fatigability affects the musculature of the limbs, facial expression, ocular movements, chewing and speech. Bulbar symptoms include dysphagia and dysarthria; difficulty with breathing is rare.
- **Signs.** The most important feature is peripheral weakness, particularly of the arms and proximal leg muscles, with wasting in longstanding cases. There is characteristically a lack of facial expression (Fig. 19.95). Ocular features are discussed below.
- **Myasthenic crisis** can be fatal due to respiratory distress if not treated promptly.

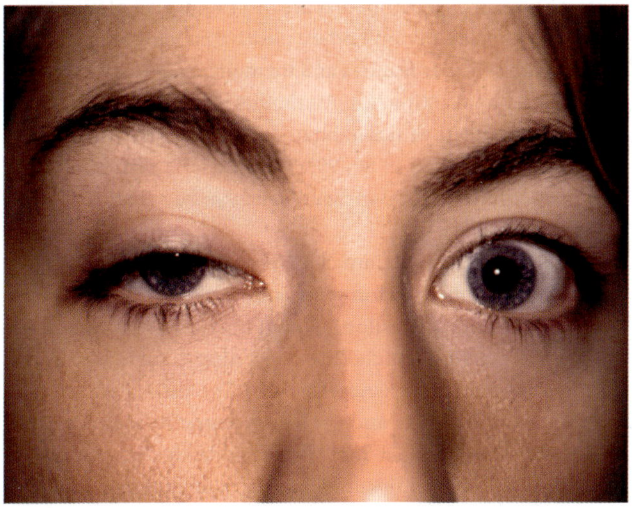

Fig. 19.96 Asymmetrical right-sided ptosis with slight left lid retraction secondary to orbicularis overaction.

Ocular myasthenia

Ocular involvement occurs in 90% of cases and is the presenting feature in 60%. Two-thirds of patients have both ptosis and diplopia.

- **Ptosis** is insidious, bilateral and frequently asymmetrical (Fig. 19.96).
  - Typically, worse at the end of the day.
  - Worse on prolonged (60 second) upgaze due to fatigue.
  - Cogan twitch sign is a brief upshoot of the eyelid as the eyes saccade from depression to the primary position.
  - If one eyelid is elevated manually as the patient looks up, the fellow eyelid may show fine oscillatory movements.
- **Diplopia** is frequently vertical, although any or all of the extraocular muscles may be affected. A pseudo-internuclear ophthalmoplegia may be seen. Patients with stable deviations may benefit from muscle surgery, botulinum toxin injection or a combination of both.

- **Nystagmoid movements** may be present on extremes of gaze. Bizarre defects of ocular motility may also occur so that MG should be considered in the differential diagnosis of any ocular motility disorder that does not fit with a recognized pattern.

Investigation

- **Ice pack test** (Fig. 19.97). This tests for an improvement after an ice pack is placed on the ptotic eyelid (or other affected muscle) for 2 minutes, as cold inhibits the breakdown of acetylcholine by acetylcholinesterase. It is around 75% sensitive but highly specific.
- **Antibody testing** supports a diagnosis of MG and predicts the likelihood of thymoma. Testing is confounded by recent (within 48 hours) general anaesthesia with muscle relaxants.
  - Acetylcholine receptor (AChR) antibodies. Present in around 90% of systemic cases but only 50–70% of patients with ocular myasthenia. Rarely present in Lambert–Eaton syndrome.
  - MuSK protein antibodies are positive in 50% of those negative for AChR antibodies; positive patients are less likely to have ocular features and thymoma.
  - Striational antibodies. Antibodies against several contractile elements of skeletal muscle (e.g. titin) may be present. They are found in 80–90% of those with thymoma – and one-third of those without – and can be a marker of more severe MG.
  - Voltage-gated calcium channel antibodies are characteristic of Lambert–Eaton syndrome.
- **Edrophonium (Tensilon) test** (Fig. 19.98). Edrophonium is a short-acting anticholinesterase that confers a transient improvement of weakness in MG. The estimated sensitivity is 85% in ocular and 95% in systemic MG. Bradycardia is uncommon and in rare instances deaths have occurred. Resuscitation facilities and appropriate expertise must be readily available on site in case of emergency and its use may be limited to cases in which less invasive tests have given equivocal results.
  - Atropine 0.3 mg is given intravenously to minimize muscarinic side effects.
  - An intravenous test dose of 0.2 ml (2 mg) edrophonium hydrochloride is given. If definite symptomatic improvement (or adverse reaction) is noted, the test is terminated.
  - The remaining 0.8 ml (8 mg) is given after 60 seconds if necessary.
  - Pre- and post-procedure measurements of ptosis and/or motility (Hess chart) are compared; the effect lasts only 5 minutes.
- **Electromyography** shows characteristic features.
- **Muscle biopsy** reveals neuromuscular junction antibodies and characteristic electron microscopy features, but is not commonly performed.
- **Thoracic imaging** (MR, CT, CT/PET) to detect thymoma, present in 15% (conversely, 30% of patients with thymoma have myasthenia). Imaging may also be used to rule out a lung tumour if Lambert–Eaton syndrome is suspected, or an intracranial mass for ocular myasthenia.

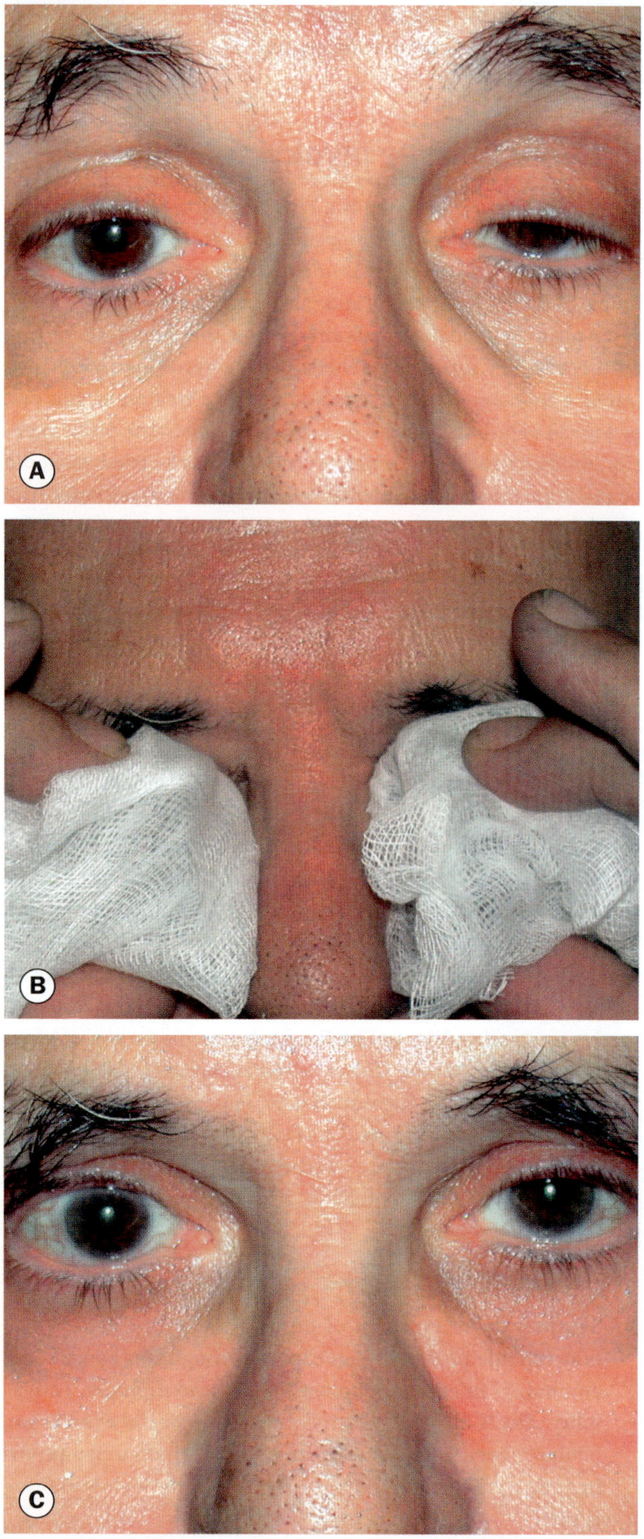

Fig. 19.97 Positive ice pack test in myasthenia gravis. **(A)** Asymmetrical ptosis; **(B)** application of ice; **(C)** improvement of ptosis. *(Courtesy of J Yangüela.)*

TIP Patients with myasthenia gravis should undergo thoracic imaging to exclude a thymoma.

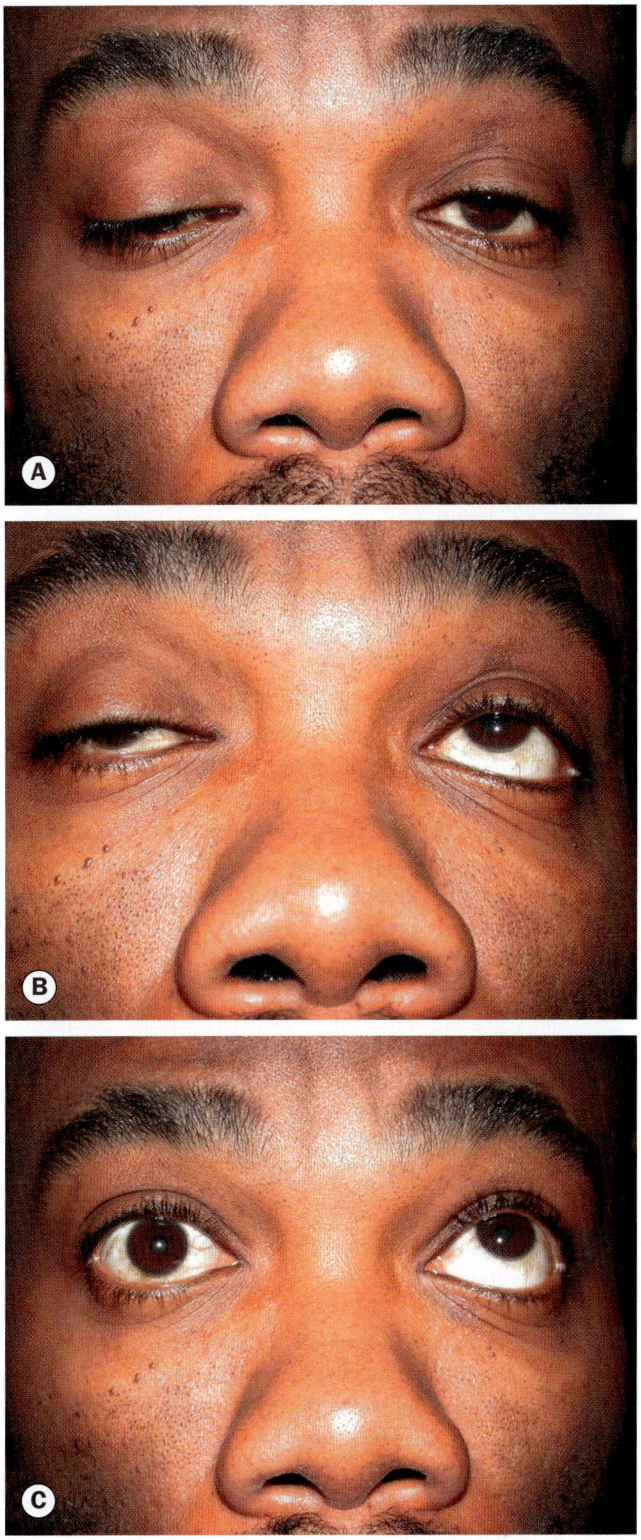

Fig. 19.98 Positive edrophonium test in myasthenia gravis. **(A)** Asymmetrical ptosis in the primary position; **(B)** defective upgaze; **(C)** following injection of edrophonium there is marked bilateral improvement of ptosis and modest improvement of left, but not right, upgaze.

- **Thyroid function testing** should be performed as autoimmune thyroid disease can be associated. There is also an association with rheumatoid arthritis, pernicious anaemia and systemic lupus erythematosus.

Treatment

An anticholinesterase agent such as pyridostigmine may be used alone in mild disease, but is usually combined with steroids and other immunosuppressive treatment (e.g. azathioprine). Plasmapheresis and intravenous immunoglobulins are short-term measures to address acute illness; emergency respiratory support is rarely required. Thymectomy is performed if a thymoma is present and leads to improvement in 75%.

Myotonic dystrophy

Introduction

Myotonic dystrophy is characterized by delayed muscular relaxation after cessation of voluntary effort (myotonia). There are two forms: the classic form, dystrophia myotonica 1 (DM1), is caused by a mutation in the dystrophia myotonica protein kinase gene *DMPK*. DM2 (proximal muscle myopathy, PROMM) involves the gene *CNBP*; DM2 has fewer systemic features (although cataract is frequent) and a better long-term prognosis, but is less common. Inheritance in both forms is AD; sporadic cases are rare. DM1 is discussed below.

Diagnosis

Successive generations tend to exhibit progressively earlier onset and greater severity of disease ('anticipation') due to a progressive increase in the size of the responsible genetic defect (a repeated trinucleotide sequence) at fertilization.

- **Symptoms** typically first occur in the third–sixth decades with weakness of the hands and difficulty in walking.
- **Systemic features**
  - Peripheral. Difficulty in releasing grip, muscle wasting and weakness.
  - Central. Mournful facial expression caused by bilateral facial wasting with hollow cheeks (myotonic facial appearance – Fig. 19.99) and slurred speech from involvement of the tongue and pharyngeal muscles.
  - Other. May include frontal baldness in males, somnolence, hypogonadism, endocrine abnormalities, cardiomyopathy, pulmonary disease, intellectual deterioration and bone changes.
- **Ophthalmic features**
  - Common. Most develop early-onset cataract, initially seen as an iridescent dust (sometimes resembling the commonly confused Christmas tree morphology) and subsequently progressing to cortical and subcapsular spokes, often in a stellate conformation. Ptosis and hypermetropia are also extremely common.
  - Uncommon. Motility dysfunction (strabismus, nystagmus, abnormal saccades and smooth pursuit), light–near dissociation, iris vascular tufts, mild pigmentary retinopathy, optic atrophy and hypotony.

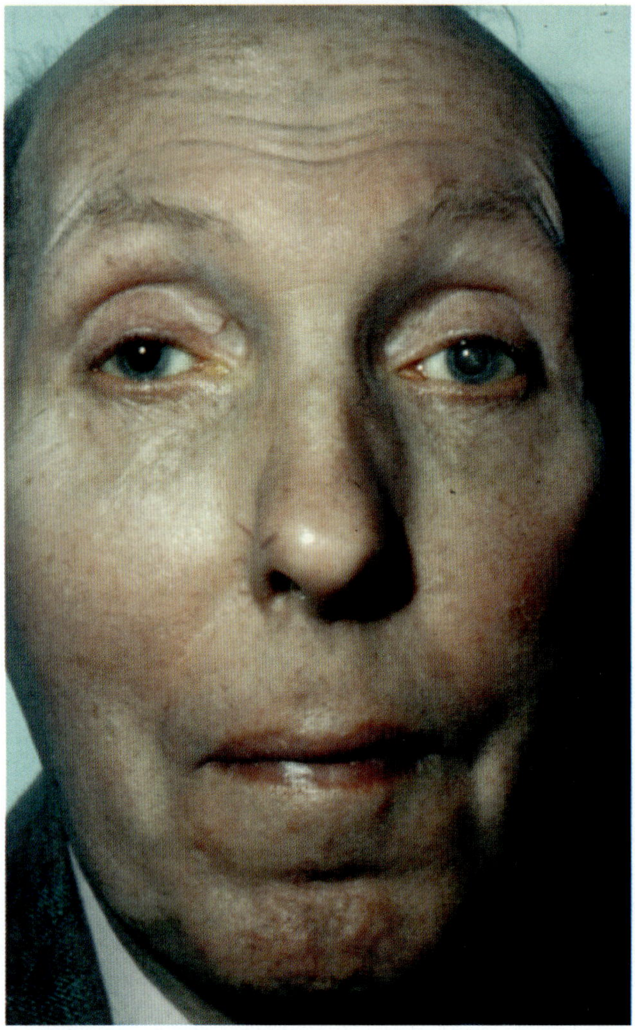

Fig. 19.99 Myotonic dystrophy. Typical facial appearance, frontal baldness and left cataract.

- **Investigation.** Genetic testing will confirm the defect and can be performed prenatally.

Treatment

Genetic counselling, cardiac monitoring and symptomatic treatment such as cataract surgery, eyelid crutches and frontalis suspension. Patients should be warned of a substantially increased risk of anaesthetic complications.

Chronic progressive external ophthalmoplegia

Chronic progressive external ophthalmoplegia (CPEO) refers to a group of disorders characterized by ptosis and slowly progressive bilateral ocular immobility. The ocular features may occur in isolation or in association with Kearns–Sayre syndrome or oculopharyngeal dystrophy.

Isolated CPEO

- **Ptosis**, usually the first sign, is bilateral and may be asymmetrical. Surgical correction may improve a compensatory head posture but does not restore normal lid movement and risks corneal exposure.
- **Pupils** are usually not involved.
- **External ophthalmoplegia** (Fig. 19.100) begins in young adulthood and is typically symmetrical. It is characterized by a progressive course without remission or exacerbation. Initially upgaze is involved and subsequently lateral gaze is affected so that the eyes may become almost totally fixed. Because of this symmetrical loss of eye movement, diplopia is rare although reading may be a problem due to inadequate convergence.
- **Investigation.** Electromyography shows myotonic and myopathic potentials; serum creatine kinase is elevated.
- **Treatment** involves exercise and prevention of contractures. A minority of patients with diplopia may benefit from surgery.

Kearns–Sayre syndrome

Kearns–Sayre is a rare myopathy associated with mitochondrial DNA deletions. These patients have a cerebral folate deficiency despite a normal serum folate level, suggesting that there is a failure of the mechanism responsible for movement of folate across the choroid plexus. Presentation is in the first and second decades with an insidious progressive external ophthalmoplegia. It is usually sporadic, though inheritance can occur. No proven treatment is currently available.

- **Clinical features**
  - The classic triad is chronic progressive external ophthalmoplegia with ptosis (Fig. 19.101A), cardiac conduction abnormalities and pigmentary retinopathy, the latter typically in a 'salt and pepper' appearance that is most striking at the macula (Fig. 19.101B). Mild visual impairment and nyctalopia may occur.
  - Fatigue, proximal muscle weakness, deafness, diabetes, cerebellar ataxia, short stature, renal disease, endocrine abnormalities and dementia may be present.
- **Investigations**
  - Genetic testing.
  - Lumbar puncture: elevation of CSF protein.
  - Electrocardiography demonstrates cardiac conduction defects and should be performed periodically; pacemaker implantation may be required.
  - Histology of extraocular muscles shows 'ragged red fibres' due to intramuscular accumulation of abnormal mitochondria.
  - Endocrine screening is important.

Oculopharyngeal dystrophy

Oculopharyngeal muscular dystrophy (OPMD) is caused by a mutation in *PABPN1*. Like myotonic dystrophy, OPMD is a trinucleotide repeat disorder; inheritance is AD or AR. Clinical onset is typically in early middle age, systemic features including

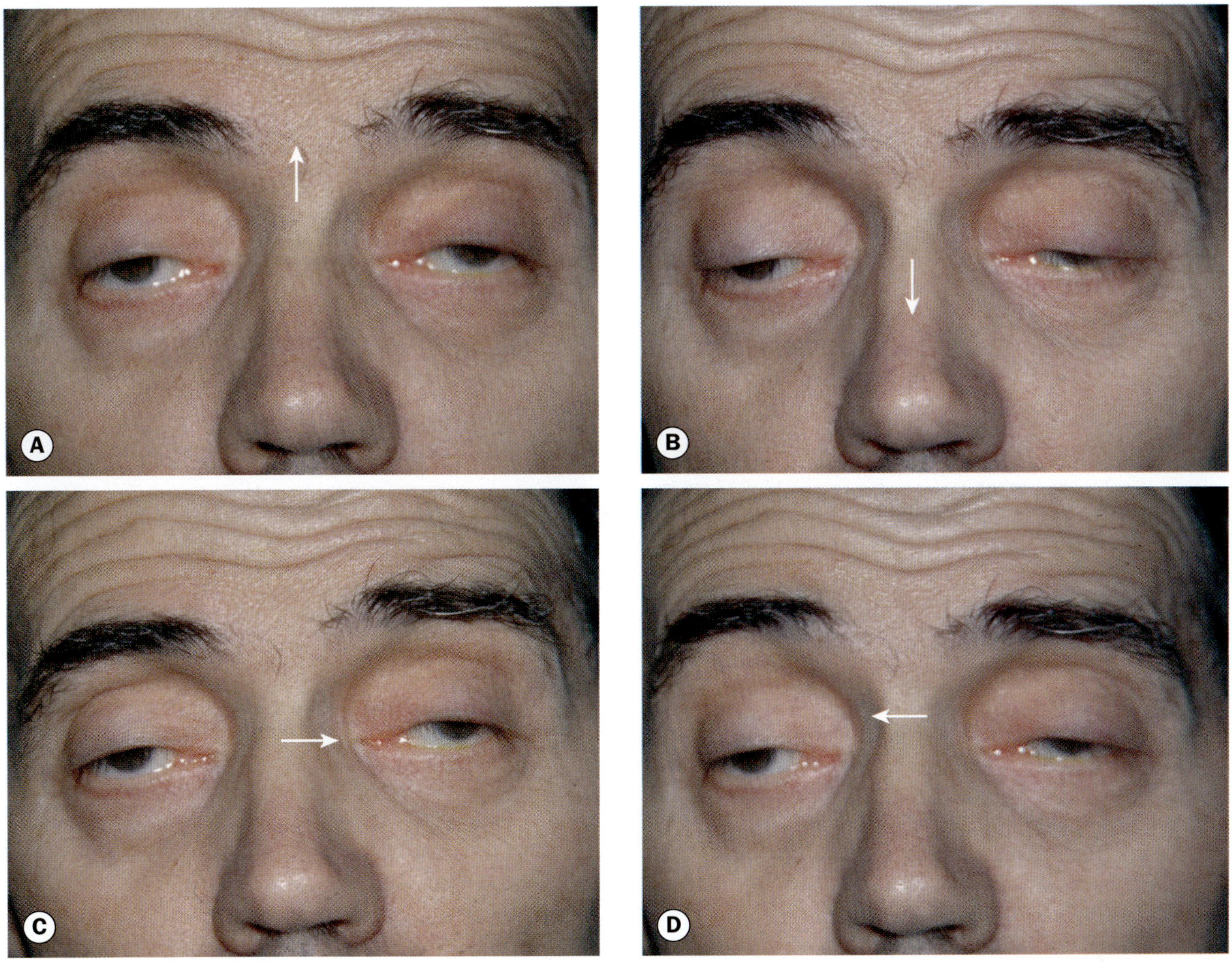

Fig. 19.100 Progressive external ophthalmoplegia. **(A)** Severe bilateral ptosis with defective upgaze; **(B)** defective downgaze; **(C)** defective left gaze; **(D)** defective right gaze. *(Courtesy of J Yangüela.)*

weakness of the pharyngeal muscles and temporalis wasting. Treatment is palliative, e.g. cricopharyngeal myotomy improves swallowing.

MILLER FISHER SYNDROME

Miller Fisher syndrome is a rare form of the acute polyneuropathy Guillain–Barré syndrome and because of its ocular features may present to an eye-care professional. It typically affects the extraocular muscles as the first manifestation, with a classic clinical triad of ophthalmoplegia, gait and trunk ataxia, and areflexia. Anti-GQ1b antibodies are present in most cases.

NEUROFIBROMATOSIS

Neurofibromatosis type 1

Neurofibromatosis is a disorder that primarily affects cell growth in neural tissues. The two main forms are neurofibromatosis type 1 (NF1) and type 2 (NF2). Both may show segmental involvement in which the features are confined to one or more body segments. NF1 (von Recklinghausen disease) is the most common phacomatosis, affecting 1:4000 individuals. Inheritance is AD with irregular penetrance and variable expressivity, though about 50% have new mutations. The *NF1* gene (neurofibromin) is on chromosome 17 and is normally involved in cell growth regulation mechanisms. Lack of neurofibromin promotes excessive cell growth, leading to deregulation and tumour formation. The presence of optic nerve glioma and Lisch nodules (iris hamartomas – see Ch. 20) are important ophthalmic diagnostic signs; genetic testing has around 95% specificity – a few positive individuals will not develop NF1. The National Institute of Health have determined specific diagnostic criteria.

Systemic features

- **Neurofibromas** may develop anywhere along the course of peripheral or autonomic nerves or on internal organs but do not occur on purely motor nerves. They appear as either

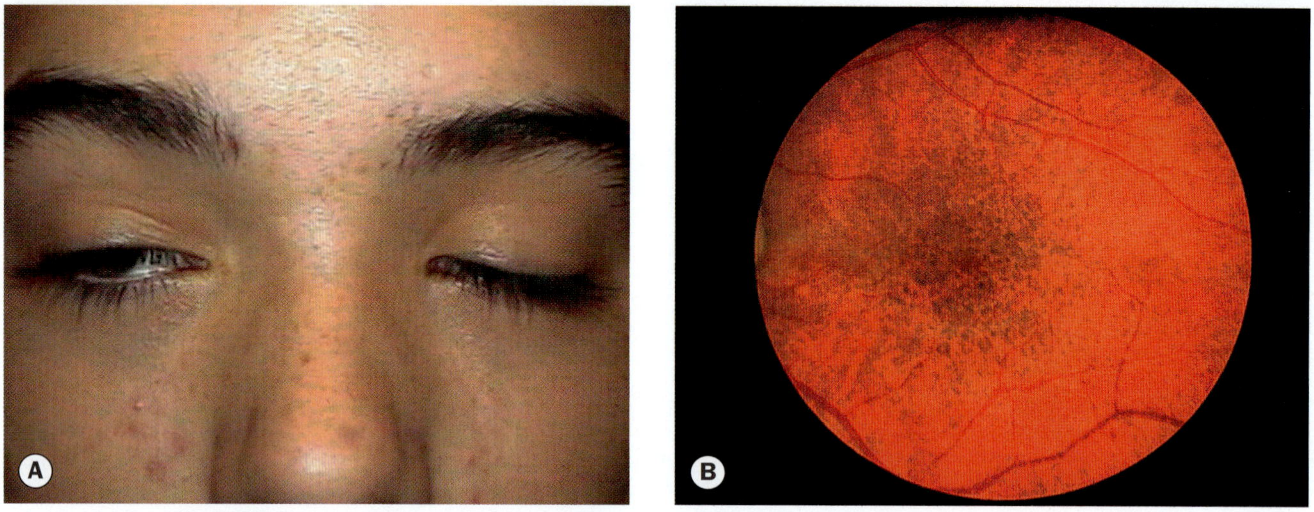

Fig. 19.101 Kearns–Sayre syndrome. (A) Chronic progressive external ophthalmoplegia with ptosis; (B) 'salt and pepper' pigmentary retinopathy.

solitary nodules (Fig. 19.102A) or more diffuse plexiform lesions, sometimes with associated soft tissue overgrowth (elephantiasis nervosa) (Fig. 19.102B) and may also involve internal organs.

- **Skin.** Café-au-lait macules are light-brown patches most commonly found on the trunk (Fig. 19.102C). They appear during the first year of life and increase in size and number throughout childhood.
- **Axillary or inguinal freckles** usually become obvious around the age of 10 years and are pathognomonic.
- **Skeletal abnormalities** may include short stature and facial hemiatrophy.
- **Intracranial tumours**, primarily meningiomas and gliomas.
- **Associations** include malignancy (especially malignant peripheral nerve sheath tumours), gastrointestinal stromal tumours, hypertension and learning difficulties. Recent research suggests that autism spectrum disorder affects nearly half of all NF1 patients.

Ophthalmic features

Regular eye examinations are critical from the time of diagnosis to detect lesions such as optic nerve glioma.

- **Eyelid plexiform neurofibroma** gives a characteristic S-shaped deformity of the upper lid (Fig. 19.103A) and classically is texturally reminiscent of a 'bag of worms'.
- **Orbital**
  - Optic nerve glioma (15–40%), a pilocytic astrocytoma, typically occurs in young children. It gives a fusiform enlargement of the nerve (see Fig. 19.103E) and may present with slowly increasing painless proptosis (see Fig. 4.39B), visual impairment (often marked), optic atrophy and strabismus. It can be bilateral and may extend posteriorly to involve the chiasm, optic tract and hypothalamus, sometimes with obstructive hydrocephalus. Slow growth is typical.
  - Other orbital neural tumours, e.g. neurilemmoma (schwannoma), plexiform neurofibroma and meningioma.
  - Spheno-orbital encephalocoele is caused by absence of the greater wing of the sphenoid bone (see Fig. 19.103F), characteristically causing a pulsating proptosis.
- **Iris lesions**
  - Bilateral Lisch nodules (at least 95%) are hamartomas that develop during the second–third decades, seen as tiny nodular pigmented lesions protruding above the iris surface (Fig. 19.103B).
  - Congenital ectropion uveae (Fig. 19.103C) is uncommon and it may be associated with glaucoma.
  - Mammillations (see Fig. 9.18D) are rare.
- **Prominent corneal nerves.**
- **Glaucoma** is not a common association. When present, it is usually unilateral and congenital and about 50% have ipsilateral neurofibroma of the upper eyelid and facial hemiatrophy.
- **Fundus**
  - Choroidal naevi may occur. NF1 patients with naevi are at increased risk of developing choroidal melanoma.
  - Retinal 'corkscrew' vessels are found in about a third of patients and do not leak.
  - Choroidal hyper-reflective nodules are multiple small, flat, pigmented lesions, which are commonly seen on OCT analysis (Fig. 19.103D). These are found in over 80% of patients and are highly sensitive and specific for NF1.
  - Other lesions that may be more common than in unaffected individuals include congenital hypertrophy of the RPE, myelinated nerve fibres, combined hamartoma of the retina and RPE (possibly increased only in NF2) and retinal astrocytic hamartoma identical to those seen tuberous sclerosis.

Neurofibromatosis type 2

Neurofibromatosis type 2 (NF2) is less common than NF1. Mutations in the *NF2* gene on chromosome 22 are causative. This gene encodes a protein (Merlin) that remodels cells and regulates cellular growth. Inheritance is AD, but 50% are sporadic. Various diagnostic criteria have been described, but often include vestibular

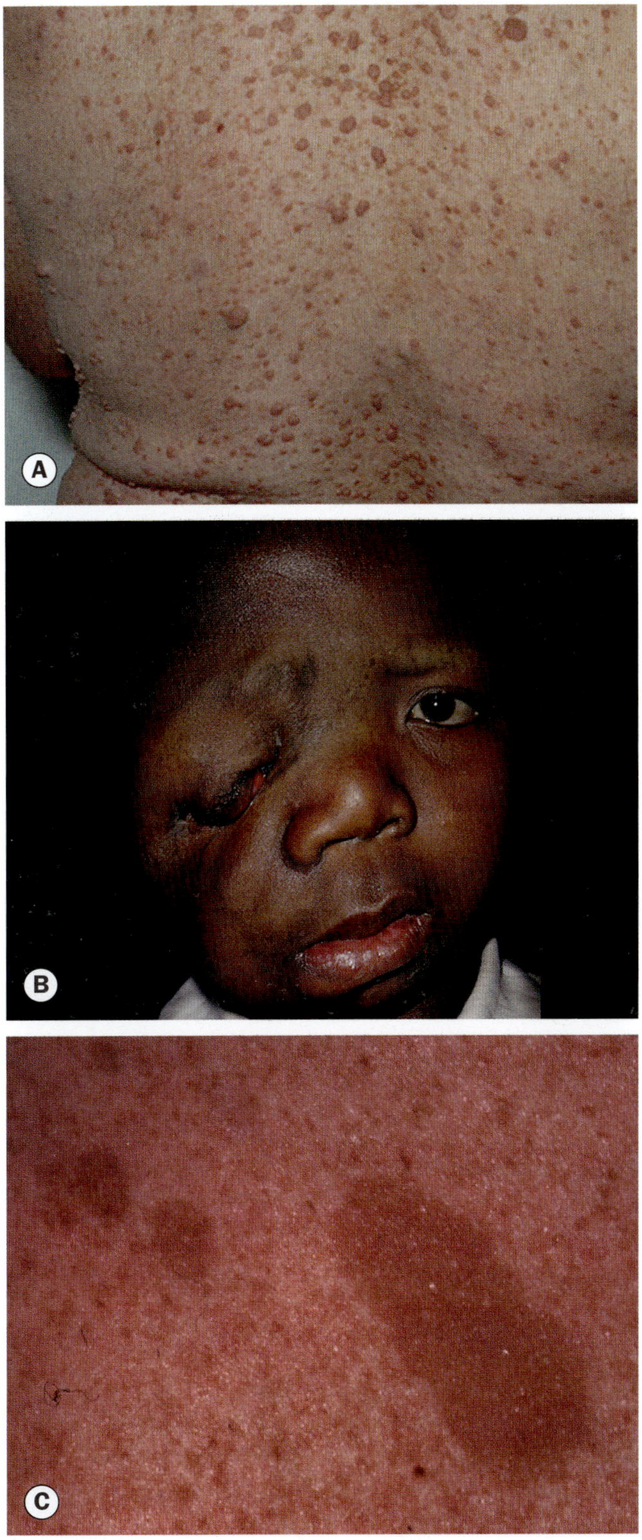

Fig. 19.102 Systemic features of neurofibromatosis type 1. **(A)** Discrete cutaneous neurofibromas; **(B)** elephantiasis nervosa; **(C)** café-au-lait macule. *(Courtesy of ADN Murray – fig. B.)*

TIP Migraine is the commonest cause of visual aura with and without headache.

schwannoma (90% – Fig. 19.104), a family history of NF2 and characteristic lesions such as juvenile cataract, neurofibroma, meningioma, glioma and schwannoma. Ocular lesions are often the first manifestations of the disease.

Ophthalmic features

- **Cataract** affects about two-thirds of patients. The opacities develop prior to the age of 30 years and may be posterior subcapsular or capsular, cortical or mixed.
- **Fundus.** Epiretinal membrane is frequent and combined hamartoma of the retina and retinal pigment epithelium is relatively common.
- **Ocular motor defects** (10%).
- **Less common.** Optic nerve sheath meningioma, optic nerve glioma, unilateral Lisch nodules, abnormal electroretinogram.

HEADACHE

Introduction

Patients with headache are commonly seen in ophthalmic practice. Any person who presents with a new, severe, unexpected headache, papilloedema, a new neurological defect or features of giant cell arteritis needs urgent investigation. Primary headache has been classified using the International Headache Society Classification Criteria (ICHD-3).

Classification

- **Migraine without aura**
- **Migraine with aura**
- **Tension-type headache**
- **Cluster headache**
- **Medication overuse headache**

Migraine

Introduction

Migraine is characterized by recurrent headaches widely variable in intensity, duration and frequency. The prevalence of migraine is higher in women (18%) than in men (6%). Migrainous headache is commonly unilateral, associated with nausea and vomiting and may be preceded by, or associated with, neurological and mood disturbances. However, all these characteristics are not necessarily present during each attack or in every patient. Migrainous aura can occur without headache and is a common presenting symptom to ophthalmologists. A family history of migraine is frequently obtained.

Migraine without aura

Migraine without aura (common migraine) is characterized by headache with autonomic nervous system dysfunction such as pallor and nausea, but without the stereotypical neurological or ophthalmic features of classical migraine (see below), such that it often goes undiagnosed. Premonitory features are often vague and may include changes in mood and poor concentration. The

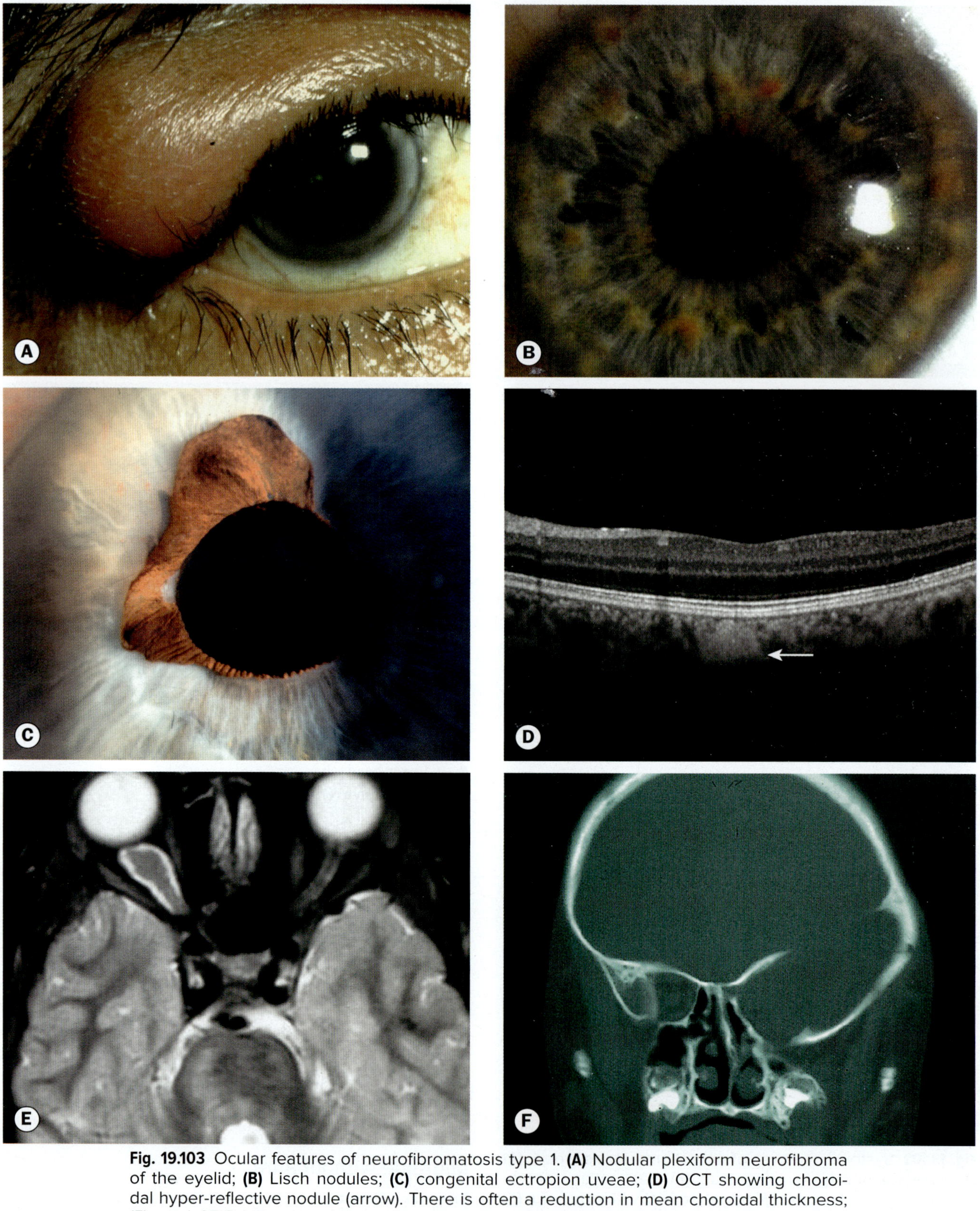

Fig. 19.103 Ocular features of neurofibromatosis type 1. **(A)** Nodular plexiform neurofibroma of the eyelid; **(B)** Lisch nodules; **(C)** congenital ectropion uveae; **(D)** OCT showing choroidal hyper-reflective nodule (arrow). There is often a reduction in mean choroidal thickness; **(E)** axial STIR MR image demonstrating a right-sided optic nerve glioma. There is myelin vacuolization in the pons; **(F)** coronal CT image showing absence of the greater wing of the left sphenoid bone. *(Courtesy of P Charbel Issa – fig. D; Ken K Nischal – fig. F.)*

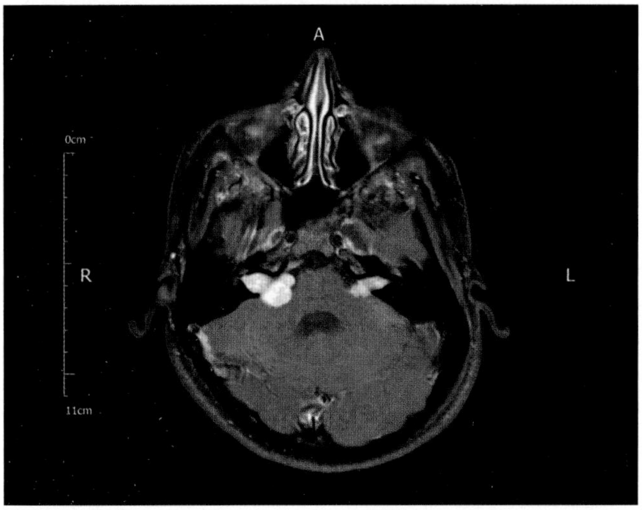

Fig. 19.104 Axial gadolinium-enhanced T1-weighted MR image through the posterior fossa showing bilateral vestibular schwannomas.

headache is unilateral pounding or throbbing, starting anywhere but usually spreading to involve one-half or the whole head. Retro-orbital pain may be mistaken for ocular or sinus disease. During the attack, which lasts from 4 hours to 3 days, the patient is frequently photophobic and phonophobic and may seek a quiet, dark environment.

Consider the diagnosis if there are at least five attacks fulfilling the following criteria:

- Headache lasting 4–72 hours.
- The headache has at least two of the following:
  - Unilateral location
  - Pulsating quality
  - Moderate or severe pain intensity
  - Aggravation by physical activity
- During the headache at least one of the following: nausea/vomiting, photophobia, phonophobia.

Migraine with aura (classical migraine)

- Migraine with aura is more readily characterized.
- An attack is heralded by a binocular visual aura that affects the central visual field on one side and typically lasts 5–30 minutes. Initially a binocular negative scotoma is commonly present, but may go unrecognized or be perceived as a vague visual disturbance. Associated positive phenomena develop after a few minutes and may consist of scintillating scotomas (zig-zags or fortification spectra), 'heat haze' distortions, or less commonly other features such as tunnel vision, progressing slowly across the field over several minutes. Full visual recovery within 30 minutes is typical.
- Other forms of aura are less common: unilateral altered or abnormal sensation (paraesthesia), weakness or disturbance of speech (dysphasia).
- Headache follows the aura and is usually hemi-cranial (on the side opposite the hemianopia) and accompanied by nausea and photophobia. It may, however, be absent, trivial or very severe, with considerable variation between attacks even in the same individual.
- Other pathology can rarely mimic a classical migrainous presentation.
- Consider this diagnosis when there are three of the following, on at least two occasions:
  - One or more **fully reversible** aura symptoms indicating focal cerebral cortical and/or brainstem dysfunction: (a) visual symptoms like zigzag lines and/or scotoma, (b) sensory symptoms like pins and needles, (c) speech and/or language symptoms like aphasia, (d) motor weakness, (e) brainstem symptoms such as vertigo.
  - At least one aura symptom develops gradually over at least 5 minutes, or two or more symptoms occur in succession.
  - At least one aura symptom is unilateral.
  - No single aura symptom lasts longer than 60 minutes.
  - Headache follows the aura within 60 minutes, but may begin before or during the aura.
- It is also important that clinical assessment does not suggest an underlying disorder or that investigation has ruled this out; for instance, very rarely a migrainous visual field defect or other aural feature may be permanent, when migraine should be a diagnosis of exclusion.
- **Occipital epilepsy** is very rare; the patient typically sees coloured circles during an attack.

Other forms of migraine

- **Chronic migraine** is defined as a headache that occurs on 15 or more days each month for more than 3 months in a patient who has at least five attacks of migraine without aura, or occurs on 8 or more days each month for more than 3 months, where the headache is relieved by triptan or ergot medication. There should be no secondary cause for the headache or evidence of medication overuse. Approximately 3% of patients with episodic migraine will progress to chronic migraine in the following year. However, up to 70% may revert from chronic to episodic migraine with effective treatment.
- **Retinal migraine** manifests with visual disturbance that may be similar to classical migraine but affects only one eye. It is a controversial entity, some authorities believing that most cases should be regarded as presumed recurrent ocular vasospasm rather than as true migraine. Young women are most commonly affected, but it is a rare condition (it is common for binocular hemifield symptoms to be misinterpreted by a patient as monocular). There is often a personal history of migraine. It may be prudent to investigate as for retinal embolization (see Ch. 13) and peripheral vasospasm (e.g. Raynaud phenomenon), with appropriate onward referral if necessary. Permanent monocular visual loss is common with recurrent episodes, probably due to vasospastic infarction and avoidance of potential precipitants and prophylactic treatment should be considered.
- **Ophthalmoplegic migraine** is rare and typically starts before the age of 10 years. It is characterized by a recurrent headache followed after a variable period by transient cranial (often

third) nerve palsy. It is now believed to be due to demyelination in most cases.

- **Familial hemiplegic** migraine is characterized by a failure of full recovery of focal neurological features after an attack of migraine subsides.
- **Basilar migraine** occurs in young females and is characterized by a typical migrainous aura associated with a variety of symptoms related to vertebrobasilar arterial insufficiency.

Treatment

- **General measures** include the elimination of conditions and agents that may precipitate an attack of migraine, such as coffee, chocolate, alcohol, cheese, oral contraceptives, stress, lack of sleep and long intervals without food. Improved hydration is associated with better migraine control.
- **Treatment of an acute attack** may be with simple analgesics and, if appropriate, an anti-emetic such as metoclopramide. Other drugs, usually reserved for patients who are refractory to analgesics, include sumatriptan and ergotamine tartrate. Occasionally intravenous agents are used.
- **Prophylaxis** should be considered for patients who experience at least six headache days per month or at least three headache days with severe impairment.
  - Most migraine prophylaxis drugs require patients to be treated for a minimum of eight weeks before response to treatment can be assessed. Treatment should be discontinued and a new option considered if the patient has an adverse side effect or if the patient does not have an adequate response.
  - Common reasons for non-response include (a) insufficient drug dosing, (b) inadequate duration of treatment and (c) untreated comorbidities that are known to exacerbate migraine.
  - The main migraine preventative drugs are antidepressants (amitriptyline), angiotensin-receptor blockers (candesartan), angiotensin-converting enzyme inhibitors (lisinopril), antiepileptic drugs (valproate and topiramate) and beta-blockers (propranolol, atenolol).
  - Start with a low dose and increase depending on results and continue for 2–3 months before changing.
  - Systemically administered monoclonal antibodies to calcitonin gene-related peptide or its receptors (erenumab, fremanezumab, galcanezumab, eptinezumab) are a novel class of preventative treatment aimed at reducing the frequency of episodic migraine, chronic migraine or cluster headaches. These drugs should not be used in pregnancy.
  - The use of botulinum toxin (BT-A) to reduce muscle spasms has been shown to be effective prophylactic treatment in some patients with chronic migraine.

Tension-type headache

This is an extremely common form of headache. The pain radiates from the back of the head, the neck and periorbital region and can cause pain behind the eyes. It typically affects both sides of the body. Consider the diagnosis if there are at least 10 episodes fulfilling the following criteria:

- Lasts between 30 minutes and 7 days.
- At least two of the following:
  - Bilateral location.
  - Pressing or tightening quality (e.g., a tight band around the forehead), of mild or moderate intensity.
  - Not aggravated by routine physical activity.
  - There must be no nausea or vomiting and no more than one episode of photophobia or phonophobia.
- Pain medication, such as aspirin and ibuprofen, is often effective treatment and tricyclic antidepressants are useful for prevention.
- Cognitive-behavioral therapy and physiotherapy can be helpful in some patients.

Medication overuse headache

- Headache occurring on at least 15 days per month associated with a pre-existing headache disorder.
- Consider this diagnosis in a patient when:
  - Medication has been used regularly for more than 3 months.
  - One or more drugs are being used for acute and/or symptomatic treatment of headache such as ergotamine, triptans, simple analgesics, or opioids.
- Patients should be counselled and warned of the risks of medication overuse.
- Triptans and non-steroidal anti-inflammatory drugs can be stopped abruptly; patients should aim to stop the offending drug for at least 1 month.
- Abrupt withdrawal of medication may precipitate a withdrawal headache, which lasts on average 3.5 days, but can last up to 10 days.

NEURALGIAS

The following conditions should be considered in the differential diagnosis of ocular or periocular pain, particularly in the absence of detectable physical signs.

- **Cluster headache** typically affects young to middle-aged men. It is of particular interest to ophthalmologists because it is associated with ocular features and may initially be misdiagnosed as a local ocular problem. The condition is characterized by a stereotyped headache accompanied by various autonomic phenomena occurring almost every day for a period of some weeks.
  - The headache is unilateral, oculotemporal, excruciating, sharp and deep.
  - It begins relatively abruptly, lasts between 10 minutes and 2 hours and then clears quickly.
  - The patient cannot keep still and is agitated, in contrast to a patient with migraine who would rather lie quietly in a dark room.
  - It may occur several times in a 24-hour period, often at consistent times, not infrequently in the early hours of the morning.
  - Once the 'cluster' is over, there may be a long headache-free interval of several years.

- Associated autonomic phenomena may include lacrimation, conjunctival injection and rhinorrhoea.
- There may be a transient or permanent postganglionic Horner syndrome.
- Acute treatment: use subcutaneous and/or nasal sumatriptan and commence inhaled oxygen (flow rate: over 10 l/min).
- Preventive treatment usually does not eliminate attacks, but reduces the frequency and intensity of symptoms. Verapamil 120 mg taken three times daily reduces the headache burden by 50% after 1–2 weeks of treatment. There is a role for topiramate, baclofen and galcanezumab in episodic cluster headache. Clinical trials have started with LSD (lysergic acid diethylamide) and psilocybin, based on anecdotal reports of long-term reduction of symptoms using sub-hallucinogenic doses for short periods (e.g. three doses).

- **SUNCT** (short-lasting, unilateral, neuralgiform headache attacks with conjunctival injection and tearing) syndrome. This consists of attacks of unilateral orbital, supraorbital or temporal stabbing or pulsating pain lasting from 5 to 240 seconds, occurring at a frequency of 3–200 per day, accompanied by marked ipsilateral conjunctival injection and lacrimation. By definition at least 20 episodes should have occurred for diagnosis. Triggers such as touching the face are common. An underlying disorder is occasionally present (secondary SUNCT).
- **Paroxysmal hemicrania** (Sjaastad syndrome). This consists of severe unilateral headache that is typically ocular, frontal and/or temporal and occurs in brief recurrent episodes (usually five or more per day) associated with one or more ipsilateral autonomic phenomena (tearing, injection, nasal congestion or watering, lid swelling or ptosis). It is more common in women and is much less common than cluster headache. The pain responds well to indomethacin, in contrast to SUNCT, which also features less severe pain, a male preponderance and more marked autonomic features.
- **Trigeminal neuralgia** is characterized by brief attacks of severe pain that start in the distribution of one of the divisions of the trigeminal (fifth) nerve. The pain is paroxysmal and sharp, usually occurring in multiple bursts in rapid succession lasting a few seconds. Attacks can be triggered either by cutaneous stimulation such as shaving or by motor activity such as chewing. Facial sensation is normal. Treatment involves antiepileptic drugs such as carbamazepine, phenytoin and sodium valproate and occasionally surgical decompression of the trigeminal nerve. A major difference from cluster headache, SUNCT syndrome and paroxysmal hemicrania is that autonomic features are sparse or absent.
- **Primary (idiopathic) stabbing headache** (comprising ophthalmodynia periodica and ice pick syndrome) is characterized by short, sharp, jabbing ocular pains, typically located around the orbit or temple, often described as similar to the sensation of being stabbed by a nail or needle and lasting from less than a second up to a few seconds. The pains may occur as isolated episodes or in brief repeated flurries. Frequency varies from a very occasional episode up to dozens per day. By definition there are no other accompanying symptoms and no causative disorder is identifiable. There is usually no trigger. It is more common in women, and children can be affected.
- **Raeder paratrigeminal syndrome** typically affects middle-aged men. It is characterized by severe unilateral headache with periocular pain in the distribution of the first division of the trigeminal nerve associated with an ipsilateral Horner syndrome. The pain may last from hours to weeks before it resolves spontaneously. Carotid dissection (blood entering the potential space between the inner and outer layers of the artery – see Fig. 19.38) must be excluded with urgency.
- **Herpes zoster ophthalmicus** frequently presents with pain 2–3 days before the onset of the characteristic vesicular rash. Zoster sine herpete denotes shingles without the development of a rash.
- **Occipital neuralgia** is characterized by attacks of pain that begin in the occipital region but may spread to the eye, temple and face.

TIP Immediate investigation is needed when the headache is new, severe and unexpected, particularly in an older person.

FACIAL SPASM

Benign essential blepharospasm

Introduction

Essential blepharospasm is an uncommon but distressing idiopathic disorder that often presents in the sixth decade and affects women more commonly than men. It is characterized by progressive bilateral involuntary spasm of the orbicularis oculi and upper facial muscles (Fig. 19.105). In severe cases blepharospasm may temporarily render the patient functionally blind. Common precipitants include stress and bright light (photophobia is a common accompanying symptom), with alleviation by relaxation and talking. It does not occur during sleep. In combination with oromandibular dystonia it comprises Meige (Fig. 19.106A) or Brueghel syndromes. There is occasionally an underlying identifiable cause, particularly basal ganglia disease, but in a clinically typical case investigation is not required.

Treatment

Prior to commencing treatment, it is important to exclude reflex blepharospasm, most commonly due to ocular surface disease and extrapyramidal conditions such as Parkinson disease. A cranial and peripheral nervous system examination should be performed.

- **Tinted spectacles** frequently provide amelioration.
- **Treating ocular surface disease** may be helpful.
- **Medical** treatment with a great variety of drugs has been reported to ameliorate specific types of blepharospasm, but their efficacy is disappointing.
- **Botulinum toxin injection** (e.g. 2.5–5 units injected subcutaneously at 3–4 periocular sites) affords relief in most (95%) patients by temporary paralysis of the injected

muscles (Fig. 19.106B); typically, repeat injections are required every 3 months. Common but temporary adverse effects include ptosis, lagophthalmos, dry eye and occasionally diplopia.

- **Surgery.** Myectomy is now rarely performed but can be considered in patients intolerant or unresponsive to botulinum toxin.

Hemifacial spasm

Hemifacial spasm is a unilateral condition that presents in the fifth–sixth decades of life. It is characterized initially by brief spasm of the orbicularis oculi that later spreads along the distribution of the facial nerve (Fig. 19.107). The condition is commonly idiopathic, but may stem from irritation of the seventh cranial nerve at any point in its course. Facial hyperkinesia may also occur several months or years after Bell palsy. Neuroimaging should be performed to exclude a compressive aetiology. Treatment is similar to that of essential blepharospasm.

DISORDERS OF CIRCADIAN RHYTHM

Introduction

A circadian rhythm is a biological process that persists in constant conditions (like darkness), is reset by exposure to light, and oscillates over a period of about 24 hours. Disorders of circadian rhythm can result in daytime sleepiness, poor sleep quality at night and reduced alertness when awake. Jet-lag is a consequence of disrupted circadian rhythm.

Anatomy

The receptors responsible for circadian rhythm are a subset of ganglion cells in the retina that contain melanopsin. Melanopsin photoreceptors respond to blue light (peak absorption around 480 nm). The resulting stimulus passes via the retinohypothalamic tract in the optic nerve to the suprachiasmic nucleus (SCN) located in the hypothalamus, then to the pineal gland, leading to

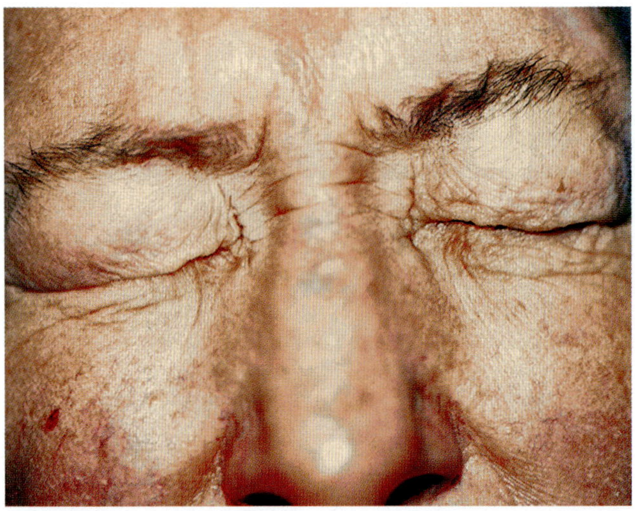

Fig. 19.105 Essential blepharospasm.

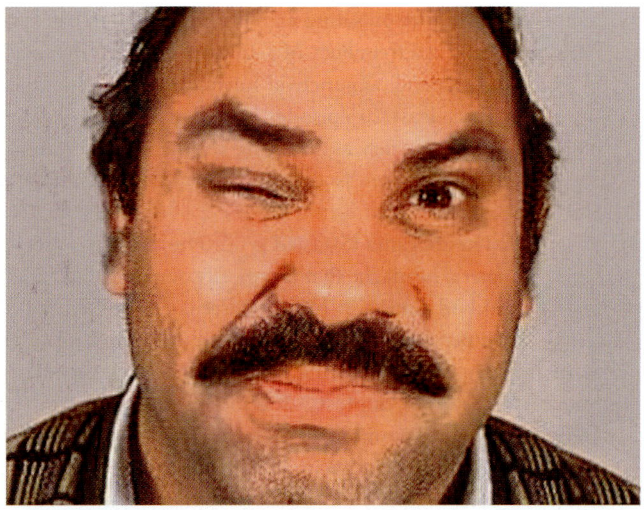

Fig. 19.107 Hemifacial spasm.

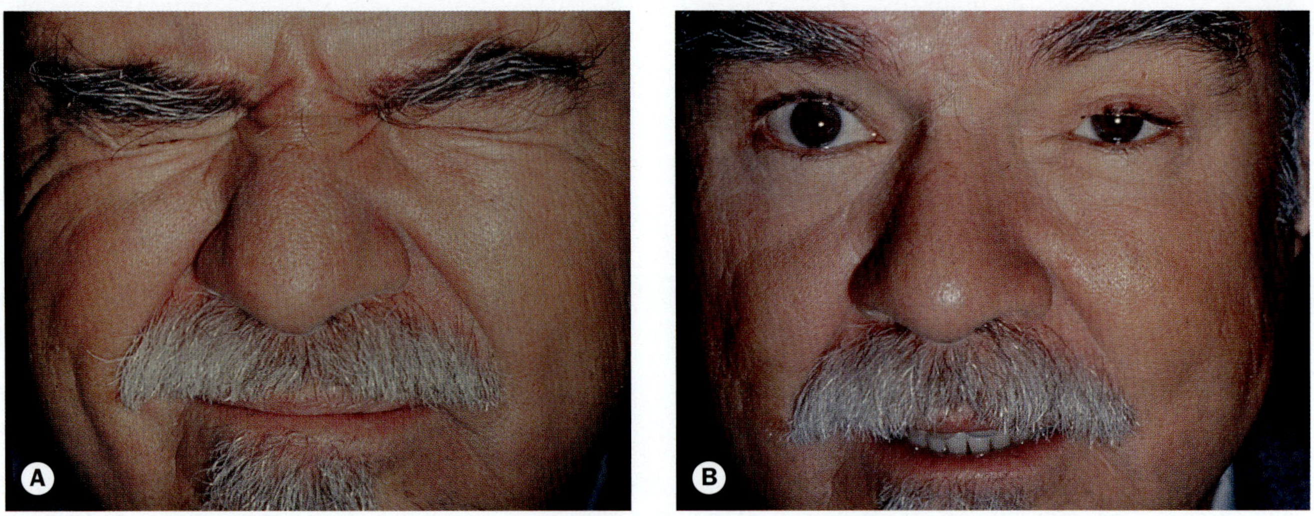

Fig. 19.106 Meige syndrome. **(A)** Blepharospasm and oromandibular dystonia; **(B)** after botulinum treatment. *(Courtesy of ADN Murray.)*

the production of melatonin. This hormone peaks at night and drops during the day.

Ocular disease causing abnormal circadian rhythm

- Bilateral ocular blindness.
- Dense cataract.
- Advanced glaucoma.
- Retinitis pigmentosa.

Treatment

The normal circadian rhythm can be reproduced with oral melatonin. Phacoemulsification with intraocular lens implantation can improve sleep quality at night and reduce daytime sleepiness in the elderly.

NEURO-OPHTHALMOLOGY OF SPACE FLIGHT

Long-duration space flight can lead to changes in the eye and optic nerve. This is known as space flight-associated neuro-ocular syndrome (SANS). Approximately two-thirds of astronauts with flights lasting more than 6 months experience a decrease in distance and near VA, which can remain unresolved for years. Optic disc oedema, globe flattening, choroidal folds and retinal cotton-wools spots have been reported. The precise cause of this syndrome is unknown, but presumably these changes occur as a consequence of orbital and cranial fluid shift brought about by prolonged exposure to microgravity. Mechanical changes in the optic nerve induced by a chronic upward shift in the brain position may also play a role.

Chapter 20 Ocular Tumours

BENIGN EPIBULBAR TUMOURS

Conjunctival naevus

Introduction

A conjunctival naevus is the most common melanocytic conjunctival tumour. The overall risk of malignant transformation is less than 1%. Treatment by excision is usually for cosmesis, but sometimes for irritation or a suspicion of malignancy. The histological appearance is similar to that of a cutaneous naevus, but as there is no conjunctival dermis, subepithelial and stromal replace dermal in the nomenclature:

- **Compound** naevus is characterized by the presence of naevus cells at the epithelial–subepithelial junction and within the subepithelial stroma, often with epithelial inclusions such as cysts and goblet cells (Fig. 20.1A).
- **Subepithelial** lesions remain localized.
- **Junctional** naevus is uncommon and consists of nests of naevus cells at the epithelial–subepithelial junction (Fig. 20.1B).

Clinical features

- **Symptoms.** The lesion is initially noticed in the first or second decade.
- **Signs**
  - A solitary slightly or moderately elevated pigmented or partially pigmented lesion of variable size, most frequently juxtalimbal. Over half contain small cysts (Fig. 20.1C and D).
  - A naevus is mobile over the underlying sclera.
  - The extent of pigmentation is variable. Absence of pigmentation is relatively common (Fig. 20.1E).
  - The plica, fornix and caruncle (Fig. 20.1F) are uncommon locations.
  - A naevus may become inflamed, especially in children and adolescents, and this may be mistaken for malignant change.
- **Signs of potential malignancy**
  - An unusual site such as the palpebral or forniceal conjunctiva.
  - Prominent feeder vessels.
  - Sudden growth or increase in pigmentation.
  - Development after the second decade.

Conjunctival papilloma

Conjunctival papillomas are strongly associated with human papillomavirus infection, especially types 6 and 11. Histopathology reveals a fibrovascular core covered by an irregular proliferation of non-keratinized stratified squamous epithelium containing goblet cells (Fig. 20.2A).

Clinical features

Lesions are sessile (wide base and flattish profile – Fig. 20.2B and C) or pedunculated (frond-like – Fig. 20.2D) and are frequently located in the juxtalimbal area, fornix or the caruncle. They are usually solitary, but may be multiple.

Large lesions may cause irritation, interfere with lid closure or encroach onto the cornea.

Treatment

Small lesions may resolve spontaneously. Large lesions are treated by excision, sometimes with cryotherapy to the base and the surrounding area. Options for recurrences include subconjunctival interferon alfa, carbon dioxide laser vaporization, topical mitomycin C and oral cimetidine.

Limbal dermoid

A limbal dermoid is a choristoma (a mass of histologically normal tissue in an abnormal location) consisting of a mass of collagenous tissue containing dermal elements, which is covered by stratified squamous epithelium (Fig. 20.3A). Presentation is in early childhood, with a smooth, yellowish, soft subconjunctival mass commonly located at the inferotemporal limbus, often with protruding hair (Fig. 20.3B). Lesions are occasionally very large and may virtually encircle the limbus (Fig. 20.3C). Treatment is indicated for cosmesis, chronic irritation, dellen formation and amblyopia from astigmatism or involvement of the visual axis. A small dermoid can undergo simple excision, but lamellar keratosclerectomy may be required for large lesions.

Systemic associations

- **Goldenhar syndrome** (oculoauriculovertebral spectrum – Fig. 20.3D) is usually sporadic.
  - Systemic features include hypoplasia of the malar, maxillary and mandibular regions, macrostomia and microtia, preauricular and facial skin tags, hemivertebrae (usually cervical), mental handicap, cardiac, renal and central nervous system (CNS) anomalies.
  - Ocular features, apart from a dermoid, include upper lid notching or coloboma, microphthalmos and disc coloboma.
- **Treacher Collins** syndrome (see Ch. 2).
- **Linear naevus sebaceous of Jadassohn.**
  - Systemic features include warty or scaly cutaneous lesions, infantile spasms, CNS anomalies and developmental delay.
  - Ocular features, apart from a dermoid, include ptosis, cloudy cornea, lid colobomas, fundus colobomas and microphthalmos.

Dermolipoma

A dermolipoma is similar in composition to a solid dermoid but also contains fatty tissue. Presentation tends to be in adult life as a soft yellowish subconjunctival mass near the outer canthus (Fig. 20.4A). The surface is usually keratinized and may exhibit hairs. Occasionally the lesion may extend into the orbit or anteriorly towards the limbus. Treatment is generally avoided because of the possibility of complications arising from the surgery, such as scarring, ptosis, dry eye and ocular motility problems. In selected cases, debulking the anterior portion may improve cosmesis with

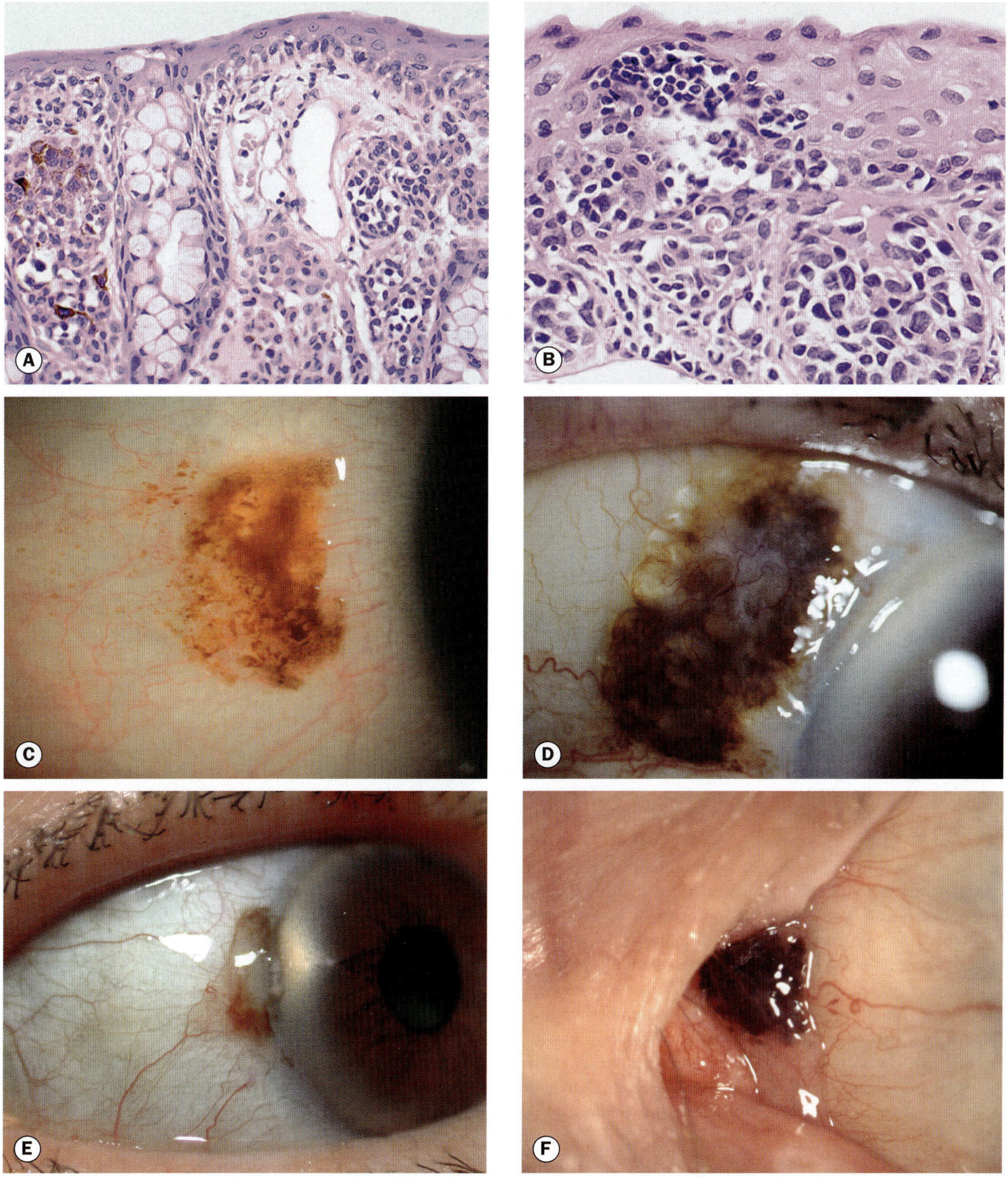

Fig. 20.1 Conjunctival naevus. **(A)** Compound naevus histology – see text; **(B)** junctional naevus histology – see text; **(C)** pigmented naevus; **(D)** cystic pigmented naevus; **(E)** partially pigmented naevus; **(F)** caruncular location. *(Courtesy of J Harry and G Misson, from* Clinical Ophthalmic Pathology, *Butterworth-Heinemann 2001 – figs A and B.)*

lower risk. It is critical to distinguish a dermolipoma from a prominent lacrimal gland lobe and from orbital fat prolapse (Fig. 20.4B). Myxoma and lymphoma can also present in a similar fashion (Fig. 20.4C and D).

Pyogenic granuloma

A pyogenic granuloma is a fibrovascular proliferative response to a conjunctival insult such as surgery or trauma, or occurs

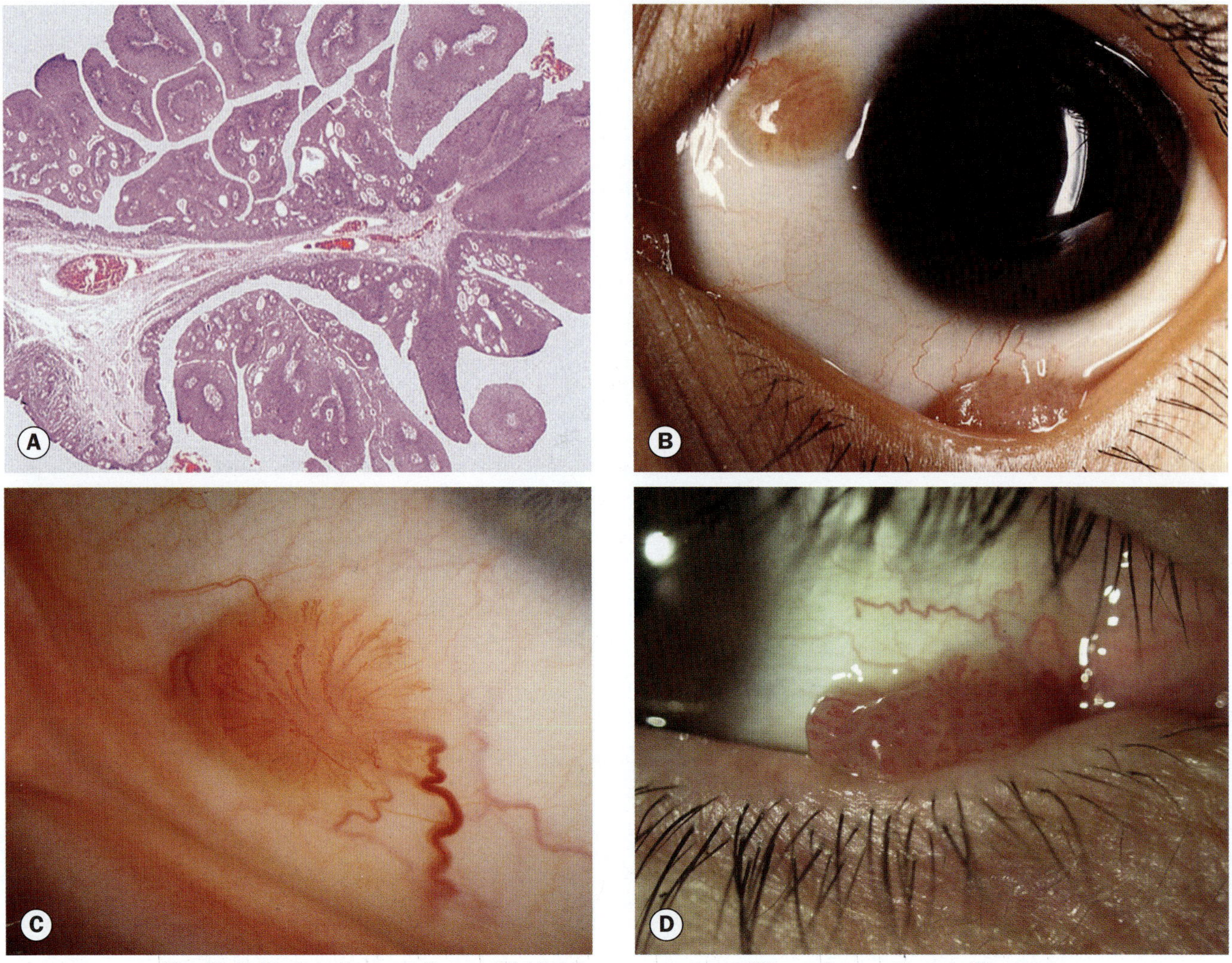

Fig. 20.2 Conjunctival papilloma. **(A)** Histology – see text; **(B)** sessile papilloma; **(C)** sessile papilloma with feeder vessels; **(D)** pedunculated papilloma.

in association with a chalazion or foreign body incarceration. Histology shows granulation tissue with both acute and chronic inflammatory cells and a proliferation of small blood vessels (the term 'pyogenic granuloma' is a misnomer as the lesion is neither pyogenic nor granulomatous). Presentation is typically a few weeks after surgery for chalazion, strabismus or enucleation, with a rapidly growing dark pink fleshy conjunctival mass (Fig. 20.5A). Treatment with topical steroids is often successful, but resistant cases require excision. The differential diagnosis includes suture granuloma (Fig. 20.5B), which can often be large and mistaken for a malignant lesion and Tenon capsule granuloma or cyst.

Miscellaneous benign epibulbar tumours

- **Epibulbar telangiectasia** (Fig. 20.6A) may be associated with Sturge–Weber syndrome.
- **Reactive pseudo-epitheliomatous hyperplasia** is a rapidly growing white juxtalimbal hyperkeratotic nodule (Fig. 20.6B) that develops secondary to irritation.
- **Melanocytoma** is a rare congenital lesion. It manifests as a slowly enlarging black lump (Fig. 20.6C) that cannot be moved freely over the globe.
- **Epibulbar angioma** is a rare late consequence of radiation treatment (Fig. 20.6D).

Benign melanosis

Benign conjunctival epithelial melanosis (conjunctival hypermelanosis) is a normal variant, more common in dark-skinned individuals (over 90% occur in Black people and 5% occur in White individuals) due to the presence of excess melanin within basal layer conjunctival epithelial melanocytes. Melanocyte numbers are normal, that is, there is no melanocytic hyperplasia. It may have a protective effect against neoplasia. Benign melanosis appears during the first few years of life and becomes static by early adulthood. Both eyes are affected but involvement may be asymmetrical. Areas of flat, patchy, brownish pigmentation may be seen throughout the conjunctiva but are often concentrated at the limbus (Fig. 20.7A) and around perforating branches of vessels or nerves as they enter the sclera (Fig. 20.7B). The pigmented epithelium moves

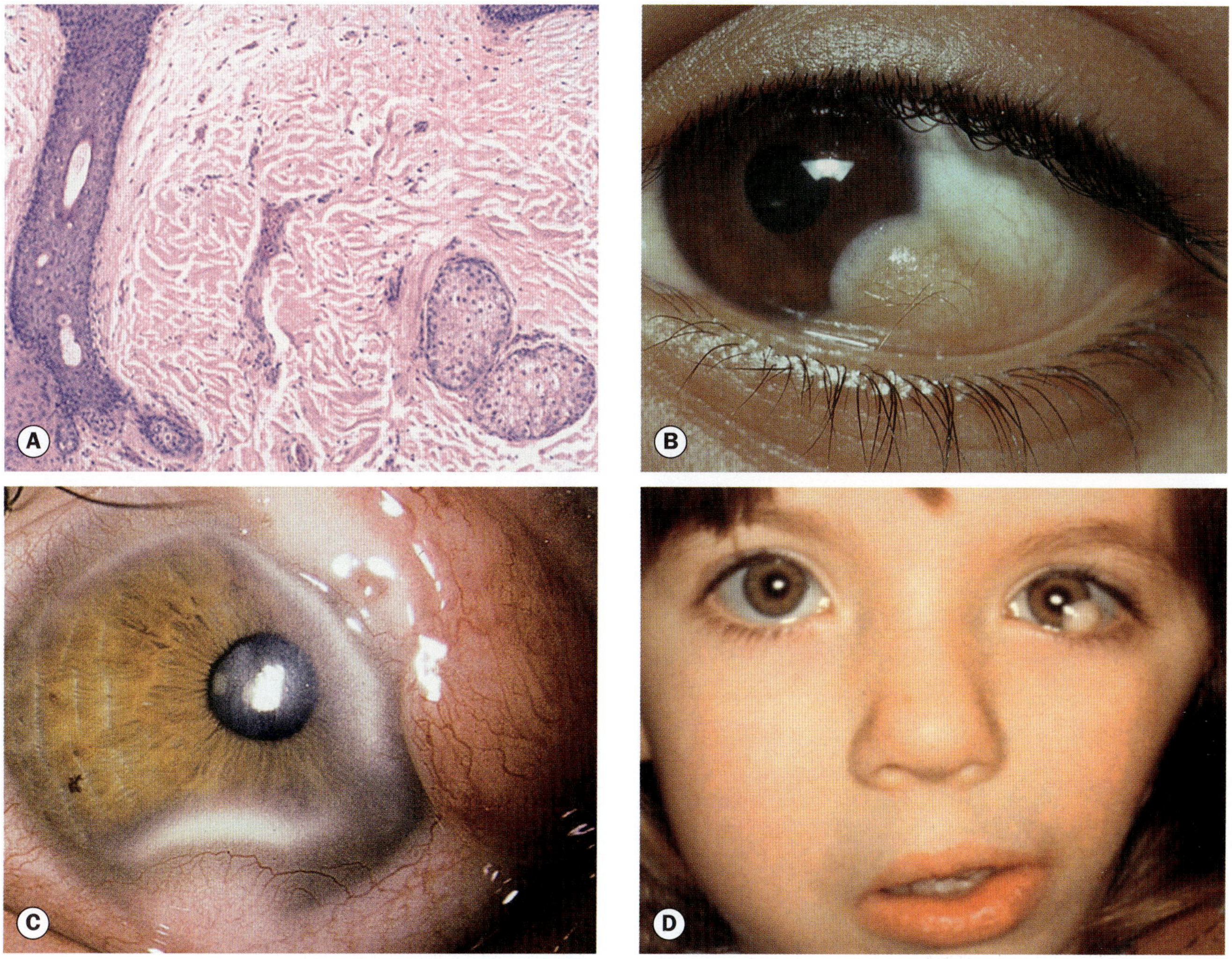

Fig. 20.3 Limbal dermoid. **(A)** Histology – see text; **(B)** typical lesion with protruding hairs; **(C)** complex dermoid; **(D)** Goldenhar syndrome. *(Courtesy of J Harry and G Misson, from* Clinical Ophthalmic Pathology, *Butterworth-Heinemann 2001 – fig. A.)*

freely over the surface of the globe. A variant is seen in which small cysts are present.

MALIGNANT AND PREMALIGNANT EPIBULBAR TUMOURS

Primary acquired melanosis/conjunctival melanocytic intraepithelial neoplasia

Introduction

Approximately 75% of conjunctival melanomas (see below) arise in areas of melanocytic hyperplasia. Recent trends in the description of pigmented conjunctival lesions have led to controversy relating to terminology. Some classifications have historically used the term primary acquired melanosis (PAM) to encompass both benign epithelial melanosis (see above) and melanocytosis/melanocytic hyperplasia (with and without atypia), whilst others have restricted its use to the latter category. To avoid this ambiguity, the term conjunctival melanocytic intraepithelial neoplasia (C-MIN) may be preferred for lesions exhibiting proliferation of melanocytes, with PAM reserved for clinical description before a histological diagnosis has been established. The differential diagnosis includes conjunctival naevus, benign melanosis, congenital ocular melanocytosis (see below), secondary pigmentation in Addison disease and pigmented squamous cell carcinoma.

- **PAM without cellular atypia or with mild atypia** is a benign intraepithelial proliferation of epithelial melanocytes (Fig. 20.8A) with little or no risk of malignant transformation.
- **PAM with severe atypia** can be regarded as melanoma *in situ* that has a substantial chance of progression to invasive melanoma over several years. The risk is higher the greater the extent of the lesion when measured in clock hours. Severe atypia is present in a minority.
- **C-MIN** is graded from 0 to 10 according to degree of atypia and spread, 0 corresponding to an absence of any melanocyte proliferation or atypia (i.e. melanosis only) and 5 to conjunctival melanoma *in situ*.

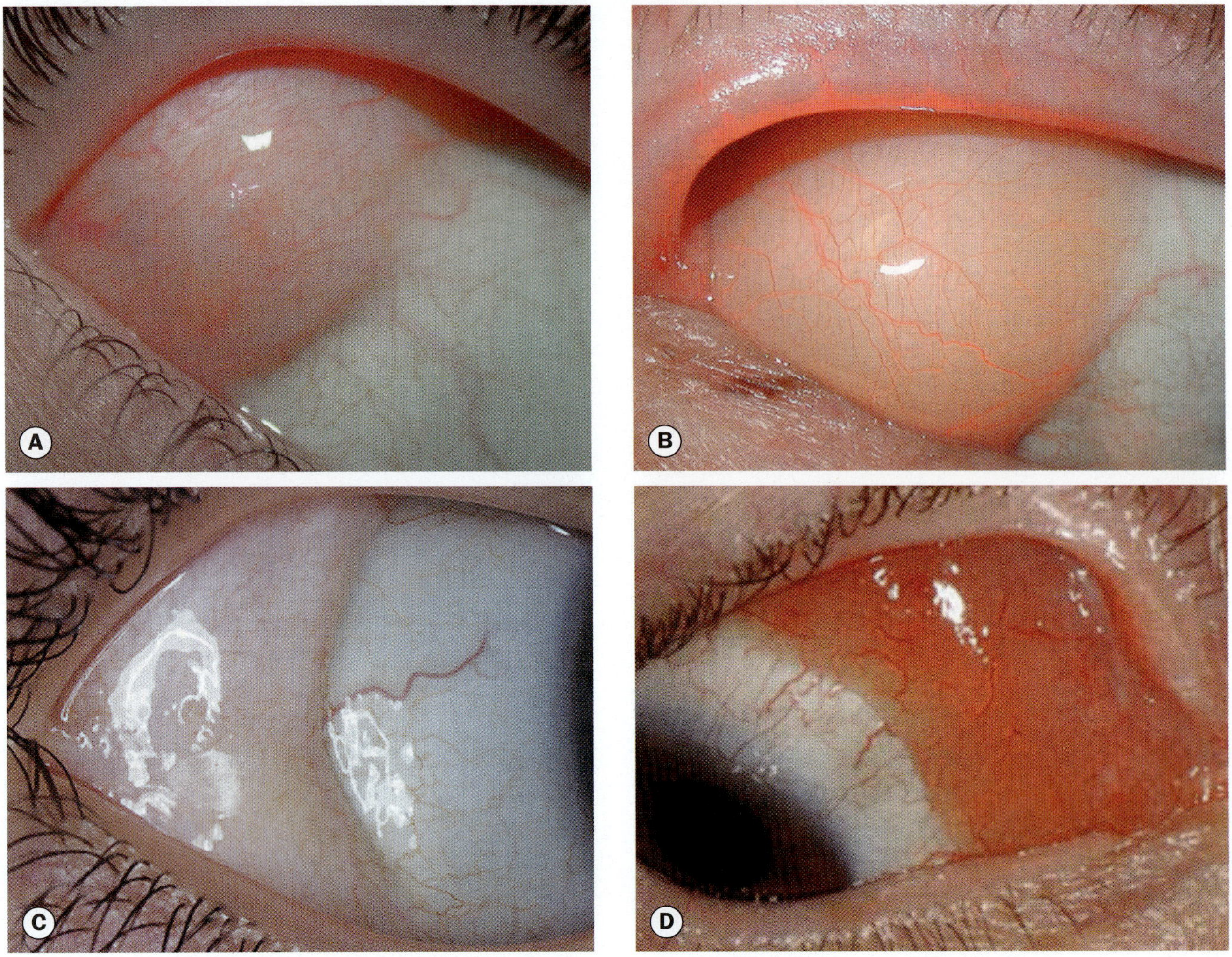

Fig. 20.4 **(A)** Dermolipoma; **(B)** orbital fat prolapse for comparison; **(C)** myxoma; **(D)** lymphoma. *(Courtesy of A Pearson – figs A and B.)*

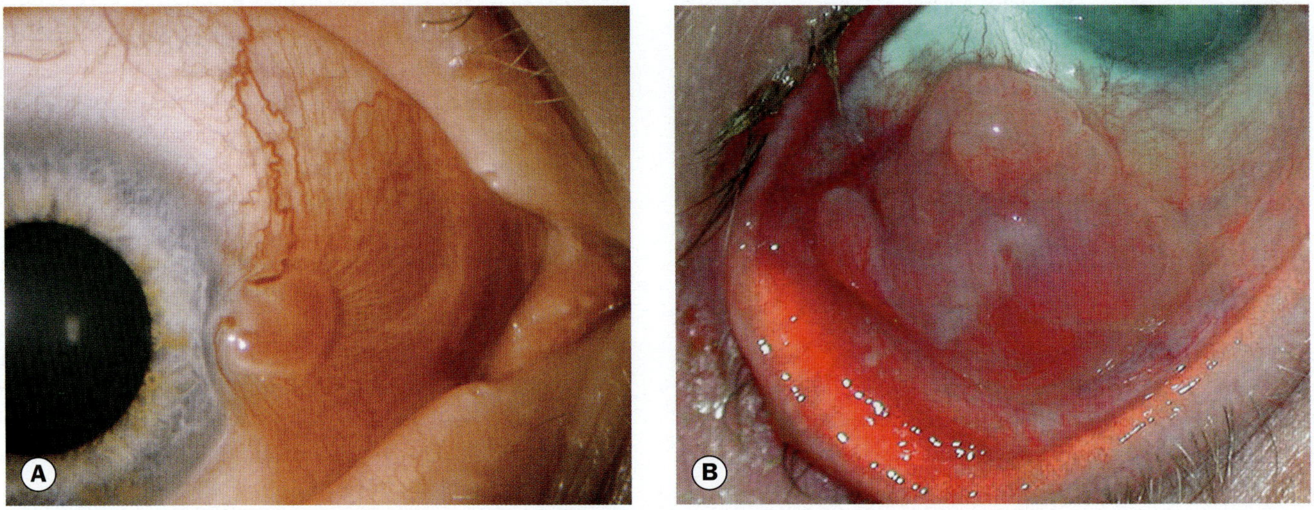

Fig. 20.5 **(A)** Pyogenic granuloma after pterygium surgery; **(B)** suture granuloma. *(Courtesy of S Chen – fig. B.)*

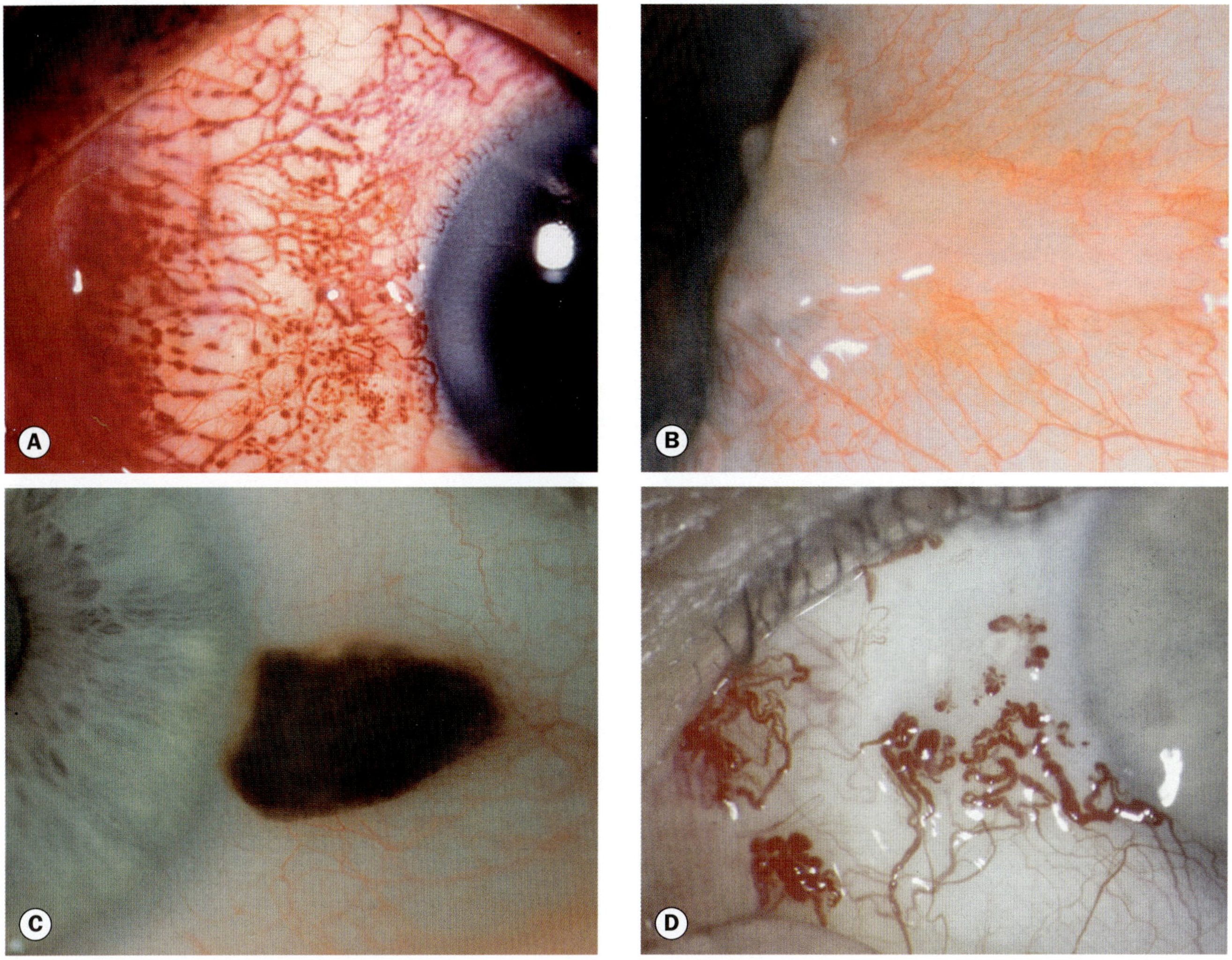

Fig. 20.6 Miscellaneous benign conjunctival tumours. **(A)** Epibulbar telangiectasia in Sturge–Weber syndrome; **(B)** reactive pseudoepitheliomatous hyperplasia; **(C)** melanocytoma; **(D)** angioma secondary to radiation. *(Courtesy of C Barry – fig. D.)*

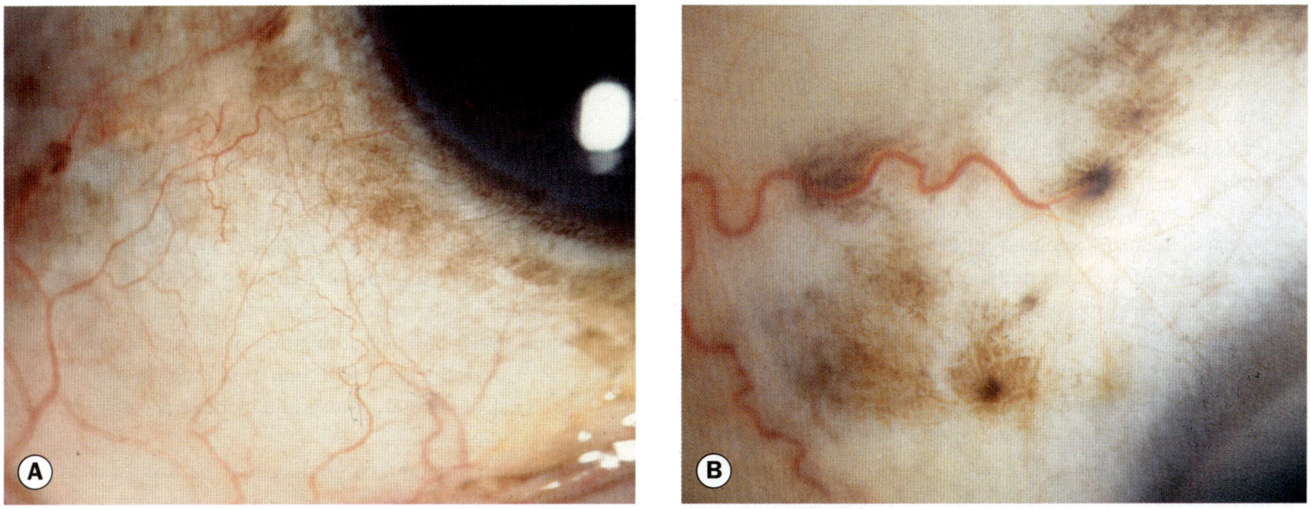

Fig. 20.7 Epithelial (racial) melanosis. **(A)** Juxtalimbal involvement; **(B)** at site of perforating vessel and nerve.

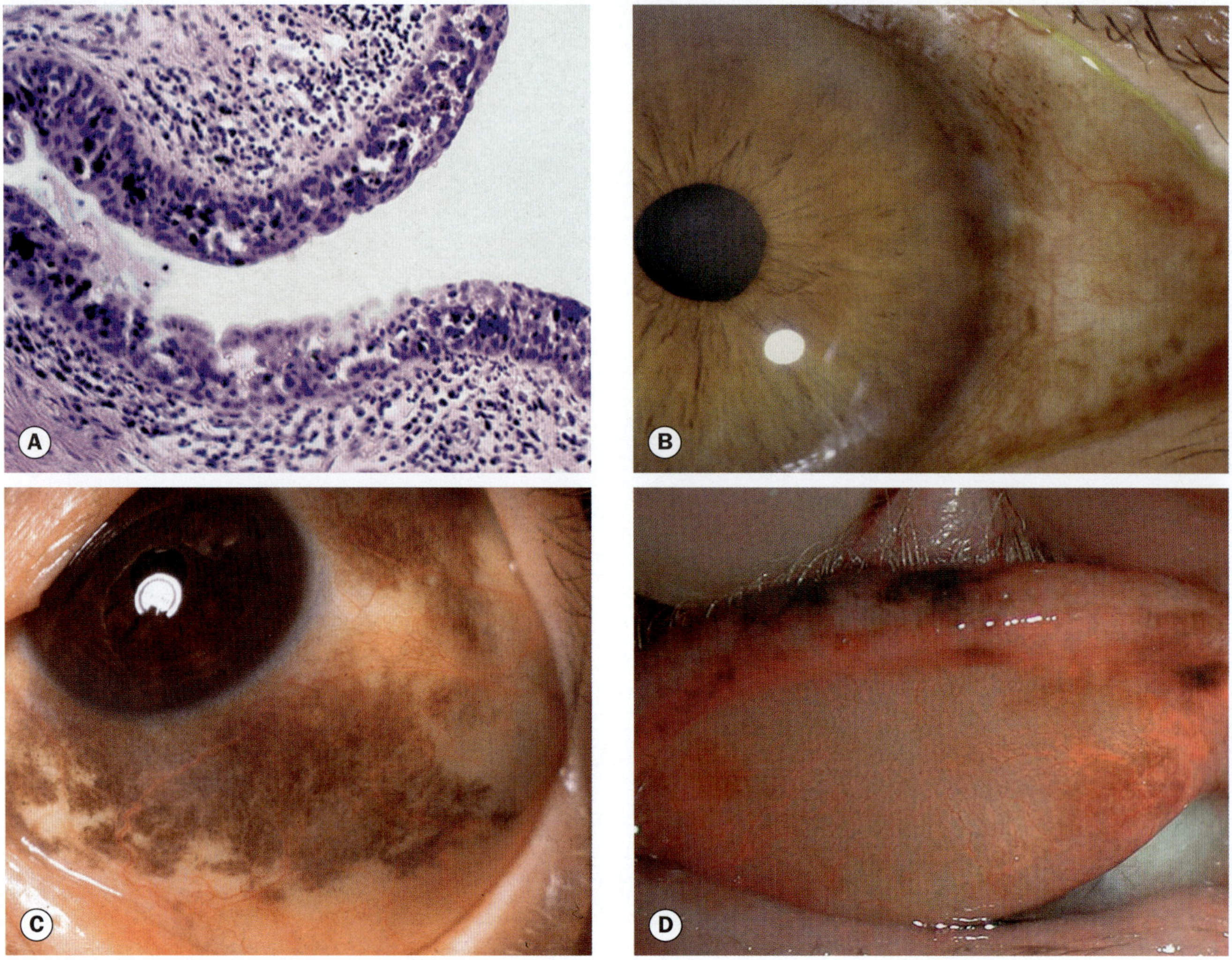

Fig. 20.8 Primary acquired melanosis (PAM). **(A)** Histology showing intraepithelial proliferation of conjunctival melanocytes; **(B)** small area of PAM; **(C)** more extensive PAM; **(D)** tarsal PAM associated with lentigo maligna of the eyelid. *(Courtesy of J Harry and G Misson, from* Clinical Ophthalmic Pathology, *Butterworth-Heinemann 2001 – fig. A; C Barry – fig. B.)*

Diagnosis

- **Symptoms.** A pigmented area is noticed on the surface of one or both (10%) eyes at a median age of 56 years, usually in a White individual.
- **Signs**
  - Uni- or multifocal flat areas of irregular golden-brown to dark chocolate-coloured epithelial pigmentation, typically involving the limbus and interpalpebral region (Fig. 20.8B and C). PAM *sine pigmento* has been reported.
  - Because any part of the conjunctiva may be affected, it is important to evert the eyelids (Fig. 20.8D). C-MIN may also extend onto the cornea.
  - Transformation to melanoma may be suggested by the appearance of nodular areas.
- **Investigation.** Careful documentation with drawing and/or photography of lesions undergoing observation is important. Immunohistochemical analysis of biopsied lesions is performed.
- **Treatment**
  - Observation of small (less than one clock hour) lesions may be appropriate, but some specialists advocate excision biopsy of every lesion.
  - Excision biopsy is generally preferred to incisional biopsy if possible (see under conjunctival melanoma below for surgical approach).
  - Double freeze–thaw cryotherapy may be administered to the excision site and/or following histological confirmation of C-MIN postoperative topical mitomycin C, e.g. four cycles of 0.04% four times daily for 7 days separated by 3-week intervals, with punctum plugs *in situ* to reduce the risk of punctal stenosis and increase drug–surface contact time.
  - Amniotic membrane grafting may be necessary for large excision sites.
  - In larger lesions, mapping using incisional biopsies can be accompanied by cryotherapy to all pigmented areas.
  - Long-term follow-up is mandatory in all cases.

- Corneal involvement: alcohol-mediated removal of the epithelium, followed by topical mitomycin C.

Conjunctival melanoma

Conjunctival melanoma is an uncommon but serious condition, accounting for about 12% of conjunctival tumours and 2% of all ocular malignancies. Around 75% arise from an area of PAM, about 25% from a pre-existing junctional or compound naevus and rarely, *de novo*. Presentation is often in the sixth decade, though patients with the rare dysplastic naevus syndrome develop multiple melanomas at a considerably younger age. The differential diagnosis includes naevus, ciliary body melanoma with extraocular extension, melanocytoma and pigmented conjunctival squamous carcinoma. The overall mortality is up to 19% at 5 years and 30% at 10 years. Metastasis occurs in 20–30%, particularly to regional lymph nodes, lung, brain and liver. Factors associated with a poor prognosis include caruncular, forniceal or lid margin location and tumour thickness of 2 mm or more.

Diagnosis

- **Histology** shows melanomatous cellular atypia with invasion of the subepithelial stroma (Fig. 20.9A).
- **Appearance.** A black or grey vascularized nodule that may be fixed to the episclera. The limbus is a common site, but a melanoma may arise anywhere in the conjunctiva (Fig. 20.9B–D). A conjunctival melanoma may extend into the eyelid (Fig. 20.9E and F). Association with PAM/C-MIN is very common.
- **Amelanotic tumours** may give rise to diagnostic difficulty.
- **B-scan ultrasonography** may be helpful in characterization of the lesion.
- **Systemic screening** consists of regular general examination, liver function testing and ultrasound, chest X-ray and possibly whole-body positron emission tomography/computed tomography (PET/CT) imaging where available.
- **Sentinel lymph node biopsy** may be helpful in staging, though its place has not yet been fully defined.

Treatment

- Circumscribed lesions are treated by excision with a wide margin. As tumour seeding can occur during excision, contact with the tumour itself should be avoided and fresh instruments used to close the conjunctival defect.
- Adjunctive radiotherapy is routinely administered by some authorities, even if histology suggests that excision is complete. Cryotherapy to the bed and surrounding tissue is an alternative. Proton beam radiotherapy can be applied if the caruncle or fornix is involved.
- Diffuse melanoma associated with extensive PAM/C-MIN is treated by excision of localized nodules with mitomycin C or cryotherapy to the diffuse component.
- Orbital recurrences are treated by local resection and radiotherapy. Exenteration may not improve survival and is therefore reserved for patients with extensive and aggressive disease when the eye cannot be preserved.
- The drug vemurafenib improves survival in patients with metastatic disease when the BRAF V600E mutation is present (50% of primary and metastatic conjunctival melanomas).
- Multifocal disease, non-limbal tumour location, tumour margin involvement and lack of adjunctive treatment are associated with a greater likelihood of recurrence.

Ocular surface squamous neoplasia

Introduction

Ocular surface squamous neoplasia (OSSN) describes a spectrum of slowly progressive, benign, premalignant and malignant epithelial lesions of the conjunctiva and cornea. Older adults are usually affected unless a predisposing systemic condition is present. Squamous carcinoma accounts for about 14% of conjunctival tumours. There is a male predominance in Europe and the USA, but in sub-Saharan Africa it is more common in women, particularly if they are HIV-positive. Risk factors include ultraviolet light exposure, a pale complexion, ciclosporin, smoking, petroleum product exposure, acquired immunodeficiency syndrome (AIDS) and xeroderma pigmentosum. Human papillomavirus infection (especially type 16) has been implicated in some cases. Metastatic disease is rare.

Diagnosis

- **Histology** shows a spectrum of abnormality. The first two are sometimes termed conjunctival–corneal intraepithelial neoplasia (CCIN):
  - Conjunctival epithelial dysplasia, where dysplastic cells are confined to the basal epithelial layers.
  - Carcinoma *in situ*, where dysplastic cells involve the full thickness of the epithelium (Fig. 20.10A).
  - Squamous cell carcinoma where there is invasion of the underlying stroma (Fig. 20.10B).
- **Symptoms.** A visible mass in one eye, sometimes accompanied by conjunctivitis-type symptoms.
- **Signs** are variable, and clinical correlation with histological severity is unreliable. Most tend to develop within the interpalpebral fissure, particularly at the limbus, although any part of the conjunctiva or cornea may be involved. The lesion may appear fleshy, gelatinous, leukoplakic or papillomatous, superficial or feeder vessels may be prominent, or the appearance may be avascular (Fig. 20.10C–F). Intraocular extension is uncommon. In patients who are heavy smokers the tumour tends to be large and in the inferior fornix.
- **Investigations** include ultrasonic biomicroscopy (UBM) or anterior segment optical coherence tomography (OCT) to estimate the depth of invasion, exfoliative cytology and impression cytology.

Treatment

- **Excision** with 2–4 mm margins and assessment for completeness of clearance has been the conventional standard approach often with intraoperative frozen section. It is important not to cut below Bowman membrane as recurrent disease can

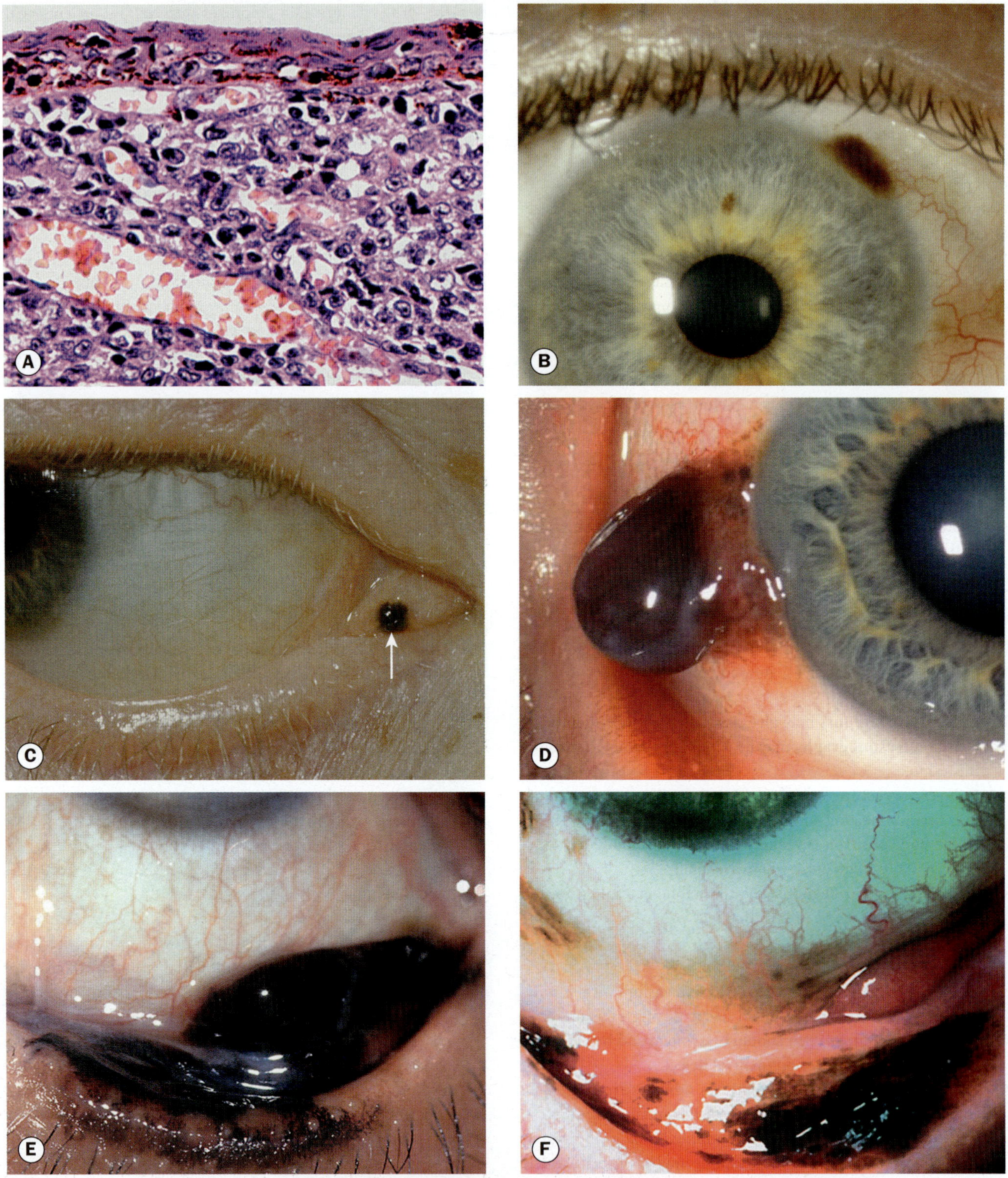

Fig. 20.9 Conjunctival melanoma. **(A)** Histology showing melanoma cells within the epithelium and subepithelial stroma; **(B)** small limbal melanoma; **(C)** small caruncular melanoma (arrow); **(D)** conjunctival melanoma with vascularization; **(E)** caruncular melanoma extending onto the eyelid margin; **(F)** conjunctival melanoma extending into the eyelid. *(Courtesy of C Barry – fig. E.)*

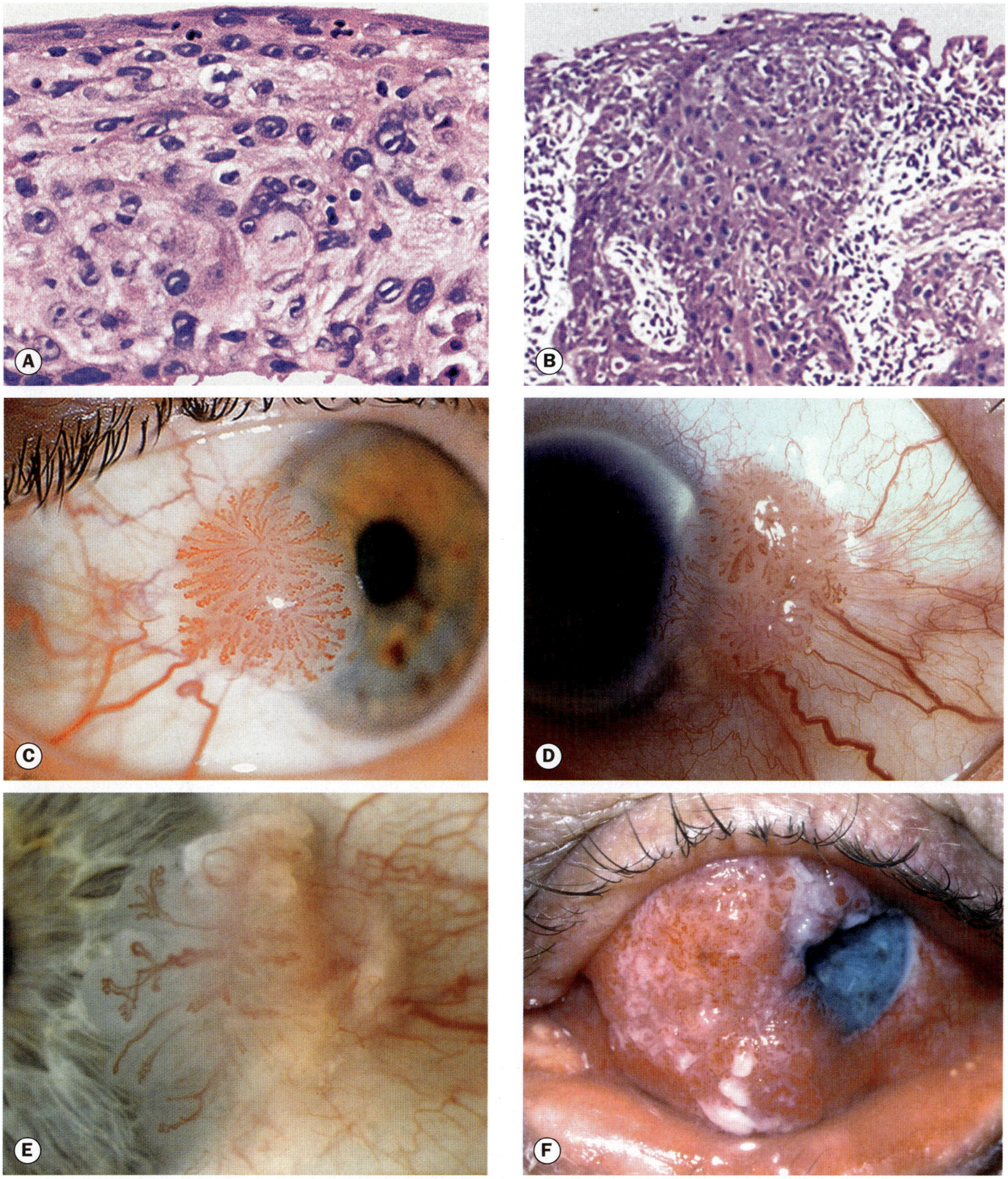

Fig. 20.10 Ocular surface squamous neoplasia. **(A)** Histology of carcinoma *in situ* showing dysplastic changes throughout the thickened epithelium; **(B)** histology of squamous cell carcinoma showing downward proliferation of irregular dysplastic epithelium with infiltration of subepithelial tissue; **(C)** nasal lesion extending onto the cornea; **(D)** large gelatinous lesion with feeder vessels; **(E)** nodular lesion; **(F)** extensive lesion in patient with AIDS.

potentially penetrate the corneal stroma. Complete histological excision may be associated with recurrence. Adjunctive measures reduce the rate of reappearance and include cryotherapy, brachytherapy or topical chemotherapy. Subconjunctival interferon injections can also be employed.

- **Topical chemotherapy.** Traditionally used as adjunctive treatment, this may also be employed as a primary modality to: (a) avoid the scarring and stem cell damage associated with extensive excision, (b) reduce tumour size prior to excision, or (c) treat recurrence.
  - 5-Fluorouracil drops can be administered four times daily for a week, followed by a 3-week resting period of no medication. These cycles are continued until complete resolution is achieved. Side effects include eyelid oedema and keratopathy. Recurrence rates are less than 10%.
  - Topical interferon alfa-2b requires refrigeration and is expensive, but is particularly effective and complete tumour resolution can be achieved in approximately 80% of patients. Subconjunctival interferon is available for patients with a superiorly located tumour. In individuals whose immune system is suppressed, a once-daily instillation of interferon drops should be used lifelong to prevent recurrence.
  - Alternatively, Mitomycin C can also be used, but it is more likely to be associated with ocular side effects than other options.

Lymphoproliferative lesions

Introduction

The most common conjunctival lymphoproliferative lesion is reactive lymphoid hyperplasia, a proliferation of both B and T cells with germinal follicle formation. Conjunctival lymphoma may arise *de novo*, by extension from orbital lymphoma or associated with systemic lymphoma at diagnosis (up to 30%). Most conjunctival lymphomas are of B-cell origin, arising from mucosa-associated lymphoid tissue (MALT) and tending to be indolent. Lymphoma accounts for about 7% of all conjunctival tumours.

Diagnosis

- **Histology** shows reactive lymphoid hyperplasia with a germinal lymphoid follicle consisting of immature lymphoid cells at the centre and mature cells at the periphery (Fig. 20.11A).
- **Symptoms.** Painless swelling, redness or irritation (which is often bilateral when systemic disease is more likely). Other possible symptoms include ptosis and diplopia.
- **Signs.** A slowly growing salmon-pink or flesh-coloured mobile infiltrate is seen on the epibulbar surface (Fig. 20.11B) or in the fornices (Fig. 20.11C and see Fig.20.4D). Rarely, a diffuse lesion (Fig. 20.11D) may mimic chronic conjunctivitis.
- **Biopsy** is taken to confirm diagnosis. The uninvolved eye should also be biopsied (inferior fornix).
- **Investigation** for systemic involvement.

Treatment

- **Systemic disease** is treated if needed.
- **External beam radiotherapy.**
- **Other options** include chemotherapy, excision of small lesions with adjuvant treatment, cryotherapy and intralesional injections of interferon alfa-2b or rituximab.
- **Prognosis** is dependent on the histological features. Patients with mantle cell lymphoma have a very poor chance of 5-year survival.

Primary amyloidosis

Amyloidosis is a heterogeneous group of diseases characterized by extracellular amyloid deposits in different organs including the orbit and periocular tissues. The most common form of local amyloidosis is caused by the deposition of monoclonal immunoglobulin light chains by a benign B-cell or plasma-cell clone. It is a rare cause of an orbital mass and can mimic lymphoma (Fig. 20.12). It presents with a wide spectrum of clinical findings, including ptosis and epiphora. Approximately 25% have periocular discomfort. The usual age of presentation is about 60 years and two-thirds are unilateral. Only 5% have systemic involvement. The diagnosis is made histologically using Congo red staining, which shows green birefringence. The usual treatment is surgical excision of the mass and observation.

Kaposi sarcoma

Kaposi sarcoma is a slowly growing tumour that is typically found in individuals with AIDS, but occasionally in the elderly and when there is long-term immunosuppression. A vascular bright red or purplish plaque or nodule is seen (Fig. 20.13), sometimes resembling (or associated with) conjunctival haemorrhage. Histology reveals a proliferation of spindle-shaped cells, vascular channels and inflammatory cells. If treatment is necessary, systemic AIDS therapy should be optimized, with local radiotherapy, excision and local or systemic chemotherapy as additional options.

IRIS TUMOURS

Iris naevus

An iris naevus consists of a proliferation of melanocytes in the superficial iris stroma and appears as a circumscribed solitary flat or variably elevated pigmented lesion (Fig. 20.14). The normal iris architecture is disrupted. A diffuse naevus characteristically occurs in congenital ocular melanocytosis and in iris naevus (Cogan–Reese) syndrome (see Ch. 11). The malignant transformation rate is up to 8% over 15 years. Risk factors include young age (under 40), inferior location, bleeding from the lesion, diffuse iris involvement, feathery margins and ectropion uveae. Observation should be lifelong and involve documentation by slit lamp examination and photography.

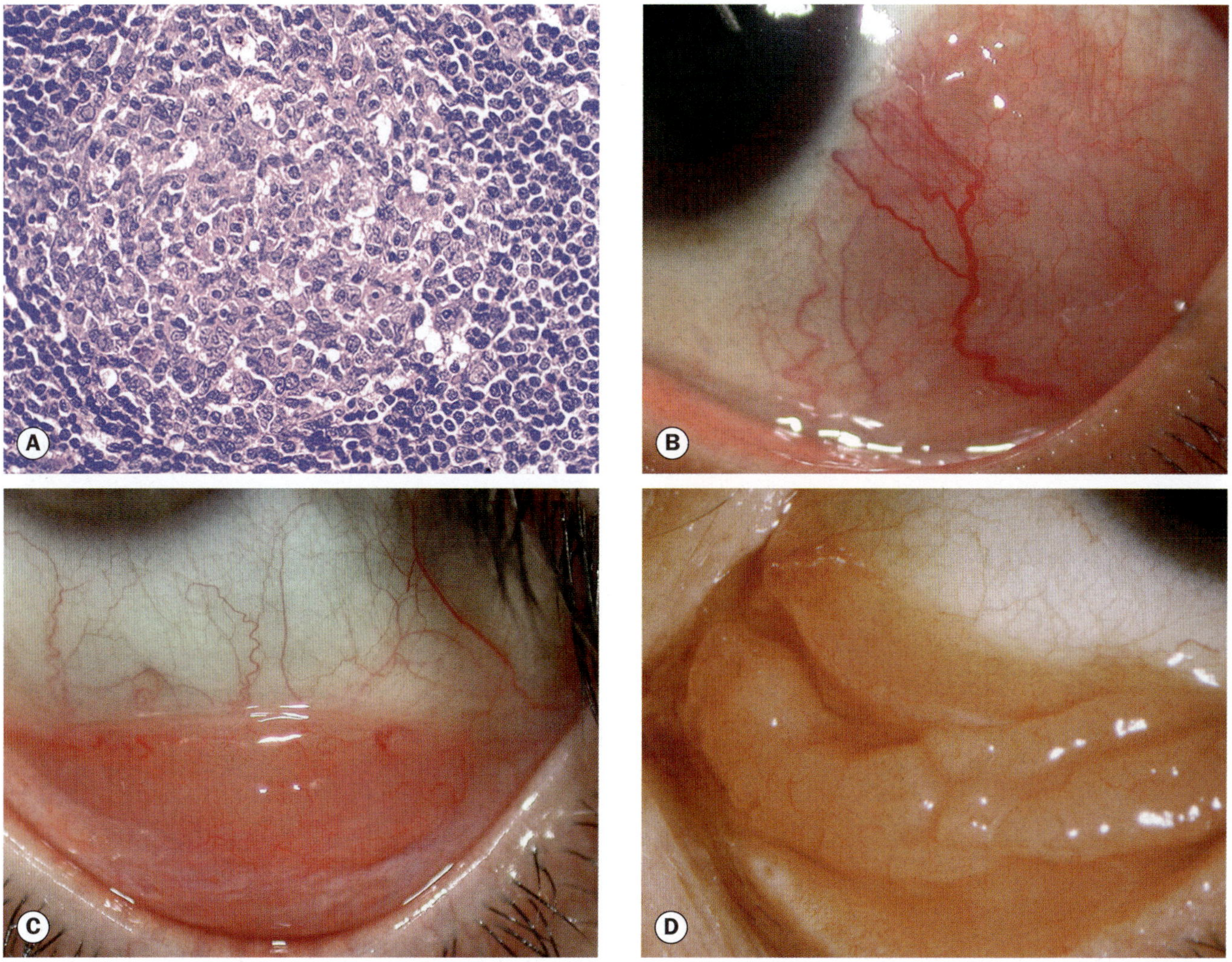

Fig. 20.11 Conjunctival lymphoproliferative lesions. **(A)** Histology shows reactive lymphoid hyperplasia with a germinal lymphoid follicle; **(B)** epibulbar lymphoma; **(C)** forniceal lymphoma; **(D)** diffuse lymphoma. *(Courtesy of J Harry and G Mission, from* Clinical Ophthalmic Pathology, *Butterworth-Heinemann 2001 – fig. A.)*

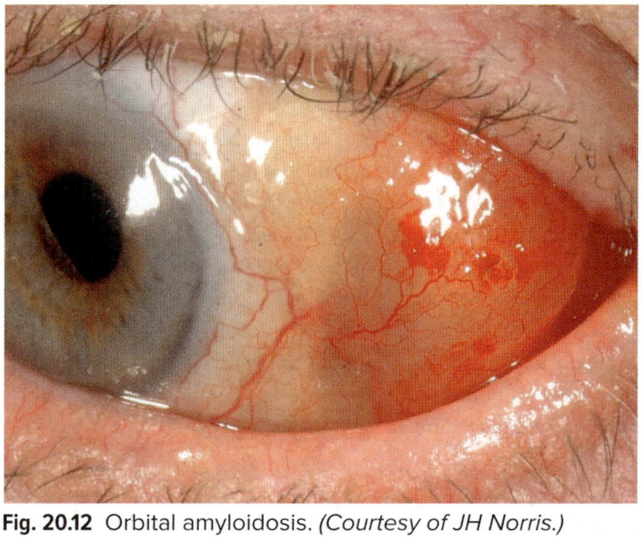

Fig. 20.12 Orbital amyloidosis. *(Courtesy of JH Norris.)*

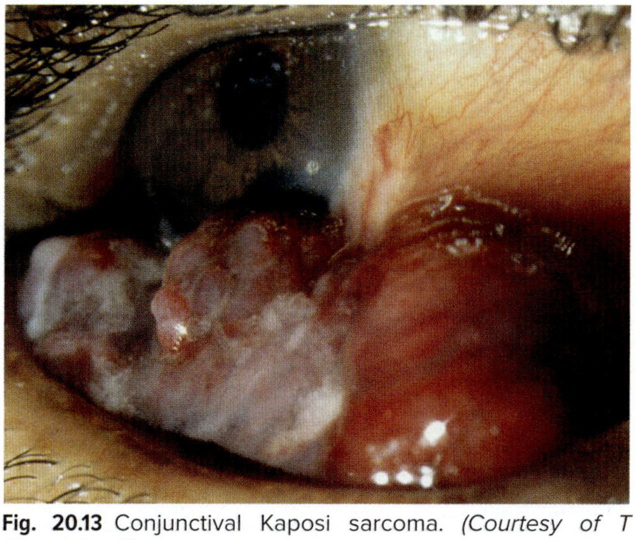

Fig. 20.13 Conjunctival Kaposi sarcoma. *(Courtesy of T Carmichael.)*

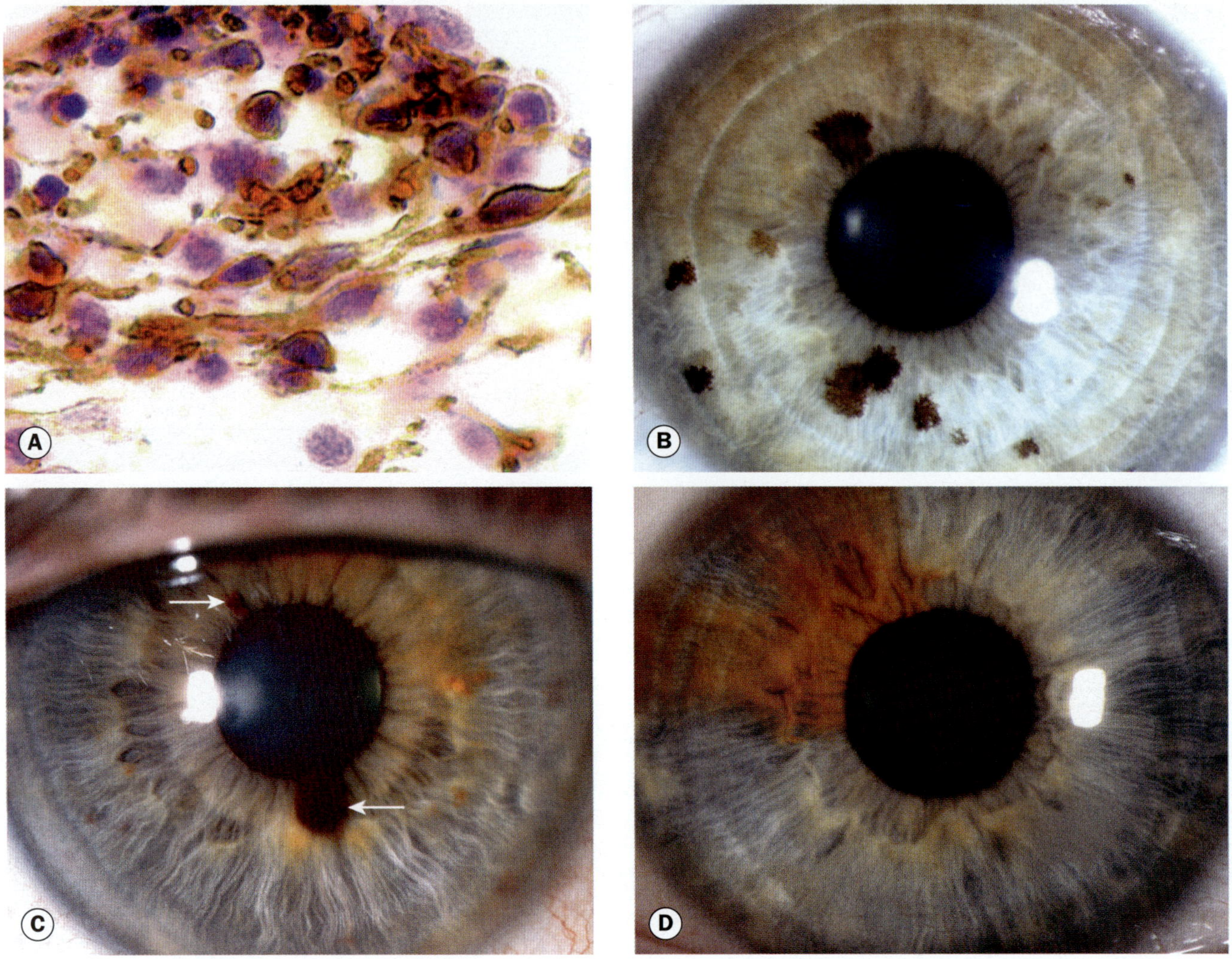

Fig. 20.14 Iris naevus. (A) Histology showing localized proliferation of melanocytes on the anterior iris stroma; (B) numerous small naevi; (C) naevi at pupil margin (arrows); (D) large naevus.

Iris freckle (ephelis)

Iris freckles are superficial lesions that are smaller than a naevus, with no elevation or distortion (Fig. 20.15A) and show increased melanocyte pigmentation with a normal number of cells.

Brushfield spots

These are small whitish peripheral iris speckles arranged in a concentric ring (Fig. 20.15B), occurring particularly in Down syndrome though also as a normal finding in blue eyes. They consist of a mildly hyperplastic focus surrounded by a ring of hypoplasia and have no malignant potential (see also Ch. 10).

Lisch nodules

These are small well-defined nodules (Fig. 20.15C and D) found in both eyes of virtually all patients with neurofibromatosis type 1 (see Ch. 19).

Iris melanoma

Introduction

About 8% of uveal melanomas arise in the iris. The prognosis is comparatively good – only about 5% of patients develop metastasis within 10 years of treatment. Conditions associated with or predisposing to uveal melanomas include fair skin and lighter iris colour, numerous and/or atypical (dysplastic) cutaneous naevi, iris or choroidal naevus, congenital ocular and oculodermal melanocytosis (naevus of Ota) and uveal melanocytoma. Chronic sunlight exposure and arc welding are environmental risk factors. Presentation is typically in middle age, a decade earlier than ciliary body and choroidal melanoma.

Diagnosis

- **Histology** usually shows diffusely infiltrating spindle cells (see below) of low-grade malignancy (Fig. 20.16A). A minority contain an epithelioid cell component and can be more aggressive.

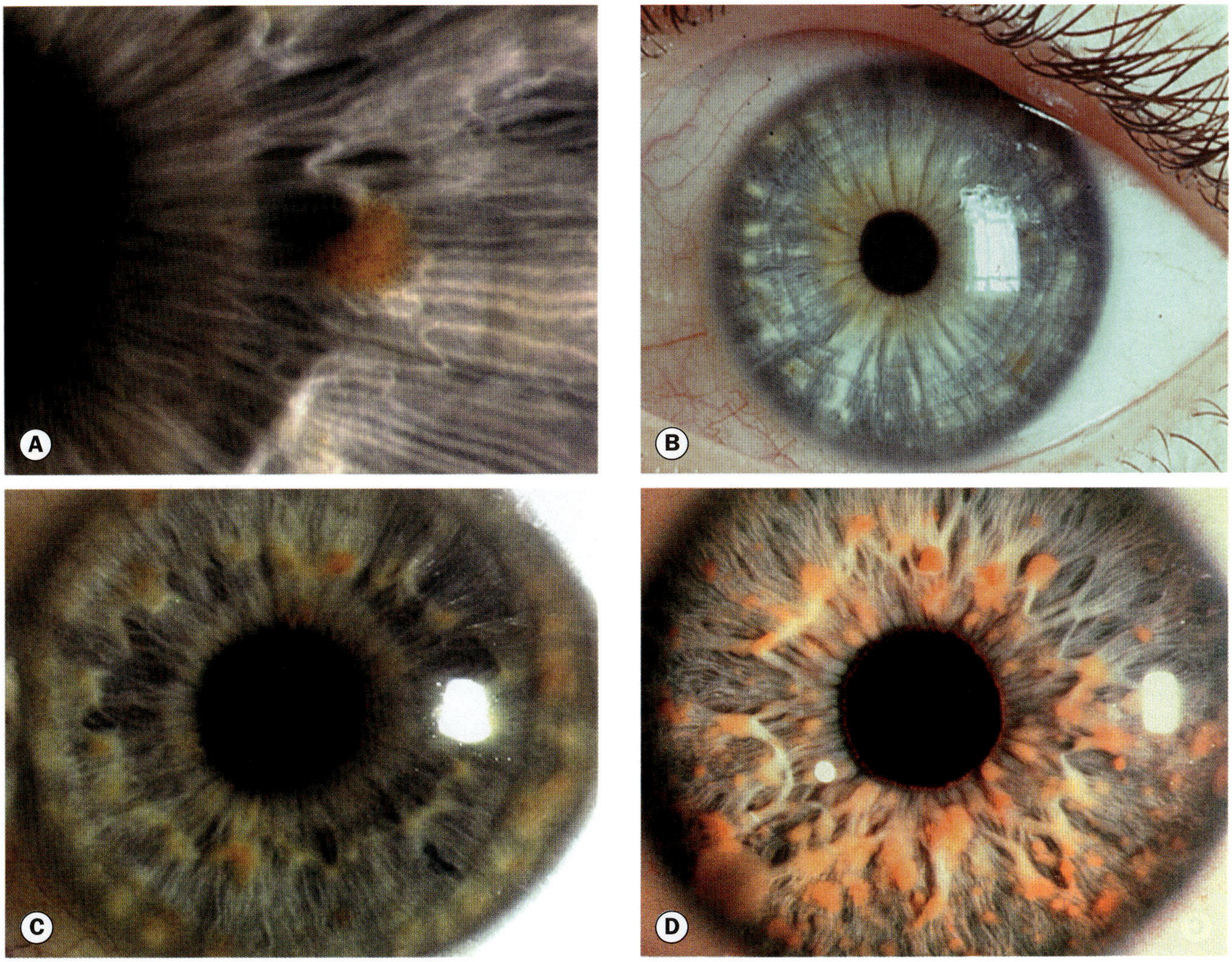

Fig. 20.15 **(A)** Iris freckle; **(B)** Brushfield spots; **(C)** Lisch nodules; **(D)** numerous Lisch nodules.

- **Symptoms.** Enlargement of a pre-existing naevus is typical, noticed either by the patient or at a routine eye examination. Signs indicative of malignant transformation include growth and the development of prominent blood vessels.
- **Signs**
  - A pigmented (Fig. 20.16B and C) nodule at least 3 mm in diameter and 1 mm thick, typically located in the inferior half of the iris and often associated with surface blood vessels.
  - Pupillary distortion, ectropion uveae (Fig. 20.16D) and occasionally localized cataract may be seen, although these can also occur with naevi.
  - A non-pigmented melanoma may occasionally be seen (Fig. 20.16E).
  - Growth is usually slow, with extension across the iris surface.
  - The angle and anterior ciliary body may be infiltrated, but extrascleral extension is rare (Fig. 20.16F).
  - Complications include hyphaema, cataract and glaucoma.
- **Ultrasound biomicroscopy** is used to rule out ciliary body involvement.
- **Fine-needle aspiration biopsy** may be employed prior to major surgical intervention.
- **Systemic investigation** should be carried out.

Treatment

- **Sector iridectomy** for small tumours and iridocyclectomy for tumours invading the angle.
- **Radiotherapy** with a radioactive plaque (brachytherapy) or external irradiation with a proton beam.
- **Enucleation** may be required for diffusely growing tumours if radiotherapy is not possible.
- **Monitoring** for recurrence and metastasis.

Metastatic tumours

Metastasis to the iris (Fig. 20.17) is rare and is characterized by one or more fast-growing white, pink or yellow masses that may be associated with anterior uveitis and occasionally hyphaema. Breast cancer, lung cancer and melanoma of the skin are among the most common primary types.

Miscellaneous iris tumours

- **Juvenile xanthogranuloma** is a rare idiopathic granulomatous disease of early childhood. Iris involvement is

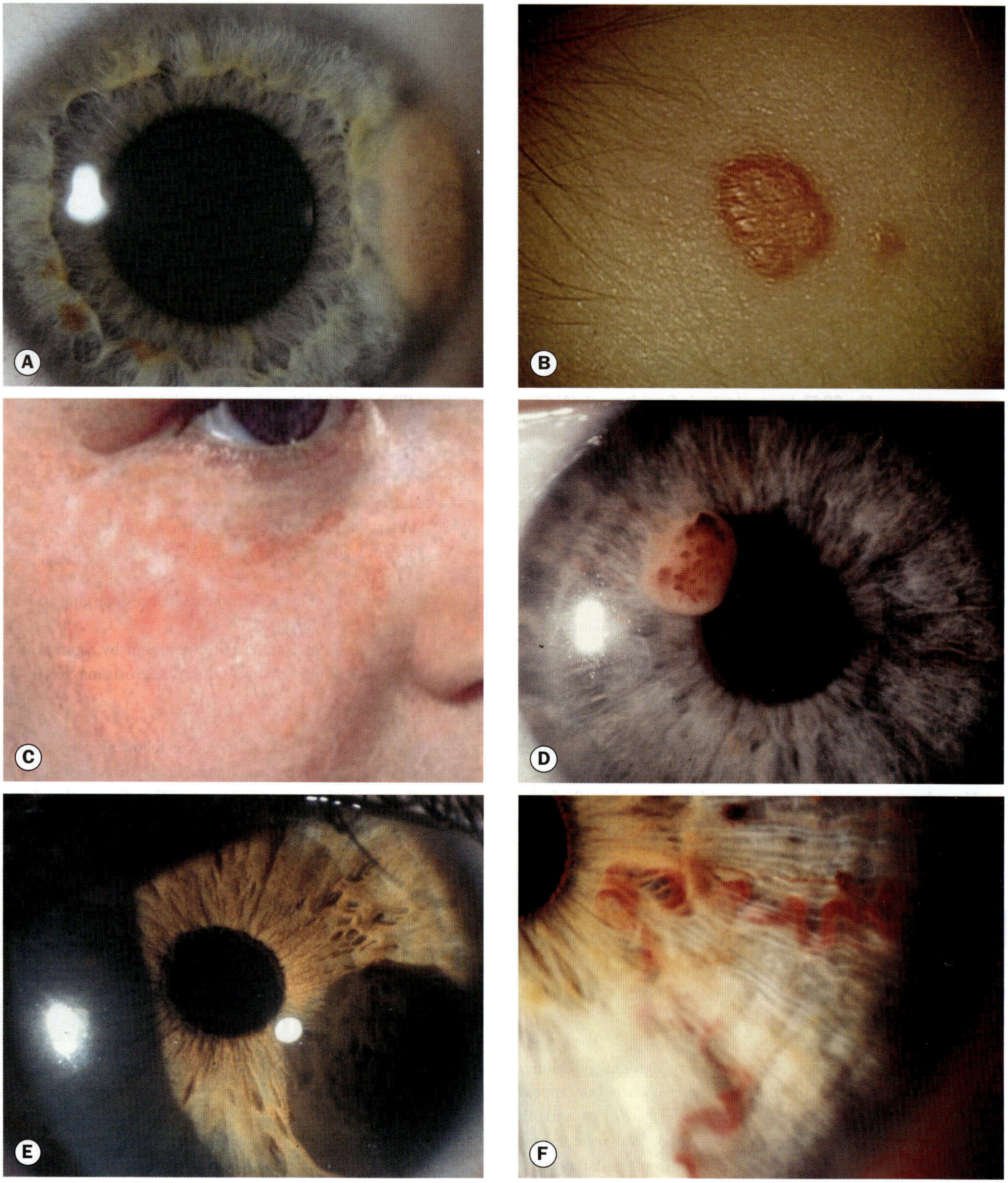

Fig. 20.18 **(A)** Juvenile iris xanthogranuloma; **(B)** xanthogranuloma of the skin; **(C)** facial skin involvement; **(D)** leiomyoma; **(E)** melanocytoma; **(F)** racemose haemangioma showing supplying and draining vessels. *(Courtesy of B Damato – figs A and D; D Hildebrand – fig. C.)*

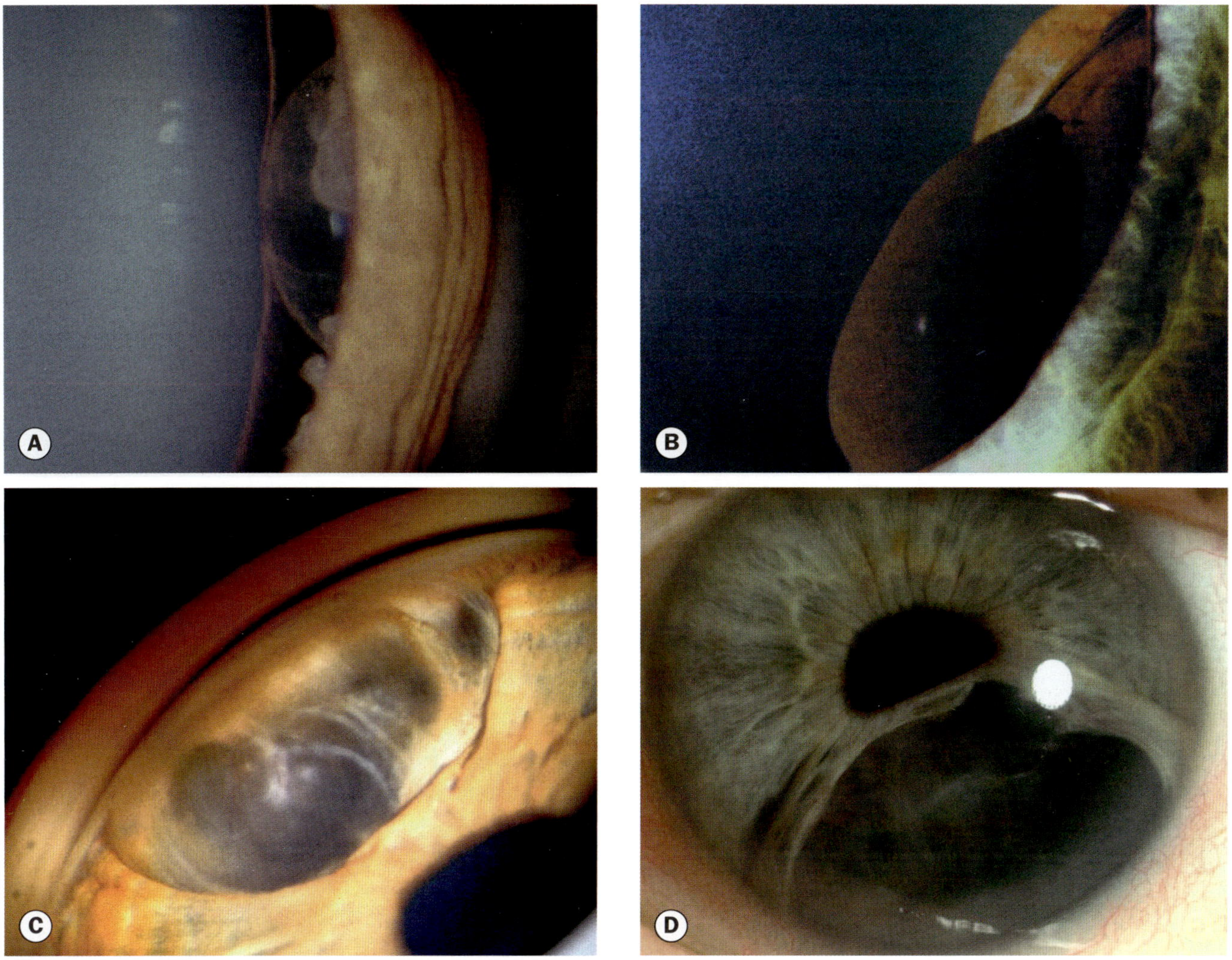

Fig. 20.19 Primary iris cysts. **(A)** Epithelial cyst; **(B)** pigmented epithelial cyst; **(C)** large stromal cyst on gonioscopy; **(D)** large stromal cyst.

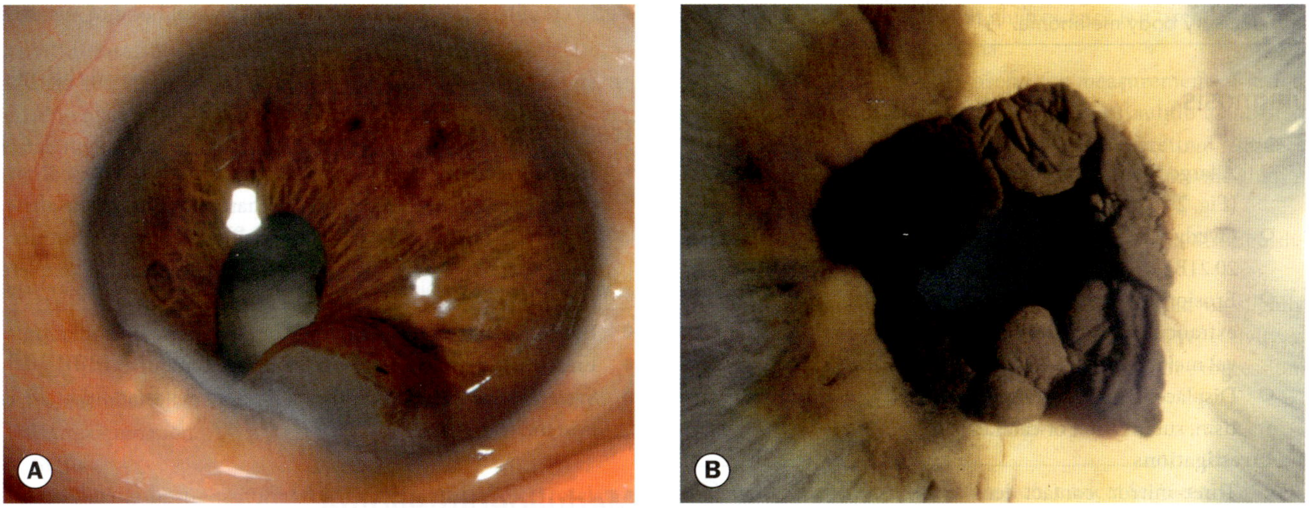

Fig. 20.20 Secondary iris cysts. **(A)** Traumatic cyst; **(B)** pigmented epithelial cysts at pupil margin secondary to prolonged miotic treatment. *(Courtesy of S Chen – fig. A.)*

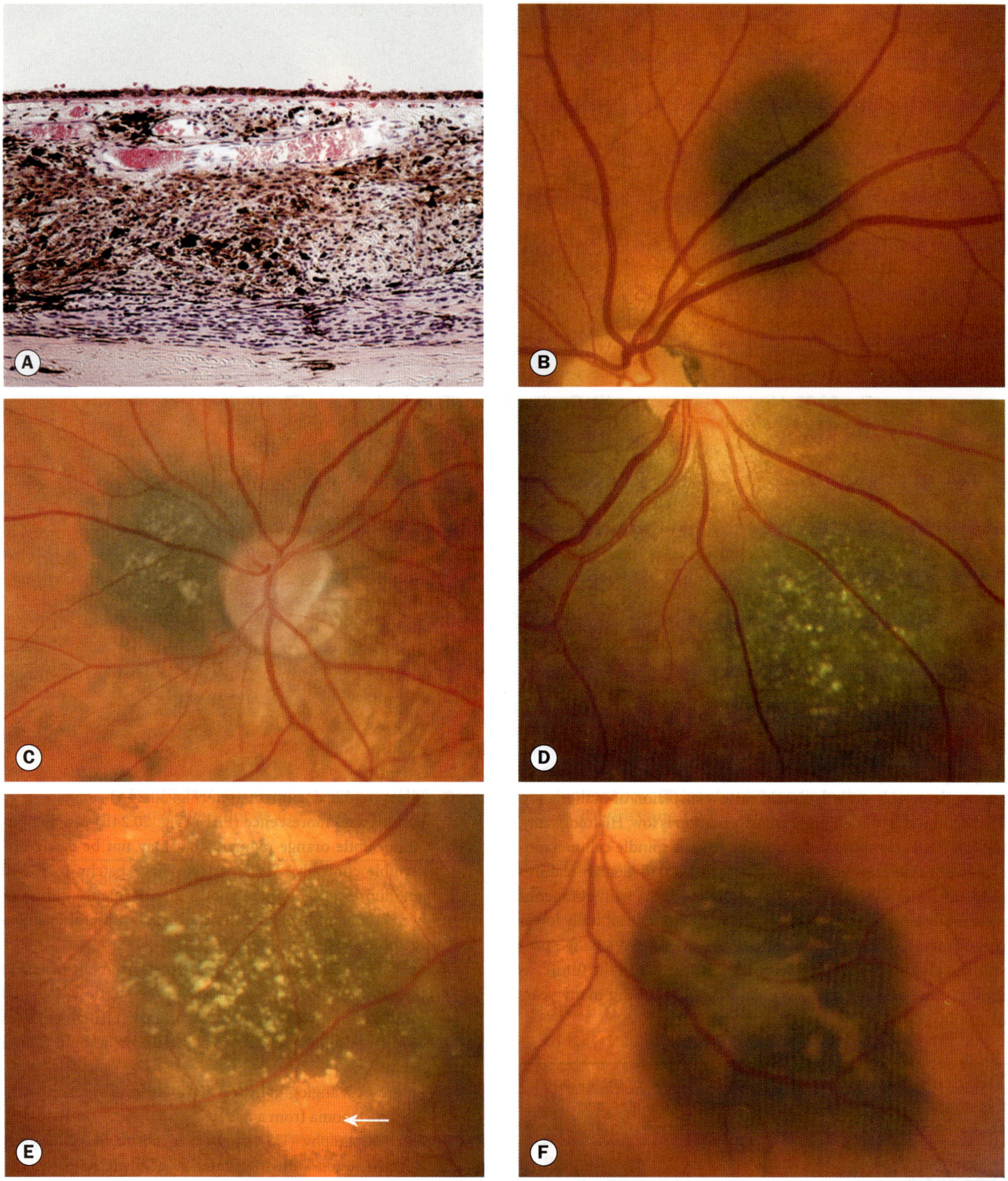

Fig. 20.23 Choroidal naevus. **(A)** Histology showing proliferation of melanocytes in the choroid, sparing the choriocapillaris; **(B)** typical flat naevus; **(C)** peripapillary naevus with overlying drusen; **(D)** larger naevus with benign features; **(E)** naevus with overlying drusen and distinct halo (arrow); **(F)** overlying orange pigment suspicious of early melanoma.

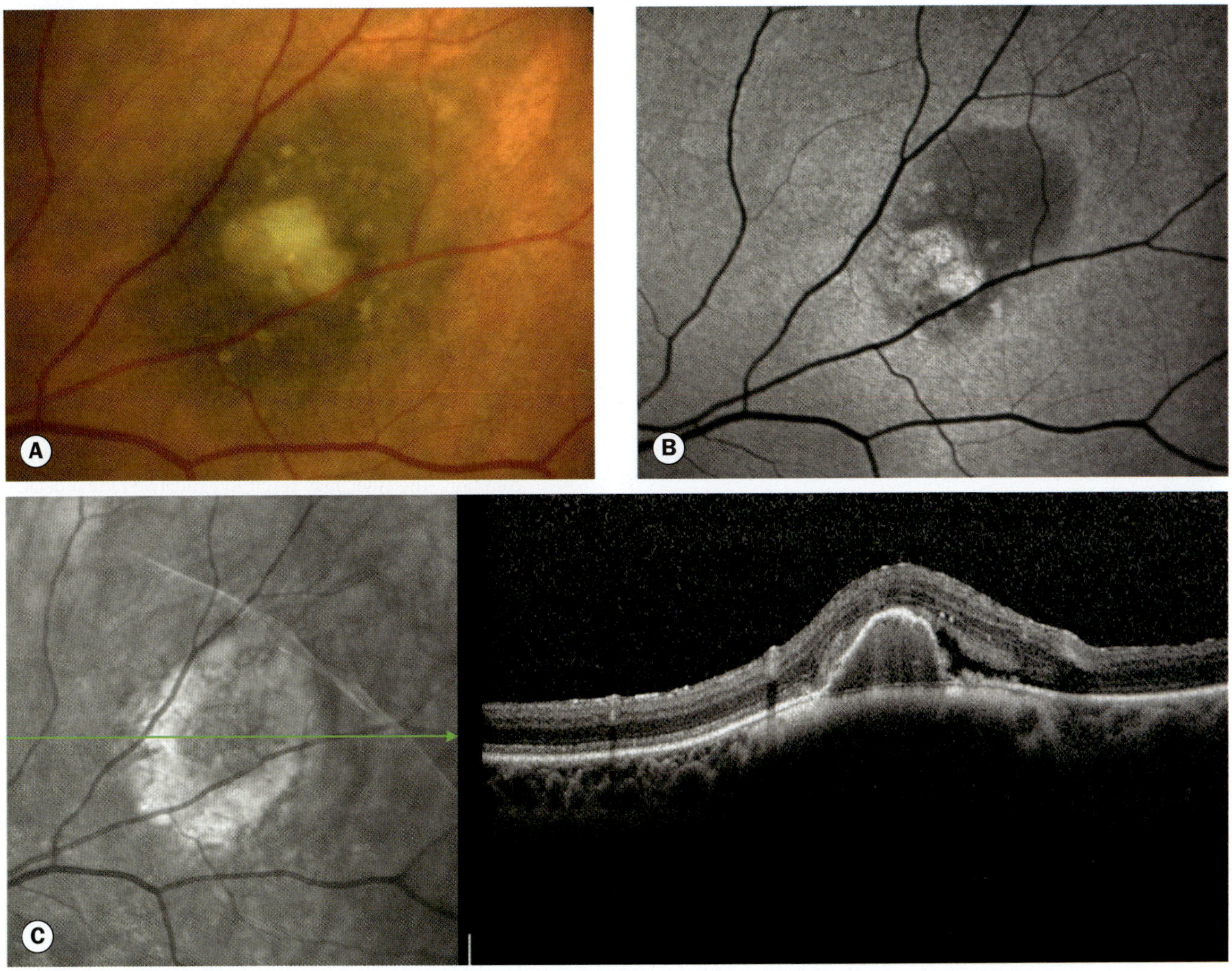

Fig. 20.24 Imaging of choroidal naevi. **(A)** Colour photograph; **(B)** fundus autofluorescence; **(C)** OCT.

Treatment

- **Baseline** fundus photography and ultrasonography or OCT, with indefinite regular review.
- **Review interval** is determined by level of suspicion:
  - No suspicious features: 6 months until stability established (e.g. 1 year), then annual review.
  - One or two suspicious features: 4–6 months.
  - Three or more suspicious features: consider referral for ocular oncology subspecialist assessment.
- **Growth.** If growth is documented or highly suspicious features are present, the lesion should generally be regarded as a melanoma and managed accordingly.

Choroidal melanoma

Choroidal melanoma is the most common primary intraocular malignancy in adults and accounts for 80% of all uveal melanomas, but it is still relatively uncommon. These tumours lack the most typical cutaneous melanoma-associated mutations and are instead characterized by a different set of genes. Predisposing factors are as for iris melanoma (above). Presentation peaks at around the age of 60 years. Most cases occur sporadically. Choroidal melanoma has distinct molecular features that differ from those found in cutaneous melanoma. Histopathology reveals spindle (Fig. 20.25A) and epithelioid (Fig. 20.25B) cell types; the former being arranged in bundles and having a better prognosis. Epithelioid cells are larger and more pleomorphic, with more frequent mitotic figures. Tumour composition is commonly exclusively spindle cell or a mixture of spindle and epithelioid. Lesions may penetrate Bruch membrane and the retinal pigment epithelium (RPE) with herniation into the subretinal space, classically assuming the shape of a collar stud (Fig. 20.25C). Scleral channel and vortex vein invasion can lead to orbital spread. Metastasis is commonly to the liver, bone and lung, but only about 1–2% of patients have detectable metastases at the time of presentation. Mortality is up to 50% at 10 years. Adverse prognostic factors include particular histological features (e.g. large numbers of epithelioid cells, mitotic activity), larger tumour dimensions, tumour genetic characteristics (e.g. somatic mutations in the tumour suppressor gene *BAP1*, present in nearly 50% of uveal melanomas, imply a greater chance of metastasis), extrascleral extension and anterior location.

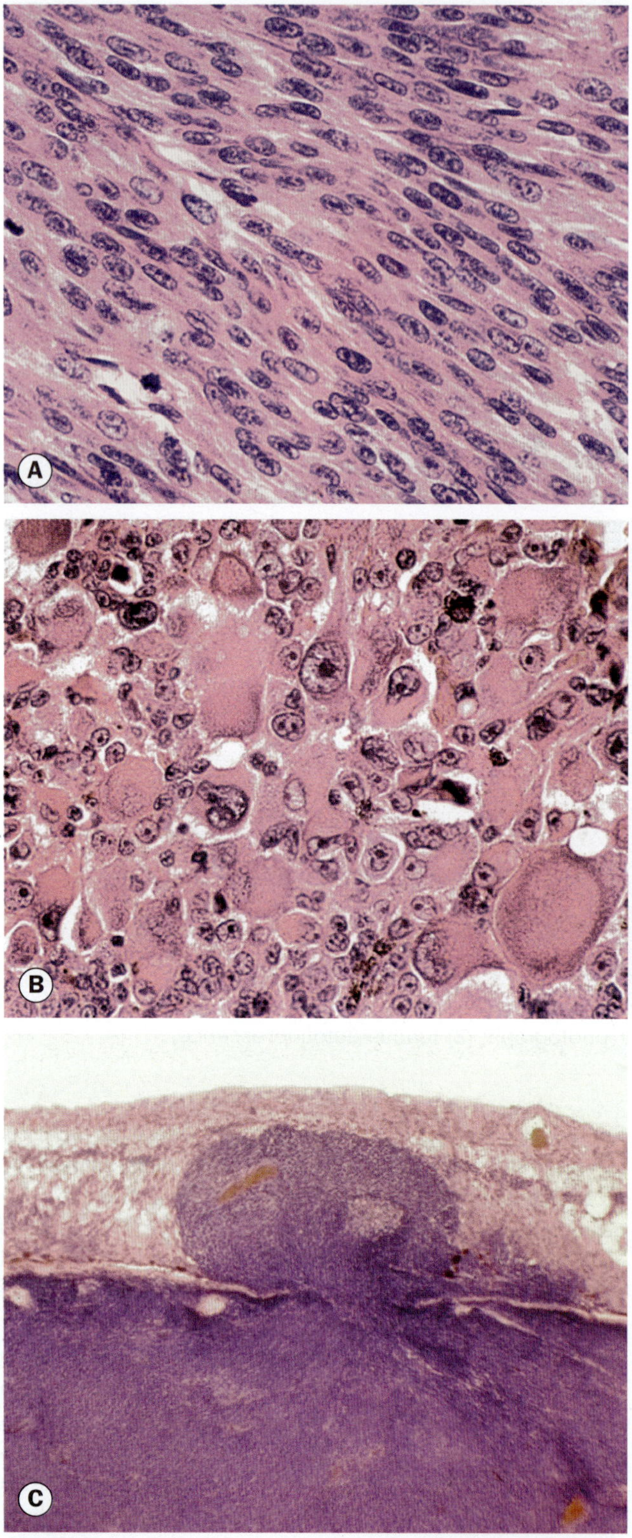

Fig. 20.25 Histology of choroidal melanoma. **(A)** Spindle cells – tightly arranged fusiform cells with indistinct cell membranes and slender or plump oval nuclei; **(B)** epithelioid cells – large pleomorphic cells with distinct cell membranes, large vesicular nuclei with prominent nucleoli, and abundant cytoplasm; **(C)** penetration of Bruch membrane in a 'collar stud' fashion. *(Courtesy of J Harry and G Misson, from* Clinical Ophthalmic Pathology, *Butterworth-Heinemann 2001 – figs A–C.)*

Diagnosis

- **Symptoms** are often absent, with a tumour detected by chance on routine fundus examination. A range of visual disturbance can occur depending on tumour characteristics.
- **Signs**
  - A solitary elevated subretinal grey-brown (Fig. 20.26A) or rarely amelanotic (Fig. 20.26B) dome-shaped mass. Diffuse infiltration is uncommon.
  - About 60% are located within 3 mm of the optic disc (Fig. 20.26C) or fovea.
  - Clumps of overlying orange pigment are common (Fig. 20.26D).
  - If the tumour breaks through Bruch membrane it acquires a 'collar stud' appearance (see Fig. 20.25C and Fig. 20.28C).
  - Associated haemorrhage and subretinal fluid (Fig. 20.26E) are common. The latter may result in exudative retinal detachment (Fig. 20.26F), which can mask the underlying lesion.
  - Other signs can include sentinel vessels (Fig. 20.27), choroidal folds, inflammation, rubeosis iridis, secondary glaucoma and cataract.

Differential diagnosis

- **Pigmented lesions**
  - A choroidal naevus usually exhibits numerous surface drusen, without serous retinal detachment and little if any orange pigment.
  - Melanocytoma is deeply pigmented and usually located at the optic disc.
  - Congenital hypertrophy of the RPE is flat, is often grey–black and has a well-defined margin with lacunae.
  - Haemorrhage in the subretinal or suprachoroidal space, for example from choroidal neovascularization or retinal artery macroaneurysm.
  - Metastatic cutaneous melanoma has a smooth surface, a light brown colour, indistinct margins, extensive retinal detachment and often a past history of malignancy.
- **Non-pigmented lesions**
  - Circumscribed choroidal haemangioma is typically posterior, pink, dome-shaped and has a smooth surface.
  - Metastasis is often associated with exudative retinal detachment.
  - Solitary choroidal granuloma, e.g. sarcoidosis, tuberculosis.
  - Posterior scleritis, which can present with a large elevated lesion. In contrast to melanoma, pain is a common feature.
  - Large elevated choroidal neovascular lesion, which can be eccentrically located, usually in the temporal pre-equatorial region, is typically associated with exudate and fresh haemorrhage, both of which rarely accompany a melanoma.
  - Prominent vortex vein ampulla is characterized by a small, smooth, brown, dome-shaped lesion, which disappears with pressure on the eye.

Investigation

Examination is sufficient for diagnosis in the majority of cases.

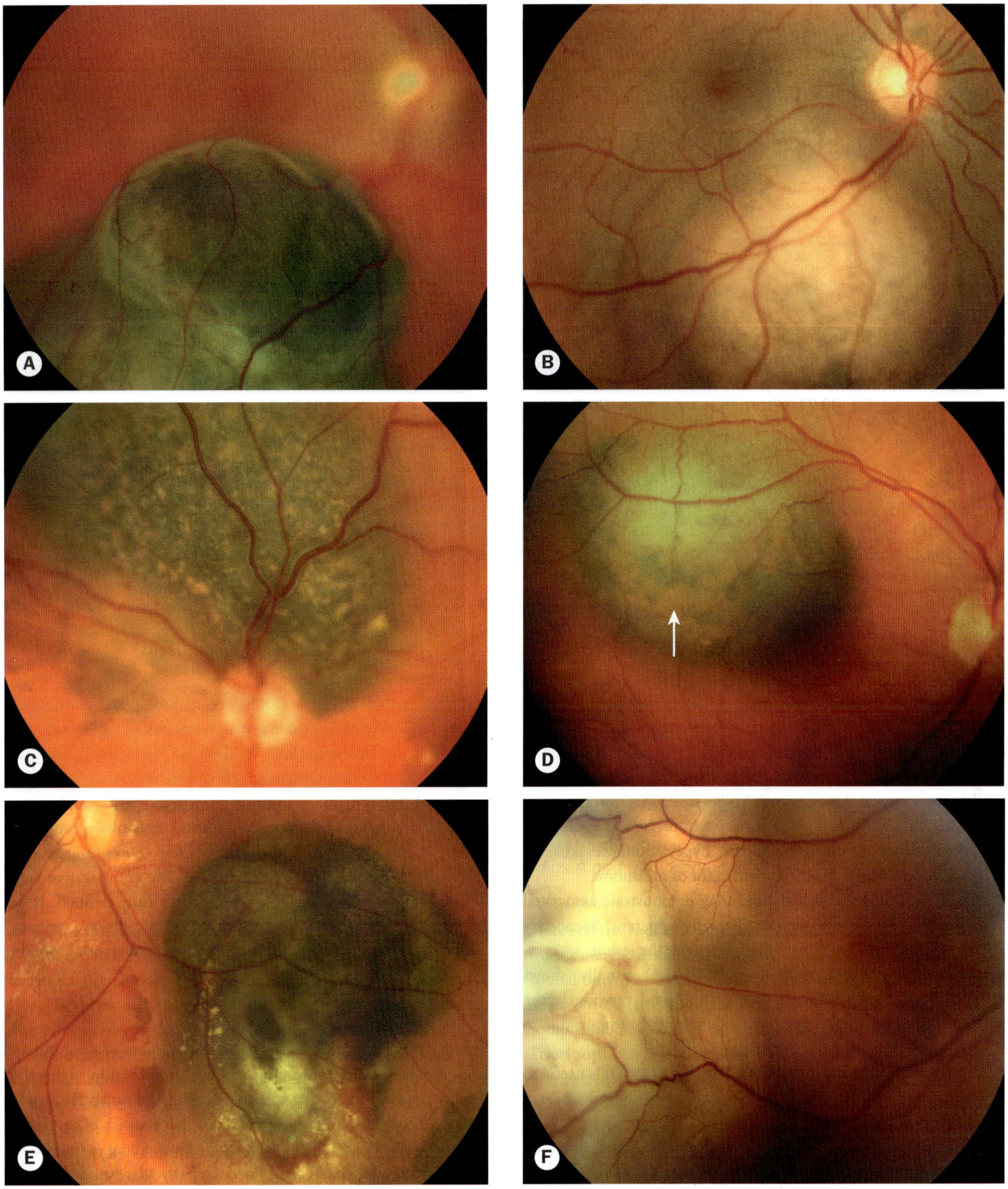

Fig. 20.26 Choroidal melanoma. **(A)** Typical pigmented melanoma; **(B)** amelanotic lesion; **(C)** choroidal melanoma adjacent to the optic disc; **(D)** overlying orange pigment (arrow); **(E)** associated haemorrhage and exudation; **(F)** peripheral melanoma with exudative retinal detachment, which may mask the underlying pathology. *(Courtesy of C Barry – figs A, E.)*

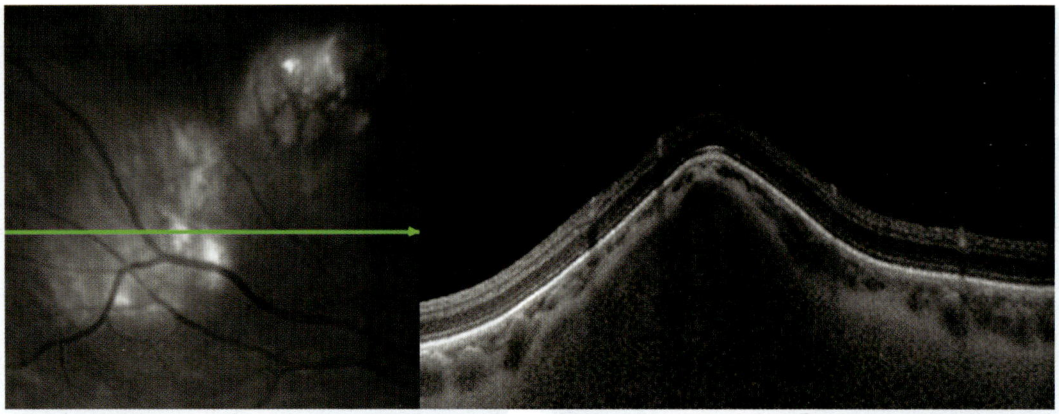

Fig. 20.36 Sclero-choroidal calcification. OCT showing a lesion arising from the sclera with abrupt elevation and a pointed surface which is compressing the choroid.

- Mammography.
- Chest radiography and sputum cytology.
- Liver function tests.
- Abdominal or whole-body scans.
- Faecal occult blood.
- Urinalysis for red blood cells.
- Abdominal ultrasound.
- Whole-body imaging, e.g. PET/CT, MRI.

Treatment

- **Observation**, if the patient is asymptomatic or receiving systemic chemotherapy, which may also be beneficial for choroidal metastases.
- **Radiotherapy**, either external beam or brachytherapy, typically for solitary lesions.
- **TTT and PDT** are useful for small tumours with minimal subretinal fluid.
- **Anti-VEGF treatment** may lead to regression of metastases in some cases, as well as addressing secondary phenomena such as subretinal fluid accumulation. It is probably more effective in small early lesions.

NEURAL RETINAL TUMOURS

Retinoblastoma

Introduction

Retinoblastoma is rare, occurring in up to 1:18 000 live births, but is the most common primary intraocular malignancy of childhood and accounts for about 3% of all childhood cancers. After uveal melanoma, it is the second most common malignant intraocular tumour. Survival rates are over 95% in specialized centres, with high rates of globe salvage and preservation of vision in many eyes, but are much lower in the developing world. The psychological impact on parents of a child with retinoblastoma is high, with many suffering from depression, anxiety and stress. Tumours are composed of small basophilic cells (retinoblasts) with large hyperchromatic nuclei and scanty cytoplasm. Many retinoblastomas are undifferentiated but varying degrees of differentiation are characterized by the formation of structures known as rosettes (Flexner–Wintersteiner, Homer–Wright and fleurettes – Fig. 20.38A). Growth (Fig. 20.38B) may be endophytic (into the vitreous) with seeding of tumour cells throughout the eye, or exophytic (into the subretinal space) leading to retinal detachment, or mixed, or the retina may be diffusely infiltrated. Optic nerve invasion (Fig. 20.38C) may occur, with spread of tumour along the subarachnoid space to the brain. Metastatic spread is to regional nodes, lung, brain and bone.

TIP Retinoblastoma needs to be excluded in a young child with leukocoria or a squint.

Genetics

The genetics of retinoblastoma are often highlighted as a paradigm illustrating the genetic basis of cancer. The tumour suppressor gene in which mutations predisposing to retinoblastoma occur is *RB1*; over 900 different mutations have been reported to date. The size of a gene deletion tends to correlate with aggressive retinoblastoma behaviour. Mutations in *RB1* or associated genes in a common pathway are also disrupted in many sporadic tumours. Modifier genes for retinoblastoma have also been identified and may constitute therapeutic targets.

- **Heritable** (hereditary, germline) retinoblastoma accounts for 40%. In heritable retinoblastoma one of the pair of alleles of *RB1* is mutated in all the cells in the body. When a further mutagenic event ('second hit' according to the 'two-hit' hypothesis proposed by Knudson) affects the second allele, the cell may then undergo malignant transformation. Because of the presence of the mutation in all cells, a large majority of these children develop bilateral and multifocal tumours. Heritable retinoblastoma patients also have a predisposition to non-ocular cancers such as pinealoblastoma ('trilateral retinoblastoma', which occurs in up to 10%, usually before the age of 5), osteosarcoma, soft tissue sarcoma and melanoma; each of these tends to occur in a particular age group. The risk of a second malignancy is about 6% but this increases five-fold if external beam irradiation has been used to treat the original tumour, the second tumour tending to arise within the irradiated field.

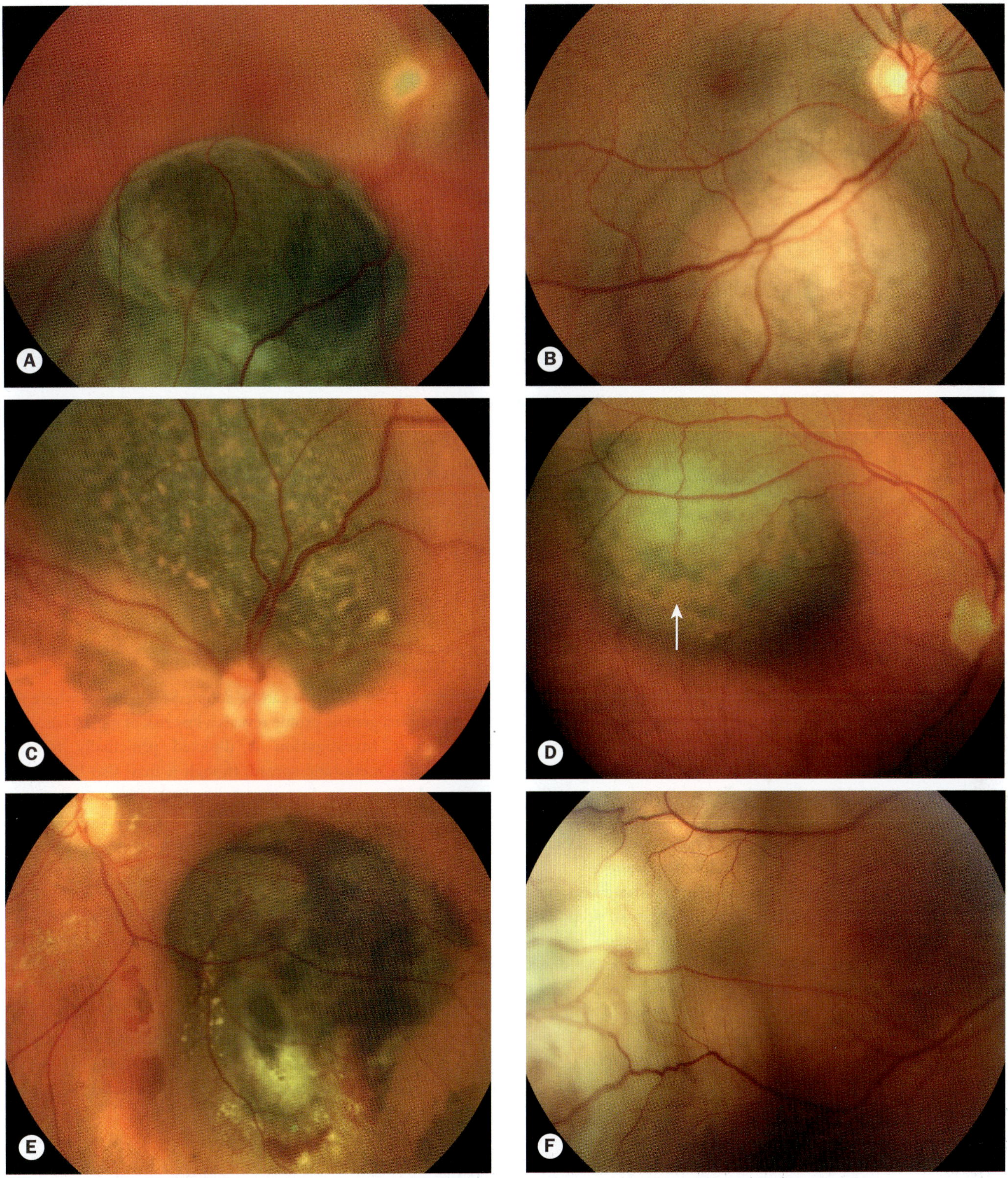

Fig. 20.26 Choroidal melanoma. **(A)** Typical pigmented melanoma; **(B)** amelanotic lesion; **(C)** choroidal melanoma adjacent to the optic disc; **(D)** overlying orange pigment (arrow); **(E)** associated haemorrhage and exudation; **(F)** peripheral melanoma with exudative retinal detachment, which may mask the underlying pathology. *(Courtesy of C Barry – figs A, E.)*

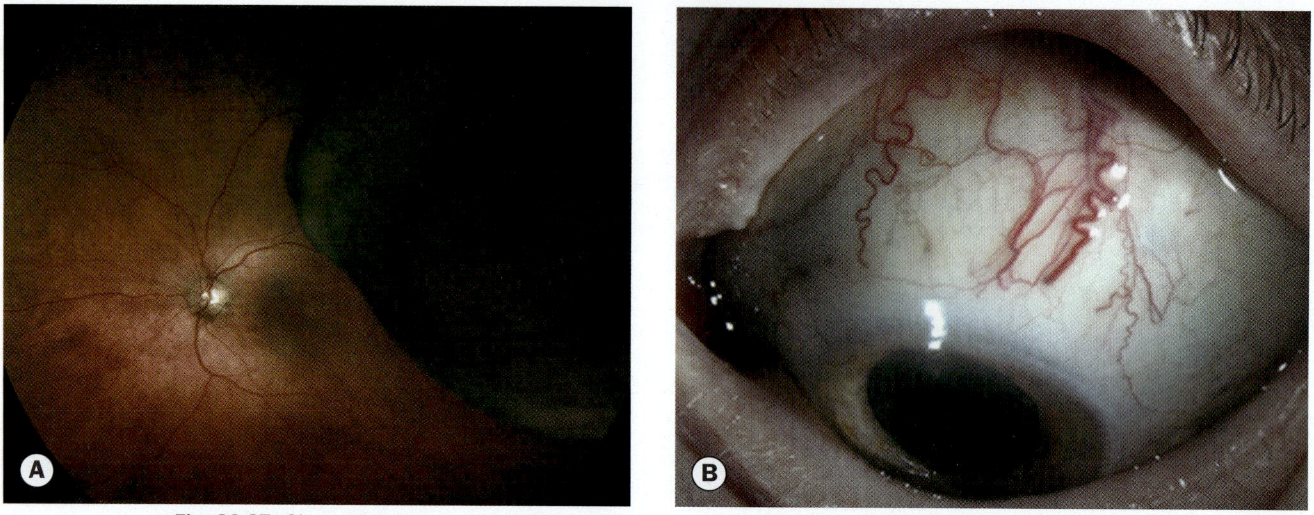

Fig. 20.27 Choroidal melanoma. **(A)** Fundal appearance; **(B)** with overlying sentinel vessels. *(Courtesy of C Barry.)*

- **FA** is of limited diagnostic value because there is no pathognomonic pattern. The most common findings are an intrinsic tumour ('dual') circulation (Fig. 20.28A), mottled fluorescence during the arteriovenous phase and late diffuse leakage and staining. FA may, however, be useful in the differential diagnosis of simulating lesions.
- **Ultrasound** is used to measure lesion dimensions and to detect tumours through opaque media and exudative retinal detachment and may also demonstrate extraocular extension. The characteristic findings are internal homogeneity with low to medium reflectivity, choroidal excavation (Fig. 20.28B) and orbital shadowing. A basal acoustically quiet zone referred to as 'acoustic hollowing' is typical and is due to the greater tissue homogeneity in this region. A 'collar stud' configuration (Fig. 20.28C) is almost pathognomonic when present.
- **FAF.** Intense diffuse or confluent hyperautofluorescence, if present, is a useful diagnostic indicator of melanoma.
- **OCT** measures dimensions and may demonstrate associated subretinal fluid, often before clinically apparent. Secondary retinal changes are often evident overlying the lesion.
- **Indocyanine green angiography (ICGA)** usually shows hypofluorescence throughout the study and provides more information than FA about the extent of the tumour, due to lower interference from the RPE.
- **Magnetic resonance imaging (MRI)** (Fig. 20.28D) is useful to demonstrate extraocular extension and may be of some help in differential diagnosis.
- **Biopsy** is useful when the diagnosis cannot be established by less invasive methods. It may be performed either with a fine needle or using the 25-gauge vitrectomy system, the latter providing a larger sample.
- **Immunocytochemistry** for PAX8 expression can help distinguish intraocular tumours with overlapping features. Melanoma and melanocytoma are PAX8-negative whereas pigmented adenocarcinomas are PAX8-positive.
- **Genetic tumour analysis** is becoming increasingly important in management, particularly with regard to prognosis, as metastasis occurs almost exclusively with certain genetic profiles. Simple chromosomal changes like the loss of one copy of chromosome 3 (M3) and changes in chromosome 8 (i8q) strongly correlate with poor outcome, especially when they occur together in the same tumour.
- **Prognostic indicators** combine anatomic findings with genetic and histopathological data. The Liverpool Uveal Melanoma Prognosticator (which is an online resource) is useful to determine prognosis for life.
- **Reduced surveillance** can be adopted for patients where the melanoma genetic profile reveals a low risk of metastasis.
- **Systemic investigation** is directed principally towards detecting metastatic spread, though it may also be used to search for a primary tumour elsewhere if choroidal metastasis is likely. Liver function testing and ultrasonography are mainstays. Chest radiography rarely shows lung secondaries in the absence of liver disease. The comparative value of whole-body PET/CT imaging is not fully defined. It has greater sensitivity for detecting metastatic disease, particularly extrahepatic lesions, but involves a substantial ionizing radiation dose.

Treatment

Treatment is performed to avoid the development of a painful and unsightly eye whilst conserving as much useful vision as possible. The extent to which ocular treatment influences survival is not yet defined, though there is some evidence that the risk of metastasis is lower with smaller earlier tumours. Management is individualized based on the characteristics of the particular tumour and the patient (e.g. general health, age, preferences, state of fellow eye). The size of the tumour (apical height and largest basal diameter) determines the treatment strategy.

- **Brachytherapy** (episcleral plaque radiotherapy) may be used for tumours less than 20 mm in basal diameter and up to 10 mm thick in which there is a reasonable chance of salvaging vision. Survival is similar to that following enucleation. A plaque is sutured to the sclera (Fig. 20.29A) for several days

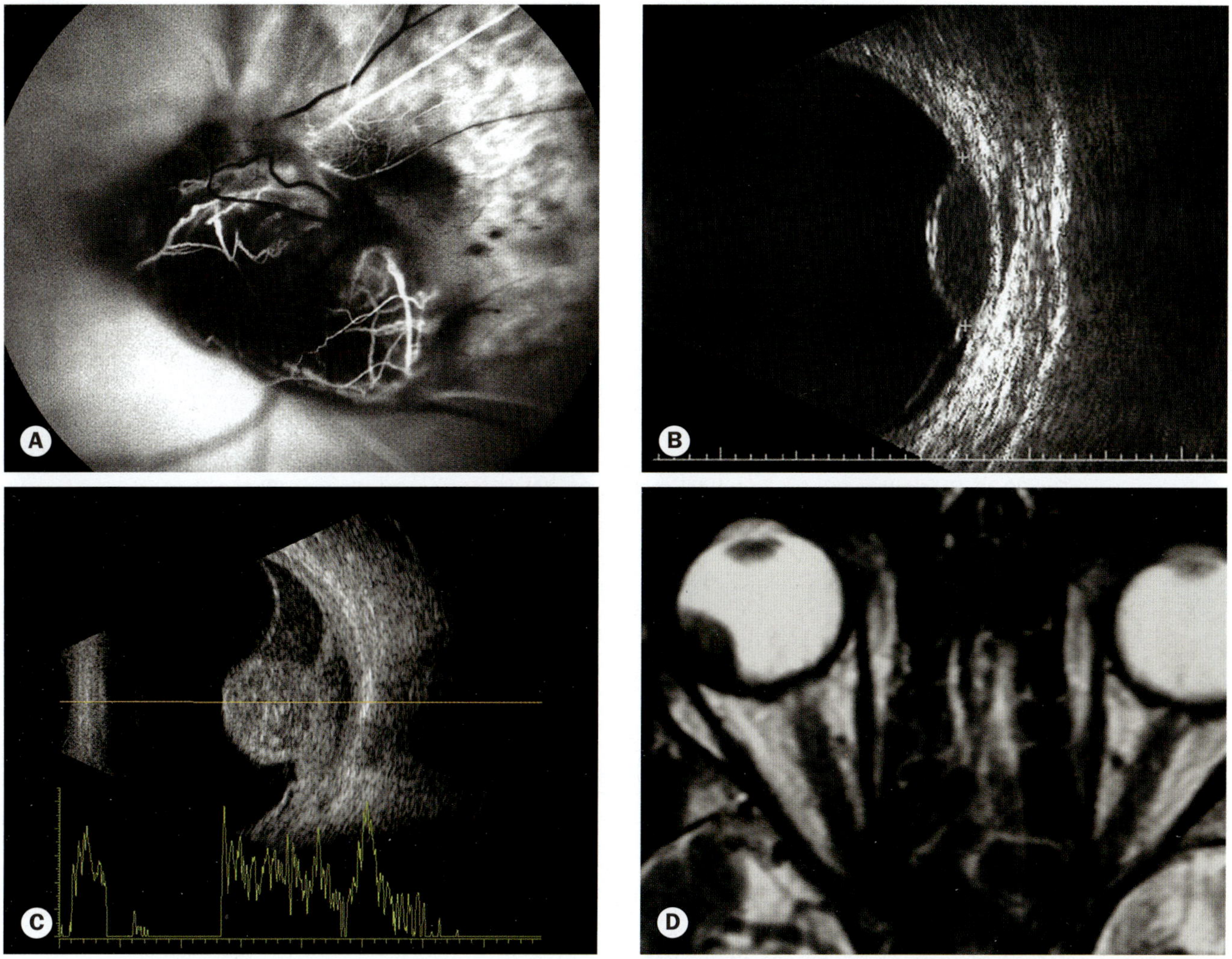

Fig. 20.28 Imaging of choroidal melanoma. **(A)** FA early phase of a 'collar stud' tumour showing a 'dual circulation'; **(B)** B-scan of a dome-shaped tumour showing choroidal excavation; **(C)** B-scan of a 'collar stud' tumour; **(D)** T2-weighted axial MRI showing a choroidal melanoma without extraocular spread. *(Courtesy of B Damato – figs A and B; G. Kontos – fig. C.)*

according to dosage requirement. Regression begins about 1–2 months after treatment and continues over several years, leaving a flat or dome-shaped pigmented scar (Fig. 20.29B). Complications include cataract, papillopathy (with or without disc neovascularization) and radiation retinopathy. Release of cytokines by the irradiated tumour can also cause retinopathy and other complications ('toxic tumour syndrome') that may need to be treated specifically (e.g. endo/exoresection, intravitreal steroid/anti-VEGF).

- **External beam radiotherapy.** Fractionated irradiation with charged particles such as protons achieves a high dose in the tumour with relative sparing of adjacent tissues and is used for tumours unsuitable for brachytherapy either because of large size or posterior location. Targeting is aided by suturing radio-opaque tantalum markers to the sclera. Regression is slower than with brachytherapy, but survival is comparable. Intraocular complications are similar, but extraocular complications such as loss of lashes, eyelid depigmentation and keratitis may be seen.
- **Stereotactic radiotherapy** uses multiple collimated beams from different directions, either concurrently or sequentially, so that only the tumour receives a high dose of radiation. It is relatively effective, though there may be a comparatively high complication rate.
- **Transpupillary thermotherapy (TTT)** uses an infrared laser beam to induce tumour cell death by hyperthermia rather than coagulation. Indications include the treatment of a small tumour when radiotherapy is considered inappropriate. It can be used as an adjunct to radiotherapy, particularly for vision-threatening exudation. Tumour response is gradual, the lesion first becoming darker and flatter and eventually disappearing to leave bare sclera (Fig. 20.30). Complications include retinal traction, retinal tear formation with rhegmatogenous detachment, vascular occlusion and neovascularization. Local recurrence is common, especially if the tumour is thick, amelanotic or involves the disc margin.
- **Trans-scleral choroidectomy.** This is a technically difficult procedure that may be used for carefully selected tumours that

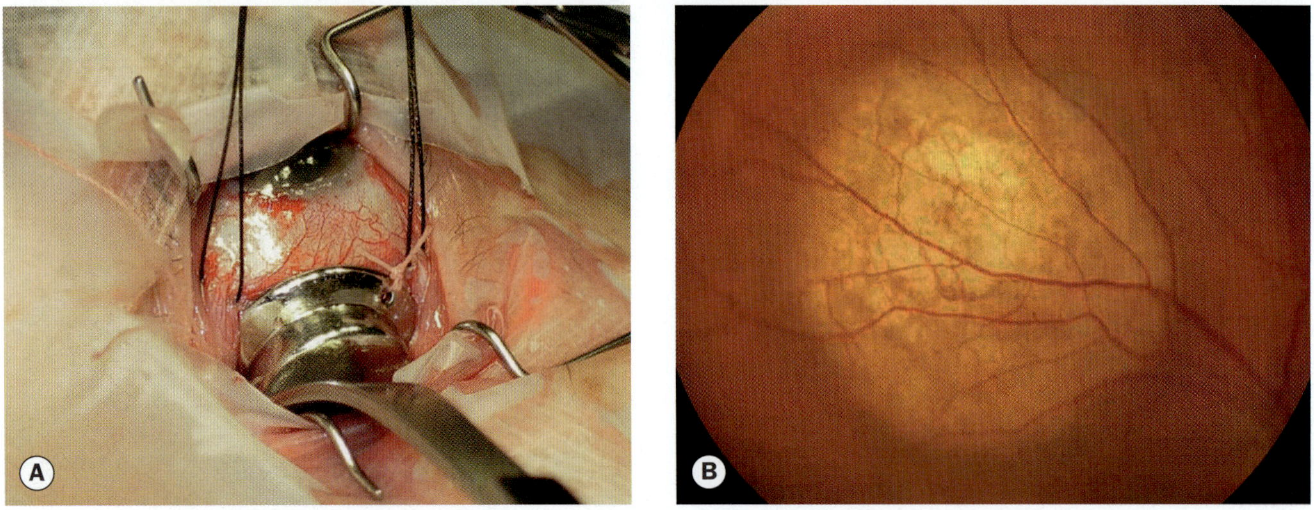

Fig. 20.29 Brachytherapy for choroidal melanoma. **(A)** Placement of plaque; **(B)** result of treatment. *(Courtesy of S Chen – fig. A.)*

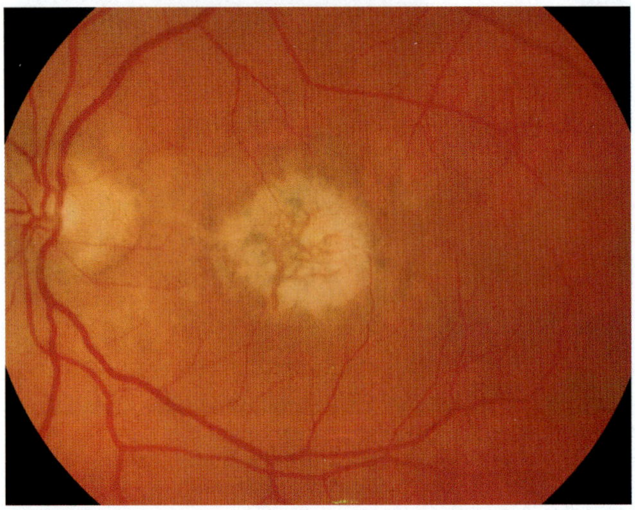

Fig. 20.30 Final result of transpupillary thermotherapy of a lesion in the macular region.

are too thick for radiotherapy but less than about 16 mm in diameter. Complications include retinal detachment, hypotony, wound dehiscence and local tumour recurrence.

- **Light-activated AU-011,** a novel treatment for small melanomas (2–3.4 mm), is showing promise in early trials. A solution of nano-particles derived from the human papilloma virus attached to an infrared fluorescent dye is injected into the vitreous cavity. These particles bind to the melanoma cells. When irradiated with infrared light the dye becomes activated and selectively causes melanoma cell necrosis.
- **Enucleation.** Indications include large tumour size, optic disc invasion, extensive involvement of the ciliary body or angle, irreversible loss of useful vision and poor motivation to keep the eye. It is essential to perform ophthalmoscopy after surgical draping to ensure that the correct eye is removed. Manipulation of the eye should be kept to a minimum. Orbital recurrence is rare if there is no extraocular tumour spread or if any such extension is completely excised.
- **There is no standard treatment for metastatic disease.** Tebentafusc, an immunotherapy drug, can be considered in some patients with metastatic choroidal melanoma and can result in a modest increase in overall survival time. Immune checkpoint inhibitors that are effective for cutaneous melanoma are **not effective** against uveal melanoma.
- **Systemic chemotherapy** has not been shown to be of benefit in cases where there is no evidence of metastatic spread.

Circumscribed choroidal haemangioma

Circumscribed choroidal haemangioma (CCH) consists of a mass of varying-sized vascular channels within the choroid. It is not associated with systemic disease. It may be dormant throughout life or may give rise to symptoms, usually in early adulthood, as a result of exudative retinal detachment. Slow enlargement can occur over many years.

TIP A choroidal haemangioma can cause an exudative retinal detachment in a young adult.

Diagnosis

- **Signs**
  - An oval orange mass at the posterior pole with indistinct margins that blend with the surrounding choroid (Fig. 20.31A and B). The median base diameter is 6 mm and median thickness 3 mm.
  - Subretinal fluid is usually present in symptomatic cases.
  - Complications include surface fibrous metaplasia (Fig. 20.31C), cystoid retinal degeneration, RPE degeneration and subretinal fibrosis.
- **OCT.** The overlying retina may be normal or show sub- and intraretinal fluid, retinoschisis and atrophy.
- **FA** reveals early spotty hyperfluorescence (see Fig. 20.31B) and late diffuse but intense hyperfluorescence.

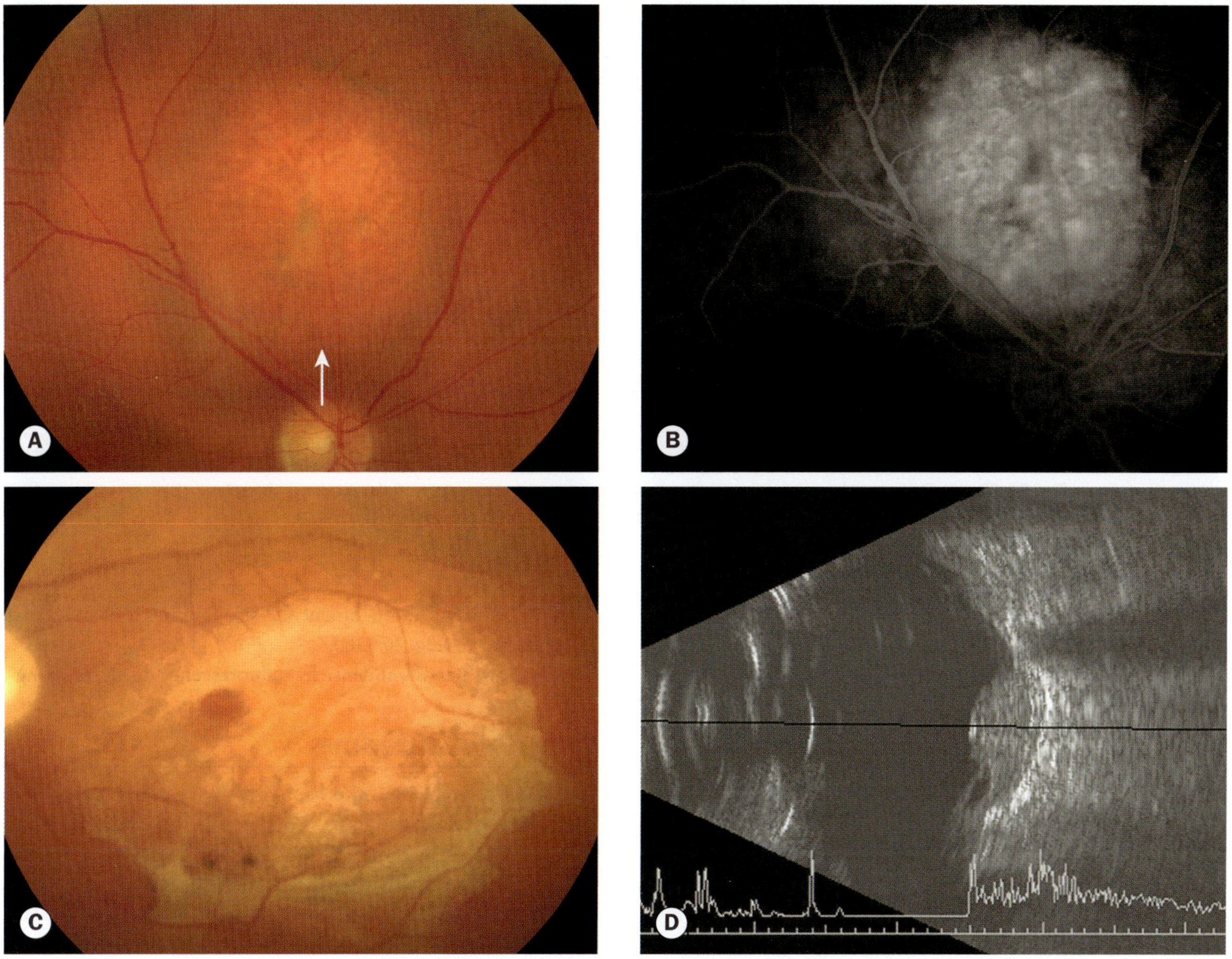

Fig. 20.31 Circumscribed choroidal haemangioma. **(A)** Clinical appearance (arrow shows the edge of the mass); **(B)** FA of **(A)** showing hyperfluorescence; **(C)** surface fibrous metaplasia; **(D)** B-scan showing an acoustically solid lesion with a sharp anterior surface and high internal reflectivity. *(Courtesy of B Damato – figs C and D.)*

- **ICGA** provides useful diagnostic information, with strongly hyperfluorescent tumour vessels evident in the arterial phase, with diffuse hypofluorescence later.
- **FAF.** The lesion itself shows little or no intrinsic autofluorescence. Associated overlying orange pigment and (fresh) subretinal fluid show hyperautofluorescence, with RPE hyperplasia and atrophy giving hypoautofluorescence.
- **Ultrasound** shows an acoustically solid lesion (high internal reflectivity) with a well-defined anterior surface (Fig. 20.31D).
- **MRI.** The tumour is iso- or hyperintense to the vitreous in T1-weighted images and isointense in T2-weighted images, with marked enhancement by gadolinium.

Treatment

The following may be used if vision is threatened. The superiority of any particular approach has not been established.

- **Photodynamic therapy (PDT)** using the same parameters as for macular neovascularization. Treatment may need to be repeated after a few months if subretinal fluid persists.
- **TTT** for lesions not involving the macula.
- **Photocoagulation** using a conventional thermal laser or micropulse treatment may be effective.
- **Radiotherapy** may be used for resistant lesions.
- **Intravitreal anti-VEGF therapy** typically reduces serous retinal detachment and can be used in combination with other modalities.
- **Oral propranolol** may be of benefit, particularly for associated exudative retinal detachment, but does not seem to consistently reduce tumour size.

Diffuse choroidal haemangioma

Diffuse choroidal haemangioma usually affects over half of the choroid and enlarges very slowly. It occurs almost exclusively in patients with Sturge–Weber syndrome ipsilateral to the naevus flammeus (see Ch. 2). The fundus has a diffuse deep red colour that is most marked at the posterior pole (Fig. 20.32A). Localized areas of thickening, simulating a circumscribed haemangioma,

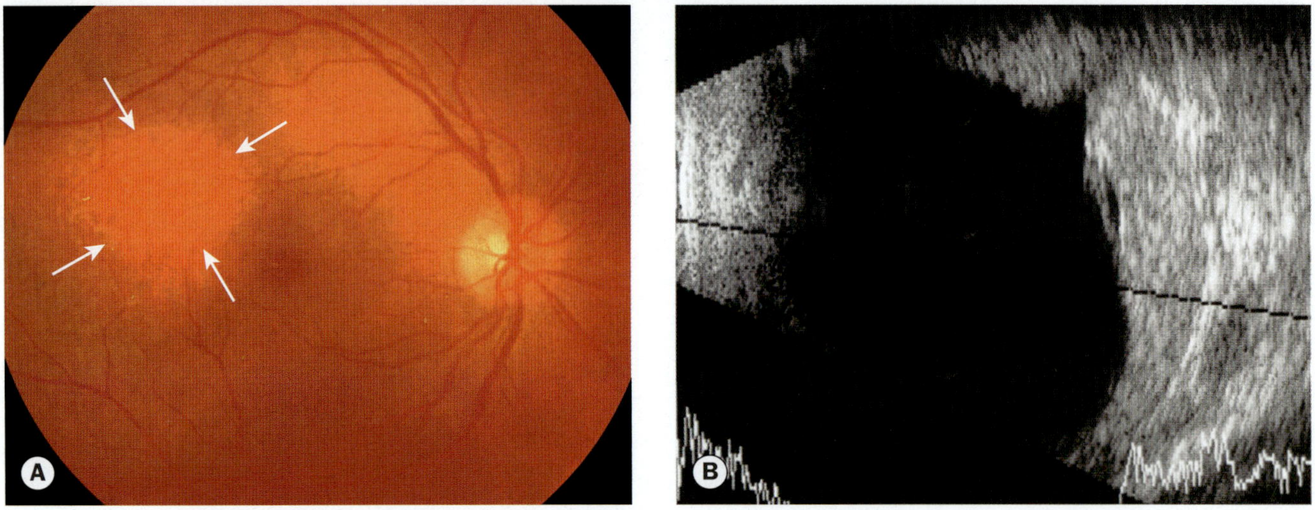

Fig. 20.32 (A) Diffuse choroidal haemangioma with localized area of thickening (arrows); **(B)** B-scan showing diffuse choroidal thickening. *(Courtesy of B Damato – fig. B.)*

may be present within the larger lesion. B-scan ultrasonography shows diffuse choroidal thickening (Fig. 20.32B). Complications include secondary retinal cystoid degeneration and exudative retinal detachment. Neovascular glaucoma can ensue if exudative detachment is not treated. Treatment of vision-threatening cases involves PDT or low-dose radiotherapy.

Optic disc melanocytoma

Melanocytoma (magnocellular naevus) is a rare, distinctive, unilateral, heavily pigmented congenital hamartoma seen most frequently in the optic nerve head (Fig. 20.33A) but may arise anywhere in the uvea. About half involve one quadrant of the optic disc. Histology shows large deeply pigmented polyhedral or spindle cells with small nuclei. In contrast to choroidal melanoma, melanocytoma is more common in dark-skinned individuals. It is discovered at an average age of 50 years and is more likely to affect women than men. Most cases have no symptoms and the condition is detected on routine examination. The tumour is generally stationary and treatment is not required except in the very rare event of malignant transformation. Other complications include spontaneous tumour necrosis, optic nerve compression and retinal vein obstruction.

Diagnosis

- A dark brown or black, flat or slightly elevated lesion with feathery edges that may extend over the edge of the disc to involve the adjacent choroid in about half of patients (Fig. 20.33B).
- Occasionally a large tumour occupies most of the disc surface and may lead to pigment dispersion into the vitreous.
- A relative afferent pupillary defect may be present, even if visual acuity (VA) is good.
- The visual field is abnormal in 90% of patients. The defect corresponds to a localised absence of the capillary network within the melanocytoma that can be shown with OCTA.
- OCT is useful to document the size and has a characteristic appearance (Fig. 20.33C).
- FA shows persistent dense hypofluorescence due to masking.

Choroidal osteoma

Choroidal osteoma is a rare benign ossifying tumour that often affects young adults and has a strong female preponderance. Both eyes are affected in about 10–20%. Histology shows mature cancellous bone, with overlying RPE atrophy. Presentation is in the second–third decades. Masquerading lesions include osseous metaplasia in association with a choroidal haemangioma and sclerochoroidal calcification, the latter characterized by multiple geographical yellow–white fundus lesions that usually involve both eyes of an older adult.

Diagnosis

- **Symptoms.** Gradual visual impairment if the macula is involved by the tumour itself, or occasionally more rapid deterioration secondary to macular neovascularization.
- **Signs**
  - Initially orange, maturing lesions appear yellow–white. They are flat or minimally elevated with well-defined, scalloped margins near the disc or at the posterior pole (Fig. 20.34A and B).
  - Spider-like fine vessels and bone-spicule RPE changes may develop.
  - Slow growth may occur over several years (Fig. 20.34C and D).
  - Spontaneous resorption and decalcification may rarely occur.
  - The visual prognosis is poor if the lesion involves the fovea.
- **FA** manifests early, irregular, diffuse mottled hyperfluorescence and late staining (Fig. 20.35A).
- **FAF** shows mainly isoautofluorescence in calcified areas and hypoautofluorescence in decalcified regions.

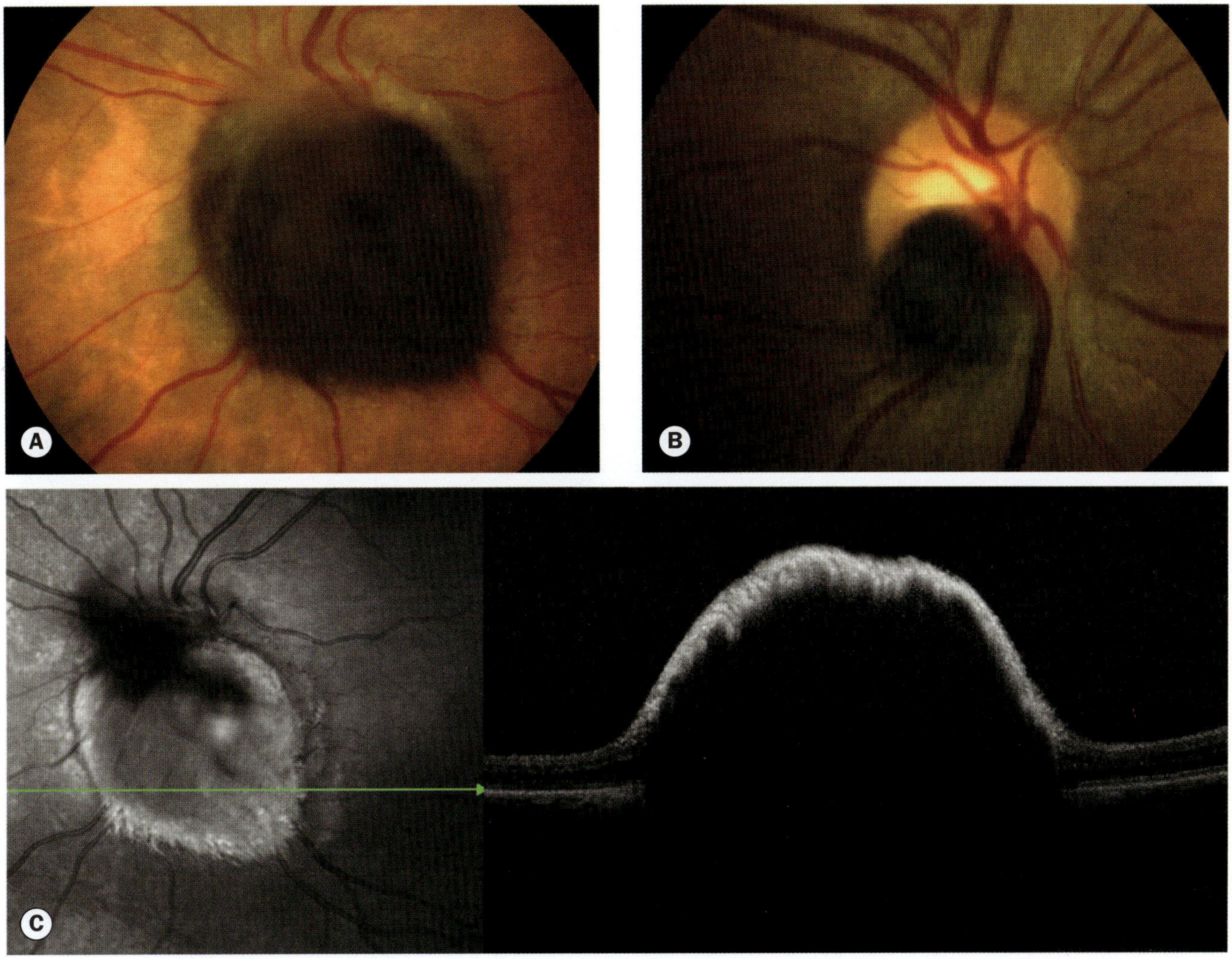

Fig. 20.33 Melanocytoma. **(A)** Clinical appearance; **(B)** infero-temporal location showing extension over the disc margin; **(C)** OCT showing a dome-shaped mass at the disc with dense posterior shadowing.

- **ICGA** shows early hypofluorescence (Fig. 20.35B) and late staining. The tumour appears larger than on clinical examination.
- **Ultrasound** shows a highly reflective anterior surface and orbital shadowing (Fig. 20.35C).
- **CT** demonstrates a dense plaque-like opacity at the level of the choroid (Fig. 20.35D).
- **OCT** demonstrates overlying retinal changes, with enhanced depth imaging showing a lattice pattern in calcified tumour similar to the appearance of cancellous bone (Fig. 20.35E).

Sclerochoroidal calcification

This is a rare condition that is usually diagnosed coincidently in asymptomatic elderly White people. The condition is commonly misdiagnosed and the visual prognosis is good as the macula is usually not involved. The placoid lesions, which measure about 3.5 mm in diameter, are flat or minimally raised, are yellowish in appearance and are found in both eyes in about 50% of patients. The calcium deposits start in the sclera and expand into the choroid. The diagnosis is made clinically and can be confirmed with OCT (Fig. 20.36). Most cases are idiopathic, but patients with calcium-phosphorus metabolic disorders are at higher risk. Parathyroid adenoma, Bartter syndrome and Gitelman syndrome should be excluded because of the systemic complications associated with these conditions.

Metastatic tumours

The choroid is by far the most common (90%) site for uveal metastases. The most frequent primary sites are the breast and bronchus. A choroidal secondary may be the initial presentation of a bronchial carcinoma, whereas a past history of breast cancer is the rule in patients with secondary spread. Other less common primary sites include the gastrointestinal tract, kidney and skin (melanoma). In patients with known systemic cancer 2–4% demonstrate ocular metastasis. Survival is poor, with a median life expectancy of 8–12 months and a 3-year survival of about one in three, depending on the primary tumour.

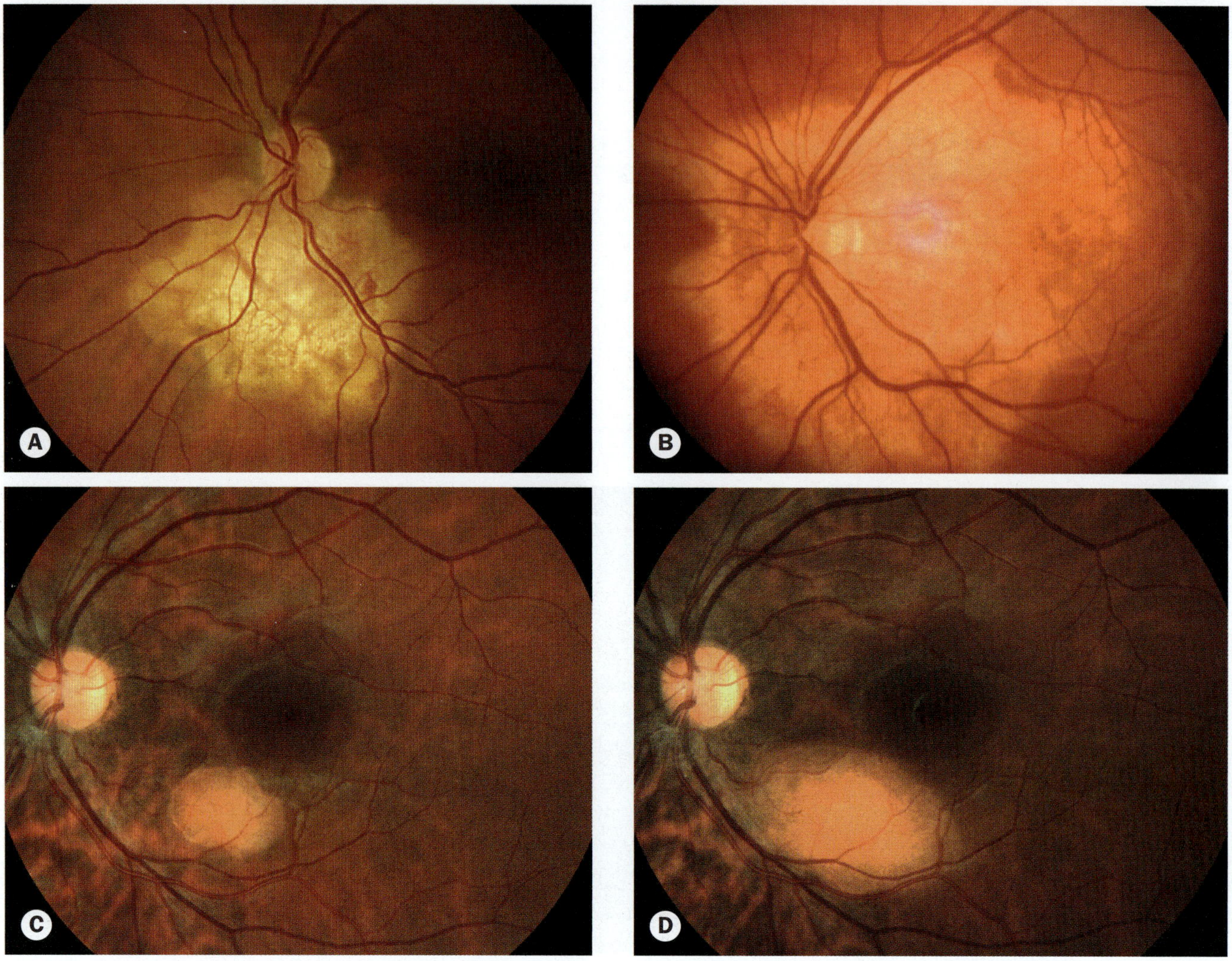

Fig. 20.34 Choroidal osteoma. **(A)** Involving parapapillary region; **(B)** large macular lesion with overlying RPE changes; **(C)** and **(D)** growth over 5 years. *(Courtesy of S Chen – figs C and D.)*

TIP Choroidal metastasis may occur secondary to bronchus or breast carcinoma and indicates a poor prognosis and short life expectancy.

Diagnosis

- **Symptoms.** Visual impairment may occur due to macular involvement by the lesion itself or associated exudative retinal detachment. A minority are discovered incidentally.
- **Signs**
  - The most common appearance is a fast-growing yellowish slightly elevated placoid lesion with indistinct margins, typically at the posterior pole and often multifocal and bilateral (10–30% – Fig. 20.37A–C). Overlying pigmentary changes are fairly common (Fig. 20.37D).
  - Melanoma secondaries are usually pigmented.
  - Secondary exudative retinal detachment is frequent and may occur in eyes with relatively small lesions.
- **Ultrasound** may be useful in detection, particularly to demonstrate a lesion underlying exudative retinal detachment. A placoid tumour shows diffuse choroidal thickening, while a larger dome-shaped lesion shows moderately high internal acoustic reflectivity (Fig. 20.37E and F).
- **OCT** shows overlying RPE thickening and photoreceptor irregularity, with subretinal fluid when present. The choroidal surface has a 'lumpy bumpy' appearance in about 2/3 patients. Enhanced depth imaging OCT shows choriocapillaris thinning overlying the tumour.
- **FA** shows early hypofluorescence and diffuse late staining, but in contrast to choroidal melanoma a dual circulation is not seen.
- **ICGA** usually shows hypofluorescence through the study and may show additional deposits not evident on clinical examination or FA.
- **Biopsy** by fine-needle aspiration or using a 25-gauge vitrectomy system may be appropriate when the primary site is unknown.
- **Systemic investigation** is directed at locating the primary tumour, if unknown, and other metastatic sites. The list below is not exhaustive.
  - Full history and physical examination.

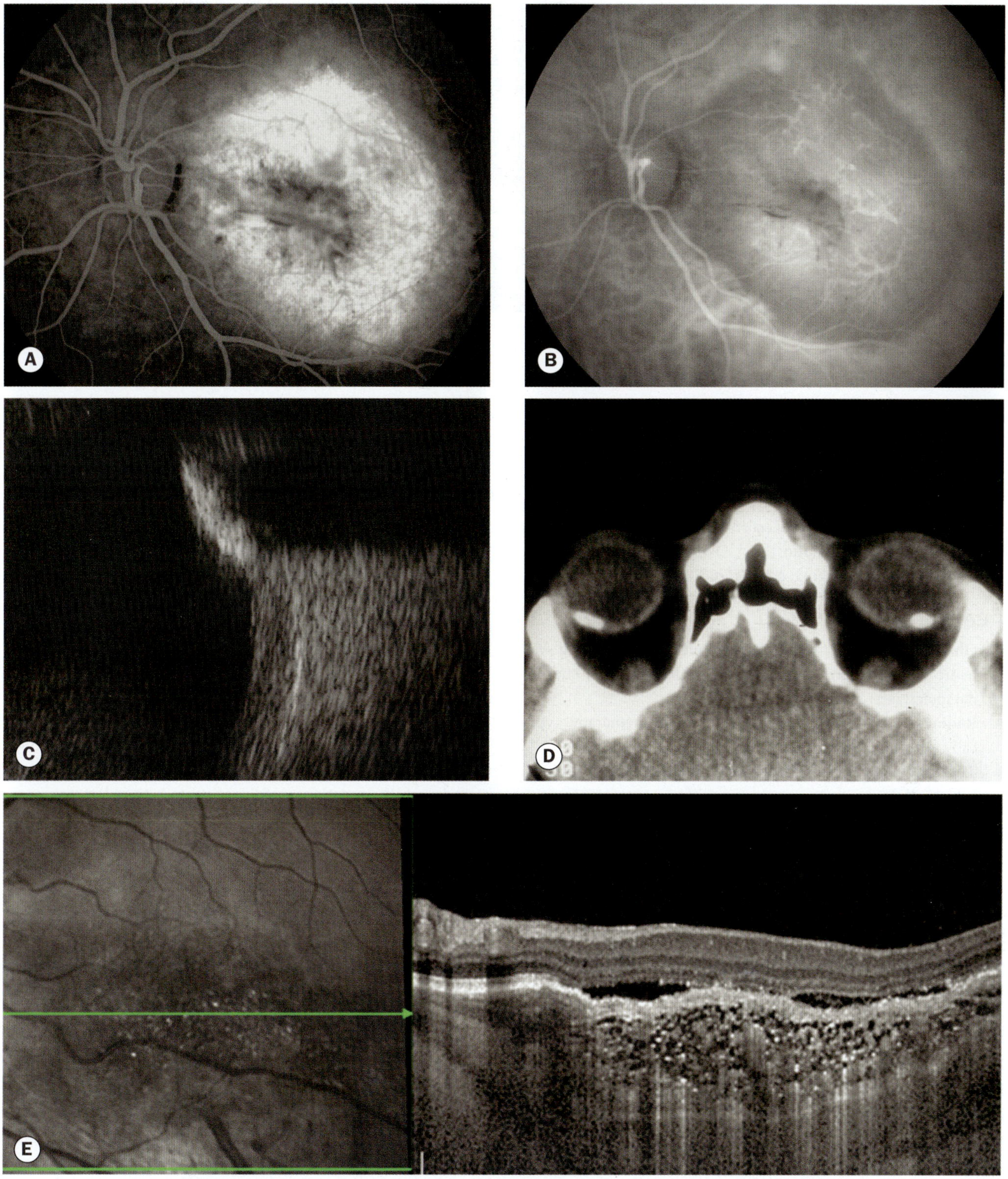

Fig. 20.35 Imaging of choroidal osteoma. **(A)** FA late phase showing mottled hyperfluorescence; **(B)** ICGA early phase showing hypofluorescence; **(C)** B-scan showing a highly reflective anterior surface and orbital shadowing; **(D)** axial CT demonstrating bilateral dense plaque-like lesions with similar consistency to bone; **(E)** OCT demonstrating overlying retinal changes, with enhanced depth imaging showing a lattice pattern in calcified tumour similar to the appearance of cancellous bone. *(Courtesy P Gili – figs A and B; T Gkika – fig. E.)*

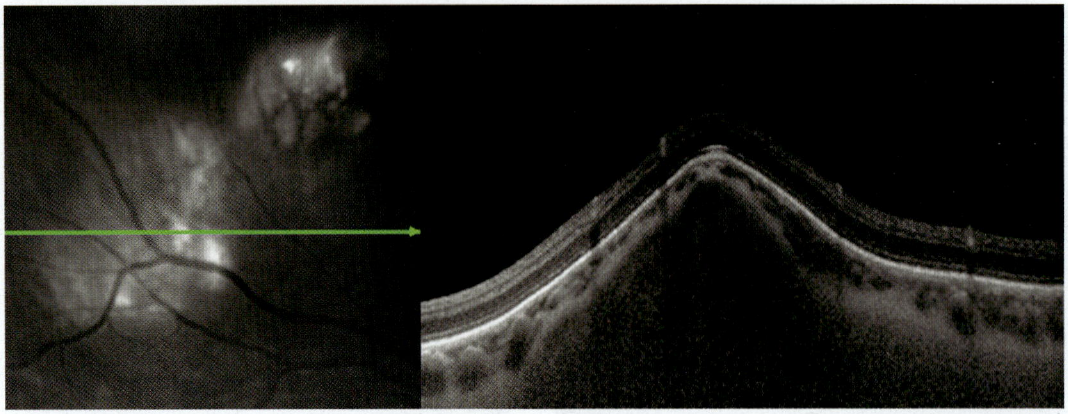

Fig. 20.36 Sclero-choroidal calcification. OCT showing a lesion arising from the sclera with abrupt elevation and a pointed surface which is compressing the choroid.

- Mammography.
- Chest radiography and sputum cytology.
- Liver function tests.
- Abdominal or whole-body scans.
- Faecal occult blood.
- Urinalysis for red blood cells.
- Abdominal ultrasound.
- Whole-body imaging, e.g. PET/CT, MRI.

Treatment

- **Observation**, if the patient is asymptomatic or receiving systemic chemotherapy, which may also be beneficial for choroidal metastases.
- **Radiotherapy**, either external beam or brachytherapy, typically for solitary lesions.
- **TTT and PDT** are useful for small tumours with minimal subretinal fluid.
- **Anti-VEGF treatment** may lead to regression of metastases in some cases, as well as addressing secondary phenomena such as subretinal fluid accumulation. It is probably more effective in small early lesions.

NEURAL RETINAL TUMOURS

Retinoblastoma

Introduction

Retinoblastoma is rare, occurring in up to 1:18 000 live births, but is the most common primary intraocular malignancy of childhood and accounts for about 3% of all childhood cancers. After uveal melanoma, it is the second most common malignant intraocular tumour. Survival rates are over 95% in specialized centres, with high rates of globe salvage and preservation of vision in many eyes, but are much lower in the developing world. The psychological impact on parents of a child with retinoblastoma is high, with many suffering from depression, anxiety and stress. Tumours are composed of small basophilic cells (retinoblasts) with large hyperchromatic nuclei and scanty cytoplasm. Many retinoblastomas are undifferentiated but varying degrees of differentiation are characterized by the formation of structures known as rosettes (Flexner–Wintersteiner, Homer–Wright and fleurettes – Fig. 20.38A). Growth (Fig. 20.38B) may be endophytic (into the vitreous) with seeding of tumour cells throughout the eye, or exophytic (into the subretinal space) leading to retinal detachment, or mixed, or the retina may be diffusely infiltrated. Optic nerve invasion (Fig. 20.38C) may occur, with spread of tumour along the subarachnoid space to the brain. Metastatic spread is to regional nodes, lung, brain and bone.

TIP Retinoblastoma needs to be excluded in a young child with leukocoria or a squint.

Genetics

The genetics of retinoblastoma are often highlighted as a paradigm illustrating the genetic basis of cancer. The tumour suppressor gene in which mutations predisposing to retinoblastoma occur is *RB1*; over 900 different mutations have been reported to date. The size of a gene deletion tends to correlate with aggressive retinoblastoma behaviour. Mutations in *RB1* or associated genes in a common pathway are also disrupted in many sporadic tumours. Modifier genes for retinoblastoma have also been identified and may constitute therapeutic targets.

- **Heritable** (hereditary, germline) retinoblastoma accounts for 40%. In heritable retinoblastoma one of the pair of alleles of *RB1* is mutated in all the cells in the body. When a further mutagenic event ('second hit' according to the 'two-hit' hypothesis proposed by Knudson) affects the second allele, the cell may then undergo malignant transformation. Because of the presence of the mutation in all cells, a large majority of these children develop bilateral and multifocal tumours. Heritable retinoblastoma patients also have a predisposition to non-ocular cancers such as pinealoblastoma ('trilateral retinoblastoma', which occurs in up to 10%, usually before the age of 5), osteosarcoma, soft tissue sarcoma and melanoma; each of these tends to occur in a particular age group. The risk of a second malignancy is about 6% but this increases five-fold if external beam irradiation has been used to treat the original tumour, the second tumour tending to arise within the irradiated field.

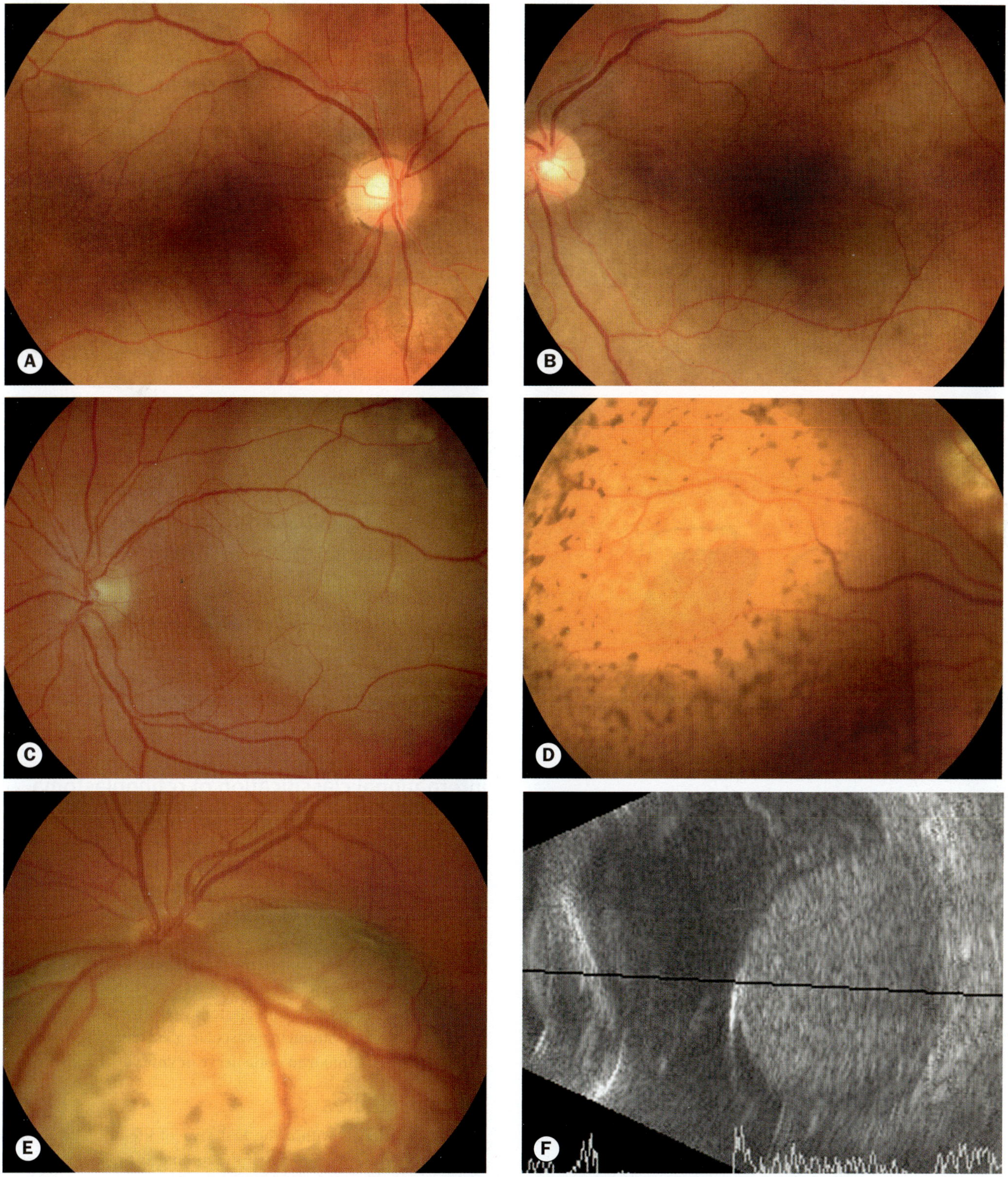

Fig. 20.37 Choroidal metastasis. **(A)** and **(B)** Bilateral multifocal metastases from a breast primary – regression in response to systemic chemotherapy is beginning in the left eye; **(C)** single metastasis from breast; **(D)** overlying pigmentary stippling; **(E)** large metastasis from bronchus; **(F)** B-scan showing internal reflectivity. *(Courtesy of C Barry – figs A and B; B Damato – fig. D.)*

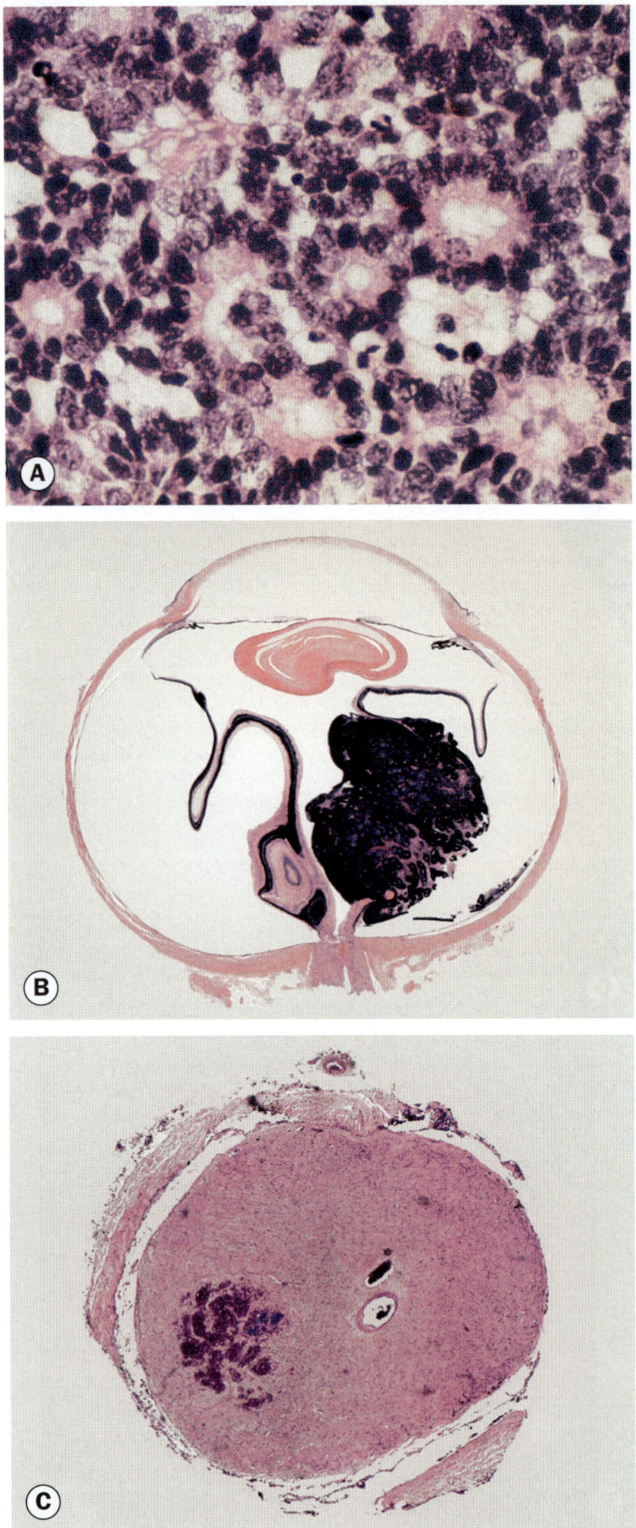

Fig. 20.38 Pathology of retinoblastoma. **(A)** Well-differentiated tumour showing abundant Flexner–Wintersteiner rosettes; **(B)** whole eye section showing both endophytic and exophytic growth; **(C)** transverse section of the cut end of an optic nerve demonstrating an area of tumour infiltration.

- **Non-heritable** (non-hereditary, somatic) retinoblastoma. The tumour is unilateral, not transmissible and does not predispose the patient to second non-ocular cancers. If a patient has a solitary retinoblastoma and no positive family history, this is almost certainly (but not conclusively) non-heritable so that the risk in each sibling and the patient's offspring is about 1%. Ninety per cent of children with unilateral retinoblastoma will have the non-hereditary form.
- **Screening of at-risk family members.** Germline mutations are autosomal dominant and so transmitted to 50%, but because of incomplete penetrance only 40% of offspring will be affected. Detection of mutations in *RB1* has approached 95% in recent years. Once identified in a particular child, the same mutation can be sought in siblings, its presence confirming their high-risk status. Siblings at risk of retinoblastoma should be screened by prenatal ultrasonography, by ophthalmoscopy soon after birth and then regularly until the age of 5–7 years. Early diagnosis correlates with a higher chance of preserving vision, salvaging the eye and preserving life. With effective screening of babies with *RB1* pathogenic variants who develop retinoblastoma, a final visual acuity of 6/6 to 6/12 can be achieved in up to 90%. If a child has heritable retinoblastoma, the risk to siblings is 2% if the parents are healthy and 40% if a parent is affected. It is important that all family members, including the parents, are examined for the presence of retinoblastoma-associated eye lesions (retinomas, calcified retinal scars, phthisis).

TIP Heritable retinoblastoma patients are predisposed to non-ocular tumours (pinealoblastoma, osteosarcoma, soft tissue sarcoma and melanoma).

International classification of retinoblastoma

- **Group A:** Small intraretinal tumours (<3 mm) away from foveola and disc.
- **Group B:** Tumours >3 mm, macular or juxtapapillary location, or with subretinal fluid.
- **Group C:** Tumour with focal subretinal or vitreous seeding within 3 mm of tumour.
- **Group D:** Tumour with diffuse subretinal or vitreous seeding > 3 mm from tumour.
- **Group E:** Extensive retinoblastoma occupying >50% of the globe with or without neovascular glaucoma, haemorrhage, extension of tumour to optic nerve or anterior chamber.

Clinical features

- **Presentation** is within the first year of life in bilateral cases and around 2 years of age if the tumour is unilateral. Careful enquiry about a family history of ocular tumours is critical.
  - Leukocoria (white pupillary reflex) is the commonest presentation (60%) (Fig. 20.39A) and may be first noticed in family photographs.
  - Strabismus is the second most common (20%). Fundus examination is therefore mandatory in all cases of childhood squint.

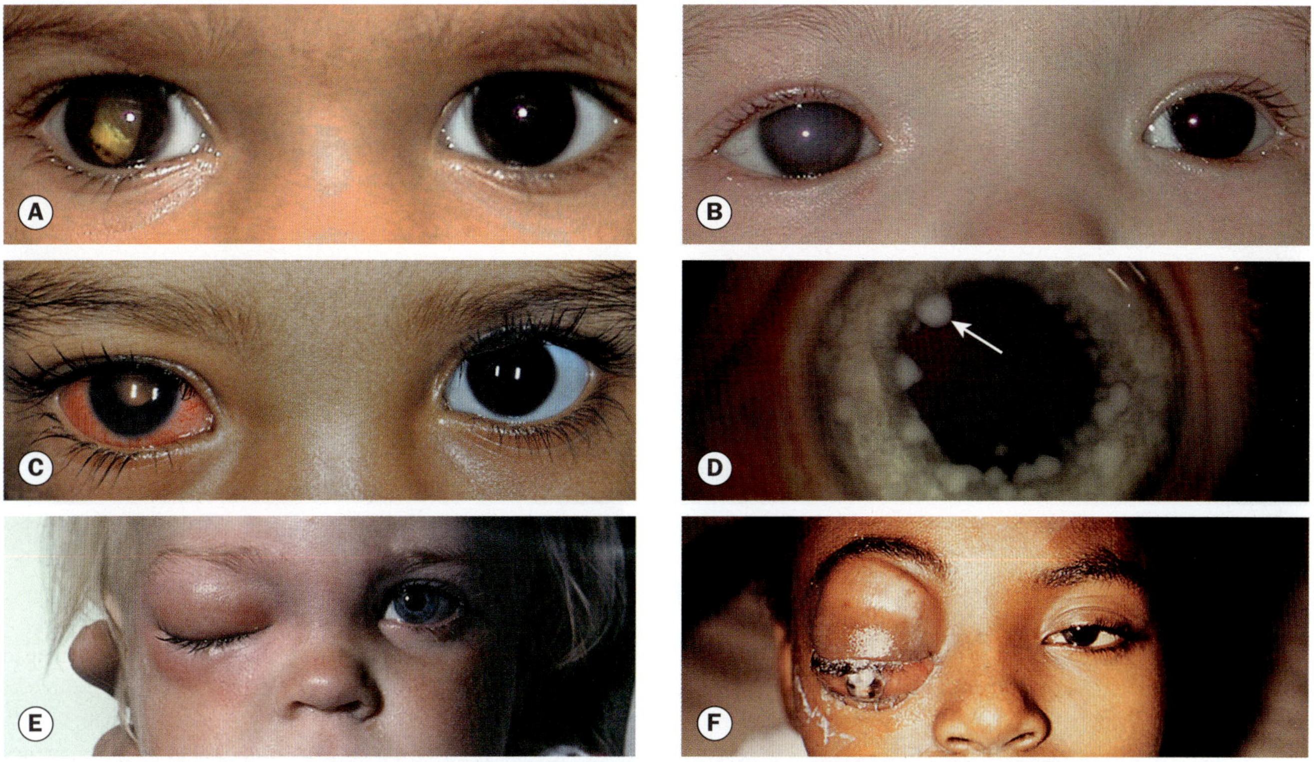

Fig. 20.39 Presentation of retinoblastoma. **(A)** Leukocoria; **(B)** secondary glaucoma and buphthalmos; **(C)** red eye due to uveitis; **(D)** iris nodules (arrow); **(E)** orbital inflammation; **(F)** orbital invasion. *(Courtesy of N Rogers – fig. B; U Raina – fig. C; M Parulekar – fig. D.)*

  - Painful red eye with secondary glaucoma, which may occasionally be associated with buphthalmos (Fig. 20.39B).
  - Poor vision.
  - Inflammation or pseudo-inflammation (Fig. 20.39C and D).
  - Routine examination of a patient known to be at risk.
  - Orbital inflammation mimicking orbital or preseptal cellulitis may occur with necrotic tumours (Fig. 20.39E).
  - Orbital invasion or visible extraocular growth may occur in neglected cases (Fig. 20.39F).
  - Metastatic disease involving regional lymph nodes and brain before the detection of ocular involvement is rare.
- **Signs**
  - An intraretinal tumour is a homogeneous, dome-shaped white lesion (Fig. 20.40A) that becomes irregular, often with white flecks of calcification.
  - An endophytic tumour projects into the vitreous as a white mass that may 'seed' into the gel (Fig. 20.40B).
  - An exophytic tumour forms multilobular subretinal white masses and causes overlying retinal detachment (Fig. 20.40C and D).

Investigation

- **Red reflex testing** with a direct ophthalmoscope is a simple screening test for leukocoria that is easily employed in the community.
- **Examination under anaesthesia** includes the following:
  - General examination for congenital abnormalities of the face and hands.
  - Tonometry.
  - Measurement of the corneal diameter.
  - Anterior chamber examination with a hand-held slit lamp.
  - Ophthalmoscopy, documenting all findings with colour drawings or photography.
  - Cycloplegic refraction.
- **Ultrasound** is used mainly to assess tumour size. It also detects calcification (Fig. 20.40E) within the tumour and is helpful in the exclusion of simulating lesions such as Coats disease.
- **Wide-field photography** (portable if necessary) is useful for both surveying and documentation and offers particular advantages in the management of retinoblastoma.
- **CT** also detects calcification (Fig. 20.40F) but entails a significant dose of radiation so is avoided by many practitioners. Plain X-rays may be used to detect calcification in resource-poor regions.
- **MRI** does not detect calcification but is useful for optic nerve evaluation, detection of extraocular extension and pinealoblastoma and to aid differentiation from simulating conditions.
- **Systemic assessment** includes physical examination and MRI scans of the orbit and skull as a minimum in high-risk cases. If these indicate the presence of metastatic disease then bone scans, bone marrow aspiration and lumbar puncture are also performed.
- **Genetic studies** on tumour tissue and blood samples from the patient and relatives.

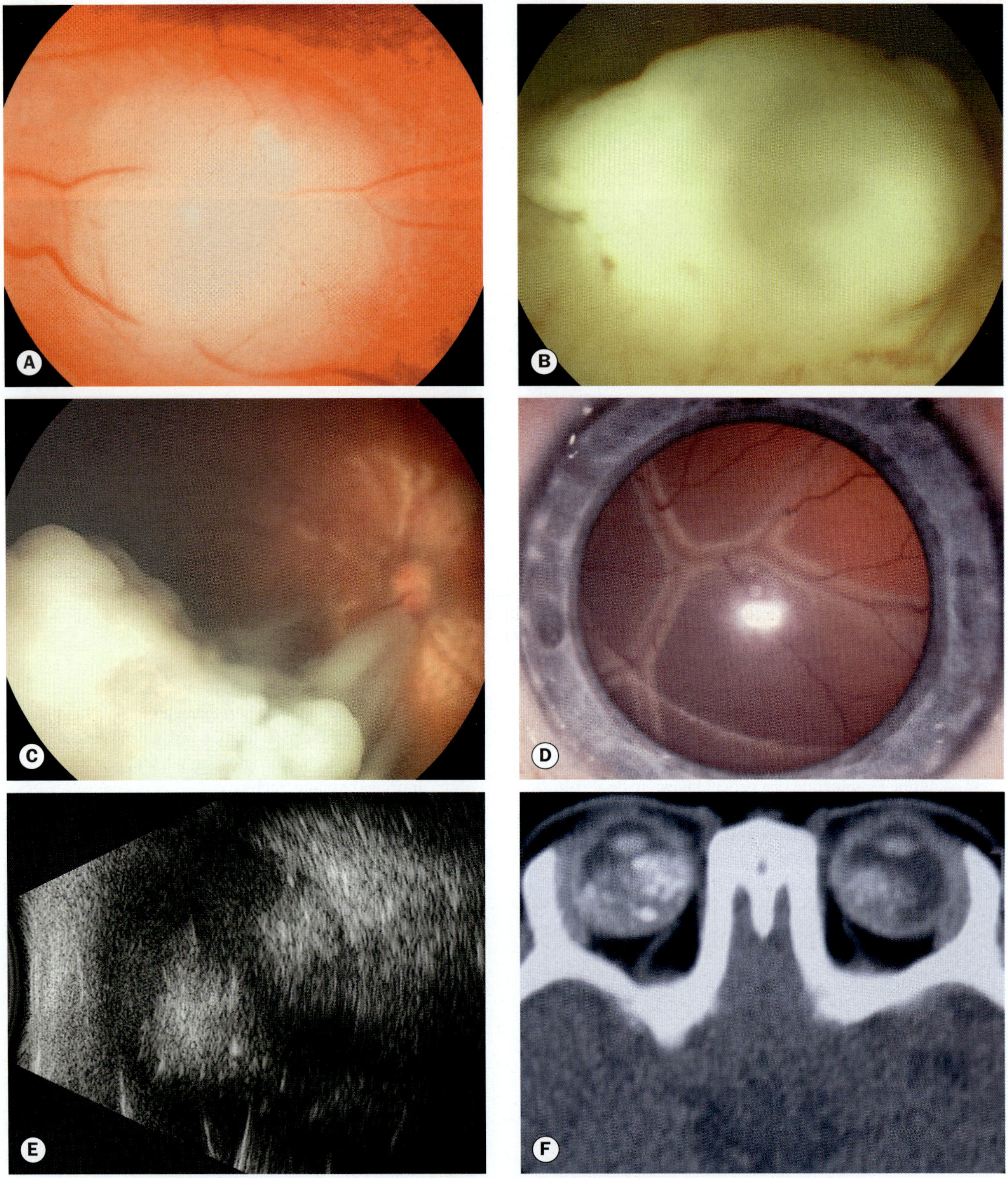

Fig. 20.40 Retinoblastoma. **(A)** Intraretinal tumour; **(B)** endophytic tumour with vitreous seeding; **(C)** mixed endophytic and exophytic growth; **(D)** total retinal detachment; **(E)** B-scan showing echoes from calcification; **(F)** axial CT showing bilateral tumours with calcification. *(Courtesy of M Parulekar – fig. C; Ken K Nischal – fig. F.)*

Treatment

A collaborative approach is required, involving the ophthalmologist, paediatric oncologist, ocular pathologist, geneticist, allied health professionals and parents. Treatment is highly individualized. The prognosis has improved significantly in recent years.

- **Chemotherapy** is the mainstay of treatment in most cases and may be used in conjunction with local treatments (focal consolidation – see below).
  - Intravenous treatment: carboplatin, etoposide and vincristine (CEV) are given in three to six cycles according to the grade of retinoblastoma. Single- (carboplatin alone) or dual-agent therapy has also given favourable results in some circumstances, such as bridging therapy to allow deferral of more aggressive measures.
  - Selective ophthalmic artery infusion: this is a promising new therapeutic option with high rates of globe salvage. The treatment offers significantly better results than intravenous treatment in eyes classified as group D. In this procedure a small-calibre cannula is introduced via the femoral artery into the opening of the ophthalmic artery. Melphalan or topotecan is then injected over about 30 minutes and is carried into the branches of the arteries that supply blood to the uvea and retina. Chorioretinal ischaemia and visual loss have been reported, but the overall safety profile is better than IV multi-drug chemotherapy.
  - Intravitreal melphalan seems to be effective for vitreous seeding, though it carries a small risk of extraocular dissemination.
  - Chemo-reduction may be followed by focal treatment with cryotherapy or TTT to consolidate tumour control.
- **TTT** achieves focal consolidation following chemotherapy, or is sometimes used as an isolated treatment. Focal techniques such as TTT and cryotherapy exert both a direct effect and probably increase susceptibility to the effects of chemotherapy.
- **Cryotherapy** using a triple freeze–thaw technique is useful for pre-equatorial tumours without either deep invasion or vitreous seeding.
- **Brachytherapy** using a radioactive plaque can be utilized for an anterior tumour if there is no vitreous seeding and in other circumstances such as resistance to chemotherapy (Fig. 20.41).
- **External beam radiotherapy** should be avoided, particularly in patients with heritable retinoblastoma, because of the risk of inducing a second malignancy. At present this option is used only for eyes with residual or relapsed retinoblastoma following previous intravenous or ophthalmic artery infusion. Adverse effects include cataract, radiation neuropathy, radiation retinopathy and hypoplasia of the bony orbit.
- **Enucleation** is generally indicated if there is neovascular glaucoma, anterior chamber infiltration, optic nerve invasion or if a tumour occupies more than half the vitreous volume (group E). It is also considered if chemo-reduction fails and is useful for diffuse retinoblastoma because of a poor visual prognosis and a high risk of recurrence with other modalities. Enucleation should be performed with minimal manipulation and it is imperative to excise a section of optic nerve to at least 10 mm.

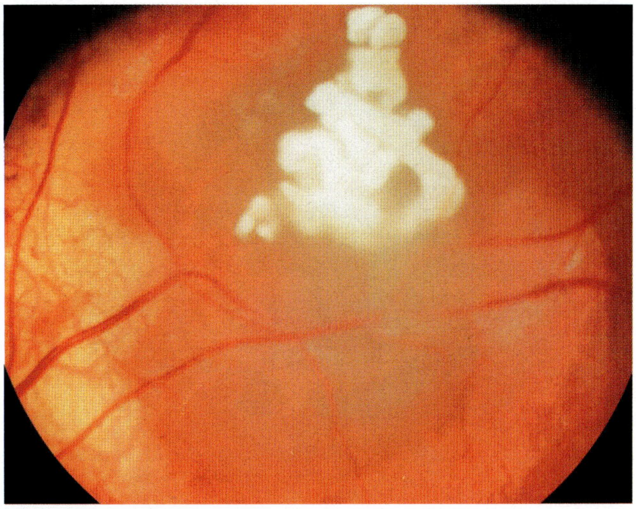

Fig. 20.41 Retinoblastoma – regression after brachytherapy.

- **Extraocular extension**
  - Adjuvant chemotherapy consisting of a 6-month course of CEV is given subsequent to enucleation at some centres if there is retrolaminar or massive choroidal spread.
  - External beam radiotherapy is indicated when there is tumour extension to the cut end of the optic nerve at enucleation, or extension through the sclera.
  - Systemic spread, especially CNS involvement, involves aggressive treatment with high-dose chemotherapy and autologous stem cell rescue.
- **Review.** Careful review at frequent intervals is generally required following treatment, in order to detect recurrence or the development of a new tumour, particularly in heritable disease.

TIP External beam radiotherapy should be avoided if possible in children with heritable retinoblastoma because of the risk of inducing a late second malignancy in the radiation field.

Differential diagnosis

- **Persistent anterior fetal vasculature** (persistent hyperplastic primary vitreous – see also Ch. 17) is confined to the anterior segment and often involves the lens.
  - Presentation is with a lens opacity (Fig. 20.42A) or leukocoria involving a retrolental mass into which elongated ciliary processes are inserted.
  - The size and density of the retrolental fibrovascular tissue is variable (Fig. 20.42B).
  - Complications include cataract and angle-closure glaucoma.
  - Early lens and vitreoretinal surgery may preserve useful vision in some cases.
- **Persistent posterior fetal vasculature** is confined to the posterior segment and the lens is usually clear.
  - Presentation is with leukocoria, strabismus or nystagmus.
  - A dense fold of condensed vitreous and retina extends from the optic disc to the ora serrata.
  - Treatment is not effective.

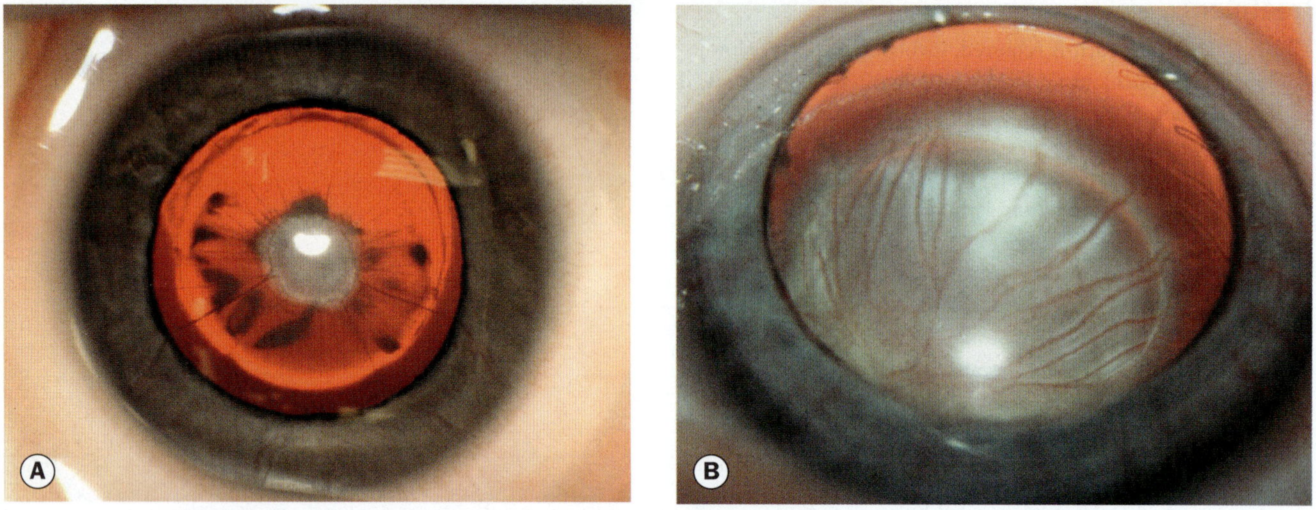

Fig. 20.42 Persistent anterior fetal vasculature. (A) Anterior polar cataract with radial vascularization; (B) retrolental vessels and less dense fibrosis. *(Courtesy of Ken K Nischal – fig. B.)*

- **Coats disease** is almost always unilateral, more common in boys and tends to present later than retinoblastoma (see Ch. 13).
- **Retinopathy of prematurity**, if advanced, may cause retinal detachment and leukocoria. Diagnosis is usually straightforward because of the history of prematurity and low birthweight (see Ch. 13).
- **Toxocariasis.** Chronic *Toxocara* endophthalmitis (see Ch. 12) may cause a cyclitic membrane and a white pupil. A granuloma at the posterior pole may resemble an endophytic retinoblastoma.
- **Uveitis** may mimic the diffuse infiltrating type of retinoblastoma seen in older children. Conversely, retinoblastoma may be mistaken for uveitis, endophthalmitis or orbital cellulitis.
- **Vitreoretinal dysplasia** is caused by faulty differentiation of the retina and vitreous that results in a detached dysplastic retina forming a retrolental mass with leukocoria (Fig. 20.43A and B). Other features include microphthalmos, shallow anterior chamber and elongated ciliary processes. Dysplasia may occur in isolation or in association with systemic abnormalities:
  - Norrie disease is an X-linked recessive disorder in which affected males are blind at birth or early infancy. It is caused by mutations in the *NDP* gene. Systemic features include cochlear deafness and mental retardation.
  - Incontinentia pigmenti is an X-linked dominant condition that is lethal *in utero* for boys. Mutations have been found in the *NEMO* gene. It is characterized by a vesiculobullous rash on the trunk and extremities (Fig. 20.43C) that with time is replaced by linear pigmentation (Fig. 20.43D). Other features include malformation of teeth, hair, nails, bones and CNS.
  - Walker–Warburg syndrome is an autosomal recessive condition characterized by absence of cortical gyri and cerebellar malformations that may be associated with hydrocephalus and encephalocele. Neonatal death is common and survivors suffer severe developmental delay. Apart from vitreoretinal dysplasia other ocular features include Peters anomaly, cataract, uveal coloboma, microphthalmos and optic nerve hypoplasia.
- **Other tumours**
  - Retinoma (retinocytoma) is a variant of retinoblastoma that generally exhibits benign behaviour but has a genetic profile indicating premalignancy – rarely, a retinoma can undergo late transformation into a rapidly growing retinoblastoma. It manifests as a smooth whitish dome-shaped lesion, which typically involutes spontaneously to a calcified mass associated with RPE alteration and chorioretinal atrophy (Fig. 20.44).
  - Retinal astrocytoma, which may be multifocal and bilateral (see below).

Retinal astrocytoma

Introduction

Astrocytoma (astrocytic hamartoma) of the retina and optic nerve head is rare. It frequently does not threaten vision or require treatment. Most are endophytic, protruding into the vitreous, but exophytic subretinal tumours can occur. An astrocytoma may be encountered as an incidental solitary lesion in normal individuals but is most frequently seen in tuberous sclerosis (see below) and occasionally in association with neurofibromatosis type 1 and retinitis pigmentosa. About 50% of patients with tuberous sclerosis have one or more astrocytomas, which may be bilateral.

Diagnosis

- **Symptoms.** Most tumours are asymptomatic and detected on screening for tuberous sclerosis. Isolated lesions, which are not associated with known systemic disease, are usually found at a routine eye examination.
- **Signs.** A yellowish or white semi-transparent plaque, nodule or mulberry-like lesion, often semi-transparent in its periphery and calcified centrally (Fig. 20.45A).

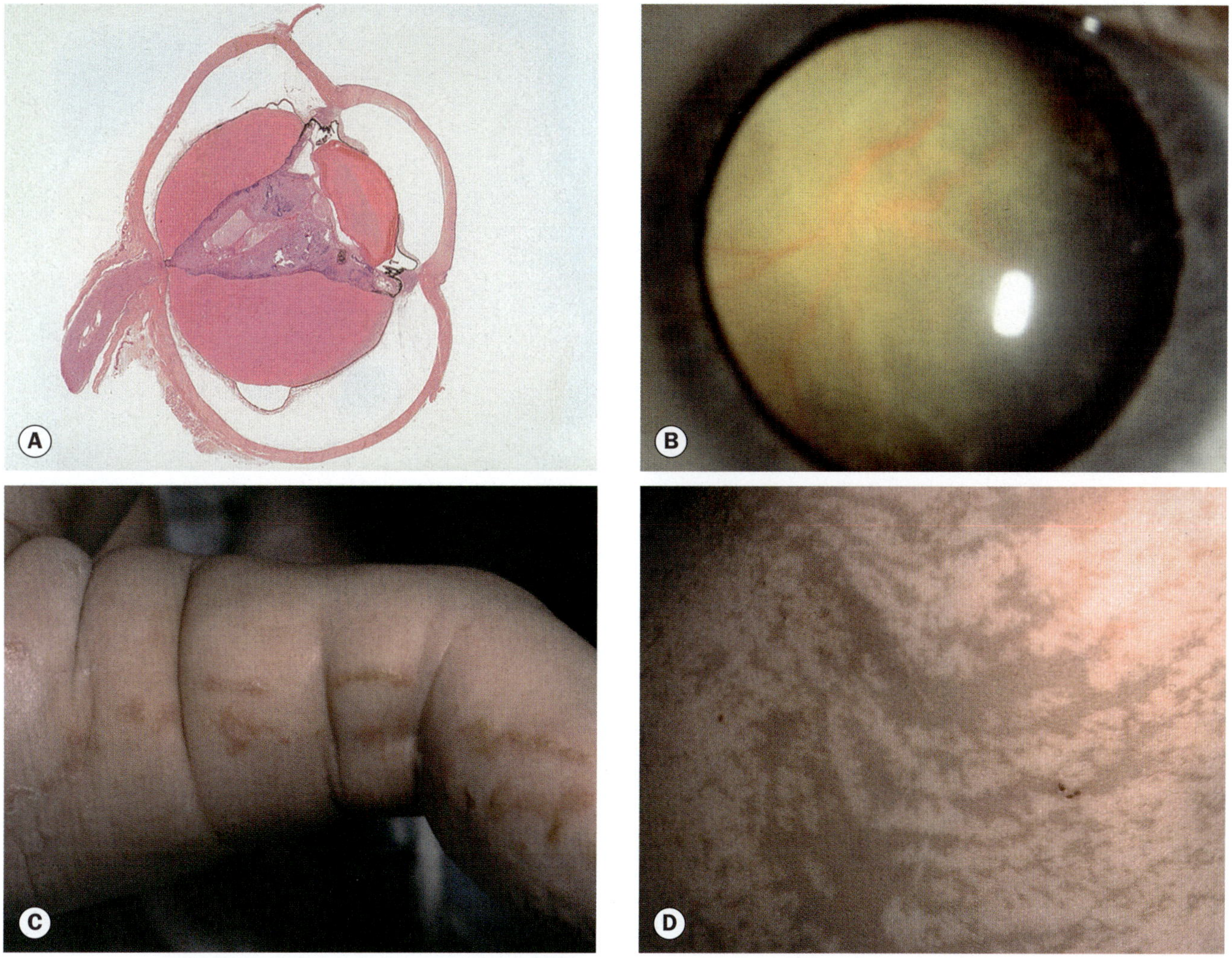

Fig. 20.43 Vitreoretinal dysplasia. (A) Pathological specimen; (B) clinical appearance; (C) vesicular-bullous rash in incontinentia pigmenti; (D) linear cutaneous pigmentation in an older child. *(Courtesy of J Harry and G Misson, from* Clinical Ophthalmic Pathology, *Butterworth-Heinemann 2001 – fig. A.)*

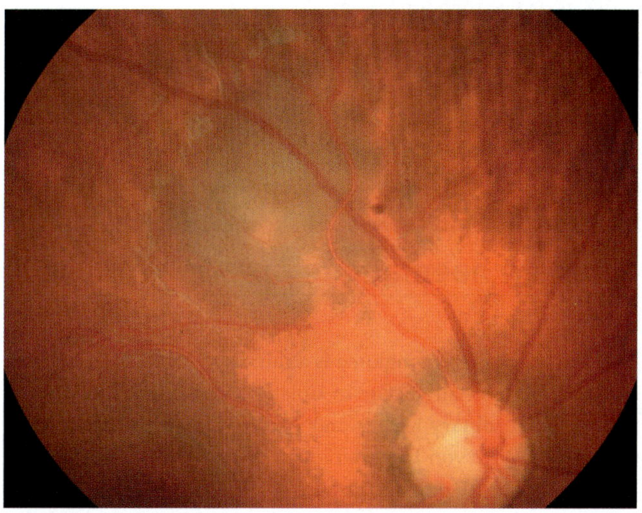

Fig. 20.44 Retinoma. *(Courtesy of M Parulekar.)*

- **Lesions can be large** (Fig. 20.45B) and/or have a cystic component (Fig. 20.45C). Growth with vision-threatening complications can occur.
- **OCT** shows a granular hyper-reflective appearance of the retinal layers with relative sparing of underlying RPE.
- **FAF** findings depend on the individual lesion's characteristics. Hyperautofluorescence is seen in seven calcified areas (Fig. 20.45D), with hypoautofluorescence elsewhere.
- **FA** shows a prominent superficial vascular network within the tumour in the arterial phase followed by late leakage and staining.
- **Systemic assessment.** With an isolated astrocytoma discovered incidentally in an older patient, the likelihood of the presence of forme fruste tuberous sclerosis is low. However, the option of genetic testing and systemic investigation may be offered.

Tuberous sclerosis

Tuberous sclerosis (Bourneville disease) is an autosomal dominant phacomatosis characterized by the development of hamartomas in multiple organ systems from all primary germ layers. The mutation is in the *TSC1* gene on chromosome 9q34 coding for hamartin, or in the *TSC2* gene on chromosome 16p13 coding for tuberin. These proteins act as suppressors of tumour growth. The classic triad of epilepsy, mental retardation and adenoma sebaceum is present in

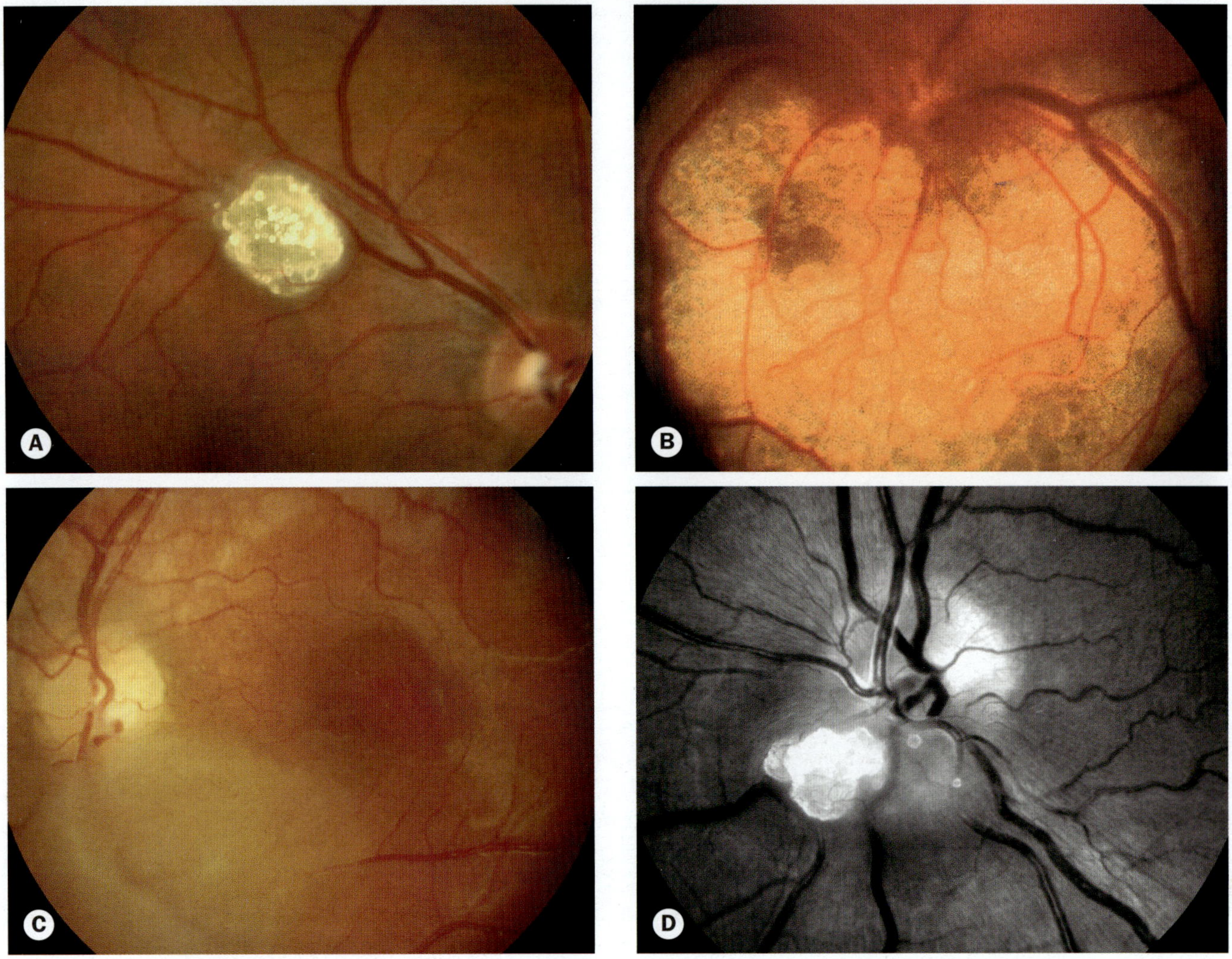

Fig. 20.45 Astrocytoma. **(A)** Yellowish mulberry-like lesion; **(B)** large diffuse lesion; **(C)** cystic variant; **(D)** red-free image of lesion infero-temporal to the disc.

only a minority of patients, but is diagnostic. About 60% of cases are sporadic and 40% are autosomal dominant.

- **Cutaneous signs**
  - Adenoma sebaceum, consisting of fibroangiomatous red papules with a butterfly distribution around the nose and cheeks (Fig. 20.46A), is universal.
  - Ash leaf spots are hypopigmented macules on the trunk, limbs and scalp (Fig. 20.46B). In infants with sparse skin pigmentation, they are best detected using ultraviolet light, under which they fluoresce (Wood lamp).
  - Shagreen patches consist of diffuse thickening over the lumbar region.
  - Subungual hamartomas (Fig. 20.46C).
  - Skin tags (molluscum fibrosa pendulum).
  - Café-au-lait spots.
- **Neurological features**
  - Intracranial paraventricular subependymal astrocytic nodules and giant cell astrocytic hamartomas.
  - Learning difficulties.
  - Seizures.
- **Visceral tumours**
  - Renal angiomyolipomas and cysts.
  - Cardiac rhabdomyomas.
  - Pulmonary lymphangiomatosis.
- **Ocular features** apart from fundus astrocytomas include patchy iris hypopigmentation and atypical iris colobomas.

RETINAL VASCULAR TUMOURS

Capillary haemangioma

Introduction

Retinal capillary haemangioma is a rare sight-threatening tumour that may occasionally occur in isolation, although about 50% of patients with solitary lesions and virtually all patients with multiple lesions have von Hippel–Lindau disease (VHL – see below). The prevalence of retinal tumours in VHL (often referred to as haemangioblastomas) is approximately 60%. Vascular endothelial growth factor (VEGF) is important in the development of retinal

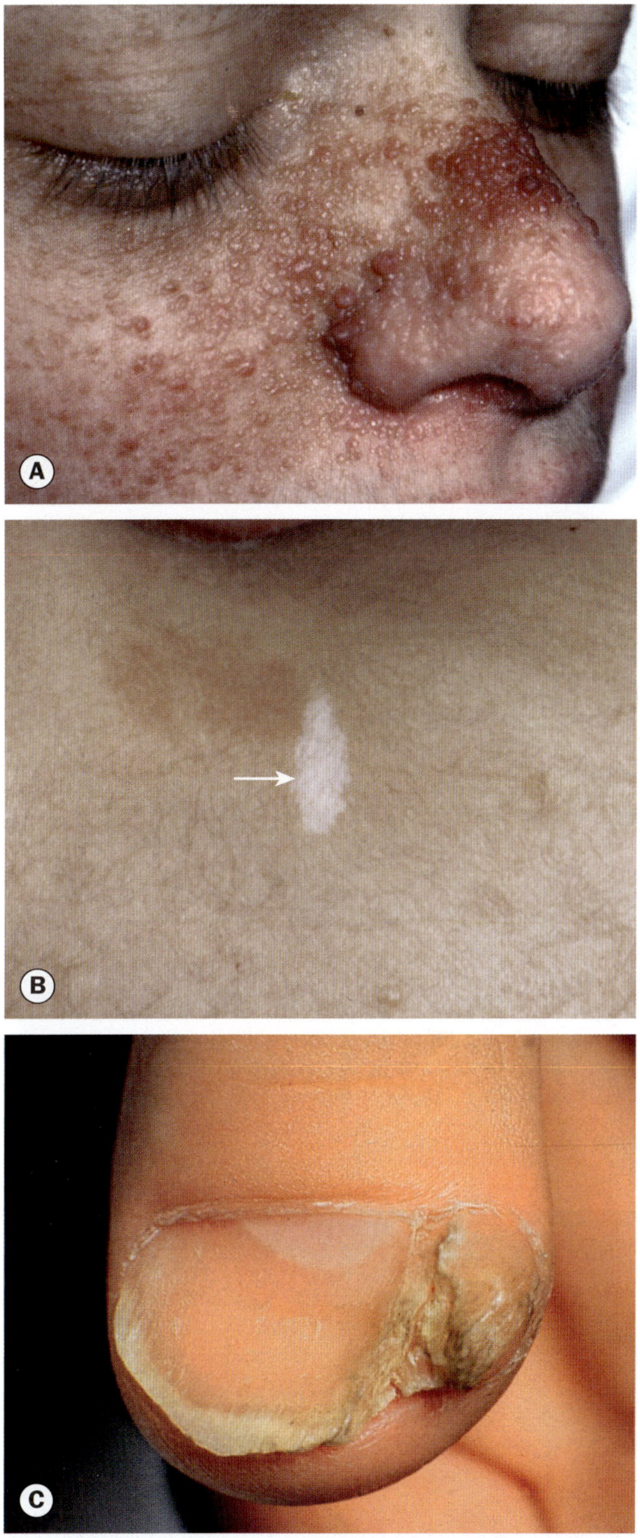

Fig. 20.46 Tuberous sclerosis. **(A)** Adenoma sebaceum; **(B)** ash leaf spot (arrow); **(C)** subungual hamartoma.

lesions, which are composed of capillary-like vascular channels between large foamy cells. The median age at haemangioma diagnosis in patients with VHL is earlier (25 years) than in those without VHL (31 years).

Diagnosis

- **Symptoms.** Tumours may be detected by screening of those at risk or because of symptoms due to macular exudates or retinal detachment.
- **Signs**
  - Early tumours appear as small red oval or round lesions located between an arteriole and venule (Fig. 20.47A).
  - A well-established tumour is seen as a round orange-red mass, usually located in the superior or inferior temporal periphery with dilatation and tortuosity of the supplying artery and draining vein extending from the optic disc (Fig. 20.47B).
  - A juxtapapillary site is common (Fig. 20.47C and D). Lesions are often on the temporal side of the disc, so that leakage can rapidly threaten the fovea.
- **Complications**
  - Leakage with exudate formation and/or haemorrhage.
  - Fibrotic bands, which can progress to tractional or rhegmatogenous retinal detachment.
  - Vitreous haemorrhage, secondary glaucoma and phthisis bulbi.
- **FA** shows early hyperfluorescence and late leakage (Fig. 20.48).

Treatment

- **Observation** is advised for asymptomatic juxtapapillary haemangiomas without exudation, because these may remain inactive for many years and because of the high risk of iatrogenic visual loss. Early peripheral lesions are not usually left untreated because they are relatively easy to ablate.
- **Laser photocoagulation** of small lesions. After closing the feeder vessels, the tumour is treated with low-energy, long-duration burns. Multiple sessions may be needed.
- **Cryotherapy** for larger peripheral lesions, especially those with exudative retinal detachment. Vigorous treatment of a large lesion may cause extensive but usually temporary exudative retinal detachment.
- **Brachytherapy** for lesions too large for cryotherapy.
- **Vitreoretinal surgery** may be required for non-absorbing vitreous haemorrhage, epiretinal fibrosis or tractional retinal detachment. If appropriate, the tumour may be destroyed by endolaser photocoagulation or surgical removal.
- **Other modalities** include photodynamic therapy (PDT), which avoids damage to adjacent tissues and anti-VEGF agents. These may be particularly appropriate for juxtapapillary tumours, which are otherwise virtually untreatable without visual loss.

Von Hippel–Lindau disease

Inherited VHL is autosomal dominant; about 20% are sporadic. The disease shows almost complete penetrance by 60 years of age. It is caused by a mutation in the *VHL* tumour suppressor gene on chromosome 3 which results in increased expression of tumour-inducing molecules.

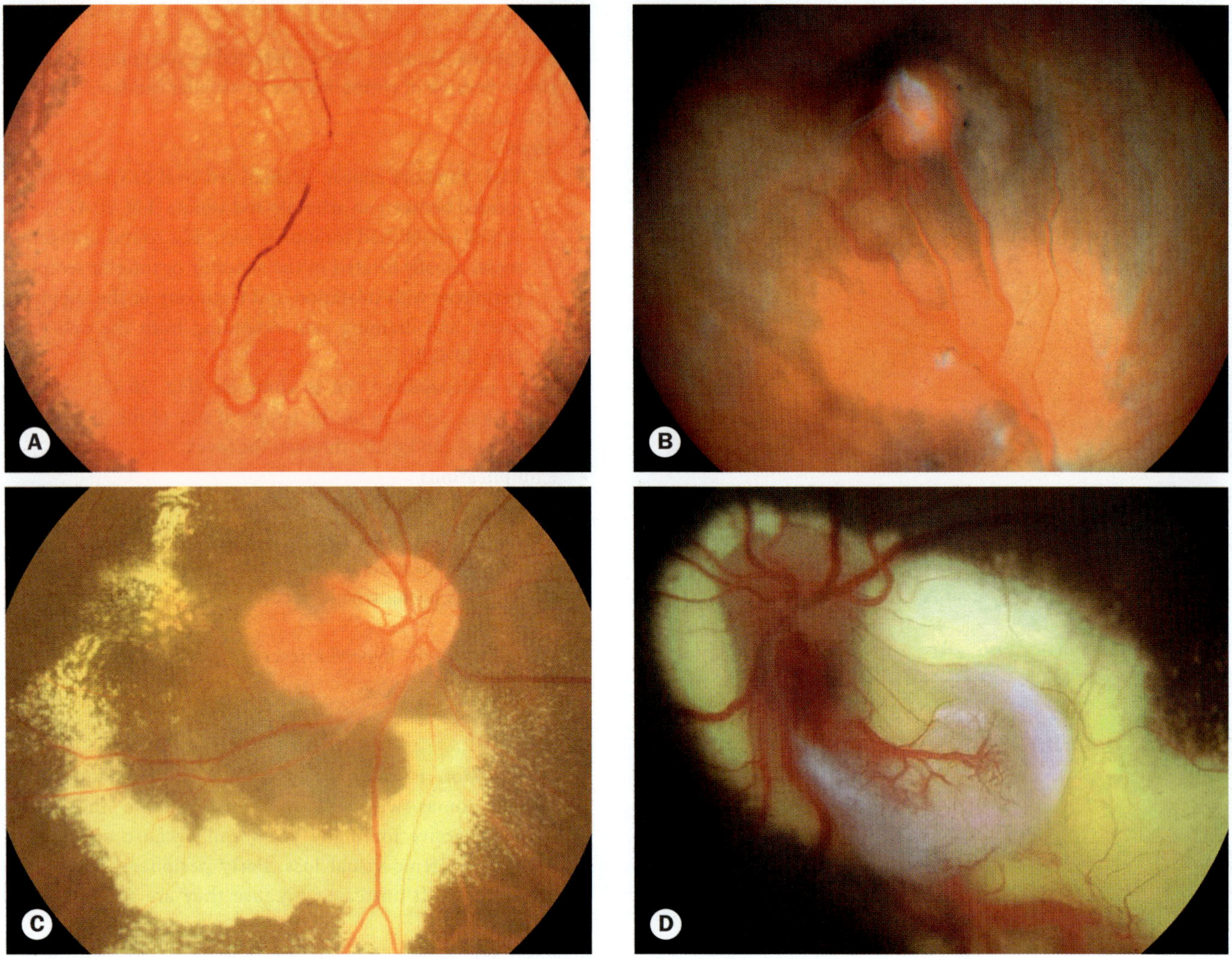

Fig. 20.47 Retinal capillary haemangioma. **(A)** Two early tumours; **(B)** more advanced lesion; **(C)** optic disc lesion with associated macular exudation; **(D)** very large optic disc lesion in von Hippel–Lindau disease. *(Courtesy of B Damato – fig. B; C Barry – fig. C.)*

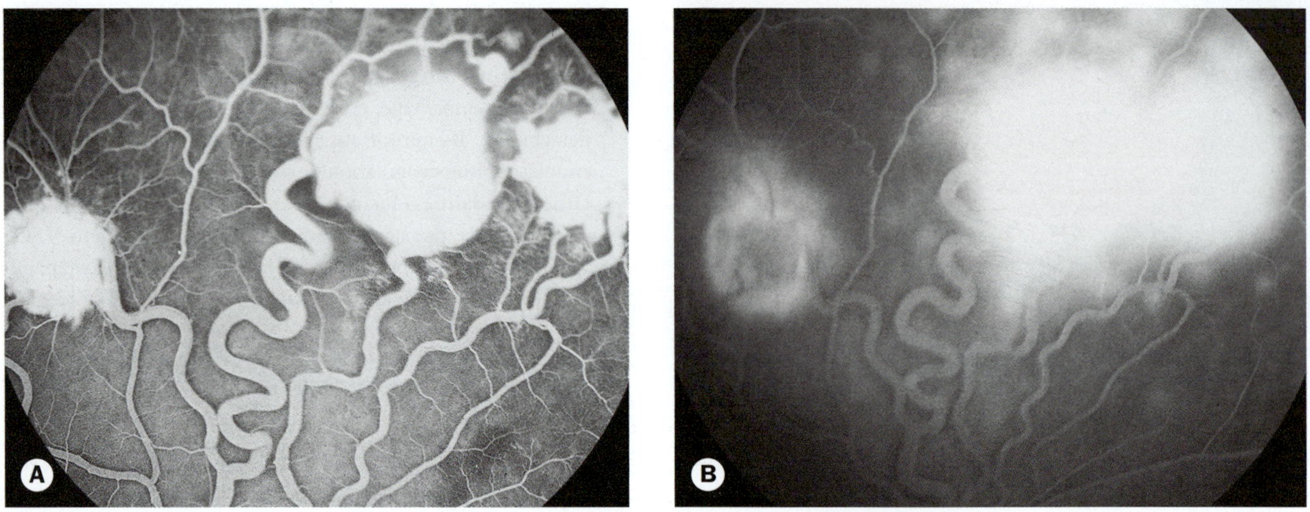

Fig. 20.48 FA of retinal capillary haemangioma. **(A)** Early filling; **(B)** late leakage.

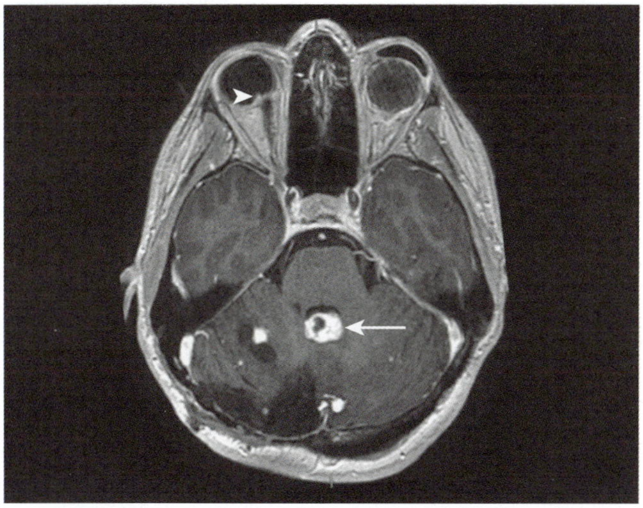

Fig. 20.49 Axial gadolinium-enhanced T1-weighted image in von Hippel–Lindau disease, showing a prosthesis in left orbit and a small haemangioma in the right fundus (arrowhead). There are eight further cerebellar haemangioblastomas, including a tumour-related cyst (arrow).

- **Clinical features**
  - Retinal haemangioblastoma is one of the first manifestations of the disease with an age of onset of about 25 years, although about 5% can present under the age of 10.
  - CNS haemangioblastoma involving the cerebellum (Fig. 20.49), spinal cord, medulla or pons affects about 25% of patients with retinal tumours.
  - Phaeochromocytoma.
  - Renal carcinoma and pancreatic islet cell carcinoma.
  - Cysts of testes, kidneys, ovaries, lungs, liver and pancreas.
  - Polycythaemia, which may be the` result of factors released by a cerebellar or renal tumour.
  - Endolymphatic sac tumours develop in the inner ear in 10%, with consequent hearing and balance difficulties.
- **Screening** is vital as it is impossible to predict which patients with retinal haemangiomas will harbour systemic lesions. Relatives should also be screened because of the dominant inheritance pattern of the disease. The following screening protocol should be regularly performed in patients with established VHL and relatives at risk.
  - Annual physical examination, retinal examination from age 2 to 5 years (6-monthly from ages 10 to 30 years), renal ultrasonography from age 15 years, 24-hour urine collection for estimation of vanillylmandelic acid and catecholamine levels from age 2 to 5 years to detect phaeochromocytoma.
  - Audiometry should be performed if there are any hearing or balance problems.
  - Two-yearly abdominal and brain MRI scans from the age of 15. If CNS lesions are symptom-free, treatment may not be required.
  - It is thought safe to discontinue screening at around age 60 years if no abnormality has been identified.
  - Genetic testing is indicated in all patients with suspected VHL and in first- and second-degree relatives. With modern techniques the likelihood of finding a mutation approaches 100% and once a mutation has been identified in the proband (initial subject) its presence can be confirmed or refuted in family members. Screening is unnecessary if the mutation is absent.

Cavernous haemangioma

Introduction

Cavernous haemangioma of the retina and optic nerve head is a rare unilateral congenital hamartoma. It is usually sporadic but occasionally can be inherited as autosomal dominant with incomplete penetrance in combination with lesions of the skin and CNS. Mutations in several different genes have been implicated. Histopathology shows multiple thin-walled dilated channels with surface gliosis.

Diagnosis

- **Symptoms** may occur secondary to vitreous haemorrhage. More frequently the lesions are detected by chance.
- **Signs**
  - Clusters of saccular aneurysms resembling a 'bunch of grapes' (Fig. 20.50A–C), with associated greyish fibrous tissue.
  - Because of sluggish flow of blood, the red cells may sediment and separate from plasma, giving rise to 'menisci' or fluid levels within the lesion.
  - A lesion occasionally involves the optic nerve head.
  - Haemorrhage and epiretinal membrane formation can occur.
- **OCT** demonstrates the aneurysmal vessels (Fig. 20.50D).
- **FA** highlights the sedimentation of erythrocytes and shows delayed filling in the venous phase and lack of leakage.

Treatment

Rarely, vitrectomy may be necessary for non-absorbing vitreous haemorrhage, but photocoagulation should be avoided as it may precipitate haemorrhage and enlargement of the tumour.

Congenital retinal arteriovenous communication (racemose haemangioma)

A congenital arteriovenous communication, the more severe forms of which are often termed racemose haemangioma, is a rare sporadic congenital malformation, with unilateral involvement in single or multiple sites of the same eye, most commonly temporally. Occasionally reported complications include haemorrhage, exudation and vascular occlusion, though the vision is commonly unaffected and the condition discovered at a routine examination. A visual field defect may be present. Some patients may harbour ipsilateral brain, facial bone and skin lesions (Wyburn-Mason syndrome), particularly those with more severe retinal changes.

- **Group 1** consists of an anastomosis with the interposition of an abnormal capillary or arteriolar plexus. A congenital retinal

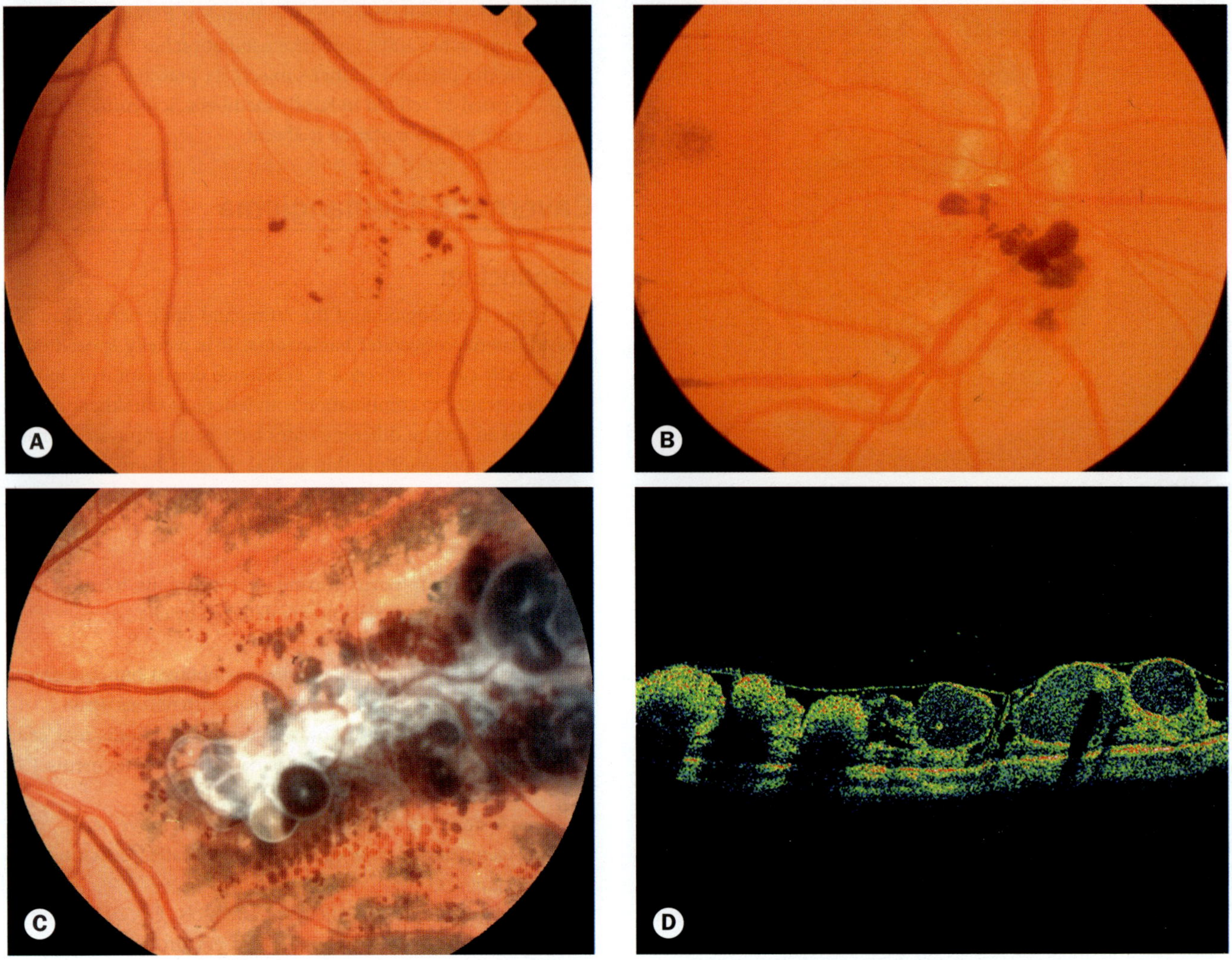

Fig. 20.50 Cavernous haemangioma. **(A)** Small peripheral lesion; **(B)** lesion adjacent to optic nerve; **(C)** larger lesion showing fibrosis; **(D)** OCT of lesion in **(C)** demonstrating aneurysms.

macrovessel is often present (Fig. 20.51A). This is an aberrant blood vessel, often larger than normal and usually a vein, located in the posterior pole; it may cross the fovea and horizontal raphe. Areas of capillary non-perfusion and foveal cysts may be seen. The anomaly is non-progressive and is usually associated with good vision.

- **Group 2.** Direct arteriovenous communication, without an intervening capillary bed. The intervening channels may be intermediate or large in size (Fig. 20.51B).
- **Group 3.** Many large-calibre tortuous anastomosing blood vessels that are often more numerous than normal, with venules and arterioles having a similar appearance. The changes extend from and are most evident in the region of the optic disc. With time the dilatation and tortuosity become more marked and sclerosis may be seen (Fig. 20.51C) but no leakage is seen on FA (Fig. 20.51D).

Vasoproliferative tumour

Retinal vasoproliferative tumour is a rare gliovascular lesion that can be primary (80%) or secondary to conditions such as intermediate uveitis, ocular trauma and retinitis pigmentosa. Secondary lesions may be multiple and occasionally bilateral depending on the underlying aetiology. Histology shows glial cells and a network of fine capillaries with some larger dilated vessels. Presentation is usually in the third to fifth decades, with blurring of vision due to macular exudation. A reddish-yellow globular gliovascular mass (Fig. 20.52A) is seen, most frequently in the inferotemporal periphery; retinal vessels may be seen entering the lesion posteriorly. Although the tumour is benign it can cause profound visual loss. Complications include subretinal exudation (Fig. 20.52B), exudative retinal detachment, macular oedema and fibrosis and haemorrhage. Treatment with cryotherapy or brachytherapy induces regression of the tumour and exudation, but the visual prognosis is poor if there is maculopathy.

PRIMARY INTRAOCULAR LYMPHOMA

Introduction

Lymphoma is a group of conditions characterized by neoplastic proliferation of cells of the immune system typified by

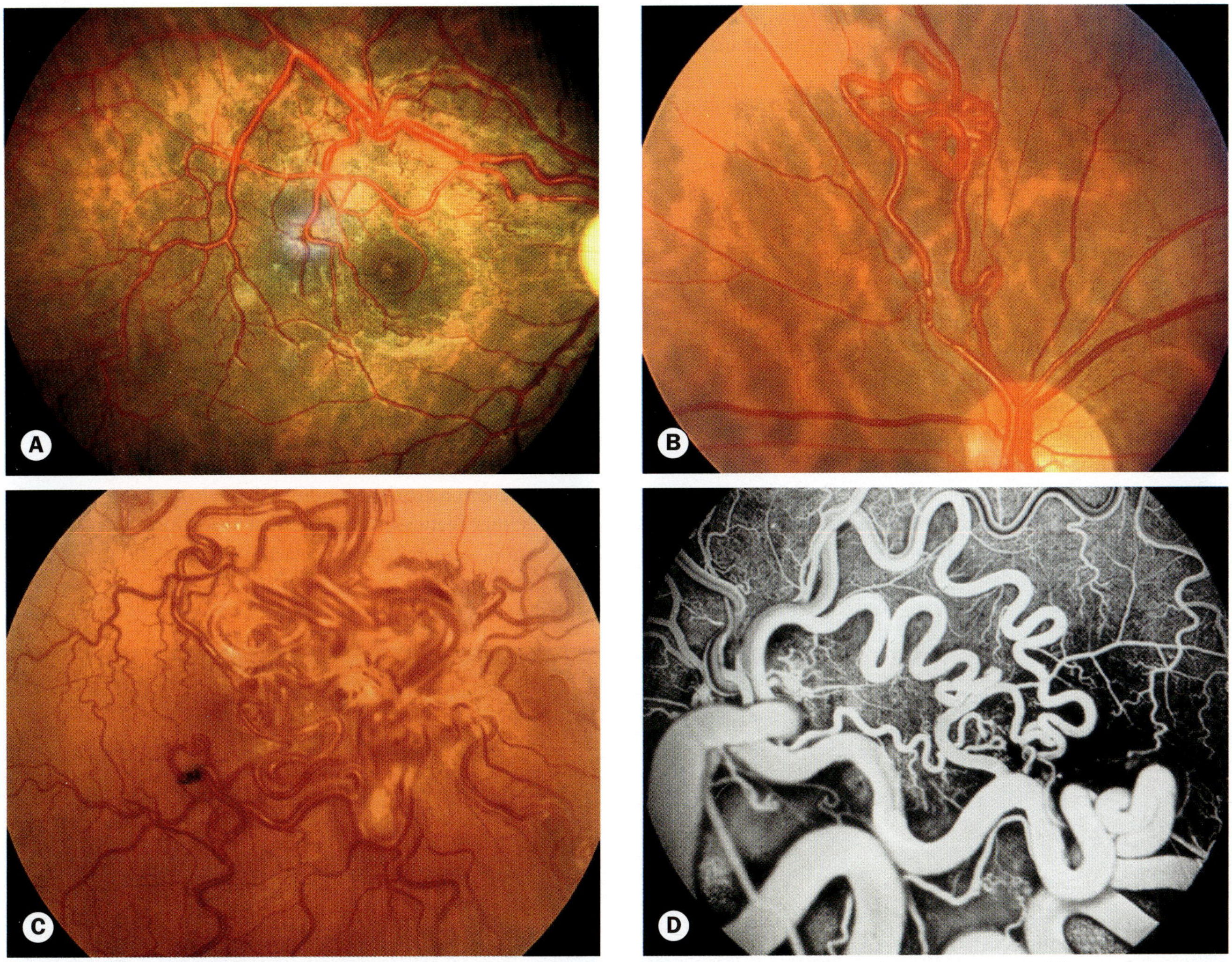

Fig. 20.51 Congenital arteriovenous communication (racemose haemangioma spectrum). **(A)** Group 1 lesion – retinal macrovessel; **(B)** group 2 – arteriovenous communication; **(C)** group 3 – typical racemose lesion with early sclerosis found in Wyburn-Mason syndrome; **(D)** FA showing hyperfluorescence but absence of leakage. *(Courtesy of C Barry – fig. B.)*

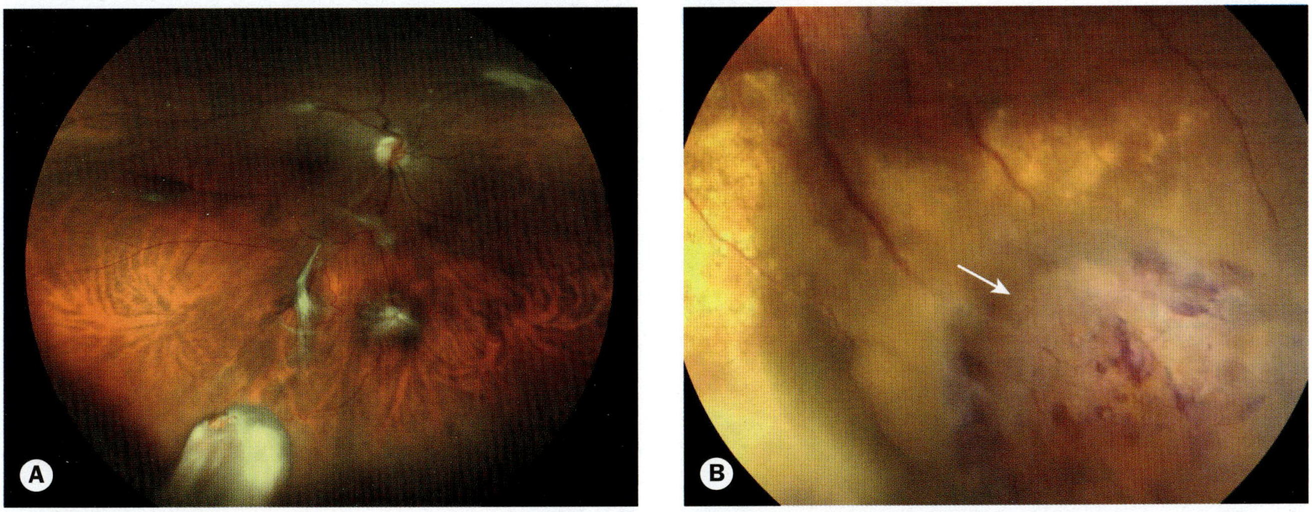

Fig. 20.52 Vasoproliferative tumour of the retina. **(A)** Yellowish peripheral glio-vascular mass; **(B)** mass (arrow) with intraretinal and subretinal exudation and haemorrhage. *(Courtesy of B Damato – fig. A.)*

lymphadenopathy, constitutional symptoms and, occasionally, CNS involvement. The main classification and ocular manifestations are as follows:

- **Hodgkin disease** may cause anterior uveitis, vitritis and multifocal fundus lesions resembling chorioretinitis.
- **Non-Hodgkin lymphoma** can manifest with conjunctival involvement, orbital involvement, Mikulicz syndrome and uveal infiltration.
- **CNS B-cell lymphoma** may be associated with intermediate uveitis and sub-RPE infiltrates.
- **Primary vitreoretinal lymphoma (PVRL)** represents a subset of primary central nervous system lymphoma (PCNSL), a variant of extranodal non-Hodgkin lymphoma. The PCNSL cells are large, pleomorphic B lymphocytes with large multilobular nuclei, prominent nucleoli and scanty cytoplasm. The tumour arises from within the brain, spinal cord and leptomeninges, is aggressive and has a poor prognosis. About 20% of patients with PCNSL have ocular manifestations, which can precede or follow neurological involvement. Most patients with PVRL subsequently develop CNS symptoms, with a mean delay of 29 months. Most of those affected are older adults.
- **Primary uveal lymphoma** is a rare entity, usually of B-cell origin, that tends to follow an extended relatively benign course and will not be considered further in this section.

Ocular features

- **Symptoms.** Unilateral floaters, blurred vision, red eye or photophobia. The symptoms frequently become bilateral after a variable interval.
- **Signs of PVRL**
  - Mild anterior uveitis with cells, flare and keratic precipitates.
  - Vitritis may impede visualization of the fundus.
  - Large, often multifocal, subretinal infiltrates (Fig. 20.53).
  - Occasionally coalescence of sub-RPE deposits may completely encircle the fundus.
  - Other features include retinal vasculitis, vascular occlusion, exudative retinal detachment and optic atrophy.

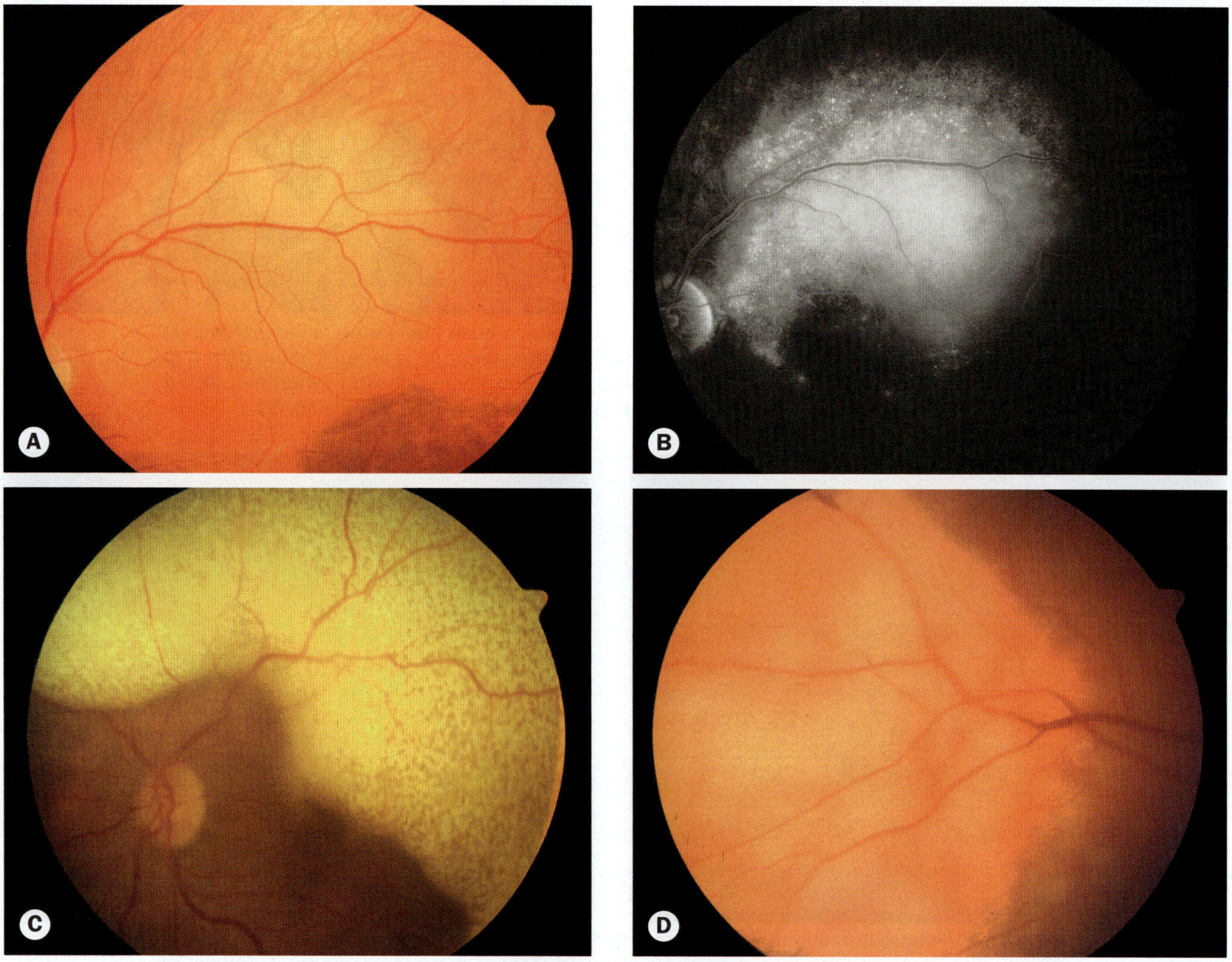

Fig. 20.53 Primary intraocular lymphoma. **(A)** Subretinal infiltrate without mottling; **(B)** FA late phase; **(C)** extensive subretinal infiltration with overlying mottling; **(D)** multifocal subretinal infiltrates without mottling. *(Courtesy of C Barry – figs A and B.)*

- Absence of cystoid macular oedema (CMO) is an important diagnostic indicator, since this is almost always present in true inflammatory vitritis.

Neurological features

- **Symptoms.** An intracranial mass may cause headache, nausea, personality change, focal deficit or seizures. Leptomeningeal disease may cause neuropathy and spinal cord involvement may cause bilateral motor and sensory deficits.
- **Clinical neurological examination** may demonstrate abnormalities such as cranial nerve palsies, hemiparesis and ataxia.

Investigation

- **OCT** will confirm an absence of CMO in most cases, aiding differentiation from vitritis and may demonstrate subretinal infiltrative lesions.
- **FA** shows blockage with a granular characteristic, due to the presence of sub-RPE accumulation of lymphomatous cells ('leopard skin spots').
- **Ultrasound** may show vitreous debris, elevated subretinal lesions, retinal detachment and thickening of the optic nerve.
- **Cytology** of vitreous samples or subretinal nodules.
- **Immunohistochemistry** based on cell-surface markers allows identification of the lymphocytic proliferation, which is of a B-cell type in most patients.
- **MRI** of head and spine with gadolinium contrast may detect one or more intracranial tumours, diffuse meningeal or periventricular lesions and/or localized intradural spinal masses.
- **Lumbar puncture** may demonstrate malignant cells in the CSF in a minority of patients with abnormal MR imaging, but a positive result avoids the need for brain or eye biopsy.

Treatment

Treatment of both the eye and the brain is often indicated. Radiotherapy and chemotherapy are the mainstays, but an optimal algorithm has not been established. Treatment limited to the eye may not improve survival, but local treatment may be preferable if there is monocular disease and no evidence of involvement elsewhere.

- **Radiotherapy** has long been the first-line treatment for PVRL, but recurrence is common and complications such as radiation retinopathy and cataract can occur. It now tends to be reserved for some cases of bilateral disease but may be associated with lower recurrence rates than chemotherapy alone. It is better tolerated by younger patients.
- **Intravitreal methotrexate** is useful for recurrent disease, but close monitoring is needed to detect ocular complications and any recurrence.
- **Systemic chemotherapy** with a variety of agents such as methotrexate can prolong survival in patients with CNS disease. This can be given in combination with whole brain irradiation but neurotoxicity is a problem. A variety of methods have been developed to overcome the blood–brain barrier. Systemic treatment is usually effective for ocular disease and this is preferred to ocular radiotherapy in some centres because in addition to avoiding radiation-induced complications it may improve survival. Monotherapy for primary intraocular lymphoma (PIOL) with ifosfamide or trofosfamide has also been successful.
- **Biologic agents involving** specific anti-B cell monoclonal antibodies (e.g. rituximab), may represent a useful alternative, but are generally given intravitreally because of poor penetration through the blood–brain barrier.

TUMOURS OF THE RETINAL PIGMENT EPITHELIUM

Congenital hypertrophy of the RPE

Introduction

Congenital hypertrophy of the retinal pigment epithelium (CHRPE) is the term used to encompass three entities with distinct features and implications: solitary CHRPE, grouped CHRPE and atypical CHRPE.

Solitary (unifocal) CHRPE

- A flat or minimally elevated dark-grey or black (Fig. 20.54A), round, oval or larger scalloped-edged lesion with well-defined margins, usually located near the equator or in the peripheral fundus.
- A depigmented halo located just inside the margin (Fig. 20.54B) and depigmented lacunae (Fig. 20.54C) are common, particularly as a lesion matures. Some lesions may become virtually totally depigmented.
- Median diameter is 4–5 mm but lesions can be much smaller or very large, especially in the far periphery (Fig. 20.54D) and may cause diagnostic difficulty unless the possibility of CHRPE is borne in mind.
- A posterior pole location is uncommon (2%).
- Histopathology shows densely packed RPE cells replete with large melanosomes – a combination of cellular hyperplasia and hypertrophy.
- Although formerly regarded as following a consistently stable course, a slight enlargement of the involved area over time is very common and the development of a presumed adenomatous or adenocarcinomatous nodule arising within the lesion (see below) occurs in around 2%. Long-term review is therefore now advised.
- Solitary CHRPE does not have an association with increased gastrointestinal malignancy risk.

Grouped (multifocal) CHRPE

- Multiple lesions, much smaller than those of solitary CHRPE and without haloes or lacunae, orientated in a pattern simulating animal footprints ('bear tracks' – Fig. 20.55A), often confined to one sector or quadrant of the fundus with the smaller spots located more centrally.
- There are typically several groups.
- Rarely the lesions may be depigmented ('polar bear tracks' – Fig. 20.55B).
- Only one eye is involved in almost all cases.

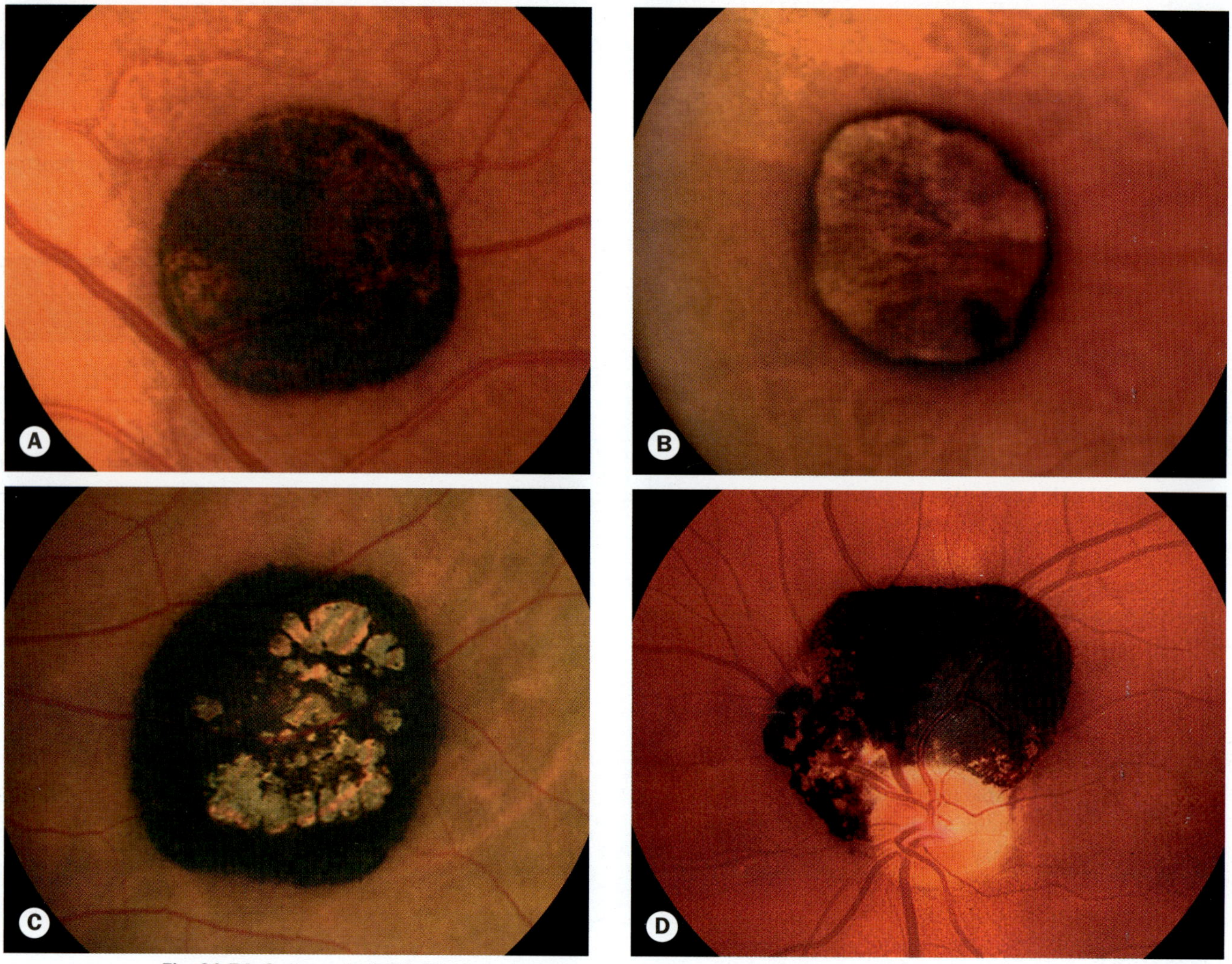

Fig. 20.54 Solitary CHRPE. **(A)** Heavily pigmented lesion; **(B)** partially depigmented lesion; **(C)** large lesion with depigmented lacunae; **(D)** peripapillary involvement.

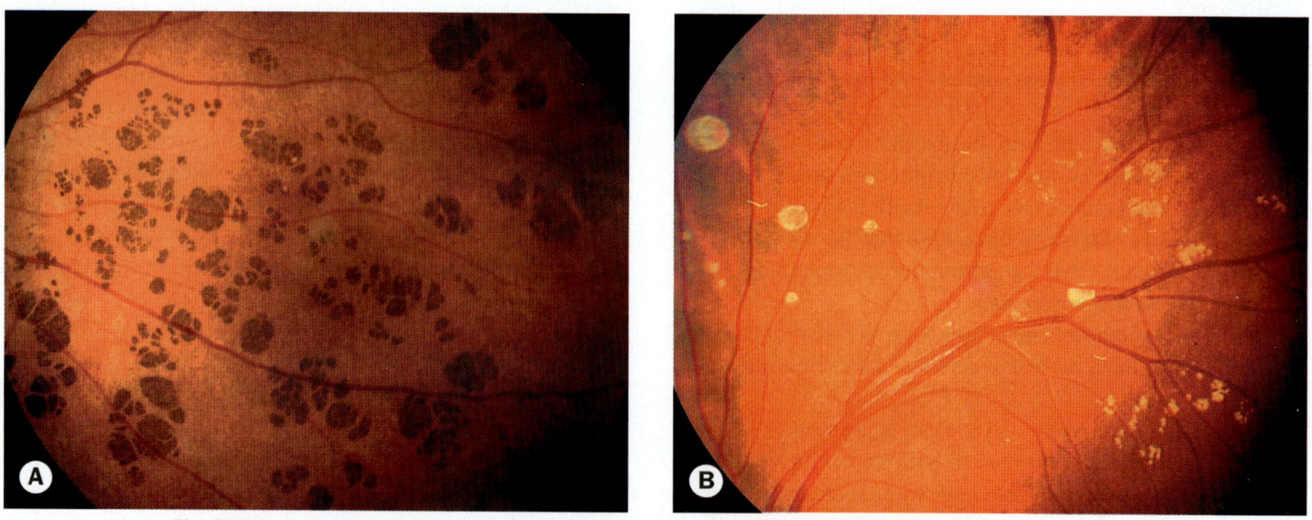

Fig. 20.55 Grouped CHRPE. **(A)** 'Bear-track' lesions; **(B)** 'polar bear-track' lesions.
(Courtesy of J Donald M Gass, from Stereoscopic Atlas of Macular Diseases, *Mosby 1997 – fig. B.)*

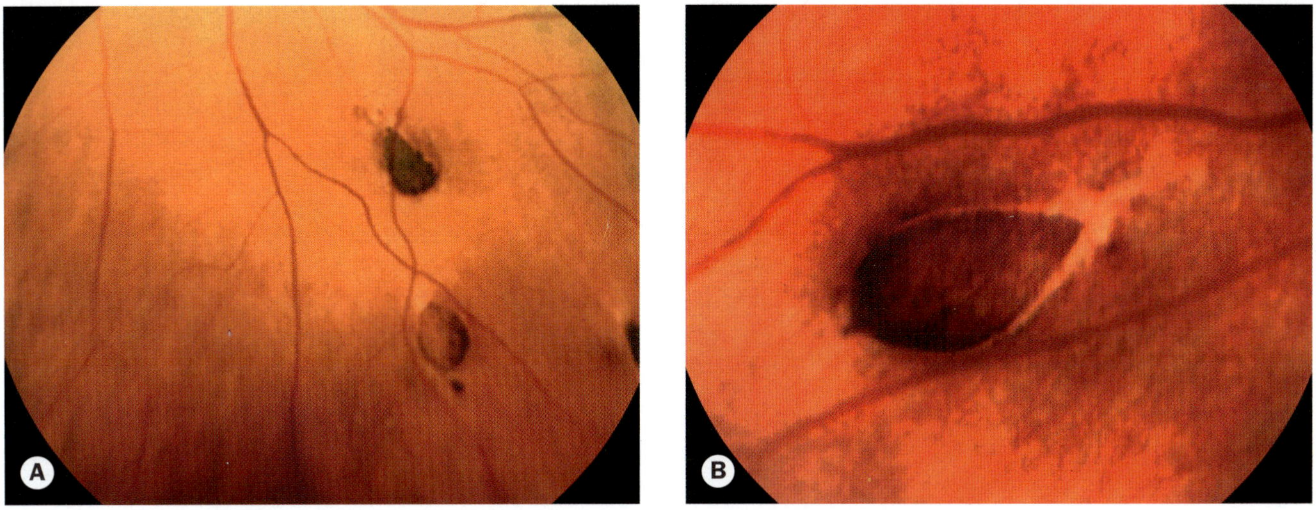

Fig. 20.56 **(A)** Atypical CHRPE; **(B)** characteristic depigmentation at one margin.

- The characteristic clinical appearance and monocular distribution serve to distinguish typical grouped CHRPE from the atypical multifocal variant associated with an increased risk of gastrointestinal malignancy (see below).

Atypical congenital hypertrophy of the RPE

- Multiple oval, spindle, comma- or fishtail-shaped lesions of very variable size associated with irregularly hypopigmented margins and perilesional areas (Fig. 20.56).
- Both eyes are involved.
- The lesions have a haphazard, not sectoral, distribution and may be pigmented, depigmented or heterogeneous.
- To emphasize the distinction with the CHRPE variants that are not associated with gastrointestinal malignancy, the alternative term 'retinal pigment epithelial hamartomas associated with familial adenomatous polyposis' (RPEH-FAP) has been proposed.
- **Systemic associations**
  - **Familial adenomatous polyposis** (FAP) is an autosomal dominant condition characterized by adenomatous polyps throughout the rectum and colon, which usually start to develop in adolescence. It results from a germline mutation in the gene *APC*; mutations falling within a certain codon range in this gene are associated with the presence of related CHRPE. Patients undergo regular colonoscopy and polyp excision. If untreated, virtually all patients with FAP develop carcinoma of the colorectal region by the age of 50 years. As a result of the dominant inheritance pattern, genetic testing and intensive survey of at-risk family members is imperative. Between 70% and 80% of patients with FAP have atypical CHRPE lesions, which are present at birth.
  - **Gardner syndrome** is characterized by FAP, osteomas of the skull, mandible and long bones, and cutaneous soft tissue tumours such as epidermoid cysts, lipomas and fibromas.
  - **Turcot syndrome** is an autosomal dominant or autosomal recessive condition characterized by FAP and tumours of the CNS, particularly medulloblastoma and glioma.

Combined hamartoma of the retina and RPE

Introduction

Combined hamartoma of the retina and RPE is a rare lesion that is probably congenital. It may be more common in males. It typically occurs sporadically in normal individuals but sometimes in association with a systemic disorder, particularly neurofibromatosis type 2, which should be considered particularly in children or if bilateral lesions are present. Histopathology shows thickening of the RPE and sensory retina with prominent glial and vascular tissue.

Diagnosis

- **Symptoms.** The most common presentation is with decreased vision or strabismus in early childhood, though symptom onset in late childhood or early adulthood is also frequent.
- **VA** is 6/60 or worse in 40–50%, usually secondary to macular involvement.
- **Fundus**
  - Slightly elevated deep grey or brown – sometimes orange, yellow or green – pigmented lesion that blends into the adjacent RPE at its margins (Fig. 20.57A).
  - Superficial whitish epiretinal membrane (ERM) formation with retinal wrinkling. Occasionally vitreoretinal interface changes are marked, sometimes with focal tractional retinal detachment.
  - Tortuosity and prominence of overlying retinal vessels, with evidence of feeder and draining vessels.
  - The lesion is usually located at the posterior pole, often in a juxtapapillary or macular site; peripheral lesions are uncommon. Dragging of the disc or macula may be present.
  - Uncommon findings include secondary macular oedema, exudation (Fig. 20.57B), choroidal and preretinal neovascularization, retinoschisis and retinal detachment.

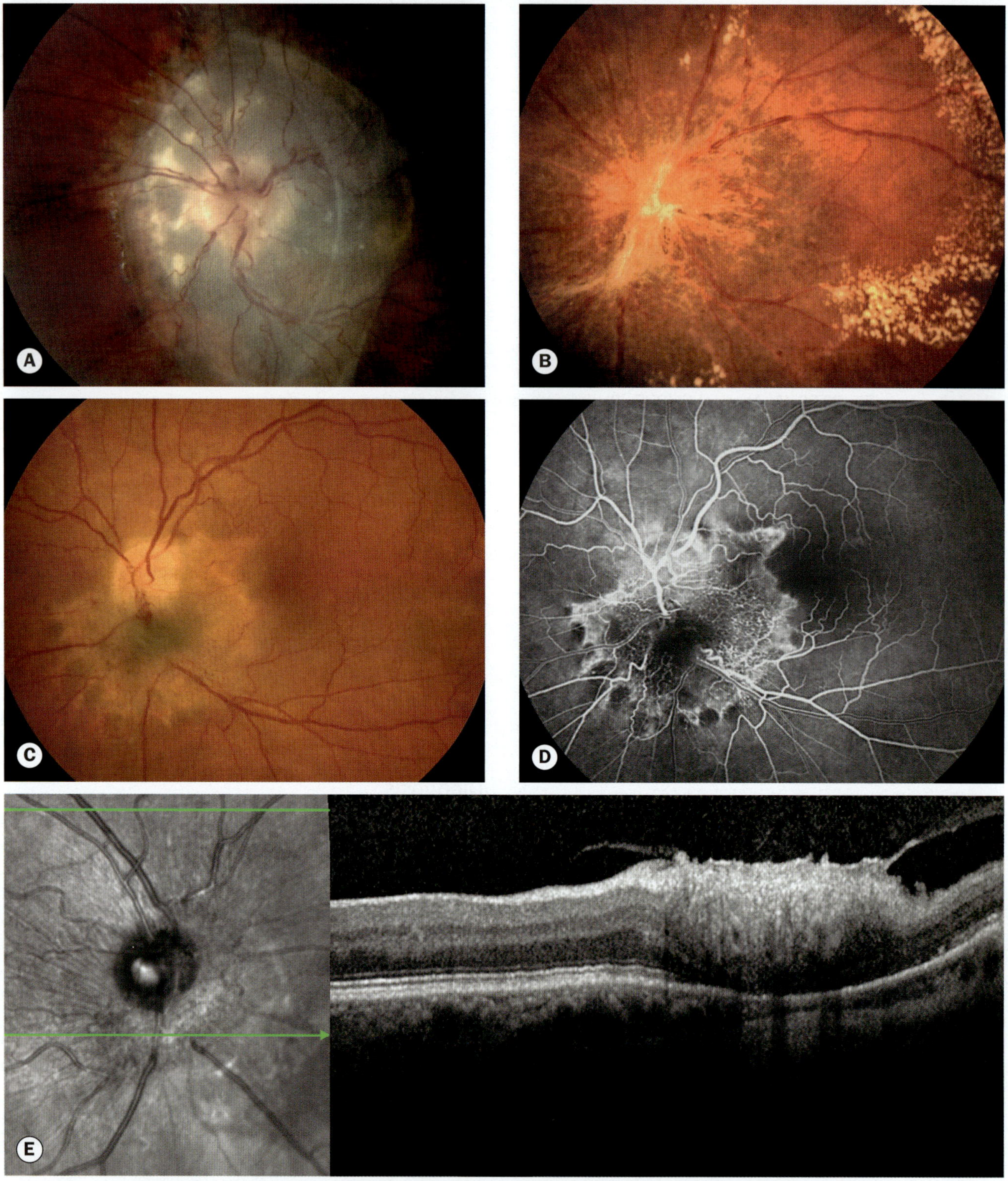

Fig. 20.57 Combined hamartoma of the retina and retinal pigment epithelium. **(A)** Lesion surrounding the optic disc; **(B)** larger peripapillary lesion with fibrosis and peripheral hard exudates; **(C)** peripapillary lesion; **(D)** FA of lesion in **(C)**; **(E)** OCT showing full-thickness retinal and RPE disorganization, associated with a saw-toothed appearance of the retinal surface secondary to an epiretinal membrane.

- **FA** shows early hyperfluorescence of the vascular abnormalities and blockage by pigment; the late phase may show leakage (Fig. 20.57C and D).
- **OCT** demonstrates localized full-thickness retinal and RPE disorganization (Fig. 20.57E). ERM formation has variously been reported as intrinsic to or distinct from the main lesion.

Treatment

- **Monitoring** for complications.
- **Amblyopia therapy** is important in young children.
- **Specific treatment** for macular neovascularization (MNV) and leakage where indicated.
- **Vitrectomy** for ERM has provided benefit in some cases.

Congenital simple hamartoma of the RPE

Congenital simple hamartoma of the RPE is a rare entity, usually incidentally diagnosed in asymptomatic children and young adults. It is typically a small (1.5 mm or less) jet-black nodular lesion, with well-defined margins, that appears to involve the full thickness of the retina and RPE and to protrude into the vitreous cavity (Fig. 20.58A). A feeding artery and draining vein are generally seen. The lesion is typically located immediately adjacent to the foveola. VA is usually normal, but is occasionally impaired as a result of central foveal involvement or traction.

Adenoma and adenocarcinoma of the RPE

Adenoma of the RPE is an oval pigmented lesion that most commonly arises in the peripheral fundus, sometimes from an area of solitary CHRPE. Associated vitreous inflammatory cells and retinal exudation are frequently present. Associated prominent feeding and draining vessels may develop. The behaviour of an adenocarcinoma is thought to be similar to that of an adenoma. Most lesions are simply observed in the absence of vision-threatening complications, as metastasis has not been reported. Fine-needle biopsy is sometimes required for diagnostic clarification.

Hyperplasia and migration of the RPE simulating uveal melanoma

Rare cases have been reported of massively proliferating RPE cells simulating a uveal melanoma, including by extraocular extension. True malignant tumours of the RPE are extraordinarily rare.

PARANEOPLASTIC SYNDROMES

Paraneoplastic retinopathies are rare diseases that might be missed or misdiagnosed by the unwary observer. Many of the patients present with visual symptoms before the primary malignancy is diagnosed. It is therefore important for clinicians to be familiar with these syndromes in order to detect the underlying malignancy as early as possible.

Bilateral diffuse uveal melanocytic proliferation

Bilateral diffuse uveal melanocytic proliferation (BDUMP) is a very rare paraneoplastic syndrome occurring usually in patients with systemic, often occult, malignancy. It is characterized by the proliferation of benign melanocytes in the outer choroid often manifesting with multiple naevus-like choroidal lesions (Fig. 20.58B), but a variety of other anterior and posterior ocular segment features have been reported, including red-grey subretinal patches, rapid-onset cataract, episcleral and conjunctival lesions. Vision can be severely diminished. The mechanism is uncertain, but a circulating factor may be responsible in many cases. Detection of an occult

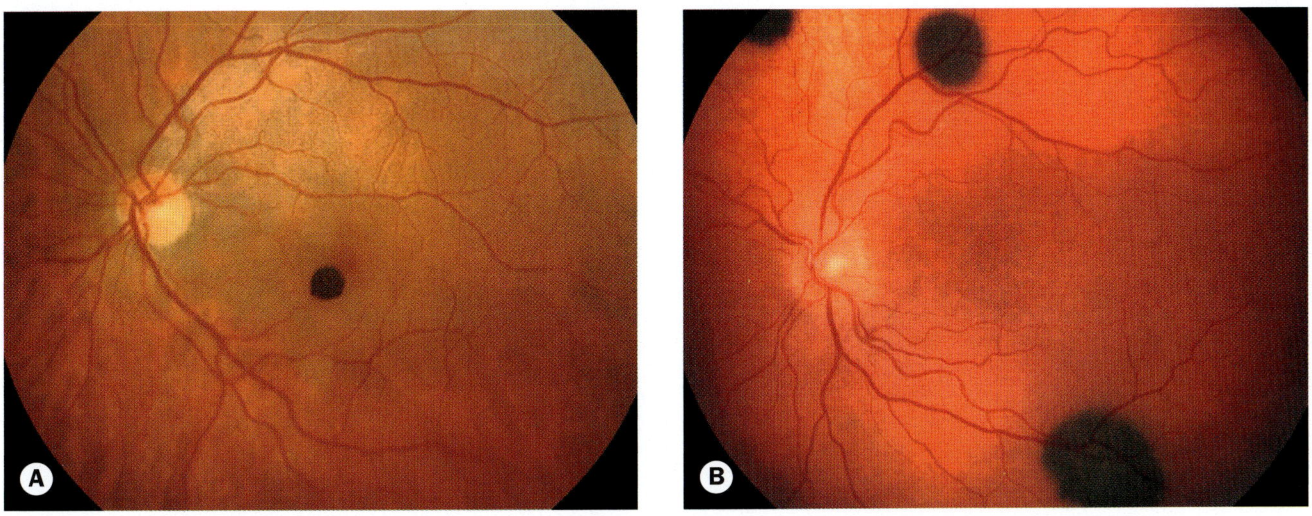

Fig. 20.58 Other pigmented lesions. **(A)** Congenital simple hamartoma of the retinal pigment epithelium; **(B)** naevus-like lesions in diffuse uveal melanocytic proliferation. *(Courtesy of A Leys.)*

primary malignancy might enable early treatment to enhance survival. Treatment of BDUMP itself is generally unrewarding – improvement with plasmapheresis has been reported – although successful treatment of the underlying primary tumour may be followed by regression of the BDUMP, but without improvement in vision.

Cancer-associated retinopathy

Cancer-associated retinopathy (CAR) is most frequently associated with small cell bronchial carcinoma. Visual symptoms precede the diagnosis of malignancy in half the cases, typically by several months but sometimes several years. Subacute visual loss occurs over weeks to months, associated with photopsia. Colour impairment, glare, photosensitivity and central scotoma are attributed to cone dysfunction. Night blindness, impaired dark adaptation, ring scotoma and peripheral field loss occur due to rod dysfunction. The fundus often appears normal on presentation, but attenuated arterioles, optic disc pallor and mild RPE changes develop as the disease progresses. The electroretinogram (ERG) is abnormal at an early stage under both photopic and scotopic conditions. As with BDUMP, CAR should prompt a thorough search for an underlying malignancy, though this is not always found and the condition is then regarded as an autoimmune retinopathy.

Melanoma-associated retinopathy

The presentation of melanoma-associated retinopathy (MAR) differs from CAR in that the visual symptoms usually arise after, rather than prior to, the diagnosis of cutaneous melanoma. There may be concurrent vitiligo. Autoantibodies from MAR sera react against bipolar cells in human retina. Clinical and electrophysiological data also implicate bipolar cells as the target in MAR. Generally, symptoms and signs are less marked than in CAR. The ERG shows marked reduction of dark-adapted and light-adapted b-wave and preservation of a-wave (normal photoreceptor function), characteristic of bipolar cell dysfunction. The prognosis for vision is usually good.

Chapter 21

Ophthalmic Side Effects of Systemic Medication

EYELIDS

- **Epidermal growth factor receptor (EGFR) inhibitors** are used for the treatment of many solid tumours. There is a dose-dependent risk of side effects. Trichomegaly is a common finding, while blepharitis and dry eye syndrome are less common. Cicatricial ectropion is rare.
- **Imatinib** is a tyrosine kinase inhibitor and is used for the treatment of chronic myeloid leukaemia and gastrointestinal stromal tumours. Up to two-thirds of patients develop periorbital oedema, usually 5–8 weeks after starting treatment. This is a mild problem and does not require discontinuation of medication. Ptosis has also been reported.
- **Dasatinib** is used for acute lymphoblastic leukemia and rarely can cause eyelash poliosis, which is reversible on stopping the medication.
- **Ipilimumab** is used for the treatment of metastatic malignant melanoma. Symptoms and signs similar to thyroid eye disease have been reported. This usually responds to systemic steroids.
- **Bortezomib** is a proteasome inhibitor which is used to treat multiple myeloma and predisposes to recurrent chalazia.
- **Isotretinoids** are used in the treatment of acne and can cause blepharoconjunctivitis, xerosis, corneal opacities, night blindness and pseudotumour. These side effects are reversible on stopping the medication.

CORNEA

Vortex keratopathy (cornea verticillata)

Clinical features

In approximately chronological order:

- Fine golden-brown opacities form an irregular horizontal line in the lower corneal epithelium of both eyes, similar to that of the common age-related Hudson–Stähli iron line.
- Several irregular branching horizontal lines form a pattern resembling the whiskers of a cat.
- With an increasing number of branches a whorled pattern develops, centred on a point below the pupil and swirling outwards, usually sparing the limbus.
- Associated pigmented clumps and iron deposition have been described.

Causes

- **Amiodarone**
  - Amiodarone is a cardiac antiarrhythmic agent.
  - Virtually all patients develop keratopathy (Fig. 21.1A), often soon after commencement. In general, the higher the dose and the longer the duration of use, the more substantial the corneal changes.
  - Vision is minimally impaired in around 5%, with loss of a single line of Snellen acuity, mild blurring and haloes. This is rarely sufficient to recommend discontinuation of the drug. The keratopathy reverses (slowly) on discontinuation.
  - Amiodarone can also cause anterior subcapsular lens deposits and optic neuropathy (see below).
- **Antimalarials**
  - Chloroquine and hydroxychloroquine are quinolones used in the treatment of certain autoimmune connective tissue diseases and in the prophylaxis and treatment of malaria.
  - In contrast to chloroquine retinopathy (see below), keratopathy bears no relationship to dosage or duration of treatment. The changes are usually reversible on cessation of therapy and sometimes clear despite continued administration.
- **Others.** Numerous other drugs have been reported as occasional causes of vortex keratopathy.
- **Fabry disease.**

Chlorpromazine

Chlorpromazine is used as a sedative and to treat psychotic mental illness. Some patients on long-term therapy may develop subtle diffuse yellowish-brown granular deposits in the corneal endothelium, Descemet membrane and deep stroma (Fig. 21.1B) within the palpebral fissure area. Anterior lens capsule deposits and retinopathy may also occur (see below).

Argyrosis

Argyrosis is a discoloration of ocular tissues secondary to silver deposits and may be iatrogenic or from occupational exposure. Keratopathy is characterized by greyish-brown granular deposits in Descemet membrane (Fig. 21.1C). The conjunctiva may also be affected.

Chrysiasis

Chrysotherapy is the therapeutic administration of gold, usually in the treatment of rheumatoid arthritis. Chrysiasis is the deposition of gold in living tissue and typically occurs only after prolonged administration. Virtually all patients who have received a total dose of gold compound exceeding 1500 mg develop corneal deposits, characterized by dust-like or glittering purple granules scattered throughout the epithelium and stroma, concentrated in the deep layers and the periphery (Fig. 21.1D). The findings are innocuous and are not an indication for cessation of therapy. In some cases, the deposits clear after stopping treatment whilst in others they may persist. Other toxic effects of gold are innocuous lens deposits and, occasionally, marginal keratitis.

Amantadine

Amantadine is an oral agent used in the treatment of Parkinson disease and related conditions. Some patients develop diffuse white punctate opacities that may be associated with epithelial oedema, 1–2 weeks after commencement of the drug, which resolve with discontinuation.

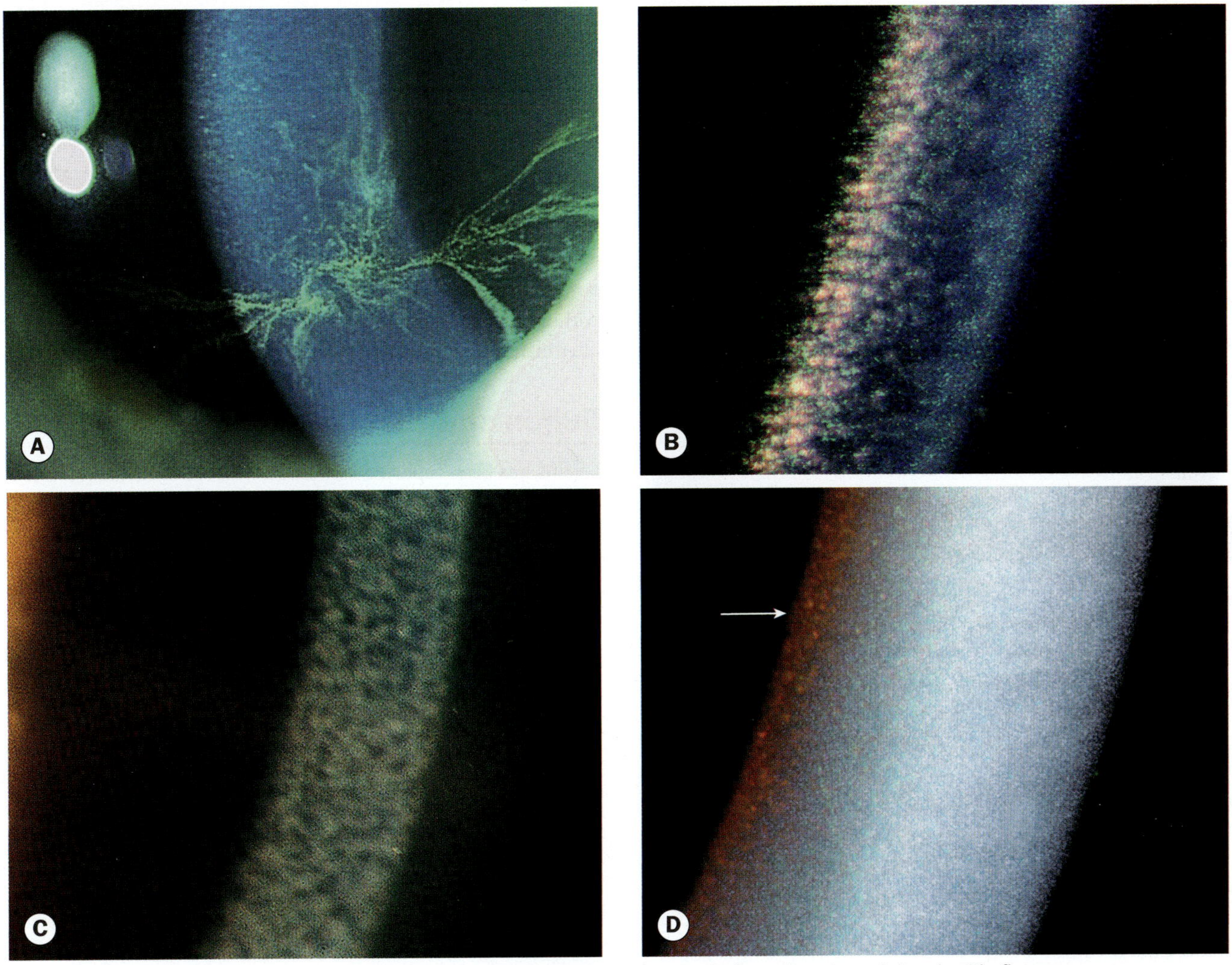

Fig. 21.1 Drug-induced keratopathies. **(A)** Amiodarone-induced vortex stained with fluorescein; **(B)** chlorpromazine; **(C)** argyrosis; **(D)** chrysiasis: characterized by dust-like granules in the deep corneal stroma and endothelium (arrow). *(Courtesy of L Zografos – fig. C.)*

Dupilumab

Dupilumab is used for eczema and atopic dermatitis and can cause conjunctivitis, refractory herpetic keratitis and uveitis.

CILIARY EFFUSION

Topiramate

Topiramate is an anticonvulsant and is also used in the treatment of migraine. It can cause acute angle closure with associated myopia secondary to ciliochoroidal effusion. A similar phenomenon has been reported with other drugs, especially other sulfonamides (including acetazolamide) and bupropion.

- **Presentation** is usually within a month of starting treatment, with blurred vision and sometimes haloes, ocular pain and redness.
- **Signs** include shallowing of the anterior chamber and raised intraocular pressure.
- **Treatment** consists of reducing the intraocular pressure and stopping the drug.
- **Prognosis** is usually good provided the complication is recognized.

TIP Topiramate is used in the treatment of migraine and may result in acute angle closure secondary to swelling of the ciliary body.

LENS

Steroids

Systemic and topical steroids can lead to cataract formation. The resultant opacities are initially posterior subcapsular (Fig. 21.2A), with subsequent anterior subcapsular involvement. Individual vulnerability seems to vary; children may be more susceptible than adults. The relationship between dose and duration and cataract formation is unclear, though higher doses and length of treatment are associated with greater risk. Early opacities may regress if steroids are discontinued, though sometimes progression may occur despite withdrawal.

TIP Excessive use of topical steroids can result in a posterior subcapsular cataract and/or secondary glaucoma.

Other drugs

- **Chlorpromazine** may cause the deposition of innocuous, fine, stellate, yellowish-brown granules on the anterior lens capsule within the pupillary area (Fig. 21.2B) in 50% of patients who have received a cumulative dose of 1000 g. The deposits persist despite discontinuation.
- **Gold** causes innocuous anterior capsular deposits in about 50% of patients on treatment for longer than 3 years.
- **Allopurinol**, used in the treatment of gout, increases the risk of cataract formation in elderly patients with a high cumulative dose or extended treatment duration.

UVEITIS

Rifabutin

Rifabutin is used mainly in the management and prophylaxis of mycobacterial infections. It may cause acute anterior uveitis (AAU), typically associated with a hypopyon. The associated vitritis may be mistaken for endophthalmitis. Concomitant use of drugs such as clarithromycin and fluconazole that inhibit the metabolism of rifabutin will increase the risk of uveitis. Treatment involves dose reduction or withdrawal of the drug.

Cidofovir

Cidofovir is used in the management of cytomegalovirus (CMV) retinitis in acquired immunodeficiency syndrome (AIDS). AAU with few cells but marked fibrinous exudate may develop following repeated intravenous infusions. Vitritis is common and hypopyon may occur with long-term administration. Treatment with topical steroids and mydriatics is usually successful, obviating the need to discontinue therapy.

Bisphosphonates

Bisphosphonates are a class of drugs that retard absorption of bone, commonly in osteoporosis but also in several other conditions. They activate a sub-group of T cells and it is thought that uveitis (usually anterior) and scleritis sometimes seen following administration is related to this. Inflammation typically occurs within 2 days of commencement of a bisphosphonate, or earlier after intravenous administration.

Sulfonamides

Uveitis has been reported associated with sulfonamide treatment, but is rare. Sulfonamides can also precipitate ciliary effusion with myopia and angle closure (see above) and are a well-documented cause of Stevens–Johnson syndrome.

Fluoroquinolones

Systemic administration of fluoroquinolone antibiotics, particularly moxifloxacin, has been associated with acute extensive anterior segment pigment dispersion (see also bilateral acute iris transillumination (BAIT) and bilateral acute depigmentation of the iris (BADI) in Ch. 11). It is not clear whether inflammation is the primary mechanism, which may be phototoxicity due to sensitization by the drug in predisposed individuals.

Tumour necrosis factor inhibitors

Although these drugs (e.g. etanercept, infliximab, adalimumab) have been adopted for the treatment of ocular inflammation, paradoxically uveitis has also been documented as an adverse effect. The induction of sarcoidosis has also been reported.

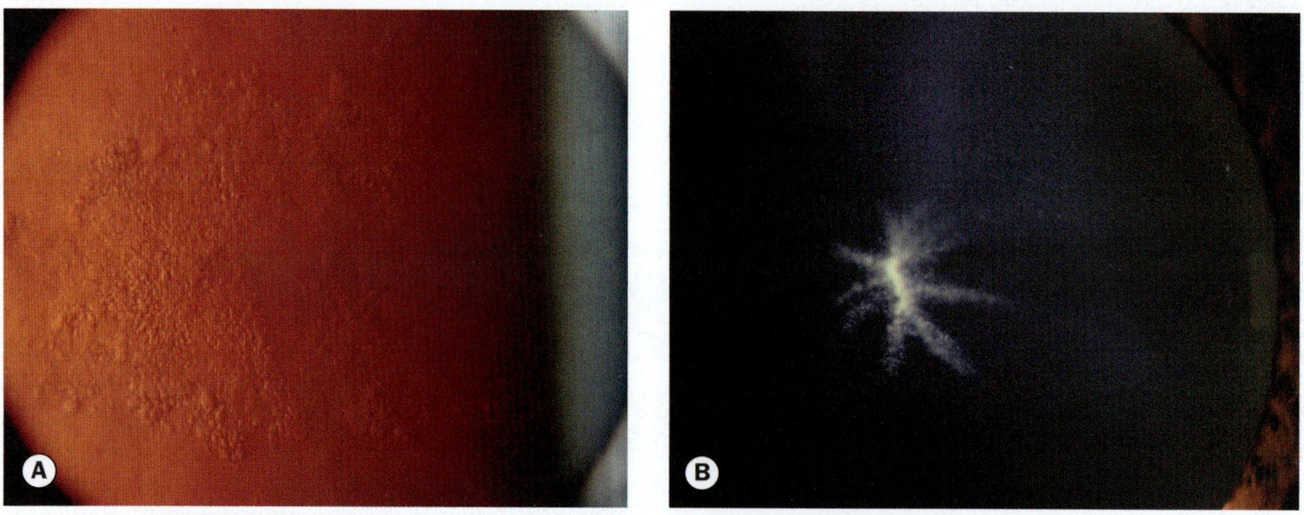

Fig. 21.2 (A) Steroid-induced posterior subcapsular cataract; **(B)** anterior capsular deposits due to chlorpromazine.

RETINA

Chloroquine and hydroxychloroquine

Introduction

Chloroquine was used to prevent and treat malaria in the past, but is less often prescribed in recent times because of resistance to the medication. Hydroxychloroquine is used to treat long-term inflammatory disorders of the joints and skin. These medications are concentrated in melanin-containing structures of the eye, such as the retinal pigment epithelium (RPE) and choroid. Hydroxychloroquine is generally safe and cost effective but can cause permanent loss of vision because of retinal toxicity, particularly if the recommended dose is exceeded. Retinal adverse effects may be more common than previously believed and progression can occur despite discontinuation of the drug. Significant damage can occur without signs on fundus examination and optical coherence tomography (OCT) scanning of the macula has therefore emerged as a key part of screening. Renal impairment and the use of tamoxifen increases the risk of toxicity. Obesity may lead to miscalculation of the safe dose, as hydroxychloroquine is not stored in fat. Vortex keratopathy may occur (see above).

- **Chloroquine** can result in retinal toxicity. The risk of toxicity increases significantly when the cumulative dose exceeds 300 g. Individual susceptibility seems highly variable.
- **Hydroxychloroquine** is much safer than chloroquine, particularly if the dose is kept to less than 5 mg/kg real weight/day. The risk of developing retinal toxicity has been reported to be 7.5% for an individual taking the medication for more than 5 years. Between 20% and 50% of people taking hydroxychloroquine for more than 20 years will have some signs of retinopathy. The risk increases with a cumulative dose over 1000 g, equating to a standard twice-daily dose of 200 mg for around 7 years.

Diagnosis

- **Premaculopathy** consists of early functional and structural changes prior to visible fundus signs. The goal of screening is to detect toxicity at this stage prior to irreversible damage.
  - High-resolution OCT imaging is relatively sensitive and shows parafoveal outer retinal lining, loss of the cone outer-segment tip-line and disruption of the inner-segment/outer-segment line as early features. The inferotemporal macula is the earliest location of hydroxychloroquine toxicity.
  - When available, multifocal electroretinography (see Ch. 15) can demonstrate early changes.
  - Subtle central visual field defects (e.g. Humphrey 10-2, Amsler grid) may be detected, but standard perimetry is less sensitive than the imaging modalities above.
  - Mild colour vision defects may be present, but the commonly used Ishihara chart is of relatively low sensitivity for this purpose.
- **Early maculopathy** is characterized by a modest reduction of visual acuity – VA (6/9–6/12) and subtle macular disturbance. Fundus autofluorescence (FAF) and macular pigment density assessment may be useful (Fig. 21.3A). With progressive loss of the perifoveal outer retina, the preserved central foveal tissue results in the 'flying saucer' sign on OCT scanning (Fig. 21.3B).
- **Progression of retinopathy** through moderate–severe reduction in VA (6/36–6/60) is associated with corresponding deterioration of the clinical appearance to give a 'bull's eye' macular lesion, characterized by a foveolar island of pigment surrounded by a depigmented zone of RPE atrophy, which is itself encircled by a hyperpigmented ring (Fig. 21.4A). A more substantial macular lesion follows, with widespread RPE atrophy surrounding the fovea (Fig. 21.4B). Retinal arterioles may become attenuated and pigment clumps can form in the peripheral retina (Fig. 21.4C). Fluorescein angiography (FA)

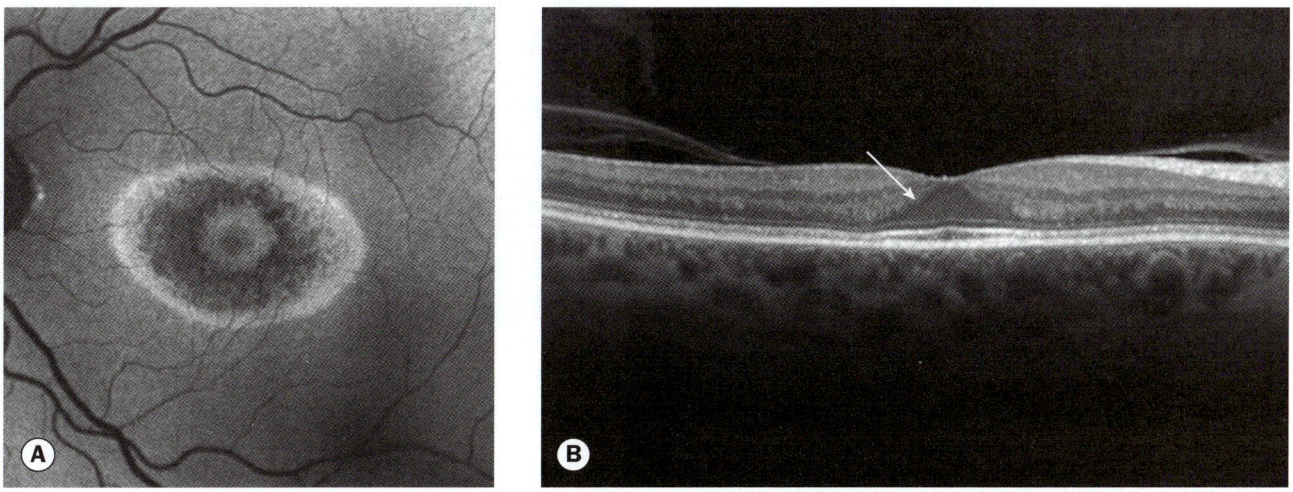

Fig. 21.3 Imaging of chloroquine retinopathy. **(A)** FAF of established maculopathy showing two oval areas of hyperautofluorescence and loss of retinal pigment epithelium in the parafovea; **(B)** OCT shows disruption of photoreceptors and loss of inner-segment/outer-segment junction in the fovea (arrow – 'flying saucer' sign). *(Courtesy of I Yusuf.)*

typically shows hyperfluorescence in a 'bull's eye' pattern. OCT has superseded the use of this investigation.

Screening

- **Patient education:** the importance of regular screening should be emphasized.
- **Baseline assessment** before or soon after commencement of treatment is advisable, including documentation of functional visual parameters together with an OCT scan of the macula. This serves as a basis for future comparison and also helps to exclude pre-existing maculopathy as a potential relative contraindication.
- **Annual review.** In the absence of special risk factors, routine annual review with ancillary testing (central visual fields, FAF and SD-OCT) should begin 5 years after starting treatment. Review one year after starting treatment: (a) in children, (b) those on chloroquine treatment or (c) if there are supplementary risk factors such as age-related maculopathy, substantial renal impairment, or tamoxifen use.
- **Discontinuation of the drug** should be discussed with the patient's rheumatologist if toxicity is suspected.

Phenothiazines

- **Thioridazine** is used to treat schizophrenia and related psychoses. The normal daily dose is 150–600 mg. Doses that exceed 800 mg/day for just a few weeks may be sufficient to cause reduced VA and impairment of dark adaptation. Progressive retinal toxicity can occur.
  - 'Salt and pepper' pigmentary disturbance involving the mid-periphery and posterior pole is an early feature (Fig. 21.5A).
  - Progression to plaque-like pigmentation and focal loss of the RPE and choriocapillaris (Fig. 21.5B).
  - Eventually, diffuse loss of the RPE and choriocapillaris is seen. FA shows punctate hyperfluorescence (Fig. 21.5C).
- **Chlorpromazine.** The normal daily dose is 75–300 mg. Retinal toxicity is a risk only if substantially larger doses are used over a prolonged period and is characterized by non-specific pigmentary granularity and clumping.
- **Digitalis (digoxin)** is used as second-line treatment for atrial fibrillation and symptomatic heart failure. It has a narrow therapeutic margin and toxicity can result in digestive, neurological and visual disturbance. A spectrum of visual abnormality may occur, including decreased visual acuity, scotomas, photophobia and dyschromatopsia, which is most commonly found on formal colour testing. Xanthopsia (yellow vision), cyanopsia (blue vision) and chloropsia (green vision) have all been reported. Electroretinogram abnormalities include delayed implicit time and reduced amplitude of the B-wave.

Drug-induced crystalline maculopathies

- **Tamoxifen** is an anti-oestrogen medication used in the treatment of some patients with breast carcinoma. The normal daily dose is 20–40 mg. Ocular complications are uncommon. Retinal toxicity with visual impairment may develop in patients on

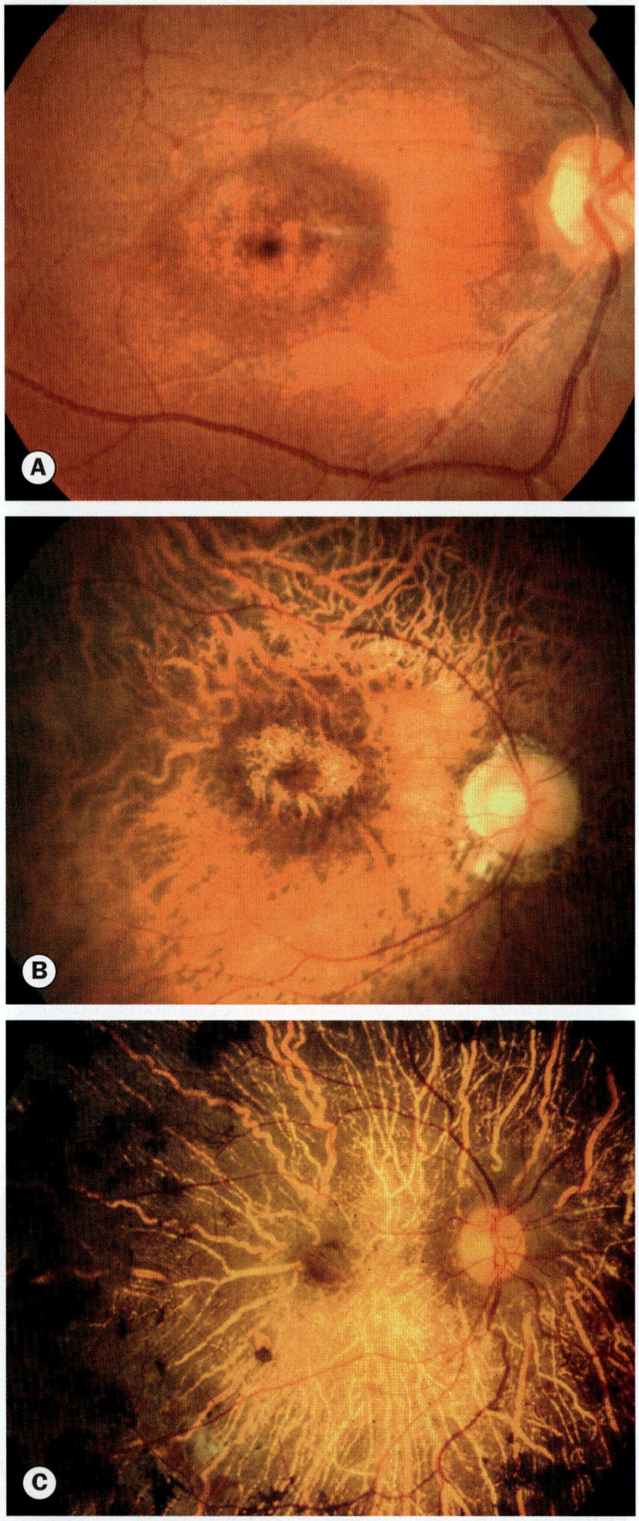

Fig. 21.4 Chloroquine retinopathy of progressive severity. **(A)** Early; **(B)** moderate; **(C)** severe.

TIP Loss of the outer retinal layer in a parafoveal distribution on OCT scanning is a sensitive method of detecting early toxicity to hydroxychloroquine.

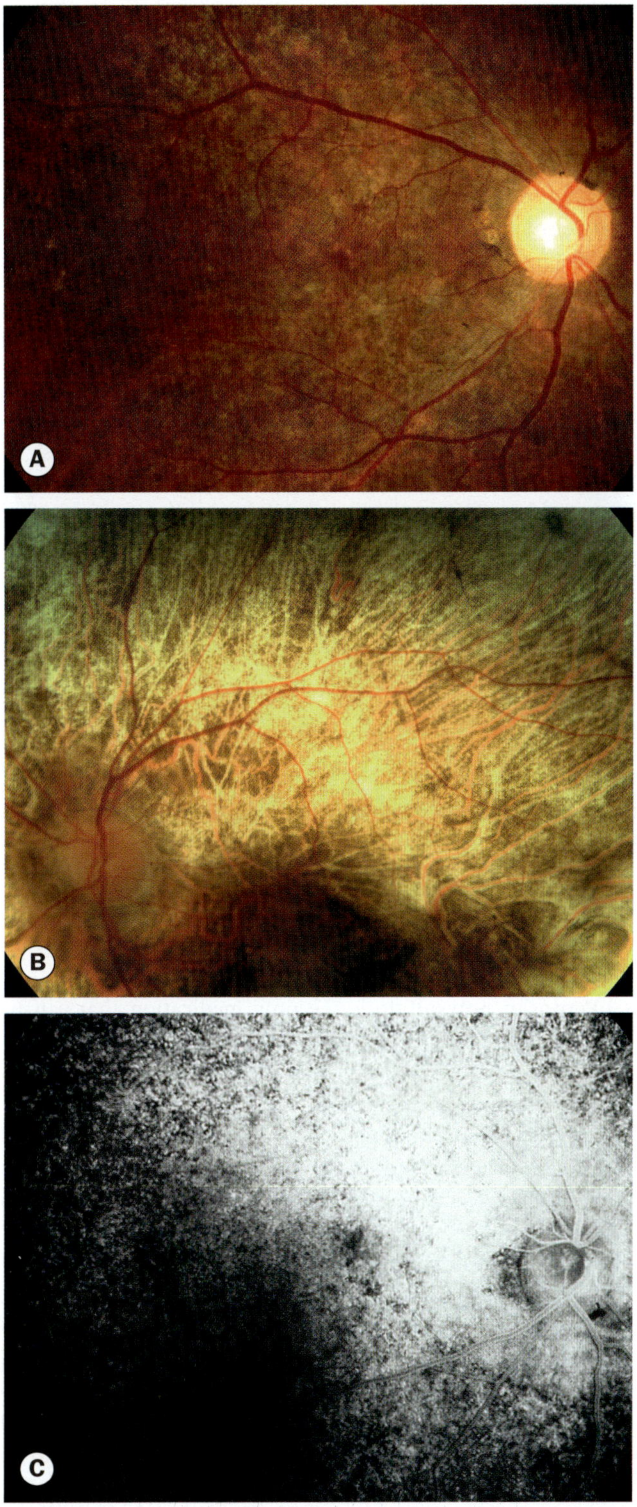

Fig. 21.5 Thioridazine retinopathy. **(A)** 'Salt and pepper' pigmentary disturbance; **(B)** pigmented plaques and atrophy of the RPE and choriocapillaris in advanced disease; **(C)** FA showing punctate hyperfluorescence. *(Courtesy of S Chen – fig. B.)*

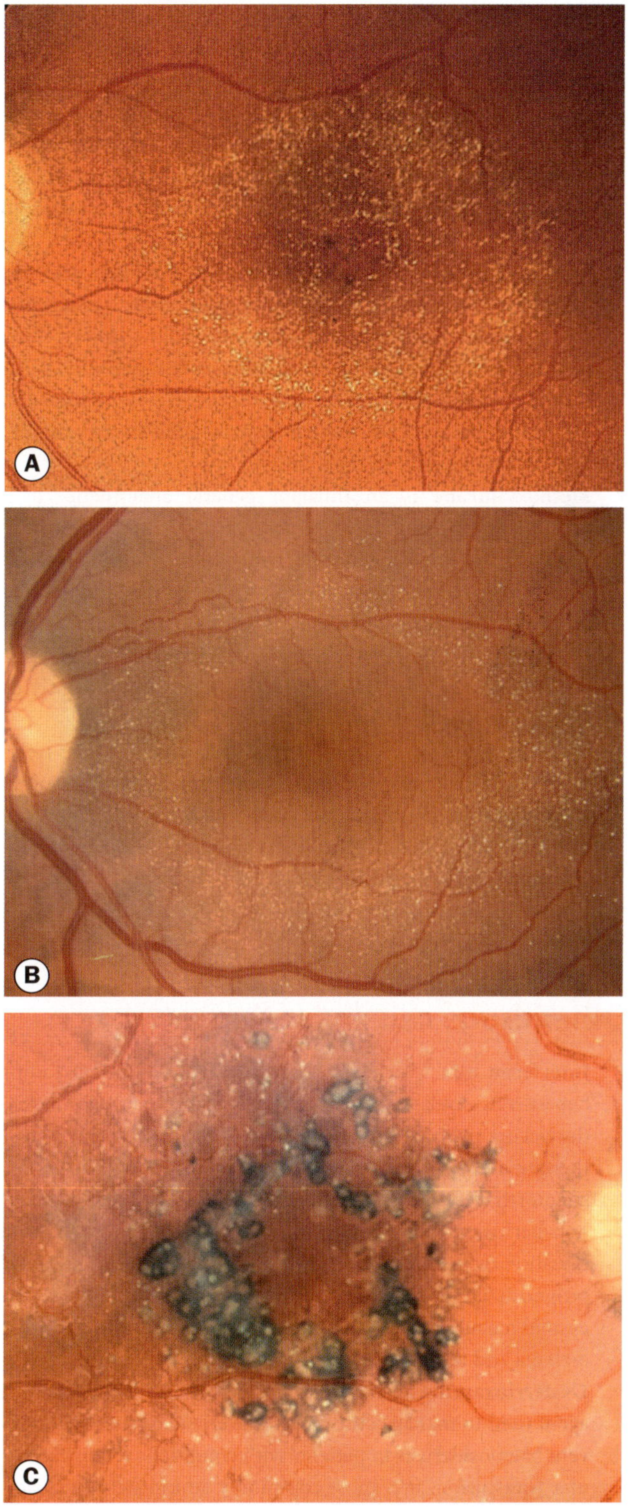

Fig. 21.6 Drug-induced crystalline retinopathies. **(A)** Tamoxifen; **(B)** canthaxanthin; **(C)** methoxyflurane (oxalosis).

higher doses, but only rarely with standard doses. Retinopathy (Fig. 21.6A) is characterized by bilateral fine yellow crystalline deposits in the inner layers of the retina and punctate grey lesions in the outer retina and RPE. Visual impairment is thought to be caused by maculopathy, including foveolar cyst formation. OCT imaging is a sensitive method of detection. A rare side effect is optic neuritis, reversible on cessation of therapy.

- **Canthaxanthin** is a carotenoid used, often in quite high doses, to simulate sun tanning. Over prolonged periods it may cause the deposition of innocuous glistening yellow inner retinal deposits in a doughnut conformation at the posterior poles (Fig. 21.6B). The deposition is slowly reversible. Because of this side effect the FDA has not approved the use of canthaxanthin 'tanning pills' in the USA.
- **Methoxyflurane** is an inhalant general anaesthetic. It is metabolized to oxalic acid, which combines with calcium to form an insoluble salt and is deposited in tissues including the RPE. Prolonged administration may lead to renal failure and secondary hyperoxalosis. Ocular involvement is characterized by calcium oxalate crystals scattered throughout the retina associated with mild visual impairment and subsequently by RPE hyperplasia at the posterior pole (Fig. 21.6C).
- **Nitrofurantoin** is an antibiotic used principally in the treatment of urinary tract infections. Long-term use may result in slight visual impairment associated with superficial and deep glistening intraretinal deposits distributed in a circinate pattern throughout the posterior pole.
- **Non-drug causes** of crystalline maculopathy are given in Table 21.1.

Table 21.1 Other Causes of Macular Crystals
Primary hyperoxaluria
Bietti corneoretinal crystalline dystrophy
Cystinosis
Sjögren–Larsson syndrome
Gyrate atrophy
Acquired parafoveal telangiectasis
Talc-corn starch emboli
West African crystalline maculopathy

Other drugs causing retinopathy

- **Interferon alfa** is used in a range of conditions, including hepatitis C and numerous malignant tumours. Retinopathy occurs in some patients, particularly those on high-dose therapy, and is characterized by cotton-wool spots and retinal haemorrhages (Fig. 21.7A). FA shows areas of focal capillary non-perfusion. Changes usually resolve spontaneously with cessation of therapy and in the majority of patients the visual prognosis is good. Less common ocular side effects include cystoid macular oedema, extraocular muscle paresis, optic disc oedema and retinal vein occlusion.
- **Desferrioxamine** (also known as deferoxamine) is a chelating agent used to manage chronic iron overload, generally to prevent haemosiderosis in patients with conditions requiring regular transfusion. It is most commonly administered via slow subcutaneous infusion. Patients present with rapid visual loss. Initially the fundi may be normal or show only mild macular greying, but within several weeks mottled pigmentary changes develop (Fig. 21.8A), associated with abnormal electrodiagnostic findings. FA shows widespread punctate hyperfluorescence (Fig. 21.8B).
- **Nicotinic acid** is a cholesterol-lowering agent. A minority of patients develop retinopathy when doses greater than 1.5 g daily are used, in the form of a cystoid maculopathy suggestive of cystoid macular oedema but without leakage on FA. The changes cause a mild reduction of VA but resolve with discontinuation of the drug.

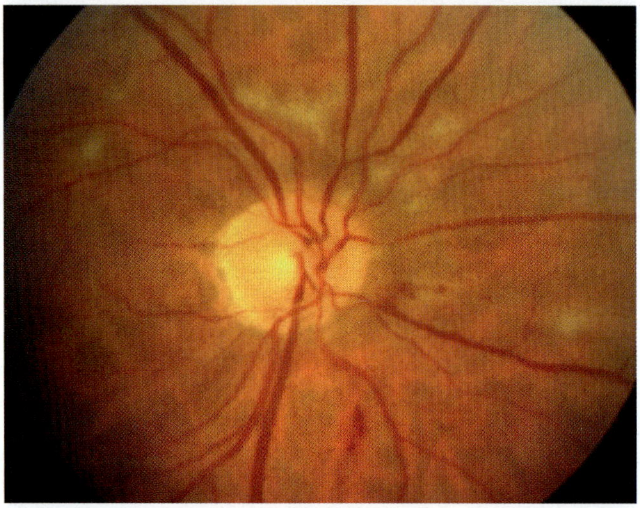

Fig. 21.7 Interferon retinopathy.

- **Pentosan polysulfate** is the only medication that can be used in the treatment of interstitial cystitis. A characteristic progressive symmetrical maculopathy may occur with long-term use (usually more than 7 years) and high cumulative exposure. Prolonged dark adaptation, nyctalopia and blurred vision are initial symptoms, followed by visual loss secondary to changes in the macular region. There is no treatment.
- **Alkyl nitrites ('poppers')** are recreational drugs used before sexual activity and can rarely cause a toxic maculopathy. The patients are usually young and present with bilateral loss of visual acuity and photopsia. Clinically a small yellow spot can be seen in the fovea, which is easily seen using autofluorescence imaging (Fig. 21.9A). OCT shows a selective defect in the foveal inner-segment ellipsoid band (Fig. 21.9B). There is no treatment, but spontaneous recovery of visual function can occur.

OPTIC NERVE

Ethambutol

Ethambutol is used in the treatment of tuberculosis, generally in a multidrug regimen. Its overall safety profile is favourable, but acute or chronic optic neuritis can occur. Toxicity is dose- and duration-dependent, with an incidence as high as 18% at a daily dose over 35

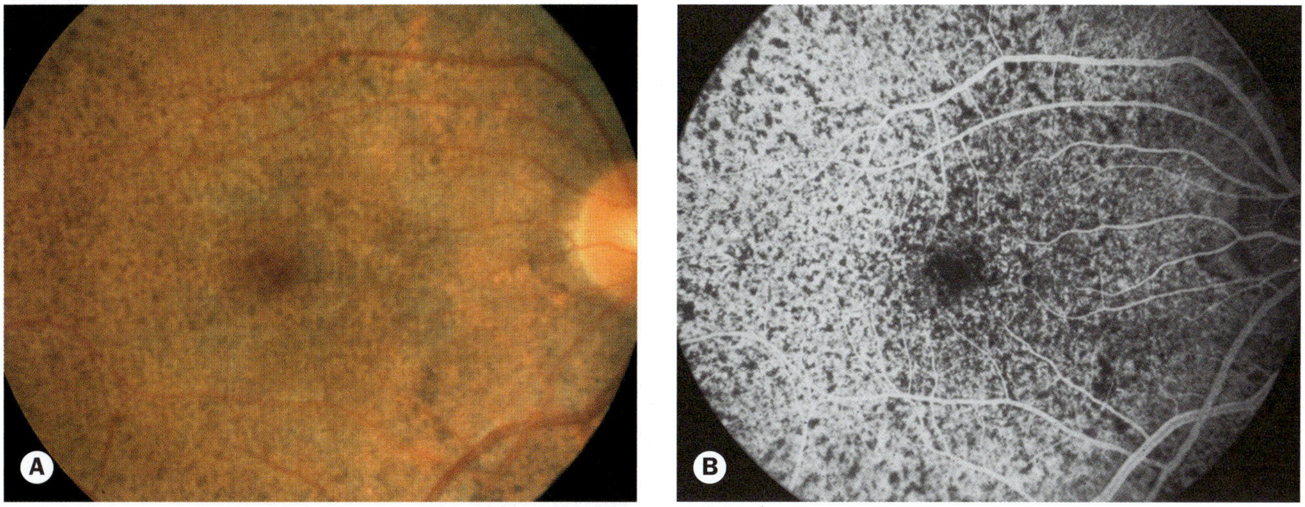

Fig. 21.8 **(A)** Desferrioxamine retinopathy; **(B)** FA showing diffuse punctate hyperfluorescence. *(Courtesy of R Smith.)*

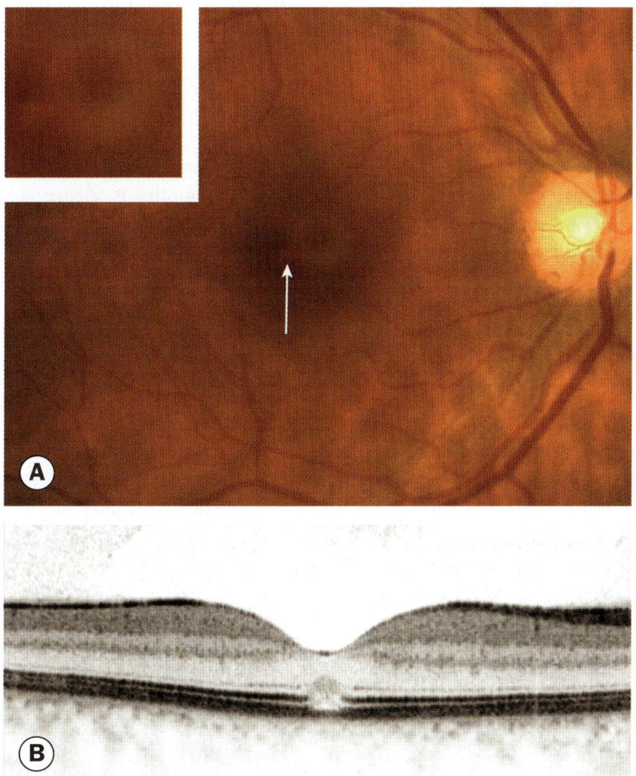

Fig. 21.9 Alkyl nitrites ('poppers'). **(A)** Clinical appearance showing yellow spot in the fovea (arrow); **(B)** OCT showing defect within the photoreceptor layer.

mg/kg daily. It is rare (<1%) with a standard daily dose of 15 mg/kg daily. Toxicity typically occurs between 3 and 6 months of starting treatment, though it has been reported after only a few days. Renal dysfunction may confer a higher risk of toxicity as ethambutol is excreted via the kidneys.

- **Symptoms** may be absent, but typically include painless bilateral blurring, usually central though sometimes paracentral or peripheral. Impairment of colour vision may be noticed.
- **Signs** include minimal to severe reduction in VA, normal or slightly swollen optic discs with splinter-shaped haemorrhages and normal or sluggish pupils. Red–green dyschromatopsia is the most common objective abnormality of colour vision, but subtle (undetectable on Ishihara testing) blue–yellow defects may be an early finding. Loss of contrast sensitivity is an early sign.
- **Visual field defects** can be central or peripheral.
- **Prognosis** is good following cessation of treatment, although recovery can take time. A minority sustain permanent visual impairment, with optic atrophy.
- **Screening.** Baseline VA and Ishihara testing are prudent prior to starting ethambutol and the patient should be advised of the necessity of reporting any visual disturbance. Repeat testing should be performed every 6 months in patients on the standard dose. Ethambutol should be stopped immediately if toxicity develops, with consideration also given to discontinuation of isoniazid if it is being used synchronously (see below).

TIP To reduce the risk of toxic optic neuropathy, the dose of ethambutol should not exceed 15 mg/kg daily.

Isoniazid

Isoniazid may very rarely cause toxic optic neuropathy. The risk is higher when given in combination with ethambutol.

Amiodarone

Optic neuropathy, probably secondary to demyelination, affects 1–2% of patients on long-term amiodarone treatment. It is almost certainly not dose-related. Distinction from non-arteritic anterior ischaemic optic neuropathy (NAION), which also affects patients with systemic vascular disease, may be difficult and it has been suggested that NAION is more common in patients on amiodarone. Differentiation is clinically important as it is key to a decision about whether to discontinue the drug. The presence of a crowded optic disc, speed of onset, bilateral involvement, duration of disc swelling and features of systemic amiodarone toxicity may be helpful in this regard.

- **Presentation** is with sudden or insidious unilateral or bilateral visual impairment, after a mean period of 6–9 months taking the drug. About one-third of patients are asymptomatic.
- **Signs** in a majority are unilateral or bilateral optic disc swelling that may persist for a few months after medication is stopped. Corneal features are discussed above.
- **Investigation**
  - Cranial imaging may be indicated when bilateral disc swelling is present.
  - Visual field defects are of varied configuration and severity and may be reversible or permanent.
  - **Prognosis** is variable; cessation of the drug usually improves vision, but 20% may deteriorate further. Final VA of worse than 6/60 occurs in around 20% of eyes.
  - **Screening** has been suggested by some authors, but no consensus exists as to its benefit. Patients should be warned of the risk and cautioned to report visual symptoms immediately.

Vigabatrin

Bilateral concentric, predominantly nasal visual field constriction occurs in many patients taking the anti-epileptic drug vigabatrin due to photoreceptor and ganglion cell damage. It is uncommon at a cumulative total dose of <1 kg, but very common at >3 kg. A maximum daily dose of 3 g is recommended in adults. Vigabatrin should be avoided in patients with pre-existing field defects and should not be prescribed in conjunction with other potentially retinotoxic drugs. The risk is higher in males than females.

- **Presentation** is usually months or years after starting treatment with bilateral concentric or binasal visual field defects. Blurring and symptoms related to the defects may occur, but there may be no symptoms, with normal VA unless scotomas are at or close to fixation.
- **Signs** may be absent but optic atrophy may be present. Other subtle signs can include peripheral atrophy, arteriolar narrowing, abnormal macular reflexes and surface wrinkling. OCT can detect peripapillary retinal nerve fibre layer atrophy, including prior to the development of field defects.
- **Prognosis.** Changes persist if treatment is stopped, but sometimes do not progress if continued.
- **Screening.** A baseline visual assessment, including visual fields and OCT, is recommended prior to starting treatment and thereafter every 3 months. In young children and others unable to perform field or OCT testing, the optimal monitoring modality has yet to be determined.

Methotrexate

Methotrexate is a very rare cause of acute or gradual visual loss due to optic neuropathy. Reduced VA, dyschromatopsia and visual field loss occur and could be linked to folic acid metabolism, levels of which should be checked. Vitamin B_{12} and folate supplementation may be helpful.

Sildenafil

Non-arteritic anterior ischaemic optic neuropathy is a rare side effect. Cyanopsia is more common, but clears spontaneously. Affected individuals report intensely blue-coloured vision, difficulty distinguishing red–green colours and photophobia.

VISUAL CORTEX

Bevacizumab

Bevacizumab is used for colon and rectal tumours and may rarely result in corticular blindness, which is not fully reversible on stopping the medication.

Chapter 22 Trauma

EYELID TRAUMA

Periocular haematoma

A 'black eye', consisting of a haematoma (focal collection of blood) and/or periocular ecchymosis (diffuse bruising) and oedema (Fig. 22.1A), is the most common blunt injury to the eyelid or forehead and is generally innocuous. It is, however, critical to exclude the following more serious conditions:

- **Trauma to the globe or orbit.** It is easier to examine the globe before the lids become oedematous. Once swelling is established, gentle sustained pressure to open the lids will often displace tissue fluid sufficiently to allow visualization of the anterior segment. It is critical not to apply any force on the globe itself until its integrity has been confirmed. Urgent imaging such as computed tomography (CT), magnetic resonance imaging (MRI) or bedside ultrasonography (taking meticulous care to avoid applying pressure on the globe) should be considered if there is suspicion of an underlying injury to the eyeball and adequate clinical visualization is not possible.
- **Orbital roof fracture**, especially if the black eye is associated with a subconjunctival haemorrhage without a visible posterior limit (which would indicate the anterior extension of a posterior bleeding point) (Fig. 22.1B).
- **Basal skull fracture**, which may give rise to characteristic bilateral ring haematomas ('panda eyes' – Fig. 22.1C).

TIP Bilateral periocular haematoma ('panda' eyes) can be a sign of a skull-base fracture.

Laceration

The presence of a lid laceration, however insignificant, mandates careful exploration of the wound and examination of the globe and adnexal structures. Any lid defect should be repaired by direct closure whenever possible, even under tension, since this affords the best functional and cosmetic result (Fig. 22.2A and B).

- **Superficial** lacerations parallel to the lid margin without gaping can be sutured with 6-0 black silk or nylon. The sutures are removed after 5–6 days.
- **Infection** is always a risk, even from a small laceration (Fig. 22.2C).
- **Lid margin** lacerations invariably gape without careful closure and to prevent notching must be sutured with optimal alignment (see Fig. 2.57C):
  - A 5-0 silk vertical mattress suture is inserted in line with the meibomian gland orifices, about 2 mm from the wound edges and 2 mm deep and left untied.
  - Tarsal plate edges are brought together with partial-thickness lamellar 5-0 absorbable (e.g. polyglactin) sutures, which are tied anteriorly.
  - The lid margin silk suture is then tied so that the cut edges slightly pucker the wound. The ends are left fairly long, e.g. 2 cm.

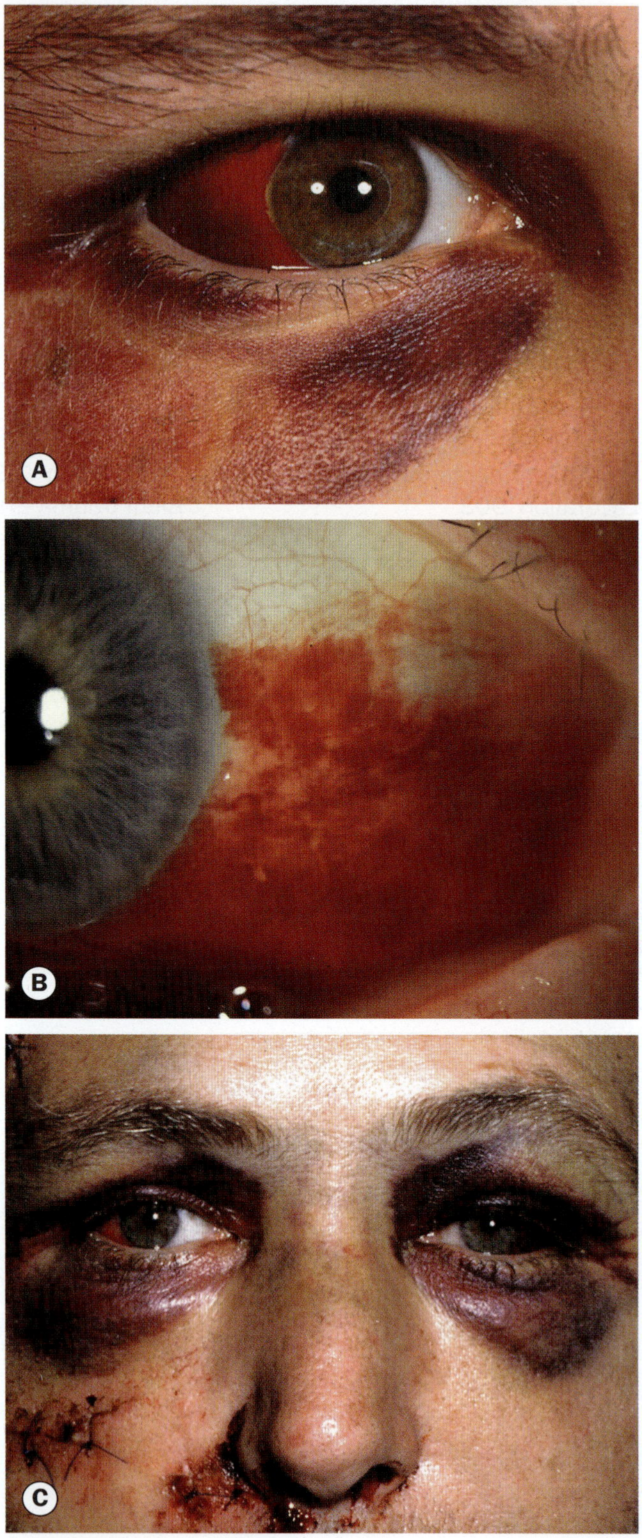

Fig. 22.1 **(A)** Lower lid haematoma with subconjunctival haemorrhage; **(B)** subconjunctival haemorrhage with no visible posterior limit; **(C)** 'panda eyes'.

The overlying skin is closed with interrupted 6-0 or 7-0 nylon or absorbable sutures, securing the ends of the silk suture to direct these and its knot away from the cornea.

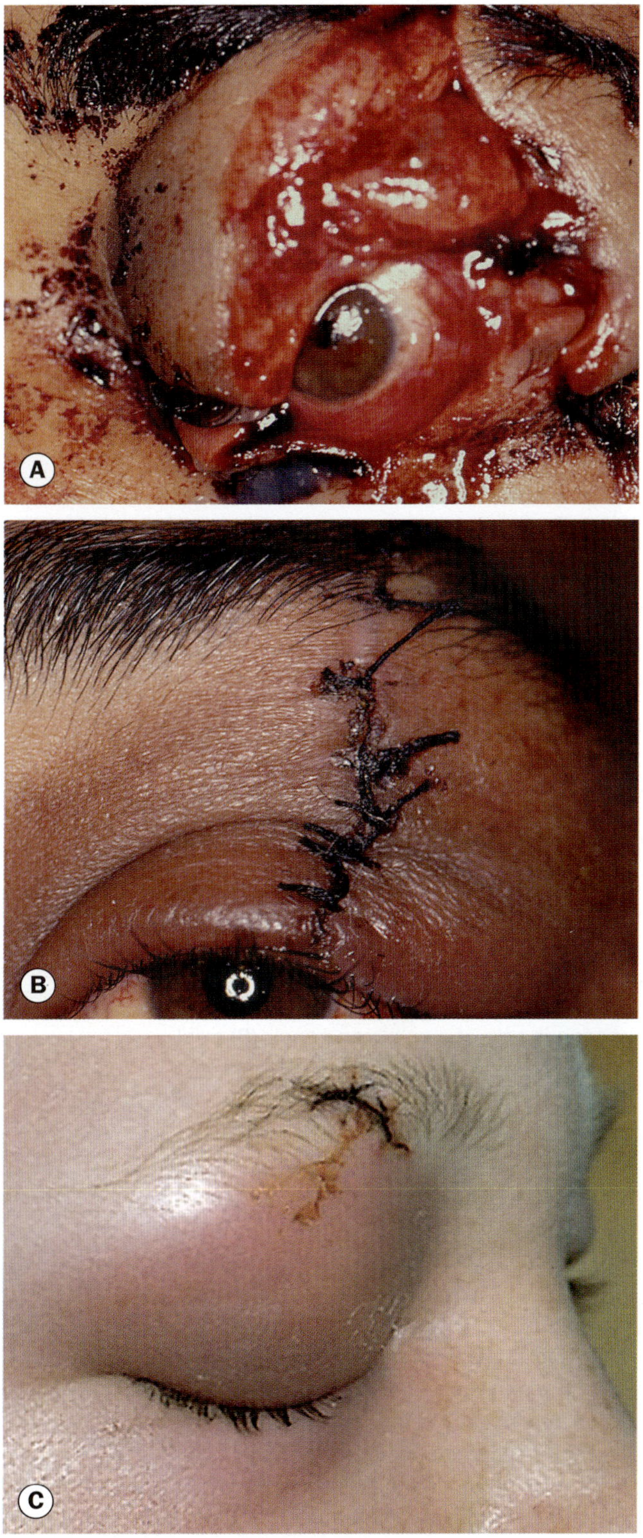

Fig. 22.2 **(A)** Lid laceration; **(B)** postoperative result; **(C)** orbital cellulitis secondary to small laceration.

- **Lacerations with mild tissue loss** just sufficient to prevent direct primary closure can usually be managed by performing a lateral cantholysis in order to increase lateral mobility.

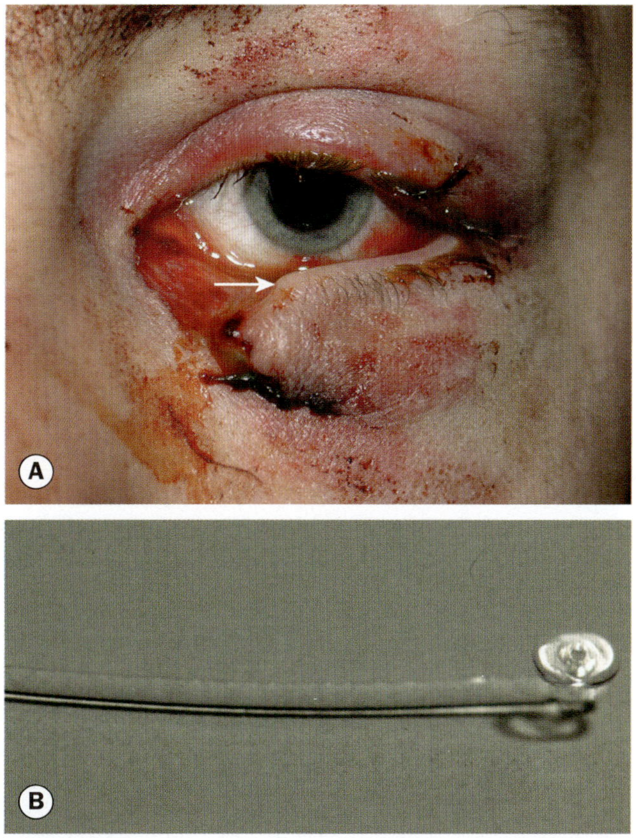

Fig. 22.3 **(A)** Lower lid laceration involving the canaliculus (arrow); **(B)** monocanalicular silicone stent needed to bridge the laceration.

- **Lacerations with extensive tissue** loss may require major reconstructive procedures similar to those used following resection of malignant tumours (see Ch. 2).
- **Canalicular lacerations** should be repaired within 24 hours (Fig. 22.3A). The laceration is bridged by silicone tubing (Crawford tube), which is threaded down the lacrimal system and tied in the nose, following which the laceration is sutured. Alternatively, repair of a single canaliculus can be performed using a monocanalicular stent (e.g. Mini Monoka – Fig. 22.3B) and, if necessary, suturing its footplate to the lid using 8-0 material. The tubing is left *in situ* for 3–6 months.
- **Tetanus status.** Ensure that the patient's tetanus immunization status is satisfactory after any injury. Without prior immunization, 250 units of human tetanus immunoglobulin are given intramuscularly (IM). If previously immunized but a booster has not been administered within the last 10 years, subcutaneous tetanus toxoid should be given.
- **Foreign body.** If there is any suspicion of a foreign body in the soft tissues of the lid or orbit (Fig. 22.4A and C), a CT scan should be undertaken (Fig. 22.4B and D).

TIP There is always a risk of orbital cellulitis after a penetrating lid laceration, particularly if there is a retained foreign body.

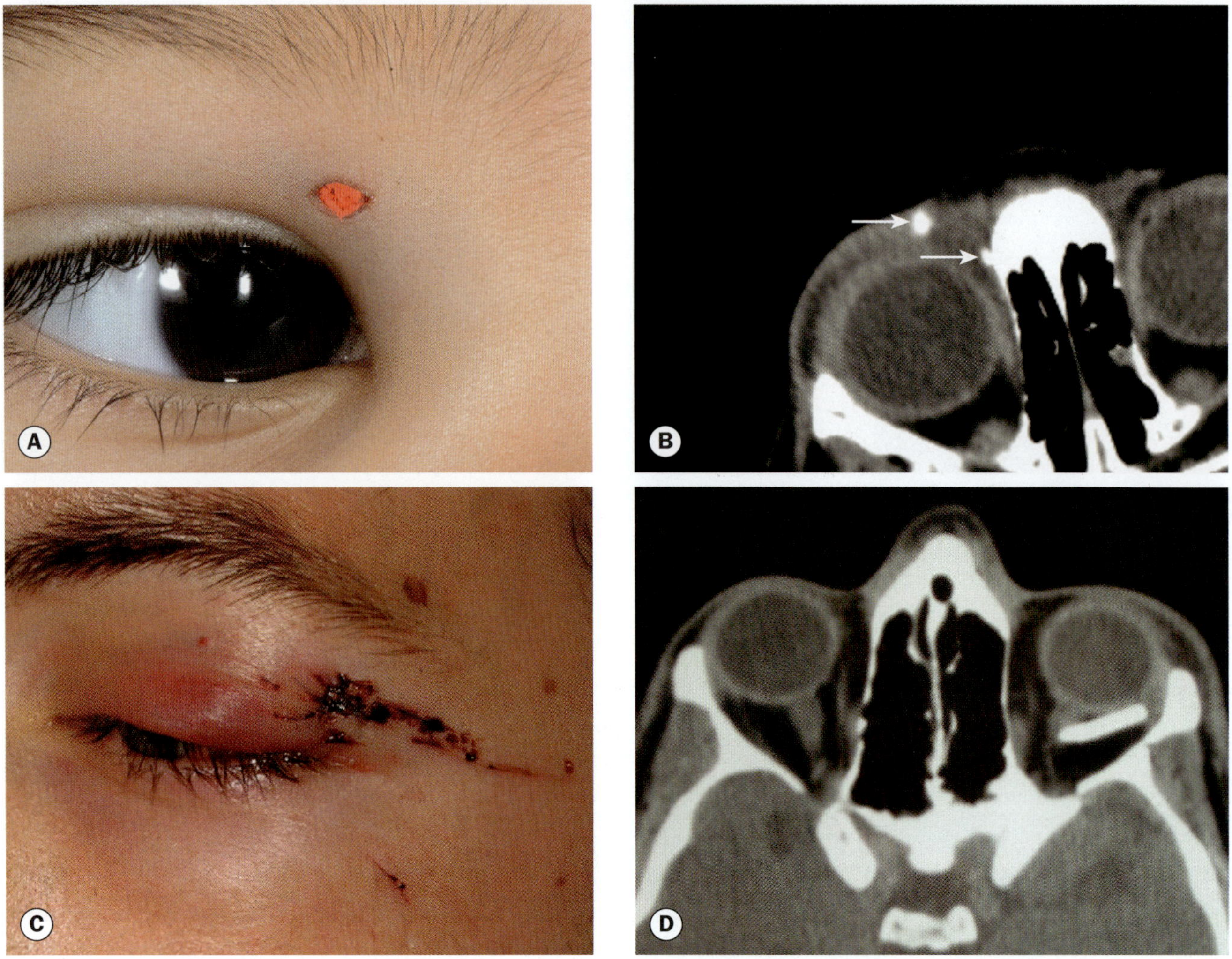

Fig. 22.4 **(A)** Small upper lid laceration in a child showing the tip of a coloured pencil; **(B)** axial CT scan showing the broken tips (arrows); **(C)** penetrating injury to the left upper lid with an intact globe; **(D)** axial CT scan showing a retrobulbar glass shard.

ORBITAL TRAUMA

Orbital floor fracture

Introduction

A blow-out fracture of the orbital floor is typically caused by a sudden increase in the orbital pressure from an impacting object that is greater in diameter than the orbital aperture (about 5 cm), such as a fist or tennis ball, so that the eyeball itself is displaced and transmits rather than absorbs the impact (Fig. 22.5A). Since the bones of the lateral wall and the roof are usually able to withstand such trauma, the fracture most frequently involves the floor of the orbit along the thin bone covering the infraorbital canal. Occasionally, the medial orbital wall may also be fractured. Fractures of the orbital rim and adjacent facial bones require appropriately tailored management. Clinical features vary with the severity of trauma and the interval between injury and examination. Care should be taken to ensure that a full evaluation for head and systemic injury has been performed and any necessary interspecialty referrals initiated.

Diagnosis

- **Visual function**, especially acuity, should be recorded and monitored.
- **Periocular signs** include variable ecchymosis, oedema (Fig. 22.5B) and occasionally subcutaneous emphysema (a crackling sensation on palpation due to air in the subcutaneous tissues).
- **Infraorbital nerve anaesthesia** involving the lower lid, cheek, side of nose, upper lip, upper teeth and gums is common as the fracture frequently involves the infraorbital canal.
- **Diplopia** may be caused by one of the following mechanisms:
  - Haemorrhage and oedema in the orbit may cause tightening of the septa connecting the inferior rectus and inferior oblique muscles to the periorbita, thus restricting movement of the globe. Ocular motility usually improves as the haemorrhage and oedema resolve.
  - Diplopia typically occurs in both upgaze (Fig. 22.6A and C) and downgaze secondary to mechanical entrapment within the fracture of the inferior rectus or inferior oblique muscle or adjacent connective tissue and fat (Fig. 22.6D).

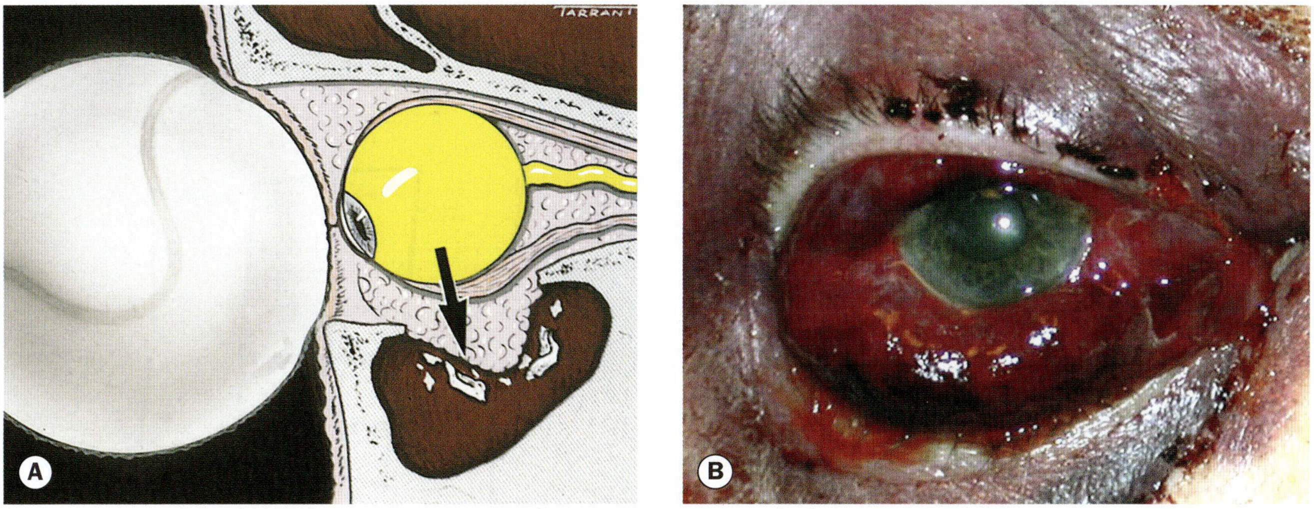

Fig. 22.5 Orbital floor blow-out fracture. (A) Diagram to illustrate the mechanism; (B) marked periocular ecchymosis, oedema and subconjunctival haemorrhage.

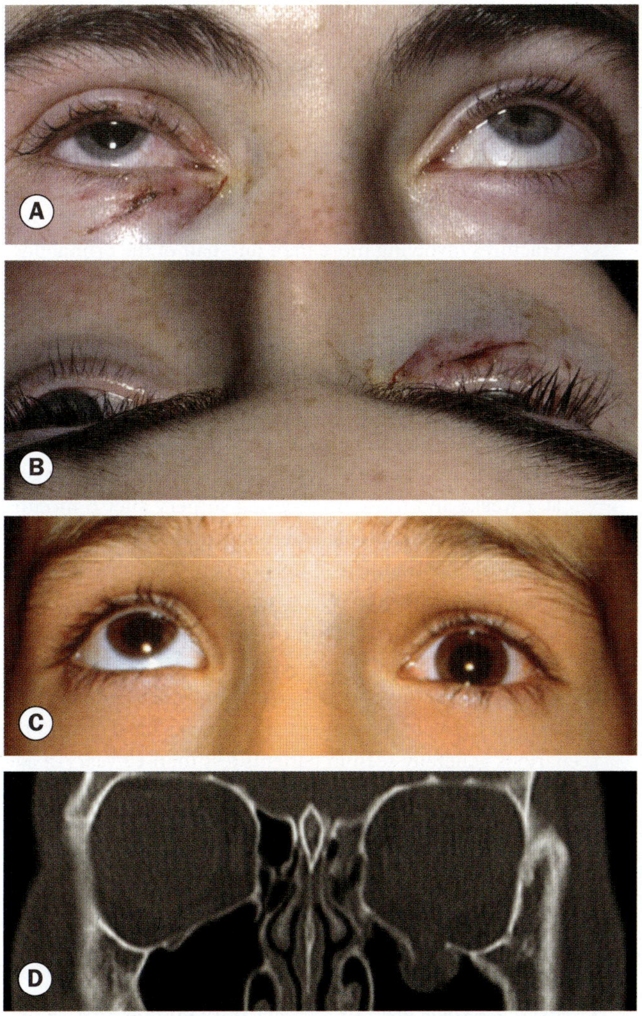

Fig. 22.6 Orbital floor blow-out fracture. (A) Restricted elevation right eye; (B) mild right enophthalmos; (C) white eye blow-out fracture of the left orbit in a child; (D) coronal CT scan showing entrapment of the left inferior rectus muscle.

  - Forced duction and the differential intraocular pressure test (increasing IOP as a restricted muscle presses on the globe) are positive. Diplopia may subsequently improve if it is mainly due to entrapment of oedematous connective tissue and fat, but usually persists if there is significant involvement of the muscles themselves.
  - Direct injury to an extraocular muscle, associated with a negative forced duction test. The muscle fibres usually regenerate and normal function often returns within about 2 months.
- **Enophthalmos** (Fig. 22.6B) may be present if the fracture is severe, although it tends to manifest only after a few days as initial oedema resolves. Late enophthalmos is uncommon, even in large fractures. Six months after a large orbital floor fracture only 20% will have enophthalmos of more than 2 mm.
- **Ocular damage** (e.g. hyphaema, angle recession, retinal dialysis) should be excluded by careful examination of the globe, although this is relatively uncommon in association with a blow-out fracture.
- **Hess chart** testing (Fig. 22.7) to map eye movements is useful in assessment and monitoring.
- **CT** with coronal sections (Fig. 22.8 and see Fig. 22.6D) aids in evaluation of the extent of a fracture and determination of the nature of maxillary antral soft tissue densities, which may represent prolapsed orbital fat, extraocular muscles, haematoma or unrelated antral polyps.

Treatment

- **Initial** treatment generally consists of observation, with the prescription of oral antibiotics. Ice packs and nasal decongestants may be helpful. The patient should be instructed not to blow his or her nose, because of the possibility of forcing infected sinus contents into the orbit. Systemic steroids are occasionally required for severe orbital oedema, particularly if this is compromising the optic nerve.

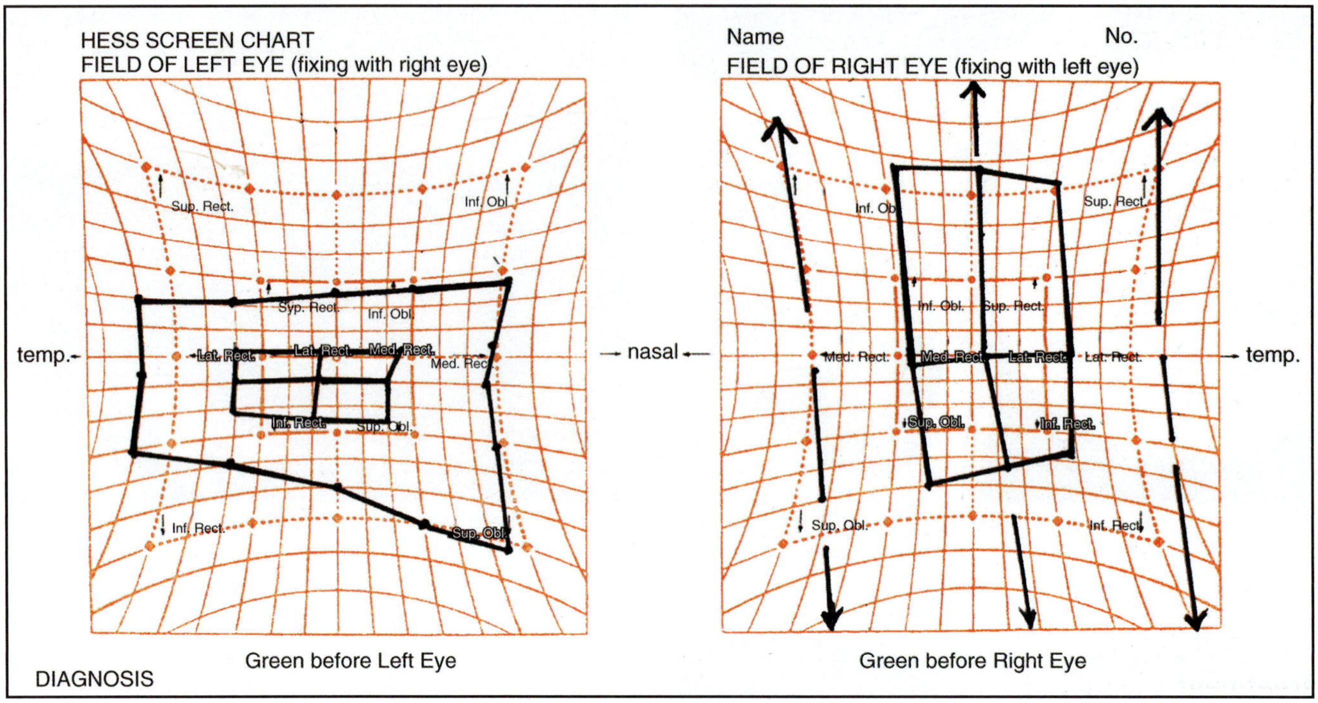

Fig. 22.7 Hess chart of a left orbital floor blow-out fracture showing restriction of left upgaze (superior rectus and inferior oblique) and restriction on downgaze (inferior rectus). There is also secondary overaction of the right eye.

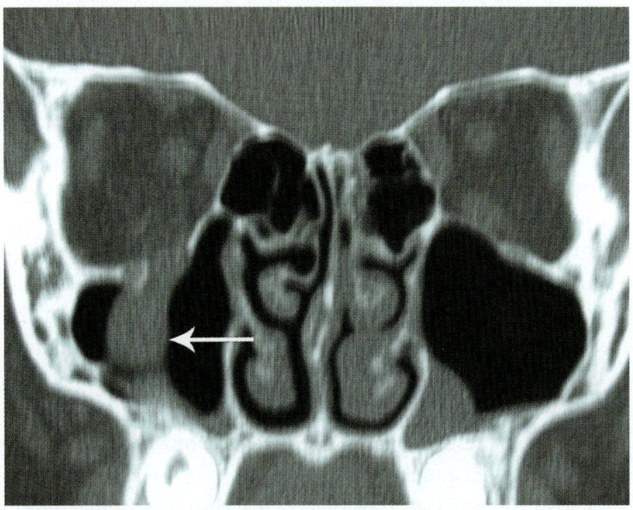

Fig. 22.8 CT of orbital floor blow-out fracture – coronal view showing a defect in the orbital floor and the 'tear drop' sign due to soft tissue prolapse into the maxillary antrum (arrow).

- **Subsequent** treatment is aimed at the prevention of permanent vertical diplopia and/or cosmetically unacceptable enophthalmos.
  - Small cracks without herniation do not require treatment as the risk of permanent complications is small.
  - Fractures involving up to one-half of the orbital floor, with little or no herniation, no significant enophthalmos and improving diplopia, also do not require treatment.
  - Fractures involving more than one-half of the orbital floor may develop enophthalmos if left untreated.
  - Fractures with entrapment of orbital contents, enophthalmos of greater than 2 mm and/or persistent and significant diplopia in the primary position should be repaired within 2 weeks. However, it has recently been reported that in patients with enophthalmos of less than 2 mm there is no difference in outcome between those undergoing surgery at 2 weeks and those undergoing surgery after 6 months. In patients with diplopia and tissue incarceration but without muscle entrapment, improvement often occurs without surgery. If the diplopia persists, delayed surgery is still likely to achieve resolution of diplopia except in extreme upgaze.
- **'White-eyed' fracture** is a subgroup for which urgent repair is required to avoid permanent neuromuscular damage. The scenario is generally seen in patients less than 18 years of age, typically with little visible external soft tissue injury and usually affects the orbital floor (see Fig. 22.6C). It involves the acute incarceration of herniated tissue in a 'trap-door' effect and occurs because of the greater elasticity of bone in younger people (see Fig. 22.6D). Patients may experience acute nausea, vomiting, headache and persistent activation of the oculocardiac reflex can occur. CT features may be subtle.
- **Surgical repair** is performed via a transconjunctival or subciliary incision or via the maxillary sinus, with elevation of the periosteum from the orbital floor, freeing of trapped orbital contents and repair of the bony defect with a synthetic implant.

Roof fracture

Introduction

Roof fractures are rarely encountered by ophthalmologists. Isolated fractures, caused by falling on a sharp object or sometimes a relatively minor blow to the brow or forehead, are most common in children and often do not require treatment. Fractures due to major trauma, with associated displacement of the orbital rim or significant disturbance of other craniofacial bones, typically affect adults.

Diagnosis

A haematoma of the upper eyelid is typical, together with periocular ecchymosis. These often develop over the course of a few hours and may progressively spread to the side opposite the fracture. Other features of orbital wall fracture as discussed above may be present. Large fractures may be associated with pulsation of the globe due to transmission of cerebrospinal fluid (CSF) pressure, best detected with applanation tonometry.

Treatment

Small fractures may not require treatment, but it is important to exclude a CSF leak, which carries a risk of meningitis. Sizeable bony defects with downward displacement of fragments usually warrant reconstructive surgery. General management is similar to that of an orbital floor fracture (see above).

Blow-out medial wall fracture

Medial wall orbital fractures are usually associated with floor fractures. It is uncommon to find an isolated fracture of the medial wall. Signs include periorbital ecchymosis and frequently subcutaneous emphysema, which typically develops on blowing the nose. Defective ocular motility involving abduction and adduction is present if the medial rectus muscle is entrapped. CT will demonstrate the fracture. Treatment involves release of incarcerated tissue and repair of the bony defect (Fig. 22.9).

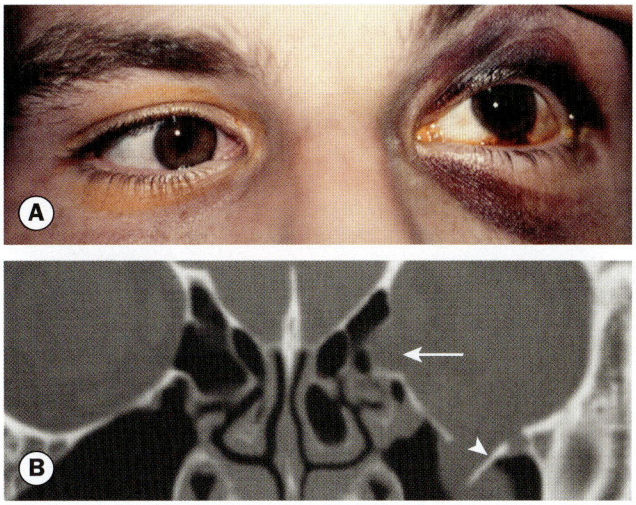

Fig. 22.9 Blow-out fracture of the left medial wall and floor. **(A)** Defective left abduction; **(B)** CT coronal view showing fractures of the medial wall (arrow) and floor (arrowhead). *(Courtesy of A Pearson.)*

Lateral wall fracture

Acute lateral wall fractures (see Fig. 22.11D) are rarely encountered by ophthalmologists. Because the lateral wall of the orbit is more solid than the other walls, a fracture is usually associated with extensive facial damage.

Orbital haemorrhage

Introduction

Orbital (retrobulbar) haemorrhage is important chiefly due to the associated risk of acute orbital compartment syndrome with compressive optic neuropathy and can lead to irreversible blindness of the affected eye in severe cases. It can occur without or in association with an orbital bony injury. Iatrogenic orbital haemorrhage is not uncommon, typically resulting from a peri- or retrobulbar local anaesthetic block performed to facilitate intraocular surgery. Rare causes include bleeding from vascular anomalies and occasionally spontaneous haemorrhage due to poor clotting.

Diagnosis

Proptosis, eyelid oedema and ecchymosis, haemorrhagic chemosis, ocular motility dysfunction, decreased visual acuity, elevated intraocular pressure, optic disc swelling and a relative afferent pupillary defect are among the possible signs.

Treatment

Treatment should be started immediately if progressive visual deterioration occurs. Canthotomy alone is rarely adequate.

- **Canthotomy.** After clamping the incision site for 60 seconds, scissors are used to make a 1–2 cm horizontal full-thickness incision under local anaesthesia (e.g. 1–2 ml lidocaine 1–2% with adrenaline) at the angle of the lateral canthus (Fig. 22.10A).
- **Cantholysis.** Following canthotomy, the lower lid is retracted downwards and the inferior crus of the lateral canthal tendon is cut (Fig. 22.10B) using blunt-tipped scissors, directed inferiorly and inserted adjacent and parallel to the lateral orbital rim between conjunctiva and skin and angled away from the eyeball. Blood is gently encouraged to drain. If necessary, the superior limb of the tendon can also be cut, but this carries a substantial risk of damage to adnexal structures.

TRAUMA TO THE GLOBE

Introduction

Terminology

- **Closed injury** is commonly due to blunt trauma. The corneoscleral wall of the globe is intact.
- **Open injury** involves a full-thickness wound of the corneoscleral envelope.

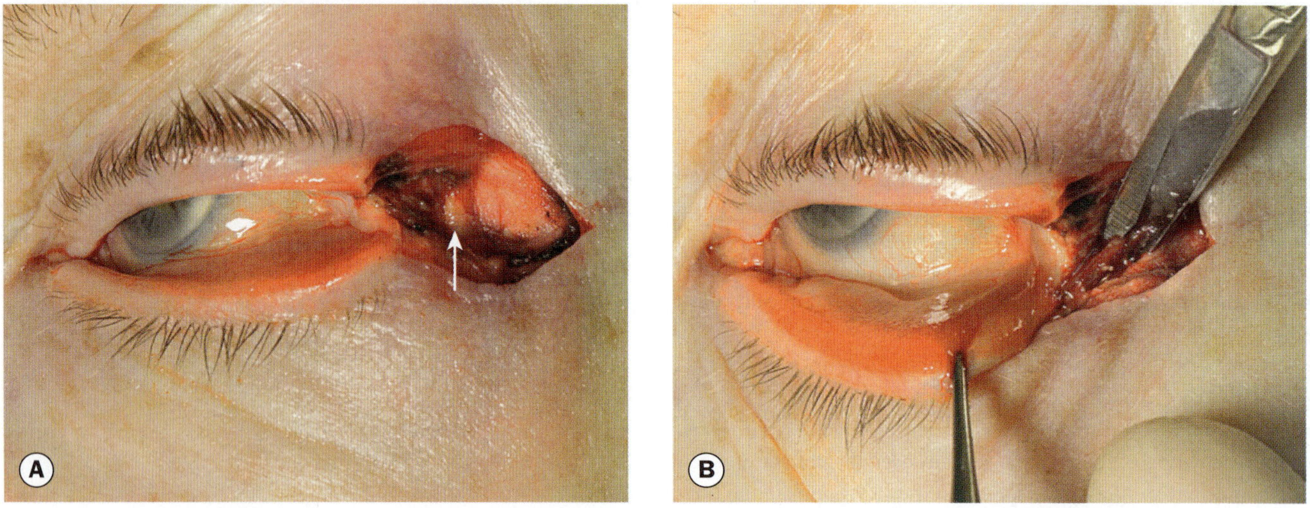

Fig. 22.10 Surgical treatment of acute retrobulbar haemorrhage. **(A)** Lateral canthotomy (arrow showing anterior orbital rim); **(B)** disinsertion of inferior crus of the lateral canthal tendon.

- **Contusion** is a closed injury resulting from blunt trauma. Damage may occur at or distant to the site of impact.
- **Rupture** is a full-thickness wound caused by blunt trauma. The globe gives way at its weakest point, which may not be at the site of impact.
- **Laceration** is a full-thickness defect in the eye wall produced by a tearing injury, usually as the result of a direct impact.
- **Lamellar laceration** is a partial-thickness laceration.
- **Incised injury** is caused by a sharp object such as glass or a knife.
- **Penetrating injury** refers to a single full-thickness wound, usually caused by a sharp object, without an exit wound. A penetrating injury may be associated with intraocular retention of a foreign body.
- **Perforation** consists of two full-thickness wounds, one entry and one exit, usually caused by a missile.

Investigation

- **Plain radiographs** may be taken when the presence of a foreign body is suspected (Fig. 22.11A). A metallic foreign body which is within the eye will move up and down if the radiographs are taken in upgaze and downgaze.
- **Ultrasonography** may be useful in the detection of intraocular foreign bodies, globe rupture, suprachoroidal haemorrhage and retinal detachment. It should be performed as gently as possible if there is a possibility of an open globe injury, taking great care not to apply pressure on the globe.
- **CT** is superior to plain radiography in the detection and localization of intraocular foreign bodies (Figs 21.11B–D). It is also of value in determining the integrity of intracranial, facial and intraocular structures (see Fig. 22.11C).
- **MRI** is more accurate than CT in the detection and assessment of injuries of the globe itself, such as an occult posterior rupture, though not for bony injury. However, MRI should not be performed if a ferrous metallic foreign body is suspected.
- **Electrodiagnostic tests** may be useful in assessing the integrity of the optic nerve and retina, particularly if some time has passed since the original injury and there is the suspicion of a retained intraocular foreign body (IOFB).

TIP MRI scanning should not be undertaken if a ferrous metallic foreign body is suspected in a patient with a penetrating injury.

Blunt trauma

The most common causes of blunt trauma are sporting injuries and assault. Severe blunt trauma to the globe results in anteroposterior compression with simultaneous expansion in the equatorial plane (Fig. 22.12) often associated with a transient but severe increase in IOP. Although the impact is primarily absorbed by the lens–iris diaphragm and the vitreous base, damage can also occur to the posterior pole. The extent of ocular damage depends on the severity of trauma. The prognosis varies, but is usually determined by the extent of retinal injury.

Cornea

- **Corneal abrasion** involves a breach of the epithelium (Fig. 22.13A) and stains with fluorescein (Fig. 22.13B). It is a painful condition, exacerbated by ocular movement. If located over the pupillary area, vision may be significantly impaired. Details of treatment are discussed under 'Recurrent corneal epithelial erosion' in Chapter 7.
- **Acute corneal oedema** may develop following blunt trauma, secondary to focal or diffuse dysfunction of the endothelium and is sometimes seen underlying a large abrasion. It is commonly associated with folds in Descemet membrane and stromal thickening, but usually clears spontaneously.
- **Tears in Descemet membrane** are usually vertical (Fig. 22.13C) and most commonly arise as the result of birth trauma.

Hyphaema

Hyphaema (haemorrhage in the anterior chamber) is a common complication of blunt ocular injury. The source of bleeding is

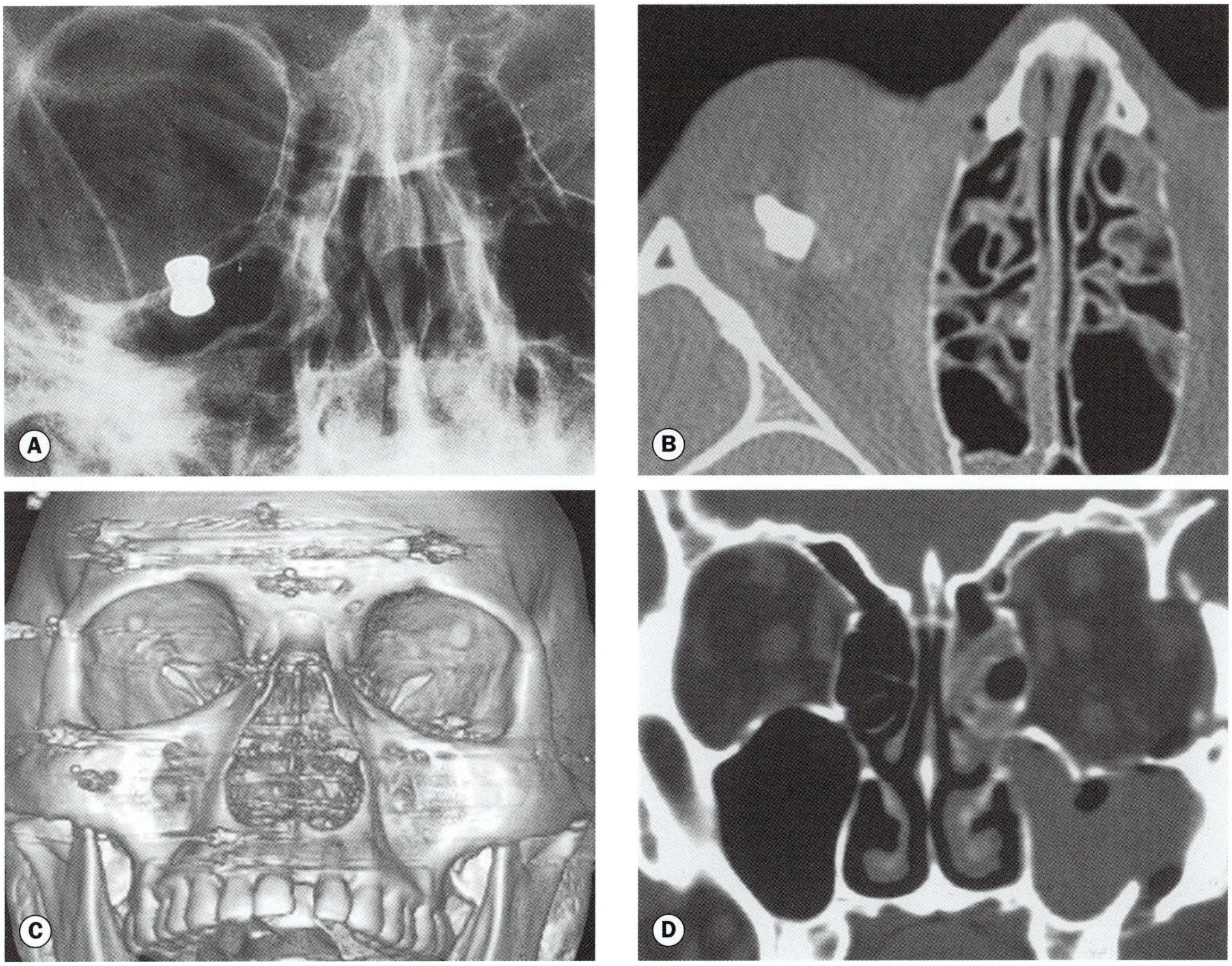

Fig. 22.11 Imaging of ocular trauma. **(A)** Plain radiograph showing a lead air gun pellet; **(B)** axial CT showing a localized intraocular foreign body in the right eye; **(C)** 3-dimensional CT reconstruction of a facial shotgun injury; **(D)** coronal CT showing left lateral orbital wall fracture. *(Courtesy of S Chen – figs B and C; A Pearson – fig. D.)*

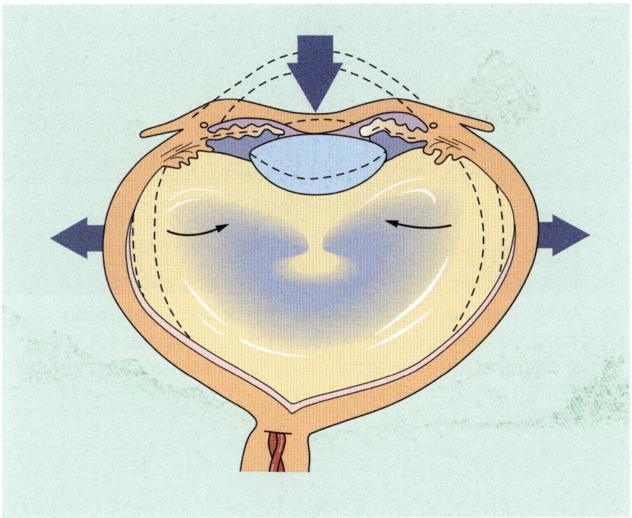

Fig. 22.12 Pathogenesis of ocular damage by blunt trauma.

typically the iris root or ciliary body face. Characteristically, the blood settles inferiorly with a resultant 'fluid level' (Fig. 22.14A), except when the hyphaema is total (Fig. 22.14B). Uncontrolled high IOP can result in ischaemic optic neuropathy and staining of the cornea (Fig. 22.14C) (see Ch. 11).

Anterior uvea

- **Pupil.** The iris may momentarily be compressed against the anterior surface of the lens by severe anteroposterior force, with resultant imprinting of pigment from the pupillary margin. Transient miosis accompanies the compression, evidenced by the pattern of pigment corresponding to the size of the constricted pupil (Vossius ring – Fig. 22.15A). Damage to the iris sphincter may result in traumatic mydriasis, which can be temporary or permanent. The pupil reacts sluggishly or not at all to both light and accommodation. Radial tears in the pupillary margin are common (Fig. 22.15B).
- **Iridodialysis** is a dehiscence of the iris from the ciliary body at its root. The pupil is typically D-shaped and the dialysis is

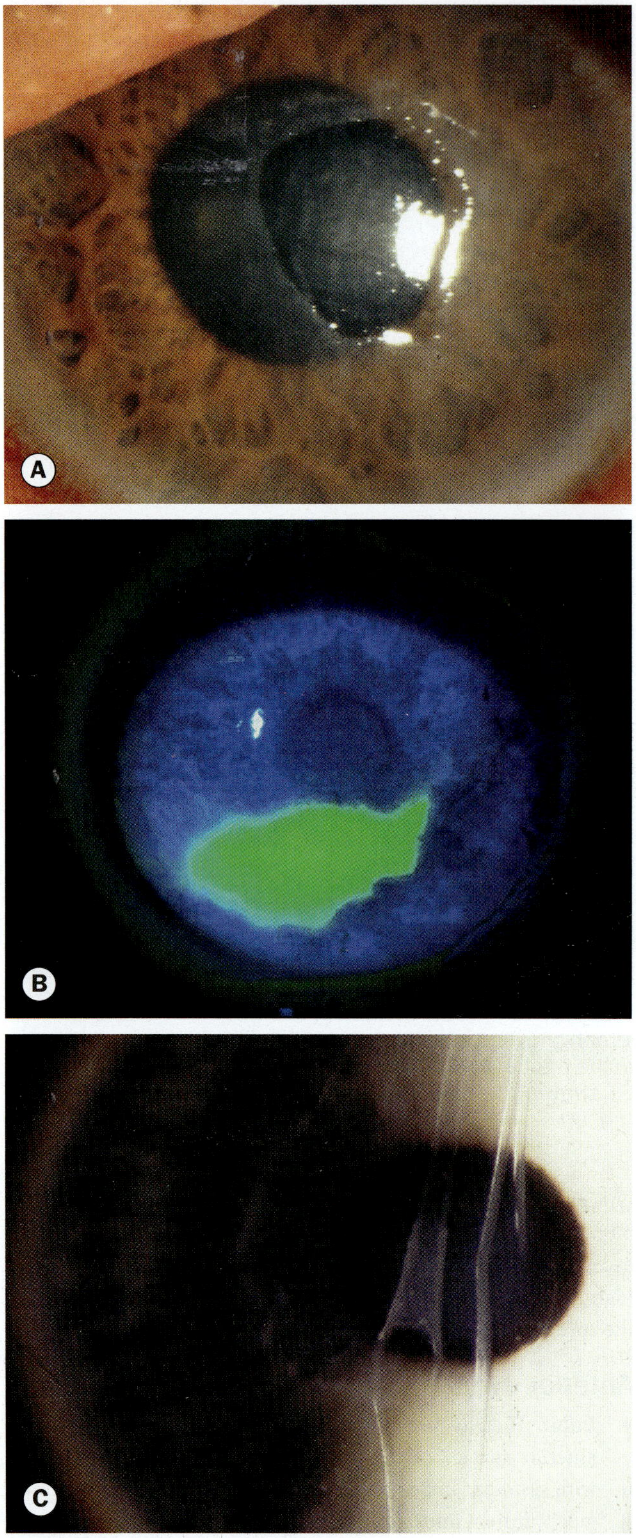

Fig. 22.13 Corneal complications of blunt trauma. **(A)** Small unstained corneal abrasion; **(B)** large corneal abrasion stained with fluorescein; **(C)** tears in Descemet membrane. *(Courtesy of C Barry – fig. B.)*

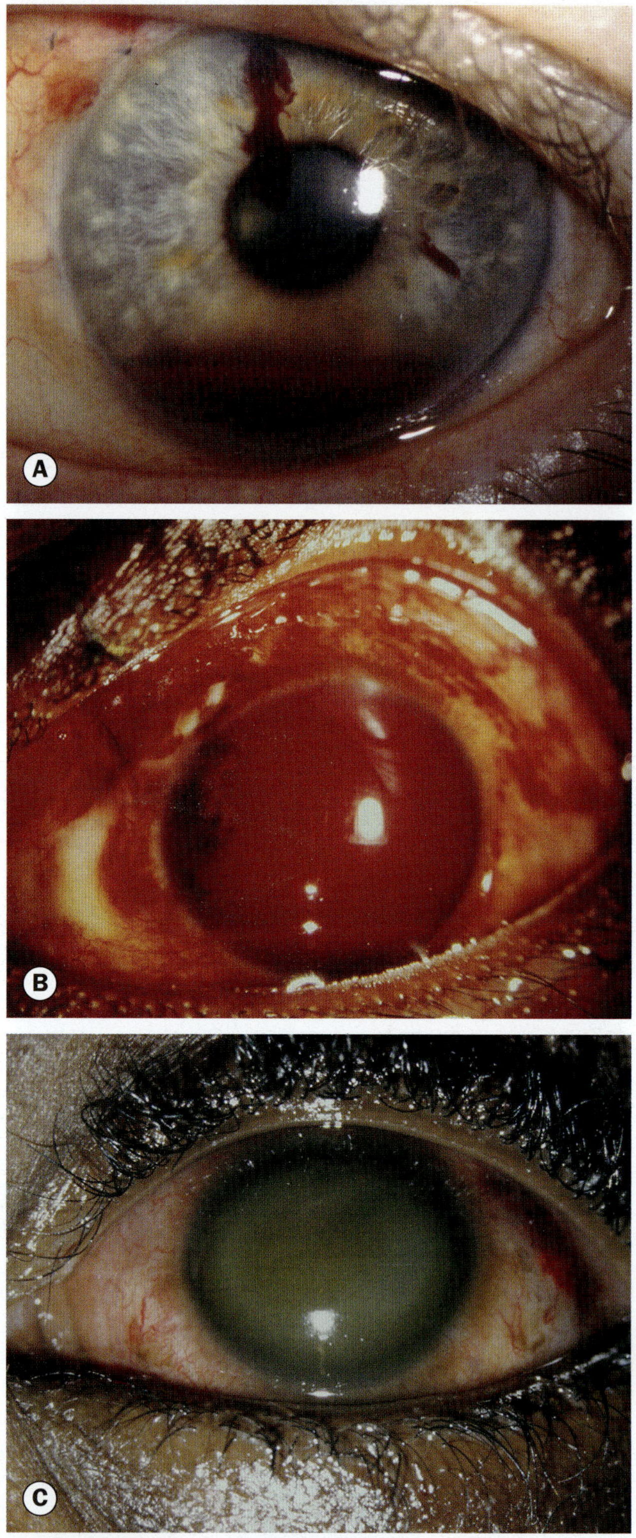

Fig. 22.14 Traumatic hyphaema. **(A)** Small hyphaema from a leaking vessel superiorly; **(B)** total hyphaema; **(C)** corneal blood staining due to sustained high intraocular pressure associated with a total hyphaema.

TIP If the intraocular pressure is low in the presence of a full hyphaema an occult posterior scleral rupture should be suspected.

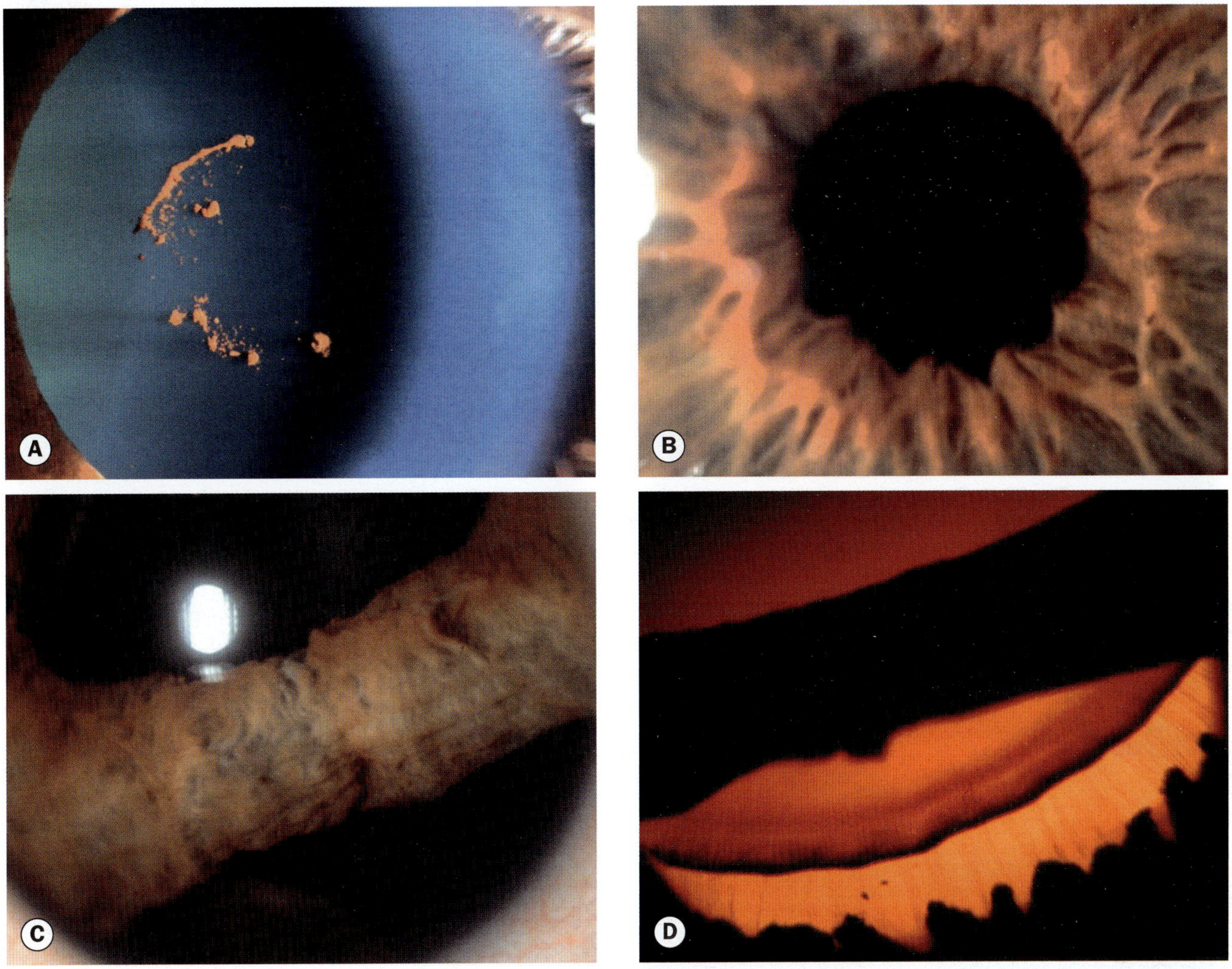

Fig. 22.15 Iris complications of blunt trauma. **(A)** Vossius ring; **(B)** radial sphincter tears; **(C)** iridodialysis; **(D)** retroillumination of iridodialysis.

seen as a dark biconvex area near the limbus (Fig. 22.15C). Retroillumination shows the extent of the injury (Fig. 22.15D). An iridodialysis may be asymptomatic if it is covered by the upper lid. However, monocular diplopia and glare sometimes ensue if the dehiscence is exposed in the palpebral aperture. Traumatic aniridia (360° iridodialysis) is rare. In a pseudophakic eye, the detached iris may be ejected through the cataract surgical incision (Fig. 22.16A). The symptoms of glare can be reduced and the cosmetic appearance can be improved by inserting a prosthetic iris (Fig. 22.16B).

- **Ciliary body** (see below).

Intraocular pressure

It is important for IOP to be monitored carefully, particularly in the early period following trauma (see Ch. 11). Elevation of IOP can occur for a variety of reasons, including hyphaema and inflammation. In the presence of hypotony, it is important to exclude an occult open injury. Tears extending into the face of the ciliary body (angle recession) are associated with a 6–9% risk of late glaucoma (Fig. 22.17).

Lens

- **Cataract** formation is a common sequel to blunt trauma. Postulated mechanisms include direct damage to the lens fibres themselves and minute ruptures in the lens capsule with an influx of aqueous humour, hydration of lens fibres and consequent opacification. A ring-shaped anterior subcapsular opacity may underlie a Vossius ring. Commonly opacification occurs in the posterior subcapsular cortex along the posterior sutures, resulting in a flower-shaped ('rosette') opacity (Fig. 22.18A) that may subsequently disappear, remain stationary or progress to maturity (Fig. 22.18B). Cataract surgery may be necessary for visually significant opacity.
- **Subluxation** of the lens may occur, secondary to tearing of the suspensory ligament. A subluxated lens tends to deviate towards the meridian of intact zonules. The anterior chamber may deepen over the area of zonular dehiscence if the lens rotates posteriorly. The edge of a subluxated lens may be visible under mydriasis (see Fig. 22.18B) and trembling of the iris (iridodonesis) or lens (phakodonesis) may be seen on ocular movement. Subluxation of magnitude sufficient to render the pupil partly aphakic may result in uniocular diplopia. Lenticular astigmatism due to tilting may occur.

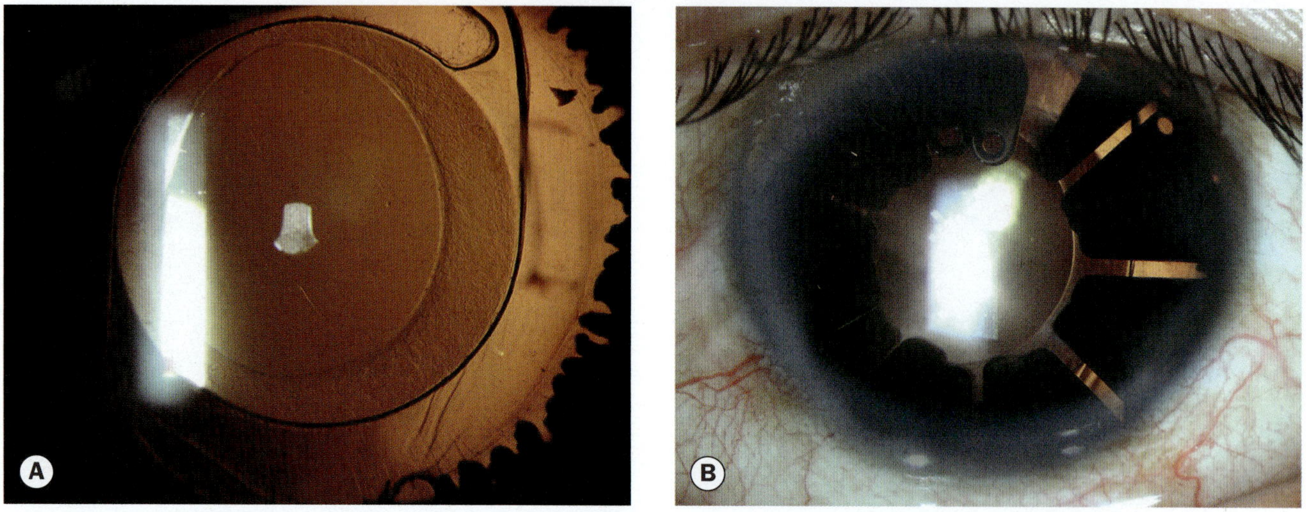

Fig. 22.16 Traumatic aniridia in a pseudophakic eye. **(A)** Retroillumination showing lens implant and ciliary processes; **(B)** prosthetic iris. *(Courtesy of C Barry.)*

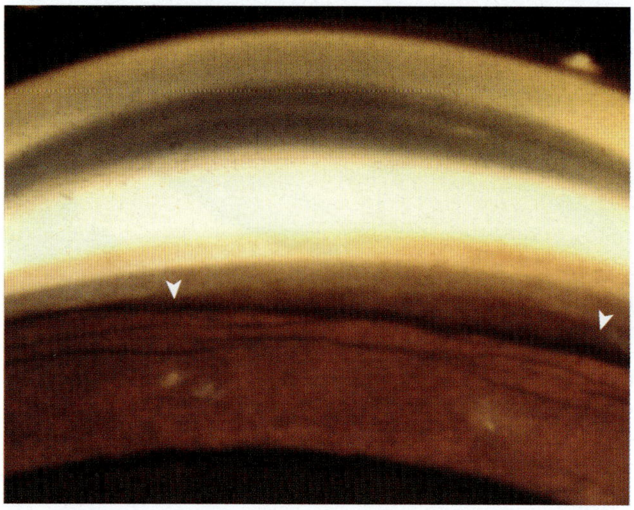

Fig. 22.17 Gonioscopic appearance of angle recession (arrowheads indicate the extent of the recession).

- **Dislocation** due to 360° rupture of the zonular fibres is rare. The lens may dislocate into the vitreous (Fig. 22.18C), or less commonly, into the anterior chamber (Fig. 22.18D). An underlying predisposing condition such as pseudoexfoliation should considered.

Globe rupture

Rupture of the globe may result from severe blunt trauma. The prognosis is poor if the initial visual level is light perception or worse. The rupture is usually anterior, in the vicinity of the Schlemm canal, with prolapse of structures such as the lens, iris, ciliary body and vitreous (Fig. 22.19A and B). An anterior rupture may be masked by extensive subconjunctival haemorrhage. Rupture at the site of a surgical wound (e.g. cataract, keratoplasty, vitrectomy) commonly follows substantial blunt force. An occult posterior rupture can be associated with little visible damage to the anterior segment, but should be suspected if there is asymmetry of anterior chamber depth. The anterior chamber of an affected eye is classically deep, with posterior rotation of the iris–lens diaphragm and IOP in the affected eye is low. The rupture is often found slightly behind the insertion of the rectus muscles where the sclera is thinnest. Gentle B-scan ultrasonography can demonstrate a posterior rupture, but CT or MRI may be necessary. The principles of repair of a rupture in the sclera are described later.

Vitreous haemorrhage

Vitreous haemorrhage may occur, commonly in association with posterior vitreous detachment. Pigment cells ('tobacco dust') can be seen floating in the anterior vitreous and though not necessarily associated with a retinal break, should always prompt careful retinal assessment.

Commotio retinae

Commotio retinae is caused by concussion of the sensory retina resulting in cloudy swelling that gives the involved area a grey appearance (Fig. 22.20A and B). It most frequently affects the temporal fundus. If the macula is involved, a 'cherry-red spot' may be seen at the fovea. Severe involvement may be associated with intraretinal haemorrhage that can involve the macula. The prognosis in mild cases is good, with spontaneous resolution in around 6 weeks. Severe commotio may result in progressive pigmentary degeneration (Fig. 22.20C) and macular hole formation.

Chorioretinitis sclopetaria

This term describes a closed globe injury that follows a high-velocity projectile passing into the orbit close to the outside of the globe. Deformation from the sudden force causes the chorioretinal layers to split and retract leaving the intact sclera exposed (Fig. 21.20D). Complications include vitreous haemorrhage and, occasionally, retinal detachment. The prognosis depends on the cause of the injury (low muzzle energy has a worse prognosis than a high muzzle injury), the location of damage and whether the macula is

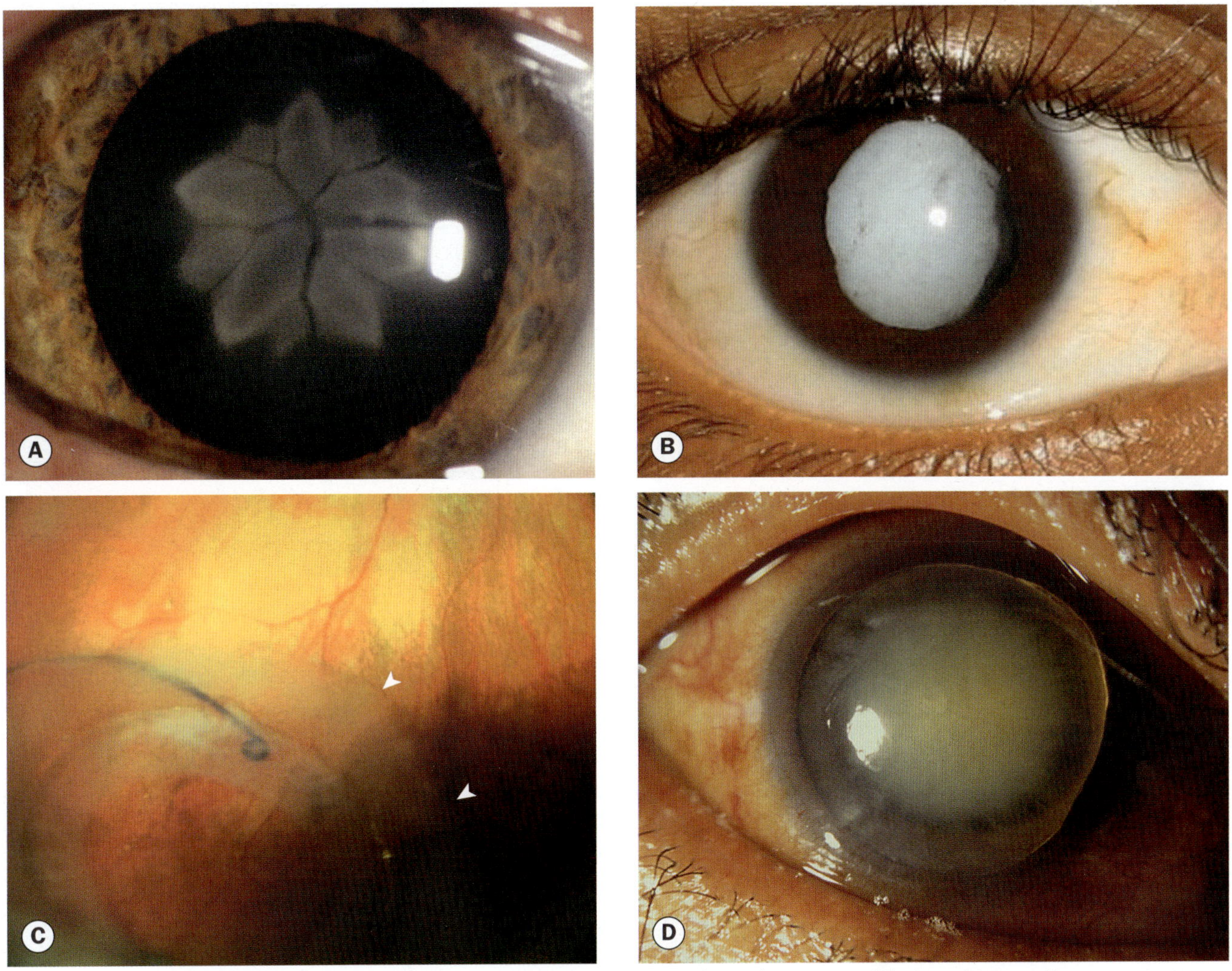

Fig. 22.18 Lens complications of trauma. **(A)** Flower-shaped cataract; **(B)** dense traumatic cataract with ruptured anterior capsule and prolapsed lens contents; **(C)** dislocation into the vitreous in a pseudophakic eye with pseudoexfoliation (arrowheads show the edge of the capsule); **(D)** dislocation into the anterior chamber.

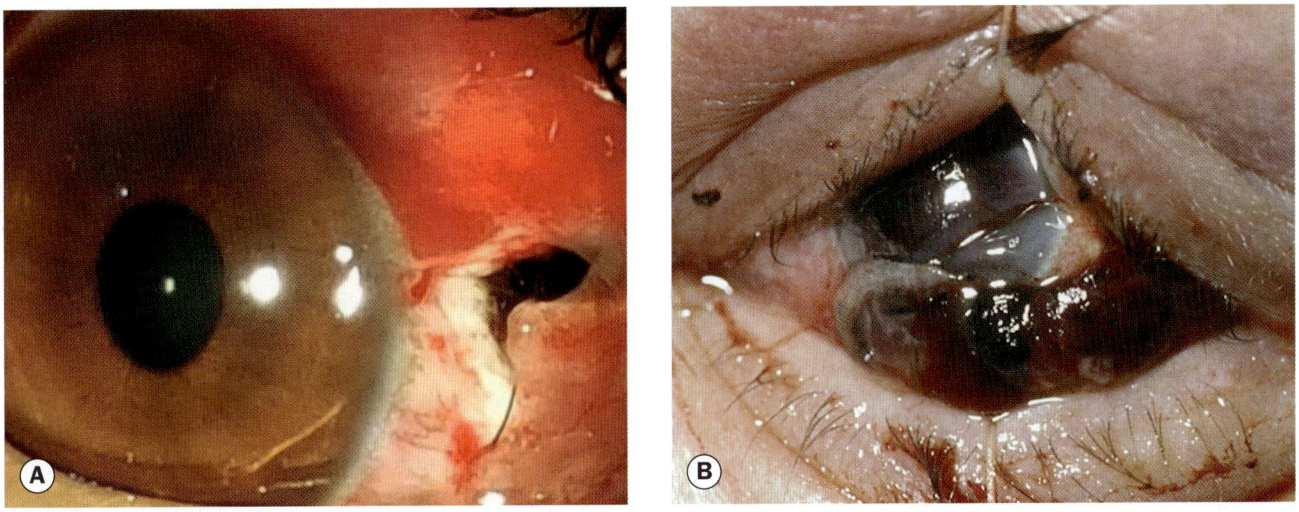

Fig. 22.19 Ruptured globe. **(A)** Localized rupture with uveal prolapse and subconjunctival haemorrhage; **(B)** large corneal rupture with significant prolapse of intraocular structures. *(Courtesy of RSR Naik – fig. A.)*

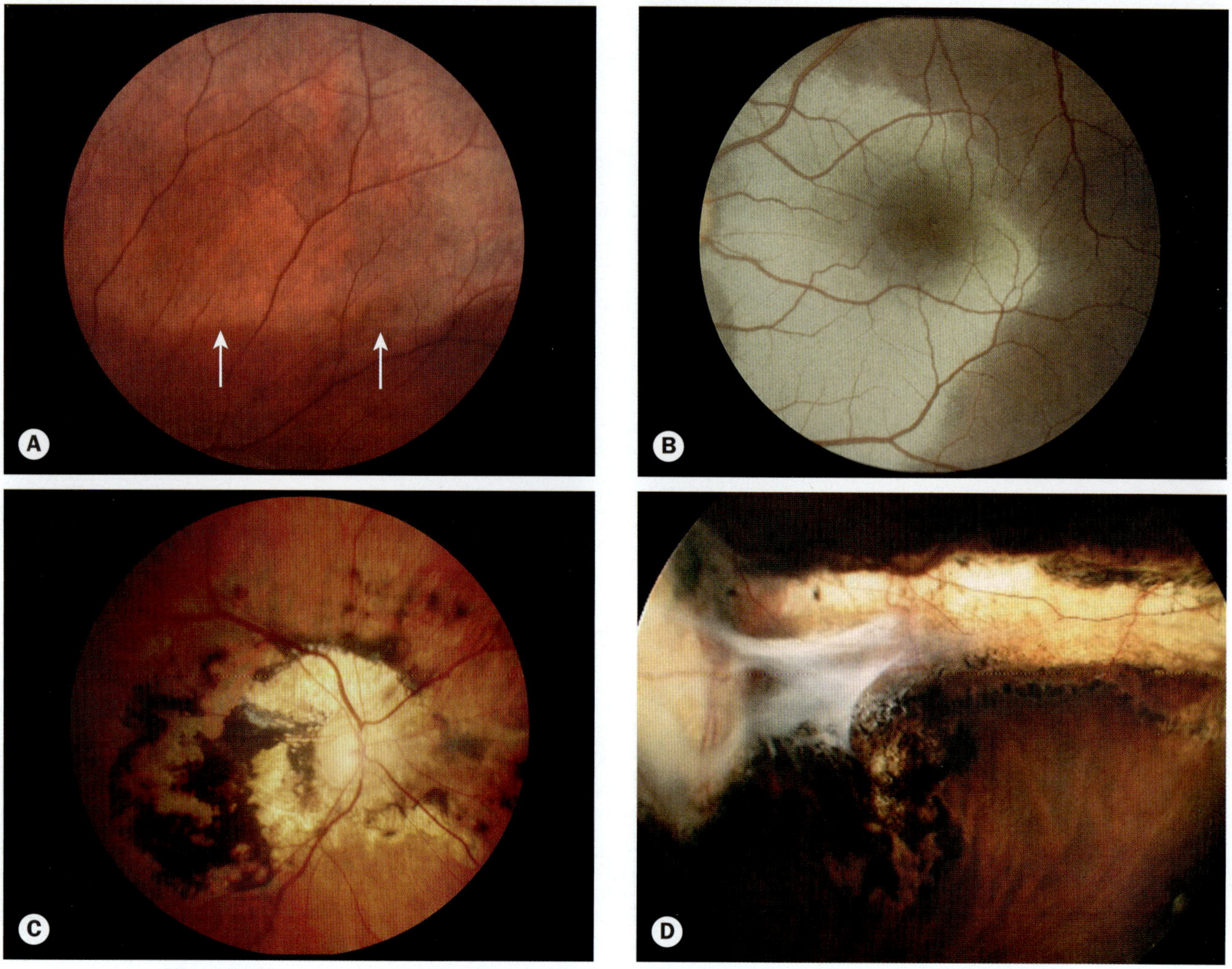

Fig. 22.20 Non-ruptured globe injuries. **(A)** Commotio retinae: acute peripheral cloudy swelling of the retina (arrows show the demarcation); **(B)** commotio retinae involving the macula; **(C)** 3 months after blunt injury in a different patient showing chorioretinal scarring and atrophy; **(D)** chorioretinitis sclopetaria showing bare sclera and chorioretinal scarring.

involved. Most patients experience improvement of vision after the injury, but only 15% achieve 6/6 vision.

Choroidal rupture

Choroidal rupture involves the choroid, Bruch membrane and retinal pigment epithelium (RPE). It may be direct or indirect. Direct ruptures are located anteriorly at the site of impact and run parallel with the ora serrata. Indirect ruptures occur opposite the site of impact. The visual prognosis is poor if the fovea is involved (Fig. 22.21A). A fresh rupture may be partially obscured by subretinal haemorrhage (Fig. 22.21B), which may break through the internal limiting membrane with resultant subhyaloid or vitreous haemorrhage. Weeks to months later, on absorption of the blood, a white crescentic vertical streak of exposed underlying sclera concentric with the optic disc becomes visible (Fig. 22.21C and D). An uncommon late complication is the development of a choroidal neovascular membrane in the region of the rupture.

Retinal breaks and detachment

Trauma is responsible for about 10% of all cases of retinal detachment (RD) and is the most common cause in children, particularly boys. A variety of breaks may develop in traumatized eyes either at the time of impact or subsequently.

- **A retinal dialysis** (Fig. 22.22A) is a break occurring at the ora serrata, caused by traction from the relatively inelastic vitreous gel along the posterior aspect of the vitreous base. The tear may be associated with avulsion of the vitreous base, giving rise to an overhanging 'bucket-handle' appearance comprising a strip of ciliary epithelium, ora serrata and the immediate post-oral retina into which basal vitreous gel remains inserted. A traumatic dialysis occurs most frequently in the superonasal and inferotemporal quadrants. Although they occur at the time of injury, they do not inevitably result in RD. In cases where detachment occurs, subretinal fluid commonly does not develop until several months later and progression is typically slow.

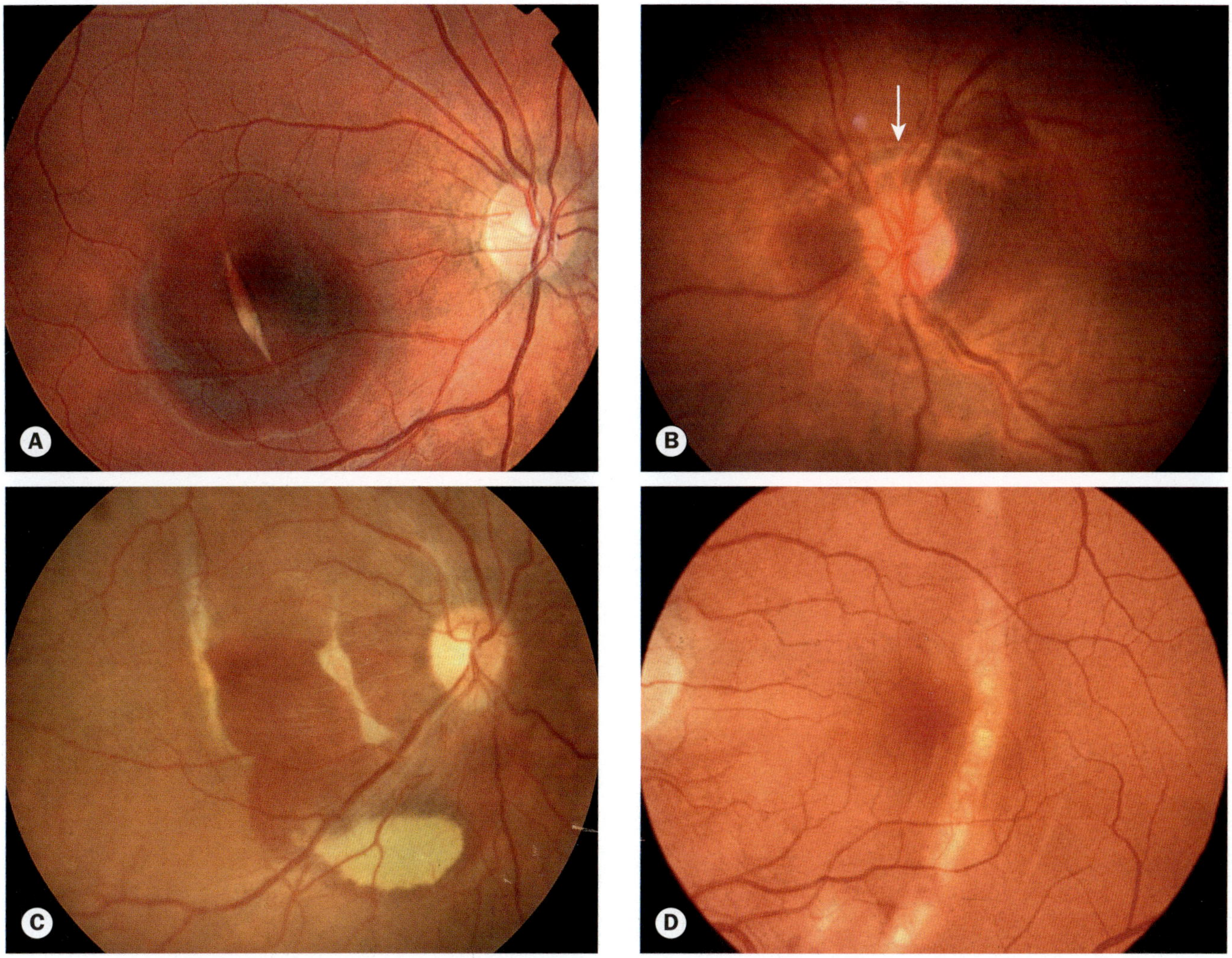

Fig. 22.21 Choroidal rupture. **(A)** Acute rupture in the macular region with subretinal haemorrhage; **(B)** acute parapapillary rupture (arrow) with subretinal haemorrhage; **(C)** foveal disruption with resorbing subretinal and sub-RPE haemorrhage; **(D)** old rupture.

- **Equatorial breaks** are less frequent and are due to direct retinal disruption at the point of scleral impact.
- **RD** secondary to a giant tear may occasionally be seen (Fig. 22.22B).
- **A macular hole** may occur either at the time of injury or following resolution of commotio retinae (Fig. 22.22C).
- **Choroidal detachment.** This can occur in a soft eye after a severe injury and needs to be distinguished from a retinal detachment (Fig. 22.22D).

Traumatic optic neuropathy

Traumatic optic neuropathy follows ocular, orbital or head trauma and presents with sudden visual loss that cannot be explained by other ocular pathology. It occurs in up to 5% of facial fractures.

- **Classification**
  - Direct, due to blunt or sharp optic nerve damage from agents such as displaced bony fragments, a projectile, or local haematoma.
  - Indirect, in which force is transmitted secondarily to the nerve without apparent direct disruption due to impacts upon the eye, orbit or other cranial structures.
- **Mechanisms** include contusion, deformation, compression or transection of the nerve, intraneural haemorrhage, shearing (acceleration of the nerve at the optic canal where it is tethered to the dural sheath, thought to rupture the microvascular supply), secondary vasospasm, oedema and transmission of a shock wave through the orbit.
- **Presentation.** Though major head injury is not unusual, associated trauma may be deceptively minor. Indirect neuropathy is considerably more common than direct. Vision is often very poor from the outset, with only perception of light in around 50%. Typically, the only objective finding is an afferent pupillary defect. The optic nerve head and fundus are initially normal, with pallor developing over subsequent days and weeks (Fig. 22.23). It is important to exclude reversible causes of traumatic visual loss such as compressive orbital haemorrhage (see above).

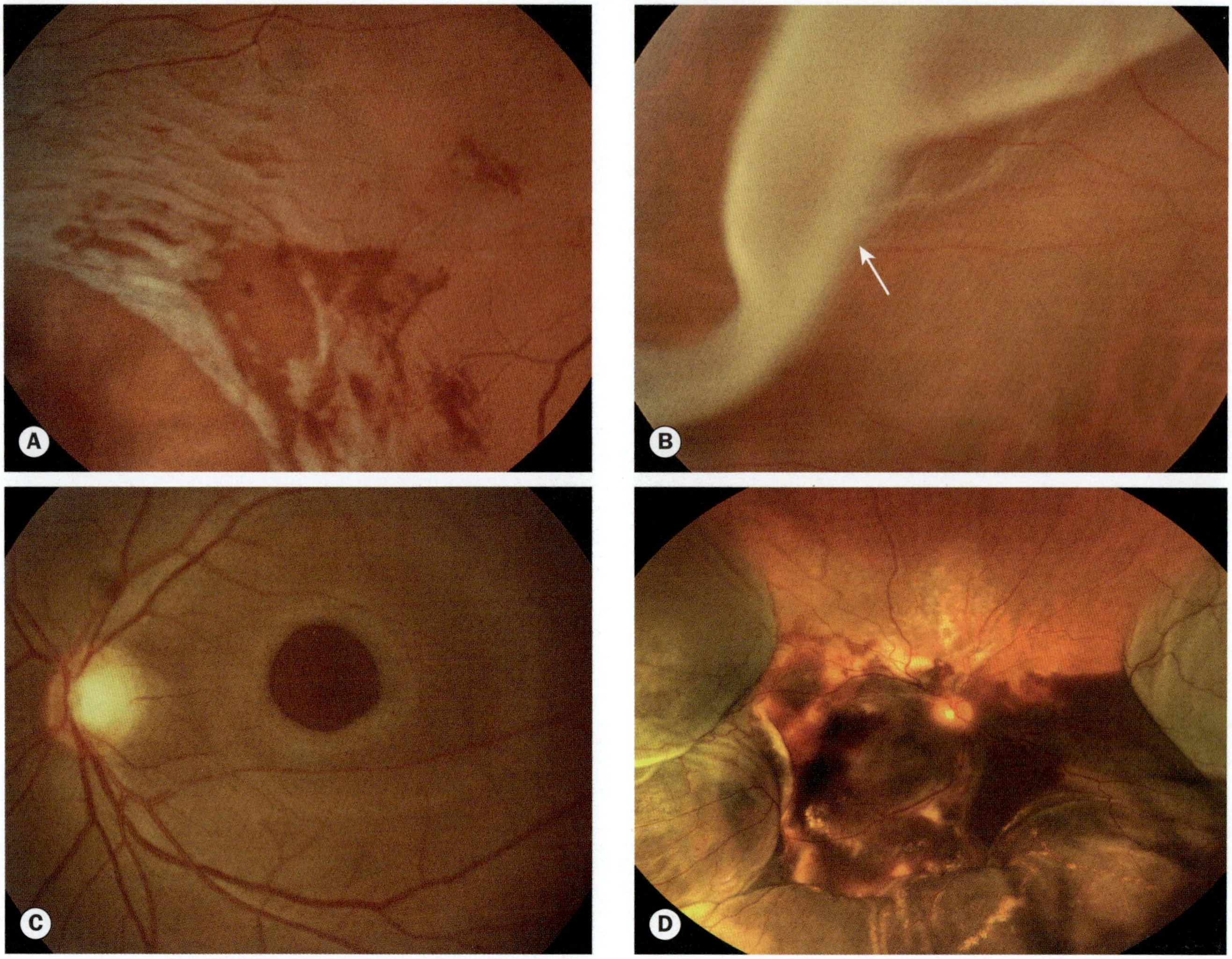

Fig. 22.22 Retinal breaks and detachment. **(A)** Dialysis with retinal detachment; **(B)** giant retinal tear (arrow showing edge of detached retina); **(C)** traumatic macular hole; **(D)** subretinal haemorrhage associated with extensive choroidal detachment.

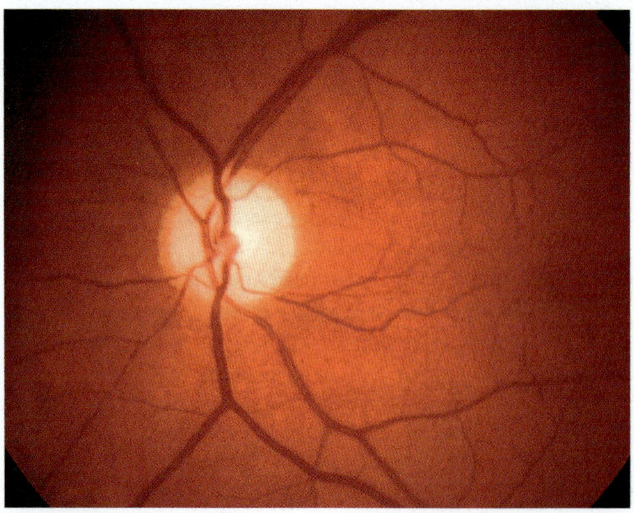

Fig. 22.23 Optic atrophy secondary to a fracture within the optic canal.

- **Investigation.** Assessment should be individualized. Some clinicians request CT, MR or both for all cases, others limit imaging to patients with observed visual decline. CT is more effective in the demonstration of bony abnormalities such as optic canal fracture, but MRI is superior for soft tissue changes (e.g. haematoma). With either modality, very thin sections are recommended.
- **Treatment.** Spontaneous visual improvement occurs in up to about half of patients with an indirect injury. However, if there is initially no light perception the prognosis is poor. Several treatment options have been advocated but no clear benefit has been shown and all carry significant risks.
  - Steroids (intravenous methylprednisolone) should be considered for otherwise healthy patients with severe visual loss or in those with delayed visual loss. If used, these should be started within the first 8 hours, but the optimal regimen has not been determined and their

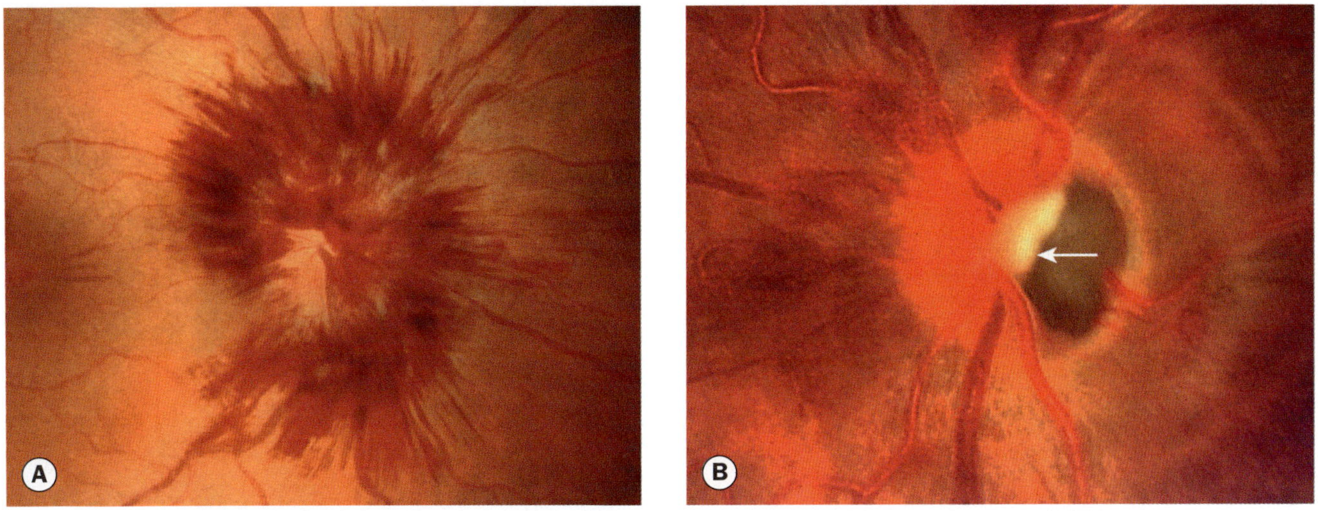

Fig. 22.24 Optic nerve avulsion. **(A)** Acute injury showing peripapillary haemorrhages; **(B)** later stage showing a cavity where the optic nerve head (arrow) has retracted from the dural sheath. *(Courtesy of J Donald M Gass, from* Stereoscopic Atlas of Macular Diseases, *Mosby 1997 – fig. B.)*

use remains controversial. In a trial of high-dose corticosteroid treatment of patients with acute brain injury (CRASH study) patients receiving steroids were at higher risk of death.

- Optic nerve decompression (e.g. endonasal, transethmoidal) may be considered if there is progressive visual deterioration despite steroids. Compression of the nerve by bony fragment or haematoma may also be an indication. However, optic canal fracture is a poor prognostic indicator and there is no evidence that surgery improves the outlook, whilst carrying a significant risk of complications.

Optic nerve avulsion

Optic nerve avulsion is rare and typically occurs when an object intrudes between the globe and the orbital wall, displacing the eye. Postulated mechanisms include sudden extreme rotation or anterior displacement of the globe. Avulsion may be isolated or occur in association with other ocular or orbital injuries. Fundus examination shows a striking cavity where the optic nerve head has retracted from its dural sheath (Fig. 22.24A and B). There is no treatment and the visual prognosis depends on whether avulsion is partial or complete.

Abusive head trauma

Abusive head trauma ('shaken baby' syndrome) is a form of physical abuse occurring typically in children under the age of 2 years. Mortality is more than 25% and it is responsible for up to 50% of deaths from child abuse. It is caused principally by violent shaking, often in association with impact injury to the head. These children should be examined in conjunction with a specialist paediatrician whenever characteristic ophthalmic features are identified. The pattern of injury results from rotational acceleration and deceleration of the head, in contrast to the linear forces generated by a fall. Direct trauma is not the main mechanism of brain damage. Brainstem traction injury causes apnoea and the consequent hypoxia leads to raised intracranial pressure and ischaemia.

TIP A small child with characteristic ophthalmic features of abusive head trauma (especially unexplained retinal haemorrhages) should be examined in conjunction with a specialist paediatrician.

- **Presentation** is frequently with irritability, lethargy and vomiting, which may be initially misdiagnosed as gastroenteritis or other infection because the history of injury is withheld.
- **Systemic features** may include signs of impact head injury, ranging from skull fractures to soft tissue bruises. Subdural and subarachnoid haemorrhage is common and many survivors suffer substantial neurological handicap. Multiple rib and long bone fractures may be present. In some cases, examination findings are limited to the ocular features.
- **Ocular features**
  - Periocular bruising and subconjunctival haemorrhages (Fig. 22.25A).
  - Retinal haemorrhages, bilateral or unilateral (20%), are the most common feature. The haemorrhages typically involve multiple layers and may also be pre- or subretinal (Fig. 22.25B). They are most obvious in the posterior pole, but often extend to the periphery.
  - Poor visual responses and afferent pupillary defects.
  - Visual loss occurs in about 20% of cases, largely as a result of cerebral damage.

Penetrating trauma

Introduction

Penetrating injuries are three times more common in males than females and typically occur in a younger age group (50% aged 15–34). The most frequent causes are assault, domestic/occupational accidents and sport. Serious eye trauma can be prevented by the appropriate use of protective eyewear. The extent of the injury is determined by the size of the object, its speed at the time of impact

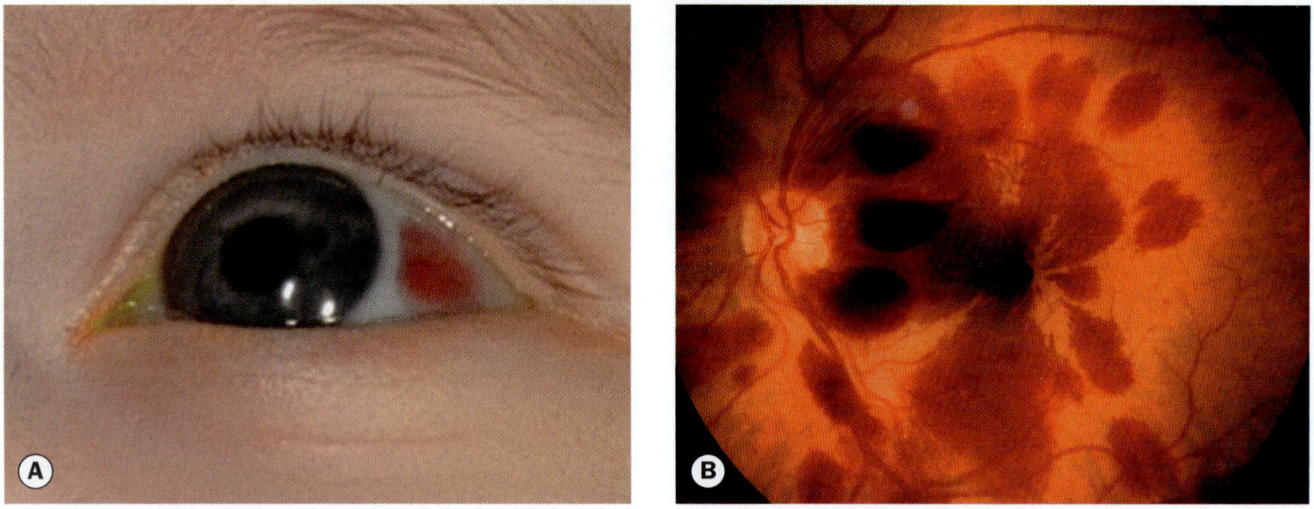

Fig. 22.25 Abusive head trauma (shaken baby syndrome). **(A)** Subconjunctival haemorrhage; **(B)** fundus haemorrhages involving different levels. *(Courtesy of G Kontos – fig. A; R Bates – fig. B.)*

and its composition. Sharp objects such as knives cause well-defined cuts in the globe. However, the extent of damage caused by flying foreign bodies is determined by their kinetic energy. For example, an air gun pellet is large and although relatively slow-moving has a high kinetic energy and can thus cause considerable ocular damage. Of paramount importance is the risk of infection that may follow any penetrating injury. Endophthalmitis or panophthalmitis, often more severe than the initial injury, may ensue with loss of the eye. Risk factors include delay in primary repair, ruptured lens capsule and a dirty wound. Prophylactic intravitreal antibiotics (see Ch. 10) should be considered; vancomycin is a common choice. As with eyelid trauma, tetanus status should be ascertained. An eye with an open injury should be covered by a protective eye shield.

TIP Most penetrating eye injuries need urgent surgical repair, usually under general anaesthesia.

Corneal

Peaking of the pupil and shallowing of the anterior chamber are key signs, though full-thickness corneal penetration may be present without these signs. The technique of primary repair depends on the extent of the wound and associated complications such as iris incarceration, flat anterior chamber and damage to intraocular contents.

- **Small shelving** wounds with a formed anterior chamber may not always require suturing as they can heal spontaneously or with the aid of a soft bandage contact lens (Fig. 22.26A).
- **Medium-sized** wounds should be sutured without delay, especially if the anterior chamber is shallow or flat. 10-0 nylon is used, with shorter stitches near the visual axis opposing perpendicular edges first and apical portions of wounds last. A postoperative bandage contact lens may be applied. The corneoscleral junction should be sutured with 9-0 nylon.
- **With iris involvement.** If possible, the iris should be carefully repositioned. However, excision of the prolapsed portion may be required, particularly if it appears necrotic or if there is a risk of contamination by foreign material (Fig. 22.26B).
- **With lens damage** (Fig. 22.26C). Wounds are treated by first suturing the laceration then removing the lens by phacoemulsification or with a vitreous cutter. Primary implantation of an intraocular lens is frequently associated with a favourable visual outcome and a low rate of postoperative complications.
- **Late scarring.** If the injury involves the visual axis (Fig. 22.26D), penetrating keratoplasty may be needed.

Scleral

Signs of an occult scleral wound are described in the section above discussing globe injury in blunt trauma.

- **Anterior** scleral lacerations have a better prognosis than those posterior to the ora serrata. A foreign body may be found in the wound (Fig. 22.27A). An anterior scleral wound may be associated with serious complications such as iridociliary prolapse (Fig. 22.27B and C) and vitreous incarceration (Fig. 22.27D). The latter, unless appropriately managed, may result in subsequent fibrous proliferation along the plane of incarcerated vitreous, with the development of tractional RD. Viable uveal tissue should be reposited and prolapsed vitreous cut flush with the wound, with subsequent vitreoretinal assessment. 8-0 nylon or 7-0 absorbable material such as polyglactin should be used for scleral suturing in this setting.
- **Posterior** scleral lacerations are frequently associated with retinal damage. Primary repair of the sclera to restore globe integrity should be the initial priority.

Prognosis

This is dependent on the severity of the injury and the complications that arise secondary to the injury. In particular, the prognosis is influenced by: (a) the initial visual acuity, (b) the presence of a relative pupillary defect, (c) the presence of an intraocular foreign

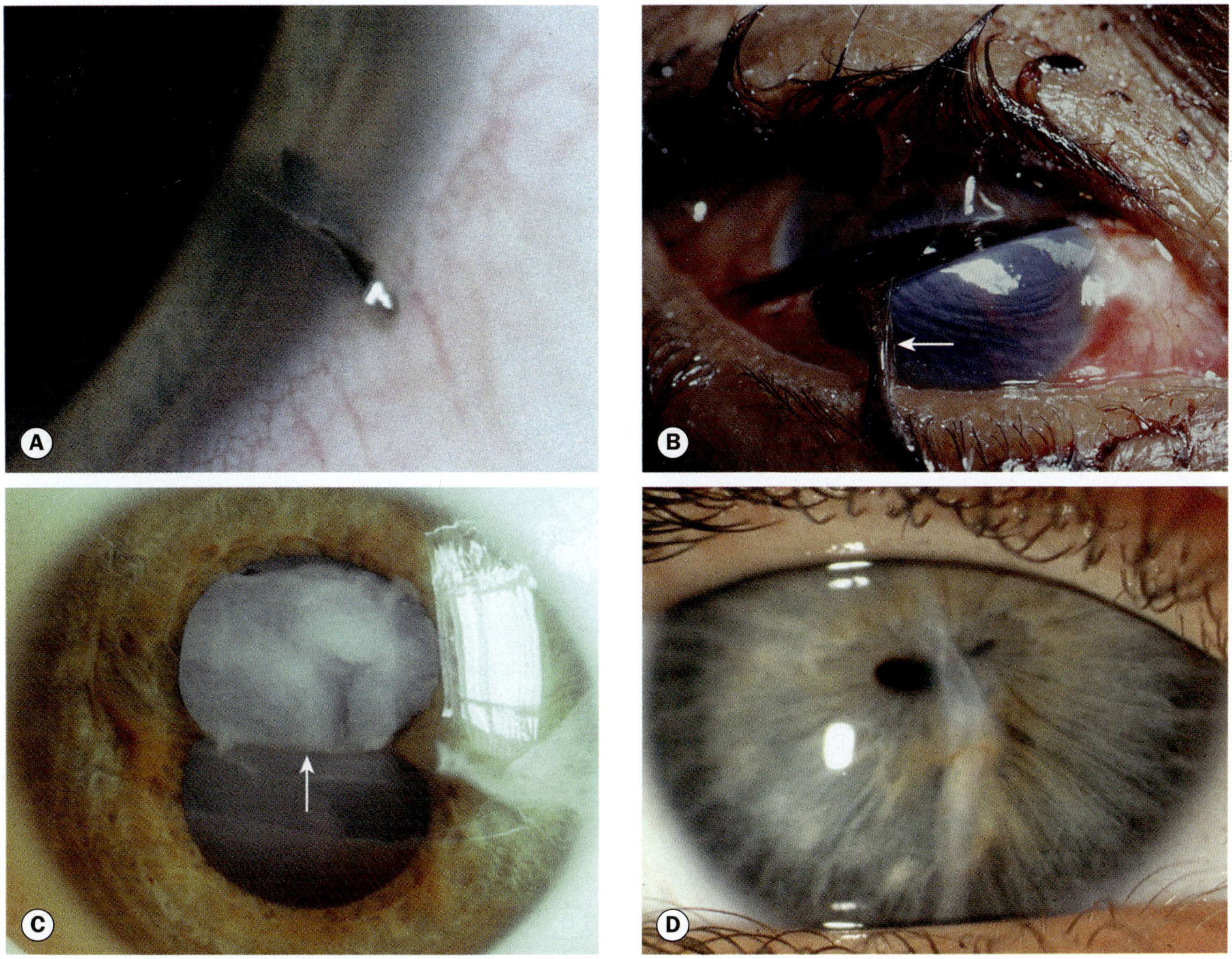

Fig. 22.26 Penetrating corneal wounds. **(A)** Small penetrating injury at the limbus. When the metallic foreign body is removed the anterior chamber may shallow and a single corneal suture may then need to be inserted; **(B)** severe corneal slicing injury with extensive iris prolapse (arrow); **(C)** associated with lens damage, showing linear cut in the lens and prolapsed lens contents (arrow); **(D)** late scarring within the visual axis.

body, (d) the presence of infection and (e) the presence of a retinal injury/detachment.

Retinal detachment

Traumatic tractional RD following a penetrating injury may result from vitreous incarceration in the wound. Subsequent fibroblastic proliferation is exacerbated by the presence of blood in the vitreous gel. Contraction of the resultant epiretinal fibrosis can progress to cause an anterior tractional RD. A retinal break may develop several weeks later, leading to a more rapidly progressing rhegmatogenous detachment.

TIP To prevent extrusion of the intraocular contents when repairing a penetrating injury, it is important not to exert any pressure on the eye.

Enucleation/evisceration

Primary enucleation or evisceration should be considered for extremely severe injuries, especially when it is impossible to repair the sclera and where there is no prospect of retention of vision (see Fig. 4.49). This usually reduces the rehabilitation time and allows a rapid return to work. Secondary enucleation or evisceration may be considered following primary repair if the eye is blind and irreversibly damaged, particularly if it is also unsightly and uncomfortable. In both instances, the surgery is safe with a low complication and infection rate. Based on anecdotal evidence, it has been recommended that if enucleation or evisceration is to be performed it should take place within 10–14 days of the original injury in order to prevent the rare complication of sympathetic ophthalmia (see Ch. 12).

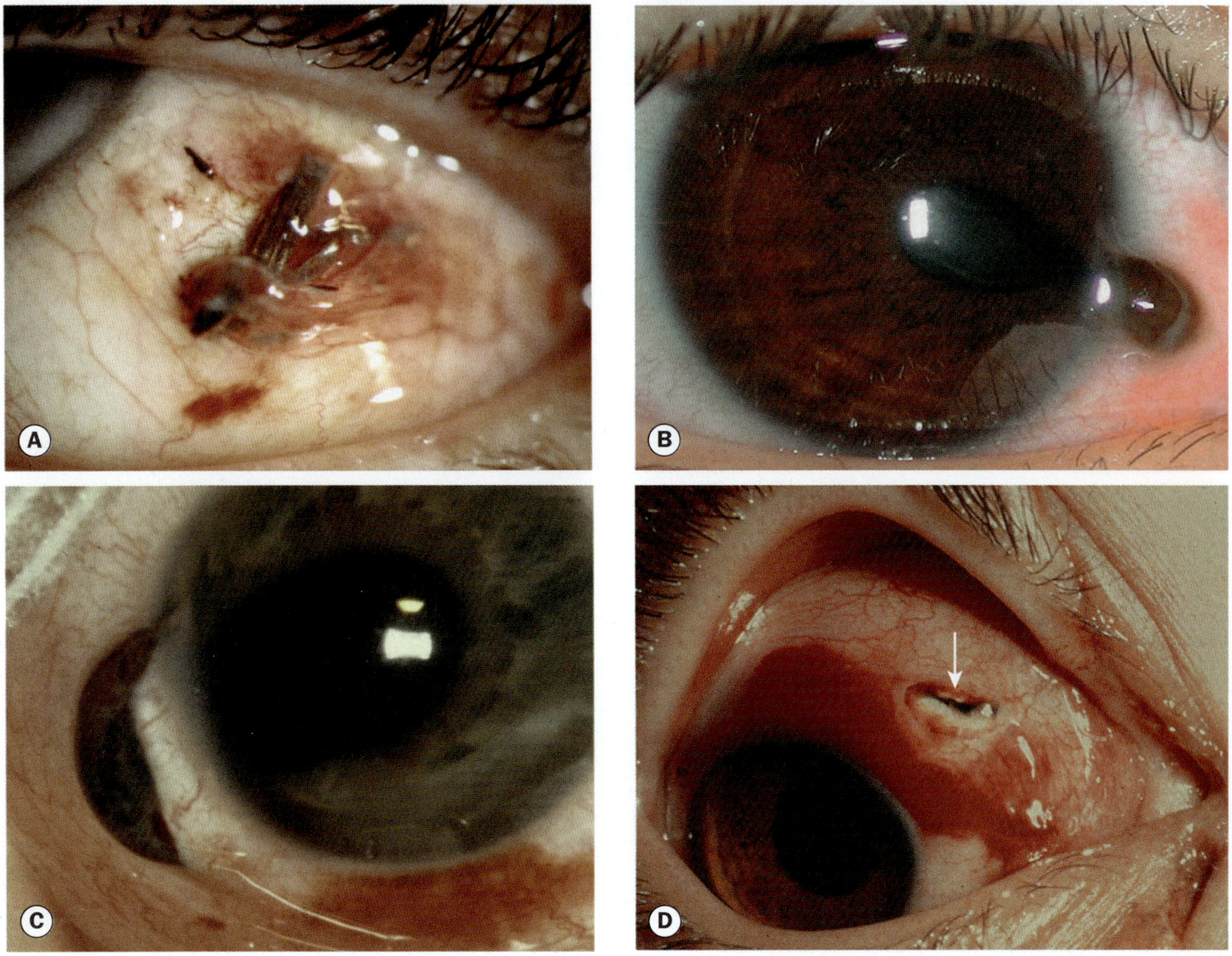

Fig. 22.27 Penetrating scleral wounds. **(A)** Scleral laceration secondary to wood splinter; **(B)** corneoscleral laceration with iris prolapse; **(C)** large scleral cut with iris prolapse; **(D)** anterior scleral laceration with vitreous prolapse (arrow).

TIP In a patient with a small lid wound who has been working with tools, always lift the lids to check for a small penetrating injury in the sclera.

Superficial foreign body

Subtarsal

A small foreign body, such as a particle of steel, coal or sand, often impacts on the corneal or conjunctival surface. This may be washed along the tear film into the lacrimal drainage system or adhere to the superior tarsal conjunctiva (Fig. 22.28A) and abrade the cornea with every blink, when a pathognomonic pattern of linear corneal abrasions may be seen (Fig. 22.28B). Occasionally a barbed foreign body, such as an insect (Fig. 22.28C) or plant material, will become deeply embedded, with resultant substantial discomfort.

TIP In a patient with a linear corneal abrasion, search for a small foreign body on the tarsal surface.

Corneal

- **Clinical features.** Marked ocular grittiness is characteristic. Magnification is often required (Fig. 22.28D). Leukocytic infiltration is typically seen around the embedded foreign body and ferrous particles *in situ* for even a few hours cause rust staining of the bed of the abrasion. Mild secondary uveitis may occur, with associated irritative miosis and photophobia.
- **Management**
    - A high index of suspicion should be maintained for the presence of an IOFB. Posterior segment examination and if necessary plain X-ray imaging can be used to help to exclude this.
    - A slit lamp is preferred to determine the position and depth of the foreign body and to guide removal using a sterile hypodermic needle (often 25-gauge).
    - A residual 'rust ring' is easiest to remove with a sterile burr.
    - Antibiotic ointment is instilled, subsequent duration of use depending on severity.
    - A cycloplegic and topical non-steroidal anti-inflammatory can be prescribed if required to promote comfort.
    - If a corneal foreign body is not removed, there is a significant risk of secondary infection and corneal ulceration.

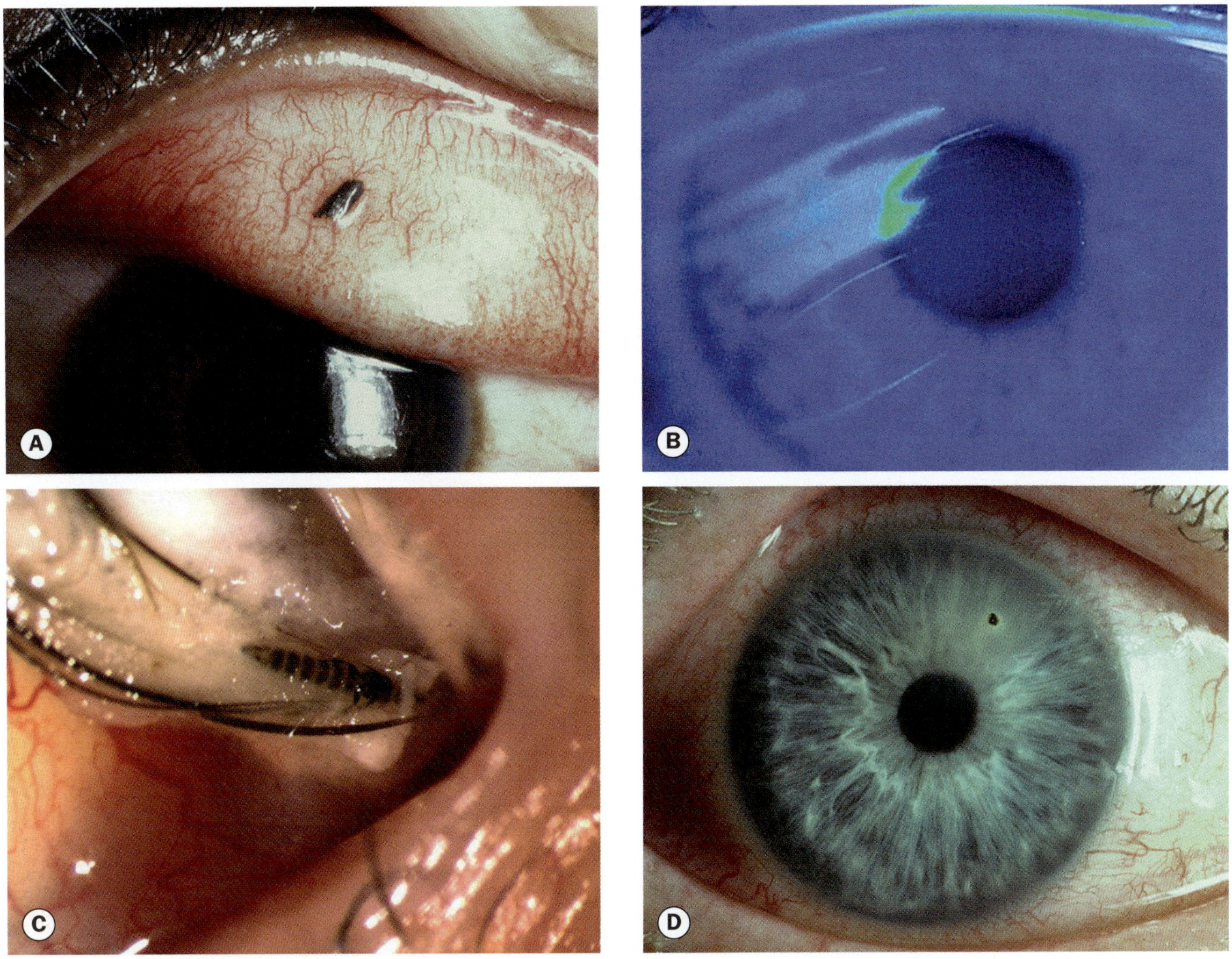

Fig. 22.28 Superficial foreign bodies. **(A)** Retained subtarsal foreign body; **(B)** linear corneal abrasion stained with fluorescein; **(C)** insect retained in the inner canthus; **(D)** recently embedded corneal foreign body.

Any discharge, infiltrate, or significant uveitis should raise suspicion of secondary bacterial infection, with subsequent management as for bacterial keratitis. Metallic particles seem to be associated with a lower risk of infection than organic and stone foreign bodies.

Intraocular foreign body

Introduction

An IOFB may traumatize the eye mechanically, introduce infection or exert other toxic effects on the intraocular structures. It may lodge in any of the structures it encounters, thus may be located anywhere in the anterior (Fig. 22.29A and B) or posterior segments (Fig. 22.29C and D). Notable mechanical effects include cataract formation secondary to capsular injury, vitreous liquefaction and retinal haemorrhages and tears. Stones and organic foreign bodies are associated with a high rate of infection. Intravitreal antibiotic prophylaxis is generally recommended. Many substances are inert, including glass, plastics, gold and silver. However, iron and copper may undergo dissociation and result in siderosis and chalcosis respectively (see below).

Diagnosis

- **History.** A careful history may be key to determining the origin and nature of the foreign material.
- **Examination** should pay special attention to possible sites of entry or exit. Topical fluorescein may be helpful to identify an entry wound. Projection from wounds may allow logical deduction of the location of a foreign body. Gonioscopy and fundoscopy must be considered, taking care to minimize pressure on the eye. Associated signs such as lid laceration and anterior segment damage should be noted.
- **CT** with axial and coronal cuts is used to detect and localize a metallic IOFB, providing cross-sectional images with a sensitivity and specificity superior to plain radiography and ultrasonography.
- **MRI** is contraindicated in the context of a metallic (specifically ferrous) IOFB.

Treatment

- **Magnetic** removal of ferrous foreign bodies involves the creation of a sclerotomy adjacent to the foreign body, with application of a magnet followed by cryotherapy to the retinal break.

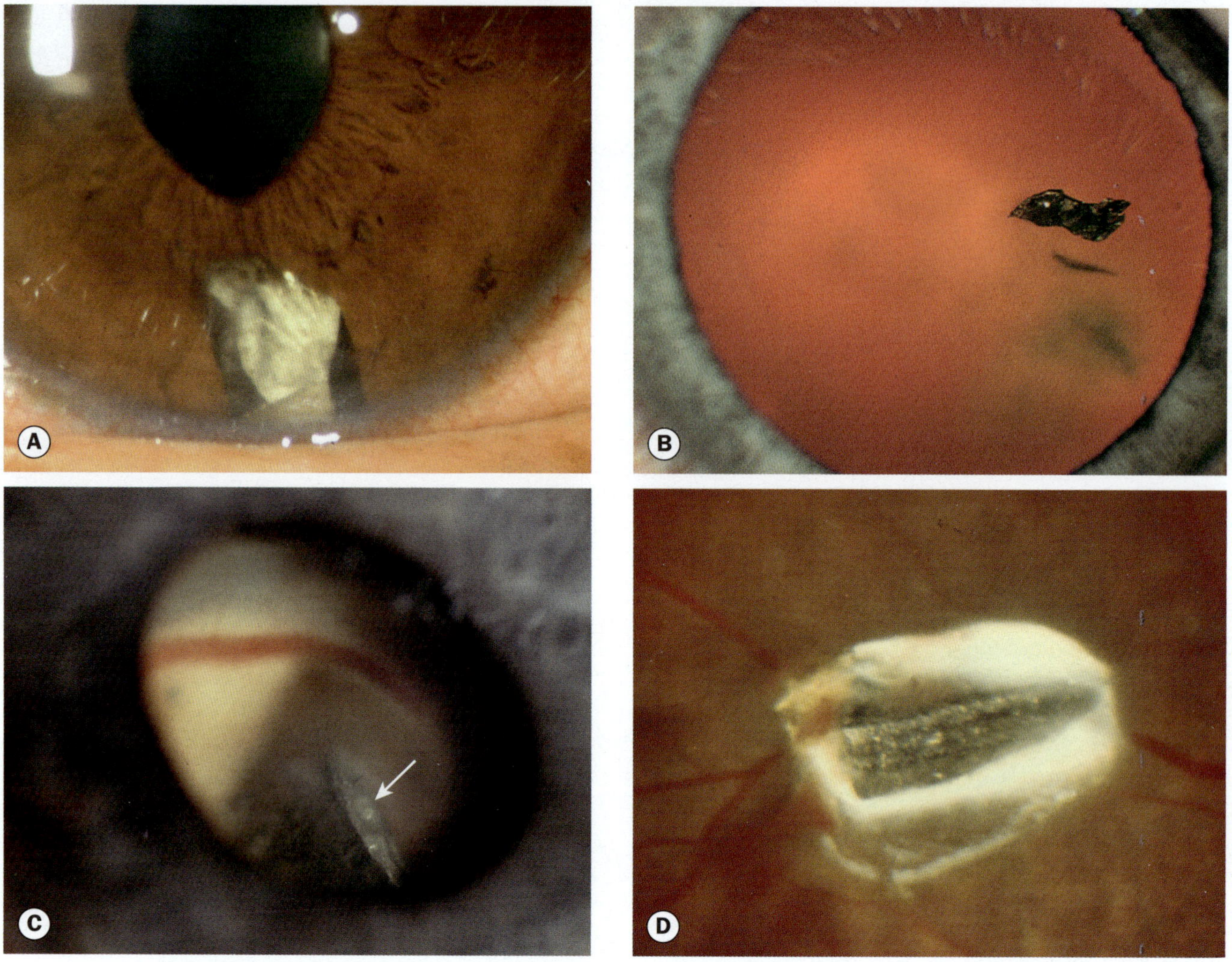

Fig. 22.29 Intraocular foreign bodies. **(A)** In the anterior chamber; **(B)** in the lens; **(C)** in the vitreous (arrow) with retinal detachment; **(D)** retinal impaction, with localized inflammation suggestive of early infection.

- **Forceps** removal may be used for non-magnetic foreign bodies and magnetic foreign bodies that cannot be safely removed with a magnet. It involves pars plana vitrectomy and removal of the foreign body with forceps either through the pars plana or limbus depending on the circumstances.
- **Prophylaxis against infection** (see below).

TIP A missed intraocular foreign body with a ferrous component can result in late visual loss secondary to siderosis.

Siderosis

Steel is the most common foreign body constituent and is typically projected into the eye by hammering or power tool use. A ferrous IOFB undergoes dissociation with the consequent deposition of iron in the intraocular epithelial structures, notably the lens epithelium, iris and ciliary body epithelium and the sensory retina. It exerts a toxic effect on cellular enzyme systems, with resultant cell death. Signs include anterior capsular cataract, consisting of radially distributed iron deposits on the anterior lens capsule (Fig. 22.30A), reddish-brown staining of the iris that may give rise to heterochromia iridis and pigmentary retinopathy followed by atrophy of the retina and RPE (Fig. 22.30B), potentially leading to profound visual loss. Trabecular damage can cause glaucoma. Electroretinography shows progressive attenuation of the b-wave over time.

Chalcosis

The ocular reaction to an IOFB with a high copper content involves a violent endophthalmitis-like picture, often with progression to phthisis bulbi. On the other hand, an alloy with a relatively low copper content such as brass or bronze, results in chalcosis. Electrolytically dissociated copper becomes deposited intraocularly, resulting in a picture similar to that seen in Wilson disease. Thus, a Kayser–Fleischer ring develops and an anterior 'sunflower' cataract. Retinal deposition results in golden plaques visible ophthalmoscopically. Since copper is less retinotoxic than iron, degenerative retinopathy does not develop and visual function may be preserved.

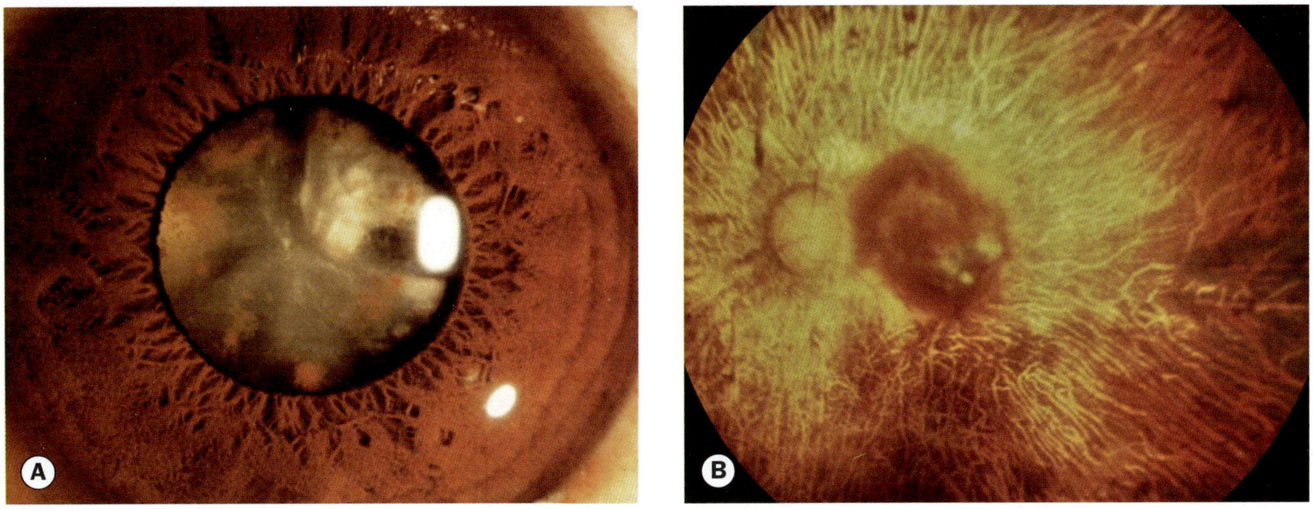

Fig. 22.30 Siderosis oculi. **(A)** Lenticular deposits; **(B)** atrophy of the retina and RPE associated with an impacted ferrous foreign body. *(Courtesy of J Donald M Gass, from* Stereoscopic Atlas of Macular Diseases, *Mosby 1997 – fig. B.)*

Bacterial endophthalmitis

Endophthalmitis develops in about 1 in 10 cases of penetrating trauma with retained foreign body.

- **Risk factors** include delay in primary repair, retained IOFB and the position and extent of wounds. Clinical signs are the same as acute postoperative endophthalmitis (see Ch. 10).
- **Pathogens.** *Staphylococcus* spp. and *Bacillus* spp. are isolated from about 90% of culture-positive cases.
- **Management**
  - Prophylactic antibiotics (e.g. ciprofloxacin 750 mg twice daily or moxifloxacin 400 mg once daily) can be given for open globe injuries, together with topical antibiotic, steroid and cycloplegia.
  - Prompt removal of a retained IOFB.
  - Prophylactic intravitreal antibiotics, especially for high-risk cases (e.g. agricultural injuries).
  - Culture of a removed IOFB.
  - Treatment for established cases is the same as for acute postoperative bacterial endophthalmitis (see Ch. 10).

CHEMICAL INJURIES

Introduction

A chemical eye injury should be considered an acute emergency that requires urgent treatment to reduce the risk of permanent visual loss. Early and appropriate treatment is fundamental to the successful management.

Aetiology

Chemical injuries range in severity from trivial to potentially blinding. The majority are accidental, but a few are due to assault. Two-thirds of accidental burns occur at work and the remainder at home. Chemical injury is the second commonest cause of work-based eye injuries at 12%, behind 'foreign body' injuries at 43%. Alkali burns are twice as common as acid burns, since alkalis are more widely used both at home and in industry. The severity of a chemical injury is related to the properties of the chemical, the area of affected ocular surface, duration of exposure (including retention of particulate chemical on the surface of the globe or under the upper lid) and related effects such as thermal damage. Alkalis tend to penetrate more deeply than acids as the latter coagulate surface proteins, forming a protective barrier. The most commonly involved alkalis are ammonia, sodium hydroxide and lime. Ammonia and sodium hydroxide characteristically produce severe damage because of rapid penetration. Hydrofluoric acid used in glass etching and cleaning also tends to rapidly penetrate the ocular tissues, whilst sulphuric acid may be complicated by thermal effects and high velocity impacts associated with car battery explosion.

Pathophysiology

- **Damage** by severe chemical injuries tends to progress as below:
  - Necrosis of the conjunctival and corneal epithelium with disruption and occlusion of the limbal vasculature. Loss of limbal stem cells may lead to conjunctivalization and vascularization of the corneal surface, or persistent corneal epithelial defects with sterile corneal ulceration and perforation. Longer-term effects include ocular surface wetting disorders, symblepharon formation and cicatricial entropion.
  - Deeper penetration causes the breakdown and precipitation of glycosaminoglycans and stromal corneal opacification.
  - Anterior chamber penetration results in iris and lens damage.
  - Ciliary epithelial damage impairs secretion of ascorbate, which is required for collagen production and corneal repair.
  - Hypotony and phthisis bulbi may ensue in severe cases.

- **Healing**
  - The epithelium heals by migration of epithelial cells originating from limbal stem cells.
  - Damaged stromal collagen is phagocytosed by keratocytes and new collagen is synthesized.

Management

Emergency treatment

A chemical burn requires urgent treatment by the first person who sees the affected person. Immediate treatment is as follows:

- **Copious irrigation** is crucial to minimize duration of contact with the chemical and to normalize the pH in the conjunctival sac as soon as possible. The speed and efficacy of irrigation is the most important prognostic factor following chemical injury. Topical anaesthetic should be instilled prior to irrigation, as this dramatically improves comfort and facilitates cooperation. A lid speculum may be helpful. Tap water should be used if necessary to avoid any delay, but a sterile balanced buffered solution, such as normal saline or Ringer lactate, should be used to irrigate the eye for 15–30 minutes or until the measured pH is neutral.
- **Double-eversion of the upper eyelid** should be performed so that any retained particulate matter trapped in the fornices is identified and removed.
- **Debridement** of necrotic areas of corneal epithelium should be performed at the slit lamp to promote re-epithelialization and remove associated chemical residue.
- **Admission** to hospital is usually required for severe injuries (grade 3 and 4 – see below) in order to ensure adequate instillation of eye drops in the early stages.

TIP The initial management of a chemical injury to the eye is immediate copious ocular irrigation. If available, instillation of a topical anaesthetic improves comfort and facilitates cooperation.

Grading of severity

Acute chemical injuries are graded in order to plan subsequent treatment and to provide an indication of the prognosis. Currently, there are two classifications used for grading chemical injuries: the Roper-Hall classification (see below) and the Dua classification. In the Roper-Hall classification, grading is performed on the basis of corneal clarity and severity of limbal ischaemia. The latter is assessed by observing the patency of the deep and superficial vessels at the limbus. The Dua classification is more detailed and is based on the number of clock hours of affected limbus and the percentage of conjunctival involvement. This provides a better prognostic predictor than the Roper-Hall classification, particularly for grade 4 cases.

- **Grade 1** (Fig. 22.31A) is characterized by a clear cornea (epithelial damage only) and no limbal ischaemia (excellent prognosis).
- **Grade 2** (Fig. 22.31 B) shows a hazy cornea but with visible iris detail and less than one-third of the limbus being ischaemic (good prognosis).
- **Grade 3** (Fig. 22.31C) manifests total loss of corneal epithelium, stromal haze obscuring iris detail and between one-third and one-half limbal ischaemia (guarded prognosis).
- **Grade 4** (Fig. 22.31D) manifests with an opaque cornea and more than half of the limbus showing ischaemia (poor prognosis).

Other features that should be noted at the initial assessment are the extent of corneal and conjunctival epithelial loss, iris changes, the status of the lens and the IOP.

Medical treatment

Most mild injuries (grade 1 and 2) are treated with topical antibiotic ointment for about a week, with topical steroids and cycloplegics if necessary. The main aims of treatment of more severe burns are to reduce inflammation, promote epithelial regeneration and prevent corneal ulceration. For moderate–severe injuries, preservative-free drops should be used.

- **Steroids** reduce inflammation and neutrophil infiltration and address anterior uveitis. However, they also impair stromal healing by reducing collagen synthesis and inhibiting fibroblast migration. For this reason, topical steroids may be used initially (usually 4–8 times daily, strength depending on injury severity) but must be tailed off after 7–10 days when sterile corneal ulceration is most likely to occur. Steroids may be replaced by topical non-steroidal anti-inflammatory drugs, which do not affect keratocyte function.
- **Cycloplegia** to improve comfort (e.g. atropine 1% twice daily).
- **Preservative-free topical antibiotic** drops are used for prophylaxis of bacterial infection (e.g. chloramphenicol four times daily).
- **Ascorbic acid** improves wound healing by promoting the synthesis of mature collagen by corneal fibroblasts. Topical sodium ascorbate 10% can be given 2-hourly in addition to a systemic dose of 1–2 g vitamin C (L-ascorbic acid) four times daily (not in patients with renal disease).
- **Citric acid** is a powerful inhibitor of neutrophil activity and reduces the intensity of the inflammatory response. Chelation of extracellular calcium by citrate also appears to inhibit collagenase. For grade 3 and 4, topical sodium citrate 10% should be instilled 2-hourly for about 10 days and may also be given orally (2 g four times daily). The aim is to eliminate the second wave of phagocytes, which normally occurs about 7 days after the injury. Ascorbate and citrate can be tapered as the epithelium heals.
- **Tetracyclines** are effective collagenase inhibitors and also inhibit neutrophil activity and reduce ulceration. They should be considered if there is significant corneal melting and can be administered both topically (tetracycline ointment four times daily) and systemically (doxycycline 100 mg twice daily tapering to once daily). Acetylcysteine 10% six times daily is an alternative anticollagenase agent given topically.
- **Symblepharon** formation should be prevented as necessary by lysis of developing adhesions with a sterile glass rod or damp cotton bud.
- **IOP** should be monitored, with treatment if necessary. Oral acetazolamide is recommended to avoid adding further to the ocular surface burden.
- **Periocular skin injury** may require a dermatology opinion.

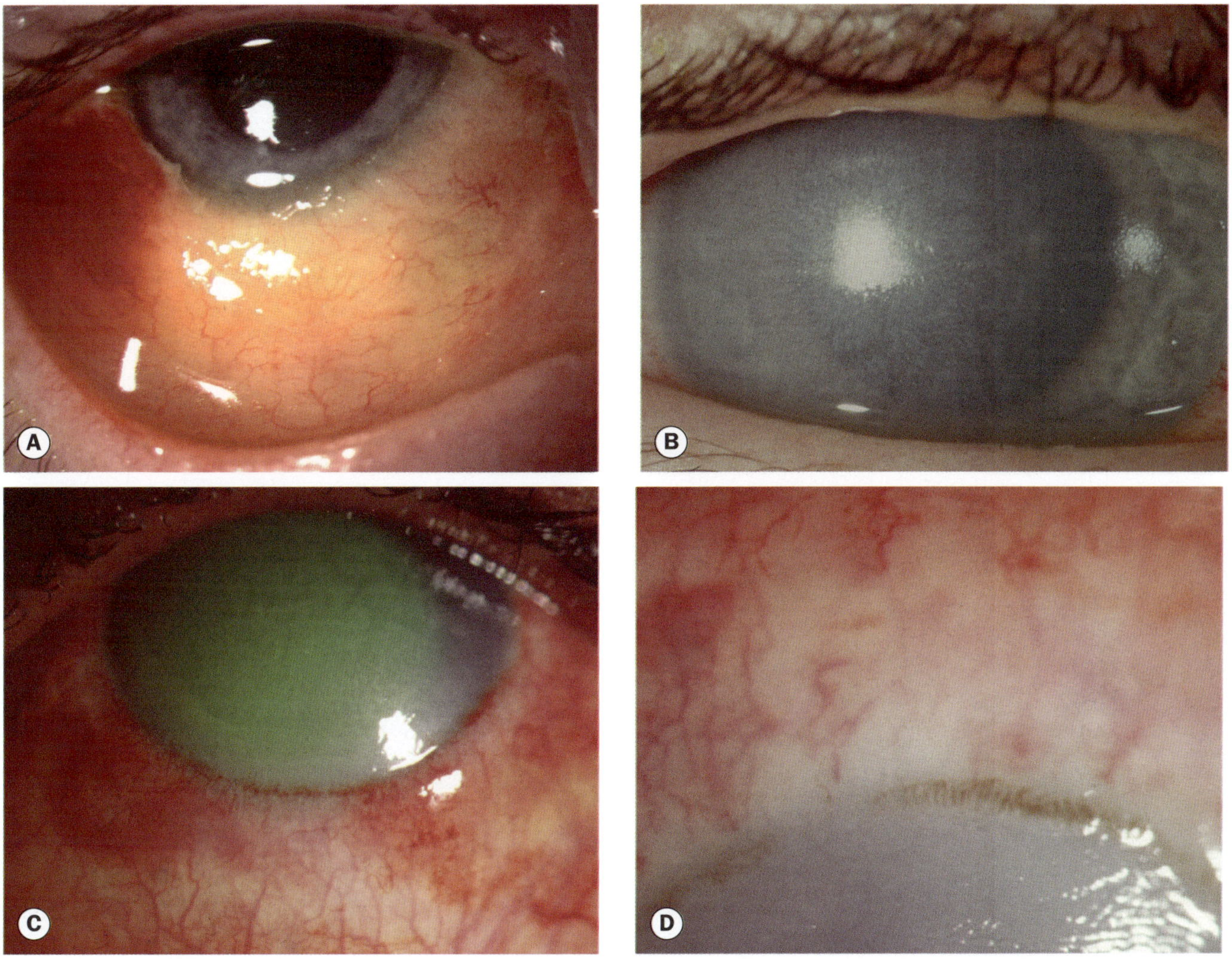

Fig. 22.31 Chemical burns. **(A)** Grade 1 – clear cornea with chemosis of the conjunctiva; **(B)** grade 2 – corneal haze but visible iris detail; **(C)** grade 3 – corneal haze obscuring iris details; **(D)** grade 4 – marked conjunctival ischaemia and an opaque cornea.

Surgery

- **Early** surgery may be necessary to promote revascularization of the limbus, restore the limbal cell population and re-establish the fornices. One or more of the following procedures may be used:
  - Advancement of Tenon capsule with suturing to the limbus is aimed at re-establishing limbal vascularity to help to prevent the development of corneal ulceration.
  - Limbal stem cell transplantation from the patient's other eye (autograft) or from a donor (allograft) is aimed at restoring normal corneal epithelium.
  - Amniotic membrane grafting to promote epithelialization and suppression of fibrosis.
  - Gluing or keratoplasty may be needed for actual or impending perforation.
- **Late** surgery may involve:
  - Division of conjunctival bands (Fig. 22.32A) and symblepharon (Fig. 22.32B).
  - Conjunctival or other mucous membrane grafting.
  - Correction of eyelid deformities such as cicatricial entropion (see Fig. 2.55B).
  - Keratoplasty for corneal scarring (Fig. 22.32C) should be delayed for at least 6 months and preferably longer, to allow maximal resolution of inflammation.
  - In a very severely damaged eye (Fig. 22.32D) a keratoprosthesis may be required (see Fig. 8.11).

THERMAL BURNS

Thermal injuries range in severity from trivial to potentially blinding. Most involve the eyelids and face, but the surface of the cornea may be burnt resulting in severe corneal scarring (Fig. 22.33A and B). Most mild injuries are treated with topical antibiotic drops for about a week with topical steroids and cycloplegics. Plastic surgery to the lids may be required if there is cicatrization and abnormal lid position. Corneal scarring will usually require keratoplasty.

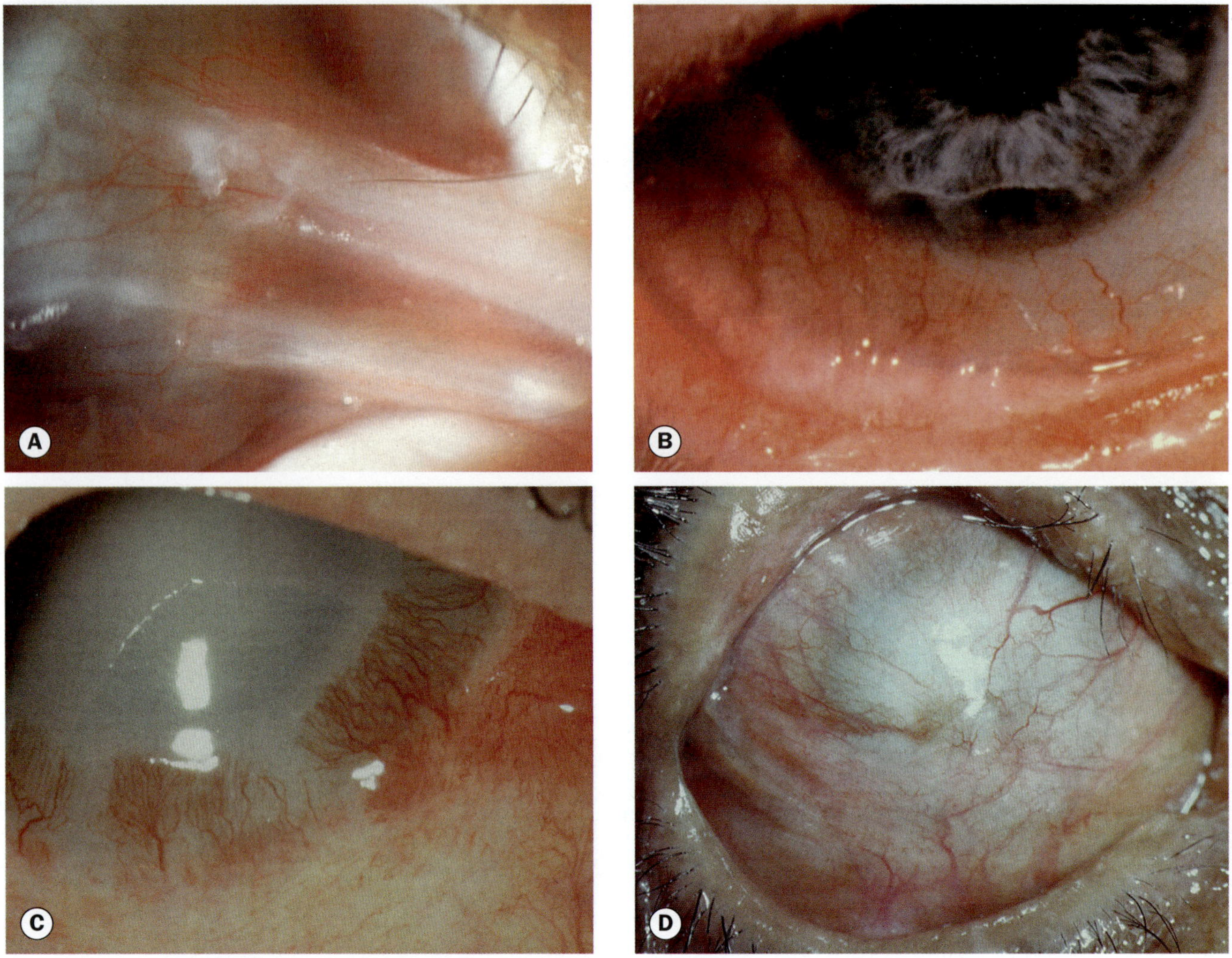

Fig. 22.32 Late sequelae of chemical injury. **(A)** Conjunctival bands; **(B)** symblepharon; **(C)** corneal scarring with pannus; **(D)** extensive cicatrization.

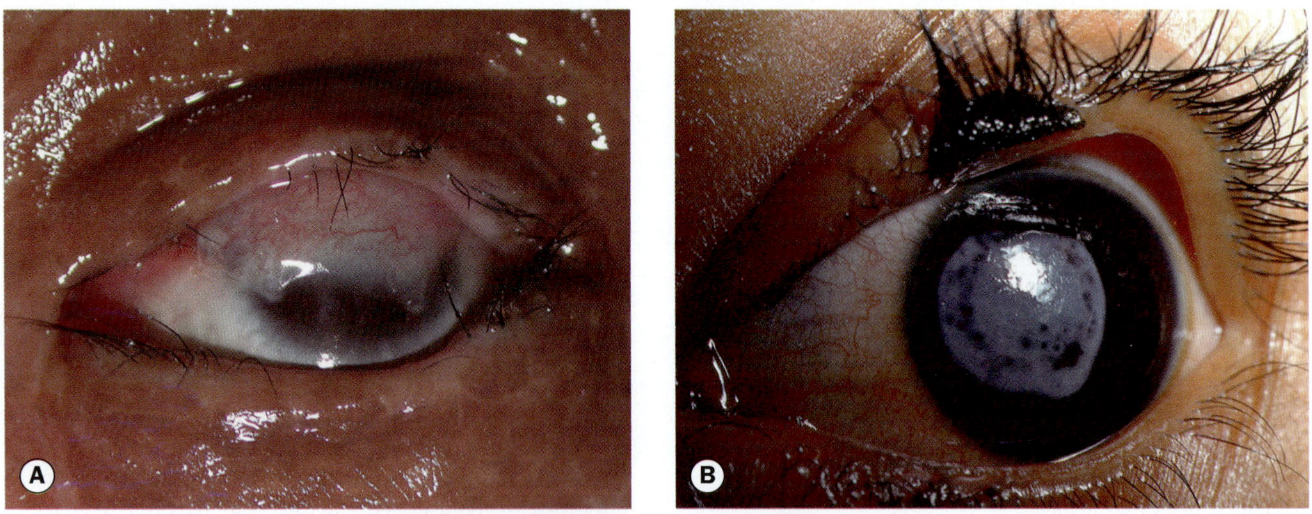

Fig. 22.33 Thermal burn. **(A)** To lids and anterior segment; **(B)** to cornea.

Index

Page numbers followed by "*f*" indicate figures, "*t*" indicate tables, and "*b*" indicate boxes.

B

C

M

N

O

P